MEDICAL-SURGICAL NURSING

Patient-Centered Collaborative Care

MEDICAL-SURGICAL NURSING

Patient-Centered Collaborative Care

EIGHTH EDITION

Donna D. Ignatavicius, MS, RN, ANEF
Speaker and Curriculum Consultant for Academic
  Nursing Programs
Founder, Boot Camp for Nurse Educators®
President, DI Associates, Inc.
Placitas, New Mexico

M. Linda Workman, PhD, RN, FAAN
Senior Volunteer Faculty
College of Nursing
University of Cincinnati
Cincinnati, Ohio;
Formerly Gertrude Perkins Oliva Professor of Oncology
Frances Payne Bolton School of Nursing
Case Western Reserve University
Cleveland, Ohio

Section Editors:

Meg Blair, PhD, MSN, RN, CEN
Professor
Nebraska Methodist College
Omaha, Nebraska

Cherie Rebar, PhD, MBA, RN, FNP, COI
Director, Division of Nursing
Chair, Prelicensure Nursing Programs
Kettering College
Kettering, Ohio

Chris Winkelman, RN, PhD, CCRN, ACNP, CNE, FCCM, FANP
Associate Professor
Frances Payne Bolton School of Nursing
Case Western Reserve University
Cleveland, Ohio

ELSEVIER

ELSEVIER

3251 Riverport Lane
St. Louis, Missouri 63043

Notices

Knowledge and best practice in this field are constantly changing. As new research and experience broaden our understanding, changes in research methods, professional practices, or medical treatment may become necessary.

Practitioners and researchers must always rely on their own experience and knowledge in evaluating and using any information, methods, compounds, or experiments described herein. In using such information or methods they should be mindful of their own safety and the safety of others, including parties for whom they have a professional responsibility.

With respect to any drug or pharmaceutical products identified, readers are advised to check the most current information provided (i) on procedures featured or (ii) by the manufacturer of each product to be administered, to verify the recommended dose or formula, the method and duration of administration, and contraindications. It is the responsibility of practitioners, relying on their own experience and knowledge of their patients, to make diagnoses, to determine dosages and the best treatment for each individual patient, and to take all appropriate safety precautions.

To the fullest extent of the law, neither the Publisher nor the authors, contributors, or editors, assume any liability for any injury and/or damage to persons or property as a matter of products liability, negligence or otherwise, or from any use or operation of any methods, products, instructions, or ideas contained in the material herein.

Previous editions copyrighted 2013, 2010, 2006, 2002, 1999, 1995, 1991

International Standard Book Number (single volume): 978-1-4557-7255-1
International Standard Book Number (2-volume set): 978-1-4557-7258-2

Executive Content Strategist: Lee Henderson
Traditional Content Development Manager: Billie C. Sharp
Senior Content Development Specialist: Rae L. Robertson
Publishing Services Manager: Deborah L. Vogel
Senior Project Manager: Jodi M. Willard
Design Direction: Margaret Reid

Printed in Canada

Last digit is the print number: 9   8   7   6   5   4   3

CONSULTANTS AND CONTRIBUTORS

CONSULTANTS

Richard Lintner, RT(R), (CV), (CT), (MR)
Clinical Instructor
Interventional Radiology
Kansas University Hospital
Kansas City, Kansas

Deanne Blach, MSN, RN
President, Nursing Education
DB Productions of NW AR, Inc.
Green Forest, Arkansas

Stephanie Ignatavicius, MA
Phoenix, Arizona

CONTRIBUTORS

Katherine L. Byar, MSN, APN, BC
Hematological Nurse Practitioner
Department of Internal Medicine/
    Oncology-Hematology
University of Nebraska Medical Center
Omaha, Nebraska

Lara L. Carver, PhD, RN, CNE
Associate Professor
Department of Nursing
National University
Las Vegas, Nevada

Robin Chard, PhD, RN, CNOR
Associate Professor
College of Nursing
Nova Southeastern University
Fort Lauderdale, Florida

Tammy Coffee, MSN, RN, ACNP
Preceptor
Department of Nursing
Case Western Reserve University;
Nurse Practitioner
Department of Surgery
MetroHealth Medical Center
Cleveland, Ohio

Janice Zeigler Cuzzell, RN, MA, CWS
Senior Rheumatology Clinical Coordinator
Immunology and Ophthalmology
Genentech, Inc.
San Francisco, California

Barbara J. Daly, PhD, RN, FAAN
Professor
School of Nursing
Case Western Reserve University;
Director
Clinical Ethics
University Hospitals Case Medical Center
Cleveland, Ohio

Laura M. Dechant, APN, MSN, CCRN, CCNS
Clinical Nurse Specialist
Heart, Vascular, and Interventional Services
Christiana Care Health System
Newark, Delaware

Cheryl Dumont, PhD, RN, CRNI
Director, Nursing Research and Vascular
    Access Team
Nursing Administration
Winchester Medical Center
Winchester, Virginia

June Eilers, PhD, APRN-CNS, BC
Research Associate Professor
College of Nursing
University of Nebraska
Omaha, Nebraska

Rachel L. Gallagher, MS, ANP-BC
Staff Officer
Physical Disability Board of Review
Diversified Technical Services, Inc.
El Paso, Texas

Nicole M. Heimgartner, RN, MSN
Assistant Professor
Division of Nursing
Kettering College
Kettering, Ohio

Stephanie Ignatavicius, MA
Phoenix, Arizona

Mary F. Justice, MSN, RN, CNE
Associate Professor
Department of Nursing
University of Cincinnati Blue Ash College
Cincinnati, Ohio

Mary Kazanowski, PhD, APRN, ACHPN
Palliative and Hospice Nurse Practitioner
VNA Hospice of Manchester and Southern
    New Hampshire
Manchester, New Hampshire;
Palliative Care Nurse Practitioner
Palliative Care Team
Concord Hospital
Concord, New Hampshire

Linda A. LaCharity, PhD, RN
Assistant Professor (Retired)
Adult Health
University of Cincinnati
Cincinnati, Ohio

Linda Laskowski-Jones, MS, RN, ACNS-BC, CEN, FAWM
Vice President
Emergency & Trauma Services
Christiana Care Health System
Wilmington, Delaware

Rona F. Levin, PhD, RN
Clinical Professor and Director, Doctor of
    Nursing Practice Program
College of Nursing
New York University;
Visiting Faculty
Quality Management Services
Visiting Nurse Service of New York
New York, New York;
Professor Emeritus
Felician College
Lodi, New Jersey

Margaret Elaine McLeod, MSN, APN, BC-ADM, ACNS-BC, CDE
Clinical Nurse Specialist
Department of Nursing
Tennessee Valley Health Care System
Nashville, Tennessee

Chris Pasero, MS, RN-BC, FAAN
Pain Management Educator and Clinical
    Consultant
El Dorado Hills, California

Jennifer Powers, MSN, FNP-BC
Clinical Assistant Professor
School of Health and Human Services
National University
San Diego, California;
Family Nurse Practitioner
Health Care Partners
Las Vegas, Nevada

Cherie Rebar, PhD, MBA, RN, FNP, COI
Director, Division of Nursing;
Chair, Prelicensure Nursing Programs
Division of Nursing
Kettering College
Kettering, Ohio

Harry C. Rees, III, MSN, ACNP-BC
Acute Care Nurse Practitioner
Cleveland Clinic Health System;
Metro Life Flight
MetroHealth Medical Center
Cleveland, Ohio

James G. Sampson, DNP, NP-C
Adjunct Assistant Professor
College of Nursing
University of Colorado
Aurora, Colorado;
Clinical Supervisor, Adult Nurse
    Practitioner
Department of Internal Medicine
Denver Health Medical Center
Denver, Colorado

Karen Toulson, RN, MSN, MBA, CEN, NE-BC
Nurse Manager
Emergency Department, Christiana Hospital
Christiana Care Health Services
Newark, Delaware

Shirley E. Van Zandt, MS, MPH, CRNP
Assistant Professor
School of Nursing
Boise State University
Boise, Idaho

Laura M. Willis, MSN, RN
Assistant Professor, Service Learning
    Coordinator
Department of Nursing, Service Learning
Kettering College
Kettering, Ohio

Chris Winkelman, RN, PhD, CCRN, ACNP, CNE, FCCM, FANP
Associate Professor
Frances Payne Bolton School of Nursing
Case Western Reserve University;
Clinical Nurse
Trauma/Critical Care
MetroHealth Medical Center
Cleveland, Ohio

Fay Wright, MS, RN, APRN-BC
Doctoral Student
The Florence S. Downs PhD Program in
    Nursing Research and Theory
    Development
New York University College of Nursing
New York, New York

CONTRIBUTORS TO TEACHING/LEARNING RESOURCES

PowerPoint® Slides

Nicole Heimgartner, RN, MSN, COI
Associate Professor of Nursing
Kettering College
Kettering, Ohio

Cherie Rebar, PhD, MBA, RN, FNP, COI
Director, Division of Nursing;
Chair, Prelicensure Nursing Programs
Division of Nursing
Kettering College
Kettering, Ohio

Laura M. Willis, MSN, APRN, FNP-C
Adjunct Professor
Kettering College
Kettering, Ohio;
Family Nurse Practitioner
The Little Clinic;
President, Connect RN2ED
Englewood, Ohio

TEACH® for Nurses Lesson Plans

Carolyn Gersch, PhDc, MSN, RN, CNE
Associate Director, Division of Nursing
Kettering College
Kettering, Ohio

Cherie Rebar, PhD, MBA, RN, FNP, COI
Director, Division of Nursing;
Chair, Prelicensure Nursing Programs
Division of Nursing
Kettering College
Kettering, Ohio

Test Bank

Meg Blair, PhD, MSN, RN, CEN
Professor
Nursing Division
Nebraska Methodist College
Omaha, Nebraska

Linda Hughes, PhD, RN, BSN, MS
Dean of Nursing
Nebraska Methodist College
Omaha, Nebraska

Tami Kathleen Little, RN, DNP, CNE
Dean of Nursing
Brookline College
Albuquerque, New Mexico

Case Studies

Candice Kumagai, RN, MSN
Formerly Clinical Instructor
University of Texas at Austin
Austin, Texas

Linda A. LaCharity, PhD, RN, MN, BSN
Adjunct Faculty
Formerly Accelerated Program Director and
    Assistant Professor
College of Nursing
University of Cincinnati
Cincinnati, Ohio

Concept Maps

Deanne A. Blach, MSN, RN
President, Nursing Education
DB Productions of NW AR, Inc.
Green Forest, Arkansas

Review Questions for the NCLEX® Examination

Lisa A. Hollett, RN, BSN, MA, MICN, Certified Forensic Nurse
Stroke Coordinator
Hillcrest Medical Center
Tulsa, Oklahoma

Mary Beth Flynn Makic, PhD, RN, CNS, CCNS, FAAN
Research Nurse Scientist
University of Colorado Hospital;
Critical Care and Associate Professor
College of Nursing
University of Colorado
Aurora, Colorado

Andrea R. Mann, MSN, RN, CNE
Interim Dean, Third Level Chair
Aria Health School of Nursing
Trevose, Pennsylvania

Denise Robinson, RN, MS, CNE
Assistant Professor of Nursing
Monroe County Community College
Monroe, Michigan

Kathryn Schartz, RN, MSN, PPCPNP-BC
Assistant Professor of Nursing
School of Nursing
Baker University
Topeka, Kansas

Mitch Seal, RN, EdD, Med-IT, BSN
Director of Strategic Planning &
    Partnerships
Medical Education and Training Campus
    Joint Base
San Antonio, Texas

Peggy Slota, DNP, RN, FAAN
Associate Professor of Nursing
Carlow University
Pittsburgh, Pennsylvania

CONTENT REVIEW PANEL

Diane K. Daddario, MSN, ACNS-BC, RN, BC, CMSRN
Adjunct Faculty, School of Nursing
Pennsylvania State University
University Park, Pennsylvania

Denise A. Foster, MSN, RN, CNE
Associate Professor
Sentara College of Health Sciences
Chesapeake, Virginia

Bradley Harrell, DNP, APRN, ACNP-BC, CCRN
Chair and Associate Professor
Germantown Undergraduate Nursing
Union University School of Nursing
Jackson, Tennessee

LaWanda Herron, PhD, MSA, MSN, FNP-BC
Director of Nursing
Holmes Community College
Grenada, Mississippi

Jamie Lynn Jones, MSN, RN, CNE
Assistant Professor
University of Arkansas at Little Rock
Little Rock, Arkansas

Tamara Kear, PhD, RN, CNS, CNN
Assistant Professor of Nursing
College of Nursing
Villanova University
Villanova, Pennsylvania

Melissa S. McNulty, PhD, ARNP
Professor
Pasco-Hernando State College
Wesley Chapel, Florida

Jason Mott, PhD, RN
Instructor of Nursing
Bellin College
Green Bay, Wisconsin

CLINICAL CHAPTER REVIEWERS

Sameeya N. Ahmed-Winston, RN, MSN, CPNP, CPHON
Pediatric Nurse Practitioner
Children's National Medical Center
Washington, D.C.

Margaret-Ann Carno, PhD, RN, MBA, CPNP, FAAN
Associate Professor of Clinical Nursing and Pediatrics
University of Rochester, School of Nursing
Rochester, New York

Laura M. Dechant, APN, MSN, CCRN, CCNS
Clinical Nursing Specialist
Christiana Care Health System
Newark, Delaware

Kathleen Sanders Jordan, DNP, MS, RN, FNP-BC, ENP-BC, SANE-P
Clinical Assistant Professor
School of Nursing
University of North Carolina Charlotte;
Nurse Practitioner
Mid-Atlantic Emergency Medicine Association
Charlotte, North Carolina

Kari Jean Ksar, RN, MS, CPNP
Pediatric Nurse Practitioner
Pediatric Gastroenterology, Hepatology, and Nutrition
Lucile Packard Children's Hospital at Stanford
Palo Alto, California

Martha E. Langhorne, MSN, RN, FNP, AOCN
Nurse Practitioner
Binghamton Gastroenterology
Binghamton, New York

Casey Norris, MSN, BSN, APRN, BC
Nursing Instructor
ITT Technical Institute
Madison, Alabama

Charles D. Rogers, MSN, RN
Assistant Professor of Nursing
Morehead State University
Morehead, Kentucky

Mark Stevens, MSN, RN, CNS, CEN, MICN
Professor of Nursing
National University
Fresno, California

Laura C. Williams, MSN, CNS, ONC, CCNS
Orthopedic Clinical Nurse Specialist
Orlando Regional Medical Center
Orlando, Florida

PREFACE

The first edition of this textbook, entitled *Medical-Surgical Nursing: A Nursing Process Approach,* was in many ways a groundbreaking work. The following six editions built on that achievement and further solidified the book's position as a major trendsetter for the practice of adult health nursing. Now in its eighth edition, "Iggy" charts an essential course for the future of adult nursing practice—a course reflected in its current title: *Medical-Surgical Nursing: Patient-Centered Collaborative Care.* The focus of this new edition continues to be to help students learn how to provide safe, quality care that is patient-centered, evidence-based, and collaborative. In addition to print formats as single- and two-volume texts, this edition is now available in a variety of electronic formats, including Pageburst on VST, Pageburst on Kno, and e-book formats for Kindle, Nook, and other e-readers.

The book's subtitle was carefully chosen to emphasize the nurse's role in providing care in collaboration with the patient, family, and members of the interdisciplinary team in both acute care and community-based settings. The Institute of Medicine (IOM), The Joint Commission, the Quality and Safety Education for Nurses (QSEN) Institute, and the 2010 IOM *Future of Nursing* report have called for all health professionals to coordinate and deliver evidence-based patient care as a collaborative care team.

KEY THEMES FOR THE 8TH EDITION

The key themes for this edition strengthen the book's focus on safety, quality care, and clinical judgment to best prepare the student for collaborative patient-centered practice in medical-surgical health settings. Each theme is outlined and described below.

- **New Focus on Concepts.** Enhanced compatibility with the concept-based nursing curriculum in pre-licensure programs and a conceptual approach to teaching and learning is the key feature that sets this edition apart. To help students connect previously-learned concepts with new information in the text, six Concept Overviews introduce groups of content units. These unique features review basic concepts learned in nursing fundamentals courses—such as oxygenation and protection—to help students make connections between foundational concepts and patient care for medical-surgical conditions. The Concept Overviews are now even more accessible with color sidebars to identify these pages. For continuity and reinforcement, a list of more specific Priority Nursing Concepts has been added at the beginning of each chapter. This placement is designed to help students better understand the role of the nurse when caring for patients with selected health problems. When these concepts are explicated in the body of each chapter, they are presented in small capital letters (e.g., OXYGENATION) to help students relate and apply essential concepts to provide more focused nursing care. Nursing Concepts and Clinical Judgment Reviews at the end of most chapters apply these same concepts to the health problems presented in the chapter.
- **Improved Focus on the Core Body of Knowledge and QSEN Competencies.** This edition not only continues to emphasize need-to-know content for the RN level of practice, but also includes an increased emphasis on Quality and Safety Education for Nurses (QSEN) Institute core competencies. Clinical practice settings emphasize the essential need for safe practices and quality improvement to provide collaborative patient-centered care that is evidence-based. Many hospitals and other health care agencies have formally adopted these QSEN competencies as core values and goals for patient care. To help prepare students for the work environment as new graduates, as well as to highlight the integration of safety and quality into all nursing actions, this edition incorporates an enhanced focus on these competencies.
- **Emphasis on Patient Safety.** Patient safety is emphasized throughout this edition, not only in the narrative but also in **Nursing Safety Priority boxes** that enable students to immediately identify the most important care needed for patients with specific health problems. These highlighted features are further classified as Action Alerts, Drug Alerts, or Critical Rescue. We also continue to include our leading-edge Best Practice for Patient Safety & Quality Care charts to emphasize the most important nursing care. Highlighted yellow text also demonstrates the application of The Joint Commission's National Patient Safety Goals initiative (http://www.joint commission.org/standards_information/npsgs.aspx) and Core Measures content into every day nursing practice.
- **Focus on Patient-Centered Care.** Patient-centered care is enhanced in the eighth edition in several ways. The eighth edition continues to use the term "patient" instead of "client" throughout. Although the use of these terms remains a subject of discussion among nursing educators, we have not defined the patient as a dependent person. Rather, the patient can be an individual, a family, or a group—all of whom have rights that are respected in a mutually trusting nurse-patient relationship. Most health care agencies and professional organizations use "patient" in their practice and publications. In addition, most nursing organizations support the term.
- **New Focus on Gender Considerations.** To increase our emphasis on patient-centered care, we delineated **Gender Health Considerations** rather than restricting our emphasis on Women's Health Considerations as we did in previous editions. To further expand that focus on differences in patient values, preferences, and beliefs, we have added new, cutting-edge **Chapter 73, Care of Transgender Patients,** dedicated to transgender patient care. Along with other individuals in the lesbian, gay, bisexual, and questioning population, the health needs of transgender patients have gained national attention through their inclusion in *Healthy People 2020* and The Joint Commission's standards. This new chapter provides tools to help prepare students and faculty to care for transgender patients who are considering or who have undergone the gender transition process.
- **Emphasis on Evidence-Based Practice.** The updated **Chapter 5, Evidence-Based Practice in Medical-Surgical Nursing** (written by evidence-based practice (EBP) experts Dr. Rona F. Levin and Fay Wright), discusses the importance of *using best current evidence in nursing practice* and how to locate and use this evidence to improve patient care. This chapter, along with the **Evidence-Based Practice boxes** throughout the book, offers a solid foundation in this

essential aspect of nursing practice. Each box summarizes a useful research article and explains the implications of its findings for practice and further research, as well as a rating of the level of evidence based on a well-respected scale.

- **New Focus on Quality Improvement.** The QSEN Institute and clinical practice agencies require that all nurses have *quality improvement* knowledge and skills. To help prepare students for that role, this edition includes new and unique **Quality Improvement boxes.** Each box summarizes a quality improvement project published in the health care literature and the implications of the project's success in improving nursing care. The inclusion of these boxes, in addition to disseminating information and research, helps students understand that quality improvement has its underpinnings in practice change at the "grass roots" level. It also emphasizes the role of the bedside nurse in identifying potential solutions to practice problems.

- **Refocused Emphasis on Clinical Judgment.** Stressing the importance of clinical judgment skills, including an enhanced emphasis on prioritization and delegation, helps to best prepare students for practice and the NCLEX® Examination. As in the seventh edition, the eighth edition emphasizes the importance of nursing judgment to make timely and appropriate clinical decisions and prioritize care. To help achieve that focus, all-new case-based **Clinical Judgment Challenges** (formerly called "Decision-Making Challenges"), based primarily on the QSEN core competencies, have been integrated throughout the text. Selected Clinical Judgment Challenges highlight ethical dilemmas and delegation and supervision issues. These exercises provide clinical situations in which students can use on-the-spot nursing judgment to help prepare them for the fast-paced world of medical-surgical nursing and become competent nurses. Suggested answer guidelines for these Clinical Judgment Challenges are provided on the book's Evolve website (http://evolve.elsevier. com/Iggy/). In addition, Dr. Christine Tanner's clinical judgment framework (Tanner, 2006) is used to help students apply selected concepts in the **Nursing Concepts and Clinical Judgment Reviews** at the end of most chapters. The components of this model include that clinical nurses use nursing judgment to provide safe, quality care by:
  - Noticing
  - Interpreting
  - Responding
  - Reflecting

- **Emphasis on Preparation for the NCLEX® Examination.** An enhanced emphasis on the NCLEX Examination and consistency with the 2013 NCLEX-RN® test plan has been refined in this edition. Like the seventh edition, the eighth edition also emphasizes "readiness"—readiness for the NCLEX® Examination, readiness for major emergencies such as those we see with all-too-frequent mass casualty events, readiness for safe drug administration, and readiness for the new and continually unfolding world of genetics and genomics. An increased number of new **NCLEX® Examination Challenges** are interspersed throughout the text to allow students the opportunity for practice in test-taking and decision-making. Answers to these Challenges are provided in the back of the book, and their rationales are provided on the Evolve website (http://evolve.elsevier.com/Iggy). As the NCLEX® Examination becomes more challenging, it is more critical than ever that students be ready to pass the licensure exam on the first try. To help both students and faculty achieve that outcome, chapter-opening **Learning Outcomes** are now more consistent with the competencies outlined in the detailed 2013 NCLEX-RN Test Plan. The eighth edition also continues to include an innovative end-of-chapter feature called **Get Ready for the NCLEX® Examination!** This unique and effective learning aid consists of a list of **Key Points** *organized by Client Needs Category* as found in the NCLEX-RN® Test Plan. Relevant QSEN competency categories are identified for selected Key Points.

- **Expanded Content on Community-Based Care.** Expanded coverage on this important nursing area, including long-term care, is included in this edition. A recent editorial article in the journal *Medical-Surgical Nursing* stated that the future of medical-surgical nurses will change to an increased role in care coordination and transition management between acute care and community-based care (Lattavo, 2014). To help students prepare for this new role, the eighth edition of our text expands coverage of community-based care, including essential collaborative management that is needed in home, long-term, rehabilitation, and ambulatory settings.

- **Collaborative Problems and NANDA-I Nursing Diagnoses.** This edition also features an improved delineation of **NANDA-I nursing diagnoses and collaborative patient problems.** As health care becomes increasingly more collaborative, nurses need to be able to communicate with other members of the health care team, including the patient and family. To help students learn how to facilitate that communication, the eighth edition identifies patient problems and specifies which actual and potential problems are NANDA-I nursing diagnoses and which are collaborative health problems.

CLINICAL CURRENCY AND ACCURACY

To ensure the book's currency and accuracy, we listened to students and faculty who have used the previous editions, focusing on their impressions of and experiences with the book. We reviewed documents crafted by a variety of health care organizations, including the Institute of Medicine (IOM), The Joint Commission (TJC), and the Institute for Healthcare Improvement (IHI). Recent nursing education publications were also examined, such as those authored by the National League for Nursing (NLN), the American Association of Colleges of Nursing (AACN), and Dr. Patricia Benner and her colleagues in their book *Educating Nurses: A Call for Radical Transformation* (2010). A thorough nursing education literature search of best current evidence helped us validate best practices and national health care trends to help shape the focus of the eighth edition.

We also commissioned in-depth reviews of every chapter by a dedicated panel of instructors and clinicians across the United States, and we used their reviews to guide us in revising the chapters into their final form. A well-respected interventional radiologist ensured the accuracy of selected diagnostic testing procedures and associated patient care.

The results of these efforts are reflected in the eighth edition's:

- Strong, consistent focus on NCLEX-RN® Examination preparation, clinical judgment, patient-centered collaborative care, pathophysiology, drug therapy, evidence-based clinical practice, and community-based care

- Foundation of relevant research and best practice guidelines
- Emphasis on the critical "need to know" information that beginning nurses must master to provide safe patient care

With today's knowledge explosion, it is easy for a book to become larger with each new edition. However, today's nursing students have a limited time to absorb and begin to apply the information essential for medical-surgical nursing care. Therefore in this eighth edition we eliminated some of the content found in previous foundation courses or other specialty textbooks. We limited our discussions to how this content is *used* in adult nursing and focused on content that was "need to know" for safe, patient-centered, quality nursing practice.

OUTSTANDING READABILITY

Today's students need to be able to read information once and understand it; they do not have time to repeatedly read the same information. To achieve this level of readability, the text employs a direct-address style (wherever appropriate) that speaks directly to the reader, and sentences are as short as possible without sacrificing essential content. In addition, we ensured that this new edition has improved consistency of difficulty level from chapter to chapter.

Reading level is highly influenced by the length of sentences and the length of words. Although we can control the length of the sentences, medical terms are often 4 to 5 syllables long and tend to skew a chapter's reading level. Nevertheless, the result of our efforts is a med-surg text of consistently outstanding readability. The average reading level is 10th to 11th grade. It is important to note that reducing the reading level of this edition did not reduce the quality or depth of content that students need to know. Instead, the content is clear, focused, and accessible.

EASE OF ACCESS

To make the text as easy to use as possible, we have maintained the previous editions' approach of smaller chapters of more uniform length. Consistent with our focus on the "need to know," we eliminated some of the less foundational content in the first unit of the last edition and added one new chapter. The more focused eighth edition contains 74 chapters.

The overall presentation of the eighth edition has been updated, including more recent and high-quality photographs for realism, and design change features to improve content access. The design of the eighth edition includes better placement of display elements (e.g., figures, tables, boxes, and charts) for a chapter flow that enhances text reading without splintering content or confusing the reader. Additional ease-of-access features for this edition include tabbed markings for the glossary, index, illustration credits, and bibliography for quick reference. To increase the smoothness of flow and reader concentration, side-turned tables and charts have been reduced throughout the text, as have tables and charts covering multiple pages. Tables and charts now feature an alternating pattern of light and dark shading to ensure essential content for a specific topic or characteristic is not confused with another topic or characteristic.

We also have maintained the unit structure of previous editions, with vital body systems (cardiovascular, respiratory, and neurologic) appearing earlier in the book. In these three units we continue to provide complex care content in separate chapters that discuss managing critically ill patients with coronary artery disease, respiratory health problems, and neurologic health problems.

To help break up long blocks of text and also to highlight key information, we continue to include streamlined yet eye-catching headings, bulleted lists, tables, charts, and in-text highlights. Key Terms are in boldface color type and are defined in the text to foster the learning of need-to-know vocabulary. A glossary is located in the back of the book. Chapter bibliographies have been moved to the back of the book to save space in chapters for need-to-know content. These current bibliographic resources include research articles, nationally accepted clinical guidelines, and other sources of evidence when available for each chapter. Classic sources from before 2011 are noted with an asterisk (*).

A PATIENT-CENTERED COLLABORATIVE CARE APPROACH

As in all previous editions, we take a collaborative care approach to patient care. We believe that in the real world of health care, nurses, patients, and other health care providers (including physicians, advanced-practice nurses, and physician's assistants) *share* responsibility for the management of patient problems. Thus we present patient care in a collaborative care framework. In this framework we make no *artificial* distinctions between medical treatment and nursing care. Instead, under each Patient-Centered Collaborative Care heading we discuss how the nurse coordinates care and interacts with members of the health care team as appropriate for the patient's health problems, including health promotion and illness prevention.

This edition includes newly redesigned patient-centered Concept Maps that underscore this collaborative care approach. Each Concept Map contains a case scenario. It then shows how a selected complex health problem is addressed. Each Concept Map spells out the steps of the nursing process and related concepts to illustrate the relationships among disease processes, priority patient problems, collaborative management, and more.

Although our approach is collaborative, the text is first and foremost a *nursing* text. We therefore use a nursing process approach as a tool to organize discussions of patient health problems and their management. Discussions of *major* health problems follow a full nursing process format using this structure:
[Health problem]
Pathophysiology
    Etiology (and Genetic Risk when appropriate)
    Incidence and Prevalence
Health Promotion and Maintenance (when appropriate)
Patient-Centered Collaborative Care
    Assessment
    Analysis
    Planning and Implementation
        [Collaborative Intervention Statement (based on priority patient problems)]
        Planning: Expected Outcomes
        Interventions
    Community-Based Care
        Home Care Management
        Self-Management Education
        Health Care Resources
Evaluation: Outcomes

The Analysis sections list the priority patient problems (collaborative problems and nursing diagnoses) associated with major health problems and disorders. This eighth edition uses official NANDA-I nursing diagnosis language where it applies; however, most health care agencies prefer to identify collaborative patient problems or needs as the basis for the interdisciplinary plan of care rather than being restricted to NANDA-I language, which addresses primarily nursing-oriented patient problems. With its more flexible interweaving of NANDA-I diagnoses and collaborative patient problems or needs, the eighth edition more closely aligns with the language of clinical practice. The nursing diagnoses used in this edition are the 2012-2014 NANDA-I diagnoses—the most recently approved diagnoses at the time of publication of this edition. Health Promotion and Maintenance sections are found in selected discussions.

Discussions of less common or less complex disorders, although not given this complete subhead structure, nonetheless follow the same basic format: a discussion of the problem itself (including pertinent information on pathophysiology) followed by a section on patient-centered collaborative care of patients with the disorder. To demonstrate our commitment to providing the content foundational to nursing education and consistent with the recommendations of Benner and colleagues through the Carnegie Foundation for the Future of Nursing Education, we highlight throughout this edition essential pathophysiologic concepts that are key to understanding the basis for collaborative management.

Integral to this collaborative care approach is a clear delineation of just who is responsible for what. When a responsibility is primarily the nurse's, the text says so. When a decision must be made jointly by the patient, nurse, physician, and physical therapist, for example, this is clearly stated. When different health care practitioners in different care settings might be involved in the patient's care, this is stated.

ORGANIZATION

The 74 chapters of *Medical-Surgical Nursing: Patient-Centered Collaborative Care* are grouped into 16 units. Unit 1, Foundations for Medical-Surgical Nursing, lays the foundation for the health care concepts incorporated throughout the text. Unit 2 consists of three chapters on concepts of emergency and trauma care and disaster preparedness.

Unit 3 consists of three chapters on the management of patients with fluid, electrolyte, and acid-base imbalances. Chapters 11 and 12 review key assessments and related patient care in a clear, concise discussion. The chapter on infusion therapy (Chapter 13) is supplemented with an online Fluids & Electrolytes Tutorial on the companion Evolve website.

Unit 4 presents the perioperative nursing content that medical-surgical nurses need to know. This content provides a solid foundation to help the student better understand the collaborative care required for the surgical patient regardless of surgical setting. Even more emphasis is placed on continuous assessment during the perioperative period to prevent complications and improve outcomes in this era of increased ambulatory care.

Unit 5 provides core content on health problems related to immune system function. This content includes normal inflammation and the immune response, altered cell growth and cancer development, and interventions for patients with

connective tissue disease, HIV infection, and other immunologic disorders, cancers, and infections.

The remaining 11 units, subdivided and introduced by the six Concept Overviews, cover medical-surgical content by body system. Each of these units begins with an Assessment chapter and continues with one or more Nursing Care chapters for patients with selected health problems in that body system. This framework is familiar to students who learn the body systems in preclinical foundational science courses such as anatomy and physiology.

MULTINATIONAL, MULTICULTURAL, MULTIGENERATIONAL FOCUS

To reflect the increasing diversity of our society, *Medical-Surgical Nursing: Patient-Centered Collaborative Care* takes a multinational, multicultural, and multigenerational focus. Addressing the needs of both U.S. and Canadian readers, we have included examples of trade names of drugs available in the United States and in Canada. Drugs that are available only in Canada are designated with a ✤ symbol. When appropriate, we identify specific Canadian health care resources, including their websites. In many areas, Canadian health statistics are combined with those of the United States for provide an accurate "North American" picture.

To help nurses provide quality care for patients whose preferences, beliefs, and values may differ from their own, numerous **Cultural Considerations** and **Gender Health Considerations** boxes highlight important aspects of culturally competent care throughout the text. In addition, a new chapter (Chapter 73) is dedicated to the special health care needs of transgender patients.

Increases in life expectancy and the "graying" of the baby-boom generation add up to a steadily increasing older adult population. To help equip nurses for this challenge, the eighth edition continues to provide thorough coverage of the care of older adults. Chapter 2 offers content on the role of the nurse and health care team in promoting health for older adults in the community. It also provides coverage of common health problems that older adults may have in the health care setting, such as falls and inadequate nutrition. The text includes many **Nursing Focus on the Older Adult charts.** Laboratory values and drug dosages typical for older patients are also included throughout the book. Charts specifying normal physiologic changes to expect in the older population are found in each Assessment chapter. In addition, **Considerations for Older Adults boxes** are included throughout the text to emphasize key points to consider when caring for these patients.

ADDITIONAL LEARNING AIDS

As in previous editions, the eighth edition continues to include a rich array of learning aids geared toward adult learners to help students quickly identify and understand key information and to serve as study aids.

- Written in "patient-friendly" language, **Patient and Family Education: Preparing for Self-Management charts** provide the types of instructions that nurses must learn to provide to patients and their families to help them cope with life changes caused by illness.
- **Laboratory Profile charts** summarize important information on laboratory tests commonly used to evaluate

health problems. Information typically includes normal ranges of laboratory values (including differences for older adults, when appropriate) and the possible significance of abnormal findings.

- **Common Examples of Drug Therapy charts** summarize important information about commonly used drugs. Most charts include both U.S. and Canadian trade names for typically used drugs, usual dosages (including dosages for older patients, as appropriate), and nursing interventions with rationales.
- **Key Features charts** highlight the clinical manifestations of important health problems based on pathophysiologic concepts.
- **Evidence-Based Practice boxes**, provided in many chapters, give synopses of recent nursing research articles and other scientific articles applicable to nursing. Each box provides a brief summary of the research, its level of evidence (LOE), and a brief commentary with implications for nursing practice and future research. The purpose of this feature is to help students identify the strengths and weaknesses of the research and to see how research guides nursing practice.
- New to this edition, **Quality Improvement boxes** offer anecdotes of recent nursing articles that focus on this important QSEN competency. These features, similar to the Evidence-Based Practice boxes, provide a brief summary of the research with commentary on the implications for nursing practice and research.
- As in the previous editions, **Home Care Assessment charts** serve as a convenient summary of essential assessment points for patients who need follow-up home health nursing care.
- Subtypes of **Clinical Judgment Challenges** (CJCs) emphasize the six QSEN core competencies: Patient-Centered Care, Teamwork and Collaboration, Evidence-Based Practice, Quality Improvement, Safety, and Informatics.

AN INTEGRATED MULTIMEDIA RESOURCE BASED ON PROVEN STRATEGIES FOR STUDENT ENGAGEMENT AND LEARNING

Medical-Surgical Nursing: Patient-Centered Collaborative Care, 8th edition, is the centerpiece of a comprehensive package of electronic and print learning resources that break new ground in the application of proven strategies for student engagement, learning, and evidence-based educational practice. This integrated multimedia resource actively engages the student in problem solving and practicing clinical decision-making skills.

Resources for Instructors

For the convenience of faculty, all Instructor Resources are available on a streamlined, secure instructor area of the Evolve website (http://evolve.elsevier.com/Iggy/). Included among these Instructor Resources are the reorganized *TEACH for Nurses* Lesson Plans. These Lesson Plans focus on the most important content from each chapter and provide innovative strategies for student engagement and learning. Lesson Plans are provided for each chapter and are categorized into several parts:
Learning Outcomes
Teaching Focus

Key Terms
Nursing Curriculum Standards
   QSEN
   Concepts
   BSN Essentials
Student Chapter Resources
Instructor Chapter Resources
Teaching Strategies
Additional Instructor Resources provided on the Evolve website include:

- A completely revised, updated, high-quality **Test Bank** consisting of more than 1750 items, both traditional multiple-choice and NCLEX-RN® "alternate" item types. Each question is coded for correct answer, rationale, cognitive level, NCLEX Integrated Process, NCLEX Client Needs Category, and new Keywords to facilitate question searches. Page references are provided for Remembering (Knowledge)- and Understanding (Comprehension)-level questions. (Questions at the Applying [Application] and above cognitive level require the student to draw on understanding of multiple or broader concepts not limited to a single textbook page, so page cross references are not provided for these higher-level critical thinking questions.) The Test Bank is provided in the Evolve Assessment Manager and in ExamView and ParTest formats.
- An electronic **Image Collection** containing all images from the book (approximately 550 images), delivered in a format that makes incorporation into lectures, presentations, and online courses easier than ever.
- **PowerPoint Presentations**—a revised collection of more than 2000 slides corresponding to each chapter in the text and highlighting key content with integrated images and Unfolding Case Studies. Audience Response System Questions (three discussion-oriented questions per chapter for use with iClicker and other audience response systems) are included in these slide presentations. Answers and rationales to the Audience Response System Questions and Unfolding Case Studies are found in the "Notes" section of each slide.

Also available for adoption and separate purchase:

- Corresponding chapter-by-chapter to the textbook, *Elsevier Adaptive Quizzing (EAQ)* integrates seamlessly into your course to help students of all skill levels focus their study time and effectively prepare for class, course exams, and the NCLEX® certification exam. *EAQ* is comprised of a bank of high-quality practice questions that allows students to advance at their own pace—based on their performance—through multiple mastery levels for each chapter. A comprehensive dashboard allows students to view their progress and stay motivated. The educator dashboard, grade book, and reporting capabilities enable faculty to monitor the activity of individual students, assess overall class performance, and identify areas of strength and weakness, ultimately helping to achieve improved learning outcomes.
- *Simulation Learning System (SLS) for Medical-Surgical Nursing* is an online toolkit designed to help you effectively incorporate simulation into your nursing curriculum, with scenarios that promote and enhance the clinical decision-making skills of students at all levels. It offers detailed instructions for preparation and implementation

of the simulation experience, debriefing questions that encourage critical thinking, and learning resources to reinforce student comprehension. Modularized simulation scenarios correspond to Elsevier's leading medical-surgical nursing texts, reinforcing students' classroom knowledge base, synthesizing lecture and clinicals, and offering remediation content that's critical to debriefing.

Resources for Students

Resources for students include a revised, updated, and retitled Clinical Nursing Judgment Study Guide, a Clinical Companion, Elsevier Adaptive Learning (EAL), Virtual Clinical Excursions (VCE), and Evolve Learning Resources.

The ***Clinical Nursing Judgment Study Guide*** has been completely revised and updated and features a fresh emphasis on clinical decision making, priorities of delegation, management of care, and pharmacology.

The pocket-sized ***Clinical Companion*** is a handy clinical resource that retains its easy-to-use alphabetical organization and streamlined format. It includes "Critical Rescue," "Drug Alert," and "Action Alert" highlights throughout based on the Nursing Safety Priority features in the textbook. National Patient Safety Goals highlights have been expanded as a QSEN feature, focusing on one of six QSEN core competencies, while still underscoring the importance of observing vital patient safety standards. This "pocket-sized Iggy" has been tailored to the special needs of students preparing for clinicals and clinical practice.

Corresponding chapter-by-chapter to the textbook, ***Elsevier Adaptive Learning (EAL)*** combines the power of brain science with sophisticated, patented Cerego algorithms to help students to learn faster and remember longer. It's fun, it's engaging, and it's constantly tracking student performance and adapting to deliver content precisely when it's needed to ensure core information is transformed into lasting knowledge.

Virtual Clinical Excursions, featuring an updated and easy-to-navigate "virtual" clinical setting, is once again available for the eighth edition. This unique learning tool guides students through a virtual clinical environment and helps them "learn by doing" in the safety of a "virtual" hospital.

Also available for students is a dynamic collection of Evolve Student Resources, available at http://evolve.elsevier.com/Iggy/. The Evolve Student Resources include the following:

- Review Questions for the NCLEX® Examination
- Answer Guidelines for NCLEX® Examination and Clinical Judgment Challenges
- Interactive Case Studies
- Concept Maps (digital versions of the 12 Concept Maps from the text)
- Concept Map Creator (a handy tool for creating customized Concept Maps)
- Fluid & Electrolyte Tutorial (a complete self-paced tutorial on this perennially difficult content)
- Key Points (downloadable expanded chapter reviews for each chapter)
- Audio Glossary
- Audio Clips and Video Clips
- Content Updates

In summary, *Medical-Surgical Nursing: Patient-Centered Collaborative Care,* 8th edition, together with its fully integrated multimedia ancillary package, provides the tools you will need to equip nursing students to meet the challenges of nursing practice both now and in an emerging healthcare environment that may look very different from today's. The only elements that remain to be added to this package are those that you alone can provide—your diligence, your commitment, your innovation, *your nursing expertise.*

Donna D. Ignatavicius
M. Linda Workman

To all the nursing educators who are passionate about teaching and all the nursing students who are passionate about learning.

Also, to my husband, Charles, who has endured countless hours of loneliness while I've worked on this project and to Stephanie, my daughter, who has educated me about the LGBTQ community's special needs. Thank you!

Donna

To students everywhere.
To John, still my one.

Linda

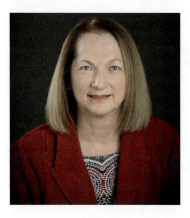

Donna D. Ignatavicius received her diploma in nursing from the Peninsula General School of Nursing in Salisbury, Maryland. After working as a charge nurse in medical-surgical nursing, she became an instructor in staff development at the University of Maryland Medical Center. She then received her BSN from the University of Maryland School of Nursing. For 5 years she taught in several schools of nursing while working toward her MS in Nursing, which she received in 1981. Donna then taught in the BSN program at the University of Maryland, after which she continued to pursue her interest in gerontology and accepted the position of Director of Nursing of a major skilled-nursing facility in her home state of Maryland. Since that time, she has served as an instructor in several associate degree nursing programs. Through her consulting activities and faculty development workshops, Donna has gained national recognition in nursing education. She is currently the President of DI Associates, Inc. (http://www.diassociates.com/), a company dedicated to improving health care through education and consultation for faculty. In recognition of her contributions to the field, she was inducted as a charter Fellow of the prestigious Academy of Nursing Education in 2007.

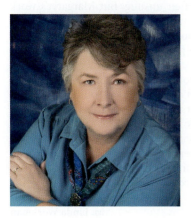

M. Linda Workman, a native of Canada, received her BSN from the University of Cincinnati College of Nursing and Health. After serving in the U.S. Army Nurse Corps and working as an Assistant Head Nurse and Head Nurse in civilian hospitals, Linda earned her MSN from the University of Cincinnati College of Nursing and a PhD in Developmental Biology from the University of Cincinnati College of Arts and Sciences. Linda's 30-plus years of academic experience include teaching at the diploma, associate degree, baccalaureate, and master's levels. Her areas of teaching expertise include medical-surgical nursing, physiology, pathophysiology, genetics, oncology, and immunology. Linda has been recognized nationally for her teaching expertise and was inducted as a Fellow into the American Academy of Nursing in 1992. She received Excellence in Teaching awards at the University of Cincinnati and at Case Western Reserve University. She is a former American Cancer Society Professor of Oncology Nursing and held an endowed chair in oncology for 5 years. In addition to authoring several textbooks and serving as a consult for major universities, she is Senior Volunteer Faculty at the College of Nursing, University of Cincinnati.

ACKNOWLEDGMENTS

Publishing a textbook and ancillary package of this depth and breadth would not be possible without the combined efforts of many people. Stephanie M. Ignatavicius assisted with literature searches. For this eighth edition, we welcomed three section editors to assist in our revision process: Meg Blair, Cherie Rebar, and Chris Winkelman. Each of these nursing educators worked with us on our seventh edition as contributors and/or ancillary material authors. For this eighth edition they updated and reviewed selected units of the text to provide their expertise.

Our contributing authors once again provided consistently excellent manuscripts in a timely fashion. Special thanks to Deanne Blach, who revised our Concept Maps, and Dr. Richard Lintner, who again provided expertise in interventional radiologic procedures and associated care. Our reviewers—expert clinicians and instructors from around the United States and Canada—provided invaluable suggestions and encouragement throughout the book's development.

The staff of Elsevier/Saunders once again provided us with crucial guidance and support throughout the planning, writing, revision, and production of the eighth edition. In particular, Executive Content Strategist Lee Henderson worked closely with us from the early stages of this edition to help us hone and focus our revision plan, and Lee coordinated the project from start to finish. Senior Content Development Specialist Rae Robertson then worked with us step-by-step to bring the eighth edition from vision to publication. Rae, Julia Curcio, and Kelly McGowan held the reins of our complex ancillary package and worked with a gifted group of writers and content experts to provide an outstanding library of resources to complement and enhance the text. Special thanks to Content Coordinators/Content Development Specialists Courtney Daniels and Samantha Taylor, who not only managed the *Clinical Companion* but also handled the countless administrative details associated with a project of this size.

Senior Project Manager Jodi Willard was once again a joy to work with. If, as is said, the mark of a good editor is that her work is invisible to the reader, then Jodi is the consummate editor. Her unwavering attention to detail, flexibility, and conscientiousness not only helped to make this edition the most consistently readable ever, but also made the entire production process incredibly smooth.

Special thanks also to Publishing Services Manager Debbie Vogel. For four editions now, Debbie has worked quietly behind the scenes to help bring the book to publication precisely on schedule and with a very high level of quality.

Designer Margaret Reid is responsible for the beautiful cover and the new interior design of the eighth edition. The praise of a book designer's work is often unsung, but Margaret's work on this edition has cast important features in exactly the right light, with neither too much nor too little emphasis, making this edition not only practical and easy to read, but also beautiful.

Our acknowledgments would not be complete without recognizing our dedicated team of Educational Solutions Consultants and other key members of the Sales and Marketing staff who helped to put this book into your hands.

Finally, we wish to thank John Danaher (President, Education) and Loren Wilson (Senior Vice President and General Manager, Content) for their ongoing vision, direction, and support for state-of-the-art educational resources for nurses.

Donna D. Ignatavicius
M. Linda Workman

CONTENTS

Unit I Foundations for Medical-Surgical Nursing

1 Introduction to Medical-Surgical Nursing Practice, 1
Donna D. Ignatavicius
 Scope of Medical-Surgical Nursing Practice, 1
 Priority Focus on Safety and Quality of Care, 2
  Protecting Five Million Lives from Harm, 2
  Quality and Safety Education for Nurses Core
   Competencies, 3
  Evidence-Based Practice, 6
  Quality Improvement, 6
  Informatics, 7
  Safety, 7

2 Common Health Problems of Older Adults, 9
Donna D. Ignatavicius
 Overview, 9
 Health Issues for Older Adults in Community-Based
  Settings, 10
  Decreased Nutrition and Hydration, 10
  Decreased Mobility, 11
  Stress and Loss, 12
  Accidents, 13
  Drug Use and Misuse, 13
  Mental Health/Behavioral Health Problems, 16
  Elder Neglect and Abuse, 19
 Health Care Issues for Older Adults in Hospitals and
  Long-Term Care Settings, 19
  Problems of Sleep, Nutrition, and Continence, 20
  Confusion, Falls, and Skin Breakdown, 20
  Care Transition from the Hospital or Long-Term
   Care Setting to Home, 22

3 Assessment and Care of Patients with Pain, 24
Chris Pasero and Donna D. Ignatavicius
 Overview, 24
 Scope of the Problem, 25
 Definitions of Pain, 25
 Categorization of Pain by Duration, 25
  Acute Pain, 25
  Chronic Pain, 26
 Categorization of Pain by Underlying
  Mechanisms, 26
  Nociceptive Pain, 26
  Neuropathic Pain, 28
 Patient-Centered Collaborative Care, 28
  Pain Assessment, 28
  Pharmacologic Management of Pain, 34
  Nonpharmacologic Management of Pain, 46
  Community-Based Care, 48

4 Genetic and Genomic Concepts for Medical-Surgical
 Nursing, 51
M. Linda Workman
 Genetic Biology Review, 51
  DNA, 52
  Gene Structure and Function, 54
  Gene Expression, 55
  Protein Synthesis, 55
  Mutations, 56

 Patterns of Inheritance, 56
  Pedigree, 57
  Autosomal Dominant Pattern of Inheritance, 57
  Autosomal Recessive Pattern of Inheritance, 58
  Sex-Linked Recessive Pattern of Inheritance, 58
  Complex Inheritance and Familial Clustering, 59
 Genetic Testing, 59
  Purpose of Genetic Testing, 59
  Benefits and Risks of Genetic Testing, 59
  Genetic Counseling, 60
  Ethical Issues, 61
 The Role of the Medical-Surgical Nurse in Genetic
  Counseling, 61
  Communication, 61
  Privacy and Confidentiality, 62
  Information Accuracy, 62
  Patient Advocacy and Support, 62

5 Evidence-Based Practice in Medical-Surgical Nursing, 64
Rona F. Levin and Fay Wright
 Overview, 64
  Definitions of Evidence-Based Practice, 64
  Steps of the Evidence-Based Practice Process, 65
 Models and Frameworks for Implementing
  Evidence-Based Practice, 68
  Iowa Model, 68
  Reavy and Tavernier Model, 69
  ARCC Model, 69
 Evidence-Based Practice Improvement (EBPI)
  Model, 70
  Steps of the EBPI Model, 70
  Application of the EBPI Model to Clinical Practice:
   A Case Study, 70

6 Rehabilitation Concepts for Chronic and Disabling
 Health Problems, 74
Donna D. Ignatavicius
 Overview, 74
  Chronic and Disabling Health Problems, 74
  Rehabilitation Settings, 75
  The Rehabilitation Team, 75

7 End-of-Life Care, 91
Mary K. Kazanowski
 Overview of Death and Dying, 91
  Death in the United States, 91
  Pathophysiology of Dying, 92
  Planning for End-of-Life and Advance Directives, 92
  Hospice and Palliative Care, 94
 Postmortem Care, 102
 The Concept of Euthanasia, 103

Unit II Concepts of Emergency Care and Disaster Preparedness

8 Concepts of Emergency and Trauma Nursing, 105
Linda Laskowski-Jones and Karen L. Toulson
 The Emergency Department Environment
  of Care, 106

xvii

Demographic Data and Vulnerable
   Populations, 106
Special Nursing Teams, 106
Interdisciplinary Team Collaboration, 106
Staff and Patient Safety Considerations, 108
Staff Safety, 108
Patient Safety, 108
Scope of Emergency Nursing Practice, 109
Core Competencies, 110
Training and Certification, 111
Emergency Nursing Principles, 111
Triage, 111
Disposition, 112
The Impact of Homelessness, 114
Trauma Nursing Principles, 114
Trauma Centers and Trauma
   Systems, 115
Mechanism of Injury, 116
Primary Survey and Resuscitation
   Interventions, 116
The Secondary Survey and Resuscitation
   Interventions, 118
Disposition, 118

**9 Care of Patients with Common Environmental
Emergencies, 120**
Linda Laskowski-Jones
Heat-Related Illnesses, 120
Heat Exhaustion, 121
Heat Stroke, 121
Snakebites, 123
North American Pit Vipers, 123
Coral Snakes, 125
Arthropod Bites and Stings, 126
Brown Recluse Spider, 126
Black Widow Spider, 127
Scorpions, 128
Bees and Wasps, 128
Lightning Injuries, 129
Cold-Related Injuries, 131
Hypothermia, 131
Frostbite, 132
Altitude-Related Illnesses, 133
Drowning, 135

**10 Concepts of Emergency and Disaster
Preparedness, 138**
Linda Laskowski-Jones
Types of Disasters, 138
Impact of External Disasters, 139
**Emergency Preparedness and
Response, 140**
Mass Casualty Triage, 140
Notification and Activation of Emergency
   Preparedness/Management Plans, 141
Hospital Emergency Preparedness: Personnel Roles
   and Responsibilities, 142
Event Resolution and Debriefing, 144
Critical Incident Stress Debriefing, 145
Administrative Review, 145
**Role of Nursing in Community Emergency
Preparedness and Response, 146**
**Psychosocial Response of Survivors to Mass Casualty
Events, 146**

Unit III Management of Patients with Fluid, Electrolyte, and Acid-Base Imbalances

**11 Assessment and Care of Patients with Fluid and
Electrolyte Imbalances, 148**
M. Linda Workman
Homeostasis, 148
**Physiologic Influences on Fluid and Electrolyte
Balance, 148**
Filtration, 149
Diffusion, 150
Osmosis, 151
Fluid Balance, 152
Body Fluids, 152
Hormonal Regulation of Fluid Balance, 153
Significance of Fluid Balance, 154
Fluid Imbalances, 155
Dehydration, 155
Fluid Overload, 158
Electrolyte Balance and Imbalances, 160
Sodium, 161
Potassium, 163
Calcium, 167
Phosphorus, 170
Magnesium, 171
Chloride, 172

**12 Assessment and Care of Patients with Acid-Base
Imbalances, 174**
M. Linda Workman
Acid-Base Balance, 174
Acid-Base Chemistry, 175
Body Fluid Chemistry, 176
Acid-Base Regulatory Actions and Mechanisms, 177
Acid-Base Imbalances, 179
Acidosis, 179
Alkalosis, 183

13 Infusion Therapy, 187
Cheryl J. Dumont
Overview, 187
Types of Infusion Therapy Fluids, 188
Prescribing Infusion Therapy, 189
Vascular Access Devices, 189
Peripheral Intravenous Therapy, 190
Short Peripheral Catheters, 190
Midline Catheters, 192
Central Intravenous Therapy, 193
Peripherally Inserted Central Catheters, 193
Nontunneled Percutaneous Central Venous
   Catheters, 194
Tunneled Central Venous Catheters, 195
Implanted Ports, 195
Hemodialysis Catheters, 196
Infusion Systems, 196
Containers, 196
Administration Sets, 197
Rate-Controlling Infusion Devices, 198
**Nursing Care for Patients Receiving Intravenous
Therapy, 200**
Educating the Patient, 200
Performing the Nursing Assessment, 200
Securing and Dressing the Catheter, 200

Changing Administration Sets and Needleless Connectors, 202
Controlling Infusion Pressure, 202
Flushing the Catheter, 202
Obtaining Blood Samples from Central Venous Catheters, 202
Removing the Vascular Access Device, 203
Documenting Intravenous Therapy, 203
Complications of Intravenous Therapy, 204
Catheter-Related Bloodstream Infection, 204
Other Complications of Intravenous Therapy, 204
IV Therapy and Care of the Older Adult, 207
Skin Care, 207
Vein and Catheter Selection, 209
Cardiac and Renal Changes, 209
Subcutaneous Infusion Therapy, 210
Intraosseous Infusion Therapy, 211
Intra-Arterial Infusion Therapy, 212
Intraperitoneal Infusion Therapy, 212
Intraspinal Infusion Therapy, 212

Unit IV Management of Perioperative Patients

14 Care of Preoperative Patients, 215
Robin Chard
Overview, 216
Categories and Purposes of Surgery, 217
Surgical Settings, 218
15 Care of Intraoperative Patients, 238
Robin Chard
Overview, 238
Members of the Surgical Team, 238
Preparation of the Surgical Suite and Team Safety, 241
Anesthesia, 244
16 Care of Postoperative Patients, 256
Robin Chard
Overview, 257

CONCEPT OVERVIEW: Protection, 274

Unit V Problems of Protection: Management of Patients with Problems of the Immune System

17 Inflammation and Immunity, 275
M. Linda Workman
Overview, 275
Self Versus Non-Self, 276
Organization of the Immune System, 276
Inflammation, 277
Infection, 278
Cell Types Involved in Inflammation, 278
Phagocytosis, 280
Sequence of Inflammation, 280
Immunity, 281
Antibody-Mediated Immunity, 281
Cell-Mediated Immunity, 285
Transplant Rejection, 286

18 Care of Patients with Arthritis and Other Connective Tissue Diseases, 290
Donna D. Ignatavicius
Osteoarthritis, 291
Rheumatoid Arthritis, 304
Lupus Erythematosus, 313
Systemic Sclerosis, 317
Gout, 319
Infectious Arthritis, 320
Lyme Disease, 320
Psoriatic Arthritis, 321
Fibromyalgia Syndrome, 321
Chronic Fatigue Syndrome, 322
Other Connective Tissue Diseases, 322
Other Disease-Associated Arthritis, 322
Mixed Connective Tissue Disease, 322
19 Care of Patients with HIV Disease and Other Immune Deficiencies, 326
James Sampson and M. Linda Workman
Acquired (Secondary) Immune Deficiencies, 326
HIV Infection and AIDS, 326
Therapy-Induced Immune Deficiencies, 344
Congenital (Primary) Immune Deficiencies, 345
Selective Immunoglobulin a Deficiency, 345
Bruton's Agammaglobulinemia, 346
Common Variable Immune Deficiency, 346
20 Care of Patients with Immune Function Excess: Hypersensitivity (Allergy) and Autoimmunity, 348
M. Linda Workman
Hypersensitivities/Allergies, 348
Type I: Rapid Hypersensitivity Reactions, 348
Type II: Cytotoxic Reactions, 355
Type III: Immune Complex Reactions, 355
Type IV: Delayed Hypersensitivity Reactions, 355
Autoimmunity, 356
Sjögren's Syndrome, 356
Goodpasture's Syndrome, 357
21 Cancer Development, 359
M. Linda Workman
Pathophysiology, 359
Biology of Normal Cells, 360
Biology of Abnormal Cells, 361
Cancer Development, 362
Carcinogenesis/Oncogenesis, 362
Cancer Classification, 363
Cancer Grading, Ploidy, and Staging, 365
Cancer Etiology and Genetic Risk, 365
Cancer Prevention, 368
Primary Prevention, 368
Secondary Prevention, 369
22 Care of Patients with Cancer, 371
June Eilers
General Disease-Related Consequences of Cancer, 371
Reduced Immunity and Blood-Producing Functions, 372
Altered GI Structure and Function, 372
Motor and Sensory Deficits, 372
Reduced Gas Exchange, 372
Cancer Management, 372
Surgery, 373
Radiation Therapy, 374
Cytotoxic Systemic Agent Therapy, 377

Oncologic Emergencies, 392
  Sepsis and Disseminated Intravascular
    Coagulation, 392
  Syndrome of Inappropriate Antidiuretic
    Hormone, 392
  Spinal Cord Compression, 393
  Hypercalcemia, 393
  Superior Vena Cava Syndrome, 393
  Tumor Lysis Syndrome, 394

23 Care of Patients with Infection, 397
Donna D. Ignatavicius
  Overview of the Infectious Process, 397
    Transmission of Infectious Agents, 398
    Physiologic Defenses for Infection, 400
    Infection Control in Health Care Settings, 400
    Methods of Infection Control and Prevention, 401
  Multidrug-Resistant Organism Infections and
    Colonizations, 405
    Methicillin-Resistant Staphylococcus aureus
      (MRSA), 405
    Vancomycin-Resistant Enterococcus (VRE), 406
    Carbapenem-Resistant Enterobacteriaceae
      (CRE), 406
  Occupational and Environmental Exposure to
    Sources of Infection, 406
  Problems From Inadequate Antimicrobial
    Therapy, 407
  Critical Issues: Emerging Infections and Global
    Bioterrorism, 411

**Unit VI Problems of Protection: Management
    of Patients with Problems of the Skin,
    Hair, and Nails**

24 Assessment of the Skin, Hair, and Nails, 415
Janice Cuzzell and M. Linda Workman
  Anatomy and Physiology Review, 415
    Structure of the Skin, 415
    Structure of the Skin Appendages, 417
    Functions of the Skin, 417
    Skin Changes Associated with Aging, 417
  Assessment Methods, 420
    Patient History, 420
    Nutrition Status, 420
    Family History and Genetic Risk, 421
    Current Health Problems, 421
    Skin Assessment, 421
    Hair Assessment, 424
    Nail Assessment, 425
    Skin Assessment Techniques for Patients with
      Darker Skin, 428
    Psychosocial Assessment, 428
    Diagnostic Assessment, 429

25 Care of Patients with Skin Problems, 432
Janice Cuzzell and M. Linda Workman
  Minor Skin Irritations, 432
    Pruritus, 432
    Urticaria, 433
  Trauma, 433
  Pressure Ulcers, 436
  Common Infections, 449

Cutaneous Anthrax, 453
Parasitic Disorders, 453
  Pediculosis, 453
  Scabies, 454
  Bedbugs, 454
Common Inflammations, 455
Psoriasis, 456
Skin Cancer, 458
Other Skin Disorders, 461
  Toxic Epidermal Necrolysis, 461
  Stevens-Johnson Syndrome, 461
Plastic Surgery, 462

26 Care of Patients with Burns, 465
Tammy Coffee
  Pathophysiology of Burn Injury, 465
    Skin Changes Resulting from Burn Injury, 465
    Vascular Changes Resulting from Burn Injuries, 469
    Cardiac Changes Resulting from Burn Injury, 470
    Pulmonary Changes Resulting from Burn Injury, 470
    Gastrointestinal Changes Resulting from Burn
      Injury, 470
    Metabolic Changes Resulting from Burn Injury, 470
    Immunologic Changes Resulting from Burn
      Injury, 470
    Compensatory Responses to Burn Injury, 470
    Etiology of Burn Injury, 470
    Incidence and Prevalence of Burn Injury, 472
  Resuscitation Phase of Burn Injury, 473
  Acute Phase of Burn Injury, 481
  Rehabilitative Phase of Burn Injury, 488

**CONCEPT OVERVIEW:
Oxygenation, 492**

**Unit VII Problems of Oxygenation: Management
    of Patients with Problems of
    the Respiratory Tract**

27 Assessment of the Respiratory System, 494
Harry Rees
  Anatomy and Physiology Review, 496
    Upper Respiratory Tract, 496
    Lower Respiratory Tract, 498
    Oxygen Delivery and the Oxygen-Hemoglobin
      Dissociation Curve, 499
    Respiratory Changes Associated with Aging, 500
  Assessment Methods, 500
    Patient History, 500
    Physical Assessment, 503
    Psychosocial Assessment, 506
    Diagnostic Assessment, 507

**28 Care of Patients Requiring Oxygen Therapy or
    Tracheostomy, 514**
Harry Rees
  Oxygen Therapy, 514
  Tracheostomy, 522

**29 Care of Patients with Noninfectious Upper Respiratory
    Problems, 531**
M. Linda Workman
  Disorders of the Nose and Sinuses, 531
    Fracture of the Nose, 531

Epistaxis, 532
Cancer of the Nose and Sinuses, 533
Facial Trauma, 534
Obstructive Sleep Apnea, 534
Disorders of the Larynx, 535
Vocal Cord Paralysis, 535
Laryngeal Trauma, 536
Other Upper Airway Disorders, 536
Upper Airway Obstruction, 536
Neck Trauma, 537
Head and Neck Cancer, 537

30 Care of Patients with Noninfectious Lower Respiratory Problems, 548
M. Linda Workman
Asthma, 548
Chronic Obstructive Pulmonary Disease, 557
Cystic Fibrosis, 567
Pulmonary Arterial Hypertension, 569
Interstitial Pulmonary Diseases, 571
Sarcoidosis, 571
Idiopathic Pulmonary Fibrosis, 571
Occupational Pulmonary Disease, 572
Bronchiolitis Obliterans Organizing Pneumonia, 572
Lung Cancer, 573

31 Care of Patients with Infectious Respiratory Problems, 583
Meg Blair
Disorders of the Nose and Sinuses, 583
Rhinitis, 583
Rhinosinusitis, 584
Disorders of the Oral Pharynx and Tonsils, 584
Pharyngitis, 584
Tonsillitis, 586
Peritonsillar Abscess, 586
Disorders of the Lungs, 586
Seasonal Influenza, 586
Pandemic Influenza, 587
Pneumonia, 588
Severe Acute Respiratory Syndrome (SARS), 594
Pulmonary Tuberculosis, 595
Lung Abscess, 599
Pulmonary Empyema, 599
Inhalation Anthrax, 599
Pertussis, 600
Coccidioidomycosis, 600

32 Care of Critically Ill Patients with Respiratory Problems, 603
Meg Blair
Pulmonary Embolism, 603
Acute Respiratory Failure, 610
Acute Respiratory Distress Syndrome, 612
The Patient Requiring Intubation and Ventilation, 614
Chest Trauma, 622
Pulmonary Contusion, 622
Rib Fracture, 623
Flail Chest, 623
Pneumothorax, 623
Tension Pneumothorax, 624
Hemothorax, 624
Tracheobronchial Trauma, 624

Unit VIII Problems of Cardiac Output and Tissue Perfusion: Management of Patients with Problems of the Cardiovascular System

33 Assessment of the Cardiovascular System, 627
Donna Ignatavicius
Anatomy and Physiology Review, 627
Heart, 627
Vascular System, 631
Cardiovascular Changes Associated with Aging, 632
Assessment Methods, 632
Patient History, 632
Nutrition History, 634
Family History and Genetic Risk, 634
Current Health Problems, 634
Functional History, 636
Physical Assessment, 636
Psychosocial Assessment, 640
Diagnostic Assessment, 640

34 Care of Patients with Dysrhythmias, 649
Laura Dechant
Review of Cardiac Conduction System, 649
Electrocardiography, 650
Lead Systems, 651
Continuous Electrocardiographic Monitoring, 652
Electrocardiographic Complexes, Segments, and Intervals, 652
Determination of Heart Rate, 654
Electrocardiographic Rhythm Analysis, 655
Overview of Normal Cardiac Rhythms, 656
Common Dysrhythmias, 656

35 Care of Patients with Cardiac Problems, 678
Laura M. Dechant
Heart Failure, 678
Valvular Heart Disease, 692
Inflammations and Infections, 697
Infective Endocarditis, 697
Pericarditis, 699
Rheumatic Carditis, 700
Cardiomyopathy, 701

36 Care of Patients with Vascular Problems, 706
Donna D. Ignatavicius
Arteriosclerosis and Atherosclerosis, 706
Hypertension, 709
Peripheral Arterial Disease, 718
Acute Peripheral Arterial Occlusion, 725
Aneurysms of Central Arteries, 726
Aneurysms of the Peripheral Arteries, 728
Aortic Dissection, 728
Other Arterial Health Problems, 728
Peripheral Venous Disease, 728
Venous Thromboembolism, 729
Venous Insufficiency, 734
Varicose Veins, 735
Vascular Trauma, 736

37 Care of Patients with Shock, 739
M. Linda Workman
Overview, 739
Review of Oxygenation and Tissue Perfusion, 739
Types of Shock, 740

Hypovolemic Shock, 742
Sepsis and Septic Shock, 749

38 Care of Patients with Acute Coronary Syndromes, 757
Laura M. Dechant
Pathophysiology, 757
Chronic Stable Angina Pectoris, 757
Acute Coronary Syndrome, 758
Etiology and Genetic Risk, 760
Incidence and Prevalence, 760
Health Promotion and Maintenance, 760
Using Complementary and Alternative Therapies, 761
Managing Metabolic Syndrome, 761
Patient-Centered Collaborative Care, 762

Unit IX Problems of Tissue Perfusion: Management of Patients with Problems of the Hematologic System

39 Assessment of the Hematologic System, 785
M. Linda Workman
Anatomy and Physiology Review, 785
Bone Marrow, 785
Blood Components, 786
Accessory Organs of Blood Formation, 787
Hemostasis and Blood Clotting, 787
Anti-Clotting Forces, 788
Hematologic Changes Associated with Aging, 788
Assessment Methods, 788
Patient History, 788
Nutrition Status, 791
Family History and Genetic Risk, 791
Current Health Problems, 792
Physical Assessment, 792
Psychosocial Assessment, 793
Diagnostic Assessment, 793

40 Care of Patients with Hematologic Problems, 798
Katherine I. Byar
Red Blood Cell Disorders, 798
Anemias Resulting From Increased Destruction of Red Blood Cells, 799
Anemias Resulting From Decreased Production of Red Blood Cells, 804
Disorders of Excess Red Blood Cells or Iron, 805
Myelodysplastic Syndromes, 806
White Blood Cell Disorders, 806
Leukemia, 806
Malignant Lymphomas, 817
Coagulation Disorders, 819
Platelet Disorders, 819
Clotting Factor Disorders, 820
Transfusion Therapy, 821
Pretransfusion Responsibilities, 821
Transfusion Responsibilities, 823
Types of Transfusions, 823
Acute Transfusion Reactions, 824
Autologous Blood Transfusions, 825

CONCEPT OVERVIEW:
Mobility, Sensory Perception, and Cognition, 828

Unit X Problems of Mobility, Sensory Perception, and Cognition: Management of Patients with Problems of the Nervous System

41 Assessment of the Nervous System, 829
Rachel L. Gallagher
Anatomy and Physiology Review, 829
Nervous System Cells: Structure and Function, 830
Central Nervous System: Structure and Function, 830
Peripheral Nervous System: Structure and Function, 833
Autonomic Nervous System: Structure and Function, 835
Neurologic Changes Associated with Aging, 836
Assessment Methods, 837
Patient History, 837
Physical Assessment, 837
Psychosocial Assessment, 844
Diagnostic Assessment, 844

42 Care of Patients with Problems of the Central Nervous System: The Brain, 853
Rachel L. Gallagher
Headaches, 853
Migraine Headache, 854
Cluster Headache, 857
Seizures and Epilepsy, 858
Infections, 863
Meningitis, 863
Encephalitis, 865
Parkinson Disease, 867
Dementia, 871
Huntington Disease, 881

43 Care of Patients with Problems of the Central Nervous System: The Spinal Cord, 884
Rachel L. Gallagher
Back Pain, 885
Low Back Pain (Lumbosacral Back Pain), 885
Cervical Neck Pain, 891
Spinal Cord Injury, 892
Spinal Cord Tumors, 902
Multiple Sclerosis, 904
Amyotrophic Lateral Sclerosis, 910

44 Care of Patients with Problems of the Peripheral Nervous System, 913
Rachel L. Gallagher
Guillain-Barré Syndrome, 913
Myasthenia Gravis, 917
Peripheral Nerve Trauma, 923
Restless Legs Syndrome, 925
Diseases of the Cranial Nerves, 926

45 Care of Critically Ill Patients with Neurologic Problems, 930
Chris Winkelman and Rachel L. Gallagher
Transient Ischemic Attack, 930
Stroke (Brain Attack), 931

Traumatic Brain Injury, 946
Brain Tumors, 957
Brain Abscess, 962
Acquired Hypoxic-Anoxic Brain Injury, 964

Unit XI Problems of Sensory Perception: Management of Patients with Problems of the Sensory System

46 Assessment of the Eye and Vision, 966
M. Linda Workman
Anatomy and Physiology Review, 966
Structure, 966
Function, 968
Eye Changes Associated with Aging, 969
Assessment Methods, 971
Patient History, 971
Physical Assessment, 972
Psychosocial Assessment, 973
Diagnostic Assessment, 973

47 Care of Patients with Eye and Vision Problems, 977
M. Linda Workman
Eyelid Disorders, 977
Entropion and Ectropion, 977
Hordeolum, 978
Chalazion, 978
Keratoconjunctivitis Sicca, 978
Conjunctival Disorders, 978
Conjunctivitis, 979
Trachoma, 980
Corneal Disorders, 980
Corneal Abrasion, Ulceration, and Infection, 980
Keratoconus and Corneal Opacities, 981
Cataract, 982
Glaucoma, 985
Retinal Disorders, 989
Macular Degeneration, 989
Retinal Holes, Tears, and Detachments, 989
Retinitis Pigmentosa, 990
Refractive Errors, 991
Trauma, 991
Foreign Bodies, 991
Lacerations, 992
Penetrating Injuries, 992
Ocular Melanoma, 992
Reduced Visual Sensory Perception, 992

48 Assessment and Care of Patients with Ear and Hearing Problems, 996
M. Linda Workman
Anatomy and Physiology Review, 996
Structure, 996
Function, 998
Ear and Hearing Changes Associated with Aging, 998
Assessment Methods, 998
Patient History, 998
Physical Assessment, 1000
General Hearing Assessment, 1001
Psychosocial Assessment, 1002
Diagnostic Assessment, 1002
Disorders of the Ear and Hearing, 1003
Conditions Affecting the External Ear, 1003
Conditions Affecting the Middle Ear, 1005
Conditions Affecting the Inner Ear, 1007
Hearing Loss, 1009

Unit XII Problems of Mobility: Management of Patients with Problems of the Musculoskeletal System

49 Assessment of the Musculoskeletal System, 1017
Donna D. Ignatavicius
Anatomy and Physiology Review, 1017
Skeletal System, 1017
Muscular System, 1019
Musculoskeletal Changes Associated with Aging, 1020
Assessment Methods, 1020
Patient History, 1020
Assessment of the Skeletal System, 1021
Assessment of the Muscular System, 1023
Psychosocial Assessment, 1024
Diagnostic Assessment, 1024

50 Care of Patients with Musculoskeletal Problems, 1029
Donna D. Ignatavicius
Metabolic Bone Diseases, 1029
Osteoporosis, 1029
Osteomalacia, 1036
Paget's Disease of the Bone, 1037
Osteomyelitis, 1039
Benign Bone Tumors, 1042
Bone Cancer, 1042
Disorders of the Hand, 1045
Dupuytren's Contracture, 1045
Ganglion, 1046
Disorders of the Foot, 1046
Foot Deformities, 1046
Morton's Neuroma, 1047
Plantar Fasciitis, 1047
Other Problems of the Foot, 1047
Scoliosis, 1047
Progressive Muscular Dystrophies, 1048

51 Care of Patients with Musculoskeletal Trauma, 1051
Donna D. Ignatavicius
Fractures, 1051
Selected Fractures of Specific Sites, 1066
Upper Extremity Fractures, 1066
Lower Extremity Fractures, 1066
Fractures of the Chest and Pelvis, 1069
Compression Fractures of the Spine, 1069
Amputations, 1069
Complex Regional Pain Syndrome, 1075
Knee Injuries, 1075
Carpal Tunnel Syndrome, 1077
Tendinopathy and Joint Dislocation, 1079
Strains and Sprains, 1079
Rotator Cuff Injuries, 1079

CONCEPT OVERVIEW:
Metabolism, 1082

Unit XIII Problems of Digestion, Nutrition, and Elimination: Management of Patients with Problems of the Gastrointestinal System

52 Assessment of the Gastrointestinal System, 1084
Donna D. Ignatavicius
　Anatomy and Physiology Review, 1084
　　Structure, 1084
　　Function, 1084
　Gastrointestinal Changes Associated with Aging, 1087
　Assessment Methods, 1087
　　Patient History, 1087
　　Nutrition History, 1087
　　Family History and Genetic Risk, 1089
　　Current Health Problems, 1089
　　Physical Assessment, 1089
　　Psychosocial Assessment, 1091
　　Diagnostic Assessment, 1091

53 Care of Patients with Oral Cavity Problems, 1099
Cherie R. Rebar, Nicole Heimgartner, Laura Willis
　Stomatitis, 1100
　Oral Tumors, 1102
　　Premalignant Lesions, 1102
　　Oral Cancer, 1102
　Disorders of the Salivary Glands, 1107
　　Acute Sialadenitis, 1107
　　Post-Irradiation Sialadenitis, 1108
　　Salivary Gland Tumors, 1108

54 Care of Patients with Esophageal Problems, 1110
Cherie R. Rebar, Nicole Heimgartner, Laura Willis
　Gastroesophageal Reflux Disease, 1110
　Hiatal Hernia, 1114
　Esophageal Tumors, 1117
　Esophageal Diverticula, 1123
　Esophageal Trauma, 1123

55 Care of Patients with Stomach Disorders, 1126
Lara Carver
　Gastritis, 1126
　Peptic Ulcer Disease, 1128
　Gastric Cancer, 1138

56 Care of Patients with Noninflammatory Intestinal Disorders, 1144
Donna D. Ignatavicius
　Irritable Bowel Syndrome, 1144
　Herniation, 1146
　Colorectal Cancer, 1148
　Intestinal Obstruction, 1157
　Abdominal Trauma, 1161
　Polyps, 1163
　Hemorrhoids, 1164
　Malabsorption Syndrome, 1165

57 Care of Patients with Inflammatory Intestinal Disorders, 1168
Donna D. Ignatavicius
　Acute Inflammatory Bowel Disorders, 1168
　　Appendicitis, 1168

　　Peritonitis, 1170
　　Gastroenteritis, 1172
　Chronic Inflammatory Bowel Disease, 1173
　　Ulcerative Colitis, 1174
　　Crohn's Disease, 1181
　　Diverticular Disease, 1186
　　Celiac Disease, 1188
　Anal Disorders, 1188
　　Anorectal Abscess, 1188
　　Anal Fissure, 1188
　　Anal Fistula, 1189
　Parasitic Infection, 1189

58 Care of Patients with Liver Problems, 1192
Jennifer Powers and Lara Carver
　Cirrhosis, 1192
　Hepatitis, 1203
　Fatty Liver (Steatosis), 1208
　Liver Trauma, 1208
　Cancer of the Liver, 1208
　Liver Transplantation, 1209

59 Care of Patients with Problems of the Biliary System and Pancreas, 1213
Lara Carver and Jennifer Powers
　Cholecystitis, 1213
　Acute Pancreatitis, 1218
　Chronic Pancreatitis, 1223
　Pancreatic Abscess, 1226
　Pancreatic Pseudocyst, 1226
　Pancreatic Cancer, 1226

60 Care of Patients with Malnutrition: Undernutrition and Obesity, 1232
Cherie R. Rebar, Nicole Heimgartner, Laura Willis
　Nutrition Standards for Health Promotion and Maintenance, 1232
　Nutrition Assessment, 1233
　　Initial Nutrition Screening, 1234
　　Anthropometric Measurements, 1234
　Malnutrition, 1236
　Obesity, 1246

Unit XIV Problems of Regulation and Metabolism: Management of Patients with Problems of the Endocrine System

61 Assessment of the Endocrine System, 1255
M. Linda Workman
　Anatomy and Physiology Review, 1256
　　Hypothalamus and Pituitary Glands, 1257
　　Gonads, 1257
　　Adrenal Glands, 1257
　　Thyroid Gland, 1259
　　Parathyroid Glands, 1260
　　Pancreas, 1260
　　Endocrine Changes Associated with Aging, 1260
　Assessment Methods, 1261
　　Patient History, 1261
　　Physical Assessment, 1262
　　Psychosocial Assessment, 1263
　　Diagnostic Assessment, 1263

62 Care of Patients with Pituitary and Adrenal Gland Problems, 1266
M. Linda Workman
  Disorders of the Anterior Pituitary Gland, 1266
    Hypopituitarism, 1266
    Hyperpituitarism, 1268
  Disorders of the Posterior Pituitary Gland, 1271
    Diabetes Insipidus, 1271
    Syndrome of Inappropriate Antidiuretic Hormone, 1272
  Disorders of the Adrenal Gland, 1273
    Adrenal Gland Hypofunction, 1273
    Adrenal Gland Hyperfunction, 1276

63 Care of Patients with Problems of the Thyroid and Parathyroid Glands, 1285
M. Linda Workman
  Thyroid Disorders, 1285
    Hyperthyroidism, 1285
    Hypothyroidism, 1291
    Thyroiditis, 1295
    Thyroid Cancer, 1295
  Parathyroid Disorders, 1296
    Hyperparathyroidism, 1296
    Hypoparathyroidism, 1298

64 Care of Patients with Diabetes Mellitus, 1300
Margaret Elaine McLeod
  Pathophysiology, 1300
    Classification of Diabetes, 1300
    The Endocrine Pancreas, 1301
    Glucose Regulation and Homeostasis, 1301
    Absence of Insulin, 1302
    Acute Complications of Diabetes, 1303
    Chronic Complications of Diabetes, 1303
    Etiology and Genetic Risk, 1306
    Incidence and Prevalence, 1307
  Health Promotion and Maintenance, 1307
  Patient-Centered Collaborative Care, 1308

CONCEPT OVERVIEW:
Urinary Elimination, 1342

Unit XV Problems of Excretion: Management of Patients with Problems of the Renal/Urinary System

65 Assessment of the Renal/Urinary System, 1344
Chris Winkelman
  Anatomy and Physiology Review, 1345
    Kidneys, 1345
    Ureters, 1350
    Urinary Bladder, 1350
    Urethra, 1350
    Kidney and Urinary System Changes Associated with Aging, 1351
  Assessment Methods, 1352
    Patient History, 1352
    Physical Assessment, 1353
    Psychosocial Assessment, 1354
    Diagnostic Assessment, 1354

66 Care of Patients with Urinary Problems, 1366
Chris Winkelman
  Infectious Disorders, 1366
    Cystitis, 1367
    Urethritis, 1373
  Noninfectious Disorders, 1373
    Urethral Strictures, 1373
    Urinary Incontinence, 1373
    Urolithiasis, 1384
    Urothelial Cancer, 1388
    Bladder Trauma, 1391

67 Care of Patients with Kidney Disorders, 1394
Chris Winkelman
  Congenital Disorders, 1394
    Polycystic Kidney Disease, 1394
  Obstructive Disorders, 1397
    Hydronephrosis, Hydroureter, and Urethral Stricture, 1397
  Infectious Disorders: Pyelonephritis, 1399
  Immunologic Kidney Disorders, 1401
    Acute Glomerulonephritis, 1402
    Rapidly Progressive Glomerulonephritis, 1403
    Chronic Glomerulonephritis, 1403
    Nephrotic Syndrome, 1404
    Immunologic Interstitial and Tubulointerstitial Disorders, 1405
  Degenerative Disorders, 1405
    Nephrosclerosis, 1405
    Renovascular Disease, 1405
    Diabetic Nephropathy, 1406
  Renal Cell Carcinoma, 1406
  Kidney Trauma, 1408

68 Care of Patients with Acute Kidney Injury and Chronic Kidney Disease, 1411
Chris Winkelman
  Acute Kidney Injury, 1412
  Chronic Kidney Disease, 1419

CONCEPT OVERVIEW:
Sexuality, 1448

Unit XVI Problems of Reproduction: Management of Patients with Problems of the Reproductive System

69 Assessment of the Reproductive System, 1449
Donna D. Ignatavicius
  Anatomy and Physiology Review, 1449
    Structure and Function of the Female Reproductive System, 1449
    Structure and Function of the Male Reproductive System, 1451
  Reproductive Changes Associated with Aging, 1452
  Assessment Methods, 1452
    Patient History, 1452
    Physical Assessment, 1454
    Psychosocial Assessment, 1454
    Diagnostic Assessment, 1454

70 Care of Patients with Breast Disorders, 1461
Mary Justice
    Benign Breast Disorders, 1461
      Fibroadenoma, 1461
      Fibrocystic Breast Condition, 1462
      Ductal Ectasia, 1462
      Intraductal Papilloma, 1463
      Issues of Large-Breasted Women, 1463
      Issues of Small-Breasted Women, 1463
      Gynecomastia, 1463
    Breast Cancer, 1464
71 Care of Patients with Gynecologic Problems, 1482
Donna D. Ignatavicius
    Endometriosis, 1482
    Dysfunctional Uterine Bleeding, 1483
    Vulvovaginitis, 1484
    Toxic Shock Syndrome, 1485
    Pelvic Organ Prolapse, 1485
    Benign Neoplasms, 1487
      Ovarian Cyst, 1487
      Uterine Leiomyoma, 1487
      Bartholin Cyst, 1491
      Cervical Polyp, 1491
    Gynecologic Cancers, 1491
      Endometrial (Uterine) Cancer, 1491
      Cervical Cancer, 1494
      Ovarian Cancer, 1495
72 Care of Patients with Male Reproductive Problems, 1499
Donna D. Ignatavicius
    Benign Prostatic Hyperplasia, 1499
    Prostate Cancer, 1506

    Prostatitis, 1512
    Erectile Dysfunction, 1512
    Testicular Cancer, 1513
    Other Problems Affecting the Testes and Adjacent
      Structures, 1516
73 Care of Transgender Patients, 1519
Donna D. Ignatavicius and Stephanie M. Ignatavicius
    Patient-Centered Terminology, 1519
    Transgender Health Issues, 1520
    Stress and Transgender Health, 1521
    Need to Improve Transgender Health Care, 1521
74 Care of Patients with Sexually Transmitted
Disease, 1530
Shirley E. Van Zandt
    Overview, 1530
    Infections Associated with Ulcers, 1531
      Syphilis, 1531
      Genital Herpes, 1535
    Infections of the Epithelial Structures, 1537
      Condylomata Acuminata (Genital Warts), 1537
      Chlamydia Infection, 1538
      Gonorrhea, 1539
    Other Gynecologic Conditions, 1541
      Pelvic Inflammatory Disease, 1541
      Vaginal Infections, 1544
    Other Sexually Transmitted Diseases, 1544

Bibliography, 1546
Glossary, 1586
NCLEX® Examination Challenges—Answer Key, AK-1
Illustration Credits, IC-1

GUIDE TO SPECIAL FEATURES

BEST PRACTICE FOR PATIENT SAFETY & QUALITY CARE

Acute Adrenal Insufficiency, 1274

AIDS, Infection Control for Home Care, 344

Alteplase, Nursing Interventions During and After Administration, 939

Altitude-Related Illnesses, Preventing, Recognizing, and Treating, 135

Alzheimer's Disease, Promoting Communication, 877

Anaphylaxis, 353

Anesthesia, Spinal and Epidural, Recognizing Serious Complications, 261

Anterior Nosebleed, 532

Anticoagulant Therapy, 732

Anticoagulant, Fibrinolytic, or Antiplatelet Therapy, 609

Prevention of Injury, 609

Arteriovenous Fistula or Ateriovenous Graft, 1435

Artificial Airway, Suctioning, 525

Aspiration Prevention During Swallowing, 528, 545

Autologous Blood Salvage and Transfusion, 251

Autonomic Dysreflexia, 899

Benzodiazepine Overdose, 266

Breast Mass Assessment, 1469

Breast Reconstruction, Postoperative Care, 1476

Breast Self-Examination, 1468

Burns, 473

Cancer, Colorectal, Screening Recommendations, 1150

Cancer, Gynecologic, Brachytherapy, 1493

Caregiver Stress Reduction, 880

Carpal Tunnel Syndrome Prevention, 1077

Catheter-Related Infection Prevention, 1368

Cervical Diskectomy and Fusion, 892

Chest Discomfort, 764

Chest Tube Drainage Systems, 579

Cognition Assessment, 839

Colonoscopy, 1096

Communicating with Patients Unable to Speak, 540

Continuous Passive Motion Machine, 302

Contracture Prevention, 487

Contrast Agent Precautions for Diagnostic Testing, 845

Contrast Media, Assessing the Patient, 1361

Dark Skin, Assessing Changes, 428

Death, Pronouncement of, 102

Dehydration, 157

Diarrhea, Skin Care, 1166

Driver Safety Improvement, Older Adults, 14

Dying Patient and the Family, Psychosocial Interventions, 101

Dysrhythmias, 658

Ear Irrigation, 1005

Eardrops Instillation, 1004

Emergency Department, Maintaining Patient and Staff Safety, 108

Endocrine Testing, 1263

Energy Conservation, 815

Extremity Fracture, 1058

Eyedrops Instillation, 975

Fall Prevention in Older Adults, 21

Feeding Tube Maintenance, 1243

Fires in Health Care Facility, Response, 139

Fluid Resuscitation for Burns, 479

Fluid Volume Management, 1426

Fundoplication, Assessment of Complications, 1116

Gait Training, 83

Gastrointestinal Health History Questions, 1088

Genetic Testing and Counseling, 60

Genital Herpes, 1537

Hand Hygiene, 401

Hearing Impairment and Communication, 1014

Heart Transplant Rejection, 703

Heat Stroke, 123

Hemodialysis, 1436

HIV, Recommendations for Preventing Transmission by Health Care Workers, 332

Home Hospice, Symptom Relief, 97

Hypertensive Crisis, 718

Hypokalemia, 165

Hypophysectomy, 1270

Hypovolemic Shock, 747

Immunosuppressed Patient, 338

Infection Risks, 401

Inflammatory Bowel Disease, Pain Control and Skin Care, 1179

Intraoperative Positioning, Prevention of Complications, 253

LGBTQ Patients, Creating a Welcoming Environment, 1523

Lumbar Spinal Surgery, Assessment and Management of Complications, 889

Magnetic Resonance Imaging, 1026

Malignant Hyperthermia, 247

Mechanical Ventilation, 617

Meningitis, 865

Minimally Invasive Inguinal Hernia Repair, Postoperative Care, 1148

Musculoskeletal Injury, Assessment of Neurovascular Status, 1057

Musculoskeletal Injury, Prevention, 890

Myasthenia Gravis, Improving Nutrition, 921

Myelosuppression, 382

Myxedema Coma, 1294

Nasogastric Tube After Esophageal Surgery, 1122

Neutropenia, 382

Nursing Database, 838

Nutritional Screening Assessment, 1234

Obstruction, Intestinal, Nursing Care, 1159

Ocular Irrigation, 991

Ophthalmic Ointment Instillation, 978

Opioid Overdose, 271

Oral Cavity Problems, 1101

Osteoporosis and Assessment of Risk Factors, 1030

Oxygen Therapy, 515

Pain, Reducing Postoperatively with Nonpharmacologic Interventions, 271

Paracentesis, 1199

Parkinson Disease, 869

Pericarditis, 700

Perineal Wound Care, 1154

Peripheral Venous Catheters, Placement, 191
Peritoneal Dialysis Catheter, 1440
Phlebostatic Axis Identification, 770
Plasmapheresis Complications, 915
Postmortem Care, 102
Postoperative Hand-off Report, 257
Post-Traumatic Stress Disorder Prevention in Staff During
    a Mass Casualty Event, 145
Pressure Ulcer Prevention, 438
Pressure Ulcers and Wound Management, 444
Prostatectomy, 1510
Pulmonary Embolism Care, 606
Pulmonary Embolism Prevention, 604
Radioactive Sealed Implants, 376
Relocation Stress in Older Adults, Minimizing Effects, 13
Reproductive Health Problems, 1453
Restraint Alternatives, 22
Sickle Cell Crisis, 802
Skin Problems, Nursing History, 429
Spinal Cord Injury and Motor Function Assessment, 897
Sports-Related Injuries, 1076
Surgical Wound Evisceration, 269
Systemic Sclerosis and Esophagitis, 318
Thrombocytopenia, 814
Thrombocytopenia, Prevention of Injury, 383
Thyroid Storm, 1291
Tonic-Clonic or Complete Partial Seizure, 861
Total Parenteral Nutrition, 1245
Tracheostomy Care, 527
Transfusion Therapy, 822
Transfusion, Older Adult, 823
Transurethral Resection of the Prostate, 1507
Tube Feeding Care and Maintenance, 1243
Urinary Incontinence Reduction with Bladder Training and
    Habit Training, 1381
Vertebroplasty or Kyphoplasty, Nursing Care, 1070
Viral Hepatitis Prevention in Health Care Workers, 1205
Vision Reduction, Care, 993
Wandering, Prevention in Hospitalized Patients, 878
Wound Monitoring, 448

COMMON EXAMPLES OF DRUG THERAPY

Adrenal Gland Hypofunction, 1276
Anaphylaxis, 354
Anthrax, Prophylaxis and Treatment, 600
Arthritis and Connective Tissue Disease, 309
Asthma, 554
Atrial Fibrillation, Nonvalvular, 668
Burns, 486
Coronary Artery Disease, 765
Diabetes Mellitus, 1312
Dysrhythmias, 658
Epilepsy, 860
Eye Inflammation and Infection, 979
Glaucoma, 988
HIV Infection, 339
Hypertension, 715
Hyperthyroidism, 1289
Hypovolemic Shock, 748
Kidney Disease, 1429
Nausea and Vomiting, Chemotherapy-Induced, 385

Osteoporosis, 1035
Pain, Postoperative, 270
Peptic Ulcer Disease, 1129
Plaque Psoriasis, 458
Pulmonary Embolism, 607
Transplant Rejection, 287
Tuberculosis, 597
Urinary Incontinence, 1378
Urinary Tract Infections, 1371
Vasodilators and Inotropes, Intravenous, 773

CONCEPT MAP

Benign Prostatic Hyperplasia, 1505
Cancer Pain, Chronic, 27
Cirrhosis, 1198
Diabetes Mellitus—Type 2, 1311
End-Stage Kidney Disease, 1425
Glaucoma, 986
Hypertension, 713
Hypovolemic Shock, 744
Multiple Sclerosis, 907
Pneumonia, Community-Acquired, 591
Pressure Ulcer, 445
Respiratory Acidosis (COPD Related), 560

EVIDENCE-BASED PRACTICE

Atrial Fibrillation and Obesity, 666
Bedside Nurse Reporting and Patient Safety, 6
Bowel Disimpaction in Spinal Cord Injury, 88
Breast Cancer and Incidence Among Night-Shift
    Workers, 1466
Cardiac Rehabilitation Enrollment and Nursing Interventions
    for Acute MI Population, 780
Colonoscopy and Best Position for Patients, 1096
Colorectal Cancer Screening Effectiveness, 1150
Complementary and Alternative Methods for Osteoarthritis
    Symptoms, 295
Depression and Despair Improvement in Older Adults
    Through Reflective Activities, 17
Diabetes and Annual Eye Care, 1304
Evidence-Based Practice or Sacred Cow?, 263
Heart Failure Education for Heart Failure Patients, 690
Heat Stroke, Predicting Non-exertional, 122
Hepatitis C and Complementary and Alternative
    Therapies, 1206
Hip Fractures and Helpfulness of Online Resources for
    Caregivers, 1068
HIV Infection Risk in Older Adults, 330
Hospice Services for Medicare Patients, 94
Inflammatory Bowel Disease and Support Groups, 1181
Nutrition and Quality of Care, 1237
Oral Care and Outcome for Patients in ICU, 1101
Oral Hygiene Methods to Prevent Ventilator-Associated
    Pneumonia, 621
Osteoporosis Risk in Men, 1031
Pain Differences in Women with Multiple Sclerosis and
    Healthy Women, 906
Pain Management and Education About Nonpharmacologic
    Methods, 46
Prostate-Specific Antigen Screening for Prostate Cancer, 1508

Reduced Hearing and Hearing Aids, 1012
Sitters, Use of in Improving Care of Older Adults with
    Dementia, 877
Strokes, Best Practice for Teaching Patients and Families, 945
Suctioning, Determining When Painful to Patient, 526
VTE Prevention, 232

FOCUSED ASSESSMENT

AIDS, 343
Cancer, Oral, Older Adults, 1106
Cataract Surgery, 984
Diabetic Foot, 1326
Diabetic Patient, Home or Clinic Visit, 1339
Hearing Loss, 1010
Hyperpituitarism, Transsphenoidal or Endoscopic Nasal
    Hypophysectomy, 1270
Hysterectomy, Total Abdominal, 1490
Infection Risk, 809
Kidney Transplant, 1445
Pneumonia, 594
Postanesthesia Care Unit Discharge to Medical-Surgical
    Unit, 258
Preoperative Patient, 225
Seizures, Nursing Observations and Documentation, 861
Sexually Transmitted Disease, 1535
Testicular Lump, 1515
Thyroid Dysfunction, 1295
Tracheostomy, 527
Urinary Incontinence, 1376

HOME CARE ASSESSMENT

Amputation, Lower Extremity, 1075
Breast Cancer Surgery, 1479
Chronic Obstructive Pulmonary Disease, 566
Colostomy, 1156
Heart Failure, 690
Inflammatory Bowel Disease, 1181
Laryngectomy, 544
Myocardial Infarction, 780
Peripheral Vascular Disease, 724
Pressure Ulcers, 449
Pulmonary Embolism, 611
Sepsis, 754
Ulcer Disease, 1138

KEY FEATURES

Acidosis, 181
Adrenal Insufficiency, 1274
AIDS, 334
Alkalosis, 184
Alzheimer's Disease, 873
Amyotrophic Lateral Sclerosis, 910
Anaphylaxis, 353
Anemia, 799
Angina and Myocardial Infarction, 762
Anthrax, 600
Asthma Control, 551
Asthma Control and Step System for Medication, 551
Autonomic Dysreflexia, 899

Bowel Obstructions, Small and Large, 1159
Brain Abscess, 963
Brain Tumors, 959
Cancer, Gastric, Early Versus Advanced, 1139
Cancer, Oral, 1103
Cancer, Pancreatic, 1227
Celiac Disease, 1188
Cervical Diskectomy and Fusion, 892
Cholecystitis, 1215
Compartment Syndrome, 1054
Cor Pulmonale, 559
Diabetes Insipidus, 1271
Endocarditis, Infective, 697
Fluid Overload, 159
Gastritis, 1128
Gastroesophageal Reflux Disease, 1111
GI Bleeding, 1132
Guillain-Barré Syndrome, 914
Heart Failure, Left-Sided, 682
Heart Failure, Right-Sided, 682
Heat Stroke, 122
Hernias, 1115
Hypercortisolism (Cushing's Disease/Syndrome), 1278
Hyperthyroidism, 1286
Hypothermia, 131
Hypothyroidism, 1292
Intracranial Pressure, Increased, 941
Kidney Disease, Chronic, Severe, 1423
Leukemia, Acute, 808
Liver Trauma, 1208
Meningitis, 864
Migraine Headaches, 855
Multiple Sclerosis, 905
Myasthenia Gravis, 918
Nephrotic Syndrome, 1404
Occupational Pulmonary Diseases, 573
Osteomyelitis, Acute and Chronic, 1040
Paget's Disease of the Bone, 1038
Pancreatitis, Chronic, 1224
Parkinson Disease, 868
Peripheral Arterial Disease, Chronic, 719
Peritonitis, 1170
Pharyngitis, Acute Viral and Bacterial, 585
Pituitary Hyperfunction, 1269
Pituitary Hypofunction, 1267
Polycystic Kidney Disease, 1396
Pressure Ulcers, 441
Pulmonary Edema, 688
Pulmonary Emboli: Fat Embolism Versus Blood Clot
    Embolism, 1055
Pulmonary Embolism, 605
Pyelonephritis, Acute, 1400
Pyelonephritis, Chronic, 1400
Renovascular Disease, 1405
Rheumatoid Arthritis, 305
Shock, 741
Skin Conditions, Inflammatory, 455
Skin Infections, 450
Spinal Cord Tumors, 903
Stroke Syndromes, 934
Strokes, Left and Right Hemisphere, 936
Systemic Lupus Erythematosus and Systemic Sclerosis, 314

Tachydysrhythmias and Bradydysrhythmias, Sustained, 657
Tonsillitis, Acute, 586
Transient Ischemic Attack, 931
Traumatic Brain Injury, 948
Tumors, Esophageal, 1118
Ulcers, Lower Extremity, 721
Uremia, 1419
Urinary Tract Infection, 1370
Valvular Heart Disease, 692

LABORATORY PROFILE

Acid-Base Assessment, 177
Acid-Base Imbalances, 182
Adrenal Gland Assessment, 1275
Anticoagulation Therapy, Blood Tests, 608
Blood Glucose Values, 1308
Burn Assessment During the Resuscitation Phase, 477
Cardiovascular Assessment, 641
Connective Tissue Disease, 307
Gastrointestinal Assessment, 1092
Hematologic Assessment, 794
Hypovolemic Shock, 747
Kidney Disease, 1415
Kidney Function Blood Studies, 1355
Musculoskeletal Assessment, 1024
Parathyroid Function, 1297
Perioperative Assessment, 223
Reproductive Assessment, 1455
Respiratory Assessment, 508
Thyroid Function, 1288
Urinalysis, 1356
Urine Collections, 24-Hour, 1359

NURSING FOCUS ON THE OLDER ADULT

Acid-Base Imbalance, 179
Burn Injury Complications, 474
Cancer, 367
Cardiovascular System Changes, 633
Cerumen Impaction, 1005
Coronary Artery Bypass Graft Surgery, 780
Coronary Artery Disease, 769
Diverticulitis, 1187
Dysrhythmias, 674
Ear and Hearing Changes, 999
Electrolyte Values, 152
Endocrine System Changes, 1261
Eye and Vision Changes, 970
Fecal Impaction, Prevention, 1161
Fluid Balance, 153
Gastrointestinal System Changes, 1088
Heat-Related Illness Prevention, 121
Hematologic Assessment, 790
Immune Function Changes, 277
Impaired Vision, Promoting Independent Living, 987
Infection, Risk Factors, 398
Integumentary System Changes, 418
Intraoperative Nursing Interventions, 251
Low Back Pain, 886
Malnutrition, Risk Assessment, 1238
Musculoskeletal System Changes, 1020

Nervous System Changes, 836
Nutrition Intake, 1240
Pain, 39
Preoperative Considerations for Care Planning, 221
Renal/Urinary System Changes, 1351
Reproductive System Changes, 1452
Respiratory Disorder, Chronic, 549
Respiratory System Changes, 501
Shock, Risk Factors, 752
Skin Care, Postoperative, 267
Spinal Cord Injury, 901
Surgical Risk Factors, 220
Thyroid Problems, 1294
Total Hip Arthroplasty, 297
Traumatic Brain Injury, 951
Urinary Incontinence, 1375

PATIENT AND FAMILY EDUCATION: PREPARING FOR SELF-MANAGEMENT

Arthritis, Energy Conservation, 312
Arthropod Bite/Sting Prevention, 126
Asthma Management, 553
Bariatric Surgery, Discharge Teaching, 1252
Beta Blocker/Digoxin Therapy, 691
Bleeding and Injury Prevention, 610
Bleeding or Injury Prevention, 384
Bleeding, Risk, 816
Brain Injury, Mild, 957
Breast Cancer Surgery, Recovery, 1478
Breathing Exercises, 563
Cancer, Dietary Habits to Reduce Risk, 367
Cancer, Skin, Prevention, 460
Cast Removal, Extremity Care, 1065
Catheter Care, Home, 1512
Central Venous Catheter, Home Care, 815
Cerumen Removal, Self-Ear Irrigation, 999
Cervical Ablation Therapy, 1495
Cervical Biopsy, 1458
Chest Pain, Home Management, 782
Cirrhosis, 1202
Condoms, 1537
Coronary Artery Disease and Activity, 781
Coronary Artery Disease Prevention, 761
Cortisol Replacement Therapy, 1281
Death, Emotional Signs of Approaching, 96
Death, Physical Signs and Symptoms of Approaching, 96
Death, Signs That Has Occurred, 102
Diabetes, Sick-Day Rules, 1335
Dry Powder Inhaler, 556
Dry Skin Prevention, 433
Dysrhythmias, How to Prevent or Decrease, 673
Ear Infection or Trauma, Prevention, 1013
Ear Surgery, Recovery, 1007
Epilepsy, Health Teaching, 861
Epinephrine Injectors, 352
Exercise, 1322
Eyedrops, 970
Foot Care Instructions, 1327
Gastritis Prevention, 1127
Gastroenteritis, Transmission Prevention, 1173
Glucosamine Supplements, 295

Halo Device, 898
Hearing Aid Care, 1011
HIV Testing Recommendations, 333
Hyperkalemia, Nutritional Management, 167
Hypoglycemia, Home Treatment, 1331
Hysterectomy, Total Abdominal, 1490
Ileostomy Care, 1181
Implantable Cardioverter-Defibrillator, 675
Infection Prevention, 338, 382, 816
Inhaler Use, 555
Insulin Administration, Subcutaneous, 1316
Joint Protection Instructions, 304
Kidney and Genitourinary Trauma, Prevention, 1408
Kidney and Urinary Problems, Prevention, 1422
Laparoscopic Nissen Fundoplication, Postoperative
    Instructions, 1116
Laryngectomy, Home Care, 545
Leg Exercises, Postoperative, 231
Lightning Strike Prevention, 130
Low Back Pain and Injury, Prevention, 886
Low Back Pain Exercises, 887
Lupus Erythematosus, Skin Protection, 316
Lyme Disease, Prevention and Early Detection, 321
Migraine Attack, Triggers, 857
Mouth Care for Mucositis, 386
MRSA, Prevention of Spread, 452
Myasthenia Gravis, Medication Teaching, 922
Ocular Compress Application, 980
Oral Cancer Care, 1107
Oral Cavity Maintenance, 1100
Osteoarthritis or Rheumatoid Arthritis Exercises, 303
Pacemakers, Permanent, 675
Pancreatitis, Chronic, Enzyme Replacement, 1225
Pancreatitis, Chronic, Prevention of Exacerbations, 1225
Peak Flow Meter, 553
Pelvic Muscle Exercises, 1377
Peripheral Neuropathy, Chemotherapy-Induced, 386
Peripheral Vascular Disease, Foot Care, 725
Pneumonia Prevention, 589
Polycystic Kidney Disease, 1397
Polycythemia Vera, 805
Postmastectomy Exercises, 1474
Radioactive Isotope, Unsealed, Safety Precautions, 1290
Reflux Control, 1113
Respiratory Care, Perioperative, 230
Sexually Transmitted Diseases, Oral Antibiotic Therapy, 1544

Sickle Cell Crisis Prevention, 803
Skin Protection During Radiation Therapy, 377
Smoking Cessation, 496
Snakebite Prevention, 123
Sperm Banking, 1515
Stretta Procedure, Postoperative Instructions, 1114
Stroke, Risk Factors, 933
Supraglottic Method of Swallowing, 543
Testicular Self-Examination, 1514
Total Hip Arthroplasty, 298
Toxic Shock Syndrome, Prevention, 1485
Urinary Calculi, 1388
Urinary Incontinence, 1383
Urinary Tract Infection Prevention, 1369
Vaginal Infections, 1485
Valvular Heart Disease, 697
Venous Insufficiency, 734
Viral Hepatitis, 1208
Viral Hepatitis, Prevention, 1205
Vulvovaginitis, Prevention, 1485
Warfarin (Coumadin), Interference of Food and
    Drugs, 733
Wellness Promotion Through Lifestyles and Practices, 10
West Nile Virus Prevention, 866

QUALITY IMPROVEMENT

Catheter Guidelines to Reduce Complications, 1440
Cathether-Associated Urinary Tract Infections,
    Reduction of, 399
Checklist Use for Patient Education, 379
Continuous Prostacyclin Therapy Error Prevention, 570
Emergency Department, Flow of Stable Patients
    Through, 113
Fall Reduction and Reduction of Harm from Falls, 885
Hand Hygiene Compliance by Nursing Staff, 402
Hemodialysis Time as a Teachable Moment, 1436
Pressure Ulcer Prevention by Team Approach, 438
Sepsis Indicators, Recognition by Nurses in Emergency
    Department, 751
Sleep Promotion by Unit-based Quality Improvement
    Project, 837
Standardization of Assessment and Communication for
    Neuroscience Patients, 843
Total Joint Replacement, Improvement in Caregiver
    Education, 300

CHAPTER 39

Assessment of the Hematologic System

M. Linda Workman

 http://evolve.elsevier.com/Iggy/

PRIORITY CONCEPTS

- CLOTTING
- PERFUSION

LEARNING OUTCOMES

Safe and Effective Care Environment
1. Protect the patient with a potential hematologic problem from injury.

Health Promotion and Maintenance
2. Teach all people how to protect the hematologic system.

Psychosocial Integrity
3. Reduce the psychological impact for the patient and family regarding the assessment and testing of the hematologic system.

Physiological Integrity
4. Explain the relationship between hematologic problems and the concepts of CLOTTING and PERFUSION.

5. Perform a focused assessment of the hematologic system, incorporating information about genetic risk and age-related changes affecting hematologic function, especially CLOTTING and PERFUSION.
6. Use knowledge of anatomy, physiology, laboratory analysis, and human development to determine whether hematologic assessment findings are normal or abnormal.
7. Explain the effects of anticoagulants, fibrinolytics, and inhibitors of platelet activity on CLOTTING and PERFUSION.
8. Prioritize nursing care for the patient after bone marrow aspiration or biopsy.

The hematologic system includes the blood, blood cells, lymph, and organs involved with blood formation or blood storage. This system is important for oxygenation (gas exchange) and tissue PERFUSION because the blood is the oxygen delivery system (Fig. 39-1). All systems depend on the blood for oxygen perfusion, and any problem of the hematologic system affects total body health. This chapter, together with Chapter 17, reviews the normal physiology of the hematologic system and assessment of hematologic status.

ANATOMY AND PHYSIOLOGY REVIEW

Bone Marrow

Bone marrow is responsible for blood formation. It produces red blood cells (RBCs, erythrocytes), white blood cells (WBCs,

leukocytes), and platelets. Bone marrow also is involved in the immune responses (see Chapter 17).

Each day the bone marrow normally releases about 2.5 billion RBCs, 2.5 billion platelets, and 1 billion WBCs per kilogram of body weight. In adults, cell-producing marrow is present only in flat bones (sternum, skull, pelvic and shoulder girdles) and the ends of long bones. With aging, fatty tissue replaces active bone marrow and only a small portion of the remaining marrow continues to produce blood in older adults (Touhy & Jett, 2014).

The bone marrow first produces **blood stem cells**, which are immature, unspecialized (undifferentiated) cells that are capable of becoming any type of blood cell, depending on the body's needs (Fig. 39-2) (McCance et al., 2014).

The next stage in blood cell production is the *committed stem cell* (or *precursor* cell). A committed stem cell enters one growth pathway and can at that point specialize (differentiate) into only one cell type. Committed stem cells actively divide but require the presence of a specific growth factor for specialization. For example, erythropoietin is a growth factor specific for the RBC. Other growth factors control WBC and platelet growth (see Chapters 17, 22, and 40 for discussion of growth factors and cytokines).

Blood Components

Blood is composed of plasma and cells. Plasma is an extracellular fluid. It is similar to the interstitial fluid found between tissue cells, but plasma contains much more protein. The three major types of plasma proteins are albumin, globulins, and fibrinogen.

Albumin maintains the osmotic pressure of the blood, preventing the plasma from leaking into the tissues (see Chapter 11). *Globulins* have many functions, such as transporting other substances and, as antibodies, protecting the body against

infection. *Fibrinogen* is activated to form fibrin, which is critical in the blood CLOTTING process.

The blood cells include RBCs, WBCs, and platelets. These cells differ in structure, site of maturation, and function.

Red blood cells (**erythrocytes**) are the largest proportion of blood cells. Mature RBCs have no nucleus and have a biconcave disk shape. Together with a flexible membrane, this feature allows RBCs to change their shape without breaking as they pass through narrow, winding capillaries. The number of RBCs a person has varies with gender, age, and general health, but the normal range is from 4,200,000 to 6,100,000/mm^3.

As shown in Figs. 39-2 and 39-3, RBCs start out as stem cells, enter the myeloid pathway, and progress in stages to mature erythrocytes. Healthy, mature, circulating RBCs have a life span of about 120 days. As RBCs age, their membranes become more fragile. These old cells are trapped and destroyed in the tissues, spleen, and liver. Some parts of destroyed RBCs (e.g., iron, hemoglobin) are recycled and used to make new RBCs.

The RBCs produce hemoglobin (Hgb). Each normal mature RBC contains hundreds of thousands of hemoglobin molecules. Each hemoglobin molecule needs iron to be able to transport up to four molecules of oxygen. *Therefore iron is an essential part of hemoglobin.* Hemoglobin also carries carbon dioxide. RBCs also help maintain acid-base balance.

The most important feature of hemoglobin is its ability to combine loosely with oxygen. Only a small drop in tissue oxygen levels increases the transfer of oxygen from hemoglobin to tissues, known as **oxygen dissociation**. See Chapter 27 for a discussion of oxygen dissociation.

The total number of RBCs a person has is carefully controlled to ensure that enough are present for good PERFUSION with oxygen and for CLOTTING without having too many cells that could "thicken" the blood and slow its flow. RBC production or **erythropoiesis** (selective growth of stem cells into mature erythrocytes) must be properly balanced with RBC destruction or loss. When balanced, this process helps tissue perfusion by ensuring adequate delivery of oxygen. The trigger

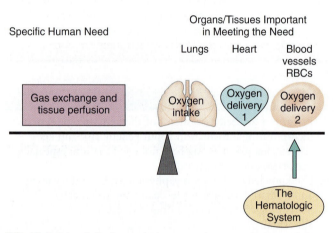

FIG. 39-1 Role of the hematologic system in gas exchange and tissue perfusion. *RBCs,* Red blood cells.

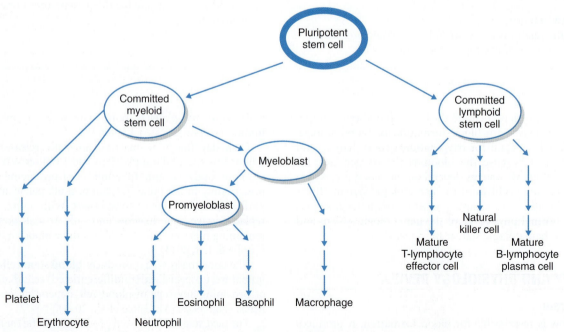

FIG. 39-2 Bone marrow cell growth and blood cell differentiation pathways.

for RBC production is an increase in the tissue need for oxygen. The kidney produces the RBC growth factor *erythropoietin* at the same rate as RBC destruction or loss occurs to maintain a constant normal level of circulating RBCs. When tissue oxygen is less than normal (**hypoxia**), the kidney releases more erythropoietin, which then increases RBC production in the bone marrow. When tissue oxygen is normal or high, erythropoietin levels fall, slowing RBC production. Synthetic erythrocyte stimulating agents (ESAs) such as Procrit, Epogen, and EPO have the same effect on bone marrow as the naturally occurring erythropoietin.

Many substances are needed to form hemoglobin and RBCs, including iron, vitamin B_{12}, folic acid, copper, pyridoxine, cobalt, and nickel. A lack of any of these substances can lead to anemia, which results in unmet tissue oxygen needs because of a reduction in the number or function of RBCs.

White blood cells (WBCs, leukocytes) also are formed in the bone marrow. The many types of WBCs all have specialized functions that provide protection through inflammation and immunity (Table 39-1). WBC function is presented in Chapter 17.

Platelets are the third type of blood cells. They are the smallest blood cells, formed in the bone marrow from megakaryocyte precursor cells. When activated, platelets stick to injured blood vessel walls and form platelet plugs that can stop the flow of blood at the injured site. They also produce substances important to blood CLOTTING and aggregate (clump together) to perform most of their functions. Platelets help keep small blood vessels intact by initiating repair after damage.

Production of platelets is controlled by the growth factor *thrombopoietin*. After platelets leave the bone marrow, they are stored in the spleen and then released slowly to meet the body's needs. Normally, 80% of platelets circulate and 20% are stored in the spleen.

Accessory Organs of Blood Formation

The spleen and liver are important accessory organs for blood production. They help regulate the growth of blood cells and form factors that ensure proper blood CLOTTING.

The spleen contains three types of tissue: white pulp, red pulp, and marginal pulp. These tissues all help balance blood cell production with blood cell destruction and assist with immunity. White pulp is filled with white blood cells (WBCs) and is a major site of antibody production. As whole blood filters through the white pulp, bacteria and old RBCs are removed. Red pulp is the storage site for RBCs and platelets. Marginal pulp contains the ends of many blood vessels.

The spleen destroys old or imperfect RBCs, breaks down the hemoglobin released from these destroyed cells, stores platelets, and filters antigens. Anyone who has had a splenectomy has reduced immune functions and has an increased risk for infection and sepsis.

The liver produces prothrombin and other blood CLOTTING factors. Also, proper liver function is important in forming vitamin K in the intestinal tract. (Vitamin K is needed to produce clotting factors VII, IX, and X and prothrombin.) Large amounts of whole blood and blood cells can be stored in the liver. The liver also stores extra iron within the protein *ferritin*.

Hemostasis and Blood Clotting

Hemostasis is the multi-stepped process of controlled blood CLOTTING. It results in localized blood clotting in damaged blood vessels to prevent excessive blood loss while blood continues to PERFUSE all other areas. This complex function balances blood clotting actions with anti-clotting actions. When

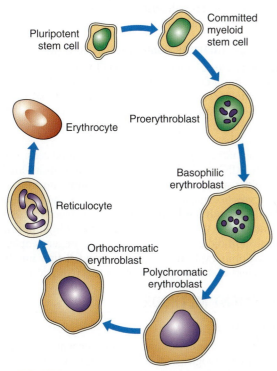

FIG. 39-3 Erythrocyte (red blood cell) growth pathway.

TABLE 39-1	**Functions of Specific Leukocytes**
LEUKOCYTE	**FUNCTION**
Inflammation	
Neutrophil	Nonspecific ingestion and phagocytosis of microorganisms and foreign protein
Macrophage	Nonspecific recognition of foreign proteins and microorganisms; ingestion and phagocytosis
Monocyte	Destruction of bacteria and cellular debris; matures into macrophage
Eosinophil	Weak phagocytic action; releases vasoactive amines during allergic reactions
Basophil	Releases histamine and heparin in areas of tissue damage
Antibody-Mediated Immunity	
B-lymphocyte	Becomes sensitized to foreign cells and proteins
Plasma cell	Secretes immunoglobulins in response to the presence of a specific antigen
Memory cell	Remains sensitized to a specific antigen and can secrete increased amounts of immunoglobulins specific to the antigen on re-exposure
Cell-Mediated Immunity	
T-lymphocyte helper/inducer T-cell	Enhances immune activity through the secretion of various factors, cytokines, and lymphokines
Cytotoxic-cytolytic T-cell	Selectively attacks and destroys non-self cells, including virally infected cells, grafts, and transplanted organs
Natural killer cell	Nonselectively attacks non-self cells, especially body cells that have undergone mutation and become malignant; also attacks grafts and transplanted organs

injury occurs, hemostasis starts the formation of a platelet plug and continues with a series of steps that eventually cause the formation of a fibrin clot. Three sequential processes result in blood clotting: platelet aggregation with platelet plug formation; the blood clotting cascade; and the formation of a complete fibrin clot.

Platelet aggregation begins forming a platelet plug by having platelets clump together, a process essential for blood CLOTTING. Platelets normally circulate as individual small cells that do not clump together until activated. Activation causes platelet membranes to become sticky, allowing them to clump together. When platelets clump, they form large, semi-solid plugs in blood vessels, disrupting local blood flow. *These platelet plugs are not clots and last only a few hours. Thus they cannot provide complete hemostasis but only start the hemostatic process.*

Substances that activate platelets and cause clumping include adenosine diphosphate (ADP), calcium, thromboxane A_2, and collagen. Platelets secrete some of these substances, and other activating substances are external to the platelet. Platelet plugs start the cascade action that ends with local blood CLOTTING and are important at most steps within the cascade. When too few platelets are present, blood clotting is impaired, increasing the risk for excessive bleeding.

Blood clotting is a cascade triggered by the formation of a platelet plug, which then rapidly amplifies the cascade (Pezzotti & Freuler, 2012). The final result is much larger than the triggering event. Thus the cascade works like a landslide—a few small pebbles rolling down a steep hill can dislodge large rocks, trees, and soil, causing an enormous movement of earth. Just like landslides, cascade reactions are hard to stop once set into motion.

Intrinsic factors are conditions, such as circulating debris or venous stasis, within the blood itself that can activate platelets and trigger the blood CLOTTING cascade (Fig. 39-4). Continuing the cascade to blood clotting requires sufficient amounts of all the clotting factors and cofactors (Table 39-2).

Extrinsic factors outside of the blood can also activate platelets. The most common extrinsic event is trauma that damages blood vessels and exposes collagen. Collagen then activates platelets to form a platelet plug within seconds. The blood clotting cascade is started sooner by this pathway because some intrinsic pathway steps are bypassed. Other blood vessel changes that can activate platelets include inflammation, bacterial toxins, or foreign proteins.

Whether the platelet plugs are formed because of abnormal blood (intrinsic factors) or by exposure to inflamed or damaged blood vessels (extrinsic factors), the end result of the cascade is the same: *formation of a fibrin clot and local blood CLOTTING (coagulation).* The cascade, from the formation of a platelet plug to the formation of a fibrin clot, depends on the presence of specific clotting factors, calcium, and more platelets at every step.

Clotting factors (see Table 39-2) are inactive enzymes that become activated in a sequence. The last part of the sequence is the activation of fibrinogen into fibrin. At each step, the activated enzyme from the previous step activates the next enzyme. The last two steps in the cascade are the activation of thrombin from prothrombin and the conversion (by thrombin) of fibrinogen into fibrin. Only fibrin molecules can begin the formation of a true clot.

Fibrin clot formation is the last phase of blood clotting. Fibrinogen is an inactive protein made in the liver. The activated enzyme *thrombin* removes the end portions of fibrinogen, converting it to active fibrin that can link together to form fibrin threads. Fibrin threads make a meshlike base to form a blood clot.

After the fibrin mesh is formed, clotting factor XIII tightens up the mesh, making it more dense and stable. More platelets stick to the threads of the mesh and attract other blood cells and proteins to form an actual blood clot. As this clot tightens (retracts), the serum is squeezed out and clot formation is complete.

Anti-Clotting Forces

Because blood CLOTTING occurs through a rapid cascade process, in theory it keeps forming fibrin clots whenever the cascade is set into motion until all blood throughout the entire body has coagulated and PERFUSION stops. Therefore, whenever the blood clotting cascade is started, anti-clotting forces are also started to limit clot formation only to damaged areas so that normal perfusion is maintained everywhere else. When blood clotting and anti-clotting actions are balanced, clotting occurs only where it is needed and normal perfusion is maintained. The anti-clotting forces both ensure that activated clotting factors are present only in limited amounts and also cause fibrinolysis to prevent over-enlargement of the fibrin clot. **Fibrinolysis** is the process that dissolves fibrin clot edges with special enzymes (Fig. 39-5). The process starts by activating plasminogen to plasmin. Plasmin, an active enzyme, then digests fibrin, fibrinogen, and prothrombin, controlling the size of the fibrin clot.

When the blood clotting cascade is activated, certain anti-clotting substances are also activated, such as protein C, protein S, and antithrombin III. Protein C and protein S increase the breakdown of clotting factors V and VIII. Antithrombin III inactivates thrombin and clotting factors IX and X. These actions prevent clots from becoming too large or forming in an area where CLOTTING is not needed. Deficiency of any anti-clotting factor increases the risk for pulmonary embolism, myocardial infarction, and strokes.

Hematologic Changes Associated with Aging

Aging changes the blood components (Touhy & Jett, 2014). The older adult has a decreased blood volume with lower levels of plasma proteins. The lower plasma protein level may be related to a low dietary intake of proteins, as well as to reduced protein production by the older liver. Chart 39-1 lists assessment tips for older adults.

As bone marrow ages, it produces fewer blood cells. Total red blood cell (RBC) and white blood cell (WBC) counts are lower among older adults, although platelet counts do not change. Lymphocytes become less reactive to antigens and lose immune function. Antibody levels and responses are lower and slower in older adults. The WBC count does not rise as high in response to infection in older people as it does in younger people.

Hemoglobin levels in men and women fall after middle age. Iron-deficient diets may play a role in this reduction.

ASSESSMENT METHODS

Patient History

Age and gender are important to consider when assessing the patient's hematologic status. Bone marrow function and immune activity decrease with age.

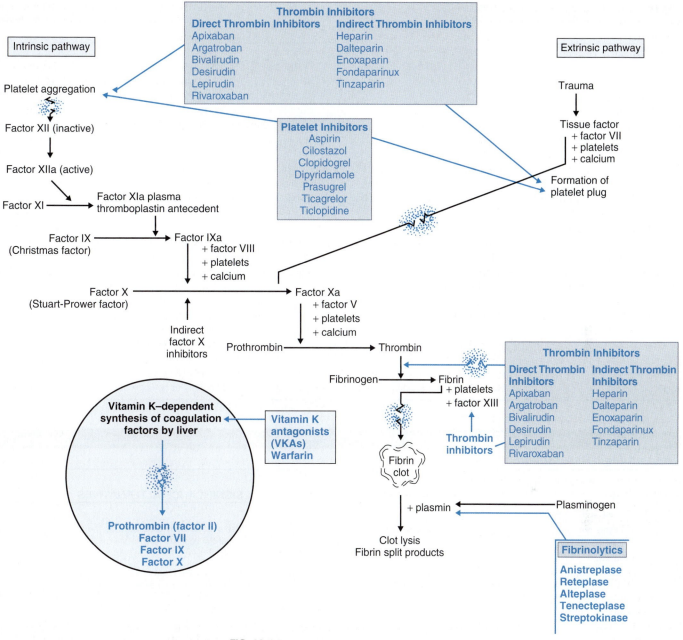

FIG. 39-4 Summary of the blood clotting cascade.

GENDER HEALTH CONSIDERATIONS

Patient-Centered Care QSEN

At all ages, women have lower blood cell counts than do men. This difference is greater during menstrual years because menstrual blood loss may occur faster than blood cell production. This difference also may be related to blood dilution caused by fluid retention from female hormones. Always assess for RBC adequacy in a woman hospitalized for any reason.

Liver function, the presence of known immunologic or hematologic disorders, current drug use, dietary patterns, and socioeconomic status are important to assess. Because the liver makes CLOTTING factors, ask about manifestations that may indicate liver problems, such as jaundice, anemia, and gallstones. Previous radiation therapy for cancer may impair hematologic function if marrow-forming bones were in the radiation path.

Ask about the patient's occupation and hobbies and whether the home is located near an industrial setting. This information may identify exposure to agents that affect bone marrow and hematologic function.

Check all drugs that the patient is using or has used in the past 3 weeks. Ask about the use of drugs listed in Table 39-3 that are known to change hematologic function. Check a drug handbook to determine whether other drugs the patient takes can affect hematologic function.

Ask the patient about use of blood "thinners" and NSAIDs, which change blood CLOTTING activity. Such drugs include anticoagulants, fibrinolytics, and platelet inhibitors. Many patients refer to these drugs as "blood thinners" although they do not

TABLE 39-2 **The Clotting Factors**

FACTOR	ACTION
I: Fibrinogen	Factor I is converted to fibrin by the enzyme *thrombin*. Individual fibrin molecules form fibrin threads, which are the mesh for clot formation and wound healing.
II: Prothrombin	Factor II is the inactive thrombin. Prothrombin is activated to thrombin by clotting factor X. Activated thrombin converts fibrinogen (clotting factor I) into fibrin and activates factors V and VIII. Synthesis is vitamin K–dependent.
III: Tissue thromboplastin	Factor III interacts with factor VII to initiate the extrinsic clotting cascade.
IV: Calcium	Calcium (Ca^{2+}), a divalent cation, is a cofactor for most of the enzyme-activated processes required in blood clotting. Calcium enhances platelet aggregation and makes red blood cells clump together.
V: Proaccelerin	Factor V is a cofactor for activated factor X, which is essential for converting prothrombin to thrombin.
VI: Discovered to be an artifact	No factor VI is involved in blood clotting.
VII: Proconvertin	Factor VII activates factors IX and X, which are essential in converting prothrombin to thrombin. Synthesis is vitamin K–dependent.
VIII: Antihemophilic factor	Factor VIII together with activated factor IX activates factor X. Factor VIII also combines with another protein (von Willebrand's factor) to help platelets adhere to capillary walls in areas of tissue injury. A lack of factor VIII is the basis for classic hemophilia (hemophilia A).
IX: Plasma thromboplastin component (Christmas factor)	Factor IX, when activated, activates factor X to convert prothrombin to thrombin. A lack of factor IX causes hemophilia B. Synthesis is vitamin K–dependent.
X: Stuart-Prower factor	Factor X, when activated, converts prothrombin into thrombin. Synthesis is vitamin K–dependent.
XI: Plasma thromboplastin antecedent	Factor XI, when activated, assists in the activation of factor IX. However, a similar factor must exist in tissues. People who are deficient in factor XI have mild bleeding problems.
XII: Hageman factor	Factor XII is critically important in the intrinsic pathway for the activation of factor XI.
XIII: Fibrin-stabilizing factor	Factor XIII assists in forming cross-links among the fibrin threads to form a strong fibrin clot.

CHART 39-1 **Nursing Focus on the Older Adult**

Hematologic Assessment

FINDINGS IN HEMATOLOGIC DISORDERS	NORMAL CHANGES IN THE OLDER ADULT	SIGNIFICANCE/ALTERNATIVES
Nail Beds (for Capillary Refill)		
Pallor or cyanosis may indicate a hematologic disorder.	Thickened or discolored nails make viewing color of nail beds impossible.	Use another body area, such as the lip, to assess central capillary refill.
Hair Distribution		
Thin or absent hair on the trunk or extremities may indicate poor circulation to a particular area.	Progressive loss of body hair is a normal facet of aging.	A relatively even pattern of hair loss that has occurred over an extended period is not significant.
Skin Moisture		
Skin dryness may indicate any of a number of hematologic disorders.	Skin dryness is a normal result of aging.	Skin moisture is not usually a reliable indicator of an underlying pathologic condition in the older adult.
Skin Color		
Skin color changes, especially pallor and jaundice, are associated with some hematologic disorders.	Pigment loss and skin yellowing are common changes associated with aging.	Pallor in an older adult may not be a reliable indicator of anemia. Laboratory testing is required. Yellow-tinged skin in an older adult may not be a reliable indicator of increased serum bilirubin levels. Laboratory testing is required.

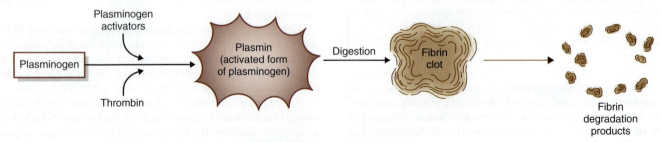

FIG. 39-5 The process of fibrinolysis.

TABLE 39-3 Drugs Impairing the Hematologic System

Drugs Causing Bone Marrow Suppression	Drugs Causing Hemolysis	Drugs Disrupting Platelet Action
• Altretamine	• Acetohydroxamic acid	• Aspirin
• Amphotericin B	• Amoxicillin	• Carbenicillin
• Azathioprine	• Chlorpropamide	• Carindacillin
• Chemotherapeutic agents	• Doxapram	• Dipyridamole
• Chloramphenicol	• Glyburide	• Ibuprofen
• Chromic phosphate	• Mefenamic acid	• Meloxicam
• Colchicine	• Menadiol diphosphate	• Naproxen
• Didanosine	• Methyldopa	• Oxaprozin
• Eflornithine	• Nitrofurantoin	• Pentoxifylline
• Foscarnet sodium	• Penicillin G benzathine	• Sulfinpyrazone
• Ganciclovir	• Penicillin V	• Ticarcillin
• Interferon alfa	• Primaquine	• Ticlopidine
• Pentamidine	• Procainamide hydrochloride	• Valproic acid
• Sodium iodide	• Quinidine polygalacturonate	
• Zalcitabine	• Quinine	
• Zidovudine	• Sulfonamides	
	• Tolbutamide	
	• Vitamin K	

change blood thickness (viscosity) (Karch, 2012). Fig. 39-4 shows where in the blood clotting cascade these agents work.

Anticoagulant drugs work by interfering with one or more steps involved in the blood CLOTTING cascade. Thus these agents *prevent* new clots from forming and limit or prevent extension of formed clots. *Anticoagulants do not break down existing clots.* These drugs are classified as direct thrombin inhibitors, indirect thrombin inhibitors, and vitamin K antagonists.

Direct thrombin inhibitors (DTIs) can be given by the parenteral route and orally. The parenteral drugs include lepirudin (Refludan), desirudin (Iprivask), bivalirudin (Angiomax), argatroban (ARGATROBAN, Acova ✦), rivaroxaban (Xarelto), and apixaban (Eliquis). The drugs prevent the conversion of prothrombin (factor X) to its active form, thrombin (factor Xa). Less thrombin disrupts the CLOTTING cascade by reducing the amount of fibrinogen that is converted to active fibrin (Karch, 2012; Straznitskas & Giarratano, 2014).

Indirect thrombin inhibitors include the heparins and heparinoids. These drugs include enoxaparin (Lovenox), dalteparin (Fragmin), tinzaparin (Innohep), and fondaparinux (Arixtra). All are given parenterally. The lower molecular weight drugs are preferred for home use. The drugs cause anticoagulation by binding to and increasing the activity of antithrombin III (AT III). By activating antithrombin III, coagulation factor Xa (thrombin) is indirectly inhibited (Karch, 2012).

Vitamin K antagonists (VKAs) decrease the synthesis of vitamin K in the intestinal tract, which then reduces the production of vitamin K–dependent CLOTTING factors II, VII, IX, and X, along with the anticoagulant proteins C and S (Karch, 2012). When the clotting factors are reduced, anticoagulation results. The most commonly used VKA is warfarin (Coumadin, Jantoven), an oral agent.

Fibrinolytic drugs (also known as *thrombolytic drugs* or "clot busters") selectively break down fibrin threads present in formed blood clots. The mechanism to start fibrin degradation is activation of the inactive tissue protein *plasminogen* to its active form, *plasmin*. Plasmin directly attacks and degrades the fibrin molecule. Common fibrinolytic drugs include alteplase (Activase), reteplase (Retavase), tenecteplase (TNKase), and urokinase (Abbokinase, Kinlytic). All are administered by the IV route. Urokinase is approved for use only in patients who have a massive pulmonary embolism.

The use of fibrinolytic drugs results in the best clot breakdown with less disruption of blood CLOTTING. These drugs are the first-line therapy for problems caused by small, localized formed clots such as myocardial infarction (MI), limited arterial thrombosis, and thrombotic strokes. For some problems, such as MI, these drugs are usually given only within the first 6 hours after the onset of symptoms. This time limitation is not related to drug activity because fibrinolytic agents can break down clots older than 6 hours. Rather, the tissue that has been anoxic for more than 6 hours as a result of an acute event is not likely to benefit from this therapy, making the risks to the patient greater than the advantages.

Platelet inhibitors or antiplatelet drugs prevent either platelet activation or aggregation (clumping). The most widely used drug for this effect is aspirin, which inhibits the production of substances that activate platelets, such as thromboxane. Other drugs change the platelet membrane, reducing its "stickiness," or prevent activators from binding to platelet receptors by inhibiting a variety of enzymes important to platelet activation (Karch, 2012). These drugs include cilostazol (Pletal), clopidogrel (Plavix), dipyridamole (Persantine), prasugrel (Effient), ticagrelor (Brilinta), and ticlopidine (Ticlid). Another group of drugs that inhibits platelets by binding to certain membrane proteins include abciximab (ReoPro), eptifibatide (Integrilin), and tirofiban (Aggrastat), which are all administered parenterally. In addition, many complementary therapy agents, such as St. John's wort and *Ginkgo biloba,* inhibit platelet activity.

Nutrition Status

Diet can alter cell quality and affect CLOTTING. Ask patients to recall what they have eaten during the past week. Use this information to assess possible iron, protein, mineral, or vitamin deficiencies. Diets high in fat and carbohydrates and low in protein, iron, and vitamins can cause many types of anemia and decrease the functions of all blood cells. Diets high in vitamin K, found in leafy green vegetables, may increase the rate of blood clotting. Assess the amount of salads and other raw vegetables that the patient eats and whether supplemental vitamins and calcium are used.

Ask about alcohol consumption because chronic alcoholism causes nutrition deficiencies and impairs the liver, both of which reduce blood CLOTTING.

Ask about personal resources, such as finances and social support. A person with a low income may have a diet deficient in iron and protein because foods containing these substances are more expensive.

Family History and Genetic Risk

Assess family history because many disorders affecting blood and blood CLOTTING are inherited. Ask whether anyone in the family has had hemophilia, frequent nosebleeds, postpartum hemorrhages, excessive bleeding after tooth extractions, or heavy bruising after mild trauma. Ask whether any family member has sickle cell disease or sickle cell trait. Although sickle cell disease is seen most often among African Americans, anyone can have the trait.

❓ NCLEX EXAMINATION CHALLENGE

Health Promotion and Maintenance

Why is it important for the nurse to teach the client starting on the anticoagulant *warfarin* (Coumadin) to limit his or her intake of leafy green vegetables?

A. These foods contain vitamin K, which can increase the effects of warfarin.

B. These foods contain vitamin K, which can reduce the effects of warfarin.

C. These foods enhance aspirin activity and increase the risk for bleeding in the person who also takes warfarin.

D. These foods reduce aspirin activity and increase the risk for pulmonary embolism in the person who also takes warfarin.

Current Health Problems

Ask about lymph nodes swelling, excessive bruising or bleeding, and whether the bleeding was spontaneous or induced by trauma. Ask about the amount and duration of bleeding after routine dental work. Ask women to estimate the number of pads or tampons used during the most recent menstrual cycle and whether this amount represents a change from the usual pattern of flow. Ask whether clots are present in menstrual blood. If menstrual clots occur, ask her to estimate clot size using coins or fruit for comparison.

Assess and record whether the patient has shortness of breath on exertion, palpitations, frequent infections, fevers, recent weight loss, headaches, or paresthesias. Any or all of these symptoms may occur with hematologic disease.

The most common manifestation of anemia is fatigue as a result of decreased oxygen delivery to cells. Cells use oxygen to produce the high-energy chemical *adenosine triphosphate (ATP)* needed to perform most cellular work. When oxygen delivery to cells is reduced, cellular work decreases and fatigue increases. Ask patients about feeling tired, needing more rest, or losing endurance during normal activities. Ask them to compare their activities during the past month with those of the same month a year ago. Determine whether other manifestations of anemia, such as vertigo, tinnitus, and a sore tongue, are present.

Physical Assessment

Assess the whole body because blood problems may reduce oxygen delivery and tissue PERFUSION to all systems (Jarvis, 2016). Some assessment findings associated with hematologic problems are less reliable when seen in the older adult (see Chart 39-1). Equipment needed for hematologic assessment includes gloves, a stethoscope, a blood pressure cuff, and a penlight. Remember to gently handle the patient suspected of having a hematologic problem to avoid causing bruising, petechiae, or excessive bleeding.

Skin Assessment

Inspect the skin and mucous membranes for pallor or jaundice. Assess nail beds for pallor or cyanosis. Pallor of the gums, conjunctivae, and palmar creases (when the palm is stretched) indicates decreased hemoglobin levels and poor tissue oxygenation. Assess the gums for active bleeding in response to light pressure or brushing the teeth with a soft-bristled brush, and assess any lesions or draining areas. Inspect for petechiae and large bruises *(ecchymoses)*. Petechiae are pinpoint hemorrhagic lesions in the skin. Bruises may cluster together. For hospitalized patients,

determine whether there is bleeding around nasogastric tubes, endotracheal tubes, central lines, peripheral IV sites, or Foley catheters. Check the skin turgor, and ask about itching because dry skin from poor perfusion itches. Assess body hair patterns. Areas with poor circulation, especially the lower legs and toes, may have sparse or absent hair, although this may be a normal finding in an older adult.

🌐 CULTURAL CONSIDERATIONS

Patient-Centered Care QSEN

Pallor and cyanosis are more easily detected in people with darker skin by examining the oral mucous membranes and the conjunctiva of the eye. Jaundice can be seen more easily on the roof of the mouth. Petechiae may be visible only on the palms of the hands or the soles of the feet. Bruises can be seen as darker areas of skin and palpated as slight swellings or irregular skin surfaces. Ask the patient about pain when skin surfaces are touched lightly or palpated. (Chapter 24 provides tips for assessing darker skin.)

Head and Neck Assessment

Check for pallor or ulceration of the oral mucosa. The tongue is smooth in pernicious anemia and iron deficiency anemia or smooth and beefy red in other nutrition deficiencies. These manifestations may occur with fissures at the corners of the mouth. Assess for scleral jaundice.

Inspect and palpate all lymph node areas. Document any lymph node enlargement, including whether palpation of the enlarged node causes pain and whether the enlarged node moves or remains fixed with palpation.

Respiratory Assessment

When blood problems reduce oxygen delivery, the lungs work harder to make adjustments that can maintain tissue PERFUSION. Assess the rate and depth of respiration while the patient is at rest and during and after mild physical activity (e.g., walking 20 steps in 10 seconds). Note whether the patient can complete a 10-word sentence without stopping for a breath. Assess whether the patient is fatigued easily, has shortness of breath at rest or on exertion, or needs extra pillows to breathe well at night. Anemia can cause these manifestations as a result of respiratory changes made as adjustments to the reduced tissue oxygen levels.

Cardiovascular Assessment

When blood problems reduce oxygen delivery, the heart works harder to make adjustments to maintain tissue PERFUSION. Pulses may become weak and thready. Observe for distended neck veins, edema, or indications of phlebitis. Use a stethoscope to listen for abnormal heart sounds and irregular rhythms. Assess blood pressure (BP). Systolic BP tends to be lower than normal in patients with anemia and higher than normal when the patient has excessive red blood cells.

Kidney and Urinary Assessment

The kidneys have many blood vessels, and bleeding problems may cause gross or occult *hematuria* (blood in the urine). Inspect urine for color. Hematuria may appear as grossly bloody red or dark brownish gold urine. Test the urine for proteins with a urine test dipstick because blood contains protein and blood in the urine increases its protein content. Keep in mind that the person with chronic kidney disease (CKD) produces less natural erythropoietin and often is anemic.

Musculoskeletal Assessment

Rib or sternal tenderness may occur with leukemia (blood cancer) when the bone marrow overproduces cells, increasing the pressure in the bones. Examine the skin over superficial bones, including the ribs and sternum, by applying firm pressure with the fingertips. Assess the range of joint motion, and document any swelling or joint pain.

Abdominal Assessment

The normal adult spleen is usually *not* palpable, but an enlarged spleen occurs with many hematologic problems. An enlarged spleen may be detected by palpation, but this is usually performed by the health care provider because an enlarged spleen is tender and ruptures easily.

> ## ! NURSING SAFETY PRIORITY (QSEN)
> ### Action Alert
>
> Do not palpate the splenic area of the abdomen for any patient with a suspected hematologic problem. An enlarged spleen ruptures easily and can lead to hemorrhage and death.

Palpating the edge of the liver in the right upper quadrant of the abdomen can detect enlargement, which often occurs with hematologic problems. The normal liver may be palpable as much as 4 to 5 cm below the right costal margin but is usually not palpable in the epigastrium.

A common cause of anemia among older adults is a chronically bleeding GI ulcer or intestinal polyp. If the ulcer is located in the stomach or the small intestine, obvious blood may not be visible in the stool or such a small amount is passed each day that the patient is not aware of it. Obtain a stool specimen for occult blood testing.

Central Nervous System Assessment

Assessing cranial nerves and testing neurologic function are important in hematologic assessment because some problems cause specific changes. Vitamin B_{12} deficiency impairs nerve function, and severe chronic deficiency may cause permanent neurologic degeneration. Many neurologic problems can develop in patients who have leukemia, because leukemia can cause bleeding, infection, or tumor spread within the brain. When the patient with a suspected bleeding disorder has any head trauma, expand the assessment to include frequent neurologic checks and checks of cognitive function (see Chapter 41).

Psychosocial Assessment

Regardless of the type of hematologic problem, each person brings his or her own coping style to the illness. Develop a rapport with the patient and learn what coping mechanisms he or she has used successfully in the past.

Ask the patient and family members about social support networks and financial resources. A problem in these areas can interfere with the patient's adherence to therapy.

Diagnostic Assessment
Laboratory Tests

Laboratory test results often provide the most definitive information about hematologic problems. Chart 39-2 lists laboratory data used to assess hematologic function. When a venipuncture is necessary, apply pressure to the site for at least 5 minutes on a patient suspected of having a hematologic problem to prevent bleeding and hematoma formation.

Tests of Cell Number and Function. *A peripheral blood smear* is made by taking a drop of blood and spreading it over a slide. It can be read by an automated calculator or by a technologist with a microscope. This rapid test provides information on the sizes, shapes, and proportions of different blood cell types within the peripheral blood.

A complete blood count (CBC) includes a number of studies: red blood cell (RBC) count, white blood cell (WBC) count, hematocrit, and hemoglobin level. The RBC count measures circulating RBCs in 1 mm^3 of blood. The WBC count measures all leukocytes present in 1 mm^3 of blood. To determine the percentages of different types of leukocytes circulating in the blood, a WBC count with differential leukocyte count is performed (see Chapter 17). The hematocrit (Hct) is the percentage of red blood cells in the total blood volume. The hemoglobin (Hgb) level is the total amount of hemoglobin in blood.

The CBC can measure other features of the RBCs. The mean corpuscular volume (MCV) measures the average volume or size of individual RBCs and is useful for classifying anemias. When the MCV is elevated, the cell is larger than normal *(macrocytic)*, as seen in megaloblastic anemias. When the MCV is decreased, the cell is smaller than normal *(microcytic)*, as seen in iron deficiency anemia. The mean corpuscular hemoglobin (MCH) is the average amount of hemoglobin by weight in a single RBC. The mean corpuscular hemoglobin concentration (MCHC) measures the average amount of hemoglobin by percentage in a single RBC. When the MCHC is decreased, the cell has a hemoglobin deficiency and is *hypochromic* (a lighter color), as in iron deficiency anemia. These three tests can help determine possible causes of low RBC counts that are not related to blood loss (Rauen, 2012).

Reticulocyte count is helpful in determining bone marrow function. A reticulocyte is an immature RBC that still has its nucleus. An elevated reticulocyte count indicates that RBCs are being produced and released by the bone marrow before they mature. Normally only about 2% of circulating RBCs are reticulocytes. An elevated reticulocyte count is desirable in an anemic patient or after hemorrhage because this indicates that the bone marrow is responding to a decrease in the total RBC level. An elevated reticulocyte count without a precipitating cause usually indicates health problems, such as polycythemia vera (a malignant condition in which the bone marrow overproduces RBCs).

A platelet count, also known as a *thrombocyte count,* reflects the number of platelets in circulation. The normal range is 150,000 to 400,000/mm^3. When this value is low *(thrombocytopenia)*, the person is at greater risk for bleeding because platelets are critical for blood clotting. Patients who have values between 40,000/mm^3 and 80,000/mm^3 may have prolonged bleeding from trauma, dental work, and surgery. Patients who have platelet values below 20,000/mm^3 may have spontaneous bleeding that is very difficult to stop.

Hemoglobin electrophoresis detects abnormal forms of hemoglobin, such as hemoglobin S in sickle cell disease. Hemoglobin A is the major type of hemoglobin in an adult.

Leukocyte alkaline phosphatase (LAP) is an enzyme produced by normal mature neutrophils. Elevated LAP levels occur during episodes of infection or stress. An elevated neutrophil

CHART 39-2 Laboratory Profile

Hematologic Assessment

TEST	REFERENCE RANGE	INTERNATIONAL REFERENCE UNITS	SIGNIFICANCE OF ABNORMAL FINDINGS
Red blood cell (RBC) count	*Females:* 4.2-5.4 million/µL *Males:* 4.7-6.1 million/µL	$4.2\text{-}5.4 \times 10^{12}$ cells/L $4.7\text{-}6.1 \times 10^{12}$ cells/L	*Decreased levels* indicate possible anemia or hemorrhage. *Increased levels* indicate possible chronic hypoxia or polycythemia vera.
Hemoglobin (Hgb)	*Females:* 12-16 g/dL *Males:* 14-18 g/dL	7.4-9.9 mmol/L 8.7-11.2 mmol/L	Same as for RBC.
Hematocrit (Hct)	*Females:* 37%-47% *Males:* 42%-52%	0.37-0.47 fraction 0.42-0.52 fraction	Same as for RBC.
Mean corpuscular volume (MCV)	80-95 fL	Same as reference range	*Increased levels* indicate macrocytic cells, possible anemia. *Decreased levels* indicate microcytic cells, possible iron deficiency anemia.
Mean corpuscular hemoglobin (MCH)	27-31 pg	Same as reference range	Same as for MCV.
Mean corpuscular hemoglobin concentration (MCHC)	32-36 g/dL	32%-36%	*Increased levels* may indicate spherocytosis or anemia. *Decreased levels* may indicate iron deficiency anemia or a hemoglobinopathy.
White blood cell (WBC) count	5000-10,000/mm³	$5.0\text{-}10.0 \times 10^9$ cells/L	*Increased levels* are associated with infection, inflammation, autoimmune disorders, and leukemia. *Decreased levels* may indicate prolonged infection or bone marrow suppression.
Reticulocyte count	0.5%-2.0% of RBCs	0.005-0.20 fraction	*Increased levels* may indicate chronic blood loss. *Decreased levels* indicate possible inadequate RBC production.
Total iron-binding capacity (TIBC)	250-460 mcg/dL	45-82 µmol/L	*Increased levels* indicate iron deficiency. *Decreased levels* may indicate anemia, hemorrhage, hemolysis.
Iron (Fe)	*Females:* 60-160 mcg/dL *Males:* 80-180 mcg/dL	11-29 µmol/L 14-32 µmol/L	*Increased levels* indicate iron excess, liver disorders, hemochromatosis, megaloblastic anemia. *Decreased levels* indicate possible iron deficiency anemia, hemorrhage.
Serum ferritin	*Females:* 10-150 ng/mL *Males:* 12-300 ng/mL	10-150 mcg/L 12-300 mcg/L	Same as for iron.
Platelet count	150,000-400,000/mm³	$150\text{-}400 \times 10^9$/L	*Increased levels* may indicate polycythemia vera or malignancy. *Decreased levels* may indicate bone marrow suppression, autoimmune disease, hypersplenism.
Hemoglobin electrophoresis	Hgb A_1: 95%-98% Hgb A_2: 2%-3% Hgb F: 0.8%-2% Hgb S: 0% Hgb C: 0% Hgb E: 0%	Same as reference range	*Variations* indicate hemoglobinopathies.
Direct Coombs' and indirect Coombs' test	Negative	Negative	*Positive findings* indicate antibodies to RBCs.
Prothrombin time (PT)	11-12.5 sec 85%-100%	Patient PT/normal PT INR 0.8-1.1	*Increased time* indicates possible deficiency of clotting factors V and VII. *Decreased time* may indicate vitamin K excess.

Data from Pagana, K., & Pagana, T. (2014). *Mosby's manual of diagnostic and laboratory tests* (5th ed.). St. Louis: Mosby.
fL, Femtoliter; *INR,* international normalized ratio; *pg,* picograms.

count without an elevation in LAP level occurs with some types of leukemia.

Coombs' tests, both direct and indirect, are used for blood typing. The direct test detects antibodies against RBCs that may be attached to a person's RBCs. Although healthy people can make these antibodies, in certain diseases (e.g., systemic lupus erythematosus, mononucleosis) these antibodies are directed against the patient's own RBCs. Excessive amounts of these antibodies can cause hemolytic anemia (Pagana & Pagana, 2014).

The indirect Coombs' test detects the presence of circulating antiglobulins. The test is used to determine whether the patient

has serum antibodies to the type of RBCs that he or she is about to receive by blood transfusion (Pagana & Pagana, 2014).

Serum ferritin, transferrin, and the total iron-binding capacity (TIBC) tests measure iron levels. Abnormal levels of iron and TIBC occur with problems such as iron deficiency anemia.

The serum ferritin test measures the amount of free iron present in the plasma, which represents 1% of the total body iron stores. Therefore the serum ferritin level provides a means to assess total iron stores. People with serum ferritin levels within 10 g of the normal range for their gender have adequate iron stores; people with levels 10 g or more lower than the normal range have inadequate iron stores and have difficulty recovering from any blood loss.

Transferrin is a protein that transports dietary iron from the intestines to cell storage sites. Measuring the amount of iron that can be bound to serum transferrin indirectly determines whether an adequate amount of transferrin is present. This test is the total iron-binding capacity (TIBC) test. Normally, only about 30% of the transferrin is bound to iron in the blood. TIBC increases when a person is deficient in serum iron and stored iron levels. Such a value indicates that an adequate amount of transferrin is present but less than 30% of it is bound to serum iron.

Tests Measuring Bleeding and Coagulation. Tests that measure bleeding and coagulation provide information that reflects the effectiveness of different aspects of blood CLOTTING. These tests are used to diagnose specific hematologic health problems, determine drug therapy effectiveness, and identify risk for excessive bleeding or clotting.

Prothrombin time (PT) measures how long blood takes to clot, reflecting the level of clotting factors II, V, VII, and X and how well they are functioning. When enough of these clotting factors are present and functioning, the PT shows blood CLOTTING between 11 and 12.5 seconds or within 85% to 100% of the time needed for a control sample of blood to clot. PT is prolonged when one or more of these clotting factors are deficient.

The PT test is now used less often to assess how fast blood clots, because control blood is taken from different people and may not be the same even in one laboratory from one day to the next. To reduce PT errors as a result of control blood variation or in some of the chemicals used in the test, the international normalized ratio is used to assess clotting time.

International normalized ratio (INR) measures the same process as the PT by establishing a normal mean or standard for PT. The INR is calculated by dividing the patient's PT by the established standard PT. A normal INR ranges between 0.7 and 1.8. When using the INR to monitor warfarin therapy, the desired outcome is usually to maintain the patient's INR between 2.0 and 3.0 regardless of the actual PT in seconds. The desired INR range for any patient, however, is individualized for specific patient factors and medical conditions.

The partial thromboplastin time (PTT) assesses the intrinsic CLOTTING cascade and the action of factors II, V, VIII, IX, XI, and XII. PTT is prolonged whenever any of these factors is deficient, such as in hemophilia or disseminated intravascular coagulation (DIC). Because factors II, IX, and X are vitamin K–dependent and are produced in the liver, liver disease can prolong the PTT. Desired therapeutic ranges for anticoagulation are usually between 1.5 and 2.0 times normal values but can be greater depending on the reason the person is receiving anticoagulation therapy.

The anti-factor Xa test measures the amount of anti-activated factor X (anti-Xa) in blood, which is affected by heparin. It is used mainly to monitor heparin levels in patients treated with either standard unfractionated heparin or low–molecular-weight heparin. For people not receiving heparin in any form, the reference range is less than 0.1 IU/mL. The usual therapeutic range for patients receiving standard heparin is 0.5 to 1.0 IU/mL, and the usual therapeutic range for patients receiving low–molecular-weight heparin is 0.3 to 0.7 IU/mL. Test results are affected by age, gender, health history, and the specific laboratory technique used for the test.

Platelet aggregation, or the ability to clump, is tested by mixing the patient's plasma with an agonist substance that should cause clumping. The degree of clumping is noted. Aggregation can be impaired in von Willebrand's disease and during the use of drugs such as aspirin, anti-inflammatory agents, psychotropic agents, and platelet inhibitors.

❓ NCLEX EXAMINATION CHALLENGE

Physiological Integrity

Which blood test result for a client being assessed for a hematologic problem indicates to the nurse that chronic anemia is likely?
A. International normalized ratio (INR) is 0.9
B. Platelet count of 180,000/mm^3
C. Reticulocyte value of 14%
D. Hematocrit of 27%

Imaging Assessment

Assessment of the patient with a suspected hematologic problem can include radioisotopic imaging. Isotopes are used to evaluate the bone marrow for sites of active blood cell formation and sites of iron storage. Radioactive colloids are used to determine organ size and liver and spleen function.

The patient is given a radioactive isotope by IV about 3 hours before the procedure. Once in the nuclear medicine department, he or she must lie still for about an hour during the scan. No special patient preparation or follow-up care is needed for these tests.

Standard x-rays may be used to diagnose some hematologic problems. For example, multiple myeloma causes classic bone destruction, with a "Swiss cheese" appearance on x-ray.

Bone Marrow Aspiration and Biopsy

Bone marrow aspiration or biopsy, which are similar invasive procedures, helps evaluate the patient's hematologic status when other tests show abnormal findings that indicate a possible problem in blood cell production or maturation. Results provide information about bone marrow function, including the production of all blood cells and platelets. In a bone marrow aspiration, cells and fluids are suctioned from the bone marrow. In a bone marrow biopsy, solid tissue and cells are obtained by coring out an area of bone marrow with a large-bore needle.

A health care provider's order and a signed informed consent are obtained before either procedure is performed. Bone marrow aspiration may be performed by a physician, an advanced practice nurse, or a physician assistant, depending on the agency's policy and regional law. The procedure may be performed at the patient's bedside, in an examination room, or in a laboratory.

After learning what specific tests will be performed on the marrow, check with the hematology laboratory to determine how to handle the specimen. Some tests require that heparin or other solutions be added to the specimen.

Patient Preparation. Most patients are anxious before a bone marrow aspiration, even those who have had one in the past. You can help reduce anxiety and allay fears by providing accurate information and emotional support. Some patients like to have their hand held during the procedure.

Explain the procedure, and reassure the patient that you will stay during the entire procedure. Occasionally a friend or family member is permitted to be present to provide emotional support. Tell the patient that the local anesthetic injection will feel like a stinging or burning sensation. Tell him or her to expect a heavy sensation of pressure and pushing while the needle is being inserted. Sometimes a crunching sound can be heard or scraping sensation felt as the needle punctures the bone. Explain that a brief sensation of painful pulling will be experienced as the marrow is being aspirated by mild suction in the syringe. If a biopsy is performed, the patient may feel more discomfort as the needle is rotated into the bone.

Assist the patient onto an examining table, and expose the site (usually the iliac crest). If this site is not available or if more marrow is needed, the sternum may be used. If the iliac crest is the site, place the patient in the prone or side-lying position. Depending on the tests to be performed on the specimen, a laboratory technician may also be present to ensure proper handling of the specimen.

Procedure. The procedure usually lasts from 5 to 15 minutes. The type and the amount of anesthesia or sedation depend on the physician's preference, the patient's preference and previous experience with bone marrow aspiration and biopsy, and the setting.

A local anesthetic agent is injected into the skin around the site. The patient may also receive a mild tranquilizer or a rapid-acting sedative, such as midazolam (Versed), lorazepam (Ativan, Apo-Lorazepam ✤, Novo-Lorazem ✤), or etomidate (Amidate). Some patients do well with guided imagery or autohypnosis.

> ### ! NURSING SAFETY PRIORITY (QSEN)
> **Action Alert**
>
> Aspiration or biopsy procedures are invasive, and sterile technique must be observed.

The skin over the site is cleaned with a disinfectant. For an aspiration, the needle is inserted with a twisting motion and the marrow is aspirated by pulling back on the plunger of the syringe. When sufficient marrow has been aspirated to ensure accurate analysis, the needle is rapidly withdrawn while the tissues are supported at the site. For a biopsy, a small skin incision is made and the biopsy needle is inserted through the skin opening. Pressure and several twisting motions are needed to ensure coring and loosening of an adequate amount of marrow tissue. Apply external pressure to the site until hemostasis is ensured. A pressure dressing or sandbags may be applied to reduce bleeding at the site.

Follow-Up Care. The nursing priority after a bone marrow aspiration or biopsy is prevention of excessive bleeding. Cover the site with a dressing after bleeding is controlled, and closely observe it for 24 hours for manifestations of bleeding and infection. A mild analgesic (aspirin-free) may be given for discomfort, and ice packs can be placed over the site to limit bruising. Instruct the patient to inspect the site every 2 hours for the first 24 hours and to note the presence of active bleeding or bruising. Advise him or her to avoid contact sports or any activity that might result in trauma to the site for 48 hours.

Information obtained from bone marrow aspiration or biopsy reflects the degree and quality of bone marrow activity present. The counts made on a marrow specimen can indicate whether different cell types are present in the expected quantities and proportions. In addition, bone marrow aspiration or biopsy can confirm the spread of cancer cells from other tumor sites.

> ### ? CLINICAL JUDGMENT CHALLENGE
> **Safety; Patient-Centered Care** (QSEN)
>
> A 52-year-old man is scheduled for a bone marrow aspiration because his white blood cell count has been persistently abnormal and his father died from chronic lymphocytic leukemia (CLL). He is very anxious this morning, and you remember him from one of his earlier visits in which you drew his blood. At that visit, he started vomiting when you placed the needle in his vein. He tells you that he is very worried about the results and the pain of the procedure. He also tells you that his daughter has a dance recital tonight and he very much wants to attend this event.
> 1. Is this patient a candidate for autohypnosis? Why or why not?
> 2. Is there any reason(s) for him to think he may also have CLL? If so, what might this be?
> 3. What will you tell him about attending the dance recital?

NURSING CONCEPTS AND CLINICAL JUDGMENT REVIEW

What might you NOTICE in a patient with adequate tissue PERFUSION related to normal hematologic function?

Vital signs:
- Heart rate and respiratory rate within normal range
- Blood pressure within normal range

Physical assessment:
- Able to speak a sentence of 12 words without stopping for breath
- Able to walk and talk without stopping for breath
- Skin color normal (no cyanosis, pallor, or jaundice)
- Oral mucous membrane and nail beds pink with rapid capillary refill
- Gums pink, no petechiae or bleeding
- Appropriate distribution of body hair, especially on legs and feet

- Warm hands and feet, no dependent edema
- Skin clear with no large bruises or petechiae
- Lower eyelid conjunctivae red
- Urine output just about equal to fluid intake
- Urine clear and yellow

Psychological assessment:
- Oriented and not confused
- Energy level good; able to engage in desired work, recreational, and personal activities

Laboratory assessment:
- Red blood cell, hemoglobin, hematocrit, white blood cell, and platelet levels within normal limits for age and gender
- Reticulocyte count less than 2%

GET READY FOR THE NCLEX® EXAMINATION!

KEY POINTS

Review these Key Points for each NCLEX Examination Client Needs Category.

Safe and Effective Care Environment

- Verify that a patient having a bone marrow aspiration or biopsy has signed an informed consent statement. **Safety** QSEN
- Handle patients with suspected hematologic problems gently to avoid bleeding or bruising. **Safety** QSEN
- Do not palpate the splenic area of any patient suspected of having a hematologic problem. **Safety** QSEN
- Maintain pressure over a venipuncture site for at least 5 minutes to prevent excessive bleeding. **Safety** QSEN

Health Promotion and Maintenance

- Teach people to avoid unnecessary contact with environmental chemicals or toxins. If contact cannot be avoided, teach people to use safety precautions.
- Instruct patients about the importance of eating a diet with adequate amounts of foods that are good sources of iron, folic acid, and vitamin B_{12}. **Patient-Centered Care** QSEN

Psychosocial Integrity

- Teach patients and family members about what to expect during procedures to assess hematologic function, including restrictions, drugs, and follow-up care. **Patient-Centered Care** QSEN
- Ask patients about their activity level and whether they are satisfied with the energy they have for activities. **Patient-Centered Care** QSEN
- Support the patient during a bone marrow aspiration or biopsy. **Patient-Centered Care** QSEN

Physiological Integrity

- Interpret blood cell counts and CLOTTING tests to assess hematologic status. **Evidence-Based Practice** QSEN
- Be aware of these facts for hematologic function:
  - Tissue oxygenation and perfusion rely on normal hematologic function for oxygen delivery.
  - The most common manifestation of a hematologic problem is fatigue.
  - A platelet plug and a fibrin clot are not the same.
  - Both CLOTTING forces and anti-CLOTTING forces are needed to maintain adequate PERFUSION.
  - Women have reduced red blood cell, hematocrit, and hemoglobin levels at all ages compared with men.
- Use the lip rather than nail beds to assess capillary refill on older adults. **Evidence-Based Practice** QSEN
- Rely on laboratory tests rather than skin color changes in older adults to assess anemia or jaundice. **Evidence-Based Practice** QSEN
- Assess the patient's endurance in performing ADLs. **Patient-Centered Care** QSEN
- Apply an ice pack to the needle site after a bone marrow aspiration or biopsy. **Patient-Centered Care** QSEN
- Check the needle insertion site at least every 2 hours after a bone marrow aspiration or biopsy. If the patient is going home, teach the patient and family how to assess the site for bleeding and when to seek help. **Patient-Centered Care** QSEN
- Instruct patients to avoid activities that may traumatize the site after a bone marrow aspiration or biopsy.

40 | CHAPTER

Care of Patients with Hematologic Problems

Katherine I. Byar

 http://evolve.elsevier.com/Iggy/

Any condition that impairs the production or function of blood cells or that causes the abnormal destruction of any type of blood cell can result in a hematologic problem. Problems of the hematologic system can affect many tissues and organs by interfering with GAS EXCHANGE and tissue PERFUSION. The type and severity of the disorder determine the impact it has on patient health. This chapter discusses mild hematologic disorders and those that are potentially life threatening, such as sickle cell disease and hematologic malignancies.

RED BLOOD CELL DISORDERS

Red blood cells (RBCs), also known as **erythrocytes**, are the major cell in the blood. As discussed in Chapter 39, tissue GAS EXCHANGE for oxygenation depends on keeping the circulating number of RBCs within the normal range for the person's age and gender and on maintaining normal RBC function. RBC disorders include problems in production, function, and destruction. Problems may result in poor function of RBCs, decreased numbers of RBCs (anemia), or an excess of RBCs (polycythemia).

Anemia is a reduction in either the number of RBCs, the amount of hemoglobin, or the **hematocrit** (percentage of packed RBCs per deciliter of blood). It is a clinical indicator, not a specific disease, because it occurs with many health problems. Anemia can result from dietary problems, genetic disorders, bone marrow disease, or excessive bleeding. GI bleeding is the most common reason for anemia in adults.

There are many types and causes of anemia (Table 40-1). Some are caused by a deficiency in one of the components needed to make fully functional RBCs. Other anemias are caused by decreased RBC production or increased RBC

TABLE 40-1	**Common Causes of Anemia**
TYPE OF ANEMIA	**COMMON CAUSES**
Sickle cell disease	Autosomal recessive inheritance of two defective gene alleles for hemoglobin synthesis
Glucose-6-phosphate dehydrogenase (G6PD) deficiency anemia	X-linked recessive deficiency of the enzyme *G6PD*
Autoimmune hemolytic anemia	Abnormal immune function in which a person's immune reactive cells fail to recognize his or her own red blood cells as self cells
Iron deficiency anemia	Inadequate iron intake caused by: • Iron-deficient diet • Chronic alcoholism • Malabsorption syndromes • Partial gastrectomy Rapid metabolic (anabolic) activity caused by: • Pregnancy • Adolescence • Infection
Vitamin B₁₂ deficiency anemia	Dietary deficiency Failure to absorb vitamin B₁₂ from intestinal tract as a result of: • Partial gastrectomy • Pernicious anemia • Malabsorption syndromes
Folic acid deficiency anemia	Dietary deficiency Malabsorption syndromes Drugs: • Oral contraceptives • Anticonvulsants • Methotrexate
Aplastic anemia	Exposure to myelotoxic agents: • Radiation • Benzene • Chloramphenicol • Alkylating agents • Antimetabolites • Sulfonamides • Insecticides Viral infection (unproven): • Epstein-Barr virus • Hepatitis B • Cytomegalovirus

CHART 40-1	**Key Features**

Anemia

Integumentary Manifestations
- Pallor, especially of the ears, the nail beds, the palmar creases, the conjunctivae, and around the mouth
- Cool to the touch
- Intolerance of cold temperatures
- Nails become brittle and become concave over time

Cardiovascular Manifestations
- Tachycardia at basal activity levels, increasing with activity and during and immediately after meals
- Murmurs and gallops heard on auscultation when anemia is severe
- Orthostatic hypotension

Respiratory Manifestations
- Dyspnea on exertion
- Decreased oxygen saturation levels

Neurologic Manifestations
- Increased somnolence and fatigue
- Headache

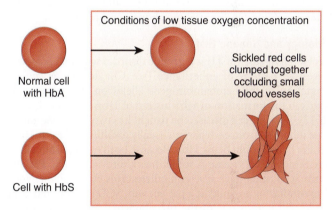

FIG. 40-1 Red blood cell actions under conditions of low tissue oxygenation. (*HbA,* Hemoglobin A; *HbS,* hemoglobin S.)

destruction. Despite the many causes, manifestations (Chart 40-1) and the nursing care needed are similar for all types of anemia.

ANEMIAS RESULTING FROM INCREASED DESTRUCTION OF RED BLOOD CELLS

SICKLE CELL DISEASE

❖ *PATHOPHYSIOLOGY*

Sickle cell disease (SCD), which used to be called *sickle cell anemia,* is a genetic disorder that results in chronic anemia, pain, disability, organ damage, increased risk for INFECTION, and early death. There is great variation among patients in how severe the disease is and when complications start.

This disorder results in the formation of abnormal hemoglobin chains. In healthy adults, the normal hemoglobin (hemoglobin A [HbA]) molecule has two alpha chains and two beta chains of amino acids. Normal adult red blood cells usually contain 98% to 99% HbA, with a small percentage of a fetal form of hemoglobin (HbF).

In SCD, at least 40% (and often much more) of the total hemoglobin is composed of an abnormal beta chain (hemoglobin S [(HbS]). HbS is sensitive to low oxygen content of the RBCs. When RBCs having large amounts of HbS are exposed to decreased oxygen conditions, the abnormal beta chains contract and pile together within the cell, distorting the cell into a sickle shape. Sickled cells become rigid and clump together, causing the RBCs to become "sticky" and fragile. The clumped masses of sickled RBCs block blood flow (Fig. 40-1), known as a *vaso-occlusive event (VOE).* VOE leads to further tissue **hypoxia** (reduced oxygen supply) and more sickle-shaped cells, which then leads to more blood vessel obstruction and ischemia in the affected tissues. Repeated episodes of ischemia cause progressive organ damage from anoxia and infarction. Conditions that cause sickling include hypoxia, dehydration, INFECTION, venous stasis, pregnancy, alcohol consumption, high altitudes, low or high environmental or body temperatures, acidosis, strenuous exercise, emotional stress, and anesthesia.

Usually sickled cells go back to normal shape when the precipitating condition is removed, the blood oxygen level is normalized, and proper tissue PERFUSION resumes. Although the cells then appear normal, some of the hemoglobin remains twisted, decreasing cell flexibility. The cell membranes are damaged over time, and cells are permanently sickled. The membranes of cells with HbS are more fragile and more easily broken. The average life span of an RBC containing 40% or more of HbS is about 10 to 20 days, much less than the 120-day life span of normal RBCs. This reduced RBC life span causes hemolytic (blood cell–destroying) anemia in patients with sickle cell disease.

The patient with SCD has periodic episodes of extensive cellular sickling, called crises. The crises have a sudden onset and can occur as often as weekly or as seldom as once a year. Many patients are in good health much of the time, with crises occurring only in response to conditions that cause local or systemic hypoxemia (deficient oxygen in the blood).

Repeated VOEs in large blood vessels cause long-term damage to tissues and organs. Most damage results from tissue hypoxia, anoxia, ischemia, and cell death. Organs begin to have small infarcted areas and scar tissue formation, and eventually organ failure results. Tissues most often affected are the spleen, liver, heart, kidney, brain, joints, bones, and retina.

Etiology and Genetic Risk

Sickle cell disease (SCD) is a genetic disorder with an autosomal recessive pattern of inheritance (see Chapter 4). A specific mutation in the hemoglobin gene alleles on chromosome 11 leads to the formation of HbS instead of HbA (Parsh & Kumar, 2012). In sickle cell disease, the patient has two HbS gene alleles, one inherited from each parent, usually resulting in 80% to 100% of the hemoglobin being HbS. Because both hemoglobin alleles are S, sickle cell disease is sometimes abbreviated "SS." Patients with SCD often have severe manifestations even when triggering conditions are mild. If a patient with SCD has children, each child will inherit one of the two abnormal gene alleles and at least have sickle cell trait.

Sickle cell trait occurs when one normal gene allele and one abnormal gene allele for hemoglobin are inherited and only half of the hemoglobin chains are abnormal. Sickle cell trait is abbreviated "AS." The patient is a carrier of the HbS gene allele (Fig. 40-2) and can pass the trait on to his or her children. However, the patient has only mild manifestations of the disease when precipitating conditions are present because less than 40% of the hemoglobin is abnormal.

Incidence and Prevalence

Sickle cell trait and different forms of SCD occur in people of all races and ethnicities but is most common among African Americans in the United States. About 72,000 people have SCD, occurring in 1 in 500 African Americans. About 1 in 12 to 1 in 15 (8%) African Americans are carriers of one sickle cell gene allele and have AS (United States National Library of Medicine, 2014).

❖ PATIENT-CENTERED COLLABORATIVE CARE

◆ Assessment

History. An adult with sickle cell disease (SCD) usually has a long-standing diagnosis of the disorder. Those with sickle cell trait usually have no manifestations or abnormal laboratory

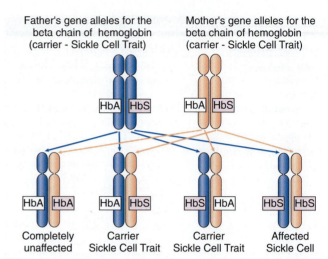

FIG. 40-2 Possible transmission of sickle cell disease and sickle cell trait when both parents are carriers. (*HbA*, Hemoglobin A; *HbS*, hemoglobin S.)

findings other than the presence of hemoglobin S. This person may be unaware that he or she has a hematologic problem until an acute illness is present or when anesthesia is administered.

Ask about previous crises, what led to the crises, severity, and usual management. Explore recent contact with ill people and activities to determine what caused the current crisis. Ask about manifestations of INFECTION.

Review all activities and events during the past 24 hours, including food and fluid intake, exposure to temperature extremes, drugs taken, exercise, trauma, stress, recent airplane travel, and ingestion of alcohol or other recreational drugs. Ask about changes in sleep and rest patterns, ability to climb stairs, and any activity that induces shortness of breath. Determine the patient's perceived energy level using a scale ranging from 0 to 10 (0 = not tired with plenty of energy; 10 = total exhaustion) to assess the degree of fatigue.

Physical Assessment/Clinical Manifestations. Pain is the most common manifestation of SCD crisis. Others vary with the site of tissue damage.

Cardiovascular changes, including the risk for high-output heart failure, occur because of the anemia. Assess the patient for shortness of breath and general fatigue or weakness. Other problems may include murmurs, the presence of an S_3 heart sound, and increased jugular-venous pulsation or distention. Assess the cardiovascular status by comparing peripheral pulses, temperature, and capillary refill in all extremities. Extremities distal to blood vessel occlusion are cool to the touch with slow capillary refill and may have reduced or absent pulses. Heart rate may be rapid and blood pressure may be low to average with anemia.

Priapism is a prolonged penile erection that can occur in men who have SCD. The cause is excessive vascular engorgement in erectile tissue. The condition is very painful and can last for hours. During the priapism episode, the patient usually cannot urinate.

Skin changes include pallor or cyanosis because of poor GAS EXCHANGE from decreased PERFUSION and anemia. Examine the lips, tongue, nail beds, conjunctivae, palms, and soles of the feet at least every 8 hours for subtle color changes. With cyanosis, the lips and tongue are gray and the palms, soles, conjunctivae, and nail beds have a bluish tinge.

Another skin manifestation of SCD is jaundice. Jaundice results from RBC destruction and release of bilirubin. To assess for jaundice in patients with darker skin, inspect the roof of the mouth for a yellow appearance. Examine the sclera closest to the cornea to assess jaundice more accurately. Jaundice often causes intense itching.

Many adults with SCD have ulcers on the lower legs that are caused by poor PERFUSION, especially on the outer sides and inner aspect of the ankle or the shin (Ladizinski et al., 2012). These lesions often become necrotic or infected, requiring débridement and antibiotic therapy. Inspect the legs and feet for ulcers or darkened areas that may indicate necrotic tissue.

Abdominal changes include damage to the spleen and liver, which often occurs early from many episodes of hypoxia and ischemia. In crisis, abdominal pain is diffuse and steady, involving the back and legs. The liver or spleen may feel firm and enlarged with a nodular or "lumpy" texture in later stages of the disease.

Kidney and urinary changes are common as a result of poor PERFUSION and decreased tissue GAS EXCHANGE. Chronic kidney disease occurs as a result of anoxic damage to the kidney nephrons. Early damage makes the kidneys less effective at filtration and reabsorption. The urine contains protein, and the patient may not concentrate urine. Eventually, the kidneys fail, resulting in little or no urine output.

Musculoskeletal changes occur because arms and legs are often sites of blood vessel occlusion. Joints may be damaged from hypoxic episodes and have necrotic degeneration. Inspect the arms and legs, and record any areas of swelling, temperature, or color difference. Ask patients to move all joints. Record the range of motion and any pain with movement.

Central nervous system (CNS) changes may occur in SCD. During crises, patients may have a low-grade fever. If the CNS has infarcts or repeated episodes of hypoxia, patients may have seizures or manifestations of a stroke. Assess for the presence of "pronator drift," bilateral hand grasp strength, gait, and coordination. See Chapter 41 for details of neurologic assessment.

Psychosocial Assessment. Often behavioral changes are early manifestations of cerebral hypoxia from poor PERFUSION. Observe the patient, and document behavior. Ask family members whether the current behavior and mental status are usual for the patient.

SCD is a painful, life-limiting disorder that can be passed on to one's children. Assess the patient's psychosocial needs in terms of new factors that might contribute to a crisis, established support systems, use of coping patterns, and disease progression.

Laboratory Assessment. The diagnosis of SCD is based on the percentage of hemoglobin S (HbS) on electrophoresis. A person who has AS usually has less than 40% HbS, and the patient with SCD may have 80% to 100% HbS. This percentage does not change during crises. Another indicator of SCD is the number of RBCs with permanent sickling. This value is less than 1% among people with no hemoglobin disease, is 5% to 50% among people with AS, and may be 90% among patients with SCD.

Other laboratory tests can indicate complications of the disease, especially during crises. The hematocrit of patients with SCD is low (between 20% and 30%) because of RBC shortened life span and RBC destruction. This value decreases even more during crises or during stress (aplastic crisis). The reticulocyte count is high, indicating anemia of long duration. The total

bilirubin level may be high because damaged RBCs release iron and bilirubin.

The total white blood cell (WBC) count is usually high in patients with SCD. This elevation is related to chronic inflammation caused by tissue hypoxia and ischemia.

Imaging Assessment. Bone changes occur as a result of chronically stimulated marrow and low bone oxygen levels. The skull may show changes on x-ray as a result of bone surface cell destruction and new growth, giving the skull a "crew cut" appearance on x-ray. X-rays of joints may show necrosis and destruction. Ultrasonography, CT, positron emission tomography (PET), and MRI may show soft-tissue and organ changes from poor PERFUSION and chronic inflammation.

Other Diagnostic Assessment. Electrocardiographic (ECG) changes document cardiac infarcts and tissue damage. Specific ECG changes are related to the area of the heart damaged. Echocardiograms may show cardiomyopathy and decreased cardiac output (low ejection fraction).

🔍 NCLEX EXAMINATION CHALLENGE

Safe and Effective Care Environment

Which new assessment finding in a client with sickle cell disease who currently is in crisis does the nurse report immediately to the health care provider?
A. Pain in the right hip with limited range of motion
B. Slow capillary refill in the toes of the right foot
C. Yellow appearance of the roof of the mouth
D. Facial drooping on the right side

◆ Analysis

The priority NANDA-I nursing diagnoses and collaborative problems for patients with sickle cell disease include:
1. Acute Pain and Chronic Pain related to poor tissue oxygenation and joint destruction (NANDA-I)
2. Potential for infection, sepsis, multiple organ dysfunction, and death

◆ Interventions

Managing Pain. The pain with sickle cell crisis is the result of tissue injury caused by poor PERFUSION and tissue GAS EXCHANGE from obstructed blood flow. Mild pain episodes can be managed at home. However, pain is often severe enough to require hospitalization and opioid analgesics. Acute pain episodes have a sudden onset, usually involving the chest, back, abdomen, and extremities. Complications of SCD can cause severe, chronic pain, requiring large doses of opioid analgesics.

Ask whether the pain is typical of past pain episodes. If not, other pain causes or disease complications must be explored. Ask the patient to rate pain on a scale ranging from 0 to 10, and evaluate the effectiveness of interventions based on the ratings.

Concerns about substance abuse can lead to inadequate pain treatment in these patients. Opioid addiction is rare, occurring in only 2% to 5% of patients with SCD. Pain management is based on past pain history, previous drug use, disease complications, and current pain assessment. Health care providers need to be aware of their own attitudes when caring for this population. If substance abuse occurs, management of addiction is incorporated into the overall treatment plan. Addicted patients in acute pain crisis still need opioids (Jenerette & Leak, 2012).

Care of the Patient in Sickle Cell Crisis

- Administer oxygen.
- Administer prescribed pain medication.
- Hydrate the patient with normal saline IV and with beverages of choice (without caffeine) orally.
- Remove any constrictive clothing.
- Encourage the patient to keep extremities extended to promote venous return.
- Do not raise the knee position of the bed.
- Elevate the head of the bed no more than 30 degrees.
- Keep room temperature at or above 72°F (22.2°C).
- Avoid taking blood pressure with external cuff.
- Check circulation in extremities every hour:
  - Pulse oximetry of fingers and toes
  - Capillary refill
  - Peripheral pulses
  - Toe temperature

Drug therapy for patients in acute sickle cell crisis often starts with at least 48 hours of IV analgesics. (Chart 40-2 lists best practices for nursing care of the patient in sickle cell crisis.) Morphine and hydromorphone (Dilaudid) are given IV on a routine schedule or by infusion pump using patient-controlled analgesia (PCA) (Myers & Eckes, 2012). Once relief is obtained, the IV dose can be tapered and the drug given orally. Avoid "as needed" (PRN) schedules because they do not provide adequate relief. Moderate pain may be managed with oral doses of opioids or NSAIDs. (See Chapter 3 for more information on pain management.)

Hydroxyurea (Droxia) may reduce the number of sickling and pain episodes by stimulating fetal hemoglobin (HbF) production. Increasing the level of HbF reduces sickling of red blood cells in patients with sickle cell disease. However, this drug is associated with an increased incidence of leukemia. Long-term complications should be discussed with the patient before this therapy is started. Hydroxyurea also suppresses bone marrow function including IMMUNITY, and regular follow-up to monitor complete blood counts (CBCs) for drug toxicity is important.

> **! NURSING SAFETY PRIORITY** QSEN
>
> **Action Alert**
>
> Hydroxyurea is **teratogenic** (can cause birth defects). Teach sexually active women of childbearing age using this drug to adhere to strict contraceptive measures while taking hydroxyurea and for 1 month after the drug is discontinued.

Hydration by the oral or IV route helps reduce the duration of pain episodes. Urge the patient to drink water or juices. Because the patient is often dehydrated and his or her blood is hypertonic, hypotonic fluids are usually infused at 250 mL/hr for 4 hours. Once the patient's blood osmolarity is down to the normal range of 270 to 300 mOsm, the IV rate is reduced to 125 mL/hr if more hydration is needed.

Complementary therapies and other measures, such as keeping the room warm, using distraction and relaxation techniques, positioning with support for painful areas, aroma therapy, therapeutic touch, and warm soaks or compresses, all help reduce pain perception.

> **? CLINICAL JUDGMENT CHALLENGE**
>
> **Ethical/Legal**
>
> A 27-year-old African-American man in sickle cell crisis is a patient on your unit. During report, one of the nurses from the previous shift mentions that she withheld the IV opioid pain medication during the night because she had taken care of this patient a year ago and feels that he is a "drug seeker."
> 1. What is your first action?
> 2. How should you approach your colleague?
> 3. Can a patient with sickle cell disease become addicted to opioids?
> 4. What can you do to prevent an incident like this one from happening again?

Preventing Sepsis, Multiple Organ Dysfunction, and Death. The patient with SCD is at greater risk for bacterial INFECTION because of decreased spleen function resulting from anoxic damage. Interventions focus on preventing infection, controlling infection, and starting treatment early for specific infections. The patient with a fever should have diagnostic testing for sepsis including CBC with differential, blood cultures, reticulocyte count, urine culture, and a chest x-ray. Usually these patients are started on prophylactic antibiotics.

Prevention and early detection strategies are used to protect the patient in sickle cell crisis from INFECTION. Frequent, thorough handwashing is of the utmost importance. Any person with an upper respiratory tract infection who enters the patient's room must wear a mask. Use strict aseptic technique for all invasive procedures.

Continually assess the patient for INFECTION, and monitor the daily CBC with differential WBC count. Inspect the mouth every 8 hours for lesions indicating fungal or viral infection. Listen to the lungs every 8 hours for crackles, wheezes, or reduced breath sounds. Inspect voided urine for odor and cloudiness, and ask about urgency, burning, or pain on urination. Take vital signs at least every 4 hours to assess for fever, or supervise this action when performed by others.

Drug therapy by prophylaxis with twice-daily oral penicillin reduces the number of pneumonia and other streptococcal infections. Urge the patient to receive yearly influenza vaccinations and to receive the pneumonia vaccine. Drug therapy for an actual INFECTION depends on the sensitivity of the specific organism, as well as on the extent of the infection.

Continued blood vessel occlusion by clumping of sickled cells increases the risk for multiple organ dysfunction. Acute chest syndrome, in which a vaso-occlusive event (VOE) causes infiltration and damage to the pulmonary system, is a major cause of death in adults with SCD. Thus preventing heart and lung damage is a priority. Management focuses on prevention of VOEs and promotion of PERFUSION.

Assess the patient admitted in sickle cell crisis for adequate PERFUSION to all body areas. Remove restrictive clothing, and instruct the patient to avoid flexing the knees and hips.

Hydration is needed because dehydration increases cell sickling and must be avoided. Assist him or her in maintaining adequate hydration. The patient in acute crisis needs an oral or IV fluid intake of at least 200 mL/hr.

Oxygen is given during crises because lack of oxygen is the main cause of sickling. Ensure that oxygen therapy is nebulized to prevent dehydration. Monitor oxygen saturation.

Prevention of Sickle Cell Crisis

- Drink at least 3 to 4 liters of liquids every day.
- Avoid alcoholic beverages.
- Avoid smoking cigarettes or using tobacco in any form.
- Contact your health care provider at the first sign of illness or infection.
- Be sure to get a "flu shot" every year.
- Ask your health care provider about taking the pneumonia vaccine.
- Avoid temperature extremes of hot or cold.
- Be sure to wear socks and gloves when going outside on cold days.
- Avoid planes with unpressurized passenger cabins.
- Avoid travel to high altitudes (e.g., cities like Denver and Santa Fe).
- Ensure that any health care professional who takes care of you knows you have sickle cell disease, especially the anesthesia provider and radiologist.
- Consider genetic counseling.
- Avoid strenuous physical activities.
- Engage in mild, low-impact exercise at least 3 times a week when you are not in crisis.

If saturation is low, evaluation of arterial blood gases (ABGs) and a chest x-ray may be needed.

Transfusion with RBCs can be helpful to increase HbA levels and dilute HbS levels, although they must be prescribed cautiously to prevent iron overload from repeated transfusions. Monitor the patient for transfusion complications (discussed on pp. 822-823 in the Acute Transfusion Reactions section).

In some treatment centers, hematopoietic stem cell transplantation (HSCT) is performed to correct abnormal hemoglobin permanently. Because HSCT is expensive and may result in life-threatening complications, its risks and benefits need to be considered for each patient.

Community-Based Care

Sickle cell disease (SCD) becomes worse over time, and a true remission is rare, although the number of crisis episodes may be reduced. Care focuses on teaching the patient and family how to prevent crises and complications (Chart 40-3). The patient with SCD may receive care in acute care, subacute care, extended or assistive care, and home care settings.

Teach the patient to avoid specific activities that lead to hypoxia and hypoxemia. Stress the recognition of the early manifestations of crisis so that interventions can be started early to prevent pain, complications, and permanent tissue damage. Teach the patient and family about the correct use of opioid analgesics at home. Counsel patients about the hereditary aspects of SCD, and provide information about birth control

GENDER HEALTH CONSIDERATIONS

Patient-Centered Care **QSEN**

Pregnancy in women with SCD may be life threatening. Barrier methods of contraception (cervical cap, diaphragm, or condoms with or without spermicides) are often recommended for women with SCD. The use of hormone-based contraceptives is controversial, because these drugs may increase clot formation, especially among smokers, predisposing them to crises. Urge women using hormone-based contraceptives to not smoke.

methods and pregnancy options. Many patients and family members can be helped by local support groups. Provide information about the closest local chapter of the Sickle Cell Foundation. Often local children's hospitals have sickle cell support groups that include adults with the disease.

GLUCOSE-6-PHOSPHATE DEHYDROGENASE DEFICIENCY ANEMIA

❖ *PATHOPHYSIOLOGY*

More than 200 forms of **hemolytic** (blood cell–destroying) anemia are present from birth as a result of defects or deficiencies of one or more enzymes in red blood cells (RBCs). Most of these enzymes are needed to complete some critical step in RBC energy production. The most common type of inherited hemolytic anemia is the deficiency of the enzyme *glucose-6-phosphate dehydrogenase* (G6PD). This disease is inherited as an X-linked recessive disorder with more severe expression in males and mild partial expression in carrier females. It affects about 10% of all African Americans and also may occur in Sephardic Jews, Greeks, Iranians, Chinese, Filipinos, and Indonesians (McCance et al., 2014).

G6PD stimulates reactions in glucose metabolism important for energy in RBCs because they contain no other way to produce adenosine triphosphate (ATP). Cells with reduced amounts of G6PD break more easily during exposure to some drugs (e.g., sulfonamides, aspirin, quinine derivatives, chloramphenicol, dapsone, high doses of vitamin C, and thiazide diuretics) and exposure to benzene and other toxins.

New RBCs have some G6PD, but the enzyme diminishes as the cells age. The patient usually does not have manifestations until exposed to triggering agents or until a severe INFECTION develops. After exposure to a precipitating cause, acute RBC breakage begins and lasts 7 to 12 days. During this acute phase, anemia and jaundice develop. The hemolytic reaction is limited because only older RBCs, containing less G6PD, are destroyed.

❖ *PATIENT-CENTERED COLLABORATIVE CARE*

Prevention is the most important therapeutic measure. Men who belong to the high-risk groups should be tested for this problem before being given drugs that can cause the hemolytic reaction.

Hydration is important during an episode of hemolysis to prevent debris and hemoglobin from collecting in the kidney tubules, which can lead to acute kidney injury (AKI). Osmotic diuretics, such as mannitol (Osmitrol), may help prevent this complication. Transfusions are needed when anemia is present and kidney function is normal (see Transfusion Therapy section, p. 819).

IMMUNOHEMOLYTIC ANEMIA

The most common types of hemolytic anemias in North America are the immunohemolytic anemias, also referred to as *autoimmune hemolytic anemias* (McCance et al., 2014). The pathophysiology is abnormal IMMUNITY that results in the excessive destruction of red blood cell membranes (*lysis*) followed by accelerated erythropoiesis. Acquired hemolytic syndromes result from increased RBC destruction occurring from trauma, viral infection, malaria, exposure to certain chemicals or drugs, and autoimmune reactions.

In immunohemolytic anemia, immune system products (e.g., antibodies) attack a person's own RBCs for unknown reasons. Regardless of the cause, RBCs are viewed as non-self by the immune system and then are attacked and destroyed.

The two types of immunohemolytic anemia are warm antibody anemia and cold antibody anemia. **Warm antibody anemia** occurs with immunoglobulin G (IgG) antibody excess. These antibodies are most active at 98.6° F (37° C) and may be triggered by drugs, chemicals, or other autoimmune problems. **Cold antibody anemia** has complement protein fixation on immunoglobulin M (IgM) and occurs most at 86° F (30° C). This problem often occurs with a Raynaud's-like response in which the arteries in the hands and feet constrict profoundly in response to cold temperatures or stress.

Management depends on disease severity. Steroid therapy to suppress IMMUNITY is temporarily effective in most patients. Splenectomy and more intense immunosuppressive therapy with chemotherapy drugs may be used if steroid therapy fails. Plasma exchange therapy with antibody removal is effective for patients who do not respond to chemotherapy drugs.

ANEMIAS RESULTING FROM DECREASED PRODUCTION OF RED BLOOD CELLS

Anemias caused by decreased RBC production occur in response to many problems. Some are caused by failure of the bone marrow to produce healthy RBCs. Anemias also are caused by failure of the body to make or absorb a substance needed for RBC production. Many substances needed for RBC production are ingested as part of a healthy diet. For some patients with anemia resulting from a dietary deficiency, diet therapy is sufficient to manage anemia.

CONSIDERATIONS FOR OLDER ADULTS

Patient-Centered Care   **QSEN**

> Older patients often have restricted diets and may be unable to eat meat because of tooth loss or economic reasons and thus are at risk for iron deficiency anemia. Ask about a family history of anemia. B_{12} deficiency anemia often occurs in patients 50 to 80 years of age and may result from an inherited genetic mutation. Because manifestations are vague, the disorder can easily be overlooked (Orton, 2012).

Iron deficiency anemia is the most common anemia worldwide, especially among women, older adults, and people with poor diets. It can result from blood loss, poor GI absorption of iron, and an inadequate diet (McCance et al., 2014). The problem is a decreased iron supply for the developing RBC.

Adults usually have between 2 and 6 g of iron, depending on the size of the person and the amount of hemoglobin in the cells. With chronic iron deficiency, RBCs are small (**microcytic**) and the patient has mild symptoms of anemia, including weakness and pallor. Other manifestations include fatigue, reduced exercise tolerance, and fissures at the corners of the mouth. Serum ferritin values are less than 10 ng/mL (normal range is 12 to 300 ng/mL).

Any adult with iron deficiency should be evaluated for abnormal bleeding, especially from the GI tract. Management of iron deficiency anemia involves increasing the oral intake of iron from food sources (e.g., red meat, organ meat, egg yolks, kidney beans, leafy green vegetables, and raisins). If iron losses are mild, oral iron supplements, such as ferrous sulfate, are started until the hemoglobin level returns to normal. Instruct patients to take the iron supplement between meals for better absorption and to reduce GI distress. When iron deficiency anemia is severe, iron solutions (iron dextran [Dexferrum, INFeD, Pri-Dextra]; ferumoxytol [Feraheme]) can be given parenterally.

Vitamin B_{12} deficiency anemia results in failure to activate the enzyme that moves folic acid into precursor RBC cells so that cell division and growth into functional RBCs can occur. These precursor cells then undergo improper DNA synthesis and increase in size. Only a few are released from the bone marrow. This type of anemia is called *megaloblastic* or **macrocytic anemia** because of the large size of these abnormal cells.

Causes of vitamin B_{12} deficiency include vegan diets or diets lacking dairy products, small bowel resection, chronic diarrhea, diverticula, tapeworm, or overgrowth of intestinal bacteria. Anemia resulting from failure to absorb vitamin B_{12} (**pernicious anemia**) is caused by a deficiency of **intrinsic factor** (a substance normally secreted by the gastric mucosa), which is needed for intestinal absorption of vitamin B_{12}.

Vitamin B_{12} deficiency anemia may be mild or severe, usually develops slowly, and manifestations include pallor and jaundice, **glossitis** (a smooth, beefy-red tongue) (Fig. 40-3), fatigue, and weight loss. Patients with pernicious anemia may also have **paresthesias** (abnormal sensations) in the feet and hands and poor balance (Simmons, 2012).

When anemia is caused by a dietary deficiency, the focus of management is to increase the intake of foods rich in vitamin B_{12} (animal proteins, fish, eggs, nuts, dairy products, dried beans, citrus fruit, and leafy green vegetables). Vitamin supplements may be prescribed when anemia is severe. Patients who have pernicious anemia are given vitamin B_{12} injections weekly at first and then monthly for the rest of their lives. Oral B_{12} preparations and nasal spray or sublingual forms of cobalamin may be used to maintain vitamin levels after the patient's deficiency has first been corrected by the traditional injection method (Orton, 2012).

Folic acid deficiency can also cause anemia with manifestations similar to those of vitamin B_{12} deficiency. However, nervous system functions remain normal because folic acid deficiency does not affect nerve function. The disease develops slowly.

Common causes of folic acid deficiency are poor nutrition, malabsorption, and drugs. Poor nutrition, especially a diet lacking green leafy vegetables, liver, yeast, citrus fruits, dried beans, and nuts, is the most common cause. Malabsorption syndromes, such as Crohn's disease, are the second most

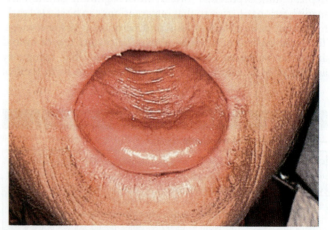

FIG. 40-3 Glossitis, a smooth tongue as a result of vitamin B_{12} deficiency anemia.

common cause. Anticonvulsants and oral contraceptives can contribute to folic acid deficiency and anemia.

Prevention begins by identifying high-risk patients, such as older, debilitated patients with alcoholism; patients at risk for malnutrition; and those with increased folic acid requirements. A diet rich in foods containing folic acid and vitamin B_{12} prevents a deficiency. This type of anemia is managed with scheduled folic acid replacement therapy.

Aplastic anemia is a deficiency of circulating red blood cells (RBCs) because of failure of the bone marrow to produce these cells. It is caused by an injury to the immature precursor cell for red blood cells. Although aplastic anemia sometimes occurs alone, it usually occurs with leukopenia (a reduction in white blood cells [WBCs]) and thrombocytopenia (a reduction in platelets), a condition known as pancytopenia. Disease onset may be slow or rapid.

The most common type of the disease is caused by long-term exposure to toxic agents, drugs (see Table 39-3 in Chapter 39), ionizing radiation, or infection, but often the cause is unknown. The disease also may follow viral infection. The most common hereditary form of the disease is Fanconi's anemia.

The patient has manifestations of severe anemia. A complete blood count (CBC) shows severe macrocytic anemia, leukopenia, and thrombocytopenia. A bone marrow biopsy may show replacement of cell-forming marrow with fat. Infection is common.

Blood transfusions are used only when the anemia causes disability or when bleeding is life threatening because of low platelet counts. Unnecessary transfusion increases the chances for developing immune reactions to platelets and shortens the life span of the transfused cell. This therapy is discontinued as soon as the bone marrow begins to produce RBCs.

Hematopoietic stem cell transplantation with donor cells is the most successful method of treatment for aplastic anemia that does not respond to other therapies. Cost, availability, and complications limit this treatment. For those patients who are unable to undergo such treatment or lack a suitable donor, immunosuppressive therapy remains the treatment of choice.

Immunosuppressive therapy helps patients who have the types of aplastic anemia with a disease course similar to that of autoimmune problems. Drugs such as prednisone, antithymocyte globulin (ATG), and cyclosporine A (Sandimmune) have resulted in partial or complete remissions. For moderate aplastic anemia, daclizumab (Zenapax) has improved both blood counts and transfusion requirements. Splenectomy may be needed for patients with an enlarged spleen that is either destroying normal RBCs or suppressing their development. (See discussion of surgical management for autoimmune thrombocytopenic purpura on p. 818.)

DISORDERS OF EXCESS RED BLOOD CELLS OR IRON

POLYCYTHEMIA VERA

❖ *PATHOPHYSIOLOGY*

In polycythemia, the number of red blood cells (RBCs) in the blood is *greater* than normal. The blood of a patient with polycythemia is hyperviscous (thicker than normal blood). The problem may be temporary (because of other conditions) or chronic.

Polycythemia vera (PV) is a disease with a sustained increase in blood hemoglobin levels to 18 g/dL, an RBC count of 6 million/mm^3, or a hematocrit of 55% or greater. PV is a cancer of the RBCs with three major hallmarks: massive production of RBCs, excessive leukocyte production, and excessive production of platelets. More than 90% of patients with PV show a mutation of the *JAK2* kinase gene in the affected cells (McCance et al., 2014). Extreme hypercellularity (cell excess) of the peripheral blood occurs in people with PV.

The patient's facial skin and mucous membranes have a dark, purple or cyanotic, flushed (plethoric) appearance with distended veins. Intense itching caused by dilated blood vessels, and poor PERFUSION is common. The thick blood moves more slowly and places increased demands on the heart, resulting in hypertension. In some areas, blood flow may be so slow that stasis occurs. Vascular stasis causes thrombosis (CLOTTING) within the smaller vessels, occluding them, which leads to tissue hypoxia, anoxia and, later, to infarction and necrosis. Tissues most at risk for this problem are the heart, spleen, and kidneys, although damage can occur in any organ or tissue.

Because the actual number of cells in the blood is greatly increased and the cells are not completely normal, cell life spans are shorter. The shorter life spans and increased cell production cause a rapid turnover of circulating blood cells. This rapid turnover increases the amount of cell debris (released when cells die) in the blood, adding to the general "sludging" of the blood. This debris includes uric acid and potassium, which cause the manifestations of gout and hyperkalemia (elevated serum potassium level).

Even though the number of RBCs is greatly increased, their oxygen-carrying capacity is impaired, and patients have poor GAS EXCHANGE with severe hypoxia. Bleeding problems are common because of platelet impairment.

❖ *PATIENT-CENTERED COLLABORATIVE CARE*

Polycythemia vera is a malignant disease that progresses in severity over time. If left untreated, few people with PV live longer than 2 years after diagnosis. With management by repeated phlebotomy with apheresis (2 to 5 times per week), the patient may live 10 to 15 years or longer. (Apheresis is the withdrawal of whole blood and removal of some of the patient's blood component, in this case RBCs. The plasma is then reinfused back into the patient.) Increasing hydration and promoting venous return help prevent clot formation. Therapy for PV also includes the use of anticoagulants. Chart 40-4 lists health tips for patients with PV.

CHART 40-4 Patient and Family Education: Preparing for Self-Management

Polycythemia Vera

- Drink at least 3 liters of liquids each day.
- Avoid tight or constrictive clothing, especially garters and girdles.
- Wear gloves when outdoors in temperatures lower than 50°F (10°C).
- Keep all health care–related appointments.
- Contact your health care provider at the first sign of infection.
- Take anticoagulants as prescribed.
- Wear support hose or stockings while you are awake and up.
- Elevate your feet whenever you are seated.
- Exercise slowly and only on the advice of your physician.
- Stop activity at the first sign of chest pain.
- Use an electric shaver.
- Use a soft-bristled toothbrush to brush your teeth.
- Do not floss between your teeth.

Aggressive IV chemotherapy is no longer recommended because of its increased risk for inducing leukemia. Aspirin therapy may be used to decrease clot formation but increases the risk for GI bleeding. Hydroxyurea, an oral chemotherapy drug, may be prescribed for severe manifestations of the disease. Interferon-alfa therapy has also shown some benefit in controlling RBC production.

HEREDITARY HEMOCHROMATOSIS

Hereditary hemochromatosis is an autosomal recessive disorder in which a mutation in both alleles of the *HFE* gene cause increased intestinal absorption of dietary iron (Beery & Workman, 2012). The excess iron is deposited in a variety of tissues and organs, including the liver, spleen, heart, joints, skin, and pancreas. The iron deposits can damage the organs, leading to organ failure. Usually the disease is more common in men and manifestations appear in men during their 40s. Women have manifestations later because the loss of menstrual blood before menopause helps remove excess iron. The most common clinical manifestations are abdominal pain, liver enlargement, hyperglycemia, and a gradual darkening of the skin. Later problems include diabetes, liver cirrhosis, endocrine gland failure, heart disease, and death.

The disorder is usually diagnosed on the basis of clinical manifestations and altered iron levels. Genetic testing is available to determine carrier status. When the disorder is identified early before organ damage, management is simple and can prevent severe organ damage and early death. Phlebotomy and removal of 500 mL of blood at a time, occurring as often as twice weekly at first, is performed to reduce the overall iron load of the blood. The desired outcome is to reduce blood ferritin levels to less than 9 to 50 micrograms per liter. Once this level has been achieved, phlebotomy frequency can be reduced to once every 2 to 4 months for maintenance.

MYELODYSPLASTIC SYNDROMES

❖ PATHOPHYSIOLOGY

Myelodysplastic syndromes (MDS) are a group of disorders caused by the formation of abnormal cells in the bone marrow. These abnormal cells are usually destroyed shortly after they are released into the blood. As a result, patients with MDS have a decrease in all blood cell types. Anemia is the most common problem with MDS, although **neutropenia** (low white blood cell count [WBC]) and **thrombocytopenia** (low platelets) are also often present.

MDS most often occurs in people ages 60 years or older. MDS has cancer-like features and is considered to be a *precancerous* state. Like cancer, it arises from a single population of abnormal cells. About 30% of all patients with MDS do eventually develop acute leukemia (McCance et al., 2014). There are a number of subtypes of MDS with different prognoses and responses to therapy. Patients are categorized into risk groups (i.e., low, intermediate [1 and 2], high) based on the severity of **pancytopenia** (low counts of all blood cell types), cytogenetic abnormalities, and numbers of blast cells (immature WBC cells) found in the bone marrow (Kurtin, 2012).

The exact cause of MDS is not clear. Risk factors include normal physiologic changes associated with aging, chemical exposures (pesticides, benzene), tobacco smoke, and exposure to radiation or chemotherapy drugs. Diagnosis is made by examination of the chromosomes and the genes within the chromosomes (cytogenetic testing) of the bone marrow cells. Peripheral blood smears are used to assess the level of cell maturation and the proportion of abnormal cells.

❖ PATIENT-CENTERED COLLABORATIVE CARE

The only potentially curative treatment for MDS is an allogeneic hematopoietic stem cell transplantation, which is often not an option because of the advanced age of many patients (Kurtin, 2012). Several alternate management strategies have demonstrated some promise. For low-risk and intermediate-1–risk MDS, the antitumor immunomodulatory agent *lenalidomide* (Revlimid) is approved for patients whose dysplastic cells have the chromosome abnormality of a deleted *5q*. Two other agents approved for intermediate-2–risk and high-risk MDS are azacitidine (Vidaza) and decitabine (Dacogen) (Kurtin, 2012). These drugs often require at least 3 to 6 months to achieve a clinical response; therefore supportive care is necessary.

Supportive care includes blood transfusions for anemia and platelet transfusions when platelet levels are very low. Erythropoiesis-stimulating agents (ESAs), such as epoetin alfa (Epogen, Procrit) or darbepoetin alfa (Aranesp), may be given in addition to transfusions.

WHITE BLOOD CELL DISORDERS

As discussed in Chapter 17, white blood cells (WBCs), or **leukocytes,** provide protection from INFECTION and cancer development. This protection depends on maintaining normal numbers and ratios of the different mature circulating WBCs. When any one type of WBC is present in either abnormal amounts (too high or too low), IMMUNITY, GAS EXCHANGE, and CLOTTING are altered to some degree, placing patients at risk for many complications. This section covers the changes and nursing care for patients with disorders involving overgrowth of specific types of WBCs. (See Chapter 19 for the problems and care needs for patients with immune deficiency.)

LEUKEMIA

❖ PATHOPHYSIOLOGY

Leukemia is cancer with uncontrolled production of immature WBCs ("blast" cells) in the bone marrow. As a result, the bone marrow becomes overcrowded with immature, nonfunctional cells and production of normal blood cells is greatly decreased. Leukemia may be **acute,** with a sudden onset, or **chronic,** with a slow onset and manifestations that persist for years.

Leukemias are classified by cell type. Leukemic cells coming from the lymphoid pathways (see Fig. 17-3 in Chapter 17) are typed as **lymphocytic** or **lymphoblastic.** Leukemic cells coming from the myeloid pathways are typed as **myelocytic** or **myelogenous**. Several subtypes exist for each of these diseases, which are classified according to the degree of maturity of the abnormal cell and the specific cell type involved. These are identified as M0 through M8. M3 is a subtype (referred to as *acute promyelocytic leukemia* [APL]) that has a specific treatment different from other AMLs. It is identified by a translocation of chromosomes 15 and 17. *Biphenotypic leukemia* is acute leukemia that shows both lymphocytic and myelocytic features.

With leukemia, cancer most often occurs in the stem cells or early precursor leukocyte cells, causing excessive growth of a specific type of immature leukocyte. In some chronic leukemias, the cancerous cells may be more mature. These cells are abnormal, and their excessive production in the bone marrow stops normal bone marrow production, leading to anemia, thrombocytopenia, and leukopenia. Often the number of immature, abnormal WBCs ("blasts") in the blood is greatly elevated, and these cells cannot provide infection protection. Leukemic cells can also be found in the spleen, liver, lymph nodes, and central nervous system. Without treatment, the patient will die of INFECTION or hemorrhage. For patients with acute leukemia, these changes occur rapidly and, without intervention, progress to death. Chronic leukemia may be present for years before changes appear.

Etiology and Genetic Risk

The exact cause of leukemia is unknown, although many genetic and environmental factors are involved in its development. The basic problem involves damage to genes controlling cell growth. This damage then changes cells from a normal to a **malignant** (cancer) state. Analysis of the bone marrow of a patient with acute leukemia shows abnormal chromosomes about 50% of the time (McCance et al., 2014). Possible risk factors for the development of leukemia include ionizing radiation, viral infection, exposure to chemicals and drugs, disorders such as myelodysplastic syndrome or Fanconi's anemia, genetic factors, immunologic factors, environmental factors, and the interaction of these factors.

Ionizing radiation exposures such as radiation therapy for cancer treatment or heavy accidental exposures increase the risk for leukemia development, particularly acute myelogenous leukemia (AML). Chemicals and drugs have been linked to leukemia development because of their ability to damage DNA. Previous treatment for cancer with some chemotherapy drugs (e.g., melphalan, doxorubicin, etoposide, and cyclophosphamide) poses risks for leukemia development about 5 to 8 years after treatment. Table 39-3 in Chapter 39 lists chemicals and drugs that damage the hematologic system.

Genetic and IMMUNITY factors influence leukemia development. There is an increased incidence of the disease among patients with genetic conditions such as Down syndrome, Bloom syndrome, Klinefelter syndrome, and Fanconi's anemia. Immune deficiencies may promote the development of leukemia. Chronic lymphocytic leukemia appears to have a familial or genetic predisposition.

Incidence and Prevalence

Leukemia accounts for 2% of all new cases of cancer and 4% of all deaths from cancer (American Cancer Society [ACS], 2014). The incidence depends on many factors, including the type of WBC affected, age, gender, race, and geographic locale.

TABLE 40-2	Classification of Leukemia Types
LEUKEMIA TYPE	**FEATURES**
Acute myelogenous leukemia (AML)	Most common in adults Has 8 subtypes
Acute promyelocytic leukemia (APL)	Subtype of AML Most curable of adult leukemias
Acute lymphocytic leukemia (ALL)	Forms about 10% of adult-onset leukemias Often is Philadelphia chromosome–positive
Chronic myelogenous leukemia (CML)	Forms about 20% of adult-onset leukemias Occurs most often after age 50 years Usually is Philadelphia chromosome–positive Has three phases: • *Chronic*—slow growing with mild manifestations that respond to therapy • *Accelerated*—more rapid growing with more severe manifestations, increased blast cells, and failure to respond to therapy • *Blast*—very aggressive leukemia with high percentage of blast and promyelocytes that spread to other organs
Chronic lymphocytic leukemia (CLL)	Most common chronic leukemia in adults; occurs most often after age 50 years Is associated with a genetic predisposition Survival time can extend to 10 years or more in patients diagnosed with early-stage disease

In the United States, about 49,000 new cases of leukemia occur each year (ACS, 2014). Leukemia is classified into four different types based on the cell type affected and how fast the disease progresses (Table 40-2).

❖ PATIENT-CENTERED COLLABORATIVE CARE

◆ Assessment

History. Ask the patient about exposure to risk factors and related genetic factors. Age is important because the risk for adult-onset leukemia increases with age. Occupation and hobbies may reveal exposure to agents that increase the risk for leukemia. Previous illnesses and the medical history may reveal exposure to ionizing radiation or drugs that increase risk.

Changes in IMMUNITY increase the risk for INFECTION in the patient with leukemia. Even when the blood count shows a normal or high level of WBCs, these cells are immature and cannot protect the patient from infection. Ask about the frequency and severity of infections, such as colds, influenza, pneumonia, bronchitis, or unexplained fevers, during the past 6 months.

Platelet function is reduced with leukemia, interfering with CLOTTING. Ask about any excessive bleeding episodes, such as:

- A tendency to bruise easily or longer after minor trauma
- Nosebleeds
- Increased menstrual flow
- Bleeding from the gums
- Rectal bleeding
- Hematuria (blood in the urine)

If the patient has experienced such an episode, ask whether this type and extent of bleeding is his or her usual response to injury or represents a change.

CHART 40-5   Key Features

Acute Leukemia

Integumentary Manifestations
- Ecchymoses
- Petechiae
- Open infected lesions
- Pallor of the conjunctivae, nail beds, palmar creases, and around the mouth

Gastrointestinal Manifestations
- Bleeding gums
- Anorexia
- Weight loss
- Enlarged liver and spleen

Renal Manifestations
- Hematuria

Musculoskeletal Manifestations
- Bone pain
- Joint swelling and pain

Cardiovascular Manifestations
- Tachycardia at basal activity levels
- Orthostatic hypotension
- Palpitations

Respiratory Manifestations
- Dyspnea on exertion

Neurologic Manifestations
- Fatigue
- Headache
- Fever

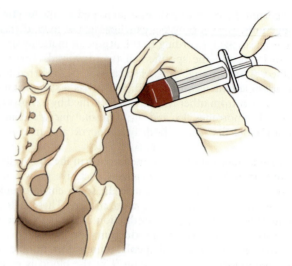

FIG. 40-4 Bone marrow aspiration from the posterior iliac crest. (*GVHD,* Graft-versus-host disease.)

The patient with leukemia often has weakness and fatigue from anemia and from the increased metabolism of the leukemic cells. Ask whether any of these problems have occurred:
- Headaches
- Behavior changes
- Increased somnolence; decreased alertness; fatigue
- Decreased attention span
- Muscle weakness
- Loss of appetite
- Weight loss

A 24-hour activity history may reveal activity intolerance, changes in behavior, and unexplained fatigue. Determine how long the patient has had any of these debilitating problems.

Physical Assessment/Clinical Manifestations. Leukemia affects all blood cells, and blood influences the health and function of all organs and systems. Thus many body areas and systems may be affected (Chart 40-5). The following manifestations occur with acute leukemia and chronic leukemia in the blast phase.

Cardiovascular changes often are related to adjustments needed when PERFUSION and GAS EXCHANGE are reduced from anemia. The heart rate is increased, and blood pressure is decreased. **Murmurs** (abnormal blood flow sounds in the heart) and **bruits** (abnormal blood flow sounds over arteries) may be heard. Capillary refill is slow. When the WBC count is greatly elevated and blood is highly viscous, blood pressure is elevated with a bounding pulse.

Respiratory changes are related to reduced GAS EXCHANGE from anemia and to INFECTION. Respiratory rate increases as anemia becomes more severe. If a respiratory infection is present, the patient may have coughing and dyspnea. Abnormal breath sounds are heard on auscultation.

Skin changes include pallor and coolness to the touch as a result of reduced PERFUSION from anemia. Pallor is most evident on the face, around the mouth, and in the nail beds. The conjunctiva of the eye also is pale, as are the creases on the palm of the hand. Petechiae may be present on any area of skin surface, especially the legs and feet. The petechiae may be unrelated to any obvious trauma. Inspect for skin infections or injured areas

that have failed to heal. Inspect the mouth for gum bleeding and any sore or lesion that may indicate infection.

Intestinal changes may be related to an increased bleeding tendency and to fatigue. Weight loss, nausea, and anorexia are common. Examine the rectal area for fissures, and test stool for occult blood. Many patients with leukemia have reduced bowel sounds and are constipated because reduced blood flow to intestinal tissue leads to decreased peristalsis. Enlargement of the liver and spleen and abdominal tenderness also may be present from leukemic cells trapped in these organs.

Central nervous system (CNS) changes include cranial nerve problems, headache, and papilledema from leukemic invasion of the CNS. Seizures and coma also may occur.

Miscellaneous changes can include bone and joint tenderness as the marrow is damaged and the bone reabsorbs. Leukemic cells invade lymph nodes, causing enlargement.

Psychosocial Assessment. The patient with newly diagnosed leukemia is very anxious and fearful of the disease outcome. Spend time with the patient and family to assess what the diagnosis means to them and what they expect in the future (Albrecht, 2014).

A diagnosis of leukemia has serious consequences for a person's lifestyle. Hospitalization for initial treatment often lasts weeks and may result in boredom, loneliness, isolation, and financial stress. Assess coping patterns, including activities that the patient finds enjoyable and methods that help him or her relax. After initial therapy, the patient may resume work, depending on the occupation. Often the patient must make adjustments for changes in functional status. He or she usually is hospitalized repeatedly for complications.

Laboratory Assessment. The patient with acute leukemia usually has decreased hemoglobin and hematocrit levels, a low platelet count, and an abnormal white blood cell (WBC) count. The WBC count may be low, normal, or elevated. The patient with a high WBC count consisting of mostly blast cells at diagnosis has a poorer prognosis.

The definitive test for leukemia is an examination of cells obtained from bone marrow aspiration and biopsy (Fig. 40-4). The bone marrow is full of leukemic **blast phase cells** (immature cells that are dividing). The proteins (**antigens**) on the surfaces of the leukemic cells are "markers" that help diagnose the type of leukemia and may indicate prognosis. These include the T11 protein, terminal deoxynucleotidyl transferase (TDT), the common acute lymphoblastic leukemia antigen (CALLA), and the CD33 antigen.

Blood CLOTTING times and factors are usually abnormal with acute leukemia. Reduced levels of fibrinogen and other clotting factors are common. Whole-blood clotting time (Lee-White clotting test) is prolonged, as is the activated partial thromboplastin time (aPTT).

Chromosome analysis (cytogenetic studies) of the leukemic cells may identify marker chromosomes to help diagnose the type of leukemia, predict the prognosis, and determine therapy effectiveness. An example is the Philadelphia chromosome, which is important in the diagnosis and treatment of some chronic myelogenous leukemia (CML) and adult acute lymphocytic leukemia (ALL). The Philadelphia chromosome is an abnormal chromosome caused by a translocation of the *ABL* gene from chromosome 9 onto the *BCR* gene of chromosome 22. The new protein produced by this mutation inhibits cell apoptosis and DNA repair, leading to further genetic abnormality (Simoneau, 2013).

Imaging Assessment. Specific manifestations determine the need for specific tests. In a patient with dyspnea, a chest x-ray is needed to determine whether leukemic infiltrates are present in the lung. Skeletal x-rays may help determine whether loss of bone minerals and bone density is present.

❓ NCLEX EXAMINATION CHALLENGE

Physiological Integrity

The blood of a client who has chronic myelogenous leukemia shows a high percentage of blast cells and promyelocytes. What is the nurse's correct interpretation of this test result?
A. The client's risk for infection is decreasing.
B. The disease has become more aggressive.
C. The drug therapy for the disease is effective.
D. The type of leukemia is now lymphocytic rather than myelogenous.

◆ Analysis

The priority NANDA-I nursing diagnoses and collaborative problems for patients with acute myelogenous leukemia (AML), the most common type of acute leukemia seen in adults, include:
1. Risk for Infection related to decreased immune response and chemotherapy (NANDA-I)
2. Risk for Injury related to thrombocytopenia and chemotherapy (NANDA-I)
3. Fatigue related to decreased tissue oxygenation and increased energy demands (NANDA-I)

◆ Planning and Implementation

Preventing Infection

Planning: Expected Outcomes. The patient with leukemia is expected to remain free from infection. Indicators include:
• Absence of fever and foul-smelling or purulent drainage
• Absence of cough, chest pain, and dyspnea
• Absence of urinary frequency, urgency, or pain and burning
• Intact skin and mucous membranes

Interventions. INFECTION *is a major cause of death in the patient with leukemia* because the white blood cells are immature

and cannot function or the cells are depleted from chemotherapy, and sepsis is a common complication. Infection occurs through both auto-contamination (normal flora overgrows and penetrates the internal environment) and cross-contamination (organisms from another person or the environment are transmitted to the patient). The most common sources of infection are the skin, respiratory tract, and intestinal tract.

Gram-negative bacteria are the most common cause of infection, although infections from other causes do occur. Interventions aim to halt infection and control infections early. Chart 40-6 lists areas to assess for the patient at risk for infection.

CHART 40-6 Focused Assessment

Patients at Risk for Infection

General Condition
• Age
• History of allergies
• History of chemotherapy, radiation therapy, or other immunosuppressive therapies, such as steroid use
• Chronic diseases
• History of febrile neutropenia and associated symptoms
• Nutrition status
• Functional status—problems with immobility
• Tobacco use—cigarettes, pipe, cigars, oral
• Recreational drug use
• Alcohol use
• Prescribed and over-the-counter drug use
• Baseline and ongoing vital signs—blood pressure, heart rate, respiratory rate, and temperature

Skin and Mucous Membranes
• Thorough inspection of all skin surfaces with attention to axillae, anorectal area, and under breasts; inspection of skin for color, vascularity, bleeding, lesions, edema, moist areas, excoriation, irritation, erythema; general condition of hair and nails, pressure areas, swelling, pain, tenderness, biopsy or surgical sites, wounds, enlarged lymph nodes, catheters, or other devices
• Inspection of oral cavity, including lips, tongue, mucous membranes, gingiva, teeth, and throat—color, moisture, bleeding, ulcerations, lesions, exudate, mucositis, stomatitis, plaque, swelling, pain, tenderness, taste changes, amount and character of saliva, ability to swallow, changes in voice, dental caries, patient's oral hygiene routine
• History of current skin or mucous membrane problems

Head, Eyes, Ears, Nose
• Pain, tenderness, exudate, crusting, enlarged lymph nodes

Cardiopulmonary
• Respiratory rate and pattern, breath sounds (presence/absence, adventitious sounds), quantity and characteristics of sputum, shortness of breath, use of accessory muscles, dysphagia, diminished gag reflex, tachycardia, blood pressure

Gastrointestinal
• Pain, diarrhea, bowel sounds, character and frequency of bowel movements, constipation, rectal bleeding, hemorrhoids, change in bowel habits, sexual practices, erythema, ulceration

Genitourinary
• Dysuria, frequency, urgency, hematuria, pruritus, pain, vaginal or penile discharge, vaginal bleeding, burning, lesions, ulcerations, characteristics of urine

Central Nervous System
• Cognition, level of consciousness, personality, behavior

Musculoskeletal
• Tenderness, pain, loss of function

Drug Therapy for Acute Leukemia. Drug therapy for patients with AML is divided into three distinctive phases: induction, consolidation, and maintenance.

Induction therapy is intense and consists of combination chemotherapy started at the time of diagnosis. The purpose of this therapy is to achieve a rapid, complete remission of all manifestations of disease. A combination of chemotherapeutic agents is usually prescribed. However, agencies and physicians differ in drugs used and the treatment schedule. One example of aggressive induction therapy is continuous IV cytosine arabinoside for 7 days together with an anthracycline for the first 3 days, sometimes referred to as a "7 plus 3" regimen. This therapy results in severe bone marrow suppression with neutropenia, making the patient even more at risk for infection. For acute promyelocytic leukemia, the agent *tretinoin* (Vesanoid) is added to the chemotherapy regimen.

Prolonged hospitalizations are common while the patient is neutropenic. Recovery of bone marrow function requires at least 2 to 3 weeks, during which the patient must be protected from life-threatening INFECTIONS. Other side effects of drugs used for induction therapy include nausea, vomiting, diarrhea, alopecia (hair loss), stomatitis (mouth sores), kidney toxicity, liver toxicity, and cardiac toxicity. (See Chapter 22 for information on effects of anticancer agents.) Older patients have a greater infection-related death rate during this phase than do younger patients. Patients with APL are at greater risk for sepsis with disseminated intravascular coagulation (DIC) during induction therapy than are patients with other subtypes of AML.

Consolidation therapy consists of another course of either the same drugs used for induction at a different dosage or a different combination of chemotherapy drugs. This treatment occurs early in remission, and its intent is to cure. Consolidation therapy may be either a single course of chemotherapy or repeated courses. Hematopoietic stem cell transplantation also may be considered, depending on the disease subtype and the patient's response to induction therapy.

Maintenance therapy may be prescribed for months to years after successful induction and consolidation therapies for acute lymphocytic leukemia (ALL) and acute promyelocytic leukemia (APL). The purpose is to maintain the remission achieved through induction and consolidation. Not all types of leukemia respond to maintenance therapy.

Drug Therapy for Chronic Leukemia. Imatinib mesylate (Gleevec) is a common first-line drug therapy for CML that is Philadelphia chromosome–positive. This oral drug is well tolerated and has been effective at inducing remission for early stages of CML. Other drugs approved for first-line therapy or for patients whose disease is resistant or intolerant to imatinib are dasatinib (Sprycel) or nilotinib (Tasigna) (Byar & Workman, 2012). Other drugs used to treat CML include interferon-alfa, which reduces the growth of leukemic cells, but its use is limited because of side effects, such as flu-like manifestations and fevers. Patient responses to therapy are evaluated on the basis of hematologic, cytogenetic, and molecular criteria.

Chronic lymphocytic leukemia (CLL) is the most prevalent form of leukemia in adults, affecting women more often than men. Cytogenetic testing is important in the prognosis. Partial deletion of chromosome 13 is associated with a benign disease course, whereas a deletion of chromosome 11 or of chromosome 17 (*p53* mutation) is associated with a poor prognosis. Treatment of CLL with standard chemotherapy can cause remissions but does not cure the disease. The decision to initiate therapy is based on disease stage, manifestations, and disease activity. Rituximab (Rituxan) is often combined with standard chemotherapy drugs or used as a single agent. Another drug approved for CLL is bendamustine (Treanda), which may be used alone or along with rituximab. Other monoclonal antibodies approved for CLL are ofatumumab (Arzerra) and alemtuzumab (Campath). Current investigational therapies for CLL include ibrutinib, oblimersen (Genasense), flavopiridol (Alvocidib), and lenalidomide (Revlimid).

Hematopoietic stem cell transplantation in patients with CLL is an option that offers curative potential or prolonged disease-free survival. However, it comes with considerable risk for mortality and is not an appropriate alternative for all patients.

Drug Therapy for Infection. Drug therapy is the main defense against INFECTIONS that develop in patients undergoing therapy for AML. Drugs used depend on the sensitivity of the organism causing the infection, as well as infection severity. Drugs for infection include antibacterial, antiviral, and antifungal agents.

Infection Protection. A major focus in caring for the patient with leukemia is protection from INFECTION. All personnel must use extreme care during all nursing procedures. Frequent, thorough handwashing is of the utmost importance. Anyone with an upper respiratory tract infection who enters the patient's room must wear a mask. Observe strict asepsis when changing dressings or accessing a central venous catheter. Maintain strict aseptic technique in the care of these catheters at all times.

If possible, ensure that the patient is in a private room to reduce cross-contamination. Other precautions are used, such as not allowing standing water in vases, denture cups, or humidifiers in the patient's room, because they are breeding grounds for organisms.

Some facilities place the immunosuppressed patient in a room with a high-efficiency particulate air (HEPA) filtration or laminar airflow system. These systems decrease the number of airborne pathogens. It is not known whether these systems benefit patients.

Continually assess the patient for the presence of INFECTION. This task is difficult because manifestations are not obvious in the patient with leukopenia. The patient with leukopenia may have a severe infection without pus and with only a low-grade fever.

Monitor the patient's daily CBC with differential WBC count and absolute neutrophil count (ANC). Inspect the mouth during every shift for lesions and mucosa breakdown. Assess the lungs every 8 hours for crackles, wheezes, and reduced breath sounds. Assess urine for odor and cloudiness. Ask about any urgency, burning, or pain on urination. Take vital signs at least every 4 hours to assess for fever.

> **! NURSING SAFETY PRIORITY** **(QSEN)**
> **_Critical Rescue_**
>
> A temperature elevation of even 1°F (or 0.5°C) above baseline is significant for a patient with leukopenia and indicates INFECTION until it has been proven otherwise. Report this finding to the health care provider at once.

Many hospital units that specialize in the care of patients with neutropenia have specific protocols for antibiotic therapy if infection is suspected. Usually the health care provider is notified immediately and specific specimens are obtained for culture. Obtain blood for bacterial and fungal cultures from peripheral IV sites and from the central venous catheter (Myers & Reyes, 2011). Obtain urine specimens, sputum specimens, and specimens from open lesions for culture. Chest x-rays are taken. After the specimens are obtained, the patient begins IV antibiotics.

Skin care is important for preventing INFECTION in the patient with leukemia because the skin may be the only intact defense. Teach him or her about hygiene, and urge daily bathing. If the patient is immobile, turn him or her every hour and apply skin lubricants.

Perform pulmonary hygiene every 2 to 4 hours. Listen to the lungs for crackles, wheezes, and reduced breath sounds. Urge the patient to cough and deep breathe or to perform sustained maximal inhalations every hour while awake.

Hematopoietic Stem Cell Transplantation. Hematopoietic stem cell transplantation (HSCT), sometimes called *bone marrow transplantation (BMT),* is standard treatment for the patient with leukemia who has a closely matched donor and who is in temporary remission after induction therapy. It is used also for lymphoma, multiple myeloma, aplastic anemia, sickle cell disease, and many solid tumors.

The bone marrow is the actual site of production of leukemic cells. It can be difficult to ensure that all leukemic cells have been eradicated during induction therapy. Therefore before an HSCT, additional chemotherapy with or without total body irradiation is given to purge (condition or clean) the marrow of leukemic cells. *These treatments are lethal to the bone marrow, and without replacement of stem cells by transplantation, the patient would die of* INFECTION *or hemorrhage.*

After conditioning, new healthy stem cells are given to the patient. The new cells go to the marrow and then begin the process of hematopoiesis, which results in normal, properly functioning blood cells and, ideally, a permanent cure.

Many hospitals have transplant units. With long-term survival increasing after HSCT, nurses can expect to be caring for these people—if not during the actual transplantation or recovery period, then after the recovery period—in a variety of health care settings.

HSCT started with the use of **allogeneic bone marrow transplantation** (transplantation of bone marrow from a sibling or matched unrelated donor) and has advanced to the use of human leukocyte antigen (HLA)–matched stem cells from the umbilical cords of unrelated donors. Transplants are classified by the source of stem cells (Table 40-3). Stem cells for transplantation may be obtained by bone marrow harvest, peripheral stem cell apheresis, or umbilical cord blood stem cell banking. Transplantation has five phases: stem cell obtainment, conditioning regimen, transplantation, engraftment, and post-transplantation recovery.

Obtaining the Stem Cells. Stem cells are taken either from the patient directly (*autologous stem cells*), an HLA-identical twin (*syngeneic stem cells*), or from an HLA-matched person (*allogeneic stem cells*). For allogeneic transplant, the best results occur when the donor is an HLA-identical sibling; however, transplant also can be successful between those with closely but not perfectly matched HLA types. The chance of matching with any given sibling is 25%. Donor registries keep records of potential donors who can provide stem cells for patients who do not have a family member HLA match. The chance of matching with an unrelated donor is 1 in 5000.

TABLE 40-3	**Classification of Transplants**
TYPE OF TRANSPLANT	**SOURCES OF STEM CELLS**
Autologous	
Self-donation	Bone marrow harvest
	Peripheral stem cell pheresis
	Umbilical cord blood
Syngeneic	
Patient's HLA identical twin	Bone marrow harvest
	Peripheral stem cell pheresis
Allogeneic	
HLA-matched relative	Bone marrow harvest
Unrelated HLA-matched donor	Peripheral stem cell pheresis
Mismatched or partially HLA-matched family member or unrelated donor (donor registries)	Umbilical cord blood

HLA, Human leukocyte antigen.

⊕ CULTURAL CONSIDERATIONS
Patient-Centered Care QSEN

About 70% of people on the bone marrow donor lists are white. The chance of finding an HLA-matched unrelated donor is estimated at 30% to 40% for white people, but for African Americans the chance is less than 20% because there are fewer African Americans among registered donors. Although blood types are common in all racial groups, tissue types can be very different among racial and ethnic groups. Nationally, efforts are made to publicize the need for donors from all cultural backgrounds. Help in this effort by providing accurate information and dispelling myths.

Bone marrow harvesting occurs after a suitable donor is identified by tissue typing. The procedure occurs in the operating room, where marrow is removed through multiple aspirations from the iliac crests, although this technique is used less often today. About 500 to 1000 mL of marrow is aspirated, and the donor's marrow regrows within a few weeks. The marrow is then filtered and, if autologous, is treated to rid the marrow of any remaining cancer cells. Allogeneic marrow is transfused into the recipient immediately. Autologous marrow is frozen for later use.

Monitor the donor for fluid loss, assess for complications of anesthesia, and manage pain. During surgery, donors may lose a large amount of fluid in addition to the volume of marrow taken. Donors are hydrated with saline infusions before and immediately after surgery. Occasionally the donor may need an RBC transfusion. Assess the harvest sites to ensure that the dressings are dry and intact and that the donor is not bleeding excessively.

Marrow donation is usually a same-day surgical procedure. Teach the donor to inspect the harvest sites for bleeding and to take analgesics for pain. Pain at the harvest sites (hips) is common and is managed with oral non–aspirin-containing analgesics. Some donors may require opioid analgesics for pain control.

Peripheral blood stem cell (PBSC) harvesting requires three phases: mobilization, collection by apheresis, and reinfusion. **PBSCs** are stem cells that have been released from the bone marrow and circulate within the blood. Although there are fewer stem cells in peripheral blood than in bone marrow, their numbers can be artificially increased. During the mobilization

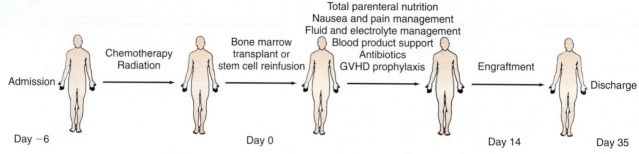

FIG. 40-5 Timing and steps of allogeneic bone marrow transplantation.

phase, chemotherapy or hematopoietic growth factors are given to the patient for an autologous collection, depending on the cancer type, and hematopoietic growth factors alone are given to the donor for an allogeneic or syngeneic collection. These agents increase the numbers of stem cells and WBCs in the peripheral blood. A new agent approved for some other types of hematologic malignancies to mobilize stem cells before harvesting in combination with hematopoietic growth factors is plerixafor (Mozobil). This drug has been shown to decrease the number of apheresis collections needed (Slater, 2012).

After mobilization, the stem cells are then collected by **apheresis** (withdrawing whole blood, filtering out the cells, and returning the plasma to the patient). One to five apheresis procedures, each lasting 2 to 4 hours, are needed to obtain enough stem cells for transplantation. The cells are frozen and stored for reinfusion after the patient's conditioning regimen is completed.

Monitor the patient or donor closely during apheresis. Complications include catheter clotting and hypocalcemia (caused by anticoagulants). Low calcium levels may cause numbness or tingling in the fingers and toes, abdominal or muscle cramping, or chest pain. Oral calcium supplements may be used to manage these symptoms. Monitor vital signs at least every hour during apheresis. The patient may become hypotensive from fluid loss during the procedure.

Cord blood harvesting involves obtaining stem cells from umbilical cord blood of newborns. This blood has a high concentration of stem cells. These cells are obtained through a simple blood draw from the placenta after birth and before the placenta detaches. The blood is then sent to the Cord Blood Registry for processing and storage. The stem cells may be used later for an unrelated recipient or stored in case the infant develops a serious illness later in life and needs them.

Conditioning Regimen. Fig. 40-5 outlines the timing and steps involved in transplantation. The day the patient receives the stem cells is day T-0. Before transplantation, the conditioning days are counted in reverse order from T-0, just like a rocket countdown. After transplantation, days are counted in order from the day of transplantation.

The patient first undergoes a conditioning regimen, which varies with the diagnosis and type of transplant to be received. The conditioning regimen serves two purposes: (1) to "wipe out" the patient's own bone marrow, thus preparing him or her for optimal graft take; and (2) to give higher-than-normal doses of chemotherapy and/or radiotherapy to rid the person of cancer cells *(myeloablation)*. Usually a period of 5 to 10 days is required. The regimen usually includes high-dose chemotherapy and, less commonly, total-body irradiation (TBI). Each conditioning regimen is individually tailored, with the patient's

specific disease, overall health, and previous treatment considered.

Because of the problems and risk for death associated with this conditioning regimen, a non-myeloablative approach may be used instead. Non-myeloablative regimens use lower doses of chemotherapy and/or lower dose of TBI that allow for recovery of a recipient's own immune system. The use of non-myeloablative conditioning regimens decreases the chemotherapy side effects but relies on the development of graft-versus-host disease (GVHD) for the control of the cancer. There are many variations of non-myeloablative conditioning regimens. In contrast, myeloablative conditioning regimens use high doses of chemotherapy with or without radiation therapy to completely destroy a recipient's bone marrow, allowing for replacement by a new immune system.

During conditioning, bone marrow and normal tissues respond immediately to the chemotherapy and radiation. *The patient has all of the expected side effects associated with both therapies (see Chapter 22). When chemotherapy is given in high doses, these side effects are more intense than those seen with standard doses.*

Late effects from the conditioning regimen may occur as late as 3 to 10 years after transplantation. These problems include veno-occlusive disease (VOD), skin toxicities, cataracts, lung fibrosis, second cancers, cardiomyopathy, endocrine complications, and neurologic complications.

Transplantation. Day T-0 is the day of transplantation. The transplantation itself is very simple. Frozen marrow, PBSCs, or umbilical cord blood cells are thawed and then infused through the patient's central catheter like an ordinary blood transfusion.

> ### ❗ NURSING SAFETY PRIORITY (QSEN)
> **Action Alert**
>
> Do not use blood administration tubing to infuse stems cells because the cells could get caught in the filter, resulting in the patient receiving fewer stem cells.

Side effects of all types of stem cell transfusions are similar. The patient may have fever and hypertension in response to the preservative used in stem cell storage. To prevent these reactions, acetaminophen (Tylenol), hydrocortisone, and diphenhydramine (Benadryl) are given before the infusion. Antihypertensives or diuretics may be needed to treat fluid volume changes.

Engraftment. The transfused PBSCs and marrow cells circulate briefly in the peripheral blood. The stems cells find their way to the marrow-forming sites of the patient's bones and establish residency there.

Engraftment, the successful "take" of the transplanted cells in the patient's bone marrow, is key to the whole transplantation process. For the stem cells to "rescue" the patient after his or her own bone marrow have been wiped out, the stem cells must survive and grow in the patient's bone marrow sites. The average time to engraftment for PBSC cells is 14 days. For bone marrow, the average time is 21 days. To aid engraftment, growth factors, such as granulocyte colony-stimulating factor or granulocyte-macrophage colony-stimulating factor, may be given. When engraftment occurs, the patient's WBC, RBC, and platelet counts begin to rise. Engraftment syndrome (ES) with fever and weight gain may occur at this time (Thoele, 2014).

Monitoring of engraftment involves checking the patient's blood for "*chimerism*," which is the presence of blood cells that show a different genetic profile or marker from those of the patient. Mixed chimerism is the presence of both the patient's cells and those from the donor. Progressive chimerism with increasing percentages of donor cells indicates engraftment. Regressive chimerism with increasing percentages of the patient's cells indicates graft failure. When engraftment is successful, only the donor's cells are present.

Prevention of Complications. The period after transplantation is difficult. INFECTION and poor CLOTTING with bleeding are severe problems because the patient remains without any IMMUNITY until the transfused cells grow and engraft. Care for this patient is the same as for the patient during induction therapy for AML. Helping the patient maintain hope through this long recovery period is difficult. Complications are often severe and life threatening. Help the patient have a positive attitude and be involved in his or her own recovery.

In addition to the problems related to the period of **pancytopenia** (too few circulating blood cells), other complications of HSCT include failure to engraft, development of graft-versus-host disease (GVHD), and veno-occlusive disease (VOD).

Failure to engraft occurs when the donated stem cells fail to grow in the bone marrow and function properly. This issue is discussed in advance with the patient and the donor. Failure to engraft occurs more often with transplants using allogeneic stem cells than with those using autologous stem cells. The causes include too few cells transplanted, attack or rejection of donor cells by the recipient's remaining immune system cells, infection of transplanted cells, and unknown biologic factors. *If the transplanted cells fail to engraft, the patient will die unless another transplant with stem cells is successful.*

Graft-versus-host disease (GVHD) occurs mostly in allogeneic transplants but also can occur in autologous transplants (Baker & McKiernan, 2011). The immunocompetent cells of the donated marrow recognize the patient's (recipient) cells, tissues, and organs as foreign and start an immunologic attack against them. The graft is actually trying to attack the host tissues and cells.

Although all host tissues can be attacked and harmed, the tissues usually damaged are the skin, eyes, intestinal tract, liver, female genitalia, lungs, immune system, and musculoskeletal system (Johnson, 2013). Fig. 40-6 shows the typical skin appearance of GVHD. About 25% to 50% of all allogeneic HSCT recipients have some degree of GVHD, and more than 15% of the patients who develop GVHD die of its complications. The presence of some GVHD indicates successful engraftment.

Management of GVHD involves limiting the activity of donor T-cells by using drugs to suppress IMMUNITY such as cyclosporine, tacrolimus, methotrexate, corticosteroids, mycophenolate

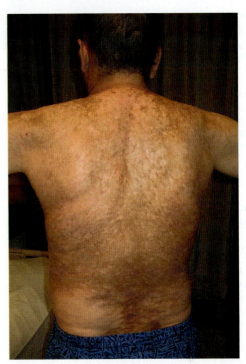

FIG. 40-6 Typical skin manifestations of graft-versus-host disease (GVHD).

mofetil (Cellcept, MMF), and antithymocyte globulin (ATG) (Baker & McKiernan, 2011). Care is taken to avoid suppressing the new immune system to the extent that either INFECTION risk increases or the new cells stop engrafting.

Veno-occlusive disease (VOD) is the blockage of liver blood vessels by CLOTTING and inflammation (phlebitis) and occurs in about one fifth of patients with HSCT. Problems usually begin within the first 30 days after transplantation. Patients who received high-dose chemotherapy, especially with alkylating agents, are at risk for life-threatening liver complications. Manifestations include jaundice, pain in the right upper quadrant, ascites, weight gain, and liver enlargement.

Because there is no way of opening the liver vessels, treatment is supportive. Early detection improves the chance for survival. Fluid management is also crucial. Assess the patient

❓ CLINICAL JUDGMENT CHALLENGE

Safety; Teamwork and Collaboration QSEN

The patient is a 44-year-old chemical plant foreman who developed acute myelogenous leukemia 6 months ago. His initial therapy was successful, and he is scheduled to have a stem cell transplant with his identical twin brother as the donor. His brother lives in the same city and is a professor at a local university. The patient is very grateful that his brother will donate bone marrow and states that he is certain that he has no risk for infection during the procedure because his brother is his identical twin.

1. What type of class of stem cell transplant would this procedure be considered?
2. Is the patient correct in assuming that he has no risk for infection because the donor is his twin brother? Provide a rationale for your response.
3. Which, if any, complications of stem cell transplantation are reduced or eliminated by having an identical sibling donate the stem cells?
4. Which, if any, complications (and why) are still possible even with a donor who is an identical sibling?

The Patient with Thrombocytopenia

- Handle the patient gently.
- Use a lift sheet when moving and positioning in bed.
- Avoid IM injections and venipunctures.
- When injections or venipunctures are necessary, use the smallest-gauge needle for the task.
- Apply firm pressure to the needle stick site for 10 minutes or until the site no longer oozes blood.
- Apply ice to areas of trauma.
- Test all urine and stool for the presence of occult blood.
- Observe IV sites every 2 hours for bleeding.
- Avoid trauma to rectal tissues:
  - Do not give enemas.
  - Administer well-lubricated suppositories with caution.
  - Advise patient not to have anal intercourse.
- Measure abdominal girth daily.
- Advise the patient to use an electric shaver.
- Teach the patient to avoid mouth trauma:
  - Use soft-bristled toothbrush or tooth sponges.
  - Do not floss between teeth.
  - Avoid dental work, especially extractions.
  - Avoid hard foods.
  - Make sure that dentures fit and do not rub.
- Encourage the patient not to blow the nose or insert objects into the nose.
- Advise the patient to avoid contact sports.
- Teach the patient to wear shoes with firm soles when ambulating.

daily for weight gain, fluid retention, increases in abdominal girth, and hepatomegaly.

Minimizing Injury. Bone marrow production of platelets is severely limited with acute myelogenous leukemia (AML), leading to thrombocytopenia. The patient is at great risk for poor CLOTTING with excessive bleeding in response to minimal trauma. Thrombocytopenia can also be caused by induction therapy for AML or high-dose chemotherapy for transplantation.

Planning: Expected Outcomes. The patient with leukemia is expected to remain free from bleeding. Indicators include:

- Maintenance of hematocrit and hemoglobin within normal limits
- Absence of visible bleeding, petechiae, or ecchymosis
- Absence of evidence of occult bleeding (e.g., abdominal swelling, tarry stools)

Interventions. The platelet count is decreased as a side effect of chemotherapy. During the period of greatest bone marrow suppression (the **nadir**), the platelet count may be less than 10,000/mm³. The patient is at extreme risk for bleeding once the platelet count falls below 50,000/mm³, and spontaneous bleeding may occur when the count is lower than 20,000/mm³.

Bleeding Precautions are used to protect the patient at increased risk for injury from bleeding (Chart 40-7). Assess at least every 4 hours for evidence of bleeding: oozing, enlarging bruises, petechiae, or purpura. Inspect all stools, urine, drainage, and vomit for blood, and test for occult blood. Measure any blood loss as accurately as possible, and measure the abdominal girth daily. Increases in abdominal girth can indicate internal hemorrhage. Institute the Bleeding Precautions listed in Chart 40-7. Platelet levels return to normal more slowly than do either WBCs or RBCs, and the patient remains at bleeding risk for weeks after discharge.

Monitor laboratory values daily, especially CBC results, to assess bleeding risk, as well as actual blood loss. The patient with a platelet count below 10,000/mm³ may need a platelet transfusion. For the patient with severe blood loss, packed RBCs may be prescribed (see discussion on p. 822 in the Red Blood Cell Transfusions section).

Conserving Energy. Production of red blood cells is limited in leukemia, causing anemia and fatigue. Also, leukemic cells have high rates of metabolism, increasing fatigue in the anemic patient. Anemia may also occur as a side effect of chemotherapy.

Planning: Expected Outcomes. The patient with leukemia is expected to have no increase in fatigue. Indicators include that the patient consistently demonstrates these behaviors:

- Participates in self-care
- Recognizes manifestations of fatigue
- Changes activity level to match energy level

Interventions. Interventions to reduce fatigue focus on conserving energy and improving RBC counts.

Nutrition therapy is needed to assist the patient to eat enough calories to meet at least basal energy requirements. However, increasing food intake can be difficult with fatigue. Collaborate with a dietitian to provide small, frequent meals high in protein and carbohydrates.

Blood transfusions are sometimes indicated for the patient with fatigue. Transfusions with packed RBCs increase the blood's oxygen-carrying capacity and replace missing RBCs. (See Chart 40-12 on p. 820 for nursing care during transfusions.)

Drug therapy with colony-stimulating growth factors may reduce the severity and duration of anemia and neutropenia after intensive chemotherapy. For anemia, erythropoiesis-stimulating agents (ESAs) that boost production of RBCs may be used. These agents now carry a warning for causing hypertension and increasing the risk for myocardial infarction. ESAs must be given with care and should be avoided in patients with myeloid malignancies. They are not used unless the hemoglobin level is lower than 10 mg/dL and are stopped when this level is reached. Assess for side effects such as hypertension, headaches, fever, **myalgia** (muscle aches), and rashes. (See Chapter 22 for information on hematopoietic growth factors.)

Activity management helps conserve the patient's energy (Chart 40-8). Examine the patient's schedule of prescribed and routine activities. Assess those activities that do not have a direct positive effect on the patient's condition in terms of their usefulness. If the benefit of an activity is less than its worsening of fatigue, coordinate with other members of the health care team about eliminating or postponing it. Activities that may be postponed include physical therapy and invasive diagnostic tests not needed for assessment or treatment of current problems.

? NCLEX EXAMINATION CHALLENGE
Safe and Effective Care Environment

The client is 3 weeks post-transplant from an allogeneic stem cell transplantation for acute lymphocytic leukemia. There is now some peeling of the client's skin on the palms of the hands and the soles of the feet. Which additional assessment data support the nurse's suspicion of possible graft-versus-host disease (GVHD)?

A. The client's temperature is slightly below normal.
B. Today's platelet count is 5,000/mm³ and the WBCs are low.
C. The client has had 6 to 10 watery stools daily for 3 days.
D. The client's urine output is less than 800 mL in 24 hours.

CHART 40-8 Best Practice for Patient Safety & Quality Care (QSEN)

Conserving Energy

- Reassure the patient that fatigue is temporary and energy levels will improve over a period of weeks to months. Stress that a return to previous energy levels may take as long as a year.
- Teach the patient that shortness of breath and palpitations are symptoms of over-activity.
- Instruct the patient to stop activity when shortness of breath or palpitations are present.
- Space care activities at least an hour apart, and avoid the time right before or right after meals.
- Schedule care activities at times when the patient has more energy (e.g., immediately after naps).
- Perform complete bed bath only every other day. In between complete baths, ensure cleansing of face, hands, axillae, and perineum.
- In collaboration with other members of the health care team, cancel or reschedule non-essential tests and activities.
- Provide four to six small, easy-to-eat meals instead of three larger ones.
- Urge the patient to drink small amounts of protein shakes or other nutritional supplements.
- During periods of extreme fatigue, encourage the patient to allow others to perform personal care.
- Help the patient identify one or two lead visitors (those designated as allowed to visit at any time and who do not disturb the patient).
- Selectively limit non–lead visitors when the patient is resting or sleeping.
- Remind families that, although independence is important, independence in ADLs during extreme fatigue can be detrimental to the patient's health.
- Monitor oxygen saturation and respiratory rate during any activity to determine patient responses and activity tolerance.

CHART 40-9 Patient and Family Education: Preparing for Self-Management

Home Care of the Central Venous Catheter

- To maintain patency, flush the catheter briskly with saline once a day and after completing infusions.
- Change the Luer-Lok cap on each catheter lumen weekly.
- Change the dressing as often as prescribed:
  - Use clean technique with thorough handwashing.
  - Clean the exit site with alcohol and povidone-iodine (Betadine) or with chlorhexidine.
  - Apply antibacterial ointment to the site, if prescribed.
  - Cover the site with dry sterile gauze dressing, taped securely, or with transparent adherent dressing.
- To prevent tension, always tape the catheter to yourself.
- Look for and report any signs of infection (redness, swelling, or drainage at the exit site).
- In case of a break or puncture in the catheter lumen, immediately clamp the catheter between yourself and the opening. *Notify your physician immediately.*

Community-Based Care

The patient with leukemia is discharged after induction chemotherapy and recovery of blood cell production. Follow-up care continues on an ambulatory care basis. Although many transplant centers discharge patients after engraftment, some centers also give high-dose chemotherapy and stem cell infusion on an ambulatory care basis. This plan involves daily clinic visits and frequent follow-up by nurses in the home care setting.

Home Care Management. Planning for home care for the patient with leukemia begins as soon as remission is achieved. Assess the available support systems. Many patients need a visiting nurse to assist with dressing changes for central venous catheters, infusions, and to answer questions. Home transfusion therapy for blood components may be needed.

Coordination of the home care team is critical for the patient receiving stem cell transplantation in the home setting. Potential candidates are evaluated in advance. Criteria include a knowledgeable caregiver, a clean home environment, location near the hospital, telephone access, and emotional stability of the patient and caregiver.

Home care nurses give chemotherapy and monitor for complications. Nurses visit the patient once or twice per day and spend between 4 and 8 hours per day in the home. The patient receives the stem cell transplant infusion in the ambulatory care clinic. Nursing care is similar to that provided in the hospital. If complications such as sepsis or veno-occlusive disease (VOD) occur, the patient is admitted to the inpatient facility.

Self-Management Education. Instruct the patient and family about the importance of continuing therapy and medical follow-up. Many patients go home with a central venous catheter in place and need instructions about its care. Chart 40-9 lists guidelines for central venous catheter care at home. These guidelines may be altered depending on the home setting, assistance available, and agency policy.

Protecting the patient from infection at home is just as important as it was during hospitalization. (See Chart 40-6 for focused assessment for the patient at risk for INFECTION.) Teach about proper hygiene and the need to avoid crowds or others with infections. Neither the patient nor any household member should receive live virus immunization (poliomyelitis, measles, or rubella) for 2 years after transplantation. Instruct the patient to continue mouth care regimens at home. Stress to the patient that he or she should immediately notify the physician if a fever or any other indications of infection develop. Chart 40-10 lists guidelines for infection prevention.

Many patients return home still at risk for bleeding because platelet recovery is slower than recovery of other cells. Reinforce safety and bleeding precautions, and emphasize that these precautions must be followed until the platelet count remains above 50,000/mm³. Teach the patient and family to assess for petechiae, avoid trauma and sharp objects, apply pressure to wounds for 10 minutes, and report blood in the stool or urine or headache that does not respond to acetaminophen. Chart 40-11 lists guidelines for patients at risk for bleeding.

Psychosocial Preparation. A diagnosis of leukemia threatens self-esteem and the family role. The patient faces the possibility of death, and treatment causes major changes in self-image. Changes occur in body image, level of independence, and lifestyle. Some feel threatened by the environment, seeing everything as infectious. Patients who are cared for in protective isolation may feel lonely and isolated. Help the patient and family define priorities, understand the illness and its treatment, and find hope. Make referrals to support groups sponsored by organizations such as the American Cancer Society or the Leukemia and Lymphoma Society of America.

One problem that lasts for a long period after transplantation is severe fatigue. Although the acute period after transplantation requires energy conservation with reduced activity, in the later recovery period, exercise provides benefits and fatigue reduction (see the Evidence-Based Practice box) (Albrecht,

CHART 40-10 Patient and Family Education: Preparing for Self-Management

Prevention of Infection

- Avoid crowds and other gatherings of people who might be ill.
- Do not share personal toilet articles, such as toothbrushes, toothpaste, washcloths, or deodorant sticks, with others.
- If possible, bathe daily.
- Wash the armpits, groin, genitals, and anal area at least twice a day with an antimicrobial soap.
- Clean your toothbrush daily by either running it through the dishwasher or rinsing it in liquid laundry bleach and then rinsing it with running water.
- Wash your hands thoroughly with an antimicrobial soap before you eat or drink, after touching a pet, after shaking hands with anyone, as soon as you come home from any outing, and after using the toilet.
- Eat a low-bacteria diet, and avoid salads, raw fruits and vegetables, and undercooked meat.
- Wash dishes between uses with hot, sudsy water, or use a dishwasher.
- Do not drink water that has been standing for longer than 15 minutes.
- Do not reuse cups and glasses without washing.
- Avoid changing pet litter boxes. If unavoidable, use gloves or wash hands immediately.
- Avoid keeping turtles and reptiles as pets.
- Do not feed pets raw or undercooked meat.
- Take your temperature at least twice a day.
- Report any of these manifestations of infection to your physician immediately:
  - Temperature greater than 100°F (38°C)
  - Persistent cough (with or without sputum)
  - Pus or foul-smelling drainage from any open skin area or normal body opening
  - Presence of a boil or abscess
  - Urine that is cloudy or foul smelling, or burning on urination
- Take all drugs as prescribed.
- Do not dig in the garden or work with houseplants.
- Avoid travel to areas of the world with poor sanitation or inadequate health care facilities.

CHART 40-11 Patient and Family Education: Preparing for Self-Management

The Patient at Risk for Bleeding

- Use an electric shaver.
- Use a soft-bristled toothbrush, and do not floss.
- Do not have dental work done without consulting your doctor.
- Do not take aspirin or any aspirin-containing products. Read the label to be sure the products do not contain aspirin or salicylates.
- Wear shoes or slippers with a sole to avoid foot injury.
- Do not participate in contact sports or any activity likely to result in your being bumped, scratched, or scraped.
- If you are bumped, apply ice to the site for at least 1 hour.
- Notify your physician if you:
  - Experience an injury and persistent bleeding results
  - Have excessive menstrual bleeding
  - See blood in your urine or bowel movement
  - Have a headache that does not respond to acetaminophen
- Avoid anal intercourse.
- Take a stool softener to prevent straining during a bowel movement.
- Do not use enemas or rectal suppositories.
- Avoid bending over at the waist.
- Do not wear clothing or shoes that are tight or that rub.
- Avoid blowing your nose or placing objects in your nose. If you must blow your nose, do so gently without blocking either nasal passage.

EVIDENCE-BASED PRACTICE QSEN

Exercise for Less Fatigue

Chiffelle, R., & Kenny, K. (2013). Exercise for fatigue management in hematopoietic stem cell transplantation recipients. *Clinical Journal of Oncology Nursing, 17*(3), 241-242.

Fatigue associated with cancer therapy has been recognized as one of the most distressing and debilitating side effects. The fatigue experienced by patients after hematopoietic stem cell transplantation (HSCT) has been found to be more severe and persist much longer than that associated with more standard therapy. Exercise, even during the treatment period, has been shown to reduce the perception of fatigue and its negative effects on performance of desired activities in patients undergoing standard chemotherapy or radiation. It is not known whether exercise would be beneficial in reducing the long-term fatigue frequently experienced after HSCT or even could have harmful effects.

Level of Evidence: 1

The results are based on a systematic review and meta-analysis of 25 previous studies related to assessing the evidence for recommending an exercise intervention for relief of cancer-related fatigue (CRF) in patients receiving traditional cancer treatments and those whose treatment additionally involved HSCT. The studies analyzed included 6 other systematic reviews, 16 randomized controlled clinical trials, 6 nonrandomized controlled trials, and 1 qualitative study. Results of this analysis do indicate that exercise for patients after HSCT is at least not harmful and has some benefit in reducing the distress of fatigue. Although not all patients universally had fatigue reduction, none experienced an increase in fatigue with exercise.

Commentary: Implications for Practice and Research

For best practice, interventions must be both effective and not harmful. Therefore this meta-analysis contributes substantial evidence that some exercise in patients after HSCT is not harmful and does provide some reduction of the distress associated with CRF. Because many patients and their families believe that the patient is much more fragile after HSCT, some are hesitant to increase activity in any way. Nurses can be instrumental in helping patients and families get past the mental barrier of fear regarding activity and can recommend low-impact exercise. However, the type of exercise (e.g., walking, cycling, low-impact aerobics) and the best timing for implementing an exercise intervention to have maximum benefit have yet to be determined.

2014; Chiffelle & Kenny, 2013). Help the patient and family understand the benefits of low-impact exercise.

Health Care Resources. The patient with limited social support may need help at home until strength and energy return. A home care aide may suffice for some patients, whereas for others a visiting nurse may be needed. The patient may also need equipment for ADLs and ambulation. Assess financial resources. Cancer treatment is expensive, and you will need to coordinate with the social services department to ensure that insurance is adequate. If the patient is uninsured, explore other sources, such as drug company–sponsored compassionate aid programs. The Leukemia and Lymphoma Society of America also offers limited financial help.

Prolonged outpatient contact and follow-up are necessary, and patients need transportation to the outpatient facility. Many local units of the American Cancer Society offer free transportation to patients with cancer, including leukemia.

Evaluation: Outcomes

Evaluate the care of the patient with leukemia based on the identified priority patient problems. The expected outcomes include that the patient will:

- Remain free of infection and sepsis
- Not experience episodes of bleeding
- Be able to balance activity and rest
- Use energy conservation techniques

Specific indicators for these outcomes are listed for each priority patient problem in the Planning and Implementation section (see earlier).

MALIGNANT LYMPHOMAS

Lymphomas are cancers of the lymphoid tissues with abnormal overgrowth of lymphocytes. Lymphomas are cancers of committed lymphocytes rather than stem cell precursors (as in leukemia). This growth occurs as solid tumors in lymphoid tissues scattered throughout the body, especially the lymph nodes and spleen, rather than in the bone marrow. The two major adult forms of lymphoma are Hodgkin's lymphoma (HL) and non-Hodgkin's lymphoma (NHL).

HODGKIN'S LYMPHOMA
❖ PATHOPHYSIOLOGY

Hodgkin's lymphoma (HL) is a cancer that can affect any age-group. However, it appears to peak in two different age-groups: (1) teens and young adults, and (2) adults in their 50s and 60s (McCance et al., 2014). HL affects younger men and women equally, but the disease is more prevalent in men in the older group.

The exact cause of HL is uncertain. Possible causes of HL include viral infections (i.e. Epstein-Barr virus [EBV], human T-cell leukemia/lymphoma virus [HTLV], and human immune deficiency virus [HIV]) and exposure to chemicals. Most cases of the disease, however, occur in people without known risk factors.

This cancer usually starts in a single lymph node or a single chain of nodes. These nodes contain a specific cancer cell type, the **Reed-Sternberg cell,** a marker for HL. HL often spreads predictably from one group of lymph nodes to the next, unlike non-Hodgkin's lymphoma.

❖ PATIENT-CENTERED COLLABORATIVE CARE
◆ Assessment

The most common assessment finding is a large but painless lymph node or nodes. The patient may also have constitutional manifestations ("B symptoms") that include: fevers (>101.5° F [>38.6° C]); heavy night sweats; and unplanned weight loss (>10% of normal body weight). The presence of these manifestations often means a poorer prognosis. Many patients have no manifestations at time of diagnosis, and specific manifestations often depend on the site and extent of disease.

Diagnosis and subtype are established when biopsy reveals Reed-Sternberg cells (McCance et al., 2014). HL is then classified into one of several different subtypes.

After diagnosis, staging is performed to determine the extent of disease. This process is detailed and must be accurate because the treatment regimen is determined by the extent of disease. Staging usually includes a history and physical examination,

TABLE 40-4	Ann Arbor Staging Criteria for Hodgkin's Lymphoma
STAGE	**MANIFESTATION CRITERIA**
Ia	Disease is present only in a single lymph node region or in only one non–lymph node site.
Ib	Disease location is the same as Ia. In addition, the patient has some or all of these manifestations: persistent fever, night sweats, weight loss of more than 10% of normal body weight.
IIa	Disease is present in two or more separate lymph node regions on the same side of the diaphragm or in two non–lymph node sites on the same side of the diaphragm.
IIb	Disease location is the same as IIa. In addition, the patient has some or all of these manifestations: persistent fever, night sweats, weight loss of more than 10% of normal body weight.
IIIa	Disease extends to lymph node regions on both sides of the diaphragm.
IIIb	Disease location is the same as IIIa. In addition, the patient has some or all of these manifestations: persistent fever, night sweats, weight loss of more than 10% of normal body weight.
IIIc	Same as IIIb along with disease present in the spleen.
IV	Disease is present in many body areas, including in one or more non-nodal tissues and organs.

CBC, electrolyte panel, kidney and liver function tests, erythrocyte sedimentation rate (ESR), bone marrow aspiration and biopsy, and computed tomography (CT) of the neck, chest, abdomen, and pelvis. Positron emission tomography (PET) may be used to assess for disease not detected by CT. PET scans are helpful after treatment to assess disease response to therapy. After staging procedures are complete, the stage of the disease is determined by the Ann Arbor Staging Criteria (Table 40-4).

◆ Interventions

HL is one of the most treatable types of cancer. For stages I and II disease, the treatment is external radiation of involved lymph node regions. With more extensive disease, radiation and combination chemotherapy are used to achieve remission. (See Chapter 22 on general care of patients receiving radiation and chemotherapy.)

Nursing management of the patient undergoing treatment for HL focuses on the acute side effects of therapy, especially:

- Drug-induced pancytopenia with increased risk for INFECTION, anemia, and bleeding
- Severe nausea and vomiting
- Skin problems at the site of radiation
- Constipation or diarrhea
- Permanent sterility for male patients receiving radiation to the lower abdomen or pelvic region in combination with specific chemotherapy drugs (The patient is informed and given the option to store sperm in a sperm bank *before* treatment.)
- Secondary cancer development and the need for long-term follow-up

NON-HODGKIN'S LYMPHOMA

❖ PATHOPHYSIOLOGY

Non-Hodgkin's lymphoma (NHL) includes all lymphoid cancers that do not have the Reed-Sternberg cell. There are over 60 subtypes of NHL divided into either indolent or aggressive lymphomas. NHL generally spreads through the lymphatic system in a less orderly fashion than HL. About 70,000 new cases are diagnosed each year in North America (ACS, 2014). The disease is more common in men and older adults.

The exact cause of NHL is unknown although the incidence is higher among patients with solid organ transplantation, immunosuppressive drug therapy, and HIV disease. Chronic infection from *Helicobacter pylori* is associated with a type of lymphoma called *mucosa-associated lymphoid tissue (MALT) lymphoma,* and Epstein-Barr viral infection has been associated with Burkitt's lymphoma. There is an increased incidence of NHL among people exposed to pesticides, insecticides, and dust.

Patients usually have swollen lymph nodes (lymphadenopathy) or tumor spread to other organs (e.g., GI tract, skin, bone marrow, sinuses, thyroid, central nervous system) at the time of diagnosis. Enlarged lymph nodes may be the only manifestation of lymphoma. Painless swelling of the cervical, axillary, inguinal, and femoral nodes is most often seen. The diagnosis of NHL is made only after the biopsy of an involved lymph node is reviewed by a hematopathologist.

Lymphoma is not a single disease but, rather, a group of diseases. The specific subtype of lymphoma must be classified because management varies with the subtype. Classification is based on cytology, immunophenotyping by flow cytometry, and genetic (chromosomal changes and molecular rearrangements) and clinical features. NHLs are broadly classified as B-cell or T-cell lymphomas, depending on the lymphocyte type that gave rise to the cancer. B-cell lymphomas are most common.

Classification of NHL is more complicated than that for Hodgkin's lymphoma and is based on the World Health Organization (WHO) classification system. In addition, lactate dehydrogenase (LDH) levels and beta-2 microglobulin levels are also evaluated to measure tumor growth rates and calculate prognosis. (High LDH levels and high beta-2 microglobulin levels are associated with a poorer prognosis.) Cerebrospinal fluid is evaluated when lymphoma is present in the CNS, around the spinal column, brain, or testes, and when HIV-related lymphoma is diagnosed.

Patients with **indolent** (slow-growing) lymphomas usually have painless lymph node swelling at diagnosis. Those with more aggressive B-cell lymphomas may have large masses at diagnosis and manifestations. Constitutional manifestations ("B symptoms"), as seen in Hodgkin's lymphoma, occur in about one third of patients with aggressive lymphomas and rarely in indolent lymphomas. Bone marrow involvement in indolent lymphomas is common.

❖ PATIENT-CENTERED COLLABORATIVE CARE

Treatment options for patients with NHL vary based on the subtype of the tumor, international prognostic index (IPI) score, stage of the disease, performance status, and overall tumor burden. Special consideration for patients with additional health problems is important, especially among older adult patients. Many new therapies have evolved over the past decade for various subtypes of NHL. These therapies include combinations of chemotherapy drugs alone or in combination with monoclonal antibodies (e.g., rituximab and alemtuzumab), localized radiation therapy, radiolabeled antibodies (^{131}I tositumomab and ^{90}Y ibritumomab tiuxetan), hematopoietic stem cell transplantation, and investigational agents (Byar & Workman, 2012).

Nursing care needs are similar to those for patients with HL, with additional organ-specific problems if the disease is widespread. With the use of biotherapy for NHL, close monitoring for infusion-related reactions is needed during and after the delivery of monoclonal antibodies (see Chapter 22 for general care of patients undergoing treatment with biotherapy). Patient and family education are important in the management and prevention of complications.

❓ CLINICAL JUDGMENT CHALLENGE

Prioritization, Delegation, and Supervision QSEN

The patient is a 52-year-old woman who has undergone an autologous stem cell transplantation for non-Hodgkin's lymphoma. She is recovering, and her white blood cell count is improving but is still very low. She remains on neutropenic precautions. The LPN reports that the patient's heart rate, respiratory rate, temperature, and blood pressure are elevated.

1. Which vital sign finding would you report to the health care provider immediately and why?
2. You must assign an unlicensed assistive personnel (UAP) to help care for this patient. Of the four UAP available, one is newly pregnant and has worked on this unit for 3 years, one has had cold symptoms for 3 days, one has not yet cared for a patient on neutropenic precautions, and one has a fear of people with cancer. Which UAP should you avoid assigning to this patient? Provide a rationale for your choice.
3. A nursing student tearfully reports to you, "I took some flowers into the patient's room to cheer him up and he told me that he didn't think he was supposed to have flowers. I took them out of the room right away and then I realized I had made a mistake." How should you respond to this student?
4. The student asks you whether a book still wrapped in shrink wrap just now brought in by a friend of the patient can be taken to the patient's room. How will you help the student know what to do in this situation?

MULTIPLE MYELOMA

❖ PATHOPHYSIOLOGY

Multiple myeloma is a white blood cell (WBC) cancer that involves a mature B-lymphocyte called a *plasma cell,* which secretes antibodies. These cells are overgrown in the bone marrow. When these cells become cancerous, they produce excessive antibodies (gamma globulins). Thus the disorder is called a "gammopathy." When myeloma cells are overproduced, fewer red blood cells (RBCs), WBCs, and platelets are produced, leading to anemia and increased risk for INFECTION and bleeding.

In addition to the excess antibodies, multiple myeloma cells also produce excess cytokines (see Chapter 17) that increase cancer cell growth and destroy bone. The excess antibodies are in the blood, increasing the serum protein levels and clogging blood vessels in the kidney and other organs. Without treatment, the disease causes progressive bone destruction, bleeding problems, kidney failure, immunosuppression, and death.

Multiple myeloma accounts for about 11,000 deaths per year in the United States (ACS, 2014). The disease is most common in people older than 65 years. The incidence is higher in American blacks than in whites, with a much higher incidence in men.

The cause of multiple myeloma is unknown. Possible risk factors include radiation exposure, chemical exposure, and INFECTION with human herpes virus-8 (HHV-8). This cancer can be distinguished by changes in immunoglobulin structure that begin within a single clone of cells even before transformation to cancer occurs. When the specifically altered immunoglobulin is present in a high enough quantity, the type can be recognized as a unique "spike" pattern on a serum electrophoresis test of plasma proteins. Because one clone of cells develops into cancer cells, the abnormal immunoglobulin produced by these cells is a *monoclonal* paraprotein.

❖ PATIENT-CENTERED COLLABORATIVE CARE

◆ Assessment

Some patients have no symptoms at time of the diagnosis. An elevation of serum total protein or a detection of a monoclonal protein (also known as *paraprotein*) in the blood or urine may be the only finding. Other common manifestations include fatigue, anemia, bone pain, pathologic fractures, recurrent bacterial INFECTIONS, and kidney dysfunction.

A positive finding of a serum monoclonal protein is not sufficient to make a diagnosis of multiple myeloma. About 1% of the population produce a monoclonal protein in the blood but do not have multiple myeloma. This condition is labeled *monoclonal gammopathy of undetermined significance* or *MGUS*, which is a premalignant condition. Follow-up of patients with MGUS is important because a small percentage eventually will develop multiple myeloma. Multiple myeloma is distinguished from MGUS by having more than 10% of the bone marrow infiltrated with plasma cells, the presence of a monoclonal protein in the serum or urine, and the presence of osteolytic bone lesions.

The staging system for multiple myeloma divides patients into stages and prognostic groups on the basis of the serum beta-2 microglobulin and albumin levels. Other factors that help determine prognosis include age, performance status, serum creatinine, serum albumin, serum calcium, lactate dehydrogenase (LDH) level, C-reactive protein, hemoglobin level, platelet count, quantitative immunoglobulins, beta-2 microglobulin, serum free light chains, serum protein electrophoresis (SPEP) with immunofixation, 24-hour urine for SPEP, and cytogenetic abnormalities found in the bone marrow biopsy (Kurtin & Faiman, 2013).

The patient usually first notices fatigue, easy bruising, and bone pain. Bone fractures, hypertension, INFECTION, hypercalcemia, and fluid imbalance may occur as the disease progresses. Diagnosis is made by x-ray findings of bone thinning with areas of bone loss that resemble Swiss cheese, high immunoglobulin and plasma protein levels, and the presence of Bence-Jones protein (protein composed of incomplete antibodies) in the urine. A bone marrow biopsy is performed to diagnose the disease and to determine chromosome changes. An abnormality of chromosome 11 predicts a longer survival, and absence of chromosome 13 is a poor prognostic factor.

◆ Interventions

Treatment options vary. For minimal disease, watchful waiting may be an option instead of chemotherapy. Standard treatment for multiple myeloma is the use of proteasome inhibitors, such as bortezomib (Velcade) or carfilzomib (Kyprolis), and immunomodulating drugs, such as thalidomide (Thalomid) or lenalidomide (Revlimid). All these agents, which are types of targeted cancer therapy (see Chapter 22), may be used alone or in combination with steroids, such as dexamethasone (Decadron). Drug selection is based on whether the patient is eligible for an autologous stem cell transplant. If eligible, drug therapy is used to reduce tumor burden before transplantation. For patients who are not eligible for an autologous stem cell transplantation, standard chemotherapy drugs such as melphalan, prednisone, vincristine, cyclophosphamide, doxorubicin, and carmustine are usually effective in controlling but not curing the disease.

Side effects and severe toxicities can occur with these agents. Myelosuppression is an expected side effect of many myeloma therapies. A nursing priority is to teach the patient about the manifestations. The risk for thromboembolic events is increased with the use of thalidomide and lenalidomide. Peripheral neuropathy can be challenging, causing pain and poor quality of life. GI side effects, such as nausea, vomiting, diarrhea, and constipation, are severe and can be life threatening if not managed properly.

Despite therapy, multiple myeloma remains largely incurable (Kurtin & Faiman, 2013). Best outcomes are seen with autologous hematopoietic stem cell transplantation, although few patients are able to pursue this option (Mangan et al., 2013). Because most patients with multiple myeloma have bone pain, analgesics and alternative approaches for pain management, such as relaxation techniques, aromatherapy, or hypnosis, are used for pain relief. The bone disease of multiple myeloma is treated with bisphosphonates (pamidronate [Aredia], zoledronic acid [Zometa], denosumab [Xgeva]), which inhibit bone resorption and can help reduce the skeletal complications.

COAGULATION DISORDERS

Coagulation disorders are bleeding disorders with increased bleeding resulting from defects in one or more components regulating blood CLOTTING. Bleeding disorders may be spontaneous or traumatic, localized or generalized, lifelong or acquired. They can arise from a defect in the clotting processes at the vascular, platelet, or clotting factor level.

PLATELET DISORDERS

As discussed in Chapter 39, CLOTTING always starts with platelets sticking together (aggregation) and forming a platelet plug. Any condition that either reduces the number of platelets or interferes with their ability to adhere (stick to one another, blood vessel walls, collagen, or fibrin threads) can result in increased bleeding. Platelet disorders are inherited, acquired, or temporarily induced by drugs that limit platelet production or inhibit aggregation.

Platelet numbers below that needed for blood CLOTTING is called **thrombocytopenia**. It may occur as a result of other conditions or treatments that suppress general bone marrow activity. The problem also can occur from limited platelet formation or an increased rate of platelet destruction in the spleen. The two thrombocytopenic conditions affecting adults are *autoimmune thrombocytopenic purpura* and *thrombotic thrombocytopenic purpura*.

AUTOIMMUNE THROMBOCYTOPENIC PURPURA

❖ PATHOPHYSIOLOGY

Autoimmune thrombocytopenic purpura is also called *idiopathic thrombocytopenic purpura (ITP)*. The number of circulating platelets is greatly reduced in ITP, even though platelet production is normal.

Patients with this disorder make an antibody against the surface of their own platelets (an antiplatelet antibody). This antibody coats the platelet surfaces, making destruction by macrophages easier (see Chapter 17). The spleen has many macrophages, and the blood vessels of the spleen are long and twisted. These conditions increase destruction of antibody-coated platelets in the spleen. When platelet destruction exceeds platelet production, the number of circulating platelets decreases and CLOTTING is impaired.

The trigger for the production of autoantibodies is unknown, but viral INFECTION is suspected. ITP is most common among women between the ages of 20 and 50 years and among people who have other autoimmune disorders (McCance et al., 2014; Radovich, 2011).

❖ PATIENT-CENTERED COLLABORATIVE CARE

◆ Assessment

Manifestations of ITP are at first seen in the skin and mucous membranes: large **ecchymoses** (bruises) or a petechial rash on the arms, legs, upper chest, and neck; mucosal bleeding occurs easily. If the patient has had significant blood loss, anemia may also be present.

A rare complication is intracranial bleeding–induced stroke. Assess for neurologic function and mental status (see Chapter 41).

ITP is diagnosed by a low platelet count and increased megakaryocytes in the bone marrow. Antiplatelet antibodies may be detected in the blood. If the patient has any episodes of bleeding, hematocrit and hemoglobin levels may be low.

◆ Interventions

As a result of the decreased platelet count, the patient is at great risk for poor CLOTTING and increased bleeding. Interventions include therapy for the underlying condition and protection from bleeding episodes. Management is often limited to those patients with platelet counts lower than 50,000/mm³, those who are bleeding, and those who are at high risk for bleeding.

Drug therapy to control ITP includes drugs that suppress immune function. Drugs such as corticosteroids, azathioprine (Imuran), eltrombopag, rituximab (Rituxan), and romiplostim are used to inhibit production of antiplatelet autoantibodies. IV immunoglobulin and IV anti-Rho can help prevent the destruction of antibody-coated platelets, although anti-Rho carries a Black Box Warning for increased risk for intravascular hemolysis and death. Aggressive therapy involves low doses of chemotherapy drugs.

Platelet transfusions are used when platelet counts are less than 10,000/mm³ or the patient has an acute life-threatening bleeding episode. Transfusions are not performed routinely because the donated platelets are just as rapidly destroyed by the spleen as the patient's own platelets. (See discussion on p. 822 in the Platelet Transfusions section.)

Maintaining a safe environment helps protect the patient from bleeding. Closely monitor the amount of bleeding that is occurring. (For nursing care actions, see the discussion of Minimizing Injury on p. 812 in the Leukemia section.)

Surgical management with a splenectomy may be needed for the patient who does not respond to drug therapy. (The spleen is the site of excessive platelet destruction.)

Depending on the size of the spleen and the risk for bleeding, splenectomy may be performed as an open abdominal surgery or as minimally invasive surgery by laparoscopy. Nursing care after surgery is the same as for any other abdominal surgery (see Chapter 16). After splenectomy, the patient is at increased risk for INFECTION because the spleen performs many protective immune functions, especially antibody generation. For this reason, vaccinations against pneumococcal, meningococcal, and *Haemophilus influenzae* are recommended either 2 weeks before a planned splenectomy or 2 weeks after the surgery. Teaching patients about their increased risk for infection, avoiding crowds and people who are ill, and consulting with the health care provider is a nursing priority.

THROMBOTIC THROMBOCYTOPENIC PURPURA

In thrombotic thrombocytopenic purpura (TTP), platelets clump together abnormally in the capillaries and too few platelets remain in circulation. The patient has inappropriate CLOTTING, yet the blood fails to clot when trauma occurs. The cause of TTP appears to be an autoimmune reaction in small blood vessel cells (endothelial cells) that starts platelet aggregation and clotting there. Tissues become ischemic, leading to kidney failure, myocardial infarction, and stroke. Untreated, this disorder is often fatal within 3 months.

Management of the patient with TTP focuses on preventing platelet clumping and stopping the autoimmune process. Plasma removal and the infusion of fresh frozen plasma reduce the clumping caused by elements of the patient's blood. Drugs that inhibit platelet clumping, such as aspirin, alprostadil (Prostin), and plicamycin, also may be helpful. Immunosuppressive therapy reduces the intensity of this disorder.

CLOTTING FACTOR DISORDERS

Coagulation or bleeding disorders can result from a CLOTTING factor defect. Defects include the inability to produce a specific clotting factor, production of low quantities of a clotting factor, or production of a less active form of a clotting factor.

Most clotting factor disorders are genetic problems of one clotting factor. A damaged liver also leads to a clotting disorder by reducing the amount of clotting factors produced. Common disorders that result from defects at the clotting factor level include hemophilias A and B and von Willebrand's disease. Disseminated intravascular coagulation (DIC) often occurs with septic shock (see Chapter 37).

HEMOPHILIA

❖ PATHOPHYSIOLOGY

Hemophilia is a hereditary bleeding disorder with two forms resulting from different CLOTTING factor deficiencies. Hemophilia A (classic hemophilia) is a deficiency of factor VIII and accounts for 80% of cases of hemophilia. Hemophilia B (Christmas disease) is a deficiency of factor IX and accounts for 20% of cases. The incidence of both disorders is 1 in 10,000 (Hitch, 2013; McCance et al., 2014).

GENETIC/GENOMIC CONSIDERATIONS

Patient-Centered Care QSEN

Hemophilia is an X-linked recessive trait. Women who are **carriers** (can pass on the gene without expressing bleeding problems) have a 50% chance of passing the hemophilia gene to their daughters (who then are carriers) and to their sons (who then have hemophilia). Hemophilia A affects mostly males, none of whose sons will have the gene for hemophilia and all of whose daughters will be carriers. About 30% of patients with hemophilia have no family history and their disease may be the result of a new gene mutation (Beery & Workman, 2012). Ensure that the family is referred to the appropriate level of genetic counseling.

The clinical pictures of hemophilias A and B are identical. The patient has abnormal bleeding in response to any trauma because of a deficiency of the specific CLOTTING factor. Hemophiliacs form platelet plugs at the bleeding site, but the clotting factor deficiency impairs the formation of stable fibrin clots. This allows excessive bleeding, which may be mild, moderate, or severe, depending on the degree of factor deficiency.

❖ PATIENT-CENTERED COLLABORATIVE CARE

Assessment of the patient with hemophilia shows:
- Excessive bleeding from minor cuts, bruises, or abrasions (from abnormal platelet function)
- Joint and muscle hemorrhages that lead to disabling long-term problems and may require joint replacement
- A tendency to bruise easily
- Prolonged and potentially fatal hemorrhage after surgery

The laboratory test results for a patient with hemophilia show a prolonged activated partial thromboplastin time (aPTT), a normal bleeding time, and a normal prothrombin time (PT). The most common problem that occurs with hemophilia is degenerating joint function as a result of chronic bleeding into the joints, especially the hip and knee.

The bleeding problems of hemophilia A are managed by either regularly scheduled infusions of synthetic factor VIII or the infusion of this substance only when injury or bleeding occurs. The cost of factor VIII replacement is prohibitive for many people with hemophilia. The source of factor VIII varies (Table 40-5), and the traditional sources, derived from pooled human serum, are no longer recommended because of the risk for transfusion-related INFECTIONS (National Hemophilia Foundation, 2014).

HEPARIN-INDUCED THROMBOCYTOPENIA

Heparin-induced thrombocytopenia (HIT) is a serious IMMUNITY-mediated CLOTTING disorder with an unexplained drop in platelet count after heparin treatment. The occurrence is increasing because of the increased use of heparin. Unlike other clotting disorders, HIT is an immune-mediated drug reaction that is caused by heparin-dependent platelet-activating immunoglobulin G (IgG) antibodies in which heparin binds with platelet factor 4 (PF4). This drug binding leads to the development of a highly reactive immune complex that activates the platelets. Once activated, platelets release procoagulants and PF4, which neutralizes heparin and increases thrombin generation from prothrombin.

HIT can occur in patients receiving any type of heparin, although it is more common after exposure to unfractionated heparin. The incidence is higher among patients with risk factors of (1) duration of heparin use longer than 1 week, (2) exposure to unfractionated heparin, (3) postsurgical thromboprophylaxis, and (4) being female.

Manifestations of HIT include venous thromboembolism (VTE) such as deep vein thrombosis and pulmonary embolism. The diagnosis is based on the patient's exposure to heparin, which can be up to 100 days before the event. Thrombocytopenia after heparin exposure is the hallmark sign of HIT. Clinical, as well as laboratory, findings need to be interpreted to properly diagnose this disorder.

Once HIT is diagnosed, anticoagulation therapy is started. Drug management for HIT management is with a direct thrombin inhibitor such as argatroban (Argatroban), lepirudin (Refludan), and bivalirudin (Angiomax).

TRANSFUSION THERAPY

Any blood component may be removed from a donor and transfused into a recipient. Blood components may be transfused individually or collectively, with varying degrees of benefit to the recipient. Table 40-6 lists indications for transfusion therapy.

Pretransfusion Responsibilities

Nursing actions during transfusions focus on prevention or early recognition of adverse transfusion reactions. Preparation of the patient for transfusion is critical, and blood product administration procedures must be carefully followed. Before infusing any blood product, review the agency's policies and procedures. Chart 40-12 lists best practices for transfusion therapy.

A health care provider's prescription is needed to administer blood components. The prescription specifies the type of component, the volume, and any special conditions. Verify the

TABLE 40-5	**Antihemophilic Drugs**	
DRUG TYPES	**SOURCES**
High purity antihemophilic factor • Alphanate • Humate-P • Koate-DIV	Pooled human serum
Monoclonal antibody purified antihemophilic factor • Hemofil-M • Monarc-M • Monoclate-P	Pooled human serum
Recombinant antihemophilic factor • Helixate FS • Kogenate FS • Recombinate	Recombinant DNA technology
B-domain deleted (BDD) recombinant antihemophilic factor • ReFacto	Recombinant DNA technology
Recombinant antihemophilic factor plasma/albumin-free method (rAHF-PFM) • Advate	Recombinant DNA technology
Recombinant antihemophilic factor plasma/albumin-free method • Xyntha	Recombinant DNA technology
Porcine factor VIII • Hyate: C	Animal serum

TABLE 40-6 **Indications for Treatment with Blood Components**

COMPONENT	VOLUME	INFUSION TIME	INDICATIONS
Packed red blood cells (PRBCs)	200-250 mL	2-4 hr	Anemia; hemoglobin <6 g/dL, 6-10 g/dL, depending on symptoms
Washed red blood cells (WBC-poor PRBCs)	200 mL	2-4 hr	History of allergic transfusion reactions Hematopoietic stem cell transplant patients
Platelets Pooled	About 300 mL	15-30 min	Thrombocytopenia, platelet count <20,000 Patients who are actively bleeding with a platelet count <50,000
Single donor	200 mL	30 min	History of febrile or allergic reactions
Fresh frozen plasma	200 mL	15-30 min	Deficiency in plasma coagulation factors Prothrombin or partial thromboplastin time 1.5 times normal
White blood cells (WBCs)	400 mL	1 hr	Sepsis, neutropenic infection not responding to antibiotic therapy

CHART 40-12 **Best Practice for Patient Safety & Quality Care** QSEN

Transfusion Therapy

NURSING ACTIONS	RATIONALES
Before Infusion	
1. Assess laboratory values.	Many institutions have specific guidelines for blood product transfusions (e.g., platelet count <20,000 or hemoglobin <6 g/dL).
2. Verify the medical prescription.	Legally, a physician's prescription is required for transfusions. The prescription should state the type of product, dose, and transfusion time.
3. Assess the patient's vital signs, urine output, skin color, and history of transfusion reactions.	Determine whether the patient can tolerate infusion. Baseline information may be needed to help identify transfusion reactions.
4. Obtain venous access. Use a central catheter or at least a 19-gauge needle if possible.	The larger-bore needle allows cells to flow more easily without occluding the lumen of the catheter.
5. Obtain blood products from a blood bank. Transfuse as soon as possible after first performing **all the required safety checks.** QSEN	Once a blood product has been released from the blood bank, the product should be transfused as soon as possible (e.g., red blood cell transfusions should be completed within 4 hours of removal from refrigeration).
6. With another registered nurse, verify the patient by name and number, check blood compatibility, and note expiration time.	Human error is the most common cause of ABO incompatibility reactions.
During Infusion	
7. Administer the blood product using the appropriate filtered tubing.	Filters are needed to remove aggregates and possible contaminants.
8. Dilute blood products with only normal saline solution.	Hemolysis occurs if some other IV solution is used.
9. Remain with the patient during the first 15 to 30 minutes of the infusion.	Hemolytic reactions occur most often within the first 50 mL of the infusion.
10. Infuse the blood product at the prescribed rate.	Fluid overload is a potential complication of rapid infusion.
11. Monitor vital signs.	Vital sign changes often indicate transfusion reactions.
After Infusion	
12. When the transfusion is completed, discontinue infusion and dispose of the bag and tubing properly.	Bloodborne pathogens may be spread inadvertently through improper disposal.
13. Document.	The patient record should indicate the type of product infused, product number, volume infused, time of infusion, and any adverse reactions.

prescription for accuracy and completeness. In many hospitals, a separate consent form must be obtained from the patient before a transfusion is performed.

A blood specimen is obtained for type and crossmatch (testing of the donor's blood and the recipient's blood for compatibility). The procedures for obtaining this specimen are specified by hospital policy. Usually a new type-and-crossmatch specimen is required at least every 72 hours.

Both Y-tubing and straight tubing sets are used for blood component infusion (Fig. 40-7). A blood filter (about 170 μm) to remove sediment from the stored blood products is included with blood administration sets and must be used to transfuse most, but not all, blood products.

Use normal saline as the solution to administer with blood products, although this practice is not evidence-based (Kessler, 2013). Ringer's lactate and dextrose in water are not used for infusion with blood products because they may cause clotting or hemolysis of blood cells, although there is not sufficient evidence of hemolysis when using hypotonic fluids (Elgin et al., 2011; Kessler, 2013; Kessler et al., 2012; Tolich et al., 2013).

! NURSING SAFETY PRIORITY QSEN

Action Alert

Never add to or infuse other drugs with blood products because they may clot the blood during transfusion.

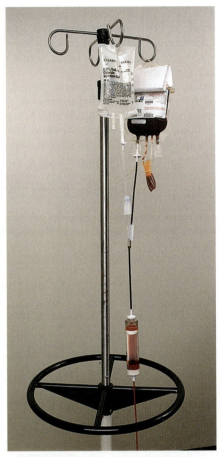

FIG. 40-7 Blood administration setup.

Before the transfusion, in compliance with recommendations by The Joint Commission's National Patient Safety Goals (NPSGs), the priority action is to determine that the blood component delivered is correct and that identification of the patient is correct. Check the physician's prescription together with another registered nurse to determine the patient's identity and whether the hospital identification band name and number are identical to those on the blood component tag. According to The Joint Commission's National Patient Safety Goals, *the patient's room number is not an acceptable form of identification.* Some facilities use a bar code–point of care (BC-POC) system, similar to drug dispensing systems, in an attempt to improve patient safety and reduce identification errors.

! NURSING SAFETY PRIORITY QSEN
Action Alert

The nurse who will be actually administering the blood products must be one of the two professionals comparing the patient's identification with the information on the blood component bag.

Examine the blood bag label, the attached tag, and the requisition slip to ensure that the ABO and Rh types are compatible with those of the patient. Check the expiration date, and inspect the product for discoloration, gas bubbles, or cloudiness, which are all indicators of bacterial growth or hemolysis.

Transfusion Responsibilities

Before starting the transfusion, explain the procedure to the patient. Assess vital signs and temperature immediately before starting the infusion. Begin the infusion slowly. *Remain with the patient for the first 15 to 30 minutes.* Any severe reaction usually occurs with infusion of the first 50 mL of blood. Ask the patient to report unusual sensations such as chills, shortness of breath, hives, or itching. Assess vital signs 15 minutes after starting the infusion for indications of a reaction. If there are none, the rate can be increased to transfuse 1 unit in 2 hours (depending on the patient's cardiac status and the facility's policy for rate of administration). Take vital signs every hour during the transfusion or as specified by the agency's policy. Some facilities are now continuously monitoring patients during transfusions using a wireless remote monitoring device (Card et al., 2012).

Blood components without large amounts of RBCs can be infused more quickly. The identification checks are the same as for RBC transfusions. It may be necessary to infuse blood products at a slower rate for older patients. Best practices related to the nursing care needs of older patients during transfusion therapy are listed in Chart 40-13.

Electrolyte imbalances are possible as a result of transfusions, especially with packed red blood cells or with whole blood. During transfusions, some cells are damaged, releasing potassium and raising the patient's serum potassium level above normal (hyperkalemia). This problem is more likely when the blood being transfused has been frozen or is several weeks old.

Types of Transfusions

At one time, transfusion with whole blood was the most common form of transfusion therapy. Today, whole-blood transfusions are extremely rare (AABB [formerly called the American Association of Blood Banks], 2013). When a whole-blood donation is made, it is centrifuged on arrival at the

TABLE 40-7 **Compatibility Chart for Red Blood Cell Transfusions**

DONOR	RECIPIENT			
	A	B	AB	O
A	X		X	
B		X	X	
AB			X	
O	X	X	X	X

blood-banking facility and separated in to various components. The individual components are then transfused according to patients' specific needs.

Red Blood Cell Transfusions

RBCs are given to replace cells lost from trauma or surgery. Patients with problems that destroy RBCs or impair RBC maturation also may receive RBC transfusions. Packed RBCs, supplied in 250-mL bags, are a concentrated source of RBCs and are the most common component given to RBC-deficient patients.

Blood transfusions are actually transplantations of tissue from one person to another. Therefore the donor and recipient blood must be carefully checked for compatibility to prevent lethal reactions (Table 40-7). Compatibility is determined by two different antigen systems (cell surface proteins): the ABO system antigens and the Rh antigen, present on the membranes of RBCs.

RBC antigens are inherited. For the ABO system, a person inherits one of these:
- A antigen (type A blood)
- B antigen (type B blood)
- Both A and B antigens (type AB blood)
- Neither A nor B antigens (type O blood)

People develop circulating antibodies against the blood type antigens they did not inherit. For example, a person with type A blood forms antibodies against type B blood. A person with type O blood has not inherited either A or B antigens and will form antibodies against RBCs with either A or B antigens. If RBCs that have an antigen are infused into a recipient who does not share that antigen, the infused blood is recognized by the recipient's antibodies as non-self and the recipient then has a reaction to the transfused products.

The Rh antigen system is slightly different. An Rh-negative person is born without the Rh-antigen on his or her RBCs and does not form antibodies unless specifically sensitized to it. Sensitization can occur with RBC transfusions from an Rh-positive person or from exposure during pregnancy and birth. Once an Rh-negative person has been sensitized and antibodies develop, any exposure to Rh-positive blood can cause a transfusion reaction. Antibody development can be prevented by giving anti-Rh-immunoglobulin (RHoGAM) as soon as exposure to the Rh antigen is suspected. *People who have Rh-positive blood can receive an RBC transfusion from an Rh-negative donor, but Rh-negative people should not receive Rh-positive blood.*

Platelet Transfusions

Platelets are given to patients with platelet counts below 10,000/mm³ and to patients with thrombocytopenia who are actively bleeding or are scheduled for an invasive procedure. Platelet transfusions are pooled from as many as 10 donors and do not

have to be of the same blood type as the patient has. For patients who are having a hematopoietic stem cell transplantation (HSCT) or who need multiple platelet transfusions, platelets from a single donor may be prescribed, which reduces the chances of allergic reactions.

Platelet infusion bags usually contain 300 mL for pooled platelets and 200 mL for single-donor platelets. Platelets are fragile and must be infused immediately after being brought to the patient's room, usually over a 15- to 30-minute period. A special transfusion set with a smaller filter and shorter tubing is used. Additional platelet filters help remove white blood cells (WBCs) from the platelets for patients who have a history of febrile reactions or who need multiple platelet transfusions.

> **! NURSING SAFETY PRIORITY** (QSEN)
> *Action Alert*
>
> When infusing platelets, do not use the standard blood administration set because the filter traps the platelets and the longer tubing increases platelet adherence to the lumen.

Take the vital signs before the infusion, 15 minutes after the infusion starts, and at its completion. A patient who has had a transfusion reaction in the past may be given diphenhydramine (Benadryl) and acetaminophen (Tylenol) before the transfusion to reduce the fever and severe chills (rigors) that often occur during platelet transfusions.

Plasma Transfusions

Plasma infusions may be given fresh to replace blood volume and CLOTTING factors. More often, plasma is frozen immediately after donation, forming fresh frozen plasma (FFP). Infuse FFP immediately after thawing while the clotting factors are still active.

ABO compatibility is required for transfusion of plasma products because the plasma contains the donor's ABO antibodies that could react with the recipient's RBC antigens. The infusion bag contains about 200 mL. Infuse FFP as rapidly as the patient can tolerate, generally over a 30- to 60-minute period, through a regular Y set or straight filtered tubing.

Granulocyte (White Blood Cell) Transfusions

Rarely, neutropenic patients with INFECTIONS receive white blood cell (WBC) replacement transfusions. WBC surfaces have many antigens that can cause severe reactions when infused into a patient whose immune system recognizes these antigens as non-self.

WBCs are suspended in 400 mL of plasma and should be infused slowly, usually over a 45- to 60-minute period depending on the concentration of cells being infused. Agency policies often require stricter monitoring of patients receiving WBCs because reactions are more common. A physician may need to be present in the hospital unit, and vital signs may need to be taken every 15 minutes throughout the transfusion. Amphotericin B infusion should be separated from WBC transfusions by 4 to 6 hours.

Acute Transfusion Reactions

Patients can develop any of these transfusion reactions: febrile, hemolytic, allergic, or bacterial reactions; circulatory overload; or transfusion-associated graft-versus-host disease (GVHD). To prevent complications, remain alert during transfusions to detect early reactions and initiate appropriate management.

Febrile transfusion reactions occur most often in the patient with anti-WBC antibodies, which can develop after multiple transfusions, white blood cell transfusions, and platelet transfusions. The patient develops chills, tachycardia, fever, hypotension, and tachypnea. Giving leukocyte-reduced blood or single-donor HLA-matched platelets reduces the risk for this type of reaction. WBC filters may be used to trap WBCs and prevent their infusion into the patient.

Hemolytic transfusion reactions are caused by blood type or Rh incompatibility. When blood containing antigens different from the patient's own antigens is infused, antigen-antibody complexes are formed in his or her blood. These complexes destroy the transfused cells and start inflammatory responses in the blood vessel walls and organs. The reaction may be mild, with fever and chills, or life threatening, with disseminated intravascular coagulation (DIC) and circulatory collapse (McCance et al., 2014). Other manifestations include:

- Apprehension
- Headache
- Chest pain
- Low back pain
- Tachycardia
- Tachypnea
- Hypotension
- Hemoglobinuria
- A sense of impending doom

The onset of a hemolytic reaction may be immediate or may not occur until subsequent units have been transfused (Kessler et al., 2012).

Allergic transfusion reactions (anaphylactic transfusion reactions) are most often seen in patients with other allergies. They may have urticaria, itching, bronchospasm, or anaphylaxis. Onset usually occurs during or up to 24 hours after the transfusion. Patients with an allergy history can be given leukocyte-reduced or washed RBCs in which the WBCs, plasma, and immunoglobulin A have been removed, reducing the possibility of an allergic reaction.

Bacterial transfusion reactions occur from infusion of contaminated blood products, especially those contaminated with a gram-negative organism. Manifestations include tachycardia, hypotension, fever, chills, and shock. The onset of a bacterial transfusion reaction is rapid. (See Chapter 37 for care of the patient with septic shock.)

Circulatory overload can occur when a blood product is infused too quickly, especially in an older adult. This is most common with whole-blood transfusions or when the patient receives multiple packed RBC transfusions. Manifestations include:

- Hypertension
- Bounding pulse
- Distended jugular veins
- Dyspnea
- Restlessness
- Confusion

You can both manage and prevent this complication by monitoring intake and output, infusing blood products more slowly, and giving diuretics. (See Chapter 11 for management of patients with fluid overload.)

Transfusion-associated graft-versus-host disease (TA-GVHD) is a rare but life-threatening problem that occurs more often in an immunosuppressed patient. Its cause in immunosuppressed patients is similar to that of GVHD that occurs with allogeneic stem cell transplantation, discussed on p. 811, in which donor T-cell lymphocytes attack host tissues.

Manifestations usually occur within 1 to 2 weeks and include thrombocytopenia, anorexia, nausea, vomiting, chronic hepatitis, weight loss, and recurrent INFECTION.

TA-GVHD has an 80% to 90% mortality rate but can be prevented by using irradiated blood products. Irradiation destroys T-cells and their cytokine products.

Transfusion-related acute lung injury (TRALI) is a life-threatening event that occurs most often when donor blood contains antibodies against the recipient's neutrophil antigens, HLA, or both (Kessler et al., 2012). Common manifestations are a rapid onset of dyspnea and hypoxia within 6 hours of the transfusion.

Acute pain transfusion reaction or APTR is a recently identified but rare event that can occur during or shortly after transfusion of any blood product. Its actual pathophysiology has not yet been elucidated. The manifestations are severe chest pain, back pain, joint pain, hypertension, and redness of the head and neck (Hardwick et al., 2013). Most patients also have anxiety. The reaction does not appear to be life threatening, and most patients respond well with drugs for pain and rigors. Although the manifestations are general, diagnosis can be supported with a positive direct antibody test (DAT), indicating that some degree of hemolysis has occurred but is not widespread. APTR management focuses on patient support and drugs to control or reduce manifestations.

Interventions for transfusion reactions occurring during transfusion (hemolytic reactions, allergic reactions, and bacterial reactions) begin with stopping the transfusion and removing the blood tubing. (For hemolytic and suspected bacterial reactions, return the component bag, labels, and all tubing to the blood bank or laboratory.) Notify the Rapid Response Team. If the patient has no other IV access, keep the access and flush with normal saline. *Do not flush the contents of the blood transfusion tubing, which would allow more of the reaction-causing blood to enter the patient.* Usually oxygen is applied and diphenhydramine (Benadryl) is administered by IV push. If manifestations of shock are present, fluid resuscitation and hemodynamic monitoring are needed. Blood pressure support with vasopressors may be needed (see Chapter 37). Other drug therapy is supportive, such as antipyretics for fever, antibiotics for suspected bacterial contamination, and meperidine for rigors.

Autologous Blood Transfusions

Autologous blood transfusions involve collection and infusion of the patient's own blood. This type of transfusion eliminates compatibility problems and reduces the risk for transmitting bloodborne diseases. The four types of autologous blood transfusions are preoperative autologous blood donation, acute normovolemic hemodilution, intraoperative autologous transfusion, and postoperative blood salvage.

Autologous blood donation before surgery is the most common type of autologous blood transfusion. It involves collecting whole blood from the patient (who must meet certain criteria), dividing it into components, and storing it for later use. As long as hematocrit and hemoglobin levels are within a safe range, the patient can donate blood on a weekly basis until the prescribed amount of blood is obtained. Fresh packed RBCs may be stored for 40 days. For patients with rare blood types, blood may be frozen for up to 10 years.

Acute normovolemic hemodilution involves withdrawal of a patient's RBCs and volume replacement just before a surgical procedure. The goal is to decrease RBC loss during surgery. The blood is stored at room temperature for up to 6 hours and reinfused after surgery. This type of autologous transfusion is not used with anemic patients or those with poor kidney function.

Intraoperative autologous transfusion and blood salvage after surgery are the recovery and reinfusion of a patient's own blood from an operative field or from a bleeding wound. Special devices collect, filter, and drain the blood into a transfusion bag. This blood is used for trauma or surgical patients with severe blood loss. The salvaged blood must be reinfused within 6 hours.

Transfuse autologous blood products using the guidelines previously described. Although the patient receiving autologous blood is not at risk for some types of transfusion reactions, circulatory overload or bacterial transfusion reactions can still occur and are managed in the same way they are managed in transfusions derived from donors.

🔑 NCLEX EXAMINATION CHALLENGE
Safe and Effective Care Environment

The nurse who just came on duty observes that the client, whose blood type is AB negative, is receiving a transfusion with type O negative packed red blood cells. What is the nurse's best first action?
A. Call the blood bank.
B. Take and record the client's vital signs.
C. Stop the transfusion and keep the IV open.
D. Document the observation as the only action.

NURSING CONCEPTS AND CLINICAL JUDGMENT REVIEW

What might you NOTICE if the patient is experiencing inadequate GAS EXCHANGE and PERFUSION as a result of hematologic problems?
- Skin cyanosis or pallor (in patients with light skin)
- Cyanosis or pallor of the lips and oral mucous membranes
- Tachycardia
- Tachypnea and dyspnea
- Slow capillary refill
- Cool to cold extremities
- Change in cognition, acute confusion
- Decreased oxygen saturation
- Decreased urine output
- Presence of bruises or petechiae
- Bleeding of gums, at IV sites, at injection sites

What should you INTERPRET and how should you RESPOND to this patient experiencing inadequate GAS EXCHANGE and PERFUSION as a result of a hematologic problem?

Perform and interpret physical assessment, including:
- Taking vital signs
- Monitoring oxygen saturation by pulse oximetry
- Checking for blood in stool, urine, emesis
- Checking for bleeding in the mouth, around IV sites, drains, urinary catheters
- Checking most recent laboratory values for hematocrit and hemoglobin levels and platelet and RBC counts
- Assessing cognition

Respond by:
- Applying oxygen
- Keeping the patient's head elevated to about 30 degrees
- Handling the patient gently
- Keeping the patient warm (blankets)
- Applying firm pressure to areas actively bleeding
- Notifying physician or Rapid Response Team
- Instituting Bleeding Precautions
- Maintaining or initiating IV therapy
- Preparing to administer blood or blood products
- Prioritizing and pacing activities to prevent fatigue

On what should you REFLECT?
- Observe patient for evidence of restored tissue perfusion (see Chapter 39)
- Think about what may have precipitated this episode and what steps could be taken to identify it earlier.

GET READY FOR THE NCLEX® EXAMINATION!

KEY POINTS

Review these Key Points for each NCLEX Examination Client Needs Category.

Safe and Effective Care Environment
- Use aseptic technique during all central line dressing changes or any invasive procedure. **Safety** QSEN
- Use good handwashing techniques before providing any care to a patient who is either immunocompromised or immune deficient. **Safety** QSEN
- Modify the environment to protect patients who have thrombocytopenia. **Safety** QSEN
- Use Bleeding Precautions for any patient with thrombocytopenia or pancytopenia (see Chart 40-7). **Safety** QSEN
- Ensure informed consent is obtained before any invasive procedure or transfusion. **Safety** QSEN
- Verify with another registered nurse prescriptions for transfusion of blood products. **Safety** QSEN
- Use at least two forms of identification for the patient who is to receive a blood product transfusion (e.g., name, birthdate, identification number). **Safety** QSEN

Health Promotion and Maintenance
- Teach patients with sickle cell disease to avoid conditions that are known to trigger crises. **Patient-Centered Care** QSEN

- Teach people to avoid unnecessary contact with environmental chemicals or toxins. If contact cannot be avoided, teach people to use safety precautions.
- Identify patients at high risk for INFECTION because of disease or therapy. **Patient-Centered Care** QSEN
- Teach the patient and family about the manifestations of INFECTION and when to seek medical advice. **Patient-Centered Care** QSEN
- Instruct patients who have anemia as a result of dietary deficiency which foods are good sources of iron, folic acid, and vitamin B_{12}. **Patient-Centered Care** QSEN
- Teach precautions to take to avoid injury (see Chart 40-11) to patients at risk for poor CLOTTING and increased bleeding. **Patient-Centered Care** QSEN

Psychosocial Integrity

- Allow the patient the opportunity to express his or her feelings regarding the diagnosis of leukemia or lymphoma or the treatment regimen. **Patient-Centered Care** QSEN
- Explain all procedures, restrictions, drugs, and follow-up care to the patient and family. **Patient-Centered Care** QSEN
- Offer alternative therapies for relaxation, pain reduction, and distraction, such as massage, music therapy, and guided imagery. **Patient-Centered Care** QSEN
- Reassure patients having pain that using opioid analgesics for needed pain relief is not drug abuse. **Patient-Centered Care** QSEN

Physiological Integrity

- Pace nonurgent health care activities to reduce the risk for fatigue among patients with anemia or pancytopenia. **Patient-Centered Care** QSEN
- Assess patients in the induction phase of chemotherapy, those after HSCT, and anyone with neutropenia every 8 hours for manifestations of INFECTION. **Evidence-Based Practice** QSEN
- Assess the skin integrity of the perianal region of a patient with leukemia or profound neutropenia after every bowel movement. **Patient-Centered Care** QSEN
- Administer analgesics on a schedule rather than PRN. **Evidence-Based Practice** QSEN
- Use normal saline as the solution infusing with blood products.
- Transfuse blood products more slowly to older patients or those who have a cardiac problem. **Patient-Centered Care** QSEN
- Remain with the patient during the first 15 minutes of infusion of any blood product. **Safety** QSEN
- Do not administer any drugs with infusing blood products. **Evidence-Based Practice** QSEN
- Make referrals to support groups sponsored by organizations such as the Sickle Cell Foundation Support Group, American Cancer Society, Leukemia and Lymphoma Society of America, and the National Hemophilia Foundation. **Teamwork and Collaboration** QSEN

Mobility, Sensory Perception, and Cognition

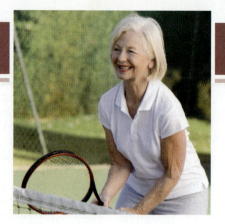

The term *mobility* means movement. When referring to physical MOBILITY, it means the ability of the body to purposely move (Giddens, 2013). MOBILITY is needed for ADL performance and many body functions, including digestion, elimination, circulation, and muscle integrity. In some cases, it helps keep a person *safe* by being able to move to prevent injury.

MOBILITY is accomplished primarily through the integration of the neurologic and musculoskeletal body systems. Risk factors for decreased MOBILITY are typically acute and chronic health problems that cause pain or injury (Giddens, 2013).

SENSORY PERCEPTION refers to receiving sensory input from the cells of the skin (feeling), eyes (seeing), and ears (hearing) and accurately interpreting this input in the neurons of the central nervous system (CNS). Therefore SENSORY PERCEPTION is also needed to keep the body *safe*. For example, if a person cannot feel water temperature, a burn may result. If vision is impaired, a fall may occur.

COGNITION refers to mental processes and intellectual function and is controlled by certain neurons in the gray matter of the brain. These cells are very sensitive to serum glucose and oxygen levels. If either of these substances falls below the amounts needed, the cells cannot function properly, resulting in diminished cognitive ability and a decreased level of consciousness.

One or all of these three concepts may be impaired as a result of disease, injury, surgery, or drugs. Problems of the neurologic, sensory, and musculoskeletal systems most commonly affect the need for MOBILITY, SENSORY PERCEPTION, and COGNITION. The interrelationship of these concepts can be compared to a computer and its parts.

As seen in Fig. 1, the computer's central processing unit (CPU), or processor, is the brain of the machine (the *cognitive* center). Much like the spinal cord, it works with the motherboard to send and receive messages (input and output). The connected pins and wires function like the spinal nerves. Peripherals such as the mouse and keyboard are similar in function to the peripheral nervous system (PNS) (SENSORY PERCEPTION) and musculoskeletal system (MOBILITY). When all of these parts are working properly, the computer functions without any problems.

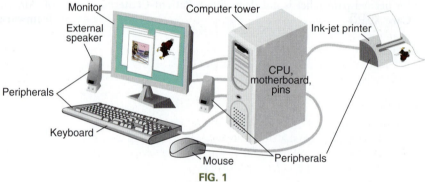

FIG. 1

However, when the CPU (brain) does not work properly (decreased COGNITION), the motherboard (spinal cord) and/or peripherals (PNS and muscles) may not function as they should (decreased MOBILITY and SENSORY PERCEPTION). If the motherboard (spinal cord) is broken, no information is sent to or from any of the other parts of the computer. In both cases, there is no display on the monitor (Fig. 2).

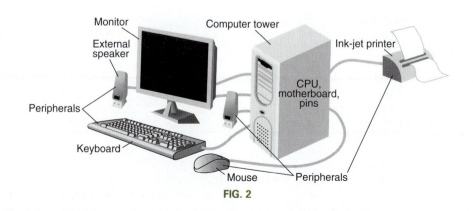

FIG. 2

CHAPTER **41**

Assessment of the Nervous System

Rachel L. Gallagher

 http://evolve.elsevier.com/Iggy/

PRIORITY CONCEPTS

- COGNITION
- MOBILITY

- SENSORY PERCEPTION

LEARNING OUTCOMES

Safe and Effective Care Environment
1. Collaborate with health care team members to establish priorities in neurologic assessment.

Health Promotion and Maintenance
2. Identify factors such as risky behaviors or lifestyle choices that place patients at risk for neurologic health problems.
3. Detect neurologic health problems early with health screening and physical assessment strategies.

Psychosocial Integrity
4. Explain psychological responses to neurologic health problems.

Physiological Integrity
5. Document findings from the neurologic history and physical examination to identify new and chronic changes in COGNITION, MOBILITY, and SENSORY PERCEPTION.

6. Perform a comprehensive and a rapid focused neurologic examination to manage conditions and promote patient safety related to impaired neurologic function.
7. Use interventions to provide assistance in the performance of activities of daily living when neurologic conditions interfere with self-care.
8. Reduce complications from diagnostic testing by determining risk factors for adverse reaction to contrast media.
9. Review neurologic anatomy and physiology to identify changes that result in health alterations.
10. Describe common physiologic changes associated with aging that affect the nervous system.

The major divisions of the nervous system are the central nervous system (CNS) and peripheral nervous system (PNS). The PNS is further divided into the somatic and autonomic systems. These systems work together to control COGNITION, MOBILITY, and SENSORY PERCEPTION. The nervous system interacts with the endocrine system to balance fluid and electrolytes. In addition, through the autonomic nervous system (ANS), it innervates many other body systems including the reproductive and digestive organs to promote their function. For example, the sacral spinal nerves (part of the ANS) stimulate the detrusor muscle to contract when the urinary bladder is full, contributing to elimination.

Health problems involving trauma and diseases of the nervous system can impair fluid and electrolyte balance, thermoregulation, elimination, and many other functions. One of the earliest and most sensitive functions that signal new-onset brain disorders is COGNITION, a term used to refer to all the processes in human thought. The primary role of the nurse is to help restore these human needs or assist the patient adapt to their deficits and avoid complications from dysfunction.

ANATOMY AND PHYSIOLOGY REVIEW

The CNS is composed of the brain and the spinal cord. The brain is contained within the cranium; the brain's role is to direct the regulation and function of the nervous system and other systems of the body. The spinal cord is lodged in the vertebral canal. From the brain, the spinal cord descends down the middle of the back and is surrounded and protected by the bony vertebral column. The spinal cord is surrounded by a clear fluid called *cerebrospinal fluid (CSF)* that protects the delicate nerve tissues against damage from banging against the inside of the vertebrae.

The PNS is composed of 12 pairs of cranial nerves, 31 pairs of spinal nerves, and the autonomic nervous system. The autonomic nervous system is further subdivided into sympathetic and parasympathetic fibers.

The nervous system contains two types of cells: neurons, which transmit or conduct nerve impulses; and neuroglia cells, which have an interdependent role with the neuron.

Nervous System Cells: Structure and Function

Two types of cells make up the nervous system: neurons and neuroglia cells. The basic unit of the nervous system, the **neuron**, transmits impulses, or "messages." Some neurons are **motor** (causing purposeful physical movement or MOBILITY), and some are **sensory** (resulting in the ability to perceive stimulation through one's sensory organs or SENSORY PERCEPTION). Some process information and some retain information. When a neuron receives an impulse from another neuron, the effect may be excitation or inhibition. Each neuron has a *cell body,* or *soma;* short, branching processes called *dendrites;* and a single *axon* (Fig. 41-1).

Afferent neurons, also known as *sensory neurons,* are specialized to send impulses toward the CNS, away from the PNS. *Efferent* neurons are motor nerve cells that carry signals from the CNS to the cells in the PNS. Each dendrite synapses with another cell body, axon, or dendrite and sends impulses along the efferent and afferent neuron pathways.

Many axons are covered by a **myelin sheath**—a white, lipid covering. Myelinated axons appear whitish and therefore are also called **white matter**. Nonmyelinated axons have a grayish cast and are called **gray matter**. Myelinated axons have gaps in the myelin called *nodes of Ranvier.* The nodes of Ranvier play a major role in impulse conduction (see Fig. 41-1). When the myelin is impaired, the impulses cannot travel from the brain to the rest of the body, such as in patients with multiple sclerosis.

The enlarged distal end of each axon is called the *synaptic* or *terminal knob.* Within the synaptic knobs are the mechanisms for manufacturing, storing, and releasing a transmitter substance. Each neuron produces a specific **neurotransmitter** chemical (e.g., acetylcholine or serotonin) that can either enhance or inhibit the impulse but cannot do both. Other substances, although not specifically identified as neurotransmitters, are considered probable transmitters or neuromodulators.

Impulses are transmitted to their eventual destination through synapses, or spaces between neurons. There are two distinct types of synapses: *neuron to neuron* and *neuron to muscle* (or gland). Between the terminal knob and the next cell is a small space called the *synaptic cleft.* The knob, the cleft, and the portion of the cell to which the impulse is being transmitted make up the **synapse.**

Neuroglia cells, which vary in size and shape, provide protection, structure, and nutrition for the neurons. They are classified into four types: astroglial cells, ependymal cells, oligodendrocytes, and microglial cells. These cells are also part of the blood-brain barrier and help regulate cerebrospinal fluid (CSF).

Central Nervous System: Structure and Function

The central nervous system (CNS) is composed of the *brain,* which directs the regulation and function of the nervous system and all other systems of the body, and the *spinal cord,* which starts reflex activity and transmits impulses to and from the brain.

Brain

The **meninges** form the protective covering of the brain and the spinal cord. The outside layer is the *dura mater.* The **subdural space** is located between the dura mater and the middle layer, the *arachnoid.* The *pia mater* is the most inner layer. Situated between the arachnoid and pia mater is the **subarachnoid space,** where CSF circulates. A potential space, referred to as the *epidural space,* is located between the skull and the outer layer of the dura mater. This area also extends down the spinal cord and is used for the delivery of epidural analgesia and anesthesia.

The dura mater also lies between the cerebral hemispheres and the cerebellum and is called the *tentorium.* It helps decrease or prevents the transmission of force from one hemisphere to another and protects the lower brainstem when head trauma occurs. Clinical references may be made to a lesion (e.g., a tumor) as being **supratentorial** (above the tentorium) or **infratentorial** (below the tentorium).

Major Parts of the Brain. The brain consists of three main areas—the brainstem, the cerebellum, and the forebrain. The *brainstem* connects the rest of the brain with the CNS. It is concerned primarily with life support and basic functions such as movement.

The *cerebellum* is concerned with coordination of movement and works together with the brainstem to focus on the functionality of the muscles. This structure is found below the occipital lobe and adjacent to the brainstem.

The *forebrain* lies above the brainstem and cerebellum and is the most advanced in evolution. This area of the brain is further divided into three areas—the diencephalon, the cerebrum, and the cerebral cortex.

The *diencephalon,* which lies below the cerebrum, includes the thalamus, hypothalamus, and epithalamus (Fig. 41-2). The **thalamus** is the major "relay station," or "central switchboard," for the CNS. The **hypothalamus** plays a major role in autonomic nervous system control (controlling temperature and other functions) and COGNITION. The epithalamus contains the roof of the third ventricle and the pineal gland. The

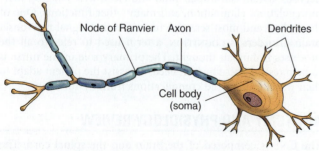

FIG. 41-1 The structure of a typical neuron.

Node of Ranvier   Axon   Dendrites

Cell body (soma)

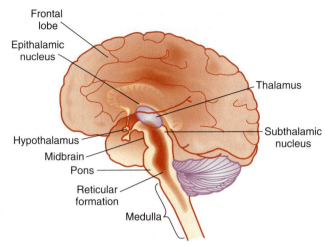

Frontal lobe
Epithalamic nucleus
Thalamus
Subthalamic nucleus
Hypothalamus
Midbrain
Pons
Reticular formation
Medulla

FIG. 41-2 The structures of the brainstem and diencephalon.

epithalamus connects the pathways to regulate emotion. Pathways through the epithalamus also contribute to smooth voluntary motor function.

The *cerebrum* is the largest part of the brain and controls intelligence, creativity, and memory. The "gray matter" of the cerebrum is the central cortex—the center that receives information from the thalamus and all the lower areas of the brain. The cerebrum consists of two halves, referred to as the *right hemisphere* and the *left hemisphere*, which are joined by the corpus callosum. The *left* hemisphere is the dominant hemisphere in most people (even in many left-handed people). Within the deeper structures of the cerebrum are the right and left lateral ventricles. At the base of the cerebrum near the ventricles is a group of neurons called the *basal ganglia*, which help regulate motor function.

The *cerebral cortex* is part of the cerebrum and is involved with almost all of the higher functions of the brain. This part of the brain processes and communicates all information coming from the peripheral nervous system (PNS). It also translates the impulses into understandable feelings and thoughts. The cerebral cortex is so complex that it is further divided into four lobes—the frontal lobe, parietal lobe, temporal lobe, and occipital lobe.

The frontal lobe is found at the front of the head near the temples and forehead. It processes voluntary muscle movements and higher functioning actions such as thought and speech. It also helps control mood, planning for the future, setting goals, and making judgments. The parietal lobe is found behind the frontal lobe. It processes spatial awareness and receives and processes information about temperature, taste, touch, and movement coming from the rest of the body. Reading and arithmetic are also processed in this lobe. The temporal lobes are located in the area of the brain parallel to the ears. They process hearing, memory, and language functions. The occipital lobe is located in the posterior of the brain and assists in the processing of visual information.

Located in the frontal lobe, the **motor cortex** controls voluntary movement. Corticospinal tracts, also called *pyramidal tracts,* begin in the motor cortex and travel through the brain before crossing in the medulla. This crossing explains how right motor cortex damage affects the movement in the left side of the body and vice versa, such as in many patients who have cerebral strokes. The cerebrum is divided into lobes by sulci

TABLE 41-1 Cerebral Lobe Main Functions

Frontal Lobe
- The primary motor area (also known as the *motor "strip"* or *cortex*)
- Broca's speech center on the dominant side
- Voluntary eye movement
- Access to current sensory data
- Access to past information or experience
- Affective response to a situation
- Regulates behavior based on judgment and foresight
- Judgment
- Ability to develop long-term goals
- Reasoning, concentration, abstraction

Parietal Lobe
- Understand sensory input such as texture, size, shape, and spatial relationships
- Three-dimensional (spatial) perception
- Important for singing, playing musical instruments, and processing nonverbal visual experiences
- Perception of body parts and body position awareness
- Taste impulses for interpretation

Temporal Lobe
- Auditory center for sound interpretation
- Complicated memory patterns
- Wernicke's area for speech

Occipital Lobe
- Primary visual center

Limbic Lobe
- Emotional and visceral patterns connected with survival
- Learning and memory

(fissures). These lobes work together and are connected by nerve fibers. The name and main functions of cerebral lobes are listed in Table 41-1.

Two important speech areas of the cerebrum are Broca's area and Wernicke's area. **Broca's area** (speech area), also located in the frontal lobe, is responsible for the formation of words, or speech. **Wernicke's area** (language area) is located in the temporal lobe and allows processing of words into coherent thought and understanding of written or spoken words.

The *hypophysis (pituitary gland)* has two lobes, each releasing specific hormones into the circulation under the regulation of the hypothalamus. The pituitary is often referred to as the "master gland" because of its control of numerous hormonal functions. However, the hypothalamus actually controls its functions.

The *cerebellum* receives immediate and continuous information about the condition of the muscles, joints, and tendons. Cerebellar function enables a person to:
- Keep an extremity from overshooting an intended target
- Move from one skilled movement to another in an orderly sequence
- Predict distance or gauge the speed with which one is approaching an object
- Control voluntary movement
- Maintain equilibrium

Unlike the motor cortex, cerebellar control of the body is **ipsilateral** (situated on the same side). The right side of the cerebellum controls the right side of the body, and the left cerebellum controls the left side of the body.

The brainstem includes the midbrain, pons, and medulla. The functions of these structures are presented in Table 41-2. Throughout the brainstem are special cells that constitute the **reticular activating system (RAS)**, which controls awareness and alertness. For example, this tissue awakens a person from sleep when presented with a stimulus such as loud noise or pain or when it is time to awaken. The reticular formation area has many connections with the cerebrum, the rest of the brainstem, and the cerebellum.

Circulation in the Brain. Circulation in the brain originates from the carotid and vertebral arteries (Fig. 41-3). The internal carotid arteries branch into the anterior cerebral artery (ACA) and middle cerebral artery (MCA), the largest ones. The two posterior vertebral arteries become the basilar artery, which then divides into two posterior cerebral arteries. The anterior, middle, and posterior cerebral arteries are joined together by small communicating arteries to form a ring at the base of the brain known as the **circle of Willis**.

The *middle* cerebral artery supplies the lateral surface of the cerebrum from about the mid-temporal lobe upward (i.e., the area for hearing and upper body motor and sensory neurons). The *anterior* cerebral artery supplies the midline, or medial, aspect of the same area (i.e., the lower body motor and sensory neurons). The *posterior* cerebral arteries supply the area from the mid-temporal region down and back (occipital lobe), as well as much of the brainstem. When blood flow is interrupted in any of these arteries (e.g., by a clot), the area of the brain being supplied is affected and may not function as it should.

The *blood-brain barrier (BBB)* seems to exist because the endothelial cells of the cerebral capillaries are joined tightly together. This barrier keeps some substances in the bloodstream out of the cerebrospinal circulation and out of brain tissue. Substances that can pass through the BBB include oxygen, glucose, carbon dioxide, alcohol, anesthetics, and water. Large molecules such as albumin, any substance bound to albumin, and many antibiotics are prevented from crossing the barrier.

Cerebrospinal fluid (CSF) also circulates, surrounds, and cushions the brain and spinal cord. While moving through the subarachnoid space, the fluid is continuously produced by the choroid plexus, reabsorbed by the arachnoid villi, and then channeled into the superior sagittal sinus. Expanded areas of subarachnoid space, where there are large amounts of CSF, are called *cisterns.* The largest one is the lumbar cistern, the site of lumbar puncture, from the level of the second lumbar vertebra to the second sacral vertebra (L2-S2).

Spinal Cord

The spinal cord controls body movement (MOBILITY); regulates organ function; processes sensory information from the extremities, trunk, and many internal organs; and transmits information to and from the brain. It contains H-shaped **gray matter** (neuron cell bodies) that is surrounded by **white matter**

TABLE 41-2	**Brainstem Functions**

Medulla
- Cardiac-slowing center
- Respiratory center
- Cranial nerves IX (glossopharyngeal), X (vagus), XI (accessory), and XII (hypoglossal) emerge from the medulla, as do portions of cranial nerves VII (facial) and VIII (vestibulocochlear)

Pons
- Cardiac acceleration and vasoconstriction centers
- Pneumotaxic center helps control respiratory pattern and rate
- Four cranial nerves originate from the pons: V (trigeminal), VI (abducens), VII (facial), and VIII (vestibulocochlear)

Midbrain
- Contains the cerebral aqueduct or aqueduct of Sylvius
- Location of periaqueductal gray, which may abolish pain when stimulated
- Cranial nerve nuclei III (oculomotor) and IV (trochlear) located here

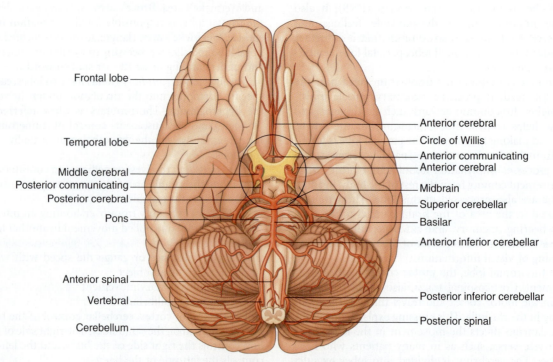

FIG. 41-3 Cerebral circulation and the circle of Willis at the base of the brain.

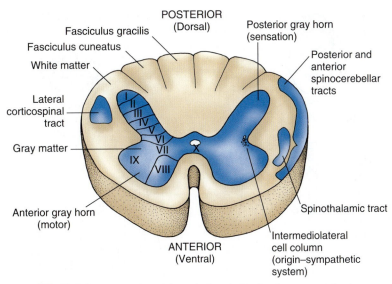

FIG. 41-4 A cross section of the spinal cord showing the common tracts.

(myelinated axons). The white matter is divided into posterior, lateral, and anterior columns. Groups of cells in the white matter (ascending and descending tracts) have been fairly well identified (Fig. 41-4).

Ascending Tracts. Ascending tracts originate in the spinal cord and end in the brain. Three groups of ascending tracts are important for understanding the patient with neurologic problems: spinothalamic tracts, spinocerebellar tracts, and fasciculi gracilis and cuneatus (posterior white columns).

As the name indicates, *spinothalamic* tracts begin in the spinal cord with most ending in the thalamus. These tracts carry SENSORY PERCEPTION of pain, temperature, light touch, and pressure. The axon fibers from the cells cross to the opposite side and then continue up to the thalamus. Some branches end in the medulla and pons.

Spinocerebellar tracts begin in the spinal cord and end in the cerebellum. The *posterior* spinocerebellar tract transmits impulses of **proprioception** (awareness of position and movements of body parts) or movement, mostly from the lower extremities. The impulses enter the posterior gray horn and synapse with tracts contained in the spinal cord. Spinocerebellar axons then connect on the *same,* or ipsilateral, side. These axons begin at the second lumbar level and ascend to the medulla and then, with additional synapses to neurons, to the cerebellum.

The *anterior* spinocerebellar tract begins lower in the lumbar spine than does the posterior tract. These fibers cross immediately and ascend as an opposite-side tract, transmitting proprioceptive impulses from the lower extremities. The fibers cross again in the midbrain on their way to the cerebellum. Because these fibers have crossed the midline twice, the sensations end on the side on which they started.

The *posterior white columns* transmit this information to the thalamus:
- The sensory perception of the position, location, and proprioception or orientation and movement of the body and its parts including muscles, joints, and tendons
- Vibratory sense
- Light touch from the skin
- Localization

Most of the fibers ascend on the *same* side as their origin to the medulla, where they cross and then synapse in the thalamus, with termination in the parietal lobe. This tract allows a person to feel an exact point of pressure on the skin. Recognition of pressure includes the shape of an object (with eyes closed), movement across the skin (a number being written), and awareness of two points of touch close together (two-point discrimination).

Descending Tracts. Descending tracts *begin* in the brain and *end* in the spinal cord. The major descending tract of importance for understanding neurologic problems is the lateral *corticospinal*, or *pyramidal*, tract. The corticospinal tract originates in the motor cortex of the frontal lobe and portions of the parietal lobe. The lateral tract fibers cross to the opposite side at the level of the medulla. After crossing, the fibers descend and synapse with interneurons of the gray matter in the spinal cord. These few fibers connect directly with lower motor neurons (LMNs). The cervical spine has a high concentration of fibers synapsing with interneurons, which possibly reflects the complexity of hand and finger movements.

The motor neurons of the other descending tracts and the basal ganglia used to be referred to as an *extrapyramidal system.* It was thought that pyramidal neurons caused voluntary muscle activity and that extrapyramidal neurons caused automatic or involuntary muscle action. However, all of the descending tracts and the basal ganglia are necessary for MOBILITY. The term *extrapyramidal* is still often used clinically, meaning *abnormal spontaneous movement.*

Peripheral Nervous System: Structure and Function

The peripheral nervous system (PNS) is composed of the spinal nerves, cranial nerves, and autonomic nervous system.

There are 31 pairs of spinal nerves (8 cervical, 12 thoracic, 5 lumbar, 5 sacral, and 1 coccygeal) exiting from the spinal cord. Each of the nerves has a posterior and an anterior branch. The posterior branch carries sensory information (SENSORY PERCEPTION) to the cord (*afferent pathway*). The anterior branch transmits motor impulses (MOBILITY) to the muscles of the body (*efferent pathway*).

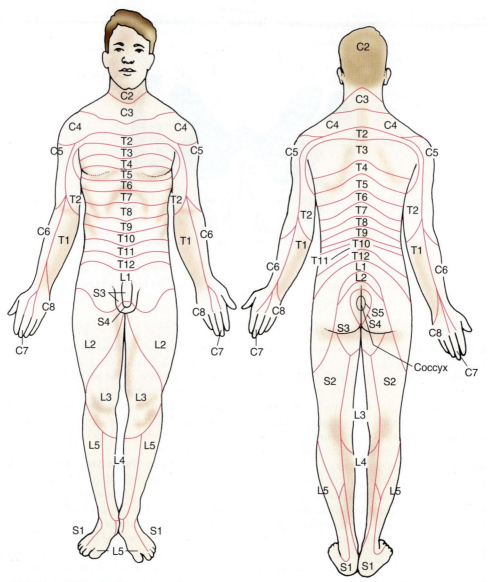

FIG. 41-5 Dermatomes (cutaneous innervation of spinal nerves). *C,* Cervical; *L,* lumbar; *S,* sacral; *T,* thoracic.

Each spinal nerve is responsible for the muscle innervation and sensory reception of a given area of the body. The cervical and thoracic spinal nerves are relatively close to their areas of responsibility, whereas the lumbar and sacral spinal nerves are some distance from theirs. Because the spinal cord ends between L1 and L2, the axons of the lumbar and sacral cord extend downward before exiting at the appropriate intervertebral foramen. The area controlled by each spinal nerve is roughly reflected in the dermatomes. Dermatomes represent sensory input from spinal nerves to specific areas of the skin (Fig. 41-5). For example, the patient with an injury to cervical spinal nerves C6 and C7 has sensory changes in the thumb, index finger, middle finger, middle of the palm, and back of the hand.

Sensory receptors throughout the body monitor and transmit impulses of pain, temperature, touch, vibration, pressure, visceral sensation, and proprioception. Sensory receptors also monitor and transmit the sensory perceptions of the special senses—vision, taste, smell, and hearing.

The cell bodies of the anterior spinal nerves are located in the anterior gray matter (anterior horn) of each level in the spinal cord. The anterior motor neurons are also referred to as *lower motor neurons.* As each nerve axon leaves the spinal cord, it joins other spinal nerves to form plexuses (clusters of nerves). Plexuses continue as trunks, divisions, and cords and finally branch into individual peripheral nerves.

The reflex arc is a closed circuit of spinal and peripheral nerves and therefore requires no control by the brain (Fig. 41-6).

Reflexes consist of sensory input from:
- Skeletal muscles, tendons, skin, organs, and special senses
- Small cells in the spinal cord lying between the posterior and anterior gray matter (interneurons)
- Anterior motor neurons, along with the muscles they innervate

There are 12 *cranial nerves.* Their number, name, origin, type, and function are summarized in Table 41-3. Cranial nerve function is an important part of the nursing assessment of the patient with a neurologic problem. For example, cranial nerves II, III, IV, and VI are important for assessment of the patient with a stroke or traumatic brain injury.

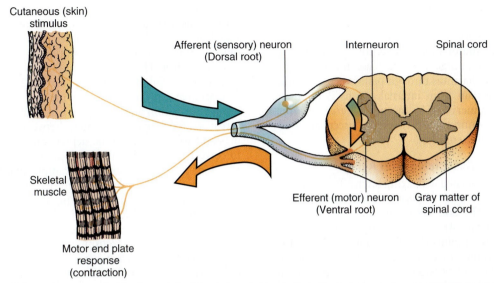

FIG. 41-6 An example of reflex activity. Stimulation of skin results in involuntary muscle contraction (reflex arc).

TABLE 41-3 Origins, Types, and Functions of the Cranial Nerves

CRANIAL NERVE	ORIGIN	TYPE	FUNCTION
I: Olfactory	Olfactory bulb	Sensory	Smell
II: Optic	Midbrain	Sensory	Central and peripheral vision
III: Oculomotor	Midbrain	Motor to eye muscles	Eye movement via medial and lateral rectus and inferior oblique and superior rectus muscles; lid elevation via the levator muscle
		Parasympathetic-motor	Pupil constriction; ciliary muscles
IV: Trochlear	Lower midbrain	Motor	Eye movement via superior oblique muscles
V: Trigeminal	Pons	Sensory	Sensory perception from skin of face and scalp and mucous membranes of mouth and nose
		Motor	Muscles of mastication (chewing)
VI: Abducens	Inferior pons	Motor	Eye movement via lateral rectus muscles
VII: Facial	Inferior pons	Sensory	Pain and temperature from ear area; deep sensations from the face; taste from anterior two thirds of the tongue
		Motor	Muscles of the face and scalp
		Parasympathetic-motor	Lacrimal, submandibular, and sublingual salivary glands
VIII: Vestibulocochlear	Pons-medulla junction	Sensory	Hearing Equilibrium
IX: Glossopharyngeal	Medulla	Sensory	Pain and temperature from ear; taste and sensations from posterior one third of tongue and pharynx
		Motor	Skeletal muscles of the throat
		Parasympathetic-motor	Parotid glands
X: Vagus	Medulla	Sensory	Pain and temperature from ear; sensations from pharynx, larynx, thoracic and abdominal viscera
		Motor	Muscles of the soft palate, larynx, and pharynx
		Parasympathetic-motor	Thoracic and abdominal viscera; cells of secretory glands; cardiac and smooth muscle innervation to the level of the splenic flexure
XI: Accessory	Medulla (anterior gray horn of the cervical spine)	Motor	Skeletal muscles of the pharynx and larynx and sternocleidomastoid and trapezius muscles
XII: Hypoglossal	Medulla	Motor	Skeletal muscles of the tongue

Autonomic Nervous System: Structure and Function

The **autonomic nervous system (ANS)** is composed of two parts: the sympathetic nervous system (SNS) and the parasympathetic nervous system. ANS functions are not usually under conscious control but may be altered in some people by using biofeedback and other methods.

The SNS cells originate in the gray matter of the spinal cord from T1 through L2 or L3. This part of the ANS is considered *thoracolumbar* because of its anatomic location. The SNS stimulates the functions of the body needed for "fight or flight" (e.g., heart and respiratory rate). It also inhibits certain functions not needed in urgent and stressful situations.

The parasympathetic cells originate in the gray matter of the sacral area of the spinal cord (from S2 through S4) plus portions of cranial nerves III, VII, IX, and X *(craniosacral)*. The parasympathetic nervous system can slow body functions when needed and contribute to digestion and reproduction ("feed and breed").

Parasympathetic fibers to the organs have some sensory ability in addition to motor function. Sensory perceptions of irritation, stretching of an organ, or a decrease in tissue oxygen are transmitted to the thalamus through pathways not yet fully understood. Because pain from internal organs is often felt below the body wall innervated by the spinal nerve, it is presumed that there are connections between the viscera and body structure that relay pain sensation.

Neurologic Changes Associated with Aging

Neurologic changes associated with aging often affect MOBILITY and SENSORY PERCEPTION. *Motor changes* in late adulthood can cause slower movement and response time and decreased sensory perception (Chart 41-1). Any problems that affect the nerves, bones, muscles, or joints also affect motor and therefore ADL ability. Determining functional status—a combination of COGNITION, MOBILITY, and SENSORY PERCEPTION—is a recommended core measure for patients with complex chronic conditions (www.cms.gov).

Sensory changes in older adults can also affect their daily activities. Pupils decrease in size, which restricts the amount of light entering the eye, and adapt more slowly. Older adults need increased lighting to see. Chapter 48 describes collaborative care for persons with hearing loss. Touch sensation decreases, which may lead to falls because the older person may not feel small objects or a step underfoot. Vibration sense may be lost in the ankles and feet. These changes can contribute to falls. (See the discussion on fall prevention in Chapter 2.)

Cognitive functions of perceiving, registering, storing, and using information often change as a normal part of aging. Therefore it is important to differentiate between these expected findings and those of dementia, depression, and delirium. Failure to correctly diagnosis pathologic cognitive problems may lead to a poor patient outcome. For example, unsafe driving can be both a cause and a result of cognitive changes. The cognitive changes may be reversible, allowing the person to continue to drive once the condition is resolved, or irreversible, indicating the health care provider may need to assist with advice or efforts to stop the person from continuing to drive (Iverson et al., 2010).

Intellect does not decline as a result of aging. However, a person with certain health problems may have a decrease in cognitive level. *Cognitive decline is frequently caused by drug interactions or toxicity or by an inadequate oxygen supply to the brain.* Some older adults may need more time than a younger person to process questions, learn and process new information, solve problems, or complete analogies.

CHART 41-1 Nursing Focus on the Older Adult

Changes in the Nervous System Related to Aging

PHYSIOLOGIC CHANGES	NURSING IMPLICATIONS	RATIONALES
Slower processing time	Provide sufficient time for the affected older adult to respond to questions and/or direction.	Allowing adequate time for processing helps differentiate normal findings from neurologic deterioration.
Recent memory loss	Reinforce teaching by repetition, using written teaching, and employing memory aids like electronic alarms or applications for electronic devices that provide recurrent alerts.	Greatest loss of brain weight is in the white matter of the frontal lobe. Intellect is not impaired, but the learning process is slowed. Repetition helps the patient learn new information and recall it when needed.
Decreased sensory perception of touch	Remind the patient to look where his or her feet are placed when walking. Instruct the patient to wear shoes that provide good support when walking. If the patient is unable, change his or her position frequently (every hour) while he or she is in bed or the chair.	Decreased sensory perception may cause the patient to fall.
Change in perception of pain	Ask the patient to describe the nature and specific characteristics of pain. Monitor additional assessment variables to detect possible health problems.	Accurate and complete nursing assessment ensures that the interventions will be appropriate for the older adult (see Chapter 2).
Change in sleep patterns	Ascertain sleep patterns and preferences. Ask if sleep pattern interferes with ADLs. Adjust the patient's daily schedule to his or her sleep pattern and preference as much as possible (e.g., evening versus morning bath).	Older adults require as much as younger adults. It is more common for older adults to fall asleep early and arise early.
Altered balance and/or decreased coordination	Instruct the patient to move slowly when changing positions. If needed, advise the patient to hold on to handrails when ambulating. Assess the need for an ambulatory aid, such as a cane.	The patient may fall if moving too quickly. Assistive and adaptive aids provide support and prevent falls.
Increased risk for infection	Monitor carefully for infection.	Older adults often have structural deterioration of microglia, the cells responsible for cell-mediated immune response in the central nervous system (CNS).
Changes in sleep patterns	Assess sleep habits. Provide usual bedtime routines. Decrease noise and light at night.	Age-related changes include more time in bed spent awake before falling asleep, reduced sleep time, daytime napping, and changes in circadian rhythm leading to "early to bed and early to rise."

Subtle memory changes can occur for many older people. Long-term memory seems better than recall (recent) or immediate (registration) memory. Older adults may need more time to retrieve information. These changes may be partly due to the loss of cerebral neurons, which is associated with the aging process.

Biorhythms vary among people. Circadian responses are reduced in older adults, and the sleep-wake cycle may become less responsive to stimuli that signal patterns of sleep. Older adults may experience changes in sleep architecture and sleeping patterns (Touhy & Jett, 2014). For example, older adults are more likely to go bed earlier and experience an earlier awakening compared with younger adults. They are also more likely to experience more periods of wakefulness lasting 30 or more minutes during the night. On average, an older person needs as much sleep as a younger person but is more likely to nap in the afternoon.

Sleep deprivation at any age can lead to significant changes in COGNITION. Sleep deprivation, common in many inpatient settings, is related to both the earlier onset and greater severity of delirium. Lack of sleep can worsen symptoms of mild dementia. Sleep deprivation can also interfere with normal immune function and wound healing. Interrupted sleep and sleep deprivation can also impair physical function and self-management. Sleep and rest are both necessary for health. Nurses can review sleep habits and promote a good sleep environment, including periods of rest and do-not-disturb during patient care (see the Quality Improvement box).

QUALITY IMPROVEMENT QSEN

Unit-based Quality Improvement Project Promotes Patient Sleep

Faraklas, I., Holt, B., Tran, S., Lin, H., Saffle, J., & Cochran, A. (2013). Impact of a nursing-driven sleep hygiene protocol on sleep quality. *Journal of Burn Care and Research, 34*(2), 249-254.

Sleep is important to cognition. In this report, a nurse-driven protocol and the use of a sound meter to monitor noise was used to evaluate patient perceptions of sleep in acutely ill and burned adults. Noise reduction, reduced lighting, and prioritizing and clustering care activities to minimize sleep interruptions between midnight and 5 AM were phased in over several months in a single unit. When the protocol was fully implemented, patient self-reports indicated an improvement in falling asleep and going back to sleep compared with self-reports before the protocol was implemented. Because it is a nurse-driven protocol, it can be implemented and adapted in quick cycles to meet quality improvement goals. For example, other studies confirm that the use of a sound meter can contribute to noise reduction. The cost of sound meters is small (less than $25), and they can be placed in high impact areas, including alarm stations or where staff commonly converse. The sound meter detects decibels providing immediate feedback to staff about high noise levels that can disrupt patient sleep.

Commentary: Implications for Practice and Research

Steps to improve patient sleep can be implemented without increasing the workload of nurses or increasing the cost of care. Both light reduction and clustering care activities require thoughtful planning and collaboration with health care team members so that the period of planned uninterrupted rest for a patient is recognized. The immediate feedback from a device to monitor decibels is helpful to noise reduction. Although this is a single unit report, the protocol can be used in a variety of inpatient settings. Phasing in interventions of light reduction, noise monitoring, and clustering activities contributes to successful changes in practice.

Mental status may be impaired as a result of infection, hypoxia, and hypoglycemia or hyperglycemia. These conditions are usually easily assessed and managed. During an acute change in mental status, assess the adult for peripheral oxygenation (Spo_2), serum glucose (fingerstick), and potential infection (e.g., fever, urine with sediment or odor, sputum production, red or draining wound). *Often a decrease in mental status is a key early sign of an infectious process in the older patient, and a urinary tract infection is a common site.*

ASSESSMENT METHODS

Patient History

Obtain information from the patient about health problems and function as outlined in Chart 41-2. During your introduction, note the patient's appearance and assess his or her speech, affect, and movement. If he or she seems to have cognitive deficits or has trouble speaking or hearing, ask a family member or significant other to stay during the interview to help obtain an accurate history. Be sure that glasses, contact lenses, and hearing aids are available if the patient wears any of these aids.

Ask the patient about his or her medical history to determine its association with the current health problem. Inquire about the ability to perform ADLs. Knowing the level of daily activity helps establish a baseline for later comparison as the patient improves or worsens. Ask whether the patient is right-handed or left-handed. This information is important for several reasons:

- The patient may be somewhat stronger on the dominant side, which is expected.
- The effects of cerebral injury or disease are more pronounced if the dominant hemisphere is involved.

Ask about family medical history such as stroke or myocardial infarction (MI) (heart attack). Some diseases occur more often in certain groups of people and may be caused by a genetic influence or other reason. For example, it has been long established that Huntington disease is inherited. A number of other neurologic diseases have a genetic basis, such as neuromuscular disorders, migraine headaches, and epilepsy. These genetic risks are described with specific neurologic diseases found later in this unit.

Physical Assessment

Compare each assessment with the patient's baseline, as well as between right and left sides and between upper and lower extremities. *Two types of neurologic assessments may be performed—a complete assessment and a focused assessment.* Some focused assessments are specifically designed to be rapid to ease repetition when recurrent neurologic assessments are needed to monitor the patient's condition over time. The type chosen depends on the information needed, the time available with the patient, and your clinical skill level. Advanced practice registered nurses (APRNs) and other health care providers usually perform the complete assessment, with selected parts done by the nurse. It is important that you understand each component of the assessment and what the results might indicate.

Complete Neurologic Assessment

A complete neurologic assessment includes a history (see Chart 41-2) and evaluation of mental status (consciousness and cognition), cranial nerves (see Table 41-3), MOBILITY and motor abnormalities at baseline or with disease progression is important. During any neurologic assessment, look for asymmetry, such as subtle unequal movement in the facial muscles.

The complete neurologic assessment is used by the health care provider to consider whether a single lesion or more than one site in the nervous system may be contributing to abnormal physical assessment findings. A complete neurologic assessment will also help establish if a lesion or injury is in the CNS, PNS, or both. If the lesion or injury is in the CNS, a complete neurologic assessment can further help the health care provider determine if abnormalities are in the cortex, below the cortex, or multifocal. These findings, along with patient history, help determine the urgency of treatment. For example, a sudden unilateral loss in motor function and sensation is an emergency requiring a stroke center and staff with expertise to diagnose and intervene during a "brain attack." A gradual unilateral loss or a variable loss (with waxing and waning symptoms) may be less urgent and not require stroke center expertise. Generally, the nurse completes a focused or rapid assessment to detect concerning changes.

Assessment of Mental Status. Mental status assessment is generally divided into assessment of *consciousness* and *cognition*. Consciousness is the ability to be aware of the environment, an object, and oneself; consciousness is often documented as level of consciousness (LOC). Consciousness usually refers to the degree of alertness or the amount of stimulation needed to engage a patient's attention and can range from *alert* to *coma*. When alert, the patient is awake and easily engaged. A patient in coma appears to be asleep and does not rouse or react despite vigorous or noxious simulation.

! NURSING SAFETY PRIORITY (QSEN)
Action Alert

Be aware that a change in level of consciousness and orientation is an early and reliable indication that central neurologic function has declined! The patient who is described as **alert** is awake and responsive. A patient may be alert but not oriented to person, place, or time. Patients who are less than alert are labeled *lethargic, stuporous,* or *comatose*. A **lethargic** patient is drowsy but is easily awakened. One who is arousable only with vigorous or painful stimulation is **stuporous**. The **comatose** patient is unconscious and cannot be aroused.

After determining alertness, the next step is to evaluate orientation. Once the patient's attention is engaged, ask him or her questions to determine orientation. Varying the sequence of questioning on repeated assessments prevents the patient from memorizing the answers. Responses that indicate orientation include ability to answer questions about person, place, and time such as:
- The patient's ability to relate the onset of symptoms
- The name of his or her physician/nurse practitioner/nurse
- The year and month
- His or her address
- The name of the referring physician or health care agency

Time of day, drug therapy, and the need for sleep, glucose, or oxygen may affect these responses, so be sure to link any changes in orientation with respiratory status, changes in drug regimens or use of intermittent drugs, time of day/sleep deprivation, or current serum glucose values. Education, occupation, interest, culture, anxiety, and depression affect performance during

system function (e.g., range, strength, posture, abnormal movements), deep tendon reflexes, sensation (e.g., pain, touch, temperature, vibration, and position), and cerebellar function (gait, balance, and coordination). Although not all components of a complete assessment are completed by the nurse, noting assessment of mental status. What is considered "normal" may not be so for a particular patient, so adaptation of questions suggested for mental status assessment may be necessary. Be alert to both *sudden* and *subtle* changes, particularly when changes are noted by family members or others who know the patient.

NCLEX EXAMINATION CHALLENGE

Physiological Integrity

During a client's neurologic assessment, the nurse finds that he is arousable after light touch combined with a loud voice. How does the nurse document this client's level of consciousness?
A. Stuporous
B. Lethargic
C. Comatose
D. Drowsy

CHART 41-3 Best Practice for Patient Safety & Quality Care QSEN

Assessment of Cognition

Perform assessment at the following care interactions:
- On admission to and discharge from an institutional care setting
- Upon transfer from one care setting to another
- Every 8 to 12 hours throughout hospitalization
- Following major changes in pharmacotherapy
- With behavior that is unusual for the person and/or inappropriate to the situation

Assess and document (noting "sometimes," "frequently," or "always" as observed):
- Does the patient respond to voice; require being shaken awake to communicate; doze off during a conversation or when no activities occur; or not respond to voice or touch?
- Is speech clear and understandable; disoriented to person, place, or time; inappropriate; or incomprehensible/garbled?
- Can the patient name the place, reason for admission or visit, month, and age?
- Can the patient follow one-step commands: open/close eyes; make fist/let go?
- Can the patient switch to a different topic or activity versus loses the thread of the conversation or is easily distracted (inattention)?
- Can the patient recognize a familiar object and its purpose or a familiar person and name relationship?
- Can the patient respond relevantly and quickly?
- Does the patient have unrealistic thoughts or act distrustful of others (e.g., does not dare to take his/her medicine; says that people are "listening," etc.)?
- Is the patient cooperative, euphoric, hostile, anxious, withdrawn, or guarded?
- Is the patient's appearance, behavior, or facial expression appropriate for the situation?

Cognition is intellectual function. It is processes of thought that embody perception, attention, visuospatial recognition, language, learning, memory and executive functions of comprehension, insight, problem solving, reasoning, decision making, creativity, and metacognition (Giddens, 2013). Cognition typically is evaluated in a rapid or focused manner using tests of memory and attention that require verbal or written ability (Chart 41-3). *Loss of memory, especially recent memory, tends to be an early sign of neurologic problems.* Three types of memory can be tested: long-term (remote) memory, recall (recent) memory, and immediate memory.

Remote, or long-term, **memory** can be tested by asking patients about their birth date, schools attended, the city of birth, or anything from the past that can be verified. Nurses often ask the name of the patient's contact person listed on the admission form.

Recall (recent) **memory** can be tested during the history and checked on the medical record:
- The accuracy of the medical history
- Dates of clinic or physician appointments
- The time of admission
- Health care providers seen within the past few days
- Mode of transportation to the hospital or clinic

Immediate (new) **memory** is tested by giving the patient three unrelated words, such as "apple," "street," and "chair," and asking him or her to repeat the words to make sure they were heard. After about 5 minutes, while continuing with the examination, ask the patient to repeat the words. An alternative to this method is to give a three-step command and observe whether it is carried out correctly. For example, "Pick up the paper, fold it in half, and draw a square on it."

To assess *attention,* ask the patient to repeat a series of three numbers, such as 4, 7, and 3. The series is increased by one number with each successful repetition until seven or eight digits are achieved. If the patient has difficulty at any level (cannot repeat the series), repeat the numbers. If the patient cannot repeat, stop the procedure. Next, ask the patient to repeat the numbers backward, starting again with three digits and increasing by one each time. Normally, a person should be able to repeat five to eight digits forward and four to six backward. The serial-seven test to determine attention may also be used. The patient is asked to count backward from 100 by 7 (the examiner stops when the patient reaches 65 successfully). An alternative approach is to ask the person to subtract by three or to add forward by five. Clinical judgment and assessment skills are used when deciding which of these tests to use.

Other assessments of cognition include examining language and executive function. Many *language* skills can be assessed during the initial interview. Language skills include understanding the spoken or written word and being able to speak or write. The patient demonstrates understanding by following directions on admission (e.g., getting undressed). If he or she hesitates, it may be the patient does not understand the vocabulary or word. When speech hesitation or performance hesitation occurs, point to objects and ask the patient to name them, such as the door or bed. Speech is assessed as being normal, slow, garbled, difficult to find words, or other impairments. If the change in speech is new and represents a deterioration from a previous ability to communicate, this change must be urgently reported to the health care provider because it may indicate a stroke, new onset of confusion, or other serious neurologic condition (Rattray et al., 2011).

The health care provider or speech-language pathologist (SLP) completes additional language tests such as reading comprehension. This is done by writing a simple command and giving it to the patient (e.g., "close your eyes"). Written language can be tested by asking the patient to write a sentence. The clinician must remember that some patients cannot read or write or may speak a language different from that of the clinician. In this case, modify the examination accordingly such as having the patient copy something that has been drawn (e.g., a cross, circle, diamond, or square).

Executive function allows for flexibility, adaptability, and goal directedness; it determines the contents of consciousness, supervises voluntary action, and is future oriented. Several approaches are used to assess executive function. Although most tests of executive function are not done by the nurse, it is important to identify and document altered executive function because this type of impairment can place the patient at risk for harm. To identify whether such a risk exists and to ensure that the need for further specialized evaluation is recognized, begin to assess the patient's judgment during the interview. Did he or she make rational decisions in dealing with his or her symptoms? Ask questions such as "What would you do if stopped for speeding?" and "What would you do if there was a fire in the wastepaper basket?" Asking the meaning of proverbs (e.g., "A stitch in time saves nine" or "A rolling stone gathers no moss") provides information about insight and abstraction. These questions might also elicit important information about a new onset of a confusional state. People from countries other than the United States or young adults may be unfamiliar with abstract proverbs. Finally, ask the patient to follow a two-step motor process such as "Show me two fingers with your right hand" (you can illustrate with your right hand) and then ask him or her to do the same thing with the other hand (removing the visual cue of your hand before asking for step two). Consult a professional interpreter to assist with language and culturally appropriate phrasing before making an evaluation of executive function to ensure that both sudden and subtle changes are identified accurately.

There are several rapid tests of cognition useful in clinical settings. One example is the Brief Interview for Mental Status (BIMS), commonly used in long-term care settings (Saliba et al., 2012). The BIMS consists of three categories. The first category is "repetition of three words." The nurse tells the patient that he or she will hear three words and then be asked to repeat them. Allow five seconds to pass between stating the words and asking for repetition. Then the three words are verbally repeated and placed into a category (e.g., blue, a color) by the assessor but not yet retested. Next, "temporal orientation" is evaluated by asking the patient to identify the year, month, and day of week. The third category of assessment is "recall." The patient is asked to name the same three words used earlier and the assessor determines if the words are recalled independently, after coaching by naming the category, or not recalled at all. Patients can achieve scores of 0 to 15 by adding across the three categories. Scores below 8 indicate severe cognitive impairment (Saliba et al., 2012). Cognitive impairment can be permanent or temporary.

An example of permanent cognitive impairment is **dementia**, an irreversible and degenerative condition described in Chapter 42. Two screening tools useful for identifying dementia that can be completed quickly are the clock drawing test and the Mini-Cog, and each require less than 3 minutes to complete. An example of a longer test is the Mini-Mental State Examination (3MS; average time to administer, 17 minutes) (Holsinger et al., 2012).

Another consideration in assessing cognition is delirium. **Delirium**, an acute confusional state, is characterized by a new and sudden cognitive impairment (Touhy & Jett, 2014). Symptoms tend to fluctuate over the course of a day and include disturbances in consciousness, attention, memory deficits, and perceptual disturbances. Delirium can also be manifested by delusional (paranoid) thoughts and behavior. Delirium is a medical emergency and specifically places geriatric patients at risk for harm and prolonged cognitive impairment. Once a patient is identified as having delirium, reassessment should be done every shift.

Early identification and targeted interventions for delirium can decrease the occurrence and severity of delirium. Delirium is associated with significant consequences such as distress (including post-traumatic distress syndrome), prolonged hospital stay, increased morbidity and mortality, and institutionalization (Touhy & Jett, 2014). Two tests to detect new onset of delirium are the Confusion Assessment Method (CAM) and the NEECHAM Confusional Scale (Adamis et al., 2010). The CAM-ICU is used for nonverbal patients (Barr et al., 2013).

Assessment of Cranial Nerves. Cranial nerves are typically tested to establish a baseline from which to compare progress or deterioration. However, they are not routinely tested unless the patient has a suspected problem affecting one or more of the cranial nerves (see Table 41-3). Adding the specific cranial nerves to be tested to the documentation record of a patient with a problem affecting the cranial nerves helps ensure continued comparison and assessment.

Testing pupils is a common cranial nerve test performed by nurses. Pupil constriction is a function of cranial nerve III, the oculomotor nerve. **P**upils should be **e**qual in size, **r**ound and **r**egular in shape, and react to **l**ight and **a**ccommodation (**PERRLA**). Estimate the size of both pupils using a millimeter ruler or a pupillometer. Patients who have had eye surgery for cataracts or glaucoma often have irregularly shaped pupils. Those using eye drops for either cataracts or glaucoma may have unequal pupils if only one eye is being treated, and the pupillary response may be altered.

To test for pupil constriction, ask the patient to close his or her eyes and dim the room lights. Bring a penlight in from the side of the patient's head, and shine the light in the eye being tested as soon as the patient opens his or her eyes. The pupil being tested should constrict (**direct response**). The other pupil should also constrict slightly (**consensual response**). To test accommodation, relight the room and ask the patient to focus on a distant object and then immediately look at an object 4 to 5 inches from the nose. The eyes should converge, and the pupils should constrict. Pinpoint, dilated, and nonreactive pupils are late signs of neurologic deterioration (Jarvis, 2016).

Assessment of Motor Function. Throughout the physical assessment, observe the patient for involuntary tremors or movements. Describe these movements as accurately as possible, such as "pill-rolling with the thumbs and fingers at rest" or "intention tremors of both hands" (tremors that occur when the patient tries to do something). These abnormalities can indicate certain diseases, such as multiple sclerosis, or the effects of selected psychotropic drugs. In addition, assess the patient for motor movements that indicate irritability, hyperactivity, or slowed movements. Measure the patient's hand *strength* by asking him or her to grasp and squeeze two fingers of each of your hands. Then compare the grasps for equality of strength. As another means of evaluating strength, try to withdraw the fingers from the patient's grasp and compare the ease or difficulty. He or she should release the grasps on command— another assessment of consciousness and the ability to follow commands.

Collaborate with the physical therapist to test the patient's strength. To test strength against resistance, ask the patient to resist the examiner's bending or straightening of the arm, hand, leg, or foot being tested (Fig. 41-7). A five-point rating scale is commonly used (see Chapter 49, Table 49-2). Always evaluate and compare strength on each side. Compare previous results with current findings, and report all decreases to the health care providers.

Cerebral motor or *brainstem* integrity may also be assessed. Ask the patient to close his or her eyes and hold the arms perpendicular to the body with the palms up for 15 to 30 seconds. If there is a cerebral or brainstem reason for muscle weakness, the arm on the weak side will start to fall, or "drift," with the palm pronating (turning inward). This is called a **pronator drift**. The same can be done for the lower extremities, with the patient lying on his or her stomach with the legs bent upward at the knees. However, it is easier for most patients to sit on the side of the bed and extend the legs outward.

Decortication is abnormal motor movement seen in the patient with lesions that interrupt the corticospinal pathways (Fig. 41-8, *A*). The patient's arms, wrists, and fingers are flexed with internal rotation and plantar flexion of the legs. **Decerebration** is abnormal movement with rigidity characterized by extension of the arms and legs, pronation of the arms, plantar flexion, and opisthotonos (body spasm in which the body is bowed forward) (Fig. 41-8, *B*). Decerebration is usually associated with dysfunction in the brainstem area.

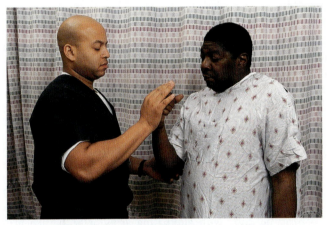

FIG. 41-7 Testing for strength against resistance.

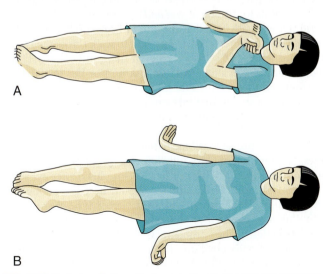

FIG. 41-8 Posturing. **A,** Decorticate posturing. **B,** Decerebrate posturing.

Assessment of Reflex Activity. The health care provider, including the APRN, may assess deep tendon reflexes (DTRs) and superficial (cutaneous) reflexes. The **deep tendon reflexes** of the biceps, triceps, brachioradialis, and quadriceps muscles and of the Achilles tendon can be tested as part of the complete neurologic assessment (Jarvis, 2016). Striking the tendon with the reflex hammer should cause contraction of the muscle. The appropriate muscle contraction indicates an intact reflex arc. The tendon is tapped quickly but not with too much force. If the patient is tensing the muscle, the reflexes will not respond. Having the patient interlock his or her hands and pull outward will help decrease muscle tensing so the reflex can be tested.

The **cutaneous (superficial) reflexes** usually tested are the plantar reflexes and sometimes the abdominal reflexes. The plantar reflex is tested with a pointed (but not sharp) object, such as the handle end of the reflex hammer or the rounded end of bandage scissors. The normal response is plantar flexion of all toes. **Babinski's sign**, a dorsiflexion of the great toe and fanning of the other toes, is abnormal in anyone older than 2 years and represents the presence of central nervous system (CNS) disease. The term "positive Babinski's sign" (abnormal response) and "negative Babinski's sign" (normal response) are clinically used terms but are not correct. Health care providers may also use the terms "upgoing" or "downgoing" to refer to the toes of the stimulated foot. "Upgoing" toes are an abnormal response that indicates the presence of pathology in the CNS. Babinski's sign can occur with drug and alcohol intoxication, after a seizure, or in patients with multiple sclerosis or liver disease.

To test the abdominal reflex, stroke the patient's abdomen in all four quadrants diagonally toward the umbilicus. The umbilicus should deviate toward the stimulus, but obesity may mask the reflex. The abdominal reflex can be absent in both upper and lower motor neuron disease.

Hyperactive reflexes indicate possible upper motor neuron disease, tetanus, or hypocalcemia. *Hypoactive* reflexes may result from lower motor neuron disease (damage to the spinal cord), disease of the neuromuscular junction, muscle disease, or health problems such as diabetes mellitus, hypothyroidism, or hypokalemia.

Asymmetry of reflexes is an important finding because it probably indicates a disease process. The results of reflex testing are recorded by the use of a stick figure and a scale of 0 to 4 (Fig. 41-9). A score of 2 is considered normal, although scores of 1 (hypoactive) or 3 (stronger than normal) may be normal for a particular patient. **Clonus** (also called *myoclonus*) is the sudden, brief, jerking contraction of a muscle or muscle group often seen in seizures.

Assessment of Sensory Function. The assessment of sensory function is done for patients with problems affecting the spinal cord or spinal nerves, such as trauma, intervertebral disk disease, Guillain-Barré syndrome (GBS), tumor, infection, stenosis, or transverse myelitis. The sensory assessment includes pain, superficial and deep sensation, light touch, and proprioception. *Pain and light touch are the most commonly assessed.*

The acuity level of the patient determines how often the sensory assessment is done. For example, patients with acute spinal cord trauma or ascending GBS are assessed every hour until stable and then every 4 hours. As the condition improves, sensory assessment may be needed only once each shift. Findings are documented according to agency protocol. A special spinal cord assessment flow sheet may be used to document

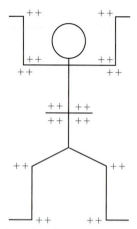

0	Absent, no response
1 (+)	Weaker than normal, hypoactive
2 (++)	Normal
3 (+++)	Stronger or more brisk than normal
4 (++++)	Hyperactive
	(Note: 1 and 3 may be normal for some individuals)

FIG. 41-9 A stick figure and scale for recording reflex activity.

sensory and/or motor findings for the patient with a spinal cord injury.

Pain and temperature sensation are transmitted by the same nerve endings. Therefore if one sensation is tested and found to be intact, it can safely be assumed that the other is intact. Testing temperature sensation can usually be accomplished using a cold reflex hammer and the warm touch of the hand for patients with known or suspected spinal problems.

Assess for *pain perception* with any sharp or dull object, such as the tips of a cotton-tipped applicator. While the patient's eyes are open, demonstrate what will be done. Then ask him or her to keep eyes closed and to indicate whether the touch is sharp or dull. The sharp and dull ends should be changed at random so he or she does not anticipate the next type of stimulus for SENSORY PERCEPTION. Not all areas need to be tested unless a spinal cord injury has occurred. If testing begins on the hands and feet, there is no need to test the other parts of the extremities because the tracts transmitting pain and temperature sensations are intact. Compare reactions on each side. A sensation reported as dull when the stimulus was actually sharp requires further testing. A patient with sensory loss as a result of diabetes mellitus or peripheral vascular disease may or may not be aware of the loss until tested. Some patients with chronic illness may report that they have had sensory losses for a long time. Prior to testing for pain, the nurse must check to determine whether the patient is on anticoagulant therapy. If the patient is on anticoagulant therapy, then any testing with a sharp object must be avoided—this can cause bleeding.

Light *touch discrimination* is likely to be normal if pain and temperature sensory tracts are intact. Touch discrimination and two-point discrimination may be assessed as part of a complete neurologic examination by the physician or APRN.

For testing **touch discrimination**, the patient closes his or her eyes. The practitioner touches the patient with a finger and asks that he or she point to the area touched. This procedure is repeated on each extremity at random rather than at sequential points. Next, the practitioner touches the patient on each side of the body on corresponding sites at the same time. The patient should be able to point to both sites.

The clinician then touches the patient in two places on the same extremity with two objects, such as cotton-tipped applicators. A person can normally identify two points fairly close together depending on the location of the stimuli. When an area is heavily innervated, the *two-point discrimination will feel closer.*

Abnormal sensory findings may have a CNS or a peripheral nervous system (PNS) cause. The neuropathies of diabetes, malnutrition, and vascular problems have a PNS cause. Damage to a specific spinal nerve may not result in significant sensory loss because the spinal nerves overlap. Injury to several nearby spinal nerves is manifested as decreased or absent SENSORY PERCEPTION in the dermatomes of those nerves.

CNS problems can occur within the spinal cord, the brainstem, the cerebellum, and the cerebral cortex. Sensory deficits from spinal cord damage vary with the location of the damage. Involvement of only the posterior column leads to lost proprioception (position sense) below the level of the damage on the same side or on both sides (if both the right and left posterior columns are involved). A lesion involving only the right spinothalamic tract results in a loss of pain and temperature sensations below the lesion on the *left* side. Problems in the brainstem, thalamus, and cortex generally result in loss of sensation on the **contralateral** (opposite) side of the body. Cerebellar lesions result in sensory deficits on the *same* side of the body.

Assessment of Cerebellar Function. Most of the assessment of cerebellar function can be performed with the patient sitting on the side of the bed or examining table. Fine *coordination* of muscle activity is tested. If cerebellar problems are suspected or diagnosed, ask the patient to perform these tasks with his or her eyes closed:

- Run the heel of one foot down the shin of the other leg and repeat with the other leg (the patient should be able to do this smoothly and keep the heel on the shin).
- Place the hands palm-up and then palm-down on each thigh, repeating as fast as possible (this can normally be done rapidly).
- With arms out at the side, touch the finger to the nose 2 or 3 times, with eyes open and then with eyes closed (this can be done with alternating arms or with each arm individually).

For the last part of the cerebellar assessment, the *ambulatory* patient stands for testing of *gait and equilibrium.* Gait and equilibrium are usually tested at the end or beginning of the entire neurologic assessment. Ask the patient to walk across the room, turn, and return. Observe for uneven steps, difficulty walking, and so forth. To evaluate balance, ask him or her to stand on one foot and then on the other. Tiptoe walking and heel-to-toe walking can also demonstrate gait problems. For patients with sciatic nerve involvement, pain may worsen when they walk on their toes or heels.

To test equilibrium, ask the patient to stand with arms at the sides, feet and knees close together, and eyes open. Check for swaying, and then ask him or her to close his or her eyes and maintain position. The examiner should be close enough to prevent falling if the patient cannot stay erect. If he or she sways with the eyes closed but not when the eyes are open (the **Romberg sign**), the problem is probably **proprioceptive** (awareness of body position). If the patient sways with the eyes both open and closed, the neurologic disturbance is probably *cerebellar* in origin.

QUALITY IMPROVEMENT (QSEN)

System-Wide Project Standardizes Assessments and Communication for Neuroscience Patients

Iacono L.A., Wells C., & Mann-Finnerty, K. (2014). Standardizing neurological assessments. *The Journal of Neuroscience Nursing, 46*(2), 125-132.

The nursing and physician leadership team at a large urban hospital identified an opportunity to improve neurologic assessment by adopting standard assessment tools. Problems during transitions in care, particularly when reporting neurologic deterioration to health care team members, alerted staff to the need to address issues in quality and safety. Assessment tools were identified and evaluated. Modifications were made to three tools to capture team-generated key components to a neurologic assessment and to improve the process for describing neurologic deterioration. The Basic Neurological Check (addressing alertness, orientation, facial palsy, and four-limb strength), the National Institutes of Health Stroke Scale (NIHSS) Neurological Check (specific for patients with stroke or suspected stroke), and the Coma Neurological Check (based on the Glasgow Coma Scale) were then incorporated into electronic documentation. An algorithm to help health care providers and nurses determine which neurologic tool to use was made available and folded into training. Mandatory training about the use of the tools was implemented. Ongoing education during orientation for new nurses as well as in-depth training of nurse educators and assistant managers to provide reinforcement and feedback also took place. Three short videos, one for each of the selected neurologic tools, were developed for staff viewing. Following implementation, nurses and physicians report that observations were more consistent and changes were more measurable. Use of the standardized neurologic assessment tools in the neuroscience patient population has helped in early identification of neurologic symptoms. Nurses verbalized more confidence in their ability to identify clinical important symptoms so that early intervention can occur. The authors emphasized the role of nurse educators in training and reinforcement of learning and outcome measures.

Commentary: Implications for Practice and Research

This quality improvement project began in a stroke unit and then was expanded to all units where patients with neurologic conditions received care. This is an example of a team working together to solve a system-wide problem. Both practice and communication issues were identified as contributing to delayed recognition of clinical deterioration in neuroscience patients and in confusion or error during hand-offs. The use of nurse educators as champions was an effective strategy of adoption and ongoing achievement of goals for care.

GLASGOW COMA SCALE*	
Eye Opening	
Spontaneous	4
To sound	3
To pain	2
Never	1
Motor Response	
Obeys commands	6
Localizes pain	5
Normal flexion (withdrawal)	4
Abnormal flexion	3
Extension	2
None	1
Verbal Response	
Oriented	5
Confused conversation	4
Inappropriate words	3
Incomprehensible sounds	2
None	1
* The highest possible score is 15	

FIG. 41-10 The Glasgow Coma Scale.

A second example of standard rapid neurologic assessment is the **Glasgow Coma Scale (GCS)** (Fig. 41-10). The GCS is used in many acute care settings to establish baseline data in each of these areas: eye opening, motor response, and verbal response. The patient is assigned a numeric score for each of these areas. The lower the score, the lower the patient's neurologic function. For patients who are intubated and cannot talk, record their score with a "t" after the number for verbal response.

The GCS is easy to teach and has demonstrated a consistent score among trained assessors. The reliability of the GCS is based on recording the patient's "best" response. If the patient does not follow commands or is unresponsive to voice, then the nurse proceeds to increasingly noxious (painful) stimuli to elicit an eye and motor response. Typically, the patient's response to central pain (brain response) is assessed first. On the basis of this response, peripheral pain may then be assessed. Failure to apply painful stimuli appropriately may lead to an incorrect conclusion about the patient's neurologic status. If the patient responds fully to voice or light touch, there is no need to progress to more vigorous or painful stimuli.

Start with the least noxious irritation or pressure and proceed to more painful stimulation if the patient does not respond. Begin each phase of the assessment by speaking in a normal voice. If no response is obtained, use a loud voice. If the patient does not respond, gently shake him or her. The shaking should be similar to that used in attempting to wake up a child. If that is unsuccessful, apply painful stimuli using one of these methods:

- Supraorbital (above eyes) pressure by placing a thumb under the orbital rim in the middle of the eyebrow and

If the patient cannot perform any of these activities smoothly, the problem is manifested on the same side as the cerebellar lesion. If both lobes of the cerebellum are involved, the incoordination affects both sides of the body (bilateral).

Rapid Neurologic Assessment

A rapid neurologic assessment, or "neuro check," is completed when the patient is admitted to a health care facility on an emergent basis. It is also part of ongoing patient assessment and performed in the event of a sudden change in neurologic status. The typical record contains data related to alertness, orientation, movement of arms and legs, and pupil size and reaction to light. *Be sure to document all aspects of the rapid neurologic assessment.* One example of a rapid neurologic assessment is the National Institutes of Health Stroke Scale, described in Chapter 45 (Table 45-2). (See the Quality Improvement box.)

pushing upward. Do not use this technique if the patient has orbital or facial fractures.

- Trapezius muscle squeeze by pinching or squeezing the trapezius muscle located at the angle of the shoulder and neck muscle.
- Mandibular (jaw) pressure to the jaw by using your index and middle fingers to pinch the lower jaw.
- Sternal (breastbone) rub by making a fist and rubbing/twisting your knuckles against the sternum.

The tissue in these areas is tender, and bruising is not unusual. Therefore do not use this technique for older adults or for patients who may experience severe bruising (e.g., recipients of anticoagulant therapy). Peripheral pain is assessed with pressure at the base of the nail on one finger and one toe and both on the right and left.

The patient may respond to painful stimuli in several ways. Although the initial response to pain may be abnormal flexion or extension, continued application of pain for no more than 20 to 30 seconds may demonstrate that he or she can localize or withdraw. If the patient does not respond after 20 to 30 seconds, stop applying the painful stimulus.

! NURSING SAFETY PRIORITY (QSEN)

Critical Rescue

A decrease of 2 or more points in the Glasgow Coma Scale total is clinically significant and should be communicated to the health care provider immediately. Other findings requiring urgent communication with the health care provider include a new finding of abnormal flexion or extension, particularly of the upper extremities (decerebrate or decorticate posturing); pinpoint, dilated, and nonreactive pupils; and sudden or subtle changes in mental status. Remember, changes in cognition are the earliest signs of changes in neurologic status. Early recognition of neurologic changes and communicating changes to the health care provider provide the best opportunity to prevent complications and preserve function.

Psychosocial Assessment

Depression can result in cognitive and behavioral changes that are similar to delirium or dementia. Depression is a common mental health disorder that is often missed in a variety of health care settings, especially in settings that care for older adults (Touhy & Jett, 2014). Consider using a depression screening tool like the Center for Epidemiological Studies Depression-Revised (CESD-R) or the Geriatric Depression Scale (short form) to identify patients with depressive symptoms, and consider referring them to the appropriate provider (both primary care and mental health care) if the screening is positive.

Patients vary in their responses to a suspected or actual health problem, often depending on whether it is acute or chronic. Response is also influenced by MOBILITY, SENSORY PERCEPTION, and/or COGNITION; these abilities can be temporarily or permanently altered as a result of neurologic disease or injury. For example, patients who have a mild stroke and no lasting neurologic deficits are less likely to be severely depressed than patients who experience a loss of independent movement or impaired communication as a result of a stroke.

Age may also be a factor in how a patient accepts the illness. For instance, a young adult who has a motorcycle crash causing a traumatic brain injury (TBI) may react differently from an older adult who has a spinal injury. In some cases, the patient's

emotional responses result from the health problem itself, especially for TBI patients.

Men may feel differently about their illness than women. Male patients who have had strokes are depressed more often than women who have had strokes. Discussions of these response differences can be found in the following chapters on specific neurologic health problems.

Regardless of what the health problem is, do not assume that everyone reacts the same way to his or her illness or injury. Consider the cultural background of the patient because this will influence his or her reaction to pain or injury. Patients experience the grieving process and may fluctuate between denial, anger, and depression. Encourage patients to express their feelings. Refer them to the appropriate support services if needed. Assess support systems, including family members and friends, if available. Document your assessment and interventions.

Diagnostic Assessment

Laboratory Assessment

Fluid, electrolyte, and glucose abnormalities can cause neurologic impairment. The basic metabolic panel and serum calcium, phosphorus, and magnesium are evaluated. Both anemia and malnutrition can contribute to neurologic disorders so a complete blood count and serum levels of albumin and minerals/vitamins (particularly B vitamins) are collected. Collection of arterial blood to evaluate pH, oxygen, and carbon dioxide levels may be done because these three results, when either too high or too low, will alter neurologic status. Serum evaluation may be required to determine the presence of a toxidrome from prescribed or illicit drugs. For patients with a neurologic problem resulting from an infection, cultures are necessary to identify the pathogen. Although the cause of infection must be determined for any patient, this is especially true for those with existing CNS disease. The blood-brain barrier is often not intact in neurologic disease, and the patient is more likely to get an infection of the nervous system, such as meningitis or encephalitis.

Imaging Assessment

Plain X-Rays. Plain *x-rays* of the skull and spine are used to determine bony fractures, curvatures, bone erosion, bone dislocation, and possible calcification of soft tissue, which can damage the nervous system. Several views are taken—anteroposterior, lateral, oblique, and, when necessary, special views of the facial bones. *In head trauma and multiple injuries, one of the first priorities is to rule out cervical spine fracture.*

Explain that the x-ray procedure for the skull and spine is similar to that for a chest x-ray. The patient must remain still during the procedure. Remind him or her that the exposure to radiation is minimal. If the patient is in traction and a portable x-ray unit is not available, the nurse may need to accompany him or her to assist with positioning. Any patient who cannot walk from a wheelchair to the x-ray table should be transferred to the radiology department on a stretcher. Hospitals may have specific procedures for transferring patients in wheelchairs or on stretchers to the radiology department. Check with your hospital on this procedure. For example, with a patient who is confused or disoriented, the hospital radiology department staff may require two or more hospital personnel to assist with the transfer. The patient is positioned for each of the desired views and is asked to not move just before each x-ray. Follow-up care is not required.

In general, for any image that involves being placed in a scanner, the nurse needs to be aware of special circumstances that can either prevent the procedure from taking place or can interfere with the procedure. If the patient is alert and claustrophobic, two options are available: one is a mild sedative such as diazepam (Valium) to calm the patient; the other option is an open scanner. The nurse must determine whether the patient has any metal prosthetics, such as heart valves or shrapnel in the part of the body to be scanned. If the patient does have any type of metal object in the body part to be examined, the nurse must notify radiology immediately because the procedure may need to be cancelled. If the patient does have a metal prosthetic or device, the nurse should ask the patient or significant other if the patient carries a medical alert card from the manufacturer. Medical device manufacturers issue cards to physicians for their patients to carry with the device number and instructions if radiologic diagnostic testing is needed.

Cerebral Angiography. Cerebral angiography (arteriography) is done to visualize the cerebral circulation to detect blockages in the arteries or veins in the brain, head, or neck. It remains the gold standard for the diagnosis of intracranial vascular disease and is required for any transcatheter therapy or for surgical intervention. Angiography may be used to identify aneurysms, traumatic injuries, strictures/occlusions, tumors, blood vessel displacement from edema, and arteriovenous (AV) malformations. Chart 41-4 lists the precautions that must be taken for patients having any test using an iodine-based contrast agent. Risk factors for adverse events must be determined before scheduling the test. Patients sensitive to iodine may be sensitive to iodinated contrast agents; as well, patients with a history of hypersensitivity in general (e.g., multiple food allergies or asthma) are more likely to have an adverse reaction compared with the general population. Seafood allergies are no longer considered an indicator of iodinated contrast allergy. Table 41-4 describes patient preparation and follow-up nursing care for cerebral angiography and other imaging tests.

The patient is placed on an examining table and made as comfortable as possible. At this time, dentures and hearing aids must be removed. He or she is then connected to cardiac monitoring throughout the procedure. Deep or moderate sedation is usually not used, although the patient may be given medication for relaxation.

The interventional radiologist or other specially trained physician numbs the area at the groin and inserts a catheter into the femoral artery. Under fluoroscopic guidance, the catheter is advanced into a carotid or vertebral artery. Then the physician injects iodinated contrast material into each vessel while recording images from different angles over the head and neck. After all the vessels have been imaged, the radiologist reviews all the images and consults with the referring physician to decide whether the patient could benefit from a therapeutic radiologic procedure or surgery to treat the problem. An arterial closure device is typically used to seal the artery and prevent bleeding.

The x-ray images are stored on a computer. With older equipment, a two-dimensional picture of the vessels is produced. Most radiographic systems now come with software to create three-dimensional images of the blood vessels in the head and/or neck. These systems can also display a "subtracted image" made from two images—one just before the contrast was injected and one with the contrast in the artery. The risks of the procedure are contrast reaction (including hives and

CHART 41-4 Best Practice for Patient Safety & Quality Care QSEN

Precautions for the Use of Iodine-Based or Gadolinium Contrast for Diagnostic Testing

Special precautions are taken for patients who will receive an iodinated or high osmolar contrast agent as part of their diagnostic test. These measures include:

- Following agency guidelines regarding informed consent.
- Screening patients at risk for developing contrast-induced kidney damage:
  - Ask the patient about all allergies (food, drug, environmental antigens), asthma, and prior reaction to contrast agents.
  - Review for the presence of these conditions:
    - Pre-existing renal disease such as a diagnosis of chronic kidney disease
    - Diabetic nephropathy
    - Heart failure
    - Dehydration
    - Older age
    - Drugs that interfere with renal perfusion such as metformin or NSAIDs
    - Administration of contrast media in the previous 72 hours
- Evaluating current kidney function. Patients with a serum creatinine greater than or equal to 1.5 mg/dL OR a calculated glomerular filtration rate (GFR) of less than 60 mL/min are at highest risk for kidney damage from contrast.
- Communicating with the health care provider before diagnostic testing when risk factors and allergic reaction to iodinated contrast are present.
  - Consider including a discussion of the patient's serum creatinine as a component of the "time-out" process prior to a diagnostic procedure.
  - Document the date, time, and name of the health care provider with whom communication of risk occurred and what actions were prescribed, if any.
  - Some diagnostic tests can be completed with a lower volume of contrast or an alternate agent.
  - Medications that are associated with kidney damage may be held for 24-48 hours before AND after the test.
- Providing adequate hydration before and after contrast administration:
  - Collaborate with the health care provider to determine whether hydration before the diagnostic test, typically with intravenous normal saline, is used. Bicarbonate with normal saline or an intravenous dose of N-acetylcysteine may be used in a high-risk patient.
  - Determine the optimal post-diagnostic intake and output. Provide sufficient hydration to flush out the contrast with oral or IV fluids over the 4-5 hours following the test.
- Re-evaluating serum creatinine and glomerular filtration rate (GFR) 24-48 hours after the diagnostic test. Communicate an increase of serum creatinine 0.5 mg/dL above baseline and a decrease in GFR >25% to the health care provider. Document communication and follow-up interventions, if any. Generally, the peak creatinine rise is at 48-72 hours after the administration of contrast.

flushing), thrombosis (clotting), and bleeding from the entry site. Patients with known contrast sensitivity are pre-treated with steroids.

Computed Tomography. Computed tomography (CT) scanning is an accurate, quick, easy, noninvasive, painless, and least-expensive method of diagnosing neurologic problems (see Table 41-4). Using x-rays (i.e., ionizing radiation), pictures are taken at many horizontal levels, or slices, of the brain or spinal cord (Schmidt, 2012). A computer then generates three-dimensional detailed anatomic pictures of tissues, typically the brain, spinal cord, or peripheral neuromuscular system in

TABLE 41-4	Preparation and Follow-Up for Selected Diagnostic Procedures	
TEST	**PATIENT CARE PREPARATION**	**PATIENT CARE FOLLOW-UP**
Sonography or Ultrasonography	No preparation is needed. This diagnostic imaging approach is noninvasive and not painful. A light and moderate touch with a probe occurs along the neck/carotid vessels.	The gel used to enhance probe images can be immediately wiped off or removed with water.
Cerebral angiography	Determine whether the patient is allergic to iodinated contrast agents, and follow the guideline in Chart 41-4. To minimize risk for aspiration, assess for the presence of nausea or recent vomiting and medicate as needed. Ensure that the patient is NPO 4 to 6 hours before the test. Reinforce these important points: • Your head is immobilized during the procedure. • Do not move during the procedure. • Contrast dye is injected through a catheter placed in the femoral artery. You will feel a warm or hot sensation when the dye is injected—this is normal. • You will be able to talk to the physician—let him or her know if you are in pain or have any concerns. Assess and document neurologic signs, vital signs, and neurovascular checks.	Follow agency policy regarding care of the injection site, which may include: • Check dressing for bleeding and swelling around site. • Apply ice pack to site. • Keep the extremity straight and immobilized. • Maintain pressure dressing for 2 hours. Check the extremity for adequate circulation to include skin color and temperature, pulses distal to the injection site, and capillary refill. If bleeding is present, maintain manual pressure on the site and notify the physician immediately. Assess vital signs with neurologic examination. Increase oral or IV fluid intake unless contraindicated. Document assessments and interventions.
Computed tomography (CT) with and without contrast CT angiography (CTA) CT myelogram	Follow the guidelines listed in Chart 41-4 if a contrast agent is to be given. Determine whether the patient is claustrophobic and whether a closed CT scan is used. Inform the radiology staff or physician to determine if pre-procedure sedation is necessary. Instruct the patient to remove hairpins, hairpieces, or wigs. Inform the patient that the scanner may make noise or knocking sounds. Reassure the patient that he or she will be able to communicate with the technician throughout the procedure. If contrast is used, the patient may feel a warm or cool sensation after the dye is injected. Occasionally the patient may report a slight metallic taste. A lumbar puncture is performed before an intrathecal contrast-enhanced CT.	Monitor the patient for a delayed allergic response if contrast medium was used.
Positron emission tomography (PET)	Follow preparation as listed for CT. Instruct the patient to withhold caffeine, alcohol, and tobacco for 24 hours before the test. Ensure that the patient has been NPO status for 4 to 12 hours before the procedure (if the patient is diabetic, no insulin is given before the test). Do not give any glucose solutions and any other drugs that alter glucose metabolism. Insert two IV lines.	The radioisotope is eliminated in the urine; no special precautions required. Encourage the patient to increase fluid intake unless contraindicated.
Single-photon emission computed tomography (SPECT)	Patient preparation is similar to that for PET/CT. Determine whether the patient has recently had other nuclear medicine screenings, which may leave traces of the radiopharmaceutical agent. Follow the guidelines listed in Chart 41-4 regarding use of a contrast agent.	The patient can return to his or her previous activity level.
Magnetic resonance imaging (MRI) Magnetic resonance angiography (MRA) Magnetic resonance spectroscopy (MRS)	Follow the information for CT scan. No metal objects may enter the MRI room. Ask the patient about any metal implants including any type of pacemaker device, implantable pumps, or stimulating devices. Instruct the patient to remove all metal objects (jewelry, earrings, body piercings, hairpins, watches, rings, pens). Check with the radiologist regarding tattoos. Do not enter the MRI room unless you have checked with the radiology technician and are sure that neither you nor the patient has any metal device. Ensure all equipment and supplies are free of metal. Gadolinium contrast is to be avoided in patients with low renal function (i.e., glomerular filtration rate <30 mL/min/1.73 m^2.)	No special post-procedure or follow-up care is required. Avoid risk for nephrogenic systemic fibrosis following gadolinium for contrast by restricting its use to patients with normal renal function or using an alternate medium during MRI with contrast diagnostic imaging.

TABLE 41-4	Preparation and Follow-Up for Selected Diagnostic Procedures—cont'd	
TEST	**PATIENT CARE PREPARATION**	**PATIENT CARE FOLLOW-UP**
Lumbar puncture	Explain the procedure, noting that some discomfort may be felt when the local anesthetic is injected or that pain may occur in the leg(s) when the spinal needle is inserted. Place the patient in the fetal position, and remind him or her to remain still. If needed, keep the patient from moving.	Obtain vital signs and complete neurologic checks. Follow agency policy regarding bedrest and remaining flat. Encourage the patient to increase fluid intake unless contraindicated. Monitor for complications, especially increased intracranial pressure (severe headache, nausea, vomiting, photophobia, and change in level of consciousness). Observe the needle insertion site for leakage. Notify the physician if it occurs. Provide drug for headache. Notify the physician if drug does not relieve pain.
Electroencephalogram (EEG)	Ensure that hair is clean and without conditioners, hair creams, lotions, sprays, or styling gels. Avoid the use of sedatives or stimulants in the 12-24 hours preceding the EEG. Instruct the patient not to fast before the test because hypoglycemia can affect the recording. Ensure a quiet room with signage to inform visitors of EEG recording in progress. Instruct the patient or family members about the reasons for periodic or continuous monitoring. The reasons for EEG monitoring include: • Determining the general activity of the cerebral hemispheres. • Determining the origin of seizure activity (epilepsy). • Determining cerebral function in epilepsy and other pathologic conditions such as tumors, abscesses, cerebrovascular disease, hematomas, injury, metabolic diseases, degenerative brain disease, and drug intoxication. • Differentiating between organic and hysterical or feigned blindness or deafness. • Monitoring cerebral activity during surgical anesthesia or sedation in the intensive care unit. • Diagnosing sleep disorders. If the EEG is related to a sleep disorder diagnosis, the patient may be asked to sleep less the night before the EEG. • Assisting in the determination of brain death.	The gel and glue used for placing electrodes can be washed out immediately after the test ends. Acetone or witch hazel will dissolve the paste. Advise the patient who has had a sleep-deprived EEG not to drive home.

neurologic testing. A contrast medium may be used to enhance the image. CT scans distinguish bone, soft tissue (e.g., the brain, vascular system, and ventricular system), and fluids such as cerebrospinal fluid (CSF) or blood. Tumors, infarctions, hemorrhage, hydrocephalus, and bone malformations can also be identified.

The patient is placed on a movable table in a head-holding device. He or she must remain completely still during the test, which may be difficult. The table is positioned in the machine—a large, donut-shaped structure. Depending on the scan, the patient may be completely enclosed or in a more open situation. A noncontrast series of pictures are taken first. Then, if needed, the patient is withdrawn from the scanner and given an injection of the iodinated contrast medium. The scan is then repeated. Each set of head scans takes less than 5 minutes in newer scanners. Spinal studies take about 10 minutes per body section (cervical, thoracic, lumbar) and are less likely to require contrast injection.

Most patients with new neurologic symptoms have both a pre-contrast and post-contrast study of the head. Contrast-enhanced CT is especially useful in locating and identifying tumor types and abscesses. For situations in which bleeding is the only concern (e.g., in trauma patients), contrast scans are not usually required.

After a standard CT scan, imaging software digitally removes images of soft tissue so that only images of bone remain. Through the use of this technology, bone deformities, trauma, and birth defects are more easily identified.

CT angiography involves administering contrast dye IV before the CT scan. It is used to identify blockages or narrowing of blood vessels, aneurysms, and other blood vessel abnormalities.

An intrathecal contrast-enhanced CT scan is performed to diagnose disorders of the spine and spinal nerve roots. A lumbar puncture is performed so that a small amount of spinal fluid can be removed and mixed with contrast dye and injected. The patient is positioned to allow for the contrast medium to move around the spinal cord and nerve roots as needed. The patient may have a headache after the procedure. Follow facility policy regarding patient positioning after the procedure.

Magnetic Resonance Imaging. Magnetic resonance imaging (MRI or MR) has advantages over CT in the diagnostic imaging of the brain, spinal cord, and nerve roots. It does not use ionizing radiation but, instead, relies on magnetic fields. Multiple sets of images are taken that are used to determine normal and abnormal anatomy. Images may be enhanced with the use of gadolinium, a non–iodine-based contrast medium. MRIs of the spine have largely replaced CT scans and myelography for evaluation. Bony structures cannot be viewed with MR; CT scans are the best way to see bones. Some facilities have a *functional MRI (fMRI)* machine that can assess blood flow to the brain rather than merely show its anatomic structure.

In addition to the traditional MRI, a *magnetic resonance angiography (MRA), magnetic resonance spectroscopy (MRS),* or *diffusion imaging (DI)* may be requested. MRA is used to evaluate blood flow and blood vessel abnormalities such as an arterial blockage, intracranial aneurysms, and AV malformations. MRS is used to detect abnormalities in the brain's biochemical processes, such as that which occurs in epilepsy, Alzheimer's disease, and brain attack (stroke). DI uses MRI techniques to evaluate ischemia in the brain to determine the location and severity of a stroke.

Newer, open-sided units ("open MRI") now produce adequate images for those patients who do not want standard MRI scanners. MRI has been contraindicated for patients with cardiac pacemakers, other implanted pumps or devices, and ion-containing metal aneurysm clips. However, extensive trials are testing ways to safely scan some patients with pacemakers. Other implanted devices, such as vascular stents, intravascular catheter (IVC) filters, and metal antiembolic devices, may be scanned immediately or after a certain period of time, depending on manufacturers' recommendations. MRI may also be contraindicated in patients who are confused or agitated, have unstable vital signs, are on continuous life support, or have older tattoos (which contain lead). New physiologic monitoring systems made specifically for the scanner allow some patients who are unstable to be scanned. A comprehensive online list of medical devices tested for MRI safety and compatibility can be found at *www.mrisafety.com*. Medical personnel must remove any medical devices they are carrying or wearing and ensure that only approved devices are allowed in the MRI room (see Table 41-4).

Positron Emission Tomography. Positron emission tomography (PET) is a diagnostic tool that is not available in all medical centers (see Table 41-4). Its benefit over a CT scan or MRI is that it provides information about the *function* of the brain, specifically glucose and oxygen metabolism and cerebral blood flow. Current CT scanners provide information about the *structure* of the central nervous system (CNS). The newest PET machines are combination CT-PET scanners that fuse images together to produce better information about the type and location of brain dysfunction.

The physician or nuclear medicine technologist injects the patient with IV deoxyglucose, which is tagged to an isotope. The isotope emits activity in the form of positrons, which are scanned and converted into a color image by computer. The more active a given part of the brain, the greater the glucose uptake. This test is used to evaluate drug metabolism and detect areas of metabolic alteration that occur in dementia, epilepsy, psychiatric and degenerative disorders, neoplasms, and Alzheimer's disease. The level of radiation is equivalent to that of five or six x-rays but much less than exposure during CT.

Teach the patient that he or she will be NPO the night before morning testing and 4 hours before afternoon testing. Patients with diabetes have their test in the morning before taking their antidiabetic drugs. During this 2- to 3-hour procedure, the patient may be blindfolded and have earplugs inserted for all or part of the test. He or she is asked to perform certain mental functions to activate different areas of the brain. Older adults and patients with mental health/behavioral health problems may be too anxious to have a PET scan.

Single-Photon Emission Computed Tomography. The limitation of PET may be overcome through the use of **single-photon emission computed tomography (SPECT)**. This test uses a radiopharmaceutical agent that enables radioisotopes to cross the blood-brain barrier. The agent is administered by IV injection. Gamma-emitting radionuclides have longer half-lives, therefore eliminating the need for a cyclotron near the scanner. Although SPECT is less expensive than PET, the resolution of the images is limited. SPECT is particularly useful in studying cerebral blood flow, amnesia, neoplasms, head trauma, or persistent vegetative state. The test is contraindicated in women who are breast-feeding.

The patient is injected with the material about 1 hour before the actual scan by the radiologist, certified nuclear medicine technologist, or specially trained RN. The patient is positioned on an x-ray table in a quiet dark room for the actual scans. Several gamma cameras scan his or her head. When completed, the images are downloaded to a computer.

Magnetoencephalography.   **Magnetoencephalography (MEG)** is a noninvasive imaging technique used to measure the magnetic fields produced by electrical activity in the brain via extremely sensitive devices such as superconducting quantum interference devices (SQUIDs). MEG is somewhat similar to electroencephalography (EEG). The advantage is greater accuracy because of the minimal distortion of the signal. This allows for more usable and reliable localization of brain function. The brain can be observed "in action" rather than just viewing a still MRI image. These machines are not widely available because of their extremely high cost.

❓ NCLEX EXAMINATION CHALLENGE
Physiological Integrity

A client with possible Parkinson disease is scheduled to have magnetic resonance imaging (MRI). The daughter asks the nurse how this test is different from a computed tomography (CT) scan. What is the nurse's best response?

A. "The MRI scan provides better contrast between normal tissue and pathologic tissue."

B. "They are not different; both use ionizing radiation."

C. "The MRI will not require contrast material and has no special precautions."

D. "The CT scan does not provide a view of deep brain structures like the region where Parkinson originates."

Other Diagnostic Assessment

Electromyography. **Electromyography (EMG)** is used to identify nerve and muscle disorders as well as spinal cord disease. (See Chapter 44 for a description of patient preparation, procedure, and follow-up care.) Electromyography and electroneurography or nerve conduction velocity studies (NCVSs) are usually used together and are referred to as *electromyoneurography.*

Electroencephalography. **Electroencephalography (EEG)** records the electrical activity of the cerebral hemispheres. Each graphic recording represents electrical impulses within the brain. The frequency, amplitude, and characteristics of the brain waves are recorded. For example, a cerebral tumor or infarct may have abnormally slow waveforms. EEGs are used both as a diagnostic test and to provide sustained monitoring, and the indications for testing and monitoring are listed in Table 41-4.

Abnormal results on an EEG test may be due to:
- An abnormal structure in the brain, such as a brain tumor
- Attention problems
- Tissue death due to a blockage in blood flow (cerebral infarction)
- Drug or alcohol intoxication
- Inflammation of the brain (encephalitis)
- Ischemia to brain tissue from low blood flow to the brain during a migraine or a surgical procedure like a carotid endarterectomy
- Seizure disorder
- Sleep disorder or sleep deprivation

Fasting is avoided before EEG testing because hypoglycemia can alter the test results. The patient is placed on a reclining chair or bed. According to an internationally accepted procedure, 16 or more electrodes are applied to the scalp with a jelly-like substance and connected to the machine. The physician or EEG technician places glue over the electrodes to prevent slippage. The patient must lie still with his or her eyes closed during the initial recording. The rest of the test engages the patient in certain activities: hyperventilation, photic stimulation, and sleep. A portable EEG may be performed at the bedside if necessary, but the preference is for the EEG to be done in a very quiet room.

Hyperventilation produces cerebral vasoconstriction and alkalosis, which increases the likelihood of seizure activity. The patient is asked to breathe deeply 20 times per minute for 3 minutes. In *photic stimulation*, a flashing bright light is placed in front of the patient. Frequencies of 1 to 20 flashes per second are used with the patient's eyes open and then closed. If the patient's seizures are photosensitive in origin, seizure activity may be seen on the EEG. A *sleep* EEG may be performed to aid in the detection of abnormal brain waves that are seen only when the patient is sleeping, such as with frontal lobe epilepsy (Pagana & Pagana, 2014).

During an EEG test, which takes 45 to 120 minutes, the recording can be stopped about every 5 minutes to allow the patient to move. If the patient moves during the recording, movement creates a change in the brain waves and the technician will note movements on the graph. Examples of unintentional movement that can affect the recordings are tongue movement, eye blinking, and muscle tensing. The technician may induce or request certain movements or sensory stimulation and record these events on the EEG record to link changes in brain waves with motor activity or sensory stimulation; these intentional movements are also documented on the EEG recording.

Evoked Potentials. Evoked potentials (also called *evoked response*) measure the electrical signals to the brain generated by sound, touch, or light. These tests are used to assess sensory nerve problems and confirm neurologic conditions including multiple sclerosis, brain tumor, acoustic neuroma (small tumors of the inner ear), and spinal cord injury. Evoked potentials are also used to test sight and hearing (especially in infants and young children), monitor brain activity in comatose patients, and confirm brain death (Wijdicks et al., 2010). During evoked potentials, a second set of electrodes is attached to the part of the body that will experience sensation. A stimulus is applied, and the amount of time it takes for the impulse generated by the stimulus to reach the brain is recorded. Under normal circumstances, the process of signal transmission is instantaneous.

Auditory evoked potentials (also called *brainstem auditory evoked response*) are used to assess high-frequency hearing loss, diagnose any damage to the acoustic nerve and auditory pathways in the brainstem, and detect acoustic neuromas. The patient sits in a soundproof room and wears headphones. Clicking sounds are delivered one at a time to one ear while a masking sound is sent to the other ear.

Visual evoked potentials detect loss of vision from optic nerve damage (in particular, damage caused by multiple sclerosis). The patient sits close to a screen and is asked to focus on the center of a shifting checkerboard pattern. Only one eye is tested at a time. The other eye is either kept closed or covered with a patch.

Somatosensory evoked potentials measure response from stimuli to the peripheral nerves and can detect nerve or spinal cord damage or nerve degeneration from multiple sclerosis and other degenerating diseases. Tiny electrical shocks are delivered by electrode to a nerve in an arm or leg.

Cerebral Blood Flow Evaluation. Cerebral blood flow (CBF) can be measured in many areas of the brain with the use of radioactive substances. It is particularly useful in evaluating cerebral vasospasm. Explain the test, and ask the physician if central nervous system (CNS) depressants and stimulants should be withheld for 24 hours before the test.

Lumbar Puncture. Lumbar puncture (spinal tap) is the insertion of a spinal needle into the subarachnoid space between the third and fourth (sometimes the fourth and fifth) lumbar vertebrae (see Table 41-4).

A lumbar puncture (LP) is used to:
- Obtain cerebrospinal fluid (CSF) pressure readings with a manometer
- Obtain CSF for analysis
- Check for spinal blockage caused by a spinal cord lesion
- Inject contrast medium or air for diagnostic study
- Inject spinal anesthetics
- Inject selected drugs

Because of the danger of sudden release of CSF pressure, a lumbar puncture is not done for patients with symptoms indicating severely increased ICP. The procedure is also not performed in patients with skin infections at or near the puncture site because of the danger of introducing infective organisms into the CSF.

Before an LP is performed, position the patient in a fetal side-lying position to separate the vertebrae and move the spinal nerve roots away from the area to be accessed. The health care provider then cleans the skin site thoroughly. The injection site is determined, and a local anesthetic is injected. In a few minutes, a spinal needle is inserted between the third and fourth lumbar vertebrae. Instruct the patient to inform the provider if there is shooting pain or a tingling sensation. After determining proper placement in the subarachnoid space by removing the stylet and seeing CSF, the patient is asked to relax as much as possible so the pressure reading will be accurate. Opening and

> **! NURSING SAFETY PRIORITY** (QSEN)
>
> **Action Alert**
>
> Be sure that the patient does not move during a lumbar puncture. If the patient is restless or cannot cooperate, two people may need to assist instead of one. The patient may need a sedative to reduce movement. Consider patient needs for additional assistance or sedation before beginning the procedure.

closing pressure readings are taken and recorded. Three to five test tubes of CSF are usually collected and numbered sequentially. After specimen collection, the needle is withdrawn, slight pressure is applied, and an adhesive bandage strip is placed over the insertion site.

Examination of CSF has been a useful diagnostic tool for some time. Recent technical advances are increasing the number of analyses that can be done on CSF. The normal characteristics of CSF and some of the more common abnormalities are given in Table 41-5. Gram-stain smears can test for particular types of meningitis, such as tubercular meningitis. CSF can be cultured, and sensitivity studies determine the best choice of antibiotic if an infection is diagnosed. A specific test for neurosyphilis is the fluorescent treponemal antibody absorption (FTA-ABS) test. Cytologic studies of CSF can identify tumor cells.

Complications of lumbar puncture, although not common, include brainstem herniation (discussed in Chapter 45), infection, CSF leakage, and hematoma formation.

Transcranial Doppler Ultrasonography. Intracranial hemodynamics can be evaluated through the use of the transcranial Doppler (TCD). It uses sound waves to measure blood flow through the arteries. The test is particularly valuable in evaluating cerebral vasospasm or narrowing of arteries. TCD is safe, can be used repeatedly for the same patient, and is an inexpensive alternative to angiography.

Muscle and Nerve Biopsies. *Muscle* or *nerve biopsies* are used to diagnose neuromuscular disorders. They may also reveal if a person is a carrier of a defective gene that could be passed on to children. Under local anesthesia, an incision is made into the skin or a hollow needle is inserted through the skin to remove a small sample of muscle or nerve. A CT scan or MRI is performed before a *brain biopsy*. This procedure involves injection of a local anesthetic into the scalp, drilling a small hole through the skull, and inserting a hollow needle into the site of the lesion. Muscle, nerve, and brain biopsy samples are analyzed under a microscope to identify abnormalities.

TABLE 41-5 Significance of Cerebrospinal Fluid Findings

FINDINGS	SIGNIFICANCE
Pressure	
More than 20 cm H_2O	Indicates increased spinal pressure, most often from bleeding, tumors, or infection within the central nervous system (CNS)
Color/Appearance	
Clear, colorless	Normal
Pink-red to orange	Red blood cells present
Yellow	Bilirubin present owing to hemolysis of red blood cells; possible causes include subarachnoid hemorrhage, jaundice, increased cerebrospinal fluid (CSF) protein, hypercarotenemia, or hemoglobinemia
Brown	Methemoglobin present, indicating previous meningeal hemorrhage
Unclear or hazy	Cell count is elevated
Cells	
0-5 small lymphocytes/mm³	Normal
More than 5 lymphocytes/mm³	Reaction to infection, tumor, chemical substance, or blood
Proteins	
Total	
15-45 mg/dL *(up to 70 mg/dL in older adults)*	Normal
45-100 mg/dL	Paraventricular tumor
50-200 mg/dL	Viral infection
More than 500 mg/dL	Bacterial infection, Guillain-Barré syndrome
Less than 15 mg/dL	Meningismus, pseudotumor cerebri, hyperthyroidism, normal finding after lumbar puncture
Immune Gamma Globulin (IgG, the most important protein)	
3%-12% of total protein	Normal
More than 12% of total protein	Multiple sclerosis, neurosyphilis, or viral infection
Albumin/Globulin Ratio	
8:1	Normal
Glucose	
50-75 mg/dL or 60%-70% of blood glucose level	Normal
Less than 50 mg/dL (usually accompanied by the presence of pathologic organisms)	May occur with bacterial, fungal, or viral meningitis; CNS leukemia; or cancer
Other Characteristics	
Lactic Acid	
10-25 mg/dL	Normal
More than 25 mg/dL	Systemic acidosis or increased CSF glucose metabolism
Glutamine	
6-15 mg/dL	Normal
More than 15 mg/dL	Hepatic coma or cirrhosis of liver
Lactate Dehydrogenase	
10% of serum level or 2.0-7.2 units/mL	Normal
More than 10% of serum level	Bacterial meningitis, inflammatory diseases of CNS

NURSING CONCEPTS AND CLINICAL JUDGMENT REVIEW

What might you NOTICE in a patient with adequate COGNITION, MOBILITY, and SENSORY PERCEPTION?

Physical assessment:
- Alert and oriented, intact short-term and long-term memory, appropriate judgment, and adequate attention span
- Communicates clearly
- Moves all four extremities without assistance and normal strength
- Performs ADLs independently
- Walks, with or without assistive devices, using normal gait

- No deficits in or unusual sensory perception
- Pupils equal in size, round and regular in shape, and reactive to light and accommodation (PERRLA)

Diagnostic assessment:
- Normal ECG
- Normal CSF
- Normal EEG
- Normal CT scan of brain
- Normal MRI scan of spinal cord

GET READY FOR THE NCLEX® EXAMINATION!

KEY POINTS

Review these Key Points for each NCLEX Examination Client Needs Category.

Safe and Effective Care Environment
- Perform a neurologic examination that may be either comprehensive or focused as determined by patient needs. **Patient-Centered Care** QSEN
- Identify key changes in the examination that need to be communicated urgently to the health care provider or other team members. **Teamwork and Collaboration** QSEN
- Collaborate with the health care provider, physical therapist, and speech-language pathologist to establish priorities in neurologic assessment. **Teamwork and Collaboration** QSEN

Health Promotion and Maintenance
- Evaluate the presence of risk factors that place patients at risk for neurologic health problems such as behaviors that result in serious harm (e.g., driving recklessly) and lifestyle choices. **Evidence-Based Practice** QSEN
- Detect neurologic changes early with health screening and physical assessment strategies that reflect the prioritized assessment. Recall that a deterioration in level of consciousness (e.g., from alert to lethargic) is the most sensitive and reliable indicator of an adverse neurologic change. Include a daily evaluation for acute confusion or delirium in hospital settings. **Evidence-Based Practice** QSEN
- Consider loss of short-term memory as a potential early sign of neurologic problems. Use findings from diagnostic imaging tests to help evaluate potential neurologic impairment (Tables 41-4 and 41-5).

Psychosocial Integrity
- Assess the reaction of the person to neurologic disease. The psychological responses to neurologic health problems can vary by age, gender, and cultural background. **Patient-Centered Care** QSEN
- Encourage patients to express their feelings, and refer them to appropriate support services as needed.

Physiological Integrity
- Take a patient history, including information listed in Chart 41-2. **Patient-Centered Care** QSEN

- Evaluate the patient's cognitive abilities on admission and regularly thereafter, using a systematic approach (Chart 41-3). **Evidence-Based Practice** QSEN
- Use the Glasgow Coma Scale for patients with new traumatic brain injury.
- Use the BIMS, CAM, CAM-ICU, or other validated tool to detect delirium, an acute confusional state.
- Assess motor and sensory function to reduce harm from acute deterioration or chronic deficits. This type of assessment is also needed for discharge planning.
- Include assessment of gait, balance, and coordination to determine risk for falls. **Safety** QSEN
- Check cranial nerve III by examining pupils for size, shape, and reaction to light. Pupils should be equal in size, round and regular in shape, and become smaller in bright light. Changes in eye signs can indicate new neurologic deterioration in nonverbal patients. **Evidence-Based Practice** QSEN
- Accommodation occurs when the eyes converge and pupils constrict as an object is moved from several feet away to within 4 to 5 inches of the nose.
- Promote independence in consultation with physical and occupational therapists and the use of assistive devices like a walker or brace. **Teamwork and Collaboration** QSEN
- Assist with the performance of daily living activities when the neurologic condition interferes with self-care. **Patient-Centered Care** QSEN
- Reduce complications for patients having neurologic diagnostic testing by providing adequate teaching and preparation as outlined in Table 41-4. **Evidence-Based Practice** QSEN
- Use serum creatinine or estimated glomerular filtration rate to identify patients with reduced kidney function. Older adults and patients with chronic kidney disease, diabetes, or heart failure are at high risk for kidney damage from iodinated and gadolinium contrast media. Provide adequate fluid intake before and after diagnostic testing to flush contrast after a diagnostic test (see Chart 41-4).
- Teach patients having an EEG to follow the precautions listed in Table 41-4.
- Check for bleeding after patients have an angiography. If bleeding is observed, call the radiologist immediately.

- Before MRI, check for implanted devices such as pacemakers, vascular stents, pumps, and aneurysm clips.
- Link abnormal neurologic function with anatomy and physiology to anticipate impaired function, prognosis, and safe, effective interventions. **Evidence-Based Practice** QSEN
- Cerebrospinal fluid (CSF) is clear and colorless with few cells. Significant changes include the presence of cells, color, and turbidity (Table 41-5).
- Use findings from diagnostic imaging tests and anatomic location of injury to locate potential neurologic impairment for a focused examination (Tables 41-1, 41-2, and 41-3).
- Decerebrate or decorticate posturing and pinpoint or dilated nonreactive pupils are late signs of neurologic deterioration.

- Recognize that older adults do not normally experience deterioration in COGNITION and memory but do experience physical and physiological changes that affect MOBILITY and SENSORY PERCEPTION (Chart 41-1). **Patient-Centered Care** QSEN
- Provide a safe environment when memory loss is part of the older adult's health status by using memory aids and assistive technology to meet teaching or self-care goals. **Safety** QSEN
- Provide safe opportunities for MOBILITY, including physical activity like walking, when caring for older adults. Mobility and physical activity promote COGNITION.

CHAPTER 42

Care of Patients with Problems of the Central Nervous System: The Brain

Rachel L. Gallagher

 http://evolve.elsevier.com/Iggy/

PRIORITY CONCEPTS

- COGNITION
- PAIN
- MOBILITY
- INFECTION

LEARNING OUTCOMES

Safe and Effective Care Environment
1. Plan with the interdisciplinary team for transitions in care including discharge to home or other setting for patients with chronic problems of the brain.
2. Implement interventions to protect patients with chronic brain conditions from injury and INFECTION, including pain management.
3. Provide written instructions about drug therapy for chronic health problems to patients and caregivers when transitioning to a new care setting.

Health Promotion and Maintenance
4. Teach patients with chronic headaches about preventive and management approaches to therapy.
5. Develop a teaching plan about drug therapy for patients with epilepsy.
6. Teach patients about vaccination to prevent meningitis.

Psychosocial Integrity
7. Include family members, patient preferences, and values in planning care, including strategies to reduce the psychosocial impact of chronic brain conditions on patients and family members.

8. Identify community resources to support caregivers or patients with chronic neurodegenerative diseases to promote cognition and mobility.

Physiological Integrity
9. Compare and contrast assessment and management for migraine and cluster headaches.
10. Differentiate the common types of seizures, including presenting clinical manifestations.
11. Prioritize evidence-based care for patients with a seizure disorder, including appropriate seizure precaution interventions.
12. Identify nursing priorities for patients with bacterial meningitis and encephalitis.
13. Identify the genetic and environmental influences on development of Parkinson disease (PD), dementia (Alzheimer's disease [AD]), and Huntington disease (HD).
14. Document a collaborative plan of care for patients with chronic brain conditions like PD, dementia, and HD based on patient values and preferences.
15. Prevent or reduce common risk factors that contribute to functional decline and decreased quality of life in adults and older adults with chronic brain disorders.

This chapter discusses five chronic and two acute neurologic conditions. All of these neurologic disorders interfere with self-management and independence; many of them contribute to chronic PAIN and reduced MOBILITY. Care of patients with chronic neurologic disorders requires coordination by nurses and significant collaboration with other members of the interdisciplinary health care team. The patient and family are the center of the collaborative team in making decisions about the plan of care (Quality and Safety Education for Nurses [QSEN], 2014).

HEADACHES

Almost everyone has had a headache at some time in his or her life. Some headaches are related to sinus congestion, allergies, or stress and are temporary. Others can be very serious and potentially life threatening. For example, an abnormal neurologic assessment together with symptoms of a cluster headache may indicate a serious neurologic problem. Patients with these symptoms are referred immediately to their health care provider or the emergency department.

Although there are many types and causes of headaches, the focus of this section is on two common types that cause people to seek medical attention: migraine headaches and cluster headaches. Patients are usually managed in the ambulatory care setting by the primary health care provider. However, it is not unusual for the person in severe PAIN to seek treatment in the emergency department. Refer to Chart 42-1 for questions to determine the pattern of headaches when assessing a patient.

CHART 42-1   Determining a Pattern of Headaches

Ask the patient:
- When do the headaches occur?
- How do they start?
- How often?
- How long do they last?
- Do you have the same type of headache all the time?
- Where do you feel the headache pain?
- Does the headache pain spread to other areas of the head?
- How does the headache pain feel: throbbing, stabbing, pounding, squeezing, or something else?
- Do you ever have accompanying symptoms with your headache, such as nausea, vomiting, diarrhea, dizziness, changes in vision, weakness?
- Do certain foods, alcohol, or other things trigger the headaches?
- Have there been any recent changes in your headaches?
- How do you treat the headaches? Does this treatment work?
- How often and what drug or herbal remedy do you take?
- Has a headache ever been severe enough to go to the emergency room for treatment?
- Have you ever been hospitalized for headache treatment?
- Have you ever seen a specialist (neurologist) for your headache?
- What do think might be causing your headaches?
- Is there a family history of headaches?
- Do you have to stop what you are doing or miss work when you get a headache?

! NURSING SAFETY PRIORITY (QSEN)

Action Alert

Encourage patients to keep a headache diary to help identify the type of headache they are experiencing and the response to medication or other intervention. Teach them to notify their health care provider if the quality, intensity, or nature of the headache increases or changes. Encourage them to report whether the headache is associated with new or unusual visual changes and whether the prescribed drug is no longer effective.

MIGRAINE HEADACHE

❖ PATHOPHYSIOLOGY

A migraine headache is a common clinical syndrome characterized by recurrent episodic attacks of head PAIN that serve no protective purpose. Migraine headache pain is usually described as throbbing and unilateral. Migraine can be accompanied by associated symptoms such as nausea or sensitivity to light, sound, or head movement. Migraine disorders are further characterized by multiple subtypes (McCance et al., 2014). Migraine pain and associated symptoms can last 4 to 72 hours. Migraines tend to be familial, and women are affected more commonly than men. Women diagnosed with migraines are more likely to have major depressive disorder (Modgill et al., 2012). Migraine sufferers are also at risk for stroke and epilepsy (McCance et al., 2014).

The cause of migraine headaches is not clear but includes a combination of neuronal hyperexcitability and vascular, genetic, hormonal, and environmental factors. In general, experts suggest that migraines are a neurogenic process with secondary cerebral vasodilation followed by a sterile brain tissue inflammation. Patients may inherit a condition of neuronal hyperexcitability from ion channel variations, particularly calcium and sodium-potassium pump channels, as well as from genetic

variations in serotonin and dopamine receptors. Following stimulation of these hyper-excitable neuronal pathways, vascular changes occur. Pain-sensing cells in the blood vessels of the brain initiate the attack. Activation of the trigeminal nerve pathways contributes to the cascade of events that activate **nociceptors**. Substances that increase sensitivity to pain such as glutamate are synthesized through the trigeminal pathway (McCance et al., 2014). As cerebral arteries dilate, **prostaglandins** are released (chemicals that cause inflammation and swelling). Vasodilation, in turn, allows prostaglandins and other intravascular molecules to leak (**extravasate**), contributing to widespread tissue swelling and the sensation of throbbing pain.

Many patients find that certain factors, or *triggers*, such as caffeine, red wine, and monosodium glutamate (MSG), tend to cause migraine headache attacks. Each patient is different regarding which environmental factors trigger headaches. For some patients, stress or a change in weather can lead to an attack. These stimuli are thought to initiate the cascade of events that cause migraines by activating hyper-excitable neurons. Neurons involved in the initiation and propagation of migraines may have an early sensitization to neurotransmitters such that patients become increasingly susceptible to triggers and to the cascade of events that culminate in migraine PAIN. Thus care includes not only managing pain but also disrupting the migraine cascade to decrease sensitization and recurrent attacks.

❖ PATIENT-CENTERED COLLABORATIVE CARE

◆ Assessment

Migraines fall into three categories: migraines with aura, migraines without aura, and atypical migraines. An **aura** is a sensation such as visual changes that signals the onset of a headache or seizure. In a migraine, the aura occurs immediately before the migraine episode. *Most headaches are migraines without aura.* The key features of migraines are listed in Chart 42-2. **Atypical migraines** are less common and include menstrual and cluster migraines. The stages of migraine may include:
- Prodromal (or prodrome) phase, in which the patient has specific symptoms such as food cravings or mood changes
- Aura phase (if present), which generally involves visual changes, flashing lights, or **diplopia** (double vision)
- Headache phase, which may last a few hours to a few days
- Termination phase, in which the intensity of the headache decreases
- Postprodrome phase, in which the patient is often fatigued, may be irritable, and has muscle pain

The diagnosis of migraine headache is based on the patient's history and on physical, neurologic, and psychological assessment. The typical migraine is described as a unilateral, fronto-temporal, *throbbing* PAIN in the head that is often worse behind one eye or ear. It is often accompanied by a sensitive scalp, anorexia, **photophobia** (sensitivity to light), **phonophobia** (sensitivity to noise), and nausea with or without vomiting. Patients tend to have the same clinical manifestations each time they have a migraine headache. Some may have to refrain from regular activities for several days if they cannot control or relieve the PAIN in its early stage.

Some physicians recommend screening patients with migraines using the Minnesota Multiphasic Personality Inventory–2 to identify personality traits and possible mental health/behavioral health problems like depression that may contribute to the headache experience (Rausa et al., 2013).

CHART 42-2 Key Features

Migraine Headaches

Phases of Migraine with Aura (Classic Migraine)

First, or Prodrome, Phase
- Aura develops over a period of several minutes and lasts no longer than 1 hour.
- Well-defined transient focal neurologic dysfunction exists.
- Pain may be preceded by:
  - Visual disturbances
    - Flashing lights
    - Lines or spots
    - Shimmering or zigzag lights
- A variety of neurologic changes, including:
  - Numbness, tingling of the lips or tongue
  - Acute confusional state
  - Aphasia
  - Vertigo
  - Unilateral weakness
  - Drowsiness

Second Phase
- Headache is accompanied by nausea and vomiting.
- Pain usually begins in the temple. It increases in intensity and becomes throbbing within 1 hour.

Third Phase
- Pain changes from throbbing to dull.
- Headache, nausea, and vomiting usually last from 4 to 72 hours. (Older patients may have aura without pain, known as a *visual migraine*.)

Migraine Without Aura (Common Migraine)
- Migraine begins without an aura before the onset of the headache.
- Pain is aggravated by performing routine physical activities.
- Pain is unilateral and pulsating.
- One of these symptoms is present:
  - Nausea and/or vomiting
  - **Photophobia** (light sensitivity)
  - **Phonophobia** (sound sensitivity)
- Headache lasts for 4 to 72 hours.
- Migraine often occurs in the early morning, during periods of stress, or in those with premenstrual tension or fluid retention.

Atypical Migraine
- Status migrainous:
  - Headache lasts longer than 72 hours.
- Migrainous infarction:
  - Neurologic symptoms are not completely reversible within 7 days.
  - Ischemic infarct is noted on neuroimaging.
- Unclassified:
  - Headache does not fulfill all of the criteria to be classified a migraine.

TABLE 42-1 Commonly Used Drugs for Migraine Headache

Nonspecific Analgesics
- Acetaminophen
- Isometheptene
- Butalbital

Nonsteroidal Anti-Inflammatory Drugs (NSAIDs)
- Ibuprofen
- Naproxen

Ergotamine Preparations
- Ergotamine with caffeine (oral or suppository) (Cafergot, Migergot)
- Ergotamine sublingual (SL) (Ergomar SL)
- Medihaler ergotamine (oral inhalation aerosol)
- Dihydroergotamine (DHE) nasal spray (Migranal)

Beta Blockers
- Propranolol
- Timolol

Calcium Channel Blockers
- Verapamil (Calan)

Triptan Preparations
- Almotriptan (Axert)
- Eletriptan (Relpax)
- Rizatriptan (Maxalt)
- Zolmitriptan (Zomig)
- Sumatriptan (Imitrex)
- Frovatriptan (Frova)

Isometheptene Combination
- Midrin

Antiepileptic Drugs (AEDs)
- Divalproex (Depakote)
- Topiramate (Topamax)

Neuroimaging such as magnetic resonance imaging (MRI) may be indicated if the patient has other neurologic findings, a history of seizures, findings not consistent with a migraine, or a change in the severity of the symptoms or frequency of the attacks.

Neuroimaging is also recommended in patients older than 50 years with a new onset of headaches, especially women. Women with a history of migraines with visual symptoms may have an increased risk for stroke, particularly if a migraine with visual symptoms occurred in the past year. Teach women older than 50 years who have migraines about the risk factors for cardiovascular disease. Encourage them to notify their health care provider if they experience symptoms such as facial drooping, arm weakness, or difficulties with speech.

◆ Interventions

The priority for care of the patient having migraines is pain management. This outcome may be achieved by abortive and preventive therapy. Drug therapy, trigger management, and complementary and alternative therapies are the major approaches to care. Provide detailed patient and family education regarding the collaborative plan of care. Effective physician/patient communication is increasingly important in managing the symptoms of migraines. Tools to help patients communicate with their health care provider and partner with their provider to manage PAIN are best practices in migraine diagnosis and treatment (Marcus, 2014).

Abortive Therapy. Abortive therapy is aimed at alleviating PAIN during the aura phase (if present) or soon after the headache has started. *Drug therapy* is prescribed to manage migraine headaches. Some of the drugs being used have major side effects, contraindications, and nursing implications. The health care provider must consider any other medical conditions that the patient has when prescribing drug therapy. In general, the patient is started on a low dose that is increased until the desired clinical effect is obtained. Table 42-1 lists commonly used drugs for migraine headaches. Many new drugs are being investigated for this painful and often debilitating health problem.

Mild migraines may be relieved by acetaminophen (APAP) (Tylenol, Abenol ✚). NSAIDs such as ibuprofen (Motrin) and naproxen (Naprosyn) may also be prescribed. In the United States, the Food and Drug Administration (FDA) has approved several over-the-counter (OTC) anti-inflammatory drugs for migraines, including Advil Migraine Capsules, Motrin Migraine Pain Caplets, and Excedrin Migraine Tablets or Caplets (contain APAP, aspirin, and caffeine). Caffeine narrows blood vessels by blocking adenosine, which dilates vessels and increases inflammation. Antiemetics may be prescribed to relieve nausea and vomiting. Metoclopramide (Reglan, Clopra) may be administered with NSAIDs to promote gastric emptying and decrease vomiting.

For more *severe* migraines, drugs such as triptan preparations, ergotamine derivatives, and isometheptene combinations are needed. A potential side effect of these drugs is rebound headache, also known as medication overuse headache, in which another headache occurs after the drug relieves the initial migraine.

Triptan preparations relieve the headache and associated symptoms by activating the 5-HT (serotonin) receptors on the cranial arteries, the basilar artery, and the blood vessels of the dura mater to produce a vasoconstrictive effect. Examples are listed in Table 42-1. For many patients, these drugs are highly effective for PAIN, nausea, vomiting, and light and sound sensitivity with few side effects. Most are contraindicated in patients with actual or suspected ischemic heart disease, cerebrovascular ischemia, hypertension, and peripheral vascular disease and in those with Prinzmetal's angina because of the potential for coronary vasospasm. Patients respond differently to drugs, and several types or combinations may be tried before the headache is relieved.

> ! **NURSING SAFETY PRIORITY** (QSEN)
>
> **Drug Alert**
>
> Teach patients taking triptan drugs to take them as soon as migraine symptoms develop. Instruct patients to report angina (chest pain) or chest discomfort to their health care providers immediately to prevent cardiac damage from myocardial ischemia. Remind them to use contraception (birth control) while taking the drugs because the drugs may not be safe for women who are pregnant. Teach them to expect common side effects that include flushing, tingling, and a hot sensation. These annoying sensations tend to subside after the patient's body gets used to the drug. Triptan drugs should not be taken with selective serotonin reuptake inhibitor (SSRI) antidepressants or St. John's wort, an herb used commonly for depression (Lilley et al., 2014).

Ergotamine preparations such as Cafergot are taken at the start of the headache. The patient may take up to six tablets in 24 hours or use a rectal suppository. Dihydroergotamine (DHE) may be given IV, IM, or as a nasal spray (Migranal) with an antiemetic if PAIN control and relief of nausea are not achieved with other drugs. DHE should not be given within 24 hours of a triptan drug.

Midrin is a combination drug containing APAP, isomeptene, and dichloralphenazone. It is the most common *isometheptene combination* given for treating migraines and is an excellent option when ergotamine preparations are not tolerated or do not work.

Other drugs that have been prescribed to relieve migraine PAIN include opioids and barbiturates. *These drugs should be avoided if at all possible because they are addictive. Some opioids actually cause a migraine.*

Preventive Therapy. Prevention drugs and other strategies are used when a migraine occurs more than twice per week, interferes with ADLs, or is not relieved with acute treatment. Unless otherwise contraindicated, the health care provider may initially prescribe an NSAID, a beta-adrenergic blocker, a calcium channel blocker, or an antiepileptic drug (AED). Propranolol (Inderal, Apo-Propranolol ♣, Novopranol ♣) and timolol (Blocadren, Apo-Timol ♣) are the only *beta blockers* approved for migraine prevention. Verapamil (Calan, Apo-Verap ♣), a *calcium channel blocking agent*, may also be used for some patients. The calcium channel and beta blockers are thought to reduce the activity of hyper-excitable neurons and act on the neurogenic causes of migraine. Both calcium channel blockers and beta blockers interfere with vasodilation, a contributing cause of migraine PAIN. Both beta-adrenergic blockers and calcium channel blocking drugs can lower blood pressure and decrease pulse rate.

> ! **NURSING SAFETY PRIORITY** (QSEN)
>
> **Drug Alert**
>
> Teach patients who take beta-adrenergic blockers or calcium channel blockers how to take their pulse. Encourage them to report bradycardia or adverse reactions such as fatigue and shortness of breath to their health care provider as soon as possible.

Topiramate (Topamax) is one of the most common *antiepileptic drugs (AEDs)* used for migraines, but it should be used in low doses of 25 to 100 mg daily. The mechanism of action is not clear, but this drug may inhibit the sodium channels, channels that may be hyper-excitable in patients with migraine. Reports of suicides have been associated with this drug when it is used in larger doses of 400 mg daily, most often with patients who have bipolar disorder.

For chronic migraine, onabotulinumtoxinA (Botox) is the only therapy approved for adults. Doses of 75 to 260 units are administered in seven specific areas of the head and neck by the health care provider. Monthly treatments for up to five treatment cycles are considered safe and effective (Diener et al., 2014; Carod-Artel, 2014).

In addition to drug therapy, *trigger avoidance and management* are important interventions for preventing migraine episodes. For example, some patients find that avoiding tyramine-containing products, such as pickled products, caffeine, beer, wine, preservatives, and artificial sweeteners, reduces their headaches. Others have identified specific factors that trigger an attack for them. Help patients identify triggers that could cause migraine episodes, and teach them to avoid them once identified (Chart 42-3). For example, at the beginning of a migraine attack, the patient may be able to reduce PAIN by lying down and darkening the room. He or she may want both eyes covered and a cool cloth on the forehead. If the patient falls asleep, he or she should remain undisturbed until awakening.

Complementary and Alternative Therapies. Many patients use complementary and alternative therapies as adjuncts to drug therapy. Yoga, meditation, massage, exercise, and biofeedback are helpful in preventing or treating migraines for some patients. Vitamin B_{12} (riboflavin), coenzyme *Q10*, and magnesium supplement to maintain normal serum values have a role in migraine prevention (Mauskop, 2012).

Acupuncture and acupressure may be effective in relieving PAIN for some patients. Some plastic surgeons have resected the

Factors That May Trigger a Migraine Attack

Teach patients to avoid factors that may trigger a migraine attack.

Foods Commonly Associated with Migraines

- Alcoholic drinks: beer, wine, and hard liquor
- Aged cheese or other foods with tyramine
- Caffeine found in beverages such as coffee, tea, cola OR caffeine withdrawal
- Chocolate
- Foods with yeast such as pastry and fresh breads
- Monosodium glutamate (MSG)
- Nitrates (meats), pickled or fermented foods
- Nuts
- Artificial sweeteners
- Smoked fish

Drugs Associated with Migraines

- Cimetidine (Tagamet)
- Estrogens
- Nitroglycerin
- Nifedipine (Procardia, Nifed)

Other Factors That Can Trigger a Migraine Attack

- Anger, conflict
- Fatigue
- Hormonal fluctuations, such as menstruation, pregnancy, and menopause
- Light glare
- Missed meals, hypoglycemia
- Psychological stress
- Sleep problems
- Smells, such as tobacco smoke
- Travel to different altitudes

trigeminal nerve to relieve chronic migraine pain. A number of herbs are also used for headaches, both for prevention and pain management. Teach patients that all herbs and nutritional remedies should be approved by their health care provider before use because they could interact with prescribed medication. At this time, there is insufficient evidence to support any herb or natural remedy, but some patients have had positive results.

❓ NCLEX EXAMINATION CHALLENGE

Health Promotion and Maintenance

The nurse is preparing a teaching plan for a client with migraine headaches. Which of these foods or food additives may trigger a migraine headache?
A. Salt
B. Sugar
C. Tyramine
D. Glutamine

CLUSTER HEADACHE

❖ PATHOPHYSIOLOGY

Cluster headaches are manifested by brief (30 minutes to 2 hours), intense unilateral PAIN that generally occurs in the spring and fall without warning. It is classified as the *most common chronic short-duration headache* with pain lasting less than 4 hours. Also referred to as *trigeminal autonomic cephalalgia*, it is far less common than migraines. Cluster headaches

typically develop in men between 20 and 50 years of age. The cause and mechanism of cluster headaches are not known but have been attributed to vasoreactivity and neurogenic inflammation (McCance et al., 2014). Neuroimaging studies suggest that cluster headaches are related to an overactive and enlarged hypothalamus.

❖ PATIENT-CENTERED COLLABORATIVE CARE

◆ Assessment

Question the patient about prescribed drugs for both the prevention and relief of the headache, as well as OTC drugs and herbal preparations he or she may be taking. Interventions used by the patient may include relaxation techniques, meditation, acupuncture, massage therapies, and avoidance of the known headache trigger. Ask the patient to recall a typical week's activities and any recent changes in lifestyle. Explore the relationship of cluster headache onset with emotional and behavioral precipitating factors such as bursts of anger, prolonged anticipation, excessive physical activity, and excitement. Ask him or her to identify bedtimes and waking times to help assess changes in activity or lack of continuity in the sleep-wake cycle.

The PAIN of these unilateral (one-sided) oculotemporal or oculofrontal headaches is often described as excruciating, boring, and *nonthrobbing*. The intense pain is felt deep in and around the eye. The headaches occur at about the same time of day for about 4 to 12 weeks (hence the term *cluster*), followed by a period of remission for 9 months to a year. This episodic form is the most common, although there is a chronic, intractable form in which there may not be a remission for more than a year.

The PAIN may radiate to the forehead, temple, or cheek. It may also radiate, but to a lesser extent, to the ear and neck. The temporal artery may be prominent and tender. The patient often paces, walks, or sits and rocks during an attack. A cluster is the only headache type in which this behavior occurs. During periods of remission, alcohol does not cause a headache (as it does during the headache period). The onset of the pain is associated with relaxation, napping, or rapid eye movement (REM) sleep.

The headache usually occurs with:

- **Ipsilateral** (same side) tearing of the eye
- **Rhinorrhea** ("runny nose") or congestion
- **Ptosis** (drooping eyelid)
- Eyelid edema
- Facial sweating
- **Miosis** (constriction of pupils)

The ptosis may become permanent. Assess for possible bradycardia, flushing or pallor of the face, increased intraocular pressure, and increased skin temperature. Nausea and vomiting may also occur. The patient may become restless and agitated from the intense pain of the headache.

◆ Interventions

Explain the need for and importance of a consistent sleep-wake cycle. The health care provider typically prescribes some of the same types of drugs used for migraines, such as triptans, ergotamine preparations, calcium channel blockers, and antiepileptic drugs (see discussion of drug therapy in the Migraine Headache section). Additional drugs include lithium and corticosteroids. OTC civamide (a capsaicin isomer), available as a nasal spray, oral melatonin, and oral glucosamine are also used by some patients. Provide health teaching about drug therapy (Lilley et al., 2014).

During the periods of attack, teach the patient to wear sunglasses and to sit facing away from the window to help decrease exposure to light and glare. For a cluster migraine, the health care provider may prescribe oxygen via high-flow mask at 12 L/min. High-flow oxygen to manage a cluster migraine is typically administered with the patient in a sitting position. Administer the oxygen for 15 to 20 minutes; most patients report relief within 15 minutes. High-flow oxygen is thought to inhibit activity of the carotid bodies and reduce the vasoreactivity of cerebral blood vessels to neurogenic stimuli. Patients may use oxygen at home. Teach them about the precautions that must be taken when oxygen is used (see Chapter 28).

Surgical intervention may be recommended for patients with *chronic* drug-resistant cluster headaches. Invasive ambulatory care procedures, such as *percutaneous stereotactic rhizotomy (PSR),* are performed with varying success rates. Information about this procedure is found in Chapter 44 in the Trigeminal Neuralgia section. Long-term high-frequency electrical stimulation of the posterior hypothalamus, also known as *deep brain stimulation,* may reduce or eliminate PAIN (see procedure discussion on p. 871 in the Parkinson Disease section). It has not been approved by the FDA but is being investigated. Both of these procedures have major complications that can cause permanent brain or nerve damage. Therefore they are done as a last resort.

SEIZURES AND EPILEPSY

❖ PATHOPHYSIOLOGY

A seizure is an abnormal, sudden, excessive, uncontrolled electrical discharge of neurons within the brain that may result in a change in level of consciousness (LOC), motor or sensory ability, and/or behavior. A single seizure may occur for no known reason. Some seizures are caused by a pathologic condition of the brain, such as a tumor. In this case, once the underlying problem is treated, the patient is often asymptomatic.

Epilepsy is defined by the National Institute of Neurological Disorders and Stroke as two or more seizures experienced by a person. It is a chronic disorder in which repeated unprovoked seizure activity occurs. It may be caused by an abnormality in electrical neuronal activity; an imbalance of neurotransmitters, especially gamma aminobutyric acid (GABA); or a combination of both (McCance et al., 2014).

Types of Seizures

The International Classification of Epileptic Seizures recognizes three broad categories of seizure disorders: generalized seizures, partial seizures, and unclassified seizures.

Five types of generalized seizures may occur in adults and involve *both* cerebral hemispheres. The *tonic-clonic seizure* lasting 2 to 5 minutes begins with a tonic phase that causes stiffening or rigidity of the muscles, particularly of the arms and legs, and immediate loss of consciousness. Clonic or rhythmic jerking of all extremities follows. The patient may bite his or her tongue and may become incontinent of urine or feces. Fatigue, acute confusion, and lethargy may last up to an hour after the seizure.

Occasionally, only tonic or clonic movement may occur. A *tonic seizure* is an abrupt increase in muscle tone, loss of consciousness, and autonomic changes lasting from 30 seconds to several minutes. The *clonic seizure* lasts several minutes and causes muscle contraction and relaxation.

The *myoclonic seizure* causes a brief jerking or stiffening of the extremities that may occur singly or in groups. Lasting for just a few seconds, the contractions may be symmetric (both sides) or asymmetric (one side).

In an *atonic (akinetic) seizure,* the patient has a sudden loss of muscle tone, lasting for seconds, followed by postictal (after the seizure) confusion. In most cases, these seizures cause the patient to fall, which may result in injury. This type of seizure tends to be most resistant to drug therapy.

Partial seizures, also called *focal* or *local* seizures, begin in a part of *one* cerebral hemisphere. They are further subdivided into two main classes: complex partial seizures and simple partial seizures. In addition, some partial seizures can become generalized tonic-clonic, tonic, or clonic seizures. Partial seizures are most often seen in adults and generally are less responsive to medical treatment when compared with other types.

Complex partial seizures may cause loss of consciousness (syncope), or "black out," for 1 to 3 minutes. Characteristic automatisms may occur as in absence seizures. The patient is unaware of the environment and may wander at the start of the seizure. In the period after the seizure, he or she may have amnesia (loss of memory). Because the area of the brain most often involved in this type of epilepsy is the temporal lobe, complex partial seizures are often called *psychomotor* seizures or *temporal lobe* seizures.

The patient with a *simple partial seizure* remains conscious throughout the episode. He or she often reports an aura (unusual sensation) before the seizure takes place. This may consist of a "déjà vu" (already seen) phenomenon, perception of an offensive smell, or sudden onset of PAIN. During the seizure, the patient may have one-sided movement of an extremity, experience unusual sensations, or have autonomic symptoms. Autonomic changes include a change in heart rate, skin flushing, and epigastric discomfort.

Unclassified, or idiopathic, seizures account for about half of all seizure activity. They occur for no known reason and do not fit into the generalized or partial classifications.

Etiology and Genetic Risk

Primary or *idiopathic epilepsy* is not associated with any identifiable brain lesion or other specific cause; however, genetic factors most likely play a role in its development. *Secondary seizures* result from an underlying brain lesion, most commonly a tumor or trauma. They may also be caused by:
- Metabolic disorders
- Acute alcohol withdrawal

- Electrolyte disturbances (e.g., hyperkalemia, water intoxication, hypoglycemia)
- High fever
- Stroke
- Head injury
- Substance abuse
- Heart disease

Seizures resulting from these problems are not considered epilepsy. Various risk factors can trigger a seizure, such as increased physical activity, emotional stress, excessive fatigue, alcohol or caffeine consumption, or certain foods or chemicals.

❖ PATIENT-CENTERED COLLABORATIVE CARE

◆ Assessment

Question the patient or family about how many seizures the patient has had, how long they last, and any pattern of occurrence. Ask the patient or family to describe the seizures that the patient has had. Clinical manifestations vary depending on the type of seizure experienced, as described earlier. Ask about the presence of an aura before seizures begin (preictal phase). Question whether the patient is taking any prescribed drugs or herbs or has had head trauma or high fever. Assess any alcohol and/or illicit drug history. Ask about any other medical condition such as a previous stroke or hypertension.

If the seizure is a new symptom, ask the patient or family if any loss of consciousness or brain injury has occurred, both in the recent and distant past. Oftentimes, patients may have had a head or brain injury sufficient to cause a loss of consciousness but may not remember this at the time of the seizure, especially if it was during their childhood.

Diagnosis is based on the history and physical examination. A variety of diagnostic tests are performed to rule out other causes of seizure activity and to confirm the diagnosis of epilepsy. Typical diagnostic tests include an electroencephalogram (EEG), computed tomography (CT) scan, MRI, or positron emission tomography (PET) scan. These tests are described in Chapter 41. Laboratory studies are performed to identify metabolic or other disorders that may cause or contribute to seizure activity.

◆ Interventions

Removing or treating the underlying condition or cause of the seizure manages *secondary* epilepsy and seizures that are not considered epileptic. *In most cases, primary epilepsy is successfully managed through drug therapy.*

Nonsurgical Management. Most seizures can be completely or almost completely controlled through the administration of antiepileptic drugs (AEDs), sometimes referred to as *anticonvulsants,* for specific types of seizures.

Drug Therapy. Drug therapy is the major component of management (Chart 42-4). The health care provider introduces one antiepileptic drug (AED) at a time to achieve seizure control. If the chosen drug is not effective, the dosage may be increased or another drug introduced. At times, seizure control is achieved only through a combination of drugs. The dosages are adjusted to achieve therapeutic blood levels without causing major side effects.

Teach patients to take their drugs on time to maintain therapeutic blood levels and maximum effectiveness. Emphasize the importance of taking their AEDs as prescribed. Instruct patients that they can build up sensitivity to the drugs as they age. If

sensitivity occurs, tell them they will need to have blood levels of this drug checked frequently to adjust the dose. In some cases, the antiseizure effects of drugs can decline and lead to an increase in seizures. Because of this potential for "drug decline and sensitivity," patients need to keep their scheduled laboratory appointments to check serum drug levels.

Be aware of drug-drug and drug-food interactions. For instance, warfarin (Coumadin, Warfilone ♣) should not be given with phenytoin (Dilantin). Document side and adverse effects of the prescribed drugs, and report to the health care provider. Patients should be taught that some citrus fruits, such as grapefruit juice, can interfere with the metabolism of these drugs. This interference can raise the blood level of the drug and cause the patient to develop drug toxicity.

Self-Management Education. Provide self-management education for the patient and family (Chart 42-5). Ask them what they understand about the disorder, and correct any misinformation. As new information is presented, be sure that the patient and family can understand it. Refer patients and families to the Epilepsy Foundation of America for more information and community support groups. Encourage patients and their significant others to utilize information from the Epilepsy Foundation website (www.epilepsy.com).

Emphasize that AEDs must not be stopped even if the seizures have stopped. Discontinuing these drugs can lead to the recurrence of seizures or the life-threatening complication of status epilepticus (discussed below). Some patients may stop therapy because they do not have the money to purchase the drugs. Refer limited-income patients to the social services department for assistance or to a case manager to locate other resources.

A balanced diet, proper rest, and stress-reduction techniques usually minimize the risk for breakthrough seizures. Encourage the patient to keep a seizure diary to determine whether there are factors that tend to be associated with seizure activity. Patients should follow state law concerning allowances for driving a motor vehicle.

All states prohibit discrimination against people who have epilepsy. Patients who work in occupations in which a seizure might cause serious harm to themselves or others (e.g., construction workers, operators of dangerous equipment, pilots) may need other employment. They may need to decrease or modify strenuous or potentially dangerous physical activity to avoid harm, although this varies with each person. Various local, state, and federal agencies can help with finances, living arrangements, and vocational rehabilitation.

CHART 42-4   Common Examples of Drug Therapy

Epilepsy

DRUG	INDICATION FOR USE	NURSING INTERVENTIONS
Carbamazepine (Tegretol, Tegretol-XR, Carbatrol)	Partial, generalized tonic-clonic seizures	Monitor for headache, dizziness, diplopia or blurred vision, N/V, and leukopenia. Monitor CBC. Do not crush or chew sustained-release capsules.
Clonazepam (Klonopin)	Absence, myoclonic, and akinetic seizures	Monitor results of liver function tests.
Clorazepate dipotassium	Adjunctive management of partial seizures	Give with food. Monitor blood pressure.
Diazepam (Valium, Apo-Diazepam ✦), lorazepam (Ativan), Diastat (diazepam rectal gel delivery system)	Status epilepticus	Monitor **a**irway, **b**reathing, **c**irculation (ABCs).
Divalproex (Depakote), valproic acid (Depakene)	All types of seizures	Monitor for hair loss, tremor, increased liver enzymes, bruising, and N/V. Monitor CBC, PT, PTT, and AST.
Ethosuximide (Zarontin)	Absence seizures	Watch for N/V, skin rash, lethargy, and anorexia. Monitor CBC and liver function tests. (Drug used infrequently.)
Felbamate (Felbatol)	Adjunctive therapy for intractable complex partial seizures	Note that aplastic anemia and liver failure are major sequelae of treatment. Patient must sign consent for use, acknowledging risk for aplastic anemia and liver failure. Monitor CBC. Monitor liver function tests. Watch for anorexia and weight loss.
Gabapentin (Neurontin)	Partial seizures	Watch for increased appetite and weight gain. Monitor for ataxia, irritability, dizziness, and fatigue.
Lamotrigine (Lamictal)	Partial seizures	Watch for diplopia, headaches, dizziness, drowsiness, ataxia, N/V, and life-threatening rash when given with valproic acid.
Levetiracetam (Keppra)	Adjunct management of partial seizures	Monitor renal function carefully. Notify health care provider for gait or coordination problems.
Oxcarbazepine (Trileptal)	Partial seizures	Monitor for hyponatremia.
Phenobarbital (Barbita, Luminal)	Generalized tonic-clonic seizures, partial seizures	Note that this is less desirable than other antiepileptic drugs (AEDs) because of sedation. Be aware that overdose can be fatal. Monitor for drowsiness, sleep disturbances, impaired cognition, and depression.
Phenytoin (Dilantin), fosphenytoin (Cerebyx)	All types, except absence, myoclonic, and atonic seizures; for status epilepticus	Monitor for gastric distress, gingival hyperplasia, anemia, ataxia, and nystagmus. Check CBC and calcium levels; monitor for therapeutic drug levels (10-20 mcg/mL) and toxic levels (>30 mcg/mL). For IV phenytoin, flush catheter with saline before and after administration. For fosphenytoin, use phenytoin equivalent for dosing.
Primidone (Mysoline, Sertan ✦)	Partial seizures, generalized tonic-clonic seizures	Monitor for vertigo and lethargy. Watch for drug interactions with phenobarbital and isoniazid.
Tiagabine (Gabitril)	Partial seizures	Monitor for dizziness, weakness, nervousness, psychomotor slowing, nystagmus, and paresthesias. Administer with food.
Topiramate (Topamax)	Adjunctive therapy for intractable partial seizures	Monitor for ataxia, confusion, dizziness, and fatigue. Be aware of increased risk for renal calculi.
Valproate (Depakote), valproate sodium injection (Depacon)	Simple and complex absence seizures Adjunct therapy for partial complex and generalized tonic-clonic seizures	Monitor for hair loss, tremor, increased liver enzymes, bruising, and N/V. Monitor CBC, PT, PTT, AST.
Zonisamide (Zonegran)	Adjunctive therapy for partial seizures	Monitor CBC, platelets, and renal function. Assess mental status, especially memory.

AST, Aspartate aminotransferase; *CBC*, complete blood count; *N/V*, nausea and vomiting; *PT*, prothrombin time; *PTT*, partial thromboplastin time.

Seizure Precautions. Precautions are taken to prevent the patient from injury if a seizure occurs. Specific seizure precautions vary depending on health care agency policy.

Siderails are rarely the source of significant injury, and the effectiveness of the use of padded siderails to maintain safety is debatable. Padded siderails may embarrass the patient and the family. Follow agency policy about the use of siderails because they may be classified as a restraint device. Other methods to

> **! NURSING SAFETY PRIORITY (QSEN)**
> **Action Alert**
>
> Seizure precautions include ensuring that oxygen and suctioning equipment with an airway are readily available. If the patient does not have an IV access, insert a saline lock, especially if he or she is at significant risk for generalized tonic-clonic seizures. The saline lock provides ready access if IV drug therapy must be given to stop the seizure.

CHART 42-5 Patient and Family Education: Preparing for Self-Management

Health Teaching for the Patient with Epilepsy

- Drug therapy information:
  - Name, dosage, time of administration
  - Actions to take if side effects occur
  - Importance of taking drug as prescribed and not missing a dose
  - What to do if a dose is missed or cannot be taken
  - Importance of having blood drawn for therapeutic or toxic levels as requested by the health care provider
- Do not take any medication, including over-the-counter drugs, without asking your health care provider.
- Wear a medical alert bracelet or necklace, or carry an identification card indicating epilepsy.
- Follow up with your neurologist, physician, or other health care provider as directed.
- Be sure a family member or significant other knows how to help you in the event of a seizure and knows when your health care provider or emergency medical services should be called.
- Investigate and follow state laws concerning driving and operating machinery.
- Avoid alcohol and excessive fatigue.
- Contact the Epilepsy Foundation (www.epilepsy.com) or other organized epilepsy group for additional information. Epilepsy Canada (www.epilepsy.ca) also provides resources and support.

CHART 42-6 Best Practice for Patient Safety & Quality Care QSEN

Care of the Patient During a Tonic-Clonic or Complete Partial Seizure

- Protect the patient from injury.
- Do not force anything into the patient's mouth.
- Turn the patient to the side to keep the airway clear.
- Loosen any restrictive clothing the patient is wearing.
- Maintain the patient's airway and suction oral secretions as needed.
- Do not restrain or try to stop the patient's movement; guide movements if necessary.
- Record the time the seizure began and ended.
- At the completion of the seizure:
  - Take the patient's vital signs.
  - Perform neurologic checks.
  - Keep the patient on his or her side.
  - Allow the patient to rest.
  - Document the seizure (see Chart 42-7).

CHART 42-7 Focused Assessment

Seizures: Nursing Observations and Documentation

- How often the seizures occur:
  - Date, time, and duration of the seizure
- Description of each seizure:
  - Tonic, clonic
  - Staring spells, blinking
  - Automatism
- Whether more than one type of seizure occurs
- Sequence of seizure progression:
  - Where the seizure began
  - Body part first involved
- Observations during the seizure:
  - Changes in pupil size and any eye deviation
  - Level of consciousness
  - Presence of apnea, cyanosis, and salivation
  - Incontinence of bowel or bladder during the seizure
  - Eye fluttering
  - Movement and progression of motor activity
  - Lip smacking or other automatism
  - Tongue or lip biting
- How long the seizures last
- When the last seizure took place
- Whether the seizures are preceded by an aura:
  - Dizziness, numbness, or visual disturbances
  - Gustatory (taste) or auditory disturbances
- What the patient does after the seizure:
  - Feels drowsy or weak
  - May resume normal behavior
  - May be unaware that the seizure took place
- How long it takes for the patient to return to pre-seizure status

consciousness. If possible, turn the patient's head to the side to prevent aspiration and allow secretions to drain. Remove any objects that might injure the patient.

It is not unusual for the patient to become cyanotic during a generalized tonic-clonic seizure. The cyanosis is generally self-limiting, and no treatment is needed. Some health care providers prefer to give the high-risk patient (e.g., older adult, critically ill, or debilitated patient) oxygen by nasal cannula or facemask during the postictal phase. He or she is not restrained because this may cause injury and may worsen the situation, causing more seizure activity. For any type of seizure, carefully observe the seizure and document assessment findings (Chart 42-7).

Emergency Care: Acute Seizure and Status Epilepticus Management. Seizures occurring in greater intensity, number, or length than the patient's usual seizures are considered *acute*. They may also appear in clusters that are different from the patient's typical seizure pattern. Treatment with lorazepam (Ativan, Apo-Lorazepam ✦) or diazepam (Valium, Meval ✦, Vivol ✦, Diastat [rectal diazepam gel]) may be given to stop the clusters to prevent the development of status epilepticus. IV phenytoin (Dilantin) or fosphenytoin (Cerebyx) may be added.

Status epilepticus is a medical emergency and is a prolonged seizure lasting longer than 5 minutes or repeated seizures over the course of 30 minutes. It is a potential complication of all types of seizures. *Seizures lasting longer than 10 minutes can cause death!* Common causes of status epilepticus include:

- Sudden withdrawal from antiepileptic drugs
- Infection
- Acute alcohol or drug withdrawal

protect the patient, such as placing a mattress on the floor, may be used instead of siderails.

Padded tongue blades do not belong at the bedside and should NEVER be inserted into the patient's mouth because the jaw may clench down as soon as the seizure begins! Forcing a tongue blade or airway into the mouth is more likely to chip the teeth and increase the risk for aspirating tooth fragments than prevent the patient from biting the tongue. Furthermore, improper placement of a padded tongue blade can obstruct the airway.

Seizure Management. The actions taken during a seizure should be appropriate for the type of seizure (Chart 42-6). For example, for a simple partial seizure, observe the patient and document the time that the seizure lasted. Redirect the patient's attention away from an activity that could cause injury. Turn the patient on the side during a generalized tonic-clonic or complex partial seizure because he or she may lose

⚠ NURSING SAFETY PRIORITY (QSEN)
Critical Rescue

Convulsive status epilepticus must be treated promptly and aggressively! Establish an airway and notify the health care provider or Rapid Response Team immediately if this problem occurs! Establishing an airway is the priority for this patient's care. Intubation by an anesthesia provider or respiratory therapist may be necessary. Administer oxygen as indicated by the patient's condition. If not already in place, establish IV access with a large-bore catheter, and start 0.9% sodium chloride. The patient is usually placed in the intensive care unit for continuous monitoring and management.

- Head trauma
- Cerebral edema
- Metabolic disturbances

Blood is drawn to determine arterial blood gas levels and to identify metabolic, toxic, and other causes of the uncontrolled seizure. Brain damage and death may occur in the patient with tonic-clonic status epilepticus. Left untreated, metabolic changes result, leading to hypoxia, hypotension, hypoglycemia, cardiac dysrhythmias, or lactic (metabolic) acidosis. Further harm to the patient occurs when muscle breaks down and myoglobin accumulates in the kidneys, which can lead to renal failure and electrolyte imbalance. *This is especially likely in the older adult.*

The drugs of choice for treating status epilepticus are IV-push lorazepam (Ativan, Apo-Lorazepam ✤) or diazepam (Valium). Diazepam rectal gel (Diastat) may be used instead. Lorazepam is usually given as 4 mg over a 2-minute period. This procedure may be repeated, if necessary, until a total of 8 mg is reached.

To prevent additional tonic-clonic seizures or cardiac arrest, a loading dose of IV phenytoin (Dilantin) is given and oral doses administered as a follow-up after the emergency is resolved. Initially, give phenytoin at no more than 50 mg/min using an infusion pump. An alternative to phenytoin is fosphenytoin (Cerebyx), a water-soluble phenytoin prodrug. It is compatible with most IV solutions. It also causes fewer cardiovascular complications than phenytoin and can be given in an IV dextrose solution. After administration, fosphenytoin converts to phenytoin in the body. Therefore the FDA requires the dosage to be written as a phenytoin equivalent (PE): 150 mg of fosphenytoin equals 100 mg of phenytoin. Give fosphenytoin at a rate of 100 to 150 mg/min IV piggyback (Lilley et al., 2014).

Serum drug levels are checked every 6 to 12 hours after the loading dose and then 2 weeks after oral phenytoin has started. Teach the patient about the side and adverse effects of any AED that is prescribed (see Chart 42-4).

❓ NCLEX EXAMINATION CHALLENGE
Safe and Effective Care Environment

A client with a history of seizures is placed on seizure precautions. What emergency equipment will the nurse provide at the bedside? **Select all that apply.**
A. Oropharyngeal airway
B. Oxygen
C. Nasogastric tube
D. Suction setup
E. Padded tongue blade

Surgical Management. Patients who cannot be managed effectively with drug therapy may be candidates for surgery, including vagal nerve stimulation (VNS) and conventional surgical procedures. VNS has been very successful for many patients with epilepsy.

Vagal Nerve Stimulation. Vagal nerve stimulation (VNS) may be performed for control of continuous simple or complex partial seizures. Patients with generalized seizures are not candidates for surgery because VNS may result in severe neurologic deficits. The stimulating device (much like a cardiac pacemaker) is surgically implanted in the left chest wall. An electrode lead is attached to the left vagus nerve, tunneled under the skin, and connected to a generator. The procedure usually takes 2 hours with the patient under general anesthesia. The stimulator is activated by the physician either in the operating room or, more commonly, 2 weeks after surgery. Programming is adjusted gradually over a period of time. The pattern of stimulation is individualized to the patient's tolerance. The generator runs continuously, stimulating the vagus nerve according to the programmed schedule.

The patient can activate the VNS with a handheld magnet when experiencing an aura, thus aborting the seizure. Patients experience a change in voice quality, which signifies that the vagus nerve has been stimulated. They usually report a relief in intensity and duration of seizures and an improved quality of life.

Observe for complications after the procedure such as hoarseness (most common), cough, dyspnea, neck pain, or dysphagia (difficulty swallowing). Teach the patient to avoid MRIs, microwaves, shortwave radios, and ultrasound diathermy (a physical therapy heat treatment).

Conventional Surgical Procedures. A small percentage of patients with epilepsy cannot be fully controlled with drug therapy or VNS. When all other options are exhausted, conventional surgery may be needed to improve the patient's quality of life. The largest group of conventional surgical candidates includes those with complex partial seizures in the frontal or temporal lobe.

Before surgery, the patient is admitted to a special inpatient observation unit. While there, he or she has continuous electroencephalogram (EEG) recording, close observation, and in many hospitals, video monitoring at all times except during personal care activities. The patient is taken off all AEDs. After the seizure area is identified, electrodes may be surgically implanted into the brain tissue to identify the extent of the focal area. This step is followed by additional continuous EEG and video monitoring, as well as close observation by the nursing staff. The area is surgically removed if vital areas of brain function will not be affected.

Preoperative care is similar to that described for patients undergoing a craniotomy (see Chapter 45). Preoperative diagnostic tests include MRI and single-photon emission computed tomography (SPECT)/positron emission tomography (PET) scans as described in Chapter 41. An intracarotid amobarbital test (Wada test) and neuropsychological testing are also done. The Wada test assesses hemispheric lateralization of language and memory after injection of amobarbital, a short-acting anesthetic. This procedure establishes the safety of surgery to preserve language memory. Neuropsychological testing evaluates memory, visuospatial function, language function, and intelligence quotient (IQ) to identify deficiencies in the brain that might correspond to areas believed to be the epileptic region. It is also used to compare preoperative and postoperative COGNITION.

Another surgical approach, the *partial corpus callosotomy,* may be used to treat tonic-clonic or atonic seizures in patients who are not candidates for other surgical procedures. The surgeon sections the anterior two thirds of the corpus callosum, preventing neuronal discharges from passing between the two hemispheres of the brain. This surgery usually reduces the number and severity of the seizures, making them more likely to respond to more conventional drug therapy. This procedure is not as commonly done as other surgeries but is very successful for some patients.

INFECTIONS

MENINGITIS

❖ PATHOPHYSIOLOGY

Meningitis is an inflammation of the meninges, specifically the pia mater and arachnoid. Bacterial and viral organisms are most often responsible for meningitis, although fungal and protozoal meningitis also occur. Cancer and some drugs, notably NSAIDs, antibiotics, and intravenous immunoglobulins, can also cause sterile meningitis. Regardless of cause of meningitis, the symptoms are similar.

The organisms responsible for meningitis enter the central nervous system (CNS) via the bloodstream or are directly introduced into the CNS. Direct routes of entry occur as a result of penetrating trauma, surgical procedures on the brain or spine, or a ruptured brain **abscess**. A basilar skull fracture may lead to meningitis as a result of the direct communication of cerebrospinal fluid (CSF) with the ear or nasal passages, manifested by **otorrhea** (ear discharge) or **rhinorrhea** (nasal discharge, or "runny nose") that is actually CSF. The infecting organisms follow the tract created by skull damage to enter the CNS and circulate in the CSF. The patient with an INFECTION in the head (i.e., eye, ear, nose, mouth) or neck has an increased risk for meningitis because of the proximity of anatomic structures. Infections linked to meningitis include otitis media, acute or chronic sinusitis, and tooth abscess; there are also reports of rare infection from a tongue piercing leading to meningitis. The immunocompromised patient (e.g., one without a spleen) receiving treatment for cancer, taking immunosuppressant drugs to manage autoimmune disease or solid organ transplant, and older adults) is also at increased risk for meningitis. The infecting organism may spread to both cranial and spinal nerves, causing irreversible neurologic damage. Increased intracranial pressure (ICP) may occur as a result of blockage of the flow of CSF, change in cerebral blood flow, or thrombus (blood clot) formation.

Viral meningitis, the most common type, is sometimes referred to as *aseptic meningitis* because no organisms are typically isolated from culture of the CSF. Common viral organisms causing meningitis are enterovirus, herpes simplex virus–2 (HSV-2), varicella zoster virus (VZV) (also causes chickenpox and shingles), mumps virus, and the human immune deficiency virus (HIV). The severity of symptoms can vary by the infecting viral agent. For example, the herpes simplex virus alters cellular metabolism, which quickly results in necrosis of the cells. HSV-2 meningitis may be accompanied by genital infections. Other viruses cause an alteration in the production of enzymes or neurotransmitters. While these alterations result in cell

dysfunction, neurologic defects are more likely to be temporary and a full recovery occurs as the inflammation resolves. Treatment may include the administration of antiviral agents.

Cryptococcus neoformans meningitis is the most common *fungal* INFECTION that affects the central nervous system (CNS) of patients with acquired immune deficiency syndrome (AIDS). Fulminant invasive fungal sinusitis is also a recognized cause of fungal meningitis. The clinical manifestations vary because the compromised immune system affects the inflammatory response. For example, some patients have fever and others do not. Treatment is symptomatic and includes IV antifungal agents.

The most frequently involved organisms responsible for bacterial meningococcal meningitis are *Streptococcus pneumoniae (pneumococcal disease)* and *Neisseria meningitidis. N. meningitidis* meningitis is also known as *meningococcal meningitis. Meningococcal meningitis is a medical emergency with a fairly high mortality rate, often within 24 hours.* Unlike other types, this disorder is highly contagious. Outbreaks of meningococcal meningitis are most likely to occur in areas of high population density, such as college dormitories, military barracks, and crowded living areas.

> ❗ **NURSING SAFETY PRIORITY** (QSEN)
>
> **Action Alert**
>
> People ages 16 through 21 years have the highest rates of INFECTION from life-threatening *N. meningitidis* meningococcal infection. The Centers for Disease Control and Prevention (CDC) recommends an initial meningococcal vaccine between ages 11 and 12 years with a booster at age 16 years (www.cdc.gov). Adults are advised to get an initial or booster vaccine if living in a shared residence (residence hall, military barracks, group home), traveling or residing in countries in which the disease is common, or are immunocompromised due to a damaged or surgically removed spleen or a serum complement deficiency. If the patient's baseline vaccination status is unclear and the immediate risk for exposure to *N. meningitidis* infection is high, the CDC recommends vaccination. It is safe to receive a booster as early as 8 weeks after the initial vaccine.

❖ PATIENT-CENTERED COLLABORATIVE CARE

◆ Assessment

Perform a complete neurologic and neurovascular assessment to detect clinical manifestations associated with a diagnosis of meningitis or suspected meningitis as outlined in Chart 42-8. Signs and symptoms of meningitis result from meningeal irritation. Clinical manifestations of meningitis include fever, **nuchal rigidity** (neck stiffness), **photophobia** (light sensitivity), **phonophobia** (noise sensitivity), headache, **myalgia** (muscle aches), nausea, and vomiting. Confusion and altered consciousness may be present. A maculopapular rash is seen when the causative organism is an enterovirus. A petechial rash is associated with *N. meningitidis* meningitis. Although the classic nuchal rigidity (stiff neck) and positive Kernig's and Brudzinski's signs have been traditionally used to diagnose meningitis, these findings occur in only a small percentage of patients with a definitive diagnosis. Older adults, patients who are immunocompromised, and those who are receiving antibiotics may not have fever. Assess the patient for complications, including increased ICP. Left untreated, increased ICP can lead to herniation of the brain and death (see Chapter 45).

CHART 42-8   Key Features

Meningitis

- Decreased (or change in) level of consciousness
- Disoriented to person, place, and year
- Pupil reaction and eye movements:
  - Photophobia
  - Nystagmus
  - Abnormal eye movements
- Motor response:
  - Normal early in disease process
  - Hemiparesis, hemiplegia, and decreased muscle tone possible later
  - Cranial nerve dysfunction, especially CN III, IV, VI, VII, VIII
- Memory changes:
  - Attention span (usually short)
  - Personality and behavior changes
  - Bewilderment
- Severe, unrelenting headaches
- Generalized muscle aches and pain
- Nausea and vomiting
- Fever and chills
- Tachycardia
- Red macular rash (meningococcal meningitis)

TABLE 42-2   Cerebrospinal Fluid Findings in Bacterial and Viral Meningitis

FINDING	BACTERIAL MENINGITIS	VIRAL MENINGITIS
Appearance	Cloudy, turbid	Clear
White blood cells	Increased	Increased
Protein	Increased	Slightly increased
Glucose	Decreased	Most often normal, but may be decreased
CSF pressure	Elevated	Normal or elevated

CSF, Cerebrospinal fluid.

A complete blood count (CBC) is performed. The white blood cell (WBC) count is usually elevated well above the normal value. Serum electrolyte values are also assessed so as to assess and maintain fluid and electrolyte balance.

X-rays of the chest, air sinuses, and mastoids are obtained to determine the presence of INFECTION. A CT or MRI scan may be performed to identify increased ICP, hydrocephalus, or the presence of a brain abscess.

Seizure activity may occur when meningeal inflammation spreads to the cerebral cortex. Inflammation can also result in abnormal stimulation of the hypothalamic area where excessive amounts of antidiuretic hormone (ADH) (vasopressin) are produced. Excess vasopressin results in water retention and dilution of serum sodium caused by increased sodium loss by the kidneys. This syndrome of inappropriate antidiuretic hormone (SIADH, Chapter 62) may lead to further increases in ICP.

Systemic inflammation (systemic inflammatory response syndrome or SIRS), a reaction to either endotoxin produced by infecting bacteria or activation of the immune cells by infecting organisms, can cause a rapidly falling blood pressure and tachycardia. Coagulopathy can occur as a result of systemic inflammation. Assess the patient's vascular status by:

- Observing the color and temperature of the extremities
- Determining the presence of peripheral pulses
- Identifying any indicators of abnormal bleeding

Thrombi may block circulation in the small vessels of the hands and feet, leading to gangrene. Coagulopathy from SIRS may lead to disseminated intravascular coagulation (DIC).

The most significant laboratory test used in the diagnosis of meningitis is the analysis of the *cerebrospinal fluid (CSF)*. Patients older than 60 years, those who are immunocompromised, or those who have signs of increased ICP usually have a CT scan before the lumbar puncture. If there will be a delay in obtaining the CSF, blood is drawn for culture and sensitivity. A broad-spectrum antibiotic should be given before the lumbar puncture. The CSF is analyzed for cell count, differential count, and protein. Glucose concentrations are determined, and culture, sensitivity, and Gram stain studies are performed. Table 42-2 compares the CSF findings in bacterial and viral meningitis.

Counterimmunoelectrophoresis (CIE) may be performed to determine the presence of viruses or protozoa in the CSF. CIE is also indicated if the patient has received antibiotics before the CSF was obtained. To identify a bacterial source of INFECTION, specimens for Gram stains and culture are obtained from the urine, throat, and nose when indicated.

◆ Interventions

Prevent meningitis by teaching people to obtain vaccination. Vaccines are available to protect against Haemophilus influenzae *type B (Hib), pneumococcal, mumps, varicella, and meningococcal organisms. Although many of these vaccines were developed to prevent respiratory illness, they have also reduced CNS infections. Mandatory vaccination programs for school enrollment and proof of vaccination as a prerequisite for group home or dormitory experiences have significantly reduced the incidence of meningitis.*

Maintain thorough handwashing. Teach visitors to wash hands before and after entering a patient's room. Preventing the transmission of infection through hand cleaning is a National Patient Safety Goal (The Joint Commission, 2014).

The most important nursing interventions for patients with meningitis are accurately monitoring and documenting their neurologic status. Best practices for nursing care are listed in Chart 42-9.

! NURSING SAFETY PRIORITY (QSEN)

Action Alert

For the patient with meningitis, assess his or her neurologic status and vital signs at least every 4 hours or more often if clinically indicated. *The priority for care is to monitor for early neurologic changes that may indicate increased ICP, such as decreased level of consciousness (LOC).* The patient is also at risk for seizure activity. Care should be provided as discussed in Interventions on pp. 859-863 in the Seizures and Epilepsy section.

Cranial nerve testing is included as part of the routine neurologic assessment because of possible cranial nerve involvement. Particular attention is given to cranial nerves III, IV, VI, VII, and VIII, nerves involved in pupillary shape and accommodation to light (see Chapter 41). *A sixth cranial nerve defect (inability to move the eyes laterally) may indicate the development of hydrocephalus (excessive accumulation of CSF within the brain's ventricles).* Other indicators of hydrocephalus include signs of increased ICP and urinary incontinence. Urinary incontinence results from decreasing LOC.

Care of the Patient with Meningitis

- Prioritize care to maintain airway, breathing, circulation.
- Take vital signs and perform neurologic checks every 2 to 4 hours, as required.
- Perform cranial nerve assessment, with particular attention to cranial nerves III, IV, VI, VII, and VIII, and monitor for changes.
- Manage pain with drug and nondrug methods.
- Perform vascular assessment, and monitor for changes.
- Give drugs and IV fluids as prescribed, and document the patient's response.
- Record intake and output carefully to maintain fluid balance and prevent fluid overload.
- Monitor body weight to identify fluid retention early.
- Monitor laboratory values closely; report abnormal findings to the physician or nurse practitioner promptly.
- Position carefully to prevent pressure ulcers.
- Perform range-of-motion exercises every 4 hours as needed.
- Decrease environmental stimuli:
  - Provide a quiet environment.
  - Minimize exposure to bright lights from windows and overhead lights.
  - Maintain bedrest with head of bed elevated 30 degrees.
- Maintain Transmission-Based Precautions per hospital policy (for bacterial meningitis).
- Monitor for and prevent complications:
  - Increased intracranial pressure
  - Vascular dysfunction
  - Fluid and electrolyte imbalance
  - Seizures
  - Shock

To avoid life-threatening complications, the health care provider prescribes a broad-spectrum antibiotic until the results of the culture and Gram stain are available. After this information is available, the appropriate anti-infective drug to treat the specific type of meningitis is given. Treatment of bacterial meningitis generally requires a 2-week course of IV antibiotics. Drug therapy should begin within 1 to 2 hours after it is prescribed. Monitor and document the patient's response.

Drugs may be used to treat increased ICP or seizures, including mannitol, a hyperosmolar agent for ICP, and antiepileptic drugs (AEDs). Controversy exists as to whether steroids are helpful in the treatment of all adults with meningitis. They are, however, recommended for patients with *S. pneumoniae* meningitis.

People who have been in close contact with a patient with *N. meningitidis* should have prophylaxis (preventive) treatment with rifampin (Rifadin, Rofact ✿), ciprofloxacin (Cipro), or ceftriaxone (Rocephin). Preventive treatment with rifampin may be prescribed for those in close contact with a patient with *H. influenzae* meningitis (Lilley et al., 2014).

Perform a complete vascular assessment every 4 hours or more often, if indicated, to detect early vascular compromise. Thrombotic or embolic complications are most often seen in circulation to the hand. Assess the patient's temperature, color, pulses, and capillary refill in the fingernails. If vascular compromise is not noticed and left untreated, gangrene can develop quickly, possibly leading to loss of the involved arm. The health care team monitors the patient for other complications, including septic shock, coagulation disorders, acute respiratory

distress syndrome, and septic arthritis. These health problems are discussed elsewhere in this textbook.

Standard Precautions are appropriate for all patients with meningitis unless the patient has a bacterial type that is transmitted by droplets, such as *N. meningitides* and *H. influenzae*.

! NURSING SAFETY PRIORITY (QSEN)
Action Alert

Place the patient with bacterial meningitis that is transmitted by droplets on Droplet Precautions *in addition to* Standard Precautions. When possible, place the patient in a private room. Stay at least 3 feet from the patient unless wearing a mask. Patients who are transported outside of the room should wear a mask (see Chapter 23). Teach visitors about the need for these precautions and how to follow them.

ENCEPHALITIS
❖ PATHOPHYSIOLOGY

Encephalitis is an inflammation of the brain tissue and often the surrounding meninges. It affects the cerebrum, the brainstem, and the cerebellum. A viral agent most often causes the disease, although bacteria, fungi, or parasites may also be involved (e.g., malaria). The virus travels to the central nervous system (CNS) via the bloodstream, along peripheral or cranial nerves, or in the meninges (e.g., varicella zoster). Therefore viral encephalitis can be life threatening or lead to persistent neurologic problems such as learning disabilities, epilepsy, memory deficits, or fine motor deficits.

After the virus invades the brain tissue, it begins to reproduce, causing an inflammatory response. Unlike in meningitis, this response does not cause exudate (pus) formation. Inflammation extends over the cerebral cortex, the white matter, and the meninges, causing degeneration of the neurons of the cortex. Demyelination of axons occurs in the involved area because the white matter is destroyed. This destruction leads to hemorrhage, edema, necrosis (cell death), and the development of small lacunae (hollow cavities) within the cerebral hemispheres. Widespread edema can cause compression of blood vessels leading to a further increase in intracranial pressure (ICP). Death may occur from herniation and increased ICP.

Arboviruses can be transmitted to humans through the bite of an infected mosquito or tick. The most common types of encephalitis caused by arboviruses are Eastern or Western equine encephalitis, St. Louis encephalitis, California encephalitis, and West Nile virus.

West Nile virus has gained attention in the United States because it has spread rapidly throughout the country and is a potentially serious illness. This INFECTION is typically mild, and usually the patient is asymptomatic. However, a small percentage of patients develop severe disease. The incubation period is 2 to 15 days after being bitten by an infected mosquito. Other possible sources of transmission include blood products, breast milk, or an organ transplant. Diagnostic tests to determine the presence of West Nile virus include enzyme-linked immunosorbent assay and West Nile virus–specific immunoglobulin M (IgM) antibody in the blood or CSF.

In mild cases of *West Nile virus,* the patient has no symptoms or has mild flu-like symptoms (e.g., fever, body aches, nausea, vomiting). Some people develop serious symptoms that may include high fever, severe headache, decreased level of consciousness, tremors, vision loss, seizures, and muscle weakness or paralysis. These manifestations may last for several weeks, and neurologic deficits may be permanent. A few patients die from the disease, especially those older than 50 years with a weakened immune system (Overstreet, 2011).

Echovirus, coxsackievirus, poliovirus, herpes zoster, and viruses that cause mumps and chickenpox are the common *enteroviruses* associated with encephalitis. *Herpes simplex virus type 1* (HSV1) encephalitis is the most common nonepidemic type of encephalitis in North America. Patients with this disease often have a history of cold sores. The mortality rates for HSV1 encephalitis are very high compared with those for other types of encephalitis.

Amebic meningoencephalitis is caused by the amebae *Naegleria* and *Acanthamoeba*. Both are found in warm freshwater areas and can enter the nasal mucosa of people swimming in ponds or lakes. The amebae may also be found in soil and decaying vegetation. Although this INFECTION has not often been seen in the past, the incidence in North America is increasing, perhaps because ponds and lakes are becoming more polluted.

❖ PATIENT-CENTERED COLLABORATIVE CARE

◆ Assessment

The typical patient with encephalitis has a high fever and reports nausea, vomiting, and a stiff neck. Assess for other clinical manifestations, including possible:

- Changes in mental status (e.g., agitation)
- Motor dysfunction (e.g., dysphagia [difficulty swallowing])
- Focal (specific) neurologic deficits
- Photophobia (light sensitivity) and phonophobia (noise sensitivity)
- Fatigue
- Symptoms of increased ICP (e.g., decreased LOC)
- Joint pain
- Headache
- Vertigo

Assess LOC using the Glasgow Coma Scale (see Chapter 41) or other agency-approved assessment tool. The patient may be lethargic, stuporous, or comatose. Mental status changes are more extensive in the patient with encephalitis than with meningitis. Changes include acute confusion, irritability, and personality and behavior changes (especially noted in the presence of herpes simplex). Signs of meningeal irritation include the presence of nuchal (neck) rigidity and motor changes that vary from a mild weakness to hemiplegia. The patient may have muscle tremors, spasticity, an ataxic gait (postencephalitic Parkinsonism), myoclonic jerks, and increased deep tendon reflexes. Seizure activity is common.

Observe for cranial nerve involvement, such as ocular palsies (paralysis), facial weakness, and nystagmus (involuntary lateral eye movements). The herpes zoster lesion affects cranial and spinal nerve root ganglia, which is clinically manifested by a rash, severe PAIN, itching, burning, or tingling in the areas innervated by these nerves.

Lumbar puncture (LP) is done to analyze the CSF for the specific offending organism. A polymerase chain reaction (PCR) test may be used to detect viral DNA or ribonucleic acid (RNA) in the CSF. Specificity and sensitivity in diagnosing encephalitis are excellent, especially with herpes simplex virus

---

CHART 42-10 Patient and Family Education: Preparing for Self-Management

Protecting the Patient and Family from West Nile Virus

- Limit your time outside between dusk and dawn when mosquitoes are out.
- Wear protective clothing, including long sleeves and pants.
- Use an insect repellent containing DEET when outdoors.
- Remove areas of standing water from flower pots, trash cans, and rain gutters.
- Check window and door screens for holes that need repair.
- Keep hot tubs and pools clean and properly chlorinated.

! NURSING SAFETY PRIORITY (QSEN)

Critical Rescue

In severe cases of encephalitis, the patient may have increased ICP resulting from cerebral edema, hemorrhage, and necrosis of brain tissue. If the patient is nonverbal or comatose at baseline, then monitoring vital signs and pupils becomes essential for detecting worsening neurologic status and increased ICP. Changes in vital signs that require an immediate notification of the health care provider are a widened pulse pressure, new bradycardia, and irregular respiratory effort. Pupils that become increasingly dilated and less responsive to light are also communicated urgently. Left untreated, increased ICP leads to herniation of the brain tissue and possibly death (see Chapter 45).

(HSV). The test is rapid and noninvasive, replacing the brain biopsy for diagnosis.

An electroencephalogram is done to evaluate brain wave activity to detect seizures. Brain imaging in the form of a CT scan with and without contrast is performed to evaluate elevated intracranial pressure (ICP) or obstructive hydrocephalus.

◆ Interventions

Teach people who live in mosquito-infested areas to protect themselves and their families from West Nile virus infections. Chart 42-10 lists measures for preventing this infection. There is no curative treatment for West Nile viral encephalitis.

Acyclovir (Zovirax) is the antiviral drug of choice for the treatment of herpes encephalitis and is associated with a significantly lower mortality rate than vidarabine (Vira-A). Drug therapy is most effective if begun early, before the patient becomes stuporous or comatose. This neurologic decline usually occurs within 4 to 6 days after the initial neurologic symptoms. No specific drug therapy is available for INFECTION by arboviruses or enteroviruses.

Nursing interventions for encephalitis are similar to those for meningitis with the exception of drug therapy. Supportive nursing care and prompt recognition and treatment of increased ICP are essential components of management. *Maintain a patent airway to prevent the development of atelectasis or pneumonia, which can lead to further brain hypoxia (lack of oxygen).*

Provide supportive nursing care for the patient who is immobile, stuporous, or comatose. Delegate and supervise unlicensed assistive personnel (UAP) to turn, cough, and deep breathe the patient at least every 2 hours. Perform deep tracheal suctioning even in the presence of increased ICP if respiratory status is compromised. Assess vital signs and neurologic signs every 2 hours or more frequently if clinically indicated. Elevate the head of the bed 30 to 45 degrees unless contraindicated (e.g., after lumbar puncture or in the patient with severe hypotension). Keep the patient's room darkened and quiet to promote comfort and decrease agitation. Remind UAP to provide safety measures such as keeping the bed in the lowest position.

Provide patient and family support. Families need health teaching to understand how to care for their loved ones. They are often fearful that the patient may not return to his or her baseline. Collaborate with a certified chaplain, social worker, or case manager to provide additional emotional support and counseling.

Patients with encephalitis and permanent neurologic deficits are usually discharged to a rehabilitation setting or a long-term care facility. Those with minimal neurologic problems are discharged to the home setting.

PARKINSON DISEASE

❖ PATHOPHYSIOLOGY

Parkinson disease (PD), also referred to as *Parkinson's disease* and *paralysis agitans,* is a progressive neurodegenerative disease that is the one of the most common neurologic disorders of older adults. It is a debilitating disease affecting motor ability and is characterized by four cardinal symptoms: tremor, muscle rigidity, **bradykinesia** or **akinesia** (slow movement/no movement), and postural instability. Most people have *primary,* or idiopathic, disease. A few patients have *secondary* parkinsonian symptoms from conditions such as brain tumors and certain anti-psychotic drugs.

Motor activity occurs as a result of integrating the actions of the cerebral cortex, basal ganglia, and cerebellum. The basal ganglia are a group of neurons located deep within the cerebrum at the base of the brain near the lateral ventricles. When the basal ganglia are stimulated, muscle tone in the body is inhibited and voluntary movements are refined. The secretion of two major neurotransmitters accomplishes this process: dopamine and acetylcholine (ACh).

Dopamine is produced in the substantia nigra, as well as in the adrenal glands, and is transmitted to the basal ganglia along a connecting neural pathway for secretion when needed. *ACh* is produced and secreted by the basal ganglia, as well as in the nerve endings in the periphery of the body. ACh-producing neurons transmit *excitatory* messages throughout the basal ganglia. Dopamine *inhibits* the function of these neurons, allowing control over voluntary movement. This system of checks and balances allows for refined, coordinated movement, such as picking up a pencil and writing.

Widespread degeneration of the *substantia nigra* then leads to a decrease in the amount of dopamine in the brain. When dopamine levels are decreased, a person loses the ability to refine voluntary movement. The large numbers of excitatory ACh-secreting neurons remain active, creating an imbalance between excitatory and inhibitory neuronal activity. The resulting excessive excitation of neurons prevents a person from controlling or initiating voluntary movement (McCance et al., 2014).

Not only does PD interfere with movement as a result of dopamine loss in the brain, it also reduces the sympathetic nervous system influence on the heart and blood vessels. This loss results in the orthostatic hypotension frequently seen in the patient with PD.

TABLE 42-3	**Stages of Parkinson Disease**
Stage 1: Initial Stage • Unilateral limb involvement • Minimal weakness • Hand and arm trembling	**Stage 3: Moderate Disease** • Postural instability • Increased gait disturbances
Stage 2: Mild Stage • Bilateral limb involvement • Masklike face • Slow, shuffling gait	**Stage 4: Severe Disability** • Akinesia • Rigidity **Stage 5: Complete ADL Dependence**

PD is separated into stages according to the symptoms and degree of disability. Stage 1 is mild disease with unilateral limb involvement, whereas the patient with stage 5 disease is completely dependent in all ADLs. Other classifications refer simply to mild, moderate, and severe disease (Table 42-3).

Although the exact cause of PD is not known, it is probably due to environmental and genetic factors. Exposure to pesticides, herbicides, and industrial chemicals and metals and drinking well water, being older than 40 years, and having reduced estrogen levels are known risk factors for the development of PD.

GENETIC/GENOMIC CONSIDERATIONS
Patient-Centered Care QSEN

Primary Parkinson disease (PD) often has a familial tendency. The disease is associated with a variety of mitochondrial DNA (mtDNA) variations that often involve deletions in the genetic sequences that are used in CNS mitochondria, the energy powerhouses of cells. These variations ultimately cause destruction of neurons that produce dopamine in the substantia nigra. Mitochondrial dysfunction is a common observation in PD and other neurodegenerative diseases, indicating there is a disorder of energy regulation that contributes to cell death (Coskun et al., 2012).

As the population ages, the number of people affected by PD is expected to dramatically increase. About 50% more men than women currently have the disease.

❖ PATIENT-CENTERED COLLABORATIVE CARE
◆ Assessment

Collect data related to the time and progression of symptoms noticed by the patient or the family. The older adult, who may assume that these behaviors are normal changes associated with aging, may ignore early signs and symptoms such as *resting* tremors, bradykinesia (slowed movement), and problems with muscular rigidity. Tremors are usually noticed in the upper extremities first and may increase with stress. Slow voluntary movements and reduced automatic movements may be manifested by a change in the patient's handwriting. Some patients report "freezing" because they feel that they are stuck to the floor. Chart 42-11 summarizes the clinical manifestations of Parkinson disease. Assess the patient for *rigidity,* or resistance to passive movement of the extremities, which is classified as:

- *Cogwheel,* manifested by a rhythmic interruption of the muscle movement
- *Plastic,* defined as mildly restrictive movement
- *Lead pipe,* or total resistance to movement

CHART 42-11   Key Features

Parkinson Disease

- Posture:
  - Stooped posture
  - Flexed trunk
  - Fingers abducted and flexed at the metacarpophalangeal joint
  - Wrist slightly dorsiflexed
- Gait:
  - Slow and shuffling
  - Short, hesitant steps
  - Propulsive gait
  - Difficulty stopping quickly
- Motor:
  - **Bradykinesia** (slow movement)
  - Muscular rigidity
  - Akinesia
  - Tremors
  - "Pill-rolling" movement
  - Masklike face
  - Difficulty chewing and swallowing
  - Uncontrolled drooling, especially at night
  - Fatigue
  - Difficulty getting into and out of bed
  - Reduced arm swinging on one side of the body when walking
  - Micrographia (change in handwriting or handwriting gets smaller)
- Speech:
  - Soft, low-pitched voice
  - **Dysarthria** (slurred speech)
  - **Echolalia** (automatic repetition of what another person says) and repetition of sentences
  - **Hypophonia** (soft voice), change in voice volume or articulation
- Autonomic dysfunction:
  - Orthostatic hypotension
  - Excessive perspiration
  - Oily skin
  - Seborrhea
  - Flushing
  - Changes in skin texture
  - Blepharospasm (eyelid spasm)
- Psychosocial assessment:
  - Emotionally labile
  - Depressed
  - Paranoid
  - Easily upset
  - Rapid mood swings
  - Impaired cognition (i.e., dementia or delirium)
  - Delayed reaction time
  - Sleep disturbances

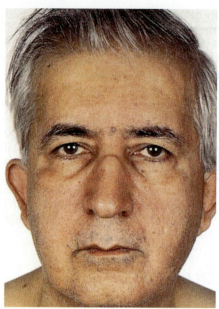

FIG. 42-1 The masklike facial expression typical of patients with Parkinson disease.

symptoms may develop because patients fear that they will not be able to cope with new situations.

Changes in speech pattern are common in PD patients. They may speak very softly, slur or repeat their words, use a monotone voice or a halting speech, hesitate before speaking, or exhibit a rapid speech pattern.

Bowel and bladder problems are commonly seen in PD due to malfunction of the autonomic nervous system, which regulates smooth muscle activity. Patients can exhibit symptoms of either urinary incontinence or difficulty urinating. Constipation can occur due to the slow motility of the GI tract or because of poor dietary habits and poor fluid intake.

The diagnosis of PD is made based on clinical findings after other neurologic diseases are eliminated as possibilities. There are no specific diagnostic tests. Analysis of cerebrospinal fluid (CSF) may show a decrease in dopamine levels, although the results of other studies are usually normal. Other diagnostic tests may be done such as an MRI, single-photon emission computed tomography (SPECT), or a positron emission tomography (PET) to rule out other CNS health problems.

Rigidity is present early in the disease process and progresses over time. Observe the patient's ability to relax a muscle or move a selected muscle group.

Changes in facial expression or a *masklike face* with wide-open, fixed, staring eyes is caused by rigidity of the facial muscles (Fig. 42-1). This rigidity can lead to difficulties in chewing and swallowing, particularly if the pharyngeal muscles are involved. As a result, the patient may have inadequate nutrition. Uncontrolled drooling may occur. Some patients develop dementia later as the disease progresses. In addition to changes in voluntary movement, many patients experience autonomic nervous system symptoms, such as excessive perspiration and orthostatic hypotension. Orthostatic hypotension is likely related to loss of sympathetic innervation in the heart and blood vessel response.

Patients can also develop emotional changes such as depression, irritability, pessimism, fear, and insecurity. These

◆ Interventions

In addition to the health care provider, physical and/or occupational therapist, speech-language pathologist, dietitian, and case manager, collaborate with the patient and family to develop a patient-centered plan of care. In some cases, palliative surgery may be performed to assist the patient to remain mobile for as long as possible. Chart 42-12 summarizes best practices for nursing management of the patient with PD.

Nonsurgical Management. Care for the patient with Parkinson disease includes drug therapy, exercise programs or physical therapy, strategies and collaboration to promote self-management, and psychosocial support. Ultimately, the goals of care are to preserve MOBILITY, COGNITION, and quality of life.

Drug Therapy. Drugs are prescribed to treat the symptoms of PD with the purpose of increasing the patient's functional abilities. An equally important desired outcome is to prescribe

CHART 42-12 Best Practice for Patient Safety & Quality Care (QSEN)

Care of the Patient with Parkinson Disease

- Allow the patient extra time to respond to questions.
- Administer medications promptly on schedule to maintain continuous therapeutic drug levels.
- Provide medication for pain, tingling in limbs, as needed.
- Monitor for side effects of medications, especially orthostatic hypotension, hallucinations, and acute confusional state (delirium).
- Collaborate with physical and occupational therapists to keep the patient as mobile and as independent as possible in ADLs.
- Allow the patient time to perform ADLs and mobility skills.
- Implement interventions to prevent complications of immobility, such as constipation, pressure ulcers, and contractures.
- Schedule appointments and activities late in the morning to prevent rushing the patient, or schedule them at the time of the patient's optimal level of functioning.
- Teach the patient to speak slowly and clearly. Use alternative communication methods, such as a communication board. Refer to speech-language pathologist.
- Monitor the patient's ability to eat and swallow. Monitor actual food and fluid intake. Collaborate with the dietitian.
- Provide high-protein, high-calorie foods or supplements to maintain weight.
- Recognize that Parkinson disease affects the patient's body image. Focus on the patient's strengths.
- Assess for depression and anxiety.
- Assess for insomnia or sleeplessness.

drugs with minimal long-term side effects. Many questions and controversies remain about which drugs to use, when to start therapy, and how to prevent complications. Drug administration is closely monitored, and the health care provider adjusts the dosage or changes therapy as the patient's condition requires. Teach the patient and family how to monitor for and report adverse effects of drug therapy.

Dopamine agonists mimic dopamine by stimulating dopamine receptors in the brain. They are typically the most effective during the first 3 to 5 years of use. The benefit of these agents is fewer incidents of **dyskinesias** (problems with movement) and "wearing off" phenomenon (loss of response to the drug) when compared with other drugs. This problem is characterized by periods of good MOBILITY ("on") alternating with periods of poor MOBILITY ("off"). Patients report that their most distressing symptom is "off time."

Examples of dopamine agonists are apomorphine (Apokyn [a morphine derivative]), pramipexole (Mirapex), and ropinirole (Requip). Another drug in this class, rotigotine, is available as a continuous transdermal patch (Neupro) to maintain a consistent level of dopamine.

! NURSING SAFETY PRIORITY (QSEN)

Drug Alert

Dopamine agonists are associated with adverse effects such as orthostatic (postural) hypotension, hallucinations, sleepiness, and drowsiness. Remind patients to avoid operating heavy machinery or driving if they have any of these symptoms. Teach them to change from a lying or sitting position to standing by moving slowly. The health care provider should not prescribe drugs in this class to older adults because of their severe adverse drug effects.

Almost all patients are on Sinemet, a combination *levodopa-carbidopa* drug, at some point in their disease. It may be the initial drug of choice if the patient's presenting symptoms are severe or interfere with work or school. Both an immediate-release (IR) and controlled-release (CR) form of Sinemet in varying doses are available. The levodopa agents are less expensive than the dopamine agonists and are better at improving motor function. Long-term use leads to dyskinesia (inability to perform voluntary movement). Teach the patient and family to give the drug before meals to increase absorption and transport across the blood-brain barrier.

Catechol O–methyltransferases (COMTs) are enzymes that inactivate dopamine. Therefore COMT *inhibitors* block this enzyme activity, thus prolonging the action of levodopa. One example is entacapone (Comtan), which is often used in combination with levodopa. Stalevo is a combination of levodopa, carbidopa, and entacapone. The benefit of these combinations is that the disease is treated in several ways with one drug. However, they are not beneficial for those patients who need more specific dosages of individual drugs.

Monamine oxidase type B (MAO-B) inhibitors (MAOIs) are more popular for use in patients with early or mild symptoms of PD. Entacapone (Comtan) and selegiline (Deprenyl, Eldepryl) are often given with levodopa for early or mild disease. A newer MAOI-B for PD is rasagiline mesylate (Azilect), which can be given as a single drug or with levodopa. This drug has been reported to decrease "freezing" episodes (Cranwell-Bruce, 2010).

The MAOI-B drugs work by slowing the main type (B) of monamine oxidase in the brain, increasing dopamine concentrations and helping reduce the clinical manifestations of PD. They may also protect neurons in the brain (Cranwell-Bruce, 2010).

! NURSING SAFETY PRIORITY (QSEN)

Drug Alert

Teach patients taking MAOIs about the need to avoid foods, beverages, and drugs that contain tyramine, including cheese and aged, smoked, or cured foods and sausage. Remind them to also avoid red wine and beer to prevent severe headache and life-threatening hypertension (Lilley et al., 2014). Patients should continue these restrictions for 14 days after the drug is discontinued.

When other drugs are no longer effective, bromocriptine mesylate (Parlodel), a *dopamine receptor agonist*, may be prescribed to promote the release of dopamine. It may be used alone or in combination with carbidopa/levodopa (Sinemet). Some providers may prescribe Parlodel early in the course of treatment. It is especially useful in the patient who has experienced side effects such as dyskinesias or orthostatic hypotension while receiving Sinemet.

Amantadine (Symmetrel) is an *antiviral drug* that has anti-Parkinson benefits. It may be given early in disease to reduce symptoms. It is also prescribed with Sinemet to reduce dyskinesias. Rivastigmine (Exelon) is a *cholinesterase inhibitor* that is used only when patients with PD have dementia. This drug works to improve the transmission of acetylcholine in the brain by delaying its destruction by the enzyme *acetylcholinesterase*.

For severe motor symptoms such as tremors and rigidity, one of the older *anticholinergic* drugs may be prescribed, but they are rarely used as primary drugs of choice for Parkinson disease

(PD) (Cranwell-Bruce, 2010). Examples are benztropine (Cogentin), trihexyphenidyl HCl (Artane), and procyclidine (Kemadrin). *These drugs should be avoided in older adults because they can cause acute confusion, urinary retention, constipation, dry mouth, and blurred vision. Newer and safer drugs are now available for this age-group.*

For the patient on any long-term drug therapy regimen, drug tolerance or *drug toxicity* often develops. Drug toxicity may be evidenced by changes in COGNITION such as delirium (acute confusion) or hallucinations and decreased effectiveness of the drug. Delirium may be difficult to assess in the patient who is already suffering from chronic dementia as a result of PD or another disease. If possible, compare the patient's current cognitive and behavioral status with his or her baseline before drug therapy began.

When drug tolerance is reached, the drug's effects do not last as long as previously. The treatment of PD drug toxicity or tolerance includes:

- A reduction in drug dosage
- A change of drug or in the frequency of administration
- A drug holiday (particularly with levodopa therapy)

During a **drug holiday,** which typically lasts up to 10 days, the patient receives no drug therapy for PD. Carefully monitor the patient for symptoms of PD during this time, and document assessment findings.

Many patients are on additional drugs to help relieve symptoms associated with the disease. For example, muscle spasms may be relieved by baclofen (Kemstro), drooling can be minimized by sublingual atropine sulfate (Atropair), and insomnia may require a sleeping aid like zolpidem tartrate (Ambien). If patients also become moderately to severely depressed, an antidepressant such as short-acting venlafaxine (Effexor) may be prescribed. This complicated drug regimen may be confusing to patients. A review by Vervloet and colleagues (2012) supports electronic reminders as effective in helping to educate patients and maintain drug adherence.

Other Interventions. *A freezing gait and postural instability are major problems for patients with PD.* Nontraditional exercise programs, such as yoga and tai chi, may help elevate mood, as well as improve MOBILITY, in the early stage of the disease. Early in the disease process, collaborate with physical and occupational therapists to plan and implement a program to keep the patient flexible, prevent falling, and retain mobility by incorporating active and passive range-of-motion (ROM) exercises, muscle stretching, and out-of-bed activity. Remind the patient to avoid concentrating on his or her feet when walking to prevent falls.

In collaboration with the rehabilitation team, encourage the patient to participate as much as possible in self-management, including ADLs. The team makes the environment conducive to independence in activity and as stress-free and safe as possible. Occupational and physical therapists provide training in ADLs and the use of adaptive devices, as needed, to facilitate independence. The occupational therapist (OT) evaluates the patient for the need for adaptive devices (e.g., special utensils for eating).

Patients with PD tend to not sleep well at night because of drug therapy and the disease itself. Some patients nap for short periods during the day and may not be aware that they have done so. This sleep misperception may put the patient at risk for injury. For example, he or she may fall asleep while driving an automobile. Therefore teach the patient and family to monitor the patient's sleeping pattern and discuss whether he or she can operate machinery or perform other potentially high-risk tasks safely.

Collaborate with the dietitian, if needed, to evaluate the patient's food intake and ability to eat. The patient's intake of calcium, vitamin K, and other nutrients is evaluated, especially in the patient who has difficulty swallowing or is susceptible to injury from falling. The dietitian considers the patient's bowel habits and adjusts the diet if constipation occurs. If the patient has trouble swallowing, collaborate with the speech-language pathologist (SLP) for an extensive swallowing evaluation. Based on these findings and the patient interview, an individualized nutritional plan is developed. Usually a soft diet and thick, cold fluids, such as milk shakes, are more easily tolerated.

Small, frequent meals or a commercial powder, such as Thick-It, added to liquids may assist the patient who has difficulty swallowing. Elevate the patient's head to allow easier swallowing and prevent aspiration. Remind UAP and teach the family to be careful when serving or feeding the patient. The SLP can be very helpful in recommending specific feeding strategies. Be sure that UAP record food intake daily or as needed. The patient loses weight because of altered food intake and the increased number of calories burned secondary to muscle rigidity. Teach the family to weigh the patient once a week so that adjustments to the diet can be made as indicated. As the disease progresses and swallowing becomes more of a problem, supplemental feedings become the main source of nutrition to maintain weight, with meals and other foods taken as the patient can tolerate.

Collaborate with the SLP if the patient has speech difficulties. Together with the interdisciplinary health care team, patient, and family, develop a communication plan. The SLP teaches exercises to strengthen muscles used for breathing, speech, and swallowing. Remind the patient to speak slowly and clearly and to pause and take deep breaths at times during each sentence. Teach the family the importance of avoiding unnecessary environmental noise to increase the listener's ability to hear and understand the patient. Ask the patient to repeat words that the listener does not understand. Have the listener watch the patient's lips and nonverbal expressions for cues as to the meaning of conversation. Remind the patient to organize his or her thoughts before speaking and use facial expression and gestures, if possible, to assist with communication. In addition, he or she should exaggerate words to increase the listener's ability to understand. If the patient cannot communicate verbally, he or she can use alternative methods of communication, such as a communication board, mechanical voice synthesizer, computer, or handheld mobile device. The SLP assesses the ability to use these devices before a decision is made about which method to use. Some older patients may not want to use electronic methods to communicate.

Psychosocial Support. Although not all patients with PD have dementia, impaired COGNITION and memory deficits are common. Some patients also experience changes in gait and tremors that are uncontrollable. In the late stages of the disease, they cannot move without assistance, have difficulty talking, have minimal facial expression, and may drool. Patients often state that they are embarrassed and tend to avoid social events or groups of people. They should not be forced into situations in which they feel ashamed of their appearance. Encourage patients to undertake activities that do not require small-muscle dexterity, such as light, modified aerobic exercises.

Collaborate with the social worker or case manager to help the family with financial and health insurance issues, as well as respite care or permanent placement if needed. Refer the patient and family to social and state agencies, as well as support groups as needed (e.g., the National Parkinson Foundation [www.pdf.org]).

Teach the family to emphasize the patient's abilities or strengths and provide positive reinforcement when he or she meets expected outcomes. The patient, the family or significant other, and the rehabilitation team mutually set realistic expected outcomes that can be achieved.

The long-term management of PD presents a special challenge in the home care setting. A case manager may be required to coordinate interdisciplinary care and provide support for the patient and family. Impaired MOBILITY affects the patient's daily lifestyle, including sexuality. The case manager or home care nurse uses a holistic approach to ensure that psychosocial, as well as physical, needs are addressed.

As the disease progresses and drug effectiveness decreases, refer the family to a palliative care organization or hospice. Referral sources can be obtained from the Center to Advance Palliative Care (www.capc.org), which advocates applying the principles of palliative care to chronic disease. Chapter 7 discusses palliative and hospice care in detail.

💡 CLINICAL JUDGMENT CHALLENGE

Informatics **QSEN**

A 68-year-old man reports shaking of his arms, hands, and head that he cannot control. He has also noticed that he walks more slowly now and thought it was part of the aging process. He is afraid that he won't be able to continue his job as an auto body worker, and he says he can't live on his monthly Social Security income. His mother had Parkinson disease for many years and died of complications before she was 70. He decided he should see his family practice physician to discuss the changes he is experiencing. He is accompanied by his wife of 45 years; they have two children who live out of town.

1. As the patient's intake nurse, what questions might you include in his history?
2. What physical assessment will you perform and why?
3. The physician places the patient on Sinemet. You realize that you need to look up information about this drug to provide accurate health teaching. What reliable resources might you use?
4. What health teaching will you need to provide for this patient and his wife regarding his drug and other aspects of his illness?

Surgical Management. Several options are available if surgery for the patient with PD is needed. Surgery is a last resort when drugs are not effective in symptom management. The most common surgeries are stereotactic pallidotomy and thalamotomy, although newer surgical procedures are being tried. Deep brain stimulation may also be done.

Stereotactic Pallidotomy/Thalamotomy. Stereotactic pallidotomy (opening into the pallidum within the corpus striatum) can be a very effective treatment for controlling the symptoms associated with PD. First, the target area within the pallidum is identified by a CT or MRI scan. Next, the stereotactic head frame is placed on the patient. IV sedation is given, and a burr hole is made into the cranium. An electrode or cylindric rod is inserted into the target area. The target area receives a mild electrical stimulation, and the patient's reaction is assessed

for reduction of tremor and rigidity. If this result does not occur or if unexpected visual, motor, or sensory symptoms appear, the probe is repositioned. When the probe is in the ideal location, a permanent lesion (scarring) is made to destroy the tissue. The patient is monitored in the postanesthesia care unit (PACU) for about 1 hour and is then returned to the inpatient unit for continuing postoperative care.

As an alternative to stereotactic pallidotomy, the surgeon may perform a **thalamotomy** (opening into the thalamus of the brain for the stimulation) for treatment of tremor through thermocoagulation (high-frequency currents to destroy tissue) of brain cells. This procedure is effective for a limited number of patients. Because bilateral procedures have increased surgical complication rates, only unilateral (one-sided) surgery is done to benefit the side of the body that is most affected by the disease.

Deep Brain Stimulation. Deep brain stimulation (DBS) is approved as a treatment for Parkinson disease. In DBS, electrodes are implanted into the brain and connected to a small electrical device called a *pulse generator* that delivers electrical current. The generator is placed under the skin similar to a cardiac pacemaker device. The generator is externally programmed to deliver an electrical current to decrease involuntary movements known as **dyskinesias**, resulting in a reduced need for levodopa and related drugs. DBS also helps to alleviate fluctuations of symptoms and to reduce tremors, slowness of movements, and gait problems (National Institute of Neurological Disorders and Stroke [NINDS], 2014).

Fetal Tissue Transplantation. Fetal tissue transplantation is an experimental and highly controversial ethical and political treatment. Fetal substantia nigra tissue, either human or pig, is transplanted into the caudate nucleus of the brain. Preliminary reports suggest that patients show clinical improvement in motor symptoms without dyskinesias after receiving the transplanted tissue. Long-term results are yet to be seen or studied.

DEMENTIA

❖ *PATHOPHYSIOLOGY*

Dementia is a loss of brain function that is chronic and progressive. Dementia affects the ability to learn new information. It also impairs language, judgment, and behavior. Alzheimer's disease (AD) is the most common type of dementia, accounting for most of the chronic confusional states that occur in people older than 65 years. Vascular dementia is the second most common dementia and is associated with stroke. When dementia occurs in people in their 40s and 50s, it is referred to as *early dementia, Alzheimer type,* or *presenile dementia.* Although symptoms of dementia can vary greatly, at least two of these cognitive functions must be significantly impaired for a diagnosis of dementia:

- Memory
- Communication and language
- Attention span or ability to focus and pay attention
- Reasoning and judgment
- Visual perception

People with dementia often have problems with short-term memory such as keeping track of keys or personal items, paying bills, preparing meals, remembering appointments, or traveling out of the neighborhood. Many dementias are progressive and result in a chronic confusional state. Severe physical deterioration occurs over time, and death is usually associated with complications of immobility.

The brain of the older adult usually weighs less and occupies less space in the cranial vault than does the brain of a younger person. Other changes in the brain that occur with aging include widening of the cerebral sulci, narrowing of the gyri, and enlargement of the ventricles. In the presence of AD and vascular dementia, these normal changes are greatly accelerated. Brain weight is reduced further. Marked atrophy of the cerebral cortex and loss of cortical neurons occur. The cerebral sulci and fissures, as well as the ventricles, are enlarged more than those of persons of the same age without AD. These areas of the brain are particularly affected:

- Precentral gyrus of the frontal lobe
- Superior temporal gyrus
- Hippocampus
- Substantia nigra

Microscopic changes of the brain found in people with AD include neurofibrillary tangles, amyloid-rich senile or neuritic plaques, and granulovascular degeneration. **Neurofibrillary tangles** are a classic finding at autopsy in the brains of patients with AD. They consist of tangled masses of fibrous tissue throughout the neurons (McCance et al., 2014).

Neuritic plaques are composed of degenerating nerve terminals and are found particularly in the hippocampus, an important part of the limbic system. Deposited within the plaques are increased amounts of an abnormal protein called *beta amyloid*. These peptides have a tendency to accumulate and form the neurotoxic plaques found in the brain (McCance et al., 2014).

Although *vascular degeneration* occurs in the normally aging brain, its presence is significantly increased in patients with dementia. Vascular degeneration accounts for at least partial loss of the ability of nerve cells to function properly. Cell deterioration and death may lead to hemorrhage. This pathologic change contributes to the mortality associated with this disorder.

In addition to the structural changes in the brain associated with AD and other dementias, abnormalities in the neurotransmitters (acetylcholine [ACh], norepinephrine, dopamine, and serotonin) may occur. High levels of beta amyloid are associated with significantly reduced ACh, which leads to a decrease in the amount of acetyltransferase in the hippocampus. This loss is major because the decrease in acetyltransferase interferes with cholinergic innervation to the cerebral cortex. This results in impaired COGNITION, recent memory, and the ability to acquire new memories. The specific role of reduced neurotransmitters in the development of AD is not well understood.

Etiology and Genetic Risk

The exact cause of AD is unknown. It is well established that *age, gender (women more than men), and family history are the most important risk factors.* Several other theories and risk factors have been studied, including chemical imbalances, environmental agents, immunologic changes, and ethnicity/race. Compared with Euro-Americans, African Americans have a greater risk for developing the disease and Hispanics tend to develop the disease earlier than other groups. The cause of these differences is not yet known.

Environmental agents, especially certain viruses such as herpes zoster and herpes simplex, and toxic metals such as zinc and copper have also been suggested as causes. Patients

GENETIC/GENOMIC CONSIDERATIONS
Patient-Centered Care QSEN

There is little doubt that many patients with AD had a genetic predisposition to the development of the disease. The inheritance pattern is highly complex with both isolated and interactive genes identified from multiple sites such as the beta-amyloid precursor *(APP)*, the presenilin1 *(PSEN1)*, and presenilin2 *(PRESN2)* genes—all involved in the formation of the distinctive plaque and neurofibrillary tangles in AD. Other genes implicated in AD are apolipoprotein E *(APOE)* and clusterin *(CLU)* genes that code for products in lipid metabolism and inflammation. A third family of genes associated with AD progression is responsible for endocytosis and vesicle trafficking—intracellular processes that help deliver neurotransmitters. These genes are phosphatidylinositol-binding clathrin assembly protein *(PICALM)* and Bridging Integrator 1 *(BIN1)* (Bettens et al., 2013). The genetic studies in AD are an example of how genetics, genomics, and proteomics are not only finding genes associated with the condition but also illustrating the mechanisms of pathology in complex conditions.

who have experienced a head injury or repeated head trauma (e.g., boxers) may be more at risk for AD and at an earlier age than others.

Incidence and Prevalence

There is a significant increase in both the incidence and prevalence of AD after 65 years of age, although it may affect anyone older than 40 years. The number of people in the United States with AD is estimated at 4.5 million and expected to triple in the next three decades (Mayeux & Stern, 2012). AD has a significant impact on health care costs, including direct and indirect medical and social service costs.

Health Promotion and Maintenance

There are no proven ways to prevent AD or other dementias. Current research activities are focusing on eating a balanced diet, eating dark-colored fruits and vegetables, using soy products, and consuming sufficient amounts of folate and vitamins B_{12}, C, and E. These substances have been reported to decrease the risk for developing AD, but study results are inconclusive and inconsistent. Walking, swimming, and other exercise not only increase tone and muscle strength but also may decrease mental decline in AD, as well as other dementias. Avoiding lifestyle factors that contribute to stroke risk, including untreated hypertension, is also advocated.

❖ PATIENT-CENTERED COLLABORATIVE CARE

◆ Assessment

History. The patient with dementia and Alzheimer's disease (AD) often presents with cognitive impairment, although many other disorders, drugs, and environmental factors can cause changes in COGNITION. A thorough history and physical examination are necessary to differentiate AD from other, possibly reversible causes of cognitive impairment (Table 42-4). Obtain information from family members or significant others because the patient may be unaware of the problems, denying their existence or covering them up. Family members often do not recognize or may deny early changes in their loved one as well.

The most important information to be obtained is the onset, duration, progression, and course of the symptoms. Question the patient and the family about changes in memory or increasing forgetfulness and about the ability to perform ADLs. Ask

TABLE 42-4   Causes of Cognitive Impairment in the Older Adult

Neurologic Causes
- Vascular insufficiency
- Infections
- Trauma
- Tumors
- Normal-pressure hydrocephalus

Cardiovascular Causes
- Myocardial infarction
- Dysrhythmias
- Heart failure
- Cardiogenic shock
- Endocarditis
- Stroke

Pulmonary Causes
- Infection
- Pneumonia
- Hypoventilation

Metabolic Causes
- Electrolyte imbalance
- Acidosis/alkalosis
- Hypoglycemia/hyperglycemia
- Kidney failure
- Fluid volume deficit
- Urinary tract infection
- Hepatic failure

Drug Intoxication
- Misuse of prescribed medications
- Side effects of medications
- Incorrect use of over-the-counter medications
- Ingestion of heavy metals

Nutritional Deficiencies
- B vitamins
- Vitamin C
- Hypoproteinemia

Environmental Causes
- Hypothermia/hyperthermia
- Unfamiliar environment
- Sensory deprivation/overload

Psychological Causes
- Depression
- Anxiety
- Pain
- Fatigue
- Grief
- Paranoia

CHART 42-13   Key Features
Alzheimer's Disease

Early (Mild), or Stage I (first symptoms up to 4 years)
- Independent in ADLs
- No social or employment problems initially
- Denies presence of symptoms
- Forgets names; misplaces household items
- Short-term memory loss; difficulty recalling new information
- Subtle changes in personality and behavior
- Loss of initiative; less engaged in social relationships
- Mild impaired cognition, problems with judgment
- Decreased performance, especially when stressed
- Unable to travel alone to new destinations
- Decreased sense of smell

Middle (Moderate), or Stage II (2 to 3 years)
- Impairment of all cognitive functions
- Problems with handling or unable to handle money and finances
- Disorientation to time, place, and event
- Possible depression, agitated
- Increasingly dependent in ADLs
- Visuospatial deficits: difficulty driving, gets lost
- Speech and language deficits: less talkative, decrease in use of vocabulary, increasingly non-fluent, and eventually aphasic
- Incontinent
- Wandering; trouble sleeping

Late (Severe), or Stage III
- Completely incapacitated; bedridden
- Totally dependent in ADLs
- Motor and verbal skills lost
- General and focal neurologic deficits
- Agnosia (loss of facial recognition)

about current employment status, work history, and ability to fulfill household responsibilities, including cleaning, grocery shopping, and preparing meals. Inquire about changes in driving ability, ability to handle routine financial transactions, and language and communication skills. In addition, document any changes in personality and behavior. Assessing functional status for complex chronic conditions such as dementia is a recommended core measure by the Centers for Medicare and Medicaid Services (www.cms.gov).

There is increasing evidence that an altered sense of smell is associated with the development of AD. Therefore ask about changes in the ability to smell or changes in the sense of smell. The history taking concludes with a review of the patient's medical history. Of particular importance is a history of head trauma, viral illness, or exposure to metal or toxic waste, as well as any family history of AD or Down syndrome.

Physical Assessment/Clinical Manifestations

Stages of Alzheimer's Disease. The clinical manifestations associated with AD can be grouped into three broad stages based on the progress of the disease (Chart 42-13). The patient does not necessarily progress from one stage to the next in an orderly fashion. A stage may be bypassed, or he or she may exhibit symptoms of one or several stages. Each patient exhibits different disease stages and clinical manifestations. Consequently, most authorities now use broader terms such as *early (mild), middle (moderate),* and *late (severe)* stages.

The primary focus of the neurologic assessment of patients with AD is to identify abnormalities in COGNITION, including language, personality, and behavior. Physical manifestations of neurologic impairment (seizures, tremors, or ataxia) tend to occur late in the disease process.

Changes in Cognition. Cognition refers to the ability of the brain to process, store, retrieve, and use information. Therefore assess the patient for deficits in these abilities:
- Attention and concentration
- Judgment and perception
- Learning and memory
- Communication and language
- Speed of information processing

One of the first symptoms of AD is short-term memory impairment. New memory and defects in information retrieval result from dysfunction in the hippocampal, frontal, or parietal region. Alterations in communication abilities, such as **apraxia** (inability to use words or objects correctly), **aphasia** (inability to speak or understand), **anomia** (inability to find words), and **agnosia** (loss of sensory comprehension), are due to dysfunction of the temporal and parietal lobes. Frontal lobe impairment causes problems with judgment, an inability to make decisions, decreased attention span, and a decreased ability to concentrate. As the disease progresses to a later stage, the patient loses all cognitive abilities, is totally unable to communicate, and becomes less aware of the environment.

To more clearly identify the nature and extent of the patient's cognitive impairment, the neurologist or psychologist administers several neuropsychological tests. The tests selected depend on clinician preference and the ability of the patient to participate in testing. All of the tests focus on cognitive ability and may be repeated over time to measure changes. Folstein's Mini-Mental State Examination (MMSE) is an example of a tool used to determine the onset and severity of cognitive impairment.

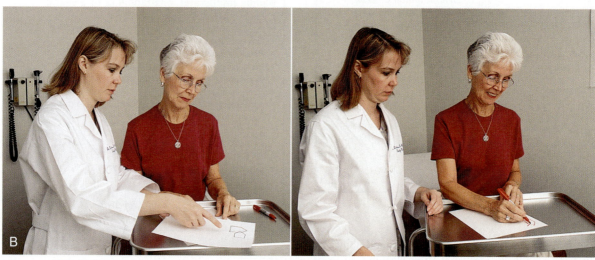

Orientation to Time
"What is the date?"

Registration
"Listen carefully, I am going to say three words. You say them back after I stop. Ready? Here they are...
HOUSE (pause), CAR (pause), LAKE (pause). Now repeat those words back to me." [Repeat up to 5 times, but score only the first trial.]

Naming
"What is this?" [Point to a pencil or pen.]

Reading
"Please read this and do what it says." [Show examinee the words on the stimulus form.]

CLOSE YOUR EYES

A

B

FIG. 42-2 A, Examples of questions that are asked on the Mini-Mental State Examination (MMSE). **B,** Copying is one of the tasks on the MMSE.

The MMSE is also known as the "mini-mental exam." The MMSE assesses five major areas—orientation, registration, attention and calculation, recall, and speech-language (including reading). Fig. 42-2 lists examples of the questions asked on this test. The patient performs certain cognitive tasks that are scored and added together for a total score of 0 to 30. The lower the score is, the greater the severity of the dementia. It is not unusual for a patient with advanced AD to score below 5.

Although the MMSE is used frequently by specialists and researchers outside of the acute care setting, it is a copyrighted tool and the patient must be able to read. For the patient who cannot read or for a quicker screening test, the "set test" can be used. The patient is asked to name 10 items in each of four sets or categories: fruits, animals, colors, and towns (FACT). Other categories can be used, if needed. The patient receives 1 point for each item for a possible maximum score of 40. Patients who score above 25 do not have dementia. Although this assessment is easy to administer, it should not be used for patients with hearing impairments or speech and language problems. Another brief tool to screen for dementia that has validity and reliability in acute care settings is the Short Blessed Test (www.mybraintest.org). In long-term care settings, the federally required Brief Interview for Mental Status (BIMS) is required as part of the Minimum Data Set 3.0 for Nursing Homes (Saliba et al., 2012).

Changes in Behavior and Personality. One of the most difficult aspects of AD and dementia that families and caregivers cope with is the behavioral changes that can occur in advanced disease. Assess the patient for:

- Aggressiveness, especially verbal and physical abusive tendencies
- Rapid mood swings
- Increased confusion at night or when light is not adequate (sundowning) or in excessively fatigued patients

The patient may wander and become lost or may go into other rooms to rummage through another's belongings. Hoarding or hiding objects is also common. For example, patients may hoard washcloths in the long-term care setting.

For some patients with dementia, emotional and behavioral problems occur with the primary disease. They may experience paranoia (suspicious behaviors), delusions, hallucinations, and depression. Document these behaviors, and ensure the patient's safety. (Refer to a mental health/behavior health nursing textbook for a complete discussion of these disorders.)

Although drug therapy is not effective in treating dementia, certain drugs may help control the emotional and psychiatric manifestations (e.g., depression, anxiety, paranoia, aggression) associated with the primary disease.

Changes in Self-Management Skills. Observe for changes in the patient's self-management skills, such as:

- Decreased interest in personal appearance
- Selection of clothing that is inappropriate for the weather or event
- Loss of bowel and bladder control
- Decreased appetite or ability to eat

Over time, the patient becomes less mobile and muscle contractures develop. He or she eventually becomes totally immobile and requires total physical care. The patient is then unable to meet the human needs of MOBILITY and COGNITION.

Psychosocial Assessment. In people with dementia, the cognitive changes and biochemical and structural dysfunctions affect personality and behavior. In the early stage, patients often recognize that they are experiencing memory or cognitive changes and may attempt to hide the problems. They begin the grieving process because of anticipated loss, experiencing denial, anger, bargaining, and depression at varying times. Older patients typically think the changes are part of "old age."

When the patient and family receive the diagnosis, one or more family members may desire genetic testing. Support the patient's/family's decisions regarding testing, and assist them in finding credible resources for testing and professional genetics counseling.

As the disease progresses, patients begin to display major changes in emotional and behavioral affect. Of particular importance is the need for an assessment of the patients' reactions to changes in routine or environment. For example, a hospital admission is very traumatic for most patients with dementia. It is not unusual for them to exhibit a catastrophic response or overreact to any change by becoming excessively aggressive or abusive. This is referred to as *traumatic relocation syndrome.*

As patients become unaware of their behavior, the focus of the psychosocial assessment shifts to the family or significant others. The health care team assesses their ability to cope with the chronicity and progression of the disease and identifies possible support systems.

Laboratory and Imaging Assessment. No laboratory test can confirm the diagnosis of AD. Definitive diagnosis is made on the basis of brain tissue examination at autopsy, which confirms the presence of neurofibrillary tangles and neuritic plaques.

Genetic testing, specifically for *apolipoprotein E4 (Apo E4),* may be helpful as an ancillary test (not a predictive test) for the differential diagnosis of AD. *Amyloid beta protein precursor (soluble)* (sBPP) may be measured for patients to diagnose AD and other types of dementia. A decrease in the patient's sBPP in the cerebrospinal fluid (CSF) supports the diagnosis because the amyloid tends to deposit in the brain and is not circulating in the CSF (Pagana & Pagana, 2014).

A variety of other laboratory tests may be performed to rule out other treatable causes of dementia or delirium, including:

- Complete blood count (CBC)
- Serum electrolyte levels, blood urea nitrogen, and glucose
- Vitamin B_{12} levels
- Folate levels
- Blood ammonia levels
- Blood gas analysis
- Cerebrospinal fluid (CSF) analysis
- Urinalysis
- Thyroid and liver function tests
- Serologic test for syphilis
- Toxicity screening tests; heavy metal screen
- Alcohol screening tests

A CT, PET, or SPECT scan may be performed to rule out other causes of disease. The CT scan typically shows cerebral atrophy and ventricular enlargement, wide sulci, and shrunken gyri in the later stages of the disease. An MRI scan can also rule out other causes of neurologic disease. The PET and SPECT scans show a significant decrease in metabolic activity in the brains of people with AD.

◆ **Analysis**

The priority NANDA-I nursing diagnoses and collaborative problems for patients with Alzheimer's disease (AD) include:

1. Chronic Confusion related to neuronal degeneration in the brain (NANDA-I)
2. Risk for Injury related to wandering or elder abuse (NANDA-I)
3. Caregiver Role Strain related to the patient's prolonged progression of disability and the patient's increasing care needs (NANDA-I)

◆ **Planning and Implementation**

The priority for interdisciplinary care is safety! Chronic confusion and physical deficits place the patient with AD at a high risk for injury.

Managing Chronic Confusion

Planning: Expected Outcomes. In the very early stages of the disease, the patient with dementia is expected to maintain the ability to perform complex mental processes. As the disease progresses, patients cannot meet this outcome. Instead, the desired outcome is to maintain cognitive function for as long as possible to keep patients safe and increase their quality of life.

Interventions. Although drug therapy may be used for patients with dementia or AD, nonpharmacologic interventions are the main focus of patient-centered collaborative management. Teach family members and significant others about the importance of being consistent in following the plan of care.

Nonpharmacologic Management. The health care provider should answer the patient's questions truthfully concerning the diagnosis of dementia or AD. In this way, the patient can more fully participate in the interdisciplinary plan of care. Interventions are the same whether he or she is cared for at home, in an adult day-care center, in an assisted-living center, in a long-term care facility, or in a hospital admitted with another medical condition. The patient with memory problems always benefits best from a structured and consistent environment (Seitz et al., 2012).

Many factors, including physical illness and environmental factors, can exacerbate (worsen) the clinical manifestations of AD (Table 42-5). The patient with dementia frequently has other medical problems such as cardiovascular disease, arthritis,

TABLE 42-5 **Factors That Can Worsen Alzheimer's Disease and Dementia**	
• Stroke	• Impaired hepatic function
• Subdural hematoma	• Infection
• Space-occupying lesion (tumor)	• Impaired vision and hearing
• Decrease in blood supply to the brain	• Sudden changes in surroundings
• Myocardial infarction	• Pain and discomfort
• Dysrhythmias	• Drugs
• Hypoglycemia	• Physical or chemical restraint
• Impaired renal function	

renal insufficiency, and pulmonary disease. Changes in vision and hearing also may be present. Managing these conditions helps the patient's functional abilities.

Approaches to managing the patient who has Alzheimer's disease include:

- Cognitive stimulation and memory training
- Structuring the environment
- Orientation and validation therapy
- Promoting self-management
- Promoting bowel and bladder continence
- Promoting communication

The purpose of *cognitive stimulation and memory training* is to reinforce or promote desirable cognitive function and facilitate memory. An individualized cognitive therapy program may provide some benefit to the patient. Training in communication can help nurses and health care team members interact with better effect and compassion (Eggenberger et al., 2013; Johnson et al., 2013).

As the disease progresses, the patient may experience **prosopagnosia,** an inability to recognize oneself and other familiar faces. Encourage the family to provide pictures of family members and close friends that are labeled with the person's name on the picture. In addition, advise the family to reminisce with the patient about pleasant experiences from the past (Subramaniam & Woods, 2012). Use *reminiscence therapy* while assisting the patient with ADLs or performing a treatment or assessment. Refer to a personal item in the room to help the patient begin to talk about its meaning in the present and in the past.

It is not unusual for the patient to talk to his or her image in the mirror. This behavior should be allowed as long as it is not harmful. If the patient becomes frightened by the mirror image, remove or cover the mirror. In some long-term care or assisted-living settings, a picture of the patient is placed on the room door to help with facial recognition and to help the patient locate his or her room. This picture also helps the staff locate the patient in case of elopement (running away).

Teach the family to keep environmental distractions and noise to a minimum. The patient's home, hospital room, or nursing home room should not have pictures on the wall or other decorations that could be misinterpreted as people or animals that could harm the patient. An abstract painting or wallpaper might look like a fire or an explosion and scare the patient. The room should have adequate, nonglare lighting and no potentially frightening shadows.

In addition to disturbed sleep, other negative effects of high noise levels include decreased nutritional intake, changes in blood pressure and pulse rates, and feelings of increased stress and anxiety. The patient with AD is especially susceptible to these changes and needs to have as much undisturbed sleep at night as possible. Fatigue increases confusion and behavioral manifestations such as agitation and aggressiveness.

! NURSING SAFETY PRIORITY (QSEN)

Action Alert

When a patient with Alzheimer's disease is in a new setting or environment, collaborate with the staff and admitting department to select a room that is in the quietest area of the unit and away from obvious exits, if possible. A private room may be needed if the patient has a history of agitation or wandering. The television should remain off unless the patient turns it on or requests that it be turned on.

Objects such as furniture, a hairbrush, and eyeglasses should be kept in the same place. Establish a daily routine, and follow it as much as possible. Arrange for a communication board for scheduled activities and other information to promote orientation such as the day of the week, the month, and the year. Pictures of people familiar to the patient can also be placed on this board.

Explain changes in routine to the patient before they occur, repeating the explanation immediately before the changes take place. Clocks and single-date calendars also help the patient maintain day-to-day orientation to the environment in the early stages of the disease process. *For the patient with early disease, reality orientation is usually appropriate.* Teach family members and health care staff to frequently reorient the patient to the environment. Remind the patient what day and time it is, where he or she is, and who you are.

For the patient in the later stages of AD or dementia, reality orientation does not work and often increases agitation. *The health care team uses validation therapy for the patient with moderate or severe AD. In* **validation therapy,** *the staff member recognizes and acknowledges the patient's feelings and concerns.* For example, if the patient is looking for his or her mother, ask him or her to talk about what Mother looks like and what she might be wearing. This response does not argue with the patient but also does not reinforce the patient's belief that Mother is still living.

As the disease progresses, altered thought processes affect the *ability to perform ADLs.* Encourage the patient to perform as much self-care as possible and to maintain independence in daily living skills as long as possible. For example, in the home setting, complete clothing outfits that can be easily removed and put on (e.g., shirt, slacks, underwear, and socks) and placed on a single hanger are preferred for patient selection. When possible, the patient should participate in meal preparation, grocery shopping, and other household routines. Many patients cannot make purposeful movements as the disease progresses.

? NCLEX EXAMINATION CHALLENGE

Psychosocial Integrity

A client with moderate dementia asks the nurse to find her brother who is deceased. What is the nurse's best response?
A. "Your brother died over 20 years ago."
B. "We can call him in a little while if you want."
C. "What did your brother look like?"
D. "I'll ask your daughter to find him for you when she comes in."

Collaborate with the occupational and physical therapists to provide a complete evaluation and assistance in helping the patient become more independent. Adaptive devices, such as grab bars in the bathtub or shower area, an elevated commode, and adapted eating utensils, may enable him or her to maintain independence in grooming, toileting, and feeding. The physical therapist prescribes an exercise program to improve physical health and functionality.

The patient may remain continent of bowel and bladder for long periods if taken to the bathroom or given a bedpan or urinal every 2 hours. Toileting may be needed more often during the day and less frequently at night. Unlicensed assistive personnel (UAP) or home caregiver encourages the patient to drink adequate fluids to promote optimal voiding. A patient

EVIDENCE-BASED PRACTICE (QSEN)

Does the Use of Sitters Improve the Care of Older Adults with Dementia in Acute Care Settings?

Moyle, W., Borbasi, S., Wallis, M., Olorenshaw, R., & Gracia, N. (2011). Acute care management of older people with dementia: A qualitative perspective. *Journal of Clinical Nursing, 20*(3-4), 420-428.

This Australian study explored management for older people with dementia in an acute hospital setting using a descriptive qualitative approach. A total of 13 nurses participated in semi-structured audio-taped interviews. All nurses worked in acute medical or surgical wards in a large South East Queensland, Australia, hospital. The authors identified an inconsistent approach to care in that the most common intervention—providing a sitter—emphasized safety at the expense of well-being and dignity. Using untrained staff (i.e., a sitter or "patient observers") to monitor a patient with dementia is a risk management strategy that reduces the use of restraints but does not incorporate other evidence-based approaches to care such as reminiscent therapy, mobility activities, or family member presence. The use of sitters does not individualize care, a hallmark of nursing care.

Level of Evidence: 3
The research was a small qualitative study.

Commentary: Implications for Practice and Research
Although this study occurred in Australia, sitters are commonly used in the United States. It may be that sitters need to be trained in communication and assisting in activities of daily living to provide safe and compassionate care that recognizes the dignity of hospitalized patients with dementia. The study needs to be repeated in the United States using a larger sample size.

CHART 42-14   Best Practice for Patient Safety & Quality Care (QSEN)

Promoting Communication with the Patient with Advanced Dementia or Alzheimer's Disease

- Ask simple, direct questions that require only a "yes" or "no" answer if the patient can communicate.
- Provide instructions with pictures in a place that the patient will see if he or she can read them.
- Use simple, short sentences and one-step instructions.
- Use gestures to help the patient understand what is being said.
- Validate the patient's feelings.
- Limit choices; too many choices cause frustration and increased confusion.
- Never assume that the patient is totally confused and cannot understand what is being communicated.
- Try to anticipate the patient's needs and interpret nonverbal communication.

may refuse to drink enough fluids because of a fear of incontinence. Assure the patient that he or she will be toileted on a regular schedule to prevent incontinent episodes.

When patients with dementia are in the hospital or other unfamiliar place, avoid the use of restraints, including siderails. Serious injury can occur when a patient with dementia attempts to get out of bed with either limb restraints or siderail use. Use frequent surveillance, toileting every 2 hours, and other strategies to prevent falls. Restraint reduction has been associated with a reduced length of stay and fewer injuries (Kwok et al., 2012). In some cases, sitters may be used to help prevent patient injury (see the Evidence-Based Practice box). Chapter 2 discusses fall prevention in detail.

Maintain a clear path between the bed and bathroom at all times. For patients who are too weak to walk to the bathroom, a bedside commode may be used. Some patients may void in unusual places, such as the sink or a wastebasket. As a reminder of where they should toilet, place a picture of the commode on the bathroom door.

Use **redirection** by attracting the patient's attention to promote communication. Keep the environment as free from distractions as possible. Speak directly to the patient in a distinct manner. Sentences should be clear and short. Remind the patient to perform one task at a time, and allow sufficient time for completion. It may be necessary to break each task down into many small steps (Chart 42-14).

As the disease progresses, the patient is unable to perform tasks when asked. Show the patient what needs to be done, or provide cues to remind him or her how to perform the task. When possible, explain and demonstrate the task that the patient is asked to perform.

Patients with dementia disorders typically have specific speech and language problems, such as:
- **Aphasia** (difficulty speaking and understanding language)
- **Anomia** (difficulty findings words to name an object)
- **Apraxia** (difficulty recognizing words)

Recognize that emotional and physical behaviors may be a form of communication. Interpret the meaning of these behaviors to address them. For example, restlessness may indicate urinary retention, PAIN, INFECTION, or hypoxia (lack of oxygen to the brain).

Drug Therapy. **Cholinesterase inhibitors** are drugs approved for treating AD symptoms. They work to improve cholinergic neurotransmission in the brain by delaying the destruction of acetylcholine (ACh) by the enzyme *acetylcholinesterase*. This action slows the onset of cognitive decline in some patients. None of these drugs alters the course of the disease. Examples include donepezil (Aricept), galantamine (Reminyl), and rivastigmine (Exelon).

Memantine (Namenda) is the first of a new class of drugs that is a low to moderate affinity **N-methyl-D-aspartate (NMDA) receptor antagonist**. Overexcitation of NMDA receptors by the neurotransmitter *glutamate* may play a role in AD. This drug therefore blocks excess amounts of glutamate that can damage nerve cells. It is indicated for advanced AD and has been shown to slow the pace of deterioration. Namenda may help maintain patient function for a few months longer. Some patients also have improved memory and thinking skills. This drug can be given with donepezil (Aricept), a cholinesterase inhibitor.

Some patients with AD develop depression and may be treated with **antidepressants**. Selective serotonin reuptake inhibitors (SSRIs), such as paroxetine (Paxil) and sertraline (Zoloft), are usually prescribed. Tricyclic antidepressants, such as amitriptyline (Elavil, Levate ✦), should not be used because of their anticholinergic effect, especially for older adults. Anticholinergic drugs frequently cause serious side effects, including increased confusion, urinary retention, and constipation.

Psychotropic drugs, also called *antipsychotic* or *neuroleptic drugs,* should be reserved for patients with emotional and behavioral health problems that sometimes accompany dementia, such as hallucinations and delusions. In clinical practice, however, these drugs are sometimes incorrectly used for agitation, combativeness, or restlessness. Psychotropic drugs are considered chemical restraints because they decrease MOBILITY and patients' self-management ability. Therefore most geriatricians recommend that these drugs be used as a last resort and with caution in low doses for a specific emotional or behavioral health problem. The specific drug prescribed depends on side effects, the condition of the patient, and expected outcomes. Follow agency policy and The Joint Commission standards concerning the use of chemical restraints.

Preventing Injury

Planning: Expected Outcomes. The patient with dementia is expected to remain free from physical harm and not injure anyone else.

Interventions. Many patients with dementia tend to wander and may easily become lost. In later stages of the disease, some patients may become severely agitated and physically or verbally abusive to others. Teach the family the importance of a patient identification badge or bracelet. The badge should include how to contact the primary caregiver. In an inpatient setting, check the patient frequently and place him or her in a room that can be monitored easily. The room should be away from exits and stairs. Some health care agencies place large stop signs or red tape on the floor in front of exits. Others have installed alarm systems to indicate when a patient is opening the door or getting out of a bed or chair.

Teach the family to enroll the patient in the Safe Return Program—a national, government-funded program of the Alzheimer's Association (www.alz.org) that assists in the identification and safe, timely return of people with dementia. The program includes registration of the patient and a 24-hour hotline to be called to assist in finding a lost patient. If a patient wanders and becomes lost, the family (or health care institution) should immediately notify the police department. An up-to-date picture of the patient makes it easier for local authorities, the public, and neighbors to identify the missing patient. Devices using radio wave beacons and a global positioning system (GPS) have been developed to help families and law enforcement officials find a lost patient more easily. These devices include shoes with a GPS unit implanted, jewelry that is hard to remove, and bracelets. Caution families that these devices are not foolproof. Just like cell phones, there are some areas where the signal from the patient may not be picked up easily if at all.

Restlessness may be decreased if the patient is taken for frequent walks. If the patient begins to wander, redirect him or her. For example, if the patient insists on going shopping for clothes, the patient is redirected to his or her closet to select clothing that will not be recognized as his or her own. This type of activity can be repeated a number of times because the patient has lost short-term memory. Best practices for preventing and managing wandering are listed in Chart 42-15.

In any setting, keep the patient busy with structured activities. In a health care agency, an activity therapist or volunteer may work with patients as a group or individually to determine the type of activity that is appropriate for the stage of the disease. Puzzles, board games, and art activities are often appropriate. Music and art therapy are nonpharmacologic approaches to managing patients with dementia (Seitz et al., 2012).

Patients with dementia may be injured because they cannot recognize objects or situations as harmful. Remove or secure all

---

CHART 42-15 Best Practice for Patient Safety & Quality Care (QSEN)

Approaches to Prevent and Manage Wandering in Hospitalized Patients

- Identify the patients most at risk for wandering through observation and history provided by family.
- Provide appropriate supervision, including frequent checks (especially at shift-change times).
- Place the patient in an area that provides maximum observation, but not in the nurses' station.
- Use family members, friends, volunteers, and sitters as needed to monitor the patient.
- Keep the patient away from stairs or elevators.
- Do not change rooms to prevent increasing confusion.
- Avoid physical or chemical restraints.
- Assess and treat pain.
- Use re-orientation methods and validation therapy, as appropriate.
- Provide frequent toileting and incontinence care as needed.
- If possible, prevent overstimulation, such as excessive noise; use soft music and nonglare lighting if possible.

! NURSING SAFETY PRIORITY (QSEN)

Action Alert

In inpatient health care agencies, use physical restraints such as waist belts and geri-chairs with lapboards only as a last resort because they often increase patient restlessness and cause agitation. Federal regulations in long-term care facilities in the United States mandate that all residents have the right to be free of both physical and chemical restraints. All health care agencies accredited by The Joint Commission are required to use alternatives to restraints before resorting to any physical or chemical restraint.

---

potentially dangerous objects (e.g., knives, drugs, cleaning solutions). Patients are often unaware that their driving ability is impaired and usually want to continue this activity even if their driver's license has been suspended or they are unsafe. Automobile keys must be secured, but the patient should be told why they were taken. (See Chapter 2 for more discussion on older adult driving.)

Late in the disease process, the patient may experience seizure activity. If he or she is cared for at home, teach caregivers what action to take when a seizure occurs. (See discussion of Interventions on pp. 859-863 in the Seizures and Epilepsy section.)

Talking calmly and softly and attempting to redirect the patient to a more positive behavior or activity are effective strategies when he or she is agitated. Use calm, positive statements, and reassure the patient that he or she is safe. Statements such as "I'm sorry that you are upset," "I know it's hard," and "I will have someone stay with you until you feel better" may help.

Actions to *avoid* when the patient is agitated include raising the voice, confrontation, arguing, reasoning, taking offense, or explaining. Teach the caregiver to not show alarm or make sudden movements out of the person's view. If the patient remains agitated, ensure his or her safety and leave the room after explaining that you will return later. Frequent visual checks must be done during this time. If the patient is connected to any type of tubing or other device, he or she may try to disconnect it or pull it out. These devices should be used cautiously in the patient with dementia. If IV access, for example, is needed,

TABLE 42-6   Minimizing Behavioral Problems for Patients with Alzheimer's Disease at Home

Carefully evaluate the patient's environment.
- Ensure environment is safe:
  - Remove small area rugs.
  - Consider replacing tile floors with non-slippery floors.
  - Arrange furniture and room decorations to maximize the patient's safety when walking.
  - Minimize clutter in all rooms in and outside of the house.
  - Install nightlights in patient's room, bathroom, and hallway.
  - Install and maintain smoke alarms, fire alarms, and natural gas detectors.
- Install safety devices in the bathroom such as handles for changing position (sit-to-stand).
- Install alarm system or bells on outside doors; place safety locks on doors and gates.
- Ensure that door locks cannot be easily opened by the patient.

Assist the patient to remain oriented.
- Place single-date calendars in patient's room and in kitchen.
- Use large-face clocks with a neutral background.

Communicate with the patient based on his or her ability to understand.
- Explain activity immediately before the patient needs to carry it out.
- Break complex tasks down to simple steps.

Encourage the patient to be as independent as possible in ADLs.
- Place complete outfits for the day on hangers; have the patient select one to wear.
- Develop and maintain a predictable routine (e.g., meals, bedtime, morning routine).

When a problem behavior occurs, divert patient to another activity.

Minimize excessive stimulation.
- Take the patient on outings when crowds are small.
- If crowds cannot be avoided, minimize the amount of time the patient is present in a crowd. For example, at family gatherings, provide a quiet room for the patient to rest throughout the visit.

Arrange for a day-care program to maintain interaction and provide respite for home caregiver.

Register the patient with the Alzheimer's Association Safe Return Program (www.alz.org).

❓ NCLEX EXAMINATION CHALLENGE
Safe and Effective Care Environment

The nurse is caring for a client with dementia. Which nursing intervention is most appropriate when caring for this client?
A. Provide a large clock and calendar at the nurses' station.
B. Use removable restraints like a roll-waist belt to prevent wandering.
C. Use incontinence pads or absorbent underwear to prevent complications from incontinence.
D. Place the patient in a room close to the nurses' station for frequent observation.

or "Do you wait long for help to the bathroom?" may be less stressful for the patient to answer.

Managing Caregiver Role Strain
Planning: Expected Outcomes. The family or other caregivers of the patient with dementia are expected to plan time to care for themselves to promote a reasonable quality of life and satisfaction (Van Mierlo et al., 2012).

Interventions. The patient with moderate or severe dementia requires continual 24-hour supervision and caregiving. Severe cognitive changes leave the patient unable to manage finances, property, or personal care. The family needs to seek legal counsel regarding the patient's competency and the need to obtain guardianship or a durable medical power of attorney when necessary. Refer the family to the local Alzheimer's or dementia support group for literature and information concerning the disease and related problems (Corbett et al., 2012).

Family members and other caregivers must be aware of their own health and stress levels. Signs of stress include anger, social withdrawal, anxiety, depression, lack of concentration, sleepiness, irritability, and health problems. When signs of stress occur, the caregiver should be referred to his or her health care provider or should seek one on his or her own. It is not unusual for the caregiver to refuse to accept help from others, even for a few brief hours. Initially, the caregiver may be more comfortable accepting help for just a few minutes a day so he or she could shower, enjoy a cup of tea, or take a brief walk. Some caregivers find that eventually they need to place their loved one into a respite setting or unit so that they can re-energize.

Refer all families to their local chapter of the Alzheimer's Association (www.alz.org) in the United States or to the Alzheimer Society of Canada (www.alzheimer.ca). These organizations provide information and support services to patients and their families, including seminars, audiovisual aids, and publications.

Community-Based Care
Home Care Management. AD is a chronic, progressive condition that eventually leaves the patient completely disoriented and totally dependent on others for all aspects of care. In the early stages, patients may be cared for at home with little need for outside intervention. Whenever possible, the patient and family should be assigned a case manager who can assess their needs for health care resources and find the best placement throughout the continuum of care.

The patient usually begins to withdraw from friends and social events as memory impairment and personality and behavior changes occur. The family may begin to decrease their own social activities as the demands of the patient's care take

the catheter or cannula is placed in an area that the patient cannot easily see or it should be covered.

Another way to manage this problem is to provide a diversion. For example, if the patient is doing an activity or holding an item such as a stuffed animal or other special item, he or she might be less likely to pay attention to medical devices. Additional strategies to minimize behavioral problems, especially at home, are listed in Table 42-6.

Drugs may be used only if other modalities fail to control the patient's agitation and the behavior may lead to the patient or other being harmed. For example, atypical psychotics like risperidone (Risperdal), quetiapine (Seroquel), and olanzapine (Zyprexa) can help with aggressive and unsafe behaviors, although not all patients respond to these drugs. Lorazepam (Ativan) should be used with particular caution because of significant sedation and reports of increased confusion.

Patients who are cared for at home are at high risk for neglect or abuse. The Joint Commission requires all patients to be assessed for neglect and abuse on admission to a health care facility. Patients with mild dementia may not report these concerns for fear of retaliation. Those with severe dementia may not have the ability to report the abuse. Asking questions such as "Who cooks for you?" "Do you get help when you need it?"

CHART 42-16 **Best Practice for Patient Safety & Quality Care** **QSEN**

Reducing Caregiver Stress

- Maintain realistic expectations for the person with Alzheimer's disease (AD).
- Take each day one at a time.
- Try to find the positive aspects of each incident or situation.
- Use humor with the person who has AD.
- Use the resources of the Alzheimer's Association, including attending local support group meetings.
- Explore alternative care settings early in the disease process for possible use later.
- Establish advance directives with the AD patient early in the disease process.
- Set aside time each day for rest or recreation away from the patient, if possible.
- Seek respite care periodically for longer periods of time.
- Take care of yourself by watching your diet, exercising, and getting plenty of rest.
- Be realistic about what you or they can do, and accept help from family, friends, and community resources.
- Use relaxation techniques.

more of their time. Emphasize to the family the importance of maintaining their own social contacts and leisure activities. Many family members experience caregiver stress, which affects their physical, mental, and emotional health. Chart 42-16 lists strategies for reducing caregiver stress. Chapter 2 discusses caregiver role strain and interventions in more detail.

It is now possible in most areas of the United States and Canada for families to arrange respite care. The patient may be placed in a respite facility or nursing home for the weekend or for several weeks to give the family a rest from the constant care demands. The family may also be able to obtain respite care in the home through a home care agency or assisted-living facility. Remind the family that respite care is for a short period—it is not permanent placement. Some health care agencies have opened adult day-care centers or specialty units for patients with AD. In the day-care center, patients spend all or part of the day at the facility and participate in activities as their condition permits. Although these centers are usually open only on weekdays, this arrangement allows the caregiver to work or participate in other activities. If patients require 24-hour care, they may be placed in a specialty unit of a long-term care or assisted-living facility.

Teach the family how to be prepared in case the patient becomes restless, agitated, abusive, or combative. In addition, the family can learn how to use reality orientation or validation therapy, depending on the stage of the disease.

Self-Management Education. Usually patients with AD and dementia are cared for in the home until late in the disease process unless they can afford private-pay care. Because health insurance coverage in the United States and family finances may not be sufficient to cover the services of a private duty nurse or home care aide, family members typically provide the care. The patient plan of care developed by the nurse or case manager, in conjunction with the family, must be reasonable and realistic for the family to implement.

Review how to assist with bathing, dressing, toileting, and other self-management activities. The occupational therapist teaches the family and the patient how to use adaptive equipment, such as a brace, a sling, a cane, or modified eating utensils.

The patient may have difficulty chewing, swallowing, or tasting foods and may not be able to eat without assistance.

The family and the dietitian should develop a diet plan to increase the patient's nutritional intake. In the late stage of AD, the patient's intake often decreases and he or she loses weight.

Provide information to the family on what to do in the event of a seizure and how to protect the patient from injury. Instruct them to notify the health care provider if the seizure is prolonged or if the patient's seizure pattern changes.

Review with the family or other caregiver the name, time, and route of administration; the dosage; and the side effects of all drugs. Remind the family to check with the health care provider before using any over-the-counter drugs or herbs because they may interact with prescribed drug therapy.

Emphasis is placed on the need for the patient to have an established exercise program to maintain MOBILITY for as long as possible, as well as to prevent complications of immobility. In collaboration with the family, the physical therapist (PT) develops an individualized exercise program. The PT may continue to work with the patient at home until goals are achieved, depending on the payer source.

Remind the family or other caregiver to take special precautions to maintain the patient safely at home. The environment must be uncluttered, consistent, and structured. All hazardous items (e.g., cooking range and oven, power tools) are removed, secured, or "locked out." All electrical sockets not in use should be covered with safety plugs. Teach families to install handrails and grab bars in the bathroom. Handrails should be along all stairways, and a guardrail should be placed around porches or open stairwells. Because the patient may have a tendency to wander, especially at night, the family may want to install alarms to all outside doors, the basement, and the patient's bedroom. All outside and basement doors should have deadbolt locks to prevent the patient from going outside unsupervised. Remind the family to adjust the temperature of the water to prevent accidental burns. Nightlights should be used in the patient's bedroom, hallway, and bathroom to prevent fear and to help with orientation.

Health Care Resources. When the patient can no longer be cared for at home, referral to an assisted-living or long-term care facility may be needed. Early in the course of the disease, advise the family that placement might be needed in the late stages of the disease or sooner. This allows the family to begin to search for an appropriate facility before a crisis develops and immediate placement is needed. A number of facilities specialize in the care of patients with AD and other dementias. These units generally have a high staff-to-patient ratio and are architecturally designed to meet the special needs of this type of patient. The national office of the Alzheimer's Association publishes an outline of criteria for a dementia unit. In the advanced stage of the disease, the patient may need referral to hospice services for total care. (See the discussion of end-of-life and hospice care in Chapter 7.)

◆ Evaluation: Outcomes

Evaluate the care of the patient with dementia based on the identified priority patient problems. The expected outcomes include that the patient and/or family will:

- Remain free from injury and have a safe home environment
- Sleep through the night and be awake at appropriate times

- Meet basic human needs (e.g., nutrition, MOBILITY)
- Have a positive perception of his or her health status and life circumstances

Specific indicators for these outcomes are listed in the Planning and Implementation section (see earlier).

⦿ CLINICAL JUDGMENT CHALLENGE

Patient-Centered Care QSEN

A middle-aged man brings his 90-year old mother to the neurologist for re-evaluation of her Alzheimer's disease (AD). The patient was diagnosed with AD 2 years ago and continues to live alone most of the time in her home. One of her sons stays with her at night, but she cannot bathe herself or prepare meals. She forgets to eat and take her medications for hypertension. Her weight is 98 pounds and she is 5'4" tall.

1. As the nurse in the neurologist office, what questions might you ask the son about his mother's health?
2. What health assessment will you perform?
3. To promote the patient's safety, what options might you recommend for her caregiving?
4. What interventions are needed to improve the patient's nutritional status?
5. What health teaching is needed for the son at this time?

HUNTINGTON DISEASE

❖ PATHOPHYSIOLOGY

Huntington disease (HD) is a hereditary disorder transmitted as an autosomal dominant trait at the time of conception. HD is called an *autosomal dominant disorder* because only one copy of the defective gene, inherited from one parent, is necessary to produce the disease. This movement disorder causes both neurologic and behavioral symptoms that usually begin between the ages of 30 and 50 years and worsen during the next one to two decades. Patients typically die from pneumonia, heart failure, or other complication of immobility (Huntington's Disease Society of America [HDSA], 2014).

⦿ GENETIC/GENOMIC CONSIDERATIONS

Patient-Centered Care QSEN

Huntington disease is a single gene disorder caused by a mutation in the HD gene *(IT15)* located on chromosome 4. The mutation is a multiple repeat of the specific base triplet *cytosine, adenine, guanine (CAG),* increasing the length of the gene. An autosomal dominant trait with high penetrance means that a person who inherits just one mutated allele has nearly a 100% chance of developing the disease (McCance et al., 2014). This gene mutation has different expressions, depending on whether it is inherited from the mother or the father. People who inherit the mutation from their father have an earlier onset and a shorter life expectancy than do those who inherit from their mother. In addition, there is some variation in the disease, depending on the size (length) of the mutation. The longer the mutation, the more severe the disease is at an earlier age.

It is estimated that 30,000 people in the United States have HD, and another 20,000 to 50,000 are thought to carry the gene (HDSA, 2014). Men and women are equally affected at a highly productive time in life. The clinical onset of HD is gradual. The two main symptoms of the disease are progressive mental status changes, leading to dementia, and **choreiform movements** (rapid, jerky movements) in the limbs, trunk, and facial muscles.

Dementia is related to the destruction of neurons within the cerebral cortex. It may also be associated with excessive amounts of dopamine found within the cerebral cortex and limbic systems of those affected. Two structures within the basal ganglia are involved in the development of HD: the caudate nucleus and the putamen. Both structures have close connections to the cerebral cortex and are closely associated with neurotransmitters. Neurotransmitters are secreted at the synapse, or junction, of one neuron with another, and it is through their specific excitation or inhibition of neurons that fine, controlled, integrated motor activity occurs.

In HD, there is a decrease in the amount of *gamma-aminobutyric acid (GABA),* an inhibitory neurotransmitter in the basal ganglia. GABA depletion causes increased activity of the thalamus and other parts of the brain. There may also be an increase in *glutamate,* a major excitatory neurotransmitter. The result of these chemical changes in the brain is brisk, jerky, purposeless movements, particularly of the hands, face, tongue, and legs, which the patient cannot stop (McCance et al., 2014).

There are three stages of HD, each lasting roughly 5 years, corresponding to the average 15-year course of the disease. Stage 1 is the onset of neurologic or psychological symptoms. Stage 2 is characterized by an increasing dependence on others for care. Stage 3 results in loss of independent function.

The diagnosis of HD is made on the basis of a family history of the disease and clinical assessment. The triad of dominant inheritance, choreoathetosis (neuromuscular symptoms), and dementia is the hallmark of the disease. The symptoms exhibited by the patient vary in range and severity, age of onset, and rate of progression. Observe for clinical manifestations, which include chorea (jerky movements), poor balance, hesitant or explosive speech, dysphagia (difficulty swallowing), impaired respiration, and bowel and bladder incontinence. Mental status changes include decreased attention span, poor judgment, memory loss, personality changes, and dementia (later in the disease process). Perform a complete neurologic assessment.

❖ PATIENT-CENTERED COLLABORATIVE CARE

There is no known cure or treatment for HD. The only way to prevent transmission of the gene is for those affected to avoid having biologic children. Genetic counseling is important for children of patients with the disease. People at risk for the disease can be tested to determine whether the gene mutation is present. Before the testing procedure is undertaken, counseling is necessary to ensure that the patient has voluntarily decided in favor of testing and is not being pressured by family or friends. In addition, counseling helps determine whether the benefits of knowing the results outweigh the risks of a positive result (e.g., depression or suicide).

The first drug to be approved to decrease chorea associated with HD is tetrabenazine (Xenazine). It is given orally and is thought to work by depleting the monoamines (e.g., dopamine, serotonin) from nerve terminals. In some patients, it may increase the risk for suicide ideations and depression. Be sure to teach them and their families to report early signs of depression, including sleeplessness, decreasing appetite, and mood changes.

In other patients, psychotropic agents may be used to manage movement abnormalities that interfere with ADLs or are functionally disabling. They are also used to help control agitation, hallucinations, or psychotic delusions. Drug therapy may be used to treat other symptoms such as depression, anxiety, or obsessive-compulsive behaviors. Many of the drugs used to treat HD may cause side effects that may be difficult to differentiate from signs of HD.

A number of clinical trials are being conducted to find other drugs or supplements that may decrease HD symptoms. Examples include the CoQ10 enzyme, growth factors, glutamate blockers, and antidepressants, such as sertraline (Zoloft).

The care of the patient with HD is managed by the collaborative efforts of the family and health care team and includes:

- Speech-language pathologist (SLP) who helps with communication, swallowing, and drooling
- Dietitian who plans meals based on the SLP's recommendations and the patient's likes and dislikes
- Physical and occupational therapists who determine exercise conditioning and assistive devices
- Nurses or home health care aides who provide supportive care
- Case manager and social worker who coordinate care and help with referrals to community resources (e.g., Huntington's Disease Society of America [www.hdsa.org]) and health care agencies for placement as needed

NURSING CONCEPTS AND CLINICAL JUDGMENT REVIEW

What might you NOTICE if the patient is experiencing PAIN, impaired MOBILITY, or altered COGNITION as a result of an acute or chronic brain disorder?

- Headache
- Acute or chronic confusion
- Sleepiness or lethargy
- Inability to perform ADLs
- Inability to ambulate or alteration in gait
- Reduced nutritional intake resulting in weight loss
- Inability to communicate effectively
- Report of photophobia or phonophobia
- One or more seizures
- Extremity tremors, rigidity, or jerky movements

What should you INTERPRET and how should you RESPOND to a patient experiencing PAIN, impaired MOBILITY, and altered COGNITION as a result of an acute CNS INFECTION or chronic brain disorder?

Perform and interpret physical assessment, including:
- Assessing neurologic status, especially level of consciousness (LOC)
- Taking vital signs (high fever may indicate infection)
- Performing a comprehensive pain assessment

- Assessing ability to communicate
- Assessing nutritional status

Respond by:
- Notifying health care provider or Rapid Response Team if seizure or sudden change in LOC or onset of an acute confusional state
- Ensuring an adequate airway
- Protecting patient from injury
- Managing pain
- Giving oxygen (during a seizure and for status epilepticus)
- Reorienting patient
- Assisting with ADLs if needed
- Collaborating with health care team members (e.g., PT, OT, SLP, dietitian)

On what should you REFLECT?
- Think about how you responded.
- Continue to monitor for improving mental status and changes in LOC.
- Assess triggers or other causes for acute event.
- Develop teaching plan for patient and family for self-management.
- Think about what resources the patient and family may need.

GET READY FOR THE NCLEX® EXAMINATION!

KEY POINTS

Review these Key Points for each NCLEX Examination Client Needs Category.

Safe and Effective Care Environment
- Provide a written summary of events during hospitalization and an oral report to the receiving caregiver during all transitions in care (e.g., from hospital to rehabilitation or home).
- Implement best practices for fall prevention and prevent injury from impaired cognition and immobility with frequent observation and interventions described in Table 42-6 and Charts 42-9, -12, -14, and -15. **Safety** `QSEN`
- Ensure that drugs have been reviewed with the patient and caregivers with each administration and that discharge drugs have been reconciled with a list of problems or indications. Provide written information about all home-going drugs. **Informatics** `QSEN`

- Collaborate with the health care team in discharge planning and health teaching for patients who have chronic seizures or neurodegenerative diseases such as PD, dementia, and HD. **Teamwork and Collaboration** `QSEN`
- Ensure a safe environment for a patient with seizure precautions by ensuring that suction and oxygen are available and that frequent observation occurs to detect seizure activity early. **Safety** `QSEN`
- Implement interventions for seizures as listed in Chart 42-6. Patients with status epilepticus have a life-threatening complication. Lorazepam and diazepam are the major drugs used for this emergency. **Evidence-Based Practice** `QSEN`
- For the patient with a chronic brain disorder, provide an environment that maximizes their MOBILITY, including consultation with physical and occupational therapy. **Teamwork and Collaboration** `QSEN`

Health Promotion and Maintenance

- Teach patients with migraine headaches about triggers that could cause an attack, such as tyramine in wine, pickled products, and aged cheeses; nitrates and nitrites in processed and grilled meats; and other dietary or environmental triggers. **Patient-Centered Care** `QSEN`
- Teach patients with cluster headaches about precipitating factors, such as anger episodes, excitement, and excessive physical activity.
- In addition to prescribed drug therapy, encourage patients with headaches to use complementary and alternative therapies to help relieve PAIN, such as ice, darkened room, and relaxation techniques. **Patient-Centered Care** `QSEN`
- Teach the patient with epilepsy to maintain seizure-free health or reduced seizure activity through using prescribed antiepileptic drugs (AEDs) and follow-up medical care. Additional instructions for the patient and family are listed in Chart 42-5.
- Document vaccination status and provide vaccination to prevent some types of infectious meningitis, particularly meningococcal vaccination to people who are in areas of high population density, such as university residences, military barracks, and crowded living areas. Vaccination is a core measure of health care effectiveness. **Evidence-Based Practice** `QSEN`

Psychosocial Integrity

- Remind caregivers of patients with chronic neurologic diseases, such as dementia, to find ways to cope with their own stress to remain physically and psychologically healthy, as suggested in Chart 42-16. **Patient-Centered Care** `QSEN`
- Teach caregivers of patients with dementia to use validation therapy rather than reality orientation. Acknowledge the patient's feelings and concerns.
- Involve families who care for patients with neurodegenerative diseases like Parkinson disease, dementia, or Huntington disease to develop a culturally appropriate continuing plan of care that reflects patient values and preferences.
- Adapt communication techniques for the patient with dementia as outlined in Chart 42-14. **Patient-Centered Care** `QSEN`
- Assist patients and family members to identify community resources that can assist with education and caregiver support, including consultation with social services or a case manager.

Physiological Integrity

- Assess patients with classic migraine headaches as listed in Chart 42-2.
- Compare migraine to cluster headache, recalling that the PAIN of cluster headaches is usually accompanied by ipsilateral (same side) eye tearing, rhinorrhea, congestion, ptosis, facial sweating, eyelid edema, and/or miosis. Migraine pain is characterized by throbbing pain that is unilateral and can be accompanied by nausea, light sensitivity, and worsening symptoms with movement.
- Recognize that generalized seizures, such as the tonic-clonic seizure, involve both cerebral hemispheres. Partial seizures, also called *focal* or *local seizures,* usually involve only one hemisphere.
- During a seizure, document the patient's body movements and other assessments as described in Chart 42-7. **Informatics** `QSEN`
- Monitor for side and adverse effects of antiepileptic drugs (AEDs) as listed in Chart 42-4. **Safety** `QSEN`
- For patients who have had one or more seizures, place on "seizure precautions," which includes having oxygen delivery and suctioning equipment available and starting or maintaining IV access. **Safety** `QSEN`
- Assess for clinical manifestations of meningitis as listed in Chart 42-8. For patients with meningitis and encephalitis, carefully monitor neurologic status, including vital signs and neurologic and vascular checks. Observe for signs and symptoms of increased intracranial pressure (ICP), and communicate changes in level of consciousness immediately to the health care provider. **Safety** `QSEN`
- Assess for key features of Parkinson disease as described in Chart 42-11. Monitor for drug toxicity when patients are taking medications for Parkinson disease, especially levodopa combinations such as Sinemet. Delirium and decreased drug effectiveness are the most common indicators of toxicity. **Safety** `QSEN`
- Communicate worsening neurologic assessment findings immediately following electrode placement for deep brain stimulation and injection of stem cells when used to control symptoms of Parkinson disease.
- Document cognitive and functional abilities of the patient with dementia, recognizing that it is a progressive condition (e.g., Alzheimer stages are listed in Chart 42-13).
- For patients with dementia, recall that a few drugs improve function and COGNITION (cholinesterase inhibitors, such as donepezil [Aricept]) or slow the disease process (Memantine) but they do not cure the disease.
- Remember that Huntington disease is a chronic, hereditary illness that is transmitted as an autosomal dominant trait at the time of conception. Refer patients with the disease for genetic counseling. **Patient-Centered Care** `QSEN`
- Foster a collaborative communication, establish outcomes for care with health care team members, and review them regularly. Document communication to reduce complications and promote quality of life in patients. **Informatics** `QSEN`

43 | CHAPTER

Care of Patients with Problems of the Central Nervous System: The Spinal Cord

Rachel L. Gallagher

 http://evolve.elsevier.com/Iggy/

PRIORITY CONCEPTS

- MOBILITY
- SENSORY PERCEPTION
- PAIN
- INFLAMMATION

- TISSUE INTEGRITY
- PALLIATION
- SEXUALITY

LEARNING OUTCOMES

Safe and Effective Care Environment

1. Use best practices to teach strategies that reduce back and neck injury and PAIN.
2. Prioritize the nursing care of the patient with an acute spinal cord injury (SCI).
3. Collaborate with other health care team members to manage care for patients with spinal cord problems.
4. Establish patient values and preferences, including integration of advance directives, PALLIATION, and managing distressing symptoms for patients with progressively debilitating spinal cord conditions.

Health Promotion and Maintenance

5. Identify with the patient behaviors that promote optimal weight.
6. Communicate with health care team members to establish outcomes for care and strategies to promote independence in ADLs.
7. Identify community resources for patients with spinal cord health problems and their families.

Psychosocial Integrity

8. Describe the impact of spinal cord conditions on the patient's SEXUALITY.
9. Use therapeutic communication to assess the need for emotional, mental, and social support of patients with spinal cord health problems and their families.

Physiological Integrity

10. Perform a comprehensive assessment of the patient with a spinal cord injury.
11. Establish priorities in care for the patient with spinal cord–related problems of MOBILITY, SENSORY PERCEPTION, elimination, and skin TISSUE INTEGRITY.
12. Apply knowledge of pathophysiology when caring for a patient having autonomic dysreflexia.
13. Explain the pathophysiology of multiple sclerosis (MS) and amyotrophic lateral sclerosis (ALS).
14. Explain the role of drug therapy in managing patients with spinal cord problems.
15. Develop an evidence-based postoperative plan of care for patients having spinal cord surgery, including monitoring for complications.

The spinal cord relays messages to and from the brain. Besides injuries, the spinal cord can develop tumors, infections such as meningitis and poliomyelitis, inflammatory and autoimmune diseases, and degenerative diseases such as amyotrophic lateral sclerosis (ALS) and spinal muscular atrophy. The spinal cord itself may be damaged, or the spinal nerves leading from the cord to the extremities may be affected, often by chronic INFLAMMATION. In some cases, both the spinal cord and the nerves are involved. Symptoms vary but often include problems with MOBILITY, SENSORY PERCEPTION, and PAIN. As

a result, the patients' ability to perform ADLs, their skin TISSUE INTEGRITY, elimination patterns, and SEXUALITY are often affected. Health care team members with expertise in symptom management can provide significant contributions to this population's quality of life by providing PALLIATION of symptoms that are chronic and often progressive. Health care team members also can promote a safe environment, preventing complications from impaired mobility and sensory perception (Forrest et al., 2012). (See the Quality Improvement box.)

QUALITY IMPROVEMENT (QSEN)

Reducing Falls and Harm from Falls

Forrest, G., Huss, S., Patel, V., Jeffries, J., Myers, D., Barber, C., et al. (2012). Falls on an inpatient rehabilitation unit: Risk assessment and prevention. *Rehabilitation Nursing, 37*(2), 56-61.

This quality improvement project had a twofold purpose. The first was to determine if a common measure of function used in a rehabilitation setting identified patients at increased risk for a fall. The second purpose was to determine if a comprehensive plan for fall reduction that used the functional assessment results to guide interventions was effective at reducing falls.

The strength of this project is the interdisciplinary team that designed the process of both assessment and care. This report also details the application of a quality improvement process to refine interventions as data became available about the usefulness of a functional assessment in identifying high-risk patients. Functional impairment was found to be associated with more falls. It is important to note that functional impairment was most often associated with Guillain-Barré, spinal cord injury, myopathy, and peripheral neuropathy. Neurologic diagnoses were then used to revise the screening tool that identified patients at increased risk for falls and develop novel interventions. Over time, falls were reduced by 50%—a significant improvement in patient safety.

Commentary: Implications for Practice and Research

This report illustrates several steps of a Plan-Do-Study-Act cycle in developing and sustaining a quality improvement project. First, the authors used information in the literature about fall reduction and then adapted that information to develop a protocol that met their patient population needs and hospital resources. Adding functional assessment provided essential information about high-risk patients in this setting. The report also illustrates the need for ongoing feedback to sustain adherence to quality improvement (protocol) interventions that were successful in reducing falls.

BACK PAIN

Back pain affects as many of 80% of adults at some time in their life. It can be recurrent, and subsequent episodes tend to increase in severity. The prevalence of both acute and chronic back pain varies with age, lifestyle factors including obesity and osteoporosis, and certain types of physical activity such as heavy physical work and lifting. Low back pain is the leading cause of work disability (Costa-Black et al., 2010).

The lumbosacral (lower back) and cervical (neck) vertebrae are most commonly affected because these are the areas where the vertebral column is the most flexible. *Acute* back PAIN is usually self-limiting. If the pain continues for 3 months or if repeated episodes of pain occur, the patient has *chronic* back pain.

LOW BACK PAIN (LUMBOSACRAL BACK PAIN)

❖ *PATHOPHYSIOLOGY*

Low back pain (LBP) occurs along the lumbosacral area of the vertebral column. Acute pain is caused by muscle strain or spasm, ligament sprain, disk (also spelled "disc") degeneration (osteoarthritis), or herniation of the center of the disk, the nucleus pulposus, past the lateral vertebral border. A herniated nucleus pulposus (HNP) in the lumbosacral area can press on the adjacent spinal nerve (usually the sciatic nerve), causing severe burning or stabbing pain down into the leg or foot (Fig. 43-1). Herniated disks occur most often between the fourth and fifth lumbar vertebrae (L4-5) but may occur at other levels. The specific area of symptoms depends on the level of herniation.

In addition to PAIN, there may be both muscle spasm and numbness and tingling (paresthesia) in the affected leg because spinal nerves have both motor and sensory fibers. The HNP may press on the spinal cord itself, causing leg weakness. Bowel and bladder incontinence or retention may occur with motor nerve involvement and because sacral spinal nerves have parasympathetic nerve fibers that help control bowel and bladder function.

Back pain may also be caused by spondylolysis, a defect in one of the vertebrae usually in the lumbar spine. Spondylolisthesis occurs when one vertebra slips forward on the one below it, often as a result of spondylolysis. This problem causes pressure on the nerve roots, leading to pain in the lower back and into the buttocks. Pain or numbness may also occur in the leg and foot. Spinal stenosis, a narrowing of the spinal canal, nerve root canals, or intervertebral foramina is typically seen in people older than 50 years. This narrowing may be caused by infection, trauma, herniated disk, arthritis, and disk degeneration. Most adults older than 50 years have some degree of degenerative disk disease, although they may not be symptomatic.

Low back pain is most prevalent during the third to sixth decades of life but can occur at any time. Acute back PAIN usually results from injury or trauma such as during a fall, vehicular crash, or lifting a heavy object. The mechanisms of injury include repetitive flexion and/or extension and

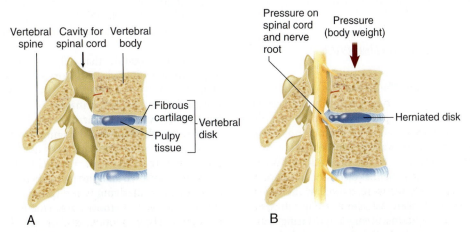

FIG. 43-1 Sagittal section of vertebrae showing (**A**) a normal disk and (**B**) a herniated disk.

CHART 43-1   Nursing Focus on the Older Adult
Factors Contributing to Low Back Pain

- Changes in support structures
  - Spinal stenosis
  - Hypertrophy of the intraspinal ligaments
  - Osteoarthritis
  - Osteoporosis
- Changes in vertebral support and malalignment
  - Scoliosis
  - Lordosis
- Vascular changes
  - Diminished blood supply to the spinal cord or cauda equina caused by arteriosclerosis
  - Blood dyscrasias
- Intervertebral disk degeneration

CHART 43-2   Patient and Family Education: Preparing for Self-Management
Prevention of Low Back Pain and Injury

- Use safe manual handling practices, with specific attention to bending, lifting, and sitting.
- Assess the need for assistance with your household chores or other activities.
- Participate in a regular exercise program, especially one that promotes back strengthening, such as swimming and walking.
- Do not wear high-heeled shoes.
- Use good posture when sitting, standing, and walking.
- Avoid prolonged sitting or standing. Use a footstool and ergonomic chairs and tables to lessen back strain. Be sure that equipment in the workplace is ergonomically designed to prevent injury.
- Keep weight within 10% of ideal body weight.
- Ensure adequate calcium intake. Consider vitamin D supplementation if serum levels are low.
- Stop smoking. If you are not able to stop, cut down on the number of cigarettes or decrease the use of other forms of tobacco.

hyperflexion or hyperextension with or without rotation. Obesity places increased stress on the vertebral column and back muscles, contributing to risk for injury. Smoking has been linked to disk degeneration, possibly caused by constriction of blood vessels that supply the spine. Congenital spinal conditions like scoliosis can also lead to LBP. Older adults are at high risk for both acute and chronic LBP. Vertebral fracture from osteoporosis contributes to LBP. Petite, Euro-American women are at high risk for both bone loss and subsequent vertebral fractures. Chart 43-1 provides a list of specific factors that can cause low back pain in the older adult. Vertebral compression fractures are discussed in detail in Chapter 51.

Health Promotion and Maintenance

Many of the problems related to acute back PAIN can be prevented by recognizing the factors that contribute to tissue injury and taking appropriate preventive measures. For example, good posture and exercise can significantly decrease the incidence of low back pain. The U.S. Occupational Safety and Health Administration (OSHA) mandated that all industries develop and implement a plan to decrease musculoskeletal injuries among their workers. One way to meet this requirement is to develop an ergonomic plan for the workplace. Ergonomics is an applied science in which the workplace is designed to increase worker comfort (thus reducing injury) while increasing efficiency and productivity. An example is a ceiling lift designed to help nurses assist patients to get out of bed. A variety of equipment can be used to decrease injury related to moving patients. Professional guidelines and legislative rules promote safe patient handling for health care workers (www.nursingworld.org/rnnoharm). Chart 43-2 summarizes various ways to help prevent LBP related to lifting objects and handling patients (ANA, 2013; Nelson et al., 2008).

❖ PATIENT-CENTERED COLLABORATIVE CARE

◆ Assessment

Physical Assessment/Clinical Manifestations. The patient's primary concern is continuous pain. Some patients have so much pain that they walk in a stiff, flexed posture or they may be unable to bend at all. They may walk with a limp, indicating possible sciatic nerve impairment. Walking on the heels or toes often causes severe pain in the affected leg, the back, or both.

Conduct a complete PAIN assessment as discussed in Chapter 3. Record the patient's current pain score, as well as the worst and best score since the PAIN began. Ask about precipitating or relieving factors such as symptoms at night or during rest. Determine if a recent injury to the back has occurred. It is not unusual for the patient to say "I just turned around and felt my back go out."

Inspect the patient's back for vertebral alignment and tenderness. Examine the surrounding anatomy and lower extremities for secondary injury (Patton & Thibodeau, 2014). Patients report stabbing, continuous PAIN in the muscle closest to the affected disk. They often describe a sharp, burning posterior thigh or calf pain that may radiate to the ankle or toes along the path of one or more spinal nerves. Pain usually does not extend the entire length of the limb. Patients may also report the same type of pain in the middle of one buttock. The pain is often aggravated by sneezing, coughing, or straining. Driving a vehicle is particularly painful.

Ask whether paresthesia (tingling sensation) or numbness is present in the involved leg. Both extremities may be checked for SENSORY PERCEPTION by using a cotton ball and a paper clip for comparison of light and deep touch. The patient may feel sensory perception in both legs but may experience a stronger sensation on the unaffected side. Ask about urinary and fecal continence and difficulty in urination or constipation.

If the sciatic nerve is compressed, severe pain occurs when the patient's leg is held straight and lifted upward. Foot, ankle, and leg weakness may accompany lower back pain. To complete the neurologic assessment, evaluate the patient's muscle tone and strength. Muscles in the extremity or lower back can atrophy as a result of severe chronic back pain. The patient has difficulty with movement, and certain movements create more pain than others.

Other information that may indicate more serious neurologic problems includes a history of fever and chills, recurrent skin or urinary tract infections, progressive motor and sensory loss, and difficulty with urination or having a bowel movement (due to involvement of sacral nerves).

Imaging Assessment. Imaging studies for patients who report mild nonspecific back PAIN may not be done depending on the nature of the pain. Patients with severe or progressive motor or SENSORY PERCEPTION deficits or who are thought to have other underlying conditions (e.g., cancer, infection) require complete diagnostic assessment. X-rays of the spine can exclude fracture, spondylosis, or neoplasm as the causative agent. Flexion-extension views can be very useful to show instability of the spine. The imaging studies of choice are magnetic resonance imaging (MRI) or computerized tomography (CT) scanning. The MRI is usually the first test of choice because it is noninvasive. A CT myelogram is done when a better delineation of the bony anatomy and the specific nerve root involvement is needed.

Electro-diagnostic testing, such as electromyography (EMG) and nerve-conduction studies, may help distinguish motor neuron diseases from peripheral neuropathies and radiculopathies (spinal nerve root involvement). These tests are especially useful in chronic diseases of the spinal cord or associated nerves. Chapter 41 describes these tests in more detail.

◆ **Interventions**

Management of patients with back PAIN varies with the severity and chronicity of the problem. Most patients with acute LBP experience a spontaneous resolution of pain and other symptoms over the short term (i.e., less than 3-6 months). Other patients need a brief treatment regimen of at-home exercise or physical therapy and drugs to manage pain. In general, return to work, if safe, is beneficial for recovery and well-being. When motor function is abruptly lost, surgery may be needed. Some patients have continuous or intermittent chronic pain that must be managed for an extended period. Referral to an interdisciplinary team that specializes in pain or back pain can provide expert long-term management.

Nonsurgical Management. Nonsurgical conservative management of LBP includes positioning, drug therapy, physical therapy, weight control, and smoking cessation.

Acute Low Back Pain. The Williams position is typically more comfortable and therapeutic for the patient with LBP from a bulging or herniated disk. In this *position,* the patient lies in the semi-Fowler's position with a pillow under the knees to keep them flexed or sits in a recliner chair. This position relaxes the muscles of the lower back and relieves pressure on the spinal nerve root. Most patients also find that they need to change position frequently. Prolonged standing, sitting, or lying down increases back PAIN. If the patient must stand for a long time for work or other reason, shoe insoles or special floor pads may help decrease pain.

The health care provider prescribes acetaminophen or NSAIDs; muscle relaxants may also be used for acute LBP. Opioid analgesics are no more effective than non-opioid analgesics and should be avoided if at all possible. If they must be used, the course of therapy should be short to prevent adverse drug events. Short-term oral steroids in tapering doses may be prescribed for some patients to rapidly reduce INFLAMMATION.

Some patients may need an epidural injection for pain relief. A corticosteroid and an anesthetic are injected to reduce INFLAMMATION in the affected area. During a facet joint injection, fluoroscopy is used to insert a needle into the epidural space surrounding the facet and a corticosteroid is injected to coat the nerve roots and outside lining of the joints.

Chronic Low Back Pain. Patients having chronic low back PAIN (LBP) are treated with NSAIDs, opioids, and/or antidepressants (as adjunctive therapy). In a recent systematic review of drug treatment, the authors reported NSAIDs and opioids provided somewhat higher relief in pain in the short term as compared with placebo. However, these drugs are associated with significant adverse drug effects. Further, there were no differences in outcomes between antidepressants and placebo in patients with nonspecific chronic LBP (Kuijpers et al., 2011).

CHART 43-3   Patient and Family Education: Preparing for Self-Management

Typical Exercises for Chronic or Postoperative Low Back Pain

Extension Exercises
- **Stomach lying:** Lie face down with a pillow under your chest; lift legs straight up (alternate legs) (may not be tolerated).
- **Upper trunk extension:** Lie face down with your arms at your sides, and lift your head and neck.
- **Prone push-ups:** Lie face down on a mat and, keeping your body stiff, push up to extend your arms.

Flexion Exercises
- **Pelvic tilt:** Lying on your back with your knees bent, tighten your abdominal muscles to push your lower back against the mat.
- **Semi–sit-ups:** Lying on your back with your knees bent, raise your upper body at a 45-degree angle and hold this position for 5 to 10 seconds.
- **Knee to chest:** Lying on your back with your knees bent, tighten your abdominal muscles to push your lower back against the mat. Now bring one or both knees to your chest and hold this position for 5 to 10 seconds.

! NURSING SAFETY PRIORITY (QSEN)

Drug Alert

Teach older adults and their families to monitor for the adverse drug effects of opioids, including constipation, drowsiness, and acute confusion. Opioids can put older adults at increased risk for falls and injury. Instruct them to notify their health care provider to report these changes, and suggest a lower dose or change to a non-opioid pain drug.

Some patients with back PAIN may have temporary relief from *heat or cold* application. Heat increases blood flow to the affected area and promotes the healing of injured nerves. Moist heat from heat packs or hot towels applied for 20 to 30 minutes at least 4 times per day is often recommended. Hot showers or baths may also be beneficial, although data are insufficient to support the use of *superficial* heat/cold applications for low back pain (van Middelkoop et al., 2011).

The physical therapist (PT) may provide *deep* heat therapy, such as ultrasound treatments and diathermy. Some patients may receive phonophoresis, which is the application of a topical drug (e.g., Xylocaine, hydrocortisone) followed by continuous ultrasound for 10 minutes. Iontophoresis is a similar procedure in which a small electrical current and dexamethasone are typically used. Both procedures push the medication into the subcutaneous tissue and provide longer-lasting pain relief.

The PT also works with the patient to develop an individualized exercise program. The type of exercises prescribed depends on the location and nature of the injury and the type of PAIN. The patient does not begin exercises until acute pain is reduced by other means. Several specific exercises for strengthening muscles to manage LBP are listed in Chart 43-3. A systematic review of 37 studies showed that there is low-quality evidence for the effectiveness of exercise for low back pain (van Middelkoop et al., 2010). Water therapy combined with exercise is helpful for some patients with chronic pain. The water also provides muscle resistance during exercise to prevent atrophy.

Weight reduction may help reduce chronic lower back PAIN by decreasing the strain on the vertebrae caused by excess weight. If the patient's weight exceeds the ideal by more than 10%, caloric restriction is recommended. Health care providers must be sensitive when reinforcing the need for patients to lose weight to prevent or to lessen chronic back pain. Behavioral approaches to weight loss and positive reinforcement are important for the nutrition plan.

Complementary and Alternative Therapies. The patient may find that nontraditional and complementary therapies provide short-term pain relief. Patients with low back muscle injuries or mild nerve involvement may find relief of pain from chiropractic therapies, although there is insufficient evidence to support consistent use of this intervention (Parkinson et al., 2013). The purpose of chiropractic or spinal manipulative therapy (SMT) is to promote alignment and prevent or treat pressure on nerve roots (Bergman & Peterson, 2011).

Imagery, acupuncture, music therapy, massage, and herbal medicines are examples of other possible pain-relief therapies for acute and chronic back pain. A systematic review of research on the effectiveness of complementary and alternative medicine (CAM) for chronic back pain supported the use of acupressure and herbal therapies for short-term pain relief (Rubinstein et al., 2010).

As many as 20% of patients with back pain may use or be prescribed weighted traction, an intervention that applies a weighted pulley system and a girdle or other device to create a pulling force along the vertebrae. However, a recent review of the evidence for this therapy suggests that weighted traction provides little or no effect on pain intensity, function, or return to work (Wegner et al., 2013).

Surgical Management

Surgery is usually performed if conservative measures fail to relieve back PAIN or if neurologic deficits continue to progress. An orthopedic surgeon and/or neurosurgeon perform these surgeries. Two major types of surgery are used depending on the severity and exact location of pain: minimally invasive surgery (MIS) and conventional open surgical procedures. MIS is not done if the disk is pressing into the spinal cord (central cord involvement).

Preoperative Care. Preoperative care for the patient preparing for lumbar surgery is similar to that for any patient undergoing surgery (see Chapter 14). Teach the patient about postoperative expectations, including:

- Techniques to get into and out of bed
- Turning and moving in bed
- Reporting immediately new SENSORY PERCEPTION, such as numbness and tingling, or new motor impairment that may occur in the affected leg or in both legs
- Home care activities and restrictions

Many patients are discharged to home within 23 to 48 hours after surgery. Therefore, before surgery, teach family members or other caregiver how to assist the patient and what restrictions the patient must follow at home.

A bone graft is done if the patient has a *spinal fusion*. The surgeon explains from where the bone for grafting will be obtained. The patient's own bone is used whenever possible, but additional bone from a bone bank may be needed. The surgeon provides verbal and written information about the type and the source of bone for surgery. Be sure that the patient signs an informed consent form before surgery. While the bone graft

heals, the patient may wear a back orthotic device for 4 to 6 weeks after surgery, but this is not common practice today. Provide information about the importance of wearing the brace as instructed during the healing process, how to take it off and put it on while maintaining spinal alignment, and how to clean it.

Operative Procedures. *Minimally invasive surgeries (MISs)* have the advantage of being associated with minimal muscle injury, decreased blood loss, and decreased postoperative pain. The primary advantage of these surgical procedures is a shortened hospital stay and the possibility of an ambulatory care (same-day) procedure. Spinal cord and nerve complications are also less likely. Several specific procedures are commonly performed.

A local anesthetic is given for the *microscopic (or surgical) endoscopic diskectomy (MED)* or *percutaneous endoscopic diskectomy (PED)*. The surgeon uses x-ray fluoroscopy to insert an endoscope (arthroscope) next to the affected disk. A special cutting tool or laser probe is threaded through the cannula for removal or destruction of the *disk pieces* that are compressing the nerve root. A newer procedure combines the PED with *laser thermodiskectomy* to also shrink the herniated disk before removal. Inpatient hospitalization is not necessary for this procedure.

A *microdiskectomy* involves microscopic surgery directly through a 1-inch incision. This procedure allows easier identification of anatomic structures, improved precision in removing small fragments, and decreased tissue trauma and pain.

Laser-assisted laparoscopic lumbar diskectomy combines a laser with modified standard disk instruments inserted through the laparoscope using an umbilical ("belly button") incision. The procedure may be used to treat herniated disks that are bulging but do not involve the vertebral canal. The primary risks of this surgery are infection and nerve root injury. The patient is typically discharged in 23 hours but may go home sooner.

The most common *conventional open procedures* are diskectomy, laminectomy, and spinal fusion. These procedures involve a surgical incision to expose anatomic landmarks for extensive muscle and soft-tissue dissection. In patients with fragile vertebrae following major spine surgery, vertebroplasty (insertion of acrylic bone cement) is sometimes performed at the levels above and below surgery. This procedure strengthens adjacent vertebral bodies that will be more stressed. Major complications from spine surgery include nerve injuries, diskitis (disk INFLAMMATION), and dural tears (tears in the dura covering the spinal cord).

As the name implies, a *diskectomy* is removal of a herniated disk. A *laminectomy* involves removal of part of the laminae and facet joints to obtain access to the disk space. When repeated laminectomies are performed or the spine is unstable, the surgeon may perform a spinal fusion (arthrodesis) to stabilize the affected area. Chips of bone are removed, typically from the iliac crest, or obtained from donor bone and are grafted between the vertebrae for support and to strengthen the back. Metal implants (usually titanium pins, screws, plates, or rods) may be required to ensure the fusion of the spine. Before closing, the surgeon may give an intrathecal (spinal) or epidural dose of long-acting morphine (Duramorph) to decrease postoperative pain.

Interbody cage fusion is a newer spinal implant. A cagelike device is implanted into the space where the disk was removed.

Bone graft tissue is packed around the device. As with instrumentation and fusion, the bone graft grows into and around the cage and creates a stable spine at that level.

An adjunct for patients for whom fusion may be difficult is the placement of an implantable **direct current stimulation (DCS)** device to promote bone fusion. External bone stimulators may also be effective for healing bone fusions.

Postoperative Care. Postoperative care depends on the type of surgery that was performed. In the postanesthesia care unit (PACU), vital signs and level of consciousness are monitored frequently, the same as for any surgery. Best practices for PACU nursing care are discussed in Chapter 16.

Minimally Invasive Surgery. Patients go home the same day or the day after surgery with a Band-Aid or Steri-Strips over their small incision. Those having a microdiskectomy may also have a clear or gauze dressing over the bandage. Most patients notice less PAIN immediately after surgery, but mild oral analgesics are needed while nerve tissue heals over the next few weeks. In collaboration with the health care provider and physical therapist, teach the patient to follow the prescribed exercise program, which begins immediately after discharge. Patients should start walking routinely every day. Complications of MIS are rare.

Conventional Open Surgery. Early postoperative nursing care focuses on preventing and assessing complications that might occur in the first 24 to 48 hours (Chart 43-4). As for any patient undergoing surgery, take vital signs at least every 4 hours during the first 24 hours to assess for fever and for hypotension, which could indicate bleeding or severe pain. Perform a neurologic assessment every 4 hours. Of particular importance are movement, strength, and SENSORY PERCEPTION in the lower extremities.

Carefully check the patient's ability to void. PAIN and a flat position in bed make voiding difficult, especially for men. An inability to void may indicate damage to the sacral spinal nerves, which control the detrusor muscle in the bladder. Opioid analgesics have also been associated with difficulty voiding. The patient with a diskectomy or laminectomy typically gets out of bed with assistance on the evening of surgery, which may help with voiding.

PAIN control may be achieved with patient-controlled analgesia (PCA) with morphine. The route is changed to oral administration after the patient is able to take fluids or the next morning.

> ### ⚠ NURSING SAFETY PRIORITY (QSEN)
> **Critical Rescue**
>
> For the patient after back surgery, inspect the surgical dressing for blood or any other type of drainage. Clear drainage may mean cerebrospinal fluid (CSF) leakage. The loss of a large amount of CSF may cause the patient to report having a sudden headache. Report signs of any drainage on the dressing to the surgeon immediately. Bulging at the incision site may be due to a CSF leak or a hematoma, both of which should also be reported to the surgeon.

Empty the surgical drain, usually a Jackson-Pratt or Hemovac, and record the amount of drainage every 8 hours. The surgeon usually removes the drain in 24 to 36 hours.

Correct turning of the patient in bed is especially important. Teach the patient to log roll every 2 hours from side to back and vice versa. In **log rolling,** the patient turns as a unit while his or her back is kept as straight as possible. A turning sheet may be

CHART 43-4 Best Practice for Patient Safety & Quality Care (QSEN)

Assessing and Managing the Patient with Major Complications of Lumbar Spinal Surgery

COMPLICATION	ASSESSMENT/INTERVENTIONS
Cerebrospinal fluid (CSF) leakage	Observe for clear fluid on or around the dressing. If leakage occurs, place patient flat. Report CSF leakage immediately to the surgeon. (The patient is usually kept on flat bedrest for several days while the dural tear heals.)
Fluid volume deficit	Monitor intake and output; monitor drain output, which should not be more than 250 mL in 8 hours during the first 24 hours. Monitor vital signs carefully for hypotension and tachycardia.
Acute urinary retention	Assist the patient to the bathroom or a bedside commode as soon as possible postoperatively. Assist male patients to stand at the bedside as soon as possible postoperatively.
Paralytic ileus	Monitor for flatus or stool. Assess for abdominal distention, nausea, and vomiting.
Fat embolism syndrome (FES) (more common in people with spinal fusion)	Observe for and report chest pain, dyspnea, anxiety, and mental status changes (particularly common in older adults). Note petechiae around the neck, upper chest, buccal membrane, and conjunctiva. Monitor arterial blood gas values for decreased PaO_2.
Persistent or progressive lumbar radiculopathy (nerve root pain)	Report pain not responsive to opioids. Document the location and nature of pain. Administer analgesics as prescribed.
Infection (e.g., wound, diskitis, hematoma)	Monitor the patient's temperature carefully (a slight elevation is normal). Increased temperature elevation or a spike after the second postoperative day is possibly indicative of infection. Report increased pain or swelling at the wound site or in the legs. Give antibiotics as prescribed if infection is confirmed. Use clean technique for dressing changes.

used for obese patients. Either turning method may require additional assistance, depending on how much the patient can assist and on his or her weight. Instruct the patient to keep his or her back straight when getting out of bed. He or she should sit in a straight-back chair with the feet resting comfortably on the floor. As with all surgical patients, prevent atelectasis and iatrogenic pneumonia with deep breathing. Follow best practices to avoid venous thromboembolism (VTE) postoperatively with early MOBILITY and intermittent sequential compression or pneumatic devices per The Joint Commission's Core Measures.

When a spinal fusion is performed in addition to a laminectomy, more care is taken with MOBILITY and positioning. The nurse or unlicensed assistive personnel (UAP) assist with log rolling the patient every 2 hours. For the conventional fusion, inspect both the iliac and spinal incision dressings for drainage and make sure they are intact. Remind the patient to avoid prolonged sitting or standing.

Community-Based Care

The patient with back PAIN who does not undergo surgery is typically managed at home. If back surgery is performed, the patient is usually discharged to home with support from family or significant others. For older adults without a community support system, a short-term stay in a nursing home or transitional care unit may be needed. Collaborate with the case manager or discharge planner, patient, and family to determine the most appropriate placement.

Home Care Management. After *conventional open back surgery*, the patient may have activity restrictions such as limited daily stair climbing. Driving, lifting objects heavier than 5 pounds, pushing, and pulling (e.g., dog walking) are also restricted during home recovery for many weeks. However, daily walking is encouraged. The duration of home-based recovery depends on the nature of the job and the extent and type of surgery. Most patients return to work after 6 weeks; some patients may not return for 3 to 6 months if their jobs are physically strenuous.

Patients having any of the *MIS procedures* may resume normal activities within a few days up to 3 weeks after surgery, depending on the specific procedure that was done and the condition of the patient. He or she may take a shower on the third or fourth day after surgery. Teach the patient to remove the outer clear or gauze dressing, if any is in place, but leave the Steri-Strips in place for removal by the surgeon or until they fall off. Instruct the patient to contact the surgeon immediately if clear drainage seeps from the incision. Clear drainage usually indicates a meningeal tear and cerebrospinal fluid is leaking.

Self-Management Education. The patient with an acute episode of back PAIN typically returns to his or her usual activities but may fear a recurrence. Remind the patient that he or she may never have another episode if caution is used. However, continuous or repeated pain can be frustrating and tiring. Encourage the patient and family members to plan short-term goals and take steps toward recovering each day.

After surgery, in collaboration with the physical therapist, instruct the patient to:
- Continue with a weight-reduction diet, if needed.
- Stop smoking, if applicable.
- Perform strengthening exercises as instructed.

The physical therapist reviews and demonstrates the principles of body mechanics and muscle-strengthening exercises. The patient is then asked to demonstrate these principles (Chart 43-5). Formal physical therapy usually begins about 2 weeks after surgery. Teach the patient the importance of keeping all appointments and following the prescribed exercise plan.

The health care provider may want the patient to continue taking anti-inflammatory drugs or, if muscle spasm is present, muscle relaxants. Remind the patient and family about the possible side effects of drugs and what to do if they occur.

In a few patients, back surgery is not successful. This situation, referred to as failed back surgery syndrome (FBSS), is a complex combination of organic, psychological, and socioeconomic factors. Repeated surgical procedures often discourage these patients, who must continue PAIN management after multiple operations. Nerve blocks, implantable spinal cord stimulators (neurostimulators), and other chronic pain management modalities may be needed on a long-term basis.

> **CHART 43-5** **Best Practice for Patient Safety & Quality Care** (QSEN)
>
> ## Prevention of Musculoskeltal Injuries
>
> **Use Best Practices to Prevent Back Injury when Moving Objects**
> - Avoid lifting objects of more than 10 pounds without assistance or aid until the surgeon approves.
> - Push objects rather than pull them.
> - Do not twist your back during movement.
> - Use handles or grips to prevent unintended shifting of the object during movement.
> - Avoid prolonged sitting or standing. Use a footstool to lessen back strain.
> - Sit in chairs with good support.
> - Avoid shoulder stooping; maintain proper posture.
> - Do not walk or stand in high-heeled shoes for prolonged periods (for women).
>
> **Use Best Practices to Prevent Back Injury when Moving a Person**
> - Establish an interdisciplinary team responsible for reviewing and implementing OSHA guidelines for the prevention of musculoskeletal disorders. Originally developed for nursing homes, these guidelines provide guidance for education and practice and programs for health care workers and other stakeholders involved in patient handling, transfers, and movement.
> - Build and support a culture of safety in health care settings that protects staff as well as patients from injury.
> - Improve communication channels among nurses, physical therapists, and family caregivers to facilitate safe patient handling and movement tasks.
> - Develop policies and procedures for the therapeutic use of patient handling equipment:
>   - Select equipment that first provides safety of patients, staff, and family caregivers.
>   - Train all staff and family caregivers in the proper and safe operation of all ergonomic-appropriate equipment.
>   - Encourage patient participation in the use of assistive equipment like sit and stand lifts that are used as an ambulation aid.
> - Develop competency-based assessments that demonstrate proficiency for use of all patient handling approaches and equipment.
> - Encourage quality improvement projects and research that support safe and effective patient handling and movement while maximizing patient-assisted or patient-independent movement. For example, investigate the cost-effectiveness of ergonomic interventions.

Spinal cord stimulation is an *invasive* technique that provides PAIN control by applying an electrical field over the spinal cord. A trial with a percutaneous epidural stimulator is conducted to determine whether or not permanent placement is appropriate. If the trial is successful, electrodes are surgically placed in the epidural space and connected to an external or implanted programmable generator. The patient is taught to program and adjust the device to maximize comfort. Spinal cord stimulation can be extremely effective in select patients but is reserved for intractable neuropathic pain syndromes that have been unresponsive to other treatments.

Ziconotide (Prialt) is a drug used for severe chronic back pain. It is given by intrathecal (spinal) infusion with a surgically implanted pump. It is the first available drug in a new class called *N-type calcium channel blockers (NCCBs).* NCCBs seem to selectively block calcium channels on those nerves that usually transmit pain signals to the brain. Ziconotide is also used for patients with cancer, acquired immune deficiency syndrome (AIDS), and unremitting pain from other nervous system disorders.

! NURSING SAFETY PRIORITY (QSEN)

Critical Rescue

For patients who have a spinal cord stimulator implanted in the epidural space, assess neurologic status below the level of insertion frequently. Monitor for early changes in SENSORY PERCEPTION, movement, and muscle strength. Ensure that the patient can void without difficulty. *If any changes occur, document and report them immediately to the surgeon!*

! NURSING SAFETY PRIORITY (QSEN)

Drug Alert

Ziconotide can be given with opioid analgesics but should *not* be given to patients with severe mental health/behavioral health problems because it can cause psychosis. *If symptoms such as hallucinations and delusions occur, teach patients to stop the drug immediately and notify their health care provider.*

? NCLEX EXAMINATION CHALLENGE

Physiological Integrity

When providing discharge teaching to a client after a lumbar laminectomy, the nurse teaches the client to engage in which activities?
A. Evening showers with hot water
B. Vigorous stair climbing
C. Return to work within 1-2 weeks
D. Daily walking

Health Care Resources. Assist the patient in identifying support systems (e.g., family, church groups, clubs) after back surgery or FBSS. For example, a spouse may help the patient with exercises or perform the exercises with the patient. Members of a church group may help run errands and do household chores. The patient with back pain may continue physical therapy on an ambulatory basis after discharge. For unresolved PAIN, the patient may be referred to pain specialists or clinics, which are usually found in large metropolitan hospitals. A case manager may be assigned to the patient to help with resource management and utilization.

CERVICAL NECK PAIN

❖ PATHOPHYSIOLOGY

Cervical neck PAIN most often results from a bulging or herniation of the nucleus pulposus (HNP) in an intervertebral disk, illustrated in Fig. 43-1. The disk tends to herniate laterally where the annulus fibrosus is weakest and the posterior longitudinal ligament is thinned. The result is spinal nerve root compression with resulting motor and sensory manifestations, typically in the neck, upper back (over the shoulder), and down the affected arm. The disk between the fifth and sixth cervical vertebrae (C5-6) is affected most often.

If the disk does not herniate, nerve compression may be caused by osteophyte (bony spur) formation from osteoarthritis. The osteophyte presses on the intervertebral foramen, which results in a narrowing of the disk and pressure on the nerve root. As with sciatic nerve compression, the patient with cervical nerve compression may have either continuous or intermittent chronic pain. When the disk herniates centrally, pressure on the spinal cord occurs.

Cervical PAIN—acute or chronic—may also occur from muscle strain, ligament sprain resulting from aging, poor posture, lifting, tumor, rheumatoid arthritis, osteoarthritis, or infection. The typical history of the patient includes a report of pain when moving the neck, which radiates to the shoulder and down the arm. The pain may interrupt sleep and may be accompanied by a headache or numbness and tingling in the affected arm. To determine the exact cause of the pain, a number of diagnostic tests may be used, including:

- Plain x-rays (show general arthritis changes and bony alignment)
- Computerized tomography (CT) scan (shows spinal bones, nerves, disks, and ligaments)
- Magnetic resonance imaging (MRI) (provides images of the spinal tissue, bones, spinal cord, nerves, ligaments, musculature, and disks)
- Bone scan (shows bone changes by injecting radioactive tracers, which attach to areas of increased bone production or show increased vascularity associated with tumor or infection)
- Myelogram/post-myelogram CT (evaluates nerve root lesions and any other mass lesion or infection of the meninges or spinal cord)
- Electromyography/nerve conduction studies (help differentiate cervical radiculopathy, ulnar or radial neuropathy, carpal tunnel syndrome, or other peripheral nerve problems)

❖ PATIENT-CENTERED COLLABORATIVE CARE

Conservative treatment for acute neck PAIN is the same as described for low back pain except the exercises focus on the shoulders and neck. The physical therapist teaches the patient the correct techniques for performing "shoulder shrug," "shoulder squeeze," and "seated rowing." Some health care providers prescribe a soft collar to stabilize the neck, especially at night. Using the collar longer than 10 days can lead to decreased muscle strength and range of motion. For that reason, some health care providers do not recommend collars for cervical disk problems. Therapeutic manipulation (chiropractic interventions) alone or in combination with other interventions does not appear to cause harm, does not consistently reduce pain or disability, but does benefit some patients (Mior et al., 2013).

If conservative treatment is ineffective, surgery may be required, most often using a *conventional open surgical approach.* A neurosurgeon usually performs this surgery because of the complexity of the nerves and other structures in that area of the spine. Depending on the cause and the location of the herniation, either an anterior or posterior approach is used. An anterior cervical diskectomy and fusion (ACDF) is commonly performed. The patient is fitted with a large neck brace before surgery. Routine preoperative and postoperative care is the same as described in Chapters 14 and 16.

! NURSING SAFETY PRIORITY (QSEN)

Critical Rescue

The priority for care in the immediate postoperative period after an ACDF is maintaining an airway and ensuring that the patient has no problem with breathing. Swelling from the surgery can narrow the trachea, causing a partial obstruction. Surgery can also interfere with cranial innervation for swallowing, resulting in a compromised airway or aspiration.

CHART 43-6   Best Practice for Patient Safety & Quality Care (QSEN)

Care of the Patient After an Anterior Cervical Diskectomy and Fusion

Postoperative Interventions

- Assess **a**irway, **b**reathing, and **c**irculation (first priority!).
- Check for bleeding and drainage at the incision site.
- Monitor vital signs and neurologic status frequently.
- Check for swallowing ability.
- Monitor intake and output.
- Assess the patient's ability to void (may be a problem secondary to opiates or anesthesia).
- Manage pain adequately.
- Assist the patient with ambulation within a few hours of surgery, if he or she is able.

Discharge Teaching

- Be sure that someone stays with the patient for the first few days after surgery.
- Review drug therapy.
- Teach care of the incision.
- Review activity restrictions:
  - No lifting
  - No driving until physician permission
  - No strenuous activities
- Walk every day.
- Call the surgeon if symptoms of pain, numbness, and tingling worsen or if swallowing becomes difficult.
- Wear brace or collar per surgeon's prescription

CHART 43-7   Key Features

Postoperative Complications of Anterior Cervical Diskectomy and Fusion

- Hoarseness due to laryngeal injury; may be temporary or permanent
- Temporary dysphagia; may last few days to several months; usually not severe
- Esophageal, tracheal, or vertebral artery injury
- Wound infection
- Injury to the spinal cord or nerve roots
- Dura mater tears with associated cerebrospinal fluid leaks
- Pseudoarthrosis caused by nonunion of fusion
- Graft and screw loosening if a fusion was performed

Chart 43-6 summarizes best practices for postoperative care and discharge planning. Complications of ACDF can occur from the brace or the surgery itself. The initial brace is worn for 4 to 6 weeks, depending on the patient. When it is removed, a soft collar is worn for several more weeks, or longer if needed. Potential complications of the anterior surgical approach can be found in Chart 43-7.

Some patients may be candidates for minimally invasive surgery (MIS), such as percutaneous cervical diskectomy through an endoscope, with or without laser thermodiskectomy to shrink the herniated portion of the disk. The care for these patients is very similar to that for the patient with low back pain who has MIS (see discussion of surgical management of patients with low back pain on pp. 888-889). Patients may also benefit from the placement of an artificial disk, a surgical option that preserves movement of the vertebrae. Artificial disks are newly approved by the U.S. Food and Drug Administration (FDA); there is evidence of their safety but the long-term effects on patient health are not yet established.

SPINAL CORD INJURY

Caring for a patient with an SCI requires both a patient-centered and family-centered collaborative approach and involves every health care team member to help meet the patient's expected outcomes. Optimally, patients with a new SCI are quickly transported to a model SCI System Center. Because of the complexity of a spinal cord injury, discharge planning needs to begin the day of admission. The rehabilitation team must be consulted on the day of admission.

❖ PATHOPHYSIOLOGY

Loss of motor function (MOBILITY), SENSORY PERCEPTION, reflex activity, and bowel and bladder control often result from an SCI. In addition, the patient may experience significant behavior and emotional problems as a result of changes in functional ability, body image, role performance, and self-concept. Addressing family member concerns and changes in family dynamics is also important to effective care

The SCIs are classified as complete or incomplete. A **complete spinal cord injury** is one in which the spinal cord has been damaged in a way that eliminates all innervation below the level of the injury. Injuries that allow some function or movement below the level of the injury are described as an **incomplete spinal cord injury**. Incomplete injuries are more common than complete SCIs.

Mechanisms of Injury

When enough force is applied to the spinal cord, the resulting damage causes many neurologic deficits. Sources of force include direct injury to the vertebral column (fracture, dislocation, and subluxation [partial dislocation]) or penetrating injury from violence (gunshot or knife wounds). Although in some cases the cord itself may remain intact, at other times the cord undergoes a destructive process caused by a contusion (bruise), compression, laceration, or transaction (severing of the cord, either complete or incomplete) (Nayduch, 2010).

The causes of SCI can be divided into primary and secondary mechanisms of injury. Five *primary* mechanisms may result in an SCI:

- Hyperflexion
- Hyperextension
- Axial loading, or vertical compression
- Excessive rotation
- Penetrating trauma

A **hyperflexion** injury occurs when the head is suddenly and forcefully accelerated (moved) forward, causing extreme flexion of the neck (Fig. 43-2). This type of injury often occurs in head-on vehicle collisions and diving accidents. Flexion injury to the lower thoracic and lumbar spine may occur when the trunk is suddenly flexed on itself, such as occurs in a fall on the buttocks. The posterior ligaments can be stretched or torn, or the vertebrae may fracture or dislocate. Either process may damage the spinal cord, causing hemorrhage, edema, and necrosis.

Hyperextension injuries occur most often in vehicle collisions in which the vehicle is struck from behind or during falls when the patient's chin is struck (Fig. 43-3). The head is suddenly accelerated and then decelerated. This stretches or tears

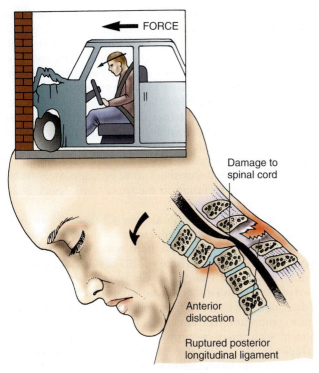

FIG. 43-2 Hyperflexion injury of the cervical spine.

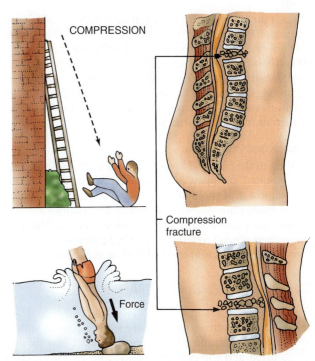

FIG. 43-4 Axial loading (vertical compression) injury of the cervical spine and the lumbar spine.

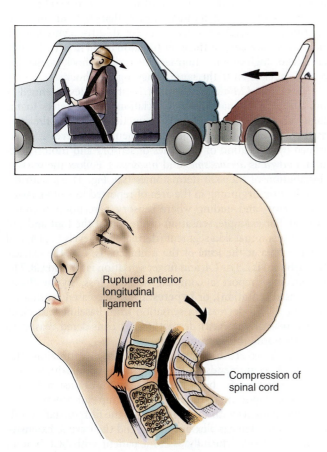

FIG. 43-3 Hyperextension injury of the cervical spine.

the anterior longitudinal ligament, fractures or subluxates the vertebrae, and perhaps ruptures an intervertebral disk. As with flexion injuries, the spinal cord may easily be damaged.

Diving accidents, falls on the buttocks, or a jump in which a person lands on the feet can cause many of the injuries attributable to **axial loading** (vertical compression) (Fig. 43-4). A blow to the top of the head can cause the vertebrae to shatter. Pieces of bone enter the spinal canal and damage the cord. **Rotation** injuries are caused by turning the head beyond the normal range.

Penetrating trauma to the spinal cord is classified by the speed of the object (e.g., knife, bullet) causing the injury. Low-speed or low-impact injuries cause damage directly at the site or local damage to the spinal cord or spinal nerves. In contrast, high-speed injuries that occur from gunshot wounds cause both direct and indirect damage.

Secondary injury worsens the primary injury. Secondary injuries include:

- Hemorrhage
- Ischemia (lack of oxygen, typically from reduced/absent blood flow)
- Hypovolemia (decreased circulating blood volume)
- Impaired tissue perfusion form neurogenic shock (a *medical emergency*)
- Local edema

Hemorrhage into the spinal cord may be manifested by contusion or petechial leaking into the central gray matter and later into the white matter. Systemic hemorrhage can result in shock and decrease perfusion to the spinal cord. Edema occurs with both primary and secondary injuries, contributing to capillary compression and cord ischemia. In neurogenic shock, loss of blood vessel tone (dilation) after *severe* cord injury may result in hypoperfusion (McCance et al., 2014).

Etiology

Trauma is the leading cause of spinal cord injuries (SCIs), with more than 35% resulting from vehicle crashes. Other leading causes are falls, acts of violence (usually gunshot wounds [GSWs]), and sport-related accidents (National Spinal Cord Injury Statistical Center, 2013). SCIs from falls are particularly likely among older adults. Spinal cord damage in adults can also result from nontraumatic vertebral fracture and diseases such as benign or malignant tumors.

Incidence and Prevalence

According to the National Spinal Cord Injury Statistical Center (2013), about 12,000 new SCIs occur every year in the United States. Almost 80% of all SCIs occur in young males, with the majority being Euro-American. Cervical cord injuries are more common than thoracic or lumbar cord injuries. The most common neurologic level of injury is C5. In paraplegia, T12 and L1 are the most common levels (Juknis et al., 2012).

❖ PATIENT-CENTERED COLLABORATIVE CARE

◆ Assessment

History. When obtaining a history from a patient with an acute SCI, gather as much data as possible about how the accident occurred and the probable mechanism of injury. Questions include the location and position of the patient immediately after the injury, the symptoms that occurred immediately with the injury, and the changes that have occurred subsequently. If possible, ask Emergency Medical Transport (EMT) rescue personnel about the type of immobilization devices used and whether any problems occurred during stabilization and transport to the hospital. Review the patient's medical record regarding the treatment given at the scene of injury or in the emergency department (ED) (e.g., drugs, IV fluids). Communicate with the ED nurse as he or she "hands off" the patient. Use the **s**ituation, **b**ackground, **a**ssessment, **r**ecommendation (SBAR) communication technique to collect valuable information for continuing patient care per The Joint Commission's National Patient Safety Goals. (See Chapter 1 for how to use SBAR.)

Obtain the patient's medical history, including a history of osteoporosis or arthritis of the spine, congenital deformities, cancer, and previous injury or surgery of the neck or back. These health problems may cause or contribute to an SCI. A detailed history of any respiratory problems is particularly important if the patient has experienced a cervical SCI.

Physical Assessment/Clinical Manifestations

Initial Assessment. Assessing the ABCs (**a**irway, **b**reathing, and **c**irculation) is the priority for any trauma patient. Therefore the first priority for the patient with an SCI is to assess the patient's airway, breathing pattern, and circulation status. The airway may be compromised because of foreign body obstruction from the tongue or teeth due to facial trauma, injury to the larynx, or mandibular (jaw) fracture. After an airway is established, assess the patient's breathing pattern. The patient with a cervical SCI is at high risk for respiratory compromise because the cervical spinal nerves (C3-5) innervate the phrenic nerve, controlling the diaphragm. A significant head injury, pneumothorax (air in the chest cavity), hemothorax (blood in the chest cavity), and/or fractured ribs may also cause respiratory distress or failure. Endotracheal intubation with mechanical ventilation may be necessary to prevent respiratory arrest.

To assess for circulation, evaluate pulse, blood pressure, and peripheral perfusion such as pulse strength and capillary refill. In the patient with traumatic SCI, multiple injuries may contribute to circulatory compromise from hemorrhage or hemorrhagic shock. Assess for indications of intra-abdominal *hemorrhage* or hemorrhage or bleeding around fracture sites. Indicators of significant blood loss compromising circulation include hypotension and tachycardia with a weak and thready pulse. In patients with known or potential cervical spinal cord injury, neurologic shock with profound vasodilation and bradycardia can occur resulting in hypotension. All symptoms of circulatory compromise or shock must be aggressively treated to preserve tissue perfusion to the spinal cord. Shock is discussed in detail in Chapter 37.

Use the Glasgow Coma Scale (see Chapter 41) or other agency-approved assessment tool to assess the patient's *level of consciousness (LOC)*. Cognitive impairment as a result of an associated traumatic brain injury (TBI) or substance abuse can occur in patients with traumatic SCIs. Perform a detailed assessment of the patient's motor function and SENSORY PERCEPTION to determine the level of injury and establish baseline data for future comparison. The level of injury is the lowest neurologic segment with intact or normal motor and sensory function. **Tetraplegia** (also called *quadriplegia*) (paralysis) and **quadriparesis** (weakness) involve all four extremities, as seen with cervical cord and upper thoracic injury. **Paraplegia** (paralysis) and **paraparesis** (weakness) involve only the lower extremities, as seen in lower thoracic and lumbosacral injuries or lesions.

Spinal shock, also called **spinal shock syndrome,** occurs immediately as the cord's response to the injury. The patient has complete but temporary loss of motor, sensory, reflex, and autonomic function that often lasts less than 48 hours but may continue for several weeks (McCance et al., 2014). Muscle spasticity, reflex activity, and bladder function begin in patients with cervical or high thoracic injuries when spinal shock is resolved. Spinal shock is NOT the same as neurogenic shock.

Sensory and Motor Assessment. Neurologic level defined by the American Spinal Injury Association (ASIA) refers to the highest neurologic level of normal function and is not the same as the anatomic level of injury. The neurologic level is determined by evaluation of the zones of sensory and motor function, known as *dermatomes* and *myotomes*. Follow the sensory distribution of the skin dermatomes (see Fig. 41-5), with the examination beginning in the area of reported loss of SENSORY PERCEPTION and ending where sensory perception becomes normal. For example, sensation of the top of the foot and calf of the leg is spinal skin segment (dermatome) levels L3, L4, and L5. The area at the level of the umbilicus is T10, the clavicle (collarbone) is C3 or C4, and finger sensation is C7 and C8. The patient may report a complete sensory loss, **hypoesthesia** (decreased sensation), or **hyperesthesia** (increased sensation). In acute SCI, a decrease in sensation from baseline, especially in a proximal (upward) dermatome, is considered reason to urgently notify the neurosurgeon.

Many scales are available to measure motor function after SCI. ASIA recommends a six-point grading scale, with 0 being no movement and 5 being normal strength against full resistance. It is important to test all muscle groups for function. For example, patients with spinal injuries at the fifth or sixth cervical vertebra often can flex but not extend their arms. Extensive training is needed to fully assess a patient with SCI (Furlan et al., 2011b). New loss of motor function in a patient with recent SCI is an emergency and requires immediate communication with the neurosurgeon.

The advanced practice nurse or health care provider may also test deep tendon reflexes (DTRs), including the biceps (C5), triceps (C7), patella (L3), and ankle (S1). It is not unusual for these reflexes, as well as all movement or sensation, to be absent immediately after the injury because of spinal shock. After shock has resolved, the reflexes may return if the lesion is incomplete.

Cardiovascular and Respiratory Assessment. *Cardiovascular* dysfunction results from disruption of sympathetic fibers of the autonomic nervous system (ANS), especially if the injury is above the sixth thoracic vertebra. Bradycardia, hypotension, and hypothermia occur because of loss of sympathetic input. These changes may lead to cardiac dysrhythmias. *A systolic blood pressure below 90 mm Hg requires treatment because lack of perfusion to the spinal cord could worsen the patient's condition.* In addition, the lack of sympathetic or hypothalamic control causes the patient to lose thermoregulatory functions. As a result, the body tends to assume the temperature of the environment and attempts to compensate by increasing extracellular fluid.

A patient with a cervical SCI is at risk for *breathing* problems resulting from an interruption of spinal innervation to the respiratory muscles. In collaboration with the respiratory therapist (RT), if available, perform a complete respiratory assessment, including pulse oximetry for arterial oxygen saturation every 8 to 12 hours. An oxygen saturation 92% or less and adventitious breath sounds may indicate a complication like atelectasis or pneumonia. Hypercarbia measured by end-tidal carbon dioxide in an intubated patient may indicate circulatory or worsening respiratory failure. The RT should also evaluate vital capacity and minute volume and repeat the tests daily and during periods of worsening oxygenation during the acute phase. Early tracheostomy is recommend if the patient is likely to need prolonged (i.e., more than 7 days) mechanical ventilation.

Gastrointestinal and Genitourinary Assessment. Assess the patient's *abdomen* for manifestations of internal bleeding, distention, or paralytic ileus. Hemorrhage may result from the trauma, or it may occur later from a stress ulcer or the administration of steroids. Monitor for abdominal pain and changes in bowel sounds. Paralytic ileus may develop within 72 hours of hospital admission. During the period of spinal shock, peristalsis decreases, leading to a loss of bowel sounds and to gastric distention. This disruption of the autonomic nervous system may lead to a hypotonic bowel.

Consult with the registered dietitian for assessment to initiate early nutrition to meet caloric and protein needs. Assess serum glucose levels to avoid complications from hypoglycemia and sustained hyperglycemia. Assess the patient for swallowing difficulties such as weak gag reflex, drooling, or cough with oral intake. Collaborate with the speech-language specialist to evaluate swallowing for patients with cervical and high thoracic injury before starting oral intake and plan for appropriate diet and treatment when **dysphagia** is present. Monitor intake and output.

Autonomic dysfunction initially causes an areflexic (neurogenic) bladder (no reflex ability for bladder contraction), which later leads to urinary retention. Assess for bladder distention and urine stasis. The patient with an indwelling urinary catheter has increased risk for urinary tract infection. Start a bowel regimen congruent with best practices for paralyzed patients. Maintain bladder and bowel programs for patients with established SCI. One source for best practices is the Paralyzed Veterans of America (www.pva.org).

Assessment of Patients for Long-Term Complications. Assess for skin TISSUE INTEGRITY with each turn or repositioning. Monitor for signs of VTE with vital signs. Monitor intake and output to maintain a normal volume of intravascular fluid (**euvolemia**). Assess glycemic and nutritional status including intake of protein, vitamins (A, C, E), zinc, and iron. Nursing management for neurogenic bowel care is usually started in rehabilitation. In patients with established SCI, assess baseline ability and encourage their participation in self-care and management (Furlan et al., 2011a). Encourage family participation in care, and support their effort to keep the patient engaged in family life.

Bones become *osteopenic* and *osteoporotic* without weight-bearing exercise, placing the long-term SCI patient at risk for fractures. Another complication of prolonged immobility is **heterotopic ossification (HO)** (bony overgrowth, often into muscle). Assess for swelling, redness, warmth, and decreased range of motion (ROM) of the involved extremity. The hip is the most common place where HO occurs (Zychowicz, 2013). Changes in the bony structure are not visible until several weeks after initial symptoms appear.

Laboratory and Imaging Assessment. The health care provider requests laboratory studies for the patient with an SCI to establish baseline data or to prepare for surgery. Arterial blood gas analysis is done to monitor the respiratory status of a patient at risk for respiratory insufficiency. The findings should be within normal limits unless the patient has a history of heavy smoking or pre-injury pulmonary disease. Respiratory failure is indicated by decreased oxygen levels, increased carbon dioxide levels, and respiratory acidosis. A complete blood count can help determine hemorrhage; blood in the urine may be another significant indication of hemorrhage. Check laboratory values for a low hemoglobin count, leukocytosis (increased white blood cells [WBCs]), lymphocytopenia (decreased lymphocytes), and thrombocytopenia (decreased platelets), which can occur in patients with cervical spine injuries. These abnormalities may be related to lack of autonomic innervation to the hematopoietic (blood-cell producing) system. Observe patients for clinical signs and symptoms of these changes, such as an increased bleeding tendency.

Computed tomography (CT) is obtained as soon as possible, especially for the patient who has sustained multiple trauma. Magnetic resonance imaging (MRI) is performed to determine the degree and extent of damage to the spinal cord and to detect the presence of blood and bone within the spinal column. The health care provider may also request a series of x-rays of the spine to identify vertebral fractures, subluxation, or dislocation.

◆ *Analysis*

The priority NANDA-I nursing diagnoses and collaborative problems for patients with an acute spinal cord injury (SCI) include:

1. Risk for respiratory distress/failure related to aspiration or diaphragmatic denervation (e.g., impaired phrenic nerve impulses in patients with cervical injury)
2. Potential for cardiovascular instability related to loss or interruption of sympathetic innervation or hemorrhage

3. Potential for secondary spinal cord injury related to hypo-perfusion, edema, or delayed spinal column stabilization
4. Impaired Physical Mobility related to spinal compression and edema (NANDA-I)
5. Spastic or flaccid bladder and bowel related to direct neurologic damage or disruption in nerve impulses
6. Risk for Compromised Resilience from injury requiring need for life change (NANDA-I)

◆ Planning and Implementation

The desired outcomes of patient-centered collaborative care following acute SCI are to stabilize the vertebral column, manage damage to the spinal cord, and prevent secondary injuries. Systemic hypothermia is an experimental approach to provide neuroprotection in the first 24 to 48 hours after SCI wherein the patient is cooled to 32° to 34° C (89° to 93.2° F) (Ahmad et al., 2013). Therapeutic hypothermia is described in Chapter 34 in conjunction with treatment for cardiac arrest. Although stem cell therapies have significant potential to treat SCI, they are not yet established as an intervention to restore damaged neurons or neuron function.

Many patients with previous spinal cord injuries (SCIs) are admitted to the acute care or long-term care setting for complications of immobility, such as pressure ulcers or fractures resulting from osteoporosis. Pressure ulcers contribute to local infection, including osteomyelitis and septicemia. Priorities in care may need to be re-evaluated as complications occur and resolve.

Nursing management strategies that promote high level of patient participation in care are associated with patient outcomes of higher life satisfaction, MOBILITY, and return to occupation (Bailey et al., 2012). Preventing complications of immobility and infection following SCI is an effort that requires patient, family, and health care team communication, collaboration, and individualized intervention.

Managing the Airway and Improving Breathing

Planning: Expected Outcomes. The patient with an SCI is expected to have a patent airway and adequate ventilation.

Interventions. *Airway management is the priority for a patient with cervical spinal cord injury!* Patients with injuries at or above T6 are especially at risk for respiratory complications and pulmonary embolus during the first 5 days after injury. These complications are due to impaired functioning of the intercostal muscles and decreased MOBILITY. Depending on the level of injury, intubation or tracheotomy with mechanical ventilation may be needed.

> ### ! NURSING SAFETY PRIORITY (QSEN)
> #### Action Alert
> Assess breath sounds every 2 to 4 hours during the first few days after SCI, and document and report any adventitious or diminished sounds. Monitor vital signs with pulse oximetry. Watch for changes in respiratory pattern or airway obstruction, and intervene when there are decreases in pulse oximetry values.

Respiratory secretions are managed with manually assisted coughing, pulmonary hygiene, and suctioning. Implement strategies to prevent ventilator-associated pneumonia (VAP) when the patient needs continuous mechanical ventilation as discussed in Chapter 32.

Teach the patient who is tetraplegic to coordinate his or her cough effort with an assistant. The nurse, or other assistant, places his or her hands on the upper abdomen over the diaphragm and below the ribs. Hands are placed one over the other, with fingers interlocked and away from the skin. If the patient is obese, an alternate hand placement is one hand on either side of the rib cage. Have the patient take a breath and cough during exhalation. The assistant locks his or her elbows and pushes inward and upwards as the patient coughs. This technique is sometimes called "assisted coughing," "quad cough," or "cough assist." Repeat the coordinated effort, with rest periods as needed, until the airway is clear.

Encourage the patient to use an incentive spirometer. The nurse and respiratory therapist perform a respiratory assessment at least every 8 hours to determine the effectiveness of these strategies. In some cases it may be necessary to perform oral or nasal suctioning if the patient cannot clear the airway of secretions effectively.

Monitoring for Neurogenic Shock and Hemorrhagic/Hypovolemic Shock

Planning: Expected Outcomes. The patient is expected to not develop neurogenic shock. If signs and symptoms of this potentially life-threatening complication occur, the patient is expected to receive prompt intervention.

Interventions. Maintain adequate hydration through IV therapy and oral fluids as appropriate, depending on the patient's overall condition. Carefully observe for manifestations of neurogenic shock, which may occur within 24 hours after injury most commonly in patients with injuries above T6. This potentially life-threatening problem results from disruption in the communication pathways between upper motor neurons and lower motor neurons.

> ### ! NURSING SAFETY PRIORITY (QSEN)
> #### Critical Rescue
> Monitor the patient with acute spinal cord injury at least hourly for:
> - Pulse oximetry (SpO$_2$) <90% or symptoms of aspiration (e.g., stridor, garbled speech, or inability to clear airway)
> - Symptomatic bradycardia, including reduced level of consciousness and deceased urine output
> - Hypotension with systolic blood pressure (SBP) <90 or mean arterial pressure (MAP) <65 mm Hg
>
> *Notify the physician immediately if these symptoms occur, because this problem is an emergency!* Respiratory compromise from aspiration may be treated with intubation or bronchial endoscopy. Neurogenic shock is treated symptomatically by providing fluids to the circulating blood volume, adding vasopressor intravenous therapy, and providing supportive care to stabilize the patient.

Preventing Secondary Spinal Cord Injury

Planning: Expected Outcomes. The patient with an *acute* SCI is expected to demonstrate adequate spinal cord stabilization as evidenced by no further deterioration in neurologic status.

Interventions. If the patient has a fractured vertebra, the primary concern of the health care team is to reduce and immobilize the fracture to prevent further damage to the spinal cord from bone fragments. Nonsurgical techniques include external fixation or orthotic devices, but surgery is usually needed to stabilize the spine and prevent further spinal cord damage.

Assessing Motor Function in the Patient with a Spinal Cord Injury

- To assess C4-5, apply downward pressure while the patient shrugs his or her shoulders upward.
- To assess C5-6, apply resistance while the patient pulls up his or her arms.
- To assess C7, apply resistance while the patient straightens his or her flexed arms.
- To assess C8, make sure the patient is able to grasp an object and form a fist.
- To assess L2-4, apply resistance while the patient lifts his or her legs from the bed.
- To assess L5, apply resistance while the patient dorsiflexes his or her feet.
- To assess S1, apply resistance while the patient plantarflexes his or her feet.

Assess the patient's neurologic status, particularly focusing on sensory and motor function, vital signs, pulse oximetry, and PAIN, at least every 1 to 4 hours depending on the patient's overall condition. See Chart 43-8 for elements of a focused motor assessment related to spinal cord injury. *Document your assessments carefully and in detail, particularly changes in motor or sensory function. Failure to do so may prevent other staff members from quickly recognizing deterioration in neurologic status.*

Regardless of the level of SCI, keep the patient in proper body alignment to prevent further cord injury or irritability. Devices such as traction, orthoses, or collars may be used to keep the spine immobilized during healing and rehabilitation.

Spinal Immobilization and Stabilization. During the immediate care of the patient with a suspected or confirmed cervical spine injury, a hard cervical collar, such as the Miami J or Philadelphia, is placed immediately and maintained until a specific order indicates it can be removed. A daily inspection of skin beneath the collar is recommended while a health care provider assists with maintaining neck alignment when the collar is removed. Padding at pressure points beneath and at the edges of the collar, particularly at the occiput, may be necessary to sustain TISSUE INTEGRITY. Until the spinal column is stabilized, a jaw-thrust maneuver is preferable to a head-tilt maneuver to open the airway should the patient need an airway intervention. Maintain spinal alignment at all times with log rolling to change position from supine to side-lying. Log rolling may also be prescribed in the initial period following surgical stabilization. Provide ongoing spinal alignment by using a slider board to transfer the patient between surfaces such as placement on a computerized tomography (CT) scanner table.

The patient may be placed in fixed skeletal traction to realign the vertebrae, facilitate bone healing, and prevent further injury, often after surgical stabilization. The most commonly used device for immobilization of the *cervical spine* is the halo fixation device, which is worn for 8 to 12 weeks. The device is affixed by the physician into the outer aspect of the skull. For patients not having surgery, the addition of traction helps reduce the fracture.

The **halo fixator** is a static traction device (Fig. 43-5). Four pins (or screws) are inserted into the skull. The metal halo ring may be attached to a plastic vest or cast when the spine is stable, allowing increased patient MOBILITY.

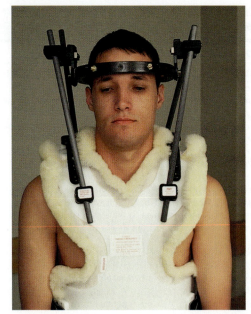

FIG. 43-5 Halo fixation device with jacket.

> ⚠ **NURSING SAFETY PRIORITY** (QSEN)
>
> **Action Alert**
>
> Never move or turn the patient by holding or pulling on the halo device. Do not adjust the screws holding it in place. Check the patient's skin frequently to ensure that the jacket is not causing pressure. Pressure is avoided if one finger can be inserted easily between the jacket and the patient's skin. Monitor the patient's neurologic status for changes in movement or decreased strength. A special wrench is needed to loosen the vest in emergencies such as cardiopulmonary arrest. Tape the wrench to the vest for easy and consistent accessibility. Do not use sharp objects (e.g., coat hangers, knitting needles) to relieve itching under the vest; skin damage and infection will slow recovery.

Common complications of the halo device are pin loosening, local infection, and scarring. More serious complications include osteomyelitis (cranial bone infection), subdural abscess, and instability. Hospital policy is followed for pin site care, which may specify the use of solutions such as saline. Vaseline dressings may also be used. *Monitor vital signs for indications of possible infection (e.g., fever, purulent drainage from the pin sites), and report any changes to the physician immediately. Discharge teaching related to halo fixator management is described in Chart 43-9.*

Nonsurgical treatment of *thoracic and lumbosacral injuries* is often challenging. Most health care providers choose to refer the patient for surgery and then immobilize the spine with lightweight, custom-fit thoracic lumbar sacral orthoses (TLSOs) to prevent prolonged periods of immobility.

> ❓ **NCLEX EXAMINATION CHALLENGE**
>
> **Safe and Effective Care Environment**
>
> A client was admitted this morning with an incomplete cervical spinal cord injury and is placed in a halo fixator. Halo fixation is used to reduce motion of the cervical spine. Which assessment finding will the nurse report immediately to the health care provider?
> A. A new-onset heart rate of 48 beats/min
> B. Mean arterial pressure of 90 mm Hg
> C. Pain level of 2 on a 0-to-10 pain scale
> D. Oxygen saturation of 95% on room air

CHART 43-9 **Patient and Family Education: Preparing for Self-Management**

Use of a Halo Device*

- Be aware that the weight of the halo device alters balance. Be careful when leaning forward or backward.
- Wear loose clothing, preferably with hook and loop (Velcro) fasteners or large openings for head and arms.
- Bathe in the bathtub, or take a sponge bath. (Some physicians allow showers.)
- Wash under the lambs wool liner of the vest to prevent rashes or sores; use powders or lotions sparingly under the vest.
- Have someone change the liner if it becomes odorous.
- Support the head with a small pillow when sleeping to prevent unnecessary pressure and discomfort.
- Try to resume usual activities to the extent possible; keep as active as possible. (The weight of the device may cause fatigue or weakness.) However, avoid contact sports and swimming.
- Do not drive because vision is impaired with the device.
- Keep straws available for drinking fluids.
- Cut meats and other food into small pieces to facilitate chewing and swallowing.
- Before going outside in cold temperatures, wrap the pins with cloth to prevent the metal from getting cold.
- Have someone clean the pin sites as recommended by physician or hospital protocol.
- Observe the pin sites daily for redness, drainage, or loosening; report changes to the physician.
- Increase fluids and fiber in the diet to prevent constipation.
- Use a position of comfort during sexual activity.

*Home care instructions may vary depending on hospital or physician preference.

Drug Therapy. *Dextran*, a plasma expander, may be used to increase capillary blood flow within the spinal cord and to prevent or treat hypotension. *Atropine sulfate* is used to treat bradycardia if the pulse rate falls below 50 to 60 beats per minute. Hypotension, if severe, is treated with continuous intravenous sympathomimetic agents such as *dopamine* or other vasoactive agent.

Centrally-acting skeletal muscular relaxants, such as *tizanidine* (Zanaflex, Sirdalud), may help control severe muscle spasticity. However, these drugs cause severe drowsiness and sedation in most patients and may not be effective in reducing spasticity. As an alternative to these drugs, *intrathecal baclofen (ITB) (Lioresal)* therapy may be prescribed. This drug is administered through a programmable, implantable infusion pump and intrathecal catheter directly into the cerebrospinal fluid. The pump is surgically placed in a subcutaneous pouch in the lower abdomen. Monitor for common adverse effects, which include sedation, fatigue, dizziness, and changes in mental status. *Seizures and hallucinations may occur if ITB is suddenly withdrawn.*

Other drugs to prevent or treat complications of immobility may be needed *later* during the rehabilitative phase. For example, celecoxib (Celebrex) may be prescribed to prevent or treat **heterotopic ossification** (bony overgrowth). Calcium and bisphosphonates may prevent the osteoporosis that results from lack of weight-bearing or resistance activity. Osteoporosis can cause fractures in later years. Early and continued exercise may help decrease the incidence of these complications.

Surgical Management. Surgery within 24 hours of injury to stabilize the vertebral spinal column, particularly if there is evidence of spinal cord compression, results in decreased secondary complications (Stahel et al., 2012). Emergent surgery also removes bone fragments, hematomas, or penetrating objects such as a bullet. Typical procedures include wiring and spinal fusion for cervical injuries and the insertion of steel or metal rods (e.g., Harrington rods) to stabilize thoracic and lumbar spinal injuries. During a cervical fusion, the surgeon reduces the fracture by placing the bone ends in proper alignment. Metal wiring is then used to secure bone chips (bone graft) taken from the patient's hip. The patient wears a halo vest to immobilize the spine during the healing process. For thoracic and lumbar fusions, metal or steel rods (e.g., Harrington rods) are used to keep the bone ends in alignment after fracture reduction. After surgery, the patient usually wears a molded plastic support (cervical or thoracic-lumbar or both) to keep the injured and operative areas immobilized during recovery. Postoperative care occurs as described in Chapter 16.

> **! NURSING SAFETY PRIORITY** (QSEN)
>
> ### Action Alert
>
> After surgical spinal fusion, assess the patient's neurologic status and vital signs at least every hour for the first 4 to 6 hours and then, if the patient is stable, every 4 hours. Assess for complications of surgery, including worsening of motor or sensory function at or above the site of surgery.

Managing Impaired Mobility

Planning: Expected Outcomes. The patient with an SCI is expected to be free from complications of immobility and perform ADLs as independently as possible with or without assistive/adaptive devices.

Interventions. The patient with an SCI is especially at risk for pressure ulcers (impaired skin TISSUE INTEGRITY), venous thromboembolism (VTE), contractures, orthostatic hypotension, and fractures related to osteoporosis. Patients with high SCIs are also at risk for orthostatic hypotension. Frequent and therapeutic positioning not only helps prevent complications but also provides alignment to prevent further spinal cord injury or irritability. Assess the condition of the patient's skin, especially over pressure points, with each turn or repositioning. Reduce pressure on any reddened area, and monitor it with the next turn. Reposition patients frequently (every 1-2 hours). When sitting in a chair, the patient is repositioned or taught to reposition himself or herself more often than every hour. Paraplegic patients usually perform frequent "wheelchair push-ups" to relieve skin pressure. Use a pressure-reducing mattress and wheel chair or chair pad to help prevent skin breakdown. Prevent pressure ulcers using best practices as described in Chapter 25. Prevent VTE including using interventions of intermittent pneumatic compression stockings and low–molecular-weight heparin (LMWH). Document pressure ulcer and VTE prophylaxis in accordance with Core Measures developed by the Centers for Medicare and Medicaid Services and The Joint Commission (www.jointcommision.org).

Contractures may be prevented or minimized with splints. Consult with the PT and occupational therapist (OT) for optimal scheduling for placing/removing splints (typically individually molded to the patient's extremity), trigger points to relieve spasticity, and positioning to maintain joint function. Administer antispasmodic drugs, and monitor the patient's response.

Patients with cervical cord injuries are especially at high risk for orthostatic (postural) hypotension, but anyone who is immobilized may have this problem. If the patient changes from a lying position to a sitting or standing position too quickly, he or she may experience hypotension, which could result in dizziness and falls. Because of interrupted sympathetic innervation caused by the spinal cord injury, the blood vessels do not constrict quickly enough to push blood up into the brain. The resulting vasodilation causes dizziness or light-headedness and possible falls with syncope ("blackout"). Consult with the registered dietitian to optimize diet for general health and to reduce osteoporosis from reduced daily weight-bearing activities. Provide out-of-bed activity in collaboration with the PT and OT. Resistance exercise, if it can be performed, promotes bone health.

Promote self-management with regular communication with the patient, family, and interdisciplinary health care team members. Help identify and set realistic expected outcomes on the basis of the patient's MOBILITY and functional level. Even patients with a cervical SCI often learn how to perform most ADLs independently in specialized rehabilitation programs, and the majority of patients with SCI return home.

Managing Risk for Autonomic Dysreflexia

Planning: Expected Outcomes. The patient with an SCI is expected to be free from episodes of autonomic dysreflexia (AD). If this complication of a high SCI occurs, the patient is expected to receive prompt interventions

Interventions. Autonomic dysreflexia (AD), sometimes referred to as *autonomic hyperreflexia,* is a potentially life-threatening condition in which noxious visceral or cutaneous stimuli cause a sudden, massive, uninhibited reflex sympathetic discharge in people with high-level SCI. AD primarily affects men more than women. The signs and symptoms of AD are listed in Chart 43-10 (Gunduz & Binak, 2012). The sudden rise in blood pressure can result in end-organ damage, including stroke.

People with a cervical or high-thoracic SCI face lifelong abnormalities in systemic arterial pressure control (Krassioukov, 2012). Be aware that the sudden rise in blood pressure in AD is usually associated with bradycardia. Normal systolic blood pressure (SBP) for SCI above T6 is 90 to 110 mm Hg; a SBP 20 to 40 mm Hg above the reference range for patients with established SCI may be a sign of AD. Patients with AD may display no symptoms other than an elevated blood pressure.

The causes of AD are typically gastrointestinal (GI), gynecologic-urologic (GU), and vascular stimulation as well as skin and bone injury. Conditions associated with AD onset are bladder distention, urinary tract infection, epididymitis or scrotal compression, bowel distention or impaction from constipation, or irritation of hemorrhoids. PAIN, circumferential constriction of the thorax, abdomen, or an extremity (e.g., tight clothing), contact with hard or sharp objects, and temperature fluctuations can also cause AD.

Certain procedures and pathologic conditions are also associated with AD. Anticipate the need for frequent assessment to detect AD early and intervene before blood pressure becomes dangerously elevated. For example, INFLAMMATION or injury in the GI system from gallstones, ulcers, gastritis, appendicitis, or other pathology is associated with the onset of AD. Stimulation of the GU system from menses, vaginitis, sexual penetration, ejaculation, and pregnancy (especially labor) can lead to AD. Venous thromboembolism can also cause AD. Acute and deep skin or mucosal injury from insect bites, blistering, pressure ulcers, and invasive instrumentation (e.g., cystoscopy, urodynamic testing, central line placement, and surgical procedures) can initiate AD. Heterotopic bone (i.e., bone tissue formed outside of the skeleton due to derangements in bone metabolism in patients confined to bed) and fractures can lead to AD. There have been case reports of ingrown toenails leading to AD.

Awareness of the causes of AD assists the nurse in prioritizing assessment and using best practices to avoid conditions that contribute to the onset and severity of AD. For example, proper bladder and bowel care to prevent fecal impaction and bladder distention are essential. *AD is a neurologic emergency and must be promptly treated to prevent a hypertensive stroke!* Chart 43-11 lists emergency care for autonomic dysreflexia.

Managing Urinary and Bowel Elimination

Planning: Expected Outcomes. The patient with an SCI is expected to achieve control of elimination of urine and stool without complications, if possible.

CHART 43-10 Key Features

Autonomic Dysreflexia

- Sudden, significant rise in systolic and diastolic blood pressure, accompanied by bradycardia
- Profuse sweating above the level of lesion—especially in the face, neck, and shoulders; rarely occurs below the level of the lesion because of sympathetic cholinergic activity
- Goose bumps above or possibly below the level of the lesion
- Flushing of the skin above the level of the lesion—especially in the face, neck, and shoulders
- Blurred vision
- Spots in the patient's visual field
- Nasal congestion
- Onset of severe, throbbing headache
- Flushing about the level of the lesion with pale skin below the level of the lesion
- Feeling of apprehension

CHART 43-11 Best Practice for Patient Safety & Quality Care QSEN

Emergency Care of the Patient Experiencing Autonomic Dysreflexia: Immediate Interventions

- Place patient in sitting position (first priority!), or return to previous safe position.
- Page/notify care provider.
- Assess for and treat the cause:
- Check for urinary retention or catheter blockage:
- Check the urinary catheter tubing (if present) for kinks or obstruction.
- If a urinary catheter is not present, check for bladder distention and catheterize immediately if indicated:
- Consider using anesthetic ointment on tip of catheter before catheter insertion to reduce urethral irritation.
- Determine if a urinary tract infection or bladder calculi (stones) are contributing to genitourinary irritation.
- Check the patient for fecal impaction or other colorectal irritation, using anesthetic ointment at rectum. Disimpact if needed.
- Examine skin for new or worsening pressure ulcer symptoms.
- Monitor blood pressures every 10 to 15 minutes.
- Give nifedipine or nitrate as prescribed:
- Patients with recurrent autonomic dysreflexia may receive an alpha blocker prophylactically.

Interventions. Patients with SCIs have reflex or neurogenic loss of bowel and bladder control. Many can become continent if they rigorously adhere to an established program. The type of program depends on the usual elimination pattern and whether the injury involved cervical or lower motor neurons (LMNs). A urologic evaluation may be needed to identify bladder type.

Patients with injuries to the lumbosacral area usually have a flaccid bladder and bowel. Patients with a flaccid bladder may achieve emptying of the bladder by performing a Valsalva maneuver or tightening the abdominal muscles. These techniques are not successful for all LMN injuries. To determine the effectiveness of these maneuvers, use a bedside bladder ultrasound or bladder scan device to measure bladder residual. This use of this device is discussed in Chapter 65.

Some patients rely on intermittent catheterization 2 or 3 times daily to empty the bladder. Obese patients and those with thoracic and cervical SCIs may need an indwelling urinary catheter for a period of time. External urinary catheters connected to a leg bag may be used for men.

The patient with *any* SCI is at risk for long-term kidney complications, such as hydronephrosis, acute and chronic kidney disease, and kidney stones. Urinary tract infections (UTIs) are common because organisms are introduced into the urinary tract by urinary catheters. Patients with an SCI may not be aware of the infection because they cannot feel dysuria, urgency, or back pain. They must rely on other signs and symptoms, such as foul-smelling urine or fever.

Teach the patient that the essential elements of a bowel program include stool softeners, fluid intake sufficient to result in clear, light yellow urine (unless medically contraindicated), high-fiber diet, and a consistent time for elimination. *Rectal digital stimulation is done only if requested by the health care provider because it could cause a vagal response, manifested by severe bradycardia and syncope.*

Adjusting to Major Life Change, Promoting Resilience

Planning: Expected Outcomes. The patient with an SCI is expected to adapt to a significant life change.

Interventions. Information obtained from the psychosocial assessment is used by the interdisciplinary team to identify strategies to help the patient adjust to the disability. Help the patient set realistic goals and verbalize feelings about the injury and his or her future. Invite the patient to ask questions, and answer them openly and honestly. Questions about prognosis and potential for complete recovery are referred to the health care provider because the timing and extent of recovery are different for each patient.

Collaborate with the case manager or discharge planner for a review of the patient's insurance and financial status. Many insurance policies cover rehabilitation services but for a limited time each year. The discharge coordinator or financial counselor may be able to assist the patient or family to locate other sources for adapting the home or funding an adapted car, such as private foundations and community organizations.

Community-Based Care

Case managers are ideal care coordinators to act as SCI patient advocates. In some settings, case managers begin working with patients in the emergency department to establish a positive image of SCI rehabilitation. Rehabilitation begins in the acute or critical care unit when patients are hemodynamically stable. They are usually transferred from the acute care setting to a rehabilitation setting, where they learn more about self-care,

MOBILITY skills, and bladder and bowel retraining. One promising therapy in rehabilitation is functional electrical stimulation (FES). FES uses small electrical pulses to paralyzed muscles to restore or improve their function. FES is commonly used for exercise but also to assist with breathing, grasping, transferring, standing, and walking.

Psychosocial adaptation is one of the critical factors in determining the success of rehabilitation. The case manager or acute care nurse can help the patient and family members prepare for discharge or transfer to a rehabilitation hospital. Assist in verbalizing feelings and fears about body image, self-concept, role performance, self-esteem, and SEXUALITY. The patient should be told about the expected reactions of those outside the security of the hospital environment. Role-playing or anticipating responses to potential problems is helpful. For example, the patient can practice answering questions from children about why he or she is in a wheelchair or cannot move certain parts of the body.

Particularly among young men, who are the most common patients with SCI, SEXUALITY is a major issue. Many patients are concerned about their ability to have sexual intercourse and have children. Most hospitals do not have psychological social workers or counselors to discuss sexuality issues. Rehabilitation programs often include a sexuality/intimacy counselor as part of the interdisciplinary team approach to patient care.

Home Care Management. If the patient is discharged home or returns home for a weekend visit from the rehabilitation setting, the environment must be assessed to ensure that it is free from hazards and can accommodate the patient's special needs (e.g., a wheelchair). The occupational or physical therapist, in collaboration with rehabilitation and the home care nurse, usually assesses the patient's temporary or permanent home environment. Ease of accessibility is particularly important at the entrance of the home as well as the bathroom, kitchen, and bedroom. The height of the patient's bed may need to be adjusted to allow a smooth transfer into and out of the bed.

All adaptive devices that the patient will use at home should be requested and delivered to the rehabilitation facility. This enables the nurse and other therapists to ensure that the items fit correctly and that the patient and family know how to use them correctly.

Self-Management Education. The teaching plan for the patient with an SCI includes:

- Mobility skills
- Pressure ulcer prevention
- ADL skills
- Bowel and bladder program
- Education about sexuality and referral for counseling to promote sexual health
- Prevention of autonomic dysreflexia with appropriate bladder, bowel, and skin care practices and recognition of early signs or symptoms of autonomic dysreflexia

This information should be reinforced with written handouts, CDs, DVDs, or other patient education material that the patient and family members can use after discharge to the home. Chart 43-12 provides information about aging for middle-aged and older adults with a spinal cord injury.

A full-time caregiver or personal assistant is sometimes required if the patient with tetraplegia returns home. The caregiver may be a family member or a nursing assistant employed to help provide care and companionship. A patient who is

CHART 43-12 Nursing Focus on the Older Adult

What Patients Need to Know About Aging with Spinal Cord Injury

NURSING INTERVENTION	RATIONALES
Follow guidelines for adult vaccination, particularly influenza and pneumococcus vaccination recommendations.	Respiratory complications are the most common cause of death after spinal cord injury (SCI). The vaccine to prevent herpes zoster (shingles) can help prevent skin breakdown.
For women, have Papanicolaou (Pap) smears and mammograms as recommended by the American Cancer Society or your health care provider.	Limitations in movement may make breast self-examination difficult.
Take measures to prevent osteoporosis, such as increasing calcium intake, avoiding caffeine, and not smoking. Exercise against resistance can maintain muscle strength and slow bone loss.	Women older than 50 years often lose bone density, which can result in fractures. Men can also have osteoporotic fractures as a result of immobility.
Practice meticulous skin care, including frequent repositioning, using pressure-reduction surfaces in bed and chairs/wheelchairs, and applying skin protective products like Mepilex.	As a person ages, skin becomes dry and less elastic, predisposing the patient to pressure ulcers.
Take measures to prevent constipation, such as drinking adequate fluids, eating a high-fiber diet, adding a stool softener or bowel stimulant daily, and establishing a regular time for bowel elimination.	Constipation is a problem for most patients with SCI, and bowel motility can slow, contributing to constipation later in life.
Modify activities if joint pain occurs; use a powered rather than a manual wheelchair. Ask the health care provider about treatment options.	Arthritis occurs in more than half of people older than 65 years. Patients with SCI are more likely to develop arthritis as a result of added stress on the upper extremities when using a wheelchair.

paraplegic is often able to function without assistance after an appropriate rehabilitation program.

ADL training for the patient with an SCI includes a structured exercise program to promote strength and endurance. The occupational therapist instructs the patient in the correct use of all adaptive equipment. In collaboration with the therapists, instruct family members or the caregiver in transfer skills, feeding, bathing, dressing, positioning, and skin care as discussed briefly in this chapter and in more detail in Chapter 6.

! NURSING SAFETY PRIORITY (QSEN)

Drug Alert

Teach the SCI patient and his or her family or other caregiver about the name, purpose, dosage, timing of administration, and side effects of all *drugs*. Make sure they understand the possible interaction of prescribed drugs with over-the-counter drugs or alcohol and illegal drugs.

SEXUALITY is associated with sexual and reproductive function. Sexual function after spinal cord injury depends on the level and extent of injury. Incomplete lesions allow some control over SENSORY PERCEPTION and motor ability. Complete lesions disconnect the messages from the brain to the rest of the body, and vice versa. However, men with injuries above T6 are often able to have erections by stimulating reflex activity. For example, stroking the penis will cause an erection. Ejaculation is less predictable and may be mixed with urine. However, urine is sterile, so the patient's partner will not get an infection. To prevent AD, prophylactic administration of a vasodilator may be needed prior to intercourse (Courtois et al., 2012).

Women with an SCI have a different challenge because they have indwelling urinary catheters more commonly than men with an SCI. However, some women do become pregnant and have full-term children. For others, ovulation stops in response to the injury. In this case, alternate methods for pregnancy, such as *in vitro* fertilization, may be an option. Some women also report vaginal dryness. Recommend a water-soluble lubricant for both partners to promote comfort.

For patients who choose not to have intercourse, intimate pleasure can be achieved in other ways, including kissing, hugging, fondling, masturbation, and oral sex. Variations in positioning may be needed to accommodate weak or paralyzed parts of the body. An understanding partner can help the patient adjust to his or her physical changes.

? CLINICAL JUDGMENT CHALLENGE

Safety; Evidence-Based Practice; Teamwork and Collaboration (QSEN)

A 52-year-old man who has had a T-10 spinal cord injury for 10 years is admitted for septicemia. He has a 3 × 2–centimeter discoloration on his left buttock that is classed as an unstageable pressure ulcer. He has an indwelling urinary catheter. The patient has been living alone and states that he has no family or friends. He has had a variety of health problems and wishes he would die. An antidepressant was prescribed for the patient 3 years ago, but he does not take it because it makes him tired.

1. What priority problems does this patient have at this time? Which problems need immediate action and why? What other data do you need to help formulate your answer?
2. With what members of the interdisciplinary and nursing team should you collaborate to provide quality care for this patient?
3. What may be causing the patient's septicemia? What are the evidence-based interventions for the care of patients with septicemia? Use a reliable electronic database to help you answer this question.
4. Use the SBAR method to communicate your concerns about this patient to another nurse who will be continuing his care.

Health Care Resources. Refer the patient and family to local, state or province, and national organizations for more information and support for patients with SCI. These organizations include the National Spinal Cord Injury Association (www.spinalcord.org) in the United States and Spinal Cord Injury Canada (www.sci-can.ca). Many excellent consumer-oriented books, journals, and DVDs are also available. Support groups may help the patient and family adjust to a changed lifestyle and provide solutions to commonly encountered problems.

The primary purpose of rehabilitation is to enable patients to function independently in their communities. However,

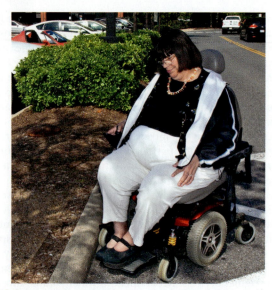

FIG. 43-6 Community physical barrier example: A curb prevents the patient in a wheelchair from getting onto the sidewalk.

many physical barriers still exist in some communities that prevent the patient in a wheelchair from finding a parking place, using sidewalks, and attending activities or utilizing resources (Fig. 43-6). The use of Photovoice (sometimes referred to as *Photo Voice*) projects can be very helpful in making positive changes in the community for people who are disabled.

Photovoice is a combination of photographs, videos, and storytelling that allows disabled people in the community to "<u>v</u>oice <u>o</u>ur <u>i</u>ndividual and <u>c</u>ollective <u>e</u>xperiences" in an organized way. This process can allow groups of patients with SCIs to work together to record and discuss their community's strengths and concerns. The collective desired outcome for Photovoice is to influence policymakers to make changes that remove or change their community's barriers. Newman (2010) described a Photovoice project to create a database of community environmental barriers and facilitators in a large city in the southeastern United States. Over 500 facilitators and over 500 barriers were identified. The authors produced a YouTube video and concluded that this type of community-based participatory project was extremely valuable to help wheelchair-bound SCI patients.

◆ Evaluation: Outcomes

Evaluate the care of the patient with an SCI based on the identified priority patient problems. The expected outcomes are that the patient:

- Exhibits no deterioration in neurologic status
- Maintains a patent airway, a physiologic breathing pattern, and adequate ventilation
- Is free from complications of immobility
- Performs basic ADLs as independently as possible with or without the use of assistive/adaptive devices
- Achieves control of regular elimination of stool and urine
- Adapts to a significant life change

SPINAL CORD TUMORS

❖ PATHOPHYSIOLOGY

Primary spinal cord tumors make up only a small percentage of all central nervous system neoplasms. Most spinal cord tumors are secondary or metastatic. Common primary cancers that metastasize (spread) to the spinal cord are lungs, breasts, prostate, colon, and uterus. Spinal cord tumors, whether primary or secondary, occur most often in the thoracic area, but they can occur in the lumbar and cervical areas. Signs and symptoms depend on the location of the tumor and its speed of growth. In addition, tumors in the spinal area can involve the vertebrae, and this location for bone cancer is usually as a result of metastasis from other areas of the body.

The pathologic effects of a spinal cord tumor are more often related to compression of the cord rather than the tumor itself. As the tumor expands, it compresses the cord or the spinal nerve roots. A large tumor may affect the blood supply to the cord causing ischemia or obstruct the normal flow of cerebrospinal fluid (CSF). Venous occlusion by the tumor may lead to spinal cord congestion and infarction (tissue death).

The appearance of neurologic signs and symptoms is related to the rate of tumor growth. With a slow-growing tumor, the cord may become significantly misshapen and displaced but the patient has surprisingly few symptoms. However, a rapidly growing tumor quickly leads to spinal cord compression, edema, and the development of neurologic symptoms, such as numbness and paralysis.

Primary spinal cord tumors can be extradural or intramedullary. Their cause is unknown. **Intramedullary tumors** are within the cord in the central gray matter or glial cells of the spinal cord. Intramedullary tumors are usually cancerous and grow rapidly and invasively. **Extramedullary tumors**, representing 90% of primary spinal cord tumors, are found within the spinal dura but outside the cord. They are further defined anatomically as extradural and intradural tumors. *Extradural or epidural* tumors occur between the vertebrae and the spinal dura. They develop in the surrounding bone and cause destruction of the vertebral bodies. *Intradural* tumors are located within the dura and originate from the pia-arachnoid, spinal roots, or ligaments. Most extramedullary tumors (e.g., schwannomas, neurofibromas, and meningiomas) do not exhibit the signs of uncontrolled growth and organ invasion of cancerous tumors.

❖ PATIENT-CENTERED COLLABORATIVE CARE

◆ Assessment

The clinical manifestations of a spinal cord tumor depend on its location (Chart 43-13) and rate of growth. The most common problem is non-mechanical back PAIN. Pain results from spinal cord compression, infiltration of the spinal tracts, or irritation of the spinal roots. Assess the quality, severity, and intensity of the pain. In addition, ask the patient to describe factors that worsen and relieve the pain. **Radicular** (nerve root) pain is stabbing or dull, with intermittent episodes of sharp, piercing pain. The pain may increase during coughing, straining, or sneezing. Lying flat may increase the pain as a consequence of stretching the involved spinal nerve roots.

Involvement of the corticospinal tract may lead to MOBILITY problems. Assess for weakness, clumsiness, spasticity, and hyperactive reflexes, and compare responses on both sides of the body. Other presenting signs include ataxia (staggered gait), hypotonia (decreased muscle tone), and a positive Babinski's reflex. Spastic paralysis occurs most often, although a flaccid paralysis may be present in a tumor that affects the spinal roots, an intramedullary tumor in the lumbosacral area, or an extramedullary tumor.

CHART 43-13	**Key Features**

Spinal Cord Tumors

General Manifestations
- Pain
- Sensory loss or impairment
- Motor loss or impairment
- Sphincter disturbance (bladder before bowel)

Cervical Manifestations

High Cervical
- Respiratory distress
- Diaphragm paralysis
- Occipital headache
- Quadriparesis
- Stiff neck
- Nystagmus
- Cranial nerve dysfunction

Low Cervical
- Pain in the arms and the shoulders
- Weakness
- Paresthesia
- Motor loss
- Horner's syndrome
- Increased reflexes

Thoracic Manifestations
- Sensory loss
- Spastic paralysis
- Positive Babinski's sign
- Bladder and bowel dysfunction
- Pain in the chest and the back
- Muscle atrophy
- Muscle weakness in the legs
- Foot drop

Lumbosacral Manifestations
- Low back pain
- Paresis
- Spastic paralysis
- Sensory loss
- Bladder and bowel dysfunction
- Sexual dysfunction
- Decreased-to-absent ankle and knee reflexes

Determine SENSORY PERCEPTION on each side of the body, and compare the responses. Early symptoms include a slowly progressive numbness or tingling, PAIN, and temperature loss. The sensory deficit is further marked by a decreased touch perception, an inability to sense vibration, and a loss of position sense. The patient often reports a tight, bandlike feeling around the trunk.

Loss of bladder control often occurs before a loss of bowel control. Assess for urinary hesitancy, dribbling, incontinence, urgency, or acute retention. Bowel dysfunction is manifested by constipation. Keep in mind that the patient is often embarrassed to admit to bladder or bowel dysfunction.

A lesion in the sacral area may cause a decrease in genital sensation and thus affect the patient's sexual function and enjoyment. Men may be unable to have an erection or to ejaculate.

Diagnostic Assessment. Radiographic examinations or scans of the spine are obtained to detect a narrowing of the spinal canal, destruction of the vertebrae, or the presence of calcification. An MRI scan with and without contrast medium provides more detail of the pathologic condition of the spinal cord than either a CT scan or myelography. Electromyography (EMG) may help make a differential diagnosis to rule out multiple sclerosis (MS) or amyotrophic lateral sclerosis (ALS) or when spinal cord symptoms indicate an incomplete block. It indicates the level, extent, and boundaries of a tumor. This test is being performed less today because of newer imaging techniques.

A biopsy may be done to diagnose the specific type of tumor using a CT/MRI–guided needle. If the tumor is malignant, a biopsy assists in determining the cancer's type, which will subsequently determine treatment options. A biopsy is not needed for tumors that result from metastases if cancer has been diagnosed in another site of the body.

◆ *Interventions*

Nursing care of the patient with a spinal cord tumor focuses on careful monitoring of vital signs and neurologic status at least every 4 hours or more often if clinically indicated.

! NURSING SAFETY PRIORITY (QSEN)

Critical Rescue

For the patient with a spinal cord tumor, report any change in motor and sensory status immediately to the physician or Rapid Response Team. Swelling or tumor invasion can damage the spinal nerves that help control the diaphragm, and respiratory failure can result.

The primary management of a spinal cord tumor is *surgery.* The desired outcome of surgical intervention is to remove as much of the tumor as possible. Often this is not possible and other treatment is needed (e.g., radiation therapy). *Emergency surgery is performed if the patient has a rapid loss of motor and sensory function or a loss of bladder and bowel control. Surgical decompression may be performed to maintain bladder, bowel, or motor function and to preserve quality of life—even with a poor prognosis.*

The neurosurgeon performs a laminectomy and surgical total or partial resection of the tumor to remove the source of spinal cord compression. Depending on the extent of the tumor, a spinal fusion may be necessary. Experts in palliative care can provide interventions to relieve pain. Rarely, a cordotomy or a palliative sectioning of sensory roots is done to control intractable pain.

After surgery, assess the patient's vital signs and neurologic status every 1 to 2 hours until they are stable and then every 4 hours. Help turn the patient as a unit (log roll) and reposition every 2 hours. Inspect the incision site for drainage, especially for cerebrospinal fluid (CSF), and signs of infection. Carefully monitor the patient with a cervical cord tumor for respiratory compromise. Postoperative nursing care for a patient undergoing a laminectomy is discussed on pp. 888-889 in the Back Pain section of this chapter.

Radiation therapy may be necessary, depending on the tumor type. It is usually used with low-grade malignant tumors that are not completely removed, with metastatic tumors, or with recurrent tumors when there is no other treatment option. The spinal cord cannot tolerate high doses of radiation. Overexposure to radiation may lead to spinal damage, which can develop as long as 6 to 12 months after therapy. Radiation overdose is manifested by progressive spinal cord degeneration and neurologic deficits. With time, the patient experiences spastic paralysis, loss of SENSORY PERCEPTION, and bowel and bladder dysfunction. Death may occur. Care of the patient undergoing radiation therapy is described in detail in Chapter 22.

The use of chemotherapy in the treatment of spinal cord tumors is very limited. The drugs that are given tend to be alkylating agents, which are effective for some CNS tumors because they cross the barrier formed in the CNS by unique capillary characteristics and glial cells similar to the blood-brain barrier in the skull. Chemotherapy may also be used as an adjunctive therapy for tumors that have metastasized to the spinal cord from other primary sites, such as the breast. Meningeal involvement may benefit from intrathecal (spinal) chemotherapy. Chapter 22 describes the general nursing care associated with giving chemotherapy.

Community-Based Care

Collaborate with the patient and his or her family members or significant others to identify and suggest ways to eliminate potential hazards in the home. If needed, make a referral to a home care nurse, social worker, or case manager to assess the need for structural alterations to the home. Alterations may be needed to accommodate ambulatory aids (e.g., a walker) and to help the patient perform ADLs.

Depending on the prognosis, some patients are discharged from the acute care hospital to a rehabilitation setting, where they can learn to function as independently as possible. Chapter 6 describes rehabilitation in detail.

The teaching plan for the patient with a spinal cord tumor depends on his or her level of dysfunction. With decompression of the tumor, the severity of the patient's symptoms often lessens. Deficits that may remain include MOBILITY and SENSORY PERCEPTION. Learning mobility skills can enable the patient to negotiate movement on sidewalks, carpeting, and other flooring surfaces. The patient must also be able to negotiate sidewalk curbs independently. The physical or occupational therapist instructs the patient in the correct use of all adaptive equipment. Review the individualized bowel and bladder program with the patient, family member, or other caregiver. Chapter 6 describes these programs and the rehabilitation process in detail.

The interventions related to SEXUALITY are usually focused on education in the acute care setting. The nurse answers questions and corrects any misinformation. Unless the nurse has had specific training or experience in sexual counseling of people with spinal cord tumors or injuries, more detailed questions should be directed to a sexual counselor.

The prognosis for the patient with malignant tumors or metastatic tumors is poor. Determine what the physician and family members have told the patient about diagnosis and prognosis. Encourage the patient to verbalize feelings and fears about prognosis, body image, self-concept, role performance, and self-esteem.

Refer patients and family members to local, state or province, and national organizations for people with spinal cord injuries. These groups often have information and support groups for patients with spinal cord tumors. Refer patients with a malignancy to the American Cancer Society (www.cancer.org). Referral to support groups may also assist families with helping the patient adapt to lifestyle changes. The Canadian Cancer Society (www.cancer.ca) offers similar services.

MULTIPLE SCLEROSIS

Multiple sclerosis (MS) is a life-long inflammatory disease of unknown etiology that affects the brain and spinal cord. It is one of the leading causes of neurologic disability in young adults. This chronic disease is characterized by periods of remission and exacerbation (flare), which is commonly referred to as a *relapsing-remitting course*. Patients progress at different rates and over different lengths of time. However, as the severity and duration of the disease progress, the periods of exacerbation become more frequent. Patients with MS have a normal life expectancy as long as the effects of the disease are treated.

A major concern reported by most patients is how long it takes to establish a diagnosis of MS. Many patients go to several health care providers, are given varying diagnoses and treatment, and/or are told that their symptoms are related to stress and anxiety. Often times, young adults will present with weakness, fatigue, or changes in vision and are diagnosed with exhaustion and advised to get more sleep. The patient and family are often relieved to have a definite diagnosis but may express anger and frustration that it took a long time to start appropriate treatment. Therefore establish open and honest communication with the patient, and allow him or her to share frustrations, anger, and anxiety.

❖ PATHOPHYSIOLOGY

Multiple sclerosis is characterized by an inflammatory process causing demyelination and axonal injury. Diffuse random or patchy areas of *plaque* in the white matter of the CNS is the definitive finding. Initially, remyelination takes place to some degree, and clinical symptoms decrease. Over time, however, new lesions develop and neuronal injury and atrophy occurs. Myelin is responsible for the electrochemical transmission of impulses between the brain and spinal cord and the rest of the body, and demyelination can result in slowed or stopped impulse transmission. The white fiber tracts that connect the neurons in the brain and spinal cord are generally involved in MS. The areas particularly affected include optic nerves, pyramidal tracts, posterior columns, brainstem nuclei, and the ventricular region of the brain. Eventually, with repeated exacerbations of the disease, damage to the axons becomes permanent.

The four major types of MS include (McCance et al., 2014):
- Relapsing-remitting
- Primary progressive
- Secondary progressive
- Progressive-relapsing

The classic picture of the relapsing-remitting type of MS (RRMS) occurs in most cases of multiple sclerosis. The course of the disease may be mild or moderate, depending on the degree of disability. Symptoms develop and resolve in a few weeks to months, and the patient returns to baseline. During the relapsing phase, the patient reports loss of function and the continuing development of new symptoms.

Primary progressive MS (PPMS) involves a steady and gradual neurologic deterioration without remission of symptoms. The patient has progressive disability with no acute attacks. Patients with this type of MS tend to be between 40 and 60 years of age at onset of the disease.

Secondary progressive MS (SPMS) begins with a relapsing-remitting course that later becomes steadily progressive. About half of all people with RRMS developed SPMS within 10 years. The current addition of disease-modifying drugs as part of disease management may decrease the development of SPMS.

Progressive-relapsing MS (PRMS) is characterized by frequent relapses with partial recovery but not a return to baseline. This type of MS is seen in only a small percentage of patients. Progressive, cumulative symptoms and deterioration occur over several years.

Etiology

The exact cause of MS remains unknown and is very complex. Research continues on viral, immunologic, genetic, and environmental etiologic factors. Viruses are well recognized as causes of demyelination and INFLAMMATION. Therefore it may be possible that a virus or other infectious agent is the triggering factor in MS. Although a number of viruses have been studied, no single virus has been identified as causing MS in genetically predisposed people. The environment may also contribute to the development of MS. The disease is seen more often in the colder climates of the northeastern, Great Lakes, and Pacific northwestern states, as well as in Canada. MS is common in areas inhabited by people of northern European ancestry (National Multiple Sclerosis Society, 2013a).

GENETIC/GENOMIC CONSIDERATIONS
Patient-Centered Care QSEN

Large genome studies of families have helped identify familial patterns of multiple sclerosis (MS). For example, having a first-degree relative such as a parent or sibling with MS increases a person's risk for developing the disease. Recent research also confirms the association of MS with the interleukin (IL)-7 and IL-2 receptor genes. Other interleukin genes, B-lymphocytes, and B-cells play a role in more progressive forms of the disease (McCance et al., 2014). These data help guide development of targeted drug therapies that may cure or better manage MS.

Incidence and Prevalence

MS usually occurs in people between the ages of 20 and 40 years, but cases may occur in those younger than 15 years and older than 50 years. About 400,000 people in the United States have MS, and women are affected about twice as often as men. The disease affects over 2 million people worldwide. Although MS tends to occur more frequently among whites, it affects people of all races (Frankel & James, 2011).

❖ PATIENT-CENTERED COLLABORATIVE CARE

◆ Assessment

History. Multiple sclerosis (MS) often looks like other neurologic diseases, which can make the diagnosis difficult and prolonged. As a result, patients often see many health care providers and undergo a variety of diagnostic tests and treatments. Obtaining a thorough history is essential for accurate diagnosis. Ask about a history of vision, MOBILITY, and SENSORY PERCEPTION changes, all of which are early indicators of MS. Symptoms are often vague and nonspecific in the early stages of the disease and may disappear for months or years before returning. Ask about the progression of symptoms. Pay particular attention to whether the symptoms are intermittent or are becoming progressively worse. Document the date (month and year) when the patient first noticed the clinical manifestations.

Next, ask about factors that aggravate the symptoms, such as fatigue, stress, overexertion, temperature extremes, or a hot shower or bath. Ask the patient and the family about any personality or behavioral changes that have occurred (e.g., euphoria [very elated mood], poor judgment, attention loss). In addition, determine whether there is a family history of MS or autoimmune disease.

Physical Assessment/Clinical Manifestations. Multiple sclerosis produces a wide variety of manifestations (Chart 43-14). Any myelinated fibers of the brain and spinal cord may be affected. To determine a patient's specific manifestations, perform a comprehensive neurologic assessment as described in Chapter 41.

First, assess the patient's ability to move. The patient often reports increased fatigue and stiffness of the extremities, particularly the legs. Fatigue is one of the most disabling manifestations, affecting almost all patients with MS. Unlike fatigue in

---

CHART 43-14   Key Features
Multiple Sclerosis

- Muscle weakness and spasticity
- Fatigue
- Intention tremors
- Dysmetria (inability to direct or limit movement)
- Numbness or tingling sensations (paresthesia)
- Hypalgesia (decreased sensitivity to pain)
- Ataxia (decreased motor coordination)
- Dysarthria (slurred speech)
- Dysphagia (difficulty swallowing)
- Diplopia (double vision)
- Nystagmus (involuntary eye movements)

- Scotomas (changes in peripheral vision)
- Decreased visual and hearing acuity
- Tinnitus (ringing in the ears), vertigo (dizziness)
- Bowel and bladder dysfunction
- Alterations in sexual function, such as impotence
- Cognitive changes, such as memory loss, impaired judgment, and decreased ability to solve problems or perform calculations
- Depression

---

other patients, MS fatigue is associated with continuous sensitivity to temperature.

Flexor spasms at night may awaken the patient from sleep. Further examination reveals increased or hyperactive deep tendon reflexes, positive Babinski's reflex, and absent abdominal reflexes. Gait may be unsteady because of leg weakness and spasticity due to cerebral motor strip damage.

Significant *cerebellar* findings include **intention tremor** (tremor when performing an activity), **dysmetria** (inability to direct or limit movement), and dysdiadochokinesia (inability to stop one motor impulse and substitute another). Motor movements are often clumsy. The patient may lose balance easily and may exhibit signs of poor coordination.

During examination of the *cranial nerves* and brainstem function, ask the patient if he or she has or has had episodes of tinnitus (ringing in the ears), vertigo (dizziness), and hearing loss. Assess for facial weakness and dysphagia. Speech problems include dysarthria, such as slurred words resulting from weak muscles of the tongue, lips, cheek, or mouth. Scanning is also a type of dysarthria common in MS. Scanning is an abnormal speech pattern with long pauses between words or syllables.

Typical clinical findings from assessment of the patient's visual acuity, visual fields, and pupils include:

- Blurred vision
- **Diplopia** (double vision)
- Decreased visual acuity
- **Scotomas** (changes in peripheral vision)
- **Nystagmus** (involuntary rapid eye movements)

Sensory findings include hypalgesia (diminished sensitivity to pain), paresthesia, facial pain, and decreased temperature perception. The patient may report numbness, tingling, burning, or crawling sensations. Some patients with RRMS, especially women, report pain (Newland, et al., 2010) (see the Evidence-Based Practice box). Perform a complete pain assessment for all patients with MS as described in Chapter 3.

If demyelination of the *spinal cord* has occurred, the patient may experience bowel and bladder dysfunctions. The patient may have an areflexic bladder or may experience frequency, urgency, or nocturia. Ask the patient if he or she has constipation or incontinence. Inquire about problems with SEXUALITY,

EVIDENCE-BASED PRACTICE (QSEN)

Are There Differences in Pain Between Women with Multiple Sclerosis and Healthy Women?

Newland, P.K., Riley, M.A., Fearing, A.D., Neath, A.A., & Gibson, D. (2010). Pain in women with relapsing-remitting multiple sclerosis and healthy women: Relationship to demographic variables. *MEDSURG Nursing, 19*(3), 177-182.

The purpose of this descriptive study was to determine if there is a relationship among aspects of pain and demographic variables in women with relapsing-remitting multiple sclerosis (RRMS) and healthy women. The researcher used data from a previous study consisting of 40 women with RRMS and 40 healthy women in the Midwest. Subjects were volunteers from one hospital. They were primarily Caucasian, married, and highly educated.

Findings revealed that pain prevalence was higher in women with RRMS when compared with healthy women. As years of education increased, prevalence and intensity of pain decreased. Pain also increased significantly in women who did not work. Conversely, for healthy women there was not a significant relationship with years of experience and pain prevalence or intensity.

Level of Evidence: 4

The study was a descriptive study that used a small convenience sample but with comparative groups.

Commentary: Implications for Practice and Research

When caring for patients with MS, especially women, medical-surgical nurses need to assess for the presence and intensity of their pain. When providing health teaching, patients may have special learning needs due to possible cognitive impairment. In addition, if possible, women should be encouraged to work or stay active to prevent increased pain.

This research used only Caucasian women in the study. Therefore the findings cannot be generalized to men or to any other racial or ethnic group. The research needs to be duplicated using male patients with MS and/or using a larger sample size of both men and women to compare with healthy men and women of mixed racial/ethnic origin.

including impotence, difficulty sustaining an erection, and decreased vaginal secretions.

Psychosocial Assessment. Assess the patient for mental status changes. Cognitive changes are usually seen late in the course of the disease and include decreased short-term memory, concentration, and ability to perform calculations; inattentiveness; and impaired judgment.

After the initial diagnosis of MS, the patient is often anxious. Apathy and emotional lability are common problems that occur later. Depression may occur at the time of diagnosis and can also occur later with disease progression. The patient may be euphoric or giddy, either as a result of the disease itself or because of the drugs used to treat the disease. Assess the patient's previously used coping and stress-management skills in preparing him or her for a chronic, usually debilitating disease. Secondary depression is the most frequent mental health disorder diagnosed in people with MS.

Assess the impact of bowel and bladder problems. Managing fecal incontinence or constipation can be time-consuming and embarrassing. The authors of a single site study found that elimination problems affected quality of life as much as MOBILITY difficulties (Norton & Chelvanayagam, 2010).

SEXUALITY can be affected in people with multiple sclerosis, and sexual dysfunction can have a major impact on quality of life. Assess the patient's fatigue level and pattern, since fatigue contributes to sexual dysfunction. Be sensitive when asking about the patient's sexual practices and orientation. Women report impaired genital sensation, diminished orgasm, and loss of sexual interest. Men most often report difficulty in achieving and maintaining an erection and delayed ejaculation. If able, answer the patient's questions, or refer the patient to a counselor or urologist with experience in the field of sexuality, intimacy, and disability.

MS affects the entire family due to the unpredictability and uncertainty of the course of the disease. Chronic fatigue and PAIN may also prevent the patient from participating in family and community activities. CNS stimulants such as amantadine (Symmetrel), aerobic exercise as tolerated, and energy-conservation strategies may help manage fatigue. Assess coping strategies of family members or other caregivers, and help them identify support systems that can assist them as they live with the patient with MS.

Laboratory Assessment. No single specific laboratory test is definitively diagnostic for MS. However, the collective results of a variety of tests are usually conclusive. Abnormal cerebrospinal fluid (CSF) findings include an elevated protein level and a slight increase in the white blood cell count. CSF electrophoresis reveals an increase in the myelin basic protein and the presence of increased immunoglobulins, especially immunoglobulin G (IgG). IgG bands are seen in most patients with MS.

Other Diagnostic Assessment. MRI of the brain and spinal cord demonstrates the presence of plaques and is considered diagnostic for MS. MRI with contrast shows active plaques and reveals older lesions not associated with current symptoms.

A complete history and physical examination is necessary to exclude other disease diagnoses. In general, assessment of cranial nerve function, coordination, strength, reflexes, and sensation are needed to diagnose MS, and a variety of neurologic tests are used to evaluate the many areas in which dysfunction from MS plaques can occur. Results of visual, auditory, and brainstem evoked potential studies are often abnormal. Electromyography (EMG) findings may be grossly abnormal in people with advanced disease.

◆ Interventions

The purpose of management is to modify the disease's effects on the immune system, prevent exacerbations, manage symptoms, and improve function. As with other spinal cord diseases, care of the patient with MS requires the collaborative efforts of the interdisciplinary team.

The patient with MS is often weak and easily fatigued. The Concept Map on p. 907 illustrates the priority problems and interventions for the patient with MS. Teach the patient the importance of planning activities and allowing sufficient time to complete activities. For example, the patient should check that all items needed for work are gathered before leaving the house. Items used on a daily basis should be easily accessible.

Drug Therapy. Current therapies are based on emerging evidence that MS is an autoimmune disorder. A variety of drugs are used to treat and control the disease, decrease specific symptoms, and attempt to slow its progression.

One or more of these drugs is recommended for treatment of relapsing types of MS:

- Interferon-beta-1a (Avonex or Rebif)—immunomodulators that *modify* the course of the disease and have antiviral effects

CONCEPT MAP

MULTIPLE SCLEROSIS

- MOBILITY
- PAIN
- SENSORY PERCEPTION

HISTORY

40-year-old Carolyn Brown is admitted with progressive relapsing MS (PRMS) after a fall. She was diagnosed last year after several years of vague and nonspecific symptoms. Married with two school-age children, she is having difficulty managing ADLs. Her marriage is struggling due to these health issues. She is experiencing generalized weakness, muscle spasms, and urinary incontinence.

Subjective Data: "I am so tired, I can hardly get around....and my legs are so stiff, I fall. I just gradually get worse. I sometimes choke when I'm eating." The patient reports weakness, muscle spasms, trouble with balance, and has periods of double vision and vertigo.

Objective Data: Slightly slurred speech. Intention tremor with eating or writing.

Ms. Brown has been diagnosed with PRMS – frequent relapses with partial recovery. Progressive, cumulative symptoms occur over many years from inflammatory damage to myelin in the brain and spinal cord.

Physical Assessment →

Data Synthesis →

Medical Diagnosis

Data Synthesis →

PATIENT PROBLEMS

MOBILITY – Difficulty managing ADLs related to generalized weakness, muscle spasms, fatigue, loss of balance, and falls
SENSORY PERCEPTION – Urinary incontinence, dysarthria, dysphagia, pain
Knowledge Deficit related to drug therapy and safety [MOBILITY, SENSORY PERCEPTION]
SEXUALITY and Psychosocial Issues – Life management of chronic illness

Planning →

EXPECTED OUTCOMES

- Participate in regular exercise to maintain mobility
- Maximize independence in ADLs.
- Manage urinary and bowel elimination
- Adhere to drug regimen to avoid complications
- Remain free of complications from ineffective airway clearance
- Use effective coping strategies for patient and family to reduce stress and enhance relationships

INTERVENTIONS

1. History and Physical Assessment

Assess history of onset and severity of signs/symptoms. Ask about their progression and about factors that aggravate or reduce symptoms. Complete a neurological assessment. *A focused history and physical assessment guides effective nursing care.*

2. Nursing Safety Priority: Action Alert!

Assist the cognitively impaired patient with orientation by placing a calendar in the room. Encourage written lists or recorded messages. Suggest keeping frequently used items in familiar places, and using mobile device "apps" for re-orientation or reminders. *Cognitive impairment impacts patient safety. Orientation helps the patient to function as safely as possible in the environment.*

3. SENSORY PERCEPTION Management

- Instruct the patient to wear an eye patch, alternating between eyes every few hours. *Relieves diplopia.*
- Teach scanning techniques. *Compensates for peripheral vision loss.*
- Encourage patient to see an ophthalmologist. *Manages changes in visual acuity that may be aided by corrective lenses.*

4. Maintaining Mobility

Collaborate with a physical/occupational therapist to maintain mobility and promote independence with ADLs. Teach patient to conserve energy and balance activities with periods of rest. Avoid common aggravating factors such as fatigue, stress, overexertion, or temperature extremes. *Maintain mobility by managing MS fatigue, the most disabling symptom. Fatigue level and pattern can contribute to immobility, dysfunction, and depression.*

5. Elimination Management

Assess for urinary hesitancy, dribbling, incontinence, urgency, and constipation. Use a bladder scanner to assess for urinary retention. Implement necessary interventions such as catheterization, bladder pacemaker, or drug therapy. Use best practices to prevent hospital acquired UTIs. *Promotes urinary continence and bowel evacuation. Dysfunction can have a major impact on quality of life.*

6. Drug and Complementary Therapies

- Review and provide written instructions of drug therapies for PAIN, inflammation, and incontinence. *Ensures patient understands drug mechanisms of action for safe administration.*
- Discuss complementary therapies such as massage, yoga, meditation, acupuncture, reflexology, and aromatherapy. *May help the patient to maintain MOBILITY and independence.*

7. Managing Dysarthria and Dysphagia

Collaborate with a speech-language pathologist for evaluation and treatment of slurred speech and swallowing difficulty. *Avoids complications resulting in ineffective airway clearance of secretions and aspiration.*

8. Maintaining Psychosocial Integrity

Assist patient in verbalizing concerns about body image, self-concept, role performance, self-esteem, and sexuality. *Helps patient cope with anxiety and depression over the progression of the disease. Depression is the most frequent mental health disorder diagnosed with MS.*

Concept Map by Deanne A. Blach, MSN, RN

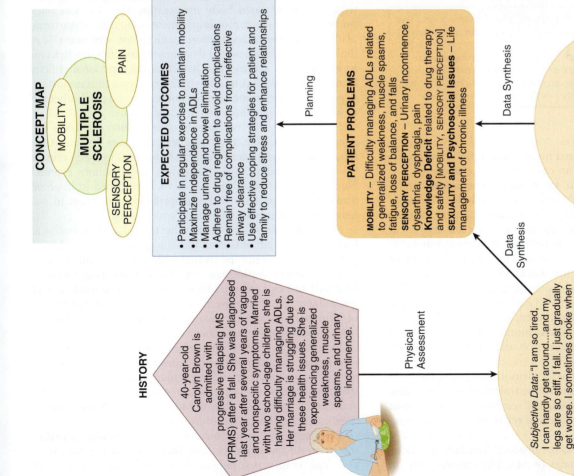

- Interferon-beta-1b (Betaseron, Extavia)—another immunomodulator with antiviral properties
- Glatiramer acetate (Copaxone)—a synthetic protein that is similar to myelin-based protein
- Mitoxantrone (Novantrone)—an antineoplastic agent and anti-inflammatory used to resolve relapses but with risks for leukemia and cardiotoxicity
- Natalizumab (Tysabri)—the first monoclonal antibody approved for MS that binds to WBCs to prevent further damage to the myelin
- Fingolimod (Gilenya), teriflunomide (Aubagio), or dimethyl fumarate (Tecfidera)—newer oral immunomodulating drugs
- Mitoxantrone (Novantrone) for patients with worsening disease or increased frequency of relapses
- Corticosteroid (methylprednisolone [Solu-Medrol], dexamethasone, or prednisone) for acute exacerbation or onset
- Other immunosuppressants (e.g., cyclophosphamide, methotrexate, azathioprine, cladribine, and cyclosporine) can reduce symptoms of MS and suppress the number of circulating immune cells to slow the autoimmune process and neuronal damage

The interferons and glatiramer acetate are subcutaneous injections that patients can self-administer.

! NURSING SAFETY PRIORITY (QSEN)

Drug Alert

Teach patients how to give and rotate the site of interferon-beta and glatiramer acetate injections because local injection site (skin) reactions are common. The first dose of these drugs is given under medical supervision to monitor for allergic response, including anaphylactic shock. Teach patients receiving these drugs to avoid crowds and people with infections. Remind them to report any sign or symptom associated with infection immediately to their health care provider.

Natalizumab, a humanized monoclonal antibody, is a controversial drug because it can cause many adverse events. It is given as an IV infusion in an infusion clinic under careful supervision. The patient is monitored carefully for allergic or anaphylactic reaction when each dose is given because the drug tends to build up in the body. *Patients receiving this drug are at a high risk for* progressive multifocal leukoencephalopathy (PML). This opportunistic viral infection leads to death or severe disability. Monitor for neurologic changes, especially changes in mental state, such as disorientation or acute confusion. PML is confirmed by an MRI and examining the cerebrospinal fluid for the causative pathogen. Natalizumab also causes damage to hepatic cells. Carefully monitor liver enzymes and teach patients to have frequent laboratory tests to assess for changes.

Mitoxantrone (Novantrone), a chemotherapy drug, has been shown to be effective in reducing neurologic disability. It also decreases the frequency of clinical relapses in patients with secondary progressive, progressive-relapsing, or worsening relapsing-remitting MS.

Fingolimod (Gilenya) was the first oral immunomodulator approved for the management of MS. The capsules may be taken with or without food. Teach patients to monitor their pulse every day because the drug can cause bradycardia, especially within the first 6 hours after taking it (Duddy et al., 2011). Two newer oral immunomodulating drugs have been approved for MS—teriflunomide (Aubagio) and dimethyl fumarate (Tecfidera). Like fingolimod, these drugs inhibit immune cells and have antioxidant properties that protect brain and spinal cord cells. Teach the patient that the two most common side effects of all the oral drugs are facial flushing and GI disturbances (Lilley et al., 2014). Remind the patient to keep follow-up appointments for laboratory monitoring of the white blood cell (WBC) count because the oral drugs can cause a decrease in WBCs, which can predispose the patient to infection.

Another oral drug, dalfampridine (also known as fampridine) (Ampyra), was approved several years ago to improve walking ability in patients with MS. However, half of patients taking the drug have experienced seizures. The FDA has issued a warning to limit patients who are eligible to take the drug. For example, patients older than 50 years, those with renal impairment, and those with a history of seizures should not take dalfampridine. For these reasons, the drug is not widely prescribed.

Immunosuppressive therapy with a combination of cyclophosphamide (Cytoxan) and methylprednisolone (Solu-Medrol) may be used for some patients to stabilize the disease process and decrease INFLAMMATION. IV adrenocorticotropic hormone (ACTH) may be given instead of methylprednisolone and tapered gradually over 2 to 4 weeks.

Promoting Mobility and Managing Symptoms. The symptoms of MS include spasticity, tremor, worsening of symptoms triggered by increased body temperature (i.e., Uhthoff phenomenon), pain, cognitive impairment, dysphagia, dysarthria, bladder and bowel dysfunction, oculomotor symptoms (e.g. diplopia, nystagmus), sexual dysfunction, and fatigue. Referral to rehabilitative services can help manage functional deficits from MS symptoms. A multidisciplinary approach is important to provide pharmacotherapy, physiotherapy, and psychotherapy as well as attain patient-centered goals for care.

For spasticity, the health care provider may prescribe baclofen (Lioresal), tizanidine (Zanaflex), diazepam (Valium, Apo-Diazepam), or dantrolene sodium (Dantrium) to lessen muscle spasticity. Dalfampridine (Ampyra), a potassium channel blocker, is a new oral drug that can be prescribed to improve walking ability and speed. Dalfampridine is not given to patients with a history of seizures or renal disease.

Severe muscle spasticity may be treated with intrathecal baclofen (ITB) administered through a surgically implanted pump. Paresthesia may be treated with carbamazepine (Tegretol) or tricyclic antidepressants. Propranolol hydrochloride (Inderal) and clonazepam (Klonopin) have been used to treat cerebellar ataxia. If fatigue cannot be controlled through the use of nonpharmacologic measures, amantadine hydrochloride (Symmetrel) may be prescribed.

In collaboration with physical and occupational therapists, plan an exercise program that includes range-of-motion (ROM) exercises and stretching and strengthening exercises to manage spasticity and tremor. Beta-blockers (e.g., propranolol [Inderal]) and neurosurgery (e.g., thalamotomy or deep brain stimulation) can provide some relief from tremors.

Emphasize the importance of avoiding rigorous activities that increase body temperature. Increased body temperature may lead to increased fatigue, diminished motor ability, and decreased visual acuity resulting from changes in the conduction abilities of the injured axons.

PAIN and paresthesia are often problems for the MS patient. Antispasmodics, antiepileptic drugs (AEDs), analgesics, NSAIDs, tranquilizers, or antidepressants may be used, depending on the cause of the pain and the patient's response. Teach patients about side and adverse effects for drugs that they may need to help increase their quality of life.

Cognitive impairment may occur early in the disease process. Many patients have some degree of neuropsychological dysfunction during the course of their disease. Areas affected include attention, memory, problem solving, auditory reasoning, handling distractions, visual perception, and use of speech.

> **! NURSING SAFETY PRIORITY** (QSEN)
>
> **Action Alert**
>
> For the patient with MS who has cognitive impairment, assist with orientation by placing a single-date calendar in his or her room. Give or encourage the patient to use written lists or recorded messages. To maintain an organized environment, encourage him or her to keep frequently used items in familiar places. Applications for handheld devices like mobile phones and electronic tablets can also be used for re-orientation, reminders, and behavioral cues.

If the patient experiences dysarthria (slurred speech), refer him or her to the speech-language pathologist (SLP) for evaluation and treatment. It is not unusual for the patient with dysarthria also to have dysphagia (difficulty swallowing). The SLP performs a swallowing evaluation, but further diagnostic testing may be indicated.

The patient may experience a variety of bladder problems. Bladder dysfunction (detrusor hyperreflexia) may be treated with anticholinergic agents. Other measures include an intermittent self-catheterization program, indwelling urinary catheter, or insertion of a bladder pacemaker. When the patient activates the control on the pacemaker, the bladder is stimulated and voiding is initiated. Patients with MS are at increased risk for urinary tract infections. Prophylactic antibiotics may be prescribed by the health care provider. Remind the patient to drink plenty of fluids unless contraindicated by other medical conditions.

Bowel symptoms can include constipation that can be treated with increased physical activity, adequate fluid intake of 1.5 to 2 liters daily, and increased dietary fiber to 25 to 35 g daily. Osmotic agents such as magnesium oxide may be used. Prokinetic agents such as lubiprostone may be used to increase motility. Enemas or suppositories may also be used.

An eye patch that is alternated from eye to eye every few hours usually relieves diplopia (double vision). For peripheral visual deficits, teach scanning techniques by having the patient move his or her head from side to side. Changes in visual acuity may be assisted by corrective lenses.

Sexual dysfunction may benefit from counseling. Prostaglandin-5 inhibitors (sildenafil, vardenafil, tadalafil) can be used to help men with erectile dysfunction. Penile prostheses are also used for men. The EROS Clitoral Therapy Device is a FDA-approved therapy for women with impaired sexual response.

Patients with MS who experience fatigue may limit their professional and social interactions. Depression can be manifested by fatigue, so screen for both of these symptoms. There are no licensed therapies for MS-related fatigue. Physiotherapy and occupational therapy can help reduce effort and fatigue. Depression can be managed with cognitive therapy and antidepressant drugs.

Complementary and Alternative Therapies. Patients with MS have reported a number of complementary and alternative medicine (CAM) therapies that have been successful in decreasing their symptoms. Consultation with a health care provider certified in palliative care may also provide strategies for effective symptom management. Some of the CAM therapies used by patients with MS are:

- Reflexology
- Massage
- Yoga
- Relaxation and meditation
- Acupuncture
- Aromatherapy

Marijuana has been used by some patients to relieve the PAIN of muscle spasms and is now legal for medical use in over 20 U.S. states and in Canada.

Community-Based Care

Home Care Management. To help the patient maintain maximum strength, function, and independence, continuity of care by an interdisciplinary team in both the rehabilitation and home setting is necessary. Admission to a rehabilitation center is brief but provides a program to improve functional ability. In collaboration with the case manager and occupational therapist, assess the patient's home before discharge for any hazards. Any items that might interfere with MOBILITY (e.g., scatter rugs) are removed. In addition, care must be taken to prevent injury resulting from vision problems. Teach the patient and family to keep the home environment as structured and as free from clutter as possible. As the disease progresses, the home may need to be adapted for wheelchair accessibility. Adaptation in the kitchen, bedroom, and bathroom may also be needed to promote self-management. Any necessary assistive/adaptive device should be readily available before discharge from the hospital.

Self-Management Education and Health Care Resources. The health care provider explains to the patient and family the development of MS and the factors that may exacerbate the symptoms. Emphasize the importance of avoiding overexertion, stress, extremes of temperatures (fever, hot baths, use of sauna baths and hot tubs, overheating, and excessive chilling), humidity, and people with infections. Explain all medications to be taken on discharge, including the time and route of administration, dosage, purpose, and side effects. Teach the patient how to differentiate expected side effects from adverse or allergic reactions, and provide the name of a resource person to call if questions or problems occur. Provide written instructions as a resource for the patient and caregivers at home.

The physical therapist develops an exercise program appropriate for the patient's tolerance level at home. The patient is instructed in techniques for self-care, daily living skills, and the use of required adaptive equipment, such as walkers and electric carts. Include information related to bowel and bladder management, skin care, nutrition, and positioning techniques. Chapter 6 describes in detail these aspects of chronic illness and rehabilitation.

Teach patients about conservation strategies that balance periods of rest and activity, including regular social interactions. Remind them to use assistive devices and modify the environment to avoid fatigue. Explore strategies to manage stress and avoid undue stress. Often patients are anxious and worry about how long the remission will last or when the disease will progress.

Because personality changes are not unusual, teach the family or significant others strategies to enable them to cope with these changes. For example, the family may develop a nonverbal signal to alert the patient to potentially inappropriate behavior. This action avoids embarrassment for the patient.

Resources required by the patient depend on the course of the disease and the complications that occur. Patients often are able to live completely independently, but they may need some assistance. In severe disease, placement in an assisted-living or long-term care facility may be the best alternative. The population of young and middle-aged residents in these settings is increasing as people with chronic, disabling diseases live longer. Refer the patient and family members or significant others to the local chapter of the National Multiple Sclerosis Society (www.nationalmssociety.org). Other community resources include meal delivery services (e.g., Meals on Wheels), transportation services for the disabled, and homemaker services.

AMYOTROPHIC LATERAL SCLEROSIS

❖ PATHOPHYSIOLOGY

Amyotrophic lateral sclerosis (ALS), also known as Lou Gehrig's disease, is an upper and lower motor neuron disease of adult onset. It is characterized by progressive weakness, muscle wasting, and spasticity that eventually lead to paralysis. Beginning in one area of the body, motor weakness and deterioration spread until the entire body is involved, including the ability to talk, swallow, and breathe. As a result of loss of lower motor neurons (LMNs) found in the spinal cord and brainstem, the muscles to which they connect weaken, atrophy, and die.

Loss or death of upper neurons (found in the brain) breaks their connections with LMNs, and spasticity occurs in the muscles. Death typically occurs within 3 years of diagnosis due to respiratory failure (McCance et al., 2014). There is no known cause, no cure, no specific treatment, no standard pattern of progression, and no method of prevention. Unlike with many other neural degenerative diseases, the sensory and autonomic nervous systems are not involved. Cognitive and behavioral dysfunction may occur, although the exact cause and extent of this has not been established.

Amyotrophic lateral sclerosis commonly affects people between the ages of 40 and 60 years, but it may also begin in younger and older age-groups. The incidence increases with each decade of life. ALS affects about 5 of every 100,000 people worldwide and is more common in men than in women. The cause of the disease is unknown but is likely due to multiple genetic and cell biologic hits and interactions of genetic, viral, and environmental factors (Ludolph et al., 2012).

❖ PATIENT-CENTERED COLLABORATIVE CARE

◆ Assessment

The clinical manifestations of ALS include fatigue, muscle atrophy, and weakness. Early symptoms are listed in Chart 43-15.

CHART 43-15   Key Features

Early Clinical Manifestations of Amyotrophic Lateral Sclerosis

- Tongue atrophy
- Weakness of the hands and arms
- Beginning muscle atrophy of the arms
- Fasciculations (twitching) of the face or tongue
- Difficulty controlling crying or laughing (emotional incontinence)
- Nasal quality of speech
- Dysarthria (slurred speech)
- Dysphagia (difficulty swallowing)
- Fatigue while talking
- Stiff or clumsy gait
- Abnormal reflexes

In addition to motor changes, cognitive changes may affect the thinking and planning processes. As the disease progresses, muscle atrophy, particularly of the trapezius and sternocleidomastoid muscles, develops. Eventually the respiratory muscles become involved, leading to respiratory compromise, pneumonia, and death.

Diagnosis is based on clinical and diagnostic test findings and by ruling out other causes of the motor changes. There is no specific test to diagnose ALS, but creatine kinase (CK) is increased. The electromyogram (EMG) demonstrates fibrillations and fasciculations of the muscles. The use of ultrasound to visualize fasciculation particularly in deep muscles can lead to earlier diagnosis (de Carvalho & Swash, 2011). A muscle biopsy specimen typically demonstrates small, angulated, atrophic fibers. Other diagnostic studies reveal motor strength deficits in serial muscle testing; abnormal pulmonary function test results, such as a decreased vital capacity (<2 L); and dysphagia (difficulty swallowing).

◆ Interventions

There is no known cure for ALS, but an interdisciplinary approach is needed for maintaining optimum functioning and end-of-life care. Interdisciplinary care can prolong survival and enhance quality of life in this population (Miller et al., 2009).

Riluzole (Rilutek) is the only drug approved by the Food and Drug Administration for use with ALS patients (Miller et al., 2012). It is not a cure, but it does extend survival time. Remind patients to take the drug when the stomach is empty. Teach the patient how to detect signs and symptoms of liver toxicity, such as vomiting and jaundice, that the drug may cause. Instruct them to have frequent liver enzyme tests, such as alanine aminotransferase (ALT) and aspartate aminotransferase (AST), as directed by the health care provider.

The health care provider also prescribes drug therapy for PAIN, fatigue, spasticity, excessive secretions, sleep disturbances, and other complications as they occur (Andersen et al., 2012). The interdisciplinary health care team collaborates with the patient and family to develop an individualized plan of care and PALLIATION of symptoms. The physical therapist and occupational therapist evaluate the patient's home and recommend modifications as the disease progresses. An exercise program is developed, and special equipment is obtained as needed to help with ADLs and MOBILITY. Other interventions are directed toward preventing complications of immobility and promoting comfort.

The speech-language pathologist (SLP) evaluates the patient for speech and swallowing problems and makes recommendations as needed. The SLP teaches patients various adaptive strategies, such as techniques to help them speak louder and more clearly. He or she works with the patient and family to develop a communication system to be used when the patient can no longer verbally communicate.

A nutrition consult may be needed to help with planning meals that the patient can swallow when dysphagia occurs. The family is taught how to ensure that the patient obtains sufficient nutrients, fiber, and fluids. When the patient can no longer swallow, a feeding tube may be placed, depending on the patient's decision or advance directives. The dietitian can recommend the appropriate enteral feedings.

For symptomatic treatment of dyspnea and/or intractable PAIN, opioids alone or in combination with benzodiazepines if anxiety is present may be prescribed. Titrating the dose against the clinical symptoms is less likely to cause life-threatening respiratory depression. For PALLIATION of terminal restlessness and confusion because of hypercapnia, neuroleptics may be used (e.g., chlorpromazine [Thorazine, Chlorpromanyl ✦] 12.5 mg orally, IV, or rectally every 4 to 12 hours).

As the patient's condition worsens, he or she will require respiratory support. Intermittent positive-pressure ventilation (IPPV) or bi-level positive airway pressure (BiPAP) may be used to aid breathing during sleep or full time. Some patients may be a candidate for diaphragmatic pacing (Scherer & Bedlack, 2012). Diaphragmatic pacing, also known as *phrenic nerve pacing*, is a pacemaker-like application of electrical impulses to the diaphragm, resulting in inhalation. Another option is invasive mechanical ventilation. None of these options prolong life. For this reason, many patients elect not to be placed on a mechanical ventilator, according to their wishes or advance directives. Teach the patient about the need for advance directives, such as a living will. Chapter 7 discusses end-of-life issues and hospice services in detail.

> **! NURSING SAFETY PRIORITY (QSEN)**
> **Action Alert**
>
> Refer the patient with amyotrophic lateral sclerosis to palliative care for symptom management. The palliative team collaborates with the health care provider to ensure that the patient has effective interventions to manage pain, fatigue, and dyspnea. Focusing care on symptom management is not restricted to patients who are at the end of life and can significantly improve quality of life in complexly ill patients and their family caregivers.

Other community resources include clinics and other support services run by the ALS Association (www.alsa.org) or the Muscular Dystrophy Association (www.mda.org).

NURSING CONCEPTS AND CLINICAL JUDGMENT REVIEW

What might you NOTICE if the patient is experiencing impaired MOBILITY and SENSORY PERCEPTION as a result of spinal cord health problems?
- Weakness or paralysis of one or more extremities
- Report of decreased sensation in one or more extremities
- Muscle spasticity or flaccidity
- Forward bent position when ambulating
- Limp or altered gait
- Bladder incontinence or retention
- Bowel incontinence or retention
- Report of pain at or above the site of injury along the spinal column and/or in one or more extremities
- Difficulty breathing

What should you INTERPRET and how should you RESPOND to a patient experiencing inadequate MOBILITY and SENSORY perception as a result of spinal cord health problems?

Perform and interpret physical assessment, including:
- Assessing airway patency and breathing pattern
- Assessing use of accessory muscles, pattern of respiratory effort, and rate and depth of breathing
- Assessing level of consciousness
- Taking vital signs
- Performing a complete physical assessment
- Performing a complete neurologic assessment

Respond by:
- Establishing an airway as needed
- Stabilizing the spine by positioning until surgery or other treatment is provided
- Preparing for imaging assessment tests
- Inserting an indwelling urinary catheter
- Collaborating with the health care team, especially the physical therapist and the occupational therapist, if needed

On what should you REFLECT?
- Monitor the patient for changes in condition, including deterioration of neurologic status.
- Consider how to best collaborate with the health care team when caring for patients with spinal cord injury or illness.
- Think about family reaction to the injury or illness and what additional resources could have been used or should be used in the future.

GET READY FOR THE NCLEX® EXAMINATION!

KEY POINTS

Review these Key Points for each NCLEX Examination Client Needs Category.

Safe and Effective Care Environment

- Use safe object and patient handling practices to prevent back injury as described in Chart 43-5. **Safety** QSEN
- Assess airway and breathing *first* for patients with an acute SCI. **Evidence-Based Practice** QSEN
- Integrate team meetings into care of patients with long-term or degenerating spinal cord conditions.
- Identify patient and family values and preferences as the foundation for regular communication and collaboration with health care team members, including the physician, physiatrist, advanced practice provider, physical therapist, occupational therapist, sexual counselor, registered dietitian, respiratory therapist, and case manager. **Teamwork and Collaboration** QSEN
- Ask the patient about advance directives and palliative care/symptom management to promote patient-centered care. **Patient-Centered Care** QSEN

Health Promotion and Maintenance

- Use community resources and behavioral strategies to assist overweight and obese patients in losing weight to reduce back PAIN and strain.
- Collaborate with physical and occupation therapy to promote self-management, including the provision of adaptive/assistive devices for independence in ADLs. **Teamwork and Collaboration** QSEN
- Include community resources in discharge planning and teaching for patients with SCI, MS, ALS, and cancer that involves the spine or vertebrae. There are specialty organizations for each of these spinal conditions.

Psychosocial Integrity

- Refer patients to appropriate resources, such as a sexual counselor or urologist, for sexual dysfunction resulting from illness or disease. Counsel them as needed about SEXUALITY. **Teamwork and Collaboration** QSEN
- Recognize that spinal cord injury and progressive neurologic diseases, such as MS, require the patient and family to make major adjustments to roles and goals. **Patient-Centered Care** QSEN
- Include the family in planning for rehabilitation and discharge when spinal disorders occur or worsen.

- Determine patient and family coping strategies to help patients adjust to spinal trauma or disease. **Patient-Centered Care** QSEN

Physiological Integrity

- Assess PAIN level in patients with back injury, including the nature of the pain and location.
- Provide complete neurologic assessment of patients with spinal cord health problems, with ongoing focused motor assessment as described in Chart 43-8.
- Implement effective drug and non-drug interventions for back PAIN, including analgesics, NSAIDs, and adjunctives such as heat and exercise.
- Implement interventions to prevent complications associated with immobility, including turning; VTE prophylaxis; early ambulation or transfers out of bed; and airway and breathing management such as bedside suctioning equipment, incentive spirometry, and Aspiration Precautions. **Safety** QSEN
- Monitor patients with cervical spinal injuries for manifestations of autonomic dysreflexia (see Chart 43-10). Provide a bowel and bladder regimen to prevent retention of stool and urine because these common problems can initiate autonomic dysreflexia. **Evidence-Based Practice** QSEN
- Provide emergency care for patients who experience autonomic dysreflexia as listed in Chart 43-11. **Safety** QSEN
- Explain that the pathophysiology of MS is a demyelination syndrome of the brain and spinal neurons.
- Explain the pathophysiology of ALS is unknown. Neurons that conduct nerve impulses from the spinal or brain to muscles degenerate. Without motor neuron input, the muscles atrophy and the patient becomes weak and then paralyzed.
- Monitor respiratory status carefully in patients with ALS. Patients experience respiratory failure as the disease progresses. **Safety** QSEN
- Assess patients with multiple sclerosis for clinical manifestations as listed in Chart 43-14. Fatigue is the most common symptom.
- For patients who have surgery to manage vertebral or spinal cord conditions, observe the incision site for bleeding and cerebrospinal fluid leakage (clear fluid).
- Log roll during repositioning, especially during acute spinal cord injury or following surgical fusion of vertebrae.
- Provide postoperative care and discharge teaching for patients having cervical neck surgery as listed in Chart 43-6.

CHAPTER 44

Care of Patients with Problems of the Peripheral Nervous System

Rachel L. Gallagher

 http://evolve.elsevier.com/Iggy/

PRIORITY CONCEPTS

- MOBILITY
- SENSORY PERCEPTION
- PAIN

- INFLAMMATION
- GAS EXCHANGE

LEARNING OUTCOMES

Safe and Effective Care Environment

1. Collaborate with interdisciplinary health care team members when providing care for patients with Guillain-Barré syndrome (GBS) and myasthenia gravis (MG) to avoid pain or complications from reduced SENSORY PERCEPTION.

Health Promotion and Maintenance

2. Provide information to patients and families on common side effects and administration of drugs for peripheral nervous system (PNS) disorders to ensure safety.
3. Identify community resources for PNS disorders for patients and families.

Psychosocial Integrity

4. Plan interventions for patients with GBS and MG for promoting communication based on patient preferences.

Physiological Integrity

5. Describe how to perform focused neurologic assessments for patients with PNS disorders.
6. Compare and contrast the pathophysiology of GBS and MG, including the roles of INFLAMMATION and autoimmunity.
7. Prioritize evidence-based nursing interventions for the patient with GBS or MG to maintain MOBILITY, reduce PAIN, and promote GAS EXCHANGE.
8. Differentiate between a myasthenic crisis and a cholinergic crisis. Assess patients having a thymectomy for postoperative complications.
9. Plan and implement evidence-based postoperative care for the patient undergoing peripheral nerve repair.
10. Compare trigeminal neuralgia and facial paralysis assessment findings.

There are over 100 peripheral nerve disorders. Although only a few require treatment in an acute care setting, many peripheral nerve disorders are present in patients admitted with an unrelated diagnosis. For example, neuropathies caused by systemic diseases like diabetes, chronic kidney disease, or cancers are common and interfere with MOBILITY, alter SENSORY PERCEPTION, and cause PAIN. Generally, peripheral nervous system disorders have symptoms that start gradually and then get worse. Often symptoms include:
- Pain, burning, or tingling
- Muscle weakness
- Either increased or reduced sensitivity to touch

The peripheral nervous system (PNS) is composed of the spinal nerves, cranial nerves, and part of the autonomic nervous system. Its function is to provide communication from the brain and spinal cord to other parts of the body. *Neuropathy* or *peripheral neuropathy (PN)* is a global word that refers to any disease, disorder, or damage to the PNS. These health problems may be acute, such as Guillain-Barré syndrome (GBS), or chronic, such as myasthenia gravis (MG). Secondary PN may result from disorders such as peripheral vascular disease and diabetes mellitus. These health problems are discussed elsewhere in this text.

GUILLAIN-BARRÉ SYNDROME

❖ PATHOPHYSIOLOGY

Guillain-Barré syndrome (GBS) is an acute inflammatory polyradiculoneuropathy that affects the axons and/or myelin of the peripheral nervous system, causing motor weakness and abnormalities in SENSORY PERCEPTION. It is an uncommon disorder, affecting males slightly more than females and peaking after age 55 years (Sejvar et al., 2011).

GBS may be referred to by a variety of other names, such as *acute idiopathic polyneuritis, acute inflammatory demyelinating polyneuropathy (AIDP), acute motor axonal neuropathy (AMAN),* and *acute motor and sensory axonal neuropathy* (Arcila-Londono & Lewis, 2012). In some forms of GBS, primarily the axons are affected. In other forms, **demyelination** (destruction of the myelin sheath) of the peripheral nerves occurs. Symptoms are the same: progressive motor weakness and abnormal SENSORY PERCEPTION. In demyelinating GBS, symptoms typically begin in the legs and spread to the arms and upper body. This is referred to as an *ascending paralysis.* Paralysis can increase in intensity until the muscles cannot be used at all and the patient is almost totally immobile. As a result, some patients require mechanical ventilation because of a weak or paralyzed diaphragm and accessory muscles for respiration. Healing occurs in reverse; the neurons affected last are the first to recover.

GBS is the result of immune-mediated pathology. Antibodies attack the myelin sheath that surrounds the axons of the peripheral nerves. On microscopic examination, groups of lymphocytes are seen at the points of myelin breakdown. In some instances, secondary damage to the cell body, the neurilemma, or the axon occurs. Neurilemma and axonal injury can delay recovery or result in permanent neurologic defects. Segmental demyelination (the destruction of myelin between the nodes of Ranvier) is the major pathologic finding in most variants of GBS. This destruction slows the transmission of impulses from node to node. Damaged motor neurons result in weakness. Damaged sensory nerves send fewer messages to the brain, affecting the patient's SENSORY PERCEPTION.

Three stages make up the *acute* course of GBS:

- The *acute or initial period* (1 to 4 weeks), which begins with the onset of the first symptoms and ends when no further deterioration occurs
- The *plateau period* (several days to 2 weeks)
- The *recovery phase* (gradually over 4 to 6 months, maybe up to 2 years), which is thought to coincide with remyelination and axonal regeneration (Some patients do not completely recover and have permanent neurologic deficits, referred to as *chronic GBS.*)

GBS is associated with bacterial infection, especially infection with *Campylobacter jejuni.* Influenza, Epstein-Barr, and cytomegalovirus viral infections have also been associated with GBS. There are other anecdotal and case reports from patients with surgery, trauma, and pregnancy who also developed GBS, but numbers are not sufficient to establish a causal relationship. There are also reports of some vaccines increasing the risk for GBS slightly, but epidemiologic evidence is weak (Centers for Disease Control and Prevention [CDC], 2014). It is believed that the precipitating infection or event sensitizes the T-cells to the patient's myelin, resulting in production of a demyelinating autoantibody.

❖ PATIENT-CENTERED COLLABORATIVE CARE

◆ Assessment

Obtain a complete health history. Ask the patient to describe GBS symptoms in chronologic order, if possible. Inquire about the presence of PAIN, numbness, and **paresthesias** (unpleasant sensations such as burning, stinging, and prickly feeling).

Although features vary, most people report a sudden onset of muscle weakness (Chart 44-1). The common symptoms of GBS are loss of reflexes in the arms and legs; low blood pressure or poor blood pressure control; muscle weakness or paralysis; numbness; uncoordinated movement, clumsiness, and falls; blurred or double vision; difficulty moving facial muscles; and palpitations (Simmons, 2010). Typically, the

---

CHART 44-1 Key Features

Guillain-Barré Syndrome

Motor Manifestations
- Ascending symmetric muscle weakness → flaccid paralysis without muscle atrophy
- Decreased or absent deep tendon reflexes (DTRs)
- Respiratory compromise (dyspnea, diminished breath sounds, decreased tidal volume, reduced peripheral oxygenation [SpO$_2$] and vital capacity) and respiratory failure
- Loss of bowel and bladder control (less common)
- Ataxia

Sensory Manifestations
- Paresthesias
- Pain (cramping)

Cranial Nerve Manifestations
- Facial weakness
- Dysphagia
- Diplopia
- Difficulty speaking

Autonomic Manifestations
- Labile blood pressure
- Cardiac dysrhythmias
- Tachycardia

---

disease does not affect level of consciousness, cognition, or pupillary constriction or dilation. The clinical variations of GBS reflect the areas of earliest or most severe involvement (Arcila-Londono & Lewis, 2012).

With any of the variants, *cranial nerve* involvement most often affects the facial nerve (cranial nerve [CN] VII). Assess the patient's ability to smile, frown, whistle, or drink from a straw. Assess the patient for dysphagia (difficulty swallowing), which involves CNs V, VII, X, XI, and XII. The patient's inability to cough, gag, or swallow results from the involvement of CNs IX and X. Monitor the patient closely for varying blood pressure (hypertensive and hypotensive episodes or orthostatic hypotension), bradycardia, heart block, and, possibly, asystole. These symptoms are part of *autonomic dysfunction,* which is linked to vagus nerve (CN X) deficit. Assess CN XI (accessory) by asking the patient to shrug the shoulders. Hypoglossal nerve (CN XII) deficit is manifested by an inability to stick the tongue out straight.

In addition to determining the usual roles and responsibilities, occupation, motivation, and available support systems, assess the patient's ability to cope with this devastating illness and the accompanying fear and anxiety. In general, GBS is self-limiting and the paralysis is temporary. It is not unusual for the patient to have depression throughout the recovery period or feel significant powerlessness.

Although no single clinical or laboratory finding confirms the diagnosis of GBS, the health care provider may perform a lumbar puncture (LP) to evaluate *cerebrospinal fluid (CSF).* An increase in CSF protein level can occur from inflammatory plasma proteins, myelin breakdown, and damage to nerve roots. However, high protein levels may not occur until after 1 to 2 weeks of illness, reaching a peak in 4 to 6 weeks. The CSF lymphocyte count is normal.

Peripheral blood tests may show a moderate *leukocytosis* early in the illness. The number of leukocytes rapidly returns to normal if there are no complications or concurrent illness.

Electrophysiologic studies (EPSs) demonstrate demyelinating neuropathy. The degree of abnormality found on testing does not always correlate with clinical severity. Within 3 weeks of symptoms, nerve conduction velocities are depressed. In some cases, denervated potentials (fibrillations) develop later in the illness. Electromyographic (EMG) findings, which reflect peripheral nerve function, are normal early in the illness.

Electrophysiologic changes appear only after denervation of muscle has been present for 4 weeks or longer. Nerve conduction velocity (NCV) testing is performed with the EMG. Nerve damage or disease may still exist despite normal NCV results. A magnetic resonance imaging (MRI) or computed tomography (CT) scan may be requested to rule out other causes of motor weakness. These tests are described in Chapter 41.

Respiratory function manifested by poor GAS EXCHANGE is often compromised in patients with GBS. Therefore vital capacity or tidal volume may be decreased and respiratory rate increased. Arterial blood gas (ABG) values may be abnormal with a decreased partial pressure of arterial oxygen (Pao_2), increased partial pressure of arterial carbon dioxide ($Paco_2$), or decreased pH.

◆ **Interventions**

Managing Drug Therapy and Plasmapheresis. The health care provider follows the most recent best practice guidelines from the American Academy of Neurology (Patwa et al., 2012) for the treatment of GBS. The patient may receive either plasma exchange (also known as *plasmapheresis* or *apheresis*) or IV immunoglobulin (IVIG). There is no benefit to combining these treatments (Rajabally, 2012). Corticosteroids are not used unless medically necessary to treat other associated diseases.

Plasmapheresis removes the circulating antibodies thought to be responsible for the disease. In this procedure, plasma is selectively separated from whole blood. The blood cells are returned to the patient without the plasma. Plasma usually replaces itself, or the patient is transfused with a colloidal substitute such as albumin. Fresh frozen plasma is generally not used because of the associated risk for infection and allergic pulmonary edema. Plasmapheresis should be done within several days after the onset of the illness, although some patients benefit up to 30 days after the onset of symptoms. The patient usually receives three or four treatments, 1 to 2 days apart. Some patients may require a second round of treatment if they deteriorate after the first plasmapheresis.

Nursing interventions for the patient undergoing plasmapheresis include providing information and reassurance, weighing the patient before and after the procedure, and caring for the shunt or venous access site and preventing complications described in Chart 44-2 (Kaplan, 2012).

> **! NURSING SAFETY PRIORITY** (QSEN)
>
> **Action Alert**
>
> If a shunt is used for plasmapheresis, be sure to:
> - Check shunt patency by assessing the presences of bruit or thrill every 2 to 4 hours
> - Keep double bulldog clamps at the bedside
> - Observe the access site for bleeding or ecchymosis (bruising)

IVIG has been shown to be as effective as plasmapheresis and is immediately available in most settings. Side effects of immunoglobulin therapy range from minor discomforts (e.g., chills, mild fever, myalgia, and headache) to major complications (e.g., anaphylaxis, aseptic meningitis, retinal necrosis, acute renal failure). Infuse IVIG slowly when it is started. Observe for and document side and adverse effects, and report their occurrence to the health care provider. The rate of administration can be increased based on the patient's tolerance and on agency protocol.

CHART 44-2 Best Practice for Patient Safety & Quality Care (QSEN)

Preventing and Managing Complications of Plasmapheresis

COMPLICATION	NURSING INTERVENTIONS
Treatment-Related Complications	
Citrate-induced hypocalcemia	Monitor electrolytes before and after therapy. Communicate abnormal results appropriately to the health care provider.
	Anticipate calcium replacement therapy (Chapter 11).
Urticarial (skin) reactions from proteins in replacement fluids	Obtain order and administer diphenhydramine (Benadryl) or corticosteroid as premedications when urticaria occurred with previous exchange.
Depletion coagulopathy	Monitor complete blood count and coagulation panel before and after treatment. Communicate abnormal values to the health care provider in an urgent time frame.
Risk for infection from immunoglobulin depletion	Assess and document vital signs, including temperature 3 times daily. Report symptoms of infection, fever, or abnormal vital signs to the health care provider promptly.
Fluid shift or depletion	Monitor fluid status and vital signs during treatment and at least twice in the first hour following treatment.
Sensitivity reaction (including potential anaphylaxis with incorrect crossmatch or administration) when fresh frozen plasma is used in replacement fluid	Follow institution policy for safe, effective administration of blood products like fresh frozen plasma.
Site-Related Complications	
Trauma to skin and blood vessels from large-bore needles for access or catheter-related trauma	Teach the patient rationale for and how to monitor access site as described below.
Bleeding, phlebitis, or infection at access site	Anchor tubing securely during treatment.
	Minimize patient agitation, if present, during treatment.
	Assess access site immediately following cessation of treatment and at regular intervals (every 4 hours or more often). Assessment includes appearance of site or dressing, palpation of thrill, and auscultation of bruit.
Clotting at access site	Report loss of thrill or bruit, uncontrolled or large volume bleeding, and presence of redness (particularly along venous pathway), drainage, and swelling to provider immediately.

Managing Respiratory and Cardiac Status. Frequent and focused monitoring of both the respiratory and cardiovascular systems can prevent complications from GBS as well as identify patients in need of critical rescue interventions.

Inability to maintain an airway is a high risk and potentially fatal consequence of rapidly ascending GBS. The priority nursing intervention of *airway management* is to promote airway patency and adequate GAS EXCHANGE. Consider implementing Aspiration Precautions that include elevating the head of the bed to 45 degrees or higher and testing for dysphagia prior to restarting oral drugs or nutrition. Have suctioning equipment available and follow institution procedure for oral or oral-tracheal suctioning if the airway becomes compromised with secretions or food. Monitor the color, consistency, and amount of secretions obtained. Chest physiotherapy, often performed by the respiratory therapist (RT), and frequent position changes are combined with breathing exercises (coughing and deep breathing) and the use of an incentive spirometer to prevent pneumonia and atelectasis. Oxygen may be administered by nasal cannula at a flow rate prescribed by the health care provider.

> ### ! NURSING SAFETY PRIORITY (QSEN)
> #### *Action Alert*
>
> In the initial phase of Guillain-Barré syndrome, monitor the patient closely with each interaction for signs of respiratory distress, such as dyspnea, air hunger, adventitious breath sounds, decreased oxygen saturation, and cyanosis. In addition, assess respiratory rate, rhythm, and depth every 1 to 2 hours. In collaboration with the respiratory therapist (RT), check vital capacity every 2 to 4 hours and auscultate the lungs at 4-hour intervals. Monitor the patient's ability to cough and swallow for any change. Assess cognitive status, especially in older adults; a decline in mental status often indicates hypoxia.

Monitor ABG values or end-tidal carbon dioxide for signs of respiratory failure; pulse oximetry reveals decreasing oxygen saturation. A decrease in vital capacity to less than 15 to 20 mL/kg (or less than two thirds of the patient's normal) and the inability to clear secretions may be indications for elective intubation.

Both the sympathetic and parasympathetic systems may be affected. A patient with acute GBS may require cardiac monitoring because of the risk for dysrhythmias. Monitor trends in vital signs closely. Report significant changes in heart rate and blood pressure to the health care provider in an urgent time frame. Hypertension is treated with a beta blocker or nitroprusside (Nitropress). Hypotension is treated with IV fluids and placing the patient in a supine position unless he or she is in extreme respiratory distress. Atropine may be prescribed to treat bradycardia.

Improving Mobility and Preventing Complications of Immobility. Collaborate with the patient, family, physical and occupational therapists (PT/OT), speech-language pathologist (SLP), and dietitian to develop interventions that prevent complications of immobility and to address deficits in self-care. Assess the patient's motor (muscle) strength every 2 to 4 hours as part of the neurologic assessment. The interventions prescribed for MOBILITY and self-management and to prevent complications depend on the degree of motor deficit. The PT and OT provide assistive devices and instructions for their use.

To ensure safety, assist the patient with walking, transfers from bed to chair, position changes, and maintenance of proper body alignment until he or she is able to perform these activities independently. Encourage maximum independence. Perform active or passive range-of-motion (ROM) exercises at least daily, or delegate this activity to unlicensed assistive personnel (UAP) with supervision. Teach family members these techniques.

See Chapter 6 for detailed discussion of ways to promote self-management and prevent complications of immobility. Monitor the patient's responses, including fatigue level. Provide adequate rest periods between activities.

Decreased gastric motility, dysphagia, and depression can cause malnutrition. Collaborate with the dietitian to develop caloric and protein intake goals. The patient may require assistance with feeding. If he or she cannot safely swallow food or liquids, enteral nutrition is prescribed. Weigh the patient 3 times a week, and monitor serum prealbumin each week to evaluate nutritional status.

Immobility and malnutrition place patients at risk for pressure ulcers. Assess skin integrity at least daily and with any assisted MOBILITY intervention. While bedbound, ensure the patient is turned a minimum of every 2 hours. Consider the use of pressure-relieving supports after a turn or special mattress or overlay. Document the skin assessment daily. Consult with the skin or wound care expert when changes occur that contribute to pressure ulcer formation (see Chapter 25).

Because venous thromboembolism (VTE) and pulmonary emboli are common complications of immobility, the health care provider may prescribe prophylactic anticoagulant therapy, such as subcutaneous low–molecular-weight heparin. Sequential pneumatic compression devices for legs may be used to promote venous return. Ensure documentation of starting and maintaining VTE prophylaxis; this is a Joint Commission Core Measure of high-quality health care delivery in acute and critical care units.

Managing Pain. Assess the severity and nature of the patient's PAIN, which is often worse at night. The patient may have paresthesia or hyperesthesia (extreme sensitivity to touch), deep muscle aches, and muscle stiffness. The typical pain experienced is severe and requires opioids at least initially for management. Other drugs that are given include gabapentin (Neurontin) or tricyclic antidepressants (Cranwell-Bruce, 2011).

> ### ! NURSING SAFETY PRIORITY (QSEN)
> #### *Drug Alert*
>
> Older adults should not receive tricyclic drugs because they cause serious anticholinergic effects such as urinary retention, blurred vision, and confusion. These adverse drug events can contribute to cognitive impairment, falls, and injury (see Chapter 2).

Other pain control measures include frequent repositioning, massage, ice, heat, relaxation techniques, guided imagery, hypnosis, and distractions (e.g., music, visitors). Chapter 3 discusses these modalities and other pain-relief measures in detail.

> ### ? NCLEX EXAMINATION CHALLENGE
> #### *Physiological Integrity*
>
> A client is admitted to the critical care unit with possible Guillain-Barré syndrome. Which symptom of neurologic impairment will require priority nursing interventions? **Select all that apply.**
> A. New adventitious breath sounds
> B. A respiratory rate of 12
> C. Rapid, shallow breathing pattern
> D. A peripheral oxygen saturation (SpO$_2$) of 90%
> E. New-onset nausea following a position change

Promoting Communication. The patient may have difficulty communicating because the muscles required for the production of speech are weak or he or she may be mechanically ventilated. In either case, collaborate with the speech-language pathologist to develop a communication system. A simple technique involves eye blinking or moving a finger to indicate "yes" and "no." A communication board or flash cards can be used with the letters of the alphabet or a list of common requests, such as the need to be repositioned or the need for pain medication. Computer or handheld mobile devices may also be used, depending on functional ability.

Providing Psychosocial Support. Teach the patient and family about the illness, and explain all diagnostic tests and treatments. Assess the patient and family for verbal and non-verbal behaviors that indicate powerlessness, anxiety, fear, and isolation (Simmons, 2010). Encourage the patient to verbalize feelings about the illness and its effects, if possible, while fostering hope. Assess previous decision-making patterns, roles, and responsibilities. To help identify personal factors that influence coping ability, ask the patient and/or family to describe their usual lifestyles and the situations in which they coped effectively. Sleep disturbances related to PAIN and altered autonomic function may affect the patient's sleep-wake cycle. Allow for regularly scheduled rest periods (Simmons, 2010).

Refer patients who need further psychosocial support to the social worker, certified hospital chaplain or appropriate spiritual resource, and local support groups. If necessary, obtain a psychological consultation for further evaluation and intervention.

Community-Based Care

The severity and course of GBS are variable, which makes the prognosis difficult to predict. The most likely residual deficits at discharge are related to MOBILITY, self-management, altered SENSORY PERCEPTION, and disturbed self-concept. For patients who have total quadriparesis (weakness in all four extremities) or respiratory paralysis, the course of the rehabilitation phase is even more variable and may require weeks to years. The expected outcome of the recovery phase is to move from dependence to independence (Khan & Amatya, 2012).

Planning for discharge begins on admission. Include a family member in the education process throughout the patient's hospitalization and in the discharge process. Provide them with both oral and written instructions to improve adherence to the plan of care and promote continuity during care transitions. The patient may transition to home or skilled care. In collaboration with the discharge planner or case manager (CM), the nurse communicates patient status and summarizes the hospital stay to provide safe transitions in care to a rehabilitation or long-term care setting. If the patient is discharged to home, consider referral to a home health care agency or support group. If assistive devices are needed at home, the CM in collaboration with the interdisciplinary health care team makes certain that the necessary equipment has been delivered after evaluating the home setting. Home care management for patients with GBS is similar to that for those who have had a stroke or spinal cord injury, depending on the nature of the neurologic deficit.

Self-help and support groups for patients with chronic illness are common. Refer the patient and family to these groups, if indicated. For example, the Guillain-Barré Syndrome Foundation International (www.gbs-cidp.org) provides resources and information for patients and their families. The psychosocial adjustment needed may be minimal or dramatic, depending on the patient's residual deficit, age, gender, usual roles and responsibilities, usual coping strategies, available support systems, and occupation. Help the patient identify other support systems, such as church members, friends, or spiritual resources.

❓ CLINICAL JUDGMENT CHALLENGE

Patient-Centered Care; Safety QSEN

A female patient is admitted to the critical care unit with Guillain-Barré syndrome. She has ascending paralysis to the level of the waist.
1. What is the priority for this patient's care?
2. What health teaching will you provide for this patient about her disease?
3. What options for treatment will she have during this acute phase?
4. What other care will you include in your health teaching?

MYASTHENIA GRAVIS

❖ PATHOPHYSIOLOGY

Myasthenia gravis (MG) is an acquired autoimmune disease characterized by muscle weakness. There are two types of MG: ocular and generalized. About two thirds of patients initially present with reports about vision that arise from disturbances of the ocular muscles. MG may take many forms—from mild disturbances of the cranial and peripheral motor neurons to a rapidly developing, generalized weakness that may lead to death from respiratory failure. MG can present at any age, and the incidence is slightly higher among men. It is a progressive disease.

MG is caused by distorted acetylcholine receptors (AChRs) in the muscle motor end plate membranes. Antibodies are attached to the AChRs. As a result, nerve impulses are reduced at the neuromuscular junction; nerve impulses do not result in muscle contraction. MG and hyperplasia (abnormal growth) of the thymus gland are related because **thymoma** (encapsulated thymus gland tumor) occurs in a few cases.

There are five main classes and several subclasses of MG (Liang & Han, 2013):

- Class I: Any ocular muscle weakness; may have weakness of eye closure; all other muscle strength is normal
- Class II: Mild weakness affecting other than ocular muscles; may also have ocular muscle weakness of any severity:
  - Class IIa: Predominantly affecting limb, axial muscles, or both; may also have lesser involvement of oropharyngeal muscles
  - Class IIb: Predominantly affecting oropharyngeal, respiratory muscles, or both; may also have lesser or equal involvement of limb, axial muscles, or both
- Class III: Moderate weakness affecting other than ocular muscles; may also have ocular weakness of any severity:
  - Class IIIb: Predominantly affecting oropharyngeal, respiratory muscles, or both; may also have lesser or equal involvement of limb, axial muscles, or both;
- Class IV: Severe weakness affecting other than ocular muscles; may also have ocular muscle weakness of any severity:
  - Class IVa: Predominantly affecting limb, axial muscles, or both; may also have lesser involvement of oropharyngeal muscles

- Class IVb: Predominantly affecting oropharyngeal, respiratory muscles, or both; may also have lesser or equal involvement of limb, axial muscles, or both; use of a feeding tube to avoid aspiration and maintain nutrition
- Class V: Defined by the need for intubation, with or without mechanical ventilation, except when used during routine postoperative management

❖ PATIENT-CENTERED COLLABORATIVE CARE

◆ Assessment

Physical Assessment/Clinical Manifestations. In addition to the biographic data and history, ask the patient about specific muscle weakness (Abbott, 2010). Although the onset of MG is usually insidious (slow), some instances of fairly rapid development have been caused by infection, pregnancy, or anesthesia. A temporary increase in weakness may be noted after vaccination, menstruation, and exposure to extremes in environmental temperature. The course of the disease may have periods of exacerbation or flares when symptoms worsen. Ask the patient when symptoms worsen, specifically noting the affected muscle groups and any limitation or inability in performing ADLs. Anticipate worsening symptoms with repetitive muscle use. Determine the reason for admission to plan care. Patients with MG are typically hospitalized for diagnostic evaluation, myasthenic or cholinergic crisis resulting in respiratory failure, or periods of exacerbation when GAS EXCHANGE is threatened.

Additional areas of inquiry include any history of **ptosis** (drooping eyelids), **diplopia** (double vision), or **dysphagia** (difficulty chewing or swallowing) and the type of diet best tolerated. Assess the patient about a history of respiratory difficulty, choking, or voice weakness. Other areas of assessment include asking about any difficulty holding up the head, brushing teeth, combing hair, or shaving. Assess for the presence of paresthesias or aching in weakened muscles. Finally, ask about a history of thymus gland tumor. The most common symptoms of MG are related to involvement of the levator palpebrae or extraocular muscles (Chart 44-3). These symptoms may last only a few days at the onset and then resolve, only to return weeks or months later. Pupillary responses to light and accommodation are usually normal.

For most patients, the muscles of facial expression, chewing, and speech are affected (**bulbar** involvement). Note the patient's smile, which may be transformed into a snarl. The jaw may hang so that the patient must prop it up with the hand. Chewing and swallowing difficulties, choking, and regurgitation of fluids through the nose may lead to considerable weight loss. Ask about the patient's nutritional intake and any recent weight loss. He or she may have more difficulty eating after talking. After extended conversations, the voice may become weaker or exhibit a nasal twang. In some patients, the tongue has fissures (ulcers).

Less often involved are the muscles of the shoulders, the flexors of the neck, and the hip flexors. Because limb weakness is more often *proximal* (closer to the body), the patient may have difficulty climbing stairs, lifting heavy objects, or raising the arms overhead. Neck weakness may be mild or severe enough to cause difficulty in holding the head erect. Among the trunk muscles, the erector spinae are most commonly affected, causing difficulty maintaining a sitting or walking posture.

In the most advanced cases of MG, all muscles are weakened, including those associated with respiratory function and the control of bladder and bowel. In these severe cases, ask about bowel and bladder function. Assess respiratory rate, depth, pattern, and Spo_2 frequently to ensure adequate GAS EXCHANGE.

Muscle atrophy, although rarely severe, occurs in a small percentage of patients with MG. The tendon reflexes should be assessed, but they are not often affected. Assess for pain, although this is seldom a major concern. Some patients report that their weakened muscles ache. If present, paresthesias (painful tingling sensations) affecting the muscles of the face, hands, and thighs are not associated with any loss of sensation. Lost or decreased sensations of smell and taste have been reported. Consciousness is not altered.

In **Eaton-Lambert syndrome**, a form of myasthenia often seen with small cell carcinoma of the lung, the muscles of the trunk and the pelvic and shoulder girdles are most commonly affected. Although weakness increases after exertion, muscle strength may temporarily increase during the first few contractions, followed by rapid decline. Diagnosis is confirmed by electromyography (EMG). Management differs somewhat from that of other types of MG. Treatment includes removing the tumor, managing the cancer, and administering drug therapy to release acetylcholine (ACh). Additional therapies may include plasmapheresis and immunosuppressive therapy (discussed later).

Diagnostic Assessment. Because the incidence of MG is rare, diagnosis may be delayed or missed (Abbott, 2010). An experienced clinician can diagnose the disease from the history and physical examination findings. MG may be immediately confirmed by the patient's response to cholinergic drugs. A standard series of laboratory studies is usually performed for patients with known or suspected MG. *Thyroid function* should be tested because **thyrotoxicosis** (excessive thyroid hormone) is present in a small number of myasthenic patients. *Serum protein electrophoresis* evaluates the patient for immunologic disorders. Immunologic-based diseases, such as rheumatoid arthritis, systemic lupus erythematous, and polymyositis, may be associated with the disease (Pagana & Pagana, 2014).

Several types of antibodies are found in the majority of patients with MG and include forms directed against the acetylcholine receptor (AChR) and the enzyme *muscle-specific receptor tyrosine kinase* (MuSK). However, whereas a positive antibody test confirms the diagnosis, a negative finding does not rule out the disease.

Some patients with MG have a thymoma, and therefore patients are assessed for this condition. The thymus, an H-shaped gland located in the upper mediastinum beneath the

---

CHART 44-3   Key Features

Myasthenia Gravis

Motor Manifestations
- Progressive (proximal) muscle weakness that worsens with repetitive use and usually improves with rest
- Poor posture
- Ocular palsies
- Ptosis; incomplete eyelid closure
- Diplopia
- Respiratory compromise
- Loss of bowel and bladder control
- Fatigue

Sensory Manifestations
- Muscle achiness
- Paresthesias
- Decreased sense of smell and taste

sternum, is where B- and T-cells interact, refining self-recognition of these white blood cells. It is hypothesized that thymic abnormalities cause the breakdown in tolerance that causes the immune-mediated attack on AChR in myasthenia gravis. A thymoma can be seen on a chest *x-ray* or a *CT scan*.

The most common electrodiagnostic test performed to detect MG is *repetitive nerve stimulation (RNS)* of proximal nerves. Each nerve studied is electrically stimulated 6 to 10 times at 2 or 3 Hertz. The compound muscle action potential (CMAP) is recorded with surface electrodes over muscle. In MG, there is a progressive decline in CMAP amplitude (force, or strength) with the first 4 or 5 stimuli. This test diagnoses most cases of generalized MG but far fewer cases of ocular MG.

During *electromyography* (EMG) to diagnose MG, a recording electrode is placed into skeletal muscle and the electrical activity of skeletal muscle can be monitored in a way similar to electrocardiography (ECG) (Pagana & Pagana, 2014). A progressive decrease in the amplitude of the electrical waveform is a classic sign of MG. This study can be combined with nerve conduction studies and may be called an *electromyoneurography*. It can be performed at the bedside by a technician.

Single-fiber EMG (SFEMG) is a newer and most sensitive form of electromyography in detecting defects of neuromuscular transmission. This test compares the stability of the firing of one muscle fiber with that of another fiber innervated by the same motor neuron. The time interval between the two firings normally shows a minor degree of variability, called *jitter*. Defective transmission increases jitter or actually blocks successive discharges. This test can diagnose almost all cases of generalized and ocular MG.

Pharmacologic tests with the cholinesterase inhibitors *edrophonium chloride (Tensilon)* and *neostigmine bromide (Prostigmin)* may be performed. This older test is often referred to as a *Tensilon challenge test*. Tensilon is used most often for testing because of its rapid onset and brief duration of action. This drug inhibits the breakdown of ACh at the postsynaptic membrane, which increases the availability of ACh for excitation of postsynaptic receptors. To perform the test, the health care provider first estimates the strength of cranial muscles. Initially, 2 mg (0.2 mL) is injected IV; if this is tolerated, an additional 8 mg (0.8 mL) is injected after 30 seconds. Within 30 to 60 seconds of the first dose, most myasthenic patients show a marked improvement in muscle tone that lasts 4 to 5 minutes. False-positive test results may be caused by increased muscle effort by the patient. False-negative findings may be seen if the tested muscle is extremely weak or refractory to the drug.

Tensilon testing may be used also to help determine whether increasing weakness in the previously diagnosed myasthenic patient is due to a cholinergic crisis (too much cholinesterase inhibitor drugs) or a myasthenic crisis (too little cholinesterase inhibitor drugs). In a cholinergic crisis, muscle tone does not improve after giving Tensilon. Instead, weakness may actually increase, and fasciculations (muscle twitching) may be seen around the eyes and face.

! **NURSING SAFETY PRIORITY** (QSEN)

Drug Alert

The Tensilon test can cause cardiac dysrhythmias and cardiac arrest, but these reactions rarely occur. Be sure that atropine sulfate, the antidote for Tensilon, is available in case these complications occur.

◆ *Interventions*

MG is one of the most treatable neurologic disorders. The classic presentation of MG is muscle weakness that increases when the patient is fatigued and limits his or her MOBILITY and ability to participate in activities. Management for this disease falls into two categories:

- Treatment that affects the symptoms of MG without influencing the actual course of the disease (anticholinesterases or cholinergic drugs)
- Therapeutic efforts for inducing remission, such as the administration of immunosuppressive drugs or corticosteroids, plasmapheresis, and thymectomy (removal of the thymus gland)

Nonsurgical Management. Although not all patients with MG have respiratory compromise, ongoing assessment and maintenance of respiratory gas exchange are nursing care priorities.

Providing Respiratory Support. Both myasthenic crisis and cholinergic crisis increase muscle weakness and the patient's risk for respiratory compromise. The diaphragm and intercostal muscles may be affected, which inhibits the patient's ability to maintain adequate GAS EXCHANGE, breathe deeply, and cough effectively. In addition, dysphagia may result in the aspiration of foods, fluids, or saliva, which worsens the respiratory problems. Because of their respiratory muscle involvement, many of these patients have an increased risk for lung infections.

The patient who cannot cough effectively may require oropharyngeal or nasopharyngeal suctioning. If needed, teach the assisted-cough technique, similar to that used by patients who are quadriplegic. Collaborate with the respiratory therapist (RT) to provide chest physiotherapy consisting of postural drainage, percussion, and vibration to mobilize secretions and improve GAS EXCHANGE.

! **NURSING SAFETY PRIORITY** (QSEN)

Critical Rescue

Keep a bag-valve-mask setup (e.g., Ambu), equipment for oxygen administration, and suction equipment at the bedside of the patient with myasthenia gravis in case of respiratory distress.

Because breathing difficulty or the inability to breathe easily is frightening, be aware of the patient's mental and emotional status during periods of respiratory compromise. Monitor his or her response to drug therapy for muscle weakness. Monitor for pulmonary congestion that can lead to respiratory complications like pneumonia and atelectasis.

Noninvasive mechanical ventilation (NIMV) can be used to support patients with acute respiratory failure from MG crisis while awaiting improvement from IV immunoglobulin (IVIG) therapy or plasma exchange. Chapter 32 explains further about NIMV.

Promoting Mobility. Assess the patient's muscle strength before and after periods of activity. Provide assistance as necessary to prevent the patient from becoming fatigued. Schedule him or her for tests, treatments, and other activities early in the day or during the energy peaks after giving the prescribed drugs. Assist the patient in planning the periods of rest.

During periods of maximum weakness, provide assistance with positioning and activity. Assess for skin breakdown with each repositioning intervention. Pressure-reducing devices or mattresses are used to help prevent pressure ulcers. Collaborate with the physical and occupational therapists to develop a program for the patient to assist with MOBILITY, self-care, and energy conservation techniques. Chapter 6 discusses rehabilitation as one strategy to improve functional ability after a period of immobility, and Chapter 25 describes strategies to prevent and manage pressure ulcers.

Administering Drug Therapy. Two groups of drugs are typically prescribed for the treatment of myasthenia gravis (MG): anticholinesterases and immunosuppressants. Be sure to *give these drugs on time to maintain blood levels and thus improve muscle strength.* Monitor and document the patient's response to drug therapy. Provide information for the patient and the family about the indications for, effectiveness of, and side effects of the drugs used in the treatment of MG.

Cholinesterase Inhibitor Drugs. Cholinesterase (ChE) inhibitor drugs are the first-line management of MG. These drugs are also referred to as *anticholinesterase drugs* or *antimyasthenics.* They enhance neuromuscular impulse transmission by preventing the decrease of ACh by the enzyme *ChE.* This increases the response of the muscles to nerve impulses and improves muscle strength. The ChE inhibitor drug of choice is pyridostigmine (Mestinon, Regonol). Expect a day-to-day variation in dosage depending on the patient's changing symptoms.

Administer ChE inhibitors with a small amount of food to help alleviate GI side effects.

⚠ NURSING SAFETY PRIORITY (QSEN)

Drug Alert

Instruct the patient to eat meals 45 minutes to 1 hour after taking ChE inhibitors to avoid aspiration. This is especially important if the patient has bulbar involvement. Drugs containing magnesium, morphine or its derivatives, curare, quinine, quinidine, procainamide, or hypnotics or sedatives should be avoided because they may increase the patient's weakness. Antibiotics such as neomycin and certain tetracyclines impair transmitter release and also increase myasthenic symptoms (Lilley et al., 2014).

A potential adverse effect of ChE inhibitors is cholinergic crisis. Sudden increases in weakness accompanied by hypersalivation, sweating, and increased bronchial secretions help identify this as a cholinergic crisis rather than a myasthenic crisis. A cholinergic crisis is more likely to be associated with nausea, vomiting, and diarrhea. Teach the patient and family to monitor for these two types of crises:

1. Myasthenic crisis—an exacerbation (flare-up or worsening) of the myasthenic symptoms caused by not enough anticholinesterase drugs
2. Cholinergic crisis—an acute exacerbation of muscle weakness caused by too many anticholinesterase drugs

Because myasthenic and cholinergic crises have many common characteristics, the type of crisis the patient is experiencing must be identified for effective treatment to be provided (Table 44-1). Monitor carefully for early detection of these emergencies if the patient is in a health care setting.

Emergency Care: Myasthenic Crisis. Myasthenic crisis is often caused by some type of infection. For other patients, increasing muscle weakness leads to an overdose of anticholinesterase drugs. As a result, the patient may experience a *mixed* crisis. The Tensilon test (described on p. 919), although not always conclusive, is an important procedure for differentiation. *Tensilon*

TABLE 44-1   Characteristics of Myasthenic and Cholinergic Crises

MYASTHENIC CRISIS	CHOLINERGIC CRISIS	FEATURES COMMON TO BOTH
Increased pulse and respiration	Flaccid paralysis	Apprehension
Rise in blood pressure	Hypersecretion: salivation, tearing, and sweating	Restlessness
Bowel and bladder incontinence	Nausea	Dyspnea
Decreased urine output	Vomiting	Dysphagia (difficult swallowing)
Absence of cough and swallow reflex	Diarrhea	Generalized weakness
Improvement of symptoms with Tensilon test*	Abdominal cramps	Respiratory failure
	Miosis, blurred vision	
	Pallor	
	Worsening of symptoms with Tensilon test	

*Tensilon test: Edrophonium (Tensilon) is given intravenously; muscle movement improves immediately in patients with myasthenia or myasthenia crisis.

produces a temporary improvement in myasthenic crisis but worsening or no improvement of symptoms in cholinergic crisis.

The priority for nursing management of the patient in myasthenic crisis is maintaining adequate respiratory function to promote GAS EXCHANGE. The acutely ill patient may need intensive nursing care for monitoring. He or she may require mechanical ventilation or other technologic support. Cholinesterase-inhibiting drugs are withheld because they increase respiratory secretions and are usually ineffective for the first few days after the crisis begins. Drug therapy is restarted gradually and at lower dosages.

Emergency Care: Cholinergic Crisis. In *cholinergic* crisis, do not give anticholinesterase drugs while the patient is maintained with mechanical ventilation. Atropine 1 mg IV may be given and repeated, if necessary. When atropine is prescribed, observe the patient carefully. Secretions can be thickened by the drug, which causes more difficulty with airway clearance and possibly the development of mucus plugs. Unless complications such as pneumonia or aspiration develop, the patient in crisis improves rapidly after the appropriate drugs have been given. Continue to provide assistance as necessary because he or she tires easily after minimal exertion.

Immunosuppressants. Immunosuppression may be accomplished with the use of corticosteroids, methotrexate, a chemotherapeutic agent, or rituximab, a biologic agent effective against B-cells (Diaz-Manera et al., 2012). B-cells are lymphocytes active in antibody formation (see Chapter 17). For ocular MG, corticosteroid treatment that does not cause significant systemic complications may significantly reduce the prevalence of generalized myasthenia gravis after 2 years on the drug. IV immunoglobulins (IVIGs) may also be used for acute disease management or as a long-term option for disease refractory to other treatment.

Other Interventions. Plasmapheresis is a method by which antibodies are removed from the plasma to decrease symptoms. This is used as short-term management of an exacerbation. Six exchanges occur over a 2-week period with follow-up exchanges weekly or monthly as needed, usually as an ambulatory care patient. Nursing management of the patient undergoing plasmapheresis is presented in the earlier discussion of Guillain-Barré syndrome, p. 915, and Chart 44-2.

Generalized weakness and fatigue affect the patient's ability to participate in ADLs. Impaired fine motor control and shoulder weakness, which results in difficulty raising the arms, can compound the problem. Self-care deficits may be complete or partial depending on the severity of the illness or the patient's response to drugs.

Assess the patient's ability to perform ADLs. Although he or she is encouraged to perform activities as independently as possible, assistance is provided as needed to avoid frustration and fatigue. *For maximizing independence and making attempts at self-management successful, plan activities to follow the administration of medication.* Monitor and document the patient's response to or tolerance of activity, providing periods of rest after an activity. *Rest is critical because repetitive movement can precipitate a crisis.* Occupational and physical therapists evaluate patients for assistive-adaptive devices. In collaboration with the nurse, they also teach the patient and family energy conservation techniques and ideas for making work and self-management easier after discharge from the hospital.

Weakness of the speech and facial muscles often results in dysarthric (slurred) and nasal speech. In collaboration with the speech-language pathologist (SLP), determine the patient's ability to communicate. Instruct the patient to speak slowly while attempting to lip-read. Repeat what the patient says to check that it is correct. Questions that can be answered with "yes" or "no" or by gestures may be used along with other communication systems such as eye blinking, notebook and pencil, computer, handheld mobile devices, and picture, letter, or word boards.

The patient with myasthenia gravis (MG) may have difficulty maintaining an adequate intake of food and fluid because the muscles needed for chewing and swallowing become weakened and tire easily. In collaboration with the dietitian, occupational therapist, and speech-language pathologist, evaluate the patient's nutritional status and his or her ability to receive adequate oral nutrition. High-calorie snacks are often well tolerated. Monitor the effectiveness of the nutrition program by recording the patient's calorie counts, intake and output, serum prealbumin levels, and daily weights (Chart 44-4). If he or she cannot swallow, a feeding tube may be used.

The patient's inability to completely close the eyes may lead to corneal abrasions and further decrease vision and comfort. During the day, apply artificial tears to keep the corneas moist and free from abrasion. A lubricant gel and shield may be applied to the eyes at bedtime to provide more extensive coverage. To help relieve diplopia, cover the eyes with a patch for 2 to 3 hours at a time, one eye at a time. At times, patients tape their eyes shut at night.

Surgical Management. For patients with MG, **thymectomy** (removal of the thymus gland) is usually performed early in the disease. The procedure is not always immediately effective. Those who have surgery within 2 years of the onset of myasthenic symptoms show the most improvement, but many patients do not experience a change in status despite thymectomy.

Provide routine preoperative care as discussed in Chapter 14. Because there is no way to predict whether remission or improvement will occur, it is important to avoid making promises but be optimistic. Immediately before surgery, pyridostigmine (Mestinon) may be given with a small amount of water to keep the patient stable during and after surgery. If steroids have been used, they are also given before surgery and are

---

CHART 44-4 Best Practice for Patient Safety & Quality Care (QSEN)

Improving Nutrition in Patients with Myasthenia Gravis

- Assess the patient's gag reflex and ability to chew and swallow.
- Provide frequent oral hygiene as needed.
- Collaborate with the dietitian, speech-language pathologist, and occupational therapist to plan and implement meals that the patient can eat and enjoy.
- Cut food into small bites or request a soft or edentulous diet, and encourage the patient to eat slowly.
- Observe the patient for choking, nasal regurgitation, and aspiration.
- Provide high-calorie snacks or supplements (e.g., puddings).
- Keep the head of the bed elevated during meals and for 30 to 60 minutes after the patient eats.
- Consider thickening liquids to avoid choking or aspiration.
- Monitor caloric and food intake.
- Weigh the patient daily.
- Monitor serum prealbumin levels.
- Administer anticholinesterase drugs as prescribed, usually 45 to 60 minutes before meals.

---

tapered during the postoperative period. Antibiotics are administered immediately before or during the surgery. Plasmapheresis may be used before and after surgery to decrease circulating antibodies.

One of two surgical approaches may be used: the transcervical incision (minimal access technique) or the sternal split. The *transcervical approach* is becoming more popular because it allows more rapid recovery with less discomfort after surgery, especially if done using the video-assisted thoracoscopic surgery (VATS) technique. However, this procedure is used only for patients who do not have a thymoma. Only a small dressing and an IV line are needed after surgery.

The older *sternal split* procedure is preferred when patients have a thymoma. It allows the surgeon to directly see the mediastinum and areas around the thymus. When thymoma is present, all surrounding involved structures (i.e., the pericardium, the innominate vein, a portion of the superior vena cava, and a portion of the lung) are removed. A single chest tube is placed in the anterior mediastinum. The patient is usually admitted to the critical care unit after surgery. Thymoma should be considered as a potentially malignant tumor requiring prolonged follow-up. The presence of myasthenic weakness can still complicate its management.

Although patients with adequate respiratory effort and GAS EXCHANGE may be extubated immediately after surgery, most require a gradual weaning from the ventilator. Prolonged ventilatory assistance is rare. *After the patient is extubated, pay special attention to respiratory status and maintaining a patent airway.* Encourage the patient to turn, breathe deeply 3 to 6 times every 15 to 30 minutes in the hours after extubation, and use incentive spirometry.

For the sternal surgical technique, provide chest tube care (see Chapter 32). Both surgical approaches require sterile technique for wound care. Observe the patient for signs of infection, such as increasing or purulent drainage; redness, warmth, or swelling around the wound; and elevated temperature. Patient and family teaching about follow-up care is needed before discharge from the hospital.

Critical Rescue

For the patient having a thymectomy, monitor respiratory effort and promote effective GAS EXCHANGE. Observe for signs of pneumothorax or hemothorax, including:
- Chest pain
- Sudden shortness of breath
- Diminished or delayed chest wall expansion
- Diminished or absent breath sounds
- Restlessness or a change in vital signs (decreasing blood pressure or a weak, rapid pulse)

If respiratory distress or symptoms of ineffective gas exchange occur, provide oxygen to the patient and raise the head of the bed to at least 45 degrees. Then report any of these signs and symptoms to the surgeon or Rapid Response Team immediately!

Community-Based Care

The patient with myasthenia gravis (MG) may be cared for in a variety of settings, including the home, long-term acute care facility, rehabilitation setting, or skilled nursing facility. The patient discharged from the hospital may require the assistance of a family member, home care nurse, physical therapist (PT), occupational therapist (OT), and/or home care aide.

Home Care Management. Patients with MG are often managed at home. Unless the patient requires new assistive devices, little preparation of the home setting is required. In collaboration with physical and occupational therapists, the case manager (CM) and nurse make certain that the necessary equipment has been delivered and properly installed. Teach the patient and family members how to use the equipment safely. If the patient becomes wheelchair dependent, the discharge planner, CM, or OT checks on any necessary modifications to the home (e.g., the installation of ramps or widening of doorways) that have been completed. Home health care can provide assistance in transitioning from acute to home care.

Self-Management Education. The patient and family need to know about the disease and the drugs used for treatment. Discuss the episodic nature of the disease, including factors that increase the risk for exacerbation, such as infection, stress, surgery, hard physical exercise, sedatives, and enemas or strong cathartics (Table 44-2). Teach the patient the importance of collaborating with the health care team to monitor muscle strength, ability to perform ADLs, and the need to evaluate and adjust drug therapy.

Stress the importance of lifestyle adaptations such as avoiding heat (e.g., sauna, hot tubs, sunbathing), crowds, overeating, erratic changes in sleep habits, or emotional extremes. Teach the signs of exacerbation, such as increased weakness, increased diplopia, ptosis, and problems with chewing or swallowing. Remind the patient to plan activities to allow for rest periods and to conserve energy.

Provide the drug regimen in a written format that includes the names, purposes, dosages, scheduled dosage times, and side effects of the drugs. Explain that the drugs are normally taken before activities such as eating, participating in sports, or working. Stress the importance of maintaining therapeutic blood levels by taking the medications on time and as prescribed and not missing or postponing doses (Chart 44-5). In addition, inform the patient of the side effects of anticholinesterase drugs and drugs that can worsen symptoms, such as corticosteroids, narcotics, antidysrhythmics, and antimalarials.

TABLE 44-2 Factors Precipitating or Worsening Myasthenia Gravis

• Various drugs, including:	• Rheumatoid arthritis
• Strong cathartics	• Alcohol
• Antidysrhythmics	• Hormonal changes
• Beta-blocking agents	• Stress
• Aminoglycosides and other antibiotics	• Infection
• Antirheumatic drugs	• Seasonal temperature changes
• Antispasmodics, including quinine	• Heat
• Antihistamines	• Surgery
• Opioids	• Enemas
• Phenytoin (Dilantin)	
• Antidepressants (tricyclics)	

CHART 44-5 Patient and Family Education: Preparing for Self-Management

Helpful Hints for Teaching Patients with Myasthenia Gravis About Drug Therapy

- Keep prescribed drugs and a glass of water at your bedside if you are weak in the morning.
- Wear a watch with an alarm function (or beeper) to remind you to take your drugs.
- Post your drug schedule so others know it.
- Plan strenuous activities, when possible, when the drug peaks.
- Keep a secure supply of drugs in your car or at work.
- Check with your health care provider before using any over-the-counter drugs.

Check with the pharmacist before starting or stopping drugs. In preparing the patient for discharge, explain the signs and symptoms of myasthenic and cholinergic crises and the need to contact the health care provider whenever either type of crisis is suspected.

Action Alert

Because respiratory compromise often occurs in myasthenic patients, encourage family members to learn resuscitation procedures. A manual resuscitation bag, suctioning equipment, and oxygen should be available in the home for patients susceptible to crises. Teach family members in the proper use of equipment.

The episodic and progressive nature of MG, the potential or actual loss of independence, and body image changes (e.g., the inability to smile) affect the patient's adjustment. During discharge planning, the CM considers factors such as age, gender, usual roles and responsibilities, available support systems, occupation, and financial status. Because the patient's and family's need for psychosocial adjustment may range from minimal to dramatic, the CM remains sensitive to their needs and provides information and support. Encourage family members or significant others to discuss their feelings with one another.

Health Care Resources. In collaboration with the health care provider, patient, and family, the staff nurse or CM may initiate referrals to home care agencies and to local self-help groups for people who have chronic illnesses and their families. The

Myasthenia Gravis Foundation (www.myasthenia.org) provides education and research programs and assistance with financial aid and community resources. Support groups are also available. Teach the patient the importance of obtaining and wearing a medical alert (MedicAlert) bracelet or necklace and to carry a medical alert identification card at all times.

PERIPHERAL NERVE TRAUMA

❖ PATHOPHYSIOLOGY

The peripheral nerves are subject to injuries associated with mechanical injury, vehicular crashes, sports, the injection of particular drugs, military conflicts or wars, and acts of violence (e.g., knife or gunshot wounds). Most commonly affected are the median, ulnar, and radial nerves of the arms and the peroneal, femoral, and sciatic nerves of the legs (Fig. 44-1). Specific mechanisms of injury to a peripheral nerve include:

- Partial or complete severance
- Contusion, stretching, constriction, or compression
- Ischemia
- Electrical, thermal, or radiation exposure

Six degrees of peripheral nerve injury can occur (Novak, 2012):

- First-degree nerve injury (neuropraxia) involves a temporary conduction block with demyelination of the nerve at the site of injury. EMG study results are normal above and below the level of injury, and no denervation muscle changes are present. Once the nerve has remyelinated at that area, complete recovery occurs. Recovery may take up to 12 weeks.
- Second-degree nerve injury (axonotmesis) results from a more severe trauma or compression. This causes degeneration distal to the level of injury and proximal axonal degeneration to at least the next node of Ranvier. In more severe traumatic injuries, the proximal degeneration may extend beyond the next node of Ranvier. EMG studies demonstrate denervation changes in the affected muscles. In cases of reinnervation, motor unit potentials (MUPs) are present. Axonal regeneration occurs at the rate of 1 mm/day or 1 inch/month and can be monitored by the physiatrist or physical therapist.
- Third-degree injury is more severe than a second-degree injury and causes degeneration. EMG studies demonstrate denervation changes with fibrillations in the affected muscles. In cases of reinnervation, MUPs are present. Regeneration occurs at 1 mm/day. However, with the increased severity of the injury, regenerating axons may not reinnervate their original motor and sensory targets. The pattern of recovery is mixed and incomplete. Reinnervation occurs only if sensory fibers grow into a different area within the nerve's sensory distribution. If

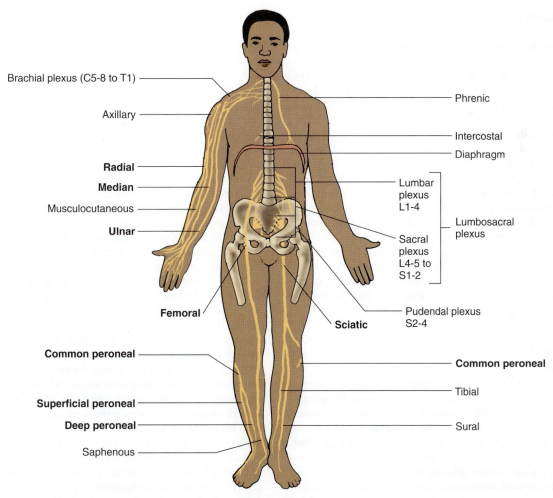

FIG. 44-1 Distribution of selected peripheral nerves in the body. The nerves most commonly affected by trauma are highlighted in bold type.

the muscle target is a long distance from the site of injury, nerve regeneration may occur. The muscle may not be completely reinnervated because of the long period of denervation.

- Fourth-degree injury results in a large scar at the site of nerve injury and prevents any axons from advancing distal to the level of nerve injury. EMG studies reveal denervation changes in the affected muscles. No improvement in motor function is noted, and the patient requires surgery to restore neural continuity, thus permitting axonal regeneration and motor and sensory reinnervation.
- Fifth-degree injury is a complete transection (cutting across) of the nerve. Similar to a fourth-degree injury, it requires surgery to restore neural continuity. EMG findings are the same as those for a fourth-degree injury.
- Sixth-degree injury describes a mixed nerve injury that combines the other degrees of injury. This commonly occurs when some fascicles of the nerve are working normally while other fascicles may be recovering. Other fascicles may require surgical intervention to permit axonal regeneration.

Injuries to the peripheral nerves may result in loss of motor function (reduced MOBILITY), sensory function (impaired SENSORY PERCEPTION), or both. After a nerve is cut or damaged, the nerve distal to the injury degenerates and retracts within 24 hours. Motor and sensory dysfunction below the injury coincides with the loss of electrical excitability. Recovery occurs as Schwann cells of the neurilemma regenerate from both the proximal and distal stumps. Dividing mitotically, these cells form neurilemmal cords, which act as guidelines for the regenerating axon. Tiny unmyelinated sprouts are generated at the proximal axon and grow daily. Some can cross a transected gap through guidance by the neurilemma and reattach to the distal stump. The better aligned the union, the more normal the physical functional ability return (Fig. 44-2). Reinnervation is always a slow process.

Successfully realigned nerves remyelinate, grow to their former size, and eventually have conduction velocities near their former capacity. Successful reinnervation is slowed by infection and increasing age. Disorganization of the nerve or mismatched realignments may result in functional weakness, unintentional muscle movements, and poor sensation.

Some SENSORY PERCEPTION may return before the regeneration process can occur. This return occurs because nerves above the injured neurons are stimulated to produce collateral innervation to the affected areas. These collaterals occur before the injured axon has regenerated sufficiently.

❖ PATIENT-CENTERED COLLABORATIVE CARE

◆ Assessment

The patient may relate a history of extremity or pelvic trauma, penetrating injury, recent surgery, or compression. Peripheral nerve trauma is especially common from combat-acquired injuries. In addition to weakness or flaccid *paralysis,* the patient may report *burning sensations* below the trauma or PAIN that increases with touch or environmental stimulation. Observe for skin and nail changes of the affected extremities.

Perform a physical assessment to determine physical function. In acute trauma, the injury should first be evaluated by the health care provider to determine whether movement is

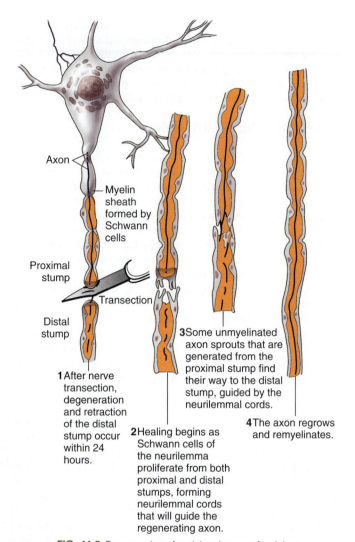

1 After nerve transection, degeneration and retraction of the distal stump occur within 24 hours.

2 Healing begins as Schwann cells of the neurilemma proliferate from both proximal and distal stumps, forming neurilemmal cords that will guide the regenerating axon.

3 Some unmyelinated axon sprouts that are generated from the proximal stump find their way to the distal stump, guided by the neurilemmal cords.

4 The axon regrows and remyelinates.

FIG. 44-2 Regeneration of peripheral nerve after injury.

contraindicated. If movement is not contraindicated, the patient's motor function is assessed by putting the limb through the normal range of motion. Any abnormal movements, tremor, atrophy, contractions, paresis or paralysis, and weak or absent deep tendon reflexes are documented. Ask the patient about abnormal sensations.

After complete denervation, the extent of vasomotor function is reflected in skin temperature, skin color, and edema. A warm phase and a cold phase have been identified. During the **warm phase,** the extremity is warm and the skin appears flushed or rosy. Over 2 to 3 weeks, this phase is gradually superseded by a **cold phase,** during which the skin appears cyanotic, mottled, or reddish blue and feels cool compared with the unaffected extremity. Use the dorsal surface of your hand to compare skin temperatures because the abundance of temperature receptors in this area provides more accurate assessments. Edema may be noted immediately after injury or later as a result of surgical procedures. Record any observations of trophic changes (e.g., scaling of skin, brittleness of nails, and loss of body hair). This initial assessment serves as the baseline for comparison during subsequent examinations, which are performed every 2 to 4 hours or less frequently as the patient's condition indicates.

◆ Interventions

Interventions for the patient with peripheral nerve trauma depend on the location as well as the type and degree of injury. If the nerve trauma results from a primary lesion, such as a tumor, the underlying problem is addressed first (Walsh, 2012).

The health care provider may prescribe immobilization of the involved area by splint, cast, or traction to provide the rest needed to limit and resolve any INFLAMMATION. The purpose of surgical management is to restore the function of the damaged nerve. There are usually no special preoperative interventions for the patient undergoing peripheral nerve repair. Chapter 14 describes the general care of the patient before surgery.

If the nerve is lacerated or transected, surgery may be indicated. Restorative procedures include resecting and suturing to realign the severed nerve ends, nerve grafts, and nerve and tendon transplants.

The timing of procedures to repair nerves has been controversial. In the past, a repair delay of 3 to 8 weeks after injury allowed associated injuries to heal, after which the surgeon could better assess the extent of nerve damage. Although microsurgery and the use of lasers now allow primary nerve repair at the time of injury, the surgeon's judgment in selecting the optimal time and surgical procedure remains crucial.

After an injury, the two severed nerve segments contract and may form scar tissue. Before surgical anastomosis, the surgeon dissects these stumps to remove any damaged nerve tissue. This further decreases the lengths of the ends to be joined. To compensate for this shortening and to avoid excessive tension on the sutured nerve, the involved extremity is positioned in exaggerated flexion. The surgeon aligns the segments under magnification, bringing the nerve fiber ends together, and then sutures the nerve tissue.

After suturing, the extremity is placed in a cast to maintain the flexed position and to avoid tension on the suture line. Ten to 14 days after nerve repair, the entire dressing is removed, the joint flexion is eased, and a new splint may be applied for an additional 2 weeks. At that time, a removable splint may be applied and physical therapy begun. Protection of the nerve sutures is continued for a minimum of 6 weeks.

If a large segment of nerve has been damaged and direct anastomosis would be impossible without stretching the nerve, the surgeon may insert a *nerve graft*. Motor and sensory axons may regenerate through the graft, joining the nerve segments through the two sites of anastomosis. The results of grafting are not usually as favorable as with direct anastomosis. Immobilization by splints or casts to facilitate healing of the surgical sites is essential.

Splints are usually held in place with elastic wrapping or hook-and-loop (Velcro) closures, which can become too tight if edema develops.

> ! **NURSING SAFETY PRIORITY** (QSEN)
>
> ### Critical Rescue
>
> Perform frequent neurovascular assessments after surgical nerve repair, including checking the skin around the splints and casts (hourly, initially) for tightness, warmth, and color. If the patient reports discomfort, tingling, or coolness or if the color is blanched, the cast or splint may be too tight (constricted). *Inform the health care provider immediately about constriction and any indication of drainage under a splint or cast!*

Skin care is essential. Atrophy of the epidermis and underlying tissue causes the skin to become more fragile and more susceptible to injury and breakdown. Decreased skin nutrition and vascularity associated with denervation cause delayed healing, which further worsens the problem. Thoroughly examine the skin for signs of irritation or injury, and assist or instruct the patient to wash and dry the involved areas carefully. If the skin is dry, lanolin or cocoa butter may be used as a lubricant. *Because sensation may be absent or inhibited, teach the patient to protect the involved areas from temperature extremes and other sources of potential trauma.*

Physical or occupational therapy is the major approach for rehabilitation after surgical repair. Reinforce and help the patient perform the exercises learned in these therapy sessions. Because the regeneration of nerves and subsequent return of sensory and motor function may be extremely slow and produce PAIN, the patient may become discouraged and depressed. If the disability is permanent, he or she needs encouragement and assistance to cope with the changes in body image, self-esteem, and lifestyle.

RESTLESS LEGS SYNDROME

❖ PATHOPHYSIOLOGY

Restless legs syndrome (RLS) is characterized by leg paresthesias (burning, prickly sensation) associated with an irresistible urge to move. Over 10% of the population in the United States have the problem, and women are affected twice as often as men (National Institute of Neurological Disorders and Stroke, 2013a). RLS occurs most often in middle-aged and older adults. Stress can exacerbate this condition. RLS is related to a dysfunction in the brain circuits that use the neurotransmitter *dopamine*. Many of those affected with *primary RLS* have a positive family history, indicating a possible genetic basis. The incidence is higher in patients who have diabetes mellitus type 2; chronic kidney disease; iron deficiency; Parkinson disease; peripheral neuropathy; use of certain medications such as caffeine, calcium channel blockers, lithium, or neuroleptics; and withdrawal from sedatives. Although not a cause of hospitalization, restless leg syndrome may be a comorbidity that complicates recovery from other conditions.

❖ PATIENT-CENTERED COLLABORATIVE CARE

◆ Assessment

The patient reports intense burning or "crawling-type" sensations in the legs and therefore feels the need to move them repeatedly. These symptoms are worse in the evening and at night and when the patient is still for a period of time. Patients feel they need to move to relieve the symptoms. Many move their legs periodically while sleeping. For that reason, they often refer to themselves as "night walkers."

◆ Interventions

The management of RLS is symptomatic and involves treating the underlying cause or contributing factor, if known. Both nonpharmacologic measures and drug therapy are used. Teach patients to avoid as many risk factors as possible or make lifestyle modifications. Examples are avoiding caffeine and alcohol, quitting smoking, losing weight, and exercising.

Strategies to relieve the symptoms of RLS include walking, stretching, moderate exercise, or a warm bath. Refer them to

The Restless Legs Foundation (www.rls.org) as an excellent resource for information and patient and family support.

Many of the drugs prescribed for RLS are also used for either Parkinson disease (PD) or epilepsy. *Dopamine agonists* such as pramipexole (Mirapex) and ropinirole (Requip) are oral drugs used extensively. Gabapentin enacarbil (Horizant) is an *antiepileptic drug (AED)* that is also approved by the U.S. Food and Drug Administration (FDA) for RLS. These agents are usually taken at bedtime because they may cause daytime sleepiness. Teach patients to be cautious of driving or operating heavy equipment when taking these drugs (Silber, 2013). Correcting iron and magnesium deficiencies can reduce RLS symptoms, and ongoing supplementation of these minerals may be needed.

Some patients have had success with *Sinemet,* a combination of levodopa and carbidopa. This drug is often given with other medications to be more effective in reducing the symptoms of the disease. Other classes of drugs for managing RLS include *benzodiazepines, such as diazepam (Valium), and opioids* as a last resort. Two other AEDs, carbamazepine (Tegretol) and gabapentin (Neurontin), have been particularly effective and are taken in divided doses throughout the day. For insomnia from RLS, *melatonin* may be effective for many people, especially older adults. However, the focus of treatment should be on RLS, not insomnia. Teach patients to inform their health care providers when adding these supplements.

DISEASES OF THE CRANIAL NERVES

Patients with cranial nerve disease may be seen in any practice setting. The cranial nerves may be affected in association with other disorders of the nervous system or as a result of trauma. The most common disorders, those affecting cranial nerves V (trigeminal) and VII (facial), are discussed here.

TRIGEMINAL NEURALGIA
❖ PATHOPHYSIOLOGY

Trigeminal neuralgia (TN) is also known as *tic douloureux.* The trigeminal nerve has three branches: the first branch controls sensation in a person's eye, upper eyelid, and forehead; the second branch controls sensation in the lower eyelid, cheek, nostril, upper lip, and upper gum; and the third branch controls sensations in the jaw, lower lip, lower gum, and some of the muscles used for chewing.

According to the National Institute of Neurological Disorders and Stroke (2013b), trigeminal neuralgia has these characteristics:

- Affects the trigeminal (fifth cranial) nerve
- Occurs more often in people older than 50 years and in women more often than men
- Causes a specific type of facial pain, which occurs in sudden, intense facial spasms
- Is usually provoked by minimal stimulation of a trigger zone (like dental procedures)
- Is unilateral (one-sided) and confined to the area innervated by the trigeminal nerve, most often the second and third branches (Fig. 44-3)
- Is familial due to an inherited pattern of blood vessel formation

The cause of trigeminal neuralgia is thought to be related to impaired inhibitory mechanisms in the brainstem caused by excessive firing of irritated fibers in the trigeminal nerve.

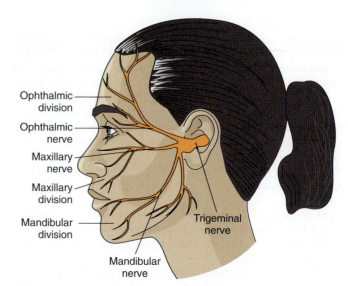

FIG. 44-3 Distribution of the trigeminal nerve and its three divisions: ophthalmic, maxillary, and mandibular.

Labels: Ophthalmic division; Ophthalmic nerve; Maxillary nerve; Maxillary division; Mandibular division; Mandibular nerve; Trigeminal nerve

Trauma and infection of the teeth, jaw, or ear may be contributing factors. Patients younger than 30 years with pain in more than one branch of the trigeminal nerve may be further evaluated to rule out the possibility of a tumor or multiple sclerosis.

❖ PATIENT-CENTERED COLLABORATIVE CARE
◆ Assessment

TN is a chronic PAIN syndrome. It can be categorized into two types of pain: classic and atypical. When describing trigeminal pain, patients use terms such as "excruciating," "sharp," "shooting," "piercing," "burning," and "jabbing." Atypical pain descriptions may include migraine-like headache. Between bursts of pain, which last from seconds to minutes, there is usually no pain. Often no sensory or motor deficits are found on examination. Pain can be initiated by light touch, a change in facial expression (e.g., smiling), or chewing. The fear of precipitating agonizing attacks often causes patients to avoid talking, smiling, eating, or attending to hygienic needs such as shaving, washing the face, and brushing the teeth. The pain can cause uncontrollable facial twitching. The course of TN involves bouts of classic pain for several weeks or months followed by spontaneous remissions. The length of these remissions may vary from days to years, but attack-free periods tend to become shorter as the patient grows older.

The patient suspected of TN usually has a CT scan and MRI to determine whether there is a reversible cause of trigeminal compression or INFLAMMATION. The diagnosis is made based on patient history and the results of these imaging tests.

◆ Interventions

The priority for care of the patient with TN is pain management. Specific interventions are determined by the amount of pain he or she is experiencing. Drug therapy is the first choice, but surgery can provide satisfactory pain relief in patients who do not respond to drug management or who experience profound adverse drug reactions (Ibrahim, 2012).

Drug Therapy and Radiosurgery. The first choice for drug therapy is carbamazepine (CBZ, Tegretol), an antiepileptic drug

(AED) (Ibrahim, 2012). Other drugs, such as gabapentin (Neurontin), pregabalin (Lyrica), and baclofen (Lioresal, Kemstro), a muscle relaxant, may be used. Some patients also achieve pain relief with complementary therapies, such as acupuncture (Lui et al., 2010).

Microvascular decompression, radiosurgery techniques such as a peripheral chemical nerve block with ropivacaine, or stereotactic radiation treatments with the Gamma Knife are surgical approaches to disrupt trigeminal neuralgia. These minimally invasive procedures prevent the complications of major surgery. Surgical interventions are often combined with drug therapy for pain management of this challenging condition.

In some cases, a **percutaneous stereotactic rhizotomy (PSR)** is performed as an ambulatory care procedure under general anesthesia. The surgeon passes a hollow needle through the inside of the patient's cheek into the trigeminal nerve fibers. A heating current (radiofrequency thermocoagulation) goes through the needle to destroy some of the fibers. As an option to heat, a balloon microcompression of the trigeminal nerve root may be performed. A glycerol injection may also be used as an option, but it is not done as commonly as thermocoagulation.

The entire nerve is not destroyed. The advantages of this procedure include long-term pain relief, absence of facial paralysis, and preservation of the sensation of touch. Puncturing the internal carotid artery is a possible complication. The affected side is permanently insensitive to pain.

After the PSR procedure, apply an ice pack to the PSR operative site on the cheek and jaw for 3 to 4 hours. Perform a focused cranial nerve assessment to assess whether other nerves have been damaged (e.g., facial nerve). Discourage the patient from chewing on the affected side until paresthesias resolve. A soft diet is usually prescribed.

> ### ⚠ NURSING SAFETY PRIORITY (QSEN)
> **Action Alert**
>
> Teach the patient who has had percutaneous stereotactic rhizotomy to avoid rubbing the eye on the affected side because the protective mechanism of pain will no longer warn of injury. Instruct him or her to inspect the eye daily for redness or irritation and report to the health care provider any change or blurred vision. Stress the importance of regular dental examinations because the absence of pain may not warn the patient of potential problems.

Surgical Management. In addition to the general preoperative care provided to all patients, the surgeon thoroughly explains the surgical benefits and any expected neurologic deficits. Ensure that the patient understands the procedure to be performed and any risks or complications.

In some patients, a small artery compresses the trigeminal nerve as it enters the pons. Surgical relocation of this artery (**microvascular decompression**) may relieve the pain of TN without compromising facial sensation. This procedure is more invasive, requiring a craniotomy. Though not common, complications include aseptic meningitis, cerebrospinal fluid leak, ataxia, **ipsilateral** (same side) hearing loss, and facial nerve damage. Older adults and patients with other medical problems may not be candidates for this procedure.

In addition to general post-craniotomy care for patients as described in Chapter 45, monitor the patient who has microvascular decompression for signs of complications including headache, cranial nerve dysfunction, and bleeding. Assess his or her corneal reflex, extraocular muscles, and facial nerve, and report abnormal findings to the surgeon. Document all changes promptly.

Psychosocial considerations for the patient with trigeminal neuralgia include disappointment with ineffective drug protocols or surgical procedures, as well as the fear that the pain may recur with any activity. The patient may fail to move the face in an attempt to prevent pain. This behavior may be misinterpreted by others as withdrawal or depression. Refer patients and their families to the TNA—Facial Pain Association (www.fpa-support.org) for more information and support. TNA of Canada (www.catna.ca) is the national organization in Canada that advocates and informs patients and their families about trigeminal neuralgia.

FACIAL PARALYSIS

❖ *PATHOPHYSIOLOGY*

Facial paralysis, or **Bell's palsy**, is an acute paralysis of cranial nerve VII but may also affect cranial nerves V (trigeminal) and VIII (vestibulocochlear [auditory]). The condition is also known as *cranial polyneuritis*. Although the incidence may be slightly higher among people with diabetes, Bell's palsy occurs in all ages; however, it is more commonly seen in young adults.

Acute maximum paralysis occurs over 2 to 5 days in almost all patients with this condition. PAIN behind the ear or on the face may occur a few hours or even days before paralysis. The disorder involves a drawing sensation and paralysis of all facial muscles on the affected side. The patient cannot close his or her eye, wrinkle the forehead, smile, whistle, or grimace. Tearing may stop or become excessive. The face appears masklike and sags. Taste is usually impaired to some degree, but this symptom seldom persists beyond the second week of paralysis. Tinnitus (ringing in the ears) may also occur. Most patients go into remission within 3 months.

The cause of Bell's palsy is believed to be the result of INFLAMMATION triggered by a formerly dormant herpes simplex virus type 1 (HSV-1). Infection, immunosuppression, or exposure to cold may trigger the HSV-1 re-activation. Patients are rarely hospitalized, but the nurse may encounter them in clinics, office settings, or emergency departments.

❖ *PATIENT-CENTERED COLLABORATIVE CARE*

Medical management usually includes corticosteroids, 30 to 60 mg daily, during the first week after the onset of symptoms. Antiviral drugs such as acyclovir (Zovirax), famciclovir (Famvir), or valacyclovir (Valtrex) may be prescribed for 7 to 10 days after symptoms begin. Mild analgesics may help relieve the PAIN. Nursing care is directed toward managing the major neurologic deficits and providing psychosocial support. Because the eye does not close, the cornea must be protected from drying and subsequent ulceration or abrasion. Teach the patient to manually close the eyelid at intervals and to instill artificial tears during the day. An ointment to supply moisture can be used at night. The eye may be patched or taped closed at bedtime.

The patient may be unable to chew, sip fluids through a straw, or control drooling on the affected side, creating difficulties at mealtimes. Encourage the patient to eat and drink using the unaffected side of the mouth. High-calorie snacks may supplement meals, and patients may require a soft diet. Explain how to use massage; the application of warm, moist heat; and facial exercises to manage pain and paralysis. In some cases, physical therapy is prescribed. As muscle tone improves, teach the patient to grimace, wrinkle the brow, force the eyes closed, whistle, and blow air out of the cheeks 3 or 4 times daily for 5 minutes.

Nerve block to manage pain may be performed, but it is not common. Surgery is reserved for patients with complete, severe Bell's palsy to decompress the facial nerve. In some cases, cosmetic surgery is done.

Although most patients recover fully within a few weeks or months, some may experience permanent neurologic deficits. For chronic PAIN, gabapentin (Neurontin) may be prescribed. Patients with Bell's palsy may require psychosocial support because body image and self-esteem are affected. Provide both information and psychosocial support. Refer patients and their families to the Bell's Palsy Research Foundation for information (www.angelfire/az/BellsPalsy.com). The Bell's Palsy Association in the United Kingdom is also a good source of web-based information (www.bellspalsy.org.uk).

> ### ❓ NCLEX EXAMINATION CHALLENGE
> #### *Safe and Effective Care Environment*
>
> The nurse is caring for a client with Bell's palsy. Which potential problem requires assessment by the nurse to ensure client safety?
> A. Risk for falls from balance impairment
> B. Risk for communication difficulties from impaired hearing
> C. Risk for eye ulceration or abrasion from inability to close eyelid
> D. Risk for adverse drug effects from pain management therapy

NURSING CONCEPTS AND CLINICAL JUDGMENT REVIEW

What might you NOTICE if a patient is experiencing impaired MOBILITY, altered SENSORY PERCEPTION, or PAIN as a result of acute or chronic peripheral nervous system disorders?

- Report of muscle weakness in face, arms, or legs
- Inability to swallow or clear the upper airway
- Changes in respiratory rate and pattern indicating respiratory compromise or failure
- Loss of sensation in face or extremities
- Report of burning, tingling sensations in face or extremities
- Report of pain in extremities or face
- Ptosis and either dry eye or excessive tearing

What should you INTERPRET and how should you RESPOND to a patient experiencing impaired MOBILITY, and/or SENSORY PERCEPTION, and/or PAIN as a result of peripheral nervous system disorders?

Perform and interpret physical assessment, including:
- Completing a neurologic assessment
- Assessing a patient's airway and breathing ability
- Performing a comprehensive pain assessment (see Chapter 3)

Respond by:
- Notifying health care provider or contacting Rapid Response Team if patient has problems with breathing or experiences a sudden change in neurologic status

- Establishing an airway and promoting ease in breathing (e.g., put patient in sitting position, provide oxygen, set up suction)
- Having emergency equipment like ventilator and tracheostomy set available for patient who has respiratory compromise
- Assisting with ADLs as needed
- Providing analgesics and other pain-relief measures

On what should you REFLECT as you assess and manage care for a patient with problems of the peripheral nervous system?
- Continue to observe patient for changes in functional ability and gas exchange.
- Consider multiple approaches to managing pain.
- Think about ways to promote independence in mobility and self-care.
- Think about health care team members with whom you will need to collaborate to improve mobility.
- Consider how to provide a safe environment for patients with decreased sensory perception.
- Develop a teaching plan for the patient and family for continuing care.

GET READY FOR THE NCLEX® EXAMINATION!

▌ KEY POINTS

Review these Key Points for each NCLEX Examination Client Needs Category.

Safe and Effective Care Environment
- Collaborate with members of the interdisciplinary team, including the health care provider, physical and occupational therapists, speech-language pathologist, and dietitian, to establish goals for care and individualized interventions for patients with Guillain-Barré syndrome (GBS) and myasthenia gravis (MG). **Teamwork and Collaboration** `QSEN`

Health Promotion and Maintenance
- Reinforce the need for patients with MG to take their drugs on time. **Safety** `QSEN`
- Assess patient response to drugs to control PAIN related to peripheral nerve conditions; opioids, AEDs, and antidepressants have the potential to cause significant adverse effects.
- Refer patients with peripheral nervous system (PNS) disorders to community support groups and health care organizations, such as The Restless Legs Syndrome Foundation and the Myasthenia Gravis Foundation.

Psychosocial Integrity

- Provide alternatives to promote communication for patients with GBS and MG, including speaking slowly, lip-reading, and using communication boards or electronic technology. **Patient-Centered Care** QSEN

Physiological Integrity

- Assess for changes related to GAS EXCHANGE and functional ability for patients with PNS disorders.
- Recall that patients with GBS have ascending paralysis, sensory changes, cranial nerve involvement, and autonomic manifestations as a result of demyelination of neurons (see Chart 44-1).
- Note that patients with MG have an autoimmune disease in which muscle weakness, including ocular symptoms, is the result of attacks on the acetylcholine receptors at neuromuscular junctions (see Chart 44-3).
- Teach patients about factors that can worsen (exacerbate) MG as listed in Table 44-2. **Evidence-Based Practice** QSEN
- Remember that the priority for care for patients with GBS and MG is respiratory monitoring and airway management. **Safety** QSEN

- Prevent complications of immobility for patients with GBS and MG, such as pressure ulcers and venous thromboembolic events.
- Teach patients on cholinesterase inhibitor drugs and their families about clinical manifestations of cholinergic and myasthenic crises as listed in Table 44-1. **Safety** QSEN
- For patients having a thymectomy, maintain adequate GAS EXCHANGE and observe for complications such as pneumothorax or hemothorax (e.g., chest pain, shortness of breath). **Evidence-Based Practice** QSEN
- Perform frequent neurovascular assessments for patients having a peripheral nerve repair.
- Teach patients with restless legs syndrome to minimize risk factors for the disorder, including exercising, losing weight, and quitting smoking. **Evidence-Based Practice** QSEN
- Recall that trigeminal neuralgia (TN) affects primarily the fifth cranial nerve (although others may be involved) and does not typically involve paralysis or changes in sensation other than excruciating pain along the cranial nerve tract. Facial paralysis (Bell's palsy) affects cranial nerve VII and involves unilateral facial muscle paralysis.
- Prioritize pain management for the care of the patient with TN. **Patient-Centered Care** QSEN

Care of Critically Ill Patients with Neurologic Problems

Chris Winkelman and Rachel L. Gallagher

 http://evolve.elsevier.com/Iggy/

PRIORITY CONCEPTS

- MOBILITY
- SENSORY PERCEPTION
- COGNITION
- PERFUSION

LEARNING OUTCOMES

Safe and Effective Care Environment

1. Prioritize airway, breathing, and circulation during the initial care of a patient with acute and critical neurologic illness to avoid complications from inadequate gas exchange or low PERFUSION
2. Explain the importance of collaborating with health care team members when planning and providing care for critically ill patients with neurologic problems.
3. Discuss strategies to provide safe, effective transitions in care following acute management of patients with a stroke, traumatic brain injury (TBI), or brain tumor.

Health Promotion and Maintenance

4. Develop a teaching plan about risk factors for having a stroke.
5. Describe strategies to prevent secondary brain injury.

Psychosocial Integrity

6. Discuss how to support the patient and family coping with life changes that result from stroke, TBI, or brain tumor.

Physiological Integrity

7. Perform a neurologic assessment of patients who are experiencing acute neurologic events of stroke, TBI, or cranial surgery, with a focus on changes in cognition, mobility, and SENSORY PERCEPTION.
8. Prioritize evidence-based care for a patient with acute neurologic changes indicating a stroke or TBI.
9. Assess the patient after fibrinolytic therapy for ischemic stroke for potential adverse effects.
10. Describe elements of care for common patient responses to acute stroke, TBI, or brain tumor.
11. Explain the role of chemotherapy, radiation, and surgery in the management of patients with a brain tumor.

Many acute neurologic problems are associated with high mortality and severe morbidity and create significant and enduring impact upon patients, their families, and the wider society. Early recognition and comprehensive care of adult patients with acute neurologic compromise by the nurse can reduce mortality and disability. Acute neurologic problems from stroke, brain trauma, and malignancy cause varying degrees of impaired MOBILITY, SENSORY PERCEPTION, COGNITION, and PERFUSION.

TRANSIENT ISCHEMIC ATTACK

Ischemic strokes often follow warning signs such as a **transient ischemic attack (TIA)**. Temporary neurologic dysfunction resulting from a *brief* interruption in cerebral blood flow is easy to ignore or miss, particularly if symptoms resolve by the time the patient reaches the emergency department (ED). Typically, symptoms of a TIA resolve within 30 to 60 minutes (Chart 45-1). TIAs may damage the brain tissue with repeated insults, as seen on MRI or CT scan. Single TIAs indicate a high stroke risk; recurrent and multiple TIAs increase the risk for permanent brain damage.

Upon admission to the ED, a complete neurologic assessment is performed and laboratory tests, electrocardiogram (ECG), and CT scan are performed. If no neurologic deficit is identified, the patient may be admitted for further diagnostic testing to evaluate the risk for stroke, including an MRI of carotid and cerebral blood vessels and brain tissue. Treatment focuses on preventing another TIA or stroke and may include:

- Reducing high blood pressure, the most common risk factor for stroke, by adding or adjusting drugs to lower blood pressure
- Taking aspirin or another antiplatelet drug (e.g., clopidogrel [Plavix]) to prevent strokes (Aw & Sharma, 2012)
- Controlling diabetes and keeping blood sugar levels in a target range, typically 100-180 mg/dL
- Promoting lifestyle changes such as quitting smoking, eating heart-healthy foods, and being more active

As part of the discharge processes to meet The Joint Commission's National Patient Safety Goals and Core Measures for Venous Thromboembolism (VTE), ensure that the patient taking antiplatelet drugs is aware of precautions and actions to

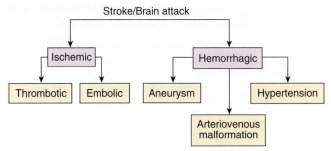

FIG. 45-1 Types of stroke/brain attack.

take if bleeding occurs. Anticoagulant therapy is discussed in detail in Chapter 36 under the VTE section. Reinforce the need to follow up with the health care provider and to complete any diagnostic tests requested on an ambulatory care basis.

STROKE (BRAIN ATTACK)

❖ PATHOPHYSIOLOGY

A **stroke** is caused by an interruption of PERFUSION to any part of the brain. The National Stroke Association uses the term **brain attack** to convey the urgency for acute stroke care similar to that provided for acute myocardial infarction. *A stroke is a medical emergency, and it should be treated immediately to reduce permanent disability.* About 14% of patients in hospitals in the United States have a stroke while in the hospital (Mink & Miller, 2011a).

Stroke is the third leading cause of death in the United States and is considered a major cause of disability worldwide. According to the Centers for Disease Control and Prevention (CDC), about 137,000 Americans die each year from stroke (CDC, 2013b) On average, one American dies from stroke every 4 minutes (CDC, 2013b).

Pathophysiologic Changes in the Brain

The brain cannot store oxygen or glucose and therefore must receive a constant flow of blood to provide these substances for normal function. In addition, blood flow is important for the removal of metabolic waste (e.g., carbon dioxide, lactic acid). If blood supply to any part of the brain is interrupted for more than a few minutes, cerebral tissue dies (**infarction**). The result is disability, depending on the location and amount of brain tissue affected. Brain metabolism and blood flow after a stroke are affected around the infarction as well as in the **contralateral** (opposite side) hemisphere. Effects of a stroke on the contralateral (nonaffected) side may be due to brain edema or global changes in PERFUSION in the brain. As a result of brain edema, patients may develop increased intracranial pressure and secondary brain damage.

Types of Strokes

Strokes are generally classified as ischemic (occlusive) or hemorrhagic (Fig. 45-1). Acute ischemic strokes are either thrombotic or embolic in origin (Table 45-1). Most strokes are ischemic.

Ischemic Stroke. An acute **ischemic stroke** is caused by the occlusion (blockage) of a cerebral artery by either a thrombus or an embolus. A stroke that is caused by a **thrombus** (clot) is referred to as a **thrombotic stroke**, whereas a stroke caused by an **embolus** (dislodged clot) is referred to as an **embolic stroke**.

Thrombotic strokes account for more than half of all strokes and are commonly associated with the development of atherosclerosis in either intracranial or extracranial arteries (usually the carotid arteries). Atherosclerosis is the process by which fatty plaques develop on the inner wall of the affected arterial vessel. Chapter 36 describes this health problem, including its pathophysiology, in detail.

Rupture of one or more plaques promotes clot formation. When the clot is of sufficient size, it interrupts blood flow to the brain tissue supplied by the vessel, causing an ischemic (occlusive) stroke. The **bifurcation** (point of division) of the common carotid artery and the vertebral arteries at their junction with the basilar artery are the most common sites involved in atherosclerotic plaque formation. Because of the gradual nature of clot formation when atherosclerotic plaque is present, thrombotic strokes tend to have a *slow* onset, evolving over minutes to hours.

An *embolic stroke* is caused by a thrombus or a group of thrombi that break off from one area of the body and travel to the cerebral arteries via the carotid artery or vertebrobasilar system. The usual source of emboli is the heart. Emboli can occur in patients with atrial fibrillation, heart valve disease, mural thrombi after a myocardial infarction (MI), or a prosthetic heart valve. Another source of emboli may be plaque or clot that breaks off from the carotid sinus or internal carotid artery. Emboli tend to become lodged in the smaller cerebral blood vessels at their point of bifurcation or where the lumen narrows.

The middle cerebral artery (MCA) is most commonly involved in an embolic stroke. As the emboli occlude the vessel, ischemia develops and the patient experiences the clinical manifestations of the stroke. However, the occlusion may be temporary if the embolus breaks into smaller fragments, enters smaller blood vessels, and is absorbed. For these reasons, embolic strokes are characterized by the *sudden* development and rapid occurrence of neurologic deficits. The symptoms may resolve over several hours or a few days. Conversion of an occlusive stroke to a hemorrhagic stroke may occur because the arterial vessel wall is also vulnerable to ischemic damage from blood

TABLE 45-1   Differential Features of the Types of Stroke

| FEATURE | ISCHEMIC | | HEMORRHAGIC |
	THROMBOTIC	EMBOLIC	
Evolution	Intermittent or stepwise improvement between episodes of worsening symptoms Completed stroke	Abrupt development of completed stroke Steady progression	Usually abrupt onset
Onset	Gradual (minutes to hours)	Sudden	Sudden, may be gradual if caused by hypertension
Level of consciousness	Preserved (patient is awake)	Preserved (patient is awake)	Deepening stupor or coma
Contributing associated factors	Hypertension Atherosclerosis	Cardiac disease	Hypertension Vessel disorders
Prodromal symptoms	Transient ischemic attack		
Neurologic deficits	Deficits during the first few weeks Slight headache Speech deficits Visual problems Confusion	Maximum deficit at onset Paralysis Expressive aphasia	Focal deficits Severe, frequent
Cerebrospinal fluid	Normal; possible presence of protein	Normal	Bloody
Seizures	No	No	Usually
Duration	Improvements over weeks to months Permanent deficits possible	Rapid improvements	Variable Permanent neurologic deficits possible

supply interruption. Sudden hemodynamic stress may result in vessel rupture, causing bleeding directly within the brain tissue.

Hemorrhagic Stroke. The second major classification of stroke is hemorrhagic stroke. In this type of stroke, vessel integrity is interrupted and bleeding occurs into the brain tissue or into the subarachnoid space.

Intracerebral hemorrhage (ICH) describes bleeding into the brain tissue generally resulting from severe or sustained hypertension. Elevated blood pressure (BP) leads to changes within the arterial wall that leave it likely to rupture. Damage to the brain occurs from bleeding, causing edema, distortion, and displacement, which are direct irritants to brain tissue. Cocaine use is one example of a trigger for sudden, dramatic blood pressure elevation leading to hemorrhagic stroke.

Subarachnoid hemorrhage (SAH) is much more common and results from bleeding into the subarachnoid space—the space between the pia mater and arachnoid layers of the meninges covering the brain. This type of bleeding is usually caused by a ruptured aneurysm or arteriovenous malformation (Mink & Miller, 2011b). It can also be caused by trauma.

An **aneurysm** is an abnormal ballooning or blister along a normal artery, which usually develops in a weak spot on the artery wall, typically along the posterior circulation such as the basilar artery, vertebral artery, or the superior cerebral artery. Larger aneurysms are more likely to rupture than smaller ones.

An **arteriovenous malformation (AVM)** is an uncommon abnormality that occurs during embryonic development. It is a tangled collection of malformed, thin-walled, dilated vessels without a capillary network (Fig. 45-2). Normally the capillary network lowers the pressure between the arterial and venous systems. In the absence of the capillary network, the thin-walled veins are subjected to arterial pressure. The abnormal vessels may eventually rupture, causing bleeding into the intracerebral tissue or spaces.

Vasospasm, a sudden and periodic constriction of a cerebral artery, often follows SAH or bleeding from an aneurysm or AVM rupture. Blood flow to distal areas of the brain supplied by the damaged cerebral vessel is markedly diminished. Reduced

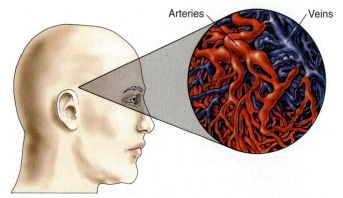

FIG. 45-2 Appearance of an arteriovenous malformation. Note the dilated, entangled blood vessels.

PERFUSION from vasospasm contributes to secondary cerebral ischemia and infarction and further neurologic dysfunction.

Etiology and Genetic Risk

As with many health problems, the causes of stroke are likely a combination of genetic and environmental risk factors. Major risk factors increase the likelihood of strokes and can be divided into those that can be modified and those that cannot (nonmodifiable factors) (see Health Promotion and Maintenance section on p. 933). Many of these factors have a familial or genetic predisposition and are discussed elsewhere in this text. For example, the first-order relative (mother, father, sister, brother) stroke risk increases with a strong family history of hypertension, atherosclerotic disease, and a diagnosis of aneurysm. Relatives of a patient with an aneurysm, regardless of vessel location, may be at higher risk for intracranial aneurysms and should consider diagnostic testing and follow-up.

Incidence and Prevalence

It is estimated that there are more than 4.7 million stroke survivors in the United States. About 795,000 Americans have strokes each year, but deaths have declined over the past 15 years. The number of strokes occurring in the younger adult population is increasing (Lee et al., 2012). Strokes are associated with illicit drug use because many street drugs cause hypercoagulability, spasm of cerebral vessels, or hypertensive crisis.

Health Promotion and Maintenance

Risk factors that contribute to stroke are divided into three groups: risk factors that cannot be changed, risk factors that can be changed with medical treatment, and risk factors that can be changed by lifestyle modification.

People with predisposing health conditions should be aware that lifestyle habits contribute to stroke. Many of these factors contribute to other health problems. Teach them the importance of seeking professional health care and adhering to the recommended treatment plan. Recommend a diet high in fruits and vegetables and low in saturated fats. Light to moderate alcohol consumption may reduce the risk for stroke, but a higher consumption may increase it. Chart 45-2 describes common risk factors that can be changed (modifiable).

⊕ CULTURAL CONSIDERATIONS
Patient-Centered Care QSEN

American Indian/Alaskan Native groups have the highest prevalence of stroke. Black men and women have more strokes than white men and women. Hispanic or Latino men have more strokes than non-Hispanic men. About half of the excess stroke risk in blacks between ages 45 and 65 years is attributable to traditional risk factors such as elevated systolic blood pressure and socioeconomic factors. These data suggest a critical need to study the role that nontraditional risk factors play in stroke development and severity in this group (Howard et al., 2011; Lakoski et al., 2011).

❓ NCLEX EXAMINATION CHALLENGE
Health Promotion and Maintenance

Which statements by a client or family member about preventing stroke indicate a need for further teaching by the nurse? **Select all that apply.**
A. "I will adjust my aspirin drug dose depending on whether I have pain."
B. "I have cut down on smoking to only a half-pack daily."
C. "I need to walk at least 30 minutes most days of the week."
D. "I need to consider salt content in the foods I eat at restaurants."
E. "I don't need to worry about fat calories in what I eat—my heart is fine!"

CHART 45-2 Patient and Family Education: Preparing for Self-Management
Common Modifiable Risk Factors for Developing a Stroke

- Smoking
- Substance use (particularly cocaine)
- Obesity
- Sedentary lifestyle
- Oral contraceptive use
- Heavy alcohol use
- Use of phenylpropanolamine (PPA), found in antihistamine drugs

---

❖ PATIENT-CENTERED COLLABORATIVE CARE
◆ Assessment

History. Although an accurate history is important in the diagnosis of a stroke, *the first priority is to ensure the patient is transported to a stroke center.* A stroke center is designated by The Joint Commission for its ability to rapidly recognize and effectively treat strokes. At the center, the patients are evaluated for their eligibility to receive fibrinolytic therapy. Obtaining a history should not delay the patient's arrival to either the stroke center or interventional radiology within the stroke center. A focused history to determine if the patient has had a recent bleeding event or is taking an anticoagulant is an important part of the rapid stroke assessment protocol.

A more extensive history, after either fibrinolytic therapy or determination that the patient is unable to receive this therapy, assists in identifying the cause of the stroke and the area of brain involved. If possible, obtain a history of the patient's activity when the stroke began. Hemorrhagic strokes tend to occur during activity. Next ask the patient or a family member how the symptoms progressed. Be sure to document the history of the stroke's onset. Symptoms of a hemorrhagic stroke tend to occur abruptly, whereas thrombotic strokes generally have a more gradual progression. Determine the severity of the symptoms, such as whether they worsened after the initial onset or began to improve.

During the interview, observe the patient's level of consciousness (LOC) and assess for indications of cognitive or memory impairments and difficulties with speech or hearing. When LOC is suddenly decreased or altered, immediately determine if hypoglycemia or hypoxia is present because these conditions may mimic emergent neurologic disorders. Hypoglycemia and hypoxia are easily treated and reversed, unlike brain injury from poor PERFUSION or trauma.

Question the patient or family member about the presence of SENSORY PERCEPTION deficits or motor changes, visual problems, problems with balance or gait, and changes in reading or writing abilities.

In addition, ask about the patient's medical history with specific attention directed toward a history of head trauma, diabetes, hypertension, heart disease, anemia, and obesity. Obtain a list of current medications, including prescribed drugs, over-the-counter (OTC) drugs, herbal and nutritional supplements, and recreational (illicit) drugs. To complete the history, obtain data about the patient's social history, including education, employment, travel, leisure activities, and personal habits (e.g., smoking, diet, exercise pattern, drug and alcohol use).

The patient with a SAH, particularly when the hemorrhage is from a leaking aneurysm, often reports the onset of a sudden, severe headache described as "the worst headache of my life." Additional symptoms of SAH or cerebral aneurysmal and AVM bleeding are nausea and vomiting, photophobia, cranial neuropathy, stiff neck, and change in mental status. There may also be a family history of aneurysms.

Physical Assessment/Clinical Manifestations. First-responder personnel (e.g., paramedics, emergency medical technicians) perform an initial neurologic examination using well-established stroke assessment tools.

Nurses also perform a complete neurologic assessment on admission to the ED. The National Institutes of Health Stroke Scale (NIHSS) is a commonly used valid and reliable assessment tool that nurses complete as soon as possible after the patient

! NURSING SAFETY PRIORITY (QSEN)

Critical Rescue

In the ED, assess the stroke patient within 10 minutes of arrival. This same standard applies to patients already hospitalized for other medical conditions who have a stroke. The priority is assessment of ABCs—**a**irway, **b**reathing, and **c**irculation. Many hospitals have designated stroke teams and centers that are expert in acute stroke assessment and management.

CHART 45-3 Key Features

Stroke Syndromes

Middle Cerebral Artery Strokes
- Contralateral hemiparesis: arm > leg
- Contralateral sensory perception deficit
- Homonymous hemianopsia
- Unilateral neglect or inattention
- Aphasia, anomia, alexia, agraphia, and acalculia
- Impaired vertical sensation
- Spatial deficit
- Perceptual deficit
- Visual field deficit
- Altered level of consciousness: drowsy to comatose

Posterior Cerebral Artery Strokes
- Perseveration (word or action repetition)
- Aphasia, amnesia, alexia, agraphia, visual agnosia, and ataxia
- Loss of deep sensation
- Decreased touch sensation
- Stupor, coma

Internal Carotid Artery Strokes
- Contralateral hemiparesis
- Sensory perception deficit
- Hemianopsia, blurred vision, blindness
- Aphasia (dominant side)
- Headache
- Bruit

Anterior Cerebral Artery Strokes
- Contralateral hemiparesis: leg > arm
- Bladder incontinence
- Personality and behavior changes
- Aphasia and amnesia
- Positive grasp and sucking reflex
- Perseveration
- Sensory perception deficit (lower extremity)
- Memory impairment
- Apraxic gait

Vertebrobasilar Artery Strokes
- Headache and vertigo
- Coma
- Memory loss and confusion
- Flaccid paralysis
- Areflexia, ataxia, and vertigo
- Cranial nerve dysfunction
- Disconjugate gaze
- Visual deficits (uniorbital) and homonymous hemianopsia
- Sensory loss: numbness

---

arrives in the ED (Table 45-2). The NIHSS includes 11 areas of assessment (Mink & Miller, 2011a).

As the patients are transitioned from the ED to other settings, the most important area to assess is the patient's level of consciousness (LOC). Use the Glasgow Coma Scale (see Fig. 41-10) to frequently monitor for changes in LOC throughout the patient's acute care. Specific patient manifestations of stroke should also be monitored. Stroke symptoms depend on the extent and location of the ischemia and the arteries involved as described in Chart 45-3.

Stroke symptoms can appear at any time of the day or night (Beal, 2010). The five most common symptoms are (CDC, 2013b):
- Sudden confusion or trouble speaking or understanding others
- Sudden numbness or weakness of the face, arm, or leg
- Sudden trouble seeing in one or both eyes
- Sudden dizziness, trouble walking, or loss of balance or coordination
- Sudden severe headache with no known cause

Cognitive Changes. The patient may have a variety of cognitive problems in addition to changes in LOC. LOC varies depending on the extent of increased intracranial pressure (ICP) caused by the stroke and on the location of the stroke. Assess for:
- Denial of the illness
- Spatial and proprioceptive (awareness of body position in space) dysfunction
- Impairment of memory, judgment, or problem-solving and decision-making abilities
- Decreased ability to concentrate and attend to tasks

Dysfunction in one or more of these areas may be severe depending on the hemisphere involved (Chart 45-4).

The *right* cerebral hemisphere is more involved with visual and spatial awareness and **proprioception** (sense of body position). A person who has a stroke involving the right cerebral hemisphere is often unaware of any deficits and may be disoriented to time and place. Personality changes include impulsivity (poor impulse control) and poor judgment. The *left* cerebral hemisphere, the dominant hemisphere in all but about 15% to 20% of the population, is the center for language, mathematic skills, and analytic thinking. Therefore a left hemisphere stroke results in **aphasia** (inability to use or comprehend language), **alexia** or **dyslexia** (reading problems), **agraphia** (difficulty with writing), and **acalculia** (difficulty with mathematic calculation). A complete assessment of these problems is performed by a speech-language pathologist (SLP).

Motor Changes. The motor examination provides information about which part of the brain is involved. A *right* **hemiplegia** (paralysis on one side of the body) or **hemiparesis** (weakness on one side of the body) indicates a stroke involving the *left* cerebral hemisphere because the motor nerve fibers cross in the medulla before entering the spinal cord and periphery. On the other hand, a *left* hemiplegia or hemiparesis indicates a stroke in the *right* cerebral hemisphere. If the brainstem or cerebellum is affected, the patient may experience hemiparesis or quadriparesis and **ataxia** (gait disturbance).

In collaboration with the physical therapist (PT) and occupational therapist (OT), assess the patient's muscle tone. The patient with **hypotonia,** or **flaccid paralysis,** cannot overcome the forces of gravity, and the extremities tend to fall to the side. The extremities feel heavy, and muscle tone is inadequate for balance, equilibrium, or protective mechanisms. **Hypertonia (spastic paralysis)** tends to cause fixed positions or contractures of the involved extremities. Range of motion (ROM) of

TABLE 45-2 **NIH Stroke Scale**	
CATEGORY AND MEASUREMENT	**SCORE***
1a. Level of Consciousness (LOC) 0 = Alert; keenly responsive. 1 = Not alert; but arousable by minor stimulation to obey, answer, or respond. 2 = Not alert; requires repeated stimulation to attend or is obtunded and requires strong or painful stimulation to make movements (not stereotyped). 3 = Responds only with reflex motor or autonomic effects or totally unresponsive, flaccid, and areflexic.	_____
1b. LOC Questions 0 = Answers two questions correctly. 1 = Answers one question correctly. 2 = Answers neither question correctly.	_____
1c. LOC Commands 0 = Performs two tasks correctly. 1 = Performs one task correctly. 2 = Performs neither task correctly.	_____
2. Best Gaze 0 = Normal. 1 = Partial gaze palsy; gaze is abnormal in one or both eyes, but forced deviation or total gaze paresis is not present. 2 = Forced deviation, or total gaze paresis not overcome by the oculocephalic maneuver.	_____
3. Visual 0 = No visual loss. 1 = Partial hemianopia. 2 = Complete hemianopia. 3 = Bilateral hemianopia (blind including cortical blindness).	_____
4. Facial Palsy 0 = Normal symmetrical movements. 1 = Minor paralysis (flattened nasolabial fold, asymmetry on smiling). 2 = Partial paralysis (total or near-total paralysis of lower face). 3 = Complete paralysis of one or both sides (absence of facial movement in the upper and lower face).	_____
5. Motor (Arm) 0 = No drift; limb holds 90 (or 45) degrees for full 10 seconds. 1 = Drift; limb holds 90 (or 45) degrees, but drifts down before full 10 seconds; does not hit bed or other support. 2 = Some effort against gravity; limb cannot get to or maintain (if cued) 90 (or 45) degrees, drifts down to bed, but has some effort against gravity. 3 = No effort against gravity; limb falls. 4 = No movement. Untestable = Amputation or joint fusion.	Right arm: _____ Left arm: _____
6. Motor (Leg) 0 = No drift; leg holds 30-degree position for full 5 seconds. 1 = Drift; leg falls by the end of the 5-second period but does not hit bed. 2 = Some effort against gravity; leg falls to bed by 5 seconds, but has some effort against gravity. 3 = No effort against gravity; leg falls to bed immediately. 4 = No movement. Untestable = Amputation or joint fusion.	Right leg: _____ Left leg: _____
7. Limb Ataxia 0 = Absent. 1 = Present in one limb. 2 = Present in two limbs. Untestable = Amputation or joint fusion.	_____
8. Sensory 0 = Normal; no sensory loss. 1 = Mild-to-moderate sensory loss; patient feels pinprick is less sharp or is dull on the affected side; or there is a loss of superficial pain with pinprick, but patient is aware of being touched. 2 = Severe-to-total sensory loss; patient is not aware of being touched in the face, arm, and leg.	_____
9. Best Language 0 = No aphasia; normal. 1 = Mild-to-moderate aphasia; some obvious loss of fluency or facility of comprehension, without significant limitation on ideas expressed or form of expression. 2 = Severe aphasia; all communication is through fragmentary expression; great need for inference, questioning, and guessing by the listener. 3 = Mute, global aphasia; no usable speech or auditory comprehension.	_____

Continued

TABLE 45-2 NIH Stroke Scale—cont'd

CATEGORY AND MEASUREMENT	SCORE*
10. Dysarthria	____
0 = Normal.	
1 = Mild-to-moderate dysarthria; patient slurs at least some words and, at worst, can be understood with some difficulty.	
2 = Severe dysarthria; patient's speech is so slurred as to be unintelligible in the absence of or out of proportion to any dysphasia, or is mute/anarthric.	
Untestable = Intubated or other physical barrier.	
11. Extinction and Inattention (Neglect)	
0 = No abnormality.	
1 = Visual, tactile, auditory, spatial, or personal inattention or extinction to bilateral simultaneous stimulation in one of the sensory modalities.	
2 = Profound hemi-inattention or extinction to more than one modality; does not recognize own hand or orients to only one side of space.	

Modified from National Institutes of Health Stroke Scale, 2013. www.ninds.nih.gov/doctors/NIH_stroke_scale.pdf.
*The patient can have a score of 0 to 40, with 0 having no neurologic deficits and 40 being the most deficits.

CHART 45-4 Key Features

Left and Right Hemisphere Strokes

FEATURE	LEFT HEMISPHERE*	RIGHT HEMISPHERE
Language	Aphasia Agraphia Alexia	Impaired sense of humor
Memory	Possible deficit	Disorientation to time, place, and person Inability to recognize faces
Vision	Inability to discriminate words and letters Reading problems Deficits in the right visual field	Visual spatial deficits Neglect of the left visual field Loss of depth perception
Behavior	Slowness Cautiousness Anxiety when attempting a new task Depression or a catastrophic response to illness Sense of guilt Feeling of worthlessness Worries over future Quick anger and frustration Intellectual impairment	Impulsiveness Lack of awareness of neurologic deficits Confabulation Euphoria Constant smiling Denial of illness Poor judgment Overestimation of abilities (risk for injury)
Hearing	No deficit	Loss of ability to hear tonal variations

*Location for speech in all but 5% to 20% of people.

the joints is restricted, and shoulder subluxation may easily occur from either spasticity or flaccidity. Also assess head and trunk control, balance, coordination, and gait. The patient who has had a stroke may also be unable to use an object correctly (agnosia) or carry out a purposeful motor activity or speech (apraxia).

Loss of neurologic control by the cerebral cortex causes a spastic (upper motor neuron) uninhibited bladder. Bowel function may also be affected. Assess the patient for incontinence (most common) or retention of urine and stool. Some patients have both problems.

Sensory Changes. The sensory examination evaluates the patient's response to touch and painful stimuli. In addition to diminished motor function, decreased sensation typically occurs on the affected side of the body.

Evaluate for indications of unilateral body neglect syndrome, which is particularly common with strokes in the *right* cerebral hemisphere. In this syndrome, the patient is unaware of the existence of his or her left or paralyzed side. The typical picture is that of the patient sitting in a wheelchair and leaning to the left with the arm caught in the wheelchair wheel. When questioned, the patient often states that everything is fine and believes that he or she is sitting up straight in the chair. The patient may wash or dress only one side of the body or eat from only one side of a plate.

Another important part of the nursing assessment focuses on visual ability. Infarction or ischemia involving the carotid artery may cause pupil constriction or dilation, ptosis (eyelid drooping), visual field deficits, or pallor and petechiae of the conjunctiva. Amaurosis fugax, a brief episode of blindness in one eye, results from retinal ischemia caused by ophthalmic or carotid artery insufficiency. Hemianopsia, or blindness in half of the visual field, results from damage to the optic tract or occipital lobe. Usually this deficit occurs as homonymous hemianopsia, in which there is blindness in the same side of both eyes (Fig. 45-3). The patient with this condition must turn his or her head to scan the complete range of vision. Otherwise, he or she does not see half of the visual field. For example, the patient eats only half of a meal because that is the only portion seen. Patients with brainstem or cerebellar damage may have abnormal eye movements, such as nystagmus (involuntary movements of the eyes).

Cranial Nerve Function. Assess the patient's ability to chew, which reflects the function of cranial nerve (CN) V. Assessment of the patient's ability to swallow reflects the function of CNs IX and X. In addition, note any facial paralysis or paresis (CN VII), absent gag reflex (CN IX), or impaired tongue movement (CN XII). The patient who has difficulty chewing or swallowing foods and liquids (dysphagia) is at risk for aspiration pneumonia and may become constipated or dehydrated from inadequate fluid intake.

Cardiovascular Assessment. Patients with embolic strokes may have a heart murmur, dysrhythmias (most often atrial fibrillation), or hypertension. It is not unusual for the patient to be admitted to the hospital with a blood pressure greater than 180 to 200/110 to 120 mm Hg. Although a somewhat higher blood pressure of 150/100 mm Hg is needed to maintain

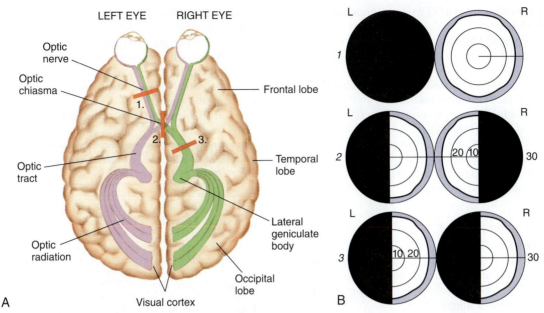

FIG. 45-3 **A,** Site of lesions causing visual loss. *1,* Total blindness left eye; *2,* Bitemporal hemianopia; *3,* Left homonymous hemianopia. **B,** Visual fields corresponding to lesions shown in **A.** *1,* Total blindness left eye; *2,* Bitemporal hemianopia; *3,* Left homonymous hemianopia.

cerebral PERFUSION after an acute ischemic stroke, pressures above these values may lead to another stroke.

Psychosocial Assessment. The typical patient with a stroke is older than 60 years, is hypertensive, and has varying degrees of motor weakness and level of consciousness. Language and cognitive deficits, as well as behavior and memory problems, may also occur.

Assess the patient's reaction to the illness, especially in relation to changes in body image, self-concept, and ability to perform ADLs. In collaboration with the patient's family and friends, identify any problems with coping or personality changes.

Ask about the patient's financial status and occupation, because they may be affected by the residual neurologic deficits of the stroke. Patients who do not have disability or health insurance may worry about how their family will cope financially with the disruption in their lives. Early involvement of social services, certified hospital chaplain, or psychological counseling may enhance coping skills.

Assess for **emotional lability,** especially if the frontal lobe of the brain has been affected. In such cases, the patient laughs and then cries unexpectedly for no apparent reason. Explain these uncontrollable emotions to the family or significant others so they do not feel responsible for these reactions.

Laboratory Assessment. Clinical history and presentation are usually enough to identify a stroke once it has occurred. No definitive laboratory tests confirm its diagnosis. Elevated hematocrit and hemoglobin levels are often associated with a severe or major stroke as the body attempts to compensate for lack of oxygen to the brain. An elevated white blood cell (WBC) count may indicate the presence of an infection, possibly subacute bacterial endocarditis, or a response to physiologic stress or inflammation. Cardiac enzymes may be elevated in patients who have a cardiac cause for their stroke.

The health care provider typically requests a prothrombin time (PT) or international normalized ratio (INR) and a partial thromboplastin time (PTT) to establish baseline information in case anticoagulation therapy is started. These diagnostic tests may also provide supportive evidence that a hemorrhagic stroke has occurred.

Imaging Assessment. Brain imaging is the most important tool for confirming the diagnosis of a stroke. *CT* without contrast is the standard for initial diagnosis (Mink & Miller, 2011b). Cerebral aneurysms or AVM may also be identified. For a patient with an ischemic or occlusive stroke, the head CT is usually initially negative, indicating a thrombotic or embolic stroke rather than intracerebral hemorrhage. After the first 24 hours, CT shows progressive changes of ischemia, infarction, and associated cerebral edema. This test establishes baseline information for future comparison in case the patient's condition deteriorates. In addition, the scan enables the physician to identify pathologic changes that may mimic a stroke, such as a brain tumor or cerebral hematoma, both of which may be unrelated to cerebrovascular disease.

MRI demonstrates ischemic brain injury earlier than CT. *Magnetic resonance angiography (MRA)* and multimodal techniques such as perfusion-weighted imaging enhance the sensitivity of the MRI to detect early changes in the brain, including confirming blood flow. *Ultrasonography* (carotid duplex scanning) and *echocardiography* help determine additional cardiovascular risks.

Other Diagnostic Assessment. To assist in the determination of a cardiac cause of a stroke, the health care provider may request a 12-lead electrocardiogram (ECG) and an evaluation of cardiac enzymes. As with other cardiovascular diseases, it is not unusual to find these changes on the ECG: inverted T wave, ST depression, and prolongation of the QT interval in the cardiac cycle.

◆ **Analysis**

The priority NANDA-I nursing diagnoses and collaborative problems for patients with a stroke include:

1. Inadequate perfusion to the brain related to interruption of arterial blood flow and a possible increase in ICP

2. Impaired Swallowing related to neuromuscular impairment (NANDA-I)
3. Impaired Physical Mobility and self-care deficit related to neuromuscular impairment or cognitive impairment (NANDA-I)
4. Aphasia or dysarthria related to decreased circulation in the brain or facial muscle weakness
5. Urinary and/or Bowel Incontinence related to reflex bladder and bowel (NANDA-I)
6. Sensory perception deficits from altered neurologic reception, transmission, and perception
7. Unilateral Neglect related to disturbed perceptual abilities or hemianopsia (NANDA-I)

◆ *Planning and Implementation*
Improving Cerebral Perfusion
Planning: Expected Outcomes. The patient with a stroke is expected to have an adequate blood flow to the brain and through the cerebral blood vessels to maintain brain function and prevent further brain injury.

Interventions. Interventions for patients experiencing strokes are determined primarily by the type and extent of the stroke. For patients having ischemic strokes, the standard of practice is to start two IV lines with non-dextrose isotonic saline (Hughes, 2011). Consider placing the patient in a supine position with a low head-of-bed elevation to maximize cerebral PERFUSION. The immediate primary role of the nurse is to manage the patient receiving treatment and continuously assess for increasing intracranial pressure.

Nonsurgical Management. Nursing interventions are initially aimed at monitoring for neurologic changes or complications associated with stroke and its treatment. The two major treatment modalities for patients with acute ischemic stroke are systemic fibrinolytic therapy and endovascular interventions. Regardless of the immediate management approach used, once the patient is stable, provide ongoing supportive care. Provide interventions to prevent and/or monitor for early signs of complications, such as hyperglycemia, urinary tract infection, and pneumonia. Implement interventions to prevent patient falls. These health problems are discussed in appropriate chapters in this textbook.

Fibrinolytic Therapy. For select patients with ischemic strokes, early intervention with systemic fibrinolytic therapy ("clot-busting drug") is the standard of practice to improve blood flow to or through the brain. The success of fibrinolytic therapy for a stroke depends on the interval between the time symptoms begin and available treatment. It also depends on where the treatment is given. Hospitals with stroke centers or specialized stroke teams who care for numerous stroke patients have lower mortality rates than those hospitals that care for fewer of these patients (Hughes, 2011).

Intravenous (systemic) fibrinolytic therapy (also called *thrombolytic therapy*) for an acute ischemic stroke dissolves the cerebral artery occlusion to re-establish blood flow and prevent cerebral infarction. Alteplase (Activase) is the only drug approved at this point for the treatment of acute ischemic stroke. It is a fibrinolytic that activates plasminogen to degrade the thrombus. The most important factor in whether or not to give alteplase is the time between symptom onset and time seen in the stroke center. In 2009, the American Stroke Association recommended an expanded time interval from 3 to 4.5 hours

to administer this fibrinolytic for patients unless they fall into these categories:

- Age older than 80 years
- Anticoagulation with an international normalized ratio greater than or equal to 1.7
- Baseline National Institutes of Health Stroke Scale score greater than 25
- History of both stroke and diabetes

GENDER HEALTH CONSIDERATONS
Patient-Centered Care QSEN

Previous studies have suggested that being a female is a risk factor for delay in recognizing early symptoms of stroke and may contribute to ineligibility for fibrinolytic therapy. Current data show that women arrive at the ED at the same speed as men after acute ischemic stroke, so the delay in treatment does not appear to be related to transport time once the emergency medical transport system is called. Woman may be less likely to demonstrate focal symptoms, leading to diagnostic or treatment delay (Beal, 2010). Women have greater functional impairments at 3 months and 12 months after stroke and stroke treatment despite similar pre-stroke functional ability and admission score of stroke severity (Knauft et al., 2010).

Fibrinolytic therapy is explained to the patient and/or family member, and informed consent is obtained. The dosage of the drug is based on the patient's actual weight. Each hospital has strict protocols for mixing and administering the fibrinolytic drug and for monitoring the patient before and after fibrinolytic drug administration.

! NURSING SAFETY PRIORITY QSEN
Drug Alert

In addition to frequent monitoring of vital signs, carefully observe for signs of intracerebral hemorrhage and other signs of bleeding during administration of fibrinolytic drug therapy. Other best practice interventions are listed in Chart 45-5.

? NCLEX EXAMINATION CHALLENGE
Physiological Integrity

A client begins to have severe epistaxis after completing a dose of alteplase. In order of priority, what are the nurse's actions?
A. Obtain vital signs.
B. Assess the airway, and set up suction at bedside.
C. Draw blood for anticoagulation studies.
D. Call the health care provider.

Endovascular Interventions. Endovascular procedures include intra-arterial thrombolysis using drug therapy, mechanical **embolectomy** (clot removal), and carotid stent placement. *Intra-arterial thrombolysis* has the advantage of delivering the fibrinolytic agent directly into the thrombus within 6 hours of the stroke's onset. It is particularly beneficial for some patients who have an occlusion of the middle cerebral artery or those who arrive in the ED after the window for rtPA. If the patient arrives in less than 8 hours, the interventional neuroradiologist may perform mechanical embolectomy using special instrumentation systems that can remove the clot by suction or other

CHART 45-5 Best Practice for Patient Safety & Quality Care QSEN

Nursing Interventions During and After IV Administration of Alteplase

- Perform a double check of the dose. Use a programmable pump to deliver the initial dose of 0.9 mg/kg (maximum dose 90 mg) over 60 minutes with 10% of the dose given as a bolus over 1 minute. Do not manually push this drug.
- Admit the patient to a critical care or specialized stroke unit.
- Perform neurologic assessments, including vital signs, every 10 to 15 minutes during infusion and every 30 minutes after that for at least 6 hours; monitor hourly for 24 hours after treatment. Be consistent regarding the device used to obtain blood pressures because blood pressures can vary when switching from a manual to a noninvasive automatic to an intra-arterial device.
- If systolic blood pressure is 180 mm Hg or greater or diastolic is 105 mm Hg or greater, give antihypertensive drugs as prescribed.
- To prevent bleeding, do not place invasive tubes, such as nasogastric (NG) tubes or indwelling urinary catheters, until the patient is stable.
- Discontinue the infusion if the patient reports severe headache or has severe hypertension, bleeding, nausea, and/or vomiting; notify the health care provider immediately.
- Obtain a follow-up CT scan after treatment before starting antiplatelet or anticoagulant drugs.

method (Mink & Miller, 2011a). Patients having either fibrinolytic therapy or endovascular interventions are admitted to the critical care setting for intensive collaborative monitoring.

Carotid artery angioplasty with stenting is common to *prevent* or, in some cases, help manage an acute ischemic stroke. This interventional radiology procedure is usually done under moderate sedation. It may be performed by a cardiovascular surgeon or interventional radiologist. A technique using a distal/embolic protection device has made this procedure very safe. The device is placed beyond the stenosis through a catheter inserted into the femoral artery (groin). The device catches any clot debris that breaks off during the procedure. Placement of a carotid stent is performed to open a blockage in the carotid artery typically at the division of the common carotid artery into the internal and external carotid arteries. Throughout the procedure, the patient's neurologic and cardiovascular statuses are assessed.

! NURSING SAFETY PRIORITY QSEN

Action Alert

Before discharge after carotid stent placement, teach the patient to report these symptoms to the health care provider as soon as possible:
- Severe headache
- Change in level of consciousness or COGNITION (e.g., drowsiness, new-onset confusion)
- Muscle weakness or motor dysfunction
- Severe neck pain
- Neck swelling
- Hoarseness or difficulty swallowing (due to nerve damage)

When the stroke is hemorrhagic and the cause is related to an AVM or cerebral aneurysm, the patient is evaluated for the optimal procedure to stop bleeding. The goal of treatment is to embolize abnormal vessels or the aneurysm itself. Some procedures can be used to prevent bleeding in an AVM or aneurysm that is discovered *prior* to symptom onset or SAH. Procedures

occur in the interventional radiology suite or operating room. The different approaches used by the interventional neuroradiologist or neurosurgeon to embolize the vessel defect and nursing implications during postprocedure recovery are summarized in Table 45-3. How a brain aneurysm or AVM is treated depends on the size of the aneurysm, whether it has ruptured (bled), where in the brain it is located, and the age and overall health of the patient. Fig. 45-4 illustrates a common approach to manage an intact (non-ruptured) AVM.

Following endovascular procedures, a rare postprocedure complication, hyperperfusion syndrome, has a high morbidity and mortality rate. This syndrome is thought to be the result of an impaired autoregulation of cerebral blood flow that results from long-standing decreased cerebral PERFUSION pressure resulting from carotid artery disease. The signs and symptoms include severe temporal headache, hypertension, seizures, and focal neurologic deficits. This syndrome may be associated with intracranial hemorrhage and may occur within 1 hour postprocedure up to 24 hours or even 1 week later (Oran & Oran, 2010).

Monitoring for Increased Intracranial Pressure. The patient is most at risk for increased ICP resulting from edema during the first 72 hours after onset of the stroke. Some patients may have worsening of their neurologic status starting within 24 to 48 hours after their endovascular procedure from increased ICP (Chart 45-6). Reassess patients with stroke and with endovascular treatment of stroke symptoms every 1 to 4 hours depending on severity of the condition. Use the approved assessment strategy and documentation tools.

! NURSING SAFETY PRIORITY QSEN

Critical Rescue

Be alert for symptoms of increased ICP in the stroke patient, and report any deterioration in the patient's neurologic status to the health care provider immediately! *The first sign of increased ICP is a declining level of consciousness (LOC).*

The best head-of-bed (HOB) positioning has not yet been determined; more studies are needed to determine best practice. A reduced head elevation of less than 25 degrees can improve perfusion pressure to damaged brain in ischemic conditions like most strokes. However, a HOB elevation greater than 30 degrees can improve oxygenation and reduce aspiration risk. Provide oxygen therapy to prevent hypoxia for patients with oxygen saturation less than 93%. Maintain the head in a midline, neutral position to help promote venous drainage from the brain. In collaboration with other team members, avoid sudden and acute hip or neck flexion during positioning. Extreme hip flexion may increase intrathoracic pressure, leading to decreased cerebral venous outflow and elevated ICP. Extreme neck flexion also interferes with venous drainage from the brain and intracranial dynamics.

Additional nursing considerations include avoiding the clustering of nursing procedures (e.g., giving a bath followed immediately by changing the bed linen). When multiple activities are clustered in a narrow time period, the effect on ICP can be dramatic elevation. Hyperoxygenating the patient before suctioning may also be appropriate to avoid even transient hypoxemia and resultant ICP elevation from dilation of cerebral arteries. Coughing and suctioning increase ICP. Careful attention to airway management can reduce unnecessary increases in ICP.

TABLE 45-3 **Surgical and Interventional Radiologic Procedures to Manage Intracranial Aneurysms and Arteriovenous Malformations**

PROCEDURE	DESCRIPTION	NURSING IMPLICATIONS
Surgical ligation or resection	A neurosurgeon performs a full or micro-craniectomy. Once the defective vessels are located, they are separated from brain tissue and removed. A graft may be placed to preserve blood flow of the parent vessel. Surgical elimination of arteriovenous malformation (AVM) or aneurysm depends on the size of the defect, the risk for major brain damage during resection, the absence of bleeding, and the condition of the patient preoperatively.	Ligation and clip placement can be done simultaneously. Preoperative and postoperative care are similar to that for patients undergoing a craniotomy as described in this chapter. Perioperative care described in Chapters 14-16 is also essential.
Clip	Clips are small devices, similar to a paperclip, that are clamped over the aneurysm base to isolate it from the parent vessel circulation. The neurosurgeon performs a full craniotomy or micro-craniotomy to visualize the aneurysm in the operating room. A contrast agent is injected into the vessel to determine the degree of aneurysm occlusion and parent vessel patency. Micro-Doppler ultrasonography can also be used to evaluate the placement of the clips intraoperatively.	Older clips have metal components, preventing use of magnetic resonance imaging postprocedure. It is possible for clips to move, and movement is greatest immediately postplacement. Movement may occur as late as 2-5 years after placement. Patients require care as outlined under the perioperative chapters with close neurologic assessment to detect early rebleeding or migration of the clip. Changes in cognition or new focal neurologic deficits must be communicated urgently to the neurosurgeon.
Coil —With stent assist —With balloon assist	Detachable coils are placed under fluoroscopy to occlude the aneurysm without interrupting main vessel flow. Coils are platinum, and some are coated with polymers to promote fibrosis. Stents are used to enhance vessel stability and are an adjunct prior to vessel rupture. Balloon-assisted coil placement is thought to enhance endovascular remodeling and decrease postprocedure rebleeding when the aneurysm is intact before the procedure.	Up to 20% of patients experience bleeding or rebleeding after coil placement, with the greatest risk for bleeding occurring in the year following the procedure. As a result, patients are advised to avoid drugs that interfere with clotting during recovery. Patients return for re-evaluation typically at 3, 6, and 12 months to determine the extent of embolization. Full embolization is the goal for this type of procedure; it is possible to undergo a second placement of coils to achieve best results. Teach the patient to maintain an ongoing relationship with the neurosurgeon to evaluate the effectiveness of the procedure over time. Perform frequent neurologic assessments in the first 24 hours postprocedure to detect intracranial bleeding early.
Flow diversion	These stent-like devices look like a braided cylindric mesh and are delivered under fluoroscopy to the neck of an aneurysm, shifting blood flow away from the vessel defect and resulting in a thrombosed (clotted) aneurysm over 5-6 months. An example is the pipeline embolization device (PED).	These are the newest devices for treatment of intracranial aneurysms. Full embolization takes 5-12 months, so ongoing monitoring by the neurosurgery staff in community health settings (office or clinic) is common postprocedure. Encourage the patient to avoid strenuous activity or situations that create hypertension while the prolonged embolization occurs.
Liquid polymer embolization	This procedure is reserved for AVMs. It is used either preoperatively to reduce the size of the AVM or as a permanent treatment for a small AVM. Treatment can occur once or over several stages to achieve maximum AVM reduction.	This procedure is often used prior to surgical ligation or stereotactic surgery to reduce the size of the AVM and decrease the number of branches of the tangled, defective vessel. Help the patient understand that this procedure may not provide definitive treatment if it is either staged or planned to precede surgery. Perform frequent neurologic assessment in the 24 hours postprocedure to detect early signs of bleeding.
Stereotactic surgery	Under the simultaneous supervision of the neurosurgeon, radiologist, and physicist, microwave or radio beams are directed to the defective vessel(s) to obliterate the defect.	Stereotactic surgery requires that the patient undergo extensive diagnostic study and be placed in a brace that will hold the head fixed while the beam is directed toward the abnormal vessel. Swelling around the beam site may alter neurologic status. Perform neurologic assessment with each opportunity to take vital signs, and inform the neurosurgeon of any deterioration in consciousness or new focal weakness or sensory changes.

A quiet environment is particularly important for the patient experiencing a headache, which is common with a cerebral hemorrhage or increased ICP. The patient may have **photophobia** (sensitivity to light). Therefore keep the room lights very low.

Close physiologic monitoring of blood pressure, heart rhythm, oxygen saturation, blood glucose, and body temperature may prevent secondary brain injury and promote good outcomes after stroke. High quality evidence is not available on how to manage blood pressure in patients with hemorrhagic strokes, but for many patients, severe hypertension is the cause

of their stroke (Mink & Miller, 2011b). Assessing vital signs (VS) regularly and communicating concerning changes from baseline promote quality and safety for both individualized and system-wide outcomes.

Monitor vital signs closely, at least every 1 to 2 hours. Notify the health care provider if the blood pressure or core temperature does not meet a prescribed range of values. Although the optimal blood pressure range after stroke is controversial, the health care provider may allow the patient with *acute ischemic stroke* to be slightly hypertensive with a systolic blood pressure (SBP) between 140 and 150 mm Hg to promote cerebral tissue

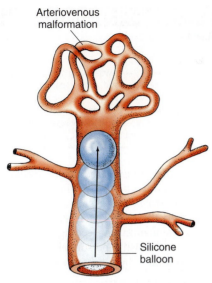

Arteriovenous malformation

Silicone balloon

FIG. 45-4 Embolization procedure to treat an arteriovenous malformation. The liquid embolic agent causes vessel thrombosis.

CHART 45-6   Key Features

Increased Intracranial Pressure (ICP)

- Decreased level of consciousness (LOC) (lethargy to coma)
- Behavior changes: restlessness, irritability, and confusion
- Headache
- Nausea and vomiting (may be projectile)
- Change in speech pattern
  - Aphasia
  - Slurred speech
- Change in sensorimotor status
  - Pupillary changes: dilated and nonreactive pupils ("blown pupils") or constricted and nonreactive pupils
  - Cranial nerve dysfunction
  - Ataxia
- Seizures (usually within first 24 hours after stroke)
- Cushing's triad
  - Severe hypertension
  - Widened pulse pressure
  - Bradycardia
- Abnormal posturing:
  - Decerebrate (extensor)
  - Decorticate (flexion)

PERFUSION. A SBP greater than 180 mm Hg or a diastolic BP greater than 110 mm Hg is generally considered dangerous, contributing to a risk for hemorrhagic stroke or rebleeding of an aneurysm (if present). Carefully monitor the patient's temperature because fever may extend the area of injury in the brain.

! NURSING SAFETY PRIORITY (QSEN)

Critical Rescue

If the stroke patient's SBP is more than 180 mm Hg, notify the health care provider immediately and anticipate prescription of an IV antihypertensive medication. Monitor the patient's BP and mean arterial pressure (MAP) every 5 minutes until the SBP is between 140 and 150 mm Hg to maintain brain PERFUSION. Avoid a sudden SBP drop to less than 120 mm Hg with drug administration.

Monitoring for Other Complications. Monitor the patient with an aneurysm or arteriovenous malformation (AVM) as well as patients following repair of these vessel malformations for signs and symptoms of hydrocephalus and vasospasm. **Hydrocephalus** (increased cerebrospinal fluid [CSF] within the ventricular and subarachnoid spaces) may occur as a result of blood in the CSF. This prevents CSF from being reabsorbed properly by the arachnoid villi. Cerebral edema, which interferes with the flow of CSF out from the ventricular system, may also develop. Eventually the ventricles become enlarged. If hydrocephalus is left untreated, increased intracranial pressure (ICP) results. Observe for clinical manifestations of hydrocephalus, which are similar to those of ICP elevation, including a change in the LOC. Clinical findings may also include headache, pupil changes, seizures, poor coordination, gait disturbances (if ambulatory), and behavior changes.

If blood is in the subarachnoid space, the patient is at risk for cerebral vasospasm. Clinical manifestations of vasospasm may include decreased LOC, motor and reflex changes, and increased neurologic deficits (e.g., cranial nerve dysfunction, motor weakness, and aphasia). The symptoms may fluctuate with the occurrence and degree of vasospasm present. Hemorrhage-related cerebral vasospasm can result in permanent vascular changes and irreversible neurologic impairment.

Rebleeding or rupture is a common complication for the patient with an aneurysm or AVM. Recurrent hemorrhage may occur within 24 hours of the initial bleed or rupture and up to 7 to 10 days later. About 20% of patients experience a second episode of bleeding after a repair of vessel malformations. Assess for severe headache, nausea and vomiting, a decreased LOC, and additional neurologic deficits. Potential consequences of a second cerebral hemorrhagic event may be catastrophic.

Patients admitted to a critical care unit are observed for dysrhythmias with cardiac monitoring. The nurse performs a cardiac assessment, with particular attention to identify the presence of cardiac murmurs or atrial fibrillation (AF). Cardiac valve disorders, manifested by a murmur or AF, place the patient at increased risk for emboli.

Both hyperglycemia and hypoglycemia are associated with new, secondary brain damage. Too high or too low blood sugar values increase the area of primary brain damage and contribute to greater disability from stroke. Monitor the patient's finger stick blood sugars (FSBS) frequently. Perform an FSBS when there is any unexplained decrease in level of consciousness for the patient admitted with a central nervous system injury or insult. Ensure daily communication with the health care team members to share desired glycemic outcomes and interventions to achieve them.

Ongoing Drug Therapy. Ongoing drug therapy depends on the type of stroke and the resulting neurologic dysfunction. In general, the purposes of drug therapy are to prevent further thrombotic episodes (anticoagulation) and to protect the neurons from hypoxia.

The use of aspirin or other antiplatelet drug is considered for treatment following acute ischemic strokes or for preventing future strokes when risk factors of prodromal symptoms (TIA) occur (Bousser, 2012). Sodium heparin and other anticoagulants, such as warfarin (Coumadin, Warfilone ✦), are used in the presence of atrial fibrillation. *Anticoagulants are high-alert drugs that can cause bleeding, including intracerebral hemorrhage.* ✦

An *initial* dose of 325 mg of aspirin (Ecotrin, Ancasal ✦) is recommended within 24 to 48 hours after stroke onset. Aspirin should not be given within 24 hours of rtPA administration. Low-dose aspirin is an antiplatelet drug and reduces blood clotting by reducing platelet adhesiveness (clumping). Aspirin can cause bruising, hemorrhage, and liver disease over a long-term period. Teach the patient to report any unusual bruising or bleeding to the health care provider.

A calcium channel blocking drug that crosses the blood-brain barrier such as nimodipine (Nimotop) may be given to treat or prevent cerebral vasospasm after a subarachnoid hemorrhage. Vasospasm, which usually occurs between 4 and 14 days after the stroke, slows blood flow to the area and worsens ischemia. Nimodipine works by relaxing the smooth muscles of the vessel wall and reducing the incidence and severity of the spasm. Neurologic functioning may improve, and further deterioration from ischemia is then prevented. In addition, this drug dilates collateral vessels to ischemic areas of the brain.

Stool softeners, analgesics for pain, and antianxiety drugs may also be prescribed as needed for symptom management. Stool softeners also prevent the Valsalva maneuver during defecation to prevent increased ICP.

Surgical Management. Few patients are candidates for immediate surgery once a stroke occurs. A neurosurgeon may perform a decompressive craniectomy (explained on p. 956) to manage refractory intracranial hypertension in a patient with a massive stroke.

Following recovery from a stroke or to prevent a TIA from progressing to a stroke, the patient may have surgery to improve cerebral circulation. In an **extracranial-intracranial bypass**, the surgeon performs a craniotomy (surgical opening into the brain through the skull) and bypasses the blocked artery by making a graft or a bypass from the first artery to the second artery. This procedure establishes blood flow around the blocked artery and re-establishes blood flow to the involved areas. The two most common techniques are the superficial temporal artery–to–middle cerebral artery (STA-MCA) graft and the occipital–to–posterior inferior cerebellar artery (PICA) bypass.

Whenever possible, an AVM is also totally removed via a craniotomy. The surgeon cuts and separates the group of vessels and removes the defect. Radiosurgery (Gamma Knife) can also be used by the neurosurgeon. Radiation delivered during surgery results in fibrous thickening of the endothelial lining of the vessels to prevent further vessel enlargement and ultimately eliminate the lesion from the cerebral circulation. Improved microsurgical techniques have significantly reduced morbidity and mortality rates, and these procedures are becoming the treatment of choice in many medical centers.

Managing Impaired Swallowing

Planning: Expected Outcomes. The patient with a stroke is expected to avoid aspiration and have adequate nutrition to promote health and prevent complications, including major weight loss.

Interventions. Aspiration is a frequent complication for patients with dysphagia (difficulty swallowing) (Hughes, 2011). Many of these aspirations are "silent" and are not recognized until pulmonary complications occur.

Observe the patient for facial drooping, drooling, impaired voluntary cough, hoarseness, incomplete mouth closure, or cranial nerve palsies. Next check the gag and cough reflexes. If the patient does not pass this swallowing screen, collaborate with the speech-language pathologist (SLP) to conduct a bedside swallowing evaluation. He or she may recommend a modified barium swallow (video fluoroscopy) to identify

---

> **⚠ NURSING SAFETY PRIORITY** (QSEN)
> ### Action Alert
>
> The best practice for all *suspected* and *diagnosed* stroke patients is to maintain a NPO status until their swallowing ability is assessed. Before the patient is given any liquids, food, or medication, he or she must be screened for the ability to swallow. Follow agency guidelines for screening or use an evidence-based bedside swallowing screening tool to determine if dysphagia is present. If dysphagia is present, develop a plan of care to prevent aspiration and support nutrition.

specific structures that are impaired during swallowing. *Ensure that the patient remains completely NPO status until the SLP determines that the patient can tolerate liquids or foods without aspirating.* Based on the complete swallowing evaluation, the SLP makes recommendations for feeding for the staff to follow. Remind all unlicensed assistive personnel (UAP) and the family about the need to follow these precautions exactly as they are written.

Some patients can swallow without difficulty but are at risk for aspiration because they are easily distracted and impulsive. These patients require a distraction-free environment with minimal disruption from television, visitors, or environmental noise. Observe for indications of fatigue, because it can significantly interfere with the patient's desire and ability to eat.

Studies indicate that as many as 50% of patients are malnourished at 2 to 3 weeks after a severe stroke. To avoid this complication, collaborate with the dietitian to provide an accurate, comprehensive nutritional assessment on admission and throughout the hospital stay (Perry et al., 2013). Implement nutritional interventions, such as an early gastrostomy or oral nutrition, by at least the third or fourth hospital day to prevent weight loss, an altered immune status, increased length of stay, and increased mortality (Hughes, 2011).

For patients who can tolerate oral foods and liquids, follow the SLP's recommendations for thickened liquids, head positioning, and patient teaching to prevent aspiration. Teach UAP and family members how to follow these instructions, and have them readily available for reference.

> **? NCLEX EXAMINATION CHALLENGE**
> ### Physiological Integrity
>
> A client with a confirmed acute ischemic stroke is comatose but breathing spontaneously. The client has an advance directive requesting limited resuscitation and is not a candidate for fibrinolytic therapy. What is the nurse's priority action on admission?
> A. Ask for palliative care consultation to assist with end-of-life decision making.
> B. Consult with the speech-language pathologist about alternative strategies for communication.
> C. Evaluate swallowing ability with an institution-specific, evidence-based protocol.
> D. Assess vital signs and determine if the advance directives need to be communicated to the health care provider.

Improving Mobility and Promoting Self-Care

Planning: Expected Outcomes. The patient with a stroke is expected to ambulate and provide self-care independently, with or without one or more assistive-adaptive devices.

Interventions. Patients who have had a stroke often have flaccid or spastic paralysis. It is not unusual for the patient to eventually have a flaccid arm and spastic leg on the affected side because the affected leg often regains function more quickly than the arm. Patients begin rehabilitation as soon as possible to regain function and prevent complications of immobility, such as pneumonia, atelectasis, and pressure ulcers.

> ### ! NURSING SAFETY PRIORITY (QSEN)
> **Action Alert**
>
> Be sure to support the affected flaccid arm of the stroke patient, and teach UAP to avoid pulling on it. Position the arm on a pillow while the patient is sitting to prevent it from hanging freely, which could cause shoulder subluxation. The physical or occupational therapist provides a sling-like device to support the arm during ambulation.

Another major complication of impaired MOBILITY is the development of venous thromboembolism (VTE), especially deep vein thrombosis (DVT) that can lead to a pulmonary embolism (PE). This risk is highest in older patients and those with a severe stroke. Per The Joint Commission's Core Measures for VTE, provide care to prevent this complication by applying intermittent sequential pneumatic devices, changing the patient's position frequently, and ambulating the patient if possible. Report any indications of DVT to the health care provider, and document assessments in the patient's record. Chapter 36 discusses VTE prevention in detail.

The rehabilitation therapists evaluate the patient's ability to perform MOBILITY skills, basic ADLs, and household tasks that will be performed at home. After a thorough evaluation, collaborate with them to develop a plan of care to promote patient independence, with or without assistive or adaptive devices. Therapy begins in the hospital setting and continues after discharge in most cases. Chapter 6 describes interventions for rehabilitation, including improving MOBILITY and promoting self-care.

Promoting Effective Communication
Planning: Expected Outcomes. The patient with a stroke is expected to receive, interpret, and express spoken, written, and nonverbal messages, if possible. However, some patients may need to develop strategies for alternative methods of communication, such as pictures or nonverbal language.

Interventions. Language or speech problems are usually the result of a stroke involving the dominant hemisphere. The left cerebral hemisphere is the speech center in most patients. Speech and language problems may be the result of aphasia or dysarthria. Whereas aphasia is caused by cerebral hemisphere damage, dysarthria (slurred speech) is due to a loss of motor function to the tongue or to the muscles of speech, causing facial weakness and slurred speech. Involvement of the speech-language pathologist (SLP) as early as possible in the hospitalization greatly increases the patient's chances for optimal recovery. Remind patients to practice their exercises for dysarthria to strengthen their facial and oral muscles.

Aphasia can be classified in a number of ways. Most commonly, it is classified as expressive, receptive, or mixed (Table 45-4). Expressive (Broca's, or motor) aphasia is the result of damage in Broca's area of the frontal lobe. It is a motor speech problem in which the patient generally understands what is said but cannot communicate verbally. He or she also has difficulty writing but may be able to write. Rote speech and automatic speech such as responses to a greeting are often intact. The

---

TABLE 45-4 Types of Aphasia

Expressive (or nonfluent)
- Referred to as *Broca's,* or *motor, aphasia*
- Difficulty speaking
- Difficulty writing

Receptive
- Referred to as *Wernicke's,* or *sensory, aphasia*
- Difficulty understanding spoken words
- Difficulty understanding written words
- Speech often meaningless
- Made-up words

Mixed
- Combination of difficulty understanding words and speech
- Difficulty with reading and writing

Global
- Profound speech and language problems
- Often no speech or sounds that cannot be understood

---

patient is aware of the deficit and may become frustrated and angry. Reassure patients, and remind them to talk slowly.

Receptive (Wernicke's, or sensory) aphasia is due to injury involving Wernicke's area in the temporoparietal area. The patient cannot understand the spoken and often the written word. Although he or she may be able to talk, the language is often meaningless. Neologisms (made-up words) are common parts of speech.

Usually the patient has some degree of dysfunction in the areas of both expression and reception. This is known as *mixed aphasia.* Reading and writing ability are equally affected. Few patients have just expressive *or* receptive aphasia. In most cases, though, one type is dominant.

To help communicate with the patient with aphasia, use these guiding principles:
- Present one idea or thought in a sentence (e.g., "I am going to help you get into the chair.").
- Use simple one-step commands rather than ask patients to do multiple tasks.
- Speak slowly but not loudly; use cues or gestures as needed.
- Avoid "yes" and "no" questions for patients with expressive aphasia, because they often give automatic responses that may be incorrect.
- Use alternative forms of communication if needed, such as a computer, communication board, or flash cards (often with pictures).

For more specific communication strategies for your patient, collaborate with the SLP.

Promoting Continence
Planning: Expected Outcomes. The patient with a stroke is expected to control elimination of urine and stool.

Interventions. The patient may be incontinent of urine and stool because of an altered level of consciousness, impaired innervation to the bladder and rectum, and/or the inability to communicate the need to urinate or defecate. Before beginning a patient education program to correct these problems, the cause must first be established. Typically, the patient who has had a stroke can regain both bowel and bladder control in time. To begin a bladder training program, place the patient on the bedpan or the commode or offer the urinal every 2 hours. Encourage a total fluid intake to maintain dilute urine and a balanced intake and output. A bedside bladder ultrasound is used to check for residual urine after voiding in the early phase of the bladder training program to ensure that the patient is emptying the bladder. Retained urine can lead to a urinary tract infection.

Before establishing a bowel training program, determine the patient's normal time for bowel elimination and any routine that helps promote a stool. This routine is followed, if possible, and the patient is placed on the commode or toilet at the same time as the previous schedule at home. Encourage the patient to drink apple or prune juice and to consume high-fiber foods to help promote bowel elimination. A stool softener (Colace) may be prescribed. Suppositories may also assist in re-establishing a bowel routine. Chapter 6 provides a discussion of bowel and bladder training programs.

If the patient has an indwelling urinary catheter, it should be removed as soon as hourly urine output is no longer essential to therapeutic decisions. The patient with a fever or an older adult who becomes increasingly confused should always be evaluated for a urinary tract infection.

Managing Changes in Sensory Perception

Planning: Expected Outcomes. The major concern of patients with SENSORY PERCEPTION deficits is adapting to neurologic deficits. Therefore the patient with a stroke is expected to adapt to sensory perception changes in vision, proprioception (position sense), and sensation and to be free from injury.

Interventions. Patients with right hemisphere brain damage typically have difficulty with visual-perceptual or spatial-perceptual tasks. They have problems with depth and distance perception and with discrimination of right from left or up from down. Because of these problems, they have difficulty performing routine ADLs. Caregivers help the patient adapt to these disabilities by using frequent verbal and tactile cues and by breaking down tasks into discrete steps. Always approach the patient from the unaffected side, which should face the door of the room.

Place objects within the patient's field of vision. A mirror may help visualize more of the environment. If the patient has **diplopia** (double vision), a patch may be placed over the affected eye. Remind the nursing staff to ensure a safe environment by removing clutter from the room.

The patient with a left hemisphere lesion generally has memory deficits and may show significant changes in the ability to carry out simple tasks. To assist with memory problems, re-orient the patient to the month, year, day of the week, and circumstances surrounding hospital admission. Establish a routine or schedule that is as structured, repetitious, and consistent as possible. Provide information in a simple, concise manner. A step-by-step approach is often most effective because the patient can master one step before moving to the next. When possible, ask the family to bring in pictures and other familiar objects.

The patient may be unable to plan and execute tasks in an organized manner. **Apraxia,** or the inability to perform previously learned motor skills or commands, may be present. Typically, the patient with apraxia exhibits a slow, cautious, and hesitant behavior style. The physical therapist (PT) assists the patient in compensating for loss of position sense.

Managing Unilateral Body Neglect

Planning: Expected Outcomes. The patient with stroke is expected to adjust and use techniques to compensate for unilateral (one-sided) body neglect.

Interventions. Unilateral neglect, or neglect syndrome, occurs most commonly in patients who have had a right cerebral stroke. However, it can occur in any patient who experiences hemianopsia, in which the vision of one or both eyes is affected. This problem places the patient at additional risk for injury, especially falls, because of an inability to recognize his or her physical impairment or because of a lack of proprioception (position sense).

Teach the patient to touch and use both sides of the body. For example, encourage the patient to wash both the affected and unaffected sides of the body. When dressing, remind the patient to dress the affected side first. If hemianopsia is present, teach the patient to turn his or her head from side to side to expand the visual field. This scanning technique is also useful when the patient is eating or ambulating.

Community-Based Care

The patient with a stroke may be discharged to home, a rehabilitation center, or a skilled nursing facility (SNF), depending on the extent of the disability and the availability of family or caregiver support. Some patients have no significant neurologic dysfunction and are able to return home and live independently or with minimal support. Other patients are able to return home but require ongoing assistance with ADLs and supervision to prevent accidents or injury. The case or care manager coordinates speech/language, physical, and/or occupational therapy services to continue in the home or on an ambulatory care basis. Patients admitted to a rehabilitation unit/facility or SNF require continued or more complex nursing care as well as extensive physical, occupational, recreational, speech-language, or cognitive therapy, which is coordinated by a case manager. The expected outcome for rehabilitation is to maximize the patient's abilities in all aspects of life. Some patients who have strokes have severe brain damage with profound neurologic impairments and require palliative care.

Home Care Management. Collaborate with the case manager to plan the patient's discharge. Coordinate with rehabilitation therapists to identify needs for assistive or adaptive and safety equipment. The extent of this assessment depends on the patient's disabilities. Teach the patient and family to ensure that the home is free from scatter rugs or other obstacles in the walking pathways. The bathtub and toilet should be equipped with grab bars. Anti-skid patches or strips should be placed in the bathtub to prevent slipping. The PT or OT works with the patient and the family or significant others to obtain all needed assistive devices and home modifications *before* the patient is discharged from the hospital, rehabilitation setting, or SNF. Appointments for ambulatory care speech, physical, and occupational therapy are arranged before discharge for continuing care.

Self-Management Education. As part of the discharge process, teach the family about depression that may occur within the 3 months after a stroke. The strongest predictors of post-stroke depression (PSD) are a history of depression, severe stroke, and post-stroke physical or cognitive impairment. Patients may not exhibit typical signs of depression because of their cognitive, physical, and emotional impairments. PSD is associated with increased morbidity and mortality, especially in older men.

The three areas that should be included in patient and family education are disease prevention, disease-specific information, and self-management (American Heart Association, 2014).

EVIDENCE-BASED PRACTICE (QSEN)

What Are the Best Practices for Teaching Patients and Their Families About Strokes?

Cameron, V. (2013). Best practices for stroke patient and family education in the acute care setting: A literature review. *MEDSURG Nursing, 22*(3), 51-55.

Many patients have strokes and are admitted to the acute care setting. Nurses need to know the most effective methods for educating these patients and their families before they are discharged from the hospital. The researcher conducted an integrative interdisciplinary review of the literature published between 2003 and 2012 to determine the best practices for patient and family education. Three areas of health teaching are needed: stroke prevention, stroke-specific education, and self-management skills. Best practices for these areas include:

- Be flexible and adapt to the health and learning needs of the patient (e.g., aphasia is/is not present).
- Use multiple types of education materials (written, audiovisual, interactive strategies).
- Focus on key points, and be repetitive; as many as five or six repetitions are associated with retention.
- Group meetings may be beneficial to patient understanding, motivation, and quality of life.
- Use reading materials with a low literacy level, large font type, and short (15 minute) learning sessions.
- Identify sources of emotional support, encourage social support, and locate community education groups for caregivers to enhance their well-being.

Level of Evidence: 1

This study provided a systematic review of literature to determine best practices for teaching patients with strokes and their families about the disease and self-management.

Commentary: Implications for Practice and Research

This review did not use statistical analysis to generate recommendations for patient and family education, an approach common to integrative reviews. The strategies are practical and accessible to nurses and health care team members in both hospital and community care settings. Nurses need to consider the specific limitations, health needs, and health literacy of patients with strokes to modify their approach to health teaching as needed.

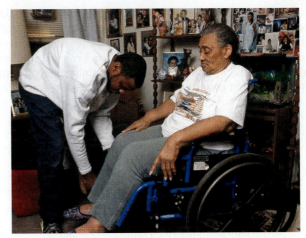

FIG. 45-5 Son adjusting his mother's wheelchair.

Families may feel overwhelmed by the continuing demands placed on them. Depending on the location of the lesion, the patient may be anxious, slow, cautious, and hesitant and lack initiative (left hemisphere lesions). As a result of right hemisphere lesions, he or she may be impulsive and seemingly unaware of any deficit. Family members and other caregivers need to spend time away from the patient on a routine basis to continue to provide full-time care without sacrificing their own physical and emotional health. Refer the family to social services or other community resources for further support, counseling, and possible respite care.

Health Care Resources. Available resources include a variety of publications from the American Heart Association (www.americanheart.org), including *Stroke: A Guide for Families* and *Stroke: Why Do They Behave That Way?* The National Stroke Association (www.stroke.org) also provides publications and videotapes for caregivers and patients. *Recovering After a Stroke: A Patient and Family Guide* is available from the Agency for Healthcare Research and Quality (www.ahrq.gov). Refer the patient and family members or significant others to local stroke support groups.

For patients who require symptom management or end-of-life care, refer the family to palliative care or hospice services. Chapter 7 gives a detailed description of end-of-life care and advance directives.

◆ Evaluation: Outcomes

Evaluate the care of the patient with stroke based on the identified priority patient problems. The expected outcomes are that the patient:

- Maintains blood pressure and blood sugar within a safe, prescribed range
- Performs self-care and MOBILITY activities independently, with or without assistive devices
- Learns to adapt to SENSORY PERCEPTION changes
- Adjusts and uses techniques to compensate for one-sided neglect
- Communicates effectively or develops strategies for effective communication
- Has adequate nutrition and avoids aspiration
- Controls elimination of urine and stool

There are eight core measures associated with the care of stroke patients (The Joint Commission, 2014). These core measures form the basis of not only individual patient goals but also

The teaching plan includes lifestyle changes, drug therapy, ambulation/transfer skills, communication skills, safety precautions, nutritional management, activity levels, and self-management skills. Health teaching should focus on tasks that must be performed by the patient and the family after hospital discharge. Provide both written and verbal instruction in all these areas (see the Evidence-Based Practice box). Return demonstrations assist in evaluating the family members' competency in tasks required for the patient's care (Fig. 45-5).

Teach patients to take their prescribed drugs to prevent another stroke and control hypertension. Instruct the patient and the family the name of each drug, the dosage, the timing of administration, how to take it, and possible side effects. In collaboration with the PT and OT, teach the patient how to climb stairs safely, if he or she is able; transfer from the bed to a chair; get into and out of a car; and use any aids for MOBILITY. The patient and family members are also taught how to use any equipment needed to increase independence in self-management skills. Provide important information regarding what to do in an emergency and who to call for nonemergency questions.

system-wide goals of care. As a result, continuous quality improvement efforts are based on these core measures. Certification as a Stroke Center is tied to consistent performance in achieving satisfactory core measures. The core measures may have additional implications in terms of reimbursement in the future. The eight core measures for Ischemic Stroke Care are:

1. Venous thromboembolism (VTE) prophylaxis
2. Discharge with antithrombotic therapy
3. Anticoagulation therapy for atrial fibrillation/flutter
4. Thrombolytic therapy (in the presence of a thrombotic stroke of <4 hours from symptom onset)
5. Antithrombotic therapy is evaluated by end of hospital day (e.g., diagnostic testing for therapeutic range of values following thrombolytic or anticoagulant therapy)
6. Discharged on statin medication
7. Stroke education provided and documented
8. Assessed for rehabilitation

Comprehensive stroke centers are required to collect data for the eight stroke core measures and submit monthly data points every quarter through the Certification Measure Information Process (CMIP). Nurses not only provide direct care to patients with ischemic stroke but also contribute to the peer review process to evaluate and monitor the care provided to patients with ischemic stroke.

TRAUMATIC BRAIN INJURY

❖ PATHOPHYSIOLOGY

Traumatic brain injury (TBI) is damage to the brain from an external mechanical force and not caused by neurodegenerative or congenital conditions. TBI can lead to temporary and permanent impairment of cognitive, physical, and psychosocial functions.

Various terms are used to describe the brain injuries that occur when a mechanical force is applied either directly or indirectly to the brain. A force produced by a blow to the head is a *direct* injury, whereas a force applied to another body part with a rebound effect to the brain is an *indirect* injury. The brain responds to these forces by movement within the rigid cranial vault. It may also rebound or rotate on the brainstem, causing diffuse axonal injury (shearing injuries). The brain may be contused (bruised) or lacerated/torn as it moves over the inner surfaces of the cranium, which are irregularly shaped and sharp.

Movement or distortion within the cranial cavity is possible because of multiple factors. The first factor is how the brain is supported by cerebrospinal fluid (CSF) within the cranial cavity. When external force is applied to the head, the brain can be injured by the internal surfaces of the skull and meninges. The second factor is the consistency of brain tissue, which is very fragile and prone to injury. Brain injury occurs from both initial forces on the head and brain and as a result of secondary derangements of physiologic stability.

The type of force and the mechanism of injury contribute to traumatic brain injury. An *acceleration* injury is caused by an external force contacting the head, suddenly placing the head in motion. A *deceleration* injury occurs when the moving head is suddenly stopped or hits a stationary object (Fig. 45-6). These forces may be sufficient to cause the cerebrum to rotate about the brainstem, resulting in shearing, straining, and distortion of the brain tissue, particularly of the axons in the brainstem and cerebellum. Small areas of hemorrhage (contusion, intracranial hemorrhage) may develop around the blood vessels that sustain

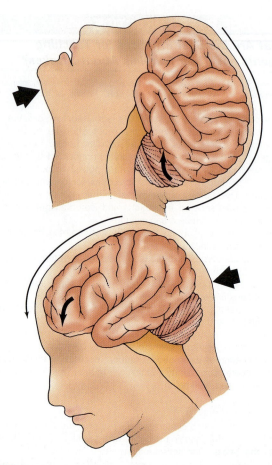

FIG. 45-6 Head movement during acceleration-deceleration injury, which is typically seen in motor vehicle crashes.

the impact of these forces (stress), with destruction of adjacent brain tissue. Particularly affected are the basal nuclei and the hypothalamus.

Primary Brain Injury

Primary brain damage occurs at the time of injury and results from the physical stress (force) within the tissue caused by blunt force. A primary brain injury may be categorized as focal or diffuse. A *focal* brain injury is confined to a specific area of the brain and causes localized damage that can often be detected with a CT scan or MRI. *Diffuse* injuries are characterized by damage throughout many areas of the brain. They initially may be at a microscopic level and not initially detectable by CT scan. MRI has greater ability to detect microscopic damage, but these areas may not be imaged until necrosis occurs.

Primary brain injuries are also classed as either open or closed. An open traumatic brain injury occurs when the skull is fractured or when it is pierced by a penetrating object. The integrity of the brain and the dura is violated, and there is exposure to environmental contaminants. Damage may occur to the underlying vessels, dural sinus, brain, and cranial nerves. In a closed traumatic brain injury, the integrity of the skull is not violated.

Open Versus Closed Traumatic Brain Injury. The types of skull fractures associated with *open traumatic brain injury* are linear, depressed, open, and comminuted. A *linear fracture* is a simple, clean break in which the impacted area of bone bends inward and the area around it bends outward. Linear fractures

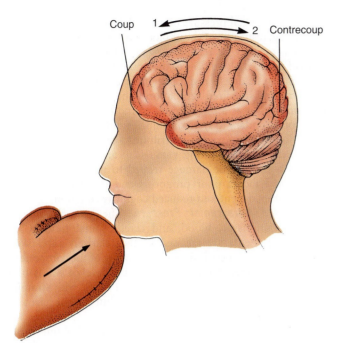

FIG. 45-7 Coup (site of impact) injury to frontal area of brain, and contrecoup injury to frontal and temporal areas of the brain.

are the most common type of skull fracture. In a *depressed fracture,* the bone is pressed inward into the brain tissue to at least the thickness of the skull. In an *open fracture,* the scalp and dura are lacerated, creating a direct opening to the brain tissue. A *comminuted fracture* involves fragmented bone with depression into the brain tissue.

A unique skull fracture is a *basilar fracture.* It occurs at the base of the skull, usually extending into the anterior, middle, or posterior fossa, and can result in cerebrospinal fluid (CSF) leakage from the nose or ears. A CSF leak increases the risk for a central nervous system (CNS) infection. A basilar skull fracture is associated with an increased risk for hemorrhage caused by damage to the internal carotid artery. Basilar skull fractures can also damage cranial nerves (CNs) I, II, VII, and VIII.

Most penetrating injuries to the brain are caused by gunshot wounds (GSWs) and knife injuries. The degree of injury to brain tissue depends on the velocity (speed), mass, shape, and direction of impact. High-velocity injuries produce the greatest damage to brain tissue. As with any open wound, the patient with a penetrating injury is at high risk for infection from the object that pierced the skull and from other environmental contaminants.

Closed traumatic brain injuries are caused by blunt force. The blunt force can be direct or a result of a blast shock wave. These forces can lead to contusions and lacerations of the brain. A **contusion** is a bruising of the brain tissue and is most commonly found at the site of impact (**coup injury**) or in a line opposite the site of impact (**contrecoup injury**) (Fig. 45-7). Contusions and lacerations are most commonly located at the base of the frontal and temporal lobes. A **laceration** causes actual tearing of the cortical surface vessels, which may lead to secondary hemorrhage and significant cerebral edema and inflammation. This condition is more serious than a contusion.

When damage to the brain is severe but without local injury such as a contusion or laceration, a closed traumatic brain injury may be diagnosed as diffuse axonal injury or widespread injury to the white matter of the brain. **Diffuse axonal injury (DAI)** is usually related to high-speed acceleration/deceleration, typically seen in motor vehicle crashes. This type of brain injury causes shearing of large nerve fibers and stretching of blood vessels in many areas of the brain. In addition to bleeding, a DAI can trigger a biochemical cascade of toxic substances in the brain during the days following the initial injury. DAI occurs throughout the brain, and the frontal and temporal lobes are particularly susceptible. Damage may also be found in the corpus callosum, midbrain, cerebellum, and upper brainstem. DAI can also occur in focal but important nerve centers (white matter tracts) causing visual field loss or weakness on one side of the body. Depending on severity, small areas of hemorrhage and changes in the lateral ventricles may be seen with a CT or MRI, but there is no specific or sensitive test to definitively diagnose DAI. The most prominent manifestation of DAI is impaired cognitive function, resulting in disorganization, impaired memory, and varying degrees of inattentiveness. Severe DAI may present with immediate coma, and most survivors require long-term care.

Mild, Moderate, and Severe Traumatic Brain Injury. TBI is further defined as mild, moderate, or severe. Generally, the determination of severity of TBI is the result of the Glasgow Coma Scale (GCS) score immediately following resuscitation, the presence (or absence) of brain damage imaged by CT or MRI following the trauma, an estimation of the force of the trauma, and symptoms in the injured person.

Mild Traumatic Brain Injury. The terms *mild traumatic brain injury (MTBI)* and *concussion* are used synonymously (Thompson & Mauk, 2011). MTBI is characterized by a blow to the head, transient confusion or feeling dazed or disoriented, and one or more of these conditions: (1) loss of consciousness for up to 30 minutes, (2) loss of memory for events immediately before or after the accident, and (3) focal neurologic deficit(s) that may or not be transient. Loss of consciousness does not have to occur for a person to be diagnosed with MTBI. With MTBI, there is no evidence of brain damage on a CT or MRI imaging scan. Subsequent to a new MTBI, symptoms can include a wide array of physical and cognitive problems that range from headache and dizziness to changes in behavior listed on Chart 45-7. These symptoms usually resolve within 72 hours. In some cases the symptoms persist and may last days, weeks, or months. For other patients, severe physical and cognitive problems remain despite relatively mild initial symptoms and normal diagnostic test findings. Persistent symptoms following MTBI are also referred to as **post-concussion syndrome**.

The incidence of *MTBI* is difficult to estimate because most cases are not reported. Further, the symptoms and diagnostic terminology (international classification diagnostic [ICD] codes) used for mild traumatic brain injury are not well established in the practice community. For example, some providers use the word *concussion* for a temporary and reversible change in COGNITION or SENSORY PERCEPTION from a blow to the head. A concussion is a MTBI. Regardless of terminology, MTBI accounts for at least 75% of all traumatic brain injuries in the United States. Estimating incidence and prevalence is also complicated because patients may not seek medical care. Some patients may not perceive any health problem from the injury. Others do not have any health insurance to assist with costs of diagnosis and care or may feel guilty or embarrassed over the circumstances of the injury.

CHART 45-7   Key Features

Mild Traumatic Brain Injury

Physical Findings
- Appears dazed or stunned
- Loss of consciousness <30 minutes (unresponsive after injury)
- Headache
- Nausea
- Vomiting
- Balance or gait problems
- Dizziness
- Visual problems
- Fatigue
- Sensitivity to light
- Sensitivity to noise

Cognitive Findings
- Feeling mentally foggy
- Feeling slowed down
- Difficulty concentrating
- Difficulty remembering
- Amnesia about the events around the time of injury

Sleep Disturbances
- Drowsiness
- Sleeping less than usual
- Sleeping more than usual
- Trouble falling asleep

Emotional Changes
- Irritability
- Sadness
- Nervousness
- More "emotional"

Moderate Traumatic Brain Injury. A moderate TBI is characterized by a period of loss of consciousness (LOC) for 30 minutes to 6 hours and a GCS score of 9 to 12. Often but not always, focal or diffuse brain injury can be seen with a diagnostic CT or MRI scan. Post-traumatic amnesia (memory loss) may last up to 24 hours. Moderate TBI may occur with either closed or open brain injury. A short acute or critical care stay may be needed for close monitoring and to prevent secondary injury from brain edema, intracranial bleeding, or inadequate cerebral PERFUSION. Additional secondary injury results from complex inflammatory processes, also known as the *biomolecular cascade* that occurs in the CNS immediately, hours, or days after primary injury (Thompson & Mauk, 2011).

Severe Traumatic Brain Injury. A severe TBI is defined by a GCS score of 3 to 8 and loss of consciousness for longer than 6 hours. Focal and diffuse damage to the brain, cerebrovascular vessels, and/or ventricles are common. Both open and closed head injuries can cause severe TBI, and injury can be focal or diffuse. When the damage is present in a localized area of the brain, it is usually extensive. CT and MRI scans can capture images of tissue damage quite early in the course of this illness. Patients with severe TBI require management in critical care, including monitoring of hemodynamics, neurologic status, and possibly, intracranial pressure (ICP). Patients with severe TBI are also at high risk for secondary brain injury from cerebral edema, hemorrhage, reduced PERFUSION, and the biomolecular cascade.

Secondary Injury

Secondary injury to brain injury includes any processes that occur *after* the initial injury and worsen or negatively influence patient outcomes. Secondary injuries result from physiologic, vascular, and biochemical events that are an extension of the primary injury. The most common secondary injuries result from hypotension and hypoxia, intracranial hypertension, and cerebral edema. Damage to the brain tissue occurs primarily because the delivery of oxygen and glucose to the brain is interrupted.

Hypotension and Hypoxia. Both hypotension, defined as a mean arterial pressure less than 70 mm Hg, and hypoxemia, defined as a partial pressure of arterial oxygen (Pao_2) less than 80 mm Hg, restrict the flow of blood to vulnerable brain tissue. Hypotension may be related to shock (Chapter 37) or other states of reduced blood flow to the brain such as clot formation. Hypoxia can be due to respiratory failure, asphyxiation, or loss of airway and impaired ventilation (Chapter 32). These problems may occur as a direct result of moderate to severe brain injury or secondary to systemic injuries and comorbidities. Low blood flow and hypoxemia contribute to cerebral edema, creating a cycle of deteriorating PERFUSION and hypoxic damage. Patients with hypoxic damage related to moderate or severe brain injury face a poor prognosis and typically experience memory impairment and reduced cognitive function.

Increased Intracranial Pressure. The cranial contents include brain tissue, blood, and cerebrospinal fluid (CSF). These components are encased in the relatively rigid skull. Within this space, there is little room for any of the components to expand or increase in volume. A normal level of ICP is 10 to 15 mm Hg. Periodic increases in pressure occur with straining during defecation, coughing, or sneezing but do not harm the uninjured brain.

As a result of brain injury, the increase in the volume of one component must be compensated for by a decrease in the volume of one of the other components. As a first response to an increase in the volume of any of these components, the CSF is shunted or displaced from the cranial compartment to the spinal subarachnoid space or the rate of CSF absorption is increased. An additional response, if needed, is a decrease in cerebral blood volume by movement of cerebral venous blood into the sinuses. As long as the brain can compensate for the increase in volume and remain compliant, increases in ICP are minimal.

Increased ICP is the leading cause of death from head trauma in patients who reach the hospital alive. It occurs when compliance no longer takes place and the brain cannot accommodate further volume changes. As ICP increases, cerebral perfusion decreases, leading to brain tissue ischemia and edema. If edema remains untreated, the brain may herniate downward toward the brainstem or laterally from a unilateral lesion within one cerebral hemisphere, causing irreversible brain damage and possibly death (brain herniation syndromes).

Three types of edema may contribute to increased ICP: vasogenic edema, cytotoxic edema, and interstitial edema. *Vasogenic edema* is caused by an abnormal permeability of the walls of the cerebral vessels, which allows protein-rich plasma infiltrate to leak into the extracellular space of the brain. The fluid collects primarily in the white matter. *Cytotoxic edema* may occur as a result of a hypoxic insult, which causes a disturbance in cellular metabolism and active ion transport. The brain is quickly depleted of available oxygen, glucose, and glycogen and converts to anaerobic metabolism. Derangements in cell membrane function result in cell edema, cell dysfunction, and cell death. Cytotoxic edema may lead to vasogenic edema and a further increase in ICP. *Interstitial edema* occurs with fluid accumulation between the cells of the brain. Interstitial edema is *associated with* elevated blood pressure or increased CSF pressure. Interstitial edema develops rapidly in the perivascular and periventricular white space and can be controlled through measures to reduce blood pressure or decrease CSF pressures.

Besides providing oxygen to decrease ischemic injury, sustaining mean arterial pressure or systolic blood pressure within a therapeutic range, and draining cerebral spinal fluid, the staff nurse manages increased intracranial pressure with attention to balancing fluid intake and output and promoting normal serum electrolyte values. When intracranial pressure monitoring is used, a desired outcome of therapy includes maintaining **cerebral perfusion pressure (CPP)**. The CPP is the pressure gradient over which the brain is perfused. CPP is determined by subtracting the mean ICP from the mean arterial pressure. *Maintenance of a CPP above 70 mm Hg is generally accepted as an expected outcome of therapy.* ICP monitoring also includes evaluating the shape and quality of the ICP waveform to determine whether compliance is compromised as manifested by an abnormal ICP waveform. Some specialized units also monitor jugular venous oxygenation saturation to evaluate the amount of hemoglobin saturated by oxygen as it drains from the cranium. A value that falls outside the range of 55% to 70% indicates inadequate delivery of oxygen to brain tissue.

Hemorrhage. Hemorrhage, which causes a brain hematoma (collection of blood) or clot, may occur as part of the primary injury and begin at the moment of impact. It may also arise later from vessel damage. Classically, bleeding is caused by vascular damage from the shearing force of the trauma or direct physical damage from skull fractures or penetrating injury. *All hematomas are potentially life threatening because they act as space-occupying lesions and are surrounded by edema.* Three major types of hemorrhage after TBI are epidural, subdural, and intracerebral hemorrhage. Subarachnoid hemorrhage may also occur.

An **epidural hematoma** results from arterial bleeding into the space between the dura and the inner skull (Fig. 45-8). It is often caused by a fracture of the temporal bone, which houses the middle meningeal artery. Patients with epidural hematomas have "lucid intervals" that last for minutes during which time the patient is awake and talking. This follows a momentary unconsciousness that occurs within minutes of the injury.

A **subdural hematoma (SDH)** results from venous bleeding into the space beneath the dura and above the arachnoid (see Fig. 45-8). It occurs most often from a tearing of the bridging veins within the cerebral hemispheres or from a laceration of

---

! NURSING SAFETY PRIORITY (QSEN)
Critical Rescue

After the initial interval, symptoms of neurologic impairment from hemorrhage can progress very quickly with potentially life-threatening ICP elevation and irreversible structural damage to brain tissue. Monitor the patient suspected of epidural bleeding frequently (every 5-10 minutes) for changes in neurologic status. The patient can become quickly and increasingly symptomatic. *A loss of consciousness from an epidural or subdural hematoma is a neurosurgical emergency!* Notify the health care provider or Rapid Response Team immediately if these changes occur. Carefully document your assessments.

---

brain tissue. *Bleeding from this injury occurs more slowly than from an epidural hematoma.* SDHs are subdivided into acute, subacute, and chronic. An acute SDH presents within 48 hours after impact; the subacute SDH, between 48 hours and 2 weeks; and the chronic SDH, from 2 weeks to several months after injury. SDHs have the highest mortality rate because they often are unrecognized until the patient presents with severe neurologic compromise.

Traumatic **intracerebral hemorrhage** (ICH) is the accumulation of blood within the brain tissue caused by the tearing of small arteries and veins in the subcortical white matter (see Fig. 45-8). It often acts as a space-occupying lesion (like a tumor) and may be potentially devastating, depending on its location. ICH may also produce significant brain edema and ICP elevations. A traumatic brainstem hemorrhage occurs as a result of a blow to the back of the head, fractures, or torsion injuries to the brainstem. Brainstem injuries have a very poor prognosis.

Hydrocephalus. Hydrocephalus is an abnormal increase in CSF volume. It may be caused by impaired reabsorption of CSF at the arachnoid villi (from subarachnoid hemorrhage or meningitis), called a **communicating hydrocephalus**. It may also be caused by interference or blockage with CSF outflow from the ventricular system (from cerebral edema, tumor, or debris). The ventricles may dilate from the relative increase in CSF

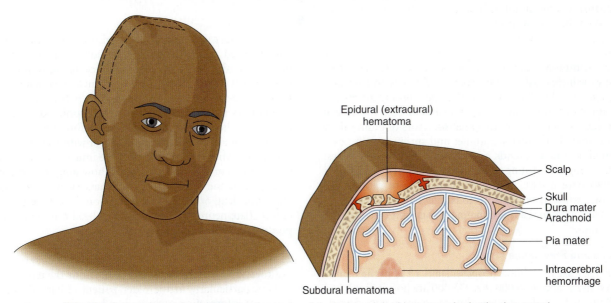

FIG. 45-8 Epidural hematoma (outside the dura mater of the brain), subdural hematoma (under the dura mater), and intracerebral hemorrhage (within the brain tissue).

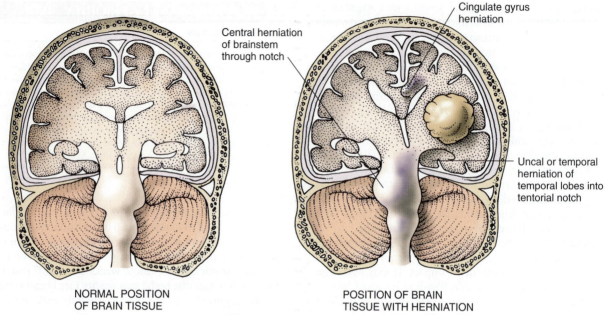

Central herniation
of brainstem
through notch

Cingulate gyrus
herniation

Uncal or temporal
herniation of
temporal lobes into
tentorial notch

NORMAL POSITION
OF BRAIN TISSUE

POSITION OF BRAIN
TISSUE WITH HERNIATION

FIG. 45-9 Herniation syndromes.

volume. Ultimately, if not treated, this increase may lead to increased ICP.

Brain Herniation. In the presence of increased ICP, the brain tissue may shift and herniate downward. Of the several types of herniation syndromes (Fig. 45-9), uncal herniation is one of the most clinically significant because it is life threatening. It is caused by a shift of one or both areas of the temporal lobe, known as the **uncus.** This shift creates pressure on the third cranial nerve. Late findings include dilated and nonreactive pupils, ptosis (drooping eyelids), and a rapidly deteriorating level of consciousness. Central herniation is caused by a downward shift of the brainstem and the diencephalon from a supratentorial lesion. It is clinically manifested by Cheyne-Stokes respirations, pinpoint and nonreactive pupils, and potential hemodynamic instability. All herniation syndromes are potentially life threatening, and the physician must be notified immediately when they are suspected.

Etiology

The most common causes of TBI in the United States are falls and motor vehicle crashes, followed by colliding with a stationary or moving object (CDC, 2013a). Alcohol and drugs are significant contributing factors to the causes of TBI. The United States is seeing increasing numbers of survivors of brain injury from wartime blast injuries. Summer and spring months, evenings, nights, and weekends are associated with the greatest number of injuries. Young males are more likely than young females to have a TBI. Men tend to play more sports, take more risks when driving, and consume larger amounts of alcohol than women. Falls are the most common cause of TBI in older adults.

Incidence and Prevalence

Annually, at least 1.4 million people sustain a TBI in the United States. Of these, about 50,000 die, 235,000 are hospitalized, and 1.1 million are treated and released from an emergency department (CDC, 2013a).

Health Promotion and Maintenance

Nurses can educate the public on ways to decrease the incidence of TBI by using safe driving practices such as not driving while impaired and wearing seat belts. Teach people at risk about how alcohol and illicit drug use affect driving ability. Promote the use of helmets for skateboarding and bicycle and motorcycle riding. Help prevent falls by providing a safe environment, especially for older adults. People need to be aware of environmental factors that may increase the likelihood of falls such as inadequate lighting and loose rugs. When possible, install safety equipment in bathtubs and showers. Evaluate balance and coordination as part of a falls prevention strategy inside the hospital and at home.

❖ PATIENT-CENTERED COLLABORATIVE CARE

◆ Assessment

History. Obtaining an accurate history from a patient who has sustained a TBI may be difficult because of either the seriousness of the injury or the presence of **amnesia** (loss of memory). It is not unusual for the patient to experience amnesia for events before or after the injury. The patient with a serious brain injury may be unconscious or in a confused and combative state. If the patient cannot provide information, the history can be obtained from first responders or witnesses to the injury. Always ask when, where, and how the injury occurred. Did the patient lose consciousness; if so, for how long? Has there been a change in the level of consciousness (LOC)? If trauma is related to drug or alcohol consumption, it may be difficult to differentiate neurologic changes from head trauma from those produced by intoxication.

Determine whether the patient had fluctuating consciousness or seizure activity and whether there is a history of a seizure disorder. Obtain precise information about the circumstances of falls, particularly in the older patient (Chart 45-8). Other pertinent information includes hand dominance, any diseases of or injuries to the eyes, and any allergies to drugs or food.

CHART 45-8 Nursing Focus on the Older Adult

Traumatic Brain Injury

- Brain injury is the fifth leading cause of death in older adults.
- The 65- to 75-year age-group has second highest incidence of brain injury of all age-groups.
- Falls and motor vehicle crashes are the most common causes of brain injury.
- Factors that contribute to high mortality are:
  - Falls causing subdural hematomas (closed head injuries), especially chronic subdural hematomas
  - Poorly tolerated systemic stress, which is increased by admission to a high-stimuli environment
  - Medical complications, such as hypotension, hypertension, and cardiac problems
  - Decreased protective mechanisms, which make patients susceptible to infections (especially pneumonia)
  - Decreased immunologic competence, which is further diminished by brain injury

! NURSING SAFETY PRIORITY (QSEN)

Critical Rescue

The upper cervical spinal nerves innervate the diaphragm to control breathing. Monitor TBI patients for respiratory problems and diaphragmatic breathing, as well as diminished or absent reflexes in the airway (cough and gag). Hypoxia and hypercapnia are best detected through arterial oxygen levels (partial pressure of arterial oxygen [PaO_2]), oxygen saturation (SpO_2), and end-tidal volume carbon dioxide measurement ($EtCO_2$). Observe chest wall movement and listen to breath sounds. Report any sign of respiratory problems immediately to the physician!

Inquire about a history of alcohol or drug use and abuse because these substances may interfere with the neurologic baseline assessment. Consider whether the patient is a victim of violence if he or she lives in residential care. The Joint Commission and the Centers for Medicare and Medicaid Services require that all patients be screened for abuse and neglect when they are admitted to any type of health care facility.

Physical Assessment/Clinical Manifestations. No two brain injuries are alike. The patient with a TBI may have a variety of manifestations depending on the severity of injury and the resulting increase in intracranial pressure (ICP) (see Chart 45-6). Assess for signs of increased ICP, hypotension, hypoxemia (decreased blood level of oxygen), or **hypercarbia** ($PaCO_2$ >40-45 mm Hg or increased partial pressure of carbon dioxide in arterial blood). Hypercarbia can cause cerebral vasodilation and contribute to elevated ICP. Determination of hypercarbia in an intubated patient can be done with an end-tidal carbon dioxide ($EtCO_2$) monitor. The early detection of changes in the patient's neurologic status enables the health care team to prevent or treat potentially life-threatening complications. Subtle changes in blood pressure, consciousness, and pupillary reaction to light can be very informative about neurologic deterioration.

Airway and Breathing Pattern Assessment. *The first priority is the assessment of the patient's ABCs—airway, breathing, and circulation.* Because TBI is occasionally associated with cervical spinal cord injuries, all patients with head trauma are treated as though they have cord injury until radiography proves otherwise. *Older adults are especially prone to cervical injuries at the first or second vertebral level, a life-threatening problem.* Assess for indicators of spinal cord injury, such as loss of motor function (MOBILITY) and SENSORY PERCEPTION, tenderness along the spine, and abnormal head tilt.

Injuries to the brainstem may cause a change in the patient's breathing pattern, such as Cheyne-Stokes respirations, central neurogenic hyperventilation, and/or apnea. In the unconscious patient, an artificial airway provides protection from aspiration as well as a route for oxygenation. Mechanical ventilation may be needed to support inadequate respiratory effort.

Spine Precautions. Patients with blunt trauma to the head or neck are typically transported from the scene of the injury to the hospital with a rigid cervical collar and a long spine board. The goal is to prevent new and secondary spine injury if there is unstable vertebrae or ligament damage. Spine precautions require placing the patient supine and aligning the spinal column in a neutral position so there is no rotation, flexion, or extension. The long spine board is removed as soon as possible upon arrival to the emergency department (ED) or intensive care unit (ICU); some EDs require this to be done within 20 minutes of arrival. The rigid cervical collar is maintained until definitive diagnostic studies to rule out cervical spine injury are completed (see Chapter 43). Skin breakdown and pressure ulcer formation are concerns when either the spine board or rigid collar are used.

Once the spine board is removed, spinal precautions are maintained until the provider indicates it is safe to bend or rotate the cervical, thoracic, and lumbar spine. Spinal precautions include: (1) bedrest; (2) no neck flexion with a pillow or roll; (3) no thoracic or lumbar flexion with head of bed elevation/bed controls (reverse Trendelenburg is acceptable); (4) manual control of the cervical spine anytime the rigid collar is removed; and (5) using a "log roll" procedure to reposition the patient. Log roll allows for maintaining the neutral anatomic alignment of the entire vertebral column while turning or moving the patient. A patient with known or suspected spine injury requires preplanning and the assistance of three or more qualified people to move the patient. One person is assigned to maintain manual control of the cervical spine, and one person is positioned on each side of the torso to turn the patient while preventing segmental rotation, flexion, extension, and/or lateral bending of the chest or abdomen during transfer of the patient. A fourth person may be assigned to check skin integrity and/or change linens and position padding. Neurologic function must be assessed after each position change.

A rigid cervical collar is used to maintain cervical spine ("c-spine") precautions as well as cervical spine immobilization with a confirmed cervical injury. If the collar is ill-fitting or soiled, it may be changed according to hospital guidelines while a second qualified person maintains c-spine immobilization.

Spine clearance is a clinical decision made by the health care provider, often in collaboration with the radiologist. Spine clearance includes determining the absence of acute bony, ligamentous, and neurologic abnormalities of the cervical spine based on history, physical examination, and/or negative radiologic studies.

Vital Signs Assessment. The mechanisms of autoregulation are often impaired as the result of a TBI. The more serious the injury, the more severe is the impact on *autoregulation* or the ability of cerebral vasculature to modify systemic pressure such that blood flow to the brain is sufficient. Monitor the patient's blood pressure and pulse. The patient may have hypotension or hypertension. Cushing's triad, a classic but late sign of increased ICP, is manifested by severe hypertension, a widened pulse pressure (increasing difference between systolic and diastolic values), and bradycardia. This triad of cardiovascular changes usually indicates imminent death.

Hypotension and tachycardia suggest hypovolemic shock. A decrease in blood volume may lead to decreased CPP and secondary brain ischemia and injury. Hypovolemic shock is usually due to bleeding outside the cranial vault such as traumatic injuries to the abdomen or chest. Cardiac dysrhythmias may result from chest trauma, bruising of the heart, or interference with the autonomic nervous system from primary or secondary injuries to the brain or spinal cord. Chapter 43 describes acute spinal cord injury manifestations and management.

Neurologic Assessment. Many hospitals use the Glasgow Coma Scale to document neurologic status (see Fig. 42-10). A change of 2 points is considered clinically important; urgent notification of the provider is advised if the change is a 2-point deterioration of GCS values.

The most important variable to assess with any brain injury is LOC! A decrease or change in LOC is typically the first sign of deterioration in neurologic status. A decrease in arousal or increased sleepiness should result in an increased aggressiveness and/or frequency in assessment. *Early* indicators of a change in LOC include behavior changes (e.g., restlessness, irritability) and disorientation, which are often subtle in nature.

Use a bright light to assess pupillary size and reaction to light. Facial trauma may swell eyelids, making this assessment difficult. Consider whether drugs that affect pupillary dilation and constriction, such as anticholinergics or adrenergics, have been used recently. Cycloplegics (eye drops to dilate the pupil) are used by ophthalmologists to evaluate eye and orbit injuries; these drugs also alter pupillary response to light.

> **! NURSING SAFETY PRIORITY** (QSEN)
>
> ***Critical Rescue***
>
> Check pupils of TBI patients for size and reaction to light, particularly if the patient is unable to follow directions to assess changes in level of consciousness. Report and document any changes in pupil size, shape, and reactivity to the health care provider immediately because they could indicate an increase in ICP.

Pupillary changes or eye signs differ depending on which areas of the brain are damaged. *Pinpoint and nonresponsive pupils are indicative of brainstem dysfunction at the level of the pons.* Of particular importance is the ovoid pupil, which is regarded as the midstage between a normal-size pupil and a dilated pupil. In some agencies, a portable automated pupillometer is used to measure pupil size and reaction rather than manual examination.

Asymmetric (uneven) pupils, loss of light reaction, or unilateral or bilateral dilated pupils are treated as herniation of the brain from increased ICP until proven differently. *Pupils that are fixed (nonreactive) and dilated are a poor prognostic sign. Patients with this problem are sometimes referred to as having "blown" pupils.*

Check gross vision if the patient's condition permits. Have the patient read any printed material (e.g., your name tag) or count the number of fingers that you hold within the patient's

visual field. Loss of vision is usually caused by either direct injury to the eye or injury to the occipital lobe. Visual loss may be temporary or permanent.

If the patient can participate, the health care provider or neurosurgical nurse tests *cranial nerves* (CNs) III, IV, and VI by asking the patient to following the sketch of an "H" in the visual field. Extraocular movements may be diminished because of injury or increased ICP. Damage to the optic chiasm or optic tract may cause visual-field deficits or diplopia (double vision). In the unconscious patient, additional oculocephalic and oculovestibular tests are performed to test the integrity of the brainstem and of CNs III, VI, and VII.

Monitor for additional late signs of increased ICP. These manifestations include severe headache, nausea, vomiting (often projectile), and seizures. The provider may evaluate for papilledema (seen by ophthalmoscopic examination). Papilledema, *also known as a* choked disc, *is edema and hyperemia (increased blood flow) of the optic disc. It is always a sign of increased ICP.* Headache and seizures are a response to the injury and may or may not be associated with increased ICP. Always remember that the patient with a brain injury is at risk for potentially devastating ICP elevations during the first hours after the event and that this risk decreases over the course of 1 to 3 days.

Assess for bilateral *motor* responses. The patient's motor loss or dysfunction usually appears contralateral (opposite side) to the site of the lesion, similar to a stroke. For example, a left-sided hemiparesis reflects an injury to the right cerebral hemisphere. Deterioration in motor function or the development of abnormal posturing (decerebrate or decorticate posturing) or flaccidity is another indicator of progressive brain injury (see Fig. 41-11 in Chapter 41). These changes are due to dysfunction within the pyramidal (motor) tracts of the spinal cord. Assess for brainstem or cerebellar injury, which may cause ataxia (loss of balance), decreased or increased muscle tone, and weakness. Remember that absence of motor function may also be an indicator of a spinal cord injury.

Carefully observe the patient's ears and nose for any signs of cerebrospinal fluid (CSF) leaks that result from a basilar skull fracture. Suspicious ear or nose fluid can be analyzed by the laboratory for glucose and electrolyte content. CSF placed on a white absorbent paper or linen can be distinguished from other fluids by the "halo" sign, a clear or yellowish ring surrounding a spot of blood. Although other body fluids can be used, a halo sign is most reliable when blood is in the center of the absorbent material since tears and saliva can also cause a clear ring in some conditions.

Palpate the patient's head gently to detect the presence of fractures or hematomas. Look for areas of ecchymosis (bruising), tender areas of the scalp, and lacerations. *Battle sign* or mastoid ecchymosis is bruising behind the ears and lower jaw indicating a fracture of the middle cranial fossa of the skull. *Raccoon's eyes* are purplish discoloration around eyes that can follow fracture of the skull's base. When CT scans are used with head and brain injury, these fractures are often visualized before bruising appears.

Psychosocial Assessment. Patients with mild brain injury may still have symptoms of disability 1 year or longer after injury, but long-term effects are not common. Patients with moderate to severe TBI may have varying degrees of psychosocial changes that persist for a lifetime. Personality changes manifested by temper outbursts, depression, risk-taking behavior, and denial of disability can occur. The patient may become talkative and develop a very outgoing personality. Memory, especially recent or short-term memory, is often affected. The patient may report difficulties in concentrating or the ability to learn new information and may have problems with insight and planning. Aggressive behavior, agitation, and sleep disorders may interfere with the ability to return to work or school. The ability to communicate and understand the spoken and written language may be altered. Changes in MOBIL-ITY and SENSORY PERCEPTION may necessitate rehabilitation or use of assistive devices. All these changes in health status may lead to difficulties within the family structure and with social and work-related interactions. Behavioral interventions are used by cognitive and brain injury rehabilitation specialists to help both the patient and family members develop adaptive strategies.

Assess family dynamics, particularly if the patient is discharged to the family's care directly from the acute care hospital. The family or significant others must also cope with changes in the patient's physical appearance and cognitive abilities. Family members may feel guilty or angry about not being able to prevent the injury or blame the patient for the personal choices that contributed to the event. The family or significant others may feel overwhelmed by the complexity of care required and the long recovery period. Help both the family and the patient identify coping strategies to deal with the role changes caused by the injury.

Laboratory Assessment. There are no established serum tests to diagnose a primary brain injury. Detection of the protein *S-100B* in serum is showing some promise as an indicator of brain injury (Defazio et al., 2013; Müller et al., 2011). Several laboratory tests are used to guide interventions and to prevent secondary brain insult. The health care provider requests arterial blood gases, complete blood count (CBC), serum glucose, osmolarity, and electrolyte levels. These tests are performed to monitor hemodynamic status, identify electrolyte imbalance, determine oxygen-carrying capacity, and detect infection. Electrolyte imbalances, hypoxia, hypovolemia, and reduced blood pressure from infection or shock can contribute to secondary injury, as well as increase the risk for seizures. A toxicology screen and an electrocardiogram (ECG) are often requested.

Imaging Assessment. The health care provider immediately requests CT of the brain to identify the extent and scope of injury. This diagnostic test can identify the presence of an injury that requires surgical intervention, such as an epidural or subdural hematoma. *Radiography* and *CT scanning* of the cervical spine and the skull are done to rule out fractures and dislocations. An *MRI* may be done to detect subtle changes in brain tissue and show more specific detail of the brain injury. MRI is particularly useful in the diagnosis of diffuse axonal injury, but it is not recommended for patients with ICP monitoring devices.

Other Diagnostic Assessment. As the patient's condition stabilizes, the physician may request other diagnostic tests to identify the extent of injury to the brain. For example, the integrity of the cerebral vessels is measured through the use of ultrasonography. *Evoked potentials* (electroencephalogram recordings with sensory stimuli) provide information on cerebral function and may be useful in predicting the patient's outcome.

◆ **Interventions**

The patient with a *severe* TBI is admitted to the critical care unit or a trauma center. Patients with *moderate* TBI are admitted to either the general nursing unit or the critical care unit, where they are closely observed for at least 24 hours. Those with *mild* TBI may be sent home from the emergency department with instructions for home-based observation and primary care provider follow-up.

Nonsurgical Management. As with any critically injured patient, priority is given to maintaining a patent airway, breathing, and circulation. Specific nursing interventions for the patient with a TBI are directed toward preventing or detecting secondary brain injury or the conditions that contribute to secondary brain injury such as increased ICP, promoting fluid and electrolyte balance, and monitoring the effects of treatments and drug therapy. Providing health teaching and emotional support for the patient and family are vital parts of the plan of care.

Preventing and Detecting Secondary Brain Injury. Take and record the patient's *vital signs* every 1 to 2 hours or more often based on patient acuity. The health care provider may prescribe IV fluids or drug therapy to prevent severe hypertension or hypotension. Dysrhythmias and nonspecific ST-segment or T-wave changes may occur, possibly in response to stimulation of the autonomic nervous system or an increase in the level of circulating catecholamines such as epinephrine. Document and report cardiac dysrhythmias, hypotension, and hypertension to the health care provider. Obtain the target range for blood pressure and heart rate from the health care provider.

The patient with a brain injury may develop a fever as a result of systemic trauma, blood in the cranium, or a generalized inflammatory response to brain injury. Fever as a consequence of infection may develop later in the course of the disease. A third cause of fever is a central fever caused by hypothalamic damage. It is manifested by an absence of sweating and no diurnal (night and day) variation. This type of fever is high and lasts several days to weeks. In addition, it responds better to cooling (e.g., cool air hypothermia, sponge bath) than to the administration of antipyretic drugs such as acetaminophen (Tylenol, Ace-Tabs ✦). *Fever from any cause is associated with higher morbidity and mortality rates.*

Therapeutic hypothermia may be started regardless of the presence of fever. The purpose of therapeutic hypothermia is to rapidly cool the patient to a core temperature of 89.6° and 93.2° F (32° to 34° C) for 24 to 48 hours after the primary injury. Rewarming to a normal core temperature requires specialized knowledge and skill because rapid fluid and electrolyte shifts can cause cardiac dysrhythmias and changes to systemic and cerebral pressures. The rationale for therapeutic hypothermia is to reduce brain metabolism and prevent the cascade of molecular and biochemical events that contribute to secondary brain injury in moderate to severe TBI.

Arterial blood gas (ABG), oxygen saturation (Spo_2), and end-tidal carbon dioxide ($EtCO_2$) values are all used to evaluate respiratory status and guide mechanical ventilation therapy. *Hyperventilation* for the intubated patient during the first 24 hours after brain injury is usually avoided because it may produce ischemia by causing cerebral vasoconstriction. The result is a decrease in cerebral blood volume. In acute elevations of ICP or neurologic deterioration, however, brief periods of hyperventilation may be used. After the first 24 hours, when a patient is mechanically ventilated and intracranial hypertension persists, the health care provider may adjust mechanical ventilation settings to reduce arterial carbon dioxide. Other interventions are used first, including diversion of CSF and manipulation of fluid intake and output. When mechanical ventilation adjustments are used, the goal is to maintain the partial pressure of arterial carbon dioxide ($Paco_2$) at 35 to 38 mm Hg. *Carbon dioxide is a very potent vasodilator that can contribute to increases in ICP.*

Prevent intermittent and sustained hypoxemia. Monitor peripheral oxygen saturation continuously in moderate to severe TBI. Hypoxemia damages brain tissue and contributes to cerebral vasodilation and increased ICP. Arterial oxygen levels (Pao_2) are maintained between 80 and 100 mm Hg to prevent secondary injury. If the patient is intubated, provide 100% oxygen before each pass of the endotracheal suction catheter. Avoid overly aggressive hyperventilation with endotracheal suctioning because of the potential for hypocarbia. Cerebral ischemia caused by even transiently decreased oxygen and either high or low carbon dioxide levels contributes to secondary brain injury. Lidocaine given IV or endotracheally may be used to suppress the cough reflex; coughing increases ICP.

Patients with moderate or severe brain injury are at risk for losing airway patency. Absence of a cough and/or gag reflex, pooled oral and nasal secretions in the pharynx, and inability to position oneself to facilitate pulmonary secretion removal all contribute to the need to manage the airway in the non-intubated brain-injured adult. Pulmonary secretions may be thick because of the diuretics or fluid intake restriction that may be used to prevent cerebral edema. Collaborate with the respiratory therapist to provide humidified air and chest physiotherapy as needed based on patient assessment. If the patient has an ICP monitor present, pay close attention to the ICP response and moderate or stop suctioning, chest vibration, or repositioning when ICP increases.

⚠ NURSING SAFETY PRIORITY (QSEN)

Action Alert

Position the TBI patient to avoid extreme flexion or extension of the neck and to maintain the head in the midline, neutral position. Log roll the patient during turning to avoid extreme hip flexion, and keep the head of the bed elevated at least 30 degrees or as recommended by the health care provider.

Generally, HOB elevation in patients with TBI is elevated at 30 to 45 degrees to prevent aspiration. However, if increasing head elevation significantly lowers systemic blood pressure, the patient does not benefit from drainage of venous blood or CSF

out of the skull from this position. If hypotension accompanies an elevated backrest position, the patient may be harmed. Adjust head elevation to sustain CPP >70 mm Hg when possible. Avoid sudden vertical changes of the head of the bed in the older patient because the dura is tightly adhered to the skull and may pull away from the brain, leading to a subdural hematoma.

Patients with *severe* TBI often die. As the physiologic deterioration begins, keep in mind that the patient may be a potential organ donor. *Before* brain death is declared, contact the local organ procurement organization. Determine if the patient consented to be an organ donor. This information is typically on a driver's license or other state-issued card or advance directive. The patient's wishes should be followed unless he or she has a medical condition that prevents organ donation. The organ donor agency representative or physician discusses the possibility of organ donation with the family. Some families may not agree with the patient's decision, which can cause an ethical dilemma. Many health care agencies have an ethics specialist of committee members who can help with these situations.

Determining Brain Death. In 2010, the American Academy of Neurology guidelines for determining brain death were updated. Four prerequisites must be met to establish a brain death diagnosis (Wijdicks et al., 2010):

- Coma of known cause as established by history, clinical examination, laboratory testing, and neuroimaging
- Normal or near-normal core body temperature (higher than 96.8° F (36°C)
- Normal systolic blood pressure (higher than or equal to 100 mm Hg)
- At least one neurologic examination (some states and health care systems require two)

No consensus has been reached on who is qualified to perform head-to-toe brain death neurologic examinations, but neurologists and critical care intensivists typically do them. Neuroimaging tests are not required to confirm brain death but are desirable. Examples of tests that may be done include cerebral angiography, bedside electroencephalography (EEG), and cerebral computed tomographic angiography (CTA).

Drug Therapy. Mannitol (Osmitrol), an osmotic diuretic, is used to treat cerebral edema by pulling water out of the extracellular space of the edematous brain tissue. It is most effective when given in boluses rather than as a continuous infusion. Furosemide (Lasix), a loop diuretic, is often used as adjunctive therapy to reduce the incidence of rebound from mannitol. It also enhances the therapeutic action of mannitol, reduces edema and blood volume, decreases sodium uptake by the brain, and decreases the production of CSF at the choroid plexus. *Glucocorticoids* (dexamethasone [Decadron, Dexasone] and methylprednisolone sodium succinate [Solu-Medrol, Medrol]) have no benefit in the management of increased ICP caused by brain injury or infarction.

Administer *mannitol* through a filter in the IV tubing or, if given by IV push, draw it up through a filtered needle to eliminate microscopic crystals. For the patient receiving either osmotic or loop diuretics, monitor for intake and output, severe dehydration, and indications of acute renal failure, weakness, edema, and changes in urine output. Serum electrolyte and osmolarity levels are measured every 6 hours. Mannitol is used to obtain a serum osmolarity of 310 to 320 mOsm/L, depending on physician preference and the desired outcome of therapy. Insert an indwelling urinary catheter to maintain strict measurement of output. Check the patient's serum and urine osmolarity daily.

Sedative agents like dexmedetomidine (Precedex, Dexdor) or propofol (Diprivan) can be used as continuous IV infusions to manage agitation and ventilatory asynchrony. They have a short duration of action and can be stopped for a daily neurologic examination. However, when a patient requires sedation for management of ICP hypertension, stopping these drugs is not advised until periods of ICP elevation are infrequent and not sustained.

Opioids such as morphine sulfate or fentanyl may be used with ventilated patients to decrease agitation and control restlessness if the agitation is caused by pain. Fentanyl has fewer effects on blood pressure and heart rate than morphine and may therefore be a safer agent to manage pain. These agents may be reversed with naloxone (Narcan), but opioid reversal should be avoided if at all possible to reduce risk for withdrawal and rebound pain and agitation.

Antiepileptic drugs, such as phenytoin (Dilantin), to prevent seizures are not recommended routinely. However, they may be given as an option to prevent early-onset seizure activity that may occur with some types of specific brain injury. Acetaminophen (Tylenol, Ace-Tabs ✦) and aspirin (acetylsalicylic acid [ASA], Ancasal ✦) are given to patients who are febrile (temperature greater than 101° F [38.3° C]) to reduce fever.

Inducing Barbiturate Coma. Barbiturate coma (coma induced by barbiturates) has been used for intracranial hypertension (increased ICP) that cannot be controlled by other means. Either pentobarbital sodium (Nembutal, Novopentobarb ✦) or thiopentone is the drug of choice. These drugs decrease the metabolic demands of the brain and cerebral blood flow, stabilize cell membranes, decrease the formation of vasogenic edema, and produce a more uniform blood supply. The health care provider adjusts the dosage to maintain complete unresponsiveness. As a consequence, it is difficult to recognize subtle or obvious neurologic changes. The patient requires mechanical ventilation, sophisticated hemodynamic monitoring, and ICP monitoring. Complications of barbiturate coma include decreased GI motility, cardiac dysrhythmias from hypokalemia, hypotension, and fluctuations in body temperature.

Maintaining Fluid and Electrolyte Management. The patient with TBI is at risk for diabetes insipidus (DI) and the syndrome of inappropriate antidiuretic hormone (SIADH) because the pituitary gland may be injured or compressed from cerebral edema (see Chapter 62). In the patient with multiple trauma, fluid overload can occur and cerebral edema can worsen from the rapid administration of IV fluids or plasma expanders. Fluid management is titrated to optimize volume resuscitation but minimize brain swelling and ICP elevation. ICP is also influenced by the response to diuretic therapy and laboratory values. Monitor serum and urine osmolarity and electrolytes at least daily when IV fluids and diuretics are used for management of the TBI patient.

Managing Nutritional Status. The patient with a brain injury may have changes in these areas:

- Coma or impaired ability to feed oneself
- Dysphagia, including swallowing difficulties or pocketing food and being unaware of the presence of food within the oral cavity
- Sense of smell
- Sense of taste

As a result, he or she is at risk for acute or chronic nutritional deficits that may interfere with the healing process. Weigh the patient daily to assess fluid and nutritional intake. Collaborate with the dietitian to determine whether caloric needs are being met.

A small-lumen nasogastric or nasoduodenal tube or a percutaneous endoscopic gastrostomy (PEG) tube can be used to provide enteral nutrition. Parenteral nutrition can be used if the patient is unable to meet caloric or protein intake goals because of GI dysfunction, which is common during acute care and immediately following trauma. Communicate with the health care provider before a nasogastric tube is placed. Do not insert anything into nasal passages in the presence of a cribriform plate fracture since this type of fracture can allow passage of the tube into the brain.

For the patient who can take food and fluids by mouth, ensure that mealtime is a pleasant experience. Position the patient to maximize swallowing ability. The speech-language pathologist (SLP) identifies strategies to prevent food from accumulating in the cheek of the affected side. In general, patients who have swallowing problems can tolerate or swallow soft or semisoft foods and liquids (mechanical soft or dental diet, junior baby foods, custards, scrambled eggs) better than thin liquids (water, juice, milk). Powdered thickener (e.g., Thick-It) may be added to increase liquid consistency to aid in swallowing effort. Commercial dietary supplements (e.g., Ensure) may be needed to meet the patient's caloric and protein requirements. Collaborate with the dietitian and SLP to create a nutritional plan appropriate for the patient with dysphagia.

Managing Sensory Perception, Cognitive, and Behavioral Changes. If a large lesion of the parietal lobe is present, the patient may experience a loss of sensation for pain, temperature, touch, and proprioception (position sense), which prevents an appropriate response to environmental stimuli. A hazard-free environment is necessary to prevent injury (e.g., from burns if the patient's coffee is too hot). In collaboration with the rehabilitation therapist, integrate a sensory stimulation program into the comatose or stuporous patient's routine care activities. Sensory stimulation is done to facilitate a meaningful response to the environment. Present visual, auditory, or tactile stimuli one at a time, and explain the purpose and the type of stimulus presented. For example, show a picture of the patient's mother and say, "This is a picture of your mother." The picture is shown several times, and the same words are used to describe the picture. If auditory tapes or DVDs are used, they should be no longer than 10 to 15 minutes. If the stimulus is presented for a longer period, it simply becomes "white" noise, or meaningless background noise.

Patients with a mild brain injury may be disoriented and have a short-term memory loss. Always introduce yourself before any interaction. Keep explanations of procedures and activities short and simple, and give them immediately before and throughout patient care. To the extent possible, maintain a sleep-wake cycle with scheduled rest periods. Orient the patient to time (day, month, and year) and place, and explain the reason for the hospitalization. Reassure the patient that he or she is safe. Ask the family to bring in familiar objects, such as pictures. Provide orientation cues within the environment, such as a large clock with numbers or a single-date calendar.

An overwhelming majority of brain injury survivors have altered COGNITION. Cognitive impairments interfere with the brain-injured patient's ability to function effectively in school,

TABLE 45-5　Advantages and Disadvantages of Intracranial Pressure Monitoring Devices

MONITORING DEVICE	ADVANTAGES	DISADVANTAGES
Intraventricular catheter (IVC)	Allows accurate measurement of intracranial pressure (ICP) Allows drainage or sampling of cerebrospinal fluid (CSF) Allows instillation of contrast media Provides reliable evaluation of cerebral compliance	Provides additional site for potential infection Most invasive method for monitoring ICP Must be balanced and recalibrated frequently Catheter can become occluded by blood or tissue Insertion can be difficult with small or collapsed ventricles CSF leakage can occur around insertion site
Subarachnoid bolt or screw	Lower infection rates than with IVC Quickly and easily placed Can be used with small or collapsed ventricles Does not penetrate brain parenchyma	Tendency for dampened waveform Less accurate at high ICP May become occluded by blood or tissue Must be balanced and recalibrated frequently (i.e., every 4 hours and whenever patient is repositioned) Baseline drift Does not provide for CSF sampling
Subdural/epidural catheter or sensor	Least invasive Decreased risk for infection Easily and quickly placed	Increasing baseline drift over time; therefore accuracy and reliability are questionable Does not provide for CSF sampling or drainage
Fiberoptic transducer-tipped catheter	Can be placed in subdural or subarachnoid space, in ventricle, or into brain tissue Easily transported Requires calibrating only once (during insertion) Baseline drift to 1 mm Hg/day Decreased risk for infection Less waveform artifact No need to adjust transducer to patient's position Easy to insert	Does not provide for CSF sampling or drainage Cannot be recalibrated after placement Probe needs periodic replacement Fragile fiberoptic cable easily damaged and broken

at work, and in his or her personal life. *Cognitive rehabilitation* is a way of helping brain-injured patients regain function in areas that are essential for a return to independence and a reasonable quality of life. However, these services are not widely available or accessible.

The patient may be at risk for seizure activity. Keep the bed in low position, and have oxygen and suction available at the bedside. For patients who exhibit poor judgment or who dislodge therapeutic lines, consider the use of hand mittens. Be sure to follow the agency's policy for caring for patients in restraints, if needed. Provide opportunities for toileting. Encourage self-care to promote function at discharge.

Surgical Management. The physician may elect to insert an intracranial pressure (ICP) monitoring device to evaluate the patient's ICP more closely (Table 45-5). All devices are inserted through a *burr hole* (also known as a *keyhole craniotomy*). Strict sterile technique is observed during placement of ICP monitoring devices, and the site is maintained subsequently with attention to sterile technique. Each device is connected to an electronic transducer and a bedside monitor that displays pressure waves and provides a digital value of the pressure. *Be sure to provide ongoing head-to-toe assessments even though the patient's ICP is being invasively monitored!*

In extreme cases in which the patient's ICP cannot be controlled, the physician may elect to perform a decompressive craniectomy (removal of a section of the skull) or craniotomy (skull opening followed by immediate skull closure) to remove ischemic brain tissue or the tips of the temporal lobes. The removal of a portion of the skull and/or nonvital brain tissue allows additional space for edema without increasing ICP. Following a craniectomy, information about side-lying restrictions may be placed in the plan of care and repeated in a sign at the head of bed; patients do not lie on the side from with the skull fragment was removed. The patient must wear protective gear

(bike or football helmet) when out of bed because an injury to the head where the skull fragment is missing will cause significant brain injury. The skull fragment can be frozen and re-implanted as late as 3 years after removal; re-implantation is planned as the patient becomes ambulatory.

A craniotomy without brain tissue removal may be performed to remove an epidural or subdural clot (hematoma). Care of the patient with a craniotomy is discussed on p. 960 under Postoperative Care in the Brain Tumors section.

Community-Based Care

The patient with a *mild* brain injury recovers at home after discharge from the emergency department (ED) or hospital (Chart 45-9). The patient with a *severe* brain injury requires long-term case management and ongoing rehabilitation after hospitalization. A number of specialized brain injury rehabilitation facilities are available in the United States and Canada. Communicate the patient's plan of care, including drug therapy (use best practices for drug reconciliation and transitions in care), to the receiving nurse or provider during each transition in care.

Home Care Management. The major desired outcome for rehabilitation after brain injury is to maximize the patient's ability to return to his or her highest level of functioning. Activities such as occupational therapy (OT), physical therapy (PT), and speech-language therapy may continue in the home after discharge from the hospital or rehabilitation facility. Adaptation of the home environment to accommodate the patient safely may be needed. For example, smoke and fire alarms must function properly because the patient with a brain injury often loses the sense of smell. Home evaluations and referrals to outside agencies are completed before discharge.

Self-Management Education. Collaborate with the case manager (CM) to provide the patient and family with both

Mild Brain Injury

- Initial neurologic assessment occurs hourly until the patient returns to baseline. The frequency of ongoing assessment for mild traumatic brain injury (MTBI) is not established.
- For a headache, give acetaminophen (Tylenol) every 4 hours as needed.
- Avoid giving the person sedatives, sleeping pills, or alcoholic beverages for at least 24 hours unless the physician instructs otherwise.
- Do not allow the person to engage in strenuous activity for at least 48 hours.
- While assessment of balance is a component of advanced nursing or medical practice, the caregiver should be aware that balance disturbances cause safety concerns and he or she should provide for monitored or assisted movement.
- If any of these symptoms occur, take the person back to the emergency department immediately:
  - Severe headache
  - Persistent or severe nausea or vomiting
  - Blurred vision
  - Drainage from the ear or nose
  - Weakness
  - Slurred speech
  - Progressive sleepiness
  - Worsening headache
  - Unequal pupil size
- Keep follow-up appointments with the health care provider.

written and verbal instructions for discharge. The teaching plan includes a review of seizure safety at home and strategies to adapt to sensory dysfunction. Discuss issues related to personality or behavior problems that may arise and how to cope with them. Explain the purpose, dosage, schedule, and route of administration of drug therapy. Teach the family to encourage the patient to participate in activities as tolerated. Demonstrations and return demonstrations of care activities help family members become more skillful. Stress the importance of regular follow-up visits with therapists and other health care providers.

Patients with personality and behavior problems respond best to a structured and consistent environment. Instruct the family to develop a home routine that provides structure, repetition, and consistency. Remind the family about the importance of reinforcing positive behaviors rather than negative behaviors.

! NURSING SAFETY PRIORITY (QSEN)

Action Alert

Teach the patient who has sustained a *mild* brain injury, sometimes called a *concussion,* that symptoms that disturb sleep, enjoyment of daily activities, work performance, mood, memory, and ability to learn new material and cause changes in personality require follow-up care. Provide the patient and family with education materials that will alert them to symptoms and management options. A good source of written instructions is *Heads Up: What to Expect After a Concussion—Patient Discharge Instruction Sheet and Getting Better (after concussion)* from the Centers for Disease Control and Prevention (CDC, 2013a).

Most patients with *moderate to severe* TBI are discharged with varied physical and cognitive disabilities. Changes in personality and behavior are very common. The family must learn

to cope with the patient's increased fatigue, irritability, temper outbursts, depression, and memory problems. These patients often require constant supervision at home, and families may feel socially isolated. Teach the family about the importance of regular respite care, either in a structured day-care respite program for the patient or through relief provided by a friend or neighbor. Family members, particularly the primary caregiver, may become depressed and have feelings of loneliness. In addition, they may feel angry with the patient because of the physical, financial, and emotional responsibilities that his or her care has placed on them. To help the family cope with these problems, suggest that they join and actively participate in a local brain injury support group.

Health Care Resources. Collaborate with the CM to refer families and patients to local chapters of the Brain Injury Association of America (BIAA) (www.biausa.org) and the National Brain Injury Foundation (www.nbif.org) for information and support. The BIAA has a number of helpful publications on preventing and living with TBI. Other resources include religious, spiritual, and cultural leaders.

BRAIN TUMORS

Brain tumors can arise anywhere within the brain structures and are named according to the cell or tissue where they are located; however, cerebral tumors are the most common. *Primary* tumors originate within the CNS and rarely metastasize (spread) outside this area. *Secondary* brain tumors result from metastasis from other areas of the body, such as the lung, breast, kidney, and GI tract.

❖ PATHOPHYSIOLOGY

Complications of Cerebral Tumors

Regardless of location, the tumor expands and invades, infiltrates, compresses, and displaces normal brain tissue. This leads to one or more of these complications:

- Cerebral edema/brain tissue inflammation
- Increased intracranial pressure (ICP)
- Neurologic deficits
- Hydrocephalus
- Pituitary dysfunction

Cerebral edema (vasogenic edema) results from changes in capillary endothelial tissue permeability that allows plasma to seep into the extracellular spaces. This leads to *increased ICP* and, depending on the location of the tumor, brain herniation syndromes. A variety of *neurologic deficits* result from edema, infiltration, distortion, and compression of surrounding brain tissue. The cerebral blood vessels may become compressed because of edema and increased ICP. This compression leads to ischemia (decreased blood flow) of the area supplied by the vessel. In addition, the tumor may enter the walls of the vessel, causing it to rupture and hemorrhage into the tumor bed or other brain tissue. Some patients who have brain tumors have seizure activity from interference with the brain's normal electrical activity.

Increased ICP may also result from *hydrocephalus* (increased cerebrospinal fluid [CSF]) related to obstruction of the flow of CSF or displacement of the lateral ventricles by the expanding lesion. Typically, a tumor obstructs the aqueduct of Sylvius or one of the ventricles or pushes into the subarachnoid space.

TABLE 45-6 **Classification of Brain Tumors**

Benign	Malignant
• Acoustic neuroma (schwannoma)	• Astrocytoma (a *glioblastoma multiforme* is a Grade 4 astrocytoma)
• Choroid plexus papilloma	
• Meningioma	• Oligodendroglioma
• Pituitary adenoma	• Ependymoma
• Astrocytoma	• Medulloblastoma
• Grade 1 (may undergo changes and become malignant)	• Chondrosarcoma
	• Glioma
• Chondroma	• Lymphoma
• Craniopharyngioma	
• Hemangioblastoma	

Pituitary dysfunction may occur as the tumor compresses the pituitary gland and causes the syndrome of inappropriate antidiuretic hormone (SIADH) or diabetes insipidus (DI). These disorders result in severe fluid and electrolyte imbalances and can be life threatening. (See Chapters 42 and 62 for a complete description.)

Classification of Tumors

Brain tumors are usually classified as benign, malignant (cancerous), or metastatic (Table 45-6). They may or may not be treated, depending on their location. Benign (noncancerous) tumors are generally associated with a favorable outcome. Malignant or metastatic tumors require more aggressive intervention including surgery, radiation, and/or chemotherapy.

A second classification system is based on location. Supratentorial tumors are located within the cerebral hemispheres. Located beneath the tentorium (fold of dura mater) is the infratentorial area—the area of the brainstem structures and cerebellum.

A third classification system depends on the cellular or anatomic origins of the tumor. The nervous system is composed of two types of cells: (1) neurons, which are responsible for nerve impulse conduction; and (2) neuroglial cells, which provide support, nourishment, and protection for neurons. Four specific types of neuroglial cells are astrocytes, oligodendroglia, ependymal cells, and microglia. When classifying gliomas according to this system, tumors are named by their cell type. For example, an astrocytoma is a tumor of astrocytes. Gliomas are *malignant* tumors.

Meningiomas, the most common *benign* tumors, arise from the coverings of the brain (the meninges). This tumor is capsular, globular, and well outlined and causes compression and displacement of nearby brain tissue. Although complete removal of the tumor is possible, it tends to recur.

Pituitary tumors that occur in the anterior lobe account for up to one fourth of brain tumors and may cause endocrine dysfunction. The most common type of pituitary tumor is the adenoma. These tumors are *benign* and often occur in young and middle-aged adults. The presenting symptoms include visual disturbances and hypopituitary signs, such as loss of body hair, diabetes insipidus (DI), infertility, visual field defects, and headaches.

Acoustic neuromas arise from the sheath of Schwann cells in the peripheral portion of cranial nerve VIII. They are also referred to as *cerebellar pontine angle (CPA) tumors* to describe their anatomic location. Acoustic neuromas compress brain tissue and tend to surround nearby cranial nerves (VII, V, IX, X), making surgical removal difficult without causing permanent cranial nerve dysfunction. Women are twice as likely as men to have acoustic neuromas. Common symptoms include hearing loss, tinnitus (ringing in the ears), and dizziness or vertigo.

Metastatic, or secondary, tumors account for many brain tumors. Cancer cells from the lung, breast, colon, pancreas, and kidney can travel to the brain via the blood and the lymphatic system. Multiple metastatic lesions are fairly common.

Brain tumors are also grouped by grade, which refers to the microscopic tissue evaluated by the histologist:

- Grade I: The tissue is benign; the cells look nearly like normal brain cells, and they grow slowly.
- Grade II: The tissue is malignant; the cells look less like normal cells than do the cells in a Grade I.
- Grade III: The malignant tissue has cells that look very different from normal cells; the abnormal cells are actively growing (anaplastic).
- Grade IV: The malignant tissue has cells that look most abnormal and tend to grow quickly.

Etiology and Genetic Risk

The exact cause of brain tumors is unknown. Several areas under investigation include genetic mutations and a variety of environmental factors. The use of cellular phones has been investigated as a cause of brain tumors, but findings are not confirmed. Brain tumors account for a small percentage of all cancer deaths. Primary brain tumors are relatively uncommon; many more patients have metastatic lesions (Cahill & Armstrong, 2011). Malignant brain tumors are seen primarily in patients 40 to 70 years of age, and the survival rate is low compared with that of other cancers.

❖ PATIENT-CENTERED COLLABORATIVE CARE

◆ Assessment

When possible, obtain a history from both the patient and the family, including current signs and symptoms. A complete neurologic assessment is needed to establish baseline data and to determine the nature and extent of neurologic deficits.

The clinical manifestations of brain tumors vary with the site of the tumor (Chart 45-10). In general, assess for these symptoms of a brain tumor:

- Headaches that are usually more severe on awakening in the morning
- Nausea and vomiting
- Visual symptoms
- Seizures or convulsions
- Facial numbness or tingling
- Loss of balance or dizziness
- Weakness or paralysis in one part or one side of the body
- Difficulty thinking, speaking, or articulating
- Changes in mentation or personality
- Papilledema (swelling of the optic disc) indicating increased ICP

Neurologic deficits result from the destruction, distortion, or compression of brain tissue. *Supratentorial (cerebral)* tumors usually result in paralysis, seizures, memory loss, cognitive impairment, language impairment, or vision problems. *Infratentorial* tumors produce ataxia, autonomic nervous system dysfunction, vomiting, drooling, hearing loss, and vision impairment. As the tumor grows, ICP increases and the symptoms become progressively more severe.

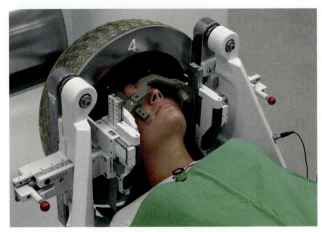

FIG. 45-10 A gamma knife treatment. The treatment beams are widely dispersed over the surface of the head to prevent damage to healthy brain tissue. The beams are intense only at the point of target.

Diagnosis is based on the history, neurologic assessment, clinical examination, and results of neurodiagnostic testing. Noninvasive diagnostic studies such as *CT, MRI,* and *skull films* are conducted first. These tests identify the size, location, and extent of the tumor. The MRI may be used for initial diagnostic evaluation and is a more sensitive diagnostic study, whereas the CT is often used for follow-up during the course of illness.

Cerebral angiography is usually not indicated to diagnose a brain tumor but may be used to provide additional information about blood supply to the tumor. *Electroencephalography (EEG), lumbar puncture (LP), brain scan,* and *positron emission tomography (PET)* may be indicated to provide further information about the size, location, and characteristics of the tumor. *To prevent brain herniation, LP should not be performed if the patient is exhibiting signs of ICP elevation.* Laboratory tests may also be requested to evaluate endocrine function, renal status, and electrolyte balance.

◆ Interventions

Interventions depend on the type, size, and location of the tumor. For example, a small benign tumor may be periodically monitored through CT and MRI scanning to assess its growth. Malignant tumors may be managed by chemotherapy, radiation, and/or surgery.

Nonsurgical Management. The desired outcomes of treatment of brain tumors are to decrease tumor size, improve quality of life, and improve survival time. The type of treatment selected depends on the tumor size and location, patient symptoms and general condition, and whether the tumor has recurred. In addition to traditional interventions, a number of experimental treatment modalities are being investigated. These include blood-brain barrier disruption, recombinant DNA, monoclonal antibodies, new chemotherapeutic drugs, and immunotherapy. Traditional *radiation therapy* may be used alone, after surgery, or in combination with chemotherapy and surgery. Chapter 22 discusses radiation treatment for patients with cancer.

Drug Therapy. The health care provider may prescribe a variety of drugs to treat the tumor, manage the patient's symptoms, and prevent complications. *Chemotherapy* may be given

alone, in combination with radiation and surgery, and with tumor progression. Although these drugs may control tumor growth or decrease tumor burden, the benefit does not last. Chemotherapy usually involves more than one agent that may be given orally, IV, intra-arterially, and/or intrathecally through an Ommaya reservoir placed in a cranial ventricle. In electro-chemotherapy, electric voltage carries agents into the tumor. When given systemically, the drug must be lipid-soluble to cross the blood-brain barrier.

Commonly used oral drugs are lomustine (CCNU), temozolomide (Temodar), procarbazine (Matulane), and methotrexate (MTX). Vincristine (Oncovin) may be given IV in combination with other drugs. Monitor for side effects of these drugs, which are similar to those of any chemotherapeutic drug. Chapter 22 describes general nursing implications for care of a patient receiving chemotherapy.

Direct drug delivery to the tumor is an emerging practice. Disk-shaped drug (Gliadel) wafers may be placed directly into the cavity created during surgical tumor removal (interstitial chemotherapy). The major drug in the wafer is carmustine (BCNU). This therapy is usually given for newly diagnosed high-grade malignant gliomas, but recurrent tumors may also be treated with this method. Other drugs used are molecularly targeted. Examples include erlotinib (Tarceva), gefitinib (Iressa), and bevacizumab (Avastin) (Lilley et al., 2014).

Analgesics, such as codeine and acetaminophen (Tylenol, Ace-Tabs ✦), are given for headache. Dexamethasone (Decadron) is usually given to control cerebral edema. Phenytoin (Dilantin) or other antiepileptic drugs may be given to prevent or treat seizure activity. Proton pump inhibitors are given to decrease gastric acid secretion and prevent the development of stress ulcers.

Stereotactic Radiosurgery. Stereotactic radiosurgery (SRS) is an alternative to traditional surgery. Several techniques are used, including the modified linear accelerator (LINAC) using accelerated x-rays, a particle accelerator using beams of protons (cyclotron), and isotope seeds implanted in the tumor (brachytherapy).

The gamma knife is an SRS procedure that uses a single high dose of ionized radiation to focus multiple beams of gamma radiation produced by the radioisotope *cobalt-60* to destroy intracranial lesions selectively without damaging surrounding healthy tissue (Fig. 45-10). Combining neurodiagnostic imaging tools—including MRI, CT, magnetic resonance angiography (MRA), and angiography—with the gamma knife allows for precise localization of deep-seated or anatomically difficult lesions. Treatment usually takes less than an hour, and patients require only overnight hospitalization. Advantages of this technique include its:

- Noninvasive nature
- Lower risk when compared with traditional craniotomy
- Surgical precision
- Decreased cost
- Decreased morbidity
- Deceased length of hospital stay
- Rapid recovery time

A disadvantage is that the device requires an uncomfortable rigid head frame. In another system, called the *CyberKnife*, no frame is needed. A third stereotactic system is the Novalis system. This radiosurgery system utilizes a small computer-controlled micro Multi Leaf Collimator (mMLC) that can produce many complicated shapes with a wide range of tumor area. Both procedures are used primarily for brain tumors or arteriovenous malformations (AVMs) that are in a difficult location and therefore not removable by craniotomy. These procedures may also be used with patients who decline conventional surgery, for patients whose age and physical condition do not allow general anesthesia, as an adjunct to radiation therapy, and for recurrent or residual AVM or tumors after embolization or craniotomy.

Surgical Management. A **craniotomy** (incision into the cranium) may be performed to remove the tumor, to improve symptoms related to the lesion, or to decrease the tumor size (debulk). The challenge for the neurosurgeon is to remove the tumor as completely as possible without damaging normal tissue. Complete removal is possible with some benign tumors, which results in a "surgical cure." Postoperatively, the patient may be admitted to the critical care unit or neurosurgical unit for frequent observation.

Preoperative Care. The patient having a craniotomy is typically very anxious about having his or her head opened and the brain exposed. Concerns are centered on the possibility of increased neurologic deficits after the surgery and the patient's self-image when part or all of the head is shaved. Provide reassurance that the surgeon will spare vital parts of the brain while removing or decreasing the size of the tumor. Teach the patient and family about what to expect immediately after surgery and throughout the recovery period. Some patients require short-term or long-term rehabilitation.

Check that the patient has not had alcohol, tobacco, anticoagulants, or NSAIDs for at least 5 days before surgery. Some neurosurgeons require a week or longer. Be sure that the patient has been NPO status for at least 8 hours. Other preoperative care is similar to that for any patient having surgery, as described in Chapter 14.

Operative Procedures. Surgery is performed under local or general anesthesia or sedation. Small tumors that are easily located may be removed by *minimally invasive surgery (MIS)*. For example, the trans-nasal approach using endoscopy can be performed for pituitary tumors. The patient has a short hospital stay and few complications after surgery. Stereotactic surgery using a rigid head frame can be done for tumors that are easily reached. This procedure requires only burr holes and local anesthesia because the brain has no sensory neurons for pain. Laser surgery can also be done.

For a *craniotomy*, the surgeon makes an incision along or behind the hairline after placing the patient's head in a skull fixation device. Several burr holes are drilled into the skull, and a saw is used to remove a piece of bone (bone flap) to expose the tumor area. The flap is stored carefully until the end of the procedure. The tumor is located using imaging technology and removed or debulked. After the tumor removal, the bone flap is replaced and held by small screws or bolts. A drain or monitoring device may be inserted. The surgeon creates a soft dressing "cap" over the top of the head to keep the surgical area clean.

Postoperative Care. The focus of postoperative care is to monitor the patient to detect changes in status and to prevent or minimize complications, especially increased intracranial pressure (ICP).

> ⚠ **NURSING SAFETY PRIORITY** (QSEN)
> ### Action Alert
>
> Assess neurologic and vital signs every 15 to 30 minutes for the first 4 to 6 hours after a craniotomy and then every hour. If the patient is stable for 24 hours, the frequency of these checks may be decreased to every 2 to 4 hours, depending on the agency's policy or the patient's condition. Report immediately and document new neurologic deficits, particularly a decreased level of consciousness (LOC), motor weakness or paralysis, aphasia (speech and/or language problems), decreased sensation, and reduced pupil reaction to light! Personality changes such as agitation, aggression, or passivity can also indicate worsening neurologic status.

Managing the Patient. Periorbital (around the eye) edema and ecchymosis of one or both eyes are not unusual and are treated with cold compresses to decrease swelling. Irrigate the affected eye with warm saline solution or artificial tears to improve patient comfort. The patient in the critical care unit has routine cardiac monitoring because dysrhythmias may occur as a result of brain–autonomic nervous system–cardiac interactions or fluid and electrolyte imbalance.

Regardless of setting, ensure recording of the patient's intake and output for the first 24 hours. Anticipate fluid restriction to 1500 mL daily if there is pituitary involvement in either the tumor or surgical site. Reposition the patient, but do not turn him or her onto the operative site. Delegate or provide repositioning and deep breathing every 2 hours. To prevent the development of VTE, maintain intermittent sequential pneumatic devices until the patient ambulates.

For patients who have undergone *supratentorial* surgery, elevate the head of the bed 30 degrees or as tolerated to promote venous drainage from the head. *Position the patient to avoid extreme hip or neck flexion and maintain the head in a midline, neutral position to prevent increased ICP.* Turn the patient side to side or supine to prevent pressure ulcers and prevent pneumonia.

Keep the patient with an *infratentorial* (brainstem) craniotomy flat and positioned side-lying, alternating sides every 2 hours, for 24 to 48 hours. This position prevents pressure on the neck-area incision site. It also prevents pressure on the internal tumor excision site from higher cerebral structures. Make sure that the patient remains NPO status for 24 hours, because edema around the medulla and lower cranial nerves may cause vomiting and aspiration.

Check the head dressing every 1 to 2 hours for signs of drainage. Mark the area of drainage once during each shift for baseline comparison, although this practice varies by health care agency. A small or moderate amount of drainage is expected. Some patients may have a Hemovac, Jackson-Pratt, or other surgical drain in place for 24 hours after surgery. Measure the drainage every 8 hours, and record the amount and color. A typical amount of drainage is 30 to 50 mL every 8 hours. Follow the manufacturer's and neurosurgeon's instructions to maintain suction within the drain.

> **! NURSING SAFETY PRIORITY** (QSEN)
> ### Critical Rescue
>
> After craniotomy, monitor the patient's dressing for excessive amounts of drainage. Report a saturated head dressing or drainage greater than 50 mL/8 hrs immediately to the surgeon! Observe for manifestations of hypovolemic shock, and position the patient flat to maintain blood pressure if needed.

The usual laboratory studies monitored postoperatively include complete blood count (CBC), serum electrolyte levels and osmolarity, and coagulation studies. The patient's hematocrit and hemoglobin concentration may be abnormally low from blood loss during surgery or elevated if the blood was replaced. Hyponatremia (low serum sodium) may occur as a result of fluid volume overload, syndrome of inappropriate antidiuretic hormone (SIADH), or steroid administration.

Hypokalemia (low serum potassium) may cause cardiac irritability. Weakness, a change in LOC, and confusion are symptoms of hyponatremia and hypokalemia. Hypernatremia may be caused by meningitis, dehydration, or diabetes insipidus (DI). It is manifested by muscle weakness, restlessness, extreme thirst, and dry mouth. Additional signs of dehydration such as decreased urinary output, thick lung secretions, and hypotension may be present. *Untreated hypernatremia can lead to seizure activity. DI should be considered if the patient voids large amounts of very dilute urine with an increasing serum osmolarity and electrolyte concentration.*

Often the patient is mechanically ventilated for the first 24 to 48 hours after surgery to help manage the airway and maintain optimal oxygen levels. If the patient is awake or attempting to breathe at a rate other than that set on the ventilator, drugs such as dexmedetomidine (Precedex) or propofol (Diprivan) and fentanyl are given to treat pain and anxiety, as well as to promote rest and comfort. Suction the patient as needed. *Remember to hyperoxygenate the patient carefully before, during, and after suctioning!*

Drugs routinely given postoperatively include antiepileptic drugs, histamine blockers or proton pump inhibitors for stress

> **? NCLEX EXAMINATION CHALLENGE**
> ### Physiological Integrity
>
> A client returns from the postanesthesia care unit (PACU) after a craniotomy for removal of a left parietal lobe tumor. How will the nurse position the client after surgery?
> A. Flex the client's knees to decrease intra-abdominal pressure and cerebral hypertension.
> B. Keep the client on the left side to prevent surgical site bleeding or cerebrospinal fluid leakage.
> C. Elevate the client's head to at least 30 degrees to promote cerebral venous drainage.
> D. Hyperextend the client's neck to maintain the airway and prevent aspiration regardless of supine or side-lying positioning.

TABLE 45-7	Postoperative Complications of Craniotomy

• Increased intracranial pressure (ICP)
 • Hematomas
   • Subdural hematoma
   • Epidural hematoma
 • Subarachnoid hemorrhage
 • Hypovolemic shock
 • Hydrocephalus
 • Respiratory complications
   • Atelectasis
   • Hypoxia
   • Pneumonia
   • Neurogenic pulmonary edema
	• Wound infection
	 • Meningitis
	 • Fluid and electrolyte imbalances
	   • Dehydration
	   • Hyponatremia
	   • Hypernatremia
	 • Seizures
	 • Cerebrospinal fluid (CSF) leak
	 • Cerebral edema

ulcer prophylaxis, and glucocorticoids, such as dexamethasone (Decadron) to reduce intracranial edema. Give acetaminophen for fever or mild pain. Some surgeons may prescribe antibiotics to prevent infection.

Preventing and Managing Postoperative Complications. Postoperative complications are listed in Table 45-7. The major complications of supratentorial surgery are increased ICP from cerebral edema or hydrocephalus and hemorrhage.

Symptoms of *increased ICP* include severe headache, deteriorating LOC, restlessness, irritability, and dilated or pinpoint pupils that are slow to react or nonreactive to light. Treatment of increased ICP is the same as that described on p. 948 under Interventions in the Traumatic Brain Injury section.

Hydrocephalus (increased CSF in the brain) is caused by obstruction of the normal CSF pathway from edema, an expanding lesion such as a hematoma, or blood in the subarachnoid space. Rapidly progressive hydrocephalus produces the classic symptoms of increased ICP. Slowly progressive hydrocephalus is manifested by headache, decreased LOC, irritability, blurred vision, and urinary incontinence. An intraventricular catheter (ventriculostomy) may be placed to drain CSF during surgery or emergently postoperatively for rapidly deteriorating neurologic function. If long-term treatment is required for chronic hydrocephalus, a surgical shunt is inserted to drain CSF to another area of the body. A major complication of the shunting procedure is a subdural hematoma from the tearing of bridging veins. An external lumbar drain may also be used temporarily. Additional information about shunts may be found in neuroscience nursing textbooks.

Subdural and epidural *hematomas and intracranial hemorrhage* are manifested by severe headache, a rapid decrease in LOC, progressive neurologic deficits, and herniation syndromes (brain tissue shifting, often downward). Bleeding into the posterior fossa may lead to sudden cardiovascular and respiratory arrest. Treatment of a hematoma requires surgical removal. An intracranial hemorrhage is treated with aggressive medical management (e.g., osmotic diuretics, ICP monitoring, CPP management).

Respiratory complications include atelectasis, pneumonia, and neurogenic pulmonary edema. Prevent atelectasis and pneumonia by turning the patient frequently and encouraging him or her to take frequent deep breaths to expand the lungs each hour. Humidified air and incentive spirometry are also useful techniques. Other treatment modalities include endotracheal or oral tracheal suctioning and chest physiotherapy.

However, these measures may cause an increase in ICP. Although not common, *neurogenic pulmonary edema* is a life-threatening complication of traumatic brain injury (TBI), brain tumors, and brain surgery. Its symptoms are the same as those of acute pulmonary edema, but there are no associated cardiac problems. In spite of aggressive treatment, most patients with neurogenic pulmonary edema do not survive.

Wound infections occur more often in older and debilitated patients and in patients with a history of diabetes, long-term steroid use, obesity, and previous infections. The patient may contribute to the problem by rubbing or scratching the wound. If infection is present, the wound appears reddened and puffy. It may begin to separate, is sensitive to touch, and feels warm. The patient may or may not be febrile. Treatment is based on the degree and extent of the infection. A localized infection may be treated by cleaning it with an antiseptic and applying a topical antibiotic. For more severe infections, systemic antibiotic administration is needed. If the underlying bone is involved, it may need to be removed.

Meningitis is an inflammation of the meninges and may occur as a result of surgery or wound infection, a cerebrospinal fluid (CSF) leak, or contamination during surgery. (See the Meningitis section in Chapter 42 for a more complete explanation of this condition.)

Complications related to *fluid and electrolyte imbalance* include DI, SIADH, and cerebral salt wasting (CSW). DI is seen most often after supratentorial surgery, especially procedures involving the pituitary gland or hypothalamus. Failure of the posterior pituitary gland to release antidiuretic hormone (ADH) leads to failure of the renal tubules to reabsorb water. The patient's urine output increases dramatically (it may be up to 10 L/day), and the urine specific gravity drops to below 1.005. Urine osmolarity decreases, whereas serum osmolarity increases. The patient may become dehydrated and hypovolemic shock may develop rapidly if this condition is left untreated. Fluid therapy to replace urinary losses and prevent dehydration may be accomplished by having the patient increase oral intake or use IV fluids. Hormonal replacement may also be necessary, especially if fluid loss is greater than 6 L/24 hr. Aqueous vasopressin is short-acting, lasting only 6 to 8 hours. Desmopressin acetate (DDAVP) may be administered for long-term replacement therapy.

Syndrome of inappropriate antidiuretic hormone (SIADH) occurs when the posterior pituitary gland releases too much ADH, causing water retention. The urine output decreases dramatically, with a urine output of less than 20 mL/hr. Sodium concentration in the urine is normal or elevated, whereas the serum sodium level falls. Other indications of SIADH are loss of thirst, weight gain, irritability, muscle weakness, and decreased LOC. SIADH is treated by fluid restriction, which is usually sufficient to correct the hyponatremia. Conivaptan (Vaprisol) and tolvaptan are vasopressin receptor antagonists used to increase water diuresis without serum electrolyte loss and may be useful in hypervolemic hyponatremic conditions. Slow, controlled IV infusion of hypertonic sodium may be needed for severe hyponatremia (<118 mEq/L).

Cerebral salt wasting (CSW) is thought to result from the influence of atrial natriuretic factor (ANF). ANF cells are located in the hypothalamus and the right atrium and regulate fluid volume. CSW is believed to be the primary cause of hyponatremia in the neurosurgical population. It is characterized by hyponatremia, decreased serum osmolarity, and decreased blood volume. Serum vasopressin and ANF levels can differentiate CSW and SIADH. CSW is treated with the replacement of sodium and isotonic fluid volume.

Patients with complications related to fluid and electrolyte imbalance undergo strict measurement of their intake and output. Be sure that an accurate weight measurement is taken every day at the same time with the same scale. Carefully assess for indications of fluid overload or dehydration during treatment. Serum electrolyte levels and osmolarity are measured daily (or more often if clinically indicated).

Community-Based Care

The patient with a brain tumor is managed at home if possible. Maintaining a reasonable quality of life is an important outcome for recovery and rehabilitation. Unless the patient has a significant degree of disability, no special preparation for home care is needed. Patients with hemiparesis need assistance to ensure that their home is accessible according to their method of MOBILITY (e.g., cane, walker, and wheelchair). The environment should be made safe to prevent falls. For example, teach caregivers to remove scatter rugs and to place grab bars in the bathroom.

Information about the selection of rehabilitation or chronic care facility, if needed, can be obtained from the case manager (CM) or discharge planner. The selected facility should have experience in providing care for neurologically impaired patients. A psychologist should be available to provide input in the evaluation of the cognitive disabilities that the patient may have.

It is very important that the patient and family fully understand the importance of any recommended follow-up health care appointments. The discharge summary should state the name of the person who has been given the follow-up information.

Health teaching includes drug therapy and who to call if adverse drug events occur. Remind the patient to avoid taking any over-the-counter drugs unless approved by the health care provider.

Teach the patient to maintain a program of regular physical exercise within the limits of any disabilities. Referral to the dietitian may be needed to ensure adequate caloric intake for the patient receiving radiation or chemotherapy.

Seizures are a potential complication that can occur at any time for as long as 1 year or more after surgery. Provide the patient and the family with information about seizure precautions and what to do if a seizure occurs.

Refer the patient and the family or significant others to the American Brain Tumor Association (www.abta.org) or the National Brain Tumor Foundation (www.braintumor.org). The American Cancer Society (www.cancer.org) is also an appropriate community resource for patients with malignant tumors. Home care agencies are available to provide both the physical and rehabilitative care that the patient may need at home. Hospice services and palliative care may be needed if he or she is terminally ill. (See Chapter 7 for additional information about end-of-life care.) Brain tumor support groups may also be a valuable asset to the patient and family.

BRAIN ABSCESS

A brain abscess is a purulent infection of the brain in which pus forms in the extradural, subdural, or intracerebral area of the brain. The causative organisms are usually bacteria that invade the brain directly or indirectly. Cerebral abscesses may be a complication of meningitis.

❖ PATHOPHYSIOLOGY

In general, organisms from the ear, sinus, or mastoid area enter the brain by traveling along the wall of the cerebral veins, and therefore they may spread to any area of the brain. The typical source is a lung infection, although it is common not to find the source of infection. Bacteria may travel from a nearby infected area such as an ear infection or a sinus infection or enter the body with a bullet, knife wound, or neurosurgery. At times, the organisms (especially those from the ear) destroy the bone, form a tract, and enter the brain directly. A portion of an abscess from a distant organ, such as the heart or tonsils, may break off and enter the systemic circulation. These septic emboli contain organisms that may become lodged in a cerebral vessel and produce a localized infection. Penetrating trauma, open head injuries, and neurosurgical procedures provide a potential means for the direct entry of an organism into the brain.

The organisms cause a local infection, and acute inflammation surrounds the involved area. Within a few days, necrosis of the tissue takes place, pus forms, and the tissue liquefies. This process is followed by the development of cerebral edema from localized vascular congestion and tissue swelling in response to inflammation. During the next few weeks, the area becomes encapsulated. The abscess usually occurs deep within the cerebral hemisphere and involves the white matter of the brain. In a few cases, it spreads through the brain tissue to the subarachnoid space and ventricular system. The organism varies with the source of the abscess. Streptococci are the most common organisms and are often found with other anaerobes such as *Bacteroides*. Enterobacteriaceae such as *Escherichia coli* and proteus organisms may also be combined with streptococcus. Yeast and fungi also cause cerebral abscess formation, particularly in patients who are immunosuppressed. *Toxoplasma gondii* is one of the most commonly seen central nervous system (CNS) opportunistic infections in the acquired immune deficiency syndrome (AIDS) population.

Most brain abscesses occur in the frontal and temporal lobes. A few affected patients have more than one abscess. Mortality rates vary up to more than one half of patients with abscesses. Those that occur in immunosuppressed patients are associated with a higher mortality rate.

❖ PATIENT-CENTERED COLLABORATIVE CARE

◆ Assessment

Physical Assessment/Clinical Manifestations. The clinical manifestations of a brain abscess begin slowly and are similar to some of the manifestations of meningitis. The patient may have headache, fever, and neurologic deficits or nonspecific signs and symptoms (Chart 45-11). Perform ongoing neurologic assessments. The patient may be mildly lethargic or somewhat confused. The pupillary response to light is normal in the early stages. As increased intracranial pressure (ICP) progresses, the pupils may become sluggish, unequal, dilated, and nonresponsive to light. The patient's level of consciousness (LOC) declines to a state in which he or she loses the ability to interact with the environment. Airway and respiratory function may also be altered.

CHART 45-11   Key Features

Brain Abscess

- Headache
- Fever
- Pain
- Motor deficits, such as hemiplegia
- Ataxia
- Sensory impairment (varies)
- Aphasia
- Seizure activity
- Visual field changes (e.g., decreased peripheral vision, nystagmus)
- *If severe*, signs of increased intracranial pressure (ICP), such as decreased level of consciousness (LOC), severe headache, bradycardia, widened pulse pressure

---

Examination of the patient's visual fields often reveals a **temporal field blindness** (decrease in peripheral vision laterally). If the abscess affects the cerebral hemispheres, nystagmus (involuntary eye movements) may be evident. Motor examination reveals a generalized weakness. More significant motor problems, such as hemiplegia, may be apparent in the presence of a frontal lobe abscess. An ataxic gait is seen with a cerebellar abscess. Sensory impairment varies, although the patient often exhibits no SENSORY PERCEPTION deficits. The patient may have varying degrees of aphasia (impaired communication ability) if he or she has a frontal or temporal lobe abscess. Seizure activity may occur because of irritation of the cortical tissue. Late in the disease process, more severe symptoms of increased ICP occur and include severe headache, decreased LOC (possibly coma), a widened pulse pressure, bradycardia, and irregular respirations. The patient with AIDS often presents with systemic infection, CNS involvement, and lymphoma.

Some patients may have atypical presentations, including older adults (age-related compromise in immune function), those receiving steroid therapy or immune-modulating drugs, and patients with later stages of human immune deficiency virus (HIV) infection (immune system compromise). In the earlier stages, the inflammatory response is responsible for much of the clinical presentation, particularly if cerebral abscess formation results from meningitis. The risk is that the patient may progress to severe abscess formation before the onset of "classic" manifestations.

Diagnostic Assessment. The white blood cell (WBC) count and erythrocyte sedimentation rate (ESR) are usually elevated, indicating the presence of infection. If the abscess is encapsulated, the WBC count may be normal. Obtain specimens for aerobic and, when possible, anaerobic cultures of the blood, ear, nose, and throat to determine the primary source of infection.

The health care provider requests a CT scan to determine the presence of cerebritis, hydrocephalus, or a midline shift. MRI is also useful in detecting the presence of an abscess early in the course of the disease. An EEG can localize the lesion in most cases and shows high-voltage, slow-wave activity; electrocerebral silence may be noted in the area of the abscess. Radiography of the sinuses and the mastoid is often indicated. A lumbar puncture may be performed if meningitis is also suspected and the patient does not have ICP elevation. A needle biopsy is performed to identify the cause of the infection.

◆ Interventions

Drug therapy is recommended if the patient has several abscesses, a small abscess (less than 2 cm), an abscess deep in the brain, an abscess and meningitis, a shunt for hydrocephalus (in some cases the shunt may need to be removed temporarily or replaced) or *Toxoplasma gondii* infection in a person with HIV. Drug therapy is prescribed by the physician to treat the abscess. Antibiotic dosing may be maximized to ensure adequate CNS penetration. Antibiotics are particularly useful in the early stages (cerebritis) of abscess formation. A combination of antibiotics is used, particularly if the infection resulted from septic emboli. Antiepileptic drugs such as phenytoin (Dilantin) may be used to prevent seizures. The drug regimen is strictly followed to maintain therapeutic blood levels. Give analgesics to treat headache.

The physician may surgically drain an encapsulated abscess via a burr hole to reduce the mass effect of the lesion. In certain cases, a craniotomy may be performed to remove the abscess. The decision to perform surgery is based on the patient's general condition, the stage of abscess development, and the site of the abscess. Provide routine preoperative and postoperative care for the patient undergoing a craniotomy, as discussed in this chapter under Surgical Management in the Brain Tumors section.

The patient with a brain abscess is discharged to home if few or no neurologic deficits are present. Patients with severe dysfunction are usually transferred to long-term care or a rehabilitation facility. Some patients have permanent neurologic deficits.

ACQUIRED HYPOXIC-ANOXIC BRAIN INJURY

Acquired hypoxic-anoxic brain injury is brain damage caused by a reduced or absent supply of oxygen. Common causes include cardiac arrest, asphyxiation from a suicide attempt (i.e., hanging), near-drowning, drug use and overdose, accidental electrocution, and severe asthma. Neurons in the brain experience ischemia, injury, and cell death within 4 minutes of a reduced oxygen supply to the brain. The reduction of oxygen can be a primary event such as asphyxiation or a secondary event such as loss of airway during a drug overdose or decreased cerebral PERFUSION from increased intracranial pressure (Smania et al., 2013). Generally hypoxic-anoxic brain injury is global with decreases in COGNITION, MOBILITY, and sensation that occur with the event and persist in an unpredictable manner following resuscitation. An MRI provides the most sensitive diagnostic test for determining hypoxic-anoxic brain injury (Muttikkal & Wintermark, 2013).

Initial interventions are generally supportive with a focus on airway, breathing, and circulation to restore the oxygen. Therapeutic hypothermia, described earlier in this chapter on p. 953, is useful when anoxia is related to a witnessed cardiac arrest. Frequent neurologic assessment is undertaken to detect and prevent secondary injury as discussed with severe traumatic brain injury in this chapter. It is not uncommon for patients to experience increased intracranial pressure from cerebral edema in the days following the initial anoxic event. Increased intracranial pressure and cerebral edema are managed similarly to severe traumatic brain injury. Because it is difficult to predict whether brain function will be restored and the course of recovery, patients and family often require emotional support to deal with uncertainty. Early physical and specialized neurocognitive rehabilitation can promote functional outcomes following this type of brain injury.

NURSING CONCEPTS AND CLINICAL JUDGMENT REVIEW

What might you NOTICE if the patient is experiencing changes in cerebral PERFUSION, MOBILITY, SENSORY PERCEPTION, and COGNITION as a result of severe acute neurologic health problems affecting the brain?

- Decreased level of consciousness (LOC)
- Inability to communicate (aphasia)
- Impaired swallowing (dysphagia)
- Weakness or paralysis of one side of the body (hemiparesis or hemiplegia)
- Alteration in gait
- Inability to perform ADLs
- Report of nausea and vomiting
- Report of impaired visual acuity or fields
- Ptosis (eyelid drooping)
- Unilateral body neglect
- Report of decreased peripheral sensation
- Inability to make appropriate judgments; confusion
- Impaired memory
- Report of severe headache

What should you INTERPRET and how should you RESPOND to a patient experiencing impaired PERFUSION, MOBILITY, SENSORY PERCEPTION, and COGNITION as a result of severe neurologic health problems affecting the brain?

Perform and interpret physical assessment, including:
- Assess airway, breathing, and circulation status.
- Assess neurologic status, especially LOC and mental state.
- Take vital signs, and establish blood pressure goals.
- Assess neurologic status with particular attention to level of consciousness and cognition.
- Assess functional status.
- Assess for swallowing and nutrition status.

Respond by:
- Notifying health care provider or Rapid Response Team of changes in the Glasgow Coma Scale value of 2 or more points, a reduction in level of consciousness or pupil reactivity to light, hypertension, hypotension, widened pulse pressure, dysrhythmias, fever, and hypoxemia (low Spo_2) urgently
- Ensuring an adequate airway
- Giving oxygen if Spo_2 <92%
- Establishing IV access
- Communicating and collaborating with health care team members efficiently to meet patient's needs
- Assisting with ADLs and mobility as needed
- Providing a safe environment to prevent harm from altered sensory perception

On what should you REFLECT?

- Evaluate the effectiveness and timeliness of health care team responses, including your own.
- Determine strategies to efficiently monitor neurologic status.
- Monitor for indications of secondary brain insult as the patient is treated.

- Plan health teaching for the patient and family.
- Initiate actions to provide emotional and spiritual support for the patient and family.
- Consider whether the patient preferences and values been incorporated into care.

GET READY FOR THE NCLEX® EXAMINATION!

▌KEY POINTS

Review these Key Points for each NCLEX Examination Client Needs Category.

Safe and Effective Care Environment

- When caring for a patient with a stroke or traumatic brain injury (TBI), assess airway, breathing, and circulation status first and implement interventions to maintain them.
- Collaborate with the interdisciplinary team members including physicians, physical therapists, respiratory therapists, occupational therapists, social workers, and dietitians to ensured shared priorities in care. **Teamwork and Collaboration** `QSEN`
- Develop electronic care pathways and document patient progress using interdisciplinary patient-centered plans for care based on patient values for the patient recovering from neurologic critical illness. **Informatics** `QSEN`

Health Promotion and Maintenance

- Identify risk factors for new or recurrent stroke and teach patients and families about modifiable risk factors for stroke as listed in Chart 45-2. **Evidence-Based Practice** `QSEN`
- Prevent secondary brain injury by protecting the airway, promoting an appropriate range of blood pressure and mean arterial pressure, maintaining fluid and electrolyte balance, promptly treating fever, avoiding sustained hypoglycemia and hyperglycemia, addressing hypoxia and hypercarbia, positioning the patient appropriately, and managing intracranial hypertension with prescribed interventions.
- Teach patients and families about community organizations, such as the National Stroke Association and the Brain Injury Association of America.

Psychosocial Integrity

- Assess the emotional reactions of families to a TBI, stroke, or brain cancer diagnosis, and help them cope by providing information and including them in planning for care. **Patient-Centered Care** `QSEN`

Physiological Integrity

- Perform a comprehensive, rapid, or focal neurologic assessment at regular intervals to identify changes in status. **Evidence-Based Practice** `QSEN`
- Recall that decreased level of consciousness is the most sensitive indicator of adverse outcome or complication from stroke, TBI, brain tumor, or craniotomy.
- Recall the differences between a transient ischemic attack and a brain attack (stroke) as described in Table 45-1 and Chart 45-1.
- Monitor patients with critical neurologic health problems for manifestations of increasing intracranial pressure (ICP) as described in Chart 45-6.
- Assess the patient's ability to swallow before providing oral intake if a stroke is suspected or diagnosed. **Safety** `QSEN`
- Assess patients with strokes for SENSORY PERCEPTION changes such as unilateral neglect and impaired vision; help patients adapt to these changes, such as turning their head from side to side to see the entire meal tray. **Patient-Centered Care** `QSEN`
- Provide alternate means of communication when expressive and/or receptive aphasia is present in patients who have had a stroke or brain injury in consultation with the speech-language expert. **Teamwork and Collaboration** `QSEN`
- Monitor the patient on fibrinolytic therapy or anticoagulants for bleeding and abnormal coagulation studies. Best practices for fibrinolytic therapy administration are listed in Chart 45-5. **Safety** `QSEN`
- Teach patients with mild traumatic brain injury and their families to monitor for neurologic changes as listed in Charts 45-7 and 45-9.
- Assess for manifestations of brain tumors as listed in Chart 45-10.
- Recognize that the desired outcome for the patient with a brain tumor is to remove it if possible. Other methods may be used to decrease its size, including chemotherapy and radiation.
- Administer antibiotic therapy to provide the most effective management of patients with brain abscess.

46 | CHAPTER

Assessment of the Eye and Vision

M. Linda Workman

ℯ http://evolve.elsevier.com/Iggy/

PRIORITY CONCEPTS

- SENSORY PERCEPTION

LEARNING OUTCOMES

Safe and Effective Care Environment
1. Prevent injury or infection of the eye to preserve visual SENSORY PERCEPTION.

Health Promotion and Maintenance
2. Teach all people about eye health and the use of eye protection equipment and strategies.

Psychosocial Integrity
3. Reduce the psychological impact for the patient and family regarding the assessment and testing of the eyes and vision.

Physiological Integrity
4. Use knowledge of anatomy, physiology, pathophysiology, and psychomotor skills when assessing the eye and vision.
5. Perform a focused assessment of visual SENSORY PERCEPTION, incorporating information about genetic risk and age-related changes affecting the eye and vision.

The eye and the brain work together to allow visual SENSORY PERCEPTION. Many people consider vision to be the most important sensory perception. It is used to assess surroundings, allow independence, warn of danger, appreciate beauty, work, play, and interact with others.

Vision begins with the eye, where light is changed into nerve impulses. These impulses are sent to the brain, where images are fully perceived (McCance et al., 2014). Many systemic conditions, as well as eye problems, change vision temporarily or permanently. Changes in the eye and vision can provide information about the patient's general health status and problems that might occur in self-care.

ANATOMY AND PHYSIOLOGY REVIEW

Structure

The eyeball, a round, ball-shaped organ, is located in the front part of the eye orbit. The **orbit** is the bony socket of the skull that surrounds and protects the eye along with the attached muscles, nerves, vessels, and tear-producing glands.

Layers of the Eyeball

The eye has three layers (Fig. 46-1). The external layer is the **sclera** (the "white" of the eye) and the transparent cornea on the front of the eye.

The middle layer, or **uvea,** is heavily pigmented and consists of the choroid, the ciliary body, and the iris. The choroid, a dark brown membrane between the sclera and the retina, lines most of the sclera. It has many blood vessels that supply nutrients to the retina.

The ciliary body connects the choroid with the iris and secretes aqueous humor. The **iris** is the colored portion of the external eye; its center opening is the **pupil.** The muscles of the iris contract and relax to control pupil size and the amount of light entering the eye.

The innermost layer is the **retina,** a thin, delicate structure made up of sensory photoreceptors that begin the transmission of impulses to the optic nerve (McCance et al., 2014). The retina contains blood vessels and two types of photoreceptors called *rods* and *cones.* The rods work at low light levels and provide peripheral vision. The cones are active at bright light levels and provide color and central vision.

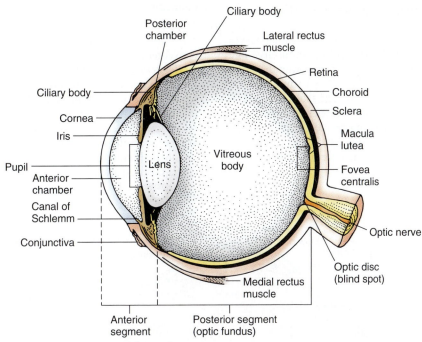

FIG. 46-1 Anatomic features of the eye.

The **optic fundus** is the area at the inside back of the eye that can be seen with an ophthalmoscope. This area contains the **optic disc**—a pink or white depressed area where the nerve fibers that synapse with the photoreceptors join together to form the optic nerve and exit the eyeball. The optic disc contains only nerve fibers and no photoreceptor cells. To one side of the optic disc is a small, yellowish pink area called the *macula lutea.* The center of the macula is the *fovea centralis,* where vision is most acute.

Refractive Structures and Media

Light waves pass through the cornea, aqueous humor, lens, and vitreous humor on the way to the retina. Each structure bends *(refracts)* the light waves to focus images on the retina. Together, these structures are the eye's *refracting media.*

The **cornea** is the clear layer that forms the external bump on the front of the eye (see Fig. 46-1). The **aqueous humor** is a clear, watery fluid that fills the anterior and posterior chambers of the eye. This fluid is continually produced by the ciliary processes and passes from the posterior chamber, through the pupil, and into the anterior chamber. This fluid drains through the canal of Schlemm into the blood to maintain a balanced intraocular pressure (IOP), the pressure within the eye (Fig. 46-2).

The **lens** is a circular, convex structure that lies behind the iris and in front of the vitreous body. It is transparent and bends the light rays entering through the pupil to focus properly on the retina. The curve of the lens changes to focus on near or distant objects. A *cataract* is a lens that has lost its transparency.

The **vitreous body** is a clear, thick gel that fills the large vitreous chamber (the space between the lens and the retina). This gel transmits light and maintains eye shape.

The eye is a hollow organ and must be kept in the shape of a ball for vision to occur. To maintain this shape, the vitreous humor gel in the posterior segment and the aqueous humor in the anterior segment must be present in set amounts that apply pressure inside the eye to keep it inflated. This pressure is the **intraocular pressure** or **IOP**. IOP has to be just right. If the pressure is too low, the eyeball is soft and collapses, preventing light from getting to the photoreceptors on the retina in the back of the eye. If the pressure becomes too high, the extra pressure compresses capillaries in the eye as well as nerve fibers. Pressure on retinal blood vessels prevents blood from flowing through them; therefore the photoreceptors and nerve fibers become hypoxic. Compression of the fine nerve fibers prevents intracellular fluid flow, which also reduces nourishment to the distal portions of these thin nerve fibers. The increased pressure and resulting hypoxia of photoreceptors and their synapsing nerve fibers is a condition called *glaucoma.* Continued hypoxia in the retina results in photoreceptor necrosis and death and permanent nerve fiber damage. When extensive photoreceptor and nerve fiber loss occur, vision is lost and the person is permanently blind.

External Structures

The eyelids are thin, movable skinfolds that protect the eyes and keep the cornea moist. The upper lid is larger than the lower one. The **canthus** is the place where the two eyelids meet at the corner of the eye.

The **conjunctivae** are the mucous membranes of the eye. The palpebral conjunctiva is a thick membrane with many blood vessels that lines the under surface of each eyelid. The thin, transparent bulbar conjunctiva covers the entire front of the eye.

Tears are produced by a small **lacrimal gland**, which is located in the upper outer part of each orbit (Fig. 46-3). Tears flow across the front of the eye, toward the nose, and into the inner canthus. They drain through the **punctum** (an opening at the nasal side of the lid edges) into the lacrimal duct and sac and then into the nose through the nasolacrimal duct.

Muscles, Nerves, and Blood Vessels

Six voluntary muscles rotate the eye and coordinate eye movements (Fig. 46-4 and Table 46-1). Coordinated eye movements ensure that both eyes receive an image at the same time so only a single image is seen.

The muscles around the eye are innervated by cranial nerves (CNs) III (oculomotor), IV (trochlear), and VI (abducens). The optic nerve (CN II) is the nerve of sight, connecting the optic disc to the brain. The trigeminal nerve (CN V) stimulates the blink reflex when the cornea is touched. The facial nerve (CN VII) innervates the lacrimal glands and muscles for lid closure.

The ophthalmic artery brings oxygenated blood to the eye and the orbit. It branches to supply blood to the retina. The ciliary arteries supply the sclera, choroid, ciliary body, and iris.

Function

The four eye functions that provide clear images and vision are refraction, pupillary constriction, accommodation, and convergence.

Refraction bends light rays from the outside into the eye through curved surfaces and refractive media and finally to the retina. Each surface and media bend (refract) light differently to focus an image on the retina. Emmetropia is the perfect refraction of the eye in which light rays from a distant source are focused into a sharp image on the retina. Fig. 46-5 shows the normal refraction of light within the eye. Images fall on the retina inverted and reversed left to right. For example, an object

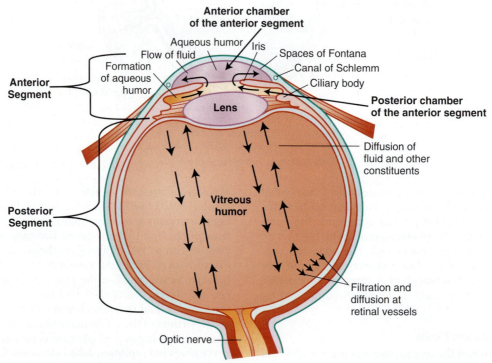

FIG. 46-2 Flow of aqueous humor.

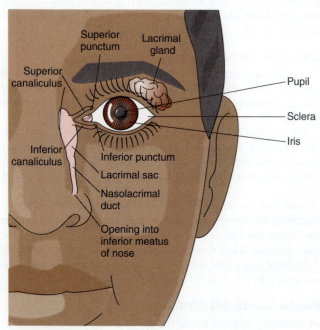

FIG. 46-3 Front view of the eye and adjacent structures.

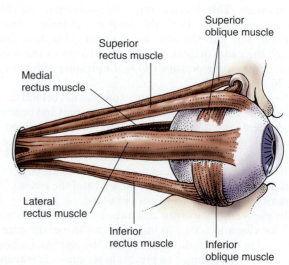

FIG. 46-4 The extraocular muscles.

in the lower nasal visual field strikes the upper outer area of the retina.

Errors of refraction are common. Hyperopia (farsightedness) occurs when the eye does not refract light enough. As a result, images actually converge behind the retina (see Fig. 46-5). With hyperopia, distant vision is normal but near vision is poor. It is corrected with a convex lens in eyeglasses or contact lenses.

Myopia (nearsightedness) occurs when the eye overbends the light and images converge in front of the retina (see Fig. 46-5). Near vision is normal, but distance vision is poor. Myopia is corrected with a biconcave lens in eyeglasses or contact lenses.

Astigmatism is a refractive error caused by unevenly curved surfaces on or in the eye, especially of the cornea. These uneven surfaces distort vision.

Pupillary constriction and dilation control the amount of light that enters the eye. If the level of light to one or both eyes is increased, both pupils constrict (become smaller). The amount of constriction depends on how much light is available and how well the retina can adapt to light changes. Pupillary constriction is called miosis, and pupillary dilation is called mydriasis (Fig. 46-6). Drugs can alter pupillary constriction.

Accommodation allows the healthy eye to focus images sharply on the retina whether the image is close to the eye or distant. The process of maintaining a clear visual image when the gaze is shifted from a distant to a near object is known as accommodation. The healthy eye can adjust its focus by changing the curve of the lens.

Convergence is the ability to turn both eyes inward toward the nose at the same time. This action helps ensure that only a single image of close objects is seen.

Eye Changes Associated with Aging

Changes inside the eye cause visual acuity to decrease with age (Touhy & Jett, 2014). Age-related changes of the nervous system and in the eye support structures also reduce visual function (Chart 46-1).

Structural changes occur with aging, including decreased eye muscle tone that reduces the ability to keep the gaze focused on a single object. The lower eyelid may relax and fall away from the eye *(ectropion),* leading to dry eye manifestations.

Arcus senilis, an opaque, bluish white ring within the outer edge of the cornea, is caused by fat deposits (see Fig. 24-4 in Chapter 24). This change does not affect vision.

The clarity and shape of the cornea change with age. The cornea flattens, and the curve of its surface becomes irregular. This change causes or worsens astigmatism and blurs vision.

TABLE 46-1	**Functions of Ocular Muscles**

Superior Rectus Muscle
- Together with the lateral rectus, this muscle moves the eye diagonally upward toward the side of the head.
- Together with the medial rectus, this muscle moves the eye diagonally upward toward the middle of the head.

Lateral Rectus Muscle
- Together with the medial rectus, this muscle holds the eye straight.
- Contracting alone, this muscle turns the eye toward the side of the head.

Medial Rectus Muscle
- Contracting alone, this muscle turns the eye toward the nose.

Inferior Rectus Muscle
- Together with the lateral rectus, this muscle moves the eye diagonally downward toward the side of the head.
- Together with the medial rectus, this muscle moves the eye diagonally downward toward the middle of the head.

Superior Oblique Muscle
- Contracting alone, this muscle pulls the eye downward.

Inferior Oblique Muscle
- Contracting alone, this muscle pulls the eye upward.

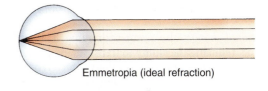

Emmetropia (ideal refraction)

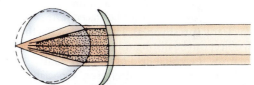

Hyperopia (hypermetropia, or farsightedness)

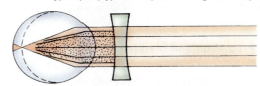

Myopia (nearsightedness)

FIG. 46-5 Refraction and correction in emmetropia, hyperopia, and myopia.

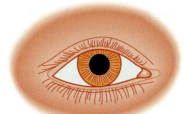

Normal pupil slightly dilated for moderate light

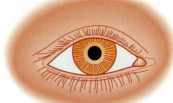

Miosis—pupil constricted when exposed to increased light or close work, such as reading

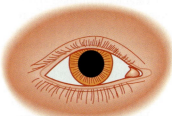

Mydriasis—pupil dilated when exposed to reduced light or when looking at a distance

FIG. 46-6 Miosis and mydriasis.

CHART 46-1 **Nursing Focus on the Older Adult**

Changes in the Eye and Vision Related to Aging

STRUCTURE/ FUNCTION	CHANGE	IMPLICATION
Appearance	Eyes appear "sunken." Arcus senilis forms. Sclera yellows or appears blue.	Do not use eye appearance as an indicator for hydration status. Reassure patient that this change does not affect vision. Do not use sclera to assess for jaundice.
Cornea	Cornea flattens, which blurs vision.	Encourage older adults to have regular eye examinations and wear prescribed corrective lenses for best vision.
Ocular muscles	Muscle strength is reduced, making it more difficult to maintain an upward gaze or maintain a single image.	Reassure patient that this is a normal happening and to re-focus gaze frequently to maintain a single image.
Lens	Elasticity is lost, increasing the near point of vision (making the near point of best vision farther away). Lens hardens, compacts, and forms a cataract.	Encourage patient to wear corrective lenses for reading. Stress the importance of yearly vision checks and monitoring.
Iris and Pupil	Decrease in ability to dilate results in small pupil size and poor adaptation to darkness.	Teach about the need for good lighting to avoid tripping and bumping into objects.
Color vision	Discrimination among greens, blues, and violets decreases.	The patient may not be able to use color-indicator monitors of health status.
Tears	Tear production is reduced, resulting in dry eyes, discomfort, and increased risk for corneal damage or eye infections.	Teach about the use of saline eyedrops to reduce dryness. Teach patient to increase humidity in the home.

Fatty deposits cause the sclera to develop a yellowish tinge. A bluish color may be seen as the sclera thins. With age, the iris has less ability to dilate, which leads to difficulty in adapting to dark environments. Older adults may need additional light for reading and other "close up" work and to avoid tripping over objects.

Functional changes also occur with aging. The lens yellows with aging, reducing the ability to transmit and focus light. The lens hardens, shrinks, and loses elasticity, which reduces accommodation. The **near point of vision** (the closest distance at which the eye can see an object clearly) increases. Near objects, especially reading material, must be placed farther from the eye to be seen clearly (**presbyopia**). The **far point** (farthest point at which an object can be distinguished) decreases. Together these changes narrow the visual field of an older adult.

General color perception decreases, especially for green, blue, and violet. More light is needed to stimulate the visual receptors. Intraocular pressure (IOP) is slightly higher in older adults.

Health Promotion and Maintenance

Vision is important for function and quality of life. Many vision and eye problems can be avoided, and others can be corrected or managed if discovered early. Teach all people about eye protection methods, adequate nutrition, and the importance of regular eye examinations.

The risks for cataract formation and for cancer of the eye (ocular melanoma) increase with exposure to ultraviolet (UV) light. Teach people to protect the eyes by using sunglasses that filter UV light whenever they are outdoors, at tanning salons, and when work involves UV exposure.

Vision can be affected by injury. Eye injury also increases the risk for both cataract formation and glaucoma. Urge all people to wear eye and head protection when working with particulate matter, fluid or blood spatter, high temperatures, or sparks. Protection also should be worn during participation in sports, such as baseball, or any activity that increases the risk for the eye being hit by objects in motion. Teach people to avoid rubbing the eyes to avoid trauma to outer eye surfaces.

CHART 46-2 **Patient and Family Education: Preparing for Self-Management**

Using Eyedrops

- Check the eyedrop name, strength, expiration date, color, and clarity.
- If both eyes are to receive the same drug and one eye is infected, use two separate bottles and label each bottle with "right" or "left" for the correct eye.
- Wash your hands.
- Remove the cap from the bottle.
- Tilt your head backward, open your eyes, and look up at the ceiling.
- Using your nondominant hand, gently pull the lower lid down against your cheek, forming a small pocket.
- Hold the eyedrop bottle (with the cap off) like a pencil, with the tip pointing down, with your dominant hand.
- Rest the wrist holding the bottle against your mouth or upper lip.
- Without touching any part of the eye or lid with the tip of the bottle, gently squeeze the bottle and release the prescribed number of drops into the pocket of your lower lid.
- Release the lower lid and gently close your eye without squeezing the lids.
- Gently press and hold the corner of the eye nearest the nose to close off the punctum and prevent the drug from being absorbed systemically.
- Gently blot away any excess drug or tears with a tissue.
- Keep the eye closed for about 1 minute.
- Place the cap back on the bottle, and store it as prescribed.
- Wash your hands again.

Eye infections can lead to vision loss. Although the eye surface is not sterile, the sclera and cornea have no separate blood supply and thus are at risk for infection. Teach everyone to wash their hands before touching the eye or eyelid. Teach people who use eyedrops about the proper technique to use these drugs (Chart 46-2), which includes not touching the eye with the bottle tip, and to not share eyedrops with others. If an eye has a discharge, teach the patient to use a separate eyedrop bottle for this eye and to wash the unaffected eye before washing the affected eye.

Other health problems, especially diabetes and hypertension, can seriously affect visual SENSORY PERCEPTION. Teach patients with these health problems about the importance of controlling blood glucose levels and managing blood pressure to reduce the risk for vision loss. Yearly evaluation by an ophthalmologist is needed to slow or prevent eye complications.

Teach all people who have a refractive error to have an eye examination yearly. Young adults without vision problems may need an eye examination only every 3 to 5 years. Adults older than 40 years should have an eye examination yearly that includes assessment of intraocular pressure and visual fields, because the risk for both glaucoma and cataract formation increases with age.

> ! **NURSING SAFETY PRIORITY** (QSEN)
>
> **Action Alert**
>
> Teach people to see a health care provider *immediately* when an eye injury occurs or an eye infection is suspected.

> ? **NCLEX EXAMINATION CHALLENGE**
>
> **Health Promotion and Maintenance**
>
> For which client does the nurse recommend annual evaluation by an ophthalmologist?
> A. 35-year-old man with asthma
> B. 21-year-old man with psoriasis
> C. 24-year-old woman with diabetes
> D. 38-year-old woman who has lost 50 pounds

ASSESSMENT METHODS

Patient History

Collect information to determine whether problems with the eye or vision have an impact on ADLs or other daily functions. *Age* is an important factor to consider when assessing visual SENSORY PERCEPTION and eye structure. The incidence of glaucoma and cataract formation increases with aging. Presbyopia commonly begins in the 40s.

Gender may be important. Retinal detachments occur more often in men, and dry eye syndromes occur more often in women.

Occupation and leisure activities can affect visual SENSORY PERCEPTION. Ask about how the eye is used at work. In occupations such as computer programming, constant exposure to monitors may lead to eyestrain. Machine operators are at risk for eye injury because of the high speeds at which particles can be thrown at the eye. Chronic exposure to infrared or ultraviolet light may cause photophobia and cataract formation. Teach the patient about the use of eye protection during work.

Ask whether the patient wears eye protection when participating in sports. A blow to the head near the eye, such as with a baseball, can damage external structures, the eye, the connections with the brain, or the area of the brain where vision is perceived.

Systemic health problems can affect vision. Check whether the patient has any condition listed in Table 46-2. Ask about past accidents, injuries, surgeries, or blows to the head that may have led to the present problem. Specifically ask about previous laser surgeries.

Drugs can affect vision and the eye (see Table 46-2). Ask about the use of any prescription or over-the-counter drugs,

TABLE 46-2 Systemic Conditions and Common Drugs Affecting the Eye and Vision

SYSTEMIC CONDITIONS AND DISORDERS	DRUGS
Diabetes mellitus	Antihistamines
Hypertension	Decongestants
Lupus erythematosus	Antibiotics
Sarcoidosis	Opioids
Thyroid problems	Anticholinergics
Acquired immune deficiency syndrome	Cholinergic agonists
Cardiac disease	Adrenergic agonists
Multiple sclerosis	Adrenergic antagonists
Pregnancy	(beta blockers)
	Oral contraceptives
	Chemotherapy agents
	Corticosteroids

especially decongestants and antihistamines, which tend to dry the eye and may increase intraocular pressure. Document the name, strength, dose, and scheduling for all drugs the patient uses. Ocular effects from drugs include itching, foreign body sensation, redness, tearing, photophobia (sensitivity to light), and the development of cataracts or glaucoma.

Nutrition History

Some eye problems are caused by or made worse with vitamin deficiencies. Ask the patient about food choices. For example, vitamin A deficiency can cause eye dryness, keratomalacia, and blindness. Some nutrients and antioxidants, such as lutein and beta carotene, help maintain retinal function. A diet rich in fruit and red, orange, and dark green vegetables is important to eye health. Teach all people to eat about 10 servings of these foods daily.

Family History and Genetic Risk

Ask about a family history of eye problems because some conditions have a familial tendency and some genetic problems lead to visual impairment. When a patient tells you that other relatives, especially first-degree relatives (parents, siblings, and children), have eye problems, document the gender of the affected person, the relationship to the patient, the exact nature of the problem, and the age that the problem was first noted.

Current Health Problems

Ask the patient about the onset of visual changes. Did the change occur rapidly or slowly? Determine whether the manifestations are present to the same degree in both eyes. Ask these questions if eye injury or trauma is involved:
- How long ago did the injury occur?
- What was the patient doing when it happened?
- If a foreign body was involved, what was its source?
- Was any first aid administered at the scene? If so, what actions were taken?

> ! **NURSING SAFETY PRIORITY** (QSEN)
>
> **Critical Rescue**
>
> Notify the ophthalmologist immediately for any patient who has a sudden or persistent loss of visual SENSORY PERCEPTION within the past 48 hours, eye trauma, a foreign body in the eye, or sudden ocular pain.

Physical Assessment

Inspection

Look for head tilting, squinting, or other actions that indicate the patient is trying to attain clear vision. For example, patients with double vision may cock the head to the side to focus the two images into one or they may close one eye to see clearly.

Assess for symmetry in the appearance of the eyes. Check the eyes to determine whether they are equal distance from the nose, are the same size, and have the same degree of prominence. Assess the eyes for their placement in the orbits and for symmetry of movement. Exophthalmos (*proptosis*) is protrusion of the eye. Enophthalmos is the sunken appearance of the eye.

Examine the eyebrows and eyelashes for hair distribution, and determine the direction of the eyelashes. Eyelashes normally point outward and away from the eyelid. Assess the eyelids for ptosis (drooping), redness, lesions, or swelling. The lids normally close completely, with the lid edges touching. When the eyes are open, the upper lid covers a small portion of the iris. The edge of the lower lid lies at the iris. No sclera should be visible between the eyelid and the iris.

Scleral and corneal assessment require a penlight. Examine the sclera for color; it is usually white. A yellow color may indicate jaundice or systemic problems. In dark-skinned people, the normal sclera may appear yellow and small, pigmented dots may be visible (Jarvis, 2016).

The cornea is best seen by directing a light at it from the side. The cornea should be transparent, smooth, shiny, and bright. Any cloudy areas or specks may indicate injury.

Assess the blink reflex by bringing a fist quickly toward the patient's face. Patients with vision will blink.

Pupillary assessment involves examining each pupil separately and comparing the results. The pupils are usually round and of equal size. About 5% of people normally have a noticeable difference in the size of their pupils, which is known as anisocoria (Jarvis, 2016). Pupil size varies in people exposed to the same amount of light. Pupils are smaller in older adults. People with myopia have larger pupils. People with hyperopia have smaller pupils. The normal pupil diameter is between 3 and 5 mm. Smaller pupils reduce vision in low light conditions.

Observe pupils for response to light. Increasing light causes constriction, whereas decreasing light causes dilation. Constriction of both pupils is the normal response to direct light and to accommodation. Assess pupillary reaction to light by asking the patient to look straight ahead while you quickly bring the beam of a penlight in from the side and direct it at the right pupil. Constriction of the right pupil is a direct response to shining the penlight into that eye. Constriction of the left pupil when light is shined at the right pupil is known as a consensual response. Assess the responses for each eye. (You may see the abbreviation "PERRLA" in a patient's medical record, which stands for **p**upils **e**qual, **r**ound, **r**eactive to **l**ight, and **a**ccommodative.)

Evaluate each pupil for speed of reaction. The pupil should immediately constrict when a light is directed at it—a *brisk* response. If the pupil takes more than 1 second to constrict, the response is *sluggish*. Pupils that fail to react are *nonreactive* or *fixed*. Compare the reactivity speed of right and left pupils, and document any difference.

Assess for accommodation by holding your finger about 18 cm from the patient's nose and move it toward the nose. The patient's eyes normally converge during this movement, and the pupils constrict equally.

Vision Testing

Visual SENSORY PERCEPTION is measured by first testing each eye separately and then testing both eyes together. Patients who wear corrective lenses are tested both without and with their lenses.

Visual acuity tests measure both distance and near vision. The Snellen eye chart measures distance vision. This chart has letters, numbers, pictures, or a single letter presented in various positions. The chart with one letter in different positions is used for patients who cannot read, who do not speak the language used at the facility, or who cannot speak but do have adequate cognition. Have the patient stand or sit 20 feet from the chart, cover one eye, and use the other eye to read the line that appears most clear. If the patient can do this accurately, ask him or her to read the next lower line. Repeat this sequence to the last line on which the patient can correctly identify most characters. Repeat the procedure with the other eye. Record findings as a comparison between what the patient can read at 20 feet and the distance that a person with normal vision can read the same line. For example, *20/50* means that the patient sees at 20 feet from the chart what a healthy eye sees at 50 feet.

For patients who cannot see the 20/400 character, assess visual acuity by holding fingers in front of their eyes and asking them to count the number of fingers. Acuity is recorded as "count fingers vision at 5 feet," or the farthest distance at which fingers are counted correctly.

Patients who cannot count fingers are tested for hand motion (HM) acuity. Stand about 2 to 3 feet in front of the patient. Ask him or her to cover the eye not being tested. Direct a light onto your hand from behind the patient. Demonstrate the three possible directions in which the hand can move during the test (stationary, left-right, or up-down). Move your hand slowly (1 second per motion), and ask the patient, "What is my hand doing now?" Repeat this procedure 5 times. Visual acuity is recorded as HM at the farthest distance at which most of the hand motions are identified correctly.

If the patient cannot detect hand motion, assess light perception (LP). Ask the patient first to cover the left eye. In a darkened room, direct the beam of a penlight at the patient's right eye from a distance of 2 to 3 feet for 1 to 2 seconds. Instruct the patient to say "on" when the beam of light is perceived and "off" when it is no longer detected. If the patient identifies the presence or absence of light 3 times correctly, acuity is documented as LP.

Near vision is tested for patients who have difficulty reading without using glasses or other means of vision correction. Use a small, handheld miniature eye chart called a *Rosenbaum Pocket Vision Screener* or a *Jaeger card*. Ask the patient to hold the card 14 inches away from his or her eyes and read the characters. Test each eye separately and then together. Document the lowest line on which the patient can identify more than half the characters.

Visual field testing determines the degree of peripheral vision. It can be performed with a computerized machine or with a "confrontation test" for a rapid check of peripheral vision. Perimetry is a computerized test. During this test, the patient is asked to look straight ahead into a viewer and then indicate, by pressing a control button, when a moving light enters the peripheral vision. This process maps the person's peripheral vision and any deficits.

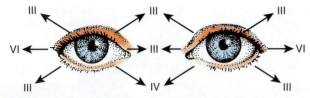

FIG. 46-7 Checking extraocular movements in the six cardinal positions indicates the functioning of cranial nerves III, IV, and VI.

During the confrontation test, sit facing the patient and ask him or her to look directly into your eyes while you look into the patient's eyes. Cover your right eye and have the patient cover his or her left eye so that you both have the same visual field. Then move a finger or an object from a nonvisible area into the patient's line of vision. The patient with normal peripheral vision notices the object at about the same time you do. Repeat this examination by covering your left eye and the patient covering his or her right eye. Document any areas in which you can see but the patient cannot.

Extraocular muscle function is assessed using the corneal light reflex and the six cardinal positions of gaze. These tests assess smoothness of eye movements and the function of cranial nerves III, IV, and VI.

The corneal light reflex determines alignment of the eyes. After asking the patient to stare straight ahead, shine a penlight at both corneas from a distance of 12 to 15 inches. The bright dot of light reflected from the shiny surface of the cornea should be in a symmetric position (e.g., at the 1 o'clock position in the right eye and at the 11 o'clock position in the left eye). An asymmetric reflex indicates a deviating eye and possible muscle weakness.

Use the six cardinal positions of gaze to assess muscle function (Fig. 46-7). The eye will not turn to a particular position if the muscle is weak or if the controlling nerve is affected. Ask the patient to hold his or her head still and to move only the eyes to follow a small object. Move the object to the patient's right (lateral), upward and right (temporal), down and right, left (lateral), upward and left (temporal), and down and left (see Fig. 46-7). While the patient moves the eyes to these positions, note whether both eyes move in a parallel manner and any deviation of movement. Nystagmus, an involuntary and rapid twitching of the eyeball, is a normal finding for the far lateral gaze. It may also be caused by abnormal nerve function or problems with the inner ear.

Color vision is usually tested using the *Ishihara chart,* which shows numbers composed of dots of one color within a circle of dots of a different color (Fig. 46-8). Test each eye separately by asking the patient what numbers he or she sees on the chart. Reading the numbers correctly indicates normal color vision.

Psychosocial Assessment

A patient with changes in visual SENSORY PERCEPTION may be anxious about possible vision loss. Patients with severe visual defects may be unable to perform ADLs. Dependency from reduced vision can affect self-esteem. Ask the patient how he or she feels about the vision changes, and assess coping techniques. Assess the family to determine available support. Provide information about local resources and services for reduced vision.

Diagnostic Assessment
Laboratory Assessment

Cultures of corneal or conjunctival swabs and scrapings help diagnose infections. Obtain a sample of the exudate for culture

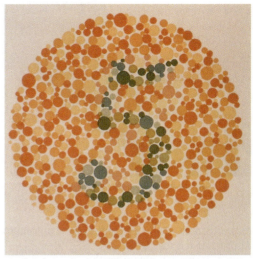

FIG. 46-8 An Ishihara chart for testing color vision.

before antibiotics or topical anesthetics are instilled. Take swabs from the conjunctivae and any ulcerated or inflamed areas.

Imaging Assessment

CT is useful for assessing the eyes, the bony structures around the eyes, and the extraocular muscles. It can also detect tumors in the orbital space. Contrast dye is used unless trauma is suspected. Tell the patient that this test is not painful but does require being in a confined space and keeping the head still.

MRI is often used to examine the orbits and the optic nerves and to evaluate ocular tumors. MRI cannot be used to evaluate injuries involving metal in the eyes. *Metal in the eye is an absolute contraindication for MRI.*

Radioisotope scanning is used to locate tumors and lesions. This test requires that the patient sign an informed consent. The patient receives a tracer dose of the radioactive isotope, either orally or by injection, and must then lie still. The scanner measures the radioactivity emitted by the radioactive atoms concentrated in the area being studied. Sedation may be used for patients who are anxious. No special follow-up care is required.

Ultrasonography is used to examine the orbit and eye with high-frequency sound waves. This noninvasive test helps diagnose trauma, intraorbital tumors, proptosis, and choroidal or retinal detachments. It is also used to determine the length of the eye and any gross outline changes in the eye and the orbit in patients with cloudy corneas or lenses that reduce direct examination of the fundus.

Inform the patient that this test is painless because the test is performed either with the eyes closed or, when the eyes must remain open, anesthetic eyedrops are instilled first. He or she sits upright with the chin in the chin rest. The probe is touched against the patient's anesthetized cornea, and sound waves are bounced through the eye. The sound waves create a reflective pattern on a computer screen that can be examined for abnormalities. No special follow-up care is needed. Remind the patient not to rub or touch the eye until the anesthetic agent has worn off.

Other Diagnostic Assessment

Many tests are used to examine specific eye structures when patients have specific risks, manifestations, or exposures. These

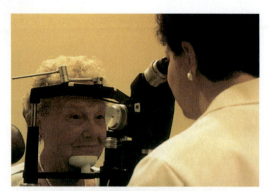

FIG. 46-9 Slit-lamp ocular examination.

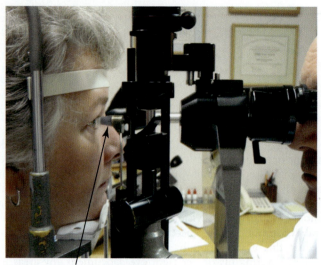

Goldman's applanation tonometer

FIG. 46-10 Use of Goldman's applanation tonometer and a slit lamp to measure intraocular pressure (IOP).

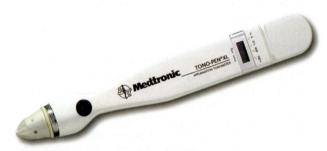

FIG. 46-11 The Tono-Pen.

tests are performed only by physicians, optometrists, or advanced practice nurses.

Slit-lamp examination magnifies the anterior eye structures (Fig. 46-9). The patient leans on a chin rest to stabilize the head. A narrow beam (slit) of light is aimed so that only a segment of the eye is brightly lighted. The examiner can then locate the position of any abnormality in the cornea, lens, or anterior vitreous humor.

Corneal staining consists of placing fluorescein or other topical dye into the conjunctival sac. The dye outlines irregularities of the corneal surface that are not easily visible. This test is used for corneal trauma, problems caused by a contact lens, or the presence of foreign bodies, abrasions, ulcers, or other corneal disorders.

This procedure is noninvasive and is performed under aseptic conditions. The dye is applied topically to the eye, and the eye is then viewed through a blue filter. Nonintact areas of the cornea stain a bright green color.

Tonometry measures intraocular pressure (IOP) using a tonometer. This instrument applies pressure to the outside of the eye until it equals the pressure inside the eye. Normal IOP readings have always been considered to range from 10 to 21 mm Hg; however, this number is not absolute and must be considered along with corneal thickness. The thickness of the cornea affects how much pressure must be applied before indentation occurs. For example, a person with a thicker cornea will have a higher tonometer reading that may falsely indicate increased IOP. A person with a thinner-than-normal cornea may have a low tonometer reading even when higher IOP is present.

About 5% of patients with healthy eyes have a slightly higher pressure. Tonometer readings are indicated for all patients older than 40 years. Adults with a family history of glaucoma should have their IOP measured once or twice a year. The most common method to measure IOP by an ophthalmologist is the Goldman's applanation tonometer used with a slit lamp (Fig. 46-10). This method involves direct eye contact. Another instrument, the Tono-Pen (Fig. 46-11), is designed for use by patients in the home to measure IOP daily.

Intraocular pressure varies throughout the day and may peak at any time of the day. Therefore always document the time of IOP measurement, and teach patients who are measuring IOP at home to perform the measurement at the same time or times each day.

Ophthalmoscopy allows viewing of the eye's external and interior structures with an instrument called an *ophthalmoscope*. This examination can be performed by any nurse but

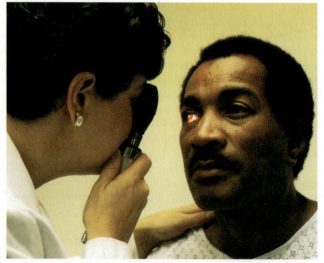

FIG. 46-12 Proper technique for direct ophthalmoscopic visualization of the retina.

usually is performed by a physician, advanced practice nurse, or physician assistant. It is easiest to examine the fundus when the room is dark, because the pupil dilates. Stand on the same side as the eye being examined. Tell the patient to look straight ahead at an object on the wall behind you. Hold the ophthalmoscope firmly against your face, and align it so that your eye sees through the sight hole (Fig. 46-12).

TABLE 46-3	Structures Assessed By Direct Ophthalmoscopy

Red Reflex
- Presence or absence

Optic Disc
- Color
- Margins (sharp or blurred)
- Cup size
- Presence of rings or crescents

Optic Blood Vessels
- Size
- Color
- Kinks or tangles
- Light reflection
- Narrowing
- Nicking at arteriovenous crossings

Fundus
- Color
- Tears or holes
- Lesions
- Bleeding

Macula
- Presence of blood vessels
- Color
- Lesions
- Bleeding

CHART 46-3   Best Practice for Patient Safety & Quality Care (QSEN)

Instillation of Eyedrops

- Check the name, strength, expiration date, color, and clarity of the eyedrops to be instilled.
- Check to see whether only one eye is to have the drug or if both eyes are to receive the drug.
- If both eyes are to receive the same drug and one eye is infected, use two separate bottles and carefully label each bottle with "right" or "left" for the correct eye.
- Wash your hands.
- Put on gloves if secretions are present in or around the eye.
- Explain the procedure to the patient.
- Have the patient sit in a chair, and you stand behind the patient.
- Ask the patient to tilt the head backward, with the back of the head resting against your body and looking up at the ceiling.
- Gently pull the lower lid down against the patient's cheek, forming a small pocket.
- Hold the eyedrop bottle (with the cap off) like a pencil, with the tip pointing down.
- Rest the wrist holding the bottle against the patient's cheek.
- Without touching any part of the eye or lid with the tip of the bottle, gently squeeze the bottle and release the prescribed number of drops into the pocket you have made with the patient's lower lid.
- Gently release the lower lid.
- Tell the patient to close the eye gently (without squeezing the lids tightly).
- Gently press and hold the corner of the eye nearest the nose to close off the punctum and prevent the drug from being absorbed systemically.
- Without pressing on the lid, gently blot away any excess drug or tears with a tissue.
- Remove your gloves, and place the cap back on the bottle.
- Ask the patient to keep the eye closed for about 1 minute.
- Wash your hands again.

When using the ophthalmoscope, move toward the patient's eye from about 12 to 15 inches away and to the side of his or her line of vision. As you direct the ophthalmoscope at the pupil, a red glare (red reflex) should be seen in the pupil as a reflection of the light on the retina. An absent red reflex may indicate a lens opacity or cloudiness of the vitreous. Move toward the patient's pupil while following the red reflex. The retina should then be visible through the ophthalmoscope. Examine the optic disc, optic vessels, fundus, and macula. Table 46-3 lists the features that can be observed in each structure.

The use of an ophthalmoscope may make a confused patient or one who does not understand the language more anxious. When working with a patient who does not speak the language used at the facility, use an interpreter, when possible, to ensure the patient's understanding and cooperation with the examination.

! NURSING SAFETY PRIORITY (QSEN)

Action Alert

Avoid using an ophthalmoscope with a confused patient.

Fluorescein angiography, which is performed by a physician or advanced practice nurse, provides a detailed image of eye circulation. Digital pictures are taken in rapid succession after the dye is given IV. This test helps assess problems of retinal circulation (e.g., diabetic retinopathy, retinal hemorrhage, and macular degeneration) or diagnose intraocular tumors.

Explain the procedure to the patient, and instill mydriatic eyedrops (cause pupil dilation) 1 hour before the test. Chart 46-3 lists the best practice for correct eyedrop installation. Check that the informed consent has been signed by the patient. Warn that the dye may cause the skin to appear yellow for several hours after the test. The stain is eliminated through the urine, which turns green.

Encourage patients to drink fluids to help eliminate the dye. Remind them that any staining of the skin will disappear in a few hours. Instruct the patient to wear dark glasses and avoid direct sunlight until pupil dilation returns to normal, because the bright light will cause eye pain.

Electroretinography graphs the retina's response to light stimulation. This test is helpful in detecting and evaluating blood vessel changes from disease or drugs. The graph is obtained by placing an electrode on an anesthetized cornea. Lights at varying speeds and intensities are flashed, and the neural response is graphed. The measurement from the cornea is identical to the response that would be obtained if electrodes were placed directly on the retina.

Gonioscopy is a test performed when a high IOP is found and determines whether open-angle or closed-angle glaucoma is present. It uses a special lens that eliminates the corneal curve, is painless, and allows visualization of the angle where the iris meets the cornea.

Laser imaging of the retina and optic nerve creates a three-dimensional view of the back of the eye. It is often used for those people with ocular hypertension or who are at risk for glaucoma from other problems. This computerized examination assesses the thickness and contours of the optic nerve and retina for changes that indicate damage as a result of high IOP. It can be used serially for a person at risk for glaucoma to detect early changes and indicate when intervention is needed.

ⓘ CLINICAL JUDGMENT CHALLENGE

Patient-Centered Care; Safety **QSEN**

The patient is a 56-year-old woman whose primary care provider has referred her to an ophthalmologist because she is having manifestations of glaucoma. She has never been evaluated by an ophthalmologist, even though she has used reading glasses for about 10 years. She seems very anxious and tells you that she cannot stand to have her eyes touched directly. She also tells you that her mother developed an eye infection and lost the vision in that eye after she had her intraocular pressure tested by an instrument with small feet that scratched her eye.

1. Will this patient's eyes be "touched" during a typical assessment of intraocular pressure?
2. What will you tell her about this procedure?
3. What assurance can you give her that she will not develop an infection from this evaluation?
4. Should you relay this patient's concerns to the ophthalmologist? Why or why not?

NURSING CONCEPTS AND CLINICAL JUDGMENT REVIEW

What might you NOTICE in a patient with adequate visual SENSORY PERCEPTION?

Physical assessment:
- Eyes are symmetric on the face on a line just about even with the tops of the ears.
- Eyes are clear with no drainage or open areas.
- Patient does not squint or tilt the head.
- Patient does not close one eye to read or see at a distance.
- Patient startles when a sudden move is made at the face.
- Patient blinks 5 to 10 times per minute.
- Pupils are the same size in each eye.
- Both pupils constrict when a light is shined at only one eye.
- Patient comments on the presence of art or unusual visual objects in the immediate environment.
- Patient walks without hesitation into a room without bumping into objects in his or her path.

Psychological assessment:
- Patient is oriented and not confused.
- Patient makes eye contact when speaking.

GET READY FOR THE NCLEX® EXAMINATION!

▌KEY POINTS

Review these Key Points for each NCLEX Examination Client Needs Category.

Safe and Effective Care Environment
- Wash your hands before moving a patient's eyelids or instilling drugs into the eye. **Safety** **QSEN**
- If a patient has discharge from one eye, examine the eye without the discharge first. **Safety** **QSEN**
- Wear gloves when examining an eye with drainage. **Safety** **QSEN**
- Avoid using an ophthalmoscope on a confused patient. **Safety** **QSEN**

Health Promotion and Maintenance
- Teach patients not to rub their eyes. **Patient-Centered Care** **QSEN**
- Identify patients at risk for eye injury as a result of work environment or leisure activities. **Patient-Centered Care** **QSEN**
- Urge all patients to wear eye protection when they are performing yard work, working in a woodshop or metal shop, using chemicals, or are in any environment in which drops or particulate matter is airborne. **Safety** **QSEN**
- Teach everyone to wear sunglasses outdoors in bright sunlight. **Patient-Centered Care** **QSEN**

Psychosocial Integrity
- Provide opportunities for the patient and family to express their concerns about a possible change in visual SENSORY PERCEPTION. **Patient-Centered Care** **QSEN**
- Explain all diagnostic procedures, restrictions, and follow-up care to the patient scheduled for tests. **Patient-Centered Care** **QSEN**

Physiological Integrity
- Ask the patient about vision problems in any other members of the family, because some vision problems have a genetic component. **Patient-Centered Care** **QSEN**
- Test the vision of both eyes immediately of any person who experiences an eye injury or any sudden change in vision. **Patient-Centered Care** **QSEN**

CHAPTER 47

Care of Patients with Eye and Vision Problems

M. Linda Workman

PRIORITY CONCEPTS

- SENSORY PERCEPTION
- INFECTION

LEARNING OUTCOMES

Safe and Effective Care Environment

1. Protect the patient with eye and vision problems from injury or INFECTION.
2. Ensure that all members of the health care team are aware of a patient's visual limitations and need for assistance.

Health Promotion and Maintenance

3. Teach people when annual eye examinations with measurement of intraocular pressure are important to receive.
4. Teach patients and family members how to correctly instill ophthalmic drops and ointment into the eye.
5. Teach patients with glaucoma the relationship between increased intraocular pressure (IOP) and their eye problems.
6. Teach the patient with reduced visual SENSORY PERCEPTION and family how to alter the home environment for patient safety.

Psychosocial Integrity

7. Reduce the psychological impact for the patient and family experiencing a potential change in visual SENSORY PERCEPTION.
8. Work with other members of the health care team to ensure that the values, preferences, and expressed needs of patients with reduced visual SENSORY PERCEPTION are respected.

Physiological Integrity

9. Prioritize care and educational needs for the patient after cataract surgery with lens replacement.
10. Prioritize care and educational needs for patients with primary open-angle glaucoma.
11. Collaborate with other health care professionals to help patients and families experiencing reduced visual sensory perception achieve their desired health outcomes.
12. Coordinate interventions for the patient with reduced visual SENSORY PERCEPTION in the community.

Many factors and problems can affect visual SENSORY PERCEPTION. Problems may have a gradual onset, such as the most common form of glaucoma or cataracts, whereas others may have a sudden onset. Any temporary or permanent change in visual sensory perception requires the patient to make some changes in function or lifestyle.

EYELID DISORDERS

The eyelid is composed of skin and small muscles to protect the eye surface and spread tears. Vision is affected by problems that change the structure, function, or position of the eyelid.

Entropion and Ectropion

An **entropion** is the turning inward of the eyelid causing the lashes to rub against the eye. It can be caused by eyelid muscle spasms or by scarring and deformity of the eyelid after trauma and is seen more often among older adults because of age-related loss of tissue support.

The patient reports "feeling something in my eye." Pain and tears may also be present. The conjunctiva is red, and corneal abrasion may result from constant irritation.

Surgery corrects eyelid position by either tightening the orbicular muscles and moving the eyelid to a normal position or by preventing inward rotation of the eyelid. After surgery, the eye is covered with a patch and the patient is discharged.

Demonstrate instillation of eyedrops, and evaluate the patient's ability to instill the drops. Teach the patient how to clean the suture line with a cotton swab and the prescribed solution. A small amount of antibiotic ointment may be applied (Fig. 47-1). Chart 47-1 describes how to apply ophthalmic ointment. Chart 47-2 lists common drugs for eye inflammation and INFECTION.

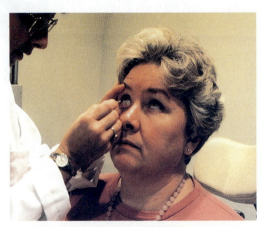

FIG. 47-1 Application of ophthalmic ointment.

> ## ! NURSING SAFETY PRIORITY QSEN
> ### *Drug Alert*
>
> Check the route of administration for ophthalmic drugs. Most are administered by the eye instillation route, not the oral route. Administering these drugs orally can cause systemic side effects in addition to not having a therapeutic effect on the eye.

An **ectropion** is the turning outward and sagging of the eyelid caused by muscle relaxation or weakness, which often occurs with aging. This lid position reduces the washing action of tears, leading to corneal drying and ulceration.

Patients often have constant tears and a sagging lower eyelid. Surgery can restore lid alignment. After surgery, the eye is covered with a patch and the patient is discharged. Nursing care is the same as for an entropion.

Hordeolum

A **hordeolum**, or *stye,* is INFECTION of the eyelid sweat glands (external hordeolum) or of the eyelid sebaceous gland (internal hordeolum). A red, swollen, painful area occurs on the skin surface side of the eyelid. The most common causative organisms are *Staphylococcus aureus, Staphylococcus epidermidis,* and *Streptococcus.* Visual SENSORY PERCEPTION is not affected.

Management includes applying warm compresses 4 times a day and an antibacterial ointment. When the lesion opens, the purulent material drains and the pain subsides.

Nursing interventions include instructing the patient how to apply compresses to the eye (Chart 47-3) and how to instill antibiotic ointment (see Chart 47-1). Remind the patient to remove the ointment from the eyes before driving or operating machinery.

Chalazion

A **chalazion** is an inflammation of a sebaceous gland in the eyelid. It begins with redness and tenderness, followed by a gradual *painless* swelling. Later, redness and tenderness are not present. Most chalazia protrude on the inside of the eyelid. The patient has eye fatigue, light sensitivity, and excessive tears.

Management includes applying warm compresses 4 times a day, followed by instillation of ophthalmic antibiotic ointment. If the chalazion is large enough to affect vision or is cosmetically displeasing, it may be removed surgically. Instruct the patient to immediately report increasing redness, purulent drainage, or reduced vision to the ophthalmologist.

> ## CHART 47-1   Best Practice for Patient Safety & Quality Care QSEN
> ### *Instillation of Ophthalmic Ointment*
>
> - Check the name, strength, and expiration date of the ointment to be instilled. Be sure it is an ophthalmic (eye) preparation and not a general topical ointment.
> - Check whether only one eye or both eyes are to receive the drug.
> - If both eyes are to receive the same drug and one eye is infected, use two separate tubes and carefully label each tube with "right" or "left" for the correct eye.
> - Wash your hands and put on gloves.
> - Explain the procedure to the patient.
> - Ask the patient to tilt the head backward and look up at the ceiling.
> - Gently pull the lower lid down against the patient's cheek, forming a small pocket.
> - Hold the tube (with the cap off) like a pencil, with the tip down.
> - Rest the wrist holding the tube against the patient's cheek.
> - Without touching any part of the eye or lid with the tip of the tube, gently squeeze the tube and release a small thin strip of ointment into the pocket of the lower lid. Start at the nose side of the pocket, and move toward the outer edge of the pocket.
> - Gently release the lower lid.
> - Tell the patient to close the eye without squeezing the lid.
> - While the eye is closed, gently wipe away excess ointment.
> - Remind the patient that vision in that eye will be blurred and to not drive or operate heavy machinery until the ointment is removed.
> - Remove your gloves, and place the cap back on the tube.
> - Ask the patient to keep the eye closed for about 1 minute.
> - Wash your hands again.
> - To remove ointment, wear gloves if drainage is present.
> - Then ask the patient to close the eye; wipe the closed lids with a clean tissue from the corner of the eye nearest the nose outward. If you are wiping the same eye twice, use a different area of the tissue or use a new one.

KERATOCONJUNCTIVITIS SICCA

The lacrimal system moistens the eye surface with tears and removes tears from the eye. Problems arise from reduced tear production, INFECTION, or inflammation in the lacrimal system.

Keratoconjunctivitis sicca, or dry eye syndrome, results from changes in tear production, tear composition, or tear distribution. Drugs (e.g., antihistamines, beta-adrenergic blocking agents, anticholinergic drugs) also can reduce tear production. Diseases associated with dry eye syndrome include rheumatoid arthritis, leukemia, sarcoidosis, and Sjögren's syndrome. Radiation or chemical burns to the eye also decrease tear production. Injury to cranial nerve VII inhibits tears. Eye dryness may follow vision-enhancing surgery.

The patient has a foreign body sensation in the eye, burning and itching eyes, and *photophobia* (sensitivity to light). The corneal light reflex is dulled. Tears contain mucus strands.

Management depends on symptom severity. Cyclosporine (Restasis) eyedrops may be prescribed to increase tear production. Artificial tears (HypoTears, Refresh) also can be used to reduce daytime dryness. A lubricating ointment (Lacri-Lube SOP, Refresh P.M.) is used at night. If the dry eye syndrome is caused by an abnormal eyelid position, surgery may be needed.

CONJUNCTIVAL DISORDERS

The conjunctiva is a thin mucous membrane that covers and protects the eye. Because of its location, the conjunctiva is subject to trauma and INFECTION.

CHART 47-2   Common Examples of Drug Therapy

Eye Inflammation and Infection

DRUG	NURSING INTERVENTIONS*†	RATIONALES
Topical Anesthetics		
Proparacaine HCl, or proxymetacaine (AK-Taine, Alcaine, Ocu-Caine, Ophthetic) Tetracaine HCl, cocaine HCl (Pontocaine)	Remind the patient not to rub or touch the eye while it is anesthetized. Patch the eye if the patient leaves the facility before the anesthetic wears off. Instruct the patient not to use discolored solution. Teach the patient to store the bottle tightly closed.	Touching may injure the eye. The use of a patch prevents injury, such as corneal abrasion. Discoloration is a sign of altered drug composition. Air may cause drug contamination and oxidation.
Topical Steroids		
Prednisolone acetate (Ocu-Pred, Ophtho-Tate ✣) Prednisolone phosphate (Inflamase) Dexamethasone (Dexair, Dexotic, Maxidex) Betamethasone (Betnesol) Fluorometholone (Fluor-Op, Liquifilm)	Tell the patient to shake the bottle vigorously before use. Teach the patient to check for corneal ulceration (pain, reduced vision, secretions). Warn the patient not to share eyedrops with others.	Drug is a suspension; shaking is required to distribute the drug evenly in the solution. Steroid use predisposes the patient to local infection. Disease transmission is possible when sharing eyedrops.
Anti-Infective Agents		
Gentamicin (Genoptic, Gentak Alcomicin ✣) Tobramycin (Tobrex) Ciprofloxacin (Ciloxan) Erythromycin (Ilotycin) Chlortetracycline (Aureomycin) Sulfisoxazole (Gantrisin) Ofloxacin (Ocuflox) Levofloxacin (Quixin) Bacitracin; Polymyxin B (Polysporin, Polytracin ophthalmic, AK-Poly-Bac)	Teach the patient the importance of using the drug exactly as prescribed, even if he or she needs to use it hourly. Teach the patient how to clean exudate from the eyes before using drops. Reinforce the importance of completing the prescribed drug regimen.	Bacterial and fungal eye infections worsen rapidly and can lead to blindness if not treated adequately. Cleansing decreases the risk for contaminating the drug and increases contact of the conjunctiva with the drug. Adherence is critical to maintain a therapeutic level of drug.
Antibiotic-Steroid Combinations		
Tobramycin with dexamethasone (TobraDex) Neomycin sulfate with polymyxin B sulfate and dexamethasone (Maxitrol)	This is the same as for the general anti-infective agents alone and for the steroids alone.	This is the same as for the general anti-infective agents alone and for the steroids alone.
Topical Antiviral Agents		
Trifluridine (Viroptic) Vidarabine (Vira-A)	Teach the patient to refrigerate the drug and protect it from light. Teach the patient to assess for itching lids and burning eyes.	Drug stability is affected by warm temperatures and light. Sensitivity to these drugs is common.
Antifungal Agents		
Amphotericin B Natamycin (Natacyn)	Teach the patient to assess for itching lids and burning eyes.	Sensitivity to these drugs is common.
Nonsteroidal Anti-Inflammatory Agents		
Flurbiprofen (Ocufen) Diclofenac (Voltaren) Bromfenac (Xibrom) Ketorolac (Acular)	Teach the patient to check for bleeding in the eye. Teach the patient not to wear soft contact lenses during therapy with these drugs.	These drugs disrupt platelet aggregation. These drugs interact with contact lens materials and increase the risk for infection.

*When instilling eyedrops, teach patients to use nasal punctal occlusion to reduce the risk for systemic absorption and side effects.
†When more than one topical ophthalmic drug is prescribed, teach patients to separate the instillation of each drug by 5-10 minutes (or package recommendations).

Conjunctivitis

Conjunctivitis is an inflammation with or without INFECTION of the conjunctiva. Inflammation occurs from exposure to allergens or irritants. Infectious conjunctivitis occurs with bacterial or viral infection and is easily transmitted from person to person.

Allergic conjunctivitis manifestations are edema, a sensation of burning, a "bloodshot" eye appearance, excessive tears, and itching (Watkinson, 2013). Management includes vasoconstrictor and corticosteroid eyedrops (see Chart 47-2). Instruct patients to avoid using makeup near the eye until all manifestations are gone.

Bacterial conjunctivitis, or "pink eye," is most often caused by *S. aureus.* Manifestations are blood vessel dilation, edema, tears, and discharge. The discharge is watery at first and then becomes thicker, with shreds of mucus.

Cultures of the drainage may be obtained to identify the organism. Ophthalmic antibiotics are prescribed to eliminate the infection. Nursing interventions focus on preventing INFECTION spread to the other eye or to other people. Remind the patient to wash his or her hands after touching the eye and before using eyedrops. Warn him or her not to touch the unaffected eye without first washing the hands and to avoid sharing washcloths and towels with others. Instruct patients to discard eye makeup and applicators used at the time the infection developed. Contact lenses worn during the infection need to be discarded to avoid reinfection.

Trachoma

Trachoma is a chronic conjunctivitis caused by *Chlamydia trachomatis*. It scars the conjunctiva and is a common cause of preventable blindness worldwide. The incidence is highest in warm, moist climates where sanitation is poor.

At first the disease resembles bacterial conjunctivitis with manifestations of tears, photophobia, and eyelid edema. Follicles form on the upper eyelid conjunctiva. As the disease progresses, the eyelid scars and turns inward, causing the eyelashes to damage the cornea.

Antibiotic therapy is used when the organism is identified. The most effective antibiotic is oral azithromycin (Zithromax). The infection also can be eliminated early in the disease with a 4-week course of tetracycline eye ointment. Nursing interventions focus on INFECTION control. Patient teaching is the same as for conjunctivitis.

! NURSING SAFETY PRIORITY (QSEN)

Action Alert

Teach patients who are prescribed oral antibiotics or antibiotic ointments to complete the entire course of antibiotics. Stopping antibiotic therapy too soon promotes INFECTION recurrence and development of antibiotic-resistant bacteria.

CORNEAL DISORDERS

For a sharp retinal image, the cornea must be transparent and intact. Corneal problems may be caused by irritation or INFECTION (keratitis) with ulceration of the corneal surface, degeneration of the cornea (keratoconus), or deposits in the cornea. All corneal problems reduce visual SENSORY PERCEPTION, and some can lead to blindness.

CORNEAL ABRASION, ULCERATION, AND INFECTION

❖ PATHOPHYSIOLOGY

A corneal abrasion is a scrape or scratch injury of the cornea. This painful condition can be caused by a small foreign body,

trauma, or contact lens use (Corneal Abrasion, 2013). Other problems contributing to corneal injury are malnutrition, dry eye syndromes, and some cancer therapies. The abrasion allows organisms to enter, leading to corneal INFECTION. Bacterial, protozoal, and fungal infections can lead to corneal ulceration, which is a deeper injury. *This problem is an emergency because the cornea has no separate blood supply and infections that can permanently impair vision develop rapidly.* Use of homemade contact lens solutions and the use of large-volume solution containers that can easily become contaminated have led to a sharp rise in the incidence of corneal ulcers infected with *Pseudomonas aeruginosa* and fungi.

❖ PATIENT-CENTERED COLLABORATIVE CARE

The patient with a corneal disorder has pain, reduced vision, photophobia, and eye secretions. Cloudy or purulent fluid may be present on the eyelids or lashes. Wear gloves when examining the eye.

The cornea looks hazy or cloudy with a patchy area of ulceration. When fluorescein stain is used, the patchy areas appear green. Microbial culture and corneal scrapings are used to determine the causative organism. Anti-infective therapy is started before the organism is identified because of the high risk for vision loss. For culture, obtain swabs from the ulcer and its edges. For corneal scrapings, the cornea is anesthetized with a topical agent and a physician or advanced practice nurse removes samples from the ulcer center and edge.

Antibiotics, antifungals, and antivirals are prescribed to eliminate the organisms. A broad-spectrum antibiotic is prescribed first and may be changed when culture results are known. Steroids may be used with antibiotics to reduce the eye inflammation. Drugs can be given topically as eyedrops, injected subconjunctivally, or injected IV. Chart 46-3 in Chapter 46 lists best practices for instilling eyedrops. The nursing priorities are to begin the drug therapy, to ensure patient understanding of the drug therapy regimen, and to prevent INFECTION spread.

Often the anti-infective therapy involves instilling eyedrops *every hour* for the first 24 hours. Teach the patient or family member how to instill the eyedrops correctly. (See Chart 46-2 in Chapter 46.)

If the eye INFECTION occurs only in one eye, teach the patient not to use the drug in the unaffected eye. Instruct him or her to wash hands after touching the affected eye and before touching or doing anything to the healthy eye. If both eyes are infected, separate bottles of drugs are needed for each eye. Teach the patient to clearly label the bottles "right eye" and "left eye" and not to switch the drugs from eye to eye. Also teach him or her to completely care for one eye, then wash the hands, and using the drugs designated for the other eye, care for that eye. Remind the patient not to wear contact lenses during the entire time that these drugs are being used because the eye is more vulnerable to infection or injury and because the drugs can cloud or damage the contact lenses.

! NURSING SAFETY PRIORITY (QSEN)

Action Alert

Stress the importance of applying the drug as often as prescribed, even at night. Stopping the infection at this stage can save the vision in the infected eye. Instruct the patient to make and keep all follow-up appointments; usually the patient is seen again in 24 hours or less.

Drug therapy may continue for 3 or more weeks to ensure eradication of the INFECTION. Warn patients to avoid using makeup around the eye until the infection has cleared (Corneal Abrasion, 2013). Instruct patients to discard all open containers of contact lens solutions and bottles of eyedrops because these may be contaminated. Patients should not wear contact lenses for weeks to months until the infection is gone and the ulcer is healed.

KERATOCONUS AND CORNEAL OPACITIES

❖ PATHOPHYSIOLOGY

The cornea can permanently lose it shape, become scarred or cloudy, or become thinner, reducing useful visual SENSORY PERCEPTION. Keratoconus, the degeneration of the corneal tissue resulting in abnormal corneal shape, can occur with trauma or may be an inherited disorder (Fig. 47-2). Inadequately treated corneal INFECTION and severe trauma can scar the cornea and lead to severe visual impairment that can be improved only by surgical interventions.

❖ PATIENT-CENTERED COLLABORATIVE CARE

For a misshaped cornea that is still clear, surgical management involves a corneal ring implant that adjusts the shape of the cornea. With this procedure, the shape of the cornea is changed by placing a flexible ring in the outer edges of the cornea (outside of the optical zone).

The procedure is performed under local anesthesia. Improvement to best vision is immediate. Removal, replacement, or adjustment of ring tightness can enhance refraction, especially when the patient's vision changes further as a result of aging. Because the ring is placed outside of the optical zone, the risk for corneal clouding or scarring is low.

Surgery to improve clarity for a permanent corneal disorder that obscures vision is a **keratoplasty** (corneal transplant), in which the diseased corneal tissue is removed and replaced with tissue from a human donor cornea. This process improves vision by removing corneal deformities and replacing them with healthy corneal tissue.

Preoperative care may be short, with little time for teaching because transplantation is performed when the donor cornea becomes available. Examine the eyes for manifestations of INFECTION, and report any redness, drainage, or edema to the ophthalmologist. Instill prescribed antibiotic eyedrops and obtain IV access before surgery.

Operative procedures are *keratoplasties* and are usually performed with local anesthesia in an ambulatory surgical setting. The transplant may involve the entire depth of corneal tissue (penetrating keratoplasty) or only certain layers of the corneal tissue (lamellar keratoplasty). The nerves around the eye are anesthetized so that the patient cannot move the eye or see out of the eye. The center 7 to 8 mm of the diseased cornea is removed with an instrument that works like a cookie cutter (Fig. 47-3). The same instrument is used to cut the tissue graft from the donor cornea so that the graft will be a perfect fit. The donor cornea is sutured into place on the eye. The procedure takes about an hour, and the patient is discharged to home within 1 to 2 hours.

Postoperative care involves extensive patient teaching. Local antibiotics are injected or instilled. Usually the eye is covered with a pressure patch and a protective shield until the patient returns to the surgeon.

Instruct the patient to lie on the nonoperative side to reduce intraocular pressure (IOP). If a patch is to be used for more

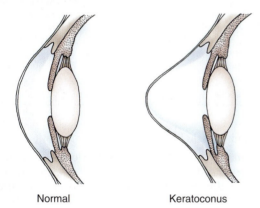

Normal	Keratoconus

FIG. 47-2 Profile of a normal cornea and one with keratoconus.

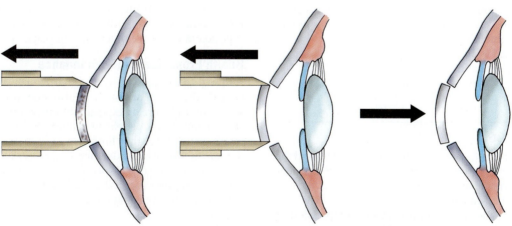

The diseased cornea is removed with a trephine.

A button, or graft, of donor cornea is removed with the same trephine so the cuts are identical.

The donor cornea is placed on the eye and stitched into place with suture material that is finer than a human hair.

FIG. 47-3 The steps involved in corneal transplantation (penetrating keratoplasty).

TABLE 47-1	Activities That Increase Intraocular Pressure	

- Bending from the waist
- Lifting objects weighing more than 10 lbs
- Sneezing, coughing
- Blowing the nose
- Straining to have a bowel movement

- Vomiting
- Having sexual intercourse
- Keeping the head in a dependent position
- Wearing tight shirt collars

than a day, teach the patient or family member how to apply it. Instruct the patient to wear the shield at night for the first month after surgery and whenever he or she is around small children or pets. Instruct him or her *not* to use an ice pack on the eye. Complications after surgery include bleeding, wound leakage, INFECTION, and graft rejection. Teach the patient how to instill eyedrops. Teach him or her to examine the eye (or have a family member do the examination) daily for the presence of infection or graft rejection. Stress that the presence of purulent discharge, a continuous leak of clear fluid from around the graft site (not tears), or excessive bleeding needs to be reported immediately to the surgeon. Other complications include decreased vision, increased reddening of the eye, pain, increased sensitivity to light, and the presence of light flashes or "floaters" in the field of vision. Teach the patient to report any of these manifestations to the surgeon if they develop after the first 48 hours and persist for more than 6 hours.

The eye should be protected from any activity that can increase the pressure on, around, or inside the eye. Teach the patient to avoid jogging, running, dancing, and any other activity that promotes rapid or jerky head motions for several weeks after surgery. Other activities that may raise intraocular pressure (IOP) and should be avoided are listed in Table 47-1.

Graft rejection can occur and starts as inflammation in the cornea near the graft edge that moves toward the center. Vision is reduced, and the cornea becomes cloudy. Topical corticosteroids and other immunosuppressants are used to stop the rejection process. If rejection continues, the graft becomes opaque and blood vessels branch into the opaque tissue.

Eye donation is a common procedure and needed for corneal transplantation. If a deceased patient is a known eye donor, follow these recommended steps:

- Raise the head of the bed 30 degrees.
- Instill prescribed antibiotic eyedrops.
- Close the eyes, and apply a *small* ice pack.

CATARACT

❖ PATHOPHYSIOLOGY

The lens is a transparent, elastic structure suspended behind the iris that focuses images onto the retina. A cataract is a lens opacity that distorts the image (Fig. 47-4). With aging, the lens gradually loses water and increases in density (Touhy & Jett, 2014). Lens density increases with drying and compression of older lens fibers and production of new fibers and lens crystals. With time, as lens density increases and transparency is lost, visual SENSORY PERCEPTION is greatly reduced. Both eyes may have cataracts, but the rate of progression in each eye is different.

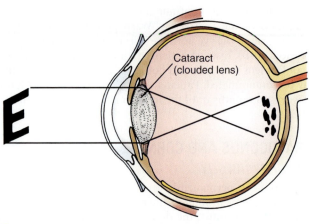

FIG. 47-4 The visual impairment produced by the presence of a cataract.

TABLE 47-2	Common Causes of Cataracts	

Age-Related Cataracts
- Lens water loss and fiber compaction

Traumatic Cataracts
- Blunt injury to eye or head
- Penetrating eye injury
- Intraocular foreign bodies
- Radiation exposure, therapy

Toxic Cataracts
- Corticosteroids
- Phenothiazine derivatives
- Miotic agents

Associated Cataracts
- Diabetes mellitus
- Hypoparathyroidism
- Down syndrome
- Chronic sunlight exposure

Complicated Cataracts
- Retinitis pigmentosa
- Glaucoma
- Retinal detachment

Etiology and Genetic Risk

Cataracts may be present at birth or develop at any time. They may be age-related or caused by trauma or exposure to toxic agents. They also occur with other diseases and eye disorders (Table 47-2).

Incidence and Prevalence

About 25 to 27 million people in North America have cataracts (National Eye Institute, 2012). The age-related cataract is the most common type. Some degree of cataract formation is expected in all people older than 70 years.

Health Promotion and Maintenance

Although most cases of cataracts in North America are age-related, the onset of cataract formation occurs earlier with heavy sun exposure or exposure to other sources of ultraviolet (UV) light. Teach people to reduce the risk for cataract by wearing sunglasses that limit exposure to UV light whenever they are outdoors in the daytime. Cataracts also may result from direct eye injury. Urge all people to wear eye and head protection during sports, such as baseball, or any activity that increases the risk for the eye being hit.

❖ PATIENT-CENTERED COLLABORATIVE CARE

◆ Assessment

History. Age is important because cataracts are most prevalent in the older adult. Ask about these predisposing factors:

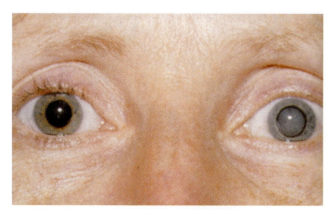

FIG. 47-5 The appearance of an eye with a mature cataract.

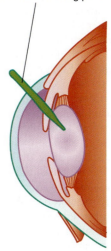

Sound wave and suctioning probe

Sound waves break up the lens, pieces are sucked out, and the capsule remains largely intact

FIG. 47-6 Cataract removal by phacoemulsification.

- Recent or past trauma to the eye
- Exposure to radioactive materials, x-rays, or UV light
- Systemic disease (e.g., diabetes mellitus, hypoparathyroidism)
- Prolonged use of corticosteroids, chlorpromazine, beta blockers, or miotic drugs
- Intraocular disease (e.g., recurrent uveitis)
- Family history of cataracts

Ask the patient to describe his or her vision. For example, you might say "Tell me what you can see well and what you have difficulty seeing."

Physical Assessment/Clinical Manifestations. Early manifestations of cataracts are slightly blurred vision and decreased color perception. At first the patient may think his or her glasses or contact lenses are smudged. As lens cloudiness continues, blurred and double vision occur and the patient may have difficulty with ADLs. Without surgical intervention, visual impairment progresses to blindness. *No pain or eye redness is associated with age-related cataract formation.*

Visual SENSORY PERCEPTION is tested using an eye chart and brightness acuity testing (see Chapter 46). Examine the lens with an ophthalmoscope, and describe any observed densities by size, shape, and location. As the cataract matures, the opacity makes it difficult to see the retina and the red reflex may be absent. When this occurs, the pupil is bluish white (Fig. 47-5).

Psychosocial Assessment. Loss of vision is gradual, and the patient may not be aware of it until reading or driving is affected. The patient often has anxiety about loss of independence. Encourage the patient and family to express concerns about reduced vision.

◆ **Planning and Implementation**

The priority problem for the patient with cataracts is reduced visual SENSORY PERCEPTION, which is a safety risk. Patients often live with reduced vision for years before the cataract is removed. Interventions for safety and independence before surgery are on pp. 993-994 in Patient-Centered Collaborative Care in the Reduced Visual Sensory Perception section.

Improving Vision

Planning: Expected Outcomes. The patient with cataracts is expected to recognize when ADLs cannot be performed safely and independently and then is expected to have cataract surgery. This procedure is covered by Medicare for patients who are 65 years or older.

Interventions. Surgery is the only "cure" for cataracts and should be performed as soon as possible after vision is reduced to the extent that ADLs are affected.

Preoperative Care. The ophthalmologist provides the patient with accurate information so that he or she can make informed decisions about treatment and obtains informed consent. Reinforce this information, and teach about the nature of cataracts, their progression, and their treatment.

Assess how the reduced vision affects ADLs, especially dressing, eating, and ambulating. Stress that care after surgery requires the instillation of different types of eyedrops several times a day for 2 to 4 weeks. Careful assessment of eye appearance is also needed. If the patient is unable to perform these tasks, help him or her make arrangements for this care.

Ask whether the patient takes any drugs that affect blood clotting, such as aspirin, warfarin (Coumadin), clopidogrel (Plavix), and dabigatran (Pradaxa). Communicate this information to the surgeon because, for some patients, these drugs may need to be discontinued before cataract surgery.

A series of ophthalmic drugs are instilled just before surgery to dilate the pupils and cause vasoconstriction. Other eyedrops are instilled to induce paralysis to prevent lens movement. When the patient is in the surgical area, a local anesthetic is injected into the muscle cone behind the eye for anesthesia and eye paralysis.

Operative Procedures. The lens is extracted by *phacoemulsification* (Fig. 47-6), in which a probe is inserted through the capsule and high-frequency sound waves break the lens into small pieces, which are then removed by suction. The replacement intraocular lens (IOL) is placed inside the capsule to be positioned so that light rays are focused in the retina. The IOL is a small, clear, plastic lens. Different types are available, and one is selected by the surgeon and patient to allow correction of a specific refractive error. Some patients have distant vision restored to 20/20 and may need glasses only for reading or close work. Some replacement lenses have multiple focal planes and may correct vision to the extent that glasses or contact lenses may not be needed.

Postoperative Care. Immediately after surgery, antibiotic and steroid ointments are instilled. The patient usually is discharged within an hour after surgery. Instruct him or her to wear dark glasses outdoors or in brightly lit environments until the pupil responds to light. Teach the patient and family members how to instill the prescribed eyedrops. (See Chart 46-2 in Chapter 46.) Work with them in creating a written schedule for the timing and the order of eyedrops administration. Stress the importance of keeping all follow-up appointments.

Remind the patient that mild eye itching is normal, as is a "bloodshot appearance." The eyelid may be slightly swollen. However, significant swelling or bruising is abnormal. Cool compresses may be beneficial. Discomfort at the site is controlled with acetaminophen (Abenol ♣, Tylenol) or acetaminophen with oxycodone (Endocet ♣, Percocet, Tylox). Aspirin is avoided because of its effects on blood clotting.

Pain early after surgery may indicate increased intraocular pressure (IOP) or hemorrhage. Instruct patients to contact the surgeon if pain occurs with nausea or vomiting.

To prevent increases in IOP, teach the patient and family about activity restrictions. Activities that can cause a sudden rise in IOP are listed in Table 47-1.

INFECTION is a potential and serious complication. Teach the patient and family to observe for increasing eye redness, a decrease in vision, or an increase in tears and photophobia. Creamy white, dry, crusty drainage on the eyelids and lashes is normal. However, yellow or green drainage indicates infection and must be reported.

Patients experience a dramatic improvement in vision within a day of surgery. Remind them that final best vision will not occur until 4 to 6 weeks after surgery.

! NURSING SAFETY PRIORITY (QSEN)

Action Alert

> Instruct the patient who has had cataract surgery to immediately report any reduction of vision after surgery in the eye that had the cataract removed.

Community-Based Care

The patient is usually discharged within an hour after cataract surgery. Nursing interventions focus on helping the patient and family plan the eyedrop schedule and daily home eye examination.

Home Care Management. If the patient has difficulty instilling eyedrops, a supportive neighbor, friend, or family member can be taught the procedure. Adaptive equipment that positions the bottle of eyedrops directly over the eye can also be purchased (Fig. 47-7).

Self-Management Education. The best outcome of cataract removal requires close adherence to the eyedrop regimen after surgery. Providing the patient or family with accurate information and demonstration of needed skills are nursing priorities. Before discharge, review these indications of complications after cataract surgery with the patient and family:
- Sharp, sudden pain in the eye
- Bleeding or increased discharge
- Green or yellow, thick drainage
- Lid swelling
- Reappearance of a bloodshot sclera after the initial appearance has cleared

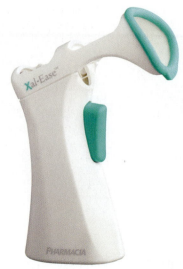

FIG. 47-7 The Ableware automatic eyedrop guide for self-administering eyedrops.

CHART 47-4   Focused Assessment

The Patient After Cataract Surgery

Assess the eye and vision:
- Visual acuity in both eyes using a handheld eye chart
- Visual fields of both eyes
- Compare operative eye with nonoperative eye for presence or absence of:
  - Redness
  - Tearing
  - Drainage

Ask the patient about:
- Pain in or around the operative eye
- Any change in vision (decreased or improved) in the operative eye
- Whether any of these has been noticed in the operative eye:
  - Dark spots
  - Increase in the number of floaters
  - Bright flashes of light

Assess the home environment for:
- Safety hazards (especially tripping and falling hazards)
- Level of room lighting

Assess patient adherence with and understanding of treatment and limitations, such as:
- Manifestations to report
- Drug regimen
- Activity restrictions
- Ability to perform ADLs

- Decreased vision
- Flashes of light or floating shapes

Remind the patient to avoid activities that might increase IOP (see Table 47-1). Some patients are prescribed to wear a light eye patch at night to prevent accidental rubbing. Instruct the patient to avoid getting water in the eye for 3 to 7 days after surgery.

Teach the patient about activity restrictions. Cooking and light housekeeping are permitted, but vacuuming should be avoided for several weeks because of the forward flexion involved and the rapid, jerky movements required. Advise him or her to refrain from driving until vision is not blurry. Chart 47-4 lists items to cover in the focused assessment of a patient at home after cataract surgery.

Health Care Resources. If the patient lives alone and has no support, arrange for a home care nurse to assess him or her and the home situation. If the patient is unable to instill eyedrops independently, a friend, neighbor, or family member can be taught this technique.

◆ *Evaluation: Outcomes*

Evaluate the care of the patient with cataracts on the basis of improving visual SENSORY PERCEPTION. The expected outcomes include that the patient after cataract surgery will:

- Have improved visual sensory perception
- Recognize manifestations of complications

Specific indicators for these outcomes are listed under the Planning and Implementation section (see earlier).

💡 NCLEX EXAMINATION CHALLENGE

Health Promotion and Maintenance

The client who had cataract surgery with a lens implant 1 week ago remarks to the home care nurse that after his daughter left to go to her home in another state yesterday, he combined all of his prescribed eyedrops together in one container so he had fewer drops to administer. What is the nurse's best response?

A. "This is not a good idea because not all of the drugs are on the same schedule."

B. "That is a good idea; just remember to not touch the dropper to your eye when giving yourself the drops."

C. "Call your surgeon immediately and get new prescriptions because together these drugs can lower your blood pressure."

D. "Call your surgeon immediately and get new prescriptions to use one at a time because these drugs cannot be mixed together."

GLAUCOMA

❖ *PATHOPHYSIOLOGY*

Glaucoma is a group of eye disorders resulting in increased IOP (intraocular pressure). As described in Chapter 46, the eye is a hollow organ. For proper eye function, the gel in the posterior segment (vitreous humor) and the fluid in the anterior segment (aqueous humor) must be present in set amounts that apply pressure inside the eye to keep it ball-shaped.

In adults the volume of the vitreous humor does not change. The aqueous humor, however, is continuously made from blood plasma by the ciliary bodies located behind the iris and just in front of the lens (see Fig. 46-2 in Chapter 46). The fluid flows through the pupil into the bulging area in front of the iris. At the outer edges of the iris beneath the cornea, blood vessels collect fluid and return it to the blood. Usually about 1 mL of aqueous humor is always present, but it is continuously made and reabsorbed at a rate of about 5 mL daily. *A normal IOP requires a balance between production and outflow of aqueous humor (McCance et al., 2014). If the IOP becomes too high, the extra pressure compresses retinal blood vessels and photoreceptors and their synapsing nerve fibers. This compression results in poorly oxygenated photoreceptors and nerve fibers. These sensitive nerve tissues become ischemic and die. When too many have died, vision is lost permanently.* Tissue damage starts in the periphery and moves inward toward the fovea centralis. Untreated, glaucoma can lead to complete loss of visual SENSORY PERCEPTION. Glaucoma is usually painless, and the patient may be unaware of gradual vision reduction.

TABLE 47-3	Common Causes of Glaucoma

Primary Glaucoma	**Secondary Glaucoma**
• Aging	• Uveitis
• Heredity	• Iritis
• Central retinal vein occlusion	• Neovascular disorders
	• Trauma
Associated Glaucoma	• Ocular tumors
• Diabetes mellitus	• Degenerative disease
• Hypertension	• Eye surgery
• Severe myopia	
• Retinal detachment	

There are several causes and types of glaucoma (Table 47-3), classified as primary, secondary, or associated. The most common type is primary glaucoma.

Primary open-angle glaucoma (POAG), the most common form of primary glaucoma, usually affects both eyes and has no manifestations in the early stages. Outflow of aqueous humor through the chamber angle is reduced. Because the fluid cannot leave the eye at the same rate it is produced, IOP gradually increases. **Primary angle-closure glaucoma** (PACG or *acute glaucoma*) has a sudden onset and is an emergency. The problem is a forward displacement of the iris, which presses against the cornea and closes the chamber angle, suddenly preventing outflow of aqueous humor.

Glaucoma is a common cause of blindness in North America. It is usually age-related, occurring in about 3.5 million people in North America (National Eye Institute, 2012).

❖ *PATIENT-CENTERED COLLABORATIVE CARE*

Primary open-angle glaucoma (POAG) develops slowly, with gradual loss of visual fields that may go unnoticed because central vision at first is unaffected. At times, vision is foggy and the patient has mild eye aching or headaches. Late manifestations occur after irreversible damage to optic nerve function and include seeing halos around lights, losing peripheral vision, and having decreased visual SENSORY PERCEPTION that does not improve with eyeglasses. The Concept Map on p. 986 addresses collaborative care issues for patients with glaucoma.

◆ *Assessment*

Physical Assessment/Clinical Manifestations. Ophthalmoscopic examination shows cupping and atrophy of the optic disc. It becomes wider and deeper and turns white or gray. In POAG the visual fields first show a small loss of peripheral vision that gradually progresses to a larger loss.

Manifestations of acute angle-closure glaucoma include a sudden, severe pain around the eyes that radiates over the face. Headache or brow pain, nausea, and vomiting may occur. Other manifestations include seeing colored halos around lights and sudden blurred vision with decreased light perception. The sclera may appear reddened and the cornea foggy. Ophthalmoscopic examination reveals a shallow anterior chamber, cloudy aqueous humor, and a moderately dilated, nonreactive pupil.

Diagnostic Assessment. An elevated intraocular pressure (IOP) is measured by tonometry. In open-angle glaucoma, the tonometry reading is between 22 and 32 mm Hg (normal is 10 to 21 mm Hg). In angle-closure glaucoma, the tonometry reading may be 30 mm Hg or higher. Visual field testing by

CONCEPT MAP

SENSORY PERCEPTION

PRIMARY OPEN-ANGLE GLAUCOMA (POAG)

INFECTION

Concept Map by Deanne A. Blach, MSN, RN

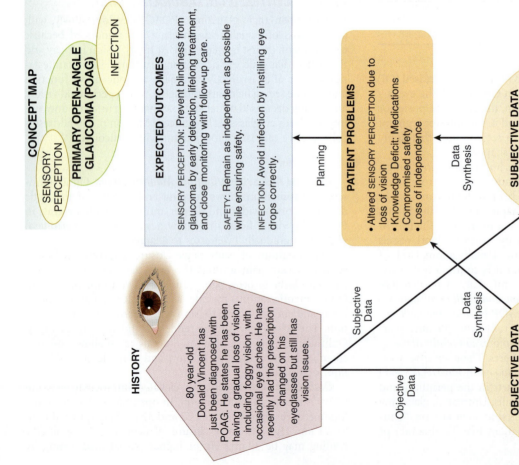

HISTORY

80 year-old Donald Vincent has just been diagnosed with POAG. He states he has been having a gradual loss of vision, including foggy vision, with occasional eye aches. He has recently had the prescription changed on his eyeglasses but still has vision issues.

OBJECTIVE DATA

- PERRL with reduced accommodation
- Tonometry reading – 28 mm Hg (N = 10-21 mm Hg)
- Cupping and atrophy of the optic disk noted
- Peripheral vision decreased
- Patient instills 1 drop of travoprost ophthalmic solution (Travatan) 0.004% to the left eye daily

SUBJECTIVE DATA

"Everything is a little bit deteriorated. I have a little double vision sometimes. I can't read very much, that's why I like to watch the news on TV. I can't see far away, I just see a figure walking, not the facial features. I have to use a magnifying glass to read the label on the eyedrop bottle."

Objective Data

Subjective Data

Data Synthesis

Data Synthesis

PATIENT PROBLEMS

- Altered sensory perception due to loss of vision
- Knowledge Deficit: Medications
- Compromised safety
- Loss of independence

Planning

EXPECTED OUTCOMES

SENSORY PERCEPTION: Prevent blindness from glaucoma by early detection, lifelong treatment, and close monitoring with follow-up care.

SAFETY: Remain as independent as possible while ensuring safety.

INFECTION: Avoid infection by instilling eye drops correctly.

INTERVENTIONS

1. Physical Assessment/Clinical Manifestations

Perform an eye exam; glaucoma will show cupping and atrophy of the optic disc. *Measures visual fields to determine the extent of peripheral vision loss (SENSORY PERCEPTION).*

2. Medication Administration

- Demonstrate how to apply eyedrops and evaluate the patient's ability to self-administer. If needed, suggest adaptive equipment that positions the bottle directly over the eye. *Provides psychomotor demonstration for verifying the skill is done correctly. Adaptive equipment used for SENSORY PERCEPTION loss.*
- Teach the patient that most eye medications initially cause tearing and mild burning with blurred vision; the sclera may become red and itchy. *Helps the patient understand these are expected effects and not to be alarmed.*
- Emphasize instilling eyedrops on time, not skipping doses, and when more than one drug is required, wait 5-10 minutes between drops. *Reinforces verbal and written instructions; prevents one drug from "washing out" or diluting the other.*

3. Nursing Safety Priority: Drug Alert!

Teach the correct technique to instill eyedrops (punctal occlusion). *Prevents drugs for glaucoma from being systemically absorbed, causing serious side effects.*

4. Providing Safe and Effective Care

Teach principles of infection control (e.g., hand hygiene), and teach the patient not to touch the tip of the eyedrop container to any part of the eye. *Protects the patient from transmission of INFECTION.*

5. Blindness Prevention Strategy

Encourage the patient to keep follow-up appointments to monitor intraocular pressure (IOP). *Monitors IOP; if it becomes too high, the extra pressure can cause sensitive nerve tissues to become ischemic and die, leading to permanent blindness.*

6. Travoprost (Travatan) Side Effects

Teach the patient to report emergent signs of allergy – hives, difficulty breathing, angioedema. Stop using drops and call the provider for serious side effects: redness, swelling, itching, eye pain, discharge, increased light sensitivity, visual changes, or chest pain. *Educates the patient and prevents medication complications.*

7. Psychosocial Integrity

Encourage the patient and family to express concerns about reduced vision. *Helps the patient and family to cope with fear of blindness and anxiety about loss of independence.*

8. Health Promotion and Maintenance

Teach the patient and family how to alter the home for patient safety. *Minimizes patient risk of injury from lack of vision.*

perimetry is performed, as is visualization by gonioscopy to determine whether the angle is open or closed. Usually the optic nerve is imaged to determine to what degree nerve damage is present. All of these diagnostic assessment techniques are described in Chapter 46.

◆ Interventions

Nonsurgical Management. Loss of visual SENSORY PERCEPTION from glaucoma can be prevented by early detection, lifelong treatment, and close monitoring. Use of ophthalmic drugs that reduce ocular pressure delays or prevents damage. Chart 47-5 lists ways to assist the patient with reduced vision to remain as independent as possible.

Drug therapy for glaucoma works to reduce IOP in several ways. Eyedrop drugs can reduce the production, increase the absorption of aqueous humor, or constrict the pupil so that the ciliary muscle is contracted, allowing better circulation of the aqueous humor to the site of absorption. *These drugs do not improve lost vision but prevent more damage by decreasing IOP.* The prostaglandins agonists drugs reduce IOP by dilating blood vessels in the trabecular mesh, which then collects and drains aqueous humor at a faster rate. The adrenergic agonists and beta-adrenergic blockers reduce IOP by limiting the production of aqueous humor and by dilating the pupil, which improves the flow of the fluid to its absorption site. Cholinergic agonists reduce IOP by limiting the production of aqueous humor and by making more room between the iris and the lens, which improves fluid outflow. Carbonic anhydrase inhibitors directly and strongly inhibit production of aqueous humor. They do not affect the flow or the absorption of the fluid. Most eyedrops cause tearing, mild burning, blurred vision, and a reddened sclera for a few minutes after instilling the drug. Specific nursing interventions are listed in Chart 47-6.

The priority nursing intervention for the patient on drug therapy for glaucoma is teaching. The benefit of drug therapy occurs only when the drugs are used on the prescribed schedule, usually every 12 hours. Teach patients the importance of instilling the drops on time and not skipping doses. When more than one drug is prescribed, teach him or her to wait 5 to 10 minutes between drug instillations to prevent one drug from "washing out" or diluting another drug. Stress the need for good handwashing, keeping the eyedrop container tip clean, and avoiding touching the tip to any part of the eye. Also teach the technique of punctal occlusion (placing pressure on the corner of the eye near the nose) immediately after eyedrop instillation to prevent systemic absorption of the drug (Fig. 47-8).

CHART 47-5 Nursing Focus on the Older Adult

Promote Independent Living in Patients with Impaired Vision

Drugs

- Having a neighbor, relative, friend, or visiting nurse visit once a week to measure the proper drugs for each day may be helpful.
  - If the patient is to take drugs more than once each day, it is helpful to use a container of a different shape (with a lid) each time. For example, if the patient is to take drugs at 9 AM, 1 PM, and 9 PM, the 9 AM drugs would be placed in a round container, the 1 PM drugs in a square container, and the 9 PM drugs in a triangular container.
  - It is helpful to place each day's drug containers in a separate box with raised letters on the side of the box spelling out the day.
- "Talking clocks" are available for the patient with low vision.
- Some drug boxes have alarms that can be set for different times.

Communication

- Telephones with large, raised block numbers may be helpful. The best models are those with black numbers on a white phone or white numbers on a black phone.
- Telephones that have a programmable automatic dialing feature ("speed dial") are very helpful. Programmed numbers should include those for the fire department, police, relatives, friends, neighbors, and 911.

Safety

- It is best to leave furniture the way the patient wants it and not move it.
- Throw rugs are best eliminated.
- Appliance cords should be short and kept out of walkways.
- Lounge-style chairs with built-in footrests are preferable to footstools.
- Nonbreakable dishes, cups, and glasses are preferable to breakable ones.
- Cleansers and other toxic agents should be labeled with large, raised letters.
- Hook-and-loop (Velcro) strips at hand level may help mark the locations of switches and electrical outlets.

Food Preparation

- Meals on Wheels is a service that many older adults find helpful. This service brings meals at mealtime, cooked and ready to eat.

The cost of this service varies, depending on the patient's ability to pay.
- Many grocery stores offer a "shop by telephone" service. The patient can either complete a computer booklet indicating types, amounts, and brands of items desired, or the store will complete this booklet over the telephone by asking the patient specific information. The store then delivers groceries to the patient's door (many stores also offer a "put away" service) and charges the patient's bank card.
- A microwave oven is a safer means of cooking than a standard stove, although many older patients are afraid of microwave ovens. If the patient has and will use a microwave oven, others can prepare meals ahead of time, label them, and freeze them for later use. Also, many microwavable complete frozen dinners that comply with a variety of dietary restrictions are available.
- Friends or relatives may be able to help with food preparation. Often relatives do not know what to give an older person for birthdays or other gift-giving occasions. One suggestion is a homemade prepackaged frozen dinner that the patient enjoys.

Personal Care

- Handgrips should be installed in bathrooms.
- The tub floor should have a nonskid surface.
- Male patients should use an electric shaver rather than a razor.
- Choosing a hairstyle that is becoming but easy to care for (avoiding parts) helps in independent living.
- Home hair care services may be available.

Diversional Activity

- Some patients can read large-print books, newspapers, and magazines (available through local libraries and vision services).
- Books, magazines, and some newspapers are available on audiotapes or discs.
- Patients experienced in knitting or crocheting may be able to create items fashioned from straight pieces, such as afghans.
- Card games, dominoes, and some board games that are available in large, high-contrast print may be helpful for patients with low vision.

CHART 47-6 Common Examples of Drug Therapy (Eyedrops)

Glaucoma

CATEGORY/DRUG	NURSING IMPLICATIONS	RATIONALES
Prostaglandins Agonists Bimatoprost (Lumigan) Latanoprost (Xalatan) Tafluprost (Zioptan) Travoprost (Travatan) Unoprostone (Rescula)	Teach the patient to check the cornea for abrasions or trauma. Remind the patient that, over time, the eye color darkens and eyelashes elongate in the eye receiving the drug. If only one eye is to be treated, teach the patient *not* to place drops in the other eye to try to make the eye colors similar. Warn the patient that using more drops than prescribed reduces drug effectiveness.	Drugs should not be used when the cornea is not intact. Knowing the side effects in advance reassures the patient that their presence is expected and normal. Using the drug in an eye with normal IOP can cause a *lower*-than-normal IOP, which reduces vision. Drug action is based on blocking receptors, which can increase in number when the drug is overused.
Adrenergic Agonists Apraclonidine (Iopidine) Brimonidine tartrate (Alphagan) Dipivefrin hydrochloride (Propine)	Ask whether the patient is taking any antidepressants from the MAO inhibitor class, such as phenelzine (Nardil) or tranylcypromine (Parnate). Teach the patient to wear dark glasses outdoors and also indoors when lighting is bright. Teach the patient not to use the eyedrops with contact lenses in place and to wait 15 minutes after using the drug to put in the lenses.	These enzyme inhibitors increase blood pressure as do the adrenergic agonists. When taken together, the patient may experience hypertensive crisis. The pupil dilates (mydriasis) and remains dilated, even when there is plenty of light, causing discomfort. These drugs are absorbed by the contact lens, which can become discolored or cloudy.
Beta-Adrenergic Blockers Betaxolol hydrochloride (Betoptic) Carteolol (Cartrol, Ocupress) Levobunolol (Betagan) Timolol (Betimol, Istalol, Timoptic) Timoptic GFS (gel-forming solution) (Timoptic-XE, Timolol-GFS)	Ask whether the patient has moderate to severe asthma or COPD. Warn diabetic patients to check their blood glucose levels more often when taking these drugs. Teach patients who also take oral beta blockers to check their pulse at least twice per day and to notify the health care provider if the pulse is consistently below 58 beats per minute.	If these drugs are absorbed systemically, they constrict pulmonary smooth muscle and narrow airways. These drugs induce hypoglycemia and also mask the hypoglycemic symptoms. These drugs potentiate the effects of systemic beta blockers and can cause an unsafe drop in heart rate and blood pressure.
Cholinergic Agonists Carbachol (Carboptic, Isopto Carbachol, Miostat) Echothiophate (Phospholine Iodide) Pilocarpine (Adsorbocarpine, Akarpine, Isopto Carpine, Ocu-Carpine, Ocusert, Piloptic, Pilostat)	Teach the patient not to use more eyedrops than are prescribed and to report increased salivation or drooling to the health care provider. Teach the patient to use good light when reading and to take care in darker rooms.	These drugs are readily absorbed by conjunctival mucous membranes and can cause systemic side effects of headache, flushing, increased saliva, and sweating. The pupil of the eye will not open more to let in more light, and it may be harder to see objects in dim light. This problem can increase the risk for falls.
Carbonic Anhydrase Inhibitors Brinzolamide (Azopt) Dorzolamide (Trusopt)	Ask whether the patient has an allergy to sulfonamide antibacterial drugs. Teach the patient to shake the drug before applying. Teach the patient not to use the eyedrops with contact lenses in place and to wait 15 minutes after using the drug to put in the lenses.	Drugs are similar to the sulfonamides, and if a patient is allergic to the sulfonamides, an allergy is likely with these drugs, even as eyedrops. Drug separates on standing. These drugs are absorbed by the contact lens, which can become discolored or cloudy.
Combination Drugs Brimonidine tartrate and timolol maleate (Combigan) Latanoprost and timolol (Xalcom)	Same as for each drug alone.	Same as for each drug alone.

COPD, Chronic obstructive pulmonary disease; *IOP*, intraocular pressure; *MAO*, monamine oxidase.

❗ NURSING SAFETY PRIORITY (QSEN)

Drug Alert

Most eyedrops used for glaucoma therapy can be absorbed systemically and cause systemic problems. It is critical to teach punctal occlusion to patients using eyedrops for glaucoma therapy.

Systemic osmotic drugs may be given for angle-closure glaucoma to rapidly reduce IOP. These agents include oral glycerin and IV mannitol (Osmitrol).

Surgical Management. Surgery is used when drugs for open-angle glaucoma are not effective at controlling IOP. Two common procedures are laser trabeculoplasty and trabeculectomy. A *laser trabeculoplasty* burns the trabecular meshwork, scarring it and causing the meshwork fibers to tighten. Tight fibers increase the size of the spaces between the fibers, improving outflow of aqueous humor and reducing IOP. *Trabeculectomy* is a surgical procedure that creates a new channel for fluid outflow. Both are ambulatory surgery procedures.

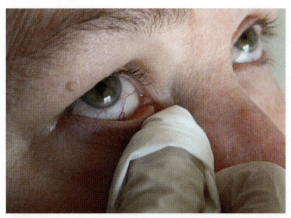

FIG. 47-8 Applying punctal occlusion to prevent systemic absorption of eyedrops.

If glaucoma fails to respond to common approaches, an implanted shunt procedure may be used. A small tube or filament is connected to a flat plate that is positioned on the outside of the eye in the eye orbit. (The plate is not visible on the front part of the eye.) The open part of the fine tube is placed into the front chamber of the eye. The fluid then drains through or around the tube into the area around the flat plate where it collects and is reabsorbed into the bloodstream. Potential complications of glaucoma surgery include choroidal hemorrhage and choroidal detachment.

❓ NCLEX EXAMINATION CHALLENGE

Safe and Effective Care Environment

Which assessment is most important for the nurse to perform before instilling travoprost (Travatan) into the client's eye?
A. Measuring the client's blood pressure
B. Measuring the client's intraocular pressure
C. Checking the cornea for abrasions or open areas
D. Assessing heart rate and rhythm for 1 full minute

RETINAL DISORDERS

MACULAR DEGENERATION
❖ PATHOPHYSIOLOGY

Macular degeneration is the deterioration of the macula (the area of central vision) and can be age-related or exudative. Age-related macular degeneration (AMD) has two types. The most common type is *dry* AMD, caused by gradual blockage of retinal capillaries, allowing retinal cells in the macula to become ischemic and necrotic. Central vision declines, and patients describe mild blurring and distortion at first. Eventually the person loses all central vision. About 2.5 million older adults in the United States and Canada have dry AMD (National Eye Institute, 2012). This loss of visual SENSORY PERCEPTION affects independence, well-being, and quality of life. It is often the reason an older adult leaves his or her independent living environment and moves into an assisted-living facility (Touhy & Jett, 2014).

Dry AMD is more common and progresses at a faster rate among smokers than among nonsmokers. Other risk factors

include hypertension, female gender, short stature, family history, and a long-term diet poor in carotene and vitamin E.

Another cause of AMD is the growth of new blood vessels in the macula, which have thin walls and leak blood and fluid (*wet* AMD). Exudative macular degeneration is also a type of wet macular degeneration but can occur at any age. The condition can occur in only one eye or in both eyes. The person with dry AMD can also develop exudative macular degeneration. Patients with exudative degeneration have a sudden decrease in vision after a detachment of pigment epithelium in the macula. Newly formed blood vessels invade this injured area and cause fluid and blood to collect under the macula (like a blister), with scar formation and visual distortion.

❖ PATIENT-CENTERED COLLABORATIVE CARE

Dry AMD has no cure. Management is focused on slowing the progression of the vision loss and helping the patient maximize remaining vision (Kerr, 2013). The risk for dry AMD can be reduced by increasing long-term dietary intake of antioxidants, vitamin B_{12}, and the carotenoids *lutein* and *zeaxanthin*. The same dietary therapy slows the progression of dry AMD.

Central vision loss reduces the ability to read, write, recognize safety hazards, and drive. Suggest alternatives (e.g., large-print books, public transportation) and referrals to community resources that provide adaptive equipment. See pp. 992-994 of Patient-Centered Collaborative Care in the Reduced Visual Sensory Perception section for discussion of patient care needs.

Management of patients with exudative or wet AMD is geared toward slowing the process and identifying further changes in visual perception. Fluid and blood may resorb in some patients. Laser therapy to seal the leaking blood vessels can limit the extent of the damage. Ocular injections with the vascular endothelial growth factor inhibitors (VEGFIs), such as bevacizumab (Avastin) or ranibizumab (Lucentis), can improve vision for the patient with wet AMD.

❓ NCLEX EXAMINATION CHALLENGE

Health Promotion and Maintenance

Which precaution is most important for the nurse to teach a 62-year-old client newly diagnosed with early-stage dry age-related macular degeneration?
A. Quit smoking
B. Quit drinking alcoholic beverages
C. Eat more dark green, red, and yellow vegetables
D. Wear dark glasses whenever he or she is outside or in bright interior lighting environments

---

RETINAL HOLES, TEARS, AND DETACHMENTS
❖ PATHOPHYSIOLOGY

A retinal hole is a break in the retina. These holes can be caused by trauma or can occur with aging. A retinal tear is a more jagged and irregularly shaped break in the retina. It can result from traction on the retina. A retinal detachment is the separation of the retina from the epithelium. Detachments are classified by the type and cause of their development.

❖ PATIENT-CENTERED COLLABORATIVE CARE

The onset of a retinal detachment is usually sudden and painless. Patients may suddenly see bright flashes of light (photopsia) or floating dark spots in the affected eye. During the initial phase of the detachment or if the detachment is partial, the patient may describe the sensation of a curtain being pulled over part of the visual field. The visual field loss corresponds to the area of detachment.

On ophthalmoscopic examination, detachments are seen as gray bulges or folds in the retina. Sometimes a hole or tear may be seen at the edge of the detachment.

If a retinal hole or tear is discovered before it causes a detachment, the defect may be closed or sealed. Closure prevents fluid from collecting under the retina and reduces the risk for a detachment. Treatment involves creating a scar that will bind the retina and choroid together around the break. Common methods to create the scar are with laser photocoagulation or with a freezing probe (cryopexy).

Spontaneous reattachment of a totally detached retina is rare. Surgical repair is needed to place the retina in contact with the underlying structures. A common repair procedure is scleral buckling.

Preoperative Care

The patient is usually anxious and fearful about a possible permanent loss of vision. *Nursing priorities include providing information and reassurance to allay fears.*

Instruct the patient to restrict activity and head movement before surgery to prevent further tearing or detachment. An eye patch is placed over the affected eye to reduce eye movement. Topical drugs are given before surgery to inhibit pupil constriction and accommodation.

Operative Procedures

The surgery is performed with the patient under general anesthesia. In scleral buckling, the ophthalmologist repairs wrinkles or folds in the retina and indents the eye surface to relieve the tugging pressure on the retina. The indentation or "buckling" is performed by placing a small piece of silicone against the outside of the sclera and holding it in place with an encircling band. This device keeps the retina in contact with the choroid for reattachment. Any fluid under the retina is drained.

A gas or silicone oil placed inside the eye can be used to promote retinal reattachment. These agents float up and against the retina to hold it in place until healing occurs.

Postoperative Care

After surgery an eye patch and shield usually are applied. Monitor the patient's vital signs, and check the eye patch and shield for any drainage.

Activity after surgery varies. If gas or oil has been placed in the eye, teach the patient to keep his or her head in the position prescribed by the surgeon to promote reattachment. Teach the patient to report any sudden increase in pain or pain occurring with nausea to the surgeon immediately. Remind the patient to avoid activities that increase intraocular pressure (IOP) (see Table 47-1).

Instruct the patient to avoid reading, writing, and close work, such as sewing, in the first week after surgery because these activities cause rapid eye movements and detachment. Teach him or her the manifestations of INFECTION and detachment (sudden reduced visual acuity, eye pain, pupil that **does not constrict** in response to light) and to notify the surgeon immediately if these manifestations occur.

CLINICAL JUDGMENT CHALLENGE

Safety; Patient-Centered Care QSEN

The patient is a 68-year-old retired college professor who was recently widowed. He lives alone with a cat. His main leisurely activities are reading, using the computer, and listening to classical music. While hiking with a friend, he pulled himself along a rope bridge, assuming a variety of positions. At the far end of the bridge, he stood up and noticed that the vision in his right eye was greatly reduced to the extent that he could see only the bottom half of the visual field. His friend insisted that the patient go immediately to the emergency department. Once there, a large partial retinal detachment is diagnosed. It is treated within the hour with laser therapy and the injection of a gas to the affected eye. He is permitted to go home and instructed to sit upright with his head bent slightly downward for the next 24 hours and then to return to the ophthalmology office. He tells you that he really likes wine and sometimes drinks as much as two bottles in an evening.

1. Should he drive himself home? Why or why not?
2. Is drinking permitted at this time? Why or why not?
3. What will you tell him about a sleeping position?
4. What suggestions and precautions do you have for him about caring for the cat?
5. Which of the leisure-time activities can he perform this evening and which ones should he avoid? Provide a rationale for your choices.

RETINITIS PIGMENTOSA

Several types of retinal disorders can cause progressive degeneration of the retina and lead to loss of visual SENSORY PERCEPTION. Retinitis pigmentosa (RP) is a condition in which retinal nerve cells degenerate and the pigmented cells of the retina grow and move into the sensory areas of the retina, causing further degeneration.

GENETIC/GENOMIC CONSIDERATIONS

Patient-Centered Care QSEN

Different forms of retinitis pigmentosa can be inherited as an autosomal dominant (AD) trait, an autosomal recessive (AR) trait, or an X-linked recessive trait (Online Mendelian Inheritance in Man [OMIM], 2014). Mutations in more than 20 genes have been identified as being responsible for retinitis pigmentosa, and gene testing for more than 800 mutations of the AR and AD forms of the problem is commercially available.

The earliest manifestation of RP is night blindness, often occurring in childhood. Over time, decreased acuity progresses to total blindness. Examination of the retina shows heavy pigmentation in a lacy pattern. Cataracts may accompany this disorder.

No current therapy is effective in preventing the degenerative process. Management strategies focus on protecting active retinal cells and slowing the progression of disease. Teach patients with RP to avoid drugs that are known to adversely affect retinal cells, such as isotretinoin (Accutane) and drugs for erectile dysfunction (e.g., sildenafil [Viagra]). Also remind them to wear eyeglasses that provide ultraviolet protection. The ingestion of 15,000 international units of vitamin A daily is recommended to slow the progression of the disorder, as is the daily ingestion of docosahexaenoic acid (DHA), an omega-3 fatty acid and antioxidant. Additional supplements that may slow the progression of RP include beta carotene, lutein, and zeaxanthin. When macular edema is present, oral acetazolamide (Diamox) can reduce the edema. Cataract surgery and lens replacement is recommended when cataracts further reduce vision. Other treatments under investigation include retinal transplantation, stem cell therapy, and gene therapy (Foundation Fighting Blindness, 2012).

REFRACTIVE ERRORS

❖ PATHOPHYSIOLOGY

The ability of the eye to focus images on the retina depends on the length of the eye from front to back and the refractive power of the lens system. Refraction is the bending of light rays. Problems in either eye length or refraction can result in refractive errors.

Myopia is nearsightedness, in which the eye over-refracts the light and the bent images fall in front of, not on, the retina. Hyperopia, also called *hypermetropia,* is farsightedness, in which refraction is too weak, causing images to be focused behind the retina. Presbyopia is the age-related problem in which the lens loses its elasticity and is less able to change shape to focus the eye for close work. As a result, images fall behind the retina. This problem usually begins in people in their 30s and 40s. Astigmatism occurs when the curve of the cornea is uneven. Because light rays are not refracted equally in all directions, the image does not focus on the retina.

❖ PATIENT-CENTERED COLLABORATIVE CARE

Refractive errors are diagnosed through a process known as refraction. The patient is asked to view an eye chart while lenses of different strengths are systematically placed in front of the eye. With each lens strength, he or she is asked whether the lenses sharpen or worsen vision. The strength of the lens needed to focus the image on the retina is expressed in measurements called *diopters.*

Nonsurgical Management

Refractive errors are corrected with eyeglass lenses or contact lenses that focus light rays on the retina (see Fig. 46-5 in Chapter 46). Hyperopic vision is corrected with a convex lens that moves the image forward. Myopic vision is corrected with a biconcave lens to move the image back to the retina.

Surgical Management

Surgery can correct some refractive errors and enhance vision. The most common vision-enhancing surgery is laser in-situ keratomileusis (LASIK). This procedure can correct nearsightedness, farsightedness, and astigmatism. The superficial layers of the cornea are lifted temporarily as a flap, and powerful laser pulses reshape the deeper corneal layers. After reshaping is complete, the corneal flap is placed back into its original position.

Usually both eyes are treated at the same time, which is convenient for the patient, although this practice has some risks. Many patients have improved vision within an hour after surgery, and complete healing to best vision takes up to 4 weeks. The outer corneal layer is not damaged, and pain is minimal.

Complications of LASIK include INFECTION, corneal clouding, chronic dry eyes, and refractive errors. Some patients have developed blurred vision, halos around lights, and other refractive errors months to years after this surgery as a result of excessive laser-thinning of the cornea. The cornea then becomes unstable and does not refract appropriately.

Another procedure, corneal ring placement, can enhance vision for nearsightedness, although this procedure is usually performed for keratoconus. For more information about the procedure, see surgical intervention for keratoconus on pp. 981-982.

TRAUMA

Trauma to the eye or orbital area can result from almost any activity. Care varies depending on the area of the eye affected and whether the globe of the eye has been penetrated.

Foreign Bodies

Eyelashes, dust, dirt, and airborne particles can come in contact with the conjunctiva or cornea and irritate or abrade the surface. If nothing is seen on the cornea or conjunctiva, the eyelid is everted to examine the conjunctivae. The patient usually has a feeling of something being in the eye and may have blurred vision. Pain occurs if the corneal surface is injured. Tearing and photophobia may be present.

Visual SENSORY PERCEPTION is assessed before treatment. The eye is examined with fluorescein, followed by irrigation with normal saline (0.9%) to gently remove the particles. Best practices for ocular irrigation are listed in Chart 47-7.

CHART 47-7 Best Practice for Patient Safety & Quality Care QSEN

Ocular Irrigation

1. Assemble equipment:
   - Normal saline IV (1000-mL bag)
   - Macrodrip IV tubing
   - IV pole
   - Eyelid speculum
   - Topical anesthetic (proparacaine hydrochloride)
   - Gloves
   - Collection receptacle (emesis basin works well)
   - Towels
   - pH paper
2. Quickly obtain a history from the patient while flushing the tubing with normal saline:
   - Nature and time of the injury
   - Type of irritant or chemical (if known)
   - Type of first aid administered at the scene
   - Any allergies to the "caine" family of medications
3. Evaluate the patient's visual acuity *before* treatment:
   - Ask the patient to read your name tag with the affected eye while covering the good eye.
   - Ask the patient to "count fingers" with the affected eye while covering the good eye.
4. Put on gloves.
5. Place a strip of pH paper in the cul-de-sac of the patient's affected eye to test the pH of the agent splashed into the eye and to know when it has been washed out.
6. Instill proparacaine hydrochloride eyedrops as prescribed.
7. Place the patient in a supine position with the head turned slightly toward the affected eye.
8. Have the patient hold the affected eye open, or position an eyelid speculum.
9. Direct the flow of normal saline across the affected eye from the nasal corner of the eye toward the outer corner of the eye.
10. Assess the patient's comfort during the procedure.
11. If both eyes are affected, irrigate them simultaneously using separate personnel and equipment.

If an eye patch is applied after the foreign body is removed, tell the patient how long the patch must be left in place. Follow-up with the ophthalmologist is needed.

Lacerations

Lacerations are caused by sharp objects and projectiles. The injury occurs most commonly to the eyelids and cornea, although any part of the eye can be lacerated.

The patient should receive medical attention as soon as possible. Initially the eye is closed and a small ice pack is applied to decrease bleeding. Minor lacerations of the eyelid can be sutured in an emergency department, an urgent care center, or an ophthalmologist's office. A microscope is needed in the operating room if the patient has a laceration that involves the eyelid margin, affects the lacrimal system, involves a large area, or has jagged edges.

Corneal lacerations are an emergency because eye contents may prolapse through the laceration. Manifestations include severe eye pain, photophobia, tearing, decreased vision, and inability to open the eyelid. If the laceration is the result of a penetrating injury, an object may be seen protruding from the eye.

> ### ! NURSING SAFETY PRIORITY (QSEN)
> #### Action Alert
> An object protruding from the eye is removed only by an ophthalmologist because it may be holding the eye structures in place. Improper removal can cause structures to prolapse out of the eye.

Antibiotics are given to reduce the risk for INFECTION. Depending on the depth of the laceration, scarring may develop. If the scar alters vision, a corneal transplant may be needed later. If the eye contents have prolapsed through the laceration or if the injury is severe, enucleation (surgical eye removal) may be indicated.

Penetrating Injuries

A penetrating eye injury often leads to permanent loss of visual SENSORY PERCEPTION. Glass, high-speed metal or wood particles, BB pellets, and bullets are common causes of penetrating injuries. The particles can enter the eye and lodge in or behind the eyeball.

The patient has eye pain and reports "I suddenly felt something hit my eye." A wound may be visible. Depending on where the object enters and rests within the eye, vision may be affected.

X-rays and CT scans of the orbit are usually performed. *MRI is contraindicated because the procedure may move any metal-containing projectile and cause more injury.*

Surgery is usually needed to remove the foreign object, and sometimes vitreal removal is needed. IV antibiotics are started before surgery, and a tetanus booster is given if necessary.

OCULAR MELANOMA

❖ PATHOPHYSIOLOGY

Melanoma is the most common malignant eye tumor in adults (American Cancer Society, 2014). This tumor occurs most often in the uveal tract among people in their 30s and 40s and is associated with exposure to ultraviolet (UV) light. Because of its rich blood supply, a melanoma can spread by extension through the sclera or invasion into nearby tissue and the brain.

❖ PATIENT-CENTERED COLLABORATIVE CARE

Manifestations of melanoma may not be readily apparent; the tumor may be discovered during a routine examination. Blurred vision may occur if the macular area is invaded. Vision is reduced if the tumor grows inward toward the center of the eye and alters the visual pathway. Increased intraocular pressure (IOP) can result if the tumor obstructs flow of aqueous humor. Iris color changes when the tumor infiltrates the iris. Sudden loss of a visual field may result from tumor invasion that causes retinal detachment.

Diagnostic tests for a melanoma depend on the size and tumor growth rate. Ultrasonography or MRI is performed to determine the tumor's location and size. Treatment depends on the tumor's size and growth rate, as well as the condition of the other eye. Small iris lesions are monitored until growth is observed. Tumors of the choroid are treated by surgical enucleation or by radiation therapy with a radioactive plaque.

Enucleation (surgical removal of the entire eyeball) is the most common surgery for ocular melanoma and is performed under general anesthesia. After the eye is removed, a ball implant is inserted as a base for the socket prosthesis, which is fitted about 1 month after surgery.

Radiation therapy is an "eye-sparing" procedure that can reduce the size and thickness of melanomas and sometimes eliminates the tumor completely. The radioactive plaque—a round, flat disk about the size of a dime and containing a radioactive material—is sutured to the sclera overlying the tumor site. The length of time the plaque remains sutured to the sclera depends on the size of the tumor and the dose of radiation to be delivered (usually 3 to 6 days).

Complications of radiation therapy include vascular changes, retinopathy, glaucoma, necrosis of the sclera, and cataract formation. Vitreous hemorrhage may develop as the tumor becomes smaller and pulls or breaks blood vessels.

While the plaque is in place, an eye patch may or may not be used. Cycloplegic eyedrops and an antibiotic-steroid combination are given. Teach the patient how to instill eyedrops.

REDUCED VISUAL SENSORY PERCEPTION

❖ PATHOPHYSIOLOGY

Different forms of reduced visual SENSORY PERCEPTION may affect color, light, image, eye movement, and acuity. Reduced vision may be temporary, such as when cataracts obscure vision but surgery has not yet been performed. Patients are legally blind if their best visual acuity with corrective lenses is 20/200 or less in the better eye or if the visual field is 20 degrees or less.

Blindness can occur in one or both eyes. When one eye is affected, the field of vision is narrowed and depth perception is impaired.

❖ PATIENT-CENTERED COLLABORATIVE CARE

Priorities for nursing involve safety and teaching the patient with reduced visual SENSORY PERCEPTION some techniques to make better use of existing vision. Moving the head slightly up and down can enhance a three-dimensional effect. When shaking hands or pouring water, the patient can line up the object and move toward it. He or she should choose a position that favors the eye with better vision. For example, people with vision in the right eye should position people and items on their right.

Nursing interventions for the patient with reduced sight focus on communication, safety, ambulation, self-care, and

CHART 47-8 Best Practice for Patient Safety & Quality Care (QSEN)

Care of the Patient with Reduced Vision

- Always knock or announce your entrance into the patient's room or area and introduce yourself.
- Ensure that all members of the health care team also use this courtesy of announcement and introduction.
- Ensure that the patient's reduced vision is noted in the medical record, is communicated to all staff, is marked on the call board, and is identified on the door of the patient's room.
- Determine to what degree the patient can see anything.
- Orient the patient to the environment, counting steps with him or her to the bathroom.
- Assist the patient in placing objects on the bedside table or in the bed and around the bed and room, and do not move them without the patient's permission.
- Remove all objects and clutter between the patient's bed and the bathroom.
- Ask the patient what type of assistance he or she prefers for grooming, toileting, eating, and ambulating, and communicate these preferences with the staff.
- Describe food placement on a plate in terms of a clock face.
- Open milk cartons; open salt, pepper, and condiment packages; and remove lids from cups and bowls.
- Unless the patient also has a hearing problem, use a normal tone of voice when speaking.
- When walking with the patient, offer him or her your arm and walk a step ahead.

support. Chart 47-8 lists ways to help patients with reduced vision to function as independently as possible.

Communication is important in helping the patient remain independent and connected to the world. Many adaptive devices are available to help the person with reduced vision maintain independence. Many cities have auditory traffic signals so that people with reduced vision can know when it is safe to cross a street. Curbs in these areas may have high-contrast color paint to let the person know when to step up or down. Libraries have large-print books and books on disc. "Talking" clocks, watches, and timers are available. Playing cards, games, restaurant menus, calendars, and instruction booklets are available in large print sizes using bold black print, sans-serif fonts, and white or yellow backgrounds (Russo & Bowden, 2013). Computer keyboards with high contrast and larger letters on the keys are available, as are large screens. Direct the patient with reduced vision to the local resources to obtain adaptive items and to learn how to use them (Warren, 2013).

Safety is a major issue for the person with reduced vision. For most patients, home is the place where they feel most safe because they are familiar with room and item location. For example, they may have counted the number of footsteps needed to move from one area to another. Stress to family members not to change item locations without input from the patient. Teach family members with vision to make these home adaptations to increase the patient's independence and safety:

- Using tape and a heavy black marker, mark the 350-degree temperature setting on the oven and mark the 70-degree temperature setting on the heating or cooling thermostat.
- Paint or mark light switches in a deep color that contrasts with the surrounding wall.
- Label canned goods with large, bold, black letters on white tape.

- Teach the patient to feel for the crease in paper milk cartons that indicates the place to open the spout.
- Differentiate different drugs by altering the shape of a bottle. Rubber bands can be wound around a bottle to change its texture. Raised symbols can be glued to caps to make identification easier.

The patient with reduced visual SENSORY PERCEPTION is most at risk for safety problems in an unfamiliar or changing environment. When he or she must be hospitalized, promote safety and independence by orienting him or her to the new environment.

Many people with reduced vision had sight at some time and have background knowledge regarding size and shape that can be used when providing information. When talking with a person who has limited vision, use a normal tone of voice unless he or she also has a hearing problem.

First orient the patient to the immediate environment, including the size of the room. Use one object in the room, such as a chair or hospital bed, as the focal point for the description. Guide the person to the focal point, and orient him or her to the environment from that point. For example, you might say "To the left of the bed is a chair." Then describe all other objects in relation to the focal point. Go with the patient to the bathroom so that he or she can learn this location. Highlight the location of the toilet, sink, and toilet paper. Use specific descriptors, and avoid gestures or vague language (Warren, 2013). For example, say "the wall to the right of the door" instead of "over there."

! NURSING SAFETY PRIORITY (QSEN)
Action Alert

Never leave the patient with reduced vision in the center of an unfamiliar room.

Patients with reduced vision prefer to establish the location of important objects, such as the call light, water pitcher, and clock. Once their location has been fixed, do not move these items without the patient's consent. Do not move the location of chairs, stools, and wastebaskets without consulting the patient.

At mealtime, set up food on the tray using clock placement. For example, "There is sliced ham at the 6 o'clock position; peas are located at the 3 o'clock position; to the right of the plate is coffee; salt and pepper are next to the coffee."

Ambulation with a patient who has reduced vision is best when he or she holds your arm at the elbow. Keep the arm close to your body so that the patient can detect your direction of movement. Alert him or her when obstacles are in the path ahead.

Patients may use a cane to detect obstacles, such as furniture, walls, or curbs. The cane is held several inches off the floor and sweeps the ground where the foot will be placed next. The laser cane sends out signals to help detect obstacles.

Self-care and the ability to control the environment are important. Knock on the door before entering the hospital room or any other environment of a patient with reduced vision. State your name and the reason for visiting when entering the room. Coordinate with other members of the health care team to ensure this etiquette is used consistently. Mark the door to the room to indicate it is occupied by a person with reduced visual SENSORY PERCEPTION.

Support is needed, especially when the reduced vision occurs suddenly and may be permanent. The reactions are similar to the reaction to loss of a body part. Allow the newly blind person a period of grieving for the "dead" (nonseeing) eye. He or she may feel hopeless and angry. The ability to cope may begin within days, but some patients mourn for months or years.

Patients benefit from the honest support that you can provide. They need to hear that it is normal to mourn, to cry, and to feel the loss. Help them move toward acceptance by encouraging the mastery of one task at a time and by providing positive reinforcement for each success.

? NCLEX EXAMINATION CHALLENGE

Safe and Effective Care Environment

Which action by a nurse is most likely to increase accurate communication with a client who has low vision?
A. Speaking slowly and loudly
B. Enhancing the talk using hand gestures
C. Being very specific with descriptions and directions
D. Marking the door of the client's room to indicate his or her vision status

NURSING CONCEPTS AND CLINICAL JUDGMENT REVIEW

What might you NOTICE if the patient is experiencing reduced visual SENSORY PERCEPTION?

Assessment:
- Patient squints or tilts the head when viewing objects or print at a distance.
- Patient closes one eye to read or see at a distance.
- Patient moves reading materials either very close to his or her face or as far away from the face as he or she can reach.
- Patient may not startle when a sudden move is made at the face.
- Pupils are unequal and may not react to light.
- Eyes do not focus on a distant object and track it as it is moved closer to the face.
- Red reflex may be absent or present in only one eye.
- Patient does not make eye contact and turns head toward sounds rather than sights.
- Patient walks with hesitation into a room or bumps into objects in his or her path.
- Patient may seem confused about time and place.

What should you INTERPRET and how should you RESPOND to a patient experiencing reduced visual SENSORY PERCEPTION?

Interpret by:
- Assessing visual acuity with an eye chart, counting fingers, hand motion, or light perception
- Asking the patient to describe the objects in the room and their colors
- Asking the patient what he or she can see well and what is more difficult to see

Respond by:
- Orienting the patient to the immediate surroundings
- Offering your arm for the patient to hold when he or she is moving to a different location
- Not leaving the patient alone in the center of a strange room
- Asking him or her what assistance is needed for independent activity
- Assessing the immediate environment for safety hazards and removing the hazard

On what should you REFLECT?
- Consider what environmental changes could make the unit safer or more manageable for a person with reduced vision.

GET READY FOR THE NCLEX® EXAMINATION!

KEY POINTS

Review these Key Points for each NCLEX Examination Client Needs Category.

Safe and Effective Care Environment
- Use aseptic technique when performing an eye examination or instilling drugs into the eye. **Safety** QSEN
- Apply the principles of INFECTION control when caring for a patient with an eye infection. **Safety** QSEN
- Avoid performing an ophthalmoscopic examination on a confused patient. **Safety** QSEN
- Orient the patient with reduced vision to his or her immediate surroundings, including how to call for help and where the bathroom is located. **Safety** QSEN
- Identify the room of a patient with reduced vision. **Safety** QSEN
- Never administer a topical ophthalmic liquid or ointment by the oral route. **Safety** QSEN

Health Promotion and Maintenance
- Identify people at risk for visual SENSORY PERCEPTION problems as a result of work environment or leisure activities, and teach them specific ways to protect the eyes. **Patient-Centered Care** QSEN
- Encourage all patients to wear eye protection when they are performing yard work, are working in a woodshop or metal shop, are using chemicals, or are in any environment in which drops or particulate matter is airborne.
- Encourage all adult patients older than 40 years and those with chronic disorders that affect the eye and vision to have an eye examination with measurement of intraocular pressure every year. **Patient-Centered Care** QSEN
- Encourage everyone to use polarizing sunglasses whenever outdoors in the daytime. **Patient-Centered Care** QSEN
- Teach all patients to wash their hands before and after touching the eyes. **Patient-Centered Care** QSEN

- Teach family members who have good vision to make the adaptations for the patient's home listed on p. 993 to increase the patient's independence and safety. **Patient-Centered Care** QSEN

Psychosocial Integrity
- Teach patients and family members about what to expect during procedures to correct visual SENSORY PERCEPTION and eye problems.
- Provide opportunities for the patient and family to express concerns about a change in visual SENSORY PERCEPTION.
- Refer the patient with reduced visual SENSORY PERCEPTION to local services, resources, and support groups for the blind and those with low vision. **Patient-Centered Care** QSEN
- Teach the patient with reduced visual SENSORY PERCEPTION techniques for performing ADLs and self-care independently. **Patient-Centered Care** QSEN
- Use a normal tone of voice to talk with a patient who has a vision problem and normal hearing.
- Knock on the door before entering the room of a patient with reduced visual SENSORY PERCEPTION and introduce yourself. **Patient-Centered Care** QSEN

Physiological Integrity
- Ask the patient about vision problems in any other members of the family, because many vision problems have a genetic component. **Evidence-Based Practice** QSEN
- Teach patients the proper techniques for self-instillation of eyedrops and eye ointment. **Safety** QSEN

- Stress the importance of completing an antibiotic regimen for an eye INFECTION. **Evidence-Based Practice** QSEN
- When instilling more than one type of eyedrop into the same eye, wait 5 to 10 minutes (or as directed by the manufacturer) between instillations. **Evidence-Based Practice** QSEN
- Teach patients who are at risk for increased intraocular pressure (IOP) what activities to avoid (see Table 47-1). **Patient-Centered Care** QSEN
- Teach patients with an INFECTION of the eye or eyelid not to rub the eye (to avoid infecting the other eye). **Evidence-Based Practice** QSEN
- Instruct the patient who has cataract surgery to report immediately any reduction in vision after initial improvement in vision in the eye that had cataract surgery. **Patient-Centered Care** QSEN
- Stress the importance of using antiglaucoma eyedrop agents exactly as prescribed to prevent IOP from increasing and to prevent complications of glaucoma drug therapy. **Patient-Centered Care** QSEN
- Never attempt to remove any object protruding from the eye. **Safety** QSEN
- Use and teach punctal occlusion technique when administering antiglaucoma eyedrops. **Safety** QSEN
- Work with the physician, occupational therapist, social worker, and other health care professionals to increase the patient's independence and safety within the home and the community. **Teamwork and Collaboration** QSEN

Assessment and Care of Patients with Ear and Hearing Problems

M. Linda Workman

ⓔ http://evolve.elsevier.com/Iggy/

PRIORITY CONCEPTS

- SENSORY PERCEPTION

LEARNING OUTCOMES

Safe and Effective Care Environment
1. Protect the patient with ear and hearing problems from injury and infection.

Health Promotion and Maintenance
2. Teach all people how to protect the ear and hearing.
3. Teach patients who need them how to use hearing assistive devices.

Psychosocial Integrity
4. Reduce the psychological impact for the patient and family experiencing a potential change in auditory SENSORY PERCEPTION.
5. Work with other members of the health care team to ensure that the values, preferences, and expressed needs of the patient with reduced auditory SENSORY PERCEPTION are respected.

Physiological Integrity
6. Perform a focused assessment of the ear and auditory SENSORY PERCEPTION, incorporating information about anatomy and physiology, genetic risk, environmental risk, and age-related changes affecting the ear and hearing.
7. Use laboratory data and clinical manifestations to evaluate and prioritize the nursing care needs for the patient with a problem of the ear or hearing.
8. Prioritize the nursing care and educational needs of the patient with Ménière's disease.
9. Prioritize nursing care and educational needs for the patient after ear surgery.
10. Collaborate with other health care professionals to help patients and families experiencing reduced auditory SENSORY PERCEPTION achieve desired health outcomes.

Together, the ear and the brain allow auditory SENSORY PERCEPTION. Hearing is one of the five senses important for cognition and communicating with others. It is used to assess surroundings, allow independence, warn of danger, appreciate music, work, play, and interact with other people.

Ear and hearing problems are common among adults of all ages. Assessment of the ear and hearing is an important skill for nurses in any care environment. Many ear and hearing problems develop over long periods and may be affected by drugs or systemic health problems. Auditory SENSORY PERCEPTION problems reduce the ability to fully communicate with the world and can lead to confusion, mistrust, and social isolation.

ANATOMY AND PHYSIOLOGY REVIEW

Structure

The ear has three divisions: the external ear, the middle ear, and the inner ear. Each part is important to hearing.

External Ear

The external ear develops in the embryo at the same time as the kidneys and urinary tract. Thus any person with a defect of the external ear should be examined for possible problems of the kidney and urinary systems.

The *pinna* is the part of the external ear that is composed of cartilage covered by skin and attached to the head at about a 10-degree angle at the level of the eyes. The external ear extends from the pinna through the external ear canal to the *tympanic membrane* (eardrum) (Fig. 48-1). The external ear includes the *mastoid process,* which is the bony ridge located over the temporal bone behind the pinna. The ear canal is slightly S-shaped and lined with cerumen-producing glands, oil glands, and hair follicles. Cerumen (ear "wax") helps protect and lubricate the ear canal. The distance from the opening of the ear canal to the eardrum in an adult is 1 to 1½ inches (2.5 to 3.75 cm).

Middle Ear

The eardrum separates the external ear and the middle ear. The middle ear consists of a compartment called the *epitympanum.*

Located in the epitympanum are the top opening of the eustachian tube and three small bones known as the *bony ossicles,* which are the *malleus* (hammer), the *incus* (anvil), and the *stapes* (stirrup) (Fig. 48-2). The bony ossicles are joined loosely, thereby moving with vibrations created when sound waves hit the eardrum.

The eardrum is a thick sheet of tissue; is transparent, opaque, or pearly gray; and moves when air is injected into the external canal. The landmarks on the eardrum include the *annulus,* the *pars flaccida,* and the *pars tensa.* These correspond to the parts of the malleus that can be seen through the transparent eardrum. The eardrum is attached to the first bony ossicle, the malleus, at the umbo (Fig. 48-3). The umbo is seen through the eardrum membrane as a white dot and is one end of the long process of the malleus. The pars flaccida is that portion of the eardrum above the short process of the malleus. The pars tensa is that portion surrounding the long process of the malleus.

The middle ear is separated from the inner ear by the round window and the oval window. The eustachian tube begins at the floor of the middle ear and extends to the throat. The tube opening in the throat is surrounded by adenoid lymphatic tissue (Fig. 48-4). The eustachian tube allows the pressure on both sides of the eardrum to equalize. Secretions from the middle ear drain through the tube into the throat.

Inner Ear

The inner ear is on the other side of the oval window and contains the semicircular canals, the cochlea, the vestibule, and the

Right tympanic membrane

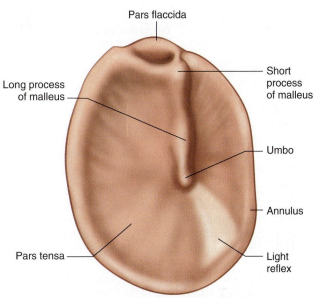

FIG. 48-3 Landmarks on the tympanic membrane.

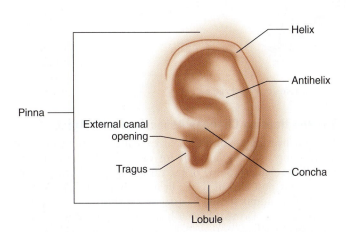

FIG. 48-1 Anatomic features of the external ear.

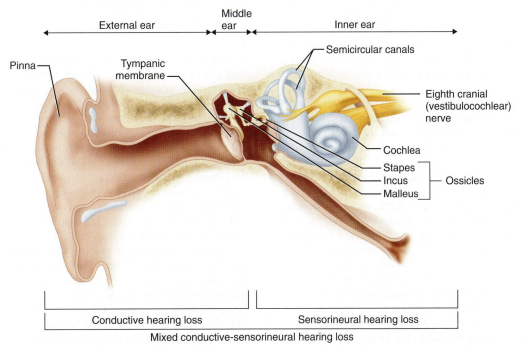

FIG. 48-2 Anatomic features of the middle and inner ear and areas involved in the three types of hearing loss.

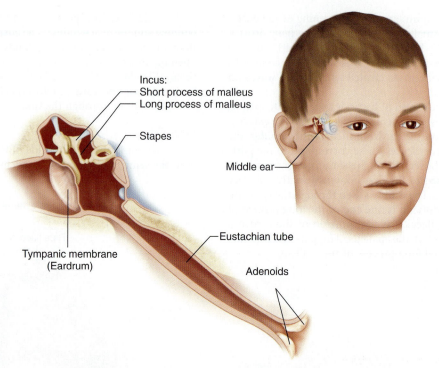

FIG. 48-4 Anatomic features and attached structures of the middle ear.

distal end of the eighth cranial nerve (see Fig. 48-2). The *semicircular canals* are tubes made of cartilage and contain fluid and hair cells. These canals are connected to the sensory nerve fibers of the vestibular portion of the eighth cranial nerve. The fluid and hair cells within the canals help maintain the sense of balance.

The *cochlea,* the spiral organ of hearing, is divided into the scala tympani, the scala media, and the scala vestibuli. The scala media is filled with *endolymph,* and the scala tympani and scala vestibuli are filled with *perilymph.* These fluids protect the cochlea and the semicircular canals by allowing these structures to "float" in the fluids and be cushioned against abrupt head movements.

The *organ of Corti* is the receptor of hearing located on the membrane of the cochlea. The cochlear hair cells detect vibration from sound and stimulate the eighth cranial nerve.

The *vestibule* is a small, oval-shaped, bony chamber between the semicircular canals and the cochlea. It contains the utricle and the saccule, organs that are important for balance.

Function

Auditory SENSORY PERCEPTION is the main function of the ear and occurs when sound is delivered through the air to the external ear canal. The sound waves strike the movable eardrum, creating vibrations. The eardrum is connected to the first bony ossicle, which allows the sound wave vibrations to be transferred from the eardrum to the malleus, the incus, and the stapes. From the stapes, the vibrations are transmitted to the cochlea. Receptors at the cochlea transduce (change) the vibrations into action potentials. The action potentials are conducted to the brain as nerve impulses by the cochlear portion of the eighth cranial (auditory) nerve. The nerve impulses are processed and interpreted as sound by the brain in the auditory cortex of the temporal lobe.

Ear and Hearing Changes Associated with Aging

Ear and hearing changes related to aging are listed in Chart 48-1, along with implications for care of older patients who have these changes. Some of the ear changes are harmless, and others may pose threats to the hearing ability of older adults.

All older adults should be screened for hearing acuity, starting by asking "Do you have a hearing problem now?" Family members may have noticed behaviors that suggest changes in a patient's hearing.

ASSESSMENT METHODS

Patient History

Hearing assessment begins while observing the patient listening to and answering questions (Jarvis, 2016). The patient's posture and responses can provide information about hearing acuity. For example, posture changes, such as tilting the head to one side or leaning forward when listening to another person speak, may indicate the presence of a hearing problem. Other indicators of hearing difficulty include frequently asking the speaker to repeat statements or frequently saying "What?" or "Huh?" Notice whether the patient responds to whispered questions and startles when an unexpected sound occurs in the environment. Also assess whether the patient's responses match the question asked. For example, when you ask the patient "How old are you?" does the patient respond with an age or does he or she say "No, I don't have a cold."

During the interview, sit in adequate light and face the patient to allow him or her to see you speak. Use short, simple language the patient is comfortable with rather than long medical terms. Obtain data on demographics, personal and family history, socioeconomic status, current health problems, and the use of remedies for ear problems.

The patient's gender is important. Some hearing disorders, such as otosclerosis, are more common in women. Other

---

CHART 48-1 Nursing Focus on the Older Adult

Age-Related Changes in the Ear and Hearing

EAR OR HEARING CHANGE	NURSING ADAPTATIONS AND ACTIONS
Pinna becomes elongated because of loss of subcutaneous tissues and decreased elasticity.	Reassure the patient that this is normal. When positioning a patient on the side, do not "fold" the ear under the head.
Hair in the canal becomes coarser and longer, especially in men.	Reassure the patient that this is normal. More frequent ear irrigation may be needed to prevent cerumen clumping.
Cerumen is drier and impacts more easily, reducing hearing function.	Teach the patient to irrigate the ear canal weekly or whenever he or she notices a change in hearing.
Tympanic membrane loses elasticity and may appear dull and retracted.	Do not use this finding as the only indication of otitis media.
Hearing acuity decreases (in some people).	Assess hearing with the voice test or the watch test. If a deficit is present, refer the patient to a specialist to determine hearing loss and appropriate intervention. Do not assume all older adults have a hearing loss!!
The ability to hear high-frequency sounds is lost first. Older adults may have particular problems hearing the *f, s, sh,* and *pa* sounds.	Provide a quiet environment when speaking (close the door to the hallway), and face the patient. If the patient wears glasses, be sure he or she is using them to enhance speech understanding. Speak slowly and in a deeper voice, and emphasize beginning word sounds. Some patients with a hearing loss that is not corrected may benefit from wearing a stethoscope while listening to you speak.

---

disorders, such as Ménière's disease, are more common in men. Age is also an important factor in hearing loss.

Personal history includes past or current manifestations of ear pain, ear discharge, **vertigo** (spinning sensation), **tinnitus** (ringing), decreased hearing, and difficulty understanding people when they talk. Ask the patient about:

- Ear trauma or surgery
- Past ear infections
- Excessive cerumen
- Ear itch
- Any invasive instruments routinely used to clean the ear (e.g., Q-tip, match, bobby pin, key)
- Type and pattern of ear hygiene
- Exposure to loud noise or music
- Air travel (especially in unpressurized aircraft)
- Swimming habits and the use of ear protection when swimming
- History of health problems that can decrease the blood supply to the ear such as heart disease, hypertension, or diabetes
- History of vitiligo (a pigment disorder that may include a loss of melanin-containing cells in the inner ear, resulting in hearing loss)
- History of smoking
- History of vitamin B_{12} and folate deficiency

If the patient uses foreign objects to clean the ear canal, explain the danger in using these objects. They can scrape the skin of the canal, push cerumen up against the eardrum, and even puncture the eardrum. If the patient says that cerumen buildup is a problem, teach him or her to use an ear irrigation syringe and proper solutions to remove it. Chart 48-2 describes techniques to teach patients how to remove cerumen safely.

! NURSING SAFETY PRIORITY (QSEN)

Action Alert

Teach patients the safe way to clean their ears, stressing that nothing smaller than his or her own fingertip should be inserted into the canal.

CHART 48-2 Patient and Family Education: Preparing for Self-Management

Self–Ear Irrigation for Cerumen Removal

- *Do not attempt to remove earwax or irrigate the ears if you have ear tubes or if you have blood, pus, or other drainage from the ear.*
- Use an ear syringe designed for the purpose of wax removal (available at most drugstores).
- The safest type of ear syringe to use is one that has a right-angle or "elbow" in the tip.
- Irrigating your ears in the shower is an easy method.
- Always use tap water that feels just barely warm to you. Water that is warmer or colder can make you feel dizzy and nauseated.
- If your earwax is thick and sticky, you may need to place a few warm commercial eardrops that soften earwax (or baby oil or mineral oil) into the ear an hour or so before you irrigate the ear.
- Fill the syringe with the lukewarm tap water.
- If you are using a syringe with an elbow tip, place only the last part of the tip into your ear and aim it toward the roof of your ear canal.
- If you are using a straight-tipped syringe, insert the tip only about $\frac{1}{2}$ to $\frac{3}{4}$ inch into your ear canal, aiming toward the roof of the canal.
- Hold your head at a 30-degree angle to the side you are irrigating.
- Use one hand to hold the syringe and the other to push the plunger or squeeze the bulb.
- Apply gentle but firm continuous pressure, allowing the water to flow against the top of the canal.
- *Do not use blasts or bursts of sudden pressure.*
- The ear canal should fill, and water will begin to flow out, bringing earwax and debris with it.
- If a dental water-pressure irrigator is used, put it on the lowest possible setting.
- This process should not be painful! If pain occurs, decrease the pressure. If pain persists, stop the irrigation.
- Continue the irrigation until at least a cup of solution has washed into and out from your ear canal. (You may have to refill the syringe.)
- Tilting your head at a 90-degree angle to the side should allow most, if not all, of the water to drain out of your ear.
- Repeat the procedure on the other ear.
- If you feel that water is still in the canal, hold a hair dryer on a low setting near the ear.
- Irrigate your ears weekly to monthly, depending on how fast your earwax collects.

If the patient uses a hearing aid, assess whether hearing is improved with its use. Obtain the date of the last hearing test, the type of test given, and the results. Ask about problems that may impair auditory SENSORY PERCEPTION such as allergies, upper respiratory infections, hypothyroidism, atherosclerosis, head trauma, and recent head, facial, or dental surgery. A thorough drug history is important because many drugs are oto- toxic (damaging to the ear), especially many antibiotics, some diuretics, NSAIDs, and many chemotherapy agents. Use a drug handbook to determine whether any of the patient's prescribed drugs are known to affect auditory SENSORY PERCEPTION.

Ask about the patient's occupation and hobbies that involve exposure to loud noise or music. Assess whether protective ear devices are used. Also ask whether any devices are consistently inserted into the ear, such as ear plugs or earpiece headsets, and for how long each day they are used. Use this opportunity to teach the patient about protecting the ears from loud noises by wearing protective ear devices, such as over-the-ear headsets or foam ear inserts, when persistent loud noises are in the environment. Also suggest the use of earplugs when engaging in water sports to prevent ear infections.

Family History and Genetic Risk

Family history, as well as personal history, is important in determining genetic risk for hearing loss. Although most hearing loss as a result of a genetic mutation is seen in childhood, some genetic problems can lead to progressive hearing loss in adults. For example, most people with Down syndrome develop hearing loss as adults. People with osteogenesis imperfecta have bilateral and progressive hearing loss by their 30s.

🧬 GENETIC/GENOMIC CONSIDERATIONS
Patient-Centered Care **QSEN**

Mutations in several different genes are associated with hearing loss. One type of hearing loss among adults has a genetic basis with a mutation in gene *GJB2* (Online Mendelian Inheritance in Man [OMIM], 2014). This mutation causes poor production of the protein *connexin-26,* which has a role in the function of cochlear hair cells. Other genetic variations in some of the genes for drug-metabolizing enzymes (cytochrome p450) family) slow the metabolism and excretion of drugs, including ototoxic drugs. This allows ototoxic drugs to remain in the body longer, thus increasing the risk for hearing loss.

Ask the patient:
- Who in your family has hearing problems?
- Are the hearing problems present in men and women equally, or are they present more in one gender?
- At what age was hearing loss diagnosed in your relative(s)?
- Are both ears affected?

Current Health Problems

Assess current ear-related problems by asking about any ear "trouble," ear pain, or discharge, including earwax. Ask about a change in hearing, such as hyperacusis (the intolerance for sound levels that do not bother other people), or tinnitus (ringing in the ears). If a change in hearing is reported, ask whether one or both ears are involved and if the change was sudden or gradual. Also ask about problems with dizziness, sensations of being "off-balance," or vertigo.

Physical Assessment

Begin the examination by having the patient sit or lie down. Remove any hearing aids before the examination. After the examination, inspect the hearing aid for cracks, debris, and a proper fit. A complete ear examination is usually performed by a physician, advanced practice nurse, or physician assistant. The brief assessment of the ear and hearing usually performed by a medical-surgical nurse is described next.

External Ear and Mastoid Assessment

Inspect the entire external ear for shape, location of attachment to the head, and condition of all visible ear structures. The normal pinna has no skin tags or deformity. It should be attached to the side of the head at a posterior angle of 10 degrees or less. The normal external canal is dry, clean, free from lesions, and not reddened.

Abnormalities of the pinna include swelling, nodules, and lesions (Jarvis, 2016). In chronic gout, collections of uric acid crystals result in hard, irregular, painless nodules called *tophi* on the pinna. Other nodules on the pinna might also be from basal cell carcinoma or rheumatoid arthritis. Small, crusted, ulcerated, or indurated lesions on the pinna that fail to heal could be squamous cell carcinoma.

Inspect the mastoid process for redness and swelling. To assess for tenderness, gently tap with one finger over the mastoid process, compress the tragus with one finger, and gently move the pinna forward and backward. Any tenderness suggests an inflammation in either the external ear or the mastoid.

Assess for and record these problems:
- Furuncles
- Large amounts of cerumen
- Scaliness
- Redness
- Swelling of the ear
- Drainage and its character

Otoscopic Assessment

The purpose of a brief otoscopic examination is to assess the patency of the external canal, identify lesions or excessive cerumen in the canal, and assess whether the tympanic membrane (eardrum) is intact or inflamed (Jarvis, 2016). An instrument called an otoscope is used to examine the ear. Many types are available. It consists of a light, a handle, a magnifying lens, and a pressure bulb for injecting air into the external canal to test mobility of the eardrum (Fig. 48-5). Specula of various diameters attach to the head of the otoscope. Select the largest speculum that most comfortably fits the patient's external canal.

⚠ NURSING SAFETY PRIORITY **QSEN**
Action Alert

Do not use an otoscope to examine the ears of any patient who is unable to hold his or her head still during the examination or who is confused.

If the patient has pain during the external ear examination, cautiously attempt an otoscopic examination. The speculum will cause extreme pain if it comes in contact with inflamed tissue in the external canal.

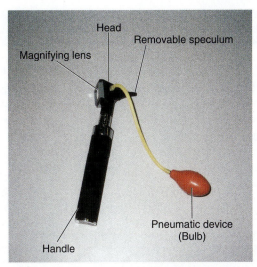

FIG. 48-5 Functional components of an otoscope.

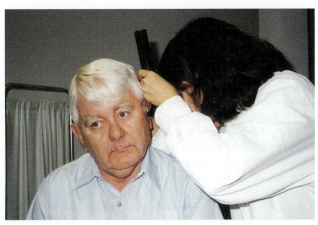

FIG. 48-6 Proper technique for an otoscopic examination.

Tilt the patient's head slightly away, and hold the otoscope upside down, like a large pen (Fig. 48-6). This position permits your hand to lie against the patient's head for support. If the patient moves, both your hand and the otoscope also move, preventing damage to the canal or eardrum. Hold the otoscope in your dominant hand, and gently pull the pinna up and back with your other hand to straighten the canal. View the ear canal while you slowly insert the speculum. Use caution to avoid causing pain by touching the speculum on the walls of the canal.

> ! **NURSING SAFETY PRIORITY** (QSEN)
>
> **Action Alert**
>
> Observe the ear canal through the otoscope as you insert the speculum into the external canal to avoid the risk for perforating the eardrum.

After the otoscope is comfortably in the external canal, assess for lesions and the amount, consistency, and color of cerumen and hair. The normal external canal is skin-colored, intact, and without lesions. It contains various amounts of soft cerumen and small, fine hairs.

Assess the eardrum for intactness and color. *The normal eardrum is always intact.* The eardrum is shiny, transparent or opaque, pearly gray, and without lesions. Redness is seen in otitis media. Reflection of the otoscope's light from the normal eardrum is the **light reflex**, and it appears as a clearly outlined triangle of light. On the right eardrum, the light reflex appears in the right lower quadrant. On the left eardrum, the light reflex appears in the left lower quadrant. The light reflex is termed **diffuse** when the light reflex is spotty or multiple because of a changed eardrum shape.

> ⊕ **CULTURAL CONSIDERATIONS**
>
> **Patient-Centered Care** (QSEN)
>
> Cerumen is generally moist and tan or brown in white people and black people. It is dry and light brown to gray in Asians and American Indians. The color of the lining of the external ear canal varies with the patient's skin tone. Variations should not be mistaken for indications of problems. Patients with more moist earwax form cerumen impactions more easily than patients with drier, flaky earwax and require more frequent ear irrigations.

General Hearing Assessment

Several rapid and simple tests for acuity of auditory SENSORY PERCEPTION can be performed at the patient's bedside. Although these tests do not determine the true extent or type of hearing loss, they can indicate a patient's functional hearing ability.

The *voice test* for hearing is conducted by asking the patient to block one external ear canal while standing 1 to 2 feet (30 to 60 cm) away. Quietly whisper a statement, and then ask the patient to repeat it. Test each ear separately. If the patient does not respond correctly, use a louder whisper. If you suspect the patient is lip-reading, use your hand to block the view of your mouth or stand behind him or her while whispering. More complex hearing tests, performed by audiologists, physicians, advanced practice nurses, specialty nurses, and physician assistants, can determine the type and extent of hearing loss.

Sound is transmitted by air conduction and bone conduction. Air conduction of sound is normally more sensitive than bone conduction. If auditory SENSORY PERCEPTION is decreased, the hearing loss is categorized as:

- **Conductive hearing loss**, resulting from obstruction of sound wave transmission such as a foreign body in the external canal, a retracted or bulging tympanic membrane, or fused bony ossicles.
- **Sensorineural hearing loss**, resulting from a defect in the cochlea, the eighth cranial nerve, or the brain. Exposure to loud noise or music causes this type of hearing loss by damaging the cochlear hair.
- **Mixed conductive-sensorineural hearing loss**, resulting from both conductive and sensorineural hearing loss.

Audioscopy testing involves the use of a handheld device to generate tones of varying intensities to test hearing. Auditory SENSORY PERCEPTION can be measured at a 40-decibel (dB) intensity at frequencies of 500, 1000, 2000, and 4000 cycles per second (cps), or hertz (Hz).

Tuning fork tests for hearing are the Weber and Rinne tests. These tests are useful, although limited, in distinguishing between conductive and sensorineural hearing losses. The frequency range of the tuning fork used for these tests corresponds to that of normal speech.

The Weber tuning fork test is performed by placing a vibrating tuning fork on the middle of the patient's head and asking him or her to indicate in which ear the sound is louder. The normal test result is sound heard equally in both ears. The term *lateralization* is used if the sound is louder in one ear. For example, lateralization to the right means that the sound is heard louder in the right ear.

The Rinne tuning fork test compares hearing by air conduction with hearing by bone conduction. Sound is normally heard 2 to 3 times longer by air conduction than by bone conduction. Perform this test by placing the vibrating tuning fork stem on the mastoid process (bone conduction) and asking the patient to indicate when the sound is no longer heard. When the patient no longer hears the sound, bring the fork quickly in front of the pinna (air conduction) without touching the patient. He or she should then indicate when this sound is no longer heard. The patient normally continues to hear the sound 2 to 3 times longer in front of the pinna after not hearing it with the tuning fork touching the mastoid process.

Psychosocial Assessment

The patient may become frustrated and depressed by an inability to hear well. Reduced or lost hearing may lead to social isolation. Be sensitive to the patient, and conduct the interview at a pace appropriate for that person.

Ask about social and work relationships to determine whether the patient is isolated because of hearing problems. Encourage the patient to express feelings related to hearing loss and discuss any changes in ADLs that have been made as a result of a change in hearing. Ask family members whether hearing problems have changed the patient's interactions.

💡 NCLEX EXAMINATION CHALLENGE

Safe and Effective Care Environment

With which client does the nurse avoid performing an otoscopic examination?
A. 34-year-old woman who is pregnant
B. 90-year-old woman who is visually impaired
C. 75-year-old man with dizziness and vertigo
D. 70-year-old man with advanced Alzheimer's disease

Diagnostic Assessment

Laboratory Assessment

Laboratory tests are helpful only when an external or internal ear infection is suspected. For an external ear infection, the typical causative organisms are known and this infection is managed without obtaining cultures. If the usual antibiotic therapy is not successful at clearing the infection, microbial culture and antibiotic sensitivity tests may be performed.

Imaging Assessment

CT, with or without contrast enhancement, shows the structures of the ear in great detail. CT is especially helpful in diagnosing acoustic tumors.

MRI most accurately reflects soft-tissue changes. Patients with older internal metal vascular clips cannot have MRI. Newer clips are made from titanium and are not a contraindication for MRI.

Specific Auditory Assessment

Audiometry. Audiometry is the most reliable method of measuring the acuity of auditory SENSORY PERCEPTION. It is

TABLE 48-1	Decibel Intensity and Safe Exposure Time for Common Sounds	
SOUND	**DECIBEL INTENSITY (dB)**	**SAFE EXPOSURE TIME***
Threshold of hearing	0	
Whispering	20	
Average residence or office	40	
Conversational speech	60	
Car traffic	70	>8 hr
Motorcycle	90	8 hr
Chain saw	100	2 hr
Rock concert, front row	120	3 min
Jet engine	140	Immediate danger
Rocket launching pad	180	Immediate danger

*For every 5-dB increase in intensity, the safe exposure time is cut in half.

performed by audiologists, audiology technicians, or nurses with special training. **Frequency** is the highness or lowness of tones (expressed in hertz). The greater the number of vibrations per second, the higher the frequency (pitch) of the sound. The fewer the number of vibrations per second, the lower the frequency (pitch).

Intensity of sound is expressed in decibels (dB). **Threshold** is the lowest level of intensity at which pure tones and speech are heard by a patient about 50% of the time. The lowest intensity at which a young, healthy ear can detect sound about 50% of the time is 0 dB. Sound at 110 dB is so intense (loud) that it is painful for most people with normal hearing. Conversational speech is around 60 dB, and a soft whisper is around 20 dB (Table 48-1). With a hearing loss of 45 to 50 dB, speech cannot be heard without a hearing aid. A person with a hearing loss of 90 dB may not be able to hear speech even with a hearing aid.

Pure tones are generated by an audiometer to determine hearing acuity. The two types of audiometry are pure-tone audiometry and speech audiometry.

Pure-Tone Audiometry. Pure-tone audiometry generates tones that are presented to the patient at frequencies for hearing speech, music, and other common sounds. The results of pure-tone audiometry are graphed on an audiogram. For some patients, the hearing of one ear is "masked" while the hearing of the other ear is tested.

Pure-tone air-conduction testing determines whether a patient hears normally or has a hearing loss. It tests air-conduction hearing sensitivity (through earphones) at frequencies ranging from 125 to 8000 Hz. The intensities for pure tones generally range from 10 to 110 dB.

The patient sits in a sound-isolated room so that background noise does not interfere with the test. Earphones are placed over his or her ears, and tones of varying frequencies and intensities are delivered through the earphones, testing one ear at a time. The patient presses a button or raises a hand to indicate when he or she hears a tone.

Pure-tone bone-conduction testing determines whether the hearing loss detected by air-conduction testing is due to conductive or sensorineural factors or to a combination of the two. It is used only when air-conduction testing results are abnormal. Testing is similar to air-conduction testing except that a bone-conduction vibrator, placed firmly behind the ear on the mastoid process, is used instead of earphones.

Interpretation of audiometric evaluation determines whether hearing is within normal limits or shows a hearing impairment and, if present, whether the hearing loss is conductive, sensorineural, or mixed. The type of loss is determined by an experienced clinician who examines the shape of the audiogram after completion of pure-tone air-conduction and bone-conduction audiometry.

Speech Audiometry. In speech audiometry, the patient's ability to hear spoken words is measured. The speech reception threshold and speech discrimination are assessed.

Speech reception threshold is the minimum loudness at which a patient can repeat simple words. This test determines how intense (or loud) a simple speech stimulus must be before the patient can hear it well enough to repeat it correctly at least 50% of the time. In one common test, lists of two-syllable words called **spondee** are used (i.e., words in which there is equal stress on each syllable, such as *airplane, railroad,* and *cowboy*).

Speech discrimination testing determines the patient's ability to discriminate among similar sounds or among words that contain similar sounds. This test assesses the patient's *understanding* of speech. An auditory SENSORY PERCEPTION loss decreases sensitivity to sound and impairs understanding of what is being said.

A standard format contains lists of 25 to 50 *monosyllabic* (one-syllable) words, such as *carve, day, toe,* and *ran,* and phonemically balanced words, and with equal word difficulty between lists. The lists are presented to the patient through earphones at a selected loudness level, generally about 30 to 40 dB above the speech reception threshold, or at the patient's most comfortable listening level. The score indicates the percentage of words repeated correctly.

Tympanometry. Tympanometry assesses mobility of the eardrum and structures of the middle ear by changing air pressure in the external ear canal. The progression or resolution of serous otitis and otitis media can be accurately monitored with this procedure.

This test is helpful in distinguishing middle ear problems, such as otosclerosis, ossicular disarticulation, otitis media, and perforation of the eardrum. It is also useful for assessing patency of the eustachian tube and for checking recovery of middle ear function after surgery.

Auditory Brainstem-Evoked Response. Auditory brainstem-evoked response (ABR) assesses hearing in patients who are unable to indicate their recognition of sound stimuli during standard hearing tests. It helps diagnose conductive and sensorineural hearing losses. Electrodes are placed on the scalp during the test. After the test, the patient's hair should be cleansed to remove the electrode gel.

Assessment of Balance

Electronystagmography (ENG) is a test to assess for central and peripheral disease of the vestibular system in the ear by detecting and recording **nystagmus** (involuntary eye movements). This response is accurate because the eyes and ears depend on each other for balance. Electrodes are taped to the skin near the eyes, and one or more procedures (caloric testing, changing gaze position, or changing head position) are performed to stimulate nystagmus. Failure of nystagmus to occur with cerebral stimulation suggests an abnormality in the vestibulocochlear apparatus, the cerebral cortex, the auditory nerve, or the brainstem.

To prepare the patient for ENG:
- Explain the procedure and its purpose. The examiners will be asking the patient to name names or do simple mathematics problems during the test to ensure he or she stays alert.
- Tell the patient to fast for several hours before the test and to avoid caffeine-containing beverages for 24 to 48 hours before the test.
- Tell patients with pacemakers that they should not have the test because pacemaker signals interfere with the sensitivity of ENG.
- Carefully introduce oral fluids after the test to prevent nausea and vomiting.

Caloric testing evaluates the vestibular (inner ear) portion of the auditory nerve. Water or air that is warmer or cooler than body temperature is infused into the ear. A normal response is the onset of vertigo and nystagmus within 20 to 30 seconds. Prepare the patient for caloric testing by:
- Explaining the procedure and its purpose
- Telling the patient to fast for several hours before the test
- Explaining that he or she will be on bedrest after the procedure with careful introduction of oral fluids to prevent nausea and vomiting

DISORDERS OF THE EAR AND HEARING

Although ear and hearing disorders are often easily managed, early recognition and intervention are necessary to prevent additional damage and to promote a maximum level of wellness. Without proper intervention, auditory SENSORY PERCEPTION can be affected.

CONDITIONS AFFECTING THE EXTERNAL EAR

The external ear is subject to outside factors that can cause problems. Disorders include congenital malformation, trauma, and infectious or noninfectious lesions of the pinna, auricle, or auditory canal. Abnormalities of the external ear range from crumpling or falling forward of the pinna to complete absence of the ear canal. Trauma can damage or destroy the auricle and external canal. Surgical reconstruction can re-form the pinna with skin grafts and plastic prostheses. Trauma to the auricle resulting in a hematoma requires the removal of blood via needle aspiration to prevent calcification and hardening, which is often referred to as a *cauliflower* or *boxer's ear.*

Benign cysts or polyps of the auricle or external canal are surgically removed if they block the canal and affect hearing. Cancer cells, usually basal cell carcinoma, can occur on the pinna. Usually treatment consists of simple excision. When the lesion becomes larger, its location near the skull and facial nerve makes treatment more difficult.

EXTERNAL OTITIS

❖ PATHOPHYSIOLOGY

External otitis is a painful condition caused when irritating or infective agents come into contact with the skin of the external ear. The result is either an allergic response or inflammation with or without infection. Affected skin becomes red, swollen, and tender to touch or movement. Swelling of the ear canal can lead to temporary hearing loss from obstruction. Allergic external otitis is often caused by contact with cosmetics, hair sprays, earphones, earrings, or hearing aids. The most common infectious organisms are *Pseudomonas aeruginosa*, *Streptococcus*, *Staphylococcus*, and *Aspergillus*.

External otitis occurs more often in hot, humid environments, especially in the summer, and is known as **swimmer's ear** because it occurs most often in people involved in water sports. Patients who have traumatized their external ear canal with sharp or small objects (e.g., hairpins, cotton-tipped applicators) or with headphones also are more susceptible to external otitis.

Necrotizing or *malignant otitis* is the most virulent form of external otitis. Organisms spread beyond the external ear canal into the ear and skull. Death from complications such as meningitis, brain abscess, and destruction of cranial nerve VII is possible.

❖ PATIENT-CENTERED COLLABORATIVE CARE

Manifestations of external otitis range from mild itching to pain with movement of the pinna or tragus, particularly when upward pressure is applied to the external canal. Patients report feeling as if the ear is plugged and hearing is reduced. The temporary hearing loss can be severe when inflammation obstructs the canal and prevents sounds from reaching the eardrum.

Treatment focuses on reducing inflammation, edema, and pain. Nursing priorities include comfort measures, such as applying heat to the ear for 20 minutes 3 times a day. This can be accomplished by using towels warmed with water and then wrapped in a plastic bag or by using a heating pad placed on a low setting. Teach the patient that minimizing head movements reduces pain.

Topical antibiotic and steroid therapies are most effective in decreasing inflammation and pain. Review best practices for instilling eardrops with the patient, as shown in Chart 48-3. Observe the patient self-administer the eardrops to make sure that proper technique is used. Oral or IV antibiotics are used in severe cases, especially when infection spreads to surrounding tissue or area lymph nodes are enlarged.

Analgesics, including opioids, may be needed for pain relief during the initial days of treatment. NSAIDs, such as acetylsalicylic acid (aspirin, Entrophen ♦) and ibuprofen (Advil), or acetaminophen (Tylenol, Abenol ♦) may relieve less severe pain.

After the inflammation has subsided, a solution of 50% rubbing alcohol, 25% white vinegar, and 25% distilled water may be dropped into the ear to keep it clean and dry and to prevent recurrence. Teach the patient to use preventive measures for minimizing ear canal moisture, trauma, or exposure to materials that lead to local irritation or contact dermatitis.

PERICHONDRITIS

Perichondritis is an infection of the **perichondrium**, a tough, fibrous tissue layer that surrounds the cartilage and shapes the pinna. This tissue supplies blood to the ear cartilage. Infection can be caused by opening an area of pus or localized infection, insect bites, trauma, and cartilage ear piercing. When infection occurs between the perichondrium and the cartilage, blood flow to the cartilage can be reduced, leading to necrosis and pinna deformity. This can occur as a complication of high helical ear piercing and may require removal of necrotic tissue.

The purposes of management are to eliminate the infection and ensure that the perichondrium stays in direct contact with the cartilage. In addition to systemic antibiotic therapy, a wide incision is made and suction drainage is used to remove pus and other fluid.

CERUMEN OR FOREIGN BODIES

❖ PATHOPHYSIOLOGY

Cerumen (earwax) is the most common cause of an impacted canal. A canal can also become impacted as a result of foreign bodies that can enter or be placed in the external ear canal, such as vegetables, beads, pencil erasers, and insects. Although uncomfortable, cerumen or foreign bodies are rarely emergencies and can be carefully removed by a health care professional. Cerumen impaction in the older adult is common, and removal of the cerumen from older adults often improves hearing.

❖ PATIENT-CENTERED COLLABORATIVE CARE

Patients with a cerumen impaction or a foreign body in the ear may have a sensation of fullness in the ear, with or without hearing loss, and may have ear pain, itching, dizziness, or bleeding from the ear. The object may be visible with direct inspection.

When the occluding material is cerumen, management options include watchful waiting, manual removal, and the use of ceruminolytic agents followed by either manual irrigation or the use of a low-pressure electronic oral irrigation device. The canal can be irrigated with a mixture of water and hydrogen peroxide at body temperature (Fig. 48-7), following best practices for proper irrigation (Chart 48-4). Removal of a cerumen obstruction by irrigation is a slow process and may take more than one sitting. When it is the cause of hearing loss, cerumen removal may improve hearing. Between 50 and 70 mL of solution is the maximum amount that the patient usually can tolerate at one sitting.

If the cerumen is thick and dry or cannot be removed easily, use a ceruminolytic product such as Cerumenex to soften the wax before trying to remove it. Another way to soften cerumen is to add 3 drops of glycerin or mineral oil to the ear at bedtime and 3 drops of hydrogen peroxide twice a day for several days. Then the cerumen is more easily removed by irrigation. In some cases, a small curette or cerumen spoon may be used by a health

---

CHART 48-3 Best Practice for Patient Safety & Quality Care (QSEN)

Instillation of Eardrops

- Gather the solutions to be administered.
- Check the labels to ensure correct dosage and time.
- Wear gloves to remove and discard any ear packing.
- Wash your hands.
- Perform a gentle otoscopic examination to determine whether the eardrum is intact.
- Irrigate the ear if the eardrum is intact (see Chart 48-4).
- Place the bottle of eardrops (with the top on tightly) in a bowl of warm water for 5 minutes.
- Tilt the patient's head in the opposite direction of the affected ear, and place the drops in the ear.
- With his or her head tilted, ask the patient to gently move the head back and forth 5 times.
- Insert a cotton ball into the opening of the ear canal to act as packing.
- Wash your hands again.

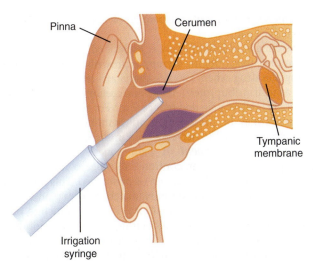

FIG. 48-7 Irrigation of the external canal. Cerumen and debris can be removed from the ear by irrigation with warm water. The stream of water is aimed above or below the impaction to allow back-pressure to push it out rather than further down the canal.

CHART 48-4   Best Practice for Patient Safety & Quality Care (QSEN)

Ear Irrigation

- Wash your hands.
- Use an otoscope to locate the impaction; ascertain that the eardrum is intact and that the patient does not have otitis media.
- Gather the equipment: basin, irrigation syringe, otoscope, towel.
- Warm tap water (or other prescribed solution) to body temperature.
- Fill a syringe with the warmed irrigating solution.
- Place a towel around the patient's neck.
- Place a basin under the ear to be irrigated.
- Place the tip of the syringe at an angle so that the fluid pushes to one side of and not directly on the impaction (to loosen it without moving it deeper into the canal).
- Apply gentle but firm continuous pressure, allowing the water to flow against the top of the canal.
- Do not use blasts or bursts of sudden pressure.
- If pain occurs, reduce the pressure. If pain persists, stop the irrigation.
- Watch the fluid return for cerumen plug removal.
- Continue to irrigate the ear with about 70 mL of fluid.
- If the cerumen does not drain out, wait 10 minutes and repeat the irrigation procedure.
- Monitor the patient for signs of nausea.
- If the patient becomes nauseated, stop the procedure.
- If the cerumen cannot be removed by irrigation, place mineral oil into the ear 3 times a day for 2 days to soften dry, impacted cerumen, after which irrigation may be repeated.
- After completion of the irrigation, have the patient turn his or her head to the side just irrigated to drain any remaining irrigation fluid.
- Wash your hands.

! NURSING SAFETY PRIORITY (QSEN)

Action Alert

Do not irrigate an ear with an eardrum perforation or otitis media because this may spread the infection to the inner ear. Also, do not irrigate the ear when the foreign object is vegetable matter, because this material expands when wet, making the impaction worse. For vegetable matter, the object needs to be physically removed by an experienced health care professional.

CHART 48-5   Nursing Focus on the Older Adult

Cerumen Impaction

- Assess the hearing of all older patients using simple voice tests.
- Perform a gentle otoscopic inspection of the external canal and eardrum of any older patient who has a problem with hearing acuity, especially the patient who wears a hearing aid.
- Use ear irrigation to remove any impacted cerumen.
- Make certain that the irrigating fluid is about 98.6° F (37° C) to reduce the chance for stimulating the vestibular sense.
- Use no more than 5 to 10 mL of irrigating fluid at a time.
- If nausea, vomiting, or dizziness develops, stop the irrigation immediately.
- Teach the patient how to irrigate his or her own ears.
- Obtain a return demonstration of ear irrigation from the patient, observing for specific areas in which the patient may need assistance.
- Encourage the patient to wash the external ears daily using a soapy, wet washcloth over the index finger (best done in the shower or while washing the hair).

---

care professional to scoop out the wax. Improper use of the curette can damage the canal or the eardrum.

Discourage the use of cotton swabs and ear candles (hollow tubes coated in wax inserted into the ear and then lighted at the far end) to clean the ears or remove cerumen. Chart 48-2 describes steps to teach patients regarding ear hygiene and self–ear irrigation. Refer to Chart 48-5 for nursing care considerations of older adult patients with cerumen impaction.

Insects are killed before removal unless they can be coaxed out by a flashlight. A topical anesthetic can be placed in the ear canal for pain relief. Mineral oil or diluted alcohol instilled into the ear can suffocate the insect, which is then removed with ear forceps.

If the patient has local irritation, an antibiotic or steroid ointment may be applied to prevent infection and reduce local irritation. Hearing acuity is tested if hearing loss is not resolved by removal of the object.

Surgical removal of the foreign object may be performed through the ear canal by a health care provider using a wire bent at a 90-degree angle. The wire is looped around the object, and the object is pulled out. Because this procedure is painful, general anesthesia is needed.

CONDITIONS AFFECTING THE MIDDLE EAR

OTITIS MEDIA

❖ *PATHOPHYSIOLOGY*

The common forms of otitis media are acute otitis media, chronic otitis media, and serous otitis media. Each type affects the middle ear but has different causes and pathologic changes. If otitis progresses or is untreated, permanent conductive hearing loss may occur.

Acute otitis media and chronic otitis media are similar. An infecting agent in the middle ear causes inflammation of the mucosa, leading to swelling and irritation of the ossicles within the middle ear, followed by purulent inflammatory exudate. Acute disease has a sudden onset and lasts 3 weeks or less. Chronic otitis media often follows repeated acute episodes, has a longer duration, and causes greater middle ear injury. It may be a result of the continuing presence of a biofilm in the middle ear. A *biofilm* is a community of bacteria working together to overcome host defense mechanisms to continue to survive and proliferate (see Chapter 23 for more information about biofilms). Therapy for complications associated with chronic otitis media usually involves surgical intervention.

The eustachian tube and mastoid, connected to the middle ear by a sheet of cells, are also affected by the infection. If the eardrum membrane perforates, the infection can thicken and scar the eardrum and middle ear if left untreated. Necrosis of the ossicles destroys middle ear structures and causes hearing loss.

❖ PATIENT-CENTERED COLLABORATIVE CARE

◆ Assessment

The patient with acute or chronic otitis media has ear pain. Acute otitis media causes more intense pain from increased pressure in the middle ear. Conductive hearing is reduced and distorted as sound wave transmission is obstructed. The patient may notice tinnitus in the form of a low hum or a low-pitched sound. Headaches and systemic manifestations such as malaise, fever, nausea, and vomiting can occur. As the pressure on the middle ear pushes against the inner ear, the patient may have dizziness.

Otoscopic examination findings vary, depending on the stage of the condition. The eardrum is initially retracted, which allows landmarks of the ear to be seen clearly. At this early stage, the patient has only vague ear discomfort. As the condition progresses, the eardrum's blood vessels dilate and appear red (Fig. 48-8). Later, the eardrum becomes red, thickened, and bulging, with loss of landmarks. Decreased eardrum mobility is evident on inspection with a pneumatic otoscope. Pus may be seen behind the membrane.

With progression, the eardrum spontaneously perforates and pus or blood drains from the ear (Fig. 48-9). Then the patient notices a marked decrease in pain as the pressure on middle ear structures is relieved. Eardrum perforations often heal if the underlying problem is controlled. Simple central perforation does not interfere with hearing unless the ossicles are damaged or the perforation is large. Repeated perforations with extensive scarring cause hearing loss.

◆ Interventions

Nonsurgical Management. Management can be as simple as putting the patient in a quiet environment. Bedrest limits head movements that intensify the pain. Application of low heat may help reduce pain.

Systemic antibiotic therapy is prescribed. Teach the patient to complete the antibiotic therapy as prescribed and to not stop taking the drug when manifestations are relieved. Analgesics such as aspirin, ibuprofen (Advil), and acetaminophen (Tylenol, Abenol ♣) relieve pain and reduce fever. For severe pain, opioid analgesics may be prescribed. Antihistamines and decongestants are prescribed to decrease fluid in the middle ear.

Surgical Management. If pain persists after antibiotic therapy and the eardrum continues to bulge, a **myringotomy** (surgical opening of the eardrum) is performed. This procedure drains middle ear fluids and immediately relieves pain.

The procedure is a small surgical incision, which is often performed in an office or clinic setting, and the incision heals rapidly. Another approach is the removal of fluid from the middle ear with a needle. For relief of pressure caused by serous otitis media and for those patients who have repeated episodes of otitis media, a small **grommet** (polyethylene tube) may be surgically placed through the eardrum to allow continuous drainage of middle ear fluids (Fig. 48-10).

Priority care after surgery includes teaching the patient to keep the external ear and canal clean and dry while the incision is healing. Instruct him or her to not wash the hair or shower for several days. Other instructions after surgery are listed in Chart 48-6.

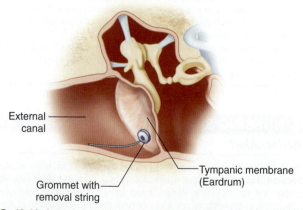

FIG. 48-9 Otoscopic view of a perforated tympanic membrane.

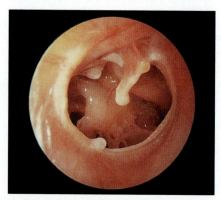

FIG. 48-8 Otoscopic view of otitis media.

External canal

Grommet with removal string

Tympanic membrane (Eardrum)

FIG. 48-10 Grommet through the tympanic membrane. A small grommet is placed through the tympanic membrane away from the margins, which allows prolonged drainage of fluids from the middle ear.

MASTOIDITIS

❖ PATHOPHYSIOLOGY

The lining of the middle ear is continuous with the lining of the mastoid air cells, which are embedded in the temporal bone. Mastoiditis is an infection of the mastoid air cells caused by progressive otitis media. Antibiotic therapy is used to treat the middle ear infection before it progresses to mastoiditis. If mastoiditis is not managed appropriately, it can lead to brain abscess, meningitis, and death.

❖ PATIENT-CENTERED COLLABORATIVE CARE

The manifestations of mastoiditis include swelling behind the ear and pain when moving the ear or the head. Pain is *not* relieved by myringotomy. Cellulitis develops on the skin or external scalp over the mastoid process, pushing the ear sideways and down. The eardrum is red, dull, thick, and immobile. Perforation may or may not be present. Lymph nodes behind the ear are tender and enlarged. Patients may have low-grade fever, malaise, and ear drainage. Hearing loss occurs, and CT scans show fluid in the air cells of the mastoid process.

Interventions focus on halting the infection before it spreads to other structures. IV antibiotics are used but do not easily penetrate the infected bony structure of the mastoid. Cultures of the ear drainage determine which antibiotics should be most effective. Surgical removal of the infected tissue is needed if the infection does not respond to antibiotic therapy within a few days. A simple or modified radical mastoidectomy with tympanoplasty is the most common treatment. All infected tissue must be removed so that the infection does not spread to other structures. A tympanoplasty is then performed to reconstruct the ossicles and the eardrum to restore hearing (see pp. 1012-1013 for care after tympanoplasty.)

TRAUMA

Trauma and damage may occur to the eardrum and ossicles by infection, by direct damage, or through rapid changes in the middle ear pressure. Objects placed in the external canal exert pressure on the eardrum and cause perforation. If the objects continue through the canal, the ossicles may be damaged. Blunt injury to the skull and ears can also damage or fracture middle ear structures. Slapping the external ear increases the pressure in the ear canal and can tear the eardrum. Excessive nose blowing and rapid changes of pressure (*barotrauma*) can increase pressure within the middle ear leading to damaged ossicles and a perforated eardrum.

Most eardrum perforations heal within a week or two without treatment. Repeated perforations heal more slowly, with scarring. Depending on the amount of damage to the ossicles, auditory SENSORY PERCEPTION may or may not return. Hearing aids can improve hearing in this type of hearing loss. Surgical reconstruction of the ossicles and eardrum through a tympanoplasty or a myringoplasty may also improve hearing. (See later discussion of nursing care on p. 1013 in the Tympanoplasty section.)

Nursing care priorities focus on teaching about trauma prevention. Caution patients to avoid inserting objects into the external canal and to follow the steps in Chart 48-2 for ear hygiene. Stress the importance of using ear protectors when blunt trauma is likely.

NEOPLASMS

Middle ear tumors are rare, and the most common type is the *glomus jugulare*, a benign vascular lesion. Malignant ear tumors also can occur. The growth of any lesion within the middle ear area disrupts conductive auditory SENSORY PERCEPTION, erodes the ossicles, and may affect the inner ear and cranial nerves.

Patients have progressive hearing loss and tinnitus. Infection and pain are rare. Otoscopic examination shows a bulging eardrum or a mass extending to the external ear canal. The blood vessels of the *glomus jugulare* tumor give the mass a reddish color and a visible pulsation.

Diagnosis is made by physical examination, tomography, and angiography. Tumors are removed by surgery, which often destroys hearing in the affected ear. Depending on the extent of the tumor, surgery can performed through the ear canal or may involve opening the cranium to remove the tumor.

Benign tumors are removed because, with continued growth, other structures can be affected, further damaging the facial or trigeminal nerve. When possible, reconstruction of the middle ear structures is performed later to restore conductive hearing.

CONDITIONS AFFECTING THE INNER EAR

TINNITUS

Tinnitus (continuous ringing or noise perception in the ear) is a common ear problem that can occur in one or both ears. Diagnostic testing cannot confirm tinnitus; however, testing is performed to assess hearing and rule out other disorders.

Manifestation range from mild ringing, which can go unnoticed during the day, to a loud roaring in the ear, which can interfere with thinking and attention span. Some patients feel as if the constant ringing could drive them mad. Factors that contribute to tinnitus include age, sclerosis of the ossicles, Ménière's disease, certain drugs (aspirin, NSAIDs, high-ceiling diuretics, quinine, aminoglycoside antibiotics), exposure to loud noise, and other inner ear problems (Ruppert & Fay, 2012).

The problem and its management vary with the underlying cause. When no cause can be found or the disorder is untreatable, therapy focuses on ways to mask the tinnitus with background sound, noisemakers, and music during sleeping hours. Ear mold hearing aids can amplify sounds to drown out the tinnitus during the day. A drug that is helpful to some patients is pramipexole (Mirapex), an antiparkinson drug. The American Tinnitus Association assists patients in coping with tinnitus. Refer patients with tinnitus to local and online support groups to help them cope with this problem.

? NCLEX EXAMINATION CHALLENGE
Physiological Integrity

The client who has tinnitus is taking these drugs daily: 1 multiple vitamin, losartan (Cozaar) 50 mg, aspirin 650 mg, and diphenhydramine (Benadryl) 25 mg. Which drug alerts the nurse to a possible cause of tinnitus?
A. Aspirin
B. Losartan
C. Multiple vitamin
D. Diphenhydramine

VERTIGO AND DIZZINESS

Vertigo and dizziness are common manifestations of many ear disorders. **Dizziness** is a disturbed sense of a person's relationship to space. Vertigo is often used interchangeably with dizziness, but the definition and cause are somewhat different. True **vertigo** is a sense of whirling or turning in space.

Because the visual system, the vestibular system, and the proprioceptive system (muscles and nerve endings) combine to give input to the brain about balance, problems in any of these areas lead to a disturbed sense of balance. Problems that cause vertigo include Ménière's disease, labyrinthitis, acoustic neuromas, motion sickness, and drug or alcohol ingestion.

Manifestations of vertigo include nausea, vomiting, falling, nystagmus, hearing loss, and tinnitus. Until the cause of the vertigo can be identified, each manifestation is treated. Teach patients these strategies to reduce manifestations:

- Restrict head motion and change position slowly
- Take drugs that reduce the vertigo effects, such as over-the counter dimenhydrinate (Dramamine, Gravol ♣) or prescription drugs such as diazepam (Valium, Apo-Diazepam ♣), meclizine (Antivert, Bonamine ♣), and scopolamine (Transderm Scop, Transderm-V ♣)

LABYRINTHITIS

Labyrinthitis is an infection of the labyrinth, which may occur as a complication of acute or chronic otitis media that spreads to the inner ear. Labyrinthitis also may result from the growth of a **cholesteatoma** (benign overgrowth of squamous cell epithelium) from the middle ear into the semicircular canal. It may follow middle ear or inner ear surgery and may follow a viral upper respiratory infection or mononucleosis.

Manifestations include auditory SENSORY PERCEPTION loss, tinnitus, nystagmus to the affected side, and vertigo with nausea and vomiting. Labyrinthitis is usually a self-limiting condition. If it does not resolve with supportive therapy, management includes systemic antibiotics. Teach the patient to complete the antibiotic therapy as prescribed and to not stop taking the drug when manifestations are no longer present because inadequate treatment may lead to meningitis. Advise patients to stay in bed in a darkened room until manifestations are reduced. Antiemetics and antivertiginous drugs, such as dimenhydrinate (Dramamine, Gravol ♣) and meclizine (Antivert, Bonamine ♣), relieve nausea and dizziness.

MÉNIÈRE'S DISEASE
❖ PATHOPHYSIOLOGY

Ménière's disease has three features: tinnitus, one-sided sensorineural auditory SENSORY PERCEPTION loss, and vertigo, occurring in attacks that can last for several days (Haynes, 2014). (Some patients have continuous manifestations of varying intensity rather than intermittent attacks.) Patients are almost totally incapacitated during an attack, and recovery takes hours to days. The pathology of Ménière's disease is an excess of endolymphatic fluid that distorts the entire inner-canal system. This distortion decreases hearing by dilating the cochlear duct, causes vertigo because of damage to the vestibular system, and stimulates tinnitus. At first, hearing loss is reversible, but repeated damage to the cochlea from increased fluid pressure leads to permanent hearing loss.

❖ PATIENT-CENTERED COLLABORATIVE CARE
◆ Assessment

Ménière's disease usually first occurs in people between the ages of 20 and 50 years. It is more common in men and affects about 615,000 people in the United States (Alm, 2012). Severe, debilitating attacks alternate with symptom-free periods. Patients often have certain manifestations before an attack of vertigo, such as headaches, increasing tinnitus, and fullness in the affected ear.

Patients describe the tinnitus as a continuous, low-pitched roar or a humming sound, which worsens just before and during an attack. Hearing loss occurs first with the low-frequency tones but progresses to include all levels and, with repeated attacks, can become permanent. The vertigo with periods of whirling may even cause patients to fall. It is so intense that even while lying down, the patient often holds the bed or ground to keep from falling. Severe vertigo usually lasts 3 to 4 hours, but he or she may feel dizzy long after the attack. Nausea and vomiting are common. Other manifestations include rapid eye movements (**nystagmus**) and severe headaches.

◆ Interventions

Nonsurgical Management. Teach patients to move the head slowly to prevent worsening of the vertigo. Nutrition and lifestyle changes can reduce the amount of endolymphatic fluid. Encourage patients to stop smoking because of the blood vessel constricting effects.

Nutrition therapy with a hydrops diet may stabilize body fluid levels to prevent excess endolymph accumulation. The basic structure of this diet involves:

- Distributing food and fluid intake evenly throughout the day and from day to day
- Avoiding foods or fluids with a high salt content
- Drinking adequate amounts of fluids daily
- Avoiding caffeine-containing fluids and foods
- Limiting alcohol intake to one serving per day
- Avoiding monosodium glutamate (MSG)

Coordinate with a dietitian for more information about diet therapy for reduction of Ménière's manifestations.

Drug therapy may reduce the vertigo and vomiting and restore normal balance. Mild diuretics are prescribed to decrease endolymph volume, which reduces vertigo, hearing loss, tinnitus, and aural fullness. Nicotinic acid has been found to be useful because of its vasodilatory effect. Antihistamines, such as diphenhydramine hydrochloride (Benadryl, Allerdryl ✦) and dimenhydrinate (Dramamine, Gravol ✦), and antivertiginous drugs, such as meclizine (Antivert, Bonamine ✦), help reduce the severity of or stop an acute attack. Antiemetics, such as chlorpromazine hydrochloride (Thorazine, Novo-Chlorpromazine✦), droperidol (Inapsine), promethazine (Phenergan), and ondansetron (Zofran), help reduce the nausea and vomiting. Diazepam (Valium, Apo-Diazepam ✦) calms the patient; reduces vertigo, nausea, and vomiting; and allows the patient to rest quietly during an attack. Intratympanic therapy with gentamycin and steroids can prevent manifestations; however, this therapy results in some hearing loss.

Pressure pulse treatments, such as the Meniett device, which use a tympanostomy tube to apply low-pressure micropulses to the inner ear several times daily, have helped reduce episodes in some patients with Ménière's disease (National Institute on Deafness and other Communication Disorders [NIDCD], 2010). This action displaces inner ear fluid and prevents or relieves manifestations.

An experimental technique to control dizziness is in clinical trials. This technique involves the use of an implant placed behind the affected ear that blocks abnormal activity of the eighth cranial nerve (Alm, 2012).

Surgical Management. When medical therapy is ineffective and the patient's general function is decreased significantly, surgery may be performed. The choice of the surgical procedure depends on the degree of usable hearing, the severity of the spells, and the condition of the opposite ear. The most radical procedure involves resection of the vestibular nerve or total removal of the labyrinth (labyrinthectomy), performed through the ear canal. This procedure results in total auditory SENSORY PERCEPTION loss on the operative side.

Another procedure performed early in the course of the disease is endolymphatic decompression with drainage and a shunt. The effectiveness of this procedure varies. The endolymphatic sac is drained, and a tube is inserted for continued fluid drainage. Some patients report relief of vertigo with retention of their hearing. Vertigo is present immediately after surgery from movement of the vestibule of the inner ear during surgery. Reassure the patient that the vertigo is a temporary result of the surgical procedure, not the disease.

💡 **NCLEX EXAMINATION CHALLENGE**

Health Promotion and Maintenance

Which lifestyle modification does the nurse suggest to the client with Ménière's disease to reduce the frequency or intensity of acute episodes?
A. Quitting cigarette smoking
B. Avoiding aspirin-containing drugs
C. Reducing the amount of saturated fats in the diet
D. Avoiding crowds and people who have upper respiratory infections

---

ACOUSTIC NEUROMA

An acoustic neuroma is a benign tumor of cranial nerve VIII that often damages other structures as it grows. Depending on the size and exact location of the tumor, damage to hearing, facial movements, and sensation can occur (McCance et al.,

2014). An acoustic neuroma can cause many neurologic manifestations as the tumor enlarges in the brain.

Manifestations begin with tinnitus and progress to gradual sensorineural hearing loss. Later, patients have constant mild to moderate vertigo. As the tumor enlarges, nearby cranial nerves are damaged.

The tumor is diagnosed with CT scanning and MRI. Cerebrospinal fluid assays show increased pressure and protein.

Surgical removal can be performed in a variety of ways. Usually a craniotomy is performed, and usually the remaining hearing is lost. Care is taken to preserve the function of the facial nerve (cranial nerve VII). Care after craniotomy is discussed in Chapter 45. Acoustic neuromas rarely recur after surgical removal.

HEARING LOSS

❖ *PATHOPHYSIOLOGY*

Loss of auditory SENSORY PERCEPTION is common and may be conductive, sensorineural, or a combination of the two (see Fig. 48-2). Conductive hearing loss occurs when sound waves are blocked from contact with inner ear nerve fibers because of external ear or middle ear disorders. If the inner ear sensory nerve that leads to the brain is damaged, the hearing loss is *sensorineural*. Combined hearing loss is *mixed conductive-sensorineural*.

The differences in conductive and sensorineural hearing loss are listed in Table 48-2. Disorders that cause conductive hearing loss are often corrected with minimal or no permanent damage. Sensorineural hearing loss is often permanent.

Etiology and Genetic Risk

Conductive hearing loss can be caused by any inflammation or obstruction of the external or middle ear. Changes in the

---

TABLE 48-2 Comparison of Features for Conductive and Sensorineural Hearing Loss

CONDUCTIVE HEARING LOSS	SENSORINEURAL HEARING LOSS
Causes	
Cerumen	Prolonged exposure to noise
Foreign body	Presbycusis
Perforation of the tympanic membrane	Ototoxic substance
	Ménière's disease
Edema	Acoustic neuroma
Infection of the external ear or middle ear	Diabetes mellitus
	Labyrinthitis
Tumor	Infection
Otosclerosis	Myxedema
Assessment Findings	
Evidence of obstruction with otoscope	Normal appearance of external canal and tympanic membrane
Abnormality in tympanic membrane	Tinnitus common
	Occasional dizziness
Speaking softly	Speaking loudly
Hearing best in a noisy environment	Hearing poorly in loud environment
Rinne test: air conduction greater than bone conduction	Rinne test: air conduction less than bone conduction
Weber test: lateralization to affected ear	Weber test: lateralization to unaffected ear

eardrum such as bulging, retraction, and perforations may damage middle ear structures and lead to conductive hearing loss. Tumors, scar tissue, and overgrowth of soft bony tissue (otosclerosis) on the ossicles from previous middle ear surgery also lead to conductive hearing loss.

Sensorineural hearing loss occurs when the inner ear or auditory nerve (cranial nerve VIII) is damaged. Prolonged exposure to loud noise damages the hair cells of the cochlea (NIDCD, 2012). Many drugs are toxic to the inner ear structures, and their effects on hearing can be transient or permanent, dose related, and affect one or both ears. When ototoxic drugs are given to patients with reduced kidney function, increased ototoxicity can occur because drug elimination is slower, especially among older patients.

Presbycusis is a sensorineural auditory SENSORY PERCEPTION loss that occurs with aging (McCance et al., 2014). It is caused by degeneration of cochlear nerve cells, loss of elasticity of the basilar membrane, or a decreased blood supply to the inner ear. Deficiencies of vitamin B_{12} and folic acid increase the risk for presbycusis. Other causes include atherosclerosis, hypertension, infections, fever, Ménière's disease, diabetes, and ear surgery (Touhy & Jett, 2014). Trauma to the ear, head, or brain also contributes to sensorineural hearing loss.

Incidence and Prevalence

Because hearing loss may be gradual and affect only some aspects of hearing, many adults are unaware that their hearing is impaired. The incidence of adult hearing loss in the United States is estimated to be 36 to 46 million, or 17% of the population, and dramatically increases among people in their 70s and 80s (NIDCD, 2014; Oyler, 2012).

Health Promotion and Maintenance

With special care to the ears, hearing can be preserved at maximum levels. Address barriers to the use of hearing protection, exposure to loud music, and other modifiable risk factors that affect hearing. Encourage everyone to have simple hearing testing performed as part of their annual health assessment.

Teach everyone the danger in using objects such as bobbypins, Q-tips, or toothpicks to clean the ear canal. These can scrape the skin of the canal, push cerumen up against the eardrum, and puncture the eardrum. If cerumen buildup is a problem, teach the person the proper technique to remove it (see Chart 48-2).

Teach all people to use protective ear devices, such as over-the-ear headsets or foam ear inserts, when exposed to persistent loud noises. Suggest using earplugs when engaging in water sports to prevent ear infections, as well as using an over-the-counter product such as Swim-Ear to assist with drying the ears after swimming.

❖ PATIENT-CENTERED COLLABORATIVE CARE

◆ Assessment

History. Ask patients how long they have noticed a change in hearing and whether the changes were sudden or gradual. Age is important, because some ear and hearing changes occur with aging. Ask about exposures to loud or continuous noises, as well as current or previous use of ototoxic drugs. Also ask about a history of ear infections and whether eardrum perforation occurred. Ask patients about any direct trauma to the ears. Because some types of hearing loss have a genetic basis, ask

---

CHART 48-7 Focused Assessment
The Patient with Suspected Hearing Loss

Assess whether the patient has any of these ear problems:
- Pain
- Feeling of fullness or congestion
- Dizziness or vertigo
- Tinnitus
- Difficulty understanding conversations, especially in a noisy room
- Difficulty hearing sounds
- The need to strain to hear
- The need to turn the head to favor one ear or the need to lean forward to hear

Assess visible ear structures, particularly the external canal and tympanic membrane:
- Position and size of the pinna
- Patency of the external canal; presence of cerumen or foreign bodies, edema, or inflammation
- Condition of the tympanic membrane: intact, edema, fluid, inflammation

Assess functional ability, including:
- Frequency of asking people to repeat statements
- Withdrawal from social interactions or large groups
- Shouting in conversation
- Failing to respond when not looking in the direction of the sound
- Answering questions incorrectly

---

whether any family members are hearing impaired. When pain occurs with acute-onset hearing loss, ask about recent upper respiratory infection and allergies affecting the nose and sinuses.

The patient with hearing loss from peripheral neuropathy may have other systemic diseases, including human immune deficiency virus (HIV) disease or diabetes. Patients undergoing cancer chemotherapy or interferon therapy are at risk for neuropathic hearing loss.

Physical Assessment/Clinical Manifestations. Chart 48-7 lists focused assessment techniques for patients with suspected loss of auditory SENSORY PERCEPTION. The loss may be sudden or gradual and often affects both ears. The ability to hear high-frequency consonants—especially *s*, *sh*, *f*, *th*, and *ch* sounds—is lost first. Patients may state that they have no problem with hearing but cannot understand specific words and that other people are mumbling. Vertigo and continuous tinnitus may be present.

Tuning fork tests help diagnose hearing loss. With the Weber test, the patient can usually hear sounds well in the ear with a conductive hearing loss because of bone conduction. With the Rinne test, the patient reports that sound transmitted by bone conduction is louder and more sustained than that transmitted by air conduction.

Otoscopic examination is used to assess the ear canal, eardrum, and middle ear structures that can be seen through the eardrum. Findings vary, depending on the cause of the hearing loss. Perform the examination as described earlier on pp. 1000-1001, and document the findings.

Psychosocial Assessment. For people with a loss of auditory SENSORY PERCEPTION, communication can be a struggle and they may isolate themselves because of the difficulty in talking and listening. Social isolation can lead to depression (Spyridakou, 2012). Be sensitive to emotional changes that may be related to reduced hearing and a decline in conversational skills. Encourage the patient and family to express their feelings and concerns about an actual or potential hearing loss.

Laboratory Assessment. No laboratory test diagnoses hearing loss. However, some laboratory findings can indicate problems that affect hearing. White blood cell counts are assessed in the patient with otitis media.

Imaging Assessment. Imaging assessment can determine some problems affecting hearing ability. Skull x-rays determine bony involvement in otitis media and the location of otosclerotic lesions. CT and MRI are used to determine soft-tissue involvement and the presence and location of tumors.

Other Diagnostic Assessment. Audiometry can help determine whether hearing loss is only conductive or whether it has a sensorineural component. This is important in determining possible causes of the hearing loss and in planning interventions.

◆ **Analysis**

The priority NANDA-I nursing diagnoses and collaborative problems for the patient with any degree of hearing impairment include:

1. Difficulty hearing related to obstruction, infection, damage to the middle ear, or damage to the auditory nerve
2. Impaired Verbal Communication related to difficulty hearing (NANDA-I)

◆ **Planning and Implementation**

Increasing Hearing

Planning: Expected Outcomes. The patient with impaired auditory SENSORY PERCEPTION is expected to either have an increase in functional hearing or maintain existing hearing levels. Indicators include:

- No or minimal loss of high-pitch tones
- No or minimal loss of ability to distinguish conversation from background noise
- Turning toward sound
- Identifying discrete sounds

Interventions. Interventions are expected to identify the problem, halt the pathologic processes, and increase usable hearing. Nursing care priorities focus on teaching the patient about the use of an appropriate assistive device, providing support to the patient and family to maintain or increase communication, and assisting patients to find support services.

Nonsurgical Management. Interventions include early detection of impaired auditory SENSORY PERCEPTION, use of appropriate therapy, and use of assistive devices to augment the patient's usable hearing.

Early detection helps correct the problem causing the hearing loss. Assess for indications of hearing loss, as listed in Chart 48-7.

Drug therapy is focused on correcting the underlying problem or reducing the side effects of problems occurring with hearing loss. Antibiotic therapy is used to manage external otitis and other ear infections. Teach the patient the importance of taking the drug or drugs exactly as prescribed and completing the entire course. Caution him or her to not stop the drug just because manifestations have improved. By treating the infection, antibiotics reduce local edema and improve hearing. When pain is also present, analgesics are used. Many ear disorders induce vertigo and dizziness with nausea and vomiting. Antiemetic, antihistamine, antivertiginous, and benzodiazepine drugs can help reduce these problems.

Assistive devices are useful for patients with permanent hearing loss. Portable amplifiers can be used while watching television to avoid increasing the volume and disturbing others. Telephone amplifiers increase telephone volume, allowing the caller to speak in a normal voice. Flashing lights activated by the ringing telephone or a doorbell alert patients visually. Some patients may have a service dog to alert them to sounds (ringing telephones or doorbells, cries of other people, and potential dangers). Provide information about agencies that can assist the hearing-impaired person.

Small, portable audio amplifiers can assist in communicating with patients with hearing loss who do not use a hearing aid. Using amplifiers or allowing patients to use a stethoscope for listening helps you communicate with anyone who requires additional volume to hear speech.

A hearing aid is a small electronic amplifier that assists patients with conductive hearing loss but is less effective for sensorineural hearing loss. Most common hearing aids are small. Some are attached to a person's glasses and are visible to other people. Another type fits into the ear and is less noticeable. Newer devices fit completely in the canal with only a fine, clear filament visible. The cost of smaller hearing aids varies with size and quality. Some people benefit from classes that explain the best use and care of these devices.

Remind patients that hearing with a hearing aid is different from natural hearing. Teach the patient to start using the hearing aid slowly, at first wearing it only at home and only during part of the day. Listening to television and the radio and reading aloud can help the patient get used to new sounds. A difficult aspect of a hearing aid is the amplification of background noise. The patient must learn to concentrate and filter out background noises. In a study of hearing aid users, the most desired feature for a hearing aid is its functionality in noisy settings (see the Evidence-Based Practice box).

Teach the patient how to care for the hearing aid (Chart 48-8). Hearing aids are delicate devices that should be handled only by people who know how to care for them properly.

Cochlear implantation may help patients with sensorineural hearing loss. Although a superficial surgical procedure is needed

---

CHART 48-8 Patient and Family Education: Preparing for Self-Management

Hearing Aid Care

- Keep the hearing aid dry.
- Clean the ear mold with mild soap and water while avoiding excessive wetting.
- Using a toothpick, clean debris from the hole in the middle of the part that goes into your ear.
- Turn off the hearing aid when not in use.
- Check and replace the battery frequently.
- Keep extra batteries on hand.
- Keep the hearing aid in a safe place.
- Avoid dropping the hearing aid or exposing it to temperature extremes.
- Adjust the volume to the lowest setting that allows you to hear, to prevent feedback squeaking.
- Avoid using hair spray, cosmetics, oils, or other hair and face products that might come into contact with the receiver.
- If the hearing aid does not work:
  - Change the battery.
  - Check the connection between the ear mold and the receiver.
  - Check the on/off switch.
  - Clean the sound hole.
  - Adjust the volume.
  - Take the hearing aid to an authorized service center for repair.

EVIDENCE-BASED PRACTICE (QSEN)

What Do People with Reduced Hearing Want Most from a Hearing Aid?

Bridges, J., Lataille, A., Buttorff, C., White, S., & Niparko, J. (2012). Consumer preference for hearing aid attributes: A comparison of rating and conjoint analysis methods. *Trends in Amplification, 16*(1), 40-48.

The number of older adults with hearing loss is increasing, although only about one in five hearing-impaired people uses a hearing aid. Several drawbacks from hearing aid use include cost, appearance, and the quality of amplification, particularly the utility of the device in noisy environments. The purpose of this study was to determine what hearing aid factors or attributes are preferred by users. There were 75 subjects with documented hearing loss followed in the ambulatory care setting of a large medical center. With the exception of income, the cohort strongly represented the typical hearing aid user (male, older). This group had a higher-than-typical education level and income level. The study built upon previous studies that identified the seven hearing aid attributes (i.e., performance in quiet settings, comfort, feedback, frequency of battery replacement, purchase price, water and sweat resistance, and performance in noisy settings) that were important in the choice and use of different models of hearing aids.

Subjects were asked to rate these attributes on a Likert-like scale and were asked to perform eight pair-comparison conjoint tasks. In addition to descriptive statistics, data were analyzed using ordinary least squares (OLS) and logit models.

Although all positive attributes (e.g., good performance, lower cost, longer battery life) were considered desirable, the attribute considered by a large margin to be most desirable and most likely to help the person continue usual activities was improved performance in noisy environments. Both methods of measurement and analysis had similar results. This result was confirmed by the subjects indicating that they would be willing to pay $2000 to $4000 more for a hearing aid that had good performance in noisy environments.

Level of Evidence: 3

This quasi-experimental study did not include randomization or a true control group. However, the identified variables were evidence-based from previous studies and the methods of statistical analysis were appropriate for the research questions posed.

Commentary: Implications for Practice and Research

A limitation to the generalizability of this study is the higher-than-average levels of income and education among the subject population. The results of this study indicated that the attribute of improving hearing in a noisy environment is very important in hearing aid selection, even when the cost of hearing aids with this attribute is considerably greater than for hearing aids that performed less well in this area. These results indicate that people with hearing loss would prefer to maintain all their social and work activities, including those in environments in which noise affects communication. Nurses and other health care professionals may have been underestimating the degree and effect of social isolation experienced by people who have reduced or lost auditory sensory perception. Until technologic advances in hearing aid performance in noisy environments are more affordable, research into the types of social activities that can be satisfying to the person with reduced hearing is needed.

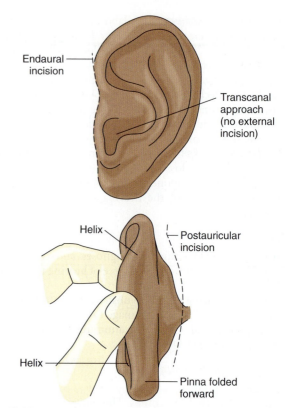

FIG. 48-11 Surgical approaches for repair of the ear and hearing structures.

have a 50% return of their hearing with this method (Holmes et al., 2012).

Surgical Management. Many surgical interventions are available for patients with specific disorders leading to hearing loss.

Tympanoplasty. Tympanoplasty reconstructs the middle ear to improve conductive hearing loss. The procedures vary from simple reconstruction of the eardrum (**myringoplasty**) to replacement of the ossicles within the middle ear (**ossiculoplasty**).

Preoperative Care. The patient requires specific instructions before surgery. Systemic antibiotics reduce the risk for infection. Teach the patient to follow other measures to decrease the risks for infection, such as avoiding people with upper respiratory infections, getting adequate rest, eating a balanced diet, and drinking adequate amounts of fluid.

Assure the patient that hearing loss immediately after surgery is normal because of canal packing and that hearing will improve when it is removed. Stress that forceful coughing increases middle ear pressure and must be avoided.

Operative Procedures. Surgery is performed only when the middle ear is free of infection. If an infection is present, the graft is more likely to become infected and not heal. Surgery of the eardrum and ossicles requires the use of a microscope and is a delicate procedure. Local anesthesia can be used, although general anesthesia is often used to prevent the patient from moving.

The surgeon can repair the eardrum with many materials, including muscle fascia, a skin graft, and venous tissue. If the ossicles are damaged, more extensive surgery is needed for repair or replacement. The ossicles can be reached in several ways—through the ear canal, with an endaural incision, or by an incision behind the ear (Fig. 48-11).

to implant the device, the procedure does not enter the inner ear and thus is not considered a surgical correction for hearing impairment. A small computer converts sound waves into electronic impulses. Electrodes are placed near the internal ear, with the computer attached to the external ear. The electronic impulses then directly stimulate nerve fibers. Some patients

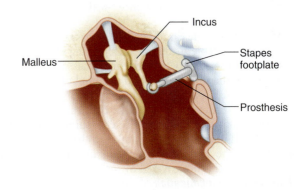

FIG. 48-12 Prosthesis used with stapedectomy. The stapes is removed, leaving the footplate. A metal or plastic prosthesis is connected to the incus and inserted through the hole to act as an artificial stapes.

The surgeon removes diseased tissue and cleans the middle ear cavity. The patient's cartilage or bone, cadaver ossicles, stainless steel wire, or special polymers (Teflon) are used to repair or replace the ossicles.

Postoperative Care. An antiseptic-soaked gauze, such as iodoform gauze (NU GAUZE), is packed in the ear canal. If a skin incision is used, a dressing is placed over it. Keep the dressing clean and dry, using sterile technique for changes. Keep the patient flat, with the head turned to the side and the operative ear facing up for at least 12 hours after surgery. Give prescribed antibiotics to prevent infection.

Patients often report hearing improvement after removal of the canal packing. Until that time, communicate as with a hearing-impaired patient, directing conversation to the unaffected ear. Instruct the patient in care and activity restrictions (see Chart 48-6).

Stapedectomy. A partial or complete stapedectomy with a prosthesis can correct some hearing loss, especially in patients with hearing loss related to otosclerosis. Although hearing usually improves after primary stapes surgery, some patients redevelop conductive hearing loss after surgery and revision surgery is needed.

Preoperative Care. To prevent infection, the patient must be free from external otitis at surgery. Teach the patient to follow measures that prevent middle ear or external ear infections (Chart 48-9).

Review with the patient the expected outcomes and possible complications of the surgery. Hearing is initially worse after a stapedectomy. The success rate of this procedure is high. However, there is always a risk for failure that might lead to total deafness on the affected side. Other possible complications include vertigo, infection, and facial nerve damage.

Operative Procedures. A stapedectomy is usually performed through the external ear canal with the patient under local anesthesia. After removal of the affected ossicles, a piston-shaped prosthesis is connected between the incus and the footplate (Fig. 48-12). Because the prosthesis vibrates with sound as the stapes did, most patients have restoration of functional hearing.

Postoperative Care. Remind the patient that improvement in hearing may not occur until 6 weeks after surgery. Drugs for pain help reduce discomfort, and antibiotics are used to prevent infection. Teach the patient about the precautions in Chart 48-6.

The surgical procedure is performed in an area where cranial nerves VII, VIII, and X can be damaged by trauma or by swelling after surgery. *Assess for facial nerve damage or muscle weakness. Indications include an asymmetric appearance or drooping of features on the affected side of the face. Ask the patient about changes in facial perception of touch and in taste.* Vertigo, nausea, and vomiting usually occur after surgery because of the nearness to inner ear structures.

Antivertiginous drugs, such as meclizine (Antivert, Bonamine ✦), and antiemetic drugs, such as droperidol (Inapsine), are given. Take care to prevent falls.

! NURSING SAFETY PRIORITY (QSEN)

Action Alert

Prevent injury by assisting the patient with ambulation during the first 1 to 2 days after stapedectomy. Keep top bed siderails up, and remind the patient to move the head slowly to avoid vertigo.

Totally Implanted Devices. Totally implanted devices, such as the Esteem, can improve bilateral moderate to severe sensorineural hearing loss without any visible part (Barbara et al., 2011). These devices have three totally implanted components: a sound processor, a sensor, and a computer. Vibrations of the eardrum and ossicles are picked up by the sensor and converted to electric signals that are processed by the sound processor. The processor is programmed to the patient's specific hearing pathology. The processor filters out some background noise and amplifies the desired sound signal. The signal is transferred to the computer, which then converts the processed signal into vibrations that are transmitted to the inner ear for auditory SENSORY PERCEPTION.

Patient criteria for totally implantable devices include:
- Bilateral stable sensorineural hearing loss
- Speech discrimination score of 40% or higher
- Healthy tympanic membrane, eustachian tube, and ossicles of the middle ear
- Large enough ear cavity to fit the device components

- At least 30 days experience with an appropriate hearing aid
- Absence of middle ear, inner ear, or mastoid infection
- Absence of Ménière's disease or recurring vertigo
- Absence of sensitivity to device materials

The devices and the surgery may lead to complications, including temporary facial paralysis, changes in taste sensation, and ongoing or new-onset tinnitus. Unlike cochlear implants, the middle ear is entered and it is considered a surgical procedure. Care before and after surgery is similar to that required with stapedectomy. The cost of the implant and procedure can exceed $30,000 and is not covered by insurance.

Maximizing Communication

Planning: Expected Outcomes. The patient with reduced auditory SENSORY PERCEPTION is expected to become proficient in hearing compensation behaviors to maintain or improve communication. Indicators include that the patient consistently demonstrates these behaviors:

- Uses hearing assistive devices
- Uses sign language, lip-reading, closed captioning, or video description (for television viewing)
- Accurately interprets messages
- Uses nonverbal language
- Exchanges messages accurately with others

Interventions. Nursing priorities focus on facilitating communication and reducing anxiety.

Use best practices that are listed in Chart 48-10 for communicating with a hearing-impaired patient. Ask the patient what type of communication tools he or she is most comfortable using, and then use that format (Shuler et al., 2013). Do not shout at the patient, because the sound may be projected at a higher frequency, making him or her less able to understand. Communicate by writing (if he or she is able to see, read, and write) or pictures of familiar phrases and objects. Many television programs are now closed captioned or video described (subtitled). When available, use the assistive devices described on p. 1011 to increase communication.

Lip-reading and *sign language* can increase communication. In lip-reading, patients are taught special cues to look for when lip-reading and how to understand body language. However, the best lip-reader still misses more than half of what is being said. Because hearing is assisted by even minimal lip-reading, urge patients to wear their eyeglasses when talking with someone to see lip movement.

Sign languages, such as American Sign Language (ASL), combine speech with hand movements that signify letters, words, and phrases. These languages take time and effort to learn, and many people are unable to use them effectively (Richardson, 2014).

Managing anxiety can increase the effectiveness of communication efforts. One source of anxiety is the possibility of permanent hearing loss. Provide accurate information about the likelihood of hearing returning. When the hearing impairment is likely to be permanent, reassure patients that communication and social interaction can be maintained.

To reduce anxiety and prevent social isolation, assist patients to use resources and communication to make social contact satisfying. Identify the patient's most satisfying activities and social interactions, and determine the effort necessary to continue them. The patient can alter activities to improve satisfaction. Instead of large gatherings, the patient might choose smaller groups. A meal at home with friends can substitute for dining in a noisy restaurant.

Community-Based Care

Lengthy hospitalization is rare for ear and hearing disorders. If surgery is needed and the procedure is completed without complications, it may be performed in an ambulatory surgery center.

Home Care Management.
Patients who have persistent vertigo are in danger of falling. Assess the home for potential hazards and to determine whether family or significant others are available to assist with meal preparation and other ADLs. A nurse case manager can coordinate with the home care nurse to assist patients and their families in determining how to maintain adequate self-care abilities, maintain a safe environment, decide about assistance needs, and provide needed care.

Self-Management Education.
Provide written instructions to the patient and family about how to take drugs and when to return for follow-up care. Teach patients how to instill eardrops (see Chart 48-3) and irrigate the ears (see Chart 48-2), and obtain a return demonstration.

To prevent infection after surgery, instruct patients to follow the suggestions in Chart 48-9. Teach patients who use a hearing aid how to use it effectively.

Health Care Resources.
If patients do not have family or friends to help before or after surgery, a referral to a home care agency is needed. Help with meal preparation, cleaning, and personal hygiene can be arranged by the case manager.

Follow-up hearing tests are scheduled when the lesions are well healed, in about 6 to 8 weeks. Audiograms done before and after treatment are compared, and evaluation for further intervention to improve hearing begins. A complication of surgery is continued disability or complete loss of hearing in the affected ear. Surgery is performed first on the ear with the greatest hearing loss. If the surgery does not improve hearing, patients must decide to either attempt surgical correction of the other ear or continue to use an amplification device. When the underlying disorder causing the hearing impairment is progressive, this decision is difficult. Support patients by listening to their concerns and giving additional information when needed.

Costs to the person with a hearing impairment can be extensive. Information and support can come from public and private agencies that specialize in counseling patients with disorders affecting auditory SENSORY PERCEPTION.

CHART 48-10 Best Practice for Patient Safety & Quality Care (QSEN)

Communicating with a Hearing-Impaired Patient

- Position yourself directly in front of the patient.
- Make sure that the room is well lighted.
- Get the patient's attention before you begin to speak.
- Move closer to the better-hearing ear.
- Speak clearly and slowly.
- Do not shout (shouting often makes understanding more difficult).
- Keep hands and other objects away from your mouth when talking to the patient.
- Have conversations in a quiet room with minimal distractions.
- Have the patient repeat your statements, not just indicate assent.
- Rephrase sentences and repeat information to aid understanding.
- Use appropriate hand motions.
- Write messages on paper if the patient is able to read.

◆ *Evaluation: Outcomes*

Evaluate the care of the patient with hearing loss or hearing impairment based on the identified priority patient problems. The expected outcomes include that the patient will:

- Have at least partial improvement of hearing
- Have minimal anxiety
- Use appropriate hearing compensation behaviors
- Communicate effectively in most situations

Specific indicators for these outcomes are listed for each priority problem under the Planning and Implementation section (see earlier).

? CLINICAL JUDGMENT CHALLENGE

Ethical/Legal

The patient is a 78-year-old man whose hearing loss has progressed to the extent that hearing aids are no longer helpful. His only other health problems are early-stage prostate cancer (for which he is undergoing "watchful waiting") and type 2 diabetes mellitus (which is well controlled by diet and exercise). He lives alone in a condominium complex with many amenities. His son has voiced concern that his father should not live alone but should go into assisted living. The patient insists that this is not necessary because he can still drive, cook, and take care of himself. He also states that he has many friends in the condo complex and wants to remain active within the social groups there.

1. What should be your question when you meet with the father and the son?
2. Are there any major concerns for the father's immediate safety or health because of the hearing loss?
3. Are there any ethical or legal considerations in play here? If so, which one(s)?
4. What accommodations or environmental alterations can you recommend that would make it easier for the father to continue to live alone?
5. What other health care professionals should you consult with or bring in to this situation?

NURSING CONCEPTS AND CLINICAL JUDGMENT REVIEW

What might you NOTICE if the patient has auditory SENSORY PERCEPTION problems?

- Person tilts head to one side or leans forward to listen when another person speaks.
- Person watches the lips of a speaker closely.
- Person does not startle when a loud or unexpected sound occurs in the environment.
- Person frequently asks the speaker to repeat statements or questions.
- Person does not verbally interact with those around him or her.
- When a sentence is whispered to the person, he or she does not accurately repeat it back to the speaker.
- Person responds inappropriately to questions.

How should you RESPOND to a patient who has auditory SENSORY PERCEPTION problems?

- Reduce the background sound when speaking to the person (close the door to the hall, use a private area, turn off televisions and radios).
- Speak slowly, distinctly, and with a deeper tone.
- Face the patient while speaking.
- Ensure that all members of the health care team are aware of the patient's impairment and use an appropriate method to communicate with him or her.
- Determine whether the patient can communicate by sign language.
- Identify safety issues specific for the patient with a hearing impairment.
- Use a certified medical interpreter when taking a history from, explaining procedures to, or teaching the patient who has a hearing impairment.

GET READY FOR THE NCLEX® EXAMINATION!

KEY POINTS

Review these Key Points for each NCLEX Examination Client Needs Category.

Safe and Effective Care Environment

- Use Contact Precautions with any patient who has drainage from the ear canal. **Safety** QSEN
- Use a separate speculum cover for each ear when conducting an otoscopic examination. **Safety** QSEN
- Slowly and gently introduce the otoscopic speculum into the external ear canal during assessment. **Safety** QSEN
- Do not perform an otoscopic examination on a confused patient. **Safety** QSEN

- Use the suggestions presented in the Patient History section (p. 998) to enhance communication with a patient who has an impairment of auditory SENSORY PERCEPTION. **Safety** QSEN
- Protect the patient with vertigo or dizziness from injury by assisting with ambulation. **Safety** QSEN
- Follow the guidelines in Chart 48-4 when irrigating the ear canal. **Safety** QSEN

Health Promotion and Maintenance

- Teach patients the proper way to clean the pinna and external ear canal and how to remove cerumen from the external canal. **Evidence-Based Practice** QSEN

- Identify patients at risk for hearing impairment as a result of work environment or leisure activities. **Patient-Centered Care** QSEN
- Encourage all patients, even if they already have a hearing impairment, to use ear protection in loud environments. **Patient-Centered Care** QSEN
- Inform all patients who smoke that smoking increases the risk for development of hearing problems. **Evidence-Based Practice** QSEN
- Teach patients how to properly care for their hearing aids. **Patient-Centered Care** QSEN
- Instruct patients to avoid closing off one naris when blowing the nose. **Patient-Centered Care** QSEN
- Remind patients who engage in water sports and who are at risk for external otitis to wear earplugs when in the water. **Patient-Centered Care** QSEN
- Teach patients the proper techniques for self-instillation of eardrops and ear irrigation. **Patient-Centered Care** QSEN

Psychosocial Integrity

- Allow the patient the opportunity to express fear or anxiety about a change in hearing status. **Patient-Centered Care** QSEN
- Explain all diagnostic and therapeutic procedures, restrictions, and follow-up care to the patient and family. **Patient-Centered Care** QSEN
- Refer patients newly diagnosed with hearing impairment or any chronic ear problem to appropriate local resources and support groups.
- Teach family members ways to communicate with a hearing-impaired patient with and without a hearing aid. **Patient-Centered Care** QSEN

- Assess the degree to which hearing problems interfere with the patient's ability to interact with others. **Patient-Centered Care** QSEN
- Remind patients having ear surgery that hearing in the affected ear may be reduced immediately after surgery because of packing, swelling, or surgical manipulation. **Patient-Centered Care** QSEN

Physiological Integrity

- Ask the patient about hearing problems in any other members of the family, because many hearing problems have a genetic component. **Patient-Centered Care** QSEN
- Check the hearing of any patient receiving an ototoxic drug for more than 5 days. **Evidence-Based Practice** QSEN
- Ask the patient about current and past drug use (prescribed, over-the-counter), and check with a pharmacist to evaluate for ototoxicity. **Patient-Centered Care** QSEN
- Avoid ear canal irrigation if the eardrum is perforated or if the canal contains vegetative matter. **Safety** QSEN
- Stress the importance of completing an antibiotic regimen for an ear infection. **Evidence-Based Practice** QSEN
- Remind patients to move the head slowly after ear surgery to prevent dizziness or vertigo. **Patient-Centered Care** QSEN
- Use upper siderails for any patient experiencing dizziness or vertigo. **Safety** QSEN
- Work with the case manager, home care nurse, speech-language pathologist, and occupational therapist to ensure safety and optimal function for the patient with a hearing or balance problem in the community setting. **Teamwork and Collaboration** QSEN

CHAPTER | 49

Assessment of the Musculoskeletal System

Donna D. Ignatavicius

 http://evolve.elsevier.com/Iggy/

PRIORITY CONCEPTS

- MOBILITY
- PAIN

- SENSORY PERCEPTION

LEARNING OUTCOMES

Safe and Effective Care Environment

1. Collaborate with the physical and occupational therapists to perform a complete musculoskeletal assessment, including functional status, as needed.

Health Promotion and Maintenance

2. Explain how physiologic aging changes of the musculoskeletal system affect care of older adults.

Psychosocial Integrity

3. Assess the patient's and family's reaction to change in body image caused by a major musculoskeletal health problem.

Physiological Integrity

4. Recall the basic anatomy and physiology of the musculoskeletal system.
5. Assess patients for MOBILITY, gait, motor skills, PAIN, SENSORY PERCEPTION, and the use of assistive devices.
6. Interpret assessment findings in a patient with a musculoskeletal health problem.
7. Explain the use of laboratory testing for a patient with a musculoskeletal health problem.
8. Develop a teaching plan to educate the patient and family about diagnostic procedures.

The musculoskeletal system is the second largest body system. It includes the bones, joints, and skeletal muscles, as well as the supporting structures needed to move them. MOBILITY (movement) is a basic human need that is essential for performing ADLs. When a patient cannot move to perform ADLs or other daily routines, self-esteem and a sense of self-worth can be diminished.

Disease, surgery, and trauma can affect one or more parts of the musculoskeletal system, often leading to decreased mobility. When MOBILITY is impaired for a long time, other body systems can be affected. For example, prolonged immobility can lead to skin breakdown, constipation, and thrombus formation. If nerves are damaged by trauma or disease, patients may also have problems with SENSORY PERCEPTION, also known as *sensation*.

ANATOMY AND PHYSIOLOGY REVIEW

Skeletal System

The skeletal system consists of 206 bones and multiple joints. The growth and development of these structures occur during childhood and adolescence and are not discussed in this text. Common physical skeletal differences among selected racial/ethnic groups are listed in Table 49-1.

Bones

Types and Structure. Bone can be classified in two ways—by shape and by structure. **Long bones,** such as the femur, are cylindric with rounded ends and often bear weight. **Short bones,** such as the phalanges, are small and bear little or no weight. **Flat bones,** such as the scapula, protect vital organs and

TABLE 49-1	Musculoskeletal Differences in Selected Racial/Ethnic Groups
GROUP	**MUSCULOSKELETAL DIFFERENCES**
African Americans	Greater bone density than Europeans, Asians, and Hispanics. Accounts for decreased incidence of osteoporosis.
Amish	Greater incidence of dwarfism than in other populations.
Chinese Americans	Bones are shorter and smaller with less bone density. Increased incidence of osteoporosis.
Egyptian Americans	Shorter in stature than Euro-Americans and African Americans.
Filipino/Vietnamese	Short in stature; adult height about 5 feet.
Irish Americans	Taller and broader than other Euro-Americans. Less bone density than African Americans.
Navajo American Indians	Taller and thinner than other American Indians.

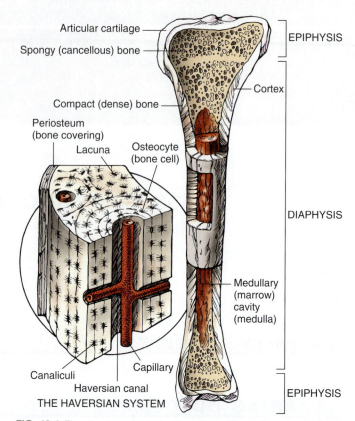

FIG. 49-1 The structure of a typical long bone. The cortex, or outer layer, is composed of dense, compact tissue. The microscopic structure of this compact cortical tissue is the haversian system.

often contain blood-forming cells. Bones that have unique shapes are known as **irregular bones.** The carpal bones in the wrist and the small bones in the inner ear are examples of **irregular bones**. The sesamoid bone is the least common type and develops within a tendon; the patella is a typical example.

The second way bone is classified is by *structure* or composition. As shown in Fig. 49-1, the outer layer of bone, or cortex, is composed of dense, compact bone tissue. The inner layer, in the medulla, contains spongy, cancellous tissue. Almost every bone has both tissue types but in varying quantities. The long bone typically has a shaft, or diaphysis, and two knoblike ends, or epiphyses.

The structural unit of the cortical compact bone is the haversian system, which is detailed in Fig. 49-1. The haversian system is a complex canal network containing microscopic blood vessels that supply nutrients and oxygen to bone, as well as lacunae, which are small cavities that house **osteocytes** (bone cells). The canals run vertically within the hard cortical bone tissue.

The softer **cancellous** tissue contains large spaces, or trabeculae, which are filled with red and yellow marrow. **Hematopoiesis** (production of blood cells) occurs in the red marrow. The yellow marrow contains fat cells, which can be dislodged and enter the bloodstream to cause fat embolism syndrome (FES), a life-threatening complication. Volkmann's canals connect bone marrow vessels with the haversian system and periosteum, the outermost covering of the bone. In the deepest layer of the periosteum are osteogenic cells, which later differentiate into **osteoblasts** (bone-forming cells) and **osteoclasts** (bone-destroying cells).

Bone also contains a matrix consisting chiefly of collagen, mucopolysaccharides, and lipids. Deposits of inorganic calcium salts (carbonate and phosphate) in the matrix provide the hardness of bone.

Bone is a very vascular tissue. Its estimated total blood flow is between 200 and 400 mL/min. Each bone has a main nutrient artery, which enters near the middle of the shaft and branches into ascending and descending vessels. These vessels supply the cortex, the marrow, and the haversian system. Very few nerve fibers are connected to bone. Sympathetic nerve fibers control dilation of blood vessels. Sensory nerve fibers transmit pain signals experienced by patients who have primary lesions of the bone, like bone tumors.

Function. The skeletal system:
- Provides a framework for the body and allows the body to be weight bearing, or upright
- Supports the surrounding tissues (e.g., muscle and tendons)
- Assists in movement through muscle attachment and joint formation
- Protects vital organs, such as the heart and lungs
- Manufactures blood cells in red bone marrow
- Provides storage for mineral salts (e.g., calcium and phosphorus)

After puberty, bone reaches its maturity and maximum growth. Bone is a dynamic tissue. It undergoes a continuous process of formation and **resorption,** or destruction, at equal rates until the age of 35 years. In later years, bone resorption increases, decreasing bone mass and predisposing patients to injury, especially older women.

Numerous minerals and hormones affect bone growth and metabolism, including:
- Calcium
- Phosphorus
- Calcitonin
- Vitamin D
- Parathyroid hormone (PTH)
- Growth hormone
- Glucocorticoids

- Estrogens and androgens
- Thyroxine
- Insulin

Bone accounts for about 99% of the *calcium* in the body and 90% of the *phosphorus*. In healthy adults, the serum concentrations of calcium and phosphorus maintain an inverse relationship. As calcium levels rise, phosphorus levels decrease. When serum levels are altered, calcitonin and PTH work to maintain equilibrium. If the calcium in the blood is decreased, the bone, which stores calcium, releases calcium into the bloodstream in response to PTH stimulation.

Calcitonin is produced by the thyroid gland and *decreases* the serum calcium concentration if it is increased above its normal level. Calcitonin inhibits bone resorption and increases renal excretion of calcium and phosphorus as needed to maintain balance in the body.

Vitamin D and its metabolites are produced in the body and transported in the blood to promote the absorption of calcium and phosphorus from the small intestine. They also seem to enhance PTH activity to release calcium from the bone. A decrease in the body's vitamin D level can result in osteomalacia (softening of bone) in the adult. Vitamin D metabolism and osteomalacia are described in Chapter 50.

When serum calcium levels are lowered, *parathyroid hormone* (PTH, or parathormone) secretion increases and stimulates bone to promote osteoclastic activity and *release* calcium to the blood. PTH reduces the renal excretion of calcium and facilitates its absorption from the intestine. If serum calcium levels increase, PTH secretion diminishes to preserve the bone calcium supply. This process is an example of the feedback loop system of the endocrine system.

Growth hormone secreted by the anterior lobe of the pituitary gland is responsible for increasing bone length and determining the amount of bone matrix formed before puberty. During childhood, an increased secretion results in gigantism and a decreased secretion results in dwarfism. In the adult, an increase causes acromegaly, which is characterized by bone and soft-tissue deformities (see Chapter 62).

Adrenal glucocorticoids regulate protein metabolism, either increasing or decreasing catabolism to reduce or intensify the organic matrix of bone. They also aid in regulating intestinal calcium and phosphorus absorption.

Estrogens stimulate osteoblastic (bone-building) activity and inhibit PTH. When estrogen levels decline at menopause, women are susceptible to low serum calcium levels with increased bone loss (osteoporosis). *Androgens,* such as testosterone in men, promote anabolism (body tissue building) and increase bone mass.

Thyroxine is one of the principal hormones secreted by the thyroid gland. Its primary function is to increase the rate of protein synthesis in all types of tissue, including bone. *Insulin* works together with growth hormone to build and maintain healthy bone tissue.

Joints

A **joint** is a space in which two or more bones come together. This is also referred to as *articulation* of the joint. The major function of a joint is to provide movement and flexibility in the body.

There are three types of joints in the body:

- Synarthrodial, or completely immovable, joints (e.g., in the cranium)

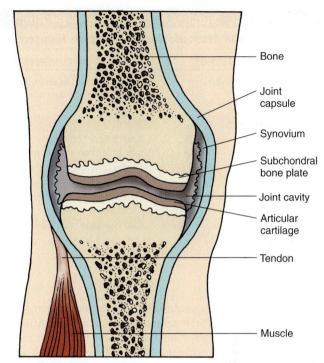

FIG. 49-2 The structure of a synovial joint. Synovium lines the joint capsule but does not extend into the articular cartilage.

- Amphiarthrodial, or slightly movable, joints (e.g., in the pelvis)
- Diarthrodial (synovial), or freely movable, joints (e.g., the elbow and knee)

Although any of these joints can be affected by disease or injury, the synovial joints are most commonly involved as discussed in Chapter 18.

The diarthrodial, or synovial, joint is the most common type of joint in the body. **Synovial joints** are the only type lined with synovium, a membrane that secretes synovial fluid for lubrication and shock absorption. As shown in Fig. 49-2, the synovium lines the internal portion of the joint capsule but does not normally extend onto the surface of the cartilage at the spongy bone ends. Articular cartilage consists of a collagen fiber matrix impregnated with a complex ground substance. Patients with inflammatory types of arthritis often have synovitis (synovial inflammation) and breakdown of the cartilage. Bursae, small sacs lined with synovial membrane, are located at joints and bony prominences to prevent friction between bone and structures adjacent to bone. These structures can also become inflamed, causing bursitis.

Synovial joints are described by their anatomic structures. *Ball-and-socket* joints (shoulder, hip) permit movement in any direction. *Hinge* joints (elbow) allow motion in one plane—flexion and extension. The knee is often classified as a hinge joint, but it rotates slightly, as well as flexes and extends. It is best described as a *condylar* type of synovial joint. The gliding movement of the wrist is characteristic of the *biaxial* joint. *Pivot* joints permit rotation only, as in the radioulnar area.

Muscular System

There are three types of muscle in the body: smooth muscle, cardiac muscle, and skeletal muscle. Smooth, or non-striated, involuntary muscle is responsible for contractions of organs

---

CHART 49-1   **Nursing Focus on the Older Adult**

Changes in the Musculoskeletal System Related to Aging

PHYSIOLOGIC CHANGE	NURSING INTERVENTIONS	RATIONALES
Decreased bone density	Teach safety tips to prevent falls. Reinforce need to exercise, especially weight-bearing exercise.	Porous bones are more likely to fracture. Exercise slows bone loss.
Increased bone prominence	Prevent pressure on bone prominences.	There is less soft tissue to prevent skin breakdown.
Kyphotic posture: widened gait, shift in the center of gravity	Teach proper body mechanics; instruct the patient to sit in supportive chairs with arms.	Correction of posture problems prevents further deformity; the patient should have support for bony structures.
Cartilage degeneration	Provide moist heat, such as a shower or warm, moist compresses.	Moist heat increases blood flow to the area.
Decreased range of motion (ROM)	Assess the patient's ability to perform ADLs and mobility.	The patient may need assistance with self-care skills.
Muscle atrophy, decreased strength	Teach isometric exercises.	Exercises increase muscle strength.
Slowed movement	Do not rush the person; be patient.	The patient may become frustrated if hurried.

---

and blood vessels and is controlled by the autonomic nervous system. Cardiac or striated involuntary muscle is also controlled by the autonomic nervous system. The smooth and cardiac muscles are discussed with the body systems to which they belong in the assessment chapters.

In contrast to smooth and cardiac muscle, skeletal muscle is striated voluntary muscle controlled by the central and peripheral nervous systems. The junction of a peripheral motor nerve and the muscle cells that it supplies is sometimes referred to as a **motor end plate**. Muscle fibers are held in place by connective tissue in bundles, or fasciculi. The entire muscle is surrounded by dense fibrous tissue, or fascia, which contains the muscle's blood, lymph, and nerve supply.

The main function of skeletal muscle is *movement* of the body and its parts. When bones, joints, and supporting structures are adversely affected by injury or disease, the adjacent muscle tissue is often involved, limiting mobility. During the aging process, muscle fibers decrease in size and number, even in well-conditioned adults. Atrophy results when muscles are not regularly exercised, and they deteriorate from disuse.

Supporting structures for the muscular system are very susceptible to injury. They include **tendons** (bands of tough, fibrous tissue that attach muscles to bones) and **ligaments**, which attach bones to other bones at joints.

MUSCULOSKELETAL CHANGES ASSOCIATED WITH AGING

Osteopenia, or decreased bone density (bone loss), occurs as one ages. Many older adults, especially white, thin women, have severe osteopenia, a disease called *osteoporosis*. This condition causes postural and gait changes and predisposes the person to fractures. Chapter 50 discusses this health problem in detail.

Synovial joint cartilage can become less elastic and compressible as a person ages. As a result of these cartilage changes and continued use of joints, the joint cartilage becomes damaged, leading to osteoarthritis (OA). Genetic defects in cartilage may also contribute to joint disease. The most common joints affected are the weight-bearing joints of the hip, knee, and cervical and lumbar spine, but joints in the shoulder and upper extremity, feet, and hands also can be affected. Refer to Chapter 18 for a complete discussion of OA.

As one ages, muscle tissue atrophies. Increased activity and exercise can slow the progression of atrophy and restore muscle strength (Touhy & Jett, 2014). Musculoskeletal changes cause decreased coordination, loss of muscle strength, gait changes, and a risk for falls with injury. (See Chapter 2 for discussion on fall prevention.) Chart 49-1 lists the major anatomic and physiologic changes and implications for nursing care.

ASSESSMENT METHODS

Patient History

In the assessment of a patient with an actual or potential musculoskeletal problem, a detailed and accurate history is helpful in identifying priority problems and nursing interventions. The history reveals information about the patient that can direct the physical assessment.

Accidents, illnesses, lifestyle, and drugs may contribute to a patient's current problem. Young men are at the greatest risk for trauma related to motor vehicle crashes. Older adults are at the greatest risk for falls that result in fractures and soft-tissue injury. When taking a personal health history, question the patient about any traumatic injuries and sports activities, no matter when they occurred. An injury to the lumbar spine 30 years ago may have caused a patient's current low back pain. A motor vehicle crash or sports injury can cause osteoarthritis years after the event.

Previous or current illness or disease may affect musculoskeletal status. For example, a patient with diabetes who is treated for a foot ulcer is at high risk for acute or chronic osteomyelitis (bone infection). In addition, diabetes slows the healing process. Ask the patient about any previous hospitalizations and illnesses or complications. Inquire about his or her ability to perform ADLs independently or if assistive/adaptive devices are used.

Current lifestyle also contributes to musculoskeletal health. Weight-bearing activities such as walking can reduce risk factors for osteoporosis and maintain muscle strength (McCance et al., 2014). High-impact sports, such as excessive jogging or running, can cause musculoskeletal injury to soft tissues and bone. Tobacco use slows the healing of musculoskeletal injuries. Excessive alcohol intake can decrease vitamins and nutrients the person needs for bone and muscle tissue growth.

When assessing a patient with a possible musculoskeletal alteration, inquire about occupation or work life. A person's occupation can cause or contribute to an injury. For instance, fractures are not uncommon in patients whose jobs require manual labor, such as housekeepers, mechanics, and industrial workers. Certain occupations, such as computer-related jobs, may predispose a person to carpal tunnel syndrome (entrapment of the median nerve in the wrist) or neck pain. Construction workers and health care workers may experience back injury from prolonged standing and excessive lifting. Amateur and professional athletes often experience acute musculoskeletal injuries (e.g., joint dislocations and fractures) and chronic disorders (e.g., joint cartilage trauma), which can lead to osteoarthritis.

Ask about allergies, particularly allergy to dairy products, and previous and current use of drugs—prescribed, over-the-counter, and illicit. Allergy to dairy products could cause decreased calcium intake. Some drugs, such as steroids, can negatively affect calcium metabolism and promote bone loss. Other drugs may be taken to relieve musculoskeletal pain. Inquire about herbs, vitamin and mineral supplements, or biologic compounds that may be used for arthritis and other musculoskeletal problems, such as glucosamine and chondroitin. Complementary and alternative therapies are commonly used by patients with various types of arthritis and arthralgias (joint aching). Chapter 18 discusses these therapies in detail.

Nutrition History

A brief review of the patient's nutrition history helps determine any risks for inadequate nutrient intake. For example, most people, especially women, do not get enough calcium in their diet. Determine if the patient has had a significant weight gain or loss.

Ask the patient to recall a typical day of food intake to help identify deficiencies and excesses in the diet. Lactose intolerance is a common problem that can cause inadequate calcium intake. People who cannot afford to buy food are especially at risk for undernutrition. Some older adults and others are not financially able to buy the proper foods for adequate nutrition.

Inadequate protein or insufficient vitamin C or D in the diet slows bone and tissue healing. Obesity places excess stress and strain on bones and joints, with resulting trauma to joint cartilage. In addition, obesity inhibits MOBILITY in patients with musculoskeletal problems, which predisposes them to complications such as respiratory and circulatory problems. People with eating disorders such as anorexia nervosa and bulimia nervosa are also at risk for osteoporosis related to decreased intake of calcium and vitamin D.

Family History and Genetic Risk

Obtaining a family history assists in identifying disorders that have a familial or genetic tendency. Osteoporosis (age-related bone loss) and gout, for instance, often occur in several generations of a family. Osteogenic sarcoma, a type of bone cancer, may be genetically influenced by *Tp53* gene mutation (Nussbaum et al., 2007). Positive family history of these types of disorders can increase risks to the patient. Chapters 18 and 50 provide a more complete description of musculoskeletal problems that have strong genetic links.

Current Health Problems

The most common reports of persons with a musculoskeletal problem are PAIN and weakness, either of which can impair MOBILITY. Collect data pertinent to the patient's presenting health problem:

- Date and time of onset
- Factors that cause or exacerbate (worsen) the problem
- Course of the problem (e.g., intermittent or continuous)
- Clinical manifestations (as expressed by the patient) and the pattern of their occurrence
- Measures that improve clinical manifestations (e.g., heat, ice)

Assessment of PAIN can present many challenges. Pain can be related to bone, muscle, or joint problems. It may be described as acute or chronic, depending on the onset and duration. Pain with movement could indicate a fracture and/or muscle or joint injury. Assess the intensity of pain by using a pain scale and asking the patient to rate the level he or she is experiencing. Quality of pain may be described as dull, burning, aching, or stabbing. Determine the location of pain and areas to which it radiates. With any assessment, it is always best if the patient describes the pain in his or her own words and points to its location, if possible. Chapter 3 describes acute and chronic pain in detail.

Weakness may be related to individual muscles or muscle groups. Determine if weakness occurs in proximal or distal muscles or muscle groups. Proximal weakness (near trunk of body) may indicate myopathy (a problem in muscle tissue), whereas distal weakness (in extremities) may indicate neuropathy (a problem in nerve tissue). Muscle weakness in the lower extremities may increase the risk for falls and injury. Weakness in the upper extremities may interfere with ADLs.

Assessment of the Skeletal System

Although bones, joints, and muscles are usually assessed simultaneously in a head-to-toe approach, each subsystem is described separately for emphasis and understanding. For physical assessment of the musculoskeletal system, use inspection, palpation, and range of motion (ROM). A general assessment is described in this chapter. More specific assessment techniques are discussed in the musculoskeletal problem chapters in this unit.

General Inspection

Observe the patient's posture, gait, and general mobility for gross deformities and impairment. Note unusual findings, and coordinate with the physical or occupational therapist for an in-depth physical assessment.

Posture and Gait. Posture includes the person's body build and alignment when standing and walking. Assess the curvature of the spine and the length, shape, and symmetry of extremities. Fig. 49-3 illustrates several common spinal deformities. Inspect muscle mass for size and symmetry.

Most patients with musculoskeletal problems eventually have a problem with *gait*. The nurse or therapist evaluates the patient's balance, steadiness, and ease and length of stride. Any limp or other asymmetric leg movement or deformity is noted. An abnormality in the stance phase of gait is called an antalgic gait. When part of one leg is painful, the patient shortens the stance phase on the affected side. An abnormality in the swing phase is called a lurch. This abnormal gait occurs when the muscles in the buttocks and/or legs are too weak to allow the person to change weight from one foot to the other. In this case, the shoulders are moved either side-to-side or front-to-back for help in shifting the weight from one leg to the other. Some patients, such as those with chronic hip pain and muscle atrophy from arthritic disorders, have a combination of an antalgic gait and lurch.

Mobility and Functional Assessment. In collaboration with the physical or occupational therapist, assess the patient's need for ambulatory devices, such as canes and walkers, during

transfer from bed to chair and while walking and climbing stairs. Observe his or her ability to perform ADLs, such as dressing and bathing. PAIN and deformity may limit physical MOBILITY and function. Coordinate with the physical and occupational therapists to assess the patient's functional status. A complete discussion of functional assessment is found in Chapter 6.

Assess major bones, joints, and muscles by inspection, palpation, and determination of ROM. Pay special attention to areas that are affected or may be affected, according to the patient's history or current problem.

A **goniometer** is a tool that may be used by rehabilitation therapists or nurses to provide an exact measurement of flexion and extension or joint ROM. Active range of motion (AROM) can be evaluated by asking the patient to move each joint through the ROM himself or herself. If the patient cannot actively move a joint through range of motion, ask him or her to relax the muscles in the extremity. Hold the part with one hand above and one hand below the joint to be evaluated and allow passive range of motion (PROM) to evaluate joint MOBILITY. Movements shown in Fig. 49-4 may be used to evaluate active and passive ROM. Circumduction is a movement that can also be evaluated in the shoulder by having the patient move the arm in circles from the shoulder joint. As long as the patient can function to meet personal needs, a limitation in ROM may not be significant. For each anatomic location, observe the skin for color, elasticity, and lesions that may relate to musculoskeletal dysfunction. For instance, redness or warmth may indicate an inflammatory process and/or pressure injury to skin.

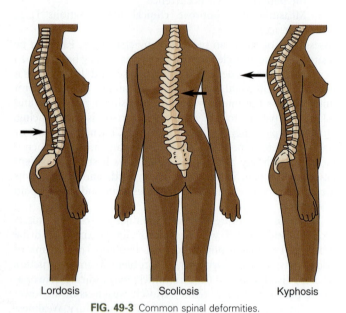

Lordosis   Scoliosis   Kyphosis

FIG. 49-3 Common spinal deformities.

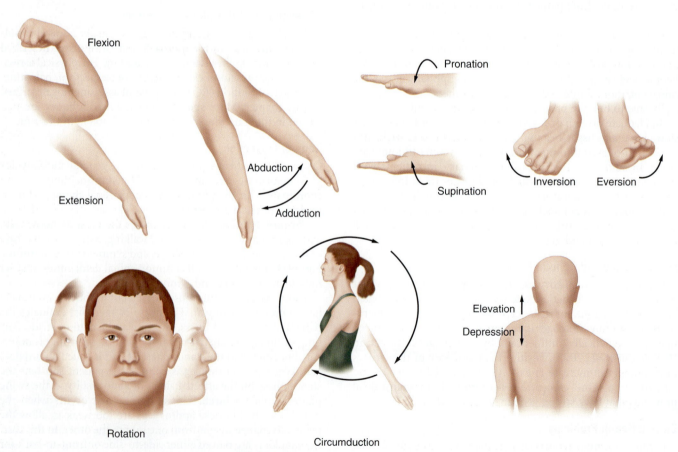

Flexion

Extension

Abduction

Adduction

Pronation

Supination

Inversion   Eversion

Rotation

Circumduction

Elevation

Depression

FIG. 49-4 Movements of the skeletal muscles.

? NCLEX EXAMINATION CHALLENGE

Health Promotion and Maintenance

A nurse is performing a musculoskeletal assessment on an older adult living independently in a senior housing apartment. What normal physiologic changes of aging does the nurse expect? **Select all that apply.**
A. Muscle contractures
B. Slowed movement
C. Lordosis
D. Antalgic gait
E. Decreased coordination

Specific Assessments

If the patient has PAIN or weakness in the *face* or *neck*, inspect and palpate this area for tenderness and masses. Ask the patient to open his or her mouth while palpating the temporomandibular joints (TMJs). Common abnormal findings are tenderness or PAIN, crepitus (a grating sound), and a spongy swelling caused by excess synovium and fluid.

Inspect and palpate each vertebra of the spine in the neck. Proceed cautiously and gently if PAIN is present. Clinical findings may include malalignment; tenderness; or inability to flex, extend, and rotate the neck as expected. Muscle and nerve pain often accompany neck pain if spinal nerves are involved.

The thoracic spine, lumbar spine, and sacral spine are evaluated in the same manner as the neck. Spinal alignment problems are common (see Fig. 49-3). Place both hands over the posterior iliac crests with the thumbs over the lumbosacral area. Apply pressure with the thumbs along the lumbosacral spine to elicit tenderness. Many patients do not have discomfort until the area is palpated. Lordosis is a common finding in adults who have abdominal obesity. During screening for scoliosis, ask the patient to flex forward from the hips and inspect for a lateral curve in the spine.

If the extremities are affected by a musculoskeletal problem, assess arms or legs at the same time for side-to-side comparisons. For example, inspect and palpate both shoulders for size, swelling, deformity, poor alignment, tenderness or PAIN, and MOBILITY. A shoulder injury may prevent the patient from combing his or her hair with the affected arm, but severe arthritis may inhibit movement in both arms. Assess the elbows and wrists in a similar way.

Because the hand has multiple joints in a single digit, assessment of hand function is perhaps the most critical part of the examination. If the hands are affected, inspect and palpate the metacarpophalangeal (MCP), proximal interphalangeal (PIP), and distal interphalangeal (DIP) joints. The same digits are compared on the right and left hands (Fig. 49-5). Determine the range of motion (ROM) for each joint by observing active movement. If movement is not possible, evaluate passive motion. For a quick and easy assessment of ROM, ask the patient to make a fist and then appose each finger to the thumb. If he or she can perform these maneuvers, ROM of the hand is not seriously restricted.

Evaluation of the hip joint relies primarily on determination of its degree of mobility, because the joint is deep and difficult to inspect or palpate. *The patient with hip pain usually experiences it in the groin or has pain that radiates to the knee.* The knee is readily accessible for physical assessment, particularly when the patient is sitting and the knee is flexed. Fluid accumulation,

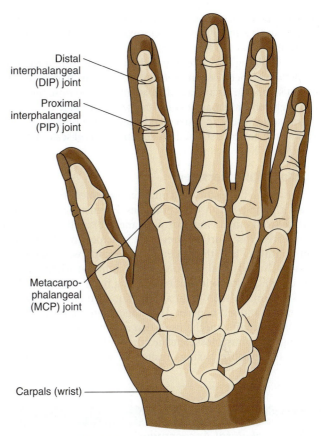

FIG. 49-5 The small joints of the hand.

or effusion, is easily detected in the knee joint. Limitations in movement with accompanying PAIN are common findings. The knees may be poorly aligned, as in genu valgum ("knock-knee") or genu varum ("bowlegged") deformities.

The ankles and feet are often neglected in the physical examination. However, they contain multiple bones and joints that can be affected by disease and injury. Observe and palpate each joint and test for ROM if feet are affected by musculoskeletal problems.

Neurovascular Assessment

While completing a physical assessment of the musculoskeletal system, perform an assessment of peripheral vascular and nerve integrity. Beginning with the injured side, always compare one extremity with the other.

! NURSING SAFETY PRIORITY (QSEN)

Action Alert

Perform a complete neurovascular assessment (also called a "circ check"), which includes *palpation of pulses in the extremities below the level of injury and assessment of sensation, movement, color, temperature, and pain in the injured part*. If pulses are not palpable, use a Doppler to find pulses in the extremities. See Chart 51-3 in Chapter 51 for more details about neurovascular assessment.

Assessment of the Muscular System

During the skeletal assessment, notice the size, shape, tone, and strength of major skeletal muscles. The circumference of each muscle may be measured and compared for symmetry for an estimation of muscle mass if abnormalities are observed.

Ask the patient to demonstrate muscle strength. Apply resistance by holding the extremity and asking the patient to move against resistance. As an option, place your hands on the patient's upper arms and ask the patient to try to raise the arms. Although movement against resistance is not easily quantified, several scales used by nurses and therapists are available for grading the patient's strength. A commonly used scale is shown in Table 49-2.

Psychosocial Assessment

The data from the history and physical assessment provide clues for anticipating psychosocial problems. For instance, prolonged absence from employment or permanent disability may cause job or career loss. Further stress may be experienced if chronic pain continues and the patient cannot cope with numerous stressors. Anxiety and depression are common when patients have chronic pain. Deformities resulting from musculoskeletal disease or injury, such as an amputation, can affect a person's body image and self-concept. Help the patient identify support systems and coping mechanisms that may be useful if he or she has long-term musculoskeletal health problems. Encourage him or her to verbalize feelings related to loss and body image

changes. Refer the patient for psychological or spiritual counseling if needed and if it is culturally appropriate.

Diagnostic Assessment
Laboratory Assessment

Chart 49-2 lists the common laboratory tests used in assessing patients with musculoskeletal disorders. There is no special

TABLE 49-2	Common Scale for Grading Muscle Strength
RATING	**DESCRIPTION**
5	Normal: ROM unimpaired against gravity with full resistance
4	Good: can complete ROM against gravity with some resistance
3	Fair: can complete ROM against gravity
2	Poor: can complete ROM with gravity eliminated
1	Trace: no joint motion and slight evidence of muscle contractility
0	Zero: no evidence of muscle contractility

ROM, Range of motion.

CHART 49-2 Laboratory Profile
Musculoskeletal Assessment

TEST	NORMAL RANGE FOR ADULTS	SIGNIFICANCE OF ABNORMAL FINDINGS
Serum calcium	9.0-10.5 mg/dL (2.25-2.75 mmol/L) *Older adults:* decreased	*Hypercalcemia* (increased calcium) • Metastatic cancers of the bone • Paget's disease • Bone fractures in healing stage *Hypocalcemia* (decreased calcium) • Osteoporosis • Osteomalacia
Serum phosphorus (phosphate)	3.0-4.5 mg/dL (0.97-1.45 mmol/L) *Older adults:* decreased	*Hyperphosphatemia* (increased phosphorus) • Bone fractures in healing stage • Bone tumors • Acromegaly *Hypophosphatemia* (decreased phosphorus) • Osteomalacia
Alkaline phosphatase (ALP)	30-120 units/L *Older adults:* slightly increased	*Elevations* may indicate: • Metastatic cancers of the bone • Paget's disease • Osteomalacia
Serum muscle enzymes Creatine kinase (CK-MM)	Total CK: *Men:* 55-170 units/L *Women:* 30-135 units/L	*Elevations* may indicate: • Muscle trauma • Progressive muscular dystrophy • Effects of electromyography
Lactic dehydrogenase (LDH)	Total LDH: 100-190 units/L LDH_1: 17%-27% LDH_2: 27%-37% LDH_3: 18%-25% LDH_4: 3%-8% LDH_5: 0% to 5%	*Elevations* may indicate: • Skeletal muscle necrosis • Extensive cancer • Progressive muscular dystrophy
Aspartate aminotransferase (AST)	0-35 units/L *Older adults:* slightly increased	*Elevations* may indicate: • Skeletal muscle trauma • Progressive muscular dystrophy
Aldolase (ALD)	3.0-8.2 units/dL	*Elevations* may indicate: • Polymyositis and dermatomyositis • Muscular dystrophy

patient preparation or follow-up care for any of these tests. Teach the patient about the purpose of the test and the procedure that can be expected. Additional tests performed for patients with connective tissue diseases, such as rheumatoid arthritis, are described in Chapter 18.

Disorders of bone and the parathyroid gland are often reflected in an alteration of the serum calcium or phosphorus level. Therefore these electrolytes, especially calcium, are monitored. A decrease in serum calcium could indicate bone density loss.

Alkaline phosphatase (ALP) is an enzyme normally present in blood. The concentration of ALP increases with bone or liver damage. In metabolic bone disease and bone cancer, the enzyme concentration rises in proportion to the osteoblastic activity, which indicates bone formation. The level of ALP is normally slightly increased in older adults (Pagana & Pagana, 2014).

The major *muscle enzymes* affected in skeletal muscle disease or injuries are:

- Creatine kinase (CK-MM)
- Aspartate aminotransferase (AST)
- Aldolase (ALD)
- Lactic dehydrogenase (LDH)

As a result of damage, the muscle tissue releases additional amounts of these enzymes, which increases serum levels.

The serum CK level begins to rise 2 to 4 hours after muscle injury and is elevated early in muscle disease, such as muscular dystrophy. The CK molecule has two subunits: M (muscle) and B (brain). Three isoenzymes have been identified. Skeletal muscle CK (CK-MM, or CK_3) is the only isoenzyme that rises in concentration with damage to skeletal muscle, such as trauma, surgery, and neuromuscular disease. This test is 90% accurate because it is affected by exercise and certain drugs, such as anticoagulants, furosemide, and statins (Kress et al., 2008).

AST is moderately elevated (3 to 5 times normal) in certain muscle diseases, such as muscular dystrophy. The levels of the isoenzymes *aldolase A (ALD-A)* and LDH_5 also increase in patients with these disorders.

Imaging Assessment

The skeleton is very visible on *standard x-rays*. Anteroposterior and lateral projections are the initial screening views used most often. Other approaches, such as oblique or stress views, depend on the part of the skeleton to be evaluated and the reason for the x-ray.

Radiography. Bone density, alignment, swelling, and intactness can be seen on x-ray. The conditions of joints can be determined, including the size of the joint space, the smoothness of articular cartilage, and synovial swelling. Soft-tissue involvement may be evident but not clearly differentiated.

Inform the patient that the x-ray table is hard and cold, and instruct him or her to remain still during the filming process. Coordinate with the radiology department or clinic to keep older adults and those at risk for hypothermia as warm as possible (e.g., by using blankets).

Myelography involves the injection of contrast medium into the subarachnoid space of the spine, usually by spinal puncture. The vertebral column, intervertebral disks, spinal nerve roots, and blood vessels can be visualized. Although this test is still performed, CT and MRI have often replaced such invasive and potentially painful and risky diagnostic techniques. The post-test care is similar to that for lumbar puncture, except that the

patient is usually placed with the head of the bed elevated 30 to 50 degrees to prevent the contrast medium from getting into the brain (see Chapter 41).

An *arthrogram* is an x-ray study of a joint after contrast medium (air or solution) has been injected to enhance its visualization. Double-contrast arthrography, which uses both air and solution, may be performed when a traumatic injury is suspected. The physician can often determine bone chips, torn ligaments, or other loose bodies within the joint. This test is not used commonly because of newer advances in diagnostic imaging. Most joints are now studied by MRI and magnetic resonance (MR) arthrography.

CT has gained wide acceptance for detecting musculoskeletal problems, particularly those of the vertebral column and joints. The scanned images can be used to create additional images from other angles or to create three-dimensional images and view complex structures from any position. The nurse or radiology technologist should ask the patient about iodine-based contrast allergies.

Nuclear Scans. The *bone scan* is a radionuclide test in which radioactive material is injected for viewing the entire skeleton. It may be used primarily to detect tumors, arthritis, osteomyelitis, osteoporosis, vertebral compression fractures, and unexplained bone pain. Bone scans are used less commonly today as more sophisticated MRI equipment becomes more available. However, it may be very useful for detecting hairline fractures in patients with unexplained bone pain and diffuse metastatic bone disease.

The *gallium* and *thallium scans* are similar to the bone scan but are more specific and sensitive in detecting bone problems. Gallium citrate (^{67}Ga) is the radioisotope most commonly used. This substance also migrates to brain, liver, and breast tissue and therefore is used in examination of these structures when disease is suspected.

For patients with osteosarcoma, thallium (^{201}Tl) is better than gallium or technetium for diagnosing the extent of the disease. Thallium has traditionally been used for the diagnosis of myocardial infarctions but can be used for additional evaluation of cancers of the bone.

Because bone takes up gallium slowly, the nuclear medicine physician or technician administers the isotope 4 to 6 hours before scanning. Other tests that require contrast media or other isotopes cannot be given during this time.

Instruct the patient that the radioactive material poses no threat because it readily deteriorates in the body. Because gallium is excreted through the intestinal tract, it tends to collect in feces after the scanning procedure.

Depending on the tissue to be examined, the patient is taken to the nuclear medicine department 4 to 6 hours after injection. The procedure takes 30 to 60 minutes, during which time the patient must lie still for accurate test results to be achieved. The scan may be repeated at 24, 48, and/or 72 hours. Mild sedation may be necessary to facilitate relaxation and cooperation during the procedure for confused older adults or those in severe pain.

No special care is required after the test. The radioisotope is excreted in stool and urine, but no precautions are taken in handling the excreta. Remind the patient to push fluids to facilitate urinary excretion.

Magnetic Resonance Imaging. MRI, with or without the use of contrast media, is commonly used to diagnose musculoskeletal disorders. It is more accurate than CT and myelography for many spinal and knee problems. MRI is most appropriate for joints, soft tissue, and bony tumors that involve soft tissue. CT is still the test of choice for injuries or pathology that involves only bone.

The image is produced through the interaction of magnetic fields, radio waves, and atomic nuclei showing hydrogen density. Simply put, the radio waves "bounce" off the body tissues being examined. Because each tissue has its own density, the computer image clearly distinguishes normal and abnormal tissues. For some tissues, the cross-sectional image is better than that produced by radiography or CT. The lack of hydrogen ions in cortical bone makes it easily distinguishable from soft tissues. The test is particularly useful in identifying problems with muscles, tendons, and ligaments.

Ensure that the patient removes all metal objects and checks for clothing zippers and metal fasteners. Although joint implants made of titanium or stainless steel are usually safe, depending on the age of the MRI equipment, pacemakers, stents, and surgical clips usually are not. Chart 49-3 lists questions that the nurse or technician should consider in preparing the patient for MRI. Open MRIs prevent the claustrophobia that occurs with the older, encased machines.

MR arthrography combines arthrography and magnetic resonance imaging. It is particularly useful for diagnosing problems of the shoulder. The patient's shoulder is injected with gadolinium contrast medium under fluoroscopy. Then the patient is taken for an MRI where the shoulder is examined. This test is particularly useful for diagnosing the type and degree of rotator cuff tears (Smith & Smith, 2010).

Ultrasonography. Sound waves produce an image of the tissue in ultrasonography. An ultrasound procedure may be used to view:

- Soft-tissue disorders, such as masses and fluid accumulation
- Traumatic joint injuries
- Osteomyelitis
- Surgical hardware placement

A jelly-like substance applied to the skin over the site to be examined promotes the movement of a metal probe. No special preparation or post-test care is necessary. A quantitative ultrasound (QUS) may be done for determining fractures or bone density. Bone density testing is discussed in Chapter 50.

Other Diagnostic Assessment

Biopsies. In a **bone biopsy**, the physician extracts a specimen of the bone tissue for microscopic examination. This invasive test may confirm the presence of infection or neoplasm, but it is not commonly done today. One of two techniques may be used to retrieve the specimen: needle (closed) biopsy or incisional (open) biopsy.

! NURSING SAFETY PRIORITY (QSEN)
Action Alert

After a bone biopsy, watch for bleeding from the puncture site and for tenderness, redness, or warmth that could indicate infection. Mild analgesics may be used.

Muscle biopsy is done for the diagnosis of atrophy (as in muscular dystrophy) and inflammation (as in polymyositis). The procedure and care for patients undergoing muscle biopsy are the same as those for patients undergoing bone biopsy.

Electromyography. Although not commonly used today, electromyography (EMG) may be performed to evaluate diffuse or localized muscle weakness. EMG is usually accompanied by nerve conduction studies for determining the electrical potential generated in an individual muscle. This test helps in the diagnosis of neuromuscular, lower motor neuron, and peripheral nerve disorders.

Inform the patient that EMG may cause temporary discomfort, especially when the patient is subjected to episodes of electrical current. For selected patients, mild sedation is prescribed. The physician may also prescribe a temporary discontinuation of skeletal muscle relaxants several days before the procedure to prevent drugs from affecting the test results.

Arthroscopy. **Arthroscopy** may be used as a diagnostic test or a surgical procedure. An arthroscope is a fiberoptic tube inserted into a joint for direct visualization of the ligaments, menisci, and articular surfaces of the joint. The knee and shoulder are most commonly evaluated. In addition, synovial biopsy and surgery to repair traumatic injury can be done through the arthroscope as an ambulatory care or same-day surgical procedure.

Patient Preparation. Arthroscopy is performed on an ambulatory care basis or as same-day surgery. The patient must have mobility in the joint being examined. Those who cannot move the joint or who have an infected joint are not candidates for the procedure.

If the procedure is done for surgical repair, the patient may have a physical therapy consultation before arthroscopy to learn the exercises that are necessary after the test. ROM exercises are also taught but may not be allowed immediately after arthroscopic surgery. The nurse in the surgeon's office or at the surgical center can teach these exercises or reinforce the information provided by the physical therapist. The nurse also reinforces the explanation of the procedure and post-test care and ensures that the patient has signed an informed consent.

Procedure. The patient is usually given local, light general, or epidural anesthesia, depending on the purpose of the procedure. As shown in Fig. 49-6, the arthroscope is inserted through a small incision less than $\frac{1}{4}$-inch (0.6 cm) long. Multiple incisions may be required to allow inspection at a variety of angles. After the procedure, a dressing may be applied, depending on the amount of manipulation during the test or surgery.

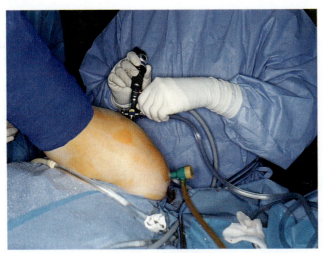

FIG. 49-6 An arthroscope is used in the diagnosis of pathologic changes in the joints. This patient is undergoing arthroscopy of the shoulder.

Postprocedure Care. The immediate care after an arthroscopy is the same for patients having the procedure for diagnostic purposes as for those having it for surgical intervention.

! NURSING SAFETY PRIORITY (QSEN)

Action Alert

The priority for postprocedure care after arthroscopy is to assess the neurovascular status of the patient's affected limb every hour or according to agency or surgeon protocol. Monitor and document distal pulses, warmth, color, capillary refill, PAIN, movement, and sensation of the affected extremity.

Encourage the patient to perform exercises as taught before the procedure, if appropriate. For the mild discomfort experienced after the diagnostic arthroscopy, the surgeon prescribes a mild analgesic, such as acetaminophen (Tylenol, Ace-Tabs ✦). If postoperative, the patient may have short-term activity restrictions, depending on the musculoskeletal problem. Ice is often used for 24 hours, and the extremity should be elevated for 12 to 24 hours. When arthroscopic surgery is performed, the health care provider usually prescribes an opioid-analgesic combination, such as oxycodone and acetaminophen (Percocet, Tylox).

Although complications are not common, monitor and teach the patient to observe for:
- Swelling
- Increased joint pain attributable to mechanical injury
- Thrombophlebitis
- Infection

Severe joint or limb PAIN after discharge may indicate a possible complication. Teach the patient to contact the physician immediately. The surgeon usually sees the patient about 1 week after the procedure to check for complications.

? NCLEX EXAMINATION CHALLENGE

Safe and Effective Care Environment

A client returns to the postanesthesia care unit (PACU) after an arthroscopy for a shoulder rotator cuff tear. What is the nurse's priority when caring for this client?
A. Perform passive range-of-motion exercises.
B. Keep the affected arm immobilized.
C. Ensure that the patient uses the patient-controlled analgesia (PCA) pump.
D. Check the neurovascular status of the affected arm.

NURSING CONCEPTS AND CLINICAL JUDGMENT REVIEW

What might you NOTICE in a patient with adequate MOBILITY and SENSORY PERCEPTION related to the musculoskeletal system?

Physical assessment:
- No gross deformities or impairments in posture or gait
- Adequate size, strength, and symmetry of muscle for age
- Can perform ADLs independently
- Can perform other routine daily activities independently
- Can ambulate with or without assistive devices
- No pain or tenderness on palpation or passive range-of-motion (ROM) of joints

- Active ROM of joints within normal limits for age
- No crepitus when moving joints
- No swelling of joints or extremities
- Equal size and alignment of extremities
- Equal sensation in extremities

Diagnostic assessment:
- Muscle enzymes (e.g., CK-MM, ALD) within normal limits for age
- Bone density adequate for age and gender
- Joint changes within normal limits for age

GET READY FOR THE NCLEX® EXAMINATION!

KEY POINTS

Review these Key Points for each NCLEX Examination Client Needs Category.

Safe and Effective Care Environment
- Collaborate with the physical and/or occupational therapist to perform a complete musculoskeletal assessment, including gait, muscle strength, and ADL ability, as indicated. **Teamwork and Collaboration** (QSEN)

Health Promotion and Maintenance
- Be aware that older adults have physiologic changes that affect their musculoskeletal system, such as decreased bone

density and joint cartilage degeneration (see Chart 49-1). **Patient-Centered Care** [QSEN]

Psychosocial Integrity
- Assess the patient's support systems and coping mechanisms when musculoskeletal trauma or disease affects his or her body image. **Patient-Centered Care** [QSEN]
- Ask about the patient's occupation, because heavy manual labor may cause back injury and other musculoskeletal trauma.

Physiological Integrity
- Assess the patient's pain intensity, quality, duration, and location.
- Assess the patient's mobility, including gait, posture, and muscle strength.

- Interpret the patient's laboratory values that are related to musculoskeletal disease (see Chart 49-2).
- Teach the patient that mild discomfort can be expected during electromyography, a test to assess the electrical potential of muscles and their innervation.
- Instruct the patient to report swelling, infection, and increased pain after an arthroscopy.
- Ask the patient questions to ensure safety before an MRI (see Chart 49-3). **Safety** [QSEN]
- Ask the patient about allergy to contrast media before diagnostic testing such as CT scans.
- Evaluate the neurovascular status of the patient's affected extremity after an arthroscopic procedure as the *priority for care*. **Safety** [QSEN]

CHAPTER 50

Care of Patients with Musculoskeletal Problems

Donna D. Ignatavicius

 http://evolve.elsevier.com/Iggy/

PRIORITY CONCEPTS

- PAIN
- MOBILITY

- INFLAMMATION
- INFECTION

LEARNING OUTCOMES

Safe and Effective Care Environment

1. Coordinate with health care team members when planning and providing high quality care for patients with musculoskeletal problems.
2. Teach the patient and family about home safety when the patient has a metabolic bone problem such as osteoporosis.

Health Promotion and Maintenance

3. Identify community resources for patients with musculoskeletal problems that impair mobility.
4. Develop a patient-centered teaching plan for all age-groups about ways to decrease the risk for osteoporosis.
5. Assess the genetic risk for patients who have parents with muscular dystrophy.

Psychosocial Integrity

6. Assess the patient's and family's responses to a bone cancer diagnosis and treatment options.

Physiological Integrity

7. Educate the patient and family about common drugs used for bone diseases, such as calcium supplements and bisphosphonates, to promote patient safety.
8. Compare and contrast osteoporosis and osteomalacia.
9. Identify key features of Paget's disease of the bone.
10. Prioritize care for patients with osteomyelitis.
11. Identify collaborative management options for treating patients with primary and metastatic bone cancer.
12. Describe common disorders of the foot, including hallux valgus and plantar fasciitis, that can affect MOBILITY.
13. Explain the role of the nurse when caring for an adult patient with muscular dystrophy.

Musculoskeletal disorders include metabolic bone diseases (e.g., osteoporosis and Paget's disease), bone tumors, and a variety of deformities and syndromes. Older adults are at the greatest risk for most of these problems, although *primary* bone cancer is most often found in adolescents and young adults. As technology advances and patients survive longer with primary cancers, metastatic lesions have become more prevalent among older adults. Almost all musculoskeletal health problems can cause the patient to have difficulty meeting the human need of MOBILITY. This chapter focuses on selected disorders not covered in Chapter 18 on arthritis and other connective tissue diseases.

METABOLIC BONE DISEASES

OSTEOPOROSIS

❖ PATHOPHYSIOLOGY

Osteoporosis is a chronic metabolic disease in which bone loss causes decreased density and possible fracture. It is often referred to as a "silent disease" or "silent thief" because the first sign of osteoporosis in most people follows some kind of a fracture (Kamienski et al., 2011). The spine, hip, and wrist are most often at risk, although any bone can fracture (National Osteoporosis Foundation [NOF], 2010).

Osteoporosis is a major health problem in the world. The estimated cost for osteoporosis-related health care alone in the United States is more than $18 billion each year with continual cost increases each year. By 2040, that number is expected to double or triple as baby boomers become older adults (NOF, 2010).

Bone is a dynamic tissue that is constantly undergoing changes in a process referred to as **bone remodeling**. Osteoporosis and **osteopenia** (low bone mass) occur when osteoclastic (bone resorption) activity is greater than osteoblastic (bone building) activity. The result is a decreased **bone mineral density (BMD)**. BMD determines bone strength and peaks between 25 and 30 years of age. Before and during the peak years, osteoclastic activity and osteoblastic activity work at the same rate. After the peak years, bone resorption activity exceeds bone-building activity and bone density decreases. BMD decreases most rapidly in postmenopausal women as serum estrogen levels diminish. Although estrogen does not build bone, it helps prevent bone loss. Trabecular, or cancellous (spongy), bone is lost first, followed by loss of cortical (compact) bone. This results in thin, fragile bone tissue that is at risk for fracture.

Standards for the diagnosis of osteoporosis are based on BMD testing that provides a T-score for the patient. A T-score represents the number of standard deviations above or below the average BMD for young, healthy adults. *Osteopenia is present when the T-score is at −1 and above −2.5. Osteoporosis is diagnosed in a person who has a T-score at or lower than −2.5.* Medicare reimburses for BMD testing every 2 years in people ages 65 years and older who (NOF, 2010):

- Are estrogen deficient
- Have vertebral abnormalities
- Receive long-term steroid therapy
- Have primary hyperparathyroidism
- Are being monitored while on osteoporosis drug therapy

Osteoporosis can be classified as generalized or regional. *Generalized* osteoporosis involves many structures in the skeleton and is further divided into two categories—primary and secondary. *Primary* osteoporosis is more common and occurs in postmenopausal women and in men in their seventh or eighth decade of life. Even though men do not experience the rapid bone loss that postmenopausal women have, they do have decreasing levels of testosterone (which builds bone) and altered ability to absorb calcium. This results in a slower loss of bone mass in men, especially those older than 75 years. *Secondary* osteoporosis may result from other medical conditions, such as hyperparathyroidism; long-term drug therapy, such as with corticosteroids; or prolonged immobility, such as that seen with spinal cord injury (Table 50-1). Treatment of the secondary type is directed toward the cause of the osteoporosis when possible.

Regional osteoporosis, an example of secondary disease, occurs when a limb is immobilized related to a fracture, injury, or paralysis. Immobility for longer than 8 to 12 weeks can result in this type of osteoporosis. Bone loss also occurs when people spend prolonged time in a gravity-free or weightless environment (e.g., astronauts).

Etiology and Genetic Risk

Primary osteoporosis is caused by a combination of genetic, lifestyle, and environmental factors. Chart 50-1 lists the major factors that contribute to the development of this disease.

TABLE 50-1 **Causes of Secondary Osteoporosis**

Diseases/Conditions	Drugs (Chronic Use)
• Diabetes mellitus	• Corticosteroids
• Hyperthyroidism	• Anti-epileptic drugs (AEDs) (e.g., phenytoin)
• Hyperparathyroidism	• Barbiturates (e.g., phenobarbital)
• Cushing's syndrome	• Ethanol (alcohol)
• Growth hormone deficiency	• Drugs that induce hypogonadism (decreased levels of sex hormones)
• Metabolic acidosis	
• Female hypogonadism	
• Paget's disease	• High levels of thyroid hormone
• Osteogenesis imperfecta	• Cytotoxic agents
• Rheumatoid arthritis	• Immunosuppressants
• Prolonged immobilization	• Loop diuretics
• Bone cancer	• Aluminum-based antacids
• Cirrhosis	
• HIV/AIDS	
• Chronic airway limitation	

AIDS, Acquired immune deficiency syndrome; *HIV*, human immune deficiency virus.

CHART 50-1 **Best Practice for Patient Safety & Quality Care** **QSEN**

Assessing Risk Factors for Primary Osteoporosis

Assess for:
- Older age in both genders and all races
- Parental history of osteoporosis, especially mother
- History of low-trauma fracture after age 50 years
- Low body weight, thin build
- Chronic low calcium and/or vitamin D intake
- Estrogen or androgen deficiency
- Current smoking (active or passive)
- High alcohol intake (3 or more drinks a day)
- Lack of physical exercise or prolonged immobility

GENETIC/GENOMIC CONSIDERATIONS

Patient-Centered Care **QSEN**

The genetic and immune factors that cause osteoporosis are very complex. Strong evidence demonstrates that genetics is a significant factor, with a heritability of 50% to 90% (Chang et al., 2010). Many genetic changes have been identified as possible causative factors, but there is no agreement about which ones are most important or constant in all patients. For example, changes in the vitamin D_3 receptor *(VDR)* gene and calcitonin receptor *(CTR)* gene have been found in some patients with the disease. Receptors are essential for the uptake and use of these substances by the cells.

The bone morphogenetic protein-2 *(BMP-2)* gene has a key role in bone formation and maintenance. Some osteoporotic patients who had fractures have changes in their *BMP-2* gene. Alterations in growth hormone-1 (GH-1) have been discovered in petite Asian-American women, those who are predisposed to developing osteoporosis.

Hormones, tumor necrosis factor (TNF), interleukins, and other substances in the body help control osteoclasts in a very complex pathway. The identification of the importance of the cytokine receptor activator of nuclear factor kappa-B ligand *(RANKL)*, its receptor *RANK*, and its decoy receptor osteoprotegerin *(OPG)* has helped researchers understand more about the activity of osteoclasts in metabolic bone disease. Disruptions in the *RANKL, RANK,* and *OPG* system can lead to increased osteoclast activity in which bone is rapidly broken down (McCance et al., 2014).

EVIDENCE-BASED PRACTICE (QSEN)

What Do Men Know About Their Risk of Osteoporosis?

Doheny, M.O., Sedlak, C.A., Estok, P.J., & Zeller, R.A. (2011). Bone density, health beliefs, and osteoporosis preventing behaviors in men. *Orthopaedic Nursing, 30*(4), 266-272.

The researchers conducted an experimental, two-group longitudinal study to examine the effect of dual-energy x-ray absorptiometry (DXA) results on osteoporosis preventing behaviors (OPB), health beliefs, and knowledge of osteoporosis of men ages 50 years or older. The sample was obtained through a community call for volunteers, and the participants were randomly assigned to either the control or experimental group. At the beginning of the study, all 196 subjects received information on osteoporosis diagnosis and management and completed a series of questionnaires. All subjects also had a free DXA test in which 50 men were found to be osteopenic or osteoporotic. Knowledge about osteoporosis was not a predictor of calcium intake or exercise. Although the osteoporotic men increased their calcium and increased their exercise, the amount of each intervention was below the national recommendations. Health beliefs predicted both calcium intake and exercise.

Level of Evidence: 2

This study used an experimental design over a period of time to determine changes in behavior.

Commentary: Implications for Practice and Research

Very little research has been done on the diagnosis and management of osteoporosis in men. This study used an experimental design to examine multiple factors. Nurses and other health care professionals need to educate men older than 50 years about the risk for and prevention of osteoporosis. The cost of DXA screening is far less than the financial, social, and health care costs of osteoporosis.

The subjects in the convenience sample were fairly well educated, almost all were white, and most were married. Further studies are needed using more diverse samples to allow generalization of the findings of this research.

GENDER HEALTH CONSIDERATIONS

Patient-Centered Care (QSEN)

Primary osteoporosis most often occurs in women after menopause as a result of decreased estrogen levels. Women lose about 2% of their bone mass every year in the first 5 years after natural or surgical (ovary removal) menopause. Obese women can store estrogen in their tissues for use as necessary to maintain a normal level of serum calcium.

Men also develop osteoporosis after the age of 50 years because their testosterone levels decrease. Testosterone is the major sex hormone that builds bone tissue. Men are often underdiagnosed, even when they become older adults (Swislocki et al., 2010; Voda, 2009b). In a large experimental study, Doheny et al. (2011) found that men lacked knowledge about osteoporosis and their risk for the disease (see the Evidence-Based Practice box).

The relationship of osteoporosis to nutrition is well established. For example, excessive caffeine in the diet can cause calcium loss in the urine. A diet lacking enough calcium and vitamin D stimulates the parathyroid gland to produce parathyroid hormone (PTH). PTH triggers the release of calcium from the bony matrix. Activated vitamin D is needed for calcium uptake in the body. Malabsorption of nutrients in the GI tract also contributes to low serum calcium levels. Institutionalized or homebound patients who are not exposed to sunlight may be at a higher risk because they do not receive adequate vitamin D for the metabolism of calcium.

Calcium loss occurs at a more rapid rate when phosphorus intake is high. (Chapter 11 describes the usual relationship between calcium and phosphorus in the body.) People who drink large amounts of carbonated beverages each day (over 40 ounces) are at high risk for calcium loss and subsequent osteoporosis, regardless of age or gender.

Protein deficiency may also reduce bone density. Because 50% of serum calcium is protein bound, protein is needed to use calcium. However, excessive protein intake may increase calcium loss in the urine. For instance, people who are on high-protein, low-carbohydrate diets, like the Atkins diet, may consume too much protein to replace other food not allowed. Dietary protein intake in healthy adults is recommended at 0.8 grams per kilogram of body weight. Protein is needed for bone healing when a fracture occurs.

Excessive alcohol and tobacco use are other risk factors for osteoporosis. Although the exact mechanisms are not known, these substances promote acidosis, which in turn increases bone loss. Alcohol also has a direct toxic effect on bone tissue, resulting in decreased bone formation and increased bone resorption. For those people who have excessive alcohol intake, alcohol calories decrease hunger and the need to take in adequate amounts of nutrients.

Incidence and Prevalence

Osteoporosis is a potential health problem for more than 44 million Americans. About 10 million people in the United States have the disease, and about 34 million people 50 years of age and older have osteopenia and are at risk for development of osteoporosis. Women remain the largest group affected by osteoporosis, although some men, especially those older than 75 years, also have the disease.

🌐 CULTURAL CONSIDERATIONS

Patient-Centered Care (QSEN)

Body build, weight, and race/ethnicity seem to influence who gets the disease. Osteoporosis occurs most often in older, lean-built Euro-American and Asian women, particularly those who do not exercise regularly. However, African Americans are at risk for decreased vitamin D, which is needed for adequate calcium absorption in the small intestines. Dietary preferences or intolerances or the inability to afford high-nutrient food may influence anyone's rate of bone loss. For example, many blacks have lactose intolerance and cannot drink regular milk or eat other dairy-based foods (NOF, 2010). Lactose-free milk (e.g., Lactaid) or soy milk provides calcium. Milk and cheese are good sources of protein, a nutrient needed to bind calcium for use by the body.

Osteoporosis results in more than 1.5 million fragility fractures each year (NOF, 2010). A woman who experiences a hip fracture has a 4 times greater risk for a second fracture. Fractures as a result of osteoporosis and falling can decrease a patient's MOBILITY and quality of life. The mortality rate for older patients with hip fractures is very high, especially within the first 6 months, and the debilitating effects can be devastating.

Health Promotion and Maintenance

Peak bone mass is achieved by about 30 years of age in most women. *Building strong bone as a young person may be the best defense against osteoporosis in later adulthood.* Young women need to be aware of appropriate health and lifestyle practices that can prevent this potentially disabling disease. Teaching should begin with young women because they begin to lose bone after 30 years of age. Nurses can play a vital role in patient education for women of any age to prevent and manage osteoporosis.

The focus of osteoporosis prevention is to decrease modifiable risk factors. For example, teach patients who do not include enough dietary calcium which foods to eat, such as dairy products and dark green leafy vegetables. Teach them to read food labels for sources of calcium content. Explain the importance of sun exposure (but not so much as to get sunburned) and adequate vitamin D in the diet. The National Osteoporosis Foundation recommends taking a vitamin D_3 supplement for all adults. Patients being treated for osteopenia or osteomalacia (vitamin D deficiency) may be prescribed high therapeutic doses up to 20,000 international units a week (NOF, 2010).

Teach the need to limit the amount of carbonated beverages consumed each day. Remind patients who have sedentary lifestyles about the importance of exercise and what types of exercise builds bone tissue. Weight-bearing exercises, such as regularly scheduled walking, are preferred. Teach high-risk people to avoid activities that cause jarring, such as horseback riding and jogging, to prevent potential vertebral compression fractures.

❖ PATIENT-CENTERED COLLABORATIVE CARE

◆ Assessment

A complete health history with assessment of risk factors is important in the prevention, early detection, and treatment of osteoporosis. Patients who have risk factors for osteoporosis are at increased risk for fractures when falls occur. Include a fall risk assessment in the health history, especially for older adults. Assess for fall risk factors as described in Chapter 2. The Joint Commission's National Patient Safety Goals (NPSGs) specify the need to reduce risk for harm to patients resulting from falls. People with osteoporosis are at an increased risk for fracture if a fall occurs.

Physical Assessment/Clinical Manifestations. When performing a musculoskeletal assessment, inspect and palpate the vertebral column. The classic "dowager's hump," or kyphosis of the dorsal spine, is often present (Fig. 50-1). The patient may state that he or she has gotten shorter, perhaps as much as 2 to 3 inches (5 to 7.5 cm) within the previous 20 years. Take or delegate height and weight measurements, and compare with previous measurements if they are available.

The patient may have back pain, which often occurs after lifting, bending, or stooping. The pain may be sharp and acute in onset. Pain is worse with activity and is relieved by rest. Palpation of the vertebrae, particularly the lower thoracic and lumbar vertebrae, can increase the patient's discomfort. Therefore palpation should be gentle.

Back pain accompanied by tenderness and voluntary restriction of spinal movement suggests one or more compression vertebral fractures—the most common type of osteoporotic fracture. Movement restriction and spinal deformity may result in constipation, abdominal distention, reflux esophagitis, and respiratory compromise in severe cases. The most likely area for spinal fracture is between T8 and L3.

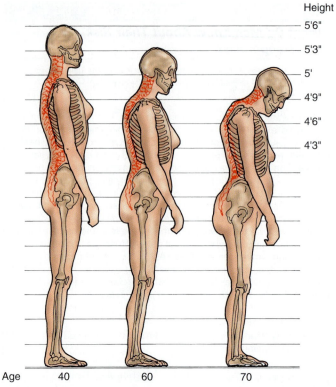

FIG. 50-1 A normal spine at age 40 years and osteoporotic changes at ages 60 and 70 years. These changes can cause a loss of as much as 6 inches in height and can result in the so-called *dowager's hump (far right)* in the upper thoracic vertebrae.

Fractures are also common in the distal end of the radius (wrist) and the upper third of the femur (hip). Ask the patient to locate all areas that are painful, and observe for signs and symptoms of fractures, such as swelling and malalignment. Fractures are discussed in Chapter 51.

Psychosocial Assessment. Women associate osteoporosis with menopause, getting older, and becoming less independent. The disease can result in suffering, deformity, and disability that can affect the patient's well-being and life satisfaction. The quality of life may be further impacted by pain, insomnia, depression, and **fallophobia** (fear of falling) (Touhy & Jett, 2014).

Assess the patient's concept of body image, especially if he or she is severely kyphotic. For example, the patient may have difficulty finding clothes that fit properly. Social interactions may be avoided because of a change in appearance or the physical limitations of being unable to sit in chairs in restaurants, movie theaters, and other places. Changes in sexuality may occur as a result of poor self-esteem or the discomfort caused by positioning during intercourse.

Because osteoporosis poses a risk for fractures, teach the patient to be extremely cautious about activities. As a result, the threat of fracture can create anxiety and fear and result in further limitation of social or physical activities. Assess for these feelings to assist in treatment decisions and health teaching. For example, the patient may not exercise as prescribed for fear that a fracture will occur.

Laboratory Assessment. No definitive laboratory tests confirm a diagnosis of primary osteoporosis, although a number of *biochemical markers* can provide information about bone resorption and formation activity. Although not commonly tested, these biochemical markers are sensitive to bone changes and can be used to monitor effectiveness of treatment for osteoporosis. *Bone-specific alkaline phosphatase (BSAP)* is found in the cell membrane of the osteoblast and indicates bone formation status. *Osteocalcin* is a protein substance in bone and increases during bone resorption activity. Pyridinium (PYD) cross-links are released into circulation during bone resorption. *N-telopeptide (NTX)* and *C-telopeptide (CTX)* are proteins released when bone is broken down. Some laboratories require a 24-hour urine collection for testing, whereas others use a double-voided specimen. Some markers, like NTX and CTX, can also be measured in the blood using immunoassay techniques. Increased levels of any of these markers indicate a risk for osteoporosis. Increased levels are found in patients with osteoporosis, Paget's disease, and bone tumors (Pagana & Pagana, 2014).

Serum calcium and vitamin D₃ levels should be routinely monitored (at least once a year) for all women and men older than 50 years who are at a high risk for the disease. These results determine the need for drug supplements.

A battery of tests can be performed to rule out secondary osteoporosis or other metabolic bone diseases, such as osteomalacia and Paget's disease. These include measurements of serum calcium, vitamin D, and phosphorus. Urinary calcium levels may also be assessed.

Imaging Assessment. Conventional x-rays of the spine and long bones show decreased bone density but only after a 25% to 40% bone loss has occurred. Fractures can also be seen on x-ray.

The most commonly used screening and diagnostic tool for measuring bone mineral density (BMD) is **dual x-ray absorptiometry** (**DXA**, or **DEXA**). The spine and hip are most often assessed when central DXA (cDXA) scan is performed. Many physicians recommend that women in their 40s have a baseline screening DXA scan so that later bone changes can be detected and compared. DXA is a painless scan that emits less radiation than a chest x-ray. *It is the best tool currently available for a definite diagnosis of osteoporosis.* A height is taken prior to performing the test. The patient stays dressed but is asked to remove any metallic objects such as belt buckles, coins, keys, or jewelry that might interfere with the test. The results are displayed on a computer graph, and a T-score is calculated. No special follow-up care for the test is required. However, the patient needs to discuss the results with the primary care provider for any decisions about possible preventive or management interventions.

A peripheral DXA (pDXA) scan assesses BMD of the heel, forearm, or finger. It is often used for large-scale screening purposes. The pDXA is commonly used for screening at community health fairs, skilled nursing facilities, and women's health centers.

Peripheral quantitative ultrasound (pQUS) is an effective and low-cost peripheral screening tool that can detect osteoporosis and predict risk for hip fracture. The heel, tibia, and patella are most commonly tested. The procedure requires no special preparation, is quick, and has no radiation exposure or specific follow-up care (Pagana & Pagana, 2014). The National Osteoporosis Foundation recommends that men older than 70 years have the pQUS as a screening tool for the disease (NOF, 2010).

◆ *Analysis*

The most common problem for patients with osteoporosis or osteopenia is *potential for fractures related to weak, porous bone tissue.*

◆ *Planning and Implementation*

Planning: Expected Outcomes. The expected outcome is that the patient avoids fractures by preventing falls, managing risk factors, and adhering to preventive or treatment measures for bone loss.

Interventions. Because the patient is predisposed to fractures, nutritional therapy, exercise, lifestyle changes, and drug therapy are used to slow bone resorption and form new bone tissue. Self-management education (SME) can help prevent osteoporosis or slow the progress.

Nutrition Therapy. The nutritional considerations for the treatment of a patient with a diagnosis of osteoporosis are the same as those for preventing the disease. Teach patients about the adequate amounts of protein, magnesium, vitamin K, and trace minerals that are needed for bone formation. Calcium and vitamin D intake should be increased. Teach patients to avoid excessive alcohol and caffeine consumption. For the patient who has sustained a fracture, adequate intake of protein, vitamin C, and iron is important to promote bone healing. People who are lactose intolerant can choose a variety of soy and rice products that are fortified with calcium and vitamin D. In addition, calcium and vitamin D are added to many fruit juices, bread, and cereal products.

A variety of nutrients are needed to maintain bone health. *The promotion of a single nutrient will not prevent or treat osteoporosis.* Help the patient develop a nutritional plan that is most beneficial in maintaining bone health; the plan should emphasize fruits and vegetables, low-fat dairy and protein sources, increased fiber, and moderation in alcohol and caffeine (NOF, 2010).

Lifestyle Changes. Exercise is important in the prevention and management of osteoporosis. It also plays a vital role in PAIN management, cardiovascular function, and an improved sense of well-being.

In collaboration with the health care provider, the physical therapist may prescribe exercises for strengthening the abdominal and back muscles for those at risk for vertebral fractures. These exercises improve posture and support for the spine. Abdominal muscle tightening, deep breathing, and pectoral stretching are stressed to increase lung capacity. Exercises for the extremity muscles include muscle-tightening, resistive, and range-of-motion (ROM) exercises. Encourage active ROM exercises, which improve joint MOBILITY and increase muscle tone, as well as prescribed exercise activities. Swimming provides overall muscle exercise.

In addition to exercises for muscle strengthening, a general weight-bearing exercise program should be implemented. Teach patients that walking for 30 minutes 3 to 5 times a week is the single most effective exercise for osteoporosis prevention.

In addition to nutrition and exercise, other lifestyle changes may be needed. Teach the patient to avoid tobacco in any form, especially cigarette smoking. Remind women not to consume more than one alcoholic drink per day (5 ounces each); instruct men not to have more than two alcoholic drinks per day.

Hospitals and long-term care facilities have risk management programs to assess for the risk for falls. For those patients at high risk, communicate this information to other members of the health care team, using colored armbands or other easy-to-recognize methods (National Patient Safety Goals). Chapter 2 discusses fall prevention in health care agencies and at home in more detail.

Drug Therapy. Drug therapy is used when the BMD T-score for the hip is below −2.0 with no other risk factors or when the T-score is below −1.5 with one or more risk factors or previous fracture (NOF, 2010). The health care provider may prescribe calcium and vitamin D₃ supplements, bisphosphonates, or estrogen agonist/antagonists (formerly called *selective estrogen receptor modulators*) or a combination of several drugs to treat or prevent osteoporosis (Chart 50-2). Estrogen and combination hormone therapy are not used solely for osteoporosis prevention or management because they can increase other health risks such as breast cancer and myocardial infarction.

Calcium and Activated Vitamin D (D₃). Intake of *calcium* alone is not a treatment for osteoporosis, but calcium is an important part of a *prevention* program to promote bone health. Most people cannot or do not have enough calcium in their diet, and therefore calcium supplements are needed. Calcium carbonate, found in over-the-counter (OTC) drugs such as Os-Cal, is one of the most cost-effective supplement formulas. Calcium citrate, available OTC as Citracal, is often recommended for those who have gastric upset when taking a calcium supplement. Teach patients to take calcium supplements with food and 6 to 8 ounces of water, although Citracal can be taken anytime. It is best to divide the daily dose, with at least one third of the daily dose being taken in the evening. Teach women to start taking supplements in young adulthood to assist in maintaining peak bone mass. Instruct patients of any age to take calcium supplements that also contain a small amount of activated vitamin D (D₃), such as Os-Cal Ultra.

Because vitamin D is needed for calcium absorption by the body, vitamin D₃ supplementation is often indicated. Both calcium and vitamin D₃ are OTC supplements. Remind patients to take these drugs under the supervision of a health care provider. Hypercalcemia (excess serum calcium) can cause serious damage to the urinary system and other body systems. Teach patients to drink plenty of fluids to prevent urinary calculi (stones). Remind them to have regular laboratory assessments of their calcium and vitamin D₃ serum levels. Chapter 11 describes the clinical manifestations of hypercalcemia.

Bisphosphonates. Bisphosphonates (BPs) slow bone resorption by binding with crystal elements in bone, especially spongy, trabecular bone tissue. They are the most common drugs used for osteoporosis, but some are also approved for Paget's disease and hypercalcemia related to cancer. Three Food and Drug Administration (FDA)–approved BPs—alendronate (Fosamax), ibandronate (Boniva), and risedronate (Actonel, Atelvia)—are commonly used for the *prevention and treatment* of osteoporosis (Lilley et al., 2014). These drugs are available as oral preparations, with ibandronate (Boniva) also available as an IV preparation.

After taking any of these drugs for 3 years, the patient has a DXA scan. If bone density has improved or is maintained, the primary care provider may discontinue the bisphosphonate until the next scan in another 3 years. At that time, the provider will determine if the drug needs to be restarted. For some patients, long-term bisphosphonate use may cause osteonecrosis (discussed below) or a long-bone fracture.

❗ NURSING SAFETY PRIORITY (QSEN)

Drug Alert

Do not confuse Fosamax with Flomax, a selective alpha-adrenergic blocker used for benign prostatic hyperplasia (BPH).

Oral BPs are commonly associated with a serious problem called **esophagitis** (inflammation of the esophagus). Esophageal ulcers have also been reported with the use of BPs, especially when the tablet is not completely swallowed.

❗ NURSING SAFETY PRIORITY (QSEN)

Drug Alert

To promote safety, teach patients to take bisphosphonates (BPs) early in the morning with 8 ounces of water and wait 30 to 60 minutes in an upright position before eating. If chest discomfort occurs, a symptom of esophageal irritation, instruct patients to discontinue the drug and contact their health care provider. Patients with poor renal function, hypocalcemia, or gastroesophageal reflux disease (GERD) should not take BPs.

The most recent additions to the bisphosphonates are IV zoledronic acid (Reclast) and IV pamidronate (Aredia). For management of osteoporosis, Reclast is needed only once a year and Aredia is given every 3 to 6 months. Both drugs have been linked to a complication called jaw **osteonecrosis** (also known as *avascular necrosis,* or *bone death*) in which infection and necrosis of the mandible or maxilla occur (Lilley et al., 2014). The incidence of this serious problem is low but can be a complication of this infusion therapy.

❗ NURSING SAFETY PRIORITY (QSEN)

Drug Alert

Teach patients to have an oral assessment and preventive dentistry before beginning any bisphosphonate therapy. To promote safety, instruct them to inform any dentist who is planning invasive treatment, such as a tooth extraction or implant, that they are taking a BP drug (Cohen, 2010).

Estrogen Agonist/Antagonists. Formerly called the *selective estrogen receptor modulators (SERMs)*, estrogen agonist/antagonists are a class of drugs designed to mimic estrogen in some parts of the body while blocking its effect elsewhere. Raloxifene (Evista) is currently the only approved drug in this class and is used for *prevention and treatment* of osteoporosis in postmenopausal women. Raloxifene increases bone mineral density (BMD), reduces bone resorption, and reduces the incidence of osteoporotic vertebral fractures. The drug should not be given to women who have a history of thromboembolism.

Monoclonal Antibodies. A newer type of drug is denosumab (Prolia, Xgeva), a monoclonal antibody that has been approved

CHART 50-2   **Common Examples of Drug Therapy**

Osteoporosis

DRUG AND USUAL DOSAGE	PURPOSE OF DRUG	NURSING INTERVENTIONS	RATIONALES
Supplements			
Calcium (with vitamin D if needed) (e.g., Os-Cal, Citracal) 1-1.5 g in divided doses orally daily	Increases calcium intake (and vitamin D if needed)	Give a third of daily dose at bedtime. Push fluids.	Calcium is most readily utilized by the body when the patient is fasting and immobile. Increased fluid intake aids in preventing the formation of calcium-based urinary stones.
		Assess for a history of urinary stones.	Calcium supplements are not given to patients who are susceptible to urinary stone formation.
		Monitor serum calcium level.	Hypercalcemia, or calcium excess, is a side effect of calcium supplementation.
		Monitor urinary calcium level (no more than 4 mg/kg in 24 hr).	The kidneys attempt to excrete excess calcium.
		Observe for signs of hypercalcemia.	Hypercalcemia can result in urinary stones, cardiac dysrhythmias, and an increase or decrease in skeletal muscle tone.
Bisphosphonates			
Alendronate (Fosamax) or (Fosamax plus D) **For Prevention:** 5 mg orally daily or 35 mg orally weekly (available as tablet or liquid) **For Treatment:** 10 mg orally daily or 70 mg orally weekly with 2800-5600 international units of vitamin D	Prevents bone loss and increases bone density	Take on an empty stomach, first thing in the morning with a full glass of water. Take 30 minutes before food, drink, or other drugs. Remain upright, sitting or standing, for 30 minutes after administration. Take liquid (75 mL) and follow with 2 ounces of water.	Difficulty swallowing, esophagitis, esophageal ulcers, and gastric ulcers can result from alendronate therapy. Any of these should be reported to a health care provider as soon as possible.
Risedronate (Actonel) or (Actonel with Calcium) 5 mg orally daily, 35 mg orally every week, or 150 mg monthly	Same as for alendronate	Follow interventions for alendronate. Observe for CNS side/adverse effects, such as drowsiness, anxiety, agitation.	Same as for alendronate. Drug can also cause CNS effects that may not be tolerated.
Ibandronate (Boniva) 150 mg orally once every month or 3.375 mg IV every 3 months	Same as for alendronate	Take on the same day each month. Take on an empty stomach, first thing in the morning with a full glass of water. Take 60 minutes before food, drink, or other drugs. Remain upright for 1 hour after administration.	Same as for alendronate.
Zoledronic acid (Reclast, Zometa) **For Prevention:** 5 mg IV once every 2 years **For Treatment:** 5 mg IV once a year	Same as for other bisphosphonates	Infuse over 15-30 minutes.	The drug should not be infused too quickly to prevent rare complications such as atrial fibrillation.
		Make sure the patient has a dental examination before starting the drug.	The drug can cause jaw or maxillary osteonecrosis, particularly if oral hygiene is poor.
		Do not give to patients who are sensitive to aspirin.	The patient may experience bronchoconstriction.
		Check serum creatinine before and after administering the drug.	The drug can cause renal insufficiency or kidney failure.
Estrogen Agonist/Antagonists*			
Raloxifene (Evista) 60 mg orally daily	Prevents bone loss and increases bone density	Teach patient signs and symptoms of VTE.	Raloxifene can cause increased risk for VTE, especially in the first 4 months of therapy.
		Monitor liver function tests (LFTs) in collaboration with health care provider.	Raloxifene can cause increased LFT values or worsen hepatic disease (should not be given to patient who has liver disease).

CNS, Central nervous system; *VTE*, venous thromboembolism.
*Formerly Selective Estrogen Receptor Modulators (SERMs).

for treatment of osteoporosis when other drugs are not effective (Lilley et al., 2014). The drug binds to a protein that is essential for the formation, function, and survival of osteoclasts and is given subcutaneously twice a year. By preventing the protein from activating its receptor, the drug decreases bone loss and increases bone mass and strength. The most common side effects of denosumab are back pain, high cholesterol, urinary tract infection, and muscle pain. The drug can also cause a decrease in serum calcium levels. Therefore patients who already have a low calcium level should not take the drug. Like other drugs used for osteoporosis, denosumab can cause fractures, especially of the femur, and jaw osteonecrosis.

CLINICAL JUDGMENT CHALLENGE

Patient-Centered Care; Evidence-Based Practice **QSEN**

A 71-year-old Caucasian (Euro-American) woman has been diagnosed with osteoporosis for over 15 years. She has been on calcium and vitamin D$_3$ supplements since her diagnosis and has been taking risedronate (Actonel) on and off for the past 12 years. According to her most recent DXA scan, the patient continues to lose bone density despite being on drug therapy. Last year she sustained a fracture of her humerus after she tripped over her small dog. When reviewing her history, you note that her mother and older sister had osteoporosis for many years. Her sister recently died less than a year after fracturing her hip. The patient expresses her fear of having another fracture and wants to be considered for Prolia therapy.

1. What risk factors does this patient have for osteoporosis? What other information do you need to do a complete assessment?
2. Is this patient a good candidate for beginning denosumab? Why or why not? Will you need more information? If so, what do you need to know?
3. If the patient begins the new drug, what health teaching will she need?
4. How will you respond to her fear of having more fractures?

TABLE 50-2 Differential Features of Osteoporosis and Osteomalacia

CHARACTERISTIC	OSTEOPOROSIS	OSTEOMALACIA
Definition	Decreased bone mass	Demineralized bone
Pathophysiology	Lack of calcium	Lack of vitamin D
Radiographic findings	Osteopenia, fractures	Pseudofractures, Looser's zones, fractures
Calcium level	Low or normal	Low or normal
Phosphate level	Normal	Low or normal
Parathyroid hormone	Normal	High or normal
Alkaline phosphatase	Normal	High

TABLE 50-3 Causes of Osteomalacia

Vitamin D Disturbance
- Inadequate production
- Lack of sunlight exposure
- Dietary deficiency
- Abnormal metabolism
- Drug therapy
  - Phenytoin (Dilantin)
  - Fluoride
  - Barbiturates
- Liver disease
- Renal disease

- Inadequate absorption
  - Postgastrectomy
  - Malabsorption syndrome
- Inflammatory bowel disease

Kidney Disease
- Chronic kidney disease
- Acute tubular disorders
  - Acidosis
  - Hypophosphatemia

Familial Metabolic Error
- Hypophosphatemia

Community-Based Care

Patients with osteoporosis are usually managed at home unless they have major fragility fractures. Osteoporosis disease-management programs managed by nurse practitioners have helped diagnose and treat the disease. Greene and Dell (2010) reported that over a 6-year period, a large osteoporosis disease-management program resulted in a 263% increase in the number of DXA scans done each year, a 153% increase in the number of patients treated with drug therapy, and a 38.1% decrease in the expected hip fracture rate.

Refer patients to the National Osteoporosis Foundation (www.nof.org) in the United States for information regarding the disease and its treatment. The Osteoporosis Society of Canada (www.osteoporosis.ca) has similar services. Large health care systems often have osteoporosis specialty clinics and support groups for patients with osteoporosis.

OSTEOMALACIA

❖ *PATHOPHYSIOLOGY*

Osteomalacia is loss of bone related to a vitamin D deficiency. It causes softening of the bone resulting from inadequate deposits of calcium and phosphorus in the bone matrix. Normal remodeling of the bone is disrupted, and calcification does not occur. Osteomalacia is the adult equivalent of **rickets**, or vitamin D deficiency, in children.

Vitamin D deficiency is the most important factor in development of osteomalacia. In its natural form, vitamin D is activated by the ultraviolet radiation of the sun and obtained from certain foods as a nutritional supplement. In combination with calcium and phosphorus, the vitamin is necessary for bone formation.

Osteomalacia may be confused with osteoporosis because of similar characteristics shared by the two disease processes. Table 50-2 compares and contrasts osteoporosis and osteomalacia.

In addition to primary disease related to lack of sunlight exposure or dietary intake, vitamin D deficiency caused by various health problems may result in osteomalacia (Table 50-3). Malabsorption of vitamin D from the small bowel is a common complication of partial or total gastrectomy and bypass or resection surgery of the small intestine. Disease of the small bowel, such as Crohn's disease, may cause decreased vitamin and mineral absorption.

Liver and pancreatic disorders disrupt vitamin D metabolism and decrease its production. Chronic kidney disease (CKD) interferes with the synthesis of calcitriol, the most active vitamin metabolite. Osteomalacia can also be caused by bone tumors (oncogenic or tumor-induced osteomalacia).

Conditions that contribute to phosphate depletion (hypophosphatemia) lead to osteomalacia because they stimulate movement from bone and prevent calcium uptake in the bone. Osteomalacia is also an adverse effect of long-term therapy with certain drugs such as antiepileptic drugs (AEDs) and barbiturates. The exact mechanism for the drug effects is not known. Genetic deviations in vitamin D or phosphate metabolism may contribute to bone changes seen in osteomalacia.

Osteomalacia is not common in the United States and Western Europe. However, it is more common in less affluent nations and in countries where famine is common. Newcomers from these countries may seek health care in the United States. Older adults are most at risk. This group may have inadequate exposure to sunlight or intake of vitamin D–fortified foods. People who adhere to very restrictive vegan diets without adequate supplement of vitamin D can also be at risk. Assess for the risk for osteomalacia in anyone who has poor nutritional intake related to homelessness, who severely abuses drugs or alcohol, or who is very poor.

Health Promotion and Maintenance

To prevent or help treat osteomalacia, teach patients to increase vitamin D through dietary intake, sun exposure, and drug supplements. Instruct the at-risk patient about foods high in vitamin D, such as milk and food that has had it added. Remind patients that cheese and yogurt rarely contain vitamin D although they are rich in calcium. Instruct them to read food labels for nutrient content. Remind patients, especially those who are homebound, about the importance of daily sun exposure (at least 5 minutes each day) for the most important source of vitamin D.

Some people are lactose intolerant or do not use dairy products because of their vegan diets. However, many products are available for people who avoid dairy products. Soy and rice milk, tofu, and soy products are substitutes, but they are expensive. Teach patients to choose those products that are fortified with vitamin D. Other foods rich in the vitamin are eggs, swordfish, chicken, and liver, as well as enriched cereals and bread products. The at-risk patient should also take vitamin D supplements as prescribed by his or her health care provider.

❖ PATIENT-CENTERED COLLABORATIVE CARE

◆ Assessment

Collect important data for the patient with osteomalacia or suspected osteomalacia, including age, ability to be exposed to sunlight, and skin pigmentation. The older adult who has been homebound or chronically institutionalized is at the greatest risk. People who have dark skin and who may consume minimal protein are more at risk than light-skinned people with the same dietary habits. Dark-skinned people may avoid the sun and need protein for calcium binding. Take a thorough nutritional history to determine the intake of foods containing vitamin D and calcium. Coordinate the assessment with the dietitian.

Assessment includes any history of chronic disease processes of the GI tract including inflammatory bowel disease, gastric or intestinal bypass surgery, or any problem that interferes with absorption from the GI tract. A history of renal or liver dysfunction may lead to ineffective metabolism of vitamin D. Drugs such as phenytoin (Dilantin) or fluoride preparations may also interfere with metabolism of vitamin D.

Osteomalacia and osteoporosis may occur at the same time (see Table 50-2). In the early stages of osteomalacia, the manifestations are nonspecific. Muscle weakness and bone pain may be misdiagnosed as arthritis or another connective tissue disorder. In some cases, proximal muscle weakness in the shoulder and pelvic girdle area is the only presenting symptom.

Muscle weakness in the lower extremities may cause a waddling and unsteady gait, which contributes to falls and subsequent fractures. Hypophosphatemia leads to an inadequate production of muscle cell adenosine triphosphate, thus resulting in a decrease in muscle cell energy. If hypocalcemia is present, muscle cramping may occur with weakness.

In collaboration with the physical therapist, assess muscle strength and observe the patient's gait. Document concerns about muscle cramps and bone pain. Skeletal discomfort is often vague and generalized. The spine, ribs, pelvis, and lower extremities are most often affected. The patient usually describes the pain as aggravated by activity and worse at night.

Palpate the affected bones for tenderness. Bone tenderness may occur when pressure is applied to the tibia or rib cage. Skeletal malalignment, like long-bone bowing or spinal deformity, may be similar to that seen in osteoporosis. In extreme cases, the pelvis narrows, so vaginal childbirth is difficult. If osteomalacia is untreated, vertebral, rib, and long-bone fractures may occur. The patient may be misdiagnosed as having bone cancer or osteoporosis.

X-rays of bone in patients with osteomalacia reveal a decrease in the cancellous bone and lack of osteoid sharpness. The classic diagnostic finding specific to the disease, however, is the presence of radiolucent bands (Looser's lines or zones). Looser's zones represent stress fractures that have not mineralized. They often appear symmetrically in the medial area of the femoral neck, ribs, and pelvis and may progress to complete fractures with minimal trauma. Bone biopsy of these areas may be needed for complete diagnosis. DXA scan may assist in diagnosis of osteomalacia.

◆ Interventions

The major treatment for osteomalacia is vitamin D in an active form, such as ergocalciferol. Vitamin D is needed to adequately absorb and utilize calcium in the body.

Nurses play a vital role in educating other health care professionals about the need to screen patients for low vitamin D levels. For all at-risk patients, teach them about which high calcium and vitamin D foods to eat and the importance of adequate daily sunlight. Additional health teaching is discussed above in the Health Promotion and Maintenance section.

PAGET'S DISEASE OF THE BONE

❖ PATHOPHYSIOLOGY

Paget's disease, or **osteitis deformans**, is a chronic metabolic disorder in which bone is excessively broken down (osteoclastic activity) and re-formed (osteoblastic activity). The result is bone that is structurally disorganized, causing bones to be weak with increased risk for bowing of long bones and fractures. Two types of Paget's disease can occur—familial and sporadic.

Three pathophysiologic phases of the disorder have been described: active, mixed, and inactive. In the first phase (the active phase), a rapid increase in osteoclasts (cells that break down bone) causes massive bone destruction and deformity. The osteoclasts of pagetic bone are large and multinuclear, unlike the osteoclasts of normal bone tissue.

In the mixed phase, the osteoblasts (bone-forming cells) react to compensate in forming new bone. The result is bone that is vascular, structurally weak, and deformed. Paget's disease occurs in one bone or in multiple sites. The most common areas of involvement are the vertebrae, femur, skull, clavicle, humerus, and pelvis.

🧬 GENETIC/GENOMIC CONSIDERATIONS
Patient-Centered Care QSEN

Because Paget's disease is often present in identical twins, an autosomal dominant pattern has been suggested. The disease has been noted in up to 30% of people with a positive family history for Paget's disease. Several complex genetic factors have been identified in families with the disease (Najat et al., 2009), including mutations in the:

- *RANKL/RANK/OPG* system, which is needed for osteoclast development and activity (see p. 1030 in the Osteoporosis section)
- Valosin-containing gene of complement binding protein (valosin-containing protein [*VCP*]), an important inflammatory factor
- Sequestosome 1 (*SQSTM1*) or *p62*, an expressed adaptor protein that can bind to ubiquitin and the atypical protein kinase C

Teach patients the importance of genetics in familial Paget's disease, and refer them to the appropriate genetics counseling resource. Ask the patient if genetic testing is desired.

When the osteoblastic activity exceeds the osteoclastic activity, the inactive phase occurs. The newly formed bone becomes sclerotic and very hard (McCance et al., 2014).

Paget's disease is second only to osteoporosis as one of the most common bone diseases in the United States, affecting about one million people. The disease is seen more frequently in people ages 50 years and older and in those of European heritage. The reason for this pattern is not known. The risk for developing Paget's disease increases as a person ages, particularly in those 80 years old and older. Men are affected twice as often as women (National Institute of Arthritis and Musculoskeletal and Skin Diseases, 2013).

❖ PATIENT-CENTERED COLLABORATIVE CARE

◆ Assessment

Physical Assessment/Clinical Manifestations. Most patients are asymptomatic, and the disease may be confined to one bone. It may be accidentally discovered during a routine laboratory or x-ray examination. In more severe disease, the manifestations are diverse and potentially fatal (Chart 50-3).

Ask the patient about a history of fracture and current bone pain. Bone PAIN, usually described as mild to moderate, may cause the patient to seek medical attention. The most common sites for pain are the hip and pelvis, but even the bones in the ear may be affected, causing hearing loss. The pain is usually described as aching, poorly defined, deep, and worsened by pressure. It is most noticeable at night or when the patient is resting. Patients may report redness and warmth at affected sites. These manifestations may be related to increased vascularity and blood flow.

The PAIN associated with the disorder may result from metabolic bone activity, secondary arthritis, impending fracture, or nerve impingement. Arthritis often occurs at the joints (cartilage) of the affected bones, resulting from bowing in the long bones of the leg. Some patients have joint replacements as a result of very painful weight-bearing joints. Nerve impingement is particularly common in the lumbosacral area of the vertebral column, presenting as back PAIN that radiates along one or both legs.

Observe posture, stance, and gait to identify gross bony deformities. Because of the enlargement of the vertebrae, loss of normal spinal curvature, and lower extremity malalignment, the patient may have decreased height. Assess for kyphosis or scoliosis of the spinal column. Note any long-bone bowing in the legs with subsequent varus (bow-leg) deformity. Long bones of the arms may also develop bowing. Flexion contracture in the hip joint is often present. Any of these deformities may be asymmetric. This weakened bone is at risk for fracture from even a minor injury. All of these problems interfere with the patient's need for independent mobility.

When performing a musculoskeletal assessment in a patient with Paget's disease, pay particular attention to the size and shape of the skull, which is typically soft, thick, and enlarged. Pressure from an enlarged temporal bone may lead to deafness and vertigo (dizziness). Basilar (in the occipital area) complications can compress any of the cranial nerves and result in neurologic problems. Assess the patient for changes in vision, swallowing, hearing, and speech. Platybasia, or basilar invagination, causes brainstem (vital sign center) damage that threatens life. In some cases, the bony enlargement of the skull blocks cerebrospinal fluid (CSF), resulting in hydrocephalus.

Fragility (pathologic) fractures may be the presenting clinical manifestation of the disorder. The femur and the tibia are most often affected, and fracture of these bones can result from minimal trauma. The fracture line is usually perpendicular to the long axis of the bone, and healing is unpredictable because of abnormal metabolic activity within the bone.

Although rare, bones affected by Paget's disease may develop malignant changes. The most dreaded complication of Paget's disease is cancer, most commonly osteogenic sarcoma. It affects the femur, humerus, and old fracture sites and has a grave prognosis because of early metastasis to the lung or extensive local invasion. When severe bone PAIN is present in a patient with Paget's disease, bone cancer is suspected.

Assess the skin for its color and temperature. In people with Paget's disease, the skin is typically flushed and warm because of increased blood flow. In addition, assess the patient's energy level because apathy, lethargy, and fatigue are common.

Other less common manifestations of Paget's disease include hyperparathyroidism and gout. Secondary hyperparathyroidism leads to an increase in serum and urinary calcium levels. In severe cases, serum calcium excess results from prolonged immobilization. Calcium deposits occur in joint spaces or as stones in the urinary tract. Hyperuricemia (serum uric acid excess) and gout occur because the increased metabolic activity of bone creates an increase in nucleic acid catabolism. Therefore kidney stones are more common in people with Paget's disease.

In a few cases, increased blood flow causes the heart to work harder to increase cardiac output, resulting in heart failure if not treated. Cardiac complications tend to occur only when more than a third of the skeleton is involved.

Diagnostic Assessment. Increases in *serum alkaline phosphatase (ALP)* and urinary hydroxyproline levels are the primary laboratory findings indicating possible Paget's disease. Overactive osteoblasts cause an altered ALP level. ALP can be further evaluated by alkaline phosphatase isoenzymes. The isoenzyme testing can further break ALP into three fractions—liver, bone, and intestinal. Elevated bone isoenzymes can help in a more definitive diagnosis of Paget's disease. Serum isoenzyme levels of bone ALP are used to monitor effectiveness of treatment (Pagana & Pagana, 2014).

The 24-hour *urinary hydroxyproline* level reflects bone collagen turnover and indicates the degree of disease severity. The higher the hydroxyproline, the more severe is the disease.

The *calcium* levels in blood and urine may be low, normal, or elevated. The immobilized patient is more likely to have an

---

CHART 50-3   Key Features

Paget's Disease of the Bone

Musculoskeletal Manifestations
- Bone and joint pain (may be in a single bone) that is aching, poorly described, and aggravated by walking
- Low back and sciatic nerve pain
- Bowing of long bones
- Loss of normal spinal curvature
- Enlarged, thick skull
- Pathologic fractures
- Osteogenic sarcoma (bone cancer)

Skin Manifestations
- Flushed, warm skin

Other Manifestations
- Apathy, lethargy, fatigue
- Hyperparathyroidism
- Gout
- Urinary or renal stones
- Heart failure from fluid overload

increase in calcium levels as a result of calcium moving from bone into the blood.

Paget's disease often causes an elevated *uric acid* because nucleic acid from overactive bone metabolism increases. This finding may be misinterpreted as primary gout.

X-rays are also used to diagnose Paget's disease. They reveal characteristic changes including the presence of osteolytic lesions and enlarged bones with radiolucent, or punched-out, appearance. Decrease in joint space may be seen with arthritic changes in joints. Malalignment deformities, fractures, and secondary arthritic changes may be present.

Radionuclide bone scan may be most sensitive in detecting Paget's disease. A radiolabeled bisphosphonate is injected IV and shows pagetic bone in areas of high bone turnover activity. This test can determine the extent of Paget's disease in the skeleton. CT and MRI are useful in the detection of cancerous tumors, changes in the skull, and spinal cord or nerve compression (Pagana & Pagana, 2014).

◆ Interventions

Nonsurgical or surgical management may be necessary to reduce pain and promote MOBILITY. Nonsurgical interventions are used first.

Drug Therapy. The primary intervention for Paget's disease is drug therapy. The purpose of *drug therapy* in Paget's disease is to relieve pain and to decrease bone resorption.

Management of mild to moderate pain may include the use of aspirin or NSAIDs such as ibuprofen (Motrin, Apo-Ibuprofen ✦). When the calcium level is more than twice the normal value and the disease is widespread, the health care provider usually prescribes more potent drugs, such as selected bisphosphonates. Treatment with these agents for Paget's disease requires dosages and duration of therapy different from those for osteoporosis. Chart 50-2 includes information about some of these commonly used drugs.

Oral bisphosphonates are a first-line treatment choice for Paget's disease when alkaline phosphatase levels are at least twice the normal serum level. Alendronate (Fosamax), risedronate (Actonel), etidronate (Didronel), or tiludronate (Skelid) is given in tablet form. When oral agents are not effective, pamidronate (Aredia) or zoledronic acid (Reclast, Zometa) is administered IV (Lilley et al., 2014). Aredia is given once every 3 months, and Reclast is given once a year as a single IV dose. These drugs are usually highly effective. To reduce the risk for hypocalcemia, patients should receive 1500 mg of calcium daily in divided doses and 800 international units of vitamin D_3 daily for at least 2 weeks after zoledronic acid infusion unless they are prone to kidney stones. Chart 50-2 provides additional information about caring for patients receiving bisphosphonates.

Denosumab (Prolia) is a monoclonal antibody that is also approved for Paget's disease. The drug binds to a protein that is essential for the formation, function, and survival of osteoclasts and is given subcutaneously twice a year. By preventing the protein from activating its receptor, the drug decreases bone loss and increases bone mass and strength. This drug is discussed in the Osteoporosis section of this chapter.

Calcitonin is a hormone that seems to reduce bone resorption and, subsequently, relieve pain. The drug often causes a dramatic decrease in the alkaline phosphatase level in a few weeks. Calcitonin is approved for subcutaneous administration in treating Paget's disease because the nasal spray is not effective. The drug binds to osteoclast receptors, therefore slowing bone breakdown (Lilley et al., 2014). The drug may be used for those patients who do not tolerate bisphosphonates. Side effects of calcitonin include nausea, flushing, and skin rash. Skin testing may be done before administration of the first dose.

Other Interventions. In addition to administering drugs, implement physical measures to reduce pain and increase MOBILITY. These measures may include application of heat and gentle massage. An exercise program may be started with the help of a physical therapist. Exercise may be difficult because of pain and danger of fracture. Non-impact exercise should be used, but the patient may benefit from strengthening and weight-bearing exercises. In collaboration with the physical therapist, teach the patient about ROM and gentle stretching. Additional interventions for pain relief, such as relaxation techniques, are discussed in Chapter 3.

Measures to promote bone health are also important and include a diet rich in calcium and vitamin D. Nutrition therapy for bone health is described on p. 1033 in the discussion of Interventions in the Osteoporosis section.

Provide the patient with information to contact the U.S. local chapter of The Paget Foundation (www.paget.org) and the Arthritis Foundation (www.arthritis.org). The Arthritis Society in Canada (www.arthritis.ca) is also an excellent service. These resources provide information and support for the patient and family or significant others.

❓ NCLEX EXAMINATION CHALLENGE

Physiological Integrity

A client is starting on risedronate (Actonel) for treatment of Paget's disease. What precaution does the nurse include in the client's health teaching about this drug?
A. "This drug can cause serious infections."
B. "Monitor the drug injection site for redness or itching."
C. "Drink a full glass of water after taking the drug."
D. "Do not take calcium and vitamin D while on the drug."

OSTEOMYELITIS

INFECTION in bony tissue can be a severe and difficult-to-treat problem. Bone infection can result in chronic recurrence of infection, loss of function and mobility, amputation, and even death.

❖ PATHOPHYSIOLOGY

Bacteria, viruses, or fungi can cause INFECTION in bone, known as osteomyelitis. Invasion by one or more pathogenic microorganisms stimulates the inflammatory response in bone tissue. The INFLAMMATION produces an increased vascular leak and edema, often involving the surrounding soft tissues. Once inflammation is established, the vessels in the area become thrombosed and release exudate (pus) into bony tissue. Ischemia of bone tissue follows and results in necrotic bone. This area of necrotic bone separates from surrounding bone tissue, and sequestrum is formed. The presence of sequestrum prevents bone healing and causes superimposed infection, often in the form of bone abscess. As shown in Fig. 50-2, the cycle repeats itself as the new infection leads to further inflammation, vessel thromboses, and necrosis.

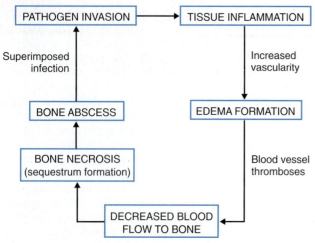

FIG. 50-2 Infection cycle of osteomyelitis.

Osteomyelitis is categorized as *exogenous*, in which infectious organisms enter from outside the body as in an open fracture, or **endogenous** (**hematogenous**), in which organisms are carried by the bloodstream from other areas of infection in the body. A third category is *contiguous*, in which bone infection results from skin infection of adjacent tissues. Osteomyelitis can be further divided into two major types: acute osteomyelitis and chronic osteomyelitis.

Each type of bone infection has its own causative factors. Pathogenic microbes favor bone that has a rich blood supply and a marrow cavity. **Acute hematogenous infection** results from bacteremia, underlying disease, or nonpenetrating trauma. Urinary tract infections, particularly in older men, tend to spread to the lower vertebrae. Long-term IV catheters (e.g., Hickman catheters) can be primary sources of INFECTION. Patients undergoing long-term hemodialysis and IV drug users are also at risk for osteomyelitis. *Salmonella* infections of the GI tract may spread to bone. Patients with sickle cell disease and other hemoglobinopathies often have multiple episodes of salmonellosis, which can cause bone infection (McCance et al., 2014).

Poor dental hygiene and periodontal (gum) INFECTION can be causative factors in **contiguous** osteomyelitis in facial bones. Minimal nonpenetrating trauma can cause hemorrhages or small-vessel occlusions, leading to bone necrosis. Regardless of the source of infection, many infections are caused by *Staphylococcus aureus*. Treatment of infection may be complicated further by the presence of methicillin-resistant *Staphylococcus aureus* (MRSA) or other multiple drug-resistant organisms (MDRO), which is very common in hospitalized and other institutionalized patients. One of the major desired outcomes in health care settings today is to reduce the number of MRSA infections from any source.

CONSIDERATIONS FOR OLDER ADULTS

Patient-Centered Care **QSEN**

Malignant external otitis media involving the base of the skull is sometimes seen in older adults with diabetes. The most common cause of contiguous spread in older adults, however, is found in those who have slow-healing foot ulcers. Multiple organisms tend to be responsible for the resulting osteomyelitis (McCance et al., 2014).

Penetrating trauma leads to acute osteomyelitis by direct inoculation. A soft-tissue infection may be present as well. Animal bites, puncture wounds, skin ulcerations, and bone surgery can result in bone INFECTION. The most common offending organism is *Pseudomonas aeruginosa*, but other gram-negative bacteria may be found.

If bone infection is misdiagnosed or inadequately treated, **chronic osteomyelitis** may develop, especially in older adults who have foot ulcers. Inadequate care management results when the treatment period is too short or when the treatment is delayed or inappropriate. About half of cases of chronic osteomyelitis are caused by gram-negative bacteria. Although bacteria are the most common causes of osteomyelitis, viruses and fungal organisms also may cause INFECTION.

❖ *PATIENT-CENTERED COLLABORATIVE CARE*

◆ *Assessment*

Bone PAIN, with or without other manifestations, is a common concern of patients with bone INFECTION. The pain is described as a constant, localized, pulsating sensation that worsens with movement.

The patient with *acute* osteomyelitis has fever, usually with temperature greater than 101°F (38.3°C). *Older adults may not have an extreme temperature elevation because of lower core body temperature and compromised immune system that occur with normal aging.* The area around the infected bone swells and is tender when palpated. Erythema (redness) and heat may also be present. When vascular compromise is severe, patients may not feel discomfort because of nerve damage from lack of blood supply.

When vascular insufficiency is suspected, assess circulation in the distal extremities. Ulcerations may be present on the feet or hands, indicating inadequate healing ability as a result of poor circulation.

Fever, swelling, and erythema are less common in those with *chronic* osteomyelitis. Ulceration resulting in sinus tract formation, localized pain, and drainage is more characteristic of chronic infection (Chart 50-4).

The patient with osteomyelitis may have an elevated white blood cell (leukocyte) count, which may be double the normal value. The erythrocyte sedimentation rate (ESR) may be normal early in the course of the disease but rises as the condition progresses. It may remain elevated for as long as 3 months after drug therapy is discontinued.

If bacteremia is present, a potentially life-threatening complication that could lead to septic shock, a blood culture identifies the offending organisms to determine which antibiotics should be used in treatment. Both aerobic and anaerobic blood cultures are collected before drug therapy begins.

Although bone changes cannot be detected early with standard x-rays, changes in blood flow can be seen early in the course of the disease by radionuclide scanning or MRI.

◆ **Interventions**

The specific treatment protocol depends on the type and number of microbes present in the infected tissue. If other measures fail to resolve the infectious process, surgical management may be needed.

Nonsurgical Management. The health care provider starts antimicrobial (e.g., antibiotic) therapy as soon as possible. In the presence of copious wound drainage, Contact Precautions are used to prevent the spread of the offending organism to other patients and health care personnel. Teach patients, visitors, and staff members how to use these precautions. (See Chapter 23 for a discussion of Contact Precautions.)

More than one agent may be needed to combat multiple types of organisms. The hospital or home care nurse gives the drugs at specifically prescribed times so that therapeutic serum levels are achieved. Observe for the actions, side effects, and toxicity of these drugs. *Teach family members or other caregivers in the home setting how to administer antimicrobials if they are continued after hospital discharge or are used only at home.*

The optimal drug regimen for patients with chronic osteomyelitis is not well established. Prolonged therapy for more than 3 months may be needed to eliminate the infection. Because of the cost of lengthy hospital stays, patients are typically cared for in the home or long-term care (LTC) setting with long-term vascular access catheters, such as the peripherally inserted central catheter (PICC), for drug administration. After discontinuation of IV drugs, oral therapy may be needed for weeks or months. Patients and families must understand the complications of inadequate treatment or failure to follow up with health care providers. Teach them that drug therapy must be continued over a long period to be effective.

! **NURSING SAFETY PRIORITY** (QSEN)

Drug Alert

Even when symptoms of osteomyelitis appear to be improved, teach the patient and family that the full course of IV and oral antimicrobials must be completed to ensure that the infection is resolved.

In addition to systemic drug therapy, the wound may be irrigated, either continuously or intermittently, with one or more antibiotic solutions. A medical technique in which beads made of bone cement are impregnated with an antibiotic and packed into the wound can provide direct contact of the antibiotic with the offending organism.

Drugs are also needed to control PAIN. Patients experience acute and chronic pain and must receive a regimen of drug therapy for control. Chapter 3 describes pharmacologic and nonpharmacologic interventions for both acute and chronic pain.

A treatment to increase tissue perfusion for patients with chronic, unremitting osteomyelitis is the use of a hyperbaric chamber or portable device to administer hyperbaric oxygen (HBO) therapy. These devices are usually available in large tertiary care centers and may not be accessible to all patients who

might benefit from them. With HBO therapy, the affected area is exposed to a high concentration of oxygen that diffuses into the tissues to promote healing. In conjunction with high-dose drug therapy and surgical débridement, HBO has proven very useful in treating a number of anaerobic infections. Other wound-management therapies are described in Chapter 25.

Surgical Management. Antimicrobial therapy alone may not meet the desired outcome of treatment. Surgical techniques may be used to minimize the disfigurement that can be a devastating result of severe osteomyelitis. Surgery is reserved for patients with chronic osteomyelitis.

Because bone cannot heal in the presence of necrotic tissue, a *sequestrectomy* may be performed to débride the necrotic bone and allow revascularization of tissue. The excision of dead and infected bone often results in a sizable cavity, or bone defect. Bone *grafts* to repair bone defects are also widely used.

When infected bone is extensively resected, reconstruction with *microvascular bone transfers* may be done. This procedure is reserved for larger skeletal defects. The most common donor sites are the patient's fibula and iliac crest. The bone graft may have an attached muscle or skin flap, if necessary. The steps of the procedure are similar to those of bone grafting in that débridement of dead or necrotic bone is done before bone transfer.

Nursing care of the patient after surgery is similar to that for any postoperative patient (see Chapter 16). However, the important difference is that neurovascular (NV) assessments must be done frequently because the patient experiences increased swelling after the surgical procedure. Elevate the affected extremity to increase venous return and thus control swelling. Assess and document the patient's NV status, including:

- Pain
- Movement
- Sensation
- Warmth
- Temperature
- Distal pulses
- Capillary refill (not as reliable as the above indicators)

! **NURSING SAFETY PRIORITY** (QSEN)

Critical Rescue

After surgery to treat osteomyelitis, frequently check for signs of neurovascular compromise, including the six *P*s: **p**ain that cannot be controlled, **p**ressure, paresis or **p**aralysis (weakness or inability to move), **p**aresthesia (abnormal, tingling sensation), **p**allor, and **p**ulselessness. If any of these findings occur, report them immediately to the surgeon.

If the bony defect is small, a *muscle flap* may be the only surgery required. Local muscle flaps are used in the treatment of chronic osteomyelitis when soft tissue does not fill the dead space, or cavity, that results from bone débridement. The flap provides wound coverage and enhances blood flow to promote healing. A split-thickness skin graft is often applied several days after the muscle flap.

When the previously described surgical procedures are not appropriate or successful and as a last resort, the affected limb may need to be amputated. The physical and psychological care for a patient who has undergone an amputation is discussed in Chapter 51.

BENIGN BONE TUMORS

❖ PATHOPHYSIOLOGY

Benign (noncancerous) bone tumors are often asymptomatic and may be discovered on routine x-ray examination or as the cause of pathologic fractures. The cause of benign bone tumors is not known. Tumors may arise from several types of tissue. The major classifications include *chondrogenic* tumors (from cartilage), *osteogenic* tumors (from bone), and *fibrogenic* tumors (from fibrous tissue and found most often in children). Although many specific benign tumors have been identified, only the common ones are described here.

The most common benign bone tumor is the *osteochondroma*. Although its onset is usually in childhood, the tumor grows until skeletal maturity and may not be diagnosed until adulthood. The tumor may be a single growth or multiple growths and can occur in any bone. The femur and the tibia are most often involved.

The *chondroma*, or endochondroma, is a lesion of mature hyaline cartilage affecting primarily the hands and the feet. The ribs, sternum, spine, and long bones may also be involved. Chondromas are slow growing and often cause pathologic fractures after minor injury. They are found in people of all ages, occur in both men and women, and can affect any bone.

The origin of the *giant cell tumor* remains uncertain. This lesion is aggressive and can be extensive and may involve surrounding soft tissue. Although classified as benign, giant cell tumors can metastasize (spread) to the lung. The peak incidence occurs in patients in their 30s.

❖ PATIENT-CENTERED COLLABORATIVE CARE

Assess for PAIN, the most common manifestation of benign bone tumors. Pain can range from mild to moderate. It can be caused by direct tumor invasion into soft tissue, compressing peripheral nerves, or by a resulting pathologic fracture.

In addition, observe and palpate the suspected involved area. When the tumor affects the lower extremities or the small bones of the hands and feet, local swelling may be detected as the tumor enlarges. In some cases, muscle atrophy or muscle spasm may be present. Carefully palpate the bone and muscle to detect these changes and elicit tenderness.

Routine x-rays and tomography are used to find bone tumors. Tumors are characterized by sharp margins, intact cortices, and smooth, uniform periosteal bone.

CT is less useful except in complex anatomic areas, such as the spinal column and sacrum. The test is helpful in evaluating the extent of soft-tissue involvement. MRI may be especially helpful in viewing problems of the spinal column.

The health care provider uses drug therapy and surgery in combination when possible. Non-drug pain-relief measures are also used. Depending on the patient's preference and tolerance, measures such as heat or cold may help relieve pain.

In addition to prescribing analgesics to reduce pain, the health care provider usually prescribes one or more NSAIDs to inhibit prostaglandin synthesis that increases pain and INFLAMMATION. Give these drugs after meals or with food to reduce GI side effects. Teach patients to report any signs of bleeding to the primary health care provider immediately.

The most common surgical procedure used for benign bone tumors is removal. If the tumor is small, surgery may not be needed. When the tumor is very extensive, as in a giant cell tumor, it is removed with care to restore or maintain the function of the adjacent joint, most often the knee. In some cases, the knee is replaced with a prosthetic device and, less often, is fused (**arthrodesis**). Bone grafting may be needed. The collaborative care for patients undergoing total knee replacement is discussed in Chapter 18.

BONE CANCER

Cancerous bone tumors may be primary or secondary (those that originate in other tissues and metastasize to bone). *Primary tumors* occur most often in people between 10 and 30 years of age and make up a small percentage of bone cancers. As for other forms of cancer, the exact cause of bone cancer is unknown but genetic and environmental factors are likely causes. *Metastatic lesions* most often occur in the older age-group and account for most bone cancers (McCance et al., 2014).

Previous radiation therapy in the anatomic area is a big risk factor. For example, bone cancer of the ribs in the path of radiation for breast cancer is fairly common.

❖ PATHOPHYSIOLOGY

Osteosarcoma, or osteogenic sarcoma, is the most common type of *primary* malignant bone tumor. More than 50% of cases occur in the distal femur, followed in decreasing order of occurrence by the proximal tibia and humerus.

The tumor is relatively large, causing acute pain and swelling. The involved area is usually warm because the blood flow to the site increases. The center of the tumor is sclerotic from increased osteoblastic activity. The periphery is soft, extending through the bone cortex in the classic sunburst appearance associated with the neoplasm. An inward spread into the medullary canal is also common. Osteosarcoma typically **metastasizes** (spreads), which results in death.

Although *Ewing's sarcoma* is not as common as other tumors, it is the most malignant. Like other primary tumors, it causes PAIN and swelling. In addition, systemic manifestations, particularly low-grade fever, leukocytosis, and anemia, characterize the lesions. The pelvis and the lower extremity are most often affected. Pelvic involvement is a poor prognostic sign. It often extends into soft tissue. Death results from metastasis to the lungs and other bones. Although the tumor can be seen in patients of any age, it usually occurs in children and young adults in their 20s. Men are affected more often than women (McCance et al., 2014). The reason for this pattern is not known.

In contrast to the patient with osteosarcoma, the patient with *chondrosarcoma* experiences dull PAIN and swelling for a long period. The tumor typically affects the pelvis and proximal femur near the diaphysis. Arising from cartilaginous tissue, it destroys bone and often calcifies. The patient with this type of tumor has a better prognosis than one with osteogenic sarcoma. Chondrosarcoma occurs in middle-aged and older people, with a slight predominance in men.

Arising from fibrous tissue, *fibrosarcomas* can be divided into subtypes, of which malignant fibrous histiocytoma (MFH) is the most malignant. Usually the clinical presentation of MFH is gradual, without specific symptoms. Local tenderness, with or without a palpable mass, occurs in the long bones of the lower extremity. As with other bone cancers, the lesion can metastasize to the lungs (McCance et al., 2014).

Primary tumors of the prostate, breast, kidney, thyroid, and lung are called *bone-seeking* cancers because they spread to the bone more often than other primary tumors. The vertebrae, pelvis, femur, and ribs are the bone sites commonly affected. Simply stated, primary tumor cells, or seeds, are carried to bone through the bloodstream. *Fragility fractures caused by metastatic bone are a major concern in patient care management.*

❖ PATIENT-CENTERED COLLABORATIVE CARE

◆ Assessment

The data collected for the patient suspected of having a malignant bone tumor are similar to the data needed for the patient with a benign growth. In addition, ask whether the patient has had previous radiation therapy for cancer and determine the status of the patient's general health.

The clinical manifestations seen in the patient with primary bone cancer or metastatic disease vary, depending on the specific type of lesion. Usually the patient has a group of nonspecific concerns, including pain, local swelling, and a tender, palpable mass. Marked disability and impaired MOBILITY may occur in those with advanced metastatic bone disease.

In a patient with Ewing's sarcoma, a low-grade fever may occur because of the systemic features of the neoplasm. For this reason, it is often confused with osteomyelitis. Fatigue and pallor resulting from anemia are also common.

In performing a musculoskeletal assessment, inspect the involved area and palpate the mass for size and tenderness. In collaboration with the physical and occupational therapists, assess the patient's ability to perform MOBILITY tasks and ADLs.

Patients with malignant bone tumors may be young adults whose productive lives are just beginning. They need strong support systems to help cope with the diagnosis and its treatment. Family, significant others, and health care professionals are major components of the needed support. Determine what systems or resources are available.

Patients often experience a loss of control over their lives when a diagnosis of cancer is made. As a result, they become anxious and fearful about the outcome of their illness. Coping with the diagnosis becomes a challenge. As patients progress through the grieving process, there may be initial denial. Identify the anxiety level, and assess the stage or stages of the grieving process. Explore any maladaptive behavior, indicating ineffective coping mechanisms. Chapter 22 further describes the psychosocial assessment for patients with cancer.

The patient with a malignant bone tumor typically shows elevated serum alkaline phosphatase (ALP) levels, indicating the body's attempt to form new bone by increasing osteoblastic activity. The patient with Ewing's sarcoma or metastatic bone cancer often has anemia. In addition, leukocytosis is common with Ewing's sarcoma. The progression of Ewing's sarcoma may be evaluated by elevated serum lactic dehydrogenase (LDH) levels.

In some patients with bone metastasis from the breast, kidney, or lung, the serum calcium level is elevated. Massive bone destruction stimulates release of the mineral into the bloodstream. In patients with Ewing's sarcoma and bone metastasis, the erythrocyte sedimentation rate (ESR) may be elevated because of secondary tissue inflammation (Pagana & Pagana, 2014).

As with benign bone tumors, routine x-rays and CT reveal malignant lesions. Metastatic lesions may increase or decrease bone density, depending on the amount of osteoblastic and osteoclastic activity. CT is helpful in determining the extent of soft-tissue damage. The patient may have an MRI for difficult-to-visualize areas such as the vertebrae.

In some cases a needle bone biopsy may be performed, usually under fluoroscopy to guide the surgeon. Needle biopsy is an ambulatory care procedure with rare complications. After biopsy, the cancer is staged for size and degree of spread. One popular method is the TNM system, based on tumor size and number (T), the presence of cancer cells in lymph nodes (N), and metastasis (spread) to distant sites (M) (see Chapter 21 for further discussion).

Another method is to correlate the tumor grade (high or low), tumor site (intracompartmental or extracompartmental), and presence of metastatic disease (positive or negative). Staging guides the health care team in their decision regarding patient-centered collaborative care.

◆ Interventions

Because the pain is often due to direct primary tumor invasion, treatment is aimed at reducing the size of or removing the tumor. The expected outcome of treating metastatic bone tumors is palliative rather than curative. Palliative therapies may prevent further bone destruction and improve patient function. A combination of nonsurgical and surgical management is used. Collaborate with members of the interdisciplinary health care team to plan high quality care to achieve positive patient outcomes.

Nonsurgical Management. In addition to analgesics for local PAIN relief, chemotherapeutic agents and radiation therapy are often administered to shrink the tumor. In patients with spinal involvement, bracing and immobilization with cervical traction may reduce back pain. Interventional radiology techniques are used to decrease vertebral pain and treat compression fractures (see Chapter 51).

Drug Therapy. The physician may prescribe *chemotherapy* to be given alone or in combination with radiation or surgery. Certain proliferating tumors, such as Ewing's sarcoma, are sensitive to cytotoxic drugs. Others, such as chondrosarcomas, are often totally drug resistant. Chemotherapy seems to work best for small, metastatic tumors and may be administered before or after surgery. In most cases the physician prescribes a combination of agents. At present, there is no one universally accepted protocol of chemotherapeutic agents. The drugs selected are determined in part by the primary source of the cancer in metastatic disease. For example, when metastasis occurs from breast cancer, estrogen and progesterone blockers may be used. Chapter 22 describes the general nursing care of patients who receive chemotherapy. *Remember that all chemotherapeutic agents are categorized as high-alert medications* (Institute for Safe Medication Practices, 2013).

Other drugs are given for specific metastatic cancers, depending on the location of the primary site. For example, biologic agents, such as cytokines, are given to stimulate the immune system to recognize and destroy cancer cells, especially in patients with renal cancer. Zoledronic acid (Zometa) and pamidronate (Aredia) are two IV bisphosphonates that are approved for bone metastasis from the breast, lung, and prostate (Lilley et al., 2014). These drugs help protect bones and prevent fractures. Inform patients that osteonecrosis of the jaw may also occur, especially in those who have invasive dental procedures. Monitor associated laboratory tests, such as serum creatinine and electrolytes, because these drugs can be toxic to the kidneys. Bisphosphonates are described earlier in the Osteoporosis section.

Denosumab (Prolia) is a monoclonal antibody that is also approved for metastatic bone disease (Lilley et al., 2014). The drug binds to a protein that is essential for the formation, function, and survival of osteoclasts and is given subcutaneously twice a year. By preventing the protein from activating its receptor, the drug decreases bone loss and increases bone mass and strength. This drug is discussed earlier in the Osteoporosis section.

Radiation Therapy. Radiation, either brachytherapy or external radiation, is used for selected types of malignant tumors. For patients with Ewing's sarcoma and early osteosarcoma, radiation may be the treatment of choice in reducing tumor size and thus pain.

For patients with metastatic disease, radiation is given primarily for palliation. The therapy is directed toward the painful sites to provide a more comfortable life. One or more treatments are given, depending on the extent of disease. With precise planning, radiation therapy can be used with minimal complications. The general nursing care for patients receiving radiation therapy is described in Chapter 22.

Interventional Radiology. Interventional radiologists can perform several noninvasive procedures to help relieve PAIN in the patient with metastasis to the spinal column. Two types of *thermal ablation techniques, radiofrequency ablation (RFA)* and *cryoablation,* can be done under moderate sedation or general anesthesia. RFA kills the targeted tissue with heat using a small needle inserted into the tumor. Most patients have pain relief or control after this ambulatory care procedure. Cryoablation is similar to RFA, but the radiologist uses an extremely cold gas through a probe into the tumor. Although this procedure has been available for years, newer surgical equipment allows a small incision and the patient can return to usual daily activities in a day or two.

The radiologist may also perform a *vertebroplasty* if the patient with spinal metastasis has pathologic compression fractures. After making a small incision, bone cement is injected through a needle into the fractured area. The cement hardens within 15 minutes. Like thermal ablation, this procedure is done in an ambulatory care setting and the patient is placed under moderate sedation.

Surgical Management. Primary bone tumors are usually reduced or removed with surgery, and surgery may be combined with radiation or chemotherapy.

Preoperative Care. In addition to the nature, progression, and extent of the tumor, the patient's age and general health state are considered. Chemotherapy may be administered preoperatively.

As for any patient preparing for cancer surgery, the patient with bone cancer needs psychological support from the nurse and other members of the health care team. Assess the level of the patient's and family's understanding about the surgery and related treatments. As an advocate, encourage the patient and family to discuss concerns and questions and provide information regarding hospital routines and procedures. Spiritual support is important to some patients. They may prefer to contact a member of the clergy or a spiritual leader or talk with a clergy member affiliated with the hospital. Offer assistance in arranging for spiritual assistance if requested.

Anticipate postoperative needs as much as possible before the patient undergoes surgery. Remind the patient what to expect postoperatively and how to help ensure adequate recovery.

Operative Procedures. Wide or radical resection procedures are used for patients with bone sarcomas to salvage the affected limb. Wide excision is removal of the lesion surrounded by an intact cuff of normal tissue and leads to cure of low-grade tumors only. A radical resection includes removal of the lesion, the entire muscle, bone, and other tissues directly involved. It is the procedure used for high-grade tumors.

Large bone defects that result from tumor removal may require either:
- Total joint replacements with prosthetic implants, either whole or partial
- Custom metallic implants
- Allografts from the iliac crest, rib, or fibula

As an alternative to total replacement, an allograft may be implanted with internal fixation for those patients who do not have metastases. This is a common procedure for sarcomas of the proximal femur. Allograft procedures for the knee are also performed, particularly in young adults. Preoperative chemotherapy is given to enhance the likelihood of success. **Allografts** with adjacent tendons and ligaments are harvested from cadavers and can be frozen or freeze-dried for a prolonged period. The graft is fixed with a series of bolts, screws, or plates.

Postoperative Care. The surgical incision for a limb salvage procedure is often extensive. A pressure dressing with wound suction is typically maintained for several days. The patient who has undergone a limb salvage procedure has some degree of impaired physical mobility and a self-care deficit. The nature and extent of the alterations depend on the location and extent of the surgery.

> ### ! NURSING SAFETY PRIORITY (QSEN)
> *Action Alert*
>
> For patients who have allografts, observe for signs of hemorrhage, infection, and fracture. Report these complications to the surgeon immediately.

After upper extremity surgery, the patient can engage in active-assistive exercises by using the opposite hand to help achieve motions such as forward flexion and abduction of the shoulder. Continuous passive motion (CPM) using a CPM machine may be initiated as early as the first postoperative day for either upper extremity or lower extremity procedures.

After lower extremity surgery, the emphasis is on strengthening the quadriceps muscles by using passive and active motion when possible. Maintaining muscle tone is an important prerequisite to weight bearing, which progresses from toe touch or partial weight bearing to full weight bearing by 3 months postoperatively. Coordinate the patient's plan of care for ambulation and muscle strengthening with the physical therapist.

The patient who has had a bone graft may have a cast or other supportive device for several months. Weight bearing is prohibited until there is evidence that the graft is incorporated into the adjacent bone tissue.

During the recovery phase, the patient may also need assistance with ADLs, particularly if the surgery involves the upper extremity. Assist if needed, but at the same time encourage the patient to do as much as possible unaided. Some patients need assistive/adaptive devices for a short period while they are healing. Coordinate the patient's plan of care for promoting independence in ADLs with the occupational therapist.

Surrounding tissues, including nerves and blood vessels, may be removed during surgery. Vascular grafting is common, but the lost nerve(s) is (are) usually not replaced. Assess the neurovascular status of the affected extremity and hand or foot every 1 to 2 hours immediately after surgery. Splinting or casting of the limb may also cause neurovascular (NV) compromise and needs to be checked for proper placement.

In addition to needing emotional support to cope with physical disabilities, the patient may need help coping with the surgery and its effects. Help identify available support systems as soon as possible.

As a result of most of the surgical procedures, the patient experiences an altered body image. Suggest ways to minimize cosmetic changes. For example, a lowered shoulder can be covered by a custom-made pad worn under clothing. The patient can cover lower extremity defects with pants.

Advocate for the patient and the family to promote the physician-patient relationship. For instance, the patient may not completely understand the medical or surgical treatment plan but may hesitate to question the physician. The nurse's intervention can increase communication, which is essential in successful management of the patient with cancer.

? CLINICAL JUDGMENT CHALLENGE

Patient-Centered Care; Teamwork and Collaboration; Safety QSEN

A 77-year-old widower reports pain in his back and abdomen. He had a radical prostatectomy for prostate cancer 5 years ago and was thought to be cancer-free until this time. A chest x-ray revealed bone metastasis in his vertebral spine. The patient is admitted to the cancer center for intensive treatment.

1. What other patient history information do you need to provide quality care for this patient and why?
2. What treatment options does this patient have to manage his bone cancer? What is the purpose of treating the cancer at this time?
3. For what major complications might this patient be most at risk, and how will you plan to help prevent them? *(Hint: see Chapter 22.)*
4. With what health care team members will you collaborate and why?
5. What are the major considerations for discharge planning?

Community-Based Care

After medical treatment for a primary malignant tumor, the patient is usually managed at home with follow-up care. The patient with metastatic disease may remain in the home or, when home support is not available, may be admitted to a long-term care facility for extended or hospice care. Coordinate the patient's discharge plan and continuity of care with the case manager and other health care team members, depending on the patient's needs.

Home Care Management. In collaboration with the occupational therapist, evaluate the patient's home environment for structural barriers that may hinder MOBILITY. The patient may be discharged with a cast, walker, crutches, or a wheelchair. Assess the patient's support system for availability of assistance if needed.

Accessibility to eating and toileting facilities is essential to promote ADL independence. Because the patient with metastatic disease is susceptible to pathologic fractures, potential hazards that may contribute to falls or injury should be removed.

Self-Management Education. For the patient receiving intermittent chemotherapy or radiation on an ambulatory care basis, emphasize the importance of keeping appointments. Review the expected side and toxic effects of the drugs with the patient and family. Teach how to treat less serious side effects and when to contact the health care provider. If the drugs are administered at home via long-term IV catheter, explain and demonstrate the care involved with daily dressing changes and potential catheter complications. Chapter 13 describes the health teaching required for a patient receiving infusion therapy at home.

If the patient has undergone surgery, he or she has a wound and limited MOBILITY. Teach the patient, family, and/or significant others how to care for the wound. Help the patient learn how to perform ADLs and mobility activities independently for self-management. Coordinate with the physical and occupational therapists to assist in ADL teaching, and provide or recommend assistive and adaptive devices, if necessary. The physical therapist also teaches the proper use of ambulatory aids, such as crutches, and exercises.

PAIN management can be a major challenge, particularly for the patient with metastatic bone disease. Discuss the various options for pain relief, including relaxation and music therapy. Emphasize the importance of those techniques that worked during hospitalization. See Chapter 3 for cancer pain assessment and management.

The patient with bone cancer may fear that the malignancy will return. Acknowledge this fear, but reinforce confidence in the health care team and medical treatment chosen. Mutually establish realistic outcomes regarding returning to work and participating in recreational activities. Encourage the patient to resume a functional lifestyle, but caution that it should be gradual. Certain activities, such as participating in sports, may be prohibited.

Help the patient with advanced metastatic bone disease prepare for death. The nurse and other support personnel assist the patient through the stages of death and dying. Identify resources that can help the patient write a will, visit with distant family members, or do whatever he or she thinks is needed for a peaceful death. Chapter 7 describes end-of-life care in detail.

Health Care Resources. In addition to family and significant others, cancer support groups are helpful to the patient with bone cancer. Some organizations, such as *I Can Cope*, provide information and emotional support. Others, such as *CanSurmount*, are geared more toward patient and family education. The American Cancer Society (www.cancer.org) and the Canadian Cancer Society (www.cancer.ca) can also provide education and resources for patients and families.

The hospital staff nurse, discharge planner, or case manager also ensures that follow-up care, including nursing care and physical or occupational therapy, is available in the home. The patient with terminal cancer may choose to become part of a hospice program as described in Chapter 7.

DISORDERS OF THE HAND

Dupuytren's Contracture

Dupuytren's contracture, or deformity, is a slowly progressive thickening of the palmar fascia, resulting in flexion contracture of the fourth (ring) and fifth (little) fingers of the hand. The third or middle finger is occasionally affected. Although

Dupuytren's contracture is a common problem, the cause is unknown. It usually occurs in older Euro-American men, tends to occur in families, and can be bilateral.

When function becomes impaired, surgical release is required. A partial or selective fasciectomy (cutting of fascia) is performed. After removal of the surgical dressing, a splint may be used. Nursing care is similar to that for the patient with carpal tunnel repair (see Chapter 51).

Ganglion

A **ganglion** is a round, benign cyst, often found on a wrist or foot joint or tendon. The synovium surrounding the tendon degenerates, allowing the tendon sheath tissue to become weak and distended. Ganglia are painless on palpation, but they can cause joint discomfort after prolonged joint use or minor trauma or strain. The lesion can rapidly disappear and then recur. Ganglia are most likely to develop in people between 15 and 50 years of age. With local or regional anesthesia in a physician's office or clinic, the fluid within the cyst can be aspirated through a small needle. A cortisone injection may follow. If the cyst is very large, it is removed using a small incision. Patients should avoid strenuous activity for 48 hours after surgery and report any signs of INFLAMMATION to their health care provider.

DISORDERS OF THE FOOT

Foot Deformities

The **hallux valgus** deformity is a common foot problem in which the great toe drifts laterally at the first metatarsophalangeal (MTP) joint (Fig. 50-3). The first metatarsal head becomes enlarged, resulting in a **bunion**. As the deviation worsens, the bony enlargement causes pain, particularly when shoes are worn. Women are affected more often than men. Hallux valgus often occurs as a result of poorly fitted shoes—in particular, those with narrow toes and high heels. Other causes include osteoarthritis, rheumatoid arthritis, and family history.

For some patients who are of advanced age or are not surgical candidates, custom-made shoes can be made to fit the deformed feet and provide comfort and support. A plaster mold is made to conform to each foot from which shoes can be made. Teach the patient to consult with a podiatrist or foot clinic to be evaluated for custom shoes.

The surgical procedure, a simple **bunionectomy,** involves removal of the bony overgrowth and bursa and realignment. When other toe deformities accompany the condition or if the bony overgrowth is large, several **osteotomies,** or bone resections, may be performed. Fusions may also be performed. Screws or wires are often inserted to stabilize the bones in the great toe and first metatarsal during the healing process. If both feet are affected, one foot is usually treated at a time. Surgery usually is performed as a same-day procedure.

Most patients are allowed partial weight bearing while wearing an orthopedic boot or shoe. Walking is difficult because the feet bear body weight. The healing time after surgery may be more than 6 to 12 weeks because the feet receive less blood flow than other parts of the body because of their distance from the heart.

Often patients have hammertoes and hallux valgus deformities at the same time. As shown in Fig. 50-4, a **hammertoe** is the dorsiflexion of any MTP joint with plantar flexion of the proximal interphalangeal (PIP) joint next to it. The second toe is most often affected. As the deformity worsens, uncomfortable corns may develop on the dorsal side of the toe and calluses may appear on the plantar surface. Patients are uncomfortable when wearing shoes and walking.

Hammertoe may be treated by surgical correction of the deformity with osteotomies (bone resections) and the insertion of wires or screws for fixation. The postoperative course is similar to that for the patient with hallux valgus repair. The patient uses crutches until full weight bearing is allowed several weeks after surgery.

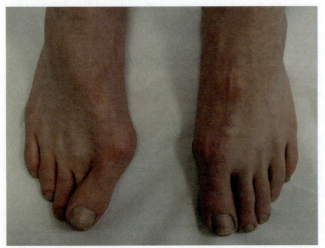

FIG. 50-3 Appearance of hallux valgus with a bunion.

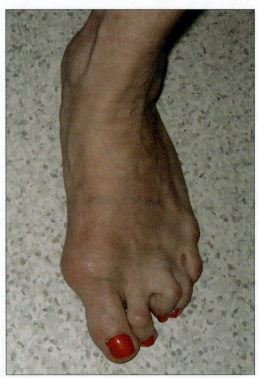

FIG. 50-4 Hammertoe of the second metatarsophalangeal joint.

Morton's Neuroma

In the patient with Morton's neuroma, or plantar digital neuritis, a small tumor grows in a digital nerve of the foot. The patient usually describes the PAIN as an acute, burning sensation in the web space. The pain involves the entire surface of the third and fourth toes. Management involves surgical removal of the neuroma and application of a pressure dressing. Ambulation is usually permitted immediately after surgery.

Plantar Fasciitis

Plantar fasciitis is an INFLAMMATION of the plantar fascia, which is located in the area of the arch of the foot. It is often seen in middle-aged and older adults, as well as in athletes, especially runners. Obesity is also a contributing factor. Patients report severe PAIN in the arch of the foot, especially when getting out of bed. The pain is worsened with weight bearing. Although most patients have unilateral plantar fasciitis, the problem can affect both feet (McCance et al., 2014).

Most patients respond to conservative management, which includes rest, ice, stretching exercises, strapping of the foot to maintain the arch, shoes with good support, and orthotics. NSAIDs or steroids may be needed to control PAIN and INFLAMMATION. If conservative measures are unsuccessful, endoscopic surgery to remove the inflamed tissue may be required. Teach the patient about the importance of adhering to the treatment plan and coordinating care with the physical therapist for instruction in exercise.

Other Problems of the Foot

Table 50-4 lists other common foot problems and how they are managed. Although patients are usually not hospitalized for these conditions, the nurse may recognize a foot disorder and alert the physician. Even small deformities or other foot deformities can be very annoying and painful for the patient and may hinder ambulation, as well as interfere with ADLs.

TABLE 50-4 **Treatment of Common Foot Problems**	
DESCRIPTION/CAUSE	**TREATMENT**
Corn	
Induration and thickening of the skin caused by friction and pressure; painful conical mass	Surgical removal by podiatrist
Callus	
Flat, poorly defined mass on the sole over a bony prominence caused by pressure	Padding and lanolin creams; overall good skin hygiene
Ingrown Nail	
Nail sliver penetration of the skin, causing inflammation	Removal of sliver by podiatrist; warm soaks; antibiotic ointment
Hypertrophic Ungual Labium	
Chronic hypertrophy of nail lip caused by improper nail trimming; results from untreated ingrown nail	Surgical removal of necrotic nail and skin; treatment of secondary infection

SCOLIOSIS

❖ PATHOPHYSIOLOGY

Scoliosis occurs when the vertebrae rotate and begin to compress. The spinal column begins to move into a lateral curve, most commonly in the right lateral thoracic area (see Fig. 49-3 in Chapter 49). As the degree of curvature increases, damage to the vertebral bodies results. The degree of the curvature increases during periods of growth, such as in adolescence. Curvature of greater than 50 degrees results in an unstable spine, and curvature of greater than 60 degrees in the thoracic spine results in compromise of cardiopulmonary function.

The exact cause of scoliosis is not well understood, yet it affects about 6 million people in the United States. The process may result from some problem in the balance mechanism located in the central nervous system. Females are affected more often than males, and onset is often in adolescence (Voda, 2009a). School health nurses screen children for scoliosis during the middle school years. Information about caring for children with scoliosis is found in most pediatric nursing textbooks. Scoliosis that occurs in childhood or early adolescence may persist into adulthood. Adults often develop scoliosis as a result of spinal degeneration.

Three types of scoliosis can be described: congenital, neuromuscular, and idiopathic; the most common curve pattern in adults is idiopathic scoliosis and the cause is unknown (Voda, 2009a). Congenital scoliosis occurs during embryonic development. Neuromuscular scoliosis can result from a neuromuscular condition in childhood or adulthood, such as cerebral palsy or spinal cord tumors. Untreated scoliosis can lead to back pain, deformity, and cardiopulmonary complications.

❖ PATIENT-CENTERED COLLABORATIVE CARE

◆ Assessment

A complete history of the patient with spinal deformity should include onset of problem, in adolescence or adulthood, and what treatments may have been used in the past. Patients who had surgery for scoliosis during adolescence are returning with progressive, debilitating back pain from degenerative disk disease below the level of vertebral fusion. A loss of lumbar curvature, or lordosis, described as "flat back" syndrome, may also be present (Voda, 2009a). Complete a thorough pain assessment for patients reporting back pain.

Observe the patient from the front and back, while standing and during forward flexion from the hips. Physical examination usually reveals asymmetry of hip and shoulder height, prominence of the thoracic ribs and scapula on one side, and visible curve in the spinal column. Observation from the side may reveal kyphosis of the thoracic spine. Assess for leg length differences as well.

Methods of managing adult scoliosis differ from those used for children. The adult spinal column is less flexible and therefore less likely to respond to exercises, weight reduction, bracing, and casting for correction of the deformity. In the adult, the disorder is progressive and can result in an additional one degree of deviation each year.

◆ Interventions

Adults with less than 50 degrees of curvature of the spine may be treated conservatively with moist heat, pain medication, and exercise. Those with greater than 50 degrees of curvature may require surgical intervention to prevent shortness of breath and fatigue, osteoarthritis, and severe back pain (Voda, 2009a).

The traditional open *surgical* reconstructive procedure consists of surgical fusion and insertion of instrumentation, including plates, screws, or rods to stabilize the spine. The surgeon performs spinal fusion by packing cancellous bone chips, usually from the iliac crest, between the affected vertebrae for support and stabilization. Both an anterior and a posterior approach may be needed. If so, the surgeon may perform both procedures during the same operative day or may stage them 7 to 10 days apart. The metal instrumentation supports the spine and immobilizes the fused area during healing.

> ### ! NURSING SAFETY PRIORITY (QSEN)
> *Action Alert*
>
> The priority for nursing care after open spinal reconstructive surgery for scoliosis is to assess the patient's respiratory status and encourage deep breathing. Teach the patient how to use the incentive spirometer to prevent atelectasis.

Either an anterior or posterior surgical thoracic or abdominal approach may be used. For anterior thoracic surgery, a chest tube is in place for about 72 hours; for anterior abdominal surgery, the patient has a nasogastric tube for 24 hours. Chapter 16 discusses general postoperative care for patients who have general anesthesia. Other nursing care is similar to that for the patient undergoing a laminectomy or spinal fusion, including teaching the patient how to log roll, keeping the body in alignment. The traditional surgery for treating scoliosis has a high percentage of complications and results in major scarring.

Several newer minimally invasive surgical (MIS) procedures are being performed at major neurosurgery centers to treat degenerative and idiopathic adult scoliosis. These surgeries are done in stages, usually several days apart, using special endoscopic instrumentation that does not require large incisions. The advantages of these procedures include shorter hospital stays, far fewer complications, less pain, and very small incisions (Voda, 2009a).

Teach patients and their families about home care, including how to care for the wound; body mechanics to prevent bending, twisting, and lifting; and how to adapt to achieve ADLs independently. Some patients may require home care nursing, physical therapy, or a home health aide for a short time after discharge if a traditional surgical approach was used (Voda, 2009a). Collaborate with the case manager to make the appropriate arrangements for continuity of care to meet the patient's needs.

For some patients, a return to work in about 3 to 6 weeks is realistic. Other surgical procedures may prevent the patient from performing these activities until 3 to 6 months postoperatively. Refer patients and their families to the National Scoliosis Foundation (www.scoliosis.org) for information and support services.

PROGRESSIVE MUSCULAR DYSTROPHIES

Many types of **muscular dystrophy (MD)** have been categorized as slowly progressive or rapidly progressive. The slowly progressive types are most commonly seen in adults. Most pediatric nursing books describe the care for patients with MD in detail. Four forms of MD are often seen in adults. Each type has its own distinct characteristics and causes, but all are progressive (Table 50-5).

The exact pathophysiologic mechanisms are unknown, but several causes are possible. These include:
- Poor blood flow to muscle resulting in reduced tissue oxygenation
- Disturbance in nerve-muscle interaction
- Loss of cell membrane integrity as a result of increased enzyme activity

Regardless of the type of MD, the primary problem is progressive muscle weakness. The major cause of death is respiratory failure caused by profound respiratory muscle weakness. Cardiac failure also occurs because dystrophin activity is needed for cardiac muscle contraction and maintenance (McCance et al., 2014).

Diagnosis of MD is often difficult because the clinical manifestations are similar to those of other muscular disorders. Muscle biopsy often confirms the diagnosis. Muscle weakness

TABLE 50-5	Differential Features of Common Muscular Dystrophies Seen in Adults		
ONSET	**GENETIC LINK**	**CLINICAL MANIFESTATIONS**	**PROGRESSION**
Becker (Benign X-Linked) Dystrophy			
5-25 yr	Sex-linked recessive; expression in males	Wasting of pelvic and shoulder muscles; normal cardiac and mental function	Gradual progression; inability to walk 25 yr after onset; usually normal life span
Limb-Girdle Dystrophy			
Usually 20s or 30s	Usually autosomal dominant; expression in either gender	Upper extremity and neck muscles and lower extremity and hip muscle weakness	Extremely variable; severe disability within 10-20 yr after onset; life span shortened by 10-20 yr
Facioscapulohumeral (Landouzy-Dejerine) Dystrophy			
Usually in 20s	Autosomal dominant; expression in either gender	Facial and shoulder girdle muscle involvement	Usually benign; normal life span
Myotonic (Steinert) Dystrophy			
Birth to 40s	Autosomal dominant; expression in either gender	Muscle atrophy with multiple organ involvement (e.g., heart, lungs, smooth muscle, and endocrine system)	Usually gradual if onset in adulthood

GENETIC/GENOMIC CONSIDERATIONS

Patient-Centered Care QSEN

The major pathologic change that occurs in most types of MD is the production or faulty action of a muscle protein called **dystrophin**. The purpose of this protein is to maintain muscle integrity by sending signals to coordinate smooth, synchronous muscle fiber contraction. The coding of this protein is by a large gene that has many parts located on the X chromosome. Different mutations of the gene where dystrophin is located determine the degree of muscle weakness. Because this protein connects with other substances for final muscle action, genetic mutations of these other substances can make dystrophin fail to work properly.

The most common forms of MD are Duchenne MD (DMD) and Becker MD (BMD). Both are X-linked recessive disorders. Women who are *carriers* (able to pass on the gene without having the disorder) have a 50% chance of passing the MD gene to their daughters, who are then carriers, and to their sons, who then have the disease. These types of MD, then, affect only males. In DMD, most patients die very young and therefore do not have children. In BMD, the patient lives longer and may have children. None of these men's sons will have the disease, but their daughters will be carriers (Nussbaum et al., 2007). Refer carriers for genetic testing and counseling.

and trophic changes are characteristic of all types of MD. Serum muscle enzyme values, such as aldolase and creatine kinase, may be elevated, and electromyographic (EMG) findings are often abnormal (Pagana & Pagana, 2014).

Collaborative care of the patient with MD is supportive and involves the entire health care team. Physical and occupational therapy help the patient maintain as much function, MOBILITY, and independence as possible. A neurologist is often the specialist who diagnoses and treats patients with MD. Refer the patient and family to the local chapter of the Muscular Dystrophy Association (www.mda.org) for support services and information.

Major organ or body system involvement is medically managed, but the life span is often shortened from these manifestations of the disease. With the exception of steroids, no drug has been found to slow the progression of the disorder, although immunosuppressive agents, anabolic steroids, and growth factors have been tried.

Nursing interventions focus on making the patient as comfortable as possible, providing supportive care, and reinforcing techniques and exercises taught in the physical therapy program. The nurse's role in caring for a patient with cardiac or other organ involvement is the same as for any patient with dysfunction of these systems.

NURSING CONCEPTS AND CLINICAL JUDGMENT REVIEW

What might you NOTICE if the patient has impaired MOBILITY as a result of chronic musculoskeletal disorders?
- Spinal deformity (e.g., kyphosis, lateral deviation)
- Bone malalignment (e.g., leg bowing)
- Muscle weakness
- Bone swelling or deformity
- Fracture
- Joint inflammation
- Flushed skin (Paget's disease)
- Fever (bone infection)
- Report of pain
- Report of weight loss

What should you INTERPRET and how should you RESPOND to a patient with impaired MOBILITY as a result of chronic musculoskeletal disorders?

Perform and interpret focused physical assessment findings, including:
- Ability to ambulate (with or without assistive device)
- ADLs ability
- Body weight
- Pain intensity and quality
- Neurovascular assessment findings
- Ability to cope with decreased mobility

Respond by:
- Providing pain control interventions, including drugs and nonpharmacologic measures

- Collaborating with members of the health care team, including physical therapist (PT), occupational therapist (OT), dietitian, as needed
- Teaching about drugs that may be needed for long-term use, including side and toxic effects
- Explaining about the need for adequate calcium and vitamin D for healthy bones and bone healing
- Assisting with ADLs and ambulation as needed, but encouraging independence when possible
- Implementing measures to prevent patient falls in the inpatient and home setting
- Encouraging the patient to discuss feelings related to disorders causing impaired mobility
- Referring patients to appropriate community resources, such as the National Osteoporosis Foundation and Paget Disease Foundation

On what should you REFLECT?
- Monitor the patient's response to pain control interventions.
- Prevent and monitor the patient for falls.
- Evaluate the patient's knowledge of nutrition and drug therapy.
- Evaluate the patient's coping ability related to disease diagnosis and treatment.
- Think about what else you might do to promote mobility.
- Decide whether you need to provide alternative interventions or additional health teaching.

GET READY FOR THE NCLEX® EXAMINATION!

KEY POINTS

Review these Key Points for each NCLEX Examination Client Needs Category.

Safe and Effective Care Environment
- Coordinate with health care team members when assessing patients with osteoporosis for risk for falls. **Safety** **QSEN**
- In coordination with the physical and occupational therapists, educate the patient and family on home safety when the patient has a metabolic bone disease, such as osteoporosis. **Teamwork and Collaboration** **QSEN**
- Refer to The Joint Commission for information about National Patient Safety Goals related to fall injury prevention.

Health Promotion and Maintenance
- Teach patients at risk for osteoporosis to minimize risk factors, such as stopping smoking, decreasing alcohol intake, exercising regularly, and increasing dietary calcium.
- Remind patients at risk for osteoporosis to have regular screening tests, such as the DXA scan.
- Instruct older adults to have at least 5 minutes of sun per day and to eat vitamin D–fortified foods to prevent osteomalacia.
- Assess the genetic risk for patients who have parents with muscular dystrophy, and refer them for genetic testing and counseling if the patient desires. **Patient-Centered Care** **QSEN**
- Refer patients with musculoskeletal problems to appropriate community resources, such as the Paget Disease Foundation and the National Osteoporosis Foundation.

Psychosocial Integrity
- Assess the patient's and family's responses to a diagnosis of bone cancer and treatment options. Be aware that they will progress through the grieving process.

Physiological Integrity
- Remind patients taking bisphosphonates (BPs) to take them early in the morning, at least 30 to 60 minutes before breakfast, with a full glass of water and to remain sitting upright during that time to prevent esophagitis, a common complication of BP therapy.
- Most patients are unaware that they have osteoporosis until they experience a fracture, the most common complication of the disease.
- Osteomalacia, the result of a deficiency in vitamin D, can be caused by the factors listed in Table 50-3.
- Priority care for patients with osteomyelitis is to treat the INFECTION and maintain Contact Precautions for open wounds. For patients having surgical intervention, assess the affected extremity for neurovascular status to ensure adequate tissue perfusion.
- For patients who have surgery for bone cancer, report postoperative manifestations of infection, dislocation, or neurovascular compromise to the surgeon promptly.
- Assess for key features of Paget's disease as summarized in Chart 50-3.
- Remember that bone tumors can be benign or malignant.
- Remember that severe chronic PAIN is a priority for patients with metastatic bone disease.
- Be aware that even minor hand and foot problems can be very painful. Common foot problems are described in Table 50-4.
- In collaboration with the health care team (physical therapist, occupational therapist, neurologist), provide supportive care for patients with muscular dystrophy and bone cancer.
- Recognize that most major types of muscular dystrophy are genetic and manifest usually in childhood. Care is supportive.
- Foot disorders can be treated with custom-made shoes or surgery to repair deformities. Recall that foot disorders are painful, and a plan for pain management is essential.

CHAPTER 51

Care of Patients with Musculoskeletal Trauma

Donna D. Ignatavicius

 http://evolve.elsevier.com/Iggy/

PRIORITY CONCEPTS

- MOBILITY
- SENSORY PERCEPTION
- PAIN
- PERFUSION
- INFECTION

LEARNING OUTCOMES

Safe and Effective Care Environment

1. Explain the importance of collaborating with the health care team when providing care for patients with fractures and amputations.

Health Promotion and Maintenance

2. Identify community resources about amputations for patients and their families.
3. Teach the public about ways to prevent fractures and other musculoskeletal injuries.
4. Plan discharge teaching for patients with fractures and amputations.

Psychosocial Integrity

5. Describe how to assess the patient's and family's reaction to changes in body image and SENSORY PERCEPTION resulting from amputation.

Physiological Integrity

6. Compare and contrast open versus closed fractures and their potential complications.

7. Assess patients with musculoskeletal trauma to prioritize interventions for their care.
8. Delineate nursing care needed to maintain casts for patients with fractures.
9. Plan nursing care needed to maintain traction and external fixation for patients with fractures.
10. Implement measures to prevent complications of fractures, including INFECTION and decreased PERFUSION.
11. Develop an evidence-based postoperative plan of care, including health teaching, for a patient after fracture repair.
12. Describe emergency care for people who have a traumatic amputation.
13. Plan postoperative care, including health teaching, after an elective amputation.
14. Describe the patient-centered care needed to manage complex regional PAIN syndrome.
15. Plan care for patients with common types of soft tissue injuries, such as carpal tunnel syndrome.

Musculoskeletal trauma accounts for about two thirds of all injuries and is one of the primary causes of disability in the United States. It ranges from simple muscle strain to multiple bone fractures with severe soft-tissue damage.

Fractures and other musculoskeletal trauma impair a patient's MOBILITY in varying degrees, depending on the severity and extent of the injury. These injuries also affect SENSORY PERCEPTION and PAIN because of pressure on nerve endings from edema. In some cases, peripheral nerves are directly damaged as a result of musculoskeletal injury.

FRACTURES

❖ PATHOPHYSIOLOGY

A **fracture** is a break or disruption in the continuity of a bone that often affects MOBILITY and SENSORY PERCEPTION. It can occur anywhere in the body and at any age. All fractures have the same basic pathophysiologic mechanism and require similar patient-centered collaborative care, regardless of fracture type or location.

Classification of Fractures

A fracture is classified by the extent of the break:

- *Complete fracture.* The break is across the entire width of the bone in such a way that the bone is divided into two distinct sections.
- *Incomplete fracture.* The fracture does not divide the bone into two portions because the break is through only part of the bone.

A fracture is described by the extent of associated soft-tissue damage as **open** (or **compound**) or **closed** (or **simple**). The skin surface over the broken bone is disrupted in a *compound*

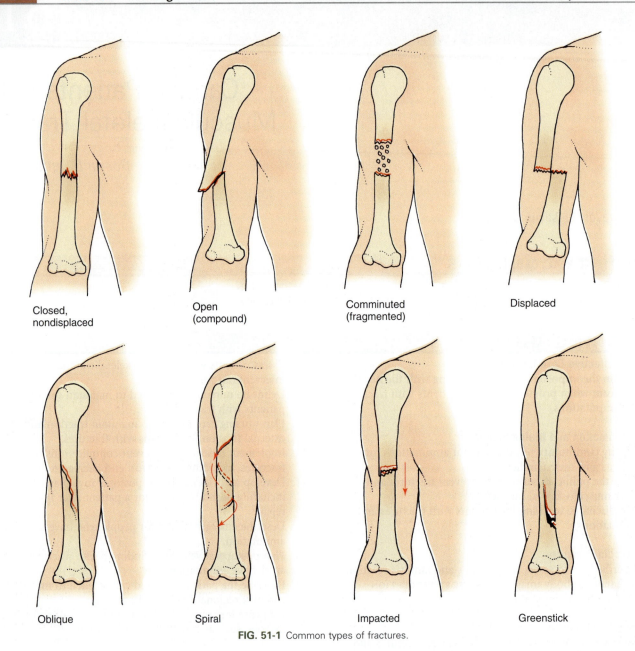

Closed, nondisplaced

Open (compound)

Comminuted (fragmented)

Displaced

Oblique

Spiral

Impacted

Greenstick

FIG. 51-1 Common types of fractures.

fracture, which causes an external wound. These fractures are often graded to define the extent of tissue damage. A *simple* fracture does not extend through the skin and therefore has no visible wound.

Fig. 51-1 shows common types of fractures. In addition to being identified by type, fractures are described by their cause. A **pathologic (spontaneous) fracture** occurs after minimal trauma to a bone that has been weakened by disease. For example, a patient with bone cancer or osteoporosis can easily have a pathologic fracture. A **fatigue (stress) fracture** results from excessive strain and stress on the bone. This problem is commonly seen in recreational and professional athletes. **Compression fractures** are produced by a loading force applied to the long axis of cancellous bone. They commonly occur in the vertebrae of older patients with osteoporosis and are extremely painful.

Stages of Bone Healing

When a bone is fractured, the body immediately begins the healing process to repair the injury and restore the body's equilibrium. Fractures heal in five stages that are a continuous process and not single stages.

- In stage one, within 24 to 72 hours after the injury, a hematoma forms at the site of the fracture because bone is extremely vascular.
- Stage two occurs in 3 days to 2 weeks when granulation tissue begins to invade the hematoma. This then prompts the formation of fibrocartilage, providing the foundation for bone healing.
- Stage three of bone healing occurs as a result of vascular and cellular proliferation. The fracture site is surrounded by new vascular tissue known as a *callus* (within 3 to 6

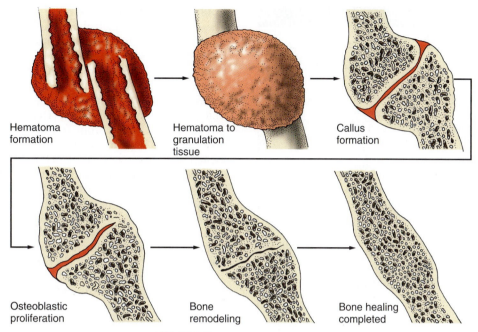

FIG. 51-2 The stages of bone healing.

Labels: Hematoma formation; Hematoma to granulation tissue; Callus formation; Osteoblastic proliferation; Bone remodeling; Bone healing completed

weeks). Callus formation is the beginning of a nonbony union.

- As healing continues in stage four, the callus is gradually resorbed and transformed into bone. This stage usually takes 3 to 8 weeks.
- During the fifth and final stage of healing, consolidation and remodeling of bone continue to meet mechanical demands. This process may start as early as 4 to 6 weeks after fracture and can continue for up to 1 year, depending on the severity of the injury and the age and health of the patient. Fig. 51-2 summarizes the stages of bone healing.

In young, healthy adult bone, healing takes about 4 to 6 weeks. In the older person who has reduced bone mass, healing time is lengthened. Complete healing often takes 3 months or longer in people who are older than 70 years. Other factors also affect healing. Examples include the severity of the trauma, the type of bone injured, how the fracture is managed, infections at the fracture site, and ischemic or avascular necrosis (AVN), also called osteonecrosis.

CONSIDERATIONS FOR OLDER ADULTS
Patient-Centered Care QSEN

Bone healing is often affected by the aging process. Bone formation and strength rely on adequate nutrition. Calcium, phosphorus, vitamin D, and protein are necessary for the production of new bone (see Chapter 50). For women, the loss of estrogen after menopause decreases the body's ability to form new bone tissue. Chronic diseases can also affect the rate at which bone heals. For instance, peripheral vascular diseases, such as arteriosclerosis, reduce arterial circulation to bone. Thus the bone receives less oxygen and fewer nutrients, both of which are needed for repair.

Complications of Fractures

Regardless of the type or location of the fracture, several limb- and life-threatening acute and chronic complications can result

from the injury. Clinical manifestations of beginning complications must be treated early to prevent serious consequences. In some cases, careful monitoring and assessment can prevent these complications:

- Acute compartment syndrome
- Crush syndrome
- Hypovolemic shock
- Fat embolism syndrome
- Venous thromboembolism
- Infection
- Chronic complications, such as ischemic necrosis and delayed union

Acute Compartment Syndrome. Compartments are areas in the body in which muscles, blood vessels, and nerves are contained within fascia. Most compartments are located in the extremities. Fascia is an inelastic tissue that surrounds groups of muscles, blood vessels, and nerves in the body. Acute compartment syndrome (ACS) is a serious condition in which increased pressure within one or more compartments reduces circulation to the area. The most common sites for this problem in patients with musculoskeletal trauma are the compartments in the lower leg (tibial fractures) and forearm (Hershey, 2013).

The pathophysiologic changes of increased compartment pressure are sometimes referred to as the *ischemia-edema cycle.* Capillaries within the muscle dilate, which raises capillary (arterial) pressure and venous pressure (Hershey, 2013). Capillaries become more permeable because of the release of histamine by the ischemic muscle tissue, and venous drainage decreases (Friedrich & Shin, 2012). As a result, plasma proteins leak into the interstitial fluid space and edema occurs. Edema increases pressure on nerve endings and causes pain. PERFUSION to the area is reduced, and further ischemia results. SENSORY PERCEPTION deficits or paresthesia generally appears before changes in vascular or motor signs. The color of the tissue pales, and pulses begin to weaken but rarely disappear. The affected area is usually palpably tense, and PAIN occurs with passive motion of the extremity. If the condition is not treated, cyanosis, tingling,

CHART 51-1   Key Features

Compartment Syndrome

PHYSIOLOGIC CHANGE	CLINICAL FINDINGS
Increased compartment pressure	No change
Increased capillary permeability	Edema
Release of histamine	Increased edema
Increased blood flow to area	Pulses present Pink tissue
Pressure on nerve endings	Pain
Increased tissue pressure	Referred pain to compartment
Decreased tissue perfusion	Increased edema
Decreased oxygen to tissues	Pallor
Increased production of lactic acid	Unequal pulses Flexed posture
Anaerobic metabolism	Cyanosis
Vasodilation	Increased edema
Increased blood flow	Tense muscle swelling
Increased tissue pressure	Tingling Numbness
Increased edema	Paresthesia
Muscle ischemia	Severe pain unrelieved by drugs
Tissue necrosis	Paresis/paralysis

numbness, paresis, necrosis, and severe pain can occur. Chart 51-1 summarizes the sequence of pathophysiologic events in compartment syndrome and the associated clinical assessment findings.

The pressure to the compartment can be from an external or internal source, but fracture is present in 75% of all cases of ACS (Hershey, 2013). Tight, bulky dressings and casts are examples of *external* pressure. Blood or fluid accumulation in the compartment is a common source of *internal* pressure. The injury or trauma causing the problem is above the compartment involved, which decreases blood flow to the more distal area of injury. ACS is not limited to patients with musculoskeletal problems. It can also occur in those with severe burns, extensive insect bites or snakebites, or massive infiltration of IV fluids. In these situations, edema increases internal pressure in one or more compartments.

Problems resulting from compartment syndrome include infection, persistent motor weakness in the affected extremity, contracture, and myoglobinuric renal failure. In extreme cases, amputation becomes necessary (Hershey, 2013).

Infection from necrosis may become severe enough that amputation of the limb is needed. *Motor weakness* from injured nerves is not reversible, and the patient may require an orthotic device for assistance in mobility. Volkmann's *contractures* of the forearm, which can begin within 12 hours of the pressure increase, result from shortening of the ischemic muscle and from nerve involvement.

Hypovolemic Shock. Bone is very vascular. Therefore bleeding is a risk with bone injury. In addition, trauma can cut nearby arteries and cause hemorrhage, resulting in rapidly developing hypovolemic shock. (The pathophysiology of hypovolemic shock is described in Chapter 37.)

Fat Embolism Syndrome. Fat embolism syndrome (FES) is another serious complication in which fat globules are released from the yellow bone marrow into the bloodstream within 12

to 48 hours after an injury or other illness (mechanical theory). These globules clog small blood vessels that supply vital organs, most commonly the lungs, and impair organ PERFUSION. The biochemical theory for FES may be considered as a separate cause or as an additive process to the mechanical theory. The embolized fat degrades into free fatty acids and C-reactive protein, which results in capillary leakage, lipid and platelet aggregation, and clot formation (Hershey, 2013).

FES usually results from fractures or fracture repair but occasionally is seen in patients who have a total joint replacement. It may also occur, although less often, in those with pancreatitis, osteomyelitis, blunt trauma, or sickle cell disease.

The problem can occur at any age or in either gender, but young men between ages 20 and 40 years and older adults between ages 70 and 80 years are at the greatest risk. Patients with fractured hips have the highest risk, but FES is also common in those with fractures of the pelvis within 24 to 72 hours after injury or surgery (Hershey, 2013).

The earliest manifestations of FES are a low arterial oxygen level (hypoxemia), dyspnea, and tachypnea (increased respirations). Headache, lethargy, agitation, confusion, decreased level of consciousness, seizures, and vision changes may follow (Hershey, 2013). Nonpalpable, red-brown **petechiae**—a macular, measles-like rash—may appear over the neck, upper arms, and/or chest. This rash is a classic manifestation but is usually the last sign to develop (Hershey, 2013).

Abnormal laboratory findings include:
- Decreased Pao_2 level (often below 60 mm Hg)
- Increased erythrocyte sedimentation rate (ESR)
- Decreased serum calcium levels
- Decreased red blood cell and platelet counts
- Increased serum level of lipids

These changes in blood values are poorly understood, but they aid in diagnosis of the condition.

The chest x-ray often shows bilateral infiltrates but may be normal. The chest CT often reveals a patchy distribution of opacities. An MRI of the brain can show evidence of neurologic deficits from hypoxemia. FES can result in respiratory failure or death, often from pulmonary edema. When the lungs are affected, the complication may be misdiagnosed as a pulmonary embolism from a blood clot (Chart 51-2).

Venous Thromboembolism. Venous thromboembolism (VTE) includes deep vein thrombosis (DVT) and its major complication, pulmonary embolism (PE). It is the most common complication of lower extremity surgery or trauma and the most often fatal complication of musculoskeletal surgery. Factors that make patients with fractures most likely to develop VTE include:
- Cancer or chemotherapy
- Surgical procedure longer than 30 minutes
- History of smoking
- Obesity
- Heart disease
- Prolonged immobility
- Oral contraceptives or hormones
- History of VTE complications
- Older adults (especially with hip fractures)

The pathophysiology and management of VTE are described in Chapter 36.

Infection. Whenever there is trauma to tissues, the body's defense system is disrupted. Wound infections are the most common type of INFECTION resulting from orthopedic trauma.

CHART 51-2 Key Features

Pulmonary Emboli: Fat Embolism Versus Blood Clot Embolism

FAT EMBOLISM	BLOOD CLOT EMBOLISM
Definition	
Obstruction of the pulmonary vascular bed by fat globules	Obstruction of the pulmonary artery by a blood clot or clots
Origin	
95% from fractures of the long bones; occurs usually within 48 hr of injury	85% from deep vein thrombosis in the legs or pelvis; can occur anytime
Assessment Findings	
Altered mental status (earliest sign)	Same as for fat embolism, except no petechiae
Increased respirations, pulse, temperature	
Chest pain	
Dyspnea	
Crackles	
Decreased SaO₂	
Petechiae (50%-60%)	
Retinal hemorrhage (not common)	
Mild thrombocytopenia	
Treatment	
Bedrest	Preventive measures (e.g., leg exercises, antiembolism stockings, SCDs)
Gentle handling	
Oxygen	
Hydration (IV fluids)	Bedrest
Possibly steroid therapy	Oxygen
Fracture immobilization	Possibly mechanical ventilation
	Anticoagulants
	Thrombolytics
	Possible surgery: pulmonary embolectomy, vena cava umbrella

SaO₂, Arterial oxygen saturation; *SCD,* sequential compression device.

They range from superficial skin infections to deep wound abscesses. Infection can also be caused by implanted hardware used to repair a fracture surgically, such as pins, plates, or rods. Clostridial infections can result in gas gangrene or tetanus and can prevent the bone from healing properly.

Bone INFECTION, or **osteomyelitis**, is most common with open fractures in which skin integrity is lost and after surgical repair of a fracture (see Chapter 50 for discussion of osteomyelitis). For patients experiencing this type of trauma, the risk for hospital-acquired infections is increased. These infections are common, and many are from multidrug-resistant organisms, such as methicillin-resistant *Staphylococcus aureus* (MRSA). Reducing MRSA infections is a primary desired outcome for all health care agencies.

Chronic Complications. Avascular necrosis and delayed bone healing are later complications of musculoskeletal trauma. Blood supply to the bone is disrupted causing decreased PERFUSION and death of bone tissue. This problem is most often a complication of hip fractures or any fracture in which there is displacement of bone. Surgical repair of fractures also can cause necrosis because the hardware can interfere with circulation. Patients on long-term corticosteroid therapy, such as prednisone, are also at high risk for ischemic necrosis.

Delayed union is a fracture that has not healed within 6 months of injury. Some fractures never achieve union; that is, they never completely heal *(nonunion)*. Others heal incorrectly *(malunion)*. These problems are most common in patients with tibial fractures, fractures that involve many treatment techniques (e.g., cast, traction), and pathologic fractures. Union may also be delayed or not achieved in the older patient. If bone does not heal, he or she typically has chronic pain and immobility from deformity.

Etiology and Genetic Risk

The primary cause of a fracture is trauma from a motor vehicle crash or fall, especially in older adults. The trauma may be a direct blow to the bone or an indirect force from muscle contractions or pulling forces on the bone. Sports, vigorous exercise, and malnutrition are contributing factors. Bone diseases, such as osteoporosis, increase the risk for a fracture in older adults (see Chapter 50). Genetic factors that increase risk for fracture are discussed with these specific health problems throughout this text.

Incidence and Prevalence

The incidence of fractures depends on the location of the injury. Rib fractures are the most common type in the adult population. Femoral shaft fractures occur most often in young and middle-aged adults. The incidence of proximal femur (hip) fractures is highest in older adults. Humeral fractures are common in adults; the older the person, usually the more proximal is the fracture. Wrist (Colles') fractures are typically seen in middle and late adulthood and usually result from a fall. Middle-aged and older adults, especially women, have a higher incidence of osteoporosis, which increases the risk for fragility fractures.

Health Promotion and Maintenance

Airbags and seat belts have decreased the number of severe injuries and deaths, but they have increased the number of leg and ankle fractures, especially in older adults. Health teaching should also focus on other risks for musculoskeletal injury, including:

- Osteoporosis screening and self-management education
- Fall prevention
- Home safety assessment and modification, if needed
- Dangers of drinking and driving
- Drug safety (prescribed, over-the-counter, and illicit)
- Older adults and driving
- Helmet use when riding bicycles, motorcycles, all-terrain vehicles (ATVs), and skateboards

These educational interventions are discussed throughout this book and in other texts. Fall prevention is discussed in detail in Chapter 2 as part of care for older adults.

❖ PATIENT-CENTERED COLLABORATIVE CARE

◆ Assessment

History. If the patient is in severe PAIN, delay the interview until he or she is more comfortable. Then ask about the cause of the fracture, which helps in developing an individualized plan of care. Certain types of force (e.g., incisional, crush, acceleration or deceleration), shearing, and friction lead to most musculoskeletal injuries. As a result, several body systems are often affected.

Incisional injuries, as from a knife wound, and *crush* injuries cause hemorrhage and decrease blood flow to major organs. *Acceleration or deceleration* injuries cause direct trauma to the spleen, brain, and kidneys when these organs are moved from their fixed locations in the body. *Shearing and friction* damage the skin and cause a high level of wound contamination.

Asking about the events leading to the injury helps identify which forces have been experienced and therefore which body systems or parts of the body to assess. For example, a forward fall often results in Colles' fracture of the wrist because the person tries to catch himself or herself with an outstretched hand. Knowing the mechanism of injury also helps determine whether other types of injury, such as head and spinal cord injury, might be present.

A drug history, including substance use, is important regardless of the patient's age. For example, a young adult may have had an excessive amount of alcohol, which contributed to a motor vehicle crash or to a fall at the work site. Many older adults also consume alcohol and an assortment of prescribed and over-the-counter drugs, which can cause dizziness and loss of balance.

A medical history may identify possible causes of the fracture and gives clues as to how long it will take for the bone to heal. Certain diseases such as bone cancer and Paget's disease cause fragility fractures that often do not achieve total healing or union.

Ask about the patient's occupation and recreational activities. Some occupations are more hazardous than others. For instance, construction work is potentially more physically dangerous than office work. Certain hobbies and recreational activities are also extremely hazardous, such as skiing. Contact sports, such as football and ice hockey, often result in musculoskeletal injuries, including fractures. Other activities do not have such an obvious potential for injury but can cause fractures nonetheless. For instance, daily jogging or running can lead to fatigue fractures.

Physical Assessment/Clinical Manifestations. The patient with a fracture often has trauma to other body systems. Therefore assess all major body systems *first* for life-threatening complications, including head, chest, and abdominal trauma. Some fractures can cause internal organ damage resulting in hemorrhage. When a pelvic fracture is suspected, assess vital signs, skin color, and level of consciousness for indications of possible hypovolemic shock. Check the urine for blood, which indicates possible damage to the urinary system, often the bladder. If the patient cannot void, suspect that the bladder or urethra has been damaged. Complete assessment of these areas is described elsewhere in this text.

The most common manifestation of fractures is moderate to often severe PAIN. Patients with severe or multiple fractures of the arms, legs, or pelvis have severe pain. Vertebral compression fractures are also extremely painful. Patients *with a fractured hip may have groin pain or pain referred to the back of the knee or lower back.* Pain is usually due to muscle spasm and edema, which result from the fracture.

For fractures of the shoulder and upper arm, the physical assessment is best done with the patient in a sitting or standing position, if possible, so that shoulder drooping or other abnormal positioning can be seen. Support the affected arm and flex the elbow to promote comfort during the assessment. For more distal areas of the arm, perform the assessment with the patient in a supine position so that the extremity can be elevated to reduce swelling.

! NURSING SAFETY PRIORITY (QSEN)
Action Alert

Patients with one or more fractured ribs have severe pain when they take deep breaths. Monitor respiratory status, which may be severely compromised from PAIN or pneumothorax (air in the pleural cavity). Assess the patient's pain level and manage pain *before* continuing the physical assessment.

Place the patient in a supine position for assessment of the legs and pelvis. A patient with an impacted hip fracture may be able to walk for a short time after injury, although this is not recommended.

When inspecting the site of a possible fracture, look for a change in bone alignment. The bone may appear deformed, a limb may be internally or externally rotated, and/or one or more bones may also be dislocated (out of their joint capsules). Observe for extremity shortening or a change in bone shape.

If the skin is intact (closed fracture), the area over the fracture may be **ecchymotic** (bruised) from bleeding into the underlying soft tissues. **Subcutaneous emphysema**, the appearance of bubbles under the skin because of air trapping, may be present but is usually seen later.

! NURSING SAFETY PRIORITY (QSEN)
Action Alert

Swelling at the fracture site is rapid and can result in marked neurovascular compromise due to decreased arterial PERFUSION. *Gently perform a thorough neurovascular assessment, and compare extremities.* Assess skin color and temperature, sensation, mobility, pain, and pulses distal to the fracture site. If the fracture involves an extremity and the patient is not in severe pain, check the nails for capillary refill by applying pressure to the nail and observing for the speed of blood return. If nails are brittle or thick, assess the skin next to the nail. Checking for capillary refill is not as reliable as other indicators of perfusion. Chart 51-3 describes the procedure for a neurovascular assessment, which evaluates **c**irculation, **m**ovement, and **s**ensation (SENSORY PERCEPTION) (CMS function).

? CLINICAL JUDGMENT CHALLENGE
Patient-Centered Care; Evidence-Based Practice (QSEN)

A 63-year-old woman fell while standing on a step ladder to reach an item on the top shelf of her closet. After calling 911, she sat in a recliner chair while protecting her swollen right arm. When the paramedics arrived, the woman was drowsy but could be awakened. She had no other apparent injury or problem. Upon arrival at the emergency department (ED), you greet the patient and help her transfer into a room. The patient continues to become very drowsy at times but stated that she did not "hit her head" when she fell.
1. What are your priority evidence-based assessments for the patient when coming into the ED?
2. What history questions will you ask the patient once her pain is controlled?
3. The patient has a fractured right distal radius and reports that she is still in pain even though the emergency medical technician (EMT) gave her IV fentanyl. How will you respond to this patient, and what action will you take?
4. The patient's husband comes to the ED and asks you if his wife's history of bone loss may have caused the fracture. How will you answer him?

CHART 51-3 **Best Practice for Patient Safety & Quality Care** QSEN

Assessment of Neurovascular Status in Patients with Musculoskeletal Injury

ASSESSMENT METHOD	NORMAL FINDINGS
Skin Color	
Inspect the area distal to the injury.	No change in pigmentation compared with other parts of the body.
Skin Temperature	
Palpate the area distal to the injury (the dorsum of the hands is most sensitive to temperature).	The skin is warm.
Movement	
Ask the patient to move the affected area or the area distal to the injury (active motion).	The patient can move without discomfort.
Move the area distal to the injury (passive motion).	No difference in comfort compared with active movement.
Sensation	
Ask the patient if numbness or tingling is present (paresthesia).	No numbness or tingling.
Palpate with a paper clip (especially the web space between the first and second toes or the web space between the thumb and forefinger).	No difference in sensation in the affected and unaffected extremities. (Loss of sensation in these areas indicates peroneal nerve or median nerve damage.)
Pulses	
Palpate the pulses distal to the injury.	Pulses are strong and easily palpated; no difference in the affected and unaffected extremities.
Capillary Refill (Least Reliable)	
Press the nail beds distal to the injury until blanching occurs (or the skin near the nail if nails are thick and brittle).	Blood returns (return to usual color) within 3 sec (5 sec for older patients).
Pain	
Ask the patient about the location, nature, and frequency of the pain.	Pain is usually localized and is often described as stabbing or throbbing. (Pain out of proportion to the injury and unrelieved by analgesics might indicate compartment syndrome.)

Psychosocial Assessment. The psychosocial status of a patient with a fracture depends on the extent of the injury, possible complications, coping ability, and the availability of support systems. Hospitalization is not required for a single, uncomplicated fracture, and the patient returns to usual daily activities within a few days. Examples include a single fracture of a bone in the finger, wrist, foot, or toe.

In contrast, a patient suffering severe or multiple traumas may be hospitalized for weeks and may undergo many surgical procedures, treatments, and prolonged rehabilitation. These disruptions in lifestyle can create a high level of stress.

The stresses that result from a long-term condition affect relationships between the patient and family members or friends. Assess the patient's feelings, and ask how he or she coped with previously experienced stressful events. Body image and sexuality may be altered by deformity, treatment modalities for fracture repair, or long-term immobilization. Assess the availability of needed support systems, such as family, church, or community groups, who can help patients during the acute and rehabilitation phases when multiple or severe fractures occur. Active patients of any age or those who are older and live alone may become depressed during the healing process. Acute and chronic PAIN can decrease energy levels and may also cause sadness, depression, and/or anxiety.

Laboratory Assessment. No special laboratory tests are available for assessment of fractures. Hemoglobin and hematocrit levels may often be low because of bleeding caused by the injury. If extensive soft-tissue damage is present, the erythrocyte sedimentation rate (ESR) may be elevated, which indicates the expected inflammatory response. If this value and the white blood cell (WBC) count increase during fracture healing, the

patient may have a bone INFECTION. During the healing stages, serum calcium and phosphorus levels are often increased as the bone releases these elements into the blood.

Imaging Assessment. The health care provider requests standard *x-rays* to confirm a diagnosis of fracture. These reveal the bone disruption, malalignment, or deformity. If the x-ray does not show a fracture but the patient is symptomatic, the x-ray is usually repeated with additional views.

The *CT* scan is useful in detecting fractures of complex structures, such as the hip and pelvis. It also identifies compression fractures of the spine. *MRI* is useful in determining the amount of soft-tissue damage that may have occurred with the fracture.

◆ *Analysis*

The priority NANDA-I nursing diagnoses and collaborative problems for patients with fractures include:
1. Acute Pain related to one or more fractures, soft-tissue damage, muscle spasm, and edema (NANDA-I)
2. Potential for neurovascular compromise related to tissue edema and/or bleeding
3. Risk for Infection related to a wound caused by an open fracture (NANDA-I)
4. Impaired Physical Mobility related to need for bone healing and/or pain (NANDA-I)

◆ *Planning and Implementation*

Managing Acute Pain

Planning: Expected Outcomes. The patient with a fracture is expected to state that he or she has adequate PAIN control after fracture reduction and immobilization.

Emergency Care of the Patient with an Extremity Fracture

1. Assess the patient's airway, breathing, and circulation, and perform a quick head-to-toe assessment.
2. Remove the patient's clothing (cut if necessary) to inspect the affected area while supporting the area above and below the injury. Do not remove shoes because this can cause increased trauma.
3. Remove jewelry on the affected extremity in case of swelling.
4. Apply direct pressure on the area if there is bleeding and pressure over the proximal artery nearest the fracture.
5. Keep the patient warm and in a supine position.
6. Check the neurovascular status of the area distal to the fracture, including temperature, color, sensation, movement, and capillary refill. Compare affected and unaffected limbs.
7. Immobilize the extremity by splinting; include joints above and below the fracture site. Recheck circulation after splinting.
8. Cover any open areas with a dressing (preferably sterile).

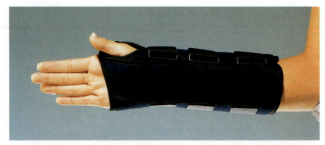

FIG. 51-3 A universal wrist and forearm splint used for immobilization.

Interventions. A fracture can happen anywhere and may be accompanied by multiple injuries to vital organs. Patient-centered collaborative care depends on the severity and extent of the injury and the number of fractures the patient has.

Emergency Care: Fracture. For any patient who experiences trauma in the community, first call 911 and assess for **a**irway, **b**reathing, and **c**irculation (ABCs, or primary survey). Then provide lifesaving care if needed before being concerned about the fracture (Chart 51-4). If cardiopulmonary resuscitation (CPR) is needed, ensure circulation first, followed by airway and breathing (see Chapter 34).

If the person is clothed, cut away clothing from the fracture site, and remove any jewelry from the affected extremity. Control any bleeding by direct pressure on the area and digital pressure over the artery above the fracture. To prevent shock, place the patient in a supine position and keep him or her warm.

After a head-to-toe assessment (secondary survey) and patient stabilization by the prehospital team, pain is managed with IV opioids such as fentanyl, hydromorphone (Dilaudid), or morphine sulfate. Cardiac monitoring for patients who are older than 50 years is established before drug administration. To prevent further tissue damage, reduce pain, and increase circulation, the prehospital or emergency team immobilizes the fracture by splinting. An air splint or any object or device that extends to the joints above and below the fracture to immobilize it can be used as a **splint**. Sterile gauze is placed loosely over open areas to prevent further contamination of the wound.

In the emergency department (ED), physician's office, or urgent care center, fracture management begins with reduction and immobilization of the fracture while attending to continued pain assessment and management.

Bone reduction, or realignment of the bone ends for proper healing, is accomplished by a closed method or an open (surgical) procedure. In some cases, dislocated bones are also reduced, such as when the distal tibia and fibula are dislocated with a fractured ankle. Immobilization is achieved by the use of bandages, casts, traction, internal fixation, or external fixation.

The health care provider selects the treatment method based on the type, location, and extent of the fracture. These interventions prevent further injury and reduce pain.

Nonsurgical Management. Nonsurgical management includes closed reduction and immobilization with a bandage, splint, cast, or traction. For some small, closed incomplete bone fractures in the hand or foot, reduction is not required. Immobilization with an orthotic device or special orthopedic shoe or boot may be the only management during the healing process.

For each modality, the primary nursing concern is assessment and prevention of neurovascular dysfunction or compromise. Assess the patient's neurovascular status every hour for the first 24 hours and every 1 to 4 hours thereafter, depending on the injury (see Chart 51-3). The patient usually reports discomfort that is unrelieved by analgesics if the bandage, splint, or cast is too tight. Elevate the fractured extremity higher than the heart, and apply ice for the first 24 to 48 hours as needed to reduce edema.

Closed Reduction and Immobilization. Closed reduction is the most common nonsurgical method for managing a simple fracture. While applying a manual pull, or traction, on the bone, the health care provider moves the bone ends so that they realign. Moderate sedation and/or analgesia is used during this procedure to decrease PAIN. The nurse monitors the patient's oxygen saturation (and possibly end-tidal carbon dioxide [EtCO$_2$] level) to ensure adequate rate and depth of respirations during the procedure. An x-ray confirms that the bone ends are approximated (aligned) before the bone is immobilized, and a splint is usually applied to keep the bone in alignment.

Splints and Orthopedic Boots/Shoes. For certain areas of the body, such as the scapula (shoulder) and clavicle (collarbone), a commercial immobilizer may be used to keep the bone in place during healing. Because upper extremity bones do not bear weight, splints may be sufficient to keep bone fragments in place for a closed fracture. Fig. 51-3 shows a wrist splint for fracture immobilization. Thermoplastic, a durable, flexible material for splinting, allows custom fitting to the patient's body part. Splints for lower extremities are also custom-fitted using flexible materials and held in place with elastic bandages (e.g., ACE wrap). When possible, splints are preferred over casts to prevent the complications that can occur with casting. Splints also allow room for extremity swelling without causing decreased arterial PERFUSION.

For foot or toe fractures, orthopedic shoes may be used to support the injured area during healing. For ankles or the lower part of the leg, padded orthopedic boots supported by multiple Velcro straps to hold the boot in place may be used. These devices are especially useful when the patient is allowed to bear weight on the affected leg.

Casts. For more complex fractures or fractures of the lower extremity, the physician or orthopedic technician may apply a cast to hold bone fragments in place after reduction. A **cast** is a rigid device that immobilizes the affected body part while

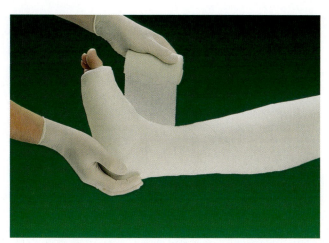

FIG. 51-4 Application of a fiberglass synthetic cast.

allowing other body parts to move. It also allows early mobility and reduces pain. Although its most common use is for fractures, a cast may be applied for correction of deformities (e.g., clubfoot) or for prevention of deformities (e.g., those seen in some patients with rheumatoid arthritis).

Fiberglass is the most common material used for casting and is typically the preferred method for immobilization with a cast (Fig. 51-4) (Satryb et al., 2011). Fiberglass can dry and become rigid within minutes and decreases the risk for skin breakdown. Waterproof casting is designed to get wet in the shower or pool and is used most commonly for athletes, especially during the summer (Satryb et al., 2011). Plaster is the traditional material used for casts but is not as commonly used today for management of most fractures. It requires application of a well-fitted stockinette under the material. If the stockinette is too tight, it may impair circulation. If it is too loose, wrinkles can lead to the development of pressure ulcers. Padding is applied over the stockinette, followed by wet plaster rolls wrapped around the extremity or other body part. The cast feels hot because an immediate chemical reaction occurs, but it soon becomes damp and cool. This type of cast takes at least 24 hours to dry, depending on the size and location of the cast. A wet cast feels cold, smells musty, and is grayish. The cast is dry when it feels hard and firm, is odorless, and has a shiny white appearance.

If the skin under the cast is open, the health care provider, orthopedic technician, or specially trained nurse cuts a window in the cast so that the wound can be observed and cared for. The piece of cast removed to make the window must be retained and replaced after wound care to prevent localized edema in the area. This is most important when a window is cut from a cast on an extremity. Tape or elastic bandage wrap may be used to keep the "window" in place. A window is also an access for taking pulses, removing wound drains, or preventing abdominal distention when the patient is in a body or spica cast.

If the cast is too tight, it may be cut with a cast cutter to relieve pressure or allow tissue swelling. The health care provider may choose to **bivalve** the cast (i.e., cut it lengthwise into two equal pieces) if bone healing is almost complete. Either half of the cast can be removed for inspection or for provision of care. The two halves are then held in place by an elastic bandage wrap (Satryb et al., 2011).

When a patient is in bed with an *arm cast,* teach him or her to elevate the arm above the heart to reduce swelling. The hand should be higher than the heart. Ice may be prescribed for the

first 24 to 48 hours. When the patient is out of bed, the arm is supported with a sling placed around the neck to alleviate fatigue caused by the weight of the cast. The sling should distribute the weight over a large area of the shoulders and trunk, not just the neck. Some health care providers prefer that the patient not use a sling after the first few days in an arm cast, particularly a short-arm cast. This encourages normal movement of the mobile joints and enhances bone healing. For many wrist fractures, a splint is used to immobilize the area instead of a cast to accommodate for edema formation.

A *leg cast* allows MOBILITY and requires the patient to use ambulatory aids such as crutches. A cast shoe, sandal, or boot that attaches to the foot or a rubber walking pad attached to the sole of the cast assists in ambulation (if weight bearing is allowed) and helps prevent damage to the cast. Teach the patient to elevate the affected leg on several pillows to reduce swelling and to apply ice for the first 24 hours or as prescribed. Table 51-1 describes specific casts that are used for various parts of the body.

Before the cast is applied, explain its purpose and the procedure for its application. With a plaster cast, warn the patient about the heat that will be felt immediately after the wet cast is applied. Do not cover the new cast. Allow for air-drying.

> **! NURSING SAFETY PRIORITY** (QSEN)
> ### Action Alert
>
> When moving a patient with a wet plaster cast, handle it with the palms of the hands to prevent indentations and resulting areas of pressure on the skin. Turn the patient every 1 to 2 hours to allow air to circulate and dry all parts of the cast. Be sure to remind unlicensed assistive personnel (UAP) and the family that the cast is wet and requires special handling. If the health care provider requests that the cast be elevated to reduce swelling, use a cloth-covered pillow instead of one encased in plastic, which could cause the cast to retain heat and prevent drying. Elevation of the casted extremity reduces edema but may impair arterial circulation to the affected limb. Therefore performing a neurovascular assessment of the limb distal to (below) the cast is very important.

> **! NURSING SAFETY PRIORITY** (QSEN)
> ### Action Alert
>
> Check to ensure that any type of cast is not too tight, and frequently monitor neurovascular status—usually every hour for the first 24 hours after application if the patient is hospitalized. You should be able to insert a finger between the cast and the skin. Teach the patient to apply ice for the first 24 to 36 hours to reduce swelling and inflammation.

Once the plaster cast is dry, inspect it at least once every 8 hours for drainage, cracking, crumbling, alignment, and fit. Plaster casts act like sponges and absorb drainage, whereas synthetic casts act like a wick pulling drainage away from the drainage site. Padding can also absorb wound drainage. Document the presence of any drainage on the cast. However, the evidence is not clear on whether drainage should be circled on the cast because it may increase anxiety and is not a reliable indicator of drainage amount. *Immediately report to the health care provider any sudden increases in the amount of drainage or change in the integrity of the cast.* After swelling decreases, it is not uncommon for the cast to become too loose and need replacement. If the patient is not admitted to the hospital, provide instructions regarding cast care.

TABLE 51-1 Types of Casts Used for Musculoskeletal Trauma	
TYPE AND CHARACTERISTICS OF CAST	**USE**
Upper Extremity Casts	
Short-arm cast (SAC) (extends from below the elbow to and including part of the hand)	Stable fractures of the wrist (metacarpals, carpals, or distal radius)
Long-arm cast (LAC) (includes the upper arm to and including part of the hand)	Unstable fractures of the wrist, distal humerus, radius, or ulna
Hanging-arm cast (same as LAC but heavier, with added loop at the mid-forearm)	Fractures of the humerus that cannot be aligned by LAC (light traction is possible while the patient is in bed or by an attached strap that extends around the neck)
Thumb spica (gauntlet) cast (similar to SAC with the thumb casted in abduction)	Fractures of the thumb
Shoulder spica cast (the shoulder is casted in abduction with the elbow flexed)	Unstable fractures of the shoulder girdle or humerus; dislocations of the shoulder
Lower Extremity Casts	
Short-leg cast (SLC) (from below the knee to the base of the toes)	Fractures of the ankle, metatarsals, or foot
Long-leg cast (LLC) (from the mid-upper thigh to the base of the toes)	Unstable fractures of the tibia, fibula, or ankle
Walking cast (a walking device on the bottom of SLC or LLC)	Same as for SLC or LLC
Leg cylinder (similar to SLC, but the ankle and foot are not casted)	Stable fractures of the tibia, fibula, or knee
Long-leg cylinder (similar to LLC, but the ankle and foot are not casted)	Stable fractures of the distal femur, proximal tibia, or knee
Cast Braces (or Brace Casts) (not as common)	
Patellar weight-bearing cast (similar to SLC or leg cylinder)	Mid-shaft or distal shaft fractures of the femur
External polycentric knee hinge cast (a hinge connects the lower and upper leg and allows 90 degrees of knee flexion)	Same as for the patellar weight-bearing cast

During hospitalization, assess for other complications resulting from casting that can be serious and life threatening, such as INFECTION, circulation impairment, and peripheral nerve damage. If the patient returns home after cast application, teach him or her how to monitor for these complications and when to notify the health care provider.

INFECTION most often results from the breakdown of skin under the cast (pressure necrosis). If pressure necrosis occurs, the patient typically reports a very painful "hot spot" under the cast and the cast may feel warmer in the affected area. Teach the patient or family to smell the area for mustiness or an unpleasant odor that would indicate infected material. If the infection progresses, a fever may develop.

Circulation impairment causing decreased PERFUSION and *peripheral nerve damage* can result from tightness of the cast. Teach the patient to assess for circulation at least daily, including the ability to move the area distal to the extremity, numbness, and increased PAIN.

The patient with a cast may be immobilized for a prolonged period, depending on the extent of the fracture and the type of cast. Assess for complications of immobility, such as skin breakdown, pneumonia, atelectasis, thromboembolism, and constipation. Before the cast is removed, inform the patient that the cast cutter will not injure the skin but that heat may be felt during the procedure.

Because of prolonged immobilization, a joint may become contracted, usually in a fixed state of flexion. Osteoarthritis and osteoporosis may develop from lack of weight bearing. Muscle can also atrophy from lack of exercise during prolonged immobilization of the affected body part, usually an extremity.

Traction. **Traction** is the application of a pulling force to a part of the body to provide reduction, alignment, and rest. It is also used as a last resort to decrease muscle spasm (thus relieving pain) and prevent or correct deformity and tissue damage. A patient in traction is often hospitalized, but in some cases, home care is possible even for skeletal traction.

Traction may be classified as running traction or balanced suspension. In *running* traction, the pulling force is in one direction and the patient's body acts as countertraction. Moving the body or bed position can alter the countertraction force. *Balanced suspension* provides the countertraction so that the pulling force of the traction is not altered when the bed or patient is moved. This allows for increased movement and facilitates care (Table 51-2).

Although not used as often today, the two most common types of traction are skin and skeletal traction. *Skin traction* involves the use of a Velcro boot (Buck's traction) (Fig. 51-5), belt, or halter, which is usually secured around the affected leg. The primary purpose of skin traction is to decrease painful muscle spasms that accompany hip fractures. A weight is used as a pulling force, which is limited to 5 to 10 pounds (2.3 to 4.5 kg) to prevent injury to the skin.

In *skeletal traction,* screws are surgically inserted directly into bone (e.g., Halo traction). These allow the use of longer traction time and heavier weights—usually 15 to 30 pounds (6.8 to 13.6 kg). Skeletal traction aids in bone realignment. Pin site care is an important part of nursing management to prevent infection.

The nurse may set up or assist in the setup of traction if specially educated. In larger or specialty hospitals or units,

! NURSING SAFETY PRIORITY (QSEN)
Action Alert

When patients are in traction, weights usually are not removed without a prescription. They should not be lifted manually or allowed to rest on the floor. Weights should be freely hanging at all times. Teach this important point to UAP on the unit, to other personnel such as those in the radiology department, and to visitors. Inspect the skin at least every 8 hours for signs of irritation or inflammation. When possible, remove the belt or boot that is used for skin traction every 8 hours to inspect under the device.

TABLE 51-2 Types of Traction Used for Musculoskeletal Trauma	
TYPE AND CHARACTERISTICS OF TRACTION	**USE**
Upper Extremity Traction	
Sidearm skin or skeletal traction (the forearm is flexed and extended 90 degrees from the upper part of the body)	Fractures of the humerus with or without involvement of the shoulder and clavicle
Overhead or 90-90 traction, skin or skeletal (the elbow is flexed and the arm is at a right angle to the body over the upper chest)	Same as above (depends on the physician's preference)
Plaster traction (pins inserted through the bone are fixed in the cast)	Fractures of the wrist
Lower Extremity Traction	
Buck's extension traction (skin) (the affected leg is in extension)	Fractures of the hip or femur preoperatively Prevention of hip flexion contractures Hip dislocation
Russell's traction (similar to Buck's traction, but a sling under the knee suspends the leg)	Fractures of the hip or distal end of the femur
Balanced skin or skeletal traction (the limb is usually elevated in a Thomas splint with Pearson's attachment, or a Böhler-Braun splint is used)	Fractures of the femur or pelvis (acetabulum)
Spinal Column and Pelvic Traction	
Cervical halter (a strap under the chin)	Cervical muscle spasms, strain/sprain, or arthritis
Cervical skeletal (e.g., halo brace)	Cervical fractures of the spine; muscle spasms
Pelvic belt (a strap around the hips at the iliac crests is attached to weights at the foot of the bed)	Pain, strain, sprain, or muscle spasms in the lower back
Pelvic sling (a wide strap around the hips is attached to an overhead bar to keep the pelvis off the bed)	Pelvic fractures; other pelvic injuries

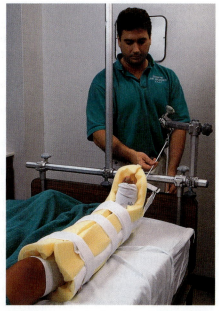

FIG. 51-5 Skin traction with a hook-and-loop fastener (Velcro) boot, commonly used for hip fractures.

Report the pain to the health care provider if body realignment fails to reduce the discomfort. Assess neurovascular status of the affected body part to detect circulatory compromise and tissue damage. The circulation is usually monitored every hour for the first 24 hours after traction is applied and every 4 hours thereafter.

❓ NCLEX EXAMINATION CHALLENGE

Physiological Integrity

A client has a new synthetic leg cast for a tibial fracture. What health care teaching does the nurse include for the client's self-management at home? **Select all that apply.**
A. "Keep your leg elevated, preferably above your heart, as much as possible."
B. "Apply ice on the cast for the first 24 hours to increase blood flow for healing."
C. "Report severe numbness or inability to move your toes to your health care provider."
D. "Take your pain medication as needed according to the prescription directions."
E. "Don't cover the cast with anything because it will stay wet for 24 hours."

orthopedic technicians or physician assistants often set up traction. Once traction is applied, maintain the correct balance between traction pull and countertraction force.

Check traction equipment frequently to ensure its proper functioning. Inspect all ropes, knots, and pulleys at least every 8 to 12 hours for loosening, fraying, and positioning. Check the weight for consistency with the health care provider's prescription. Sometimes one of the weights is accidentally removed by a staff member or visitor who bumps into it. Replace the weights if they are not correct, and notify the health care provider or orthopedic technician.

If the patient reports severe pain from muscle spasm, the weights may be too heavy or the patient may need realignment.

Drug Therapy. After fracture treatment, the patient often has pain for a prolonged time during the healing process. The health care provider commonly prescribes opioid and non-opioid analgesics, anti-inflammatory drugs, and muscle relaxants.

For patients with chronic, severe PAIN, opioid and non-opioid drugs are alternated or given together to manage pain both centrally in the brain and peripherally at the site of injury. For severe or multiple fractures, patient-controlled analgesia (PCA) with morphine, fentanyl, or hydromorphone (Dilaudid) is used. *Meperidine (Demerol) should never be used for older adults because it has toxic metabolites that can cause seizures and other complications. Most hospitals no longer use this drug for patients of any age.* Oxycodone and oxycodone with acetaminophen (Percocet) are common oral opioid drugs that are very effective for most patients with fracture pain. NSAIDs are given to decrease associated tissue inflammation.

For patients who have less severe injury, the analgesic may be given on an as-needed basis. Collaborate with the patient regarding the best times for the strong analgesics to be given (e.g., before a complex dressing change, after physical therapy sessions, and at bedtime). Assess the effectiveness of the analgesic and its side effects. Constipation is a common side effect of opioid therapy, especially for older adults. Assess for frequency of bowel movements, and administer stool softeners as needed. Encourage fluids and activity as tolerated. Chapter 3 discusses the various methods of PAIN management, including epidural analgesia and patient-controlled analgesia.

Some patients experience a long-term, intense burning PAIN and edema that are associated with *complex regional pain syndrome (CRPS).* This syndrome often results from fractures and other musculoskeletal trauma and is discussed on p. 1075 later in this chapter.

Surgical Management. For some types of fractures, closed reduction is not sufficient. Surgical intervention may be needed to realign the bone for the healing process.

Preoperative Care. Teach the patient and family what to expect during and after the surgery. The preoperative care for a patient undergoing orthopedic surgery is similar to that for anyone having surgery with general or epidural anesthesia. (See Chapter 14 for a thorough discussion of preoperative nursing care.)

Operative Procedures. Open reduction with internal fixation (ORIF) is one of the most common methods of reducing and immobilizing a fracture. External fixation with closed reduction is used when patients have soft-tissue injury (open fracture). Although nurses do not decide which surgical technique is used, understanding the procedures enhances patient teaching and care.

Because ORIF permits early MOBILITY, it is often the preferred surgical method. **Open reduction** allows the surgeon to directly view the fracture site. **Internal fixation** uses metal pins, screws, rods, plates, or prostheses to immobilize the fracture during healing. The surgeon makes one or more incisions to gain access to the broken bone(s) and implants one or more devices into bone tissue after each fracture is reduced. A cast, boot, or splint is placed to maintain immobilization during the healing process, depending on the body part affected.

After the bone achieves union, the metal hardware may be removed, depending on the location and type of fracture. Hardware is removed most frequently in ankle fractures, depending on the severity of the injury. If the metal implants are not bothersome, they remain in place. Specific types of internal fixation devices are discussed later in the Selected Fractures of Specific Sites section.

An alternative modality for the management of fractures is the external fixation apparatus, as shown in Fig. 51-6. **External fixation** is a system in which pins or wires are inserted through the skin and affected bone and then connected to a rigid external frame. The system may be used for upper or lower extremity fractures or for fractures of the pelvis, especially for open fractures when wound management is needed. After a fixator is removed, the patient may be placed in a cast or splint until healing is complete.

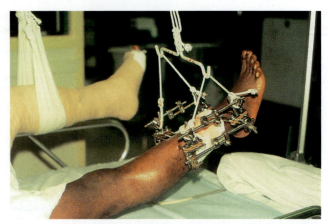

FIG. 51-6 The Hex-Fix external fixation system for tibia-fibula fractures.

External fixation has several advantages over other surgical techniques:
- There is minimal blood loss compared with internal fixation.
- The device allows early ambulation and exercise of the affected body part while relieving pain.
- The device maintains alignment in closed fractures that will not maintain position in a cast and stabilizes comminuted fractures that require bone grafting.

In open fractures, in which skin and tissue trauma accompany the fracture, the device permits easy access to the wound while the bone heals. This method is usually preferred over the use of a window in a cast for wound care.

A disadvantage of external fixation is an increased risk for pin site INFECTION. Pin site infections can lead to osteomyelitis, which is serious and difficult to treat (see Chapter 50).

Postoperative Care. The postoperative care for a patient undergoing ORIF or external fixation is similar to that provided for any patient undergoing surgery (see Chapter 16). Because bone is a vascular, dynamic body tissue, the patient is at risk for complications specific to fractures and musculoskeletal surgery. IV ketorolac (Toradol) is often given in the postanesthesia care unit (PACU) or soon after discharge to the post-surgical area to reduce inflammation and pain. Aggressive pain management starts as soon as possible after surgery to prevent the development of chronic pain and promote early mobility.

Additional information about postoperative care is found beginning on p. 1066 in the Selected Fractures of Specific Sites section. Depending on the fractures that are repaired, some ORIF procedures are performed as same-day surgeries. Patients stay in the hospital up to 23 hours after surgery.

For patients with an **external fixator**, pay particular attention to the pin sites for signs of inflammation or infection. In the first 48 to 72 hours, *clear* fluid drainage or weeping is expected. Although no standardized method or evidence-based protocol for pin site care has been established, recommendations have been made based on the evidence available regarding pin site care. Because the pins go through the skin and into bone, the risk for infection is high. Monitor the pin sites at least every 8 to 12 hours for drainage, color, odor, and severe redness, which indicate inflammation and possible infection. Follow agency policy for how to clean the pin site areas.

The patient with an external fixator may have a disturbed body image. The frame may be large and bulky, and the affected area may have massive tissue damage with dressings.

Be sensitive to this possibility in planning care. Teach about alterations to clothing that may be required while the fixator is in place.

The Ilizarov technique of circular external fixation is sometimes used to treat new fractures (closed, comminuted fractures and open fractures with bone loss), as well as malunion or nonunion of fractures. It may also be used to treat congenital bone deformities, especially in "little people" (e.g., dwarfs).

The circular external fixation device is used to gently pull apart the cortex of the bone and stimulate new bone growth. Unlike the traditional fixator, the Ilizarov external fixator promotes rotation, angulation, lengthening, or widening of bone to correct bony defects and allows for healing of any soft-tissue defect. The nursing care associated with this device is similar to the care of the patient with other external fixation systems with one major exception. If the device is being used for filling bone gaps, teach the patient how to manually turn the four-sided nuts (also called *clickers*) up to 4 times a day. Daily distraction rates vary, but 1 mm daily is common. Screening and teaching are particularly important because the patient adjusts and cares for the apparatus over a long period of up to 6 months to 1 year. PAIN control is a priority outcome for patients using this device.

Procedures for Nonunion. Some management techniques are not successful because the bone does not heal. Several additional options are available to the physician to promote bone union, such as electrical bone stimulation, bone grafting, and ultrasound fracture treatment.

For selected patients, *electrical bone stimulation* may be successful. This procedure is based on research showing that bone has electrical properties that are used in healing. The exact mechanism of action is unknown. A noninvasive, external **electrical bone stimulation** system delivers a small continuous electrical charge directed toward the non-healed bone. There are no known risks with this system, although patients with pacemakers cannot use this device on an arm. Implanted direct-current stimulators are placed directly in the fracture site and have no external apparatus. Both systems require several months of treatment.

Another method of treating nonunion is *bone grafting*. A bone graft may also replace diseased bone or increase bone tissue for joint replacement. In most cases, chips of bone are taken from the iliac crest or other site and are packed or wired between the bone ends to facilitate union. Allografts from cadavers may also be used. These grafts are frozen or freeze-dried and stored under sterile conditions in a bone bank.

Bone banking from living donors is becoming increasingly popular. If qualified, patients undergoing total hip replacement may donate their femoral heads to the bank for later use as bone grafts for others. Careful screening ensures that the bone is healthy and that the donor has no communicable disease. The bone cannot be donated without written consent.

One of the newest modalities for fracture healing is **low-intensity pulsed ultrasound** (Exogen therapy). Used for slow-healing fractures or for new fractures as an alternative to surgery, ultrasound treatment has had excellent results. The patient applies the treatment for about 20 minutes each day. It has no contraindications or adverse effects.

Physical Therapy. Many patients with musculoskeletal trauma, including fractures, are referred by their health care provider for rehabilitation therapy with a physical therapist (PT). The timing for this referral depends on the nature, severity, and treatment modality of the fracture(s).

For example, some patients who have an ORIF for one or more ankle fractures may begin therapy when the incisional staples or Steri-Strips are removed and an orthopedic boot is fitted. Based on the initial evaluation, the PT performs gentle manipulative exercises to increase range of motion. The therapist may also begin to help the patient with laterality, a concept to help the brain identify the injured foot from the uninjured foot. Computer programs and mirror-box therapy can help reprogram the brain as part of cognitive retraining. In mirror-box therapy for an injured foot, the patient covers his or her affected foot while looking at and moving the uninjured foot in front of the mirror. The brain perceives the foot in the mirror as the injured foot.

Stimulation by touch also helps the brain acknowledge the injured foot. The PT teaches the patient to have someone frequently touch the injured area and use various materials and objects against the skin to desensitize it. These interventions decrease the risk for complex regional pain syndrome, discussed later in this chapter.

When weight bearing begins about 6 weeks after surgery, the PT teaches the patient how to begin with toe-touch or partial weight bearing using crutches or a walker. Muscle strengthening exercises of the affected leg help with ambulation because atrophy begins shortly after injury.

The PT also assists with PAIN control and edema reduction by using ice/heat packs, electrical muscle stimulation ("e-stim"), and special treatments such as dexamethasone iontophoresis. **Iontophoresis** is a method for absorbing dexamethasone, a synthetic steroid, through the skin near the painful area to decrease inflammation and edema. A small device delivers a minute amount of electricity via electrodes that are placed on the skin. The patient may describe the sensation as a pinch or slight sting. The electrical current increases the ability of the skin to absorb the drug from a topical patch into the affected soft tissue.

The success of rehabilitation is affected by the patient's motivation and willingness to perform prescribed exercises and activities between PT visits. Rehabilitation for ankle surgery, for example, may take several months, depending on the severity of the injury and the age and general health of the patient.

Preventing and Monitoring for Neurovascular Compromise

Planning: Expected Outcomes. The patient with a fracture is expected to have no compromise in neurovascular status as evidenced by adequate circulation, movement, and SENSORY PERCEPTION (CMS). If severe compromise occurs, the patient is expected to have early and prompt emergency treatment to prevent severe tissue damage.

Interventions. Perform neurovascular (NV) assessments (also known as "circ checks" or CMS assessments) frequently before and after fracture treatment. Patients who have extremity casts, splints with elastic bandage wraps, and open reduction with internal fixation (ORIF) or external fixation are especially at risk for NV compromise. If blood flow to the distal extremity is impaired, the patient reports increased PAIN and decreased SENSORY PERCEPTION and movement. If these symptoms are allowed to progress, patients are at risk for acute compartment syndrome (ACS).

Early recognition of the signs and symptoms of ACS can prevent loss of function or loss of a limb. Identify patients who may be at risk, and monitor them closely. ACS can begin in 6 to 8 hours after an injury or take up to 2 days to appear. If it is suspected, notify the health care provider immediately, and if possible, implement interventions to relieve the pressure. For example, for the patient with tight, bulky dressings, loosen the bandage or tape. If the patient has a cast, follow agency protocol about who may cut the cast.

! NURSING SAFETY PRIORITY (QSEN)

Critical Rescue

Monitor for early signs of ACS. Assess for the "six Ps" including **p**ain, **p**ressure, **p**aralysis, **p**aresthesia, **p**allor, and **p**ulselessness (rare). PAIN is increased even with passive motion and may seem out of proportion to the degree of injury. Analgesics that had controlled pain become less effective. Numbness and tingling or paresthesias are often one of the first signs of the problem. The affected extremity then becomes pale and cool as a result of decreased arterial perfusion to the affected area. Capillary refill is an important assessment of PERFUSION but may not be reliable in an older adult because of arterial insufficiency. Losses of movement and function and decreased pulses or pulselessness are late signs of ACS! Fortunately, ACS is not common, but it creates an emergency situation when it does occur.

In a few cases, compartment pressure may be monitored on a one-time basis with a handheld device with a digital display, or pressure can be monitored continuously. Monitoring is recommended for comatose or unresponsive high-risk patients with multiple trauma and fractures.

If ACS is verified, the surgeon may perform a **fasciotomy**, or opening in the fascia, by making an incision through the skin and subcutaneous tissues into the fascia of the affected compartment. This procedure relieves the pressure and restores circulation to the affected area. No consensus exists on what pressure requires fasciotomy (normal is 0 to 8 mm Hg). Compartment pressures must be considered in relation to the patient's hemodynamic status. After fasciotomy, the open wound is packed and dressed daily or more often until secondary closure occurs, usually in 4 to 5 days, depending on the patient's healing ability. Some surgeons use negative pressure wound therapy (e.g., Wound Vac) over a fasciotomy to decrease edema until the wound is closed. For other patients, a skin graft may be used to promote healing.

Preventing Infection

Planning: Expected Outcomes. The patient with a fracture is expected to be free of wound or bone INFECTION as evidenced by no fever, no increase in white blood cell count, and negative wound culture (if wound is present).

Interventions. When caring for a patient with an open fracture, use clean or aseptic technique for dressing changes and wound irrigations. Check agency policy for specific protocols. *Immediately notify the health care provider if you observe inflammation and purulent drainage.* Other infections, such as pneumonia and urinary tract infection, may occur several days after the fracture. Monitor the patient's vital signs every 4 to 8 hours because increases in temperature and pulse often indicate systemic infection.

CONSIDERATIONS FOR OLDER ADULTS

Patient-Centered Care (QSEN)

Older adults may not have a temperature elevation even in the presence of severe infection. An acute onset of confusion (delirium) often suggests an infection in the older adult patient.

For most patients with an open fracture, the health care provider prescribes one or more broad-spectrum antibiotics prophylactically and performs surgical débridement of any wounds as soon as possible after the injury. First-generation cephalosporins, clindamycin (Cleocin), and gentamycin are commonly used. In addition to systemic antibiotics, local antibiotic therapy through wound irrigation is commonly prescribed, especially during débridement.

A very effective treatment is negative pressure wound therapy (e.g., vacuum-assisted closure [VAC] system) as a method of increasing the rate of wound healing for open fractures. This device allows quicker wound closure, which decreases the risk for INFECTION.

When the bone is surgically repaired, hardware and/or bone grafts have typically been implanted. However, they are limited in their use. The U.S. Food and Drug Administration (FDA) approved the use of recombinant human bone morphogenetic protein-2 (rhBMP-2) for tibial and spinal fractures. This implanted genetically engineered substance increases wound healing, decreases hardware failure, and decreases the risk for infection.

Improving Physical Mobility

Planning: Expected Outcomes. The patient with a fracture is expected to increase physical MOBILITY and be free of complications associated with impaired mobility. The patient is also expected to move purposefully in his or her own environment independently with or without an ambulatory device unless restricted by traction or other modality.

Interventions. The interventions necessary for this diagnosis can be grouped into two types: those that help increase MOBILITY and those that prevent complications of impaired mobility.

Promoting Mobility. The use of crutches or a walker increases MOBILITY and assists in ambulation. The patient may progress to using a walker or cane after crutches.

Crutches are the most commonly used ambulatory aid for many types of lower extremity musculoskeletal trauma (e.g., fractures, sprains, amputations). In most agencies, the physical therapist or emergency department/ambulatory care nurse fits the patient for crutches and teaches him or her how to ambulate with them. Reinforce those instructions, and evaluate whether the patient is using the crutches correctly.

Walking with crutches requires strong arm muscles, balance, and coordination. For this reason, crutches are not often used for older adults. Walkers and canes are preferred for the older adult. Crutches can cause upper extremity bursitis or axillary nerve damage if they are not fitted or used correctly. For that reason, the top of each crutch is padded. To prevent pressure on the axillary nerve, there should be two to three fingerbreadths between the axilla and the top of the crutch when the crutch tip is at least 6 inches (15 cm) diagonally in front of the foot. The crutch is adjusted so that the elbow is flexed no more than 30 degrees when the palm is on the handle (Fig. 51-7). The distal tips of each crutch are rubber to prevent slipping.

There are several types of gaits for walking with crutches. The most common one for musculoskeletal injury is the three-point gait, which allows little weight bearing on the affected leg. The procedure for these gaits is discussed in fundamentals of nursing books.

A *walker* is most often used by the older patient who needs additional support for balance. The physical therapist assesses the strength of the upper extremities and the unaffected leg. Strength is improved with prescribed exercises as needed.

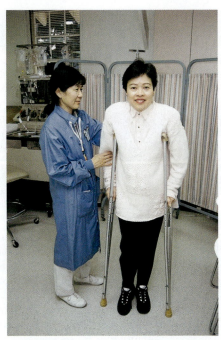

FIG. 51-7 Assisting the patient with crutch walking. Note how the therapist guards the patient and how the patient's elbows are at no more than 30 degrees of flexion.

A *cane* is sometimes used if the patient needs only minimal support for an affected leg. The straight cane offers the least support. A hemi-cane or quad-cane provides a broader base for the cane and therefore more support. The cane is placed on the *unaffected* side and should create no more than 30 degrees of flexion of the elbow. The top of the cane should be parallel to the greater trochanter of the femur or stylus of the wrist. Chapter 6 and fundamentals textbooks describe these ambulatory devices in more detail.

Preventing Complications of Immobility. The nurse plays a vital role in preventing and assessing for complications in immobilized patients with fractures. Additional information about nursing care for preventing problems associated with immobility is found in Chapter 6.

Community-Based Care

The patient with an *uncomplicated* fracture is usually discharged to home from the emergency department or urgent care center. Older adults with hip or other fractures or patients with multiple traumas are hospitalized and then transferred to home, a rehabilitation setting, or a long-term care facility for rehabilitation. Collaborate with the case manager or the discharge planner in the hospital to ensure continuity of care. Be sure to communicate the plan of care clearly to the health care agency receiving the patient.

Home Care Management. If the patient is discharged to home, the nurse, therapist, or case manager (CM) may assess the home environment for structural barriers to mobility, such as stairs. Be sure that the patient has easy access to the bathroom. Ask about scatter rugs, waxed floors, and walkway areas that could increase the risk for falls. If the patient needs to use a wheelchair or ambulatory aid, make sure that he or she can use it safely and that there is room in the house to ambulate with these devices. The physical therapist may teach the patient how to use stairs, but older adults or those using crutches may

---

CHART 51-5 Patient and Family Education: Preparing for Self-Management

Care of the Extremity After Cast Removal

- Remove scaly, dead skin carefully by soaking; do not scrub.
- Move the extremity carefully. Expect discomfort, weakness, and decreased range of motion.
- Support the extremity with pillows or your orthotic device until strength and movement return.
- Exercise slowly as instructed by your physical therapist.
- Wear support stockings or elastic bandages to prevent swelling (for lower extremity).

---

experience difficulty performing this task. Depending on the age and condition of the patient, a home health care nurse may make one or two visits to check that the home is safe and that the patient and family are able to follow the interdisciplinary plan of care.

Self-Management Education. The patient with a fracture may be discharged from the hospital, emergency department, office, or clinic with a bandage, splint, cast, or external fixator. Provide verbal and written instructions on the care of these devices. Chart 51-5 describes care of the affected extremity after removal of the cast.

The patient may also need to continue wound care at home. Instruct the patient and family about how to assess and dress the wound to promote healing and prevent INFECTION. Teach them how to recognize complications and when and where to seek professional health care if complications occur. Additional educational needs depend on the type of fracture and fracture repair.

Encourage patients and their families to ensure adequate foods high in protein and calcium that are needed for bone and tissue healing. For patients with lower extremity fractures, less weight bearing on long bones can cause anemia. The red bone marrow needs weight bearing to simulate red blood cell production. Encourage foods high in iron content. Teach the patient to take a daily iron-added multivitamin (take with food to prevent possible nausea).

Health Care Resources. Arrange for follow-up care at home. A social worker may need to help the patient apply for funds to pay medical bills. If there is severe bone and tissue damage, be realistic and help the patient and family understand the long-term nature of the recovery period. Multiple treatment techniques and surgical procedures required for complications can be mentally and emotionally draining for the patient and family. A vocational counselor may be needed to help the patient find a different type of job, depending on the extent of the fracture.

An older or incapacitated patient may need assistance with ADLs, which can be provided by home care aides if family or other caregiver is not available. In collaboration with the case manager, anticipate the patient's needs and arrange for these services.

◆ Evaluation: Outcomes

Evaluate the care of the patient with one or more fractures based on the identified priority patient problems. The expected outcomes include that the patient:

- States that he or she has adequate PAIN control
- Has adequate blood flow to maintain tissue PERFUSION and function

- Is free of INFECTION
- Is free of physiologic consequences of impaired MOBILITY
- Ambulates or moves independently with or without an assistive device (if not restricted by traction or other device)

SELECTED FRACTURES OF SPECIFIC SITES

Upper Extremity Fractures

In addition to the general care discussed in the previous section, management of upper extremity fractures includes specific interventions related to the location and nature of the injury.

Fractures of the *proximal humerus,* particularly impacted or displaced fractures, are common in the older adult. An impacted injury is usually treated with a sling or other device for immobilization. A displaced fracture often requires ORIF with pins or a prosthesis. Humeral shaft fractures are generally corrected by closed reduction and a hanging-arm cast or splint. If necessary, the fracture is repaired surgically (with an intramedullary rod or metal plate and screws) or with external fixation.

The most common upper extremity (UE) fracture is the *distal radius fracture (DRF),* which occurs in both younger and older adults. Younger adults experience this injury from high-energy (high-impact) trauma as a result of motor vehicle crashes and sports. Older adults, particularly women with osteopenia, typically have low-impact DRFs as a result of falls (Voda, 2011).

Various names are used to classify DRFs, including Colles' and Smith fractures. A Colles' fracture can occur when a person attempts to break a fall by landing on the heel of the hand when the wrist is extended. The resulting deformity is often called a "dinner fork" injury (Fig. 51-8). Seen less commonly, a Smith fracture occurs from a fall on a flexed wrist (Voda, 2011).

Initial nursing interventions for a patient with a DRF include:

- Removing jewelry on the affected hand and wrist before edema worsens (Walsh, 2013)
- Performing a neurovascular assessment of the affected UE
- Immobilizing the affected wrist and hand
- Elevating the affected UE
- Applying ice to the affected area
- Managing pain

After initial stabilization, the most common treatment for a DRF is closed reduction. The health care provider realigns the bone ends while the patient is moderately sedated. A splint is applied and held in place with an elastic bandage. The splint may be replaced several days later with a cast after edema decreases.

For more complicated DRFs, an ORIF with pins and plates may be performed. The patient may have surgery in an ambulatory care or same-day surgical setting using general anesthesia,

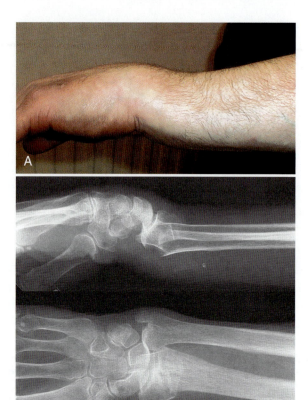

FIG. 51-8 Colles' wrist fracture showing "dinner fork" deformity.

a peripheral nerve block, or a combination of both. The nerve block is often given as a single injection of levobupivacaine (Chirocaine) or bupivacaine (Marcaine), which provides pain relief for 12 to 20 hours (Guarin, 2013). Teach patients having a peripheral nerve block (e.g., supraclavicular block) that temporarily they will not be able to move their affected arm. Also observe, report, and document signs and symptoms of pneumothorax, including tachypnea, decreased breath sounds, or respiratory distress (Guarin, 2013).

For all patients who experience a DRF, assess for nerve compression, especially the radial and median nerves. Be sure to perform frequent neurovascular assessment with special attention to the presence of decreased SENSORY PERCEPTION (e.g., numbness) or decreased movement.

Fractures of the *metacarpals* and *phalanges (fingers)* are usually not displaced, which makes their treatment less difficult than that of other fractures. Metacarpal fractures are immobilized for 3 to 4 weeks. Phalangeal fractures are immobilized in finger splints for 10 to 14 days.

Lower Extremity Fractures
Fractures of the Hip

Hip fracture is the most common injury in older adults and one of the most frequently seen injuries in any health care setting or community. It has a high mortality rate as a result of multiple complications related to surgery, depression, and prolonged immobility. Over half of older adults experiencing a hip fracture are unable to live independently, and many die within the first year (Sweitzer et al., 2013).

Hip fractures include those involving the upper third of the femur and are classified as **intracapsular** (within the joint

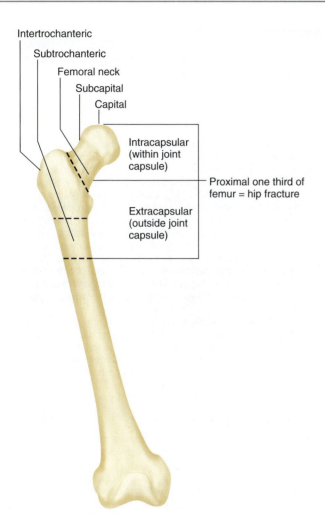

Intertrochanteric
Subtrochanteric
Femoral neck
Subcapital
Capital

Intracapsular (within joint capsule)

Proximal one third of femur = hip fracture

Extracapsular (outside joint capsule)

FIG. 51-9 Types of hip fractures.

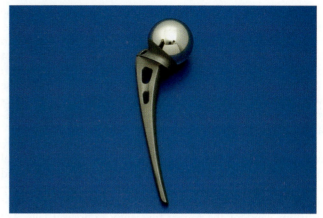

FIG. 51-10 A hip prosthesis used for fractures.

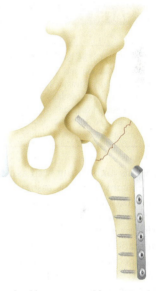

FIG. 51-11 A compression hip screw used for open reduction with internal fixation (ORIF) of the hip.

capsule) or **extracapsular** (outside the joint capsule). These types are further divided according to fracture location (Fig. 51-9). In the area of the femoral neck, disruption of the blood supply to the head of the femur is a concern, which can result in ischemic or avascular necrosis (AVN) of the femoral head. AVN causes death and necrosis of bone tissue and results in pain and decreased mobility. This problem is most likely in patients with displaced fractures.

Osteoporosis is the biggest risk factor for hip fractures (see Chapter 50). This disease weakens the upper femur (hip), which causes it to break and then causes the person to fall. The number of people with hip fracture is expected to continue to increase as the population ages, and the associated health care costs will be tremendous.

The treatment of choice is surgical repair by ORIF, when possible, to reduce PAIN and allow the older patient to be out of bed and ambulatory. Skin (Buck's) traction may be applied before surgery to help decrease pain associated with muscle spasm. Depending on the exact location of the fracture, an ORIF may include an intramedullary rod, pins, prostheses (for femoral head or femoral neck fractures), or a compression screw. Figs. 51-10 and 51-11 illustrate examples of these devices. Epidural or general anesthesia is used. Occasionally a patient will be so debilitated that surgery cannot be done. In these cases, nonsurgical options include pain management and bedrest to allow natural fracture healing.

CONSIDERATIONS FOR OLDER ADULTS
Patient-Centered Care QSEN

Teach older adults about the risk factors for hip fracture including physiologic aging changes, disease processes, drug therapy, and environmental hazards. Physiologic changes include sensory changes such as diminished visual acuity and hearing; changes in gait, balance, and muscle strength; and joint stiffness. Disease processes like osteoporosis, foot disorders, and changes in cardiac function increase the risk for hip fracture. Drugs, such as diuretics, antihypertensives, antidepressants, sedatives, opioids, and alcohol, are factors that increase the risks for falling in older adults. Use of three or more drugs at the same time drastically increases the risk for falls. Throw rugs, loose carpeting, inadequate lighting, uneven walking surfaces or steps, and pets are environmental hazards that also cause falls.

The older adult with hip fracture usually reports groin pain or pain behind the knee on the affected side. In some cases, the patient has pain in the lower back or has no pain at all. However, the patient is not able to stand. X-ray or other imaging assessment confirms the diagnosis.

Patients usually receive IV morphine after admission to the emergency department and PCA morphine or epidural analgesia after surgery. In some cases, a femoral nerve block may also be performed during surgery to help relieve pain for up to 24 hours after surgery (Guarin, 2013). Meperidine (Demerol) should not be used due to its toxic metabolites that can cause seizures and other adverse drug events, especially in the older adult population. Chapter 3 discusses the nursing care associated with pain management in detail.

After a hip repair, older adults frequently experience acute confusion, or delirium. They may pull at tubes or the surgical dressing or attempt to climb out of bed, possibly falling and causing self-injury. Other patients stay awake all night and sleep during the day. Keep in mind that some patients have a quiet delirium. Monitor the patient frequently to prevent falls. Ask the family or other visitors to let staff know if the patient is attempting to get out of bed. Chapter 2 describes fall prevention strategies and delirium management in detail.

! NURSING SAFETY PRIORITY (QSEN)
Action Alert

Patients who have an ORIF are at risk for hip dislocation or subluxation. Be sure to prevent hip adduction and rotation to keep the operative leg in proper alignment. Regular pillows or abduction devices can be used for patients who are confused or restless. If straps are used to hold the device in place, check the skin for signs of pressure. Perform neurovascular assessments to ensure that the device is not interfering with arterial circulation or peripheral nerve conduction.

The patient begins ambulating with assistance the day after surgery to prevent complications associated with immobility (e.g., pressure ulcers, atelectasis, venous thromboembolism). Early MOBILITY and ambulation also decrease the chance of INFECTION and increase surgical site healing.

Special considerations for the patient having a hip repair also include careful inspection of skin including areas of pressure, especially the heels. Use of skin traction to reduce muscle spasms may increase the period of bedrest before surgery. Decreased MOBILITY after surgery can increase the risk for pressure injury in this area within 24 hours.

! NURSING SAFETY PRIORITY (QSEN)
Action Alert

Be sure that the patient's heels are up off the bed at all times. Inspect the heels and other high-risk bony prominence areas every 8 to 12 hours. Delegate turning and repositioning every 1 to 2 hours to unlicensed assistive personnel (UAP), and supervise this nursing activity.

Other postoperative interventions to prevent complications, such as venous thromboembolism, are similar to those for total hip replacement (see Chapter 16).

Many patients recover fully from hip fracture repair and regain their functional ability. They are typically discharged to their home, rehabilitation unit or center, or a skilled nursing facility for physical and occupational therapy. However, some patients are not able to return to their pre-fracture ADLs and MOBILITY level. Family caregivers often have unexpected responsibilities caring for patients during their recovery. Hip fracture resource centers can be very useful in providing caregiver support (see the Evidence-Based Practice box).

EVIDENCE-BASED PRACTICE (QSEN)
Are Online Resources Helpful for Caregivers of Patients After Hip Fracture?

Nahm, E-S., Resnick, B., Plummer, L., & Park, B.K. (2013). Use of discussion boards in an online hip fracture resource center for caregivers. *Orthopaedic Nursing, 32*(2), 89-96.

Family caregivers (CGs) are important for the successful recovery of patients who have hip fracture repair. In a previous study the authors found that CGs lacked knowledge in understanding how to provide care during the rehabilitation and recovery phase. The purpose of this qualitative study was to explore the experiences of CGs while they were using an online hip resource center over an 8-week period. The majority of the 27 caregivers in the study were female and white. Most had some college education, and their average age was 55.5 years. Each CG posted comments related to specific topics posted on the online discussion boards. Examples of topics included the roles of therapists, awareness of bone health, and caregiver stress. Three coders recorded and analyzed the data using well-established coding rules to ensure validity and reliability.

The analysis revealed common themes, such as need for adjustment to the fracture event, and three categories: types of care provided by the CGs, strategies used by CGs to prevent fractures, and coping mechanisms used to handle stress. The researchers concluded that discussion boards (DBs) can serve as a useful medium for CGs to share their experiences. They also noted that DBs can assist health care providers identify ways to support CGs.

Level of Evidence: 4
This study was a well-designed qualitative study to gain specific information about the needs of caregivers of patients with hip fractures.

Commentary: Implications for Practice and Research
Although this study was limited to a small sample size, the researchers were very careful to ensure validity and reliability of the coding process for data analysis. Additional studies with larger sample sizes that are more diverse are needed to provide generalization of results. Nurses caring for patients having surgical hip repair need to help families locate resources to provide information and support during the patients' rehabilitation and recovery period.

Other Fractures of the Lower Extremity

Other fractures of the lower extremity may or may not require hospitalization. However, if the patient has severe or multiple fractures, especially with soft-tissue damage, hospital admission is usually required. Patients who have surgery to repair their injury may also be hospitalized. Coordinate care with the physical therapist regarding mobility, transfers, positioning, and ambulation. Collaborate with the case manager regarding placement after discharge. Most patients go home unless there is no support system or additional rehabilitation is needed. Health teaching and ensuring continuity of care are essential.

Fractures of the *lower two thirds of the femur* usually result from trauma, often from a motor vehicle crash. A femur fracture is seldom immobilized by casting because the powerful muscles of the thigh become spastic, which causes displacement of bone ends. Extensive hemorrhage can occur with femur fracture.

Surgical treatment is ORIF with nails, rods, or a compression screw. In a few cases in which extensive bone fragmentation or severe tissue trauma is found, external fixation may be employed. Healing time for a femur fracture may be 6 months or longer.

Skeletal traction, followed by a full-leg brace or cast, may be used in nonsurgical treatment.

Trauma to the lower leg most often causes fractures of both the *tibia* and the *fibula,* particularly the lower third, and is often referred to as a "tib-fib" fracture. The major treatment techniques are closed reduction with casting, internal fixation, and external fixation. If closed reduction is used, the patient may wear a cast for 6 to 10 weeks. Because of poor PERFUSION to parts of the tibia and fibula, delayed union is not unusual with this type of fracture. Internal fixation with nails or a plate and screws, followed by a long-leg cast for 4 to 6 weeks, is another option. When the fractures cause extensive skin and soft-tissue damage, the initial treatment may be external fixation, often for 6 to 10 weeks, usually followed by application of a cast until the fracture is completely healed. The patient uses ambulatory aids, usually crutches.

Ankle fractures are described by their anatomic place of injury. For example, a bimalleolar (Pott's) fracture involves the medial malleolus of the tibia and the lateral malleolus of the fibula. The small talus that makes up the rest of the ankle joint may also be broken. An ORIF is usually performed using two incisions—one on the medial (inside) aspect of the ankle and one on the lateral (outer) side. Several screws or nails are placed into the tibia, and a compression plate with multiple screws keeps the fibula in alignment. Weight bearing is restricted until the bone heals.

Treatment of fractures of the foot or phalanges (toes) is similar to that of other fractures. Phalangeal fractures may be more painful but are not as serious as most other types of fractures. Crutches are used for ambulation if weight bearing is restricted, but many patients can ambulate while wearing an orthopedic shoe or boot while the bone heals.

Fractures of the Chest and Pelvis

Chest trauma may cause fractures of the ribs or sternum. The major concern with rib and sternal fractures is the potential for puncture of the lungs, heart, or arteries by bone fragments or ends. *Assess airway, breathing, and circulation status first for any patient having chest trauma!* Fractures of the lower ribs may damage underlying organs, such as the liver, spleen, or kidneys. These fractures tend to heal on their own without surgical intervention. Patients are often uncomfortable during the healing process and require analgesia. They also have a high risk for pneumonia because of shallow breathing caused by pain on inspiration. Encourage them to breathe normally if possible.

Because the pelvis is very vascular and is close to major organs and blood vessels, associated internal damage is the major focus in fracture management. After head injuries, pelvic fractures are the second most common cause of death from trauma. In young adults, pelvic fractures typically result from motor vehicle crashes or falls from buildings. Falls are the most common cause in older adults. The major concern related to pelvic injury is venous oozing or arterial bleeding. Loss of blood volume leads to hypovolemic shock.

Assess for internal abdominal trauma by checking for blood in the urine and stool and by monitoring the abdomen for the development of rigidity or swelling. The trauma team may use peritoneal lavage, CT scanning, or ultrasound for assessment of hemorrhage. Ultrasound is noninvasive, rapid, reliable, and cost-effective and can be done at the bedside.

There are many classification systems for pelvic fractures. A system that is particularly useful divides fractures of the pelvis into two broad categories: non–weight-bearing fractures and weight-bearing fractures.

When a *non–weight-bearing* part of the pelvis is fractured, such as one of the pubic rami or the iliac crest, treatment can be as minimal as bedrest on a firm mattress or bed board. This type of fracture can be quite painful, and the patient may need stool softeners to facilitate bowel movements because of hesitancy to move. Well-stabilized fractures usually heal in 2 months.

A *weight-bearing* fracture, such as multiple fractures of the pelvic ring creating instability or a fractured acetabulum, necessitates external fixation or ORIF or both. Progression to weight bearing depends on the stability of the fracture after fixation. Some patients can fully bear weight within days of surgery, whereas others managed with traction may not be able to bear weight for as long as 12 weeks. For complex pelvic fractures with extensive soft-tissue damage, external fixation may be required.

Compression Fractures of the Spine

Most vertebral fractures are associated with osteoporosis, metastatic bone cancer, and multiple myeloma. Compression fractures result when trabecular or cancellous bone within the vertebra becomes weakened and causes the vertebral body to collapse. The patient has severe PAIN, deformity (kyphosis), and occasional neurologic compromise. As discussed in the Osteoporosis section of Chapter 50, the patient's quality of life is reduced by the impact of this problem.

Nonsurgical management includes bedrest, analgesics, nerve blocks, and physical therapy to maintain muscle strength. Vertebral compression fractures (VCFs) that remain painful and impair mobility may be surgically treated with **vertebroplasty** or kyphoplasty. These procedures are minimally invasive techniques in which bone cement is injected through the skin (percutaneously) directly into the fracture site to provide stability and immediate pain relief. **Kyphoplasty** includes the additional step of inserting a small balloon into the fracture site and inflating it to contain the cement and to restore height to the vertebra. This procedure is preferred because it reduces the complication of leaking of bone cement outside the vertebral body and it may restore height to decrease kyphosis.

Minimally invasive surgeries can be done in an operating or interventional radiology suite by a surgeon or interventional radiologist. They can be done with moderate sedation or general anesthesia. IV ketorolac (Toradol) may be given before the procedure to reduce inflammation. Large-bore needles are placed into the fracture site using fluoroscopy or CT guidance. Then the deflated balloon is inserted through the needles and inflated in the fracture site, and the cement is injected.

Patients may have the procedures in an ambulatory care setting and return home after 2 to 4 hours or be admitted to the hospital for an overnight stay. Chart 51-6 describes the preoperative and postoperative care for percutaneous interventions for vertebral compression fractures.

Before discharge, teach the patient to report any signs or symptoms of infection from puncture sites. Remind him or her to not soak in a bath for 1 week, use analgesics as needed, resume activity, and contact the health care provider for questions or concerns.

AMPUTATIONS

An **amputation** is the removal of a part of the body. Advances in microvascular surgical procedures, better use of antibiotic

Nursing Care for Patients Having Vertebroplasty or Kyphoplasty

Provide *preoperative care* including:
- Check the patient's coagulation laboratory test results; platelet count should be more than 100,000/mm^3.
- Make sure that all anticoagulant drugs were discontinued as requested by the physician.
- Assess and document the patient's neurologic status, especially extremity movement and sensation.
- Assess the patient's pain level.
- Assess the patient's ability to lie prone for at least 1 hour.
- Establish an IV line, and take vital signs.

Provide *postoperative care* including:
- Place the patient in a flat supine position for 1 to 2 hours or as requested by the physician.
- Monitor and record vital signs and frequent neurologic assessments; report any change immediately to the physician.
- Apply an ice pack to the puncture site if needed to relieve pain.
- Assess the patient's pain level, and compare it with the preoperative level; give mild analgesic as needed.
- Monitor for complications such as bleeding at the puncture site or shortness of breath; report these findings immediately if they occur.
- Assist the patient with ambulation.

Before discharge, teach the patient and family the following:
- The patient should avoid driving or operating machinery for the first 24 hours because of drugs used during the procedure.
- Monitor the puncture site for signs of infection, such as redness, pain, swelling, or drainage.
- Keep the dressing dry, and remove it the next day.
- The patient should begin usual activities, including walking the next day, and should slowly increase activity level over the next few days.

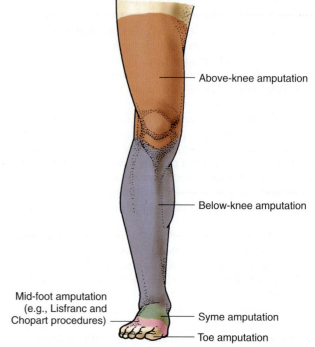

FIG. 51-12 Common levels of lower extremity amputation.

therapy, and improved surgical techniques for traumatic injury and bone cancer have reduced the number of elective amputations. The psychosocial aspects of the procedure are as devastating as the physical impairments that result. The loss is complete and permanent and causes a change in body image and self-esteem. Collaborate with members of the health care team, including prosthetists, rehabilitation therapists, psychologists, case managers, and physiatrists (rehabilitation physicians), when providing care to the patient who has an amputation.

❖ PATHOPHYSIOLOGY

Types of Amputation

Amputations may be elective or traumatic. Most are *elective* and are related to complications of peripheral vascular disease and arteriosclerosis. These complications result in ischemia in distal areas of the lower extremity. Diabetes mellitus is often an underlying cause. Amputation is considered only after other interventions have not restored circulation to the lower extremity, sometimes referred to as *limb salvage procedures* (e.g., percutaneous transluminal angioplasty [PTA]). These procedures are discussed elsewhere in this text.

Traumatic amputations most often result from accidents or war and are the primary cause of *upper extremity* amputation. A person may clean lawn mower blades or a snow blower without disconnecting the machine. A motor vehicle crash or industrial machine accident may also cause an amputation. The number of traumatic amputations also increases during war as a result of hidden land mines and bombs (e.g., in Iraq and Afghanistan). Multiple limbs or parts of limbs may be amputated as a result of these devices. Thousands of veterans of war in the United States are amputees and have had to adjust to major changes in their lifestyles.

Levels of Amputation

Elective lower extremity (LE) amputations are performed much more frequently than upper extremity amputations. Several types of LE amputations may be performed (Fig. 51-12).

The loss of any or all of the small toes presents a minor disability. Loss of the great toe is significant because it affects balance, gait, and "push off" ability during walking. Midfoot amputations and the Syme amputation are common procedures for peripheral vascular disease. In the Syme amputation, most of the foot is removed but the ankle remains. The advantage of this surgery over traditional amputations below the knee is that weight bearing can occur without the use of a prosthesis and with reduced pain.

An intense effort is made to preserve knee joints with below-the-knee amputation (BKA). When the cause for the amputation extends beyond the knee, above-knee or higher amputations are performed. Hip disarticulation, or removal of the hip joint, and hemipelvectomy (removal of half of the pelvis with the leg) are more common in younger patients than in older ones who cannot easily handle the cumbersome prostheses required for ambulation. The higher the level of amputation, the more energy is required for mobility. These higher-level procedures are typically done for cancer of the bone, osteomyelitis, or trauma as a last resort.

An amputation of any part of the upper extremity is generally more incapacitating than one of the leg. The arms and hands are necessary for ADLs such as feeding, bathing, dressing, and driving a car. In the upper extremity, as much length as possible is saved to maintain function. Early replacement with a prosthetic device is vital for the patient with this type of amputation.

🌐 CULTURAL CONSIDERATIONS
Patient-Centered Care QSEN

The incidence of lower extremity amputations is greater in black and Hispanic populations because the incidence of major diseases leading to amputation, such as diabetes and arteriosclerosis, is greater in these populations (Lowe & Tariman, 2008). Limited access to health care or lack of health insurance for these minority groups may also play a major role in limb loss. Language barriers may also be an obstacle to seeking health care providers.

Complications of Amputation

The most common complications of elective or traumatic amputations are:

- Hemorrhage
- INFECTION
- Phantom limb PAIN
- Neuroma
- Flexion contractures

When a person loses part or all of an extremity either by surgery or by trauma, major blood vessels are severed, which causes *bleeding.* If the bleeding is uncontrolled, the patient is at risk for hypovolemic shock and possibly death.

As with any surgical procedure or trauma, INFECTION can occur in the wound or the bone (osteomyelitis). The older adult who is malnourished and confused is at the greatest risk because excreta may soil the wound or he or she may remove the dressing and pick at the incision. Preventing infection is a major emphasis in hospitals and other health care settings.

PAIN is a frequent complication of amputation. Sensation is felt in the amputated part immediately after surgery and usually diminishes over time. When this sensation persists and is unpleasant or painful, it is referred to as **phantom limb pain (PLP)**. PLP is more common in patients who had chronic limb pain before surgery and less common in those who have traumatic amputations. The patient reports pain in the removed body part shortly after surgery, usually after an above-the-knee amputation (AKA). The pain is often described as intense burning, crushing, or cramping. Some patients report that the removed part is in a distorted, uncomfortable position. They experience numbness and tingling, referred to as *phantom limb sensation,* as well as pain. Others state that the most distal area of the removed part feels as if it is retracted into the residual limb end. For most patients, the PAIN is triggered by touching the residual limb or by temperature or barometric pressure changes, concurrent illness, fatigue, anxiety, or stress. Routine activities such as urination can trigger the pain. If pain is long-standing, especially if it existed before the amputation, any stimulus can cause it, including touching any part of the body.

Neuroma—a sensitive tumor consisting of damaged nerve cells—forms most often in amputations of the upper extremity but can occur anywhere. The patient may or may not have pain. It is diagnosed by sonography and can be treated either surgically or nonsurgically. Surgery to remove the neuroma may be performed, but it often regrows and is more painful than before the surgery. Nonsurgical modalities include peripheral

nerve blocks, steroid injections, and cognitive therapies such as hypnosis.

Flexion contractures of the hip or knee are seen in patients with amputations of the lower extremity. This complication must be avoided so that the patient can ambulate with a prosthetic device. Proper positioning and active range-of-motion exercises help prevent this complication.

Health Promotion and Maintenance

The typical patient undergoing elective amputation is a middle-aged or older man with diabetes and a lengthy history of smoking. He most likely has not cared for his feet properly, which has resulted in a nonhealing, infected foot ulcer and possibly gangrene. Therefore adherence to the disease management plan may help prevent the need for later amputation. Lifestyle habits like maintaining a healthy weight, regular exercise, and avoiding smoking can help prevent chronic diseases like diabetes and poor blood circulation.

The second largest group who have amputations comprise young men who have motorcycle or other vehicular crashes or who are injured by industrial equipment or by combat or accidents in war. These men may either experience a traumatic amputation or undergo a surgical amputation because of a severe crushing injury and massive soft-tissue damage. Teach young male adults the importance of taking safety precautions to prevent injury at work and to avoid speeding or driving while drinking alcohol. An increasing number of young women also tend to speed and drive while drinking, which endangers themselves and others around them.

❖ PATIENT-CENTERED COLLABORATIVE CARE

◆ Assessment

Physical Assessment/Clinical Manifestations. Monitor neurovascular status in the affected extremity that will be amputated. When the patient has peripheral vascular disease, check circulation in both legs. Assess skin color, temperature, sensation, and pulses in both affected and unaffected extremities. Capillary refill can be difficult to determine in the older adult related to thickened and opaque nails. In this situation, the skin near the nail bed can be used (see Chart 51-3). Capillary refill may not be as reliable as other indicators. Observe and document any discoloration of the skin, edema, ulcerations, presence of necrosis, and hair distribution on the lower extremities.

Psychosocial Assessment. People react differently to the loss of a body part. Be aware that an amputation of only a portion of one finger, especially the thumb, can be traumatic to the patient. The thumb is needed for hand activities. Therefore the loss must not be underestimated. Patients undergoing amputation face a complete, permanent loss. Evaluate their psychological preparation for a planned amputation, and expect them to go through the grieving process. Adjusting to a traumatic, unexpected amputation is often more difficult than accepting a planned one. The young patient may be bitter, hostile, and depressed. In addition to loss of a body part, the patient may lose a job, the ability to participate in favorite recreational activities, or a social relationship if other people cannot accept the body change.

The patient has an altered self-concept. The physical alteration that results from an amputation affects body image and self-esteem. For example, a patient may think that an intimate relationship with a partner is no longer possible. An older adult may feel a loss of independence. Assess the patient's feelings about himself or herself to identify areas in which he or she needs emotional support. Consult with the certified hospital chaplain, other spiritual leader, or hospital social worker if the patient is hospitalized. Counseling resources are also available in the community.

Attempt to determine the patient's willingness and motivation to withstand prolonged rehabilitation after the amputation. Asking questions about how he or she has dealt with previous life crises can provide clues. Adjustment to the amputation and rehabilitation is less difficult if the patient is willing to make needed changes.

In addition to assessing the patient's psychosocial status, assess the family's reaction to the surgery or trauma. Their response usually correlates directly with the patient's progress during recovery and rehabilitation. Expect the family to grieve for the loss, and allow them time to adjust to the change.

Assess the patient's and family's coping abilities, and help them identify personal strengths and weaknesses. Assess the patient's religious, spiritual, and cultural beliefs. Certain groups require that the amputated body part be stored for later burial with the rest of the body or be buried immediately. Other cultural customs and rituals may apply, depending on the group with which the patient associates.

Diagnostic Assessment. The surgeon determines which tests are performed to assess for viability of the limb based on blood flow. A large number of noninvasive techniques are available for this evaluation. For complete accuracy, the health care provider does not rely on any single test.

One procedure is measurement of segmental limb blood pressures, which can also be used by the nurse at the bedside. In this test, an ankle-brachial index (ABI) is calculated by dividing ankle systolic pressure by brachial systolic pressure. A normal ABI is 0.9 or higher.

Blood flow in an extremity can also be assessed by other noninvasive tests, including Doppler ultrasonography or laser Doppler flowmetry and transcutaneous oxygen pressure (TcPO$_2$). The ultrasonography and laser Doppler measure the speed of blood flow in the limb. The TcPO$_2$ measures oxygen pressure to indicate blood flow in the limb and has proved reliable for predicting healing.

◆ **Interventions**

A traumatic amputation requires rapid emergency care to possibly save the severed body part for reattachment and to prevent hemorrhage.

Emergency Care: Traumatic Amputation. For a person who has a traumatic amputation in the community, first call 911. Assess the patient for airway or breathing problems. Examine the amputation site, and apply direct pressure with layers of dry gauze or other cloth, using clean gloves if available. Many nurses carry gloves and first aid kits for this type of emergency. Elevate the extremity above the patient's heart to decrease the bleeding. Do not remove the dressing to prevent dislodging the clot.

The fingers are the most likely part to be amputated and replanted. The current recommendation for prehospital care is to wrap the completely severed finger in dry sterile gauze (if available) or a clean cloth. Put the finger in a watertight, sealed plastic bag. *Place the bag in ice water, never directly on ice, at 1 part ice and 3 parts water.* Avoid contact between the finger and the water to prevent tissue damage. Do not remove any

semidetached parts of the digit. Be sure that the part goes with the patient to the hospital.

Collaborative Care for the Patient with an Amputation. Patient care depends on the type and location of the amputation. For example, an above-the-knee amputation (AKA) has the potential for more postoperative complications than does a partial foot amputation. Regardless of where the amputation occurs, collaborate with the rehabilitation therapists to improve ambulation and/or enable the patient to be independent in ADLs. For many amputations, prostheses can be used to substitute for the missing body part.

Patients undergoing lower extremity amputation today are not usually confined to a wheelchair. Advancements in the design of prosthetics have enabled them to become independent. Therefore complications from extended bedrest are not common, even for older adults.

Assessing Tissue Perfusion and Managing Pain. The nurse's primary focus is to monitor for signs indicating that there is sufficient tissue PERFUSION and no hemorrhage. The skin flap at the end of the residual (remaining) limb should be pink in a light-skinned person and not discolored (lighter or darker than other skin pigmentation) in a dark-skinned patient. The area should be warm but not hot. Assess the closest proximal pulse for presence and strength, and compare it with that in the other extremity. If the patient has bilateral vascular disease, however, comparison of limbs may not be an accurate way of measuring blood flow. Use a Doppler device to determine if the affected side is being perfused.

All patients experience PAIN as a result of either a traumatic or surgical (elective) amputation. Some patients also report pain in the missing body part (PLP). Be sure to determine which type the patient has, because they are managed very differently.

! **NURSING SAFETY PRIORITY** (QSEN)

Action Alert

If the patient reports PLP, recognize that the PAIN is real and should be managed promptly and completely! It is not therapeutic to remind the patient that the limb cannot be hurting because it is missing. To prevent increased pain, handle the residual limb carefully when assessing the site or changing the dressing.

Opioid analgesics are not as effective for PLP as they are for residual limb pain. IV infusions of calcitonin (Miacalcin, Calcimar) during the week after amputation can reduce phantom limb pain. The health care provider prescribes other drugs on the basis of the type of PLP the patient experiences. For instance, beta-blocking agents such as propranolol (Inderal, Apo-Propranolol ✦, Detensol ✦) are used for constant, dull, burning pain. Antiepileptic drugs such as pregabalin (Lyrica) and gabapentin (Neurontin) may be used for knifelike or sharp burning pain. Antispasmodics such as baclofen (Lioresal) may be prescribed for muscle spasms or cramping. Some patients improve with antidepressant drugs.

Other pain management modalities are described in Chapter 3. Incorporate them into the plan of care if agreeable with the patient by collaborating with specialists who are trained to perform them. For example, physical therapists often use massage, heat, transcutaneous electrical nerve stimulation (TENS), and ultrasound therapy for pain control. Consult with the certified hospital chaplain or social worker to provide emotional support. A psychologist may be needed to provide psychotherapy.

? NCLEX EXAMINATION CHALLENGE

Psychosocial Integrity

A client who had an elective above-the-knee amputation (AKA) reports pain in the foot that was amputated. What is the nurse's best response to the client's pain?
A. "The pain will go away in a few days or so."
B. "That's phantom limb pain and every amputee has that."
C. "On a scale of 0 to 10, how would you rate your pain?"
D. "The pain is not real, so we don't treat it."

Preventing Infection. The surgeon typically prescribes a broad-spectrum prophylactic antibiotic immediately before elective surgery to prevent INFECTION. These may be continued for patients with *traumatic* amputations or for those who have open wounds on the residual limb. The initial pressure dressing and drains are usually removed by the surgeon 36 to 48 hours after surgery. Inspect the incision or wound for signs of infection. Record the appearance, amount, and odor of drainage, if present. The surgeon may want the incision open to air until staples or sutures are removed or may want the residual limb to have a continuous soft or rigid dressing made of fiberglass. A soft dressing is secured by an elastic bandage wrapped firmly around the residual limb.

Promoting Mobility and Preparing for Prosthesis. Collaborate with the physical therapist to begin exercises as soon as possible after surgery. If the amputation is planned, the therapist may work with the patient before surgery to start muscle-strengthening exercises and evaluate the need for ambulatory aids, such as crutches. If the patient can practice with these devices before surgery, learning how to ambulate after surgery is much easier.

For patients with AKAs or BKAs, teach range-of-motion (ROM) exercises for prevention of flexion contractures, particularly of the hip and knee. A trapeze and an overhead frame aid in strengthening the arms and allow the patient to move independently in bed. Teach the patient how to perform range-of-motion exercises. Be sure to turn the patient every 2 hours, or teach the patient to turn independently. Move the patient slowly to prevent muscle spasms (Pullen, 2010).

A firm mattress is essential for preventing contractures with a leg amputation. Assist the patient into a prone position every 3 to 4 hours for 20- to 30-minute periods if tolerated and not contraindicated. This position may be uncomfortable initially but helps prevent hip flexion contractures. Instruct the patient to pull the residual limb close to the other leg and contract the gluteal muscles of the buttocks for muscle strengthening. After staples are removed, the physical therapist may begin resistive exercises, which should also be done at home.

For above- and below-the-knee amputations, teach the patient how to push the residual limb down toward the bed while supporting it on a soft pillow at first. Then instruct him or her to continue this activity using a firmer pillow and then progress to a harder surface. This activity helps prepare the residual limb for prosthesis and reduces the incidence of phantom limb pain and sensation (Pullen, 2010).

Elevation of a lower-leg residual limb on a pillow while the patient is in a supine position is controversial. Some practitioners advocate avoiding this practice at all times because it promotes hip or knee flexion contracture. Others allow elevation for the first 24 to 48 hours to reduce swelling and subsequent discomfort. Inspect the residual limb daily to ensure that it lies completely flat on the bed.

Before an elective amputation, the patient often sees a certified prosthetist-orthotist (CPO) so that planning can begin for the postoperative period. Arrangements for replacing an arm part are especially important so that the patient can achieve self-management. Some patients are fitted with a temporary prosthesis at the time of surgery. Others, particularly older patients with vascular disease, are fitted after the residual limb has healed.

The patient being fitted for a leg prosthesis should bring a sturdy pair of shoes to the fitting. The prosthesis will be adjusted to that heel height.

Several devices help shape and shrink the residual limb in preparation for the prosthesis. Rigid, removable dressings are preferred because they decrease edema, protect and shape the limb, and allow easy access to the wound for inspection. The Jobst air splint, a plastic inflatable device, is sometimes used for this purpose. One of its disadvantages is air leakage and loss of compression. Wrapping with elastic bandages can also be effective in reducing edema, shrinking the limb, and holding the wound dressing in place.

For wrapping to be effective, reapply the bandages every 4 to 6 hours or more often if they become loose. *Figure-eight wrapping prevents restriction of blood flow. Decrease the tightness of the bandages while wrapping in a distal-to-proximal direction.* After wrapping, anchor the bandages to the highest joint, such as above the knee for BKAs (Fig. 51-13).

The design of and materials for prostheses have improved dramatically over the years. Computer-assisted design and manufacturing (CAD-CAM) is used for a custom fit. One of the most important developments in lower extremity prosthetics is the ankle-foot prosthesis, such as the Flex-Foot for more active amputees.

Promoting Body Image and Lifestyle Adaptation. The patient often experiences feelings of inadequacy as a result of losing a body part, especially the older adult who was in poor health before surgery and men who are often the main providers for their families. If possible, arrange for him or her to meet with a rehabilitated amputee who is about the same age as the patient.

Use of the word *stump* for referring to the remaining portion of the limb (residual limb) continues to be controversial. Patients have reported feeling as if they were part of a tree when the term was used. However, some rehabilitation specialists who routinely work with amputees believe the term is appropriate because it forces the patient to realize what has happened and promotes adjustment to the amputation. *Assess the patient to determine what term he or she prefers.*

Assess the patient's verbal and nonverbal references to the affected area. Some patients behave euphorically (extremely happy) and seem to have accepted the loss. *Do not jump to the conclusion that acceptance has occurred.* Ask the patient to describe his or her feelings about changes in body image and self-esteem. He or she may verbalize acceptance but refuse to look at the area during a dressing change. This inconsistent behavior is not unusual and should be documented and shared with other health care team members.

A patient who seems to adjust to the amputation during hospitalization may realize that it is difficult to cope with the

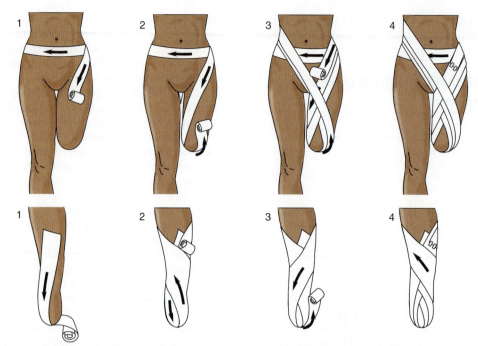

FIG. 51-13 A common method of wrapping an amputation stump. *Top,* Wrapping for above-knee amputation. *Bottom,* Wrapping for below-knee amputation.

loss after discharge from the hospital. Teach the patient and family about available resources and support from organizations such as the Amputee Coalition of America (ACA) (www.amputee-coalition.org) and the National Amputation Foundation (NAF) (www.nationalamputation.org). The NAF was originally started for veterans but has since expanded to offer services to civilians.

With advancements in prostheses and surgical techniques, most patients can return to their jobs and other activities. Professional athletes who use prostheses are often quite successful in sports. Patients with amputations ski, hike, golf, bowl, and participate in other physically demanding activities. Many amputees participate actively in organized and recreational sports.

If a job or career change is necessary, collaborate with a social worker or vocational rehabilitation specialist to evaluate the patient's skills. A supportive family or significant other is important for the adjustment to this change. The patient may also think that an intimate relationship is no longer possible because of physical changes. Discuss sexuality issues with the patient and his or her partner as needed. Professional assistance from a sex therapist, intimacy coach, or psychologist may be needed.

Help the patient and family set realistic desired outcomes and take one day at a time. Help them recognize personal strengths. If the desired outcomes are not realistic, frustration and disappointment may decrease motivation during rehabilitation. Basic principles of rehabilitation are discussed in Chapter 6.

Community-Based Care

The patient is discharged directly to home or to a skilled facility or rehabilitation facility, depending on the extent of the amputation. When rehabilitation is not feasible as in the debilitated or demented older adult, he or she may be discharged to a

❓ CLINICAL JUDGMENT CHALLENGE

Patient-Centered Care; Teamwork and Collaboration; Informatics **QSEN**

A 45-year-old man attempted to remove excess grass from his electric lawn mower blades while the mower continued to run. As a result, he severed part of his right hand. The amputated hand parts are mangled and cannot be salvaged. His wife called 911, and he was admitted to the emergency department (ED). He rates his pain as a 9 on a 0-to-10 pain intensity scale on admission.
1. As his nurse, what is your priority action when assessing this patient?
2. What other assessments will you perform and document in the electronic medical record (EMR)?
3. A hand surgeon evaluates the patient and finds that he will require surgery to débride and close the wound. What preoperative teaching will the patient require?
4. His wife is very concerned that he will lose his job if he cannot return to work soon. What is your best response at this time?
5. With what members of the health care team will you consult and collaborate?

long-term care facility. Coordinate this transfer with the case manager or discharge planner to ensure continuity of care.

At home, the patient with a leg amputation needs to have enough room to use a wheelchair if the prosthesis is not yet available. He or she must be able to use toileting facilities and have access to areas necessary for self-management, such as the kitchen. Structural home modifications may be required before the patient goes home.

After the sutures or staples are removed, the patient begins residual limb care. A home care nurse may be needed to teach the patient and/or family how to care for the limb and the prosthesis if it is available (Chart 51-7). The limb should be rewrapped 3 times a day with an elastic bandage applied in a figure-eight manner (see Fig. 51-13). For many patients, a shrinker stocking or sock is easier to apply. After the limb is healed, it is cleaned each day with the rest of the body during bathing with soap and water. Teach the patient and/or family to inspect it every day for signs of inflammation or skin breakdown.

! NURSING SAFETY PRIORITY (QSEN)

Action Alert

Collaborate with the prosthetist to teach the patient about prosthesis care after amputation to ensure its reliability and proper function. These devices are custom made, taking into account the patient's level of amputation, lifestyle, and occupation. Proper teaching regarding correct cleansing of the socket and inserts, wearing the correct liners, assessing shoe wear, and a schedule of follow-up care is essential before discharge. This information may need to be reviewed by the home care nurse.

COMPLEX REGIONAL PAIN SYNDROME

❖ PATHOPHYSIOLOGY

Complex regional pain syndrome (CRPS), formerly called **reflex sympathetic dystrophy (RSD)**, is a poorly understood dysfunction of the central and peripheral nervous systems that leads to severe, chronic PAIN. Genetic factors may play a role in the development of this devastating complication. CRPS most often results from fractures or other traumatic musculoskeletal injury and commonly occurs in the feet and hands. In some cases, specific nerve injuries are present, but in others, no injury can be identified. A triad of clinical manifestations is present, including abnormalities of the autonomic nervous system (changes in color, temperature, and sensitivity of skin over the affected area, excessive sweating, edema), motor symptoms (paresis, muscle spasms, loss of function), and SENSORY PERCEPTION symptoms (intense burning pain that becomes intractable [unrelenting]).

Over time, spotty and diffuse osteoporosis can be seen on x-ray examination. Timing of diagnosis is important because the syndrome is more difficult to treat when diagnosed in the later stages.

❖ PATIENT-CENTERED COLLABORATIVE CARE

The first priority of management is pain relief. Little research has been done to demonstrate the best practices for caring for a patient with CRPS (Hsu, 2009). Therefore a combination of interventions is used. Nurses play an important role in patient management, which includes drug therapy and a variety of nonpharmacologic modalities. Many classes of drugs may be used to manage the intense pain. These include topical analgesics, antiepileptic drugs, antidepressants, corticosteroids, bisphosphonates, and analgesics. Chapter 3 discusses pain management in detail.

In collaboration with the physical and occupational therapists, assist in maintaining adequate ROM and function. The skin of a patient with CRPS tends to alternate between warm, swollen, and red to cool, clammy, and bluish. Skin care needs to be gentle with minimal stimulation.

Peripheral or spinal cord neurostimulation using an external or internal implanted device delivers electrical pulses to block pain from getting to the brain where pain is perceived. The external or acupuncture method requires weekly sessions or a short-term continuous trial before the device is surgically implanted. Complications of implantable neurostimulators include spinal cord damage from hematoma or edema formation or other neurologic dysfunction.

A chemical sympathetic nerve block may be used. This procedure can be done by an IV infusion of phentolamine (Regitine), a drug that blocks sympathetic receptors, or by injecting an anesthetic agent next to the spine to block sympathetic nerves.

Minimally invasive surgical **sympathectomy**, or cutting of the sympathetic nerve branches via endoscopy through a small axillary incision, may be required. Topical skin adhesive is used to close the very small incision. The patient is discharged to home a few hours later with a follow-up examination the next day with the health care provider. Usual activities can resume a few days later.

Assist the patient in coping with CRPS because it often has a profound psychological effect. A referral for psychological counseling or psychotherapy may be indicated. The Reflex Sympathetic Dystrophy Syndrome Association (RSDSA) (www.rsds.org) and National Pain Association (www.nationalpainassociation.org) are available to help patients and their families organize or locate support groups and other resources.

? NCLEX EXAMINATION CHALLENGE

Physiological Integrity

The nurse is concerned that a client who had an ankle open reduction and internal fixation is at risk for complex regional pain syndrome. What assessment findings at the affected area are common when a client has this complication? **Select all that apply.**
A. Burning pain
B. Increase in sweating
C. Muscle weakness
D. Absent pedal pulse
E. Edema

KNEE INJURIES

In addition to the bone and muscle problems already discussed, trauma can cause cartilage, ligament, and tendon injury. Many musculoskeletal injuries are the result of playing sports (professional and recreational) or doing other strenuous physical activities. The popularity of all-terrain vehicles (ATVs) and skateboarding has increased injuries in younger patients. Sports

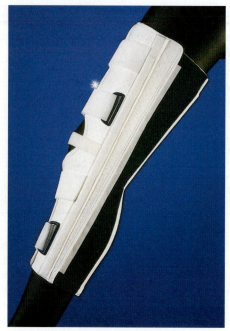

FIG. 51-14 A knee immobilizer.

injuries have become so common that large metropolitan hospitals have sports medicine clinics and physicians who specialize in this field.

The principles of injury to one part of the body are similar to those of other sports injuries and accidents. For example, a tendon rupture in a knee is cared for in the same manner as a tendon rupture in the wrist. Chart 51-8 lists general emergency measures for sports-related injuries. All patients require frequent neurovascular monitoring.

Because the knee is most often injured, it is discussed as a typical example of other areas of the body. Trauma to the knee results in internal derangement, a broad term for disturbances of an injured knee joint. When surgery is required to resolve the problem, most surgeons prefer to perform the procedure through an arthroscope when possible. A description of arthroscopy is presented in Chapter 49.

Patellofemoral pain syndrome (PFPS) is the most common diagnosis in patients who have knee PAIN. It occurs most often in people who are runners or who overuse their knee joints. For that reason, it is sometimes referred to as "runner's knee." Patients with this problem describe pain as being behind or around their patella (knee cap) in one or both knees. Swelling is not common although stiffness may be present, especially when the knee is flexed. Management usually involves rest, physical therapy, bracing or splinting, and mild analgesics. For patients who have pain lasting for more than 12 months, arthroscopic surgery is performed.

The patient with a torn meniscus (medial or lateral) typically has pain, swelling, and tenderness in the knee. A clicking or snapping sound can often be heard when the knee is moved. For a locked knee resulting from the tear, the treatment may be manipulation followed by splinting or casting for 3 to 6 weeks. If the problem recurs, a partial or total meniscectomy is performed through an arthroscope as a same-day surgical procedure. As described in Chapter 49, an arthroscope is a metal tubular instrument used for examination or surgery of joints. One or more small incisions (less than ¼-inch [0.6-cm] long) are made in the knee for insertion of the arthroscope. The surgeon threads a cutting device through the arthroscope for removal of the torn cartilage while the knee is irrigated. The surgeon may use a laser during the procedure, depending on the type and severity of the injury. A bulky pressure dressing is applied after the procedure, and the affected leg is wrapped in elastic bandages.

As for any postoperative patient, check the surgical dressing for bleeding and monitor vital signs after the patient is admitted to the same-day surgical unit. Perform neurovascular checks as outlined in Chart 51-3, usually every hour for the first few hours and then every 4 hours. Teach the patient and family what signs and symptoms to watch for after surgery and when to notify the health care provider.

The patient begins exercises immediately after surgery to strengthen the leg, prevent venous thromboembolism, and reduce swelling. Quadriceps setting, in which the patient straightens the leg while pushing the knee against the bed, is done in sets of 10 or more. Straight-leg raises are also performed. ROM exercises are usually not started for several days.

To prevent bending the affected knee, the health care provider often requests a knee immobilizer, such as the one shown in Fig. 51-14. Elevate the leg on one or two pillows according to the physician's preference, and apply ice to reduce postoperative swelling. Full weight bearing is restricted for several weeks, depending on the amount of cartilage removed. The patient is usually discharged from the hospital with crutches in less than 23 hours.

The cruciate and collateral ligaments in the knee are predisposed to injury, often from sports or vehicular crashes. The most common ligament injury is an *anterior cruciate ligament (ACL) tear*. Athletes often get these injuries during skiing, skating, or gymnastics. Women have ACL tears more often than men, possibly related to hormonal influences, biomechanical factors, and anatomic differences. Proper athletic shoes and learning how to land when jumping can help prevent this injury.

When the ACL is torn, the patient feels a snap and the knee gives way because of ACL laxity. Within hours, the knee is swollen, stiff, and painful. Examination by the health care provider shows positive ligament laxity. The diagnosis of an ACL tear is best confirmed by MRI (Pagana & Pagana, 2014).

Treatment may be nonsurgical or surgical, depending on the severity of the injury and the activity of the patient. Exercises, bracing, and limits on activities while the ligament heals may be sufficient. If medical management is not effective or the tear is severe, surgery may be needed.

The surgeon repairs the tear by reattaching the torn portions of the ligament through arthroscopy. The leg is placed in a brace or immobilizer. If the ligament cannot be repaired, reconstructive surgery may be performed with autologous grafts. A ligament from another part of the body is used to replace the torn knee ligament. Another option is artificial knee implants such as the GORE-TEX ligament.

Complete healing of knee ligaments after surgery can take 6 to 9 months or longer. These patients may use a continuous passive motion (CPM) machine at home. Teach the patient how to use and care for the machine. CPM use is discussed in Chapter 16 with the postoperative care of the patient who has had a total knee replacement.

CARPAL TUNNEL SYNDROME

❖ PATHOPHYSIOLOGY

Carpal tunnel syndrome (CTS) is a common condition in which the median nerve in the wrist becomes compressed, causing PAIN and numbness. The carpal tunnel is a rigid canal that lies between the carpal bones and a fibrous tissue sheet. A group of tendons surround the synovium and share space with the median nerve in the carpal tunnel. When the synovium becomes swollen or thickened, this nerve is compressed.

The median nerve supplies motor, sensory, and autonomic function for the first three fingers of the hand and the palmar aspect of the fourth (ring) finger. Because the median nerve is close to other structures, wrist flexion causes nerve impingement and extension causes increased pressure in the lower portion of the carpal tunnel.

CTS usually presents as a chronic problem. Acute cases are rare. Excessive hand exercise, edema or hemorrhage into the carpal tunnel, or thrombosis of the median artery can lead to acute CTS. *Patients with hand burns or a Colles' fracture of the wrist are particularly at risk for this problem.* In most cases, the cause may not result in nerve deficit for years.

CTS is also a common complication of certain metabolic and connective tissue diseases. For example, synovitis (inflammation of the synovium) occurs in patients with rheumatoid arthritis (RA). The hypertrophied synovium compresses the median nerve. In other chronic disorders such as diabetes mellitus, inadequate blood supply can cause median nerve neuropathy or dysfunction, resulting in CTS.

CTS is the most common type of repetitive stress injury (RSI). RSIs are the fastest growing type of occupational injury. People whose jobs require repetitive hand activities such as pinching or grasping during wrist flexion (e.g., factory workers, computer operators, jackhammer operators) are predisposed to CTS. It can also result from overuse in sports activities such as golf, tennis, or racquetball.

In a few cases, CTS may be a familial or congenital problem that manifests in adulthood. Space-occupying growths such as ganglia, tophi, and lipomas can also result in nerve compression.

Women, especially those older than 50 years, are much more likely than men to experience CTS, probably due to the higher prevalence of diseases such as RA in women. The problem usually affects the dominant hand but can occur in both hands simultaneously. CTS is beginning to be found in children and adolescents as a result of the increased use of computers and handheld devices.

> **CHART 51-9   Best Practice for Patient Safety & Quality Care** QSEN
>
> ### Health Promotion Activities to Prevent Carpal Tunnel Syndrome
>
> - Become familiar with federal and state laws regarding workplace requirements to prevent repetitive stress injuries such as carpal tunnel syndrome (CTS).
> - When using equipment or computer workstations that can contribute to developing CTS, assess that they are ergonomically appropriate, including:
>   - Specially designed wrist rest devices
>   - Geometrically designed computer keyboards
>   - Chair height that allows good posture
> - Take regular short breaks away from activities that cause repetitive stress, such as working at computers.
> - Stretch fingers and wrists frequently during work hours.
> - Stay as relaxed as possible when using equipment that causes repetitive stress.

Health Promotion and Maintenance

Most businesses recognize the hazards of repetitive motion as a primary cause of occupational injury and disability. Both men and women in the labor force are experiencing increasing numbers of RSIs. Occupational health nurses have played an important role in ergonomic assessments and in the development of ergonomically designed furniture and various aids to decrease CTS and other musculoskeletal injuries.

U.S federal and state legislation has been passed to ensure that all businesses, including health care organizations (HCOs), provide *ergonomically appropriate workstations* for their employees (Occupational Safety and Health Administration [OSHA]). The Joint Commission also requires that hospitals and other HCOs provide a safe work environment for all staff. In Canada, each province requires the work setting to have joint health and safety committees in which employees are actively involved in setting safety standards (Canadian Centre for Occupational Health and Safety). Chart 51-9 lists best practices for preventing CTS in the health care setting.

❖ PATIENT-CENTERED COLLABORATIVE CARE

◆ Assessment

A medical diagnosis is often made based on the patient's history and report of hand pain and numbness and without further assessment. Ask about the nature, intensity, and location of the PAIN. Patients often state that the pain is worse at night as a result of flexion or direct pressure during sleep. The pain may radiate to the arm, shoulder and neck, or chest.

In addition to reports of numbness, patients with carpal tunnel syndrome (CTS) may also have paresthesia (painful tingling). *Sensory* changes usually occur weeks or months before *motor* manifestations.

The health care provider performs several tests for abnormal sensory findings. Phalen's wrist test, sometimes called Phalen's maneuver, produces paresthesia in the median nerve distribution (palmar side of the thumb, index and middle fingers, and half of the ring finger) within 60 seconds due to increased internal carpal pressure. The patient is asked to relax the wrist into flexion or to place the back of the hands together and flex both wrists at the same time. The Phalen's test is positive in most patients with CTS (Jarvis, 2016) (Fig. 51-15).

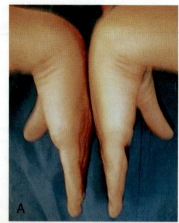

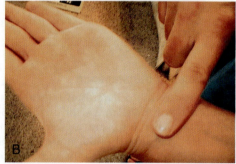

FIG. 51-15 Testing the patient for positive Phalen's sign (A) and Tinel's sign (B).

The same sensation can be created by tapping lightly over the area of the median nerve in the wrist (**Tinel's sign**). If the test is unsuccessful, a blood pressure cuff can be placed on the upper arm and inflated to the patient's systolic pressure (tourniquet). This often causes pain and tingling (Jarvis, 2016).

Motor changes in CTS begin with a weak pinch, clumsiness, and difficulty with fine movements. These changes progress to muscle weakness and wasting, which can impair self-management. If desired, test for pinching ability and ask the patient to perform a fine-movement task, such as threading a needle. Strenuous hand activity worsens the pain and numbness (McCance et al., 2014).

In addition to inspecting for muscle atrophy and task performance, observe the wrist for swelling. Gently palpate the area and note any unusual findings. Autonomic changes may be evidenced by skin discoloration, nail changes (e.g., brittleness), and increased or decreased hand sweating.

◆ **Interventions**

The health care provider uses conservative measures before surgical intervention. However, CTS can recur with either type of treatment. Management depends on the patient, but established best practices have not been determined (Uchiyama et al., 2010).

Nonsurgical Management. Aggressive drug therapy and immobilization of the wrist are the major components of nonsurgical management. Teach the patient the importance of these modalities in the hope of preventing surgical intervention.

NSAIDs are the most commonly prescribed drugs for the relief of PAIN and inflammation, if present. In addition to or instead of systemic medications, the physician may inject

corticosteroids directly into the carpal tunnel. If the patient responds to the injection, several additional weekly or monthly injections are given. Teach him or her to take NSAIDs with or after meals to reduce gastric irritation.

A splint or hand brace may be used to immobilize the wrist during the day, during the night, or both. Many patients experience temporary relief with these devices. The occupational therapist places the wrist in the neutral position or in slight extension.

Laser or ultrasound therapy may also be helpful. Some patients report fewer symptoms after beginning yoga or other exercise routine.

Surgical Management. Surgery is necessary in about half of patients with CTS. Surgery can relieve the pressure on the median nerve by providing nerve decompression. Major surgical complications are rare after CTS surgery. In some cases, however, CTS recurs months to years after surgery.

The nurse in the physician's office or same-day surgical center reinforces the teaching provided by the surgeon regarding the nature of the surgery. Postoperative care is reviewed so the patient knows what to expect. Chapter 14 describes general preoperative care in detail.

Whatever the cause of nerve compression, the surgeon removes it either by cutting or by laser. The most common surgery is the endoscopic carpal tunnel release (ECTR). In this procedure, the surgeon makes a very small incision (less than ½ inch [1.2 cm]) through which the endoscope is inserted. The surgeon then uses special instruments to free the trapped median nerve. Although ECTR is less invasive and costs less than the open procedure, the patient may have a longer period of postoperative pain and numbness compared with recovery from open carpal tunnel release (OCTR). A recent systematic review showed that surgical treatment seems to be more effective than conservative measures over the long term. However, there was no evidence that one type of procedure, open or endoscopic, was more effective than the other (Huisstede et al., 2010).

After surgery, monitor vital signs and check the dressing carefully for drainage and tightness. If ECTR has been performed, the dressing is very small. The surgeon may require that the patient's affected hand and arm be elevated above heart level for several days to reduce postoperative swelling. Check the neurovascular status of the fingers every hour during the immediate postoperative period, and encourage the patient to move them frequently. Offer pain medication, and assure him or her that a prescription for analgesics will be provided before discharge.

Hand movements, including lifting heavy objects, may be restricted for 4 to 6 weeks after surgery. The patient can expect weakness and discomfort for weeks or perhaps months. Teach him or her to report any changes in neurovascular status, including increased PAIN, to the surgeon's office immediately (Huisstede et al., 2010).

Remind the patient and family that the surgical procedure might not be a cure. For instance, synovitis may recur with rheumatoid arthritis and may recompress the median nerve. Multiple surgeries and other treatments are common with CTS.

The patient may need assistance with self-management activities during recovery. Ensure that assistance in the home is available before discharge; this is usually provided by the family or significant others.

TENDINOPATHY AND JOINT DISLOCATION

Other injuries can affect any synovial joint. The nursing management of each of these is similar to the collaborative care previously discussed for knee injuries. One of the most common injuries seen in general and sports medicine is Achilles tendon–related injuries (tendinopathy). *Rupture of the Achilles tendon* is common in adults who participate in strenuous sports or in women who wear high heels regularly. It can also occur after taking fluoroquinolone antibiotics, such as levofloxacin (Levaquin) and ciprofloxacin (Cipro) (Barry, 2010).

In the older adult, quadriceps tendon rupture may occur from a fall down several steps. Most cases of Achilles tendinopathy can be treated with RICE (see Chart 51-8):

- **R**est
- **I**ce
- **C**ompression
- **E**levation

Some evidence supports the use of NSAIDs, and changes in activity and shoes may be helpful (Chang et al., 2010). Ultrasound treatments may also be effective.

For severe damage and as a last resort, the tendon is surgically repaired and the leg is immobilized in a cast or brace for at least 6 to 8 weeks. If the tendon is beyond repair, a **tendon transplant** (also known as *tendon reconstruction*) may be performed. A tendon is removed from one part of the body and transplanted to the affected area, or a cadaver donor is used.

Dislocation of a joint occurs when the ends of two or more bones are moved away from each other. If the dislocation is not complete, the joint is partially dislocated, or **subluxed**. It can occur in any diarthrodial (synovial) joint but is most common in the shoulder, hip, knee, and fingers. This injury is usually the result of trauma but can be congenital or pathologic and can result from joint disease, such as arthritis.

The typical manifestations of dislocation are:

- Pain
- Decreased mobility
- Alteration in contour of the joint
- Deviation in length of the extremity
- Rotation of the extremity

The health care provider performs a closed reduction of the joint and moves the joint surfaces back into their normal anatomic position. The patient requires light anesthetic or moderate sedation. The joint is immobilized by a cast, splint, brace, or immobilizer until healing occurs.

Recurrent dislocations are common in the knee and shoulder. For this problem, the joint may be fixed with wires or other device to prevent further displacement. A cast, splint, or traction is applied for 3 to 6 weeks.

STRAINS AND SPRAINS

A **strain** is excessive stretching of a muscle or tendon when it is weak or unstable. Strains are sometimes referred to as *muscle pulls*. Falls, lifting a heavy item, and exercise often cause this injury.

Strains are classified according to their severity:

- A first-degree (mild) strain causes mild inflammation but little bleeding. Swelling, ecchymosis (bruising), and tenderness are usually present.
- A second-degree (moderate) strain involves tearing of the muscle or tendon fibers without complete disruption. Muscle function may be impaired.

- A third-degree (severe) strain involves a ruptured muscle or tendon with separation of muscle from muscle, tendon from muscle, or tendon from bone. Severe pain and disability result from severe strains.

Management usually involves cold and heat applications, exercise, and activity limitations. The health care provider may prescribe anti-inflammatory drugs to decrease inflammation and pain. Muscle relaxants may also be used. In third-degree strains, surgical repair of the ruptured muscle or tendon may be needed.

A **sprain** is excessive stretching of a ligament. Twisting motions from a fall or sports activity typically cause the injury. Sprains are also classified according to severity. Pain and swelling result from ligament injuries. The treatment for *mild (first-degree)* sprains includes RICE (rest, ice, compression, elevation) (see Chart 51-8).

Second-degree sprains require immobilization, such as elastic bandage and an air stirrup ankle brace or splint, and partial weight bearing while the tear heals. For severe ligament damage (*third-degree* sprain), immobilization for 4 to 6 weeks is necessary. Arthroscopic surgery may be done, particularly for chronic joint instability.

ROTATOR CUFF INJURIES

The musculotendinous, or rotator, cuff of the shoulder functions to stabilize the head of the humerus in the glenoid cavity during shoulder abduction. Young adults usually sustain a tear of the cuff by substantial trauma, such as may occur during a fall, while throwing a ball, or with heavy lifting. Older adults tend to have small tears related to aging, repetitive motions, or falls, and the tears are usually painless.

The patient with a torn rotator cuff has shoulder PAIN and cannot easily abduct the arm at the shoulder. When the arm is abducted, he or she usually drops the arm because abduction cannot be maintained (drop arm test). Pain is more intense at night and with overhead activities. Partial-thickness tears are more painful that full-thickness tears, but full-thickness tears result in more weakness and loss of function. Muscle atrophy is commonly seen, and MOBILITY is reduced. Diagnosis is confirmed with x-rays, MRI, ultrasonography, and/or CT scans.

The health care provider usually treats the patient with partial-thickness tears conservatively with NSAIDs, intermittent steroid injections, physical therapy, and activity limitations while the tear heals. Physical therapy treatments may include ultrasound, electrical stimulation, ice, and heat (Smith & Smith, 2010).

For patients who do not respond to conservative treatment in 3 to 6 months or for those who have a complete (full-thickness) tear, the surgeon repairs the cuff using mini-open or arthroscopic procedures. An interscalene nerve block may be used to extend analgesia for an open repair (Guarin, 2013). If a peripheral nerve block is used, remind the patient that the arm will feel numb and cannot be moved for up to 20 or more hours after surgery. Observe, report, and document complications of respiratory distress and neurovascular compromise.

After surgery the affected arm is usually immobilized for several weeks. Pendulum exercises are started on the third or fourth postoperative day and progress to active exercises in about 2 weeks. Patients then begin rehabilitation in the ambulatory care occupational therapy department. Teach them that they may not have full function for several months.

NURSING CONCEPTS AND CLINICAL JUDGMENT REVIEW

What might you NOTICE if the patient has impaired MOBILITY and SENSORY PERCEPTION as a result of acute musculoskeletal trauma?
- Extremity swelling, bleeding, bruising, shortening, malalignment, and/or rotation
- Report of severe pain
- Break in skin integrity
- Report of decreased or unusual sensation in extremity
- Inability or decreased ability to move extremity
- Difficulty breathing (rib trauma)
- Severe kyphosis (compression fractures)

What should you INTERPRET and how should you RESPOND to a patient with impaired MOBILITY and SENSORY PERCEPTION as a result of acute musculoskeletal trauma?

Perform and interpret focused physical assessment findings, including:
- ABC (**a**irway, **b**reathing, **c**irculation) ability (first action!)
- Pain intensity and quality
- Vital signs
- Neurovascular assessment ("circ check")

Respond by:
- First, establishing ABCs if problem exists
- If skin is not intact, covering wound with dry, sterile dressing, if available, using clean cloth as an option; applying pressure to proximal pulse if patient is bleeding; for traumatic amputation, applying direct pressure to the residual body part
- Implementing measures to prevent hypovolemic shock if patient is bleeding, including having patient lie flat, keeping him or her warm, and elevating the bleeding part
- Splinting the extremity (in community setting) to prevent movement and further damage
- If in hospital setting, assisting health care provider in splinting
- Providing pain control interventions by drug therapy as soon as possible
- Providing emotional assurance for the patient by being present and comforting

On what should you REFLECT?
- Monitor the patient's response to pain control interventions.
- Think about what else you could do to prevent complications.
- Determine what health teaching will be needed, depending on the treatment that is provided (e.g., surgery, cast).

GET READY FOR THE NCLEX® EXAMINATION!

KEY POINTS

Review these Key Points for each NCLEX Examination Client Needs Category.

Safe and Effective Care Environment
- Collaborate with physical and occupational therapists for care of patients with extremity fractures to improve MOBILITY and muscle strength. **Teamwork and Collaboration** QSEN
- Collaborate with the prosthetist, physical and occupational therapists, psychologist, and sex therapist or intimacy coach for care of patients with amputations to improve MOBILITY, muscle strength, ADLs, and self-image. **Teamwork and Collaboration** QSEN

Health Promotion and Maintenance
- Teach people to avoid musculoskeletal injury by treating or preventing osteoporosis (see Chapter 50), being cautious when walking to prevent a fall, wearing supportive shoes, avoiding dangerous sports or activities, and decreasing time spent doing repetitive stress activities, such as using a computer keyboard.
- Several community organizations, such as the Amputee Coalition of America, are available to help patients and their families cope with the loss of a body part.
- Teach patients and their family members and significant others how to care for casts or traction at home.
- Reinforce teaching for ambulating with crutches, walkers, or canes.
- Provide special care for older adults with hip fractures, including preventing heel pressure ulcers and promoting early ambulation to prevent complications of immobility.

- Teach exercises to patients with leg amputation to prevent hip flexion contractures.

Psychosocial Integrity
- Be aware that patients with severe musculoskeletal trauma may have a prolonged hospitalization and recovery period.
- For patients with severe trauma or amputation, assess coping skills and encourage verbalization. **Patient-Centered Care** QSEN
- Recognize that the patient having an amputation may need to adjust to an altered lifestyle; however, new custom prosthetics improve mobility.
- Help the patient with an amputation or other musculoskeletal trauma and family to set realistic expected outcomes and take one day at a time.

Physiological Integrity
- Be aware that open fractures cause a higher risk for infection than do closed fractures; use strict aseptic technique when providing wound management.
- Assess the risk for and implement interventions to prevent complications of immobility in patients having musculoskeletal injury or surgery (e.g., pressure ulcers, venous thromboembolism [VTE]).
- Assess patients with fractures for complications, such as VTE, INFECTION, and acute compartment syndrome.
- Recognize that fat embolism syndrome is different from pulmonary (blood clot) embolism as outlined in Chart 51-2.
- Provide emergency care of the patient with a fracture as described in Chart 51-4.

- Identify the patient at risk for acute compartment syndrome; loosen bandages, or request that the patient's cast be cut if neurovascular compromise is noted. **Evidence-Based Practice** QSEN

- As a priority, document neurovascular status frequently in patients with musculoskeletal injury, traction, or cast as described in Chart 51-3 and manage PAIN adequately. **Informatics** QSEN

- Provide evidence-based appropriate cast care, depending on the type of cast (plaster or synthetic); check for pressure necrosis under the cast by feeling for heat, assessing the patient's pain level, and smelling the cast for an unpleasant odor. **Evidence-Based Practice** QSEN

- Provide pin care for patients with skeletal traction or external fixation; assess for manifestations of INFECTION at the pin sites.

- Provide postoperative care for the patient having a fracture repair, including promoting MOBILITY and monitoring for complications of immobility.

- Provide care for patients having a vertebroplasty or kyphoplasty as described in Chart 51-6.

- Provide emergency care for a patient having a traumatic amputation in the community: Call 911, assess the patient for ABCs, apply direct pressure on the amputation site, and elevate the extremity above the patient's heart to decrease bleeding. For finger parts, wrap the amputated part with a clean cloth and place in a sealed bag, which is lowered into ice water. **Evidence-Based Practice** QSEN

- Observe for postoperative hemorrhage and INFECTION in the patient having an amputation.

- Postoperatively, assess for and promptly manage phantom limb PAIN in the patient who has an amputation; collaborate with specialists to incorporate complementary and alternative therapies and drug therapy into the patient's plan of care.

- Provide emergency care for patients with a sports-related injury as outlined in Chart 51-8.

- Recall that carpal tunnel syndrome (CTS) is the most common type of repetitive stress injury (RSI) caused by certain occupations such as computer operators and factory workers.

- Many acute musculoskeletal injuries are initially treated by RICE: rest, ice, compression, and elevation.

- The priority for managing complex regional pain syndrome (CRPS) is prompt and effective PAIN relief. Consult with PT, OT, and the pharmacist/pain specialist to determine the most effective pain management plan based on the patient's and family's preferences, values, and beliefs. **Patient-Centered Care** QSEN

CONCEPT OVERVIEW

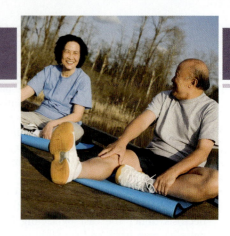

Metabolism

The word *metabolism* means to change or transform. Humans transform the energy stored within food into the types of energy needed to make the body work. Thus maintaining homeostasis of metabolism involves balancing the concepts of NUTRITION and ELIMINATION—in this instance, bowel elimination (Giddens, 2013).

As shown in Fig. 1, NUTRITION is complex and involves ingesting all of the macronutrients and micronutrients needed for optimal cellular metabolism (Giddens, 2013). As humans, we ingest many types of foods that contain proteins, carbohydrates, fats, vitamins, and minerals. Once inside the GI tract, the processes of digestion break down food into its basic elements, which then are absorbed into the blood and delivered to cells. Through metabolism, cells convert these basic elements into chemical energy, mostly adenosine triphosphate (ATP). Different cells then use metabolism to further transform ATP into heat energy, mechanical energy, chemical energy, and electrical energy. The transformation of chemical energy into other types of energy within the human body is *irreversible*. It is lost from the body in the form of heat and work. Thus bringing food into the body on a daily basis is important in meeting the human needs of nutrition and metabolism.

Heat energy helps maintain the core body temperature at or near 98.6° F—the ideal temperature for important physiologic reactions. When environmental temperatures are low, more NUTRITION intake is needed to maintain body temperature. When environmental temperatures are high, less food is needed to maintain body temperature. Therefore, in general, more calories need to be consumed per day in the winter than in the summer.

Mechanical energy is used for cell and tissue movement, cell shape changes, and whole body movement. *Electrical energy* generates the action potentials that allow nerves to transmit impulses and muscles to contract. *Chemical energy* is used to drive every chemical reaction in the body. As long as it remains alive, the body continuously needs to change food into these different energies.

Bowel ELIMINATION is the excretion of waste products so that the body rids itself of those food components that cannot be absorbed into the blood and converted into energy, such as fiber and cellulose (Giddens, 2013). If these components remained in the GI tract, they would soon fill it to the point that no nutrients could be ingested.

Consider Fig. 1 as representing the entire NUTRITION, metabolism, and bowel ELIMINATION of a person throughout his or her lifetime. The energy ingested in the form of food exactly matches the energy transformed by metabolism and is used for all the different types of internal and external "work" of the body. When this ideal situation exists, the person always has the right amount of nutrients and neither stores excess nutrients nor breaks down body tissues to use for energy.

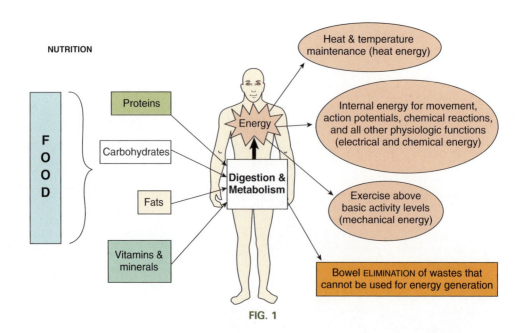

FIG. 1

In Fig. 2, the person is not ingesting enough nutrients to meet metabolic energy needs. As a result, the different types of work are less efficient and the person metabolizes his or her own body tissues to provide needed energy. If this situation continues, it will lead to death.

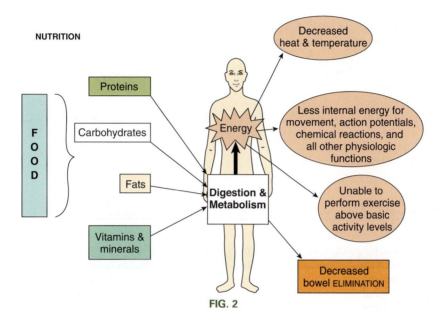

FIG. 2

In Fig. 3, the person's NUTRITION intake is greater than is needed to meet energy needs. As a result, these extra energy compounds are converted first into glycogen and eventually into fat. Although fat represents stored energy, excessive fat can harm the body. Thus excessive NUTRITION is not necessarily adequate or healthy and does not represent a balanced metabolic state. In addition, when NUTRITION is excessive, metabolism and work energies are not increased. Only heat and bowel ELIMINATION increase.

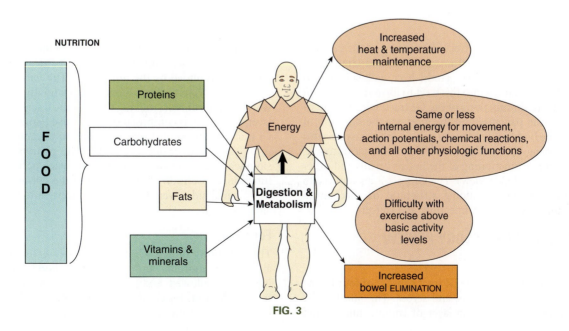

FIG. 3

52 | CHAPTER

Assessment of the Gastrointestinal System

Donna D. Ignatavicius

🅔 http://evolve.elsevier.com/Iggy/

PRIORITY CONCEPTS

- NUTRITION
- ELIMINATION

LEARNING OUTCOMES

Safe and Effective Care Environment

1. Assess patients for complications of esophagogastroduodenoscopy (EGD).

Health Promotion and Maintenance

2. Identify factors that place patients at risk for GI problems.
3. Teach pre-test and post-test care for diagnostic GI testing to patients and families to promote safety and comfort.

Psychosocial Integrity

4. Identify common psychological responses to GI health problems and diagnostic testing.

Physiological Integrity

5. Briefly review the anatomy and physiology of the GI system.
6. Describe NUTRITION and ELIMINATION changes associated with aging.
7. Perform focused physical assessment for patients with suspected or actual GI health problems.
8. Explain and interpret common laboratory tests for a patient with a GI health problem.
9. Describe care for patients having selected GI diagnostic tests.

The GI system includes the GI tract (alimentary canal), consisting of the mouth, esophagus, stomach, small and large intestines, and rectum. The salivary glands, liver, gallbladder, and pancreas secrete substances into this tract to form the GI system (Fig. 52-1). The main functions of the GI tract, with the aid of organs such as the pancreas and the liver, are the *digestion* of food to meet the body's *nutritional* needs and the ELIMINATION of waste resulting from digestion. Adequate NUTRITION is required for proper functioning of the body's organs and other cells (see the Concept Overview). The GI tract is susceptible to many health problems, including structural or mechanical alterations, impaired motility, infection, and cancer.

ANATOMY AND PHYSIOLOGY REVIEW

Structure

The lumen, or inner wall, of the GI tract consists of four layers: mucosa, submucosa, muscularis, and serosa. The *mucosa,* the innermost layer, includes a thin layer of smooth muscle and specialized exocrine gland cells. It is surrounded by the *submucosa,* which is made up of connective tissue. The *submucosa* layer is surrounded by the muscularis. The *muscularis* is composed of both circular and longitudinal smooth muscles, which work to keep contents moving through the tract. The outermost layer, the *serosa,* is composed of connective tissue. Although the GI tract is continuous from the mouth to the anus, it is divided into specialized regions. The mouth, pharynx, esophagus, stomach, and small and large intestines each perform a specific function. In addition, the secretions of the salivary, gastric, and intestinal glands; liver; and pancreas empty into the GI tract to aid digestion.

Function

The functions of the GI tract include secretion, digestion, absorption, motility, and elimination. Food and fluids are ingested, swallowed, and propelled along the lumen of the GI tract to the anus for elimination. The smooth muscles contract to move food from the mouth to the anus. Before food can be

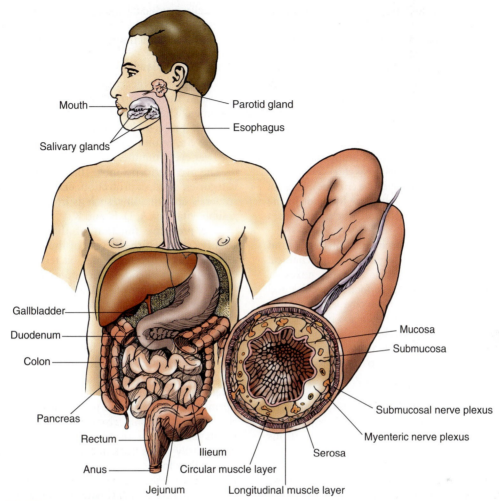

FIG. 52-1 The gastrointestinal system (GI tract) can be thought of as a tube (with necessary structures) extending from the mouth to the anus for a 25-foot length. The structure of this tube *(shown enlarged)* is basically the same throughout its length.

absorbed, it must be broken down to a liquid, called **chyme.** **Digestion** is the mechanical and chemical process in which complex foodstuffs are broken down into simpler forms that can be used by the body. During digestion, the stomach secretes hydrochloric acid, the liver secretes bile, and digestive enzymes are released from accessory organs, aiding in food breakdown. After the digestive process is complete, absorption takes place. **Absorption** is carried out as the nutrients produced by digestion move from the lumen of the GI tract into the body's circulatory system for uptake by individual cells (Jarvis, 2016).

Oral Cavity

The oral cavity (mouth) includes the buccal mucosa, lips, tongue, hard palate, soft palate, teeth, and salivary glands. The buccal mucosa is the mucous membrane lining the inside of the mouth. The tongue is involved in speech, taste, and **mastication** (chewing). Small projections called *papillae* cover the tongue and provide a roughened surface, permitting the movement of food in the mouth during chewing. The hard palate and the soft palate together form the roof of the mouth.

Adults have 32 permanent teeth: 16 each in upper and lower arches. The different types of teeth function to prepare food for digestion by cutting, tearing, crushing, or grinding the food. Swallowing begins after food is taken into the mouth and chewed. Saliva is secreted in response to the presence of food in the mouth and begins to soften the food. Saliva contains mucin and an enzyme called *salivary amylase* (also known as *ptyalin*), which begins the breakdown of carbohydrates.

Esophagus

The esophagus is a muscular canal that extends from the pharynx (throat) to the stomach and passes through the center of the diaphragm. Its primary function is to move food and fluids from the pharynx to the stomach. At the upper end of the esophagus is a sphincter referred to as the **upper esophageal sphincter (UES).** When at rest, the UES is closed to prevent air into the esophagus during respiration. The portion of the esophagus just above the gastroesophageal (GE) junction is referred to as the **lower esophageal sphincter (LES).** When at rest, the LES is normally closed to prevent reflux of gastric contents into the esophagus. If the LES does not work properly, gastroesophageal reflux disease (GERD) can develop (see Chapter 54).

Stomach

The stomach is located in the midline and left upper quadrant (LUQ) of the abdomen and has four anatomic regions (McCance et al., 2014). The *cardia* is the narrow portion of the stomach that is below the gastrocsophageal (GE) junction. The *fundus* is the area nearest to the cardia. The main area of the stomach is referred to as the *body* or *corpus*. The *antrum* (pylorus) is the distal (lower) portion of the stomach and is separated from the duodenum by the pyloric sphincter. Both ends of the stomach are guarded by sphincters (cardiac [LES] and pyloric), which aid in the transport of food through the GI tract and prevent backflow.

Smooth muscle cells that line the stomach are responsible for gastric motility. The stomach is also richly innervated with intrinsic and extrinsic nerves. Parietal cells lining the wall of the stomach secrete hydrochloric acid, whereas chief cells secrete pepsinogen (a precursor to pepsin, a digestive enzyme). Parietal cells also produce intrinsic factor, a substance that aids in the absorption of vitamin B_{12}. Absence of the intrinsic factor causes pernicious anemia.

After ingestion of food, the stomach functions as a food reservoir where the digestive process begins, using mechanical movements and chemical secretions. The stomach mixes or churns the food, breaking apart the large food molecules and mixing them with gastric secretions to form chyme, which then empties into the duodenum. The *intestinal phase* begins as the chyme passes from the stomach into the duodenum, causing distention. It is assisted by secretin, a hormone that inhibits further acid production and decreases gastric motility.

Pancreas

The pancreas is a fish-shaped gland that lies behind the stomach and extends horizontally from the duodenal C-loop to the spleen (Jarvis, 2016). The pancreas is divided into portions known as the *head,* the *body,* and the *tail* (Fig. 52-2).

Two major cellular bodies (exocrine and endocrine) within the pancreas have separate functions. The *exocrine* part consists of cells that secrete enzymes needed for digestion of carbohydrates, fats, and proteins (trypsin, chymotrypsin, amylase, and lipase). The *endocrine* part of the pancreas is made up of the islets of Langerhans, with alpha cells producing glucagon and beta cells producing insulin. These hormones produced are essential in the regulation of *metabolism.* Chapter 64 describes the endocrine function of the pancreas in detail.

Liver and Gallbladder

The *liver* is the largest organ in the body (other than skin) and is located mainly in the right upper quadrant (RUQ) of the abdomen. The right and left hepatic ducts transport bile from the liver. It receives its blood supply from the hepatic artery and portal vein, resulting in about 1500 mL of blood flow through the liver every minute.

The *liver* performs more than 400 functions in three major categories: storage, protection, and metabolism. It *stores* many minerals and vitamins, such as iron, magnesium, and the fat-soluble vitamins A, D, E, and K.

The *protective* function of the liver involves phagocytic Kupffer cells, which are part of the body's reticuloendothelial system. They engulf harmful bacteria and anemic red blood cells. The liver also detoxifies potentially harmful compounds (e.g., drugs, chemicals, alcohol). Therefore the risk for drug toxicity increases with aging because of decreased liver function.

The liver functions in the *metabolism* of proteins considered vital for human survival. It breaks down amino acids to remove ammonia, which is then converted to urea and is excreted via the kidneys (McCance et al., 2014). In addition, it synthesizes several plasma proteins, including albumin, prothrombin, and fibrinogen. The liver's role in carbohydrate metabolism involves storing and releasing glycogen as the body's energy requirements change. The organ also synthesizes, breaks down, and temporarily stores fatty acids and triglycerides.

The liver forms and continually secretes bile, which is essential for the breakdown of fat. The secretion of bile increases in response to gastrin, secretin, and cholecystokinin. Bile is secreted into small ducts that empty into the common bile duct and into the duodenum at the sphincter of Oddi. However, if the sphincter is closed, the bile goes to the gallbladder for storage.

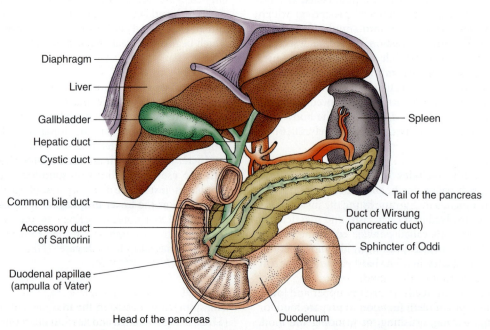

FIG. 52-2 The anatomy of the pancreas, the liver, and the gallbladder.

The *gallbladder* is a pear-shaped, bulbous sac that is located underneath the liver. It is drained by the cystic duct, which joins with the hepatic duct from the liver to form the common bile duct (CBD). The gallbladder collects, concentrates, and stores the bile that has come from the liver. It releases the bile into the duodenum via the CBD when fat is present.

Small Intestine

The small intestine is the longest and most convoluted portion of the digestive tract, measuring 16 to 19 feet (5 to 6 m) in length in an adult. It is composed of three different regions: duodenum, jejunum, and ileum. The *duodenum* is the first 12 inches (30 cm) of the small intestine and is attached to the distal end of the pylorus. The common bile duct and pancreatic duct join to form the ampulla of Vater, emptying into the duodenum at the duodenal papilla. This papillary opening is surrounded by muscle known as the sphincter of Oddi. The 8-foot (2.5-m) portion of the small intestine that follows the sphincter of Oddi is the *jejunum*. The last 8 to 12 feet (2.5 to 4 m) of the small intestine is called the *ileum*. The ileocecal valve separates the entrance of the ileum from the cecum of the large intestine (McCance et al., 2014).

The inner surface of the small intestine has a velvety appearance because of numerous mucous membrane fingerlike projections. These projections are called *intestinal villi*. In addition to the intestinal villi, the small intestine has circular folds of mucosa and submucosa, which increase the surface area for digestion and absorption.

The small intestine has three main *functions:* movement (mixing and peristalsis), digestion, and absorption. Because the intestinal villi increase the surface area of the small intestine, it is the major organ of absorption of the digestive system. The small intestine mixes and transports the chyme to mix with many digestive enzymes. It takes an average of 3 to 10 hours for the contents to be passed by peristalsis through the small intestine. Intestinal enzymes aid in the digestion of proteins, carbohydrates, and lipids.

Large Intestine

The large intestine extends about 5 to 6 feet in length from the ileocecal valve to the anus and is lined with columnar epithelium that has absorptive and mucous cells. It begins with the *cecum,* a dilated, pouchlike structure that is inferior to the ileocecal opening. At the base of the cecum is the vermiform appendix, which has no known digestive function. The large intestine then extends upward from the cecum as the colon. The colon consists of four divisions: ascending colon, transverse colon, descending colon, and sigmoid colon (McCance et al., 2014). The sigmoid colon empties into the rectum.

Following the sigmoid colon, the large intestine bends downward to form the rectum. The last 1 to 1½ inches (3 to 4 cm) of the large intestine is called the *anal canal,* which opens to the exterior of the body through the anus. Sphincter muscles surround the anal canal.

The large intestine's *functions* are movement, absorption, and ELIMINATION. Movement in the large intestine consists mainly of segmental contractions, like those in the small intestine, to allow enough time for the absorption of water and electrolytes. In addition, peristaltic contractions are triggered by colonic distention to move the contents toward the rectum, where the material is stored until the urge to defecate occurs. Absorption of water and some electrolytes occurs in the large intestine to reduce the fluid volume of the chyme. This process creates a more solid material, the feces, for elimination.

GASTROINTESTINAL CHANGES ASSOCIATED WITH AGING

Physiologic changes occur in the GI system as people age, especially ages 65 years and older. Changes in digestion and ELIMINATION that can affect NUTRITION are common (McCance et al., 2014). For example, decreased gastric hydrochloric acid (HCl) can lead to decreased absorption of essential minerals like iron. Chart 52-1 lists common GI changes and nursing implications when caring for older adults.

ASSESSMENT METHODS

Patient History

The purpose of the health history is to determine the events related to the current health problem (Chart 52-2). Focus questions about changes in appetite, weight, and stool. Determine the patient's pain experience.

Collect data about the patient's age, gender, and culture. This information can be helpful in assessing who is likely to have particular GI system disorders. For instance, older adults are more at risk for stomach cancer than are younger adults. Younger adults are more at risk for inflammatory bowel disease (IBD). The exact reasons for these differences continue to be studied.

Question the patient about previous GI disorders or abdominal surgeries. Ask about prescription medications being taken, including how much, when the drugs are taken, and why they have been prescribed. Inquire if the patient takes over-the-counter (OTC) drugs, herbs, and/or supplements. In particular, ask whether aspirin, NSAIDs (e.g., ibuprofen), laxatives, herbal preparations, or enemas are routinely taken. Large amounts of aspirin or NSAIDs can predispose the patient to peptic ulcer disease and GI bleeding. Long-term use of laxatives or enemas can cause dependence and result in constipation and electrolyte imbalance. Some herbal preparations, especially ayurvedic herbs, can affect appetite, absorption, and ELIMINATION. Determine if the patient smokes or has ever smoked cigarettes, cigars, or pipes. Smoking is a major risk factor for most GI cancers. Chewing tobacco is a major cause of oral cancer.

Finally, investigate the patient's travel history. Ask whether he or she has traveled outside of the country recently. This information may provide clues about the cause of symptoms like diarrhea.

Nutrition History

A NUTRITION history is important when assessing GI system function. Many conditions manifest themselves as a result of alterations in intake and absorption of nutrients. The purpose of a nutritional assessment is to gather information about how well the patient's needs are being met. Inquire about any special diet and whether there are any known food allergies. Ask the patient to describe the usual foods that are eaten daily and the times that meals are taken.

Health problems can also affect NUTRITION, so explore any changes that have occurred in eating habits as a result of illness. Anorexia (loss of appetite for food) can occur with GI disease. Assess changes in taste and any difficulty or pain with swallowing (dysphagia) that could be associated with esophageal

CHART 52-1 Nursing Focus on the Older Adult

Changes in the Gastrointestinal System Related to Aging

PHYSIOLOGIC CHANGE	DISORDERS RELATED TO CHANGE	NURSING INTERVENTIONS	RATIONALES
Stomach			
Atrophy of the gastric mucosa is characterized by a decrease in the ratio of gastrin-secreting cells to somatostatin-secreting cells. This change leads to decreased hydrochloric acid levels (hypochlorhydria).	Decreased hydrochloric acid levels lead to decreased absorption of iron and vitamin B_{12} and to proliferation of bacteria. Atrophic gastritis occurs as a consequence of bacterial overgrowth.	Encourage bland foods high in vitamins and iron. Assess for epigastric pain.	Bland foods help prevent gastritis. Assessment helps detect gastritis.
Large Intestine			
Peristalsis decreases, and nerve impulses are dulled.	Decreased sensation to defecate can result in postponement of bowel movements, which leads to constipation and impaction.	Encourage a high-fiber diet and 1500 mL of fluid intake daily (if not contraindicated). Encourage as much activity as tolerated.	These interventions increase the sensation of needing to defecate.
Pancreas			
Distention and dilation of pancreatic ducts change. Calcification of pancreatic vessels occurs with a decrease in lipase production.	Decreased lipase level results in decreased fat absorption and digestion. Steatorrhea, or excess fat in the feces, occurs because of decreased fat digestion.	Encourage small, frequent feedings. Assess for diarrhea.	Small, frequent feedings help prevent steatorrhea. Diarrhea may be steatorrhea. Excessive diarrhea can lead to dehydration.
Liver			
A decrease in the number and size of hepatic cells leads to decreased liver weight and mass. This change and an increase in fibrous tissue lead to decreased protein synthesis and changes in liver enzymes. Enzyme activity and cholesterol synthesis are diminished.	Decreased enzyme activity depresses drug metabolism, which leads to accumulation of drugs—possibly to toxic levels.	Assess for adverse effects of all drugs.	Assessment can help detect drug toxicity.

CHART 52-2 Best Practice for Patient Safety and Quality Care [QSEN]

Questions for Gastrointestinal Health History

- What is your typical daily food intake? Do you take any supplements? If so, what are they?
- How is your appetite? Any recent change?
- Have you lost or gained weight recently? If so, was the weight loss or gain intentional?
- Are you on a special diet?
- Do you have any difficulty chewing or swallowing?
- Do you wear dentures? How well do they fit?
- Do you ever experience indigestion or "heartburn"? How often? What seems to cause it? What helps it?
- Have you had any GI disorders or surgeries? If so, what are they?
- Is there a family history of GI health problems?
- What medications are you taking? Be sure to include prescription and over-the-counter (OTC) drugs.

- Do you smoke or have you ever smoked? Do you chew or have you ever chewed tobacco?
- Do you drink alcoholic beverages? If so, how many each week?
- Do you have pain, diarrhea, gas, or any other problems? Do any specific foods cause the problem?
- Have you traveled out of the country recently? If so, where?
- What is your usual bowel elimination pattern? Frequency? Character? Discomfort? Laxatives?
- Do you have any pain or bleeding associated with bowel movements?
- Have you experienced any changes in your usual bowel pattern or stool?
- Have you ever had an endoscopy or a colonoscopy?

⊕ CULTURAL CONSIDERATIONS

Patient-Centered Care [QSEN]

Cultural and religious patterns are important in obtaining a complete nutritional history. Ask if certain foods pose a problem for the patient. For example, the spices or hot pepper used in cooking in many cultures can aggravate or precipitate GI tract symptoms such as indigestion. Note religious patterns such as fasting or abstinence.

Many black people are lactose intolerant. A much smaller percentage of white people also have this problem. Lactose intolerance causes bloating, cramping, and diarrhea as a result of lack of the enzyme *lactase* (McCance et al., 2014). Lactase is needed to convert lactose in milk and other dairy products to glucose and galactose.

disorders. Also ask if abdominal pain or discomfort occurs with eating and whether the patient has experienced any nausea, vomiting, or **dyspepsia** (indigestion or heartburn). Unknown food allergies often cause these symptoms. Inquire about any unintentional weight loss, because some cancers of the GI tract may present in this manner. Assess for alcohol and caffeine consumption, because both substances are associated with many GI disorders, such as gastritis and peptic ulcer disease.

The patient's socioeconomic status may have a profound impact on his or her NUTRITION. For example, people who have limited budgets, such as some older adults or the unemployed, may not be able to purchase foods required for a balanced diet.

In addition, they may substitute less expensive and perhaps less effective OTC medications or herbs for prescription drugs. Necessary medical care may be delayed, and patients may not seek health care until conditions are well advanced.

Family History and Genetic Risk

Ask about a family history of GI disorders. Some GI health problems have a genetic predisposition. For example, familial adenomatous polyposis (FAP) is an inherited autosomal dominant disorder that predisposes the patient to colon cancer (McCance et al., 2014). Specific genetic risks are discussed with the GI problems in later chapters.

Current Health Problems

Because GI clinical manifestations are often vague and difficult for the patient to describe, it is important to obtain a chronologic account of the current problem, symptoms, and any treatments taken. Furthermore, ask about the location, quality, quantity, timing (onset, duration), and factors that may aggravate or alleviate each symptom (see Chart 52-2).

For example, a change in bowel habits is a common assessment finding. Obtain this information from the patient:
- Pattern of bowel movements
- Color and consistency of the feces
- Occurrence of diarrhea or constipation
- Effective action taken to relieve diarrhea or constipation
- Presence of frank blood or tarry stools
- Presence of abdominal distention or gas

An unintentional weight gain or loss is another symptom that needs further investigation. Assess the patient's:
- Normal weight
- Weight gain or loss
- Period of time for weight change
- Changes in appetite or oral intake

Pain is a common concern of patients with GI tract disorders. The mnemonic **PQRST** may be helpful in organizing the current problem assessment (Jarvis, 2016):

P: Precipitating or palliative. What brings it on? What makes it better? Worse? When did you first notice it?

Q: Quality or quantity. How does it look, feel, or sound? How intense/severe is it?

R: Region or radiation. Where is it? Does it spread anywhere?

S: Severity scale. How bad is it (on a scale of 0 to 10)? Is it getting better, worse, or staying the same?

T: Timing. Onset—Exactly when did it first occur? Duration—How long did it last? Frequency—How often does it occur?

Abdominal pain is often vague and difficult to evaluate. Ask the patient to describe the type of pain, such as burning, gnawing, or stabbing. The location of the pain can be determined by asking him or her to point to the involved site. Ask about the relationship of food intake to the onset or worsening of pain. For example, a high-fat meal may cause gallbladder pain.

Changes in the skin may result from several GI tract disorders, such as liver and biliary system obstruction. Ask about whether these clinical manifestations have occurred, or assess whether they are present:
- Skin discolorations or rashes
- Itching
- **Jaundice** (yellowing of skin caused by bilirubin pigments)

- Increased bruising
- Increased tendency to bleed

Physical Assessment

Physical assessment involves a comprehensive examination of the patient's nutritional status, mouth, and abdomen. Nutritional assessment is discussed in detail in Chapter 60. Oral assessment is described in Chapter 53.

In preparation for examination of the *abdomen*, ask the patient to empty his or her bladder and then to lie in a supine position with knees bent, keeping the arms at the sides to prevent tensing of the abdominal muscles.

The abdominal examination usually begins at the patient's right side and proceeds in a systematic fashion (Fig. 52-3):
- Right upper quadrant (RUQ)
- Left upper quadrant (LUQ)
- Left lower quadrant (LLQ)
- Right lower quadrant (RLQ)

Table 52-1 lists the organs that lie in each of these areas.

If areas of pain or discomfort are noted from the history, this area is examined last in the examination sequence. This sequence should prevent the patient from tensing abdominal muscles because of the pain, which would make the examination difficult. Examine any area of tenderness cautiously, and instruct the patient to state whether it is too painful. Observe his or her face for signs of distress or pain.

The abdomen is assessed by using the four techniques of examination, but in a sequence different from that used for other body systems: inspection, auscultation, percussion, and then palpation. This sequence is preferred so that palpation and percussion do not increase intestinal activity and bowel sounds. As a nurse generalist, perform inspection, auscultation, and light palpation. Percussion and deep palpation may be done by

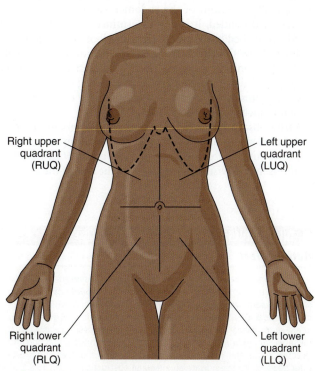

Right upper quadrant (RUQ)

Left upper quadrant (LUQ)

Right lower quadrant (RLQ)

Left lower quadrant (LLQ)

FIG. 52-3 A topographic division of the abdomen into quadrants.

TABLE 52-1   Location of Body Structures in Each Abdominal Quadrant and Midline

Right Upper Quadrant (RUQ)
- Most of the liver
- Gallbladder
- Duodenum
- Head of the pancreas
- Hepatic flexure of the colon
- Part of the ascending and transverse colon

Left Upper Quadrant (LUQ)
- Left lobe of the liver
- Stomach
- Spleen
- Body and tail of the pancreas
- Splenic flexure of the colon
- Part of the transverse and descending colon

Midline
- Abdominal aorta
- Uterus (if enlarged)
- Bladder (if distended)

Right Lower Quadrant (RLQ)
- Cecum
- Appendix
- Right ureter
- Right ovary and fallopian tube
- Right spermatic cord

Left Lower Quadrant (LLQ)
- Part of the descending colon
- Sigmoid colon
- Left ureter
- Left ovary and fallopian tube
- Left spermatic cord

primary health care providers, including advanced practice nurses (APNs), or specialty nurses. If appendicitis or an abdominal aneurysm is suspected, palpation is not done.

Inspection

Inspect the skin, and note any of these findings:
- Overall asymmetry of the abdomen
- Presence of discolorations or scarring
- Abdominal distention
- Bulging flanks
- Taut, glistening skin

Observe the shape of the abdomen by observing its contour and symmetry. The contour of the abdomen can be rounded, flat, concave, or distended. It is best determined when standing at the side of the bed or treatment table and looking down on the abdomen. View the abdomen at eye level from the side. Note whether the contour is symmetric or asymmetric. Asymmetry of the abdomen can indicate problems affecting the underlying body structures (see Table 52-1). Note the shape and position of the umbilicus for any deviations.

Finally, observe the patient's abdominal movements, including the normal rising and falling with inspiration and expiration, and note any distress during movement. Occasionally, pulsations may be visible, particularly in the area of the abdominal aorta.

! NURSING SAFETY PRIORITY (QSEN)

Action Alert

If a bulging, pulsating mass is present during assessment of the abdomen, do not touch the area because the patient may have an abdominal aortic aneurysm, a life-threatening problem. Notify the health care provider of this finding immediately! Peristaltic movements are rarely seen unless the patient is thin and has increased peristalsis. If these movements are observed, note the quadrant of origin and the direction of peristaltic flow. Report this finding to the health care provider because it may indicate an intestinal obstruction.

Auscultation

Auscultation of the abdomen is performed with the diaphragm of the stethoscope, because bowel sounds are usually high pitched. Place the stethoscope lightly on the abdominal wall while listening for bowel sounds in all four quadrants, beginning in the RLQ at the ileocecal valve area.

Bowel sounds are created as air and fluid move through the GI tract. They are normally heard as relatively high-pitched, irregular gurgles every 5 to 15 seconds, with a normal frequency range of 5 to 30 per minute (Jarvis, 2016). Bowel sounds are characterized as normal, hypoactive, or hyperactive. They are diminished or absent after abdominal surgery or in the patient with peritonitis or paralytic ileus.

For many years, nurses have been taught to count the number of bowel sounds in each quadrant as part of routine and postoperative abdominal assessment to assess for peristalsis. However, the best, most reliable method for assessing the return of peristalsis after abdominal surgery is to ask the patient if he or she has passed flatus within the past 8 hours or a stool within the past 12 to 24 hours.

Increased bowel sounds, especially loud, gurgling sounds, result from increased motility of the bowel (**borborygmus**). These sounds are usually heard in the patient with diarrhea or gastroenteritis or above a complete intestinal obstruction.

When auscultating the abdomen, also listen for vascular sounds or **bruits** ("swooshing" sounds) over the abdominal aorta, the renal arteries, and the iliac arteries. A bruit heard over the aorta usually indicates the presence of an aneurysm. *If this sound is heard, do not percuss or palpate the abdomen. Notify the health care provider of your findings!*

Percussion

Percussion may be used by APNs and other health care providers to determine the size of solid organs; to detect the presence of masses, fluid, and air; and to estimate the size of the liver and spleen. The percussion notes normally heard in the abdomen are termed *tympanic* (the high-pitched, loud, musical sound of an air-filled intestine) or *dull* (the medium-pitched, softer, thudlike sound over a solid organ, such as the liver).

The liver and spleen can be percussed. An enlarged liver is called **hepatomegaly.** Dullness heard in the left anterior axillary line indicates enlargement of the spleen (**splenomegaly**). Mild to moderate splenomegaly can be detected before the spleen becomes palpable.

Palpation

The purpose of palpation is to determine the size and location of abdominal organs and to assess for the presence of masses or tenderness. Palpation of the abdomen consists of two types: light palpation and deep palpation. Only physicians and APNs, such as clinical nurse specialists and nurse practitioners, should perform deep palpation. Deep palpation is used to further determine the size and shape of abdominal organs and masses.

The technique of *light palpation* is used to detect large masses and areas of tenderness. Place the first four fingers of the palpating hand close together and then place them lightly on the abdomen and proceed smoothly and systematically from quadrant to quadrant. Depress the abdomen to a depth of $\frac{1}{2}$ to 1 inch (1.25 to 2.5 cm). Proceed with a rotational movement of the palpating hand. Note any areas of tenderness or guarding because these areas will be examined last and cautiously during deep palpation. While performing light palpation, notice signs of rigidity, which, unlike voluntary guarding, is a sign of peritoneal inflammation.

Psychosocial Assessment

Psychosocial assessment focuses on how the GI health problem affects the patient's life and lifestyle. Remember that patients are often reluctant to discuss elimination problems, which may be very personal and embarrassing. The interview focus is on whether usual activities have been interrupted or disturbed, including employment. Question the patient about recent stressful events. Emotional stress has been associated with the development or exacerbation (flare-up) of irritable bowel syndrome (IBS) and other GI disorders. If the patient is diagnosed with cancer, he or she is expected to experience the phases of the grieving process. Patients may be depressed, angry, or in denial. More specific psychosocial assessments are included in later GI chapters as part of each disease discussion.

Diagnostic Assessment
Laboratory Assessment

To make an accurate assessment of the many possible causes of GI system abnormalities, laboratory testing of blood, urine, and stool specimens may be performed.

Serum Tests. A *complete blood count (CBC)* aids in the diagnosis of anemia and infection. It also detects changes in the blood's formed elements. In adults, GI bleeding is the most frequent cause of anemia. It is associated with GI cancer, peptic ulcer disease, diverticulitis, and inflammatory bowel disease.

Because the liver is the main site of all proteins involved in coagulation, *prothrombin time (PT)* is useful in evaluating the levels of these clotting factors. PT measures the rate at which prothrombin is converted to thrombin, a process that depends on vitamin K–associated clotting factors. Severe acute or chronic liver damage leads to a prolonged PT secondary to impaired synthesis of clotting proteins (Pagana & Pagana, 2014).

Many *electrolytes* are altered in GI tract dysfunction. For example, calcium is absorbed in the GI tract and may be measured to detect malabsorption. Excessive vomiting or diarrhea causes sodium or potassium depletion, thus requiring replacement.

Assays of serum enzymes are important in the evaluation of liver damage. *Aspartate aminotransferase (AST)* and *alanine aminotransferase (ALT)* are two enzymes found in the liver and other organs. These enzymes are elevated in most liver disorders, but they are highest in conditions that cause necrosis, such as severe viral hepatitis and cirrhosis.

Elevations in serum *amylase* and *lipase* may indicate acute pancreatitis. In this disease, serum amylase levels begin to elevate within 24 hours of onset and remain elevated for up to 5 days. Serum amylase and lipase are not elevated when extensive pancreatic necrosis is present because there are few pancreatic cells manufacturing the enzymes (Pagana & Pagana, 2014).

Bilirubin is the primary pigment in bile, which is normally conjugated and excreted by the liver and biliary system. It is measured as total serum bilirubin, conjugated (direct) bilirubin, and unconjugated (indirect) bilirubin. These measurements are important in the evaluation of jaundice and in the evaluation of liver and biliary tract functioning. Elevations in direct and indirect bilirubin levels can indicate impaired secretion.

The serum level of *ammonia* may also be measured to evaluate hepatic function. Ammonia is normally used to rebuild amino acids or is converted to urea for excretion. Elevated levels are seen in conditions that cause severe hepatocellular injury, such as cirrhosis of the liver or fulminant hepatitis (Pagana & Pagana, 2014).

Two primary *oncofetal antigens*—CA19-9 and *CEA*—are evaluated to diagnose cancer, monitor the success of cancer therapy, and assess for the recurrence of cancer in the GI tract. These antigens may also be increased in benign GI conditions. Chart 52-3 lists blood tests commonly used by the health care provider in the diagnosis of GI disorders.

Additional serum tests are described in other chapters of this GI health unit.

Urine Tests. The presence of amylase can be detected in the urine. In acute pancreatitis, renal clearance of amylase is increased. Amylase levels in the urine remain high even after serum levels return to normal. This becomes an important finding in patients who are symptomatic for 3 days or longer (Pagana & Pagana, 2014).

Urine *urobilinogen* is a form of bilirubin that is converted by the intestinal flora and excreted in the urine. Its measurement is useful in the evaluation of hepatic and biliary obstruction, because the presence of bilirubin in the urine often occurs before jaundice is seen.

Stool Tests. The American Cancer Society screening guidelines (2014) recommend yearly guaiac fecal occult blood test (gFOBT) or yearly fecal immunochemical test (FIT) at unspecified intervals to detect colorectal cancer early when it can be treated. These tests use a take-home, multi-sample method rather than having the test done during a digital rectal examination.

The traditionally used **FOBT** (e.g., Hemoccult II) requires an active component of guaiac and is therefore more likely than the FIT (e.g., HemeSelect) to yield false-positive results. In addition, patients having the guaiac-based test must avoid certain foods before the test, such as raw fruits and vegetables and red meat. Vitamin C–rich foods, juices, and tablets must also be avoided. Anticoagulants, such as warfarin (Coumadin), and NSAIDs should be discontinued for 7 days before testing begins. Patient compliance is likely to be higher with the FIT method because drugs and food do not interfere with the test results.

Stool samples may also be collected to test for *ova and parasites* to aid in the diagnosis of parasitic infection. They may also be tested for *fecal fats* when **steatorrhea** (fatty stools) or malabsorption is suspected. Fat is normally absorbed in the small intestine in the presence of biliary and pancreatic secretions. In malabsorption, fat is abnormally excreted in the stool.

Other common stool tests—stool cytotoxic assay and stool culture—detect the presence of infectious agents, especially

CHART 52-3   Laboratory Profile

Gastrointestinal Assessment

TEST (SERUM)	NORMAL RANGE FOR ADULTS	SIGNIFICANCE OF ABNORMAL FINDINGS
Calcium (total)	9.0-10.5 mg/dL (values decrease in older adults)	*Decreased* values indicate possible: Malabsorption Kidney failure Acute pancreatitis
Potassium	3.5-5.0 mEq/L or 3.5-5.0 mmol/L	*Decreased* values indicate possible: Vomiting Gastric suctioning Diarrhea Drainage from intestinal fistulas
Albumin	3.5-5.0 g/dL	*Decreased* values indicate possible: Hepatic disease
Alanine aminotransferase (ALT)	4-36 units/L (may be slightly higher in older adults)	*Increased* values indicate possible: Liver disease Hepatitis Cirrhosis
Aspartate aminotransferase (AST)	0-35 units/L (may be slightly higher in older adults)	*Increased* values indicate possible: Liver disease Hepatitis Cirrhosis
Alkaline phosphatase	30-120 units/L (may be slightly higher in older adults)	*Increased* values indicate possible: Cirrhosis Biliary obstruction Liver tumor
Bilirubin (total)	0.3-1.0 mg/dL	*Increased* values indicate possible: Hemolysis Biliary obstruction Hepatic damage
Conjugated (direct) bilirubin	0.1-0.3 mg/dL	*Increased* values indicate possible: Biliary obstruction
Unconjugated (indirect) bilirubin	0.2-0.8 mg/dL	*Increased* values indicate possible: Hemolysis Hepatic damage
Ammonia	10-80 mg/dL	*Increased* values indicate possible: Hepatic disease such as cirrhosis
Xylose absorption	20-57 mg/dL (60-minute plasma) 30-58 mg/dL (20-minute plasma)	*Decreased* values in blood and urine indicate possible: Malabsorption in the small intestine
Serum amylase	30-220 units/L	*Increased* values indicate possible: Acute pancreatitis
Serum lipase	0-160 units/L	*Increased* values indicate possible: Acute pancreatitis
Cholesterol	<200 mg/dL	*Increased* values indicate possible: Pancreatitis Biliary obstruction *Decreased* values indicate possible: Liver cell damage
Carbohydrate antigen 19-9 (CA19-9)	<37 units/mL	*Increased* values indicate possible: Cancer of the pancreas, stomach, colon Acute pancreatitis Inflammatory bowel disease
Carcinoembryonic antigen (CEA)	<5 ng/mL	*Increased* values indicate possible: Colorectal, stomach, pancreatic cancer Ulcerative colitis Crohn's disease Hepatitis Cirrhosis

Clostridium difficile. Patients who are suspected of having *C. difficile* are usually symptomatic. Prolonged antibiotic therapy, especially in older adults, depresses the natural intestinal flora, causing an overgrowth of the pathogen. The bacterium releases a toxin that causes colonic epithelium necrosis resulting in severe diarrhea that is easily transmitted from person to person via the fecal-oral route.

A stool culture takes a longer time to get results and is not the test of choice. Instead, the cytotoxic assay is considered the most reliable because it has a high sensitivity (Keske & Letizia,

2010). However, the results may not be available for up to 3 days. The most common test to detect *C. difficile* is the enzyme-linked immunosorbent assay (ELISA) toxin A+B. It is easy to use, and the results are usually available in 2 to 6 hours (Keske & Letizia, 2010).

Imaging Assessment

Radiographic examinations and similar diagnostic procedures are useful in detecting structural and functional disorders of the GI system. Teach the patient how to prepare for the examination, provide an explanation of the procedure, and teach the required postprocedure care.

A *plain film of the abdomen* may be the first x-ray study that the health care provider requests when diagnosing a GI problem. This film can reveal abnormalities such as masses, tumors, and strictures or obstructions to normal movement. Patterns of bowel gas appear light on the abdominal film and can be useful in detecting an obstruction (ileus). No preparation is required except to wear a hospital gown and remove any jewelry or belts, which may interfere with the film.

When abdominal pain is severe or when bowel perforation is suspected, an *acute abdomen series* may be requested. This procedure consists of a chest x-ray, supine abdomen film, and an upright abdomen film. The chest x-ray may reveal a hiatal hernia, and an upright abdomen film may show air in the peritoneum from a bowel perforation. Today CT and MRI scans or ultrasound scans are used more often than abdominal x-rays.

An **upper GI radiographic series** is an x-ray visualization from the mouth to the duodenojejunal junction. It may be done to detect disorders of structure or function of the esophagus (barium swallow), stomach, or duodenum. An extension of the upper GI series, the *small bowel follow-through* (SBFT), continues tracing the barium through the small intestine—up to and including the ileocecal junction—to detect disorders of the jejunum or ileum. These tests are seldom performed today because endoscopy procedures allow for direct visualization of the internal GI tract.

A double-contrast barium enema examination, also known as a lower GI series, is an x-ray of the large intestine. The 2014 American Cancer Society screening guidelines include this test every 5 years as an option to determine the presence of colorectal cancer and polyps for people older than 50 years. The other options include:

- Flexible sigmoidoscopy every 5 years, or
- CT colonography (virtual colonoscopy) every 5 years, or
- Colonoscopy every 10 years

Patient preparation is similar to that for colonoscopy. After the study is completed, the patient expels the barium. The radiology nurse or technician teaches the patient to drink plenty of fluids to assist in eliminating the barium and prevent an intestinal obstruction. A laxative is given to help remove the barium from the intestinal tract. Stools are chalky white for about 24 to 72 hours, until all barium is passed. If the patient has positive results, he or she is scheduled for a colonoscopy.

Percutaneous transhepatic cholangiography (PTC) is an x-ray of the biliary duct system using an iodinated dye instilled via a percutaneous needle inserted through the liver into the intrahepatic ducts. This procedure may be performed when a patient has jaundice or persistent upper abdominal pain, even after cholecystectomy, but is rarely done as a diagnostic procedure today. Better information about dilated biliary ducts can be obtained using ultrasound scans and endoscopic retrograde cholangiopancreatography (ERCP) (discussed on p. 1094).

CT, also referred to as a *CT scan,* provides a noninvasive cross-sectional x-ray view that can detect tissue densities and abnormalities in the abdomen, including the liver, pancreas, spleen, and biliary tract. It may be performed with or without contrast medium. If contrast medium is to be used, ask about allergies to seafood and iodine. The patient is NPO for at least 4 hours before the test if a contrast medium is to be used. IV access will be required for injection of the contrast medium. Advise the patient that he or she may feel warm and flushed upon injection. The patient who is mildly claustrophobic may require a mild sedative to tolerate the study. The radiologic technician instructs the patient to lie still and to hold his or her breath when asked, as the technician takes a series of images. The test takes about 30 minutes.

Like other parts of the body, the abdomen and its organs may also be evaluated by *MRI, such as magnetic resonance cholangiopancreatography (MRCP).* For many patients with abdominal symptoms, this may be the first diagnostic test requested by the health care provider.

❓ NCLEX EXAMINATION CHALLENGE

Health Promotion and Maintenance

A client is provided with materials to obtain three fecal occult blood tests (Hemoccult). What health teaching does the nurse provide? **Select all that apply**.
A. "Avoid red meat and raw vegetables for a week before getting the samples."
B. "Drink a gallon of GoLYTELY before you collect the first sample."
C. "Do not take food or fluids for 24 hours before the test."
D. "Do not take ibuprofen for a week before obtaining the samples."
E. "Avoid vitamin C tablets, foods, and juices a week before getting the samples."

Other Diagnostic Assessment

Endoscopy is direct visualization of the GI tract using a flexible fiberoptic endoscope. It is commonly requested to evaluate bleeding, ulceration, inflammation, tumors, and cancer of the esophagus, stomach, biliary system, or bowel. Obtaining specimens for biopsy and cell studies (e.g., *Helicobacter pylori*) is also possible through the endoscope. There are several types of endoscopic examinations. The patient must sign an informed consent form before having these invasive studies.

One of the challenges with endoscopic procedures is proper cleaning of equipment between patients to prevent the transmission of bacterial biofilms and *C. difficile* (see Chapter 23). Teach patients that these infections are possible but are not common (Muscarella, 2010).

Esophagogastroduodenoscopy. **Esophagogastroduodenoscopy (EGD)** is a visual examination of the esophagus, stomach, and duodenum. This procedure has largely replaced upper GI series testing. If GI bleeding is found during an EGD, the physician can inject a sclerotherapy or other type agent into the affected area to stop the bleeding. If the patient has an esophageal stricture, it can be dilated during an EGD. In addition, gastric lesions and celiac disease can be diagnosed using this procedure.

Teach the patient preparing for an upper GI endoscopic examination to remain NPO for 6 to 8 hours before

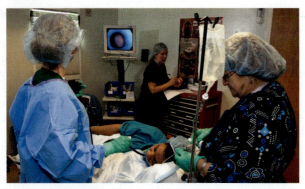

FIG. 52-4 Esophagogastroduodenoscopy allows visualization of the esophagus, the stomach, and the duodenum. If the esophagus is the focus of the examination, the procedure is called *esophagoscopy*. If the stomach is the focus, the procedure is called *gastroscopy*.

the procedure. Usual drug therapy for hypertension or other diseases may be taken the morning of the test. However, diabetic patients should consult their health care provider for special instructions. Patients are also usually asked to avoid anticoagulants, aspirin, or other NSAIDs for several days before the test unless it is absolutely necessary. Tell the patient that a flexible tube will be passed down the esophagus while he or she is under moderate sedation. Midazolam hydrochloride (Versed), fentanyl (Fentanyl, Sublimaze), and/or propofol (Diprivan) are commonly used drugs for sedation. *These drugs can depress the rate and depth of the patient's respirations.* Atropine may be administered to dry secretions. In addition, a local anesthetic is sprayed to inactivate the gag reflex and facilitate passage of the tube. Explain that this anesthetic will depress the gag reflex and that swallowing will be difficult. If the patient has dentures, they are removed.

After the drugs are given, the patient is placed in a position with the head of the bed elevated. A bite block is inserted to prevent biting down on the endoscope and to protect the teeth. The physician passes the tube through the mouth and into the esophagus (Fig. 52-4). The procedure takes about 20 to 30 minutes.

During the test, the endoscopy nurse monitors the patient's respirations for rate and depth and the oxygen saturation level via pulse oximetry. Some agencies require the use of capnography to monitor the amount of carbon dioxide that the patient exhales (Welliver, 2012). Shallow respirations decrease the amount of carbon dioxide that the patient exhales. *If the patient's respiratory rate is below 10 breaths per minute or the exhaled carbon dioxide level falls below 20%, the nurse typically uses a stimulus such as a sternal rub to encourage deeper and faster respirations.*

After the test, the endoscopy nurse or technician checks vital signs frequently (usually every 30 minutes) until the sedation begins to wear off. The siderails of the bed are raised during this time. The patient remains NPO until the gag reflex returns

(usually in 30 to 60 minutes). Intravenous fluids that were started before the procedure are discontinued when the patient is able to tolerate oral fluids without nausea or vomiting.

Because the EGD is most often performed as an ambulatory care (outpatient) procedure requiring moderate sedation, be sure that the patient has someone to drive him or her home. Remind the patient to not drive for at least 12 to 18 hours after the procedure because of sedation. Teach him or her that a hoarse voice or sore throat may persist for several days after the test. Throat lozenges can be used to relieve throat discomfort. A few patients may also experience bruising around their eyes (periorbital ecchymosis), which usually resolves in about a week (Tas, 2013).

Endoscopic Retrograde Cholangiopancreatography. Endoscopic retrograde cholangiopancreatography (ERCP) includes visual and radiographic examination of the liver, gallbladder, bile ducts, and pancreas to identify the cause and location of obstruction. It is commonly used today for therapeutic purposes rather than for diagnosis. After a cannula is inserted into the common bile duct, a radiopaque dye is instilled and then several x-ray images are obtained. The physician may perform a **papillotomy** (a small incision in the sphincter around the ampulla of Vater) to remove gallstones. If a biliary duct stricture is found, plastic or metal stents may be inserted to keep the ducts open. Biopsies of tissue are also frequently taken during this test.

The patient prepares for this test in the same manner as for an EGD, including being NPO for 6 to 8 hours before the test. The patient requires IV access for moderate sedation drugs. Ask about prior exposure to x-ray contrast media and any sensitivities or allergies. If the patient has dentures, they are removed.

Ask the patient if he or she has an implantable medical device, such as a cardiac pacemaker. Electrocautery cannot be used with this type of device (Brueschoff, 2010). Perform medication reconciliation to determine if the patient is taking anticoagulants, NSAIDs, antiplatelet drugs, or antihyperglycemic agents. The physician decides which of these drugs are safe to take and whether any will need to be stopped before the test.

The endoscopic procedure and nursing care for a patient having an ERCP are similar to those for the EGD procedure, except that the endoscope is advanced farther into the duodenum and into the biliary tract. Once the cannula is in the common duct, contrast medium is injected and x-rays are taken to view the biliary tract. A tilt table assists in distributing the contrast medium to all areas to be assessed. The patient is placed in a left lateral position for viewing the common bile duct. Once the cannula is placed, he or she is put in a prone position. After examination of the biliary tree, the cannula is directed into the pancreatic duct for examination. The ERCP lasts from 30 minutes to 2 hours, depending on the treatment that may be done.

After the test, assess vital signs frequently, usually every 15 minutes, until the patient is stable. To prevent aspiration, check to ensure that the gag reflex has returned before offering fluids or food. Discontinue intravenous fluids that were started before the procedure when the patient is able to tolerate oral fluids without nausea or vomiting.

Colicky abdominal pain can result from air instilled during the procedure. Instruct the patient to report abdominal pain, fever, nausea, or vomiting that fails to resolve after returning home. Be sure that the patient has someone to drive him or her home if the test was done on an ambulatory care basis. Remind the patient to not drive for at least 12 to 18 hours after the procedure because of sedation.

Small Bowel Capsule Endoscopy.
Small bowel endoscopy, or enteroscopy, provides a view of the small intestine. Capsule video endoscopy (M2A) is a small bowel enteroscopy that visualizes the entire small bowel, including the distal ileum. It is used to evaluate and locate the source of GI bleeding. Before the development of the M2A Capsule Endoscope, viewing the small intestine was inadequate. The capsule battery lasts around 8 hours, so it is not used to view the colon.

Prepare the patient by explaining the procedure, the purpose, and what to expect during the testing. The patient must fast (water only) for 8 to 10 hours before the test and be NPO for the first 2 hours of the testing.

At the time of the procedure, the patient's abdomen is marked for the location of the sensors, and the eight-lead sensors (Sensor Array) are applied. The patient wears an abdominal belt that houses a data recorder to capture the transmitted images. After the capsule is swallowed with a glass of water, the patient may return to normal activity for the remainder of the study. He or she can resume a normal diet 4 hours after swallowing the capsule. At the end of the procedure, the patient returns to the facility with the capsule equipment for downloading to a central computer. The procedure lasts about 8 hours.

Because the M2A Capsule Endoscope is a single-use device that moves through the GI tract by peristalsis and is excreted naturally, explain to the patient that the capsule will be seen in the stool. No other follow-up is necessary.

Colonoscopy.
Colonoscopy is an endoscopic examination of the entire large bowel. The American Cancer Society recommends that, beginning at age 50 years, all healthy men and women should have a colonoscopy every 10 years or choose another equally effective recommended screening option (ACS, 2014). The colonoscopy, however, is considered the gold standard test for detecting colon cancer. Those at high risk for cancer (e.g., family history) or those who had polyps removed should have the test more often. The physician may also obtain tissue biopsy specimens or remove polyps through the colonoscope. A colonoscopy can also evaluate the cause of chronic diarrhea or locate the source of GI bleeding. A sclerotherapy drug may be injected at the site to manage bleeding.

An alternative to this invasive procedure is the *CT colonography (virtual colonoscopy),* which is not invasive and uses a CT scanner to view the colon. Patient preparation for this alternative is the same as that for the traditional colonoscopy and should be performed every 5 years.

Patient Preparation.
Patients who have their first colonoscopy are often very anxious. Provide information about the procedure, and reassure them that pain will be controlled with medication as needed (Mikocka-Walus et al., 2012).

To help cleanse the bowel, teach the patient to stay on a clear liquid diet the day before the scheduled colonoscopy. Instruct him or her to avoid red, orange, or purple (grape) beverages and to drink an abundant amount of Gatorade or other sports drink to replace electrolytes that are lost during bowel preparation. The patient should be NPO (except water) 4 to 6 hours before the procedure.

Remind patients to avoid aspirin, anticoagulants, and antiplatelet drugs for several days before the procedure. Diabetic patients should check with their health care provider about drug therapy requirements on the day of the test because they are NPO.

The patient may be required to drink an oral liquid preparation for cleaning the bowel (e.g., sodium phosphate [Phospho-Soda]) the evening before the examination and may repeat that procedure the morning of the study. Some physicians prescribe a gallon of GoLYTELY to cleanse the bowel the day before. *This regimen should not be used for older adults to prevent excessive fluid and electrolyte loss.* All solutions should be chilled to improve their taste. Remind the patient to drink them quickly to prevent nausea. Watery diarrhea usually begins in about an hour after starting the bowel preparation process. In some cases, the patient may also require laxatives, suppositories (e.g., bisacodyl [Dulcolax]), or one or more small-volume cleansing enemas (e.g., Fleet's).

Up to 25% of patients do not have an adequate bowel preparation, which prevents complete visualization of the entire colon. An integrative review of studies on bowel preparation procedures showed that split-dose preparations (the day before and the morning of the test) were better than bowel preparations done only on the day before the test (Van Dongen, 2012).

Procedure.
IV access is necessary for the administration of moderate sedation. The physician prescribes drugs to aid in relaxation, usually IV midazolam hydrochloride (Versed), propofol (Diprivan), and/or an opiate, such as Fentanyl. Complementary and alternative therapies, such as Reiki, have been found to decrease the amount of pain medication needed during the procedure (Bourque et al., 2012).

Initially, the patient is placed on the left side with the knees drawn up while the endoscope is placed into the rectum and moved to the cecum. Air may be instilled for better visualization. The entire procedure lasts about 30 to 60 minutes. Atropine sulfate is kept available in case of bradycardia resulting from vasovagal response.

During the test, the endoscopy nurse monitors the patient's respirations for rate and depth and the oxygen saturation level via pulse oximetry. Shallow respirations decrease the amount of carbon dioxide that the patient exhales. *If the patient's respiratory rate is below 10 breaths per minute or the exhaled carbon dioxide level falls below 20%, the nurse typically uses a stimulus such as a sternal rub to encourage deeper and faster respirations.*

Follow-Up Care.
Check vital signs every 15 minutes until the patient is stable. Keep the siderails up until the patient is fully alert, and maintain NPO status. Ask the patient to lie on his or her left side to promote comfort and encourage passing flatus (see the Evidence-Based Practice box). Observe for signs of perforation (causes severe pain) and hemorrhage, such as a rapid drop in blood pressure. Reassure the patient that a feeling of fullness, cramping, and passage of flatus are expected for several hours after the test. Fluids are permitted after the patient

passes flatus to indicate that peristalsis has returned. Discontinue intravenous fluids that were started before the procedure when the patient is able to tolerate oral fluids without nausea or vomiting.

EVIDENCE-BASED PRACTICE QSEN

What Position Is Best for Patients after Undergoing a Colonoscopy?

Devitt, J., Shellman, L., Gardner, K., & Wernett, L. (2011). Using positioning after a colonoscopy for patient comfort management. *Gastroenterology Nursing, 34*(2), 93-100.

This study compared the effect of patient positioning on comfort and passage of flatus after a colonoscopy. After having a colonoscopy, 512 patients were randomly assigned to one of three body positions: left lateral, right lateral, and supine (168-174 patients per position). The patients' position, pain, bloating, and passage of flatus were assessed and rated every 15 minutes.

The results of the study found significant differences in pain and passage of flatus among the three groups of patients. The researchers concluded that patients who were positioned in the left lateral position had less discomfort and quicker passage of flatus when compared with the other two groups.

Level of Evidence: 2

This study used a large sample of patients who were randomly assigned to one of three study groups.

Commentary: Implications for Practice and Research

Nurses caring for patients who have a colonoscopy should teach patients about the need to be in a left lateral position after the procedure. Although the study used a convenience sample, patients were randomly assigned to one of three groups to compare the effect of body position on comfort and flatus passage. The study used a large sample size from which a conclusion can be generalized for best practice in nursing and health care.

If a polypectomy or tissue biopsy was performed, there may be a *small* amount of blood in the first stool after the colonoscopy. Complications of colonoscopy are not common. However, splenic injury may occur during the procedure and is difficult to diagnose (Bittler, 2011). *Report excessive bleeding or severe pain to the health care provider immediately* (Chart 52-4).

As with other endoscopic procedures, the patient will need someone to provide transportation home if the procedure was done in an ambulatory care setting. Remind the patient to avoid driving for 12 to 18 hours after the procedure because of the effects of sedation.

Virtual Colonoscopy. A noninvasive imaging procedure to obtain multi-dimensional views of the entire colon is the *CT colonography*, most popularly known as the **virtual colonoscopy**. The bowel preparation and dietary restrictions are similar to those for traditional colonoscopy. However, if a polyp is detected during a virtual colonoscopy or bleeding is found, the patient must have a follow-up invasive colonoscopy for treatment. Therefore the advantage of the traditional colonoscopy is that both diagnostic testing and minor surgical procedures can be done at the same time.

Sigmoidoscopy. Proctosigmoidoscopy, often referred to as a *sigmoidoscopy*, is an endoscopic examination of the rectum and sigmoid colon using a flexible scope. The purpose of this test is to screen for colon cancer, investigate the source of GI bleeding, or diagnose or monitor inflammatory bowel disease. If

CHART 52-4 Best Practice for Patient Safety & Quality Care QSEN

Care of the Patient after a Colonoscopy

- Do not allow the patient to take anything by mouth until sedation wears off and he or she is alert and passes flatus.
- Take vital signs every 15 to 30 minutes until the patient is alert.
- Keep patient in left lateral position to promote passing of flatus.
- Keep the top siderails up until the patient is alert.
- Assess for rectal bleeding or severe pain.
- Remind the patient that fullness and mild abdominal cramping are expected for several hours.
- Assess for manifestations of bowel perforation, including *severe* abdominal pain and guarding. Fever may occur later.
- Assess for manifestations of hypovolemic shock, including dizziness, light-headedness, decreased blood pressure, tachycardia, pallor, and altered mental status (may be the first sign in older adults).
- If the procedure is performed in an ambulatory care setting, arrange for another person to drive the patient home.

⚲ CLINICAL JUDGMENT CHALLENGE

Safety; Evidence-Based Practice QSEN

A 50-year-old man has his first screening colonoscopy today. You are assigned as his preprocedure and postprocedure nurse. When you take the patient's vital signs before the procedure, his blood pressure is 148/86 mm Hg. The patient states that he has a history of hypertension that is being well controlled with medication and diet. He tells you that he took his amlodipine (Norvasc) this morning with a small amount of water.

1. Why do you suspect his blood pressure is increased? What other assessment data will you collect?
2. What actions might you consider to decrease his blood pressure?
3. After the procedure, the patient asks for something to drink. How will you respond to him and why? What evidence supports this decision?
4. What evidence-based position should the patient be in after the procedure and why?
5. The patient tells you that he had a polyp removed. What health teaching about colorectal cancer screening will you provide?

sigmoidoscopy is used as an alternative to colonoscopy for colorectal cancer screening, it is recommended that screening begin at 50 years of age and should be done every 5 years thereafter (American Cancer Society, 2014). Patients at high risk for cancer may require more frequent screening.

The patient should have a clear liquid diet for at least 24 hours before the test. A cleansing enema or sodium biphosphate (Fleet's) enema is usually required the morning of the procedure. A laxative may also be prescribed the evening before the test.

The patient is placed on the left side in the knee-chest position. No moderate sedation is required. The endoscope is lubricated and inserted into the anus to the required depth for viewing. Tissue biopsy may be performed during this procedure, but the patient cannot feel it. The examination usually lasts about 30 minutes.

Inform the patient that mild gas pain and flatulence may be experienced from air instilled into the rectum during the examination. If a biopsy was obtained, a small amount of bleeding may be observed. Instruct the patient that excessive bleeding should be reported immediately to the health care provider.

Gastric Analysis. Although not commonly performed, gastric analysis measures the hydrochloric acid and pepsin content for evaluation of aggressive gastric and duodenal disorders (e.g., Zollinger-Ellison syndrome). There are two tests in gastric analysis: basal gastric secretion and gastric acid stimulation. Basal gastric secretion measures the secretion of hydrochloric acid between meals. If only small amounts of secretion are collected, a follow-up gastric stimulation test is given.

The patient is NPO for at least 12 hours before the test. Teach patients to avoid alcohol, tobacco, and drugs that may affect gastric secretion for 24 hours before the study. A nasogastric (NG) tube is inserted, and gastric residual contents are aspirated and discarded.

The NG tube is attached to suctioning equipment for collecting the contents at 15-minute intervals for 1 hour. Samples are collected and labeled with basal acid output (BAO), time, and volume of each specimen.

For the gastric acid stimulation test, the NG tube is left in place and a drug that stimulates gastric acid secretion (e.g., pentagastrin or betazole dihydrochloride [Histalog]) is given. Fifteen minutes after injection of the drug, specimens are again collected at 15-minute intervals for 1 hour. Samples are collected and labeled with maximal acid output (MAO), time, and volume of each specimen. Depressed levels of gastric secretion suggest the presence of gastric cancer. Increased levels of gastric secretion may indicate one or more duodenal ulcers (see Chapter 55).

After the test is completed, the NG tube is removed and the patient can resume normal eating patterns. No other follow-up is necessary.

Ultrasonography. Ultrasonography (US) is a technique in which high-frequency, inaudible vibratory sound waves are passed through the body via a transducer. The echoes created by the sound waves are then recorded and converted into images for analysis. US is commonly used to view soft tissues, such as the liver, the spleen, the pancreas, and the biliary system. The advantages of this test are that it is painless and noninvasive and requires no radiation.

The patient may be fasting, depending on the abdominal organs to be examined. Inform the patient that it will be necessary to lie still during the study.

The patient is usually placed in a supine position. The technician applies insulating gel to the end of the transducer and on the area of the abdomen under study. This gel allows airtight contact of the transducer with the skin. The technician moves the transducer back and forth over the skin until the desired images are obtained. The study takes about 15 to 30 minutes. No follow-up care is necessary.

Endoscopic Ultrasonography. Endoscopic ultrasonography (EUS) provides images of the GI wall and high-resolution images of the digestive organs. The ultrasonography is performed through the endoscope. This procedure is useful in diagnosing the presence of lymph node tumors, mucosal tumors, and tumors of the pancreas, stomach, and rectum. The patient preparation and follow-up care are similar to the preparation and follow-up care for both endoscopy and ultrasonography.

Liver-Spleen Scan. A liver-spleen scan uses IV injection of a radioactive material that is taken up primarily by the liver and secondarily by the spleen. The scan evaluates the liver and the spleen for tumors or abscesses, organ size and location, and blood flow.

Teach the patient about the need to lie still during the scanning. Assure the patient that the injection has only small amounts of radioactivity and is not dangerous. Ask female patients of childbearing age if they may be pregnant or are currently breast-feeding. The radionuclide can be found in breast milk, and radiation from x-rays or scans should be avoided in pregnancy.

The technician or the physician gives the radioactive injection through an IV line, and a wait of about 15 minutes is necessary for uptake. The patient is placed in many different positions while the scanning takes place. Tell the patient that the radionuclide is eliminated from the body through the urine in 24 hours. Careful handwashing after toileting decreases the exposure to any radiation present in the urine.

NURSING CONCEPTS AND CLINICAL JUDGMENT REVIEW

What might you NOTICE in a patient with adequate nutrition and ELIMINATION related to the GI system?

Physical assessment:
- No nausea or vomiting
- Sufficient appetite
- No intentional weight loss
- No dyspepsia (indigestion)
- No jaundice
- Abdomen soft and not tender
- Normoactive bowel sounds present is all quadrants
- No change in bowel habits

- No abdominal pain
- Normal brown, formed stool
- No frequent diarrhea or constipation

Diagnostic assessment:
- No occult blood in stool
- Normal liver enzymes, such as ALT
- Normal bilirubin levels
- Serum and urine amylase within normal limits
- Serum ammonia level within normal limit
- Serum albumin within normal limit
- Electrolytes within normal limits

GET READY FOR THE NCLEX® EXAMINATION!

KEY POINTS

Review these Key Points for each NCLEX Examination Client Needs Category.

Safe and Effective Care Environment

- Remember that the priority for care is to check for the return of the gag reflex after an upper endoscopic procedure before offering fluids or food; aspiration may occur if the gag reflex is not intact. **Safety** `QSEN`

Health Promotion and Maintenance

- If an endoscopic procedure on an ambulatory care basis is scheduled, remind the patient to have someone available to drive him or her home because of the effects of moderate sedation. **Safety** `QSEN`
- Teach patients having invasive colon diagnostic procedures to follow instructions carefully for the bowel preparation before testing; the bowel must be clear to allow visualization of the colon.
- Instruct the patient to drink plenty of fluids and take a laxative as prescribed to eliminate barium if used during diagnostic testing. **Evidence-Based Practice** `QSEN`

Psychosocial Integrity

- Remember that problems of digestion, nutrition, and elimination can markedly affect lifestyle.

- Recall that patient responses to GI health problems such as cancer or peptic ulcer can include anger, denial, and depression.

Physiological Integrity

- The GI tract is continuous from the mouth to the anus. It is responsible for food digestion and bowel elimination; the secretions of the liver, pancreas, and gallbladder empty into the GI tract to aid in digestion.
- Perform a focused abdominal assessment using inspection, auscultation, and light palpation.
- Do not palpate or auscultate any abdominal pulsating mass because it could be a life-threatening aortic aneurysm. **Safety** `QSEN`
- Be aware that aging causes changes in the GI system as summarized in Chart 52-1. **Patient-Centered Care** `QSEN`
- Assess and report any major complications of GI testing to the health care provider.
- Review and interpret laboratory results, and report abnormal findings to the health care provider (see Chart 52-3).
- Monitor vital signs carefully for the patient having any endoscopic procedure and moderate sedation.
- Assess patients who have endoscopies for bleeding, fever, and severe pain. **Safety** `QSEN`
- For patients who have had a colonoscopy, check for passage of flatus before allowing fluids or food (see Chart 52-4).

CHAPTER 53

Care of Patients with Oral Cavity Problems

Cherie R. Rebar, Nicole Heimgartner, Laura Willis

PRIORITY CONCEPTS

- INFECTION
- NUTRITION
- GAS EXCHANGE
- PAIN

LEARNING OUTCOMES

Safe and Effective Care Environment

1. Use principles of INFECTION control when caring for a patient with oral cavity problems to promote safety.
2. Collaborate with health care professionals to help patients and families experiencing oral cavity problems achieve their desired health outcomes.
3. Identify appropriate community resources for patients with oral cavity problems.

Health Promotion and Maintenance

4. Teach all people how to prevent oral cancer and maintain good oral health.
5. Develop a teaching plan for patients with stomatitis to promote digestion and NUTRITION and to minimize PAIN.
6. Teach patients with oral cancer about community-based resources.

Psychosocial Integrity

7. Reduce the psychological impact for the patient and family regarding changes in the appearance or function of any part of the oral cavity.

8. Refer patients with oral cancer to appropriate support groups.

Physiological Integrity

9. Perform a complete assessment of any oral cavity changes, lesions, and wounds.
10. Prioritize postoperative care for patients undergoing surgery for oral cancer to maintain GAS EXCHANGE and prevent aspiration.
11. Describe collaborative interventions to promote NUTRITION for postoperative patients having extensive oral surgery.
12. Identify methods to help patients communicate effectively after oral surgery.
13. Plan care for patients who have disorders of the salivary glands.
14. Identify evidence-based practice for teaching or providing oral care for patients.
15. Coordinate continuity of care between the hospital and community-based agencies for patients having oral surgery.

Digestion of food begins in the oral cavity. Within the mouth, teeth tear, grind, and crush food into small particles to promote swallowing. The enzymes in saliva begin the breakdown of carbohydrates. If a person cannot take food or fluid into the mouth, cannot chew food, or cannot swallow, the basic human need for NUTRITION may not be met by use of the GI tract. Adequate intake of fluids and nutrients into the body is vital to promote function of every body organ and system.

The pharynx (throat) is located just behind the mouth and has a role in both digestion and GAS EXCHANGE (oxygenation). The pharynx is the portal between the mouth and the GI tract, where nutrients are broken down. The pharynx also is a portal for GAS EXCHANGE, as inhaled air passes through the nose, into the pharynx, and down into the trachea. A blockage of the posterior oral cavity, such as a tumor, can interfere with GAS EXCHANGE and digestion.

Oral cavity disorders, then, can severely affect NUTRITION and GAS EXCHANGE, as well as speech, body image, and self-esteem. These disorders commonly affect people who (World Health Organization, 2014):

- Have developmental delays or mental health disorders
- Are homeless or have less (decreased) access to care
- Reside in institutions
- Use tobacco and/or alcohol
- Consume an unhealthy diet
- Have an oral cancer

This chapter discusses the most common oral health problems. As a nurse, you will play an important role in maintaining and restoring oral health through nursing interventions, including patient and family education. Chart 53-1 lists ways to help maintain a healthy oral cavity.

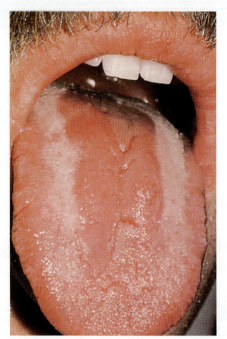

FIG. 53-1 Oral candidiasis.

STOMATITIS

❖ PATHOPHYSIOLOGY

Stomatitis is a broad term that refers to inflammation within the oral cavity and may present in many different ways. Painful single or multiple ulcerations (called *aphthous ulcers* or "canker sores") that appear as inflammation and erosion of the protective lining of the mouth are one of the most common forms of stomatitis. The sores cause PAIN, and open areas place the person at risk for bleeding and INFECTION. Mild erythema (redness) may respond to topical treatments. Extensive stomatitis may require treatment with opioid analgesics and/or antifungal medications, depending on the source of inflammation. Stomatitis is classified according to the cause of the inflammation. *Primary stomatitis,* the most common type, includes **aphthous** (noninfectious) **stomatitis**, herpes simplex stomatitis, and traumatic ulcers. *Secondary stomatitis* generally results from INFECTION by opportunistic viruses, fungi, or bacteria in patients who are immunocompromised. It can also result from drugs, such as chemotherapy. (See Chapter 22 for discussion of chemotherapy-induced stomatitis.)

A common type of secondary stomatitis is caused by *Candida albicans. Candida* is sometimes present in small amounts in the mouth, especially in older adults. Long-term antibiotic therapy

destroys other normal flora and allows the *Candida* to overgrow. The result can be **candidiasis**, also called *moniliasis,* a fungal INFECTION that is very painful. Candidiasis is also common in those undergoing immunosuppressive therapy, such as chemotherapy, radiation, and steroids.

Stomatitis can result from INFECTION, allergy, vitamin deficiency (complex B vitamins, folate, zinc, iron), systemic disease, and irritants such as tobacco and alcohol. Infectious agents, such as bacteria and viruses, may have a role in the development of recurrent stomatitis. Certain foods such as coffee, potatoes, cheese, nuts, citrus fruits, and gluten may trigger allergic responses that cause aphthous ulcers. In some cases, strict diets have resulted in the improvement of ulcers.

❖ PATIENT-CENTERED COLLABORATIVE CARE

◆ Assessment

When performing an oral assessment, ask about a history of recent infections, NUTRITION changes, oral hygiene habits, oral trauma, and stress. Also collect a drug history, including over-the-counter (OTC) drugs and NUTRITION and herbal supplements. Document the course of the current outbreak, and determine if stomatitis has occurred frequently. Ask the patient if the lesions interfere with swallowing, eating, or communicating.

The symptoms of stomatitis range in severity from a dry, painful mouth to open ulcerations, placing the patient at risk for INFECTION. These ulcerations can alter NUTRITION status because of difficulty with eating or swallowing. When they are severe, stomatitis and edema have the potential to obstruct the airway.

In oral candidiasis, white plaque-like lesions appear on the tongue, palate, pharynx (throat), and buccal mucosa (inside the cheeks) (Fig. 53-1). When these patches are wiped away, the underlying surface is red and sore. Patients may report pain, but others describe the lesions as dry or hot.

While examining the mouth, wear gloves, use a penlight to ensure adequate lighting, and use a tongue blade to aid examining the oral cavity. Assess the mouth for lesions, coating, and cracking. Document characteristics of the lesions including their location, size, shape, odor, color, and drainage.

If lesions are seen along the pharynx and the patient reports dysphagia (pain on swallowing), the lesions might extend down the esophagus. To establish a definitive diagnosis, the primary care provider may prescribe additional swallowing studies.

The physical assessment also includes palpating the cervical and submandibular lymph nodes for swelling. Advanced practice nurses and other primary care providers usually perform this part of the examination.

! NURSING SAFETY PRIORITY (QSEN)
Action Alert

When assessing the patient with stomatitis, be alert for signs and symptoms of dysphagia, such as coughing or choking when swallowing, a sensation of food "sticking" in the pharynx, or difficulty initiating the swallowing process. If dysphagia is suspected, document all findings and report these to the health care provider because dysphagia can cause numerous problems, including airway obstruction, aspiration pneumonia, and malnutrition.

◆ Interventions

Interventions for stomatitis are targeted toward health promotion and reduced risk for INFECTION through careful *oral hygiene* (see the Evidence-Based Practice box) and food selection. When providing mouth care for the patient, you may delegate oral care to unlicensed assistive personnel (UAP). Because you are accountable for the delegated task, remind UAP to use a soft-bristled toothbrush or disposable foam swabs to stimulate gums and clean the oral cavity and to use toothpaste that is free of sodium lauryl sulfate (SLS), if possible, because this ingredient has been associated with stomatitis. Teach the patient to rinse the mouth every 2 to 3 hours with a sodium bicarbonate solution or warm saline solution (may be mixed with hydrogen peroxide). He or she should avoid most commercial mouthwashes because they have high alcohol content, causing a burning sensation in irritated or ulcerated areas. Health food stores sell more natural mouthwashes that are not alcohol-based. Teach the patient to check the labels for alcohol content. Frequent, gentle mouth care promotes débridement of ulcerated lesions and can prevent superinfections. Chart 53-2 lists measures for special oral care.

Drug therapy used for stomatitis includes antimicrobials, immune modulators, and symptomatic topical agents. Complementary and alternative therapies may also be tried.

Antimicrobials, including antibiotics, antivirals, and antifungals, may be necessary for control of INFECTION. Tetracycline syrup may initially be prescribed, especially for recurrent aphthous ulcers (RAUs). The patient rinses for 2 minutes and swallows the syrup, thus obtaining both topical and systemic therapy. Minocycline swish/swallow and chlorhexidine mouthwashes may also be used.

A regimen of IV acyclovir (Zovirax) is prescribed for immunocompromised patients who contract herpes simplex stomatitis. Patients with healthy immune systems may be given acyclovir in oral or topical form.

CHART 53-2 Best Practice for Patient Safety & Quality Care (QSEN)
Care of the Patient with Problems of the Oral Cavity

- Remove dentures if the patient has severe stomatitis or oral pain.
- Encourage the patient to perform oral hygiene or provide it after each meal and as often as needed.
- Increase mouth care to every 2 hours or more frequently if stomatitis is not controlled.
- Use a soft toothbrush or gauze for oral care.
- Encourage frequent rinsing of the mouth with warm saline, sodium bicarbonate (baking soda) solution, or a combination of these solutions.
- Teach the patient to avoid commercial mouthwashes, particularly those with high alcohol content, and lemon-glycerin swabs.
- Assist the patient in selecting soft, bland, and nonacidic foods.
- Apply topical analgesics or anesthetics as prescribed by the health care provider, and monitor their effectiveness.

EVIDENCE-BASED PRACTICE (QSEN)
Does Providing Standard or Comprehensive Oral Care Result in the Best Outcomes for ICU Patients?

Prendergast, V., Jakobsson, U., Renvert, S., & Hallberg, I. (2012). Effects of a standard versus comprehensive oral care protocol among intubated neuroscience ICU patients: Results of a randomized controlled trial. *Journal of Neuroscience Nursing, 44*(3), 134-146.

Evidence shows that proper oral care is essential to prevent infections such as aspiration pneumonia and ventilator-associated pneumonia (VAP). In this study, a 2-year randomized clinical trial (RCT) involving 56 patients was conducted to compare the effect of standard oral care (manual toothbrushing) with that of comprehensive oral care (tongue scraping, electric toothbrushing, and moisturizing) on oral health of intubated neuroscience ICU patients.

Oral health was evaluated based on a standardized tool (Eilers' Oral Assessment Guide) at certain points during patients' hospitalizations. The results of this RCT demonstrated that comprehensive oral care protocols were more effective in maintaining oral health throughout intubation and after extubation when compared with standard oral care protocols.

Level of Evidence: 2

The study was a randomized controlled trial (RCT), which was also part of a larger RCT, comparing the effects of standard versus comprehensive oral care on ventilator-associated pneumonia among patients in a neuroscience ICU.

Commentary: Implications for Practice and Research

The findings of this research clearly indicate that delivery of comprehensive oral care was more effective than delivery of standard oral care in maintaining oral health of neuroscience patients who were intubated in the ICU setting. The review of literature also indicated that existing information about the specific ways in which to deliver oral care to this patient population is lacking. Be aware of best practices to deliver the most effective, evidence-based care to yield optimal patient outcomes. Further studies using larger and more diverse subjects need to be conducted.

For fungal infections like yeast, nystatin (Mycostatin) oral suspension swish/swallow is most commonly prescribed. Ice pop troches (lozenges) of the antifungal preparation allow the drug to slowly dissolve, and the cold provides an analgesic effect. Topical triamcinolone in benzocaine (Kenalog in

Orabase) and oral dexamethasone elixir used as a swish/expectorate preparation are commonly used for stomatitis, especially RAU.

Immune-modulating agents that may be prescribed as second-line therapy include:

- Topical amlexanox (Aphthasol)
- Topical granulocyte-macrophage colony-stimulating factor (GM-CSF)
- Thalidomide

The exact mechanism for how these drugs work is not clear. However, they may inhibit release of mediators that contribute to the inflammation seen in patients with RAU.

Over-the-counter (OTC) benzocaine anesthetics (e.g., Orabase, Anbesol) and camphor phenol (Campho-Phenique) can also control PAIN. Viscous lidocaine may also be prescribed to use as a gargle or mouthwash. "Magic mouthwash," a mixture of lidocaine, Benadryl, Maalox, Carafate, glucocorticoids, and other ingredients, is also commonly prescribed for those with oral pain due to cancer treatments.

! NURSING SAFETY PRIORITY (QSEN)

Drug Alert

Teach patients to use viscous lidocaine with extreme caution because its anesthetizing effect may cause burns from hot liquids in the mouth and/or increase the risk for choking.

Dietary changes may also help decrease PAIN. Cool or cold liquids can be very soothing, whereas hard, spicy, salty, and acidic foods or fluids can further irritate the ulcers. Include foods high in protein and vitamin C to promote healing, including scrambled eggs, bananas, custards, puddings, and ice cream, unless the patient has lactose intolerance.

? NCLEX EXAMINATION CHALLENGE

Physiological Integrity

Viscous lidocaine is prescribed for a client. What client teaching does the nurse provide?

A. "Be certain your food's temperature is not too hot."
B. "This medication will kill bacteria found within your mouth."
C. "You may use this drug as many times during the day as you wish."
D. "Viscous lidocaine is the most effective medication to treat fungal infections."

ORAL TUMORS

Oral cavity tumors can be benign, precancerous, or cancerous. Whether benign or malignant, tumors of the mouth affect many daily functions, including swallowing, chewing, and speaking. PAIN accompanying the tumor can also limit daily activities and self-care. Oral tumors affect body image, especially if treatment involves removal of the tongue or part of the mandible (jaw) or requires a tracheostomy.

PREMALIGNANT LESIONS

Leukoplakia presents as slowly developing changes in the oral mucous membranes causing thickened, white, firmly attached patches that cannot easily be scraped off. These patches appear slightly raised and sharply rounded. Most of these lesions are benign. However, a small percentage of them become cancerous. Although leukoplakia can be found anywhere on the oral mucosa, lesions on the lips or tongue are more likely to progress to cancer.

Leukoplakia results from mechanical factors that cause long-term oral mucous membrane irritation, such as poorly fitting dentures, chronic cheek nibbling, or broken or poorly repaired teeth. In addition, oral hairy leukoplakia (OHL) can be found in patients with human immune deficiency virus (HIV) INFECTION. The Joint Commission (TJC) Core Measures TOB-1 requires asking about tobacco use, because tobacco products (smoked, dipped, or chewed) have also been implicated in the development of leukoplakia, sometimes referred to as "smoker's patch." Oral leukoplakia can be confused with oral candidal INFECTION. However, unlike candidal infection, leukoplakia cannot be removed by scraping.

Leukoplakia is the most common oral lesion among adults. OHL is associated with Epstein-Barr virus (EBV) and can be an early manifestation of HIV INFECTION. When associated with HIV infection, the appearance of OHL is highly correlated with progression from HIV infection to acquired immune deficiency syndrome (AIDS). Leukoplakia not associated with HIV infection is more often seen in people older than 40 years. The incidence of leukoplakia is two times higher in men than in women; however, this ratio is changing because increasing numbers of women are smoking.

Erythroplakia appear as red, velvety mucosal lesions on the surface of the oral mucosa. There are more malignant changes in erythroplakia than in leukoplakia; therefore erythroplakia is often considered "precancerous" in presentation. As such, these lesions should be regarded with suspicion and analyzed by biopsy. Erythroplakia is most commonly found on the floor of the mouth, tongue, palate, and mandibular mucosa. It can be difficult to distinguish from inflammatory or immune reactions.

ORAL CANCER

Dentists and physicians systematically screen patients for oral cancer. Oral assessment has become a part of the routine dental examination. People should visit a dentist at least twice a year for professional dental hygiene and oral cancer screening, which includes inspecting and palpating the mouth for lesions.

Prevention strategies for oral cancer include minimizing sun and tanning bed exposure, tobacco cessation, and decreasing alcohol intake. Most dentists use digital technology instead of x-rays when performing the annual or biannual dental examination, because excessive, prolonged radiation from x-rays has been associated with head and neck cancer (Oral Cancer Foundation [OCF], 2014). Teach patients to follow the guidelines in Chart 53-1 to maintain oral health.

❖ PATHOPHYSIOLOGY

More than 90% of oral cancers are *squamous cell carcinomas* that begin on the surface of the epithelium. Over a period of many years, premalignant (or dysplastic) changes begin. Cells begin to vary in size and shape. Alterations in the thickness of the lining of the epithelium develop, resulting in atrophy. These tumors usually grow slowly, and the lesions may be large before the onset of symptoms unless ulceration is present. *Mucosal erythroplasia is the earliest sign of oral carcinoma. Oral lesions that appear as red, raised, eroded areas are suspicious for cancer.*

A lesion that does not heal within 2 weeks or a lump or thickening in the cheek is a symptom that warrants further assessment (OCF, 2013).

Squamous cell cancer can be found on the lips, tongue, buccal mucosa, and oropharynx. The major risk factors in its development are increasing age, tobacco use, and alcohol use. Most oral cancers occur in people older than 40 years. Tobacco use in any form (e.g., smoking or chewing tobacco) can increase the risk for cancer. A person who frequently consumes alcohol and uses tobacco in any form is at the highest risk.

GENETIC/GENOMIC CONSIDERATIONS

Patient-Centered Care QSEN

Genetic changes in patients with oral cancer have been found, especially the mutation of the *TP53* gene (McCance et al., 2014). The *TP53* gene is nicknamed the "guardian of the genome" because tumor protein *p53* is essential for cell division regulation and prevention of tumor formation (National Institutes of Health, 2014). Because mutations in this gene are linked to various cancers, always ask about a personal and family history of **any** type of cancer when assessing the patient with oral cavity problems.

An increased rate of squamous cell cancer is found in people with occupations such as textile workers, plumbers, and coal and metal workers, mainly due to prolonged exposure to polycyclic aromatic hydrocarbons (PAHs). People with **periodontal** (gum) **disease** in which mandibular (jaw) bone loss has occurred are especially at risk for cancer of the mouth. Additional factors, such as sun exposure, poor NUTRITION habits, poor oral hygiene, and INFECTION with the human papilloma virus (HPV16) may also contribute to oral cancer (OCF, 2013).

Research indicates a correlation between specific strains of the human papilloma virus (HPV) and oral cancer. Oral cancer associated with HPV appears in the tonsillar area or along the base of the tongue in younger people. Because HPV-positive oral cancers account for a large number of oral cancer diagnoses, routine oral assessment is essential. Oral cavity inspection combined with neck palpation is recommended yearly to aid in early detection (OCF, 2013).

Basal cell carcinoma of the mouth occurs primarily on the lips. The lesion is asymptomatic and resembles a raised scab. With time, it evolves into a characteristic ulcer with a raised, pearly border. Basal cell carcinomas do not metastasize (spread) but can aggressively involve the skin of the face. The major risk factor for this type of cancer is excessive sunlight exposure.

Basal cell carcinoma occurs as a result of the failure of basal cells to mature into keratinocytes. It is the second most common type of oral cancer, but it is much less common than squamous cell carcinoma.

Kaposi's sarcoma is a malignant lesion in blood vessels, appearing as a raised, purple nodule or plaque, which is usually painless. In the mouth, the hard palate is the most common site of Kaposi's sarcoma, but it can be found also on the gums, tongue, or tonsils. It is most often associated with AIDS. (See Chapter 19 for a complete discussion of Kaposi's sarcoma.)

As a group, oral cancers account for about 3% of all cancers in men and 2% of all cancers in women in the United States. Over 42,000 new cases are diagnosed each year, with almost 8000 deaths (OCF, 2013). Most cancers occur in middle-aged and older people, although in recent years, younger adults have been affected, probably as a result of sun exposure and HPV.

CHART 53-3 Key Features

Oral Cancer

- Bleeding from the mouth
- Poor appetite
- Difficulty chewing
- Difficulty swallowing
- Poor nutrition status and weight loss
- Thick or absent saliva
- Painless oral lesion that is red, raised, or eroded
- Thickening or lump in cheek

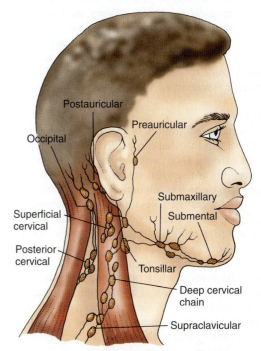

FIG. 53-2 The lymph nodes of the cervical region.

Labels: Postauricular, Preauricular, Occipital, Superficial cervical, Posterior cervical, Submaxillary, Submental, Tonsillar, Deep cervical chain, Supraclavicular

❖ PATIENT-CENTERED COLLABORATIVE CARE

◆ Assessment

Begin by assessing the patient's routine oral hygiene regimen and use of dentures or oral appliances, which might add to discomfort or mechanically irritate the mucosa. Ask about oral bleeding, which might indicate an ulcerative lesion or periodontal (gum) disease. Determine the patient's past and current appetite and NUTRITION state, including difficulty with chewing or swallowing. A continuing trend of weight loss may be related to metastasis, heavy alcohol intake, difficulty in eating or chewing, or an underlying health problem (Chart 53-3).

An examination of the oral cavity requires adequate lighting. Thoroughly inspect the oral cavity for any lesions, evidence of PAIN, or restriction of movement. Gently using a tongue blade and penlight, examine all areas of the mouth. Carefully note any change in speech caused by tongue movement. Notice any change in voice or swallowing, and assess for thick or absent saliva. After inspection, the advanced practice nurse, specialty nurse, or other health care provider uses bimanual palpation of any visible nodules to determine size and fixation. The cervical lymph nodes are also palpated (Fig. 53-2).

The functioning and appearance of the mouth are strongly linked with body image and quality of life. Therefore it is important to assess the impact of oral lesions on the patient's self-concept. In addition, assess for any educational or cultural needs that might affect health teaching or treatment. Evaluate the patient's support system and past coping mechanisms.

OralCDx is a diagnostic procedure usually performed by a dentist during a routine dental examination. The procedure involves brushing of a lesion and is helpful in determining whether the lesion is precancerous (OralCDx, 2013). However, biopsy is the definitive method for diagnosis of oral cancer. The physician obtains a needle biopsy specimen of the abnormal tissue to assess for malignant or premalignant changes. Incisional biopsies may also be performed. An intraoral biopsy can be done under local anesthesia. In very small lesions, an excisional biopsy can permit complete tumor removal. MRI is useful in detecting perineural involvement and in evaluating thickness in cancers of the tongue. Both CT and MRI can be used to determine spread to the liver or lungs if further staging of the disease is warranted.

◆ Interventions

Both the presence of tumors of the oral cavity and the effects of their treatment threaten the integrity of the oral mucosa and the patient's airway. Oral cavity lesions can be treated by surgical excision, by nonsurgical treatments such as radiation or chemotherapy, or by a combination of treatments (referred to as *multimodal therapy*). Chemotherapy is currently not used independently in the treatment of oral cancers but is used in addition to other modes of treatment to sensitize malignant cells to radiation, to shrink a malignancy before surgery, or to decrease the potential for malignancy (OCF, 2013). Multimodal therapy is the most costly treatment option yet is more frequently used (OCF, 2013). *If the patient has extensive tumor involvement and copious, tenacious (thick and "stringy") secretions, maintaining an open airway is your priority for care to promote GAS EXCHANGE.* Other nursing interventions focus on restoring and maintaining oral health.

Nonsurgical Management. Implement interventions to *manage the patient's airway* by increasing air exchange, removing secretions, and preventing aspiration as needed. Assess for dyspnea resulting from the tumor obstruction or from excessive secretions. Assess the quality, rate, and depth of respirations. Auscultate the lungs for adventitious sounds, such as wheezes caused by aspiration. Listen for stridor caused by partial airway obstruction. Promote deep breathing to help produce an effective cough to mobilize the patient's secretions.

To promote GAS EXCHANGE, place the patient in a semi-Fowler's or high-Fowler's position. If the patient is able to swallow and gag reflexes are intact, it is beneficial to encourage fluids to liquefy secretions for easier removal. Chest physiotherapy also increases air exchange as well as promotes effective coughing. If available, collaborate with the respiratory therapist about performing this procedure. If needed, use oral suction equipment with a dental tip or a tonsil tip (Yankauer catheter) to remove secretions that obstruct the airway. Teach the patient and family to use the catheters as needed.

If edema occurs with oral cavity lesions, the patient may receive steroids to reduce inflammation. Antibiotics may be prescribed if INFECTION is present because it can increase inflammation and edema. A cool mist supplied by a face tent may assist with oxygen transport and control of edema.

It is important to work with the patient to *establish an oral hygiene routine.* Perform oral hygiene every 2 hours for ulcerated lesions, INFECTION, or in the immediate postoperative period. Modifications might be needed because of oral

> **! NURSING SAFETY PRIORITY** (QSEN)
> **Action Alert**
>
> Aspiration Precautions prevent or reduce the risk factors for aspiration. Assess the patient's level of consciousness (LOC), gag reflex, and ability to swallow. To prevent aspiration, place the patient sitting upright at 90 degrees (high-Fowler's position). As a precaution, keep suction equipment nearby. For patients at high risk, assess the gag reflex before giving any fluids. Remind UAP to feed patients at risk for aspiration in small amounts. Teach visitors to speak with you before offering any type of food or drink to the patient. Provide thickened liquids as an aid to prevent aspiration. Referral to the speech/language pathologist can be beneficial for patients who are experiencing aspiration with swallowing. A swallow study may be needed to fully assess the risk for aspiration.

discomfort, bleeding, or edema. Oral care with a soft-bristled toothbrush is preferred. If the platelet count falls below 40,000/mm^3, switch the patient to an ultrasoft "chemobrush." The use of "Toothettes" or a disposable foam brush is discouraged because these products may not adequately control bacteremia-promoting plaque and may further dry the oral mucosa. Lubricant can be applied to moisten the lips and oral mucosa as needed.

Teach patients and their families that the patient should avoid using commercial mouthwashes and lemon-glycerin swabs. Commercial mouthwashes contain alcohol, and lemon-glycerin swabs are acidic. These substances can cause a burning sensation and contribute to dry oral mucous membranes. Encourage frequent rinsing of the mouth with sodium bicarbonate solution or warm saline (see also Chart 53-2). Follow hospital or health care provider protocol if available.

Radiation therapy for oral cancers can be given by external beam or interstitial implantation to reduce the size of the tumor before surgery. *External-beam* radiation passes through the skin or mucous membrane to the tumor site. Typically, treatments are given as five daily treatments per week, with a 2-day break each week, over a 6- to 9-week period. Each treatment lasts only about 10 to 15 minutes, with more time being dedicated to undertaking special precautions to minimize the dose of radiation to the brain or spinal cord (OCF, 2013).

Another option is the implantation of radioactive substances (*interstitial radiation therapy* or *brachytherapy*) either to boost the dosage or to deliver a radiation dose close to the tumor bed. This form of implant therapy can be curative in early-stage lesions in the floor of the mouth or anterior tongue. It may also add a boost of radiation to a tumor that received external-beam radiation.

With the exception of radioactive seeds, which have a low level of emission, patients receiving interstitial radiation are usually hospitalized for the duration of treatment. *Place patients on radiation transmission precautions while the materials are active or in place.* Patients need to be placed in a private room with lead-lined walls or moveable panels. When permitted, visitors may stay only 30 minutes or less each day and must sit or stand away from the patient in designated areas. Pregnant women and children younger than 18 years should not be permitted to visit. A tracheostomy may be required with interstitial implants because of edema and increased oral secretions. (See Chapter 22 for general nursing care of patients undergoing radiation therapy.)

Teach the patient undergoing *chemotherapy* and family members about the side effects of these agents, which vary with each drug. Give antiemetics as prescribed, and provide other comfort measures as needed. (See Chapter 22 for general care of patients receiving chemotherapy.)

> ! **NURSING SAFETY PRIORITY** (QSEN)
>
> **Drug Alert**
>
> Patients who are undergoing radiation and/or chemotherapy treatment may experience a decreased ability to tolerate prescribed and over-the-counter medications due to being immunocompromised. Teach patients about expected side effects, and remind them to not take any medication (including over-the-counter medications, herbs, or vitamin supplements) without first discussing them with their health care provider.

One of the most recent advances in the use of drugs for oral cancer is targeted therapy. Hormone-like substances known as *growth factors (GFs)* occur in the body's cells. Oral tumor cells, along with other types of cancers, grow quickly because they have more GF receptors than does normal healthy tissue. One of these GFs is called *epidermal growth factor (EGF)*, which has been associated with oral cancers. Newer drugs that can target and block EGF receptors (EGF-R) are being tested, and more than a dozen have been approved, including cetuximab (Erbitux), erlotinib (Tarceva), and panitumumab (Vectibix). (Chapter 22 describes targeted molecular therapy.)

> ? **NCLEX EXAMINATION CHALLENGE**
>
> **Physiological Integrity**
>
> A male client is admitted with a diagnosis of oral cancer. Which statement by the nursing assistant indicates a need for further teaching by the nurse about this client's oral care?
> A. "I need to do oral care at least every 2 hours."
> B. "I'll use a soft-bristled toothbrush to prevent bleeding."
> C. "I'll remind him to use mouthwash after brushing."
> D. "I'll tell him to rinse his mouth frequently with sodium bicarbonate."

Surgical Management. The physician can often remove small, noninvasive lesions of the oral cavity in an ambulatory surgical center with local anesthesia. The surgical defect is usually small enough to be closed by sutures. These smaller lesions may also be responsive to carbon dioxide laser therapy or **cryotherapy** (extreme cold application), as well as photodynamic therapy. These procedures can be performed as an ambulatory care procedure in a surgical center but may require general anesthesia.

Small oral cancers are equally responsive to radiation or photodynamic therapy and to surgery. More invasive lesions (stages III and IV) require more extensive surgical excision and result in a greater loss of function and disfigurement. Not all lesions can be excised by the peroral approach (through the mouth). The goal of surgical resection is removal of the tumor with a surgical margin that is free of cancer cells.

Preoperative Care. Before excision of a lesion in the oral cavity, assess and document the patient's level of understanding of the disease process, the rationale for the surgery, and the planned intervention. Problems associated with cancer therapy can be reduced or optimally managed by collaborating with the patient and family regarding preparation and instruction. Reinforce information as needed. Include family members

or other caregivers in the health teaching unless culturally inappropriate.

For small, local excisions, postoperative restrictions include a liquid diet for a day and then advancing as tolerated. There are no activity limitations, and postoperative analgesics are prescribed.

Instructions for the patient undergoing large surgical resections may include but are not limited to these expectations after surgery:

- Placement of a temporary tracheostomy, oxygen therapy, and suctioning
- Temporary loss of speech because of the tracheostomy
- Frequent monitoring of postoperative vital signs
- NPO status until intraoral suture lines are healed
- Need to have IV lines in place for drug delivery and hydration
- Postoperative drug therapy and activity (out of bed on the day or surgery or first postoperative day)
- Possibility of surgical drains

Because communication is interrupted, assess the patient's ability to read, write, and draw pictures to communicate. In coordination with the patient, select the method of communication to use after surgery with staff and family members (e.g., Magic Slate, handheld mobile device, computer, picture board, or pad and pencil). Preprinted flashcards may be used to communicate the patient's needs, such as "I am tired," "I am in pain," or "I am hungry." Urge the patient to practice the chosen method before surgery to reduce frustration after surgery.

Operative Procedures. Three factors influence the extent of surgery performed for oral cancers: the size and location of the tumor, tumor invasion into the bone, and whether there has been metastasis (cancer spread) to neck lymph nodes. Small, noninvasive tumors can be removed perorally (through the mouth). Otherwise, an external approach may be used. The most extensive oral operations are composite resections, which combine partial or total **glossectomy** (tongue removal) and partial **mandibulectomy** (jaw removal). In the **commando** (co-mandible) **procedure** (**COM**bined neck dissection, **MAN**-**D**ibulectomy, and **O**ropharyngeal resection), the surgeon removes a segment of the mandible with the oral lesion and performs a radical neck dissection (see Chapter 29).

Metastasis to cervical lymph nodes usually indicates a poor prognosis for patients with cancer of the oral cavity. In those with cervical node metastasis, a neck dissection may also be performed. A radical neck dissection usually involves the removal of all cervical lymph nodes on the affected side, along with cranial nerve XI (the accessory nerve), the internal jugular vein, and the sternocleidomastoid (front neck) muscle. Modified and selective neck dissections may be performed in patients with minimal lymph node involvement.

Postoperative Care. The patient may have a temporary or permanent tracheostomy, requiring intensive nursing care to promote airway clearance. In addition, care must be taken to protect the surgical incision site from mechanical damage and INFECTION (see Chapter 29). Nursing interventions to relieve PAIN or discomfort and promote NUTRITION are also important. Older adults are a special risk for surgery and need to be monitored very carefully (Chart 53-4).

Ensure that the predetermined method of communication is available for the patient, family members, and staff. When the patient has an adequate airway and can effectively clear secretions by coughing, the tracheostomy tube may be removed.

CHART 53-4 **Focused Assessment**

The Postoperative Older Adult with Oral Cancer

- Assess the mouth and surrounding tissues for candidiasis, mucositis, and pain; assess for loss of appetite and taste.
- Monitor the patient's weight.
- Monitor nutrition and fluid intake.
- Assess for difficulty in eating or speech.
- Assess pain status and measures used to control pain.
- Monitor the patient's response to medications.
- Identify psychosocial problems, such as depression, anxiety, and fear.
- Assess the patient's overall physiologic condition and how this may affect pharmacologic therapy.

! NURSING SAFETY PRIORITY (QSEN)

Action Alert

After extensive excision or resection for oral cancer, the most important nursing intervention is maintaining the patient's airway to promote GAS EXCHANGE! Upon awakening from anesthesia, the patient may not recall, or realize, that a tracheostomy tube is in place and may initially panic because of the inability to speak. Remind the patient why he or she cannot speak, and provide reassurance that the vocal cords are intact (unless a total laryngectomy has been performed, in which case the loss of voice is permanent).

When the tube is removed, an airtight dressing is placed over the site and the tracheostomy incision heals without the need for sutures.

Patients who have undergone extensive resection may have slurred speech or difficulty in speaking as a result of nerve damage or tongue removal. Collaborate with the speech-language pathologist if speech is altered.

Protect the incision site to avoid infection. Provide gentle mouth care for cleaning away thick secretions and stimulating the flow of saliva. The delivery of oral care depends on the nature and extent of the surgical procedure. Give oral care at least every 4 hours in the early postoperative phase. The presence of unusual odors from the mouth can indicate INFECTION; therefore continual assessment of the oral cavity is very important. In the early postoperative phase, take care to avoid disruption of the suture line during oral hygiene.

Elevate the head of the bed to assist in decreasing edema by gravity. If skin grafting was done, inspect the donor site (generally on the anterior thigh) every 8 hours for bleeding or signs of INFECTION. (See Chapter 29 for specific nursing care of the patient with a radical neck dissection.)

To provide optimal *pain relief* in the postoperative period, rely on subjective and objective data to assess the need for analgesics and their effectiveness. The desired outcome of drug therapy during this period is relief of PAIN while allowing the patient to function at an optimal level. Those who have undergone surgery for oral cancer describe their PAIN as throbbing or pounding. IV morphine is usually the initial pain medication given with acetaminophen or ibuprofen to decrease inflammation. Tylox or Percocet (oxycodone plus acetaminophen) may be used for systemic relief of moderate pain after the IV morphine is discontinued.

Patients who have undergone extensive resections of the oral cavity remain on NPO status for several days. This time allows

---

! NURSING SAFETY PRIORITY (QSEN)

Action Alert

When oral fluid intake is started, assess for and document signs of difficulty swallowing, aspiration, or leakage of saliva or fluids from the suture line. Monitor daily weights and hydration. NUTRITION supplementation may be used to improve the patient's quality of life. Patients who have weight loss or who are having difficulty maintaining hydration may be candidates for the placement of a gastrostomy tube. Coordinate NUTRITION care with the dietitian.

---

healing in the oral cavity before food comes in contact with the incision. Nasogastric feeding or total parenteral NUTRITION may be needed until oral nutrition can begin (see Chapter 60).

Encourage the patient to perform swallowing exercises. Collaborate with the speech-language pathologist to assist with swallowing techniques. Thickened fluids may be needed to prevent aspiration. A swallowing impairment may be temporary or permanent.

Community-Based Care

Continuing care for the patient with an oral tumor depends on the severity of the tumor, its collaborative care, and available support systems. Most patients are maintained at home during follow-up care. Ongoing NUTRITION management remains a vital part of the treatment plan. In addition, the patient and family may benefit from a community-based support group for cancer patients.

Home Care Management. If radiation therapy is part of the patient's treatment plan, home care considerations include health teaching and management strategies. Complications due to radiation to the head or neck can be acute or delayed. Acute effects include treatment-related mucositis, stomatitis, and alterations in taste. Long-term effects such as **xerostomia** (excessive mouth dryness) and dental decay require ongoing oral care, the use of saliva substitutes, and follow-up dental visits. Although ongoing dental care is important, the possible adverse effects that radiation has on bone make elective oral surgical procedures, such as tooth extraction, impossible in the area of the radiation. Fatigue is a common side effect of radiation and chemotherapy.

The patient whose tracheostomy tube has been removed is often placed on a soft diet by mouth before discharge. Occasionally, however, patients are discharged from the hospital while still requiring tracheostomy suction, oral suction, and nasogastric feedings. Suction equipment, NUTRITION supplies, and nursing care can be provided by home care companies. (See Chapter 60 for home care preparation for the patient receiving home parenteral nutrition and Chapter 28 for home care preparation for the patient with a tracheostomy.)

Self-Management Education. Before hospital discharge, teach the patient and family about drug therapy, NUTRITION therapies, any treatments (e.g., tracheostomy care, suture line care, dressing changes), and early symptoms of INFECTION (Chart 53-5). Alterations in taste and dysphagia make maintaining adequate nutrition a challenge for the oral cancer patient. Alterations in taste occur when the taste buds are included in the radiation treatment field. Taste sensation may begin to return several weeks after the completion of treatment. Some types of chemotherapy can also affect the patient's taste. Sometimes the loss of taste is permanent.

CHART 53-5 Patient and Family Education: Preparing for Self-Management

Care of the Patient with Oral Cancer at Home

- Follow the treatment plan for cancer therapies.
- Remember that taste sensation may be decreased; add non-spicy seasonings to food to better enjoy it.
- Use a thickening agent for liquids if dysphagia is present.
- Eat soft foods if stomatitis occurs.
- Inspect the mouth every day for changes, such as redness or lesions.
- Continue meticulous oral hygiene at home using a chemobrush and frequent rinsing; clean brush after every use.
- Use saliva substitute as prescribed.
- Avoid sun or tanning bed exposure if radiation is part of therapy.
- Clean with a gentle, nondeodorant soap, such as Ivory.

Changes in taste include dislike of meat, such as beef or pork, and metallic tastes in the mouth. Teach patients to add seasonings to foods, to use gravies or sauces to make foods more palatable, and to use high-protein foods such as cheeses, milk, eggs, puddings, and legumes in place of meat. Instruct patients with dysphagia in swallowing exercises. Recommend thickened liquids because thin liquids, such as water, are difficult to control during swallowing. Collaborate with the dietitian to teach the family how to assess the NUTRITION intake of the patient who is just beginning to eat. Liquid dietary supplements are usually recommended at this time. If bleeding or stomatitis is present, recommend soft foods to prevent further injury to the mucous membranes.

Teach the patient or family members to inspect the oral cavity daily for areas of redness, which can indicate the onset of stomatitis. Meticulous oral hygiene should be continued at home, especially with adjuvant chemotherapy or radiation. Reinforce the oral hygiene routine, emphasizing the need for frequent mouth rinsing to reduce the number of microorganisms and to maintain adequate hydration. The patient should use a chemobrush (an extra-soft type of toothbrush), rinse the chemobrush with hydrogen peroxide and water or with a diluted bleach solution after each use, and change chemobrushes weekly. The brush may also be cleaned in a dishwasher.

Saliva production is greatly reduced as a consequence of radiation. The resulting xerostomia (dry mouth) causes the inability to eat dry foods and may be permanent. Teach the patient regarding the use of saliva substitutes.

Skin reactions are also a common side effect of radiation. Instruct the patient to avoid sun exposure, to avoid perfumed lotions and powders, and to cleanse the face and neck area with a gentle nondeodorant soap. Teach male patients to use an electric razor for shaving and to avoid alcohol-based aftershave lotions to prevent further skin irritation.

Health Care Resources. Patients who have undergone composite resection often require community services because they have both physical and psychosocial needs. Depression related to a change in body image is common. Excision of a portion of the jaw can leave a facial defect that may be difficult to hide. Assess for depression and other behavioral responses. A social worker or other health care professional may be needed for patient and family counseling. Those who have undergone a total glossectomy may be able to speak with special training and the use of an intraoral prosthesis created by a maxillofacial prosthodontist. The prosthesis is similar to dentures.

Collaborate with the case manager to provide assistance in obtaining special equipment or NUTRITION resources needed by the patient at home. The case manager assesses the patient's financial needs and makes referrals to government, community, and religious organizations as needed. Refer the patient to the American Cancer Society (ACS) (www.cancer.org), the Oral Cancer Foundation (www.oralcancerfoundation.org), and/or the Canadian Cancer Society (www.cancer.ca/en/region-selector-page/) for local support groups and resources, including additional information. The ACS often provides dressing supplies and transportation to and from follow-up visits or medical treatments.

❓ CLINICAL JUDGMENT CHALLENGE

Teamwork and Collaboration; Patient-Centered Care QSEN

A 50-year-old businessman has just undergone oral surgery to remove a large oral tumor. Documentation of assessment of the oral cavity shows that the patient has poor oral hygiene. You are preparing to teach the patient methods of self-care management.

1. As the patient's nurse, what is your priority for his care immediately after surgery?
2. As you develop his plan of care, for what complications is this patient most at risk?
3. What would you teach the patient that would be most helpful to improve his oral hygiene?
4. Considering that he is a businessman, what psychosocial or sociocultural concerns would you anticipate he may experience?
5. What follow-up care is most important for this patient?

DISORDERS OF THE SALIVARY GLANDS

ACUTE SIALADENITIS

❖ PATHOPHYSIOLOGY

Acute sialadenitis, the inflammation of a salivary gland, can be caused by infectious agents, irradiation, or immunologic disorders. Salivary gland inflammation can have a bacterial or viral cause, such as INFECTION with cytomegalovirus (CMV). The most common bacterial organisms are *Staphylococcus aureus*, *Staphylococcus pyogenes*, *Streptococcus pneumoniae*, and *Escherichia coli*. This disorder most commonly affects the parotid or submandibular gland in adults.

A decrease in the production of saliva (as in dehydrated or debilitated patients or in those who are on NPO status postoperatively for an extended time) can lead to acute sialadenitis. The bacteria or viruses enter the gland through the ductal

❓ NCLEX EXAMINATION CHALLENGE

Safe and Effective Care Environment

A client has completed chemotherapy and radiation therapy for an oral tumor and is being discharged to home. Which client statements require further teaching by the nurse? **Select all that apply.**

A. "Radiation therapy will not affect my sense of taste."
B. "I am likely to be fatigued after radiation."
C. "It is important for me to keep my oral cavity very clean."
D. "I will avoid tanning beds and sun exposure."
E. "I am eager to use my perfume soon after radiation therapy."
F. "My chemobrush should be replaced monthly."

opening in the mouth. Systemic drugs, such as phenothiazines and the tetracyclines, can also trigger an episode of acute sialadenitis. Untreated infections of the salivary glands can evolve into abscesses, which can rupture and spread INFECTION into the tissues of the neck and the mediastinum.

Patients who receive radiation for the treatment of cancers of the head and neck or thyroid may develop decreased salivary flow, predisposing them to acute or persistent sialadenitis. The effect of radiation on the salivary glands is rapid and dose related. Immunologic disorders such as HIV INFECTION can cause enlargement of the parotid gland that results from secondary infection. Sjögren's syndrome, an autoimmune disorder, is characterized by chronic salivary gland enlargement and inflammation that cause a very dry mouth (see Chapter 20).

❖ PATIENT-CENTERED COLLABORATIVE CARE

During the initial interview, assess for any predisposing factors for sialadenitis, such as ionizing radiation to the head or neck area. Collect a thorough drug history, and ask about systemic illnesses, such as HIV infection.

Dehydration can be assessed by examining the oral membrane for dryness and the skin for turgor. Other assessment findings include PAIN and swelling of the face over the affected gland. Assess facial function because the branches of cranial nerve VII (the facial nerve) lie close to the salivary glands. Fever and general malaise also occur, and purulent drainage can often be massaged from the affected duct in the oral cavity.

Collaborative care includes the administration of IV fluids and measures such as these to treat the underlying cause and increase the flow of saliva:

- Hydration
- Application of warm compresses
- Massage of the gland
- Use of a saliva substitute
- Use of **sialagogues** (substances that stimulate the flow of saliva)

Sialagogues include lemon slices and citrus-flavored and other fruit-flavored candy. Massage is accomplished by milking the edematous gland with the fingertips toward the ductal opening. Elevation of the head of the bed promotes gravity drainage of the edematous gland.

Acute sialadenitis is best prevented by adherence to routine oral hygiene. This practice prevents INFECTION from ascending to the salivary glands from the mouth.

POST-IRRADIATION SIALADENITIS

The salivary glands are sensitive to ionizing radiation, such as from radiation therapy or radioactive iodine treatment of thyroid cancers. Exposure of the glands to radiation produces a type of sialadenitis known as **xerostomia** (very dry mouth caused by a severe reduction in the flow of saliva) within 24

hours. Radiation to the salivary glands can also produce PAIN and edema, which generally abate after several days.

Xerostomia may be temporary or permanent, depending on the dose of radiation and the percentage of total salivary gland tissue irradiated. Little can be done to relieve the patient's dry mouth during the course of radiation therapy. Frequent sips of water and frequent mouth care, especially before meals, are the most effective interventions. After the course of radiation therapy has been completed, saliva substitutes may provide moisture for 2 to 4 hours at a time. Over-the-counter solutions are available, or methylcellulose (Cologel), glycerin, and saline may be mixed to form a solution.

SALIVARY GLAND TUMORS

Of all oral tumors, those of the salivary glands are relatively rare. Initially, malignant tumors present as slow-growing, painless masses. Involvement of the facial nerve results in facial weakness or paralysis (partial or total) on the affected side.

Collect information about any prior radiation exposure, because radiation to the head and neck areas is associated with the occurrence of salivary gland tumors. Salivary gland tumors present as localized, firm masses. Submandibular and minor salivary gland tumors may be tender or painful. Tumor invasion of the hypoglossal nerve causes impaired movement of the tongue, and a loss of sensation can follow. *Pay particular attention to assessment of the facial nerve because of its proximity to the salivary glands.* Assess the patient's ability to:

- Wrinkle the brow
- Raise the eyebrows
- Squeeze and hold the eyes shut while you gently pull upwards on the eyebrows and cheeks beneath the orbit to check for symmetry
- Wrinkle the nose
- Pucker the lips
- Puff out the cheeks
- Grimace or smile

Be aware of any asymmetry when the patient performs these motions. The treatment of choice for both benign and malignant tumors of the salivary glands is surgical excision. However, radiation therapy is often used for salivary gland cancers that are large, have recurred, show evidence of residual disease after excision, or are highly malignant.

Patients who have undergone **parotidectomy** (surgical removal of the parotid glands) or submandibular gland surgery are at risk for weakness or loss of function of the facial nerve because the nerve courses directly through the gland. Facial nerve repair with grafting can be done at the time of surgery. A combination of surgery followed by radiation is common for advanced disease. Care for patients after parotidectomy is similar to that required for those having oral cancer surgery, described on pp. 1105-1106.

NURSING CONCEPTS AND CLINICAL JUDGMENT REVIEW

What might you NOTICE if the patient has inadequate digestion and GAS EXCHANGE as a result of oral cavity problems?
- Dysphagia (difficulty swallowing)
- Dyspnea
- Stridor or wheezes
- Changes in speech or voice
- Copious, thickened oral secretions
- Excessive coughing during meals

What should you INTERPRET and how should you RESPOND to a patient experiencing inadequate digestion and GAS EXCHANGE as a result of oral cavity problems?

Perform and interpret focused physical assessment findings, including:
- Breath sounds
- Oxygen saturation by pulse oximetry

- Ability to cough and clear the airway
- Ability to manage excessive oral secretions
- Ability to chew food and swallow

Respond by:
- Placing the patient with the head elevated to at least 30 degrees
- Applying oxygen as needed
- Suctioning the oral cavity as needed
- Encouraging deep breathing and coughing every 2 hours
- Increasing fluids to liquefy secretions, depending on swallowing ability
- Notifying the respiratory therapist or Rapid Response Team if interventions are not successful in restoring gas exchange (oxygenation).

On what should you REFLECT?
- Observe patient for evidence of increased gas exchange (oxygenation), including increased ease of breathing.
- Observe patient for evidence of increased ability to swallow.
- Observe patient for evidence of increased ability to manage oral secretions.
- Consider follow-up interventions to manage patient, including coordinating care with dietitian and speech-language pathologist.
- Think about what else you might do to promote digestion and nutrition.

GET READY FOR THE NCLEX® EXAMINATION!

KEY POINTS

Review these key points for each NCLEX Examination Client Needs Category.

Safe and Effective Care Environment
- Be aware that airway management is the priority for care for patients having surgery for oral cancer. **Safety** QSEN
- Place patients having oral cancer surgery in a high-Fowler's position to facilitate breathing and prevent aspiration. **Safety** QSEN
- Be sure to assess for swallowing ability to prevent aspiration by checking the gag reflex before offering liquids or food to the patient who has had oral cancer surgery. **Safety** QSEN
- Plan continuity of care to meet patients' needs when they are transferred from the hospital to community-based agencies. **Teamwork and Collaboration** QSEN

Health Promotion and Maintenance
- Teach patients to seek medical or dental attention for oral lesions that do not heal; these lesions could be oral carcinomas.
- Remind patients to visit their dentist regularly for dental hygiene and oral examination.
- Follow the best practice recommendations for maintaining oral health as listed in Chart 53-1.
- Instruct patients to avoid harsh commercial mouthwashes if they have oral lesions.
- In keeping with The Joint Commission (TJC) Core Measures TOB-2, teach patients to avoid tobacco, alcohol, and sun exposure to decrease their chance of having oral cancer.
- Instruct patients with acute sialadenitis to use sialagogues to stimulate saliva, such as citrus foods or candies.

Psychosocial Integrity
- Identify the patient's and family's response to an oral cancer diagnosis.

- Assist the patient and family in identifying and using coping mechanisms to deal with possible changes in body image and altered self-esteem. **Patient-Centered Care** QSEN
- Recognize that patients with stomatitis are often unable to eat or swallow without discomfort.
- Refer patients with oral cancer to support groups, such as those available through the American Cancer Society.

Physiological Integrity
- Remember that stomatitis usually manifests as painful single or multiple ulcerations within the mouth.
- Recognize that stomatitis can be caused by a variety of organisms; *Candida* INFECTIONS are very common in patients who receive antibiotic therapy and in those who are immunocompromised.
- Provide gentle oral care for patients with oral lesions, including using chemobrushes and warm saline or sodium bicarbonate solution. **Safety** QSEN
- Be aware that patients with stomatitis receive antimicrobials, anti-inflammatory agents, immune modulators, and topical agents for relief of symptoms, including PAIN. **Evidence-Based Practice** QSEN
- Differentiate leukoplakia and erythroplakia: leukoplakia presents as thin, white patches; and erythroplakia presents as red, velvety lesions.
- Be aware that patients with oral cancer may have chemotherapy, radiation, surgery, or a combination of these treatment methods.
- Be aware that sialadenitis can occur as a result of radiation therapy.
- For patients with salivary gland tumors, assess for facial nerve involvement.
- Remember that a parotidectomy involves the removal of the salivary glands; postoperative care is similar to that for patients who have oral cancer surgery.

Care of Patients with Esophageal Problems

Cherie R. Rebar, Nicole Heimgartner, Laura Willis

 http://evolve.elsevier.com/Iggy/

PRIORITY CONCEPTS

- INFECTION
- NUTRITION
- PAIN

LEARNING OUTCOMES

Safe and Effective Care Environment

1. Collaborate with health care team members when providing care to patients with esophageal health problems that impair swallowing or limit NUTRITION.

Health Promotion and Maintenance

2. Teach patients about lifestyle changes that decrease gastroesophageal reflux disease (GERD) and the PAIN associated with hiatal hernias.
3. Describe special considerations for the older adult with GERD.
4. Teach patients with esophageal health problems about community-based resources.

Psychosocial Integrity

5. Reduce the psychological impact for the patient and family who have received a diagnosis and treatment of esophageal cancer.

Physiological Integrity

6. Perform focused assessments for patients with esophageal health problems.
7. Evaluate the impact of esophageal cancer on the patient's NUTRITION status, including the risk for aspiration.
8. Apply knowledge of pathophysiology to anticipate complications of GERD and esophageal surgical procedures.
9. Teach patients how to reduce the physiological impact of esophageal health problems.
10. Develop an evidence-based teaching plan for the patient and family about postoperative care after esophageal surgery.
11. Plan community-based care for patients diagnosed with esophageal cancer.

Partially digested food is moved by the esophagus from the mouth to the stomach. If food cannot reach the stomach, the patient cannot meet the basic human need for NUTRITION. Nutrients in food are necessary for normal body cell function. Common problems of the esophagus that can interfere with digestion and NUTRITION are caused by inflammation, structural defects or obstruction, and cancer. Patient-centered collaborative care requires dietary and lifestyle changes, as well as medical and surgical therapies.

GASTROESOPHAGEAL REFLUX DISEASE

❖ PATHOPHYSIOLOGY

Gastroesophageal reflux disease (GERD) is the most common upper GI disorder in the United States. It occurs most often in middle-aged and older adults but can affect people of any age. **Gastroesophageal reflux (GER)** occurs as a result of backward flow of stomach contents into the esophagus. GERD

is the chronic and more serious condition that arises from persistent GER.

Reflux produces symptoms by exposing the esophageal mucosa to the irritating effects of gastric or duodenal contents, resulting in inflammation. A person with acute symptoms of inflammation is often described as having mild or severe **reflux esophagitis** (McCance et al., 2014).

The reflux of gastric contents into the esophagus is normally prevented by the presence of two high-pressure areas that remain contracted at rest. A 1.2-inch (3-cm) segment at the proximal end of the esophagus is called the *upper esophageal sphincter (UES)*, whereas another small portion at the gastroesophageal junction (near the cardiac sphincter) is called the **lower esophageal sphincter (LES)**. The function of the LES is supported by its anatomic placement in the abdomen, where the surrounding pressure is significantly higher than in the low-pressure thorax. Sphincter function is also supported by the acute angle (angle of His) that is formed as the esophagus enters the stomach.

The most common cause of GERD is excessive relaxation of the LES, which allows the reflux of gastric contents into the esophagus and exposure of the esophageal mucosa to acidic gastric contents. Patients who are overweight or obese are at highest risk for development of GERD because increased weight increases intra-abdominal pressure, which contributes to reflux of stomach contents into the esophagus. Nighttime reflux tends to cause prolonged exposure of the esophagus to acid because lying supine decreases peristalsis and the benefit of gravity. Hiatal hernias also increase the risk for development of GERD due to the creation of increased intra-abdominal pressure. *Helicobacter pylori* may contribute to reflux (McCance et al., 2014) by causing gastritis and thus poor gastric emptying. This increases frequency of GER events and acid exposure to the esophagus.

A person having reflux may be asymptomatic. However, the esophagus has limited resistance to the damaging effects of the acidic GI contents. The pH of acid secreted by the stomach ranges from 1.5 to 2.0, whereas the pH of the distal esophagus is normally neutral (6.0 to 7.0).

Refluxed material is returned to the stomach by a combination of gravity, saliva, and peristalsis. The inflamed esophagus cannot eliminate the refluxed material as quickly as a healthy one, and therefore the length of exposure increases with each reflux episode. Hyperemia (increased blood flow) and erosion (ulceration) occur in the esophagus in response to the chronic inflammation. Gastric acid and pepsin injure tissue. Minor capillary bleeding often occurs with erosion, but hemorrhage is rare.

During the process of healing, the body may substitute Barrett's epithelium (columnar epithelium) for the normal squamous cell epithelium of the lower esophagus. Although this new tissue is more resistant to acid and therefore supports esophageal healing, it is considered premalignant and is associated with an increased risk for cancer in patients with prolonged GERD. The fibrosis and scarring that accompany the healing process can produce esophageal stricture (narrowing of the esophageal opening). The stricture leads to progressive difficulty swallowing. Uncontrolled esophageal reflux also increases risk for other complications such as asthma, laryngitis, dental decay, cardiac disease, and serious concerns for hemorrhage and aspiration pneumonia.

Gastric distention caused by eating very large meals or delayed gastric emptying predisposes the patient to reflux. Certain foods and drugs, as well as smoking and alcohol, influence the tone function of the LES (Table 54-1).

Patients who have a nasogastric tube also have decreased esophageal sphincter function. The tube keeps the cardiac sphincter open and allows acidic contents from the stomach to enter the esophagus. Other factors that increase intra-abdominal and intragastric pressure (e.g., pregnancy, wearing tight belts or girdles, bending over, ascites) overcome the gastroesophageal pressure gradient maintained by the LES and allow reflux to occur. Many patients with obstructive sleep apnea report frequent episodes of GERD. People with hiatal hernias often have reflux because the upper portion of the stomach protrudes through the diaphragm into the thorax, which allows acid to reach the esophagus (see later discussion of hiatal hernia).

❖ PATIENT-CENTERED COLLABORATIVE CARE

◆ Assessment

Ask the patient about a history of heartburn or atypical chest PAIN associated with the reflux of GI contents. Ask whether he or she has been newly diagnosed with asthma or has experienced morning hoarseness or pneumonia, because these symptoms may indicate severe reflux reaching the pharynx or mouth or pulmonary aspiration.

Physical Assessment/Clinical Manifestations. Dyspepsia, also known as "indigestion," and regurgitation are the main symptoms of GERD, although symptoms may vary in severity (Chart 54-1). Symptoms associated with "indigestion" may include abdominal discomfort, feeling uncomfortably full, nausea, and burping. Because indigestion might not be viewed as a serious concern, patients may delay seeking treatment. The symptoms typically worsen when the patient bends over, strains, or lies down. If the indigestion is severe, the PAIN may radiate to the neck or jaw or may be referred to the back, mimicking cardiac pain. Patients may come to the emergency department (ED) fearing that they are having a myocardial infarction ("heart attack").

With severe GERD, PAIN generally occurs after each meal and lasts for 20 minutes to 2 hours. Discomfort may worsen when the patient lies down. Drinking fluids, taking antacids, or maintaining an upright posture usually provides prompt relief.

Regurgitation (backward flow into the throat) of food particles or fluids is common. Risk for aspiration is increased if regurgitation occurs when the patient is lying down. Even if the patient is in an upright position, he or she may experience warm fluid traveling up the throat without nausea. If the fluid reaches the level of the pharynx, he or she notes a sour or bitter taste in the mouth. A reflex salivary hypersecretion known as water brash occurs in response to reflux. Water brash is different from regurgitation. The patient reports a sensation of fluid in the throat, but unlike with regurgitation, there is no bitter or sour taste.

TABLE 54-1	Factors Contributing to Decreased Lower Esophageal Sphincter Pressure
• Caffeinated beverages, such as coffee, tea, and cola • Chocolate • Citrus fruits • Tomatoes and tomato products • Smoking and use of other tobacco products • Calcium channel blockers	• Nitrates • Peppermint, spearmint • Alcohol • Anticholinergic drugs • High levels of estrogen and progesterone • Nasogastric tube placement

CHART 54-1 Key Features

Gastroesophageal Reflux Disease

- Dyspepsia (indigestion)
- Regurgitation (may lead to aspiration or bronchitis)
- Coughing, hoarseness, or wheezing at night
- Water brash (hypersalivation)
- Dysphagia
- Odynophagia (painful swallowing)
- Epigastric pain
- Generalized abdominal pain
- Belching
- Flatulence
- Nausea
- Pyrosis (heartburn)
- Globus (feeling of something in back of throat)
- Pharyngitis
- Dental caries (severe cases)

Ask the patient if he or she experiences eructation (belching), flatulence (gas), and bloating after eating; these are other common manifestations. Nausea and vomiting rarely occur; unplanned weight loss is not common.

Assess for crackles in the lung, which can be an indication of associated aspiration. Patients who have had long-term regurgitation may experience coughing, hoarseness, or wheezing at night, which may be associated with bronchitis.

Chronic GERD can cause dysphagia (difficulty swallowing). Dysphagia usually indicates a narrowing of the esophagus because of stricture or inflammation. Assess the patient for degree of dysphagia, whether ingesting solids and/or liquids induces dysphagia, and whether dysphagia occurs intermittently or with each swallowing effort.

Odynophagia (painful swallowing) can also occur with chronic GERD, but it is rare in people with uncomplicated reflux disease. Severe and long-lasting chest PAIN may be present if esophageal spasms cause the muscle to contract with excess force. The resulting PAIN can be agonizing and may last for hours.

Other manifestations include atypical chest PAIN, symptoms of asthma, and chronic cough that occurs mostly at night or when the patient is lying down. Cough and symptoms of asthma occur when refluxed acid is spilled over into the tracheobronchial tree. *Atypical chest pain* is thought to be caused by stimulation of PAIN receptors in the esophageal wall and by esophageal spasm. This type of chest PAIN can mimic angina and needs to be carefully distinguished from cardiac PAIN.

CONSIDERATIONS FOR OLDER ADULTS

Patient-Centered Care QSEN

Older adults are at risk for developing severe complications associated with GERD due to age-related physiologic changes, medication side effects, and an increased prevalence of hiatal hernias (Solomon & Reynolds, 2012). Instead of heartburn associated with GERD, this population experiences more severe complications of the disease such as atypical chest pain; ear, nose, and throat infections; and pulmonary problems, such as aspiration pneumonia, sleep apnea, and asthma. Barrett's esophagus and esophageal erosions are also more common in older adults (Chait, 2010).

Diagnostic Assessment. A definitive diagnostic test for GERD does not exist; however, health care providers may use one or more options to attempt to establish a diagnosis when GERD is suspected (The Ohio State University Wexner Medical Center [OSUWMC], 2014).

Patients may drink a solution and then have x-rays performed as part of a *barium swallow,* which shows hiatal hernias, strictures, and other structural or anatomic esophageal problems. Although this test, when conducted by itself, does not confirm GERD, it can be helpful when used in combination with other diagnostic procedures.

Upper endoscopy (also called esophagogastroduodenoscopy [EGD]) involves insertion of an endoscope (a flexible plastic tube equipped with a light and lens) down the throat, which allows the health care provider to see the esophagus and look for abnormalities. A biopsy can be taken while the patient undergoes endoscopy (see Chapter 52) (OSUWMC, 2013). This test requires the use of moderate sedation during the procedure, and patients must have someone accompany them home after recovery.

A pH monitoring examination is the most accurate method of diagnosing GERD. This involves either (1) placing a small catheter through the nose into the distal esophagus or (2) temporarily attaching a small capsule to the wall of the esophagus during an upper endoscopy (the 48-hour Bravo esophageal ph test). The patient is asked to keep a diary of activities and symptoms over 24 to 48 hours (depending on diagnostic method), and the pH is continuously monitored and recorded. Ambulatory pH monitoring is especially useful in diagnosing patients with atypical symptoms. A wireless monitoring device may be used to promote patient comfort (OSUWMC, 2014).

Although not as common, *esophageal manometry,* or motility testing, may be performed when the diagnosis is uncertain. Water-filled catheters are inserted in the patient's nose or mouth and slowly withdrawn while measurements of LES pressure and peristalsis are recorded. When used alone, manometry is not sensitive or specific enough to establish a diagnosis of GERD (National Institutes of Health, 2013). A Gastric Emptying Study can also be done while a patient is in the radiology/nuclear medicine department. He or she is given a meal mixed with radiolucent dye, and imaging is performed to determine how well the stomach empties over the next few hours. If food stays too long in the stomach, it can reflux back into the esophagus, causing symptoms (OSUWMC, 2014). Imaging of the lungs can also be conducted 24 hours later to visualize whether the patient has aspirated stomach contents.

◆ Interventions

Nonsurgical Management. The purpose of treatment for GERD is to relieve symptoms, treat esophagitis, and prevent complications such as strictures or Barrett's esophagus. For most patients, GERD can be controlled by NUTRITION therapy, lifestyle changes, and drug therapy. *The most important role of the nurse is patient and family education. Teach the patient that GERD is a chronic disorder that requires ongoing management. The disease should be treated more aggressively in older adults (Chait, 2010).*

Nonpharmacologic Interventions. NUTRITION therapy is used to relieve symptoms in patients with relatively mild GERD. Ask about the patient's basic meal patterns and food preferences. Coordinate with the dietitian, patient, and family about how to adapt to changes in eating that may decrease reflux symptoms.

Teach the patient to limit or eliminate foods that decrease LES pressure and that irritate inflamed tissue, causing heartburn, such as peppermint, chocolate, alcohol, fatty foods (especially fried), caffeine, and carbonated beverages. The patient should also restrict spicy and acidic foods (e.g., orange juice, tomatoes) until esophageal healing can occur. Patients who are smartphone users may find different types of applications ("apps") that can help them follow a healthier diet, such as MyFitnessPal (www.myfitnesspal.com). In keeping with The Joint Commission Core Measures, teach patients that smoking and alcohol use should also be avoided, because these can also decrease LES pressure. Explore the possibility and methods for smoking cessation, and make appropriate referrals. Ask the patient about his or her use of alcoholic beverages, and if appropriate, assist the patient in finding alcohol-cessation programs.

Large meals increase the volume of and pressure in the stomach and delay gastric emptying. Remind the patient to eat four to six small meals each day rather than three large ones. Encourage patients to avoid eating at least 3 hours before going to bed because reflux episodes are most damaging at night. Advise the patient to eat slowly and chew thoroughly to facilitate digestion and prevent eructation (belching).

The control of GERD involves *lifestyle changes* to promote health and control reflux (Chart 54-2). Teach the patient to elevate the head by 6 to 12 inches for sleep to prevent nighttime reflux. This can be done by placing blocks under the head of the bed or by using a large, wedge-style pillow instead of a standard pillow. Teach the patient to sleep in the right side-lying position to promote oxygenation and frequent swallowing to clear the esophagus. Assist the patient in examining approaches to weight reduction. Decreasing intra-abdominal pressure often reduces reflux symptoms. Teach the patient to avoid wearing constrictive clothing, lifting heavy objects or straining, and working in a bent-over or stooped position. Emphasize that these general adaptations are an essential and effective part of disease management and can produce prompt results in uncomplicated cases.

Obese patients often have obstructive sleep apnea, as well as GERD. Those who receive continuous positive airway pressure (CPAP) treatment report improved sleeping and decreased episodes of reflux at night. See Chapter 29 for a discussion of CPAP.

Some drugs lower LES pressure and *cause* reflux, such as oral contraceptives, anticholinergic agents, sedatives, NSAIDs (e.g., ibuprofen), nitrates, and calcium channel blockers. The possibility of eliminating those drugs causing reflux should be explored with the health care provider.

Drug Therapy. Drug therapy for GERD management includes three major types—antacids, histamine blockers, and proton pump inhibitors. These drugs, which are also used for peptic ulcer disease, have one or more of these functions (see Chapter 55, Chart 55-3):

- Inhibit gastric acid secretion
- Accelerate gastric emptying
- Protect the gastric mucosa

In uncomplicated cases of GERD, *antacids* may be effective for *occasional* episodes of heartburn. Antacids act by elevating the pH level of the gastric contents, thereby deactivating pepsin. They are not helpful in controlling frequent symptoms because their length of action is too short and their nighttime

effectiveness is minimal. These drugs also *increase* LES pressure and therefore are not given for long-term use.

Antacids containing aluminum hydroxide or magnesium hydroxide may be used. Maalox and Mylanta consist of a combination of these two agents. Patients often tolerate them better because they produce fewer side effects, such as constipation and diarrhea. Liquid forms of these medications are preferred, since they coat the esophagus to provide pain relief and to buffer acid. Teach the patient to take the antacid 1 hour before and 2 to 3 hours after each meal.

Gaviscon, a combination of alginic acid and sodium bicarbonate, is often a very effective drug for GERD. It forms thick foam that floats on top of the gastric contents and theoretically decreases the incidence of reflux. If reflux occurs, the foam enters the esophagus first and buffers the acid in the refluxed material. Remind the patient to take this drug when food is in the stomach.

Histamine receptor antagonists, commonly called *histamine blockers,* such as famotidine (Pepcid) and ranitidine (Zantac), decrease acid, are long acting, have fewer side effects, and allow less-frequent dosing. Although these drugs do not affect the occurrence of reflux directly, they do reduce gastric acid secretion, improve symptoms, and promote healing of inflamed esophageal tissue. With these drugs available over the counter (OTC) and widely advertised for heartburn, many patients self-medicate before seeking professional assistance from their primary care provider. Encourage patients to speak with their primary care provider to determine whether long-term use of these medications is appropriate.

Proton pump inhibitors (PPIs), such as omeprazole (Prilosec), rabeprazole (AcipHex), pantoprazole (Protonix), and esomeprazole (Nexium), are the *main* treatment for more severe GERD. Some PPIs are available as OTC drugs. These agents provide effective, long-acting inhibition of gastric acid secretion by affecting the proton pump of the gastric parietal cells. PPIs reduce gastric acid secretion and can be given in a single daily dose. If once-a-day dosing fails to control symptoms, twice-daily dosing may be used (National Guideline Clearinghouse [NGC], 2013). A newer PPI, omeprazole/sodium bicarbonate (Zegerid), is the first immediate-release PPI and is designed for short-term use. Another newer PPI, dexlansoprazole (Kapidex), is a dual-release (delayed-release) drug that is available in several dosages but tends to be associated with more side and adverse effects than some of the other PPIs.

Some PPIs, such as Nexium and Protonix, may be administered in IV form for short-term use to treat or to prevent stress ulcers that can result from surgery. PPIs promote rapid tissue healing, but recurrence is common when the drug is stopped. Long-term use may mask reflux symptoms, and stopping the drug determines if reflux has been resolved. Long-term use may also cause community-acquired pneumonia and GI infections such as those caused by *Clostridium difficile.*

CONSIDERATIONS FOR OLDER ADULTS
Patient-Centered Care [QSEN]

Research has also found that long-term use of proton pump inhibitors may increase the risk for hip fracture, especially in older adults. PPIs can interfere with calcium absorption and protein digestion and therefore reduce available calcium to bone tissue. Decreased calcium makes bones more brittle and likely to fracture, especially as people age (Chait, 2010).

Endoscopic Therapies. The Stretta procedure, a nonsurgical method, can replace surgery for GERD when other measures are not effective. Patients who are very obese or have severe symptoms may not be candidates for this procedure. In the Stretta procedure, the physician applies radiofrequency (RF) energy through the endoscope using needles placed near the gastroesophageal junction. The RG energy decreases vagus nerve activity, thus reducing discomfort for the patient. Postoperative instructions for patients who have undergone the Stretta procedure can be found in Chart 54-3.

Surgical Management. A very small percentage of patients with GERD require anti-reflux surgery. It is usually indicated for otherwise healthy patients who have failed to respond to medical treatment or have developed complications related to GERD. Various surgical procedures may be used through conventional open techniques or laparoscope.

Laparoscopic Nissen fundoplication (LNF) is a minimally invasive surgery (MIS) and is the standard surgical approach for treatment of severe GERD (Buckley & Roberts, 2014). Information about this procedure can be found in the next section (Hiatal Hernia) in the Surgical Management discussion. Patients who have surgery are encouraged to continue following the basic anti-reflux regimen of antacids and NUTRITION therapy because the rate of recurrence is high (University of Michigan Health System, 2012).

HIATAL HERNIA

Hiatal hernias, also called *diaphragmatic hernias,* involve the protrusion of the stomach through the esophageal hiatus of the diaphragm into the chest. The esophageal hiatus is the opening in the diaphragm through which the esophagus passes from the thorax to the abdomen. Most patients with hiatal hernias are asymptomatic, but some may have daily symptoms similar to those with GERD (McCance et al., 2014).

❖ *PATHOPHYSIOLOGY*

The two major types of hiatal hernias are sliding hernias (which are most common) and paraesophageal (rolling) hernias. The esophagogastric junction and a portion of the fundus of the stomach slide upward through the esophageal hiatus into the chest, usually as a result of weakening of the diaphragm (Fig. 54-1). The hernia generally moves freely and slides into

---

CHART 54-3 Patient and Family Education: Preparing for Self-Management

Postoperative Instructions for Patients Having Stretta Procedure

- Remain on clear liquids for 24 hours after the procedure.
- After the first day, consume a soft diet, such as custard, pureed vegetables, mashed potatoes, and applesauce.
- Avoid nonsteroidal anti-inflammatory drugs (NSAIDs) and aspirin for 10 days.
- Continue drug therapy as prescribed, usually proton pump inhibitors.
- Use liquid medications whenever possible.
- Do not allow nasogastric tubes for at least 1 month because the esophagus could be perforated.
- Contact the health care provider immediately if these problems occur:
  - Chest or abdominal pain
  - Bleeding
  - Dysphagia
  - Shortness of breath
  - Nausea or vomiting

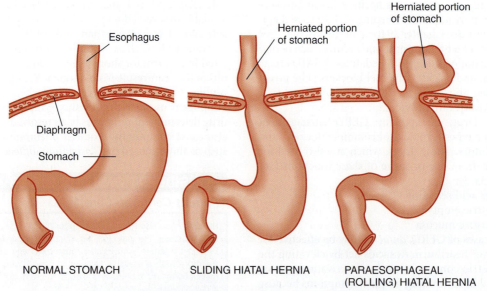

Esophagus

Diaphragm

Stomach

Herniated portion of stomach

Herniated portion of stomach

NORMAL STOMACH   SLIDING HIATAL HERNIA   PARAESOPHAGEAL (ROLLING) HIATAL HERNIA

FIG. 54-1 A comparison of the normal stomach and sliding and paraesophageal (rolling) hiatal hernias.

and out of the chest during changes in position or intra-abdominal pressure. Although volvulus (twisting of a GI structure) and obstruction do occur rarely, the major concern for a sliding hernia is the development of esophageal reflux and associated complications (see Gastroesophageal Reflux Disease section earlier in this chapter). The development of reflux is related to chronic exposure of the lower esophageal sphincter (LES) to the low pressure of the thorax, which significantly reduces the effectiveness of the LES. Symptoms associated with decreased LES pressure are worsened by positions that favor reflux, such as bending or lying supine. Coughing, obesity, and ascites also increase reflux symptoms.

With *rolling hernias,* also known as *paraesophageal hernias,* the gastroesophageal junction remains in its normal intra-abdominal location but the fundus (and possibly portions of the stomach's greater curvature) rolls through the esophageal hiatus and into the chest beside the esophagus (see Fig. 54-1). The herniated portion of the stomach may be small or quite large. In rare cases, the stomach completely inverts into the chest. Reflux is not usually present because the LES remains anchored below the diaphragm. However, the risks for volvulus (twisting of a GI structure), obstruction (blockage), and strangulation (stricture) are high. The development of iron deficiency anemia is common because slow bleeding from venous obstruction causes the gastric mucosa to become engorged and ooze. Significant bleeding or hemorrhage is rare.

Rolling hernias are thought to develop from an anatomic defect occurring when the stomach is not properly anchored below the diaphragm rather than from muscle weakness. They can also be caused by previous esophageal surgeries, including sliding hernia repair.

❖ PATIENT-CENTERED COLLABORATIVE CARE

◆ Assessment

Ask the patient if he or she has heartburn, regurgitation (backward flow of food into the throat), PAIN, dysphagia (difficulty swallowing), and eructation (belching). Assess general physical appearance and NUTRITION status. Note the location, onset, duration, and quality of PAIN, as well as factors that relieve it or make it worse. The primary symptoms of sliding hiatal hernias are associated with reflux. Auscultate the lungs because pulmonary symptoms similar to asthma may be triggered by episodes of aspiration, particularly at night. A detailed history is crucial in attempting to differentiate angina from noncardiac chest PAIN caused by reflux. Symptoms resulting from hiatal hernia typically worsen after a meal or when the patient is in a supine position (Chart 54-4).

In those with rolling hernias, assess for symptoms related to stretching or displacement of thoracic contents by the hernia. Patients may report a feeling of fullness after eating or have breathlessness or a feeling of suffocation if the hernia interferes with breathing. Some may experience chest PAIN associated with reflux that mimics angina.

The *barium swallow study with fluoroscopy* is the most specific diagnostic test for identifying hiatal hernia. Rolling hernias are usually clearly visible, and sliding hernias can often be observed when the patient moves through a series of positions that increase intra-abdominal pressure. To visualize sliding hernias, an esophagogastroduodenoscopy (EGD) may be performed to view both the esophagus and gastric lining (see Chapter 52).

CHART 54-4 Key Features

Hiatal Hernias

Sliding Hiatal Hernias	Paraesophageal Hernias
• Heartburn	• Feeling of fullness after eating
• Regurgitation	• Breathlessness after eating
• Chest pain	• Feeling of suffocation
• Dysphagia	• Chest pain that mimics angina
• Belching	• Worsening of manifestations in a recumbent position

---

◆ Interventions

Patients with hiatal hernias may be managed either medically or surgically. Collaborative care is based on the severity of symptoms and the risk for serious complications. Sliding hiatal hernias are most commonly treated medically. Large rolling hernias can become strangulated or obstructed; therefore early surgical repair is preferred.

Nonsurgical Management. The collaborative interventions for patients with hiatal hernia are similar to those for GERD and include drug therapy, NUTRITION therapy, and lifestyle changes. The health care provider typically recommends antacids and a proton-pump inhibitor such as lansoprazole (Prevacid), omeprazole (Prilosec), or esomeprazole (Nexium) in an attempt to control reflux and its symptoms (Harvard Health Publications, 2011). NUTRITION therapy is also important and follows the guidelines discussed earlier for GERD.

⚠ NURSING SAFETY PRIORITY (QSEN)

Action Alert

The most important role of the nurse in caring for a patient with a hiatal hernia is health teaching. Encourage the patient to avoid eating in the late evening and to avoid foods associated with reflux. Teach the patient and family that the patient should follow a restricted diet and should exercise regularly. Reducing body weight is beneficial because obesity increases intra-abdominal pressure and worsens both the hernia and the symptoms of reflux. Teach about positioning, including:
• Sleep at night with the head of the bed elevated 6 inches
• Remain upright for several hours after eating
• Avoid straining or excessive vigorous exercise
• Refrain from wearing clothing that is tight or constrictive around the abdomen

---

Surgical Management. Surgery may be required when the risk for complications is high or when damage from chronic reflux becomes severe.

Preoperative Care. If the surgery is not urgent, the surgeon instructs patients who are overweight to lose weight before surgery. They are also advised to quit or significantly reduce smoking. As part of preoperative teaching, reinforce the surgeon's instructions and prepare the patient for what to expect after surgery.

Operative Procedures. Several types of hiatal hernia repair procedures are used, each of which involves reinforcement of the lower esophageal sphincter (LES) by fundoplication. The surgeon wraps a portion of the stomach fundus around the distal esophagus to anchor it and reinforce the LES (Fig. 54-2).

Laparoscopic Nissen fundoplication (LNF) is a minimally invasive surgery commonly used for hiatal hernia repair (Buckley & Roberts, 2014). Complications after LNF occur less

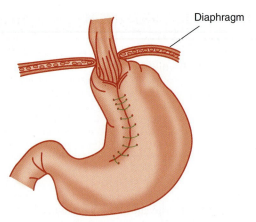

Diaphragm

FIG. 54-2 Open surgical approach for Nissen fundoplication for gastro-esophageal reflux disease or hiatal hernia repair.

frequently compared with those seen in patients having the more traditional open surgical approach. A small percentage of patients are not candidates for LNF and therefore require a conventional open fundoplication.

For the trans-thoracic surgical approach, teach the patient about chest tubes. Inform the patient that a nasogastric tube will be inserted during surgery and will remain in place for several days. Oral intake is started gradually with clear liquids after peristalsis is re-established or to stimulate peristalsis. Instruct the patient how to deep breathe and use the incentive spirometer. These measures are essential to prevent postoperative respiratory complications. The high incision makes deep breathing extremely painful. Teach the patient about postoperative pain, and assure him or her that adequate postoperative analgesic will be given promptly. PAIN levels must be continuously monitored.

In paraesophageal repair (a laparoscopic surgery), several ½-inch incisions are made in the abdomen, through which the hernia is closed and is typically reinforced using mesh. Less commonly, a conventional open procedure is used in which the surgeon uses a high trans-thoracic approach that requires a large chest incision for access to the surgical area.

Postoperative Care. Patients having the *LNF procedure* or paraesophageal repair via laparoscope are at risk for bleeding and infection, although these problems are not common. *The nursing care priority is to observe for these complications and provide health teaching as described in* Chart 54-5.

Postoperative care after *conventional open repair* closely follows that required after any esophageal surgery. Complications after open surgery are more common and potentially serious. Carefully assess for complications of open fundoplication surgery, described next, and report any complications to the health care provider (Chart 54-6).

! NURSING SAFETY PRIORITY (QSEN)

Action Alert

The primary focus of care after conventional surgery for a hiatal hernia repair is the prevention of respiratory complications. Elevate the head of the patient's bed at least 30 degrees to lower the diaphragm and promote lung expansion. Assist the patient out of bed and begin ambulation as soon as possible. Be sure to support the incision during coughing to reduce PAIN and to prevent excessive strain on the suture line, especially with obese patients.

CHART 54-5   Patient and Family Education: Preparing for Self-Management

Postoperative Instructions for Patients Having Laparoscopic Nissen Fundoplication (LNF) or Paraesophageal Repair via Laparoscope

- Stay on a soft diet for about a week, including mashed potatoes, puddings, custard, and milkshakes; avoid carbonated beverages, tough foods, and raw vegetables that are difficult to swallow.
- Remain on anti-reflux medications as prescribed for at least a month.
- Do not drive for a week after surgery; do not drive if taking opioid pain medication.
- Walk every day, but do not do any heavy lifting.
- Remove small dressings 2 days after surgery, and shower; do not remove Steri-Strips until 10 days after surgery.
- Wash incisions with soap and water, rinse well, and pat dry; report any redness or drainage from the incisions to your surgeon.
- Report fever above 101° F (38.3° C), nausea, vomiting, or uncontrollable bloating or pain. For patients older than 65 years, report elevations above 100° F (37.8° C).
- Schedule an appointment for follow-up with your surgeon in 3 to 4 weeks.

CHART 54-6   Best Practice for Patient Safety & Quality Care (QSEN)

Assessment of Postoperative Complications Related to Fundoplication Procedures

COMPLICATION	ASSESSMENT FINDINGS
Temporary dysphagia	The patient has difficulty swallowing when oral feeding begins.
Gas bloat syndrome	The patient has difficulty belching to relieve distention.
Atelectasis, pneumonia	The patient experiences dyspnea, chest pain, or fever.
Obstructed nasogastric tube	The patient experiences nausea, vomiting, or abdominal distention. The nasogastric tube does not drain.

Incentive spirometry and deep breathing are routinely used after surgery to maintain patency of the airways and lung expansion. Adequate PAIN control with analgesics is essential for postoperative deep breathing and coughing. Patients with a smoking history or chronic airway limitation (e.g., chronic obstructive pulmonary disease, asthma) require more aggressive management by the respiratory therapist to prevent atelectasis and pneumonia. Patients with large hiatal hernias are at the highest risk for developing respiratory complications.

The patient having the conventional surgery usually has a large-bore (diameter) nasogastric (NG) tube to prevent the fundoplication wrap from becoming too tight around the esophagus. Initially the NG drainage should be dark brown with old blood. The drainage should become normal yellowish green within the first 8 hours after surgery. Check the NG tube every 4 to 8 hours for proper placement in the stomach. The tube should be properly anchored so it is not displaced, because re-insertion could perforate the fundoplication. Follow the surgeon's directions for care of the patient with an NG tube.

Monitor patency of the NG tube to keep the stomach decompressed. This prevents retching or vomiting, which can strain or rupture the stomach sutures. The NG tube is irritating.

Therefore provide frequent oral hygiene to increase comfort. Assess the patient's hydration status regularly, including accurate measures of intake and output. Adequate fluid replacement helps thin respiratory secretions.

After open fundoplication, the patient may begin clear fluids when peristalsis is re-established or in an effort to stimulate peristalsis. Some surgeons create a temporary gastrostomy for feeding to allow for undisturbed healing of the repair. The patient gradually progresses to a near-normal diet during the first 4 to 6 weeks. Some foods, especially caffeinated or carbonated beverages and alcohol, are either restricted or eliminated. The food storage area of the stomach is reduced by the surgery, and meals need to be both smaller and more frequent.

Carefully supervise the first oral feedings because temporary dysphagia is common. Continuous dysphagia usually indicates that the fundoplication is too tight, and dilation may be required.

Another common complication of this surgery is *gas bloat syndrome,* in which patients are unable to voluntarily eructate (belch). The syndrome is usually temporary but may persist, even in those who have the laparoscopic approach. Teach the patient to avoid drinking carbonated beverages and to avoid eating gas-producing foods (especially high-fat foods), chewing gum, and drinking with a straw.

Other patients have *aerophagia* (air swallowing) from attempting to reverse or clear acid reflux. Teach them to relax consciously before and after meals, to eat and drink slowly, and to chew all food thoroughly. Air in the stomach that cannot be removed by belching can be extremely uncomfortable. Frequent position changes and ambulation are often effective interventions for eliminating air from the GI tract. If gas PAIN is still present, patients are taught to take simethicone, which dissolves in the mouth.

Community-Based Care

Patients undergoing one of the open surgical repairs require activity restrictions during the 3- to 6-week postoperative recovery period. For laparoscopic surgery, activity is typically restricted for a shorter time and the patient can return to his or her usual lifestyle more quickly, usually in a few days to a week.

For long-term management, teach the patient and family about appropriate NUTRITION modifications. The use of stool softeners or bulk laxatives is recommended for the first postoperative weeks until healing is complete. Instruct the patient to avoid straining and to prevent constipation. Teach him or her to inspect the healing incision daily and to notify the health care provider if swelling, redness, tenderness, discharge, or fever occurs. According to The Joint Commission National Patient Safety Goals for 2014, advise the patient to avoid contact with people with a respiratory INFECTION and to contact the health care provider if symptoms of a cold or influenza develop. Continuous coughing can cause the incision or the fundoplication to dehisce ("break open"). Per The Joint Commission Core Measures to decrease tobacco use, advise the patient to avoid smoking. Provide information about smoking-cessation methods, if appropriate.

If needed, collaborate with the dietitian to educate the patient and family about dietary changes. Encourage the patient to eat smaller and more frequent meals. Few ongoing diet restrictions are needed, but overeating or eating the wrong types of foods can produce discomfort if the patient cannot belch. Instruct the patient to report reflux symptoms to the health care provider.

Although severe surgical complications are rare, conditions such as gas bloat syndrome and dysphagia may continue. Prepare the patient for these problems and for the potential that reflux may not be completely controlled or may occur again. Although surgery controls the condition, a cure is rare and lifestyle modifications need to be ongoing.

ESOPHAGEAL TUMORS

❖ PATHOPHYSIOLOGY

Although esophageal tumors can be benign, most are malignant (cancerous) and the majority arise from the epithelium. Squamous cell carcinomas of the esophagus are located in the upper two thirds of the esophagus. Adenocarcinomas are more commonly found in the distal third and at the gastroesophageal junction and are now the most common type of esophageal cancer (McCance et al., 2014). Esophageal tumors grow rapidly because there is no serosal layer to limit their extension. Because the esophageal mucosa is richly supplied with lymph tissue, there is early spread of tumors to lymph nodes. Esophageal tumors can protrude into the esophageal lumen and can cause thickening or invade deeply into surrounding tissue. In rare cases, the lesion may be confined to the epithelial layer (in situ). In most cases, the tumor is large and well established on diagnosis. More than half of esophageal cancers metastasize (spread throughout the body).

Primary risk factors associated with the development of esophageal cancer are smoking and obesity. The compounds in tobacco smoke may be responsible for the genetic mutations seen in many squamous cell carcinomas of the esophagus. "Obesity poses a sixteen-fold increased risk of esophageal adenocarcinoma" (American Cancer Society [ACS], 2012, p. 29). Increased abdominal pressure associated with obesity is linked to reflux as well as Barrett's esophagus (a pre-malignant condition). Both conditions can contribute to changes in cellular structure in the esophagus increasing the potential for adenocarcinoma of the esophagus (ACS, 2012). In addition to these primary risk factors, malnutrition, untreated gastroesophageal reflux disease (GERD), and excessive alcohol intake are also associated with esophageal cancer. Barrett's esophagus results

---

🧬 GENETIC/GENOMIC CONSIDERATIONS

Patient-Centered Care QSEN

Certain genetic factors may have a role in the development of esophageal cancers. It is thought that these cancers result from mutations in tumor suppressor genes. Tumor suppressor genes are normal genes that control cell growth and division. When this type of gene is mutated and does not work properly, cells are unable to stop growing and dividing and tumors can result. (See Chapter 21 for a more complete discussion.)

Overexpression and mutations of the *Tp53, Tp16,* and *Tp17* tumor suppressor genes have been found in people with esophageal cancer (Nussbaum et al., 2007). In addition, the presence of the mutated *Tp53* gene may be an indication of advanced disease, especially in patients with adenocarcinomas.

Overexpression of *cyclin D1,* a protein that promotes cell growth and division, has also been found in patients with esophageal squamous cell cancers. Cyclins are products of oncogenes, which are normal genes involved in cell division and are controlled by suppressor genes. Prolonged exposure to carcinogens, such as tobacco, can cause oncogenes to escape the control of suppressor genes, leading to overexpression of cyclins and uncontrolled cell growth (cancer).

NCLEX EXAMINATION CHALLENGE

Health Promotion and Maintenance

Over the past 3 months, a client with a history of gastroesophageal reflux disease and obesity has implemented lifestyle changes. What lifestyle changes does the nurse recognize as important for the client to decrease chances of development of cancer of the esophagus? **Select all that apply.**

A. Lost 10 pounds
B. Sleeps with two pillows
C. Has quit eating processed foods
D. Drinks a glass of wine every night
E. Uses a nicotine patch instead of smoking

from exposure to acid and pepsin, which leads to the replacement of normal distal squamous mucosa with columnar epithelium as a response to tissue injury. This tissue undergoes dysplasia (cell appearance changes) and, ultimately, becomes cancerous. In parts of the world where esophageal cancer is more common, the incidence of squamous cell carcinoma appears to be linked to high levels of nitrosamines (which are found in pickled and fermented foods) and foods high in nitrate. Diets that are chronically deficient in fresh fruits and vegetables have also been implicated in the development of squamous cell carcinoma.

PATIENT-CENTERED COLLABORATIVE CARE

Assessment

History. Assess for risk factors related to the development or symptoms of esophageal cancer, such as gender, history of alcohol consumption, tobacco use, dietary habits, and other esophageal problems (e.g., dysphagia, reflux). In the United States, adenocarcinoma of the esophagus is more common than squamous cell carcinoma (National Cancer Institute at the National Institutes of Health, 2013). Men, regardless of race or ethnicity, have higher incidence and mortality rates associated with esophageal cancer (National Cancer Institute, 2013). Ask the patient about consumption of smoked and/or pickled foods, changes in appetite, changes in taste, or weight loss.

Physical Assessment/Clinical Manifestations. Cancer of the esophagus is a silent tumor in its early stages, with few observable signs. By the time the tumor causes symptoms, it usually has spread extensively.

Dysphagia *(difficulty swallowing) is the most common symptom of esophageal cancer, but it may not be present until the esophageal opening has gotten much smaller.* Dysphagia is persistent and progressive when **stricture** (narrowing) occurs. It is initially associated with swallowing solids, particularly meat, and then progresses rapidly over a period of weeks or months to difficulty in swallowing soft foods and liquids. Late in the disease, even saliva can cause choking. Patients usually report a sensation of food sticking in the throat or in the substernal area. Careful assessment of dysphagia is important because dysphagia associated with other esophageal disorders is not usually continuous. Weight loss often accompanies dysphagia and can exceed 20 pounds over several months.

Odynophagia (painful swallowing) is reported by many patients as a steady, dull, substernal PAIN that may radiate. It occurs most often when the patient drinks cold liquids. The presence of severe or persistent PAIN often indicates tumor invasion of the mediastinal structures. Assess for regurgitation, vomiting, **halitosis** (foul breath), and chronic hiccups, which often accompany advanced disease. In most patients, pulmonary problems develop. Assess for chronic cough, increased secretions, and a history of recent infections. Tumors in the upper esophagus may involve the larynx and thus cause hoarseness. Chart 54-7 summarizes the common clinical manifestations of esophageal tumors.

CHART 54-7 Key Features

Esophageal Tumors

- Persistent and progressive dysphagia (most common feature)
- Feeling of food sticking in the throat
- Odynophagia (painful swallowing)
- Severe, persistent chest or abdominal pain or discomfort
- Regurgitation
- Chronic cough with increasing secretions
- Hoarseness
- Anorexia
- Nausea and vomiting
- Weight loss (often more than 20 pounds)
- Changes in bowel habits (diarrhea, constipation, bleeding)

Psychosocial Assessment. The diagnosis of esophageal cancer causes high patient anxiety. The disease is accompanied by distressing symptoms and is often terminal. The fear of choking can place unusual stress, especially at mealtimes. The loss of pleasure and social aspects of eating may affect relationships with family and friends. Assess the patient's response to the diagnosis and prognosis. Ask about his or her usual coping strengths and resources. Assess the impact of the disease on the patient's usual daily activity routine. Determine the availability of support systems and the potential financial impact of the disease and its treatment. Refer the patient and family members to psychological counseling, pastoral care, and/or the social worker or case manager as needed. Chapter 7 describes end-of-life care for patients in the terminal stage of the disease.

Diagnostic Assessment. A *barium swallow* study with fluoroscopy may be the first diagnostic test requested to evaluate dysphagia. In a barium swallow, the margins of a tumor may be seen. The definitive diagnosis of esophageal cancer is made by *esophageal ultrasound (EUS)* with fine needle aspiration to examine the tumor tissue. An *esophagogastroduodenoscopy (EGD)* may also be performed to inspect the esophagus and obtain tissue specimens for cell studies and disease staging. A complete cancer staging workup is performed to determine the extent of the disease and plan appropriate therapy.

Positron emission tomography (PET) may identify metastatic disease with more accuracy than a CT scan. PET can also help evaluate response to chemotherapy to treat the cancer.

Analysis

The most specific common problem for patients with esophageal cancer is *decreased* NUTRITION *intake related to impaired swallowing and possible metastasis.* Many patients with cancer also have pain and are fearful because of the diagnosis of cancer. Chapter 22 describes problems that are typically seen with any patient with cancer.

Planning and Implementation

Promoting Nutrition

Planning: Expected Outcomes. The major concern for a patient with esophageal cancer is weight loss secondary to dysphagia. Therefore he or she is expected to maintain adequate nutrient intake and weight either orally or via an alternative method.

Interventions. Interventions to maintain or improve NUTRITION status focus on treatments that remove or shrink the obstructive tumor. Methods to reduce the effects of treatment that can impact NUTRITION are also a priority. Surgery is the most definitive intervention for esophageal cancer.

Nonsurgical treatment options for cancer of the esophagus that can assist in both disease and NUTRITION management include:

- Nutrition therapy
- Swallowing therapy
- Chemotherapy
- Radiation therapy
- Chemoradiation
- Targeted therapies
- Photodynamic therapy
- Esophageal dilation
- Endoscopic therapies

Nonsurgical Management. The treatment of esophageal cancer often involves a combination of therapies. Patients with cancer of the esophagus experience many physical problems, and symptom management becomes essential.

Nutrition and Swallowing Therapy. The purpose of NUTRITION therapy is to administer food and fluids to support the patient who is malnourished or at high risk for becoming malnourished. Conduct a screening assessment to provide information about the patient's NUTRITION status. The dietitian determines the caloric needs of the patient to meet daily requirements. Be sure the patient is weighed daily before breakfast on the same scale each day. To keep the esophagus patent, careful positioning is essential for a patient who is experiencing frequent reflux or who has tubes. Teach the patient to remain upright for several hours after meals and to avoid lying completely flat. Remind unlicensed assistive personnel (UAP) and other health care team members to keep the head of the bed elevated to a 30-degree angle or more to prevent reflux.

Semisoft foods and thickened liquids are preferred because they are easier to swallow. Record the amount of food and fluid intake every day to monitor progress in meeting desired NUTRITION outcomes. Liquid NUTRITION supplements (e.g., Boost, Ensure) are used between feedings to increase caloric intake. Ongoing efforts are made to preserve the ability to swallow, but enteral feedings (tube feedings) may be needed temporarily when dysphagia is severe. In patients with complete esophageal obstruction or life-threatening fistulas, the surgeon may create a gastrostomy or jejunostomy for feeding. Encourage the patient and family to meet with the dietitian for diet teaching and planning. Chapter 60 describes care for patients receiving enteral feeding.

Collaborate with the speech-language pathologist (SLP) to assist the patient with oral exercises to improve swallowing *(swallowing therapy)* and with the occupational therapist (OT) for feeding therapy. Ask the patient to suck on a lollipop to enhance tongue strength. Teach the patient to reach for food particles on the lips or chin using the tongue. In preparation for swallowing, remind the patient to position the head in forward flexion (chin tuck). Then tell him or her to place food at the back of the mouth. Monitor him or her for sealing of the lips and for tongue movements while eating. Check for pocketing of food in the cheeks after swallowing.

> ! **NURSING SAFETY PRIORITY** (QSEN)
> ***Critical Rescue***
>
> When the patient with an esophageal tumor is eating or drinking, monitor for signs and symptoms of aspiration, such as choking or coughing. Food aspiration can cause airway obstruction, pneumonia, or both, especially in older adults. In coordination with the SLP, teach family members and caregivers how to feed the patient, if needed. Teach them how to monitor for aspiration and implement appropriate measures if choking occurs.

Chemotherapy and Radiation. The use of *chemotherapy* in the treatment of esophageal cancer has been only moderately effective. It can be given as a primary treatment if the patient is not a candidate for surgery or given for palliation (control of symptoms). In most cases, however, chemotherapy is given in combination with radiation therapy to provide the patient the best chance of cure. The rationale for this approach is to shrink the primary tumor and eliminate any other tumor that may be in the local lymph nodes, improving the odds for a complete surgical resection. The most commonly used paired chemotherapeutic agents for esophageal cancer are carboplatin and paclitaxel (Taxol) or cisplatin and 5-fluorouracil (5-FU). These drugs are often combined with radiation because they make the tumor cells more sensitive to radiation effects (American Cancer Society [ACS], 2014a). Because chemotherapeutic drugs affect healthy cells as well as cancer cells, they have many side effects that cause discomfort to the patient. Chapter 22 describes chemotherapy in detail and discusses the role of the nurse in caring for patients receiving these drugs.

Radiation therapy to manage esophageal cancer is only moderately effective and can be used alone or in combination with other treatments. Radiation alone can provide palliation of symptoms by shrinking the tumor. It is contraindicated for patients with tracheoesophageal fistula, mediastinitis, mediastinal hemorrhage, or infiltration of the cancer to the trachea or bronchus. Normal esophageal tissue is very sensitive to the effects of radiation. Although high doses of radiation demonstrate the best results for tumor shrinkage, esophageal stricture or stenosis can result in many patients, which then requires esophageal dilation. Chapter 22 describes radiation methods and the general nursing care for the patient having radiation therapy.

Chemoradiation is a treatment for esophageal cancer that involves the use of chemotherapy at the same time as radiation therapy. One cycle of chemotherapy is given during the first week of radiation and another is delivered during the fifth week of radiation. Additional drug cycles are given after radiation therapy is complete.

Other Therapies. Targeted therapies may be used in combination with radiation and chemotherapy. Unlike chemotherapy, these therapies interfere with cancer cell growth in a variety of ways with less impact on healthy cells. Many of these drugs focus on proteins that are involved in signaling cells when to grow and divide. A key to success with targeted therapy is that the cancer cells must overexpress the targeted protein. Thus each patient's cancer cells are first examined for the overexpression to determine if targeted therapy is appropriate and which drug to use. Trastuzumab (Herceptin) is a commonly used drug that is used for patients whose esophageal cancer tests positive for an excess of the *HER2* protein on the cell surface. It is given by IV injection once every 3 weeks, in addition to chemotherapy (ACS, 2014b). Chapter 22 describes targeted therapies in detail, including nursing implications for patient safety and quality care.

Photodynamic therapy (PDT) is used as a palliative treatment for patients with advanced esophageal cancer who are not candidates for surgery. It may be used also as a cure for patients who have very small, localized tumors. The patient is injected with porfimer sodium (Photofrin), a light-sensitive drug that collects in cancer cells. Two days after the injection, a fiberoptic probe with a light at the tip is threaded into the esophagus through an endoscope. The light activates the Photofrin, destroying only cancer cells. PDT is far less invasive than surgery and is performed on an ambulatory care basis under moderate sedation. Endoscopy nurses observe the patient's rate and depth of respirations and monitor the patient's oxygen saturation and end-tidal (exhaled) carbon dioxide to ensure adequate oxygenation.

The side effects of Photofrin are rare but include nausea, fever, and constipation. Before the procedure, the patient is given written guidelines concerning photosensitivity measures. Remind the patient to avoid exposure to sunlight for 1 to 3 months. Sunglasses and protective clothing that covers all exposed body areas are essential. The patient may experience chest PAIN secondary to tissue damage and will require PAIN relief with opioid analgesics for a short time. Teach the patient to follow a clear liquid diet for 3 to 5 days after the procedure and advance to full liquids as tolerated. Warn the patient that tissue particles may release from the tumor site and be present in the sputum. Chapter 22 describes in detail the health teaching needed to promote patient safety associated with PDT.

Esophageal dilation may be performed as necessary throughout the course of the disease to achieve temporary but immediate relief of dysphagia. It is usually performed on an ambulatory care basis. Dilators are used to tear soft tissue, thereby widening the esophageal lumen (opening). In most cases, malignant tumors can be dilated safely, but perforation remains a significant risk. Large metal stents may be used to keep the esophagus open for longer periods. A stent covered with graft material can be used to seal a perforation. Bacteremia can also occur. To reduce the risk for endocarditis, antibiotics are given. The treatment is repeated as often as needed to preserve the patient's ability to swallow. Prolonged stent embedment into benign esophageal tissue can cause ulceration, bleeding, fistula, dysphagia, and formation of new stricture if the stent is not removed (Patel & Siddiqui, 2013).

When patients are not candidates for surgery or the tumor is too large to remove surgically, laser therapy or electrocoagulation using endoscopy may be performed as a palliative measure. Both of these methods destroy some cancer cells and reduce tumor size to improve swallowing. The procedures are done in ambulatory care settings or same-day surgery centers using moderate sedation.

Surgical Management. The purposes of surgical resection vary from palliation to cure. **Esophagectomy** is the removal of all or part of the esophagus. An **esophagogastrostomy** involves the removal of part of the esophagus and proximal stomach. The remaining stomach may be "pulled up" to take the place of the esophagus, or a section of the jejunum or colon may be placed as a conduit. Conventional open surgical techniques are lengthy and are associated with many complications or death. Fistula formation between the trachea and esophagus, abscess, and respiratory complications are common.

For patients with early-stage cancer, a laparoscopic-assisted **minimally invasive esophagectomy (MIE)** may be performed. However, most patients require the conventional open surgery because of tumor size and metastasis by the time they are diagnosed with the disease.

Preoperative Care. Preoperative preparation for patients undergoing esophagectomy or esophagogastrostomy can be quite extensive, especially before conventional techniques. Advise the patient to stop smoking 2 to 4 weeks before surgery to enhance pulmonary function. Patient preparation may include 5 days to 2 to 3 weeks of NUTRITION support to decrease the risk for postoperative complications. Ideally this supplementation is given orally, but many patients require tube feeding or parenteral NUTRITION. Teach the patient and family to monitor the patient's weight and intake and output. A preoperative evaluation may be required to treat dental disease. Teach the patient to use meticulous oral care 4 times daily to decrease the risk for postoperative INFECTION.

Preoperative nursing care focuses on teaching and on psychological support regarding the surgical procedure and preoperative and postoperative instructions. Teach the patient about:

* The number and sites of all incisions and drains
* The placement of a jejunostomy tube for initial enteral feedings
* The need for chest tubes if the pleural space is entered
* The purpose of the nasogastric tube
* The need for IV infusion

Teach the patient about routines for turning, coughing, deep breathing, and chest physiotherapy. Emphasize the crucial nature of postoperative respiratory care. If colon interposition (resecting a piece of colon and creating an esophagus) is planned, the patient also has a complete bowel preparation before surgery.

The patient facing a serious illness and extensive surgery can be expected to have feelings of grief and anxiety. Encourage the patient to talk about personal feelings and fears, and involve the family or significant others in all preoperative teaching and discussions. A social worker, certified hospital chaplain, or case manager can be extremely helpful in providing continuity of care and support to the entire family.

Operative Procedures. In the MIE procedure, the surgeon makes four or five small incisions in the chest and abdomen using a video-assisted thoracoscope and laparoscope. The lower esophagus and gastric fundus are removed. The remaining portion of the esophagus is then anastomosed (reconnected) to the stomach.

For most patients, the surgeon performs an open subtotal or total esophagectomy because tumors are often large and involve distant lymph nodes. For a subtotal (partial) removal, the diseased portion of the esophagus is removed and the cervical portion is anastomosed (connected) to the stomach (Fig. 54-3). A **pyloromyotomy** is done by cutting and suturing the pylorus. Finally, a jejunostomy tube may be placed for postoperative enteral feeding.

For patients with early-stage tumors of the lower third of the esophagus, a transhiatal esophagectomy is the preferred surgical approach. The surgery is performed through an upper midline cervical incision. With this approach, the pleural space is not entered, reducing respiratory complications. For patients with tumors in the upper esophagus, a radical neck dissection and laryngectomy may also be needed if the disease has spread to the larynx. Chapter 29 discusses the care of patients having these procedures.

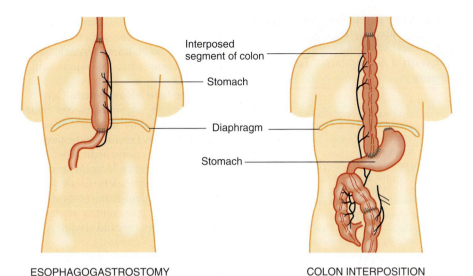

ESOPHAGOGASTROSTOMY   COLON INTERPOSITION

FIG. 54-3 Open surgical approaches to the treatment of esophageal cancer.

The surgeon may perform a **colon interposition** when the tumor involves the stomach or the stomach is otherwise unsuitable for anastomosis. A section of right or left colon is removed and brought up into the thorax to substitute for the esophagus (see Fig. 54-3).

Postoperative Care. The patient requires intensive postoperative care and is at risk for multiple serious complications. The patient having an MIE has the same risk for postoperative complications as one having the open procedure. The advantages of MIE, though, include:

- Less blood loss during surgery; fewer blood transfusions
- Decreased healing and recovery time
- Decreased trauma to the body
- No large incisions
- Less postoperative PAIN
- Shorter hospital stay (5 to 7 days rather than 7 to 10 days)

> **! NURSING SAFETY PRIORITY** (QSEN)
>
> **Action Alert**
>
> Respiratory care is the highest postoperative priority for patients having an esophagectomy. For those who had traditional surgery, intubation with mechanical ventilation is needed for at least the first 16 to 24 hours. Pulmonary complications include atelectasis and pneumonia. The risk for postoperative pulmonary complications is increased in the patient who has received preoperative radiation. Once the patient is extubated, begin deep breathing, turning, and coughing every 1 to 2 hours. Assess the patient for decreased breath sounds and shortness of breath every 1 to 2 hours. Provide incisional support and adequate analgesia for effective coughing.

Remind nursing and other staff to keep the patient in a semi-Fowler's or high-Fowler's position to support ventilation and prevent reflux. The health care provider prescribes prophylactic antibiotics and supplemental oxygen. *Ensure the patency of the chest tube drainage system, and monitor for changes in the volume or color of the drainage.*

Cardiovascular complications, particularly hypotension during surgery, can occur as a result of pressure placed on the posterior heart and usually respond well to IV fluid administration.

> **! NURSING SAFETY PRIORITY** (QSEN)
>
> **Action Alert**
>
> Monitor for manifestations of fluid volume overload, particularly in older patients and in those who have undergone lymph node dissection. Assess for edema, crackles in the lungs, and increased jugular venous pressure. In the immediate postoperative phase, the patient is often admitted to the intensive care unit. Critical care nurses assess hemodynamic parameters such as cardiac output, cardiac index, and systemic vascular resistance every 2 hours to monitor for myocardial ischemia. Observe for atrial fibrillation that results from irritation of the vagus nerve during surgery, and manage according to agency protocol.

The patient with poor NUTRITION or prior radiation or chemotherapy is at risk for INFECTION. For those who undergo more radical surgical procedures, there is a serious risk for leakage at the anastomosis (surgical connection) sites. This situation is especially true with colon interpositions because several sites are stressed by the effects of tension, poor blood supply, and delayed healing. *Mediastinitis* (inflammation of the mediastinum) resulting from an anastomotic leak can lead to fatal sepsis.

Wound management is another major postoperative concern for conventional surgery because the patient typically has multiple incisions and drains. *Provide direct support to the incision during turning and coughing to prevent dehiscence.* Wound INFECTION can occur 4 to 5 days after surgery. Leakage from the site of anastomosis is a dreaded complication that can appear 2 to 10 days after surgery. If an anastomotic leak occurs, all oral intake is discontinued and is not resumed until the site of the leak has healed.

> **! NURSING SAFETY PRIORITY** (QSEN)
>
> **Critical Rescue**
>
> After esophageal surgery, carefully assess for fever, fluid accumulation, signs of inflammation, and symptoms of early shock (e.g., tachycardia, tachypnea). Report any of these findings to the surgeon **or** Rapid Response Team immediately!

Managing the Patient with a Nasogastric Tube after Esophageal Surgery

- Check for tube placement every 4 to 8 hours.
- Ensure that the tube is patent (open) and draining; drainage should turn from bloody to yellowish green by the end of the first postoperative day.
- Secure the tube well to prevent dislodgment.
- Do not irrigate or reposition the tube without a physician's request.
- Provide meticulous oral and nasal hygiene every 2 to 4 hours.
- Keep the head of the bed elevated to at least 30 degrees.
- When the patient is permitted to have a small amount of water, place him or her in an upright position and observe for dysphagia (difficulty swallowing).
- Observe for leakage from the anastomosis site, as indicated by fever, fluid accumulation, and manifestations of early shock (tachycardia, tachypnea, altered mental status).

A nasogastric (NG) tube is placed intraoperatively to decompress the stomach to prevent tension on the suture line. Monitor the NG tube for patency, and carefully secure the tube to prevent dislodgment, which can disrupt the sutures at the anastomosis. *Do not irrigate or reposition the NG tube in patients who have undergone esophageal surgery unless requested by the surgeon!* The initial nasogastric drainage is bloody but should change to a greenish yellow color by the end of the first postoperative day. The continued presence of blood may indicate internal bleeding at the suture line. Commonly, an antacid will be prescribed to support the patient's healing. Provide oral hygiene for the patient every 2 to 4 hours while the tube is in place, or delegate and supervise this activity (Chart 54-8).

NUTRITION management of the patient who has undergone esophageal surgery is an early postoperative concern. After conventional surgery, on the second postoperative day, initial feedings usually begin through the jejunostomy tube (J tube). Do not aspirate for residual, because this increases the risk for mucosal tearing. Feedings are slowly increased over the next several days. Feeding by this method can be discontinued once the patient is taking adequate oral NUTRITION.

Before beginning oral feedings, a cine-esophagram study is performed to detect any anastomotic leaks, strictures, or signs of aspiration. If no leaks are seen, a liquid diet is started. If liquids are well tolerated, the patient's diet is advanced to include semi-solid foods and then solid foods.

Place the patient in an upright position, and supervise all initial swallowing efforts. The food storage area of the stomach has been radically decreased, and gravity is the only defense against reflux. *Teach the patient and/or family the importance of the patient eating six to eight small meals per day. Fluids should be taken between, rather than with, meals to prevent diarrhea.* Diarrhea can occur 20 minutes to 2 hours after eating and can be managed with loperamide (Imodium) before meals. The diarrhea is thought to be the result of *vagotomy syndrome,* which develops as a result of interrupted vagal fibers to the abdominal organs during surgery.

Community-Based Care

Patients with esophageal cancer have many challenges to face once they are discharged home. The combination treatment regimens cause long-lasting side effects, such as fatigue and weakness. These complex treatments also require the patient and family to be knowledgeable about symptom management and to know when to report concerns to the health care provider.

Home Care Management. *Once the patient is discharged to home, ongoing respiratory care remains a priority.* Give the patient and family instructions for ambulation and incentive spirometer use. Encourage the patient to be as active as possible and to avoid excessive bedrest because this can lead to complications of immobility. In accordance with The Joint Commission National Patient Safety Goals for 2014, teach the family to protect the patient from INFECTION and to contact the health care provider immediately if signs of respiratory INFECTION develop. Patients should stay away from people with infections and avoid large crowds.

Self-Management Education. Remind the patient and family to wash their hands frequently, and teach them to inspect the incisions daily for redness, tenderness, swelling, odor, and discharge because proper wound healing is still a concern at the time of discharge. Instruct them to report a temperature greater than 101° F (38.3° C), or 100° F (37.8° C) for older adults, which may be a sign of INFECTION. Prepare written instructions about the signs of anastomosis leakage. *Teach the patient or family to immediately report to the health care provider the presence of fever and a swollen, painful neck incision.*

NUTRITION support is important. Encourage the patient to continue increasing oral feedings as tolerated. Remind him or her to eat small, frequent meals containing high-calorie, high-protein foods that are soft and easily swallowed. Teach the value of using supplemental milkshakes between meals, and instruct the patient to eat slowly. Patients who have undergone esophageal resection can lose up to 10% of their body weight. Teach the patient to monitor his or her weight at home and to report a weight loss of 5 pounds or more in 1 month. If sufficient oral intake is not possible, the patient and family may need instruction about tube feedings or parenteral NUTRITION at home.

Emphasize the importance of remaining upright after meals. Dysphagia or odynophagia may recur because of stricture, reflux, or cancer recurrence. These symptoms should be promptly reported to the health care provider. Despite radical surgery, the patient with cancer of the esophagus often still has a terminal illness and a relatively short life expectancy. Emphasis is placed on maximizing quality of life. Realistic planning is important as the patient's condition eventually worsens, and patient and family are assisted to plan for the future together. Assist family members in exploring formal and informal sources of support. Help the family or significant others arrange for hospice care when it is needed. Chapter 7 describes end-of-life care, including hospice.

Health Care Resources. Referrals to community or home care organizations assist the family in providing care in the home. The patient may need transportation to the radiation treatment center 5 times per week for up to 6 weeks. Oncology nursing care may be needed to monitor and evaluate the patient who is receiving chemotherapy at home through venous access devices or portable infusion pumps. Inform the patient and family about the services available through the American Cancer Society (www.cancer.org), including support groups and transportation. Familiarize the family with area hospice services for future planning. Coordinate resource referrals with the case manager or home care agency.

◆ *Evaluation: Expected Outcomes*

Evaluate the care of the patient with esophageal cancer based on the identified priority patient problems. The major expected outcome is that the patient will be able to consume adequate NUTRITION and maintain a stable weight.

CLINICAL JUDGMENT CHALLENGE

Teamwork and Collaboration; Safety; Evidence-Based Practice QSEN

A 55-year-old patient has undergone a partial esophagectomy. He has a history of alcoholism and states that he quit drinking when he found out about his diagnosis. Just prior to discharge, you are preparing to teach him and his family about self-management.

1. For what postoperative complications will you monitor, and why could they occur after this surgery?
2. Of all potential postoperative complications, which signs and symptoms should the patient and family be instructed to *immediately* report?
3. Why is the patient's history of alcoholism significant? What referrals would you provide to support his choice to discontinue using alcohol?
4. The patient's life partner tells you that the patient is the family's primary provider of income. His life partner is concerned that the patient may not recover well enough to return to work. How might you respond to his concern?
5. To what community agencies would you refer the patient and his family?

ESOPHAGEAL DIVERTICULA

Diverticula are sacs resulting from the herniation of esophageal mucosa and submucosa into surrounding tissue. They may develop anywhere along the length of the esophagus. No environmental risk factors are known to be involved in their development. The incomplete or late opening of swallowing muscles can cause high pressure in the hypopharynx and lead to *Zenker's diverticula,* the most common form. This type occurs most often in older adults. Patients report dysphagia (difficulty swallowing), regurgitation (reflux), nocturnal cough, and halitosis (bad breath). They can also be at risk for perforation because the mucosa is without the protection of the normal esophageal muscle layer.

Esophageal diverticula are diagnosed most often by *esophagogastroduodenoscopy (EGD).* This procedure must be performed with strict care because of the risk for perforation. NUTRITION therapy and positioning are the major interventions for controlling symptoms related to diverticula. Collaborate with the dietitian to assist the patient in exploring variations in the size and frequency of meals and in food texture and consistency. Semisoft foods and smaller meals are often best tolerated and may reduce or relieve the symptoms of pressure and reflux. Nocturnal reflux associated with diverticula is managed by teaching the patient to sleep with the head of the bed elevated and to avoid the supine position for at least 2 hours after eating. Advise the patient to avoid vigorous exercise after meals. Teach him or her to avoid restrictive clothing and frequent stooping or bending.

Surgical management is aimed at removing the diverticula. Postoperatively, the patient is NPO status for several days to promote healing. During that period, the patient receives IV fluids for hydration and tube feedings; after that, he or she is

TABLE 54-2	**Common Causes of Esophageal Perforation**
• Straining	• Instrument or tubes
• Seizures	• Chemical injury
• Trauma	• Complications of esophageal surgery
• Foreign objects	• Ulcers

given oral fluid and food. Provide PAIN relief measures, and monitor for complications such as bleeding or perforation. *A nasogastric (NG) tube is placed during surgery for decompression and is not irrigated or repositioned unless specifically requested by the surgeon.*

Community-based care includes teaching the patient and family about:

- Nutrition therapy
- Positioning guidelines to prevent reflux
- Warning signs of complications, such as bleeding or infection

ESOPHAGEAL TRAUMA

Trauma to the esophagus can result from blunt injuries, chemical burns, surgery or endoscopy (rare), or the stress of continuous severe vomiting (Table 54-2). Trauma may affect the esophagus directly, impairing swallowing and NUTRITION, or it may create problems in related structures such as the lungs or mediastinum. The incidence of most forms of esophageal trauma is low in adults. When excessive force is exerted on the esophageal mucosa, it may perforate or rupture, allowing the caustic acid secretions to enter the mediastinal cavity. These tears are associated with a high mortality rate related to shock, respiratory impairment, or sepsis.

Chemical injury is usually a result of the accidental or intentional ingestion of caustic substances. The damage to the mouth and esophagus is rapid and severe. Acid burns tend to affect the superficial mucosal lining, whereas alkaline substances cause deeper penetrating injuries. Strong alkalis can cause full perforation of the esophagus within 1 minute. Additional problems may include aspiration pneumonia and hemorrhage. Esophageal strictures may develop as scar tissue forms.

Patients with esophageal trauma are initially evaluated and treated in the emergency department. Assessment focuses on the nature of the injury and the circumstances surrounding it. *Assess for airway patency, breathing, chest pain, dysphagia, vomiting, and bleeding as the priorities for patient care.* If the risk for extending the damage is not excessive, an endoscopic study may be requested to evaluate tears or perforation. A CT scan of the chest can be done to assess for the presence of mediastinal air.

After the injury, keep the patient NPO to prevent further leakage of esophageal secretions. Esophageal and gastric suction can be used for drainage and to rest the esophagus. Esophageal rest is maintained for more than a week after injury to allow for initial healing of the mucosa. Total parenteral NUTRITION (TPN) is prescribed to provide calories and protein for wound healing while the patient is not eating.

To prevent sepsis, the health care provider prescribes broad-spectrum antibiotics. High-dose corticosteroids may be administered to suppress inflammation and prevent strictures (esophageal narrowing). In addition, opioid and non-opioid analgesics are prescribed for PAIN management. When caustic burns involve the mouth, topical agents such as lidocaine (Xylocaine Viscous) may be used for analgesia and local anti-inflammatory action.

If nonsurgical management is not effective in healing traumatized esophageal tissue, the patient may need surgery to remove the damaged tissue. Those with severe injuries may require resection of part of the esophagus with a gastric pull-through and repositioning or replacement by a bowel segment; also, gastrostomy tube (G-tube) placement may be needed to meet NUTRITION needs while healing.

NURSING CONCEPTS AND CLINICAL JUDGMENT REVIEW

What might you NOTICE if the patient has inadequate digestion and NUTRITION as a result of chronic esophageal problems?
- Dysphagia (difficulty swallowing)
- Odynophagia (painful swallowing)
- Dyspepsia (indigestion)
- Regurgitation (reflux)
- Eructation (belching)
- Chronic cough
- Choking
- Halitosis (foul breath)
- Weight loss
- Vomiting
- Chest pain

What should you INTERPRET and how should you RESPOND to a patient experiencing inadequate digestion and NUTRITION as a result of chronic esophageal problems?

Perform and interpret focused physical findings, including:
- Assessing ability to chew and swallow food
- Assessing chest pain (dyspepsia) for quality, location, and intensity

- Assessing body weight change
- Auscultating lungs
- Assessing readiness to learn

Respond by:
- Providing semi-solid or thickened liquids if solid foods cannot be swallowed comfortably
- Collaborating with the dietitian and occupational therapist (OT) for swallowing evaluation and training
- Monitoring for aspiration of secretions or food
- Teaching lifestyle changes, such as foods to avoid, smoking and alcohol cessation, weight reduction (if obese), and importance of drug therapy to control symptoms
- Monitoring weight
- Monitoring for increased dysphagia

On what should you REFLECT?
- Evaluate for rapid weight changes (decrease if obese, and increase if severe weight loss has occurred).
- Monitor for manifestations of aspiration.
- Observe patient for improvement in GI symptoms.
- Evaluate effectiveness of health teaching.
- Consider ways to promote digestion and nutrition.

GET READY FOR THE NCLEX® EXAMINATION!

▌ KEY POINTS

Review these Key Points for each NCLEX Examination Client Needs Category.

Safe and Effective Care Environment
- Consult with the dietitian, patient, and family regarding NUTRITION restrictions for patients with GERD. **Teamwork and Collaboration** `QSEN`
- Collaborate with the health care team for the patient with impaired swallowing and/or limited NUTRITION. **Teamwork and Collaboration** `QSEN`
- Teach the patient and family to recognize the symptoms of dysphagia. **Safety** `QSEN`
- Remain with the dysphagic patient during meals to prevent or assist with choking episodes. **Safety** `QSEN`

Health Promotion and Maintenance
- Teach the patient oral exercises aimed at improving swallowing.
- Stress the importance of recognizing and controlling reflux through NUTRITION therapy and medications to avoid further esophageal damage that could lead to Barrett's esophagus.
- Teach the patient to elevate the head of the bed by 6 inches for sleep to prevent nighttime reflux.

- Instruct the patient to sleep in the right side-lying position to minimize the effects of nighttime episodes of reflux.
- Teach the patient with esophageal cancer to monitor his or her body weight and to notify the health care provider of weight loss.
- Teach the patient to avoid alcoholic beverages, smoking, and other substances as listed in Chart 54-2 because they lead to increased gastroesophageal reflux.
- Teach the patient to prevent gas bloat syndrome by avoiding drinking carbonated beverages, eating gas-producing foods, chewing gum, and drinking with a straw.
- Review postprocedure instructions for patients having the Stretta procedure for GERD as outlined in Chart 54-3.

Psychosocial Integrity
- Allow the patient the opportunity to express fear or anxiety regarding the diagnosis of esophageal cancer and related treatment regimen of surgery, chemotherapy, and radiation. **Patient-Centered Care** `QSEN`
- Explain all procedures, restrictions, drug therapy, and follow-up care to the patient and family.
- Refer the patient or family members to psychological counseling, hospice, pastoral care, and the case manager as needed. **Teamwork and Collaboration** `QSEN`

Physiological Integrity

- For patients with GERD, teach the importance of strict adherence to anti-reflux agents in preventing esophageal damage (see Chapter 55, Chart 55-3).
- Be aware that laparoscopic Nissen fundoplication (LNF) and laparoscopic paraesophageal repairs are common surgical procedures for patients with GERD and hiatal hernia.
- Assess for complications and provide postoperative care for patients having the LNF procedure, as described in Chart 54-6. **Safety** QSEN
- Be sure to frequently monitor the NUTRITION status of the patient with esophageal cancer.

- Teach the patient having open conventional esophageal surgery about incisions, drains, and jejunostomy tube placement before he or she undergoes surgery for esophageal cancer.
- For the patient with a nasogastric (NG) tube, check the NG tube every 4 to 8 hours for proper placement and anchorage; follow guidelines as outlined in Chart 54-8.
- Assess the patient after esophageal surgery for pulmonary and cardiac complications of surgery, and report changes to the health care provider. **Safety** QSEN
- Assess patients for key features of esophageal tumors as listed in Chart 54-7.

Care of Patients with Stomach Disorders

Lara Carver

PRIORITY CONCEPTS

- NUTRITION
- PAIN
- INFLAMMATION
- INFECTION

LEARNING OUTCOMES

Safe and Effective Care Environment

1. Describe the importance of collaborating with members of the health care team when caring for patients with gastric (stomach) disorders.

Health Promotion and Maintenance

2. Identify community resources for patients with gastric disorders.
3. Develop a teaching plan for patients about complementary and alternative therapies that have been used to help manage gastritis and peptic ulcer disease (PUD).
4. Plan interventions to promote GI health and prevent gastritis.

Psychosocial Integrity

5. Identify the need for end-of-life care for patients with advanced gastric cancer.

Physiological Integrity

6. Compare assessment findings of acute and chronic gastritis.
7. Compare and contrast assessment findings associated with gastric and duodenal ulcers.
8. Identify the most common medical complications that can result from PUD.
9. Describe the purpose and adverse effects of drug therapy for gastritis and PUD.
10. To promote patient safety and quality care, monitor patients with PUD and gastric cancer for signs of upper GI bleeding.
11. Prioritize evidence-based interventions for patients with upper GI bleeding.
12. To prevent complications, develop a collaborative preoperative and postoperative plan of care for the patient undergoing gastric surgery.

Although only a few diseases affect the stomach, they can be very serious and in some cases life threatening. The most common disorders include gastritis, peptic ulcer disease, and gastric cancer. Each of these health problems can result in impaired or altered *digestion* and NUTRITION. In addition, INFLAMMATION and INFECTION associated with these problems can cause PAIN. The stomach is part of the upper GI system that is responsible for a large part of the digestive process. Patient-centered collaborative care for stomach disorders often includes therapies to meet the patient's need for adequate nutrition.

GASTRITIS

Gastritis is the INFLAMMATION of gastric mucosa (stomach lining). It can be scattered or localized and can be classified according to cause, cellular changes, or distribution of the lesions. Gastritis can be erosive (causing ulcers) or nonerosive. Although the mucosal changes that result from *acute* gastritis typically heal after several months, this is not true for *chronic* gastritis.

❖ PATHOPHYSIOLOGY

Prostaglandins provide a protective mucosal barrier that prevents the stomach from digesting itself by a process called acid autodigestion. If there is a break in the protective barrier, mucosal injury occurs. The resulting injury is worsened by histamine release and vagus nerve stimulation. Hydrochloric acid can then diffuse back into the mucosa and injure small vessels. This back-diffusion causes edema, hemorrhage, and erosion of the stomach's lining. The pathologic changes of gastritis include vascular congestion, edema, acute inflammatory cell infiltration, and degenerative changes in the superficial epithelium of the stomach lining.

Types of Gastritis

INFLAMMATION of the gastric mucosa or submucosa after exposure to local irritants or other causes can result in acute gastritis. The early pathologic manifestation of gastritis is a thickened, reddened mucous membrane with prominent rugae, or folds. Various degrees of mucosal necrosis and inflammatory reaction occur in acute disease. The diagnosis cannot be based solely on clinical symptoms. Complete regeneration and healing usually occur within a few days. If the stomach muscle is not involved, complete recovery usually occurs with no residual evidence of gastric inflammatory reaction. If the muscle is affected, hemorrhage may occur during an episode of acute gastritis.

Chronic gastritis appears as a patchy, diffuse (spread out) INFLAMMATION of the mucosal lining of the stomach. As the disease progresses, the walls and lining of the stomach thin and atrophy. With progressive gastric atrophy from chronic mucosal injury, the function of the parietal (acid-secreting) cells decreases and the source of intrinsic factor is lost. Intrinsic factor is critical for absorption of vitamin B_{12}. When body stores of vitamin B_{12} are eventually depleted, pernicious anemia results. The amount and concentration of acid in stomach secretions gradually decrease until the secretions consist of only mucus and water.

Chronic gastritis is associated with an increased risk for gastric cancer. The persistent INFLAMMATION extends deep into the mucosa, causing destruction of the gastric glands and cellular changes. Chronic gastritis may be categorized as type A, type B, or atrophic (McCance et al., 2014).

Type A (nonerosive) chronic gastritis refers to an INFLAMMATION of the glands as well as the fundus and body of the stomach. Type B chronic gastritis usually affects the glands of the antrum but may involve the entire stomach. In atrophic chronic gastritis, diffuse inflammation and destruction of deeply located glands accompany the condition. Chronic atrophic gastritis affects all layers of the stomach, thus decreasing the number of cells. The muscle thickens, and inflammation is present. Chronic atrophic gastritis is characterized by total loss of fundal glands, minimal inflammation, thinning of the gastric mucosa, and intestinal metaplasia (abnormal tissue development). These cellular changes can lead to peptic ulcer disease (PUD) and gastric cancer (McCance et al., 2014).

Etiology and Genetic Risk

The onset of INFECTION with *Helicobacter pylori* can result in acute gastritis. *H. pylori* is a gram-negative bacterium that penetrates the mucosal gel layer of the gastric epithelium. Although less common, other forms of bacterial gastritis from organisms such as staphylococci, streptococci, *Escherichia coli*, or salmonella can cause life-threatening problems such as sepsis and extensive tissue necrosis (death).

Long-term NSAID use creates a high risk for acute gastritis. NSAIDs inhibit prostaglandin production in the mucosal barrier. Other risk factors include alcohol, coffee, caffeine, and corticosteroids. Acute gastritis is also caused by local irritation from radiation therapy and accidental or intentional ingestion of corrosive substances, including acids or alkalis (e.g., lye and drain cleaners).

Type A chronic gastritis has been associated with the presence of antibodies to parietal cells and intrinsic factor. Therefore an autoimmune cause for this type of gastritis is likely. Parietal cell antibodies have been found in most patients with pernicious anemia and in more than one half of those with type A gastritis. A genetic link to this disease, with an autosomal dominant pattern of inheritance, has been found in the relatives of patients with pernicious anemia (McCance et al., 2014).

The most common form of chronic gastritis is type B gastritis, caused by *H. pylori* infection. A direct correlation exists between the number of organisms and the degree of cellular abnormality present. The host response to the *H. pylori* infection is activation of lymphocytes and neutrophils. Release of inflammatory cytokines, such as interleukin (IL)-1, IL-8, and tumor necrosis factor (TNF)–alpha, damages the gastric mucosa (McCance et al., 2014).

Chronic local irritation and toxic effects caused by alcohol ingestion, radiation therapy, and smoking have been linked to chronic gastritis. Surgical procedures that involve the pyloric sphincter, such as a pyloroplasty, can lead to gastritis by causing reflux of alkaline secretions into the stomach. Other systemic disorders such as Crohn's disease, graft-versus-host disease, and uremia can also precipitate the development of chronic gastritis.

Atrophic gastritis is a type of chronic gastritis that is seen most often in older adults. It can occur after exposure to toxic substances in the workplace (e.g., benzene, lead, nickel) or *H. pylori* infection, or it can be related to autoimmune factors. Atrophic gastritis can lead to two types of cancer: gastric cancer and gastric mucosa-associated lymphoid tissue (MALT) lymphoma. See p. 1138 for a more detailed explanation of gastric cancer.

Health Promotion and Maintenance

Gastritis is a very common health problem in the United States. A balanced diet, regular exercise, and stress-reduction techniques can help prevent it (Chart 55-1). A balanced diet includes following the recommendations of the U.S. Department of Agriculture (USDA) and limiting intake of foods and spices that can cause gastric distress, such as caffeine, chocolate, mustard, pepper, and other strong or hot spices. Alcohol and tobacco should also be avoided. Regular exercise maintains peristalsis, which helps prevent gastric contents from irritating the gastric mucosa. Stress-reduction techniques can include aerobic exercise, meditation, reading, and/or yoga, depending on individual preferences.

Excessive use of aspirin and other NSAIDs should also be avoided. If a family member has *H. pylori* INFECTION or has had it in the past, patient testing should be considered. This test can identify the bacteria before they cause gastritis.

❖ PATIENT-CENTERED COLLABORATIVE CARE

◆ Assessment

Symptoms of *acute* gastritis range from mild to severe. The patient may report epigastric discomfort or PAIN, anorexia,

---

CHART 55-1 Patient and Family Education: Preparing for Self-Management

Gastritis Prevention

- Eat a well-balanced diet.
- Avoid drinking excessive amounts of alcoholic beverages.
- Use caution in taking large doses of aspirin, other NSAIDs (e.g., ibuprofen), and corticosteroids.
- Avoid excessive intake of coffee (even decaffeinated).
- Be sure that foods and water are safe, to avoid contamination.
- Manage stress levels using complementary and alternative therapies such as relaxation and meditation techniques.
- Stop smoking.
- Protect yourself against exposure to toxic substances in the workplace such as lead and nickel.
- Seek medical treatment if you are experiencing symptoms of esophageal reflux (see Chapter 54).

CHART 55-2 Key Features

Gastritis

Acute Gastritis	Chronic Gastritis
• Rapid onset of epigastric pain or discomfort	• Vague report of epigastric pain that is relieved by food
• Nausea and vomiting	• Anorexia
• Hematemesis (vomiting blood)	• Nausea or vomiting
• Gastric hemorrhage	• Intolerance of fatty and spicy foods
• Dyspepsia (heartburn)	
• Anorexia	• Pernicious anemia

---

cramping, nausea, and vomiting (Chart 55-2). Assess for abdominal tenderness and bloating, **hematemesis** (vomiting blood), or **melena** (dark, sticky feces, as evidence of blood in the stool). Symptoms last only a few hours or days and vary with the cause. Aspirin/NSAID–related gastritis may result in **dyspepsia** (heartburn). Gastritis or food poisoning caused by endotoxins, such as staphylococcal endotoxin, has an abrupt onset. Severe nausea and vomiting often occur within 5 hours of ingestion of the contaminated food. *In some cases gastric hemorrhage is the presenting symptom, which is a life-threatening emergency.*

Chronic gastritis causes few symptoms unless ulceration occurs. Patients may report nausea, vomiting, or upper abdominal discomfort. Periodic epigastric pain may occur after a meal. Some patients have anorexia (see Chart 55-2).

Esophagogastroduodenoscopy (EGD) via an endoscope with biopsy is the gold standard for diagnosing gastritis. (See Chapter 52 for discussion of nursing care associated with this diagnostic procedure.) The physician performs a biopsy to establish a definitive diagnosis of the type of gastritis. If lesions are patchy and diffuse, biopsy of several suspicious areas may be necessary to avoid misdiagnosis. A *cytologic examination* of the biopsy specimen is performed to confirm or rule out gastric cancer. Tissue samples can also be taken to detect *H. pylori* INFECTION using *rapid urease testing.* The results of these tests are more reliable if the patient has discontinued taking antacids for at least a week (Pagana & Pagana, 2014).

Interventions

Patients with gastritis are not often seen in the acute care setting unless they have an exacerbation ("flare-up") of acute or chronic gastritis that results in fluid and electrolyte imbalance, bleeding, or increased PAIN. Collaborative care is directed toward supportive care for relieving the symptoms and removing or reducing the cause of discomfort.

Acute gastritis is treated symptomatically and supportively because the healing process is spontaneous, usually occurring within a few days. When the cause is removed, PAIN and discomfort usually subside. If bleeding is severe, a blood transfusion may be necessary. Fluid replacement is prescribed for patients with severe fluid loss. Surgery, such as partial gastrectomy, pyloroplasty, and/or vagotomy, may be needed for patients with major bleeding or ulceration. Treatment of *chronic* gastritis varies with the cause. The approach to management includes the elimination of causative agents, treatment of any underlying disease (e.g., uremia, Crohn's disease), avoidance of toxic substances (e.g., alcohol, tobacco), and health teaching.

Eliminating the causative factors, such as *H. pylori* INFECTION if present, is the primary treatment approach. Drugs and nutritional therapy are also used. In the *acute* phase the health care provider prescribes drugs that block and buffer gastric acid secretions to relieve pain.

H₂-receptor antagonists, such as famotidine (Pepcid) and nizatidine (Axid), are typically used to block gastric secretions. Sucralfate (Carafate, Sulcrate ♣), a *mucosal barrier fortifier,* may also be prescribed. *Antacids* used as buffering agents include aluminum hydroxide combined with magnesium hydroxide (Maalox) and aluminum hydroxide combined with simethicone and magnesium hydroxide (Mylanta). Antisecretory agents (**proton pump inhibitors [PPIs]**) such as omeprazole (Prilosec) or pantoprazole (Protonix) may be prescribed to suppress gastric acid secretion (see Chart 55-3).

⚠ NURSING SAFETY PRIORITY (QSEN)

Drug Alert

Teach the patient to monitor for symptom relief and side effects of drugs to treat gastritis and to notify the health care provider of any adverse effects or worsening of gastric distress. The dose, frequency, or type of drug may need to be changed if symptoms of gastric irritation appear or persist. *Remind patients not to take additional over-the-counter (OTC) drugs such as Pepcid AC or Axid AR if they are taking similar prescribed drugs.*

Patients with *chronic* gastritis may require vitamin B₁₂ for prevention or treatment of pernicious anemia. If *H. pylori* is found, the health care provider treats the infection. Current practice for INFECTION treatment is described on p. 1134 in the discussion of Drug Therapy in the Peptic Ulcer Disease section.

The nurse, primary care provider, or pharmacist teaches patients to avoid drugs and other irritants that are associated with gastritis episodes, if possible. These drugs include corticosteroids, erythromycin (E-Mycin, Erythromid ♣), ASA (aspirin), and NSAIDs such as naproxen (Naprosyn) and ibuprofen (Motrin, Advil, Amersol ♣, Novo-Profen ♣). NSAIDs are also available as OTC drugs and should not be used. Teach patients to read all OTC drug labels because many preparations contain aspirin or other NSAID.

Instruct the patient to limit intake of any foods and spices that cause distress, such as those that contain caffeine or high acid content (e.g., tomato products, citrus juices) or those that are heavily seasoned with strong or hot spices. Bell peppers and onions are also commonly irritating foods. Most patients seem to progress better with a bland, non-spicy diet and smaller, more frequent meals. Alcohol and tobacco should also be avoided.

Teach the patient about various techniques that reduce stress and discomfort, such as progressive relaxation, cutaneous stimulation, guided imagery, and distraction. Table 55-1 lists commonly used complementary and alternative therapies for gastritis and peptic ulcer disease.

PEPTIC ULCER DISEASE

A **peptic ulcer** is a mucosal lesion of the stomach or duodenum. **Peptic ulcer disease (PUD)** results when mucosal defenses become impaired and no longer protect the epithelium from the effects of acid and pepsin.

TABLE 55-1	**Commonly Used Complementary and Alternative Therapies for Gastritis and Peptic Ulcer Disease (PUD)**
Herbs and Vitamins	**Homeopathy**
• Cranberry	• Carbo vegetabilis
• DGL (deglycyrrhizinated licorice)	• Ipecacuanha
• Ginger	• Nux vomica
• Probiotics	• Pulsatilla
• Slippery elm	
• Vitamin C	

❖ PATHOPHYSIOLOGY

Types of Ulcers

Three types of ulcers may occur: gastric ulcers, duodenal ulcers, and stress ulcers (less common). Most gastric and duodenal ulcers are caused by *H. pylori* INFECTION. Although it is not certain about how *H. pylori* is transmitted, it is believed to be spread through contaminated food or water. Studies have also suggested that contact with stool, vomit, and sometimes saliva of an infected person can spread the infection (National Digestive Diseases Information Clearinghouse, 2012).

As a response to the bacteria, cytokines, neutrophils, and other substances are activated and cause epithelial cell necrosis. These bacteria produce substances that damage the mucosa. Urease produced by *H. pylori* breaks down urea into ammonia, which neutralizes the acidity of the stomach. Urease can be detected through laboratory testing to confirm the *H. pylori* infection. Also, the helical shape of *H. pylori* allows the bacterium to burrow into the mucus layer of the stomach and become undetectable by the body's immune cells. Although this bacterium does not cause illness in most people, it is a major risk factor for peptic and duodenal ulcers and gastric cancer (McCance et al., 2014).

Gastric ulcers usually develop in the antrum of the stomach near acid-secreting mucosa. When a break in the mucosal barrier occurs (such as that caused by *H. pylori* INFECTION), hydrochloric acid injures the epithelium. Gastric ulcers may then result from back-diffusion of acid or dysfunction of the pyloric sphincter (Fig. 55-1). Without normal functioning of the pyloric sphincter, bile refluxes (backs up) into the stomach. This reflux of bile acids may break the integrity of the mucosal barrier, which leads to mucosal INFLAMMATION. Toxic agents and bile then destroy the membrane of the gastric mucosa.

Gastric emptying is often delayed in patients with gastric ulceration. This causes regurgitation of duodenal contents, which worsens the gastric mucosal injury. Decreased blood flow to the gastric mucosa may also alter the defense barrier and thereby allow ulceration to occur. Gastric ulcers are deep and penetrating, and they usually occur on the lesser curvature of the stomach, near the pylorus (Fig. 55-2).

Most *duodenal ulcers* occur in the upper portion of the duodenum. They are deep, sharply demarcated lesions that penetrate through the mucosa and submucosa into the muscularis propria (muscle layer). The floor of the ulcer consists of a necrotic area residing on granulation tissue and surrounded by areas of fibrosis (McCance et al., 2014).

The main feature of a duodenal ulcer is high gastric acid secretion, although a wide range of secretory levels are found. In patients with duodenal ulcers, pH levels are low (excess acid) in the duodenum for long periods. Protein-rich meals, calcium,

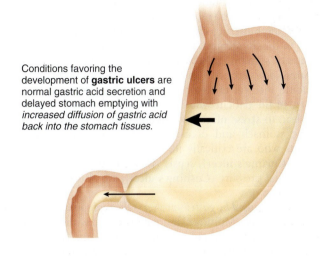

Conditions favoring the development of **gastric ulcers** are normal gastric acid secretion and delayed stomach emptying with *increased diffusion of gastric acid back into the stomach tissues.*

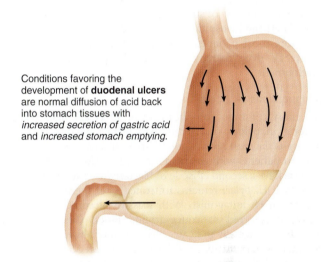

Conditions favoring the development of **duodenal ulcers** are normal diffusion of acid back into stomach tissues with *increased secretion of gastric acid and increased stomach emptying.*

FIG. 55-1 The pathophysiology of peptic ulcer.

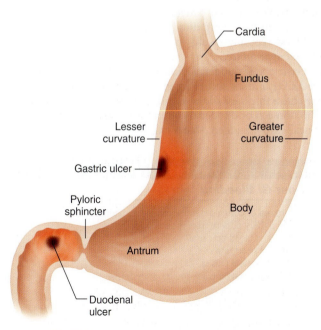

FIG. 55-2 The most common sites for peptic ulcers.

and vagus nerve excitation stimulate acid secretion. Combined with hypersecretion, a rapid emptying of food from the stomach reduces the buffering effect of food and delivers a large acid bolus to the duodenum. Inhibitory secretory mechanisms and pancreatic secretion may be insufficient to control the acid load.

Stress ulcers are acute gastric mucosal lesions occurring after an acute medical crisis or trauma, such as sepsis or a head injury. In the patient who is NPO for major surgery, gastritis may lead to **stress ulcers**, which are multiple shallow erosions of the stomach and occasionally the proximal duodenum. Patients who are critically ill, especially those with extensive burns (**Curling's ulcer**), sepsis (ischemic ulcer), or increased intracranial pressure (**Cushing's ulcer**), are also susceptible to these ulcers.

Bleeding caused by gastric erosion is the main manifestation of acute stress ulcers. Multifocal lesions associated with stress ulcers occur in the stomach and proximal duodenum. These lesions begin as areas of ischemia and evolve into erosions and ulcerations that may progress to massive hemorrhage. Little is known of the exact etiology of stress ulcers. Stress ulcers are associated with lengthened hospital stay and increased mortality rates. Therefore most patients who have major trauma or surgery receive IV drug therapy (e.g., PPI) to prevent stress ulcer development.

Complications of Ulcers

The most common complications of PUD are hemorrhage, perforation, pyloric obstruction, and intractable disease. *Hemorrhage is the most serious complication.* It tends to occur more often in patients with *gastric* ulcers and in older adults. Many patients have a second episode of bleeding if underlying INFECTION with *H. pylori* remains untreated or if therapy does not include an H_2 antagonist. With massive bleeding the patient vomits bright red or coffee-ground blood (**hematemesis**). Hematemesis usually indicates bleeding at or above the duodenojejunal junction (upper GI bleeding) (Chart 55-3).

Minimal bleeding from ulcers is manifested by occult blood in a dark, "tarry" stool (**melena**). The digestion of blood within the duodenum and small intestine may result in this black stool. Melena may occur in patients with gastric ulcers but is more common in those with duodenal ulcers. Gastric acid digestion of blood typically results in a granular dark vomitus (*coffee-ground appearance*).

Gastric and duodenal ulcers can perforate and bleed (Fig. 55-3). *Perforation* occurs when the ulcer becomes so deep that the entire thickness of the stomach or duodenum is worn away. The stomach or duodenal contents can then leak into the peritoneal cavity. Sudden, sharp PAIN begins in the midepigastric

region and spreads over the entire abdomen. The amount of pain correlates with the amount and type of GI contents spilled. The classic pain causes the patient to be apprehensive. The abdomen is tender, rigid, and boardlike (**peritonitis**). The patient often assumes a "fetal" position to decrease the tension on the abdominal muscles. He or she can become severely ill within hours. Bacterial septicemia and hypovolemic shock follow. Peristalsis diminishes, and paralytic ileus develops. *Peptic ulcer perforation is a surgical emergency and can be life threatening!*

Pyloric (gastric outlet) obstruction (blockage) occurs in a small percentage of patients and is manifested by vomiting caused by stasis and gastric dilation. Obstruction occurs at the pylorus (the gastric outlet) and is caused by scarring, edema, INFLAMMATION, or a combination of these factors.

Symptoms of obstruction include abdominal bloating, nausea, and vomiting. When vomiting persists, the patient may have hypochloremic (metabolic) alkalosis from loss of large quantities of acid gastric juice (hydrogen and chloride ions) in the vomitus. Hypokalemia may also result from the vomiting or metabolic alkalosis.

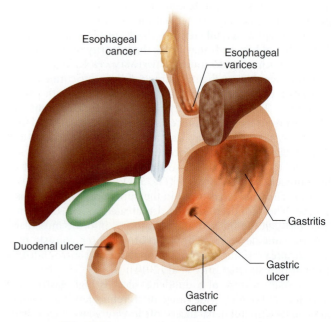

FIG. 55-3 Common causes of upper GI bleeding.

Esophageal cancer

Esophageal varices

Gastritis

Duodenal ulcer

Gastric ulcer

Gastric cancer

> **CHART 55-3** **Key Features**
> **Upper GI Bleeding**
>
> * Bright red or coffee-ground vomitus (hematemesis)
> * Melena (tarry or dark, sticky) stools
> * Decreased blood pressure
> * Increased heart rate
> * Weak peripheral pulses
> * Acute confusion (in older adults)
> * Vertigo
> * Dizziness or light-headedness
> * Syncope (loss of consciousness)
> * Decreased hemoglobin and hematocrit

Many patients with ulcers have a single episode with no recurrence. However, *intractability* may develop from complications of ulcers, excessive stressors in the patient's life, or an inability to adhere to long-term therapy. He or she no longer responds to conservative management, or recurrences of symptoms interfere with ADLs. In general, the patient continues to have recurrent pain and discomfort despite treatment. Those who fail to respond to traditional treatments or who have a relapse after discontinuation of therapy are referred to a gastroenterologist.

Etiology and Genetic Risk

Peptic ulcer disease is caused most often by bacterial INFECTION with *H. pylori* and NSAIDs. NSAIDs (e.g., ibuprofen) break down the mucosal barrier and disrupt the mucosal protection mediated systemically by cyclooxygenase (COX) inhibition. COX-2 inhibitors (celecoxib [Celebrex]) are less likely to cause mucosal damage but place patients at high risk for cardiovascular events, such as myocardial infarction. In addition, NSAIDs cause decreased endogenous prostaglandins, resulting in local gastric mucosal injury (Lilley et al., 2014). GI complications from NSAID use can occur at any time, even after long-term uncomplicated use. NSAID-related ulcers are difficult to treat, even with long-term therapy, because these ulcers have a high rate of recurrence.

Certain substances may contribute to gastroduodenal ulceration by altering gastric secretion, which produces localized damage to mucosa and interferes with the healing process. For example, corticosteroids (e.g., prednisone), theophylline (Theo-Dur), and caffeine stimulate hydrochloric acid production. Patients receiving radiation therapy may also develop GI ulcers. Other risk factors for PUD are the same as for gastritis (see Chart 55-1).

Incidence and Prevalence

PUD affects millions of people across the world. However, health care provider visits, hospitalizations, and the mortality rate for PUD have decreased in the past few decades. The use of proton pump inhibitors and *H. pylori* treatment may explain these declines.

❖ PATIENT-CENTERED COLLABORATIVE CARE

◆ Assessment

History. Collect data related to the causes and risk factors for peptic ulcer disease (PUD). Question the patient about factors that can influence the development of PUD, including alcohol intake and tobacco use. Note if certain foods such as tomatoes or caffeinated beverages precipitate or worsen symptoms. Information regarding actual or perceived daily stressors should also be obtained.

A history of current or past medical conditions focuses on GI problems, particularly any history of diagnosis or treatment for *H. pylori* INFECTION. Review all prescription and OTC drugs the patient is taking. Specifically inquire whether the patient is taking corticosteroids, chemotherapy, or NSAIDs. Also ask whether he or she has ever undergone radiation treatments. Assess whether the patient has had any GI surgeries, especially a partial gastrectomy, which can cause chronic gastritis.

A history of GI upset, PAIN and its relationship to eating and sleep patterns, and actions taken to relieve pain are also important. Inquire about any changes in the character of the pain, because this may signal the development of complications. For example, if pain that was once intermittent and relieved by food and antacids becomes constant and radiates to the back or upper quadrant, the patient may have ulcer perforation. However, many people with active duodenal or gastric ulcers report having no ulcer symptoms.

Physical Assessment/Clinical Manifestations. Physical assessment findings may reveal epigastric tenderness, usually located at the midline between the umbilicus and the xiphoid process. *If perforation into the peritoneal cavity is present, the patient typically has a rigid, boardlike abdomen accompanied by rebound tenderness and pain.* Initially, auscultation of the abdomen may reveal hyperactive bowel sounds, but these may diminish with progression of the disorder.

Dyspepsia *(indigestion) is the most commonly reported symptom associated with PUD.* It is typically described as sharp, burning, or gnawing PAIN. Some patients may perceive discomfort as a sensation of abdominal pressure or of fullness or hunger. Older adults often have more nausea and vomiting rather than abdominal discomfort (DeRanieri, 2013). Specific differences between gastric and duodenal ulcers are listed in Table 55-2.

Gastric ulcer PAIN often occurs in the upper epigastrium with localization to the left of the midline and is aggravated by food. *Duodenal* ulcer pain is usually located to the right of or below the epigastrium. The pain associated with a duodenal ulcer occurs 90 minutes to 3 hours *after* eating and often awakens the patient at night (McCance et al., 2014). Pain may also be exacerbated (made worse) by certain foods (e.g., tomatoes, hot spices, fried foods, onions, alcohol, caffeine drinks) and certain drugs (e.g., NSAIDs, corticosteroids). Perform a comprehensive pain assessment.

Nausea and vomiting may be symptoms accompanying ulcer disease, most commonly with pyloric sphincter dysfunction. It may result from gastric stasis associated with pyloric obstruction. Appetite is generally maintained in patients with a peptic ulcer unless pyloric obstruction is present.

To assess for fluid volume deficit that occurs from bleeding, take orthostatic blood pressures and monitor for signs and symptoms of dehydration. Also assess for dizziness, especially when the patient is upright, because this is a symptom of fluid volume deficit. Older adults often experience dizziness when they get out of bed and are at risk for falls.

> ### ? NCLEX EXAMINATION CHALLENGE
> #### *Physiological Integrity*
>
> When taking a history of a client diagnosed with a gastric ulcer, which assessment findings does the nurse expect? **Select all that apply**.
> A. Vomiting
> B. Weight loss
> C. Epigastric pain at night
> D. Relief of epigastric pain after eating
> E. Melena

Psychosocial Assessment. Assess the impact of ulcer disease on the patient's lifestyle, occupation, family, and social and leisure activities. Evaluate the impact that lifestyle changes will have on the patient and family. This assessment may reveal information about the patient's ability to adhere to the prescribed treatment regimen and to obtain the needed social support to alter his or her lifestyle.

TABLE 55-2 **Differential Features of Gastric and Duodenal Ulcers**

FEATURE	GASTRIC ULCER	DUODENAL ULCER
Age	Usually 50 yr or older	Usually 50 yr or older
Gender	Male/female ratio of 1.1:1	Male/female ratio of 1:1
Blood group	No differentiation	Most often type O
General nourishment	May be malnourished	Usually well nourished
Stomach acid production	Normal secretion or hyposecretion	Hypersecretion
Occurrence	Mucosa exposed to acid-pepsin secretion	Mucosa exposed to acid-pepsin secretion
Clinical course	Healing and recurrence	Healing and recurrence
Pain	Occurs 30-60 min after a meal; at night: rarely Worsened by ingestion of food	Occurs 1½-3 hr after a meal; at night: often awakens patient between 1 and 2 AM Relieved by ingestion of food
Response to treatment	Healing with appropriate therapy	Healing with appropriate therapy
Hemorrhage	Hematemesis more common than melena	Melena more common than hematemesis
Malignant change	Perhaps in less than 10%	Rare
Recurrence	Tends to heal, and recurs often in the same location	60% recur within 1 yr; 90% recur within 2 yr
Surrounding mucosa	Atrophic gastritis	No gastritis

Laboratory Assessment. There are three simple, noninvasive tests to detect *H. pylori* in the patient's blood, breath, or stool. Although the breath and stool tests are considered more accurate, *serologic testing* for *H. pylori* antibodies is the most common method to confirm *H. pylori* INFECTION. The *urea breath test* involves swallowing a capsule, liquid, or pudding that contains urea with a special carbon atom. After a few minutes the patient exhales, and if the special carbon atom is found, the bacterium is present. The *stool antigen test* is performed on a stool sample provided by the patient and is tested for *H. pylori* antigens. Patients who have venous bleeding from a peptic ulcer may have *decreased hemoglobin and hematocrit* values. The *stool* may also be positive for occult (not seen) blood if bleeding is present (Pagana & Pagana, 2014).

Imaging Assessment. If perforation is suspected, the health care provider may request a *chest and abdomen x-ray series,* but other diagnostic tests are more helpful in diagnosis.

Other Diagnostic Assessment. *The major diagnostic test for PUD is esophagogastroduodenoscopy (EGD), which is the most accurate means of establishing a diagnosis.* Direct visualization of the ulcer crater by EGD allows the health care provider to take specimens for *H. pylori* testing and for biopsy and cytologic studies for ruling out gastric cancer. The rapid urease test can confirm a quick diagnosis because urease is produced by the bacteria in the gastric mucosa. EGD may be repeated at 4- to 6-week intervals while the health care provider evaluates the progress of healing in response to therapy. Chapter 52 describes this test in more detail.

GI bleeding may be tested using a *nuclear medicine scan*. No special preparation is required for this scan. The patient is injected with a contrast medium (usually Tc99m), and the GI system is scanned for the presence of bleeding after a waiting period. A second scan may be done 1 to 2 days after the bleeding is treated to determine if the interventions were effective.

◆ **Analysis**

The priority NANDA-I nursing diagnoses and collaborative problems for patients with peptic ulcer disease (PUD) include:
1. Acute Pain or Chronic Pain related to gastric and/or duodenal ulceration (NANDA-I)
2. Upper GI bleeding related to perforation

◆ **Planning and Implementation**

Managing Acute Pain or Chronic Pain

Planning: Expected Outcomes. The patient with PUD is expected to report PAIN control as evidenced by no more than a 3 on a 0-to-10 pain intensity scale.

Interventions. PUD causes significant discomfort that impacts many aspects of daily living. Interventions to manage PAIN focus on drug therapy and dietary changes.

Drug Therapy. The primary purposes of drug therapy in the treatment of PUD are to (1) provide PAIN relief, (2) eliminate *H. pylori* INFECTION, (3) heal ulcerations, and (4) prevent recurrence. Several different regimens can be used. In selecting a therapeutic drug regimen, the health care provider considers the efficacy of the treatment, the anticipated side effects, the ability of the patient to adhere to the regimen, and the cost of the treatment.

Although numerous drugs have been evaluated for the treatment of *H. pylori* INFECTION, no single agent has been used successfully against the organism. A common drug regimen for *H. pylori* infection is PPI–triple therapy, which includes a proton pump inhibitor (PPI) such as lansoprazole (Prevacid) plus two antibiotics such as metronidazole (Flagyl, Novonidazol ✦) and tetracycline (Ala-Tet, Panmycin, Nu-Tetra ✦) or clarithromycin (Biaxin, Biaxin XL) and amoxicillin (Amoxil, Amoxi ✦) for 10 to 14 days. Some health care providers may prefer to use quadruple therapy, which contains combination of a proton pump inhibitor (PPI), any two commonly used antibiotics as described above, with the addition of bismuth (Pepto-Bismol). Bismuth therapy is often used in patients who are allergic to penicillin-based medications.

CONSIDERATIONS FOR OLDER ADULTS

Patient-Centered Care QSEN

Many older adults have *H. pylori* infection that is undiagnosed because of vague symptoms associated with physiologic changes of aging and comorbidities that mask dyspepsia. Because the average age of gastric cancer diagnosis is 70 years, it is important to teach older adults about the symptoms of PUD and to consider *H. pylori* screening. Early detection and aggressive treatment can prevent PUD and gastric cancer.

Hyposecretory drugs reduce gastric acid secretions and are therefore used for both peptic ulcer disease (PUD) and gastritis management. The primary prescribed drugs include proton pump inhibitors and H_2-receptor antagonists (Chart 55-4).

Proton pump inhibitors (PPIs) is the drug class of choice for treating patients with acid-related disorders. Examples include omeprazole (Prilosec), lansoprazole (Prevacid), rabeprazole (Aciphex), pantoprazole (Protonix), and esomeprazole (Nexium). These drugs suppress the H,K–ATPase enzyme

CHART 55-4 Common Examples of Drug Therapy
Peptic Ulcer Disease

DRUG AND USUAL DOSAGE	PURPOSE OF DRUG	NURSING INTERVENTIONS	RATIONALES
Antacids			
Magnesium hydroxide with aluminum hydroxide (Maalox, Mylanta) 50-80 mEq orally 1 hr and 3 hr after meals and at bedtime	Increases pH of gastric contents by deactivating pepsin	Give 2 hr after meals and at bedtime.	Hydrogen ion load is high after ingestion of foods.
		Use liquid rather than tablets.	Suspensions are more effective than chewable tablets.
		Do not give other drugs within 1-2 hr of antacids.	Antacids interfere with absorption of other drugs.
		Assess patients for a history of renal disease.	Hypermagnesemia may result.
			These antacids have a high sodium content.
			These antacids contain magnesium, which cannot be excreted by poorly functioning kidneys, thus causing toxicity.
		Assess the patient for a history of heart failure.	Inadequate renal perfusion from heart failure decreases the ability of the kidneys to excrete magnesium, thus causing toxicity.
		Observe the patient for the side effect of diarrhea.	Magnesium often causes diarrhea.
Aluminum hydroxide (Amphojel) 50-80 mEq orally 1 hr and 3 hr after meals and at bedtime		Give 1 hr after meals and at bedtime.	Hydrogen ion load is high after ingestion of food.
		Use liquid rather than tablets if palatable.	Suspensions are more effective than chewable tablets.
		Do not give other drugs within 1-2 hr of antacids.	Antacids interfere with absorption of other drugs.
		Observe patients for the side effect of constipation. If constipation occurs, consider alternating with magnesium antacid.	Aluminum causes constipation, and magnesium has a laxative effect.
		Use for patients with renal failure.	Aluminum binds with phosphates in the GI tract.
			This antacid does not contain magnesium.
H_2 Antagonists (Blockers)			
Ranitidine (Zantac) 150 mg orally twice daily or 300 mg orally at bedtime; 50 mg IV every 6 hr or 8 mg/hr IV (continuous)	Decreases gastric acid secretions by blocking histamine receptors in parietal cells	Give single dose at bedtime for treatment of GI ulcers, heartburn, and PUD. **NOTE:** IV famotidine or IV ranitidine may also be given to prevent surgical stress ulcers.	Bedtime administration suppresses nocturnal acid production.
Famotidine (Pepcid) 40 mg orally once daily or in two divided doses; 20 mg IV every 12 hr			
Nizatidine (Axid) 150 mg orally twice daily or 300 mg at bedtime			
Mucosal Barrier Fortifiers			
Sucralfate (Carafate, Sulcrate ✦) 1 g orally four times daily or 2 g twice daily	Binds with bile acids and pepsin to protect stomach mucosa	Give 1 hr before and 2 hr after meals and at bedtime.	Food may interfere with drug's adherence to mucosa.
		Do not give within 30 min of giving antacids or other drugs.	Antacids may interfere with effect.
Bismuth Subsalicylate (Pepto-Bismol) 525 mg (30 mL) orally four times daily	Stimulates mucosal protection and prostaglandin production Inhibits *H. pylori* from binding to mucosal lining	Patients cannot take aspirin while on this drug. **NOTE:** May cause the stools to be discolored black.	Aspirin is a salicylic acid and will lead to overdose of aspirin.

Continued

CHART 55-4   Common Examples of Drug Therapy—cont'd

Peptic Ulcer Disease

DRUG AND USUAL DOSAGE	PURPOSE OF DRUG	NURSING INTERVENTIONS	RATIONALES
Proton Pump Inhibitors			
Omeprazole (Prilosec, Losec ♣) 20-40 mg orally daily	Suppresses H,K–ATPase enzyme system of gastric acid secretion Indications for short-term and long-term use for PUD, symptomatic heartburn, and *H. pylori* treatment	Have patients take capsule whole; do not crush. Give 30 minutes before the main meal of the day.	Delayed-release capsules allow absorption after granules leave the stomach. The proton pump is activated by the presence of food. Therefore the drug needs a chance to work before the patient eats.
Lansoprazole (Prevacid) 15-30 mg orally daily		Give 30 min before the main meal of the day.	The proton pump is activated by the presence of food. Therefore the drug needs a chance to work before the patient eats.
Rabeprazole (Aciphex) 20 mg orally once daily		Take after the morning meal. Do not crush capsule.	Drug promotes healing and symptom relief of duodenal ulcers. Drug is a sustained-release capsule.
Pantoprazole (Protonix) 40 mg orally or IV daily for 7-10 days		Do not crush. IV form must be given on a pump with a filter and in a separate line. Do not give Protonix IV with other IV drugs. **NOTE:** This medication may have several adverse drug interactions. Be aware of the patient's other medications.	Drug is enteric-coated. Given IV, drug precipitates easily. The IV form is not compatible with most other drugs. This medication will alter how other drugs are metabolized, either increasing or decreasing their effectiveness.
Esomeprazole (Nexium) 20 or 40 mg orally daily (or IV daily for 7-10 days)		Assess for hepatic impairment. Do not give Nexium IV with other IV drugs. **NOTE:** This medication may have several adverse drug interactions. Be aware of the patient's other medications.	Patients with severe hepatic problems need a low dose. The IV form is not compatible with most other drugs. This medication will alter how other drugs are metabolized, either increasing or decreasing the effectiveness.
Prostaglandin Analogs			
Misoprostol (Cytotec) 200 mcg orally four times daily	Synthetic prostaglandin that stimulates mucosal protection and decreases gastric acid secretions Helps resist mucosal injury in patients taking NSAIDs and/or high-dose corticosteroids	Avoid magnesium-containing antacids. **NOTE:** Do not use in pregnant women.	Both misoprostol and magnesium-containing antacids can cause diarrhea. Can cause abortion, premature birth, or birth defects.
Antimicrobials			
Clarithromycin (Biaxin) 500 mg orally three times daily	Treats *H. pylori* infection	Be aware that the drug should be given with caution to patients with renal impairment; monitor renal function lab values.	The drug can increase the patient's BUN level and should be monitored.
Amoxicillin (Amoxil) 1 g orally twice daily	Treats *H. pylori* infection	Teach patients to take the drug with food or immediately after a meal.	The drug can cause GI disturbances, including nausea, vomiting, and diarrhea.
Tetracycline 500 mg orally four times daily	Treats *H. pylori* infection	Teach patients to take the drug at least 1 hour before meals or 2 hours after meals. Teach patients to avoid direct sunlight and wear sunscreen when outdoors.	Dairy products and other foods may interfere with drug absorption. The drug can cause the skin to burn due to photosensitivity.
Metronidazole (Flagyl) 250 mg orally three times daily and at bedtime	Treats *H. pylori* infection	Teach patients to take the drug with food. Teach patients to avoid alcohol during drug therapy and for at least 3 days after therapy is completed.	The drug can cause GI disturbances, especially nausea. The patient can experience a drug-alcohol reaction, including severe nausea, vomiting, and headache.

system of gastric acid production, and several of them are available as over-the-counter (OTC) drugs (Lilley et al., 2014).

Omeprazole, lansoprazole, and esomeprazole are each available as delayed-release capsules designed to release their contents after they pass through the stomach. Omeprazole and lansoprazole may be dissolved in a sodium bicarbonate solution and given through any feeding tube. Bicarbonate protects the dissolved omeprazole and lansoprazole granules in gastric acid. Therefore the drugs are still absorbed correctly. These capsules can also be opened. The enteric-coated capsules can be put in apple juice or orange juice and given through a large-bore feeding tube. Rabeprazole (Aciphex) and pantoprazole (Protonix) are enteric-coated tablets that quickly dissolve after the tablet has moved through the stomach and should not be crushed before giving them. Several of the PPIs are also available in an IV form, which may be helpful for patients who are NPO.

Some patients use these PPIs for years and perhaps a lifetime. However, these drugs should not be used for a prolonged period because, over time, they may contribute to osteoporotic-related fractures, especially spinal fractures in older women (Kwok et al., 2010). Omeprazole (Prilosec and Prilosec OTC) reduces the effect of clopidogrel (Plavix), an antiplatelet drug. Teach patients to tell their health care provider if they are taking clopidogrel. PPIs should not be discontinued abruptly to prevent rebound activation of the proton pump. Therefore, a step-down approach over several days is recommended (Zarowitz, 2011).

H₂-receptor antagonists are drugs that block histamine-stimulated gastric secretions. These drugs may also be used for indigestion and gastritis. Lower-dose forms are available in over-the-counter (OTC) products. H₂-receptor antagonists block the action of the H₂ receptors of the parietal cells, thus inhibiting gastric acid secretion. Two of the most common drugs are famotidine (Pepcid) and nizatidine (Axid) and are available as Pepcid OTC and Axid AR in OTC form. These drugs are typically administered in a single dose at bedtime and are used for 4 to 6 weeks in combination with other therapy.

Antacids buffer gastric acid and prevent the formation of pepsin. They may help small duodenal ulcers heal but are usually not used alone as drug therapy. Liquid suspensions are the most therapeutic form, but tablets may be more convenient and enhance adherence. The most widely used preparations are mixtures of aluminum hydroxide and magnesium hydroxide. This combination overcomes the unpleasant GI side effects of either of these preparations when used alone. Mylanta and Maalox are examples of this type of combination antacid formulation. The aluminum and magnesium hydroxide combination products neutralize well at small doses. These products must be administered cautiously to patients with renal impairment because elimination is reduced and excessive amounts are retained in the body.

! NURSING SAFETY PRIORITY (QSEN)
Drug Alert

Teach the patient that to achieve a therapeutic effect, sufficient antacid must be ingested to neutralize the hourly production of acid. For optimal effect, take antacids about 2 hours after meals to reduce the hydrogen ion load in the duodenum. Antacids may be effective from 30 minutes to 3 hours after ingestion. If taken on an empty stomach, they are quickly evacuated. Thus the neutralizing effect is reduced (Lilley et al., 2014).

Calcium carbonate (Tums) is a potent antacid, but it triggers gastrin release, causing a rebound acid secretion. Therefore its use in acid inhibition is not recommended.

Antacids can interact with certain drugs such as phenytoin (Dilantin), tetracycline (Ala-Tet, Nu-Tetra ♣), and ketoconazole (Nizoral) and interfere with their effectiveness. Ask what other drugs the patient is using before a specific antacid is prescribed. Other drugs are given 1 to 2 hours before or after the antacid. Inform the patient that flavored antacids, especially wintergreen, should be avoided. The flavoring increases the emptying time of the stomach. Thus the desired effect of the antacid is negated.

Teach the patient with past or present heart failure to avoid antacids with high sodium content, such as aluminum hydroxide, magnesium hydroxide, sodium bicarbonate, and simethicone combination products (Gelusil and Mylanta). Magaldrate (Riopan) has the lowest sodium concentration.

Sucralfate (Carafate) is a *mucosal barrier fortifier* (protector) that forms complexes with proteins at the base of a peptic ulcer. This protective coat prevents further digestive action of both acid and pepsin. Sucralfate does not inhibit acid secretion. Rather, it binds bile acids and pepsins, reducing injury from these substances. The drug may be used in conjunction with H₂-receptor antagonists and antacids but should not be administered within 1 hour of the antacid. Sucralfate is given on an empty stomach 1 hour before each meal and at bedtime. The main side effect of this drug is constipation.

Bismuth subsalicylate (Pepto-Bismol) inhibits *H. pylori* from binding to the mucosal lining and stimulates mucosal protection and prostaglandin production. Teach patients they cannot take aspirin while on this drug because aspirin is a salicylic acid and could cause an overdose of salicylates. Patients should also be taught that this medication may cause the stools to be discolored black. This discoloration is temporary and harmless.

Nutrition Therapy. The role of diet in the management of ulcer disease is controversial. There is no evidence that dietary restriction reduces gastric acid secretion or promotes tissue healing, although a bland diet may assist in relieving symptoms. Food itself acts as an antacid by neutralizing gastric acid for 30 to 60 minutes. An increased rate of gastric acid secretion, called *rebound,* may follow.

! NURSING SAFETY PRIORITY (QSEN)
Action Alert

Teach the patient with peptic ulcer disease to avoid substances that increase gastric acid secretion. This includes caffeine-containing beverages (coffee, tea, cola). Both caffeinated and decaffeinated coffees should be avoided, because coffee contains peptides that stimulate gastrin release (McCance et al., 2014).

Teach the patient to exclude any foods that cause discomfort. A bland, nonirritating diet is recommended during the acute symptomatic phase. Bedtime snacks are avoided because they may stimulate gastric acid secretion. Eating six smaller meals daily may help, but this regimen is no longer a regular part of therapy. No evidence supports the theory that eating six meals daily promotes healing of the ulcer. This practice may actually stimulate gastric acid secretion. Patients should avoid alcohol and tobacco because of their stimulatory effects on gastric acid secretion.

Complementary and Alternative Therapies. Teach patients about complementary and alternative therapies that can reduce stress, including hypnosis and imagery. For example, the use of yoga and meditation techniques has demonstrated a beneficial effect on anxiety disorders. Many have suggested that GI disorders result from the dysfunction of both the GI tract itself and the brain. This means that emotional stress is thought to worsen GI disorders such as peptic ulcer disease. Yoga may alter the activities of the central and autonomic nervous systems.

Many herbs, such as powders of slippery elm and marshmallow root, quercetin, and licorice, are used commonly by patients with gastritis and PUD. These herbs may help heal inflamed tissue and increase blood flow to the gastric mucosa. Other substances include zinc, vitamin C, essential fatty acids, acidophilus, vitamin A, and glutamine. Table 55-1 provides a list of therapies that have been used by many patients with gastric disorders. Many of them have been scientifically supported in animal studies but have not been thoroughly studied in humans.

> ### ! NURSING SAFETY PRIORITY (QSEN)
> #### Action Alert
>
> Teach the patient who has peptic ulcer disease to seek immediate medical attention if experiencing any of these symptoms:
> - Sharp, sudden, persistent, and severe epigastric or abdominal PAIN
> - Bloody or black stools
> - Bloody vomit or vomit that looks like coffee grounds

Managing Upper GI Bleeding

Planning: Expected Outcomes. The patient with upper GI bleeding (often called *upper GI hemorrhage* or *UGH*) is expected to have bleeding promptly and effectively controlled and vital signs within normal limits.

Interventions. Blood loss from PUD results in high morbidity and mortality. Fluid volume loss secondary to vomiting can lead to dehydration and electrolyte imbalances. Interventions aimed at managing complications associated with PUD include prevention and/or management of bleeding, perforation, and gastric outlet obstruction. In some cases surgical treatment of complications becomes necessary.

Nonsurgical Management. Because prevention or early detection of complications is needed to obtain a positive clinical outcome, monitor the patient carefully and immediately report changes to the health care provider. The type of intervention selected will depend on the type and severity of the complication.

Emergency: Upper GI Bleeding. The patient who is actively bleeding has a life-threatening emergency. He or she needs supportive therapy to prevent hypovolemic shock and possible death.

> ### ! NURSING SAFETY PRIORITY (QSEN)
> #### Critical Rescue
>
> *The first priority for care of the patient with upper GI bleeding is to maintain **a**irway, **b**reathing, and **c**irculation (ABCs). Provide oxygen and other ventilatory support as needed. Start two large-bore IV lines for replacing fluids and blood. Monitor vital signs, hematocrit, and oxygen saturation.*

The purpose of managing hypovolemia is to expand intravascular fluid in a patient who is volume depleted. Carefully monitor the patient's fluid status, including intake and output. *Fluid replacement in older adults should be closely monitored to prevent fluid overload.* Serum electrolytes are also assessed because depletions from vomiting or nasogastric suctioning must be replaced. Volume replacement with isotonic solutions (e.g., 0.9% normal saline solution, lactated Ringer's solution) should be started immediately. The health care provider may prescribe blood products such as packed red blood cells to expand volume and correct a low hemoglobin and hematocrit. For patients with active bleeding, fresh frozen plasma may be given if the prothrombin time is 1.5 times higher than the midrange control value.

Continue to monitor the patient's hematocrit, hemoglobin, and coagulation studies for changes from the baseline measurements. With mild bleeding (less than 500 mL), slight feelings of weakness and mild perspiration may be present. When blood loss exceeds 1 L/24 hr, manifestations of shock may occur, such as hypotension, chills, palpitations, diaphoresis, and a weak, thready pulse.

A combination of several different treatments, including nasogastric tube (NGT) placement and lavage, endoscopic therapy, interventional radiologic procedures, and acid suppression, can be used to control acute bleeding and prevent rebleeding. If the patient is actively bleeding at home, he or she is usually admitted to the emergency department for GI lavage. If the patient is already a patient in the hospital, lavage can be done at the bedside. After the bleeding has stopped, H_2-receptor antagonists, proton pump inhibitors, and antacids are the primary drugs used.

Nasogastric Tube Placement and Lavage. Upper GI bleeding often requires the primary care provider or nurse to insert a large-bore nasogastric tube (NGT) to:
- Determine the presence or absence of blood in the stomach
- Assess the rate of bleeding
- Prevent gastric dilation
- Administer lavage

Although not performed as commonly today, **gastric lavage** requires the insertion of a large-bore NGT with instillation of a room-temperature solution in volumes of 200 to 300 mL. There is no evidence that sterile saline or sterile water is better than tap water for this procedure. Follow agency protocol for the solution that is required. The solution and blood are repeatedly withdrawn manually until returns are clear or light pink and without clots. Instruct the patient to lie on the left side during this procedure. The NGT may remain in place for a few days or be removed after lavage.

Endoscopic Therapy. Endoscopic therapy via an esophagogastroduodenoscopy (EGD) can assist in achieving homeostasis during an acute hemorrhage by isolating the bleeding artery to embolize (clot) it. A physician can insert instruments through the endoscope during the procedure to stop bleeding in three different ways: (1) inject chemicals into the bleeding site; (2) treat the bleeding area with heat, electric current, or laser; or (3) close the affected blood vessels with a band or clip. During the EGD, a specialized endoscopy nurse and technician assist the physician with the procedure.

Pre-EGD nursing care involves inserting one or two large-bore IV catheters if they are not in place. A large catheter allows the patient to receive IV moderate sedation (e.g., midazolam

[Versed] and an opioid) and possibly a blood transfusion. Keep the patient NPO for 4 to 6 hours before the procedure. This prevents the risk for aspiration and allows the endoscopist to view and treat the ulcer. A patient must sign a consent form before the EGD *after* the physician informs him or her about the procedure.

> ## ! NURSING SAFETY PRIORITY (QSEN)
> ### *Action Alert*
>
> After esophagogastroduodenoscopy (EGD), monitor vital signs, heart rhythm, and oxygen saturation frequently until they return to baseline. In addition, frequently assess the patient's ability to swallow saliva. The patient's gag reflex may initially be absent after an EGD because of anesthetizing (numbing) the throat with a spray before the procedure. *After the procedure, do not allow the patient to have food or liquids until the gag reflex is intact!*

Endoscopic therapy is beneficial for most patients with active bleeding. However, ulcers that continue to bleed or continue to rebleed despite endoscopic therapy may require an interventional radiologic procedure or surgical repair.

Interventional Radiologic Procedures. For patients with persistent, massive upper GI bleeding or those who are not surgical candidates, catheter-directed embolization may be performed. This endovascular procedure is usually done if endoscopic procedures are not successful or available. A femoral approach is most often used, but brachial access may be used. An arteriogram is performed to identify the arterial anatomy and find the exact location of the bleeding. The physician injects medication or other material into the blood vessels to stop the bleeding. Post-arteriogram nursing care should be provided after the procedure as described in Chapter 36.

Acid Suppression. Aggressive acid suppression is used to prevent rebleeding. When acute bleeding is stopped and clot formation has taken place within the ulcer crater, the clot remains in contact with gastric contents. Acid-suppressive agents are used to stabilize the clot by raising the pH level of gastric contents. Several types of drugs are used. H_2-receptor antagonists prevent acid from being produced by parietal cells. Proton pump inhibitors prevent the transport of acid across the parietal cell membrane, whereas antacids buffer acid produced in the stomach.

Perforation is managed by immediately replacing fluid, blood, and electrolytes, administering antibiotics, and keeping the patient NPO. Maintain nasogastric suction to drain gastric secretions and thus prevent further peritoneal spillage. Carefully monitor intake and output and check vital signs at least hourly. Monitor the patient for clinical manifestations of septic shock, such as fever, pain, tachycardia, lethargy, or anxiety.

Pyloric obstruction is caused by edema, spasm, or scar tissue. Symptoms of obstruction related to difficulty in emptying the stomach include feelings of fullness, distention, or nausea after eating, as well as vomiting copious amounts of undigested food.

Treatment of obstruction is directed toward restoring fluid and electrolyte balance and decompressing the dilated stomach. Obstruction related to edema and spasm generally responds to medical therapy. First, the stomach must be decompressed with nasogastric suction. Next, interventions are directed at correcting metabolic alkalosis and dehydration. The NGT is clamped after about 72 hours. Check the patient for retention of gastric contents. If the amount retained is not more than 50 mL in 30

minutes, the health care provider may allow oral fluids. In some cases, surgical intervention may be required to treat PUD.

Surgical Management. Evidence-based guidelines for the treatment of PUD that include *H. pylori* treatment and the development of nonsurgical means of controlling bleeding have led to a decline in the need for surgical intervention. In PUD, surgical intervention may be used to:

- Treat patients who do not respond to medical therapy or other nonsurgical procedures
- Treat a surgical emergency that develops as a complication of PUD, such as perforation

Two general surgical approaches are available for PUD—minimally invasive surgery and conventional open surgery.

Minimally invasive surgery (MIS) via laparoscopy (a type of endoscope) may be used to remove a chronic gastric ulcer or treat hemorrhage from perforation. Several small incisions allow access to the stomach and duodenum. The patient may have partial stomach removal (subtotal gastrectomy), pyloroplasty (to open the pylorus), and/or a vagotomy (vagus nerve cutting) to control acid secretion. Acid-reduction surgery may not be necessary due to the increased use of PPIs and endoscopic procedures in the treatment of PUD. The advantages of MIS over traditional open surgical procedures include a shorter hospital stay, fewer complications, less pain, and better, quicker recovery.

> ## ? CLINICAL JUDGMENT CHALLENGE
> ### *Prioritization, Delegation, and Supervision*
>
> A 67-year-old man drove himself to the emergency department (ED) after vomiting bright red blood twice within 6 hours. He is alert and oriented and admits to having a few drinks last weekend. He takes some medicine for his stomach, but he cannot recall the name of the drug. He reports intermittent dizziness and fatigue over the past 2 days. His skin is dry and pale, and his abdomen is slightly distended. He reports pain (4/10) in the mid-epigastric area. His BP is 140/90, heart rate is 110/min, respirations are 24/min, and temperature is 98.9° F.
>
> 1. What actions are appropriate in the care of this patient in the ED? As the nurse in the ER, what additional questions will you ask his wife?
> 2. What data will you document?
> 3. Which task is most appropriate to assign to the nursing assistant working with you?
> 4. You are performing additional assessment and history on the patient. Which finding should you immediately report to the health care provider?
> 5. What medication is the physician most likely to prescribe for emergency treatment of acute and severe bleeding of the patient's ulcer?

Community-Based Care

Patients may be discharged from the hospital as long as there is no evidence of ongoing bleeding, orthostatic changes, or cardiopulmonary distress or compromise. Those discharged after treatment for peptic ulcer disease (PUD) and/or complications secondary to the disease must face several challenges to manage the disease successfully. Long-term adherence to drug therapy may require the patient to take several drugs each day. Permanent lifestyle alterations in nutrition habits must also be made.

Home Care Management. Most patients are discharged to the home to continue their recovery. Those who have had major surgery or have had complications, such as hemorrhage, may require one or two visits from a home care nurse to assess clinical progress, especially if the patient is an older adult (Chart 55-5).

Self-Management Education. The primary focus of home care preparation is patient and family teaching regarding risk factors for the recurrence of PUD. Teach them how to recognize new complications and what to do if they occur, especially abdominal pain; nausea and vomiting; black, tarry stools; and weakness or dizziness.

Teach the patient and family about risk factors for recurring peptic ulcers. Help them plan ways to make needed lifestyle changes. For postsurgical patients, especially those who have undergone partial stomach removal, smaller meals may be required. Other postoperative nutrition changes are described on p. 1142 in the discussion of Self-Management Education in the Gastric Cancer section.

! NURSING SAFETY PRIORITY (QSEN)

Action Alert

Teach the patient who has had surgery for PUD to avoid any OTC product containing aspirin or other NSAID. Emphasize the importance of following the treatment regimen for *H. pylori* infection and healing the ulcer. Emphasize the importance of keeping all follow-up appointments. Help the patient identify situations that cause stress, describe feelings during stressful situations, and develop a plan for coping with stressors.

Health Care Resources. If needed, refer the patient and family to the National Digestive Diseases Information Clearinghouse (www.digestive.niddk.nih.gov/). This group provides information and support to patients who have digestive disorders.

◆ **Evaluation: Outcomes**

Evaluate the care of the patient with peptic ulcer disease (PUD) based on the identified priority patient problems. The expected outcomes are that the patient:

- Does not have active PUD or associated complications
- Verbalizes PAIN relief or control
- Adheres to the drug regimen and lifestyle changes to prevent recurrence and heal the ulcer
- Does not experience an upper GI bleed; if bleeding occurs, it will be promptly and effectively managed

GASTRIC CANCER

Most cancers of the stomach are adenocarcinomas. This type of cancer develops in the mucosal cells that form the innermost lining of any portion or all of the stomach. *Often there are no symptoms in the early stages and the disease is advanced when detected.*

❖ **PATHOPHYSIOLOGY**

Gastric cancer usually begins in the glands of the stomach mucosa. Atrophic gastritis and intestinal metaplasia (abnormal tissue development) are precancerous conditions. Inadequate acid secretion in patients with atrophic gastritis creates an alkaline environment that allows bacteria (especially *H. pylori*) to multiply. This INFECTION causes mucosa-associated lymphoid tissue (MALT) lymphoma, which starts in the stomach (McCance et al., 2014).

Gastric cancers spread by direct extension through the gastric wall and into regional lymphatics, which carry tumor deposits to lymph nodes. Direct invasion of and adherence to adjacent organs (e.g., the liver, pancreas, and transverse colon) may also result. Hematogenous spread via the portal vein to the liver and via the systemic circulation to the lungs and bones is the most common mode of metastasis. Peritoneal seeding of cancer cells from the tumor areas to the omentum, peritoneum, ovary, and pelvic cul-de-sac can also occur.

In people with *advanced* gastric cancer, there is invasion of the muscularis (stomach muscle) or beyond. These lesions are not cured by surgical resection. The overall 5-year survival rate of people with stomach cancer in the United States is poor because most patients have no symptoms until the disease advances.

Etiology and Genetic Risk

INFECTION with *H. pylori* is the largest risk factor for gastric cancer because it carries the cytotoxin-associated gene A *(CagA)* gene. Patients with pernicious anemia, gastric polyps, chronic atrophic gastritis, and achlorhydria (absence of secretion of hydrochloric acid) are 2 to 3 times more likely to develop gastric cancer.

The disease also seems to be positively correlated with eating pickled foods, nitrates from processed foods, and salt added to food. The ingestion of these foods over a long period can lead to atrophic gastritis, a precancerous condition. A low intake of fruits and vegetables is also a risk factor for cancer (McCance et al., 2014).

Gastric surgery seems to increase the risk for gastric cancer because of the eventual development of atrophic gastritis, which results in changes to the mucosa. Patients with Barrett's esophagus from prolonged or severe gastroesophageal reflux disease (GERD) have an increased risk for cancer in the cardia (at the point where the stomach connects to the esophagus).

Incidence and Prevalence

Generally, stomach cancer rates are about twice as high in males as in females. Over 70% of new cases and gastric cancer deaths occur in developing countries (Jemal et al., 2011). The highest incidence rates are in Eastern Asia, Eastern Europe, and South America, and the lowest rates are in North America and parts of Africa (Jemal et al., 2011). The average age for developing gastric cancer is 70 years (American Cancer Society, 2014).

Nurses are uniquely positioned to improve gastric cancer survival rates by ensuring that patients with high risk and suspicious symptoms are assessed and diagnosed early (Bailey, 2011). Maintaining functional status and quality of life during gastric cancer care is a priority for nursing care.

Health Promotion and Maintenance

Teach patients with gastritis and/or *H. pylori* INFECTION to follow the treatment regimen to ensure that gastritis heals and *H. pylori* infection is eliminated. *Stress the need for eating a well-balanced diet and limiting pickled foods, salted foods, and processed foods to help prevent gastric cancer.*

❖ PATIENT-CENTERED COLLABORATIVE CARE

◆ Assessment

Question the patient about known risk factors for the development of gastric cancer. Ask about preferred foods, especially pickled, salted, or smoked foods. Inquire whether the patient has ever been diagnosed with or treated for *H. pylori* INFECTION, gastritis, or pernicious anemia. Note whether he or she has a history of gastric surgery or polyps. Also ask whether any of the patient's immediate relatives have gastric cancer.

Although patients with *early* gastric cancer may be asymptomatic, indigestion (heartburn) and abdominal discomfort are the *most* common symptoms (Chart 55-6). These symptoms are often ignored, however, or a change in diet or use of antacids relieves them. As the tumor grows, these symptoms become more severe and do not respond to nutrition changes or antacids. Epigastric or back PAIN is also an early symptom that may go unrecognized.

In *advanced* gastric cancer, progressive weight loss, nausea, and vomiting can occur. Vomiting represents pronounced dilation, thickening of the stomach wall, or pyloric obstruction. Obstructive symptoms appear earlier with tumors located near the pylorus than with those in the fundus. Patients with advanced disease may have weakness, fatigue, and anemia. Physical assessment findings in advanced disease may be absent, or a palpable epigastric mass may suggest hepatomegaly (liver enlargement) from metastatic disease. Hard, enlarged lymph nodes in the left supraclavicular chain, left axilla, or umbilicus

---

CHART 55-6 Key Features

Early Versus Advanced Gastric Cancer

Early Gastric Cancer*	Advanced Gastric Cancer
• Indigestion	• Nausea and vomiting
• Abdominal discomfort initially relieved with antacids	• Obstructive symptoms
	• Iron deficiency anemia
• Feeling of fullness	• Palpable epigastric mass
• Epigastric, back, or retrosternal pain	• Enlarged lymph nodes
	• Weakness and fatigue
	• Progressive weight loss

*NOTE: Many patients with early gastric cancer have no clinical manifestations.

---

result from metastasis from gastric cancer. Masses on the right suggest metastasis in the perigastric lymph nodes or liver.

In patients with advanced disease, anemia is evidenced by *low hematocrit* and hemoglobin values. Patients may have macrocytic or microcytic anemia associated with decreased iron or vitamin B_{12} absorption. *The stool may be positive for occult blood.* Hypoalbuminemia and *abnormal results of liver tests* (e.g., bilirubin and alkaline phosphatase) occur with advanced disease and with hepatic metastasis. The level of carcinoembryonic antigen (CEA) is elevated in advanced cancer of the stomach (Pagana & Pagana, 2014).

The health care provider uses esophagogastroduodenoscopy (EGD) with biopsy for definitive diagnosis of gastric cancer. (See Chapter 52 for a discussion of nursing care associated with this diagnostic test.) The lesion can be viewed directly, and biopsies of all visible lesions can be obtained to determine the presence of cancer cells. During the endoscopy, an endoscopic (endoluminal) ultrasound (EUS) of the gastric mucosa can also be performed. This technology allows the health care provider to evaluate the depth of the tumor and the presence of lymph node involvement, which permits more accurate staging of the disease. CT, positron emission tomography (PET), and MRI scans of the chest, abdomen, and pelvis are used in determining the extent of the disease and planning therapy.

◆ Interventions

Management of gastric cancer includes drug therapy, radiation, and/or surgery. Drug therapy and radiation may be used instead of surgery or as an adjunct before and/or after surgery.

Nonsurgical Management. The treatment of gastric cancer depends highly on the stage of the disease. Radiation and chemotherapy commonly prolong survival of patients with advanced gastric disease.

Combination *chemotherapy* with multiple cycles of drugs such as cisplatin (Platinol) and epirubicin (Elience) before and after surgery may be given. Bone marrow suppression, nausea, and vomiting are common adverse drug effects. Chapter 22 discusses the general nursing care of patients receiving chemotherapy.

Although gastric cancers are somewhat sensitive to the effects of radiation, the use of this treatment is limited because the disease is often widely spread to other abdominal organs on diagnosis. Organs such as the liver, kidneys, and spinal cord can endure only a limited amount of radiation. Intraoperative radiotherapy (IORT) is available in large tertiary care health care systems. Radiation may be used for palliative management when surgery is not an option.

The most common side effects of radiation include impaired skin integrity, fatigue, and anorexia. Nausea, vomiting, and diarrhea may occur about 1 week after treatment is initiated and diminish a month or more after treatment ends. (See Chapter 22 for more information on radiation therapy.)

Surgical Management. Surgical resection by removing the tumor is the preferred method for treating gastric cancer. The primary surgical procedures for the treatment of gastric cancer are total gastrectomy and subtotal (partial) gastrectomy. In early stages, laparoscopic surgery (minimally invasive surgery [MIS]) plus adjuvant chemotherapy or radiation may be curative. Patients having MIS have less PAIN, shorter hospital stays, rare postoperative complications, and quicker recovery. However, MIS is seldom performed because very few patients are diagnosed in the early stage of the disease.

Most patients with advanced disease are candidates for palliative surgical treatment. Metastasis in the supraclavicular lymph nodes, inguinal lymph nodes, liver, umbilicus, or perirectal wall indicates that the opportunity for cure by resection has been lost. Palliative resection may significantly improve the quality of life for a patient suffering from obstruction, hemorrhage, or PAIN.

Preoperative Care. Before conventional open-approach surgery, a nasogastric tube (NGT) is often inserted and connected to suction to remove secretions and empty the stomach. This allows surgery to take place without contamination of the peritoneal cavity by gastric secretions. The NGT remains in place for a few days *postoperatively* to prevent the accumulation of secretions, which may lead to vomiting or GI distention and pressure on the incision. Patients having laparoscopic surgery (minimally invasive surgery [MIS]) do not require an NGT.

Because weight loss is problematic for patients with gastric cancer, NUTRITION therapy is a vital aspect of preoperative and postoperative management. Preoperatively, compression by the tumor can prevent adequate nutritional intake. To correct malnutrition before surgery, the health care provider may prescribe enteral supplements to the diet and/or total parenteral nutrition (TPN). Vitamin, mineral, iron, and protein supplements are essential to correct nutritional deficits.

Other preoperative nursing measures for the patient undergoing open gastric surgery are the same as those for any patient undergoing abdominal surgery and general anesthesia (see Chapter 14).

Operative Procedures. The surgeon usually removes part or all of the stomach to take out the tumor. When the tumor is located in the mid-portion or distal (lower) portion of the stomach, a subtotal (partial) gastrectomy is typically performed. The omentum, spleen, and relevant nodes are also removed. The surgery may be performed as an MIS procedure or as an open conventional surgical technique, with or without robotic assistance.

For the patient with a removable growth in the proximal (upper) third of the stomach, a total gastrectomy is performed (Fig. 55-4). In this procedure the surgeon removes the entire stomach along with the lymph nodes and omentum. The surgeon sutures the esophagus to the duodenum or jejunum to reestablish continuity of the GI tract. More radical surgery involving removal of the spleen and distal pancreas is controversial, although the Whipple procedure may be used to prolong life. However, the complications of this drastic surgery are very serious and common. For patients with advanced disease, total gastrectomy is performed only when gastric bleeding or obstruction is present.

Patients with tumors at the gastric outlet who are not candidates for subtotal or total gastrectomy may undergo gastroenterostomy for palliation. The surgeon creates a passage between the body of the stomach and the small bowel, often the duodenum.

Postoperative Care. Provide the usual postoperative care for patients who have had general anesthesia to prevent atelectasis, paralytic ileus, wound infection, and peritonitis (see Chapter 16). Document and report any signs and symptoms of these complications immediately to the surgeon. Patients who have the laparoscopic surgery usually have less postoperative PAIN, fewer complications, and a shorter stay in the hospital.

Auscultate the lungs for adventitious sounds (crackles or reduced breath sounds), and monitor for the return of bowel sounds. Take vital signs as appropriate to detect signs of INFECTION or bleeding. Aggressive pulmonary exercises and early ambulation can help prevent respiratory complications and deep vein thrombosis. Also inspect the operative site every 8 to 12 hours for the presence of redness, swelling, or drainage, which indicates wound infection. Keep the head of the bed elevated to prevent aspiration from reflux.

Decreased patency caused by a clogged NGT can result in *acute gastric dilation* after surgery. This problem is manifested by epigastric PAIN and a feeling of fullness, hiccups, tachycardia, and hypotension. Irrigation or replacement of the NGT by request of the surgeon can relieve these symptoms.

Dumping syndrome is a term that refers to a group of vasomotor symptoms that occur after eating. This syndrome is believed to occur as a result of the rapid emptying of food contents into the small intestine, which shifts fluid into the gut, causing abdominal distention. Observe for *early* manifestations of this syndrome, which typically occur within 30 minutes of eating. Symptoms include vertigo, tachycardia, syncope, sweating, pallor, palpitations, and the desire to lie down. Report these manifestations to the surgeon, and encourage the patient to lie down. Monitor the patient for late symptoms.

Late dumping syndrome, which occurs 90 minutes to 3 hours after eating, is caused by a release of an excessive amount of insulin. The insulin release follows a rapid rise in the blood glucose level that results from the rapid entry of high-carbohydrate food into the jejunum. Observe for manifestations, including dizziness, light-headedness, palpitations, diaphoresis, and confusion.

Dumping syndrome is managed by nutrition changes that include decreasing the amount of food taken at one time and eliminating liquids ingested with meals. In collaboration with the dietitian, teach the patient to eat a high-protein, high-fat, low- to moderate-carbohydrate diet (Table 55-3). Acarbose may be used to decrease carbohydrate absorption. A somatostatin analog, octreotide (Sandostatin), 50 mcg subcutaneously 2 or 3 times daily 30 minutes before meals may be prescribed in severe cases. This drug decreases gastric and intestinal hormone secretion and slows stomach and intestinal transit time.

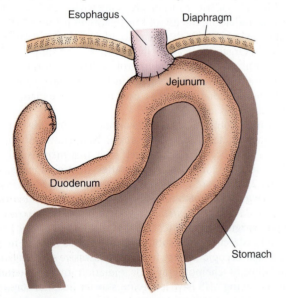

Esophagus
Diaphragm
Jejunum
Duodenum
Stomach

FIG. 55-4 Total gastrectomy with anastomosis of the esophagus to the jejunum (esophagojejunostomy) is the principal surgical intervention for extensive gastric cancer.

TABLE 55-3	**Diet for Dumping Syndrome**		
FOOD GROUP	FOODS ALLOWED OR ENCOURAGED	FOODS TO USE WITH CAUTION	FOODS THAT MUST BE EXCLUDED
Soups		Fluids 1 hr before and after meals	Spicy soups
Meat and meat substitutes	8 oz or more per day: fish, poultry, beef, pork, veal, lamb, eggs, cheese, and peanut butter		Spicy meats or meat substitutes
Potatoes	Potato, rice, pasta, starchy vegetables (small amount)		Highly spiced potatoes or potato substitutes
Bread and cereal	White bread, rolls, muffins, crackers, and cereals (small amount)	Whole-grain bread, rolls, crackers, and cereals	Breads with frosting or jelly, sweet rolls, and coffee cake
Vegetables	Two or more cooked vegetables	Gas-producing vegetables, such as cabbage, onions, broccoli, or raw vegetables	
Fruits	Limit three per day: unsweetened cooked or canned fruits	Unsweetened juice or fruit drinks 30-45 min after meals; fresh fruit	Sweetened fruit or juice
Beverages	Dietetic drinks	Limit to 1 hr after meals; caffeine-containing beverages, such as coffee, tea, and cola; if tolerated, diet carbonated beverages	Milk shakes, malts, and other sweet drinks; regular carbonated beverages and alcohol
Fats	Margarine, oils, shortening, butter, bacon, and salad dressings	Mayonnaise	Any fats with milk products
Desserts	Fruit (see Fruits)	Sugar-free gelatin, pudding, and custard	All sweets, cakes, pies, cookies, candy, ice cream, and sherbet
Seasonings and miscellaneous	Diet jelly, diet syrups, sugar substitutes	Excessive amounts of salt	Excessive amounts of spices, sugar, jelly, honey, syrup, or molasses

General Principles
- Several small meals daily
- Relatively high fat and protein content
- Low roughage
- Relatively low carbohydrate content
- No milk, sweets, or sugars
- Liquid between meals *only*

Alkaline reflux gastropathy, also known as *bile reflux gastropathy*, is a complication of gastric surgery in which the pylorus is bypassed or removed. Endoscopic examination reveals regurgitated bile in the stomach and mucosal hyperemia. Symptoms include early satiety (satisfied quickly with little food), abdominal discomfort, and vomiting.

Delayed gastric emptying is often present after gastric surgery and usually resolves within 1 week. Edema at the anastomosis (surgical connection areas) or adhesions (scar tissue) obstructing the distal loop may cause mechanical blockage. Metabolic causes (e.g., hypokalemia, hypoproteinemia, or hyponatremia) should be considered. The edema is resolved with nasogastric suction, maintenance of fluid and electrolyte balance, and proper nutrition.

Several problems related to NUTRITION develop as a result of partial removal of the stomach, including deficiencies of vitamin B_{12}, folic acid, and iron; impaired calcium metabolism; and reduced absorption of calcium and vitamin D. These problems are caused by a reduction of intrinsic factor. The decrease results from the resection and from inadequate absorption because of rapid entry of food into the bowel. In the absence of intrinsic factor, clinical manifestations of pernicious anemia may occur. Assess for the development of atrophic glossitis secondary to vitamin B_{12} deficiency. In atrophic glossitis, the tongue takes on a shiny, smooth, and "beefy" appearance. The patient may also have signs of anemia secondary to folic acid and iron deficiency. Monitor the complete blood count (CBC) for signs of megaloblastic anemia (low red blood cell [RBC] level) and leukopenia (low white blood cell [WBC] level). These manifestations are corrected by the administration of vitamin B_{12}. The health care provider may also prescribe folic acid or iron preparations.

💡 NCLEX EXAMINATION CHALLENGE
Physiological Integrity

A client has undergone a subtotal (partial) gastrectomy for gastric cancer and is scheduled to begin radiation therapy. What is the most important information for the nurse to include in the teaching plan for this client?
A. Management of alopecia
B. Medication management
C. Nutritional intake
D. Skin care

Community-Based Care

Patients who have undergone total gastrectomy and those who are debilitated with advanced gastric cancer are discharged to home with maximal assistance and support or to a transitional care unit or skilled nursing facility. Patients who have undergone subtotal gastrectomy and are not debilitated may be discharged to home with partial assistance for ADLs. Recurrence of cancer is common, and patients need regular follow-up examinations and imaging assessments. Collaborate with the case manager (CM) to ensure continuity of care and thorough follow-up with diagnostic testing.

Home Care Management. Gastric cancer is a life-threatening illness. Therefore the patient and family members require physical and emotional care. Assess their ability to cope with the disease and the possible need for end-of-life care. The adverse effects of gastric cancer treatment can be debilitating, and patients need to learn symptom management strategies. Hospice programs can help both the patient and the family cope with these physical and emotional needs.

Patients may fear returning home because of their inability for self-management. Enlisting family and health care resources for the patient may ease some of this anxiety. Provide the family with adequate information about community support systems to make the transition to home care easier. If the prognosis is poor, they need continued professional support from case managers, social workers, and/or nurses to cope with death and dying. (See Chapter 7 for a discussion of end-of-life care.)

Self-Management Education. Educate the patient and family about any continuing needs, drug therapy, and nutrition therapy. If patients are discharged to home with surgical dressings, teach the patient and family how to change them. Review the manifestations of incisional infection (e.g., fever, redness, and drainage) that they should report to their surgeon.

Patients who will be receiving radiation therapy or chemotherapy require instructions related to the side effects of these treatments. Nausea and vomiting are common side effects of chemotherapy, and instruction in the use of prescribed antiemetics may be needed. (See Chapter 22 for health teaching for patients receiving chemotherapy or radiation therapy.)

In collaboration with the dietitian, teach the patient and family about the type and quantity of foods that will provide optimal nutritional value. Interventions to minimize dumping syndrome and decrease gastric stimulants are also emphasized (see Table 55-3). Remind the patient to:

- Eat small, frequent meals
- Avoid drinking liquids with meals
- Avoid foods that cause discomfort
- Eliminate caffeine and alcohol consumption
- Begin a smoking-cessation program, if needed
- Receive B_{12} injections, as prescribed
- Lie flat after eating for a short time

Health Care Resources. A home care referral provides continued assessment, assistance, and encouragement to the patient and family. A home care nurse can help with care procedures and provide valuable psychological support. Additional referrals to a dietitian, professional counselor, or clergy/spiritual leader may be necessary. Referral to a hospice agency can be of great assistance for the patient with advanced disease. Hospice care may be delivered in the home or in an institutional setting. Appropriate support groups (e.g., I Can Cope, provided by the American Cancer Society [www.cancer.org/treatment/supportprogramsservices/i-can-cope]) can be a major resource.

NURSING CONCEPTS AND CLINICAL JUDGMENT REVIEW

What might you NOTICE if the patient is experiencing impaired digestion and NUTRITION as a result of a stomach disorder?
- Report of epigastric pain or indigestion before or after a meal
- Report of inability to tolerate certain foods
- Nausea and/or vomiting (with or without blood)
- Melena or frank blood in stools

What should you INTERPRET and how should you RESPOND to a patient experiencing impaired digestion and NUTRITION as a result of a stomach disorder?

Perform and interpret physical assessment, including:
- Taking vital signs
- Observing and documenting assessment findings
- Interpreting laboratory values and other diagnostic findings:

- Presence of *H. pylori*
- Decreased hemoglobin and hematocrit

Respond by:
- Maintaining **a**irway, **b**reathing, and **c**irculation (ABCs)
- Placing the patient in a sitting position or on the left side to prevent aspiration if vomiting
- Preparing to assist with gastric lavage if hematemesis is present

On what should you REFLECT?
- Think about what else you could do to care for this patient.
- Consider with whom you should collaborate to improve or maintain digestion and nutrition for this patient.
- After patient interventions, monitor for changes in vital signs, hematocrit, and hemoglobin.

GET READY FOR THE NCLEX® EXAMINATION!

KEY POINTS

Review these Key Points for each NCLEX Examination Client Needs Category.

Safe and Effective Care Environment
- When caring for patients with gastric health problems, collaborate with the pharmacist, dietitian, health care provider, and/or case manager. **Teamwork and Collaboration** QSEN

Health Promotion and Maintenance
- Refer the patient to the American Cancer Society if gastric cancer is the diagnosis.
- Identify patients at risk for gastritis and PUD, especially older adults who take large amounts of NSAIDs and those with *H. pylori*. **Safety** QSEN
- Teach patients behaviors to prevent PUD, such as avoiding large consumption of caffeine, alcohol, coffee, aspirin, and other NSAIDs. Also teach them to avoid contaminated foods

and water and to avoid smoking (Chart 55-1). **Evidence-Based Practice** QSEN

- Teach patients the importance of adhering to *H. pylori* treatment to prevent the risk for gastric cancer.

Psychosocial Integrity

- Allow patients with gastric cancer to express feelings of grief, fear, and anxiety. **Patient-Centered Care** QSEN
- For patients with advanced gastric cancer, identify the need for end-of-life care, including referral to hospice care.

Physiological Integrity

- Recall that *acute* gastritis causes a rapid onset of epigastric PAIN and dyspepsia; *chronic* gastritis causes vague epigastric PAIN (usually relieved with food) and an intolerance to fatty and spicy foods (Chart 55-2).
- Be aware that assessment findings vary depending on whether the patient has a gastric or duodenal ulcer: patients with gastric ulcers may be malnourished and have PAIN that is worsened by ingestion of food; patients with duodenal ulcers are usually well nourished, have PAIN that is relieved by ingestion of food, and usually awaken with PAIN during the night (Table 55-2).
- For patients who have undergone a gastrectomy, collaborate with the dietitian and instruct the patient regarding diet changes to avoid abdominal distention and dumping syndrome. **Teamwork and Collaboration** QSEN
- Teach patients with abnormal symptoms (e.g., abdominal tenderness, abdominal PAIN that is relieved by food, or PAIN

that becomes worse 3 hours after eating, dyspepsia, melena, and/or distention) to consult with their physician immediately for a prompt diagnosis and treatment.

- Teach patients that hematemesis is a medical emergency and that they should go to the emergency department for prompt treatment. **Safety** QSEN
- Teach the proper administration of antacids (one or two after meals). Tell patients that antacids can interfere with the effectiveness of certain drugs, such as phenytoin (Dilantin).
- Teach the proper administration of H$_2$ antagonists. Explain that they should be given at bedtime (Chart 55-3).
- Teach the proper administration of antisecretory agents, noting that most cannot be crushed because they are sustained-release or enteric-coated tablets.
- Monitor patients with ulcers for any of the signs and symptoms of upper GI bleeding that are listed in Chart 55-4. Report any of these symptoms if noted to a physician immediately.
- After an EGD, monitor the patient's vital signs, heart rhythm, and oxygen saturation frequently until they return to baseline. To prevent aspiration, assess the gag reflex and ensure that it is intact before giving the patient food or fluids. **Safety** QSEN
- Observe the patient for signs and symptoms of dumping syndrome after gastric surgery; teach the manifestations and management of this syndrome. Advise the patient to eat six small meals per day and to consume a diet high in protein and fat but low in carbohydrate-rich foods. Liquids should not be taken with meals. **Evidence-Based Practice** QSEN

Care of Patients with Noninflammatory Intestinal Disorders

Donna D. Ignatavicius

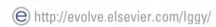

http://evolve.elsevier.com/Iggy/

PRIORITY CONCEPTS

- ELIMINATION
- NUTRITION
- PAIN
- FLUID AND ELECTROLYTE BALANCE

LEARNING OUTCOMES

Safe and Effective Care Environment

1. Prioritize nursing care for the patient with abdominal trauma.
2. Describe the importance of collaborating with health care team members to provide care for patients with colorectal cancer (CRC).

Health Promotion and Maintenance

3. Identify community-based resources for patients with CRC.
4. Teach people health promotion practices to prevent noninflammatory intestinal disorders.
5. Plan health teaching for patients to promote self-management when caring for a colostomy based on patient preferences and values.

Psychosocial Integrity

6. Assess patient and family response to a diagnosis of CRC.

Physiological Integrity

7. Develop a plan of care for a patient undergoing a minimally invasive inguinal hernia repair.
8. Interpret assessment findings for patients with CRC.
9. Explain the role of the nurse in managing the patient with CRC.
10. Develop an evidence-based perioperative plan of care for a patient undergoing a colon resection and colostomy.
11. Explain the differences between assessment findings associated with small-bowel and large-bowel obstructions.
12. Describe the postoperative care for a patient having a hemorrhoid surgical procedure.
13. Identify collaborative interventions for patients with malabsorption disorders.

Intestinal health problems may be inflammatory or noninflammatory. This chapter describes those disorders that are noninflammatory in origin. Noninflammatory intestinal problems often cause rectal bleeding, changing bowel patterns, and abdominal pain. If not diagnosed and managed early, some intestinal problems can lead to inadequate absorption of vital nutrients and therefore affect the need for NUTRITION and ELIMINATION. If these disorders become severe or progress, PAIN and problems with FLUID AND ELECTROLYTE BALANCE may occur.

IRRITABLE BOWEL SYNDROME

❖ PATHOPHYSIOLOGY

Irritable bowel syndrome (IBS) is a functional GI disorder that causes chronic or recurrent diarrhea, constipation, and/or abdominal pain and bloating. It is sometimes referred to as *spastic colon, mucous colon,* or *nervous colon* (Fig. 56-1). *IBS is the most common digestive disorder seen in clinical practice and*

may affect as many as one in five people in the United States (McCance et al., 2014).

In patients with IBS, bowel motility changes and increased or decreased bowel transit times result in changes in the normal *bowel* ELIMINATION pattern to one of these classifications: diarrhea (IBS-D), constipation (IBS-C), alternating diarrhea and constipation (IBS-A), or a mix of diarrhea and constipation (IBS-M). Symptoms of the disease typically begin to appear in young adulthood and continue throughout the patient's life.

The etiology of IBS remains unclear. Research suggests that a combination of environmental, immunologic, genetic, hormonal, and stress factors play a role in the development and course of the disorder. Examples of environmental factors include foods and fluids like caffeinated or carbonated beverages and dairy products. Infectious agents have also been identified. Several studies have found that patients with IBS often have small-bowel bacterial overgrowth, which causes bloating and abdominal distention. Multiple normal flora and pathogenic agents have been identified, including *Pseudomonas*

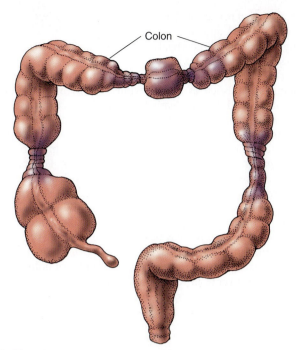

FIG. 56-1 Spastic contractions of the colon as they occur with irritable bowel syndrome.

aeruginosa (Kerckhoffs et al., 2011). Other researchers believe that these agents are less causative and serve as measurable biomarkers for the disease (Malinen et al., 2010).

Immunologic and genetic factors have also been associated with IBS, especially cytokine genes, including pro-inflammatory interleukins (IL), such as IL-6, and tumor necrosis factor (TNF)–alpha (Barkhordari et al., 2010). These findings may provide the basis of targeted drug therapy for the disease.

In the United States, women are 2 times more likely to have IBS than are men. This difference may be the result of hormonal differences. However, in other areas of the world, this distribution pattern may not occur. For example, researchers found that there is not a female predominance for the disease in Asian countries (Gwee et al., 2010).

Considerable evidence relates the role of stress and mental or behavioral illness, especially anxiety and depression, to IBS. Many patients diagnosed with IBS meet the criteria for at least one primary mental health disorder. Some researchers suggest that psychosocial problems may be a cause for IBS (Nicholl et al., 2008). However, the pain and other chronic symptoms of the disease may lead to secondary mental health disorders. For example, when diarrhea is predominant, patients fear that there will be no bathroom facilities available and can become very anxious. As a result, they may not want to leave their homes or travel on trips where bathrooms are not available at all times. The long-term nature of dealing with a chronic disease for which there is no cure can lead to secondary depression in some patients.

❖ PATIENT-CENTERED COLLABORATIVE CARE

◆ Assessment

Ask the patient about a history of weight change, fatigue, malaise, abdominal pain, changes in the bowel pattern (constipation, diarrhea, or an alternating pattern of both) or consistency of stools, and the passage of mucus. Patients with IBS do not usually lose weight. Ask whether the patient has had any GI infections. Collect information on all drugs the patient is taking, because some of them can cause symptoms similar to those of IBS. Ask about the NUTRITION history, including the use of caffeinated drinks or beverages sweetened with sorbitol or fructose, which can cause bloating or diarrhea.

The course of the illness is specific to each patient. Most patients can identify factors that cause exacerbations, such as diet, stress, or anxiety. Food intolerance may be associated with IBS. Dairy products (e.g., for those with lactose intolerance), raw fruits, and grains can contribute to bloating, **flatulence** (gas), and abdominal distention. Patients may keep a food diary to record possible triggers for IBS symptoms.

A flare-up of worsening cramps, abdominal pain, and diarrhea and/or constipation may bring the patient to the health care provider. One of the *most common concerns of patients with IBS is pain in the left lower quadrant of the abdomen.* Assess the location, intensity, and quality of the PAIN. Some patients have internal visceral (organ) hypersensitivity that can cause or contribute to the pain. Nausea may be associated with mealtime and defecation. The constipated stools are small and hard and are generally followed by several softer stools. The diarrheal stools are soft and watery, and mucus is often present in the stools. Patients with IBS often report belching, gas, anorexia, and bloating.

The patient generally appears well, with a stable weight, and nutritional and fluid status are within normal ranges. Inspect and auscultate the abdomen. Bowel sounds vary but are generally within normal range. With constipation, bowel sounds may be hypoactive; with severe diarrhea, they may be hyperactive.

Routine laboratory values (including a complete blood count [CBC], serum albumin, erythrocyte sedimentation rate [ESR], and stools for occult blood) are normal in IBS. Some health care providers request a *hydrogen breath test* (Lindberg, 2009). When small-intestinal bacterial overgrowth or malabsorption of nutrients is present, excess hydrogen is produced. Some of this hydrogen is absorbed into the bloodstream and travels to the lungs where it is exhaled. Patients with IBS often exhale an increased amount of hydrogen.

Teach the patient that he or she will need to be NPO (may have water) for at least 12 hours before the hydrogen breath test. At the beginning of the test, the patient blows into a hydrogen analyzer. Then, small amounts of test sugar are ingested, depending on the purpose of the test, and additional breath samples are taken every 15 minutes for 1 hour or longer (Pagana & Pagana, 2014).

◆ Interventions

The patient with IBS is usually managed on an ambulatory care basis and learns self-management strategies. Interventions include health teaching, drug therapy, and stress reduction. Some patients also use complementary and alternative therapies. A holistic approach to patient care is essential for positive outcomes (Bengtsson et al., 2010).

Dietary fiber and bulk help produce bulky, soft stools and establish regular bowel ELIMINATION habits. The patient should ingest about 30 to 40 g of fiber each day. Eating regular meals, drinking 8 to 10 cups of liquid each day, and chewing food slowly help promote normal bowel function.

Drug therapy depends on the main symptom of IBS. The health care provider may prescribe bulk-forming or antidiarrheal agents and/or newer drugs to control symptoms.

For the treatment of *constipation-predominant IBS (IBS-C),* bulk-forming laxatives, such as *psyllium* hydrophilic mucilloid (Metamucil), are generally taken at mealtimes with a glass of water. The hydrophilic properties of these drugs help prevent dry, hard, or liquid stools. *Lubiprostone* (Amitiza) is an oral laxative approved for women with IBS-C, which increases fluid in the intestines to promote bowel ELIMINATION. Teach the patient to take the drug with food and water. Linaclotide (Linzess) is the newest drug for IBS-C, which works by simulating receptors in the intestines to increase fluid and promote bowel transit time. The drug also helps relieve PAIN and cramping that are associated with IBS. Teach patients to take this drug once a day about 30 minutes before breakfast.

Diarrhea-predominant IBS (IBS-D) may be treated with antidiarrheal agents, such as loperamide (Imodium), and psyllium (a bulk-forming agent). *Alosetron* (Lotronex), a selective serotonin (5-HT3) receptor antagonist, may be used with caution in women with IBS-D as a last resort when they have not responded to conventional therapy. Patients taking this drug must agree to report symptoms of colitis or constipation early because it is associated with potentially life-threatening bowel complications, including ischemic colitis (lack of blood flow to the colon).

> **⚠ NURSING SAFETY PRIORITY** (QSEN)
> ### *Drug Alert*
> Before the patient begins alosetron, take a thorough drug (including herbs) history, both prescribed and over the counter, because it interacts with many drugs in a variety of classes. Remind patients that they should not take psychoactive drugs and antihistamines while taking alosetron. Teach patients to report severe constipation, fever, increasing abdominal pain, increasing fatigue, darkened urine, bloody diarrhea, or rectal bleeding as soon as it occurs and stop the drug immediately (Lilley et al., 2014).

Many patients with IBS who have bloating and abdominal distention without constipation have success with *rifaximin* (Xifaxan), an antibiotic that works locally with little systemic absorption (Pimental et al., 2011). Although the drug has been approved for "traveler's diarrhea" and other illnesses, the U.S. Food and Drug Administration (FDA) has not yet approved its use for patients with IBS.

A newer group of drugs called *muscarinic-receptor antagonists* also inhibit intestinal motility. Some of these agents have been approved for people with overactive bladders but have not yet received FDA approval for IBS. Examples in this group currently undergoing clinical trials for IBS are darifenacin (Enablex) and fesoterodine (Toviaz).

For IBS in which PAIN is the predominant symptom, tricyclic antidepressants such as amitriptyline (Elavil) have also been successfully used. It is unclear whether their effectiveness is due to the antidepressant or anticholinergic effects of the drugs. If patients have postprandial (after eating) discomfort, they should take these drugs 30 to 45 minutes before mealtime.

Complementary and Alternative Therapies. For patients with increased intestinal bacterial overgrowth, recommend daily probiotic supplements. *Probiotics* have been shown to be effective for reducing bacteria and successfully alleviating GI symptoms of IBS (Lyra et al., 2010). There is also evidence that peppermint oil capsules may be effective in reducing symptoms for patients with IBS (Pirotta, 2009).

Stress management is also an important part of holistic care. Suggest relaxation techniques, meditation, and/or yoga to help the patient decrease GI symptoms. If the patient is in a stressful work or family situation, personal counseling may be helpful. Based on patient preference, make appropriate referrals or assist in making appointments if needed. The opportunity to discuss problems and attempt creative problem solving is often helpful. Teach the patient that regular exercise is important for managing stress and promoting regular bowel ELIMINATION.

HERNIATION

❖ *PATHOPHYSIOLOGY*

A hernia is a weakness in the abdominal muscle wall through which a segment of the bowel or other abdominal structure protrudes. Hernias can also penetrate through any other defect in the abdominal wall, through the diaphragm, or through other structures in the abdominal cavity.

The most important elements in the development of a hernia are congenital or acquired muscle weakness and increased intra-abdominal pressure. The most significant factors contributing to increased intra-abdominal pressure are obesity, pregnancy, and lifting heavy objects.

The most common types of abdominal hernias (Fig. 56-2) are indirect, direct, femoral, umbilical, and incisional (McCance et al., 2014).

- An indirect inguinal hernia is a sac formed from the peritoneum that contains a portion of the intestine or

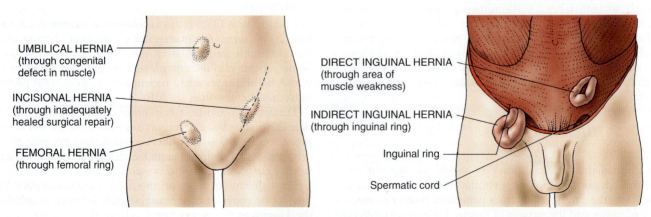

FIG. 56-2 Types of abdominal hernias.

omentum. The hernia pushes downward at an angle into the inguinal canal. In males, indirect inguinal hernias can become large and often descend into the scrotum.

- **Direct inguinal hernias,** in contrast, pass through a weak point in the abdominal wall.
- **Femoral hernias** protrude through the femoral ring. A plug of fat in the femoral canal enlarges and eventually pulls the peritoneum and often the urinary bladder into the sac.
- **Umbilical hernias** are congenital or acquired. Congenital umbilical hernias appear in infancy. Acquired umbilical hernias directly result from increased intra-abdominal pressure. They are most commonly seen in people who are obese.
- **Incisional,** or **ventral, hernias** occur at the site of a previous surgical incision. These hernias result from inadequate healing of the incision, which is usually caused by postoperative wound infections, inadequate nutrition, and obesity.

Hernias may also be classified as reducible, irreducible (incarcerated), or strangulated. A hernia is **reducible** when the contents of the hernial sac can be placed back into the abdominal cavity by gentle pressure. An **irreducible** (incarcerated) hernia cannot be reduced or placed back into the abdominal cavity. *Any hernia that is not reducible requires immediate surgical evaluation.*

A hernia is **strangulated** when the blood supply to the herniated segment of the bowel is cut off by pressure from the hernial ring (the band of muscle around the hernia). If a hernia is strangulated, there is ischemia and obstruction of the bowel loop. *This can lead to necrosis of the bowel and possibly bowel perforation. Signs of strangulation are abdominal distention, nausea, vomiting, pain, fever, and tachycardia.*

Indirect inguinal hernias, the most common type, occur mostly in men because they follow the tract that develops when the testes descend into the scrotum before birth. Direct hernias occur more often in older adults. Femoral and adult umbilical hernias are most common in obese or pregnant women. Incisional hernias can occur in people who have undergone abdominal surgery.

❖ PATIENT-CENTERED COLLABORATIVE CARE

◆ Assessment

The patient with a hernia typically comes to the health care provider's office, clinic, or the emergency department with a report of a "lump" or protrusion felt at the involved site. The development of the hernia may be associated with straining or lifting.

Perform an abdominal assessment inspecting the abdomen when the patient is lying and again when he or she is standing. If the hernia is reducible, it may disappear when the patient is lying flat. The advanced practice nurse or other health care provider asks the patient to strain or perform the Valsalva maneuver and observes for bulging. Auscultate for active bowel sounds. *Absent bowel sounds may indicate obstruction and strangulation, which is a medical emergency!*

To palpate an inguinal hernia, the health care provider gently examines the ring and its contents by inserting a finger in the ring and noting any changes when the patient coughs. *The hernia is never forcibly reduced; that maneuver could cause strangulated intestine to rupture.*

If a male patient suspects a hernia in his groin, the health care provider has him stand for the examination. Using the right hand for the patient's right side and the left hand for the patient's left side, the examiner pushes in the loose scrotal skin with the index finger, following the spermatic cord upward to the external inguinal cord. At this point, the patient is asked to cough and any palpable herniation is noted.

◆ Interventions

The type of treatment selected depends on patient factors such as age, as well as the type and severity of the hernia.

Nonsurgical Management. If the patient is not a surgical candidate (often an older man with multiple health problems), the health care provider may prescribe a truss for an inguinal hernia, usually for men. A **truss** is a pad made with firm material. It is held in place over the hernia with a belt to help keep the abdominal contents from protruding into the hernial sac. If a truss is used, it is applied only after the physician has reduced the hernia if it is not incarcerated. The patient usually applies the truss upon awakening. Teach him to assess the skin under the truss daily and to protect it with a light layer of powder.

Surgical Management. Most hernias are inguinal, and surgical repair is the treatment of choice. Surgery is usually performed on an ambulatory care basis for patients who have no pre-existing health conditions that would complicate the operative course. In same-day surgery centers, anesthesia may be regional or general and the procedure is typically laparoscopic. More extensive surgery, such as a bowel resection or temporary colostomy, may be necessary if strangulation results in a gangrenous section of bowel. Patients undergoing this extensive surgery are hospitalized for a longer period.

A **minimally invasive inguinal hernia repair (MIIHR)** through a laparoscope, also called **herniorrhaphy,** is the surgery of choice. A conventional open herniorrhaphy may be performed when laparoscopy is not appropriate. Patients having minimally invasive surgery (MIS) recover more quickly, have less PAIN, and develop fewer postoperative complications compared with those having the conventional surgery.

In addition to patient education about the procedure, the most important preoperative preparation is to teach the patient to remain NPO for the number of hours before surgery that the surgeon specifies. If same-day surgery is planned, remind the patient to arrange for someone to take him or her home and be available for the rest of the day at home. For patients having an open surgical approach, provide general preoperative care as described in Chapter 14.

During an MIIHR, the surgeon makes several small incisions, identifies the defect, and places the intestinal contents back into the abdomen. During a traditional herniorrhaphy, the surgeon makes an abdominal incision to perform this procedure. When a **hernioplasty** is also performed, the surgeon reinforces the weakened outside abdominal muscle wall with a mesh patch.

The patient who has had MIIHR is discharged from the surgical center in 3 to 5 hours, depending on recovery from anesthesia. Teach him or her to avoid strenuous activity for several days before returning to work and a normal routine. A stool softener may be needed to prevent constipation. Caution patients who are taking oral opioids for pain management to not drive or operate heavy machinery. Teach them to observe incisions for redness, swelling, heat, drainage, and increased pain and promptly report their occurrence to the surgeon. Remind patients that soreness and discomfort rather than severe, acute pain are common after MIS. Be sure to make a follow-up telephone call on the day after surgery to check on the patient's status.

General postoperative care of patients having a hernia repair is the same as that described in Chapter 16 *except that they should avoid coughing.* To promote lung expansion, encourage deep breathing and ambulation. With repair of an indirect inguinal hernia, the physician may suggest a scrotal support and ice bags applied to the scrotum to prevent swelling, which often contributes to pain. Elevation of the scrotum with a soft pillow helps prevent and control swelling.

In the immediate postoperative period, male patients who have had an inguinal hernia repair may experience difficulty voiding. Encourage them to stand to allow a more natural position for gravity to facilitate voiding and bladder emptying. Urine output of less than 30 mL per hour should be reported to the surgeon. Techniques to stimulate voiding such as allowing water to run may also be used. A fluid intake of at least 1500 to 2500 mL daily prevents dehydration, maintains urinary function, and minimizes constipation. A "straight" or intermittent ("in and out") catheterization is required if the patient cannot void. Chart 56-1 summarizes best nursing practices for postoperative care after an MIIHR.

Most patients have uneventful recoveries after a hernia repair. Surgeons generally allow them to return to their usual activities after surgery, with avoidance of straining and lifting for several weeks while subcutaneous tissues heal and strengthen.

Provide oral instructions and a written list of symptoms to be reported, including fever, chills, wound drainage, redness or separation of the incision, and increasing incisional pain. Teach

the patient to keep the wound dry and clean with antibacterial soap and water. Showering is usually permitted in a few days (see Chart 56-1).

COLORECTAL CANCER

❖ PATHOPHYSIOLOGY

Colorectal refers to the colon and rectum, which together make up the large intestine, also known as the *large bowel.* Colorectal cancer (CRC) is cancer of the colon or rectum and is a major health problem worldwide. In the United States it is one of the most common malignancies. Patients often consider a diagnosis of cancer as a "death sentence," but colon cancer for many patients is highly curable.

Tumors occur in different areas of the colon, with about two thirds occurring within the rectosigmoid region as shown in Fig. 56-3. Most CRCs are **adenocarcinomas,** which are tumors that arise from the glandular epithelial tissue of the colon. They develop as a multi-step process affecting immunity, resulting in a number of molecular changes. These changes include loss of key tumor suppressor genes and activation of certain oncogenes that alter colonic mucosa cell division. The increased proliferation of the colonic mucosa forms polyps that can transform into malignant tumors. Most CRCs are believed to arise from adenomatous polyps that present as visible protrusions from the mucosal surface of the bowel (McCance et al., 2014).

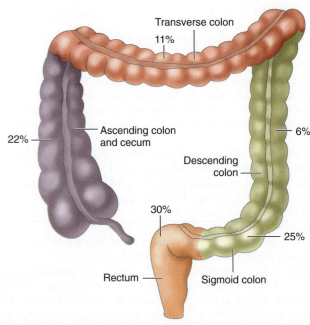

FIG. 56-3 The incidence of cancer in relation to colorectal anatomy.

CHART 56-1 **Best Practice for Patient Safety & Quality Care** (QSEN)

Nursing Care of the Postoperative Patient Having a Minimally Invasive Inguinal Hernia Repair (MIIHR)

- Monitor vital signs, especially blood pressure, for indications of internal bleeding.
- Assess and manage incisional pain with oral analgesics; report and document severe pain that does not respond to drug therapy immediately.
- Encourage deep breathing after surgery; avoid excessive coughing.
- Encourage ambulation with assistance as soon as possible after surgery (within the first few hours).
- Apply ice packs as prescribed to the surgical area.
- Assist the patient to void by standing the first time after surgery.
- Teach patients at discharge to:
  - Rest for several days after surgery.
  - Observe the incision sites for redness or drainage, and report these findings to the surgeon.
  - Shower after 24 to 36 hours after removing any bandage (do not remove Steri-Strips); be aware that the Steri-Strips will fall off in about a week.
  - Monitor temperature for the first few days, and report the occurrence of a fever.
  - Do not lift more than 10 pounds until allowed by the surgeon.
  - Avoid constipation by eating high-fiber foods and drinking extra fluids.
  - Return to work when allowed by the surgeon, usually in 1 to 2 weeks, depending on the patient's work responsibilities.

CRC can metastasize by direct extension or by spreading through the blood or lymph. The tumor may spread locally into the four layers of the bowel wall and into neighboring organs. It may enlarge into the lumen of the bowel or spread through the lymphatics or the circulatory system. The circulatory system is entered directly from the primary tumor through blood vessels in the bowel or via the lymphatic system. The liver is the most common site of metastasis from circulatory spread. Metastasis to the lungs, brain, bones, and adrenal glands may also occur. Colon tumors can also spread by peritoneal seeding during surgical resection of the tumor. Seeding may occur when a tumor is excised and cancer cells break off from the tumor into the peritoneal cavity. For this reason, special techniques are used during surgery to decrease this possibility.

Complications related to the increasing growth of the tumor locally or through metastatic spread include bowel obstruction or perforation with resultant peritonitis, abscess formation, and fistula formation to the urinary bladder or the vagina. The tumor may invade neighboring blood vessels and cause frank bleeding. Tumors growing into the bowel lumen can gradually obstruct the intestine and eventually block it completely. Those extending beyond the bowel wall may place pressure on neighboring organs (uterus, urinary bladder, and ureters) and cause symptoms that mask those of the cancer. Chapter 21 discusses cancer pathophysiology in more detail.

Etiology and Genetic Risk

The major risk factors for the development of colorectal cancer (CRC) include being older than 50 years, genetic predisposition, personal or family history of cancer, and/or diseases that predispose the patient to cancer such as familial adenomatous polyposis (FAP), Crohn's disease, and ulcerative colitis (McCance et al., 2014). Only a small percentage of colorectal cancers are familial and transmitted genetically.

GENETIC/GENOMIC CONSIDERATIONS

Patient-Centered Care QSEN

People with a first-degree relative (parent, sibling, or child) diagnosed with colorectal cancer (CRC) have 3 to 4 times the risk for developing the disease. An autosomal dominant inherited genetic disorder known as *familial adenomatous polyposis (FAP)* accounts for 1% of CRCs. FAP is the result of one or more mutations in the adenomatous polyposis coli (APC) gene (McCance et al., 2014). In these very young patients, thousands of adenomatous polyps develop over the course of 10 to 15 years and have nearly a 100% chance of becoming malignant. By 20 years of age, most patients require surgical intervention, usually a colectomy with ileostomy or ileoanal pull-through, to prevent cancer. Chemotherapy may also be used for cancer prevention.

Hereditary nonpolyposis colorectal cancer (HNPCC) is another autosomal dominant disorder and accounts for a small percentage of all colorectal cancers. HNPCC is also caused by gene mutations, including *MLH1* and *MLH2*. People with these mutations have an 80% chance of developing CRC at an average of 45 years of age. They also tend to have a higher incidence of endometrial, ovarian, stomach, and ureteral cancers (Nussbaum et al., 2007). Genetic testing is available for both of these familial CRC syndromes. Refer patients for genetic counseling and possible testing if the patient prefers.

The role of infectious agents in the development of colorectal and anal cancer continues to be investigated. Some lower GI cancers are related to *Helicobacter pylori*, *Streptococcus bovis*, John Cunningham (JC) virus, and human papilloma virus (HPV) infections.

There is also strong evidence that long-term smoking, obesity, physical inactivity, and heavy alcohol consumption are risk factors for colorectal cancer (American Cancer Society [ACS], 2014). A high-fat diet, particularly animal fat from red meats, increases bile acid secretion and anaerobic bacteria, which are thought to be carcinogenic within the bowel. Diets with large amounts of refined carbohydrates that lack fiber decrease bowel transit time.

Incidence and Prevalence

Colorectal cancer (CRC) is the third most common cause of cancer death in the United States (ACS, 2014). It is not common before 40 years of age, but the incidence in younger adults is slowly increasing, most likely due to increases in HPV infections (Stubenrauch, 2010). The overall incidence of CRC has decreased over the past 20 years, probably as a result of increased cancer screenings (Wilkes, 2013). The disease is most common in African Americans, and their survival rate is lower than that of Euro-Americans (Caucasians). The possible reasons for this difference include less use of diagnostic testing (especially colonoscopy), decreased access to health care, lack of health insurance, cultural beliefs, and lack of education about the need for early cancer detection (Good et al., 2010; Oliver et al., 2012).

Health Promotion and Maintenance

People at risk can take action to decrease their chance of getting CRC and/or increase their chance of surviving it. For example, those whose family members have had hereditary CRC should be genetically tested for FAP and HNPCC. If gene mutations are present, the person at risk can collaborate with the health care team to decide what prevention or treatment plan to implement.

Teach people about the need for diagnostic screening. An integrative review by Rawl et al. (2012) found that most efforts to increase CRC screening interventions have focused on Euro-Americans. However, other groups are more at risk than Euro-Americans (see the Evidence-Based Practice box).

When an adult turns 40 years of age, he or she should discuss with the health care provider the need for colon cancer screening. The interval depends on level of risk. People of average risk who are 50 years of age and older and without a family history should undergo regular CRC screening. The screening includes fecal occult blood testing (FOBT) and colonoscopy every 10 years or double-contrast barium enema every 5 years. People who have a personal or family history of the disease should begin screening earlier and more frequently. Teach all patients to follow the American Cancer Society recommendations for CRC screening listed in Chart 56-2.

Teach people, regardless of risk, to modify their diets as needed to decrease fat, refined carbohydrates, and low-fiber foods. Encourage baked or broiled foods, especially those high in fiber and low in animal fat. Remind people to eat increased amounts of brassica vegetables, including broccoli, cabbage, cauliflower, and sprouts. These foods help protect the intestinal mucosa from colon cancer (ACS, 2014).

Teach people the hazards of smoking, excessive alcohol, and physical inactivity. Refer patients as needed for smoking- or alcohol-cessation programs, and recommend ways to increase regular physical exercise. These programs are discussed elsewhere in this text.

CHART 56-2   Best Practice for Patient Safety & Quality Care QSEN

Screening Recommendations for Men and Women Ages 50 Years and Older at Average Risk for Colorectal Cancer

PROCEDURE: CHOICE OF ONE OF THE FOLLOWING	INTERVAL AFTER SCREENING INITIATED AT AGE 50 YEARS	COMMENTS
FOBT and sigmoidoscopy	Every 5 years	FOBT procedure: two or three samples from three consecutive bowel movements obtained at home; tested by physician or nurse
OR Double-contrast barium enema	Every 5 years	
OR Colonoscopy	Every 10 years	

FOBT, Fecal occult blood testing.

EVIDENCE-BASED PRACTICE QSEN

How Effective are Interventions to Promote Colorectal Cancer Screening?

Rawl, S.M., Menon, U., Burness, A., & Breslau, E.S. (2012). Interventions to promote colorectal cancer screening: An integrative review. *Nursing Outlook, 60*(4), 172-181.

The researchers reviewed and evaluated 33 randomized trials of colorectal cancer screening (CRC) interventions that were published between 1997 and 2007 using a modified version of TREND criteria to draw conclusions. Significant effects of interventions were reported in 6 of the 10 trials that studied fecal occult blood testing, 4 of the 7 trials that focused on colonoscopy or sigmoidoscopy interventions, and 9 of the 16 trials that included any type of recommended CRC screening method. Most of these trials studied effectiveness of interventions in Euro-Americans (Caucasians). The authors concluded that further research is needed to examine factors that contribute to successful CRC screening. Other groups in addition to Euro-Americans should also be studied, especially given their risk for the disease.

Level of Evidence: 1
This study was an integrative review and evaluation of multiple randomized trials.

Commentary: Implications for Practice and Research
Nurses should continue to teach people about the need for and effectiveness of screening to detect CRC early for the best possible outcome. Further research is needed to explore the factors that enable many patients to have regular screening for CRC. This research should include diverse subjects for comparison and analysis.

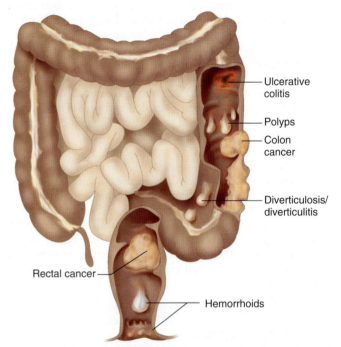

FIG. 56-4 Common causes of lower gastrointestinal bleeding.

Labels: Ulcerative colitis; Polyps; Colon cancer; Diverticulosis/diverticulitis; Rectal cancer; Hemorrhoids

❖ PATIENT-CENTERED COLLABORATIVE CARE

◆ Assessment

History. When taking a history, ask the patient about major risk factors, such as a personal history of breast, ovarian, or endometrial cancer (which can spread to the colon); ulcerative colitis; Crohn's disease; familial polyposis or adenomas; polyps; or a family history of CRC. Also assess the patient's participation in age-specific cancer screening guidelines. Ask about whether the patient uses tobacco and/or alcohol. Assess the patient's usual physical activity level.

Ask whether vomiting and changes in bowel ELIMINATION habits, such as constipation or change in shape of stool with or without blood, have been noted. The patient may also report

fatigue (related to anemias), abdominal fullness, vague abdominal PAIN, or unintentional weight loss. These symptoms suggest advanced disease.

Physical Assessment/Clinical Manifestations. The clinical manifestations of CRC depend on the location of the tumor. *However, the most common signs are rectal bleeding, anemia, and a change in stool consistency or shape.* Stools may contain microscopic amounts of blood that are not noticeably visible, or the patient may have mahogany (dark)-colored or bright red stools (Fig. 56-4). Gross blood is not usually detected with tumors of the right side of the colon but is common (but not massive) with tumors of the left side of the colon and the rectum.

Tumors in the transverse and descending colon result in symptoms of obstruction as growth of the tumor blocks the passage of stool. The patient may report "gas pains," cramping, or incomplete evacuation. Tumors in the rectosigmoid colon are associated with **hematochezia** (the passage of red blood via the rectum), straining to pass stools, and narrowing of stools. Patients may report dull pain. Right-sided tumors can grow quite large without disrupting bowel patterns or appearance because the stool consistency is more liquid in this part of the colon. These tumors ulcerate and bleed intermittently, so stools can contain mahogany (dark)-colored blood. A mass may be palpated in the lower right quadrant, and the patient often has anemia secondary to blood loss.

Examination of the abdomen begins with assessment for obvious distention or masses. Visible peristaltic waves accompanied by high-pitched or "tinkling" bowel sounds may indicate a partial bowel obstruction from the tumor. Total absence of bowel sounds indicates a complete bowel obstruction. Palpation and percussion are performed by the advanced practice nurse or other health care provider to determine whether the spleen or liver is enlarged or whether masses are present along the colon. The examiner may also perform a digital rectal examination to palpate the rectum and lower sigmoid colon for masses. Fecal occult blood screening should not be done with a specimen from a rectal examination because it is not reliable. A positive result could occur as a result of tissue trauma during the examination.

Psychosocial Assessment. The psychological consequences associated with a diagnosis of colorectal cancer (CRC) are many. Patients must cope with a diagnosis that instills fear and anxiety about treatment, feelings that life has been disrupted, a need to search for ways to deal with the diagnosis, and concern about family. They also have questions about why colon cancer affected them, as well as concerns about PAIN, possible body changes, and possible death. In addition, if the cancer is believed to have a genetic origin, there is anxiety concerning implications for immediate family members.

Laboratory Assessment. Hemoglobin and hematocrit values are often decreased as a result of the intermittent bleeding associated with the tumor. For some patients, that may be the first indication that a tumor is present. CRC that has metastasized to the liver causes liver enzymes to be elevated.

A positive test result for occult blood in the stool (**fecal occult blood test [FOBT]**) indicates bleeding in the GI tract. These tests can yield false-positive results if certain vitamins or drugs are taken before the test. Remind the patient to avoid aspirin, vitamin C, and red meat for 48 hours before giving a stool specimen. Also assess whether the patient is taking anti-inflammatory drugs (e.g., ibuprofen, corticosteroids, or salicylates). These drugs should be discontinued for a designated period before the test. Two or three separate stool samples should be tested on 3 consecutive days. Negative results do not completely rule out the possibility of CRC.

Carcinoembryonic antigen (CEA), an oncofetal antigen, is elevated in many people with CRC. The normal value is less than 5 ng/mL (Pagana & Pagana, 2014). This protein is not specifically associated with the colorectal cancer, and it may be elevated in the presence of other benign or malignant diseases and in smokers. CEA is often used to monitor the effectiveness of treatment and to identify disease recurrence.

Imaging Assessment. A *double-contrast barium enema* (air and barium are instilled into the colon) or colonoscopy provides better visualization of polyps and small lesions than does a barium enema alone. These tests may show an occlusion in the bowel where the tumor is decreasing the size of the lumen.

CT or *MRI* of the chest, abdomen, pelvis, lungs, or liver helps confirm the existence of a mass, the extent of disease, and the location of distant metastases. CT-guided virtual colonoscopy is growing in popularity and may be more thorough than

traditional colonoscopy. However, treatments or surgeries cannot be performed when a virtual colonoscopy is used.

Other Diagnostic Assessment. A *sigmoidoscopy* provides visualization of the lower colon using a fiberoptic scope. Polyps can be visualized, and tissue samples can be taken for biopsy. Polyps are usually removed during the procedure. A *colonoscopy* provides views of the entire large bowel from the rectum to the ileocecal valve. As with sigmoidoscopy, polyps can be seen and removed and tissue samples can be taken for biopsy. *Colonoscopy is the definitive test for the diagnosis of colorectal cancer. These procedures and associated nursing care are discussed in Chapter 52.*

◆ Analysis

The priority NANDA-I nursing diagnoses and collaborative problems for patients with colorectal cancer (CRC) include:
1. Potential for colorectal cancer metastasis
2. Grieving related to cancer diagnosis (NANDA-I)

◆ Planning and Implementation

The primary approach to treating CRC is to remove the entire tumor or as much of the tumor as possible to prevent or slow metastatic spread of the disease. A patient-centered collaborative care approach is essential to meet the desired outcomes.

Preventing or Controlling Metastasis

Planning: Expected Outcomes. The patient with colorectal cancer (CRC) is expected to not have the cancer spread to vital organs. Thus the patient's life expectancy will be increased and the quality of life will be improved. However, if metastasis is present, the desired outcome is to ensure that the patient is as comfortable as possible and PAIN is well-managed.

Interventions. Although surgical resection is the primary method used to control the disease, several adjuvant (additional) therapies are used. Adjuvant therapies are administered before or after surgery to achieve a cure and prevent recurrence, if possible.

Nonsurgical Management. The type of therapy used is based on the pathologic staging of the disease. Several staging systems may be used.

The administration of preoperative *radiation therapy* has not improved overall survival rates for colon cancer, but it has been effective in providing local or regional control of the disease. Postoperative radiation has not demonstrated any consistent improvement in survival or recurrence. However, as a palliative measure, radiation therapy may be used to control PAIN, hemorrhage, bowel obstruction, or metastasis to the lung in advanced disease. For rectal cancer, unlike colon cancer, radiation therapy is almost always a part of the treatment plan. Reinforce information about the radiation therapy procedure to the patient and family, and monitor for possible side effects (e.g., diarrhea, fatigue). Chapter 22 describes the general nursing care of patients undergoing radiation therapy.

Adjuvant *chemotherapy* after primary surgery is recommended for patients with stage II or stage III disease to interrupt the DNA production of cells and destroy them. The drugs of choice are IV 5-fluorouracil (5-FU) with leucovorin (LV) (folinic acid) (5-FU/LV), capecitabine (Xeloda), or a combination of drugs referred to as *FOLFOX4*. The most frequently used FOLFOX4 combination for metastatic CRC is fluorouracil (5-FU), leucovorin (LV), and oxaliplatin (Eloxatin), a platinum analog. These drugs cannot discriminate between cancer and healthy cells. Therefore common side effects are diarrhea, mucositis, leukopenia, mouth ulcers, and peripheral neuropathy (Lilley et al., 2014).

Bevacizumab (Avastin) and panitumumab (Vectibix) are antiangiogenesis drugs, also known as *vascular endothelial growth factor (VEGF) inhibitors,* approved for advanced CRC. These drugs reduce blood flow to the growing tumor cells, thereby depriving them of necessary nutrients needed to grow (Wilkes, 2013). A VEGF inhibitor is usually given in combination with other chemotherapeutic agents.

Cetuximab (Erbitux), a monoclonal antibody known as an *epidermal growth factor receptor (EGFR) antagonist,* may also be given in combination with other drugs for advanced disease (Wilkes, 2013). This drug works by blocking factors that promote cancer cell growth.

Intrahepatic arterial chemotherapy, often with 5-FU, may be administered to patients with liver metastasis. Patients with CRC also receive drugs for relief of symptoms, such as opioid analgesics and antiemetics. Chapter 22 describes care of patients receiving chemotherapy in detail.

Surgical Management. Surgical removal of the tumor with margins free of disease is the best method of ensuring removal of CRC. The size of the tumor, its location, the extent of metastasis, the integrity of the bowel, and the condition of the patient determine which surgical procedure is performed for colorectal cancer (Table 56-1). Many regional lymph nodes are removed and examined for presence of cancer. The number of lymph nodes that contain cancer is a strong predictor of prognosis. The most common surgeries performed are **colon resection** (removal of the tumor and regional lymph nodes) with reanastomosis, **colectomy** (colon removal) with *colostomy (temporary or permanent) or ileostomy/ileoanal pull-through,* and **abdominoperineal (AP) resection**. A **colostomy** is the surgical creation of an opening of the colon onto the surface of the abdomen. An AP resection is performed when rectal tumors are present. The surgeon removes the sigmoid colon, rectum, and anus through combined abdominal and perineal incisions.

For patients having a colon resection, minimally invasive surgery (MIS) via laparoscopy is commonly performed today. This procedure results in shorter hospital stays, less pain, fewer complications, and quicker recovery compared with the conventional open surgical approach (Kapritsou et al., 2013).

Preoperative Care. Reinforce the physician's explanation of the planned surgical procedure. The patient is told as accurately as possible what anatomic and physiologic changes will occur with surgery. The location and number of incision sites and drains are also discussed.

Before evaluating the tumor and colon during surgery, the surgeon may not be able to determine whether a colostomy (or less commonly, an ileostomy) will be necessary. The patient is told that a colostomy is a possibility. If a colostomy is planned, the surgeon consults a certified wound, ostomy, continence nurse (CWOCN) to recommend optimal placement of the ostomy. The CWOCN teaches the patient about the rationale and general principles of ostomy care. In many settings, he or she marks the patient's abdomen to indicate a potential ostomy site that will decrease the risk for complications such as interference of the undergarments or a prosthesis with the ostomy appliance. Table 56-2 describes the role of the CWOCN.

The patient who requires low rectal surgery (e.g., AP resection) is faced with the risk for postoperative sexual dysfunction and urinary incontinence after surgery as a result of nerve damage during surgery. The surgeon discusses the risk for these problems with the patient before surgery and allows him or her to verbalize concerns and questions related to this risk. Reinforce teaching about abdominal surgery performed for the patient under general anesthesia, and review the routines for turning and deep breathing (see Chapter 14). Teach the patient about the method of PAIN management to be used after surgery such as IV patient-controlled analgesia (PCA), epidural analgesia, or other method.

If the bowel is not obstructed or perforated, elective surgery is planned. The patient may be instructed to thoroughly clean the bowel, or "bowel prep," to minimize bacterial growth and prevent complications. Mechanical cleaning is accomplished with laxatives and enemas or with "whole-gut lavage." The use of bowel preps is controversial, and some surgeons do not recommend it because of patient discomfort. Older adults may become dehydrated from this process.

TABLE 56-1   Surgical Procedures for Colorectal Cancers in Various Locations

Right-Sided Colon Tumors
- Right hemicolectomy for smaller lesions
- Right ascending colostomy or ileostomy for large, widespread lesions
- Cecostomy (opening into the cecum with intubation to decompress the bowel)

Left-Sided Colon Tumors
- Left hemicolectomy for smaller lesions
- Left descending colostomy for larger lesions

Sigmoid Colon Tumors
- Sigmoid colectomy for smaller lesions
- Sigmoid colostomy for larger lesions
- Abdominoperineal resection for large, low sigmoid tumors (near the anus) with colostomy (the rectum and the anus are completely removed, leaving a perineal wound)

Rectal Tumors
- Resection with anastomosis or pull-through procedure (preserves anal sphincter and normal elimination pattern)
- Colon resection with permanent colostomy
- Abdominoperineal resection with colostomy

TABLE 56-2   Preoperative Assessment by the CWOCN Prior to Ostomy Surgery

Key Points of Psychosocial Assessment
- Patient's and family's level of knowledge of disease and ostomy care
- Patient's educational level
- Patient's physical limitations (particularly sensory)
- Support available to patient
- Patient's type of employment
- Patient's involvement in activities such as hobbies
- Financial concerns regarding purchase of ostomy supplies

Key Points of Physical Assessment
- Before marking the placement for the ostomy, the nurse specialist considers:
  - Contour of the abdomen in lying, sitting, and standing positions
  - Presence of skinfolds, creases, bony prominences, and scars
  - Location of belt line
  - Location that is easily visible to the patient
  - Possible location in the rectus muscle

CWOCN, Certified wound, ostomy, continence nurse.

To reduce the risk for infection, the surgeon may prescribe one dose of oral or IV antibiotics to be given before the surgical incision is made. Teach patients that a nasogastric tube (NGT) may be placed for decompression of the stomach after surgery. A peripheral IV or central venous catheter is also placed for fluid and electrolyte replacement while the patient is NPO after surgery. Patients having minimally invasive surgeries do not need an NGT.

The patient with colorectal cancer faces a serious illness with long-term consequences of the disease and treatment. A case manager or social worker can be very helpful in identifying patient and family needs, as well as ensuring continuity of care and support.

Operative Procedures. For the conventional open surgical approach, the surgeon makes a large incision in the abdomen and explores the abdominal cavity to determine whether the tumor can be removed. For a colon resection, the portion of the colon with the tumor is excised and the two open ends of the bowel are irrigated before **anastomosis** (reattachment) of the colon. If an anastomosis is not feasible because of the location of the tumor or the bowel is inflamed, a colostomy is created.

A temporary or permanent colostomy may be created in the ascending, transverse, descending, or sigmoid colon (Fig. 56-5). One of several techniques is used to construct a colostomy. A loop **stoma** (surgical opening) is made by bringing a loop of colon to the skin surface, severing and everting the anterior wall, and suturing it to the abdominal wall. Loop colostomies are usually performed in the transverse colon and are usually temporary. An external rod may be used to support the loop until the intestinal tissue adheres to the abdominal wall. Care must be taken to avoid displacing the rod, especially during appliance changes.

An end stoma is often constructed, usually in the descending or sigmoid colon, when a colostomy is intended to be permanent. It may also be done when the surgeon oversews the distal stump of the colon and places it in the abdominal cavity, preserving it for future reattachment. An end stoma is constructed by severing the end of the proximal portion of the bowel and bringing it out through the abdominal wall.

The least common colostomy is the **double-barrel stoma**, which is created by dividing the bowel and bringing both the proximal and distal portions to the abdominal surface to create two stomas. The proximal stoma (closest to the patient's head) is the functioning stoma and eliminates stool. The distal stoma (farthest from the head) is considered nonfunctioning, although it may secrete some mucus. The distal stoma is sometimes referred to as a *mucous fistula.*

MIS colon resection or total colectomy allows complete tumor removal with an adequate surgical margin and removal of associated lymph nodes. Several small incisions are made, and a miniature video camera is placed within the abdomen to help see the area that is involved. This technique takes longer than the conventional procedure and requires specialized training. However, blood loss is less.

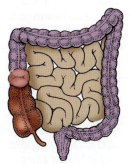

The **ascending colostomy** is done for right-sided tumors.

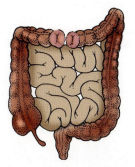

The **transverse (double-barrel) colostomy** is often used in such emergencies as intestinal obstruction or perforation because it can be created quickly. There are two stomas. The proximal one, closest to the small intestine, drains feces. The distal stoma drains mucus.

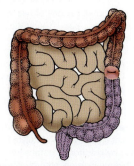

The **descending colostomy** is done for left-sided tumors.

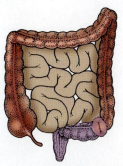

The **sigmoid colostomy** is done for rectal tumors.

FIG. 56-5 Different locations of colostomies in the colon.

Postoperative Care. Patients who have an *open colon resection* without a colostomy receive care similar to that of those having any abdominal surgery (see Chapter 16). Other patients have surgeries that also require colostomy management. They typically have a nasogastric tube (NGT) after open surgery and receive IV PCA for the first 24 to 36 hours. After NGT removal, the diet is slowly progressed from liquids to solid foods as tolerated. The care of patients with an NGT is found on p. 1159 in the discussion of Interventions in the Intestinal Obstruction section.

By contrast, patients who have *laparoscopic (MIS) surgery* can eat solid foods very soon after the procedure. Because they usually have less PAIN, they are able to ambulate earlier than those who have the conventional approach. The hospital stay is usually shorter for the patient with MIS—less than 23 hours or 1 to 2 days, depending on the patient's age and general condition.

Colostomy Management. The patient who has a colostomy may return from surgery with a clear ostomy pouch system in place. A clear pouch allows the health care team to observe the stoma. If no pouch system is in place, a petrolatum gauze dressing is usually placed over the stoma to keep it moist. This is covered with a dry, sterile dressing. In collaboration with the CWOCN, place a pouch system as soon as possible. The colostomy pouch system, also called an *appliance,* allows more convenient and acceptable collection of stool than a dressing does.

Assess the color and integrity of the stoma frequently. A healthy stoma should be reddish pink and moist and protrude about ¾ inch (2 cm) from the abdominal wall (Fig. 56-6). During the initial postoperative period, the stoma may be slightly edematous. A small amount of bleeding at the stoma is common.

! **NURSING SAFETY PRIORITY** (QSEN)

Action Alert

Report any of these problems related to the colostomy to the surgeon:
- Signs of ischemia and necrosis (dark red, purplish, or black color; dry)
- Unusual bleeding
- Mucocutaneous separation (breakdown of the suture line securing the stoma to the abdominal wall)

Also assess the condition of the peristomal skin (skin around the stoma), and frequently check the pouch system for proper fit and signs of leakage. The skin should be intact, smooth, and without redness or excoriation.

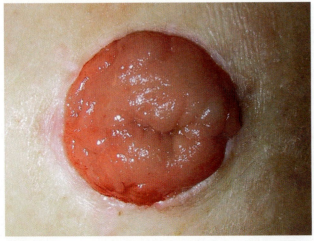

FIG. 56-6 A mature colostomy.

The colostomy should start functioning in 2 to 3 days postoperatively. When it begins to function, the pouch may need to be emptied frequently because of excess gas collection. It should be emptied when it is one-third to one-half full of stool. Stool is liquid immediately postoperatively but becomes more solid, depending on where in the colon the stoma was placed. For example, the stool from a colostomy in the ascending colon is liquid, the stool from a colostomy in the transverse colon is pasty, and the stool from a colostomy in the descending colon is more solid (similar to usual stool expelled from the rectum).

Wound Management. For an AP resection, the perineal wound is generally surgically closed and two bulb suction drains such as Jackson-Pratt drains are placed in the wound or through stab wounds near the wound. The drains help prevent drainage from collecting within the wound and are usually left in place for several days, depending on the character and amount of drainage. These drains are described in more detail in Chapter 16.

Monitoring drainage from the perineal wound and cavity is important because of the possibility of infection and abscess formation. Serosanguineous drainage from the perineal wound may be observed for 1 to 2 months after surgery. Complete healing of the perineal wound may take 6 to 8 months. This wound can be a greater source of discomfort than the abdominal incision and ostomy, and more care may be required. The patient may experience phantom rectal sensations because sympathetic innervation for rectal control has not been interrupted. Rectal PAIN and itching may occasionally occur after healing. Interventions may include use of antipruritic drugs, such as benzocaine, and warm compresses. Continually assess for signs of infection, abscess, or other complications, and implement methods for promoting wound drainage and comfort (Chart 56-3).

CHART 56-3 **Best Practice for Patient Safety & Quality Care** (QSEN)

Perineal Wound Care

Wound Care
- Place an absorbent dressing (e.g., abdominal pad) over the wound.
- Instruct the patient that he or she may:
  - Use a feminine napkin as a dressing
  - Wear jockey-type shorts rather than boxers

Comfort Measures
- If prescribed, soak the wound area in a sitz bath for 10 to 20 minutes 3 or 4 times per day or use warm/hot compresses or packs.
- Administer pain medication as prescribed, and assess its effectiveness.
- Instruct the patient about permissible activities. The patient should:
  - Assume a side-lying position in bed; avoid sitting for long periods
  - Use foam pads or a soft pillow to sit on whenever in a sitting position
  - Avoid the use of air rings or rubber donut devices

Prevention of Complications
- Maintain fluid and electrolyte balance by monitoring intake and output and by monitoring output from the perineal wound.
- Observe incision integrity, and monitor wound drains; watch for erythema, edema, bleeding, drainage, unusual odor, and excessive or constant pain.

NCLEX EXAMINATION CHALLENGE

Physiological Integrity

A nurse is assigned to care for a client who had an open partial colectomy and descending colostomy this morning. What assessment findings are expected for the client? **Select all that apply.**
A. The colostomy stoma is purple and dry.
B. The nasogastric tube is draining yellowish green fluid.
C. The client has pain that is controlled by analgesics.
D. The colostomy is not draining any stool.
E. The perineal incision is covered with a surgical dressing.

NURSING SAFETY PRIORITY (QSEN)

Action Alert

Refer patients who are at risk for or have familial CRC for genetic counseling. Specially trained nurses can discuss the purposes and goals of genetic testing. Ensure privacy and confidentiality. A review of the family history may provide important information concerning the pattern of colorectal cancer inheritance. To make an informed decision, the patient and family need information about the advantages, risks, and costs of appropriate genetic tests. Monitor the patient's response regarding genetic risk factors.

Assisting with the Grieving Process

Planning: Expected Outcomes. The expected outcomes are that the patient will verbalize feelings about the diagnosis and treatment and progress through the normal stages of grief.

Interventions. The patient and family are faced with a possible loss of or alteration in body functions. Medical and surgical interventions for the treatment of colorectal cancer may result in cure, disease control, or palliation. Interventions are designed to assist the patient and family in planning effective strategies for expressing feelings of grief and developing coping skills. Families and significant others may request that patients not be informed of the diagnosis of cancer, particularly if the patient is an older adult.

Observe and identify:
- The patient's and family's current methods of coping
- Effective sources of support used in past crises
- The patient's and family's present perceptions of the health problem
- Signs of anticipatory grief, such as denial, crying, anger, and withdrawal from usual relationships

Encourage the patient and family to verbalize feelings about the diagnosis, treatment, and anticipated alteration in body functions if a colostomy is planned. (See discussion of Operative Procedures on p. 1153 in the Surgical Management section.) Denial, sadness, anger, feelings of loss, and depression are normal responses to this change in body function. The patient will need to learn new methods for toileting and how to cope with these changes.

If a colostomy is planned, instruct the patient on what to expect about the appearance and care of the colostomy. Post-operatively, encourage him or her to look at and touch the stoma. When the patient is physically able, ask him or her to participate in colostomy care. Participation helps restore the patient's sense of control over his or her lifestyle and thus facilitates improved self-esteem. If culturally appropriate, encourage participation of family or other caregivers in colostomy care.

Assist the patient in identifying the nature of and reaction to the loss. Encourage the patient and family to verbalize feelings and identify fears to help move them through the appropriate phases of the grief process. Establish a trusting, ongoing relationship with the patient and family, and provide support through the personal grieving stages.

In collaboration with the social worker or chaplain, assist the patient in identifying personal coping strategies. Encourage him or her to implement cultural, religious, and social customs associated with the loss, and identify sources of community support. Modifications in lifestyle are needed for patients with CRC. Help the patient and family identify these changes and how best to make them. The chaplain, social worker, or case manager assists in discussions and decisions with them concerning treatment, the prognosis, and end-of-life decisions as appropriate.

Community-Based Care

Patients undergoing a colon resection by open approach are typically hospitalized for 2 to 3 days or longer, depending on the age of the patient and any complications or concurrent health problems. Collaborate with the case manager to assist patients and their families in coping with the immediate post-operative phase of recovery. After hospitalization for surgery, the patient is usually managed at home. Radiation therapy or chemotherapy is typically done on an ambulatory care basis. For the patient with advanced cancer, hospice care may be an option (see Chapter 7).

Home Care Management. Assess all patients for their ability for self-management within limitations. For those requiring assistance with care, home care visits by nurses or assistive nursing personnel can be provided.

For the patient who has undergone a colostomy, review the home situation to aid the patient in arranging for care. Ostomy products should be kept in an area (preferably the bathroom) where the temperature is neither hot nor cold (skin barriers may become stiff or melt in extreme temperatures) to ensure proper functioning. The home care nurse or CWOCN or enterostomal therapist (ET) may serve as a consultant after the patient is discharged home to ensure continuity of care (per The Joint Commission's National Patient Safety Goals).

No changes are needed in sleeping accommodations. A moisture-proof covering may initially be placed over the bed mattress if patients feel insecure about the pouch system. They may consume their usual diet on discharge.

Self-Management Education. Before discharge, teach the patient to avoid lifting heavy objects or straining on defecation to prevent tension on the anastomosis site. If he or she had the open surgical approach, the patient should avoid driving for 4 to 6 weeks while the incision heals. Patients who have had laparoscopy can usually return to all usual activities in 1 to 2 weeks.

NURSING SAFETY PRIORITY (QSEN)

Action Alert

A stool softener may be prescribed to keep stools at a soft consistency for ease of passage. Teach patients to note the frequency, amount, and character of the stools. In addition to this information, teach those with colon resections to watch for and report clinical manifestations of intestinal obstruction and perforation (e.g., cramping, abdominal pain, nausea, vomiting). Advise the patient to avoid gas-producing foods and carbonated beverages. Four to six weeks may be required to establish the effects of certain foods on bowel patterns.

Colostomy Care. Rehabilitation after surgery requires that patients and family members learn how to perform colostomy care. Provide adequate opportunity before discharge for patients to learn the psychomotor skills involved in this care. Plan sufficient practice time for learning how to handle, assemble, and apply all ostomy equipment. Teach patients and families or other caregivers about:

- The normal appearance of the stoma
- Signs and symptoms of complications
- Measurement of the stoma
- The choice, use, care, and application of the appropriate appliance to cover the stoma
- Measures to protect the skin adjacent to the stoma
- Nutrition changes to control gas and odor
- Resumption of normal activities, including work, travel, and sexual intercourse

The appropriate pouch system must be selected and fitted to the stoma. Patients with flat, firm abdomens may use either flexible (bordered with paper tape) or nonflexible (full skin barrier wafer) pouch systems. A firm abdomen with lateral creases or folds requires a flexible system. Patients with deep creases, flabby abdomens, a retracted stoma, or a stoma that is flush or concave to the abdominal surface benefit from a convex appliance with a stoma belt. This type of system presses into the skin around the stoma, causing the stoma to protrude. This protrusion helps tighten the skin and prevents leaks around the stoma opening onto the peristomal skin.

Measurement of the stoma is necessary to determine the correct size of the stomal opening on the appliance. The opening should be large enough not only to cover the peristomal skin but also to avoid stomal trauma. The stoma will shrink within 6 to 8 weeks after surgery. Therefore it needs to be measured at least once weekly during this time and as needed if the patient gains or loses weight. Teach the patient and family caregiver to trace the pattern of the stomal area on the wafer portion of the appliance and to cut an opening about $\frac{1}{8}$- to $\frac{1}{16}$-inch larger than the stomal pattern to ensure that stomal tissue will not be constricted.

Skin preparation may include clipping peristomal hair or shaving the area (moving from the stoma outward) to achieve a smooth surface, prevent unnecessary discomfort when the wafer is removed, and minimize the risk for infected hair follicles. Advise the patient to clean around the stoma with mild soap and water before putting on an appliance. He or she should avoid using moisturizing soaps to clean the area because the lubricants can interfere with adhesion of the appliance.

! NURSING SAFETY PRIORITY (QSEN)

Action Alert

Teach the patient and family to apply a skin sealant (preferably without alcohol) and allow it to dry before application of the appliance (colostomy bag) to facilitate less painful removal of the tape or adhesive. If peristomal skin becomes raw, stoma powder or paste or a combination may also be applied. The paste or other filler cream is also used to fill in crevices and creases to create a flat surface for the faceplate of the colostomy bag. If the patient develops a fungal rash, an antifungal cream or powder should be used.

Control of gas and odor from the colostomy is often an important outcome for patients with new ostomies. Although a leaking or inadequately closed pouch is the usual cause of

odor, flatus can also contribute to the odor. Remind the patient that although generally no foods for ostomates are forbidden, certain foods and habits can cause flatus or contribute to odor when the pouch is open. Broccoli, beans, spicy foods, onions, Brussels sprouts, cabbage, cauliflower, cucumbers, mushrooms, and peas often cause flatus, as does chewing gum, smoking, drinking beer, and skipping meals. Crackers, toast, and yogurt can help prevent gas. Asparagus, broccoli, cabbage, turnips, eggs, fish, and garlic contribute to odor when the pouch is open. Buttermilk, cranberry juice, parsley, and yogurt help prevent odor. Charcoal filters, pouch deodorizers, or placement of a breath mint in the pouch helps eliminate odors. The patient should be cautioned to not put aspirin tablets in the pouch because they may cause ulceration of the stoma. Vents that allow release of gas from the ostomy bag through a deodorizing filter are available and may decrease the patient's level of self-consciousness about odor.

The patient with a sigmoid colostomy may benefit from colostomy irrigation to regulate elimination. However, most patients with a sigmoid colostomy can become regulated through diet. An irrigation is similar to an enema but is administered through the stoma rather than the rectum.

In addition to teaching the patient about the clinical manifestations of obstruction and perforation, ask the patient to report any fever or sudden onset of pain or swelling around the stoma. Other home care assessment is listed in Chart 56-4.

Psychosocial Concerns. The diagnosis of cancer can be emotionally immobilizing for the patient and family or significant others, but treatment may be welcomed because it may provide hope for control of the disease. Explore reactions to the illness and perceptions of planned interventions.

The patient's reaction to ostomy surgery may include:

- Fear of not being accepted by others
- Feelings of grief related to disturbance in body image
- Concerns about sexuality

Encourage the patient and family to verbalize their feelings. By teaching how to physically manage the ostomy, help them begin to restore self-esteem and improve body image. Inclusion of family and significant others in the rehabilitation process may help maintain relationships and raise self-esteem. Anticipatory

---

CHART 56-4 Home Care Assessment

The Patient with a Colostomy

Assess gastrointestinal status, including:
- Dietary and fluid intake and habits
- Presence or absence of nausea and vomiting
- Weight gain or loss
- Bowel elimination pattern and characteristics and amount of effluent (stool)
- Bowel sounds

Assess condition of stoma, including:
- Location, size, protrusion, color, and integrity
- Signs of ischemia, such as dull coloring or dark or purplish bruising

Assess peristomal skin for:
- Presence or absence of excoriated skin, leakage underneath drainage system
- Fit of appliance and effectiveness of skin barrier and appliance

Assess the patient's and family's coping skills, including:
- Self-care abilities in the home
- Acknowledgment of changes in body image and function
- Sense of loss

instruction includes information on leakage accidents, odor control measures, and adjustments to resuming sexual relationships.

Health Care Resources. Several resources are available to maintain continuity of care in the home environment and provide for patient needs that the nurse is not able to meet. Make referrals to community-based case managers or social workers, who can provide further emotional counseling, aid in managing financial concerns, or arrange for services in the home or long-term care facility as needed.

Provide information about the United Ostomy Associations of America, Inc. (www.uoaa.org), a self-help group of people who have ostomies. This group has literature such as the organization's publication (Ostomy Quarterly) and information about local chapters. The organization conducts a visitor program that sends specially trained visitors (who have an ostomy [ostomate]) to talk with patients. After obtaining consent, make a referral to the visitor program so that the volunteer ostomate can see the patient both preoperatively and postoperatively. A physician's consent for visitation may be necessary.

The local division or unit of the American Cancer Society (ACS) (www.cancer.org) can help provide necessary medical equipment and supplies, home care services, travel accommodations, and other resources for the patient who is having cancer treatment or surgery. Inform the patient and family of the programs available through the local division or unit. Other excellent web resources include Cancer Care (www.cancercare.org), Colon Cancer Alliance (www.ccalliance.org), and the National Cancer Institute (www.nci.gov).

Because of short hospital stays, patients with new ostomies receive much health teaching from nurses working for home health care agencies. This resource also helps provide physical care needs, medication management, and emotional support. If the patient has advanced colorectal cancer, a referral for hospice services in the home, nursing home, or other long-term care setting may be appropriate. The home health care nurse informs the patient and family about what ostomy supplies are needed and where they can be purchased. Price and location are considered before recommendations are made.

? CLINICAL JUDGMENT CHALLENGE

Prioritization, Delegation, and Supervision

A 56-year-old woman returns from the postanesthesia care unit (PACU) after an open colon resection and colostomy for ascending colon cancer. She has IV fluids running at 100 mL/hr and is receiving morphine PCA. An NGT is in place connected to low suction, and she is NPO. Her abdominal dressing is dry and intact, and her oxygen saturation is 95% on 2 L/min of oxygen via nasal cannula. She is allowed out of bed to the bathroom or chair today. You are assigned to care for this patient for the rest of the day shift.

1. Upon the patient's admission to your unit at 11 AM, should you delegate taking the patient's vital signs to an experienced nursing technician? Why or why not?
2. At 5 PM, the patient states that she needs to go to the bathroom. Will you delegate this activity to the nursing technician? Why or why not?
3. While the patient was in the bathroom, her oxygen saturation level decreased to 88%. What is your best action at this time?
4. The patient's husband asks you about his wife's prognosis regarding her cancer survival. What is your best response at this time?

◆ Evaluation: Outcomes

Evaluate the care of the patient with colorectal cancer based on the identified priority patient problems. The expected outcomes are that the patient:

- Adjusts to actual or impending loss
- Is free of complications or metastasis associated with CRC
- States he or she has well-controlled pain and is as comfortable as possible (if metastasis is present)

INTESTINAL OBSTRUCTION

❖ PATHOPHYSIOLOGY

Intestinal obstructions can be partial or complete and are classified as mechanical or nonmechanical. In **mechanical obstruction,** the bowel is physically blocked by problems outside the intestine (e.g., adhesions), in the bowel wall (e.g., Crohn's disease), or in the intestinal lumen (e.g., tumors). **Nonmechanical obstruction** (also known as **paralytic ileus** or *adynamic ileus*) does not involve a physical obstruction in or outside the intestine. Instead, peristalsis is decreased or absent as a result of neuromuscular disturbance, resulting in a slowing of the movement or a backup of intestinal contents (McCance et al., 2014).

Intestinal contents are composed of ingested fluid, food, and saliva; gastric, pancreatic, and biliary secretions; and swallowed air. In both mechanical and nonmechanical obstructions, the intestinal contents accumulate at and above the area of obstruction. Distention results from the intestine's inability to absorb the contents and move them down the intestinal tract. To compensate for the lag, peristalsis increases in an effort to move the intestinal contents forward. This increase stimulates more secretions, which then leads to additional distention. The bowel then becomes edematous, and increased capillary permeability results. Plasma leaking into the peritoneal cavity and fluid trapped in the intestinal lumen decrease the absorption of fluid and electrolytes into the vascular space. Reduced circulatory blood volume (hypovolemia) and electrolyte imbalances typically occur. Hypovolemia ranges from mild to extreme (hypovolemic shock).

Specific problems related to FLUID AND ELECTROLYTE BALANCE and acid-base balance result, depending on the part of the intestine that is blocked. An obstruction high in the small intestine causes a loss of gastric hydrochloride, which can lead to *metabolic alkalosis.* Obstruction below the duodenum but above the large bowel results in loss of both acids and bases, so that acid-base balance is usually not compromised. Obstruction at the end of the small intestine and lower in the intestinal tract causes loss of alkaline fluids, which can lead to *metabolic acidosis* (McCance et al., 2014).

If hypovolemia is severe, renal insufficiency or even death can occur. Bacterial peritonitis with or without actual perforation can also result. Bacteria in the intestinal contents lie stagnant in the obstructed intestine. This is not a problem unless the blood flow to the intestine is compromised. However, with *closed-loop obstruction* (blockage in two different areas) or a **strangulated obstruction** (obstruction with compromised blood flow), the risk for peritonitis is greatly increased. Bacteria without blood supply can form and release an endotoxin into the peritoneal or systemic circulation and cause septic shock. With a strangulated obstruction, major blood loss into the intestine and the peritoneum can occur. Sepsis and bleeding can result in an increased intra-abdominal pressure (IAP) or acute

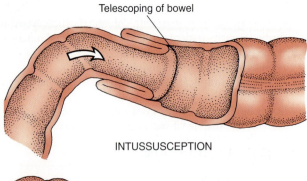

INTUSSUSCEPTION

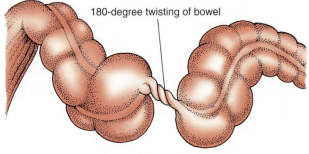

VOLVULUS

FIG. 56-7 Two major types of mechanical obstruction.

compartment syndrome (Lee, 2012). (See later discussion of IAP on p. 1163 of this chapter.)

Intestinal obstruction is a common and serious disorder caused by a variety of conditions and is associated with significant morbidity. It can occur anywhere in the intestinal tract, although the ileum in the small intestine (the narrowest part of the intestinal tract) is the most common site.

Mechanical obstruction can result from:

- Adhesions (scar tissue from surgeries or pathology)
- Benign or malignant tumor
- Complications of appendicitis
- Hernias
- Fecal impactions (especially in older adults)
- Strictures due to Crohn's disease or previous radiation therapy
- **Intussusception** (telescoping of a segment of the intestine within itself) (Fig. 56-7)
- **Volvulus** (twisting of the intestine) (see Fig. 56-7)
- Fibrosis due to disorders such as endometriosis
- Vascular disorders (e.g., emboli and arteriosclerotic narrowing of mesenteric vessels)

In people ages 65 years or older, diverticulitis, tumors, and fecal impaction are the most common causes of obstruction (McCance et al., 2014).

Postoperative ileus (POI) (paralytic ileus), or *nonmechanical* obstruction, is most commonly caused by handling of the intestines during abdominal surgery. In patients with POI, intestinal function is lost for a few hours to several days. Electrolyte disturbances, especially hypokalemia, predispose the patient to this problem. The ileus can also be a consequence of **peritonitis**, because leakage of colonic contents causes severe irritation and triggers an inflammatory response and infection (see discussion of peritonitis on p. 1170 in Chapter 57). Vascular insufficiency to the bowel, also referred to as *intestinal ischemia,* is another potential cause of an ileus. It results when arterial or venous

thrombosis or an embolus decreases blood flow to the mesenteric blood vessels surrounding the intestines, as in heart failure or severe shock. Severe insufficiency of blood supply can result in infarction of surrounding organs (e.g., bowel infarction).

❖ PATIENT-CENTERED COLLABORATIVE CARE

◆ Assessment

History. Collect information about a history of gastrointestinal disorders, surgeries, and treatments. Question the patient about recent nausea and vomiting and the color of emesis. Perform a thorough PAIN assessment with particular attention to the onset, aggravating factors, alleviating factors, and patterns or rhythms of the pain. Severe pain that then stops and changes to tenderness on palpation may indicate perforation and should be reported promptly to the physician. Ask about the passage of flatus and the time, character, and consistency of the last bowel movement. Singultus (hiccups) is common with all types of intestinal obstruction. When an obstruction is suspected, keep the patient NPO and contact the physician promptly for further direction.

Assess for a family history of colorectal cancer (CRC), and ask about blood in the stool or a change in bowel pattern. Body temperature with uncomplicated obstruction is rarely higher than 100° F (37.8° C). A temperature higher than this, with or without guarding and tenderness, and a sustained elevation in pulse could indicate a strangulated obstruction or peritonitis. A fever, tachycardia, hypotension, increasing abdominal pain, abdominal rigidity, or change in color of skin overlying the abdomen should be reported to the attending physician immediately.

Physical Assessment/Clinical Manifestations. The patient with *mechanical* obstruction in the *small intestine* often has mid-abdominal PAIN or cramping. The pain can be sporadic, and the patient may feel comfortable between episodes. If strangulation is present, the pain becomes more localized and steady. Vomiting often accompanies obstruction and is more profuse with obstructions in the proximal small intestine. The vomitus may contain bile and mucus or be orange-brown and foul smelling as a result of bacterial overgrowth with low ileal obstruction. Prolonged vomiting can result in a disruption in FLUID AND ELECTROLYTE BALANCE. **Obstipation** (no passage of stool) and failure to pass flatus accompany complete obstruction. Diarrhea may be present in partial obstruction.

Mechanical colonic obstruction causes a milder, more intermittent colicky abdominal PAIN than is seen with small-bowel obstruction. Lower abdominal distention and obstipation may be present, or the patient may have ribbon-like stools if obstruction is partial. Alterations in bowel patterns and blood in the stools accompany the obstruction if colorectal cancer or diverticulitis is the cause.

On examination of the abdomen, observe for abdominal distention, which is common in all forms of intestinal obstruction. Peristaltic waves may also be visible. Auscultate for proximal high-pitched bowel sounds (**borborygmi**), which are associated with cramping early in the obstructive process as the intestine tries to push the mechanical obstruction forward. In later stages of mechanical obstruction, bowel sounds are absent, especially distal to the obstruction. Abdominal tenderness and rigidity are usually minimal. The presence of a tense, fluid-filled bowel loop mimicking a palpable abdominal mass may signal a closed-loop, strangulating small-bowel obstruction.

CHART 56-5 Key Features
Small-Bowel and Large-Bowel Obstructions

SMALL-BOWEL OBSTRUCTIONS	LARGE-BOWEL OBSTRUCTIONS
Abdominal discomfort or pain possibly accompanied by visible peristaltic waves in upper and middle abdomen	Intermittent lower abdominal cramping
Upper or epigastric abdominal distention	Lower abdominal distention
Nausea and early, profuse vomiting (may contain fecal material)	Minimal or no vomiting
Obstipation	Obstipation or ribbon-like stools
Severe fluid and electrolyte imbalances	No major fluid and electrolyte imbalances
Metabolic alkalosis	Metabolic acidosis (not always present)

CHART 56-6 Best Practice for Patient Safety & Quality Care QSEN
Nursing Care of Patients Who Have an Intestinal Obstruction

- Monitor vital signs, especially blood pressure, for indications of fluid balance.
- Assess the patient's abdomen at least twice a day for bowel sounds, distention, and passage of flatus.
- Monitor fluid and electrolyte status, including laboratory values.
- Manage the patient who has a nasogastric tube (NGT):
  - Monitor drainage.
  - Ensure tube patency.
  - Check tube placement.
  - Irrigate tube as prescribed.
  - Maintain the patient on NPO status.
  - Provide frequent mouth and nares care.
  - Maintain the patient in a semi-Fowler's position.
- Give analgesics for pain as prescribed.
- Give alvimopan (Entereg) as prescribed for patients with a postoperative ileus.
- Maintain parenteral nutrition if prescribed.

In most types of *nonmechanical* obstruction, the PAIN is described as a constant, diffuse discomfort. Colicky cramping is not characteristic of this type of obstruction. Pain associated with obstruction caused by vascular insufficiency or infarction is usually severe and constant. On inspection, abdominal distention is typically present. On auscultation of the abdomen, note and document decreased bowel sounds in early obstruction and absent bowel sounds in later stages. Vomiting of gastric contents and bile is frequent, but the vomitus rarely has a foul odor and is rarely profuse. Obstipation may or may not be present. Chart 56-5 compares small-bowel and large-bowel obstructions.

Diagnostic Assessment. There is no definitive laboratory test to confirm a diagnosis of mechanical or nonmechanical obstruction. *White blood cell (WBC) counts* are normal unless there is a strangulated obstruction, in which case there may be leukocytosis (increased WBCs). *Hemoglobin, hematocrit, creatinine, and blood urea nitrogen (BUN)* values are often elevated, indicating dehydration. Serum sodium, chloride, and potassium are decreased. Elevations in serum amylase levels may be found with strangulating obstructions, which can damage the pancreas.

The health care provider obtains an *abdominal CT scan* as soon as an obstruction is suspected. Distention with fluid and gas in the small intestine with the absence of gas in the colon indicates an obstruction in the small intestine.

The diagnostic examination chosen depends on the suspected location of the obstruction. As an initial assessment, the health care provider may prescribe an *abdominal ultrasound* to evaluate the potential cause of the obstruction. The physician may perform endoscopy (sigmoidoscopy or colonoscopy) to determine the cause of the obstruction, except when perforation or complete obstruction is suspected.

◆ Interventions

Interventions are aimed at uncovering the cause and relieving the obstruction. Intestinal obstructions can be relieved by nonsurgical or surgical means. If the obstruction is partial and there is no evidence of strangulation, nonsurgical management may be the treatment of choice (Chart 56-6).

Nonsurgical Management. Paralytic ileus responds well to nonsurgical methods of relieving obstruction. Nonsurgical

approaches are also preferred in the treatment of patients with terminal disease associated with bowel obstruction. In addition to being NPO, patients typically have a nasogastric tube (NGT) inserted to decompress the bowel by draining fluid and air. The tube is attached to suction.

Nasogastric Tubes. Most patients with an obstruction have an NGT unless the obstruction is mild. A **Salem sump tube** is inserted through the nose and placed into the stomach. It is attached to low continuous suction. This tube has a vent ("pigtail") that prevents the stomach mucosa from being pulled away during suctioning. Levin tubes do not have a vent and therefore should be connected to low intermittent suction. They are used much less often than the Salem sump tubes.

! NURSING SAFETY PRIORITY QSEN
Action Alert

At least every 4 hours, assess the patient with an NGT for proper placement of the tube, tube patency, and output (quality and quantity). Monitor the nasal skin around the tube for irritation. Use a device that secures the tube to the nose to prevent accidental removal. Assess for peristalsis by auscultating for bowel sounds with the suction disconnected (suction masks peristaltic sounds).

Question the patient about the passage of flatus, and record flatus and the character of bowel movements daily. Flatus or stool means that peristalsis has returned. Assess for nausea, and ask the patient to report this manifestation.

Monitor any NGT for proper functioning. Occasionally NGTs move out of optimal drainage position or become plugged. In this case, note a decrease in gastric output or stasis of the tube's contents. Assess the patient for nausea, vomiting, increased abdominal distention, and placement of the tube. If the NGT is repositioned or replaced, confirmation of proper placement may be obtained by x-ray before use. After appropriate placement is established, aspirate the contents and irrigate the tube with 30 mL of normal saline every 4 hours or as requested by the health care provider.

Other Nonsurgical Interventions. Most types of nonmechanical obstruction respond to nasogastric decompression with medical treatment of the primary disorder. Incomplete mechanical obstruction can sometimes be successfully treated without surgery. Obstruction caused by lower fecal impaction usually resolves after disimpaction and enema administration. Intussusception may respond to hydrostatic pressure changes during a barium enema.

For patients with a postoperative ileus (POI), alvimopan (Entereg) may be given for short-term use. This drug is an oral, peripherally acting mu opioid receptor antagonist that increases GI motility (Russell et al., 2012).

IV fluid replacement and maintenance are indicated for all patients with intestinal obstruction because the patient is NPO and FLUID AND ELECTROLYTE BALANCE is lost (particularly potassium) through vomiting and nasogastric suction. On the basis of serum electrolytes and blood urea nitrogen (BUN) levels, the health care provider prescribes aggressive fluid replacement with 2 to 4 L of normal saline or lactated Ringer's solution with potassium added. Use care with patients who are susceptible to fluid overload (e.g., older adults with a history of heart or kidney failure). Monitor lung sounds, weight, and intake and output daily. Weight is the most reliable indicator of fluid balance. Blood replacement may be indicated in strangulated obstruction because of blood loss into the bowel or peritoneal cavity.

Monitor vital signs and other measures of fluid status (e.g., urine output, skin turgor, mucous membranes) every 2 to 4 hours, depending on the severity of the patient's symptoms. In collaboration with the dietitian, the physician may prescribe parenteral nutrition (PN), especially if the patient has had chronic nutritional problems and has been NPO for an extended period. Chapter 60 discusses the nursing care of patients receiving PN.

The patient with intestinal obstruction is usually thirsty, although some older adults have a decreased thirst response. Delegate frequent mouth care to unlicensed assistive personnel (UAP) to help maintain moist mucous membranes. Be sure to supervise this activity. A few ice chips may be allowed if the patient is not having surgery. Follow agency protocol or the physician's request regarding ice chips.

Abdominal distention can cause a great deal of discomfort, especially when it is severe. The colicky, crampy pain that comes and goes with mechanical obstruction and the nausea, vomiting, dry mucous membranes, and thirst contribute to the patient's discomfort. Continually assess the character and location of the pain, and immediately report any PAIN that significantly increases or changes from a colicky, intermittent type to a constant discomfort. These changes can indicate perforation of the intestine or peritonitis.

Opioid analgesics may be temporarily withheld in the diagnostic workup period so that clinical manifestations of perforation or peritonitis are not masked. Explain to the patient and family the rationale for not giving analgesics. In addition, if analgesics such as morphine are given, they may slow intestinal motility and can cause vomiting. Be alert to this side effect because nausea and vomiting are also signs of NG tube obstruction or worsening bowel obstruction.

Help the patient obtain a position of comfort with frequent position changes to promote increased peristalsis. A semi-Fowler's position helps alleviate the pressure of abdominal distention on the chest. This position is for comfort and promotion of thoracic excursion to facilitate breathing.

Discomfort is generally less with nonmechanical obstruction than with mechanical obstruction. With both types of obstruction, discomfort is aggravated by taking in food or fluids.

If strangulation is thought to be likely, the health care provider prescribes IV broad-spectrum antibiotics. In addition, in cases of partial obstruction or paralytic ileus, drugs that enhance gastric motility such as octreotide acetate (Sandostatin) may be used.

Surgical Management. In patients with complete mechanical obstruction and in some cases of incomplete mechanical obstruction, surgical intervention is necessary to relieve the obstruction. A strangulated obstruction is complete, and surgical intervention is always required. An **exploratory laparotomy** (a surgical opening of the abdominal cavity to investigate the cause of the obstruction) is initially performed for many patients with obstruction. More specific surgical procedures depend on the cause of the obstruction.

Preoperative Care. Provide general preoperative teaching for both the patient and family as discussed in Chapter 14. In cases of complete obstruction, the patient may feel too ill to want the information. Reinforce the information with the family or other caregiver. Depending on the cause and severity of the obstruction, as well as the expertise of the surgeon, patients have either minimally invasive surgery (MIS) via laparoscopy or a conventional open approach.

Operative Procedures. In the *conventional open surgical approach,* the surgeon makes a large incision, enters the abdominal cavity, and explores for obstruction and its cause, if possible (exploratory laparotomy). If adhesions are found, they are lysed (cut and released). Obstruction caused by a tumor or diverticulitis requires a colon resection with primary anastomosis or a temporary or permanent colostomy. If obstruction is caused by intestinal infarction, an embolectomy, thrombectomy, or resection of the gangrenous small or large bowel may be necessary. In severe cases a colectomy (removal of the entire colon) may be needed.

For the *MIS* approach, the specially trained surgeon makes several small incisions in the abdomen and places a video camera to view the abdominal contents to determine the extent of the obstruction. A laparoscope (type of endoscope) with a lighted end is inserted along with various surgical instruments to remove the problem. This procedure takes longer than the open approach, but blood loss is less and healing is faster. Robotic assistance may be used, depending on the experience of the surgeon and available equipment.

Postoperative Care. General postoperative care for the patient undergoing an *exploratory laparotomy* with lysis of adhesions, colon resection, thrombectomy, or embolectomy is similar to that described in Chapter 16. In addition, patients who had an open surgical approach have an NGT in place until peristalsis resumes. A clear liquid diet may be prescribed to encourage peristalsis return. As liquids are started, the NGT can be disconnected from suction and capped for 1 to 2 hours after the patient has taken clear liquids to determine if he or she is able to tolerate them. If the patient vomits after liquids, the suction is resumed. When the patient has return of peristalsis, the NGT suction is discontinued and the tube is clamped for a scheduled amount of time. If the patient does not experience nausea while the NGT is clamped, the tube is removed.

Most patients today have laparoscopic surgery (MIS) for mechanical intestinal obstructions. They usually do *not* have an NGT and can recover more quickly than those with the open surgical approach. The hospital stay for those having MIS to remove tumors, adhesions, and other obstructions may be as short as 1 to 2 days compared with 3 days or longer for the conventional surgical patients. Recovery is much quicker because there is less pain and there are fewer postoperative complications among those who had laparoscopic surgery.

❓ CLINICAL JUDGMENT CHALLENGE

Patient-Centered Care; Teamwork and Collaboration; Informatics QSEN

An 82-year-old woman had open abdominal surgery 36 hours ago for removal of a large uterine tumor. As her nurse, you note that she continues to have no bowel sounds and has not passed flatus. Her abdomen is moderately distended and hard. She has reported several episodes of severe nausea and has no appetite but states that she has no pain. You suspect that the patient has a postoperative ileus but need more data before calling the surgeon.

1. What questions do you need to ask the patient and her family related to her current problem?
2. What other objective assessment data do you need before contacting the surgeon?
3. Using SBAR and data that you provide, how will you communicate the information about this patient to the surgeon?
4. What evidence-based collaborative interventions are appropriate for this patient immediately? Support your answer with Internet resources.
5. What information will you document in the electronic health record?
6. What electrolyte imbalances would you expect? How might her presentation be somewhat different from that of a younger adult and why?

Community-Based Care

All patients with intestinal obstruction are hospitalized for monitoring and treatment. The length of stay varies according to the type of obstruction, the treatment, and the presence of complications. Patients who have complicated obstruction, such as strangulation or incarceration, are at greater risk for peritonitis, sepsis, and shock.

Patients with nonmechanical (adynamic) intestinal obstruction are less likely to require a lengthy hospitalization because of the obstruction alone. Adynamic obstruction generally responds to NG suction and possible drug therapy within a few days. However, if the ileus occurs as a complication of an abdominal surgery, the hospital stay could be lengthy.

Home Care Management. For the patient who has had an intestinal obstruction, preparation for home care depends on the cause of the obstruction and the treatment required. Those who have resolution of obstruction without surgical intervention are assessed for their knowledge of strategies to avoid recurrent obstruction. For example, if fecal impaction was the cause of the obstruction, assess the patient's ability to carry out a bowel regimen independently (Chart 56-7). For those who have had surgery, evaluate their ability to function at home with the added tasks of incision care and possibly colostomy care.

CHART 56-7 Nursing Focus on the Older Adult

Preventing Fecal Impaction

- Teach the patient to eat high-fiber foods, including plenty of raw fruits and vegetables and whole-grain products.
- Encourage the patient to drink adequate amounts of fluids, especially water.
- Do not routinely administer a laxative; teach the patient that laxative abuse decreases abdominal muscle tone and contributes to an atonic colon.
- Encourage the patient to exercise regularly, if possible. Walking every day is an excellent exercise for promoting intestinal motility.
- Use natural foods to stimulate peristalsis, such as warm beverages and prune juice.
- Take bulk-forming products, such as Metamucil, to provide fiber.
- Check the patient's stool for amount and frequency; oozing of soft or diarrheal stool often indicates a fecal impaction.
- Have the patient sit on a toilet or bedside commode rather than on a bedpan for elimination.

Self-Management Education. Instruct the patient to report any abdominal pain or distention, nausea, or vomiting, with or without constipation, because these symptoms might indicate recurrent obstruction. The patient should be reassured, however, that recurrent paralytic ileus is not common.

Teach the patient who has had surgery about incision care, drug therapy, and activity limitations. Drug therapy consists of an oral opioid analgesic, such as oxycodone hydrochloride with acetaminophen (Tylox, Percocet, Endocet ✦), to be taken as needed for incisional discomfort. As with any opioid therapy, an over-the-counter laxative with a softener (e.g., Docusate with Senna) or polyethylene glycol (MiraLax) may be added to prevent constipation and possible recurrent obstruction.

The patient who had curative treatment of the underlying cause most likely requires less support than one who had treatment of obstruction related to a serious disease that will require further management. Encourage the patient to express fears and concerns about the future. Assess the patient's understanding and needs with regard to treatment plans.

Health Care Resources. The need for follow-up appointments depends on the cause of the obstruction and the treatment required. In collaboration with the case manager, make arrangements for a home care nurse if the patient needs help with incision or colostomy care.

ABDOMINAL TRAUMA

❖ PATHOPHYSIOLOGY

Abdominal trauma is defined as injury to the structures located between the diaphragm and the pelvis that occurs when the abdomen is subjected to blunt or penetrating forces. Organs injured may include the large or small bowel, liver, spleen, duodenum, pancreas, kidneys, and urinary bladder.

At least one half of all *blunt abdominal traumas* occur from motor vehicle crashes. Other causes of blunt trauma include falls, aggravated assaults, and contact sports. The spleen is the most commonly injured organ from *blunt* abdominal trauma. *Penetrating abdominal trauma* is caused by gunshot wounds (GSWs), stabbing, or impalement with an object. The liver is the most commonly injured organ from penetrating abdominal trauma. *Trauma is the leading cause of death in adults younger than 40 years in the United States.*

❖ PATIENT-CENTERED COLLABORATIVE CARE

◆ Assessment

First, assess any patient experiencing trauma for **a**irway, **b**reathing, and **c**irculation (ABCs).

❗ NURSING SAFETY PRIORITY (QSEN)

Critical Rescue

Once the patient with abdominal trauma has been assessed for airway, breathing, and circulation, focus on the risks for hemorrhage, shock, and peritonitis. Mental status, vital signs, and skin perfusion are *priority* nursing assessments, with skin perfusion being the most reliable clinical guide in assessing hypovolemic shock:

- In a person with mild shock, the skin is pale, cool, and moist.
- With moderate shock, diaphoresis is more marked and urine output ceases.
- With severe shock, changes in mental status are manifested by agitation, disorientation, and recent memory loss.

Assess for abdominal trauma by asking the patient about the presence, location, and quality of pain. Inspect the abdomen, flanks, back, genitalia, and rectum for contusions, abrasions, lacerations, ecchymosis, penetrating injuries, and asymmetry. All of the patient's clothes must be removed for this examination.

Inspection of the abdomen may reveal distention. To perform an adequate inspection, turn the patient while maintaining spinal immobilization. *Ecchymosis (bruising) may indicate internal bleeding. Ecchymosis present in the distribution of a lap seat belt should be reported to the health care provider immediately because the bowel or other major organ may be injured.*

Auscultate the abdomen for bowel sounds. Absent or diminished bowel sounds may be caused by the presence of blood, bacteria, or a chemical irritant in the abdominal cavity. Also auscultate for bruits in the abdomen, which could indicate renal artery injury.

Injury to the spleen is present in many people with left lower rib fractures. Liver injury may be present in those with right lower rib fractures. Dullness over hollow organs that normally contain gas, such as the stomach and the large and small intestines, may indicate the presence of blood or fluid. Light abdominal palpation identifies areas of tenderness, rebound tenderness, guarding, rigidity, and spasm. A palpated mass may be blood or a fluid collection.

The patient without obvious significant bleeding or definite signs of peritoneal irritation undergoes abdominal ultrasound, **diagnostic peritoneal lavage (DPL)**, and CT. For DPL, the physician inserts a large-bore catheter into the abdomen and allows fluid to enter the abdominal cavity. If the return drainage from the abdomen is pink or grossly bloody, the health care team prepares for surgery. Abdominal ultrasound or *focused abdominal sonography for trauma (FAST)* is used to diagnose blunt abdominal trauma and may replace CT and DPL for diagnosis. Patients with hemodynamic instability or peritonitis are candidates for immediate laparotomy.

◆ Interventions

Nonsurgical and surgical interventions are aimed at preserving or restoring hemodynamic stability, preventing or decreasing blood loss, and preventing complications. Patients with abdominal trauma from a vehicle crash often have other injuries such as multiple fractures. *The priority for care is to establish and maintain the ABCs.*

Emergency Care: Abdominal Trauma. Nursing interventions include placement of at least two large-bore IV catheters in the upper extremities. IV catheters are not used in the lower extremities; if the vasculature has been injured, fluid can pool in the abdomen. The health care provider may insert a central venous catheter to assist with rapid fluid volume infusion. IV fluids include saline, crystalloids, and possibly blood. Be sure that the patient is typed and crossmatched for as many as 4 to 8 units of packed red blood cells.

These laboratory values are monitored:

- Arterial blood gases
- Complete blood count (CBC)
- Serum electrolyte, glucose and amylase, and blood urea nitrogen (BUN) determinations
- Liver function tests
- Coagulation studies

Measuring arterial blood gases may help determine the severity of shock. Hemoglobin and hematocrit values do not initially reflect true blood loss; values can be skewed because of hemoconcentration from volume loss or the dilutional effects of IV fluids. Serial hemoglobin and hematocrit measurements may be more accurate in determining true blood loss. An elevated white blood cell (WBC) count may indicate a ruptured spleen or intestinal injury. Elevated levels of serum transaminases may indicate liver injury. Elevation of serum amylase activity may signal injury to the pancreas or the bowel. All laboratory work is compiled so that values can be compared and trended.

Continuous hemodynamic monitoring is begun in the emergency department. Insert an indwelling urinary (Foley) catheter unless there is blood at the urinary meatus. Initially and hourly thereafter, evaluate urine output for bleeding and specific gravity. Laboratory tests indicate the amount of blood and protein in the urine. If there is an open abdominal wound or evisceration, cover it with a sterile dry dressing unless the physician requests otherwise. Unless it is contraindicated, as in the case of a skull fracture, the physician or nurse inserts a nasogastric tube (NGT) to identify bleeding and minimize the risk for vomiting and aspiration. Antibiotics may be administered as prescribed to reduce the risk for peritonitis.

If the patient with known abdominal trauma has no definite clinical manifestations of active bleeding or organ injury, he or she is admitted to the hospital for observation. Many patients are admitted to the critical care unit. Blunt trauma can cause active, but often not obvious, damage.

❗ NURSING SAFETY PRIORITY (QSEN)

Critical Rescue

For the patient who has sustained abdominal trauma, assess for abdominal or referred pain and nausea. Every 15 to 30 minutes in the early postinjury period and then hourly, evaluate:

- Mental status
- Vital signs
- Clinical findings, such as vomiting, guarding, rigidity, or rebound tenderness
- Bowel sounds
- Urine output

Report any change immediately to the health care provider! It is more important to recognize the high risk for an active abdominal injury and assess for general signs of organ injury (e.g., hemorrhage and peritonitis) than to identify the exact nature of the abdominal injury. Opioid analgesics are given for pain after the physician's initial assessment is complete. Explain to the patient and family the rationale for delaying analgesics.

Intra-Abdominal Pressure Monitoring. Some patients are monitored for intra-abdominal pressure (IAP) using a continuous monitoring system. As the name implies, **intra-abdominal pressure** is pressure within the abdominal cavity. The normal IAP in healthy adults is 0 to 5 mm Hg, but obese patients often have a higher normal value (Lee, 2012). Increased IAP commonly occurs in patients with abdominal trauma. Other causes of IAP elevation include sepsis, burns, abdominal hemorrhage, and mechanical intestinal obstruction.

Nursing interventions to help *prevent* increased IAP in high-risk patients include (Lee, 2012):

- Record bowel movements.
- Check daily for fecal impaction.
- Provide measures to prevent constipation (e.g., increased fluids if tolerated, daily stool softener).
- Provide fluid replacement with hypertonic saline, crystalloids (e.g., 0.9% saline), or colloids (e.g., albumin, Dextran) as prescribed to expand plasma volume.
- Document intake and output.
- Monitor residuals for patients being tube-fed.
- Elevate the head of the bed to 20-30 degrees, depending on the patient's condition.
- Manage pain adequately.

When IAP becomes higher than the central venous pressure, the inferior vena cava and other abdominal vessels are compressed. This leads to impaired venous return, increased afterload, and decreased preload. The patient is then at risk for deep vein thrombosis and pulmonary embolism (PE). The patient has tachycardia and hypotension. As the IAP increases further, acidosis and ischemia occur. A sustained or repeated IAP of 12 mm Hg or higher is considered **intra-abdominal hypertension (IAH)**. **Abdominal acute compartment syndrome (AACS)** results when the IAP is sustained at greater than 20 mm Hg. Untreated AACS results in damage to the intestine and increases the risk for sepsis, multiple organ dysfunction syndrome (MODS), and death. Almost every body system can be affected (Lee, 2012).

For patients with abdominal trauma or other high-risk factors, the health care provider may request continuous or intermittent IAP monitoring in the critical care unit using a urinary manometer or transducer system. *Report any increase in IAP immediately to the health care provider.* AACS has a rapid onset after abdominal trauma (especially blunt trauma) and must be treated immediately using either a nonsurgical (vasopressor drugs and fluids) or surgical approach (fasciotomy). Surgery is risky because it increases the chance of embolic stroke and PE.

Surgical Management. For the patient with severe abdominal trauma, the surgeon performs an *exploratory laparotomy* and repairs abdominal injuries immediately if there are definite signs of peritoneal irritation. These signs include rebound tenderness, significant blood loss, evisceration, or a gunshot wound (GSW) with possible peritoneal involvement. After surgery, many of these patients are admitted to a critical care unit and mechanically ventilated.

Most stab wounds and GSWs require exploratory laparotomy. The surgeon explores and cleans superficial penetrating wounds. The patient does not require an exploratory laparotomy for superficial wounds.

Patients with multiple trauma stay in the hospital for a prolonged period. Before discharge from the hospital, teach the patient and family the signs and symptoms of abdominal bleeding whether or not surgery has been performed. Instruct them to report abdominal pain, nausea, vomiting, bloody or black stools, fever, weakness, and dizziness.

Hemorrhage can occasionally occur weeks after blunt abdominal trauma, despite medical evaluation or treatment. For the patient who has surgery or exploration of wounds, provide instructions on wound care before discharge from the hospital. Provide additional health teaching as the patient's overall condition requires.

? NCLEX EXAMINATION CHALLENGE

Physiological Integrity

A client is admitted to the emergency department in severe pain with a gunshot wound to the right upper abdomen. Admitting vital signs are TPR 98-96-28; BP 118/70; oxygen saturation 94%. What is the nurse's priority when monitoring this client?
A. Open the airway to improve breathing.
B. Give oxygen via nasal cannula at 2 L/min.
C. Monitor vital signs frequently.
D. Determine how the client was shot and by whom.

POLYPS

❖ PATHOPHYSIOLOGY

Polyps in the intestinal tract are small growths covered with mucosa and attached to the surface of the intestine. Although most are benign, they are significant because some have the potential to become malignant.

Polyps are identified by their tissue type. Although only a very small number of adenomas progress to cancer, almost all colorectal cancers develop from an adenoma. Adenomas are further classified as villous or tubular. Of these, villous adenomas pose a greater cancer risk.

Familial adenomatous polyposis (FAP) and hereditary nonpolyposis colorectal cancer (HNPCC) are inherited syndromes characterized by progressive development of colorectal adenomas. Unless these syndromes are treated, colorectal cancer (CRC) inevitably occurs by the fourth to fifth decade of life. These conditions were discussed on p. 1149 in the Genetic/Genomic Considerations feature in the Colorectal Cancer section.

❖ PATIENT-CENTERED COLLABORATIVE CARE

Polyps are usually asymptomatic and are discovered during routine colonoscopy screening. However, they can cause gross rectal bleeding, intestinal obstruction, or intussusception (telescoping of the bowel). Biopsy specimens of polyps can be obtained and the entire polyp can be removed (polypectomy) with the use of a snare that fits through the sigmoidoscope or colonoscope. This often eliminates the need for abdominal surgery to remove a suspicious or definitely malignant polyp. The patient with FAP often requires a total colectomy (colon removal) to prevent the development of cancer.

Nursing care focuses on patient education. Instruct the patient about:

- The nature of the polyp
- Clinical manifestations to report to the health care provider
- The need for regular, routine monitoring or screening

If the patient has had a polypectomy, follow-up sigmoidoscopic or colonoscopic examinations are needed because there is an increased risk for developing multiple polyps.

Nursing care of the patient after a polypectomy of the colorectal area includes monitoring for abdominal distention and pain, rectal bleeding, mucopurulent drainage from the rectum, and fever. A small amount of blood might appear in the stool after a polypectomy, but this should be temporary.

HEMORRHOIDS

❖ PATHOPHYSIOLOGY

Hemorrhoids are unnaturally swollen or distended veins in the anorectal region. The veins involved in the development of hemorrhoids are part of the normal structure in the anal region. With limited distention, the veins function as a valve overlying the anal sphincter that assists in continence. Increased intra-abdominal pressure causes elevated systemic and portal venous pressure, which is transmitted to the anorectal veins. Arterioles in the anorectal region shunt blood directly to the distended anorectal veins, which increases the pressure. With repeated elevations in pressure from increased intra-abdominal pressure and engorgement from arteriolar shunting of blood, the distended veins eventually separate from the smooth muscle surrounding them. The result is prolapse of the hemorrhoidal vessels.

Hemorrhoids can be internal or external (Fig. 56-8). **Internal hemorrhoids,** which cannot be seen on inspection of the perineal area, lie above the anal sphincter. **External hemorrhoids** lie below the anal sphincter and can be seen on inspection of the anal region. Prolapsed hemorrhoids can become thrombosed or inflamed, or they can bleed (McCance et al., 2014).

Hemorrhoids are common and not significant unless they cause pain or bleeding. Caused by increased abdominal pressure, the condition worsens during pregnancy, constipation with straining, obesity, heart failure, prolonged sitting or standing, and strenuous exercise and weight lifting. Decreased fluid intake can also cause hemorrhoids because of the development of hard stool and subsequent constipation. Straining while evacuating stool causes them to enlarge.

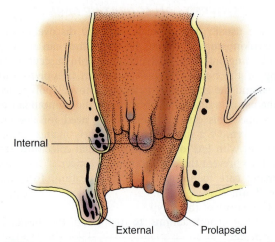

FIG. 56-8 Internal, external, and prolapsed hemorrhoids. *Internal hemorrhoids* lie above the anal sphincter and cannot be seen on inspection of the anal area. *External hemorrhoids* lie below the anal sphincter and can be seen on inspection of the anal region. Hemorrhoids that enlarge, fall down, and protrude through the anus are called *prolapsed hemorrhoids*.

Health Promotion and Maintenance

Prevention of constipation is the most important preventive measure. It can be prevented by increasing fiber in the diet, such as eating more whole grains and raw vegetables and fruits. Encourage patients to drink plenty of water unless otherwise contraindicated (e.g., kidney disease, heart disease). Remind the patient to avoid straining at stool. Remind him or her to exercise regularly with a gradual buildup in intensity. Maintaining a healthy weight also helps prevent hemorrhoids.

❖ PATIENT-CENTERED COLLABORATIVE CARE

◆ Assessment

The most common symptoms of hemorrhoids are bleeding, swelling, and prolapse (bulging). Blood is characteristically bright red and is present on toilet tissue or streaked in the stool. PAIN is a common symptom and is often associated with thrombosis, especially if thrombosis occurs suddenly. Other symptoms include itching and a mucous discharge. Diagnosis is usually made by inspection and digital examination.

◆ Interventions

Interventions are typically conservative and are aimed at reducing symptoms with a minimum of discomfort, cost, and time lost from usual activities. Local treatment and NUTRITION therapy are used when symptoms begin. Cold packs applied to the anorectal region for a few minutes at a time beginning with the onset of pain and tepid sitz baths 3 or 4 times per day are often enough to relieve discomfort, even if the hemorrhoids are thrombosed.

Topical anesthetics, such as lidocaine (Xylocaine), are useful for severe pain. Dibucaine (Nupercainal) ointment and similar products are available over the counter and may be applied for mild to moderate PAIN and itching. This ointment should be used only temporarily, however, because it can mask worsening symptoms and delay diagnosis of a severe disorder. If itching or inflammation is present, the health care provider prescribes a steroid preparation, such as hydrocortisone. Cleansing the anal area with moistened cleansing tissues rather than standard toilet tissue helps avoid irritation. The anal area should be cleansed gently by dabbing, rather than by wiping.

Diets high in fiber and fluids are recommended to promote regular bowel movements without straining. Stool softeners, such as docusate sodium (Colace), can be used temporarily. Irritating laxatives are avoided, as are foods and beverages that can make hemorrhoids worse. Spicy foods, nuts, coffee, and alcohol can be irritating. Remind patients to avoid sitting for long periods. The health care provider may prescribe mild oral analgesics for pain if the hemorrhoids are thrombosed.

Conservative treatment should alleviate symptoms in 3 to 5 days. If symptoms continue or recur frequently, the patient may require surgical intervention.

The surgeon can perform several procedures in an ambulatory care setting to remove symptomatic hemorrhoids (**hemorrhoidectomy**). The type of surgery (e.g., ultrasound or laser removal) depends on the degree of prolapse, whether there is thrombosis, and the overall condition of the patient. Complications of these procedures include PAIN, thrombosis of other hemorrhoids, infection, bleeding, and abscess formation. If the hemorrhoid is prolapsed, a circular stapling device may be used to excise a band of mucosa above the prolapse and restore the hemorrhoidal tissue back into the anal canal.

Teach patients with hemorrhoids about the need to eat high-fiber, high-fluid diets to promote regular bowel patterns before and after surgery. Advise them to avoid stimulant laxatives, which can be habit forming.

For patients who undergo any type of surgical intervention, monitor for bleeding and PAIN postoperatively and teach them to report these problems to their health care provider. Using moist heat (e.g., sitz baths or warm compresses) 3 or 4 times per day can help promote comfort.

! NURSING SAFETY PRIORITY (QSEN)
Action Alert

Tell the patient who has had surgical intervention for hemorrhoids that the first postoperative bowel movement may be very painful. Be sure that someone is with or near the patient when this happens. Some patients become light-headed and diaphoretic and may have syncope ("blackout").

The physician usually prescribes stool softeners such as docusate sodium (Colace) to begin preoperatively and continue after surgery. Analgesics and anti-inflammatory drugs are prescribed. A mild laxative should be administered if the patient has not had a bowel movement by the third postoperative day.

MALABSORPTION SYNDROME
❖ PATHOPHYSIOLOGY

Malabsorption is a syndrome associated with a variety of disorders and intestinal surgical procedures. It interferes with the ability to absorb nutrients and is a result of a generalized flattening of the mucosa of the small intestine. With various disorders, physiologic mechanisms limit absorption of nutrients because of one or more of these abnormalities:
- Bile salt deficiencies
- Enzyme deficiencies
- Presence of bacteria
- Disruption of the mucosal lining of the small intestine
- Altered lymphatic and vascular circulation
- Decrease in the gastric or intestinal surface area

The nutrient involved in malabsorption depends on the type and location of the abnormality in the intestinal tract.

Deficiencies of bile salts can lead to malabsorption of fats and fat-soluble vitamins. Bile salt deficiencies can result from decreased synthesis of bile in the liver, bile obstruction, or alteration of bile salt absorption in the small intestine.

Enzymes normally found in the intestine split disaccharides (complex sugars) to monosaccharides (simple sugars). Examples of these enzymes are lactase, sucrase, maltase, and isomaltase. Lactase deficiency is the most common disaccharide enzyme deficiency. Without sufficient amounts of this enzyme, the body is not able to break down lactose. Lactase deficiency can be due to genetic inheritance, injury to intestinal mucosa from viral hepatitis, or excessive bacteria in the intestine. Deficiencies of the other disaccharide enzymes are rare.

Pancreatic enzymes are also necessary for absorption of vitamin B_{12}. With destruction or obstruction of the pancreas or insufficient pancreatic stimulation, this nutrient is not well absorbed. Chronic pancreatitis, pancreatic carcinoma, resection of the pancreas, and cystic fibrosis can cause these malabsorption problems.

Loops of bowel can accumulate intestinal contents, resulting in bacterial overgrowth, when peristalsis is decreased. Bacteria at these sites break down bile salts, and fewer salts are available for fat absorption. They can also ingest vitamin B_{12}, which contributes to vitamin B_{12} deficiency. This process can occur after a gastrectomy.

Obstruction to lymphatic flow in the intestine can lead to loss of plasma proteins along with loss of minerals (e.g., iron, copper, calcium), vitamin B_{12}, folic acid, and lipids. Lymphatic obstruction can be caused by many conditions. Certain cancers such as lymphoma, inflammatory states, radiation enteritis, Crohn's disease, heart failure, and constrictive pericarditis are causes of lymphatic obstruction.

Interference with blood flow to the intestinal mucosa results in malabsorption. With intestinal surgery, there is loss of the surface area needed to facilitate absorption. Resection of the ileum results in vitamin B_{12}, bile salt, and other nutrient deficiencies. Gastric surgery is one of the most common causes of malabsorption and maldigestion. Other conditions associated with poor digestion and malabsorption include small-bowel ischemia and radiation enteritis.

❖ PATIENT-CENTERED COLLABORATIVE CARE
◆ Assessment

Chronic diarrhea is a classic symptom of malabsorption. It occurs as a result of unabsorbed nutrients, which add to the bulk of the stool, and unabsorbed fat. **Steatorrhea** (greater than normal amounts of fat in the feces) is a common sign. It is a result of bile salt deconjugation, nonabsorbed fats, or bacteria in the intestine. Not all patients with malabsorption have diarrhea. Instead, some have an increased stool mass. Other clinical manifestations include:
- Unintentional weight loss
- Bloating and flatus (carbohydrate malabsorption)
- Decreased libido
- Easy bruising (purpura)
- Anemia (with iron and folic acid or vitamin B_{12} deficiencies)
- Bone pain (with calcium and vitamin D deficiencies)
- Edema (caused by hypoproteinemia)

Serum laboratory studies reveal a decrease in mean corpuscular volume (MCV), mean corpuscular hemoglobin (MCH), and mean corpuscular hemoglobin concentration (MCHC). These decreases indicate hypochromic microcytic anemia resulting from iron deficiency. Increased MCV and variable MCH and MCHC values indicate macrocytic anemia resulting from vitamin B_{12} and folic acid deficiencies. Serum iron levels are low in protein malabsorption because of insufficient gastric acid for use of iron. Serum cholesterol levels may be low from decreased absorption and digestion of fat. Low serum calcium levels may indicate malabsorption of vitamin D and amino acids. Low levels of serum vitamin A (retinol) and carotene, its precursor, indicate a bile salt deficiency and malabsorption of fat. Serum albumin and total protein levels are low if protein is lost.

A quantitative *fecal fat analysis* is often elevated in either malabsorption or maldigestive disorders (Pagana & Pagana, 2014).

A *lactose tolerance test* is a type of disaccharidase analysis that may show an inability to digest foods and beverages that contain lactose. A hydrogen breath test can also be performed to detect this problem. The D-xylose absorption test can reveal low urine and serum D-xylose levels if malabsorption in the small intestine is present (Pagana & Pagana, 2014).

The *Schilling test* measures urinary excretion of vitamin B$_{12}$ for diagnosis of pernicious anemia and a variety of other malabsorption syndromes. The *bile acid breath test* assesses the absorption of bile salt. If the patient has bacterial overgrowth, the bile salts will become deconjugated and the carbon dioxide level in the breath will peak earlier than expected.

Ultrasonography is used to diagnose pancreatic tumors and tumors in the small intestine that are causing malabsorption. X-rays of the GI tract reveal pancreatic calcifications, tumors, or other abnormalities that cause malabsorption. A CT scan may also be done.

◆ Interventions

Interventions for most malabsorption syndromes focus on (1) avoidance of substances that aggravate malabsorption and (2) supplementation of nutrients. Surgical management of the primary disease may be indicated. Drug therapy may also improve or resolve malabsorption.

Nutrition management includes a low-fat diet for patients who have gallbladder disease, severe steatorrhea, or cystic fibrosis. A low-fat diet may or may not be indicated for pancreatic insufficiency because this disorder improves with enzyme replacement. Some clinicians believe that limitation of fat intake is not necessary with enzyme replacement. Dietary intake of fat is actually beneficial to the patient because it has a high number of calories. After a total gastrectomy, a high-protein, high-calorie diet and small, frequent meals are recommended. Lactose-free or lactose-restricted diets are available for patients with lactase deficiency, and gluten-free diets are available for those with celiac disease, discussed in Chapter 57.

The health care provider prescribes nutritional supplements according to the specific deficiency. Common supplements include:

- Water-soluble vitamins, such as folic acid and vitamin B complex
- Fat-soluble vitamins, such as vitamin A, vitamin D, and vitamin K
- Minerals, such as calcium, iron, and magnesium
- Pancreatic enzymes, such as pancrelipase (Pancrease, Viokase)

CHART 56-8   **Best Practice for Patient Safety & Quality Care**   **QSEN**

Special Skin Care for Patients with Chronic Diarrhea

- Use medicated wipes or premoistened disposable wipes rather than toilet tissue to clean the perineal area.
- Clean the perineal area well with mild soap and warm water after each stool; rinse soap from the area well.
- If the physician allows, provide a sitz bath several times per day.
- Apply a thin coat of A+D Ointment or other medicated protective barrier, such as aloe products, after each stool.
- Keep the patient off the affected buttock area.
- For open areas, cover with thin DuoDerm or Tegaderm occlusive dressing to promote rapid healing.
- Observe for fungal or yeast infections, which appear as dark red rashes with "satellite" lesions. Obtain prescription for medication if this problem occurs.

Antibiotics are used to treat disorders involving bacterial overgrowth. Bacterial overgrowth can be caused by a variety of disorders but is often treated with tetracycline and metronidazole (Flagyl, Novonidazol ✚).

Drug therapy is used to control the clinical manifestations of malabsorption. Antidiarrheal agents, such as diphenoxylate hydrochloride and atropine sulfate (Lomotil, N-Lomotil ✚), are often used to control diarrhea and steatorrhea. Anticholinergics, such as dicyclomine hydrochloride (Bentyl, Bentylol ✚), may be given before meals to inhibit gastric motility. IV fluids may be necessary to replenish fluid losses associated with diarrhea.

Provide special measures to protect the skin when chronic diarrhea occurs (Chart 56-8). Conduct an ongoing assessment for clinical manifestations of malabsorption, and relate these to activities and dietary intake. For example, patients with steatorrhea are monitored for FLUID AND ELECTROLYTE BALANCE and are encouraged to drink electrolyte-rich liquids liberally. Teach them the rationale for dietary, drug, and surgical management of nutritional deficiencies, and evaluate interventions on the basis of changes in or resolution of clinical manifestations.

NURSING CONCEPTS AND CLINICAL JUDGMENT REVIEW

What might you NOTICE if the patient has impaired absorption and inadequate NUTRITION as a result of noninflammatory intestinal disorders?

- Rectal bleeding
- Report of change in bowel habits
- Diarrhea or report of constipation
- Fatigue
- Vomiting
- Abdominal pain
- Change in bowel sounds (decreased or increased)
- Weight loss

What should you INTERPRET and how should you RESPOND to a patient with impaired absorption and inadequate NUTRITION as a result of noninflammatory intestinal disorders?

Perform and interpret focused physical assessment findings, including:

- Vital signs
- Complete pain assessment
- Abdominal assessment
- Current weight compared with previous weight

Respond by:

- Decreasing abdominal pain by placing patient in sitting position
- Starting IV (large-bore catheter) to replace fluids and electrolytes
- Giving blood transfusion as prescribed
- Providing rest
- Providing privacy and dignity

- Assisting with hygiene as needed
- Inserting nasogastric tube and connecting to low suction as needed
- Checking laboratory values of hemoglobin and hematocrit
- Checking stool for occult or frank blood
- Giving antidiarrheal drugs if prescribed
- Recording intake and output
- Assisting with ADLs and ambulation as needed

On what should you REFLECT?

- Continue to monitor for vomiting and diarrhea and for changes in pain.
- Think about what you need to document. Decide when you might need to call the health care provider or Rapid Response Team.
- Determine what health teaching and community resources may be needed for the patient and family.
- Think about what you can do to help prevent complications of the health problem.

GET READY FOR THE NCLEX® EXAMINATION!

KEY POINTS

Review these Key Points for each NCLEX Examination Client Needs Category.

Safe and Effective Care Environment

- Prioritize care for patients experiencing abdominal trauma: first assess **a**irway, **b**reathing, and **c**irculation (ABCs), and then monitor vital signs, mental status, and skin perfusion to assess for hypovolemic shock. **Safety** QSEN
- Collaborate with the certified wound, ostomy, continence nurse (CWOCN) or enterostomal therapist (ET) when a patient is scheduled for or has a new colostomy. **Teamwork and Collaboration** QSEN
- Collaborate with the case manager/discharge planner, health care provider, and CWOCN to plan care for the patient with CRC. **Teamwork and Collaboration** QSEN

Health Promotion and Maintenance

- Refer patients with familial CRC syndromes for genetic counseling and testing. **Patient-Centered Care** QSEN
- Refer ostomy patients to the United Ostomy Associations of America, Inc. and the American Cancer Society for additional information and support groups. **Patient-Centered Care** QSEN
- Teach patients with irritable bowel syndrome (IBS) to avoid GI stimulants, such as caffeine, alcohol, and milk and milk products, and to manage stress. **Evidence-Based Practice** QSEN
- Instruct patients on dietary modifications to decrease the occurrence of colorectal cancer (CRC), such as eating a diet high in fiber and avoiding red meat. **Evidence-Based Practice** QSEN
- Teach adults 50 years and older to have routine screening for CRC as listed in Chart 56-2; people with genetic predispositions should have earlier and more frequent screening. **Evidence-Based Practice** QSEN
- Teach people to prevent or manage constipation to help avoid hemorrhoids; teach patients the importance of maintaining a healthy weight to decrease the risk for hemorrhoids. **Evidence-Based Practice** QSEN
- Teach patients and caregivers how to provide colostomy care, including dietary measures, skin care, and ostomy products. **Patient-Centered Care** QSEN

Psychosocial Integrity

- Assist the patient with CRC with the grieving process. **Patient-Centered Care** QSEN

- Be aware that having a colostomy is a life-altering event that can severely impact one's body image; issues related to sexuality and fear of acceptance should be discussed. **Patient-Centered Care** QSEN

Physiological Integrity

- Be aware that minimally invasive inguinal hernia repair is an ambulatory care procedure done via laparoscopy; postoperative management requires health teaching regarding rest for a few days and inspection of incisions for signs of infection (see Chart 56-1). **Evidence-Based Practice** QSEN
- Be aware that a strangulated hernia can cause ischemia and bowel obstruction, requiring immediate intervention. **Safety** QSEN
- Monitor patients who have conventional open herniorrhaphy for ability to void. **Safety** QSEN
- Recall that changes in bowel habits or stool characteristics and/or rectal bleeding are often associated with a diagnosis of CRC. **Safety** QSEN
- Keep the peristomal skin clean and dry; observe for leakage around the pouch seal. **Evidence-Based Practice** QSEN
- Provide meticulous perineal wound care for patients having an abdominoperineal (AP) resection, as described in Chart 56-3. **Safety** QSEN
- Document the characteristics of the colostomy stoma, which should be reddish pink and moist; report abnormalities such as ischemia and necrosis (purplish or black) or unusual bleeding to the surgeon. **Informatics** QSEN
- Recall that bowel sounds are altered in patients with obstruction; absent bowel sounds imply total obstruction. **Safety** QSEN
- Assess the patient's nasogastric tube for proper placement, patency, and output at least every 4 hours. **Safety** QSEN
- Monitor patients with bowel obstruction for signs and symptoms of fluid, electrolyte, and acid-base imbalances; patients with small bowel obstruction are at greater risk for problems with FLUID AND ELECTROLYTE BALANCE. **Safety** QSEN
- Teach patients having hemorrhoid surgery to take stool softeners before and after surgery to decrease discomfort during ELIMINATION. **Evidence-Based Practice** QSEN
- Provide comfort measures for the patient who has chronic diarrhea associated with malabsorption as described in Chart 56-8. **Patient-Centered Care** QSEN
- Reinforce teaching regarding supplements or dietary restrictions needed for malabsorption management. **Evidence-Based Practice** QSEN

Care of Patients with Inflammatory Intestinal Disorders

Donna D. Ignatavicius

ⓔ http://evolve.elsevier.com/Iggy/

PRIORITY CONCEPTS

- ELIMINATION
- INFLAMMATION
- NUTRITION

- PAIN
- INFECTION
- FLUID AND ELECTROLYTE BALANCE

LEARNING OUTCOMES

Safe and Effective Care Environment
1. Describe the importance of collaborating with health care team members to provide care for patients with inflammatory bowel disease (IBD).

Health Promotion and Maintenance
2. Develop a health teaching plan for patients to promote self-management when caring for ileostomy or other surgical diversion.
3. Identify community resources for patients and families regarding IBD.
4. Discuss ways that gastroenteritis can be prevented.

Psychosocial Integrity
5. Identify expected body image changes associated with having an ileostomy or other surgical diversion.

Physiological Integrity
6. Differentiate common types of acute inflammatory bowel disorders.

7. Develop an evidence-based collaborative plan of care for the patient who has appendicitis or peritonitis.
8. Compare and contrast the pathophysiology and clinical manifestations of ulcerative colitis and Crohn's disease.
9. Identify priority problems for patients with ulcerative colitis.
10. Explain the purpose of and nursing implications related to drug therapy for patients with IBD.
11. Plan evidence-based postoperative care for a patient undergoing surgery for IBD.
12. Develop a hospital discharge teaching plan for patients who have IBD.
13. Explain the role of NUTRITION therapy in managing the patient with diverticular disease.
14. Describe the comfort measures to relieve PAIN that the nurse can implement for the patient with anal disorders.

Inflammatory bowel health problems affect the small intestine, large intestine (colon), or both. Together, these organs are called the *intestinal tract*. Continued digestion of food and absorption of nutrients occur primarily in the small intestine (bowel) to meet the body's needs for energy. Water is reabsorbed in the large intestine to help maintain a fluid balance and promote the passage of waste products. When the intestinal tract and its nearby structures become inflamed, NUTRITION may be inadequate to meet a patient's needs. Bowel ELIMINATION changes, PAIN, INFECTION, and/or problems with FLUID AND ELECTROLYTE BALANCE can result from inflammatory bowel diseases that are chronic.

ACUTE INFLAMMATORY BOWEL DISORDERS

Appendicitis, gastroenteritis, and peritonitis are the most common acute inflammatory bowel problems. These disorders are potentially life threatening and can have major systemic complications if not treated promptly.

APPENDICITIS

❖ PATHOPHYSIOLOGY

Appendicitis is an acute INFLAMMATION of the vermiform appendix that occurs most often among young adults. It is the most common cause of right lower quadrant (RLQ) PAIN. The appendix usually extends off the proximal cecum of the colon just below the ileocecal valve. Inflammation occurs when the lumen (opening) of the appendix is obstructed (blocked), leading to infection as bacteria invade the wall of the appendix. The initial obstruction is usually a result of fecaliths (very hard pieces of feces) composed of calcium phosphate–rich mucus and inorganic salts. Less common causes are malignant tumors, helminthes (worms), or other INFECTIONS (McCance et al., 2014).

When the lumen is blocked, the mucosa secretes fluid, increasing the internal pressure and restricting blood flow, which results in PAIN. If the process occurs slowly, an abscess may develop, but a rapid process may result in peritonitis (INFLAMMATION and INFECTION of the peritoneum). *All complications of peritonitis are serious. Gangrene and sepsis can occur within 24 to 36 hours, are life threatening, and are some of the most common indications for emergency surgery. Perforation may develop within 24 hours, but the risk rises rapidly after 48 hours.* Perforation of the appendix also results in peritonitis with a temperature of greater than 101°F (38.3°C) and a rise in pulse rate.

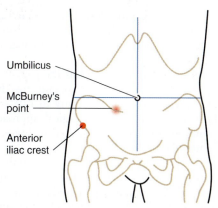

FIG. 57-1 McBurney's point is located midway between the anterior iliac crest and the umbilicus in the right lower quadrant. This is the classic area for localized tenderness during the later stages of appendicitis.

CONSIDERATIONS FOR OLDER ADULTS
Patient-Centered Care QSEN

Appendicitis is relatively rare at extremes in age. However, perforation is more common in older people, causing a higher mortality rate. The diagnosis of appendicitis is difficult to establish in older adults because symptoms of pain and tenderness may not be as pronounced in this age-group. This difference results in treatment delay and an increased risk for perforation, peritonitis, and death.

appendix. An *ultrasound* study may show the presence of an enlarged appendix. If symptoms are recurrent or prolonged, a CT scan can be used for diagnosis and may reveal the presence of a fecalith.

◆ Interventions

All patients with suspected or confirmed appendicitis are hospitalized and most have surgery to remove the inflamed appendix.

Nonsurgical Management. Keep the patient with suspected or known appendicitis on NPO to prepare for the possibility of surgery and to avoid making the INFLAMMATION worse.

❗ NURSING SAFETY PRIORITY QSEN
Action Alert

For the patient with suspected appendicitis, administer IV fluids as prescribed to maintain FLUID AND ELECTROLYTE BALANCE and to replace fluid volume. If tolerated, advise the patient to maintain a semi-Fowler's position so that abdominal drainage, if any, can be contained in the lower abdomen. Once the diagnosis of appendicitis is confirmed and surgery is scheduled, administer opioid analgesics and antibiotics as prescribed. *The patient with suspected or confirmed appendicitis should not receive laxatives or enemas, which can cause perforation of the appendix. Do not apply heat to the abdomen because this may increase circulation to the appendix and result in increased inflammation and perforation!*

❖ PATIENT-CENTERED COLLABORATIVE CARE
◆ Assessment

History taking and tracking the sequence of symptoms are important because nausea or vomiting before abdominal pain can indicate gastroenteritis. Abdominal PAIN followed by nausea and vomiting can indicate appendicitis. Ask about risk factors such as age, familial tendency, and intra-abdominal tumors. Classically, patients with appendicitis have cramplike pain in the epigastric or periumbilical area. Anorexia is a frequent symptom with nausea and vomiting occurring in many cases.

Perform a complete pain assessment. Initially, PAIN can present anywhere in the abdomen or flank area. As the INFLAMMATION and INFECTION progress, the pain becomes more severe and steady and shifts to the RLQ between the anterior iliac crest and the umbilicus. This area is referred to as *McBurney's point* (Fig. 57-1). *Abdominal pain that increases with cough or movement and is relieved by bending the right hip or the knees suggests perforation and peritonitis.* An advanced practice nurse or other health care provider assesses for muscle rigidity and guarding on palpation of the abdomen. The patient may report pain after release of pressure. This is referred to as "rebound" tenderness.

Laboratory findings do not establish the diagnosis, but often there is a moderate elevation of the *white blood cell (WBC) count* (leukocytosis) to 10,000 to 18,000/mm³ with a "shift to the left" (an increased number of immature WBCs). A WBC elevation to greater than 20,000/mm³ may indicate a perforated

Surgical Management. Surgery is required as soon as possible. An **appendectomy** is the removal of the inflamed appendix by one of several surgical approaches. Uncomplicated appendectomy procedures are done via laparoscopy. A **laparoscopy** is a minimally invasive surgical (MIS) procedure with one or more small incisions near the umbilicus through which a small endoscope is placed. Patients having this type of surgery for appendix removal have few postoperative complications (see Chapter 15). A newer procedure known as natural orifice transluminal endoscopic surgery (NOTES) (e.g., transvaginal endoscopic appendectomy) does not require an external skin incision. In this procedure the surgeon places the endoscope into the vagina or other orifice and makes a small incision to enter the peritoneal space. Patients having any type of laparoscopic procedures are typically discharged the same day of surgery with less pain and few complications after discharge. Most patients can return to usual activities in 1 to 2 weeks.

If the diagnosis is not definitive but the patient is at high risk for complications from suspected appendicitis, the surgeon may perform an exploratory laparotomy to rule out appendicitis. A **laparotomy** is an open surgical approach with a large abdominal incision for complicated or atypical appendicitis or peritonitis.

Preoperative teaching is often limited because the patient is in PAIN or may be transferred quickly to the operating suite for emergency surgery. The patient is prepared for general anesthesia and surgery as described in Chapter 14. After surgery, care of the patient who has undergone an appendectomy is the same as that required for anyone who has received general anesthesia (see Chapter 16).

If complications such as peritonitis or abscesses are found during *open* traditional surgery, wound drains are inserted and a nasogastric tube may be placed to decompress the stomach and prevent abdominal distention. Administer IV antibiotics and opioid analgesics as prescribed. Help the patient out of bed on the evening of surgery to help prevent respiratory complications, such as atelectasis. He or she may be hospitalized for as long as 3 to 5 days and return to normal activity in 4 to 6 weeks.

PERITONITIS

Peritonitis is a life-threatening, acute INFLAMMATION and INFECTION of the visceral/parietal peritoneum and endothelial lining of the abdominal cavity. Primary peritonitis is rare and indicates the peritoneum is infected via the bloodstream. This problem is not discussed here.

❖ PATHOPHYSIOLOGY

Normally the peritoneal cavity contains about 50 mL of sterile fluid (transudate), which prevents friction in the abdominal cavity during peristalsis. When the peritoneal cavity is contaminated by bacteria, the body first begins an inflammatory reaction walling off a localized area to fight the INFECTION. This local reaction involves vascular dilation and increased capillary permeability, allowing transport of leukocytes and subsequent phagocytosis of the offending organisms. If this walling-off process fails, the INFLAMMATION spreads and contamination becomes massive, resulting in diffuse (widespread) peritonitis.

Peritonitis is most often caused by contamination of the peritoneal cavity by bacteria or chemicals. Bacteria gain entry into the peritoneum by perforation (from appendicitis, diverticulitis, peptic ulcer disease) or from an external penetrating wound, a gangrenous gallbladder, bowel obstruction, or ascending infection through the genital tract. Less common causes include perforating tumors, leakage or contamination during surgery, and INFECTION by skin pathogens in patients undergoing continuous ambulatory peritoneal dialysis (CAPD). Common bacteria responsible for peritonitis include *Escherichia coli*, *Streptococcus*, *Staphylococcus*, *Pneumococcus*, and *Gonococcus*. Chemical peritonitis results from leakage of bile, pancreatic enzymes, and gastric acid (McCance et al., 2014).

When diagnosis and treatment of peritonitis are delayed, blood vessel dilation continues. The body responds to the continuing infectious process by shunting extra blood to the area of INFLAMMATION (hyperemia). Fluid is shifted from the extracellular fluid compartment into the peritoneal cavity, connective tissues, and GI tract (*"third spacing"*). This shift of fluid can result in a significant decrease in circulatory volume and *hypovolemic shock*. Severely decreased circulatory volume can result in insufficient perfusion of the kidneys, leading to acute kidney injury with impaired FLUID AND ELECTROLYTE BALANCE (McCance et al., 2014). Assess for clinical manifestations of these life-threatening problems.

Peristalsis slows or *stops* in response to severe peritoneal INFLAMMATION, and the lumen of the bowel becomes distended with gas and fluid. Fluid that normally flows to the small bowel and the colon for reabsorption accumulates in the intestine in volumes of 7 to 8 L daily. The toxins or bacteria responsible for the peritonitis can also enter the bloodstream from the peritoneal area and lead to bacteremia or **septicemia** (bacterial invasion of the blood).

Respiratory problems can occur as a result of increased abdominal pressure against the diaphragm from intestinal distention and fluid shifts to the peritoneal cavity. PAIN can interfere with respirations at a time when the patient has an increased oxygen demand because of the infectious process.

❖ PATIENT-CENTERED COLLABORATIVE CARE

◆ Assessment

Ask the patient about abdominal PAIN, and determine the character of the pain (e.g., cramping, sharp, aching), location of the pain, and whether the pain is localized or generalized. Ask about a history of a low-grade fever or recent spikes in temperature.

Physical findings of peritonitis (Chart 57-1) depend on several factors: the stage of the disease, the ability of the body to localize the process by walling off the infection, and whether the INFLAMMATION has progressed to generalized peritonitis. The patient most often appears acutely ill, lying still, possibly with the knees flexed. Movement is guarded, and he or she may report and show signs of pain (e.g., facial grimacing) with coughing or movement of any type. During inspection, observe for progressive abdominal distention, often seen when the inflammation markedly reduces intestinal motility. Auscultate for bowel sounds, which usually disappear with progression of the inflammation.

CHART 57-1 Key Features

Peritonitis

- Rigid, boardlike abdomen (classic)
- Abdominal pain (localized, poorly localized, or referred to the shoulder or chest)
- Distended abdomen
- Nausea, anorexia, vomiting
- Diminishing bowel sounds
- Inability to pass flatus or feces
- Rebound tenderness in the abdomen
- High fever
- Tachycardia
- Dehydration from high fever (poor skin turgor)
- Decreased urine output
- Hiccups
- Possible compromise in respiratory status

The cardinal signs of peritonitis are abdominal pain, tenderness, and distention. In the patient with *localized* peritonitis, the abdomen is tender on palpation in a well-defined area with rebound tenderness in this area. With *generalized* peritonitis, tenderness is widespread.

! NURSING SAFETY PRIORITY (QSEN)
Action Alert

For patients with peritonitis, assess for abdominal wall rigidity, which is a classic finding that is sometimes referred to as a "boardlike" abdomen. Monitor the patient for a high fever because of the infectious process. Assess for tachycardia occurring in response to the fever and decreased circulating blood volume. Observe whether he or she has dry mucous membranes and a low urine output seen with third spacing. Nausea and vomiting may also be present. Hiccups may occur as a result of diaphragmatic irritation. Be sure to document all assessment findings.

White blood cell (WBC) counts are often elevated to 20,000/mm³ with a high neutrophil count. *Blood culture* studies may be done to determine whether septicemia has occurred and to identify the causative organism to enable appropriate therapy. The health care provider requests laboratory tests to assess FLUID AND ELECTROLYTE BALANCE and renal status, including blood urea nitrogen (BUN), creatinine, hemoglobin, and hematocrit. Oxygen saturation and end–carbon dioxide monitoring may be obtained to assess respiratory function and acid-base balance.

Abdominal x-rays can assess for free air or fluid in the abdominal cavity, indicating perforation. The x-rays may also show dilation, edema, and inflammation of the small and large intestines. An *abdominal ultrasound* may also be performed.

◆ Interventions

Patients with peritonitis are hospitalized because of the severe nature of the illness. If complications are extensive, the patients are often admitted to a critical care unit. Nursing interventions focus on the early identification of complications.

Nonsurgical Management. The health care provider prescribes hypertonic IV fluids and broad-spectrum antibiotics immediately after establishing the diagnosis of peritonitis. IV fluids are used to replace fluids collected in the peritoneum and bowel. Monitor daily weight and intake and output carefully. A nasogastric tube (NGT) decompresses the stomach and the intestine, and the patient is NPO. Apply oxygen as prescribed and according to the patient's respiratory status and oxygen saturation via pulse oximetry (e.g., Spo₂ less than 93%). Administer analgesics, and monitor for pain control. Document all PAIN assessments and interventions thoroughly.

Surgical Management. Abdominal surgery may be needed to identify and repair the cause of the peritonitis. If the patient is so critically ill that surgery would be life threatening, it may be delayed. Surgery focuses on controlling the contamination, removing foreign material from the peritoneal cavity, and draining collected fluid.

Exploratory laparotomy (surgical opening into the abdomen) or laparoscopy is used to remove or repair the inflamed or perforated organ (e.g., appendectomy for an inflamed appendix; a colon resection, with or without a colostomy, for a perforated diverticulum). Before the incision(s) is closed, the surgeon irrigates the peritoneum with antibiotic solutions. Several catheters may be inserted to drain the cavity and provide a route for irrigation after surgery.

The preoperative care is similar to that described in Chapter 14 for patients having general anesthesia. Chapter 16 describes general postoperative care for exploratory laparotomy. Multi-system complications can occur with peritonitis. Loss of fluids and electrolytes from the extracellular space to the peritoneal cavity, NGT suctioning, and NPO status require that the patient receives IV fluid replacement. Be sure that unlicensed assistive personnel (UAP) carefully measure intake and output. Fluid rates may be changed frequently based on laboratory values and patient condition.

! NURSING SAFETY PRIORITY (QSEN)
Action Alert

Monitor the patient's level of consciousness, vital signs, respiratory status (respiratory rate and breath sounds), and intake and output at least hourly immediately after abdominal surgery. Maintain the patient in a semi-Fowler's position to promote drainage of peritoneal contents into the lower region of the abdominal cavity. This position helps increase lung expansion.

If an open surgical procedure is needed, the INFECTION may slow healing of an incision or the incision may be partially open to heal by second or third intention. These wounds require special care involving manual irrigation or packing as prescribed by the surgeon. If the surgeon requests peritoneal irrigation through a drain, *maintain sterile technique during manual irrigation.* Assess whether the patient retains the fluid used for irrigation by comparing the amount of fluid returned with the amount of fluid instilled. Fluid retention could cause abdominal distention or pain.

Community-Based Care

The length of hospitalization depends on the extent and severity of the infectious process. Patients who have a localized abscess drained and who respond to antibiotics and IV fluids without multi-system complications are discharged in several days. Others may require mechanical ventilation or hemodialysis with longer hospital stays. Some patients may be transferred to a transitional care unit to complete their antibiotic therapy and recovery. Convalescence is often longer than for other surgeries because of multi-system involvement.

When discharged home, assess the patient's ability for self-management at home with the added task of incision care and a reduced activity tolerance. Provide the patient and family with written and oral instructions to report these problems to the health care provider immediately:

- Unusual or foul-smelling drainage
- Swelling, redness, or warmth or bleeding from the incision site
- A temperature higher than 101° F (38.3° C)
- Abdominal PAIN
- Signs of wound dehiscence or ileus

Patients with large incisions heal by second or third intention and may require dressings, solution, and catheter-tipped syringes to irrigate the wound. A home care nurse may be needed to assess, irrigate, or pack the wound and change the dressing as needed until the patient and family feel comfortable with the procedure. If the patient needs assistance with ADLs, a home care aide or temporary placement in a skilled care facility may be indicated. Collaborate with the case manager (CM) to determine the most appropriate setting for seamless continuing care in the community.

Review information about antibiotics and analgesics. For patients taking oral opioid analgesics such as oxycodone with acetaminophen (Tylox, Percocet, Endocet ✦) for any length of time, a stool softener such as docusate sodium (Colace, Regulex ✦) may be prescribed. Older adults are especially at risk for constipation from codeine-based drugs. Remind patients to avoid taking additional acetaminophen (Tylenol) to prevent liver toxicity.

Teach patients to refrain from any lifting for *at least* 6 weeks after an open surgical procedure. Other activity limitations are made on an individual basis with the physician's recommendation. Patients who have laparoscopic surgery can resume activities within a week or two and may not have any major restrictions.

⚡ NCLEX EXAMINATION CHALLENGE

Safe and Effective Care Environment

A client had a bowel resection yesterday for colorectal cancer. Which assessment finding does the nurse report immediately to the surgeon?

A. Abdominal discomfort
B. Mild abdominal distention
C. Distended, board-like abdomen
D. Minimal abdominal bowel sounds

GASTROENTERITIS

❖ PATHOPHYSIOLOGY

Gastroenteritis is a very common health problem worldwide that causes diarrhea and/or vomiting as a result of INFLAMMATION of the mucous membranes of the stomach and intestinal tract. It affects mainly the small bowel and can be caused by either viral or bacterial INFECTION. Viral gastroenteritis is the most common (Krenzer, 2012). Table 57-1 lists common types of gastroenteritis and their primary characteristics.

Norovirus (also known as Norwalk-like viruses) is the leading foodborne disease that causes gastroenteritis. It occurs most often between November and April because it is resistant to low temperatures and has a long viral shedding before and after the illness. Norovirus is transmitted (spread) through the fecal-oral route from person to person and from contaminated food and water. Infected people can also contaminate surfaces and objects in the environment. Vomiting causes the virus to become airborne. The incubation time is 1 to 2 days.

In most cases of gastroenteritis, the illness is self-limiting and lasts about 3 days. However, in people who are immunosuppressed or in older adults, dehydration and hypovolemia can occur as complications requiring medical attention and possibly hospitalization.

TABLE 57-1	Common Types of Gastroenteritis and Their Characteristics
TYPE	**CHARACTERISTICS**
Viral Gastroenteritis	
Epidemic viral	Caused by many parvovirus-type organisms
	Transmitted by the fecal-oral route in food and water
	Incubation period 10-51 hrs
	Communicable during acute illness
Norovirus (Norwalk viruses)	Transmitted by the fecal-oral route and possibly the respiratory route (vomitus)
	Incubation in 48 hrs
	Affects adults of all ages
	Older adults can become hypovolemic and experience electrolyte imbalances
Bacterial Gastroenteritis	
Campylobacter enteritis	Transmitted by the fecal-oral route or by contact with infected animals or infants
	Incubation period 1-10 days
	Communicable for 2-7 wks
Escherichia coli diarrhea	Transmitted by fecal contamination of food, water, or fomites
Shigellosis	Transmitted by direct and indirect fecal-oral routes
	Incubation period 1-7 days
	Communicable during the acute illness to 4 wk after the illness
	Humans possibly carriers for months

Health Promotion and Maintenance

Outbreaks of norovirus have occurred in prisons, cruise ships, nursing homes, college dormitories, and other places where large groups of people are in close proximity. Handwashing and sanitizing surfaces and other environmental items help prevent the spread of the illness. Hand sanitizers are often placed in public areas so that hands can be cleaned when washing with soap and water is inconvenient. Proper food and beverage preparation is also important to prevent contamination.

❖ PATIENT-CENTERED COLLABORATIVE CARE

◆ Assessment

The patient history can provide information related to the potential cause of the illness. Ask about recent travel, especially to tropical regions of Asia, Africa, or Central or South America. Some areas of Mexico may also be the source of gastroenteritis.

Also inquire if the patient has eaten at any restaurant in the past 24 to 36 hours. Some people have acquired gastroenteritis from eating in "fast food" restaurants or from food items purchased at a farmer's market or grocery store. Bacterial INFECTIONS have caused large outbreaks that resulted from contaminated spinach and lettuce in the United States.

The patient who has gastroenteritis usually looks ill. Nausea and vomiting typically occur first, followed by abdominal cramping and diarrhea.

For patients who are older or for those who have inadequate immune systems, weakness and cardiac dysrhythmias may occur from loss of potassium (hypokalemia) from diarrhea. Monitor for and document manifestations of hypokalemia and hypovolemia (dehydration).

Action Alert

For patients with gastroenteritis, note any abdominal distention and listen for hyperactive bowel sounds. Depending on the amount of fluids and electrolytes lost through diarrhea and vomiting, patients may have varying degrees of dehydration manifested by:
- Poor skin turgor
- Fever (not common in older adults)
- Dry mucous membranes
- Orthostatic blood pressure changes (which can cause falls, especially for older adults)
- Hypotension
- Oliguria (scant urinary output)

In some cases, dehydration may be severe. Dehydration occurs rapidly in older adults. Monitor mental status changes, such as acute confusion, that result from hypoxia in the older adult. These changes may be the only clinical manifestation of dehydration in older adults.

◆ Interventions

For any type of gastroenteritis, encourage fluid replacement. The amount and route of fluid administration are determined by the patient's hydration status and overall health condition. Teach patients to drink extra fluids to replace fluid lost through vomiting and diarrhea. Oral rehydration therapy (ORT) may be needed for some patients to replace fluids and electrolytes. Examples of ORT solutions include Gatorade, Pedialyte, and Powerade. Depending on the patient's age and severity of dehydration, he or she may be admitted to the hospital for gastroenteritis or may stay in the emergency department or urgent care center until adequate hydration is restored.

Drugs that suppress intestinal motility may not be given for bacterial or viral gastroenteritis. *Use of these drugs can prevent the infecting organisms from being eliminated from the body.* If the health care provider determines that antiperistaltic agents are necessary, an initial dose of loperamide (Imodium) 4 mg can be administered orally, followed by 2 mg after each loose stool, up to 16 mg daily.

Drug Alert

Diphenoxylate hydrochloride with atropine sulfate (Lomotil, Lomanate) reduces GI motility but is used sparingly because of its habit-forming ability. *The drug should not be used for older adults because it also causes drowsiness and could contribute to falls.*

Treatment with antibiotics may be needed if the gastroenteritis is due to bacterial infection with fever and severe diarrhea. Depending on the type and severity of the illness, examples of drugs that may be prescribed include ciprofloxacin (Cipro), levofloxacin (Levaquin), or azithromycin (Zithromax). If the gastroenteritis is due to shigellosis, anti-infective agents such as trimethoprim/sulfamethoxazole (Septra DS, Bactrim DS, Roubac ♣) or ciprofloxacin (Cipro) are prescribed.

Frequent stools that are rich in electrolytes and enzymes, as well as frequent wiping and washing of the anal region, can irritate the skin. Teach the patient to avoid toilet paper and harsh soaps. Ideally, he or she can gently clean the area with warm water or an absorbent material, followed by thorough but gentle drying. Cream, oil, or gel can be applied to a damp, warm washcloth to remove stool that sticks to open skin. Special prepared skin wipes can also be used. Protective barrier cream can be applied to the skin between stools. Sitz baths for 10 minutes 2 or 3 times daily can also relieve discomfort.

If leakage of stool is a problem, the patient can use an absorbent cotton or panty liner and keep it in place with snug underwear. For patients who are incontinent, remind unlicensed assistive personnel (UAP) to keep the perineal and buttock areas clean and dry. The use of incontinent pads at night instead of briefs allows air to circulate to the skin and prevents irritation.

During the acute phase of the illness, teach the patient and family about the importance of fluid replacement. Teaching the patient and family about reducing the risk for transmission of gastroenteritis is also important (Chart 57-2).

CHRONIC INFLAMMATORY BOWEL DISEASE

Ulcerative colitis and Crohn's disease are the two most common inflammatory bowel diseases (IBDs) that affect adults. Comparisons and differences are listed in Table 57-2. Viral and bacterial gastroenteritis can cause symptoms similar to those of

---

CHART 57-2 Patient and Family Education: Preparing for Self-Management
Preventing Transmission of Gastroenteritis

Advise the patient to:
- Wash hands well for at least 30 seconds with an antibacterial soap, especially after a bowel movement, and maintain good personal hygiene.
- Restrict the use of glasses, dishes, eating utensils, and tubes of toothpaste for his or her own use. In severe cases, disposable utensils may be wise.
- Maintain clean bathroom facilities to avoid exposure to stool.
- Inform the health care provider if symptoms persist beyond 3 days.
- Do not prepare or handle food that will be consumed by others. If you (the patient) are employed as a food handler, the public health department should be consulted for recommendations about the return to work.

TABLE 57-2 Differential Features of Ulcerative Colitis and Crohn's Disease

FEATURE	ULCERATIVE COLITIS	CROHN'S DISEASE
Location	Begins in the rectum and proceeds in a continuous manner toward the cecum	Most often in the terminal ileum, with patchy involvement through all layers of the bowel
Etiology	Unknown	Unknown
Peak incidence at age	15-25 yr and 55-65 yr	15-40 yr
Number of stools	10-20 liquid, bloody stools per day	5-6 soft, loose stools per day, non-bloody
Complications	Hemorrhage Nutritional deficiencies	Fistulas (common) Nutritional deficiencies
Need for surgery	Infrequent	Frequent

IBD, and other problems must be ruled out before a definitive diagnosis is made.

The approach to each patient is individualized. Encourage patients to self-manage their disease by learning about the illness, treatment, drugs, and complications.

ULCERATIVE COLITIS

❖ PATHOPHYSIOLOGY

Ulcerative colitis (UC) creates widespread INFLAMMATION of mainly the rectum and rectosigmoid colon but can extend to the entire colon when the disease is extensive. Distribution of the disease can remain constant for years. UC is a disease that is associated with periodic remissions and exacerbations (flare-ups) (McCance et al., 2014). Many factors can cause exacerbations, including intestinal INFECTIONS. Older adults with UC are at high risk for impaired FLUID AND ELECTROLYTE BALANCE as a result of diarrhea, including dehydration and hypokalemia.

The intestinal mucosa becomes hyperemic (has increased blood flow), edematous, and reddened. In more severe INFLAMMATION, the lining can bleed and small erosions, or ulcers, occur. Abscesses can form in these ulcerative areas and result in tissue necrosis (cell death). Continued edema and mucosal thickening can lead to a narrowed colon and possibly a partial bowel obstruction. Table 57-3 lists the categories of the severity of UC.

The patient's stool typically contains blood and mucus. Patients report tenesmus (an unpleasant and urgent sensation to defecate) and lower abdominal colicky PAIN relieved with defecation. Malaise, anorexia, anemia, dehydration, fever, and weight loss are common. Extraintestinal manifestations such as migratory polyarthritis, ankylosing spondylitis, and erythema nodosum are present in a large number of patients. The common complications of UC, including extraintestinal manifestations, are listed in Table 57-4.

Etiology and Genetic Risk

The exact cause of UC is unknown, but a combination of genetic, immunologic, and environmental factors likely contributes to disease development. A genetic basis of the disease has been supported because it is often found in families and twins. Immunologic causes, including autoimmune dysfunction, are likely the etiology of extraintestinal manifestations of the disease. Epithelial antibodies in the immunoglobulin G (IgG) class have been identified in the blood of some patients with UC (McCance et al., 2014).

With long-term disease, cellular changes can occur that increase the risk for colon cancer. Damage from pro-inflammatory cytokines, such as specific interleukins (ILs) (e.g., IL-1, IL-6, IL-8) and tumor necrosis factor (TNF)–alpha, have cytotoxic effects on the colonic mucosa (McCance et al., 2014).

Incidence and Prevalence

Chronic inflammatory bowel disease (IBD) affects about 1.4 million people in the United States and is split about equally between ulcerative colitis (UC) and Crohn's disease (discussed later). Peak age for being diagnosed with UC is between 30 and

---

TABLE 57-3 American College of Gastroenterologists Classification of UC Severity

SEVERITY	STOOL FREQUENCY	SIGNS/SYMPTOMS
Mild	<4 stools/day with/without blood	Asymptomatic Laboratory values usually normal
Moderate	>4 stools/day with/without blood	Minimal symptoms Mild abdominal pain Mild intermittent nausea Possible increased C-reactive protein* or ESR†
Severe	>6 bloody stools/day	Fever Tachycardia Anemia Abdominal pain Elevated C-reactive protein* and/or ESR†
Fulminant	>10 bloody stools/day	Increasing symptoms Anemia may require transfusion Colonic distention on x-ray

UC, Ulcerative colitis.
*C-reactive protein is a sensitive acute-phase serum marker that is evident in the first 6 hours of an inflammatory process.
†ESR (erythrocyte sedimentation rate) may be helpful but is less sensitive than C-reactive protein.

TABLE 57-4 Complications of Ulcerative Colitis and Crohn's Disease

COMPLICATION	DESCRIPTION
Hemorrhage/perforation	Lower gastrointestinal bleeding results from erosion of the bowel wall.
Abscess formation	Localized pockets of infection develop in the ulcerated bowel lining.
Toxic megacolon	Paralysis of the colon causes dilation and subsequent colonic ileus, possibly perforation.
Malabsorption	Essential nutrients cannot be absorbed through the diseased intestinal wall, causing anemia and malnutrition (most common in Crohn's disease).
Nonmechanical bowel obstruction	Obstruction results from toxic megacolon or cancer.
Fistulas	In Crohn's disease in which the inflammation is transmural, fistulas can occur anywhere but usually track between the bowel and bladder resulting in pyuria and fecaluria.
Colorectal cancer	Patients with ulcerative colitis with a history longer than 10 years have a high risk for colorectal cancer. This complication accounts for about one third of all deaths related to ulcerative colitis.
Extraintestinal complications	Complications include arthritis, hepatic and biliary disease (especially cholelithiasis), oral and skin lesions, and ocular disorders, such as iritis. The cause is unknown.
Osteoporosis	Osteoporosis occurs especially in patients with Crohn's disease.

40 years and again at 55 to 65 years. Women are more often affected than men in their younger years, but men have the disease more often as middle-aged and older adults (McCance et al., 2014).

CULTURAL CONSIDERATIONS
Patient-Centered Care QSEN

Ulcerative colitis is more common among Jewish persons than among those who are not Jewish and among whites more than non-whites (McCance et al., 2014). The reasons for these cultural differences are not known.

❖ PATIENT-CENTERED COLLABORATIVE CARE

◆ Assessment

History. Collect data on family history of IBD, previous and current therapy for the illness, and dates and types of surgery. Obtain a NUTRITION history, including intolerance of milk and milk products and fried, spicy, or hot foods. Ask about usual bowel ELIMINATION pattern (color, number, consistency, and character of stools), abdominal pain, tenesmus, anorexia, and fatigue. Note any relationship between diarrhea, timing of meals, emotional distress, and activity. Inquire about recent (past 2 to 3 month) exposure to antibiotics suggesting *Clostridium difficile* infection. Has the patient traveled to or emigrated from tropical areas? Ask about recent use of NSAIDs that can cause a flare-up of the disease. Ask about any extraintestinal symptoms such as arthritis, mouth sores, vision problems, and skin disorders.

Physical Assessment/Clinical Manifestations. Symptoms vary with an acuteness of onset. Vital signs are usually within normal limits in mild disease. In more severe cases, the patient may have a low-grade fever (99° to 100°F [37.2° to 37.8°C]). The physical assessment findings are usually nonspecific, and in milder cases the physical examination may be normal. Viral and bacterial infections cause symptoms similar to those of UC.

Note any abdominal distention along the colon. Fever associated with tachycardia may indicate peritonitis, dehydration, and bowel perforation. Assess for clinical manifestations associated with extraintestinal complications, such as inflamed joints and lesions inside the mouth.

Psychosocial Assessment. Many patients are very concerned about the frequency of stools and the presence of blood. *The inability to control the disease symptoms, particularly diarrhea, can be disruptive and stress producing.* Severe illness may limit the patient's activities outside the home with fear of fecal incontinence resulting in feeling "tied to the toilet." Severe anxiety and depression may result. Eating may be associated with pain and cramping and an increased frequency of stools. Mealtimes may become unpleasant experiences. Frequent visits to health care providers and close monitoring of the colon mucosa for abnormal cell changes can be anxiety provoking.

Assess the patient's understanding of the illness and its impact on his or her lifestyle. Encourage and support the patient while exploring:

- The relationship of life events to disease exacerbations
- Stress factors that produce symptoms
- Family and social support systems

- Concerns regarding the possible genetic basis and associated cancer risks of the disease
- Internet access for reliable education information

Laboratory Assessment. As a result of chronic blood loss, hematocrit and hemoglobin levels may be low, which indicates anemia and a chronic disease state. *An increased WBC count, C-reactive protein, or erythrocyte sedimentation rate (ESR) is consistent with inflammatory disease.* Blood levels of sodium, potassium, and chloride may be *low* as a result of frequent diarrheal stools and malabsorption through the diseased bowel (Pagana & Pagana, 2014). Hypoalbuminemia (decreased serum albumin) is found in patients with extensive disease from losing protein in the stool.

Other Diagnostic Assessment. *Magnetic resonance enterography (MRE)* is the major examination used to study the bowel in patients who have IBD. Teach the patient that he or she will need to fast for 4 to 6 hours prior to the test. To have the test, the patient drinks a contrast medium, which can cause diarrhea. The patient has the opportunity to go to the restroom before positioning on the MRI table. The patient then lies prone while the first of two doses of glucagon are given subcutaneously. This substance helps to slow the bowel's activity and motility (Grossman, 2011).

A *colonoscopy* may be done to aid in diagnosis, but the bowel prep can be especially uncomfortable for patients with inflammatory bowel disease (IBD). Frequent colonoscopies are recommended when patients have longer than a 10-year history of UC involving the entire colon because they are at high risk for colorectal cancer. In some cases, a *CT scan* may be done to confirm the disease or its complications. *Barium enemas* with air contrast can show differences between UC and Crohn's disease and identify complications, mucosal patterns, and the distribution and depth of disease involvement. In early disease, the barium enema may show incomplete filling as a result of inflammation and fine ulcerations along the bowel contour, which appear deeper in more advanced disease.

◆ Analysis

The priority NANDA-I nursing diagnoses and collaborative problems for patients with ulcerative colitis include:

1. Diarrhea related to inflammation of the bowel mucosa (NANDA-I)
2. Acute Pain and Chronic Pain related to inflammation and ulceration of the bowel mucosa and skin irritation (NANDA-I)
3. Potential for lower GI bleeding and resulting anemia

◆ Planning and Implementation

Decreasing Diarrhea

Planning: Expected Outcomes. The major concern for a patient with ulcerative colitis is the occurrence of frequent, bloody diarrhea and fecal incontinence from tenesmus. Therefore, with treatment, the patient is expected to have decreased diarrhea, formed stools, and control of bowel movements.

Interventions. Many measures are used to relieve symptoms and to reduce intestinal motility, decrease INFLAMMATION, and promote intestinal healing. Nonsurgical and/or surgical management may be needed.

Nonsurgical Management. Nonsurgical management includes drug and NUTRITION therapy. The use of physical and emotional rest is also an important consideration. Teach the patient to record color, volume, frequency, and consistency of stools to determine severity of the problem.

Monitor the skin in the perianal area for irritation and ulceration resulting from loose, frequent stools. Stool cultures may be sent for analysis if diarrhea continues. Have the patient weigh himself or herself 1 or 2 times per week. If the patient is hospitalized, remind unlicensed assistive personnel to weigh him or her on admission and daily in the morning before breakfast and document all weights.

⚡ NCLEX EXAMINATION CHALLENGE

Physiological Integrity

The nurse is caring for an older client who experiences an exacerbation of ulcerative colitis with severe diarrhea. What is the nurse's priority for care?
A. Monitor skin for breakdown.
B. Monitor heart rate and rhythm.
C. Maintain intake and output records.
D. Auscultate bowel sounds frequently.

Drug Therapy. Common drug therapy for UC includes aminosalicylates, glucocorticoids, antidiarrheal drugs, and immunomodulators. Teach patients about side effects and adverse drug events (ADEs) and when to call their health care provider.

The *aminosalicylates* are drugs commonly used to treat mild to moderate UC and/or maintain remission. Several aminosalicylic acid compounds are available. These drugs, also called *5-ASAs*, are thought to have an anti-inflammatory effect by inhibiting prostaglandins and are usually effective in 2 to 4 weeks.

Sulfasalazine (Azulfidine, Azulfidine EN-tabs), the first aminosalicylate approved for UC, is metabolized by the intestinal bacteria into 5-ASA, which delivers the beneficial effects of the drug, and sulfapyridine, which is responsible for unwanted side effects.

Glucocorticoids, such as prednisone and prednisolone, are corticosteroid therapies prescribed during exacerbations of the disease. Prednisone (Deltasone, Winpred) 40 to 65 mg daily is typically prescribed, but the dose may be increased as acute flare-ups occur. Once clinical improvement occurs, the corticosteroids are tapered because of the adverse effects that commonly occur with long-term steroid therapy (e.g., hyperglycemia,

Drug Alert

Teach patients taking sulfasalazine to report nausea, vomiting, anorexia, rash, and headache to the health care provider. With higher doses, hemolytic anemia, hepatitis, male infertility, or agranulocytosis can occur. This drug is in the same family as sulfonamide antibiotics. Therefore assess the patient for an allergy to sulfonamide or other drugs that contain sulfa *before* the patient takes the drug. The use of a thiazide diuretic is also a contraindication for sulfasalazine (Lilley et al., 2014).

Mesalamine (Asacol, Pentasa, Rowasa, Apriso, Canasa) is better tolerated than sulfasalazine because none of its preparations contain sulfapyridine. Asacol is an enteric-coated drug and is released in the terminal ileum and right side of the colon. Pentasa and Apriso are delayed- and extended-release drugs that work throughout the colon and rectum. Rowasa can be given as an enema, and Canasa can be given as a suppository. These preparations have minimal systemic absorption and therefore have fewer side effects. Table 57-5 lists commonly used 5-ASA drugs.

osteoporosis, peptic ulcer disease, increased risk for infection). For patients with rectal INFLAMMATION, topical steroids in the form of small retention enemas may be prescribed.

To provide symptomatic management of diarrhea, *antidiarrheal drugs* may be prescribed. These drugs are given very cautiously, however, because they can cause colon dilation and toxic megacolon. Common antidiarrheal drugs include diphenoxylate hydrochloride and atropine sulfate (Lomotil) and loperamide (Imodium).

Immunomodulators are drugs that alter a person's immune response. Alone, they are often not effective in the treatment of ulcerative colitis. However, in combination with steroids, they may offer a synergistic effect to a quicker response, thereby decreasing the amount of steroids needed. Biologic response modifiers (BRMs) used for UC (and Crohn's disease, discussed later in this chapter) include infliximab (Remicade) and adalimumab (Humira). Although not approved as a first-line therapy for ulcerative colitis, *infliximab* (Remicade) may be used for refractory disease or for severe complications, such as **toxic megacolon** (massive dilation of the colon that can lead to gangrene and peritonitis) and extraintestinal manifestations. Remicade is an immunoglobulin G (IgG) monoclonal antibody that reduces the activity of tumor necrosis factor (TNF) to decrease INFLAMMATION. Adalimumab (Humira) is another monoclonal antibody approved for refractory (not responsive to other therapies) cases. BRMs are used more commonly in management

---

TABLE 57-5   Recommended Doses for 5-ASA Medications

GENERIC NAME	TRADE NAME	DOSAGE AVAILABLE	RECOMMENDED DOSE
Sulfasalazine	Azulfidine Azulfidine En-tabs Azulfidine oral suspension (50 mg/mL)	500 mg tablets 250 mg/5 mL liquid	3-4 g daily in divided doses Children >2 yr: 30 mg/kg/day not to exceed 2 g/day
Mesalamine	Asacol Pentasa Rowasa enemas Rowasa suppository	400 mg tablets 500 mg tablets 4 g/60 mL 1000 mg/supp	800 mg three times daily 1 g four times daily At bedtime Twice daily or at bedtime
Olsalazine (rarely used)	Dipentum	250 mg tablets	1 g daily in two divided doses
Balsalazide	Colazal	750 mg tablets	3 tablets three times daily

5-ASA, 5-aminosalicylic acid.

of Crohn's disease. These drugs cause immunosuppression and should be used with caution. *Teach the patient to report any signs of a beginning* INFECTION, *including a cold, and to avoid large crowds or others who are sick!*

Several newer monoclonal antibodies are awaiting FDA approval for use in patients with IBD. One of these drugs, vedolizumab, is an intestinal-specific leukocyte traffic inhibitor in that it prevents white blood cells from migrating to inflamed bowel tissue.

Nutrition Therapy and Rest. Patients with severe symptoms who are hospitalized are kept NPO to ensure bowel rest. The physician may prescribe total parenteral NUTRITION (TPN) for severely ill and malnourished patients during severe exacerbations. Chapter 60 describes this therapy in detail. Patients with less severe symptoms may drink elemental formulas such as Vivonex PLUS or Vivonex T.E.N, which are absorbed in the small bowel and reduce bowel stimulation.

Diet is not a major factor in the inflammatory process, but some patients with ulcerative colitis (UC) find that caffeine and alcohol increase diarrhea and cramping. For some patients, raw vegetables and other high-fiber foods can cause GI symptoms. Lactose-containing foods may be poorly tolerated and should be reduced or eliminated. Teach patients that carbonated beverages, pepper, nuts and corn, dried fruits, and smoking are common GI stimulants that could cause discomfort. Each patient differs in his or her food and fluid tolerances.

During an exacerbation of the disease, patient activity is generally restricted because rest can reduce intestinal activity, provide comfort, and promote healing. Ensure that the patient has easy access to a bedpan, bedside commode, or bathroom in case of urgency or tenesmus.

Complementary and Alternative Therapies. In addition to dietary changes, complementary and alternative therapies may be used to supplement traditional management of ulcerative colitis. Examples include herbs (e.g., flaxseed), selenium, and vitamin C. Biofeedback, hypnosis, yoga, acupuncture, and ayurveda (a combination of diet, yoga, herbs, and breathing exercises) may also be helpful. These therapies need further study to validate their effectiveness, but some patients find them helpful.

Surgical Management. Some patients with ulcerative colitis require surgery to help manage their disease when medical therapies alone are not effective. In some cases, surgery is performed for complications of UC such as toxic megacolon, hemorrhage, dysplastic biopsy results, and colon cancer.

Preoperative Care. General preoperative teaching related to abdominal surgery is described in Chapter 14. If a temporary or permanent ileostomy is planned, provide an in-depth explanation to the patient and family. An **ileostomy** is a procedure in which a loop of the ileum is placed through an opening in the abdominal wall (**stoma**) for drainage of fecal material into a pouching system worn on the abdomen. The external pouching system consists of a solid skin barrier (wafer) to protect the skin and a fecal collection device (pouch), similar to the system used for patients with colostomies (discussed in Chapter 56).

If an ileostomy is planned, the surgeon consults with a certified wound, ostomy, continence nurse (CWOCN) before surgery for recommendations on the best location of the stoma. A visit from an **ostomate** (a patient with an ostomy) may be helpful before surgery. Parenteral antibiotics are given within 1 hour of surgical opening based on current best evidence and per The Joint Commission's National Patient Safety Goals.

Operative Procedures. Any one of several surgical approaches may be used for the patient with UC. Minimally invasive procedures, such as laparoscopic, laparoscopic-assisted, hand-assisted, and robotic-assisted surgery, are common for patients with ulcerative colitis in large tertiary care centers (Kessler et al., 2011). Laparoscopic surgery usually involves one or several small incisions but often takes longer to perform than the open surgical approach. A newer procedure, natural orifice transluminal endoscopic surgery (NOTES), can be performed via the anus or vagina for selected patients if the surgeon has been trained in the procedure. Patients may have moderate sedation or general anesthesia for minimally invasive surgical procedures and are not typically admitted to critical care units for continuing postoperative care.

Patients who are obese, have had previous abdominal surgeries, or have dense scar tissue (adhesions) may not be candidates for laparoscopic procedures. The conventional open surgical approach involves an abdominal incision and is done under general anesthesia. Patients with open procedures are typically admitted to critical care units for short-term stabilization.

Restorative Proctocolectomy with Ileo Pouch–Anal Anastomosis (RPC-IPAA). This procedure has become the gold standard for patients with UC. In some centers, the surgery is performed via laparoscopy (laparoscopic RPC-IPAA). It is usually a two-stage procedure that includes the removal of the colon and most of the rectum (Fig. 57-2). The anus and anal sphincter remain intact. The surgeon then surgically creates an internal pouch (reservoir) using the last 1½ feet of the small intestine. The pouch, sometimes called a *J-pouch, S-pouch,* or *pelvic pouch,* is then connected to the anus. A temporary ileostomy through the abdominal skin is created to allow healing of the internal pouch and all anastomosis sites. It also allows for an increase in the capacity of the internal pouch. In the *second* surgical stage, the loop ileostomy is closed. The time interval between the first and second stages varies, but many patients have the second surgical stage to close the ileostomy within 1 to 2 months of the first surgery.

Usually bowel continence is excellent after this procedure, but some patients have leakage of stool during sleep. They may take antidiarrheal drugs to help control this problem.

Total Proctocolectomy with a Permanent Ileostomy. Total proctocolectomy with a permanent ileostomy is done for patients who are not candidates for or do not want the ileo-anal pouch. The procedure involves the removal of the colon, rectum, and anus with surgical closure of the anus (Fig. 57-3, *A*). The surgeon brings the end of the ileum out through the abdominal wall and forms a stoma, or **ostomy.**

> **! NURSING SAFETY PRIORITY** (QSEN)
> **Critical Rescue**
>
> The ileostomy stoma (Fig. 57-3, *B*) is usually placed in the right lower quadrant of the abdomen below the belt line. It should not be prolapsed or retract into the abdominal wall. *Assess the stoma frequently. It should be pinkish to cherry red to ensure an adequate blood supply. If the stoma looks pale, bluish, or dark, report these findings to the health care provider immediately!*

With an ileostomy, initially after surgery the output is a loose, dark green liquid that may contain some blood. Over time, a process called "ileostomy adaptation" occurs. The small intestine begins to perform some of the functions that had

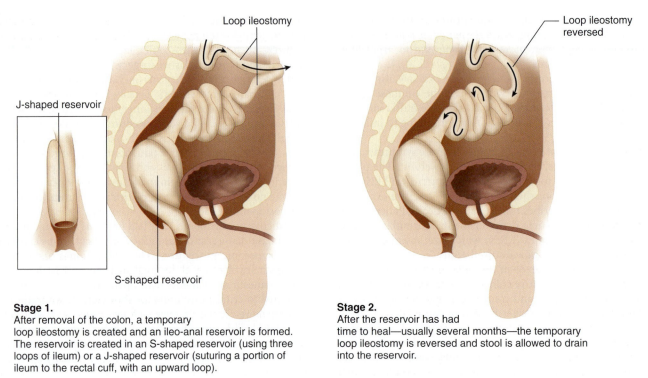

Stage 1.
After removal of the colon, a temporary
loop ileostomy is created and an ileo-anal reservoir is formed.
The reservoir is created in an S-shaped reservoir (using three
loops of ileum) or a J-shaped reservoir (suturing a portion of
ileum to the rectal cuff, with an upward loop).

Stage 2.
After the reservoir has had
time to heal—usually several months—the temporary
loop ileostomy is reversed and stool is allowed to drain
into the reservoir.

FIG. 57-2 The creation of an ileo-anal reservoir.

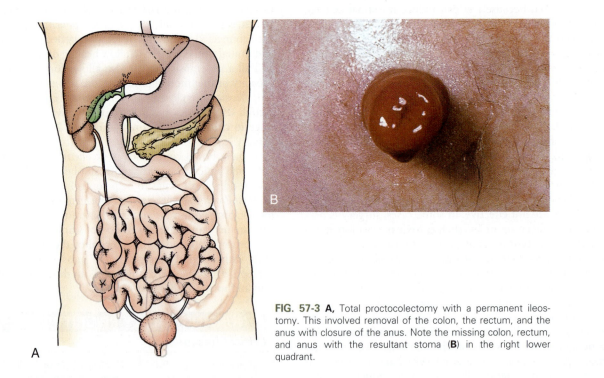

FIG. 57-3 A, Total proctocolectomy with a permanent ileostomy. This involved removal of the colon, the rectum, and the anus with closure of the anus. Note the missing colon, rectum, and anus with the resultant stoma (**B**) in the right lower quadrant.

previously been done by the colon, including the absorption of increased amounts of sodium and water. Stool volume decreases, becomes thicker (pastelike), and turns yellow-green or yellow-brown. The effluent (fluid material) usually has little odor or a sweet odor. Any foul or unpleasant odor may be a symptom of a problem such as blockage or infection.

The ostomy drains frequently, and the stool is irritating. *The patient must wear a pouch system at all times.* The stool from the small intestine contains many enzymes and bile salts, which can quickly irritate and excoriate the skin. *Skin care around the stoma is a priority!* A pouch system with a skin barrier (gelatin or pectin) provides sufficient protection for most patients. Other products are also available.

Postoperative Care. Provide general postoperative care after surgery, as described in Chapter 16. The few patients requiring open-approach surgery for ulcerative colitis have a large abdominal incision. At first they are NPO and a nasogastric tube (NGT) is used for suction. The tube is removed in 1 to 2 days as the drainage decreases, and fluids and food are slowly introduced. The patient having minimally invasive surgery (MIS) usually does not have an NGT.

In collaboration with the CWOCN, help the patient adjust and learn the required care. The ileostomy usually begins to drain within 24 hours after surgery at more than 1 L per day. Be sure that fluids are replaced by adding an additional 500 mL or more each day to prevent dehydration. After about a week of high-volume output, the drainage slows and becomes thicker. During this period, some patients need antidiarrheal drugs.

The hospital stay is usually from 1 to 4 days, depending on whether the patient has laparoscopic or conventional open surgery. Patients having MIS have less pain from surgery and faster restoration of bowel function when compared with other surgical patients, but the incidence of complications is about the same (Fajardo et al., 2010).

For those who have the RPC-IPAA procedure, remind them that the internal pouch can become inflamed. This problem is usually effectively treated with metronidazole (Flagyl) for 7 to 10 days. Teach patients that after the second stage of surgery, they might have burning during bowel ELIMINATION because gastric acid cannot be well absorbed by the ileum. Also instruct them to omit foods that can cause odors or gas, such as cabbage, asparagus, Brussels sprouts, and beans. Teach patients to eliminate foods that cannot be well digested, such as nuts and corn. Each patient differs in which foods he or she can tolerate.

Surgery for UC may result in altered body image. However, it may be viewed as positive because the patient will have fewer symptoms and feel more comfortable than before the procedure. Patients have to adjust to having an ostomy before they can resume their presurgery activities.

Minimizing Pain

Planning: Expected Outcomes. The desired outcome for the patient is that he or she will verbalize decreased PAIN as a result of collaborative, evidence-based pain management interventions.

Interventions. Pain control requires pharmacologic and nonpharmacologic measures. Physical discomfort can contribute to emotional distress. A variety of symptom-reducing interventions and supportive measures are used. Surgery also reduces pain for many patients.

The purpose of pain management is alleviation of pain or a reduction in pain to a level of comfort that is acceptable to the patient. Increases in PAIN may indicate the development of complications such as peritonitis (see earlier discussion in this chapter). Assist the patient in reducing or eliminating factors that can cause or increase the pain experience. For example, he or she may benefit from NUTRITION changes to decrease abdominal discomfort such as cramping and bloating.

Antidiarrheal drugs may be needed to control diarrhea, thus reducing the discomfort. However, they must be used with caution and for a short time because toxic megacolon can develop.

Perineal skin can be irritated by contact with loose stools and frequent cleaning. Explain special measures for skin care. Use of medicated wipes is soothing if the rectal area is tender or sensitive from the use of toilet tissue (Chart 57-3). A number of ostomy manufacturers (e.g., Hollister, ConvaTec) produce a system for skin care that may help prevent and heal perineal skin irritation. These systems usually include a skin-cleaning solution, a moisturizing and healing cream, and a petroleum jelly–like barrier that prevents contact of moisture and stool with the skin.

Monitoring for Lower GI Bleeding

Planning: Expected Outcomes. For patients who experience GI bleeding, the patient with UC is expected to have a reduction in or cessation of bleeding with prompt collaborative care. If possible, patients are expected to remain free of complications of the disease that can cause bleeding, such as perforation.

Interventions. The primary nursing priority is to monitor the patient closely for signs and symptoms of GI bleeding resulting from the disease or its complications.

CHART 57-3 Best Practice for Patient Safety & Quality Care (QSEN)

Pain Control and Skin Care for Patients with Inflammatory Bowel Disease

PATIENT PROBLEM	INTERVENTIONS
Abdominal pain (particularly with exacerbations of the disease)	Administer analgesics. Assist with frequent positioning. Identify foods that increase pain. Perform a comprehensive pain assessment. Observe for signs and symptoms of peritonitis. Evaluate effectiveness of pain management. Teach music therapy, guided imagery.
Skin excoriation and/or irritation from frequent bowel movements	Encourage good skin care with a mild soap and water after each bowel movement. Gently pat the area dry. Identify foods that increase diarrhea. Sitz baths may be of benefit. Apply a thin coat of A+D Ointment or aloe cream. Use medicated wipes instead of tissue. Ensure appropriate ostomy supplies that fit well. Antidiarrheal medications may help, but use with caution. Observe for symptoms related to megacolon (fever, leukocytosis, tachycardia, distended abdomen with 3-view abdominal x-ray noting an enlarged colon).

If the patient has lower GI bleeding of more than 0.5 mL per minute, a *GI bleeding scan* may be useful to localize the site of the bleeding (Pagana & Pagana, 2014). This test cannot indicate the cause of the bleeding, however, and may take several hours to administer. Patients in the critical care unit are not candidates for the test because they must leave the unit for the test.

Community-Based Care

Home Care Management. The patient with ulcerative colitis provides self-management at home but may require hospitalization during severe exacerbations or surgery. In addition, those who have extraintestinal problems often need ongoing collaborative care for joint and/or skin problems.

Home care management focuses on controlling clinical manifestations and monitoring for complications. For patients returning home or transferring to nursing home or transitional care after surgery, ongoing respiratory care, incision care (if applicable), ostomy care, and PAIN management should be continued.

Self-Management Education. Teach the patient about the nature of ulcerative colitis, including its acute episodes, remissions, and symptom management. Also stress that even though the cause is unknown, relapses can be prevented with proper health care. Teach patients taking immunosuppressive drugs, such as corticosteroids and biologic response modifiers (monoclonal antibodies), to report signs of possible infection, such as sore throat, to the health care provider. Remind them to avoid crowds and anyone who has an INFECTION. Review the purpose of drug therapy, when drugs should be taken, side effects, and adverse drug events.

Instruct the patient about measures to reduce or control abdominal PAIN, cramping, and diarrhea. Also teach the patient and family about symptoms associated with disease exacerbation that should be reported to the health care provider, such as fever higher than 101°F (38.3°C), tachycardia, palpitations, and an increase in diarrhea, abdominal pain, or nausea/vomiting. Provide written information and contact numbers for the health care provider.

There is no special diet for a patient with an ileostomy. However, teach the patient to avoid any foods that cause gas. Examples include high-fiber foods like nuts, raw cabbage, corn, celery, apples with peels, and popcorn. The patient needs to learn what foods he or she tolerates best and adjust the diet accordingly.

If the patient has undergone a temporary or permanent surgical diversion, collaborate with the CWOCN to explain and demonstrate required care so that the patient can self-manage or the family/caregiver can assist. Also teach the importance of including adequate amounts of salt and water in the diet because the ileostomy increases the loss of these substances. Urge the patient to be cautious in situations that lead to heavy sweating or fluid loss, such as strenuous physical activity, high environmental heat, and episodes of diarrhea and vomiting.

Finding the best ostomy pouching system is a major issue for many patients. An effective system is one that:

- Protects the skin
- Contains the effluent (drainage) and reduces odor, if any
- Remains securely attached to the skin for a dependable period of time

Most patients desire an adhesive barrier that will last for 3 to 7 days. The barrier must create a solid seal to prevent the enzymes in the drainage from irritating the skin. Solid barriers are classified as "regular wear" or "extended wear." A person with a high output may want an extended-wear barrier. A special cream can be used to help fill any uneven skin surfaces and provide a consistent seal. Pouches are also individualized by the patient. Large pouches can hold more but are heavy when full. Patients also have to consider the costs of the various systems and if or how much their insurance will pay for them. Chart 57-4 describes the main aspects of ileostomy care, including skin care.

A patient with an ileostomy may have many concerns about management at home and about sexual and social adjustments. Considering possible sexual issues helps the patient identify and discuss these concerns with the sex partner. For example, a change in positioning during intercourse may alleviate apprehension. Social situations may cause anxiety related to decreased self-esteem and a disturbance in body image. Encourage the patient to discuss possible concerns in addressing and resolving these potentially stressful events. Clinical depression is common among patients with ulcerative colitis. Refer patients to appropriate mental health resources if depression is suspected.

Some hospitals provide community support groups for their patients with inflammatory bowel disease (IBD). These groups help patients and their families cope with the psychological impact of IBD and educate them about NUTRITION and complementary and alternative therapies (see the Evidence-Based Practice box).

Health Care Resources. If the patient needs assistance with self-management at home, collaborate with the case manager or social worker to arrange the services of a home care aide or nurse. A home care nurse can provide assessment and guidance in integrating ostomy care into the patient's lifestyle. The nurse may also teach about wound care, including the monitoring of wound healing, if needed (Chart 57-5). The patient and family need to know where to purchase ostomy supplies, along with the name, size, and manufacturer's order number.

For patients with a permanent ileostomy, locate a community ostomy support group by contacting the United Ostomy Associations of America (www.uoaa.org). The United Ostomy Association of Canada serves the needs of Canadian patients (www.ostomycanada.ca). A local support group or the Crohn's and Colitis Foundation of America (www.ccfa.org) may be helpful in obtaining supplies and providing education for ostomates. Inform the patient and family of available ostomy ambulatory care clinics and ostomy specialists. If the patient agrees,

CHART 57-4   Patient and Family Education: Preparing for Self-Management

Ileostomy Care

Skin Protection

• Use a skin barrier to protect your skin from contact with contents from the ostomy.
• Use skin care products, such as skin sealants and ostomy skin creams. If your skin continues to come into contact with ostomy contents, select a product to fill in problem areas and provide an even skin surface.
• Watch your skin for any irritation or redness.

Pouch Care

• Empty your pouch when it is one-third to one-half full.
• Change the pouch during inactive times, such as before meals, before retiring at night, on waking in the morning, and 2 to 4 hours after eating.
• Change the entire pouch system every 3 to 7 days.

Nutrition

• Chew food thoroughly.
• Be cautious of high-fiber and high-cellulose foods. You may need to eliminate these from the diet if they cause severe problems (diarrhea, constipation, or blockage). Examples include corn, peanuts, coconut, Chinese vegetables, string beans, tough-fiber meats, shrimp and lobster, rice, bran, and vegetables with skins (tomatoes, corn, and peas).

Drug Therapy

• Avoid taking enteric-coated and capsule medications.
• Inform any health care provider who is prescribing medications for you that you have an ostomy. Before having prescriptions filled, inform your pharmacist that you have an ostomy.
• Do not take any laxative or enemas. You should usually have loose stool and should contact a physician if no stool has passed in 6 to 12 hours.

Symptoms to Watch for

• Report any drastic increase or decrease in drainage to your health care provider.
• If stomal swelling, abdominal cramping, or distention occurs or if ileostomy contents stop draining:
  ▪ Remove the pouch with faceplate.
  ▪ Lie down, assuming a knee-chest position.
  ▪ Begin abdominal massage.
  ▪ Apply moist towels to the abdomen.
  ▪ Drink hot tea.
  ▪ If none of these maneuvers is effective in resuming ileostomy flow or if abdominal pain is severe, call your health care provider right away.

CHART 57-5   Home Care Assessment

The Patient with Inflammatory Bowel Disease

Assess gastrointestinal function and nutritional status, including:
  ▪ Abdominal cramping or pain
  ▪ Bowel elimination pattern, specifically frequency, characteristics, and amount of stools and presence or absence of blood in stools
  ▪ Food and fluid intake (include relationship of specific foods to cramping and stools)
  ▪ Weight gain or loss
  ▪ Signs and symptoms of dehydration
  ▪ Presence or absence of fever, rectal tenesmus, or urgency
  ▪ Bowel sounds
  ▪ Condition of perianal skin, including presence or absence of perianal fistula or abscess

Assess patient's and family's coping skills, including:
  ▪ Current and ongoing stress level and coping style
  ▪ Availability of support system

Assess home environment, including:
  ▪ Adequacy and availability of bathroom facilities
  ▪ Opportunity for rest and relaxation

Assess ability to self-manage therapeutic regimen, including:
  ▪ Drug therapy
  ▪ Signs and symptoms to report
  ▪ Nutrition therapy
  ▪ Availability of community resources
  ▪ Importance of follow-up care

EVIDENCE-BASED PRACTICE (QSEN)

Is a Support Group for Patients with Inflammatory Bowel Disease Helpful?

McMaster, K., Aguinaldo, L., & Parekh, N.K. (2012). Evaluation of an ongoing psychoeducational inflammatory bowel disease support group in an adult outpatient setting. *Gastroenterology Nursing, 35*(6), 383-390.

In this study, researchers evaluated the use of an ongoing open psychoeducational support group for adult patients with inflammatory bowel disease (IBD) in an outpatient tertiary care setting. The sample was 18 adults who attended more than two meetings of the support group. The support group focused on diet and nutrition, psychological impact of IBD, and complementary and alternative medicine. Subjects completed several tools, including the Client Satisfaction Questionnaire, Multidimensional Support Scale, demographic data tool, and a brief open-ended qualitative questionnaire developed by the researchers.

The results showed that the participants in the support group were very satisfied with the support group and the peer support they received. The study demonstrated that the support group for IBD clients was effective.

Level of Evidence: 5

This study was a very small descriptive study that collected both quantitative and qualitative data.

Commentary: Implications for Practice and Research

Patients who have IBD need ongoing support and education in the community to cope with their disease. Nurses are in a prime position to facilitate these groups and help patients gain knowledge as well as emotional support as they learn to cope with their disease. This research was a small pilot study that needs a larger sample in a multi-setting research design.

---

a visit from an ostomate can be continued after discharge to home.

◆ Evaluation: Outcomes

Evaluate the care of the patient with ulcerative colitis based on the identified priority patient problems. Expected outcomes may include that the patient will:

• Verbalize decreased PAIN
• Gain control over bowel elimination
• Not experience lower GI bleeding
• Self-manage the ileostomy (temporary or permanent)
• Maintain peristomal skin integrity
• Demonstrate behaviors that integrate ostomy care into his or her lifestyle if a permanent ileostomy is performed

CROHN'S DISEASE

❖ PATHOPHYSIOLOGY

Crohn's disease (CD) is a chronic inflammatory disease of the small intestine (most often), the colon, or both. It can affect the

GI tract from the mouth to the anus but most commonly affects the terminal ileum. CD is a slowly progressive and unpredictable disease with involvement of multiple regions of the intestine with normal sections in between (called "skip lesions" on x-rays). Like ulcerative colitis (UC), this disease is recurrent with remissions and exacerbations.

Crohn's disease presents as INFLAMMATION that causes a thickened bowel wall. Strictures and deep ulcerations (cobblestone appearance) also occur, which put the patient at risk for developing bowel fistulas (abnormal openings between two organs or structures). The result is severe diarrhea and malabsorption of vital nutrients. Anemia is common, usually from iron deficiency or malabsorption issues (McCance et al., 2014).

The complications associated with Crohn's disease are similar to those of ulcerative colitis (see Table 57-4). Hemorrhage is more common in ulcerative colitis, but it can occur in CD as well. Severe malabsorption by the small intestine is more common in patients with CD because UC may not involve the small bowel to any significant extent. *Therefore patients with CD can become very malnourished and debilitated.*

Rarely, cancer of the small bowel and colon develop but can occur after the disease has been present for 15 to 20 years. Fistula formation is a common complication of CD but is rare in UC. Fistulas can occur between segments of the intestine or manifest as cutaneous fistulas (opening to the skin) or perirectal abscesses. They can also extend from the bowel to other organs and body cavities, such as the bladder or vagina (Fig. 57-4). Some patients develop intestinal obstruction, which at first is secondary to INFLAMMATION and edema. Over time, fibrosis and scar tissue develop and obstruction results from a narrowing of the bowel. Most patients with CD require surgery at some time.

Almost a million people in the United States have Crohn's disease. Most have symptoms and are diagnosed as adolescents or young adults.

❖ PATIENT-CENTERED COLLABORATIVE CARE

◆ Assessment

Crohn's disease is made worse by bacterial INFECTION. A detailed history is needed to identify manifestations specific to the disease. Ask about recent unintentional weight loss, the frequency and consistency of stools, the presence of blood in the stool, fever, and abdominal pain.

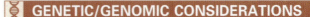

GENETIC/GENOMIC CONSIDERATIONS
Patient-Centered Care QSEN

The exact cause of CD is unknown. A combination of genetic, immune, and environmental factors may contribute to its development. About 10% to 20% of patients have a positive family history for the disease (Nussbaum et al., 2007). The discovery of a mutation in the *NOD2/CARD15* gene on chromosome 16 seems to be associated with some patients who have CD. This gene is found in monocytes that normally recognize and destroy bacteria.

Pro-inflammatory cytokines, such as tumor necrosis factor–alpha (TNF-alpha) and interleukins (ILs) (e.g., IL-6 and IL-8), are immunologic factors that contribute to the etiology of CD (McCance et al., 2014). Many of the drugs used for the disease inhibit or block one or more of these factors.

Other risk factors include tobacco use, Jewish ethnicity, and living in urban areas (McCance et al., 2014). CD is more common in people of Ashkenazi Jewish background than in any other group (Nussbaum et al., 2007). The reasons for these factors have not been established. It was once thought that stress and nutrition play a role in the *development* of CD, but these factors have not been proven. However, inadequate NUTRITION can worsen the patient's symptoms.

Perform a thorough abdominal assessment. Assess for manifestations of the disease, and evaluate the patient's NUTRITION and hydration status.

When inspecting the abdomen, assess for distention, masses, or visible peristalsis. Inspection of the perianal area may reveal ulcerations, fissures, or fistulas. During auscultation, bowel sounds may be decreased or absent with severe inflammation or obstruction. An increase in high-pitched or rushing sounds may be present over areas of narrowed bowel loops. Muscle guarding, masses, rigidity, or tenderness may be noted on palpation by the advanced practice nurse or other health care provider.

The clinical presentation of Crohn's disease varies greatly from person to person. Most patients report diarrhea, abdominal pain, and low-grade fever. Fever is common with fistulas, abscesses, and severe INFLAMMATION. If the disease occurs in only the ileum, diarrhea occurs 5 or 6 times per day, often with a soft, loose stool. Steatorrhea (fatty diarrheal stools) is common. Rarely, stools may contain bright red blood.

Abdominal pain from the inflammatory process is usually constant and often located in the right lower quadrant. The patient also may have PAIN around the umbilicus before and

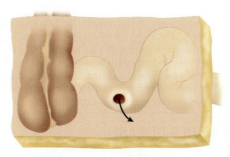

External enterocutaneous
(between skin and intestine)

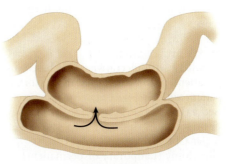

Enteroenteric
(between intestine and intestine)

FIG. 57-4 The types of fistulas that are complications of Crohn's disease.

after bowel movements. If the lower colon is diseased, pain is common in both lower abdominal quadrants.

Most patients with Crohn's disease have *weight loss*. Nutritional problems are the result of increased catabolism from chronic INFLAMMATION, anorexia, malabsorption, or self-imposed dietary restrictions. These problems result in impaired FLUID AND ELECTROLYTE BALANCE and vital nutrient deficiencies.

The inflammatory bowel changes decrease the small bowel's ability to absorb nutrients, which may be made worse by surgery and fistulas.

! NURSING SAFETY PRIORITY (QSEN)

Action Alert

For the patient with Crohn's disease, be especially alert for manifestations of peritonitis (discussed earlier in this chapter), small-bowel obstruction, and nutritional and fluid imbalances. Early detection of a change in the patient's status helps reduce these life-threatening complications.

The patient who has Crohn's disease (CD) needs a complete psychosocial assessment. The chronic nature of the problem and the associated complications can greatly affect patients and their families. Lifestyle changes are necessary to cope with such a disruptive and painful chronic illness. Assess the patient's coping skill, and help identify support systems. Similar to problems associated with other chronic diseases, clinical depression and severe anxiety disorders are common among patients with CD.

The health care provider requests many laboratory studies for patients with Crohn's disease. The results of laboratory tests often indicate the extent and severity of INFLAMMATION or complications that occur with the disease.

Anemia is common as a result of slow bleeding and poor nutrition. Serum levels of folic acid and vitamin B_{12} are generally low because of malabsorption, further contributing to anemia. Amino acid malabsorption and protein-losing enteropathy may result in *decreased albumin* levels. C-reactive protein and ESR may be elevated to indicate INFLAMMATION. White blood cells (WBCs) in the urine may show INFECTION (pyuria), which is caused by ureteral obstruction or an enterovesical (bowel to bladder) fistula. If severe diarrhea or fistula is present, the patient may have fluid and electrolyte losses, particularly potassium and magnesium. Assess the patient for clinical manifestations that can occur as a result of electrolyte losses (see Chapter 11).

X-rays show the narrowing, ulcerations, strictures, and fistulas common with Crohn's disease. *Magnetic resonance enterography (MRE)* is performed to determine bowel activity and motility as discussed on p. 1175 in this chapter. An *abdominal ultrasound or CT* scan may also be performed. In acute illness, these tests may be deferred until the risk for perforation lessens. If the patient has lower GI bleeding of more than 0.5 mL per minute, a *GI bleeding scan* may be useful to localize the site of the bleeding (Pagana & Pagana, 2014).

◆ Interventions

Collaborative care for patients with Crohn's disease is similar to that described on p. 1175 in the Nonsurgical Management

discussion in the Ulcerative Colitis section. Specific interventions vary with the severity of disease and the complications that are present.

Drug Therapy. Drugs used to manage Crohn's disease (CD) are similar to those used in the treatment of ulcerative colitis (UC). For mild to moderate disease, 5-ASA drugs may be very effective (see p. 1183 in the Drug Therapy discussion in the Ulcerative Colitis section).

Most patients have moderate to severe disease and need stronger drug therapy to control their symptoms. Two agents that may be prescribed for CD are azathioprine (Imuran) and mercaptopurine (Purinethol). These drugs suppress the immune system and can lead to serious INFECTIONS. Methotrexate (MTX) may also be given to suppress immune activity of the disease.

A group of biologic response modifiers (BRMs), also known as *monoclonal antibody drugs*, have been approved for use in Crohn's disease when other drugs have been ineffective. These drugs inhibit tumor necrosis factor (TNF)–alpha, which decreases the inflammatory response. Examples of commonly used drugs for patients with CD include infliximab (Remicade), adalimumab (Humira), natalizumab (Tysabri), and certolizumab pegol (Cimzia). These agents are not given to patients with a history of cancer, heart disease, or multiple sclerosis.

! NURSING SAFETY PRIORITY (QSEN)

Drug Alert

Both infliximab and certolizumab pegol must be given in a health care setting, such as a physician's office, via parenteral routes. Adalimumab (Humira) is self-administered by subcutaneous injection every other week. If needed, instruct patients on how to give themselves a subcutaneous injection. Teach patients to report injection site reactions, including redness and swelling. Remind them that headache, abdominal pain, and nausea and vomiting are common side effects. Teach them to avoid crowds, such as malls and large shopping centers, and people with infection. Reinforce the need to report any INFECTION, including a cold or sore throat, to the health care provider immediately.

Natalizumab is given IV under medical supervision every 4 weeks for moderate to severe CD and is given when other drugs are not effective. Although the use of this drug has decreased the length of hospital stays (Dudley-Brown et al., 2009), natalizumab can cause **progressive multifocal leukoencephalopathy** (PML), a deadly infection that affects the brain. Before giving the drug, be sure that the patient is free of all INFECTIONS. Teach patients the importance of reporting any cognitive, motor, or sensory changes immediately to the health care provider.

Although glucocorticoids can be effective for patients with Crohn's disease, sepsis can result from abscesses or fistulas that may be present. These drugs mask the symptoms of infection. Therefore they must be used with caution. Monitor the patient closely for signs of infection. Metronidazole (Flagyl, Novonidazol ✦) has been helpful in patients with fistulas.

Nutrition Therapy. Long-standing nutritional deficits can have severe consequences for the patient with Crohn's disease. Poor NUTRITION can lead to inadequate fistula and wound healing, loss of lean muscle mass, decreased immune responses, and increased morbidity and mortality. During severe exacerbations of the disease, the patient may be hospitalized to provide bowel rest and nutritional support with total parenteral nutrition (TPN). For less severe exacerbations, an elemental or semi-elemental product such as Vivonex PLUS may be prescribed to induce remission. These products are absorbed in the jejunum and therefore permit the distal small intestine and colon to rest. Nutritional supplements such as Ensure or Sustacal can be added then to provide nutrients and more calories. Teach the patient to avoid GI stimulants, such as caffeinated beverages and alcohol.

Fistula Management. Fistulas (abnormal tracts between two or more body areas) are common with acute exacerbations of Crohn's disease. They can be between the bowel and bladder (enterovesical), between two segments of bowel (enteroenteric), between the skin and bowel (enterocutaneous), or between the bowel and vagina (enterovaginal) (see Fig. 57-4). The patient with one or more fistulas often has complications such as systemic infections, skin problems, malnutrition, and impaired FLUID AND ELECTROLYTE BALANCE. Treatment of the patient with a fistula is complicated and includes nutrition and electrolyte therapy, skin care, and prevention of infection.

! NURSING SAFETY PRIORITY (QSEN)

Action Alert

Adequate NUTRITION and FLUID AND ELECTROLYTE BALANCE are priorities in the care of the patient with a fistula. GI secretions are high in volume and rich in electrolytes and enzymes. The patient is at high risk for malnutrition, dehydration, and hypokalemia (decreased serum potassium). Assess for these complications, and collaborate with the health care team to manage them. Monitor urinary output and daily weights. A decrease indicates possible dehydration, which should be treated immediately by providing additional fluids.

The patient requires at least 3000 calories daily to promote healing of the fistula. If he or she cannot take adequate oral fluids and nutrients, total enteral nutrition (TEN) or TPN may be prescribed. For patients who do not require TEN or TPN, collaborate with the dietitian to:

- Carefully monitor the patient's tolerance to the prescribed diet.
- Assist the patient in selecting high-calorie, high-protein, high-vitamin, low-fiber meals.
- Offer enteral supplements, such as Ensure and Vivonex PLUS.
- Record food intake for accurate calorie counts.

Providing enteral supplements, recording intake and output, and taking daily weights may be delegated to unlicensed assistive personnel (UAP) under the supervision of the RN.

Collaborate with the certified wound, ostomy, and continence nurse (CWOCN) to select the most appropriate wound management for each patient.

! NURSING SAFETY PRIORITY (QSEN)

Action Alert

For patients with fistulas, preserving and protecting the skin is the nursing priority. Be sure that wound drainage is not in direct contact with skin because intestinal fluid enzymes are caustic! Clean the skin promptly to prevent skin breakdown or fungal infection, which can cause major discomfort for the patient.

Enzymes and bile in the stool contribute to the problem of skin irritation and excoriation. Skin irritation needs to be prevented. This may be accomplished through the use of skin barriers, pouching systems, and insertion of drains (Fig. 57-5). Skin barriers or dressings are used when the fistula drainage is less than 100 mL in 24 hours. A pouch is used for heavily draining fistulas to reduce the risk for skin breakdown and measure the effluent (drainage). However, they are very challenging because of location and drainage amount. Treatment with an antifungal powder applied to the skin around the fistula is often very helpful to prevent or treat *Candida* infection.

For some fistulas, pouching may not be possible because of their location. Drainage may need to be managed using regulated wall suction or a negative-pressure wound therapy device. Continuous low wall suction is attached to a suction catheter in the wound bed of the fistula, not into the fistula tract. These systems are not meant for long-term management.

Negative-pressure wound therapy (e.g., VAC therapy) promotes wound healing by secondary intention as it prepares the wound bed for closure, reduces edema, promotes granulation and perfusion, and removes exudate and infectious material. It should not be used for patients who are at risk for bleeding or only for the purpose of drainage containment. Chapter 25 describes this therapy in detail.

Patients with fistulas are also at high risk for intra-abdominal abscesses and sepsis. Antibiotic therapy is commonly prescribed. Observe for signs of sepsis (systemic INFECTION), such as fever, abdominal pain, or a change in mental status. Monitor for increased WBC levels that could indicate a systemic infection.

Other helpful interventions for the patient with CD are those that relax the patient and soothe the GI tract. Such therapies may include naturopathy, herbs (e.g., ginger), acupuncture, hypnotherapy, and ayurveda (a combination of diet, herbs, yoga, breathing exercises). The evidence supporting the use of these substances for CD is lacking, but many patients find them helpful for overall physical and emotional health. Teach patients about the availability of these therapies, and recommend that they include them in their collaborative plan of care.

? CLINICAL JUDGMENT CHALLENGE

Patient-Centered Care; Teamwork and Collaboration; Informatics (QSEN)

A young woman has an exacerbation of Crohn's disease with multiple diarrheal stools each day. She has been taking adalimumab (Humira) for the past 2 years to control the disease. However, she has been especially stressed in her doctoral program because she is applying for an internship for clinical psychology. The process is very competitive, and she is concerned that she may not be successful in finding a suitable internship site. She is worried that her flare-up will put her behind in her program.

1. What is your best response to the patient at this time?
2. What patient assessments will you perform on admission and why?
3. Based on the patient data provided, what priority problems do you identify?
4. Using best current evidence, how will you plan care with other members of the health care team? What members of the health care team will be involved in this patient's care and why?

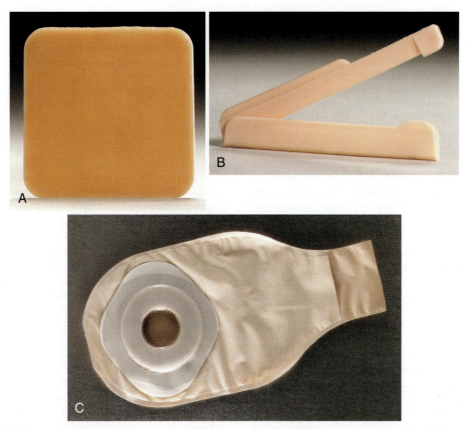

FIG. 57-5 Skin barriers, such as wafers **(A)** are cut to fit ⅛ inch around the fistula. A drainable pouch **(B)** is applied over the wafer and clamped **(C)** until the pouch is to be emptied. Effluent should drain into the bag and not contact the skin.

Surgical Management. Surgery for Crohn's disease may be performed for those patients who have not improved with medical management or for those who have complications from the disease. Surgery to manage CD is not as successful as that for ulcerative colitis because of the extent of the disease. The patient with a fistula may undergo resection of the diseased area. Other indications for surgical treatment include perforation, massive hemorrhage, intestinal obstruction or strictures, abscesses, or cancer.

In some cases, a resection (removal of part of the small bowel) can be performed as minimally invasive surgery (MIS) via laparoscopy. This surgery involves one or more small incisions, less pain, and a quicker surgical recovery when compared with traditional open surgery. Both small-bowel resection (usually the ileum) and ileocecal resection can be done using this procedure. For other patients, an open surgical approach is used to allow for better visual access to the bowel.

Stricturoplasty may be performed for bowel strictures related to Crohn's disease. This procedure increases the bowel diameter. Care before and after each of these surgical procedures is similar to care for patients undergoing other types of abdominal surgery (see Chapters 14 and 16).

Community-Based Care

The discharge care plan for the patient with Crohn's disease is similar to that for the patient with ulcerative colitis (see p. 1180 in the discussion of Community-Based Care in the Ulcerative Colitis section). Collaborate with the case manager and CWOCN or wound nurse to help the patient plan self-management.

The interventions that were started to manage the disease are continued. Reinforce measures to control the disease and related symptoms and manage nutrition. Teach the patient and family to make arrangements for the patient to have easy access to the bathroom, as well as privacy to perform fistula care, if needed.

The health teaching plan for Crohn's disease is similar to that for the patient with ulcerative colitis. Teach the patient about the usual course of the disease, symptoms of complications, and when to notify the health care provider. Provide health teaching for drug therapy, including purpose, dose, and side effects. In addition to other drugs, vitamin supplements, including monthly vitamin B_{12} injections, may be needed because of the inability of the ileum to absorb these nutrients. In collaboration with the dietitian, instruct the patient to follow a low-residue, high-calorie diet and to avoid foods that cause discomfort, such as milk, gluten (wheat products), and other GI stimulants like caffeine.

Remind the patient to take rest periods, especially during exacerbations of the disease. If stress appears to increase symptoms of the disease, recommend stress management techniques, counseling, and/or physical activity to improve quality of life (Crumbock et al., 2009). For long-term follow-up, teach the patient about the increased risk for bowel cancer and the importance of having frequent colonoscopies.

If a patient has a fistula, explain and demonstrate wound care. Provide the opportunity for the patient to practice this care in the hospital. Ideally, he or she should be independent in fistula care before leaving the hospital. However, because of location of the fistula (perirectal or vaginal) or a large abdomen, assistance may be needed. If this is the case, teach a family member or other caregiver how to manage the wound. Patients may be transferred to a transitional or skilled nursing unit for collaborative care.

Patients who are discharged to home after undergoing resection and anastomosis may require visits from a home care nurse to assess the surgical wound and monitor for complications (see Chart 57-5). Assess the patient's and family's ability to monitor the progress of fistula healing and to watch for indications of INFECTION and sepsis. A home care aide or other service might be helpful for the patient who cannot meet nutritional needs or who needs help with grocery shopping and meal preparation.

In collaboration with the CM, assist with obtaining the equipment and supplies for fistula care, such as skin barriers and wound drainage bags. A support group sponsored by the United Ostomy Associations of America (www.uoaa.org) or a local hospital in the community may also be available to help with meeting physical and psychosocial needs.

DIVERTICULAR DISEASE

Diverticula are pouchlike herniations of the mucosa through the muscular wall of any portion of the gut but most commonly the colon. Diverticulosis is the presence of many abnormal pouchlike herniations (diverticula) in the wall of the intestine. Acute diverticulitis is the INFLAMMATION of diverticula.

❖ PATHOPHYSIOLOGY

Diverticula can occur in any part of the small or large intestine but usually occur in the sigmoid colon (Fig. 57-6). The muscle of the colon hypertrophies, thickens, and becomes rigid, and herniation of the mucosa and submucosa through the colon wall is seen. Diverticula seem to occur at points of weakness in the intestinal wall, often at areas where blood vessels interrupt the muscle layer. Muscle weakness develops as part of the aging process or as a result of a lack of fiber in the diet.

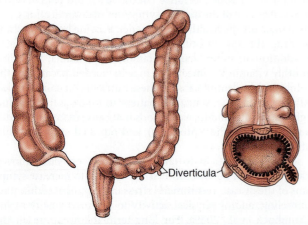

FIG. 57-6 Several abnormal outpouchings, or herniations, in the wall of the intestine, which are diverticula. These can occur anywhere in the small or large intestine but are found most often in the colon. Diverticulitis is the inflammation of a diverticulum that occurs when undigested food or bacteria become trapped in the diverticulum.

Without INFLAMMATION, diverticula cause few problems. If undigested food or bacteria become trapped in a diverticulum, however, blood supply to that area is reduced. Bacteria invade the diverticulum, resulting in diverticulitis, which then can perforate and develop a local abscess. A perforated diverticulum can progress to an intra-abdominal perforation with peritonitis (inflammation of the peritoneum). Lower GI bleeding may also occur.

High intraluminal pressure forces the formation of a pouch in the weakened area of the mucosa, frequently near blood vessels. Diets low in fiber that cause less bulky stool and constipation have been implicated in the formation of diverticula. Retained undigested food in diverticula is suggested to be one cause of diverticulitis. The retained food reduces blood flow to that area and makes bacterial invasion of the sac easier (McCance et al., 2014).

The exact incidence of diverticulosis is unknown, but millions of people are affected by the problem. It is found in two thirds of adults older than 80 years, with more men than women affected. African Americans have more diverticular disease than do Caucasians (Hall, 2011). The causes for these differences are not known.

❖ PATIENT-CENTERED COLLABORATIVE CARE

◆ Assessment

The patient with *diverticulosis* usually has no symptoms. Unless pain or bleeding develops, the condition may go undiagnosed. Diverticula are most often diagnosed during routine colonoscopy. Occasionally, diverticulosis will cause symptoms. For the patient with uncomplicated diverticulosis, ask about intermittent pain in the left lower quadrant and a history of constipation. If diverticulitis is suspected, ask about a history of low-grade fever, nausea, and abdominal PAIN. Inquire about recent bowel ELIMINATION patterns because constipation may develop as a result of intestinal INFLAMMATION. Also ask about any bleeding from the rectum.

The patient with *diverticulitis* may have abdominal PAIN, most often localized to the left lower quadrant. It is intermittent at first but becomes progressively steady. Occasionally, pain may be just above the pubic bone or may occur on one side. Abdominal pain is generalized if peritonitis has occurred. Nausea and vomiting are common. The patient's temperature is elevated, ranging from a low-grade fever to 101°F (38.3°C). Chills may be present. Often an increased heart rate (tachycardia) occurs with fever.

CONSIDERATIONS FOR OLDER ADULTS
Patient-Centered Care QSEN

The first sign of peritonitis in older adults may be a sudden change in mental status (e.g., acute confusion). For those who have dementia, the confusion worsens. Fever and chills may not be present due to normal physiologic changes associated with aging.

On examination of the abdomen, observe for distention. The patient may report tenderness over the involved area. Localized muscle spasm, guarded movement, and rebound tenderness may be present with peritoneal irritation. If generalized peritonitis is present, profound guarding occurs; rebound tenderness is more widespread; and sepsis, hypotension, or hypovolemic shock can occur. If the perforated diverticulum is close to the rectum, the health care provider may palpate a tender mass during the rectal examination. Blood pressure checks may show orthostatic changes. *If bleeding is massive, the patient may have hypotension and dehydration that result in shock.*

For the patient with uncomplicated diverticulosis, laboratory studies are not indicated. The patient with diverticulitis, however, has an *elevated white blood cell (WBC) count. Decreased hematocrit and hemoglobin* values are common if chronic or severe bleeding occurs. Stool tests for occult blood, if requested, are sometimes positive. Abdominal x-rays may be done to evaluate for free air and fluid indicating perforation. A CT scan may be performed to diagnose an abscess or thickening of the bowel related to diverticulitis.

Abdominal ultrasonography, a noninvasive test, may also reveal bowel thickening or an abscess. The health care provider may recommend a colonoscopy 4 to 8 weeks *after the acute phase* of the illness to rule out a tumor in the large intestine, particularly if the patient has rectal bleeding.

◆ Interventions

Patients are managed on an ambulatory care basis if the symptoms are mild. Monitor the patient for any prolonged or increased fever, abdominal PAIN, or blood in the stool. The patient with moderate to severe diverticulitis may be hospitalized, especially if the patient is older or has complications. Manifestations suggesting the need for admission are a temperature higher than 101°F (38.3°C), persistent and severe abdominal PAIN for more than 3 days, and/or lower GI bleeding.

Nonsurgical Management. A combination of drug and nutrition therapy with rest is used to decrease the INFLAMMATION associated with diverticular disease. Broad-spectrum antimicrobial drugs, such as metronidazole (Flagyl) plus trimethoprim/sulfamethoxazole (TMZ) (Bactrim or Bactrim DS, Septra) or ciprofloxacin (Cipro), are often prescribed. A mild analgesic may be given for PAIN. Chart 57-6 lists nursing interventions needed for care of older adults with diverticulitis.

The patient with more severe PAIN may be admitted to the hospital for IV fluids to correct dehydration and IV drug

therapy. For patients with moderate to severe diverticulitis, an opioid analgesic may alleviate pain.

Laxatives and enemas are avoided because they increase intestinal motility. Assess the patient on an ongoing basis for manifestations of impaired FLUID AND ELECTROLYTE BALANCE.

Teach the patient to rest during the acute phase of illness. Remind him or her to refrain from lifting, straining, coughing, or bending to avoid an increase in intra-abdominal pressure, which can result in perforation of the diverticulum. NUTRITION therapy should be restricted to low fiber or clear liquids based on symptoms. The patient with more severe symptoms is NPO. A nasogastric tube (NGT) is inserted if nausea, vomiting, or abdominal distention is severe. Infuse IV fluids as prescribed for hydration. In collaboration with the dietitian, the patient increases dietary intake slowly as symptoms subside. When INFLAMMATION has resolved and bowel function returns to normal, a fiber-containing diet is introduced gradually.

Surgical Management. Diverticulitis can result in rupture of the diverticulum with peritonitis, pelvic abscess, bowel obstruction, fistula, persistent fever or PAIN, or uncontrolled bleeding. The surgeon performs emergency surgery if peritonitis, bowel obstruction, or pelvic abscess is present. Colon resection, with or without a colostomy, is the most common surgical procedure for patients with diverticular disease. Chapter 56 discusses the nursing care for patients with this procedure.

Community-Based Care

The length of stay for patients hospitalized for diverticulitis ranges from 1 to 4 days, depending on the response to treatment and if surgery is performed. Discharge plans vary according to the treatment. The patient who has surgical intervention has the added responsibilities of incision care and possibly colostomy care with temporary limitations placed on activities.

Patients with diverticular disease need education regarding a high-fiber diet. Encourage the patient with *diverticulosis* to eat a diet high in cellulose and hemicellulose types of fiber. These substances can be found in wheat bran, whole-grain breads, and cereals. Teach the patient to eat at least 25 to 35 g of fiber per day. Fresh fruits and vegetables with high fiber content are added to provide bulk to stools.

If not accustomed to eating high-fiber foods, teach the patient to add them to the diet gradually to avoid flatulence and abdominal cramping. If he or she cannot tolerate the recommended fiber requirement, a bulk-forming laxative, such as psyllium hydrophilic mucilloid (Metamucil), can be taken to increase fecal size and consistency. Teach the patient to drink plenty of fluids to help prevent bloating that may occur with a high-fiber diet. Alcohol should be avoided because it irritates the bowel. Foods containing seeds or indigestible material that may block a diverticulum, such as nuts, corn, popcorn, cucumbers, tomatoes, figs, and strawberries, may be eliminated. Teach the patient that dietary fat intake should not exceed 30% of the total daily caloric intake.

Teach the patient to avoid all fiber when symptoms of *diverticulitis* are present, because high-fiber foods are then irritating. As INFLAMMATION resolves, fiber can gradually be added until progression to a high-fiber diet is established. The patient who has undergone surgery is usually taking solid food by the time of discharge from the hospital.

Provide oral and written instructions on incision care and the signs and symptoms to report to the health care provider for the patient who had abdominal surgery. If a colostomy

---

CHART 57-6 Nursing Focus on the Older Adult

Diverticulitis

- Provide antibiotics, analgesics, and anticholinergics as prescribed. Observe older patients carefully for side effects of these drugs, especially confusion (or increased confusion), urinary retention or failure, and orthostatic hypotension.
- Do not give laxatives or enemas. Teach the patient and the family about the importance of avoiding these measures.
- Encourage the patient to rest and to avoid activities that may increase intra-abdominal pressure, such as straining and bending.
- While diverticulitis is active, provide a *low-*fiber diet. When the inflammation resolves, provide a *high-*fiber diet. Teach the patient and family about these diets and when they are appropriate.
- Because older patients do not always experience the typical pain or fever expected, observe carefully for other signs of active disease, such as a sudden change in mental status.
- Perform frequent abdominal assessments to determine distention and tenderness on palpation.
- Check stools for occult or frank bleeding.

created, reinforce ostomy care as needed. Encourage the patient to express concerns about body image. Allow time and address sexual concerns regarding the changed body image.

Instruct the patient with any type of diverticular disease, orally and in writing, about the manifestations of acute diverticulitis, including fever, abdominal PAIN, and bloody, mahogany, or tarry stools. Advise patients to avoid the use of laxatives (other than bulk-forming types) and enemas. Reassure them that this disorder should not cause problems if a proper diet is followed.

In collaboration with the case manager, arrange for a home care nurse, if needed, to assess wound healing and proper functioning of the ostomy and the appliance. If the patient is interested, arrange for a visit from an ostomy volunteer (ostomate) or an ostomy nurse. For information about other community resources, remind the patient to contact the United Ostomy Associations of America (www.uoaa.org).

NCLEX EXAMINATION CHALLENGE

Physiological Integrity

The nurse is teaching a client about nutrition and diverticulitis. Which statement by the client indicates a need for further teaching?
A. "I should eat more foods low in fiber."
B. "I will not drink any alcohol."
C. "I can have any fruits that I want."
D. "I need to avoid nuts and corn."

CELIAC DISEASE

Celiac disease (CD) was once thought to be a rare disease, but many cases in adults between 30 and 50 years old have been diagnosed in the past 10 years. CD is a multi-system autoimmune disease with an estimated incidence of about 3 million Americans; most are not diagnosed (Strauch & Cotter, 2011). Patients who have other autoimmune diseases, such as rheumatoid arthritis and diabetes mellitus type 1, are at the highest risk for the disease.

CD is a chronic INFLAMMATION of the small intestinal mucosa that can cause bowel wall atrophy and malabsorption. Like many inflammatory disorders, it is thought to be caused by a combination of genetic, immunologic, and environmental factors. The primary complication of CD is cancer, specifically non-Hodgkin's lymphoma or GI cancers.

Patients with CD have varying clinical manifestations with cycles of remission and exacerbation (flare-up). Classic symptoms include anorexia, diarrhea and/or constipation, steatorrhea (fatty stools), abdominal PAIN, abdominal bloating and distention, and weight loss. Some patients have no symptoms. Still others have atypical symptoms that affect every body system (Chart 57-7).

Dietary management is the only available treatment for achieving disease remission. In most cases, a gluten-free diet (GFD) results in healing the intestinal mucosa after about 2 years (Strauch & Cotter, 2011). Gluten is the primary substance in wheat and wheat-based products. Teach patients to carefully check for hidden sources of gluten that are in foods, food additives, drugs, and cosmetics. Patients often take vitamin and mineral supplements to replace those lost in avoiding gluten foods.

CHART 57-7 Key Features

Celiac Disease

Classic Symptoms	Atypical Symptoms
• Weight loss	• Osteoporosis
• Anorexia	• Joint pain and inflammation
• Diarrhea and/or constipation	• Lactose intolerance
• Steatorrhea	• Iron deficiency anemia
• Abdominal pain and distention	• Depression
• Vomiting	• Migraines
	• Epilepsy
	• Autoimmune disorders
	• Stomatitis
	• Early menopause
	• Protein-calorie malnutrition

ANAL DISORDERS

ANORECTAL ABSCESS

Anorectal abscess is a localized area of induration and pus caused by INFLAMMATION of the soft tissue near the rectum or anus. It is most often the result of obstruction of the ducts of glands in the anorectal region. Feces, foreign bodies, or trauma can be the cause of the obstruction and stasis, leading to INFECTION that spreads into nearby tissue.

Rectal PAIN is often the first symptom. There may be no other manifestations at first, but local swelling, redness, and tenderness are present within a few days after the onset of pain. If the abscess becomes chronic, discharge, bleeding, and pruritus (itching) may exist. Fever occurs if larger abscesses are present.

Anorectal abscesses are managed by surgical incision and drainage (I&D). The physician can often excise (surgically remove) simple perianal and ischiorectal abscesses using a local anesthetic. For patients with more extensive abscesses, a regional or general anesthetic may be needed. Systemic antibiotics are given only for patients who are immunocompromised, are diabetic, have valvular disease or a prosthetic valve, or are obese.

NURSING SAFETY PRIORITY (QSEN)

Action Alert

For patients with an anorectal abscess, nursing interventions are focused on comfort and helping the patient maintain optimal perineal hygiene. Encourage the use of warm sitz baths, analgesics, bulk-producing agents, and stool softeners after the surgery until healing occurs. *Stress the importance of good perineal hygiene after all bowel movements and the maintenance of a regular bowel pattern with a high-fiber diet.*

Patients are often embarrassed about having anal problems. Provide privacy and maintain the patient's dignity during the examination and treatment.

ANAL FISSURE

An anal fissure is a tear in the anal lining, which can be very painful. Smaller fissures occur with straining to have a stool, such as with diarrhea or constipation. Larger, deeper fissures may occur as a result of another disorder (e.g., Crohn's disease, tuberculosis, leukemia, neoplasm) or from trauma (e.g., from a foreign body, anal intercourse, perirectal surgery).

An *acute* anal fissure is superficial and usually resolves on its own or heals quickly with conservative treatment. *Chronic* fissures recur, and surgical treatment may be needed. Pain during and after defecation and bright red blood in the stool are the most common symptoms. Other manifestations include pruritus, urinary frequency or retention, dysuria, and dyspareunia (painful intercourse).

The diagnosis is made by stretching and inspecting the perianal skin. If the patient is having pain at the time of the examination, diagnostic testing is usually limited to inspection. If he or she is not in severe PAIN, a digital examination and possibly a sigmoidoscopy are performed. When painless or multiple fissures are present, a colonoscopy may be performed to rule out any inflammatory bowel disorder.

Management of an acute fissure is usually aimed at local PAIN relief and softening of stools to reduce trauma to the area. Teach the patient to use warm sitz baths, analgesics, and bulk-producing agents (e.g., psyllium hydrophilic mucilloid [Metamucil]) to help minimize the pain from defecation. Topical anti-inflammatory agents (hydrocortisone creams and suppositories) may be helpful for some patients.

Explain PAIN control measures to the patient. Remind him or her to notify the health care provider if pain is not relieved within a few days. If fissures do not respond to management within several days to weeks, surgical repair under a local anesthetic may be needed. Teach the patient to report any drainage or bleeding from the rectum to the health care provider.

ANAL FISTULA

An anal fistula, or *fistula in ano,* is an abnormal tract leading from the anal canal to the perianal skin. Most anal fistulas result from anorectal abscesses, which are caused by obstruction of anal glands (see Anorectal Abscess, p. 1188). Fistulas can also occur with tuberculosis, Crohn's disease, or cancer. Intermittent discharge is usually noted over the perianal area.

The patient with an anal fistula has pruritus (itching), purulent discharge, and tenderness or PAIN that is worsened by bowel movements. A proctoscope may be used to identify the source of symptoms and to locate the fistula. Because fistulas do not heal spontaneously, surgery is necessary. To perform a fistulotomy, the surgeon opens the tissue over the tract and scrapes the base. The incision site then heals by secondary intention. For a fistula higher in the anus, a special surgical technique is used to preserve important sphincters. After surgery, instruct the patient about sitz baths, analgesics, and the use of bulk-producing agents or stool softeners to reduce pain.

PARASITIC INFECTION

❖ *PATHOPHYSIOLOGY*

Parasites can enter and invade the GI tract and cause INFECTION. They commonly enter through the mouth (oral-fecal transmission) from contaminated food or water, oral-anal sexual practices, or contact with feces from a contaminated person. Common parasites that cause infection in humans are *Giardia lamblia,* which causes giardiasis; *Entamoeba histolytica,* which causes amebiasis (amebic dysentery); and *Cryptosporidium. Handwashing is the best way to prevent the spread of parasitic infections.*

G. lamblia is a protozoal parasite that causes superficial invasion, destruction, and INFLAMMATION of the mucosa in the small intestine. This organism occurs in cysts and trophozoites (sporozoan parasites). Trophozoites die rapidly after they leave the body in stool. Cysts, however, can remain alive in the right type of environment for weeks or months. Humans who eliminate cysts are infectious. Flies can spread the cysts, and the problem is more common in areas that use human excrement for fertilizer. Humans are hosts to this organism, but beavers and dogs may be reservoirs for infection.

Giardiasis is a well-recognized problem in international travelers, campers, and immunosuppressed patients. In the United States, giardiasis is prevalent and is the most common parasitic INFECTION. This disorder affects only the intestinal system, causing acute diarrhea, chronic diarrhea, or malabsorption syndrome. The acute phase usually is self-limiting, lasting days or weeks. The chronic phase can last for years. Diarrhea is usually mild in both forms, but it can be severe. As stools increase in frequency, they become more watery, greasy, frothy, and malodorous with mucus. Weight loss and weakness are also common. Malabsorption can occur with diarrhea that continues for longer than 3 weeks. Manifestations result from malabsorption of fat, protein, and vitamin B_{12} and lactase deficiency.

Humans are the only known hosts for *E. histolytica* (also known as *amebiasis*). This organism also occurs in cysts and trophozoites. Amebiasis occurs worldwide, but it is most common in tropical areas. Prevalence rates are high in areas with poor sanitation, crowding, and poor nutrition. Amebiasis causes tens of thousands of deaths annually worldwide. The disease causes less severe symptoms and often goes undiagnosed in temperate climates.

E. histolytica either feeds on bacteria in the intestine or invades and ulcerates the mucosa of the large intestine. The parasite can be limited to the GI tract (intestinal amebiasis), or it can extend outside the intestines (extraintestinal amebiasis). People can have intestinal amebiasis without having any symptoms, or symptoms can range from mild to severe.

Cryptosporidium is manifested by diarrhea. This INFECTION occurs most commonly in immunosuppressed patients, particularly those with human immune deficiency virus (HIV). It can also occur in children and older adults from contaminated swimming pools. (See Chapter 19 for a discussion of HIV infection.)

Chagas disease is caused by the *Trypanosoma cruzi* parasite, which is most commonly transmitted to people in poverty areas of Latin America by the triatomine (kissing) bug. Patients first develop an acute infection, followed by an intermediate asymptomatic period and a chronic infection. Patients with chronic Chagas disease often develop cardiac dysrhythmias or heart failure, as well as colon or esophagus dilation causing impaired digestion and bowel elimination. An estimated 300,000 people in the United States have the disease (most in the southern areas of the United States), which can be transmitted through blood transfusions and organ transplantations. The CDC has targeted Chagas disease as one of five neglected parasitic infections that require public health action as the number of cases is expected to increase (CDC, 2014).

❖ *PATIENT-CENTERED COLLABORATIVE CARE*

◆ Assessment

A thorough history can help determine potential sources of exposure to parasitic INFECTION. A history of travel to parts of the world where such infections are prevalent increases suspicion for infection with parasites. GI symptoms related to travel may be delayed as long as 1 to 2 weeks after the return home. Immigrants (newcomers) may have the infection upon entering a new country. A NUTRITION history is especially helpful if several people in a group become ill. Common water supplies or bodies of water may be infected with *Giardia* or *Cryptosporidium*. Trichinosis should be considered if the patient has eaten pork products.

Mild to moderate *E. histolytica* infestation causes the daily passage of several strongly foul-smelling stools, possibly with mucus but without blood, accompanied by abdominal cramping, flatulence (gas), fatigue, and weight loss.

The infected patient usually experiences remissions and recurrences. Severe amebic dysentery is manifested by frequent, more liquid, and foul-smelling stools with mucus *and* blood. Fever up to 104° F (40° C), tenesmus (feeling the urge to defecate), generalized abdominal tenderness, and vomiting can also occur. The ulcerations of invading amebiasis that occur in the colon can cause pain, bleeding, and obstruction. Ulcerations can also occur in the rectum, resulting in formed stool with blood. Complications are rare but include appendicitis and bowel perforation.

Extraintestinal amebiasis can occur without symptoms of intestinal INFECTION. The most common form is amebic liver abscess, which causes symptoms of fever, PAIN, and an enlarged liver. The abscess can rupture, and death can result if the infection and complications are not treated.

The diagnosis of *amebiasis* is made by examining the stool for parasites. Because *E. histolytica* is difficult to detect, serial stool examinations are needed if the disease is suspected. The use of sigmoidoscopy may detect ulcerations in the rectum or colon. Exudate obtained during sigmoidoscopic examination is studied for the parasite. The white blood cell (WBC) count can be very high when severe dysentery is present.

The diagnosis of *giardiasis* is also confirmed by the presence of parasites in the stool. Because organisms may not be detected for at least 1 week after symptoms appear, multiple stool samples should be examined.

◆ **Interventions**

Treatment for all types of *amebiasis* involves the use of amebicide drugs. Metronidazole (Flagyl, Novonidazol ♣) and diloxanide furoate (Entamide) or diloxanide furoate and tetracycline

hydrochloride (Sumycin) followed by chloroquine are commonly prescribed. The patient with severe dysentery requires IV fluid replacement and possibly opiates, such as diphenoxylate hydrochloride and atropine sulfate (Lomotil), to control bowel motility. The patient with extraintestinal amebiasis or severe dehydration is hospitalized, especially the older adult. The patient with asymptomatic, mild, or moderate disease is treated with drug therapy on an ambulatory care basis. Therapy effectiveness is based on the examination of at least three stools at 2- to 3-day intervals, starting 2 to 4 weeks after drug therapy has been completed. *Teach patients the importance of keeping their follow-up appointments and taking all drugs as prescribed.*

Treatment for *giardiasis* is drug therapy. Metronidazole is the drug of choice, 250 mg orally 3 times daily for 5 days. Tinidazole (Fasigyn) can be used as an alternative. Stools are examined 2 weeks after treatment to assess for drug effectiveness.

> **! NURSING SAFETY PRIORITY (QSEN)**
>
> **Action Alert**
>
> Explain modes of transmission of parasitic infections and means to avoid the spread of INFECTION and recurrent contact with parasitic organisms. *Inform the patient that the infection can be transmitted to others until amebicides effectively kill the parasites. Teach the patient to:*
> - Avoid contact with stool.
> - Keep toilet areas clean.
> - Wash hands meticulously with an antimicrobial soap after bowel movements.
> - Maintain good personal hygiene by bathing or showering daily.
> - Avoid stool from dogs and beavers.
>
> Advise the patient to avoid sexual practices that allow rectal contact until drug therapy is completed. *All household and sexual partners should have stool examinations for parasites.* If the water supply is suspected as the source, a sample is obtained and sent for analysis. Multiple infections are common in households, often as a result of contaminated water supplies. Well water and water from areas with inadequate or no filtration equipment can be sources of contamination.

Infection with *Cryptosporidium* is usually self-limiting in people who have normal immune function. Drug therapy for patients who are immunosuppressed may include paromomycin (Paromycin), an aminoglycoside antibiotic. Teach patients that this drug can cause dizziness.

NURSING CONCEPTS AND CLINICAL JUDGMENT REVIEW

What might you NOTICE if the patient has impaired digestion and inadequate NUTRITION as a result of inflammatory intestinal problems?
- Report of nausea
- Vomiting
- Report of epigastric or abdominal pain
- Diarrhea (sometimes bloody)
- Elevated temperature
- Weakness

What should you INTERPRET and how should you RESPOND to a patient with impaired digestion and inadequate NUTRITION as a result of inflammatory intestinal problems?

Perform and interpret focused physical assessment findings, including:
- Vital signs
- Complete pain assessment
- Skin turgor and mucous membrane dryness
- Abdominal assessment
- Current and previous weight
- History of recent food intake
- History of recent travel

Respond by:
- Preventing pain and aspiration by placing the patient in a sitting position

- Placing an IV catheter (large-bore) to replace fluids
- Providing privacy, and assisting with hygiene
- Providing rest
- Checking laboratory values for hemoglobin and hematocrit (anemia)
- Checking serum electrolytes (dehydration, hypokalemia)
- Giving antidiarrheal drugs if prescribed
- Recording intake and output
- Assisting with ADLs and ambulation as needed

On what should you REFLECT?

- Continue to monitor for vomiting and diarrhea and changes in pain level.
- Think about what you need to document.
- Decide when you might need to call the health care provider or Rapid Response Team (for hospitalized patients).
- Determine what health teaching and community resources may be needed for this patient and family.
- Think about what you can do to help prevent complications of the health problem.

GET READY FOR THE NCLEX® EXAMINATION!

KEY POINTS

Review these Key Points for each NCLEX Examination Client Needs Category.

Safe and Effective Care Environment

- Collaborate with a CWOCN, health care provider, and case manager to plan care for patients with IBD. **Teamwork and Collaboration** QSEN

Health Promotion and Maintenance

- Teach patients to use INFECTION control measures to prevent transmission of gastroenteritis as stated in Chart 57-2.
- Teach patients how to self-manage an ileostomy or other surgical diversion, including skin care, pouch management, and stoma assessment (see Chart 57-4).
- Remind patients and families about community resources for IBD, including the United Ostomy Associations of America and the Crohn's and Colitis Foundation of America.

Psychosocial Integrity

- Be aware that all inflammatory bowel diseases (acute and chronic) are very disruptive to one's daily routine; living with IBD requires a lifetime of modifications.
- Recognize that having a chronic bowel disease or an ileostomy impacts the patient's body image and self-esteem; assess for coping strategies that the patient has previously used, and identify personal support systems, such as family members, to assist in coping.

Physiological Integrity

- Assess for the classic clinical manifestations of appendicitis, which include abdominal pain, nausea and vomiting, and abdominal tenderness upon palpation (McBurney's point); some patients also have leukocytosis.
- Recognize that perforation (rupture) of the appendix requires prompt intervention and can result in peritonitis.
- Assess for the key features of peritonitis as listed in Chart 57-1.
- Assess for signs and symptoms of dehydration in patients who have acute and chronic inflammatory bowel disorders.
- Administer antidiarrheal medications as prescribed to decrease stools and therefore prevent dehydration in patients with acute and chronic inflammatory bowel disorders.
- Be aware that there are two major types of chronic inflammatory bowel disease (IBD): ulcerative colitis (UC) and Crohn's disease; both have similarities but also have differences (see Table 57-2).
- Be alert for GI bleeding in the patient with chronic inflammatory bowel disease (IBD).
- Be aware that patients with Crohn's disease are at high risk for malnutrition as a result of an inability to absorb nutrients via the small intestine.
- Priority problems for patients with ulcerative colitis include diarrhea, pain, and potential for lower GI bleeding.
- Monitor for complications of UC as listed in Table 57-4.
- Provide nursing interventions for patients with IBD as listed in Chart 57-3.
- Teach patients with IBD to avoid GI stimulants, such as alcohol and caffeine; each patient's response to foods differs.
- Administer 5-aminosalicylic acid (5-ASA) drugs as prescribed (e.g., Pentasa) to decrease inflammation in patients with UC; most of these same drugs are also used for Crohn's disease management.
- Administer infliximab (Remicade) or other monoclonal antibody agent as prescribed for patients with Crohn's disease; these drugs may also be useful for those with UC in selected cases.
- Observe for manifestations of lower GI bleeding in patients with chronic inflammatory and diverticular disease.
- Teach patients with diverticulosis to eat a high-fiber diet; diverticulitis requires a low-fiber diet.
- Teach older patients how to self-manage diverticulitis as outlined in Chart 57-6.
- Instruct patients with diverticulosis about NUTRITION modifications, such as avoiding nuts, foods with seeds, and GI stimulants.
- Be aware that patients with celiac disease (CD) vary in their clinical manifestations; some have no symptoms, some have classic symptoms, and some have atypical symptoms (see Chart 57-7).
- Teach patients with CD about the need to consume a strict gluten-free diet, which avoids wheat and wheat-based products.
- Be aware that GI problems, including diarrhea, may also be caused by parasites and food poisoning.
- Instruct patients with anorectal disorders to use sitz baths, bulk-forming agents (e.g., Metamucil), and stool softeners to decrease pain.

Care of Patients with Liver Problems

Jennifer Powers and Lara Carver

http://evolve.elsevier.com/Iggy/

PRIORITY CONCEPTS

- INFLAMMATION
- INFECTION

- PAIN
- FLUID AND ELECTROLYTE BALANCE

LEARNING OUTCOMES

Safe and Effective Care Environment
1. Describe the need to collaborate with health care team members to provide care for patients with liver INFLAMMATION and necrosis.
2. Identify community resources for patients with chronic liver disease.

Health Promotion and Maintenance
3. Develop a health teaching plan for patients and families to prevent hepatitis and its spread to others.
4. Develop a health teaching plan for patients and families to prevent or slow the progress of alcohol-induced cirrhosis.

Psychosocial Integrity
5. Explain the psychosocial needs of patients with liver problems.

Physiological Integrity
6. Identify risk factors for developing hepatic cirrhosis.

7. Interpret laboratory test findings commonly seen in patients with cirrhosis.
8. Analyze assessment data from patients with cirrhosis to determine priority patient problems.
9. Develop an evidence-based collaborative plan of care for the patient with late-stage cirrhosis.
10. Describe the role of the nurse in monitoring for and managing potentially life-threatening complications of cirrhosis.
11. Identify emergency interventions for the patient with bleeding esophageal varices.
12. Explain the role of the nurse when assisting with a paracentesis procedure.
13. Describe treatment options for patients with cancer of the liver.
14. Describe the interventions to prevent complications that result from liver transplantation, including INFECTION.

The liver is the largest and one of the most vital internal organs, performing more than 400 functions and affecting every system in the body. When the liver is diseased or damaged, it cannot accomplish these functions. As a result, *digestion, nutrition, and metabolism* can be severely affected. Liver diseases range in severity from mild hepatic INFLAMMATION to chronic end-stage cirrhosis.

CIRRHOSIS

Cirrhosis is extensive, irreversible scarring of the liver, usually caused by a chronic reaction to hepatic INFLAMMATION and necrosis. The disease typically develops slowly and has a progressive, prolonged, destructive course resulting in end-stage liver disease. The most common causes for cirrhosis in the United States are chronic alcoholism, chronic viral hepatitis, nonalcoholic steatohepatitis (NASH), bile duct disease, and genetic diseases (Table 58-1).

❖ *PATHOPHYSIOLOGY*

Cirrhosis is characterized by widespread fibrotic (scarred) bands of connective tissue that change the liver's normal makeup. INFLAMMATION caused by either toxins or disease results in extensive degeneration and destruction of hepato-cytes (liver cells). As cirrhosis develops, the tissue becomes nodular. These nodules can block bile ducts and normal blood flow throughout the liver. Impairments in blood and lymph flow result from compression caused by excessive fibrous tissue. In early disease, the liver is usually enlarged, firm, and hard. As the pathologic process continues, the liver shrinks in size, resulting in decreased liver function, which can occur in weeks to years. Some patients with cirrhosis have no symptoms until serious complications occur. The impaired liver function results in elevated serum liver enzymes (Pagana & Pagana, 2014).

Cirrhosis of the liver can be divided into several common types, depending on the cause of the disease (McCance et al., 2014):

TABLE 58-1	**Common Causes of Cirrhosis**
• Alcoholic liver disease	• Drugs and chemical toxins
• Viral hepatitis	• Gallbladder disease
• Autoimmune hepatitis	• Metabolic/genetic causes
• Steatohepatitis (from fatty liver)	• Cardiovascular disease

- Postnecrotic cirrhosis (caused by viral hepatitis [especially hepatitis C] and certain drugs or other toxins)
- Laennec's or alcoholic cirrhosis (caused by chronic alcoholism)
- Biliary cirrhosis (also called *cholestatic;* caused by chronic biliary obstruction or autoimmune disease)

Complications of Cirrhosis

Common problems and complications associated with hepatic cirrhosis depend on the amount of damage sustained by the liver. In compensated cirrhosis, the liver is scarred but can still perform essential functions without causing major symptoms. In decompensated cirrhosis, liver function is impaired with obvious manifestations of liver failure.

The loss of hepatic function contributes to the development of metabolic abnormalities. Hepatic cell damage may lead to these common complications:

- Portal hypertension
- Ascites and esophageal varices
- Coagulation defects
- Jaundice
- Portal-systemic encephalopathy (PSE) with hepatic coma
- Hepatorenal syndrome
- Spontaneous bacterial peritonitis

Portal Hypertension. Portal hypertension, a persistent increase in pressure within the portal vein greater than 5 mm Hg, is a major complication of cirrhosis (Minano & Garcia-Tsao, 2010). It results from increased resistance to or obstruction (blockage) of the flow of blood through the portal vein and its branches. The blood meets resistance to flow and seeks collateral (alternative) venous channels around the high-pressure area.

Blood flow backs into the spleen, causing splenomegaly (spleen enlargement). Veins in the esophagus, stomach, intestines, abdomen, and rectum become dilated. Portal hypertension can result in ascites (excessive abdominal [peritoneal] fluid), esophageal varices (distended veins), prominent abdominal veins (caput medusae), and hemorrhoids.

Ascites and Gastroesophageal Varices. Ascites is the collection of free fluid within the peritoneal cavity caused by increased hydrostatic pressure from portal hypertension (McCance et al., 2014). The collection of plasma protein in the peritoneal fluid reduces the amount of circulating plasma protein in the blood. When this decrease is combined with the inability of the liver to produce albumin because of impaired liver cell functioning, the serum colloid osmotic pressure is decreased in the circulatory system. The result is a fluid shift from the vascular system into the abdomen, a form of "third spacing." As a result, the patient may have hypovolemia and edema at the same time.

Massive ascites may cause renal vasoconstriction, triggering the renin-angiotensin system. This results in sodium and water retention, which increases hydrostatic pressure and the vascular volume and leads to more ascites.

As a result of portal hypertension, the blood backs up from the liver and enters the esophageal and gastric veins. Esophageal varices occur when fragile, thin-walled esophageal veins become distended and tortuous from increased pressure. The potential for varices to bleed depends on their size; size is determined by direct endoscopic observation. Varices occur most often in the distal esophagus but can be present also in the stomach and rectum.

Bleeding esophageal varices is a life-threatening medical emergency. Severe blood loss may occur, resulting in shock from hypovolemia. The bleeding may be either hematemesis (vomiting blood) or melena (black, tarry stools). Loss of consciousness may occur before any observed bleeding. Variceal bleeding can occur spontaneously with no precipitating factors. However, any activity that increases abdominal pressure may increase the likelihood of a variceal bleed, including heavy lifting or vigorous physical exercise. In addition, chest trauma or dry, hard food in the esophagus can cause bleeding.

Patients with portal hypertension may also have portal hypertensive gastropathy. This complication can occur with or without esophageal varices. Slow gastric mucosal bleeding occurs, which may result in chronic slow blood loss, occult-positive stools, and anemia.

Splenomegaly (enlarged spleen) results from the backup of blood into the spleen. The enlarged spleen destroys platelets, causing thrombocytopenia (low serum platelet count) and increased risk for bleeding. Thrombocytopenia is often the first clinical sign that a patient has liver dysfunction.

Biliary Obstruction. In patients with cirrhosis, the production of bile in the liver is decreased. This prevents the absorption of fat-soluble vitamins (e.g., vitamin K). Without vitamin K, clotting factors II, VII, IX, and X are not produced in sufficient quantities and the patient is susceptible to bleeding and easy bruising. These abnormalities are confirmed by coagulation studies. Some patients have a genetic predisposition to obstruction of the bile duct that leads to biliary cirrhosis—usually from gallbladder disease or an autoimmune form of the disease called *primary biliary cirrhosis (PBC).*

Jaundice (yellowish coloration of the skin) in patients with cirrhosis is caused by one of two mechanisms: hepatocellular disease or intrahepatic obstruction (Fig. 58-1). *Hepatocellular* jaundice develops because the liver cells cannot effectively excrete bilirubin. This decreased excretion results in excessive circulating bilirubin levels. *Intrahepatic obstructive* jaundice results from edema, fibrosis, or scarring of the hepatic bile channels and bile ducts, which interferes with normal bile and bilirubin excretion. Patients with jaundice often report pruritus (itching).

Hepatic Encephalopathy. Hepatic encephalopathy (also called portal-systemic encephalopathy [PSE]) is a complex cognitive syndrome that results from liver failure and cirrhosis. Patients report sleep disturbance, mood disturbance, mental status changes, and speech problems early as this complication begins. Hepatic encephalopathy may be reversible with early intervention. Later neurologic symptoms include an altered level of consciousness, impaired thinking processes, and neuromuscular problems.

Hepatic encephalopathy may develop slowly in patients with chronic liver disease and go undetected until the late stages. Symptoms develop rapidly in acute liver dysfunction. Four stages of development have been identified (Table 58-2). The patient's symptoms may gradually progress to coma or fluctuate among the four stages.

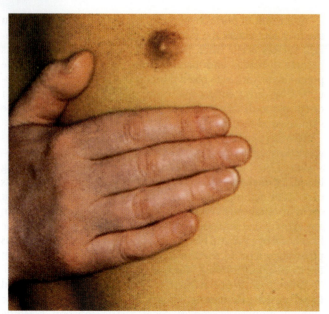

FIG. 58-1 Jaundice as a result of liver dysfunction such as cirrhosis and hepatitis.

TABLE 58-2 **Stages of Hepatic Encephalopathy**	
Stage I • Subtle manifestations that may not be recognized immediately • Personality changes • Behavior changes (agitation, belligerence) • Emotional lability (euphoria, depression) • Impaired thinking • Inability to concentrate • Fatigue, drowsiness • Slurred or slowed speech • Sleep pattern disturbances **Stage II** • Continuing mental changes • Mental confusion • Disorientation to time, place, or person • Asterixis (hand flapping)	**Stage III** • Progressive deterioration • Marked mental confusion • Stuporous, drowsy but arousable • Abnormal electroencephalogram tracing • Muscle twitching • Hyperreflexia • Asterixis (hand flapping) **Stage IV** • Unresponsiveness, leading to death in most patients progressing to this stage • Unarousable, obtunded • Usually no response to painful stimulus • No asterixis • Positive Babinski's sign • Muscle rigidity • Fetor hepaticus (characteristic liver breath—musty, sweet odor) • Seizures

The exact mechanisms causing hepatic encephalopathy are not clearly understood but probably are the result of the shunting of portal venous blood into the central circulation so that the liver is bypassed. As a result, substances absorbed by the intestine are not broken down or detoxified and may lead to metabolic abnormalities, such as elevated serum ammonia and gamma-aminobutyric acid (GABA). Elevated serum ammonia results from the inability of the liver to detoxify protein by-products and is common in patients with hepatic encephalopathy. However, it is not a clear indicator of the presence of encephalopathy. Some patients may have major impairment without high elevations of serum ammonia, and elevations of ammonia can occur without evidence of encephalopathy.

Factors that may lead to hepatic encephalopathy in patients with cirrhosis include:
• High-protein diet
• INFECTION
• Hypovolemia (decreased fluid volume)
• Hypokalemia (decreased serum potassium)
• Constipation
• GI bleeding (causes a large protein load in the intestines)
• Drugs (e.g., hypnotics, opioids, sedatives, analgesics, diuretics, illicit drugs)

The prognosis depends on the severity of the underlying cause, the precipitating factors, and the degree of liver dysfunction.

Other Complications. The development of **hepatorenal syndrome (HRS)** indicates a poor prognosis for the patient with liver failure. It is often the cause of death in these patients. This syndrome is manifested by:
• A sudden decrease in urinary flow (<500 mL/24 hr) (oliguria)
• Elevated blood urea nitrogen (BUN) and creatinine levels with abnormally decreased urine sodium excretion
• Increased urine osmolarity

HRS often occurs after clinical deterioration from GI bleeding or the onset of hepatic encephalopathy. It may also complicate other liver diseases, including acute hepatitis and fulminant liver failure.

Patients with cirrhosis and ascites may develop acute *spontaneous bacterial peritonitis (SBP)*. Those who are particularly susceptible are patients with very advanced liver disease. This may be the result of low concentrations of proteins; proteins normally provide some protection against bacteria.

The bacteria responsible for SBP are typically from the bowel and reach the ascitic fluid after migrating through the bowel wall and transversing the lymphatics. Clinical manifestations vary but may include fever, chills, and abdominal PAIN and tenderness. However, manifestations can also be minimal with only mild symptoms in the absence of fever. Worsening encephalopathy and increased jaundice may also be present without abdominal symptoms.

The diagnosis of SBP is made when a sample of ascitic fluid is obtained by paracentesis for cell counts and culture. An ascitic fluid leukocyte count of more than 250 polymorphonuclear (PMN) leukocytes may indicate the need for treatment.

Etiology and Genetic Risk

Hepatitis C is the second leading cause of cirrhosis and liver failure in the United States. It is an infectious bloodborne illness that usually causes chronic disease. INFLAMMATION caused by INFECTION over time leads to progressive scarring of the liver. It usually takes decades for cirrhosis to develop, although alcohol use in combination with hepatitis C may speed the process.

Hepatitis B and hepatitis D are the most common causes of cirrhosis worldwide. Hepatitis B also causes INFLAMMATION and low-grade damage over decades that can ultimately lead to cirrhosis. Hepatitis D virus can infect the liver but only in people who already have hepatitis B (see discussion of hepatitis on p. 1203).

Cirrhosis may also occur as a result of nonalcoholic fatty liver disease (NAFLD), a rapidly growing health care concern. NAFLD is associated with obesity, diabetes mellitus type 2, and metabolic syndrome. It is the most common cause of liver disease in the world (World Gastroenterology Organisation, 2012). This disease can progress to liver cancer, cirrhosis, or failure, causing a premature death. Up to 25% of Americans may have NAFLD (American Liver Foundation, 2010) (see p. 1208). The Patatin-like phospholipase domain-containing 3 gene (PNPLA3) has been identified as a risk gene for the disease. Hispanics have this gene more often than other ethnic groups and are therefore at the highest risk for NAFLD (Houghton-Rahrig et al., 2014).

Another common cause of cirrhosis is excessive and prolonged alcohol use. Alcohol has a direct toxic effect on the hepatocytes and causes liver inflammation (**alcoholic hepatitis**). The liver becomes enlarged, with cellular degeneration and infiltration by fat, leukocytes, and lymphocytes. Over time, the inflammatory process decreases and the destructive phase increases. Early scar formation is caused by fibroblast infiltration and collagen formation. Damage to the liver tissue progresses as malnutrition and repeated exposure to the alcohol continue. If alcohol is withheld, the fatty infiltration and INFLAMMATION are reversible. If alcohol use continues, widespread scar tissue formation and fibrosis infiltrate the liver as a result of cellular necrosis. The long-term use of illicit drugs, such as cocaine, has similar effects on the liver.

GENDER HEALTH CONSIDERATIONS

Patient-Centered Care QSEN

The amount of alcohol necessary to cause cirrhosis varies widely from person to person, and there are gender differences. In women, it may take as few as two or three drinks per day over a minimum of 10 years. In men, perhaps six drinks per day over the same time period may be needed to cause disease. However, a smaller amount of alcohol over a long period of time can increase memory loss from alcohol toxicity of the cerebral cortex. Binge drinking can increase risk for hepatitis and fatty liver.

Incidence and Prevalence

The American Liver Foundation (2011) released the following statistics on the prevalence of liver disease in the United States:

- More than 30 million people in the United States have liver disease—or 1 in 10 Americans.
- Four million Americans have hepatitis C, and more than 1 million Americans have hepatitis B.

Combined, the incidence of chronic liver disease and cirrhosis are the twelfth most common cause of death in the United States, and about 28,000 adults die from them each year.

❖ PATIENT-CENTERED COLLABORATIVE CARE

◆ Assessment

History. Obtain data from patients with suspected cirrhosis, including age, gender, and employment history, especially history of exposure to alcohol, drugs (prescribed and illicit), and chemical toxins. Keep in mind that all exposures are important regardless of how long ago they occurred. Determine whether there has ever been a needle stick injury. Sexual history and orientation may be important in determining an infectious cause for liver disease, because men having sex with men (MSM) are at high risk for hepatitis A, hepatitis B, and hepatitis C. People with hepatitis can develop cirrhosis (American Liver Foundation, 2011).

Inquire about whether there is a family history of alcoholism and/or liver disease. Ask the patient to describe his or her alcohol intake, including the amount consumed during a given period. Is there a history of illicit drug use, including oral, IV, and intranasal forms? Is there a history of tattoos? If so, when and where were they done? Has the patient been in the military or in prison? Is the patient a health care worker, firefighter, or police officer? For patients previously or currently in an alcohol or drug recovery program, how long have they been sober? This information is sensitive and often difficult for the patient to answer. Be sure to establish why you are asking these questions, and accept answers in a nonjudgmental manner. Provide privacy during the interview. For many people, the behaviors causing the liver disease occurred years before the onset of their current illness and they are regretful and often embarrassed.

Ask the patient about previous medical conditions, such as an episode of jaundice or acute viral hepatitis, biliary tract disorders (such as cholecystitis), viral INFECTIONS, surgery, blood transfusions, autoimmune disorders, obesity, altered lipid profile, heart failure, respiratory disorders, or liver injury.

Physical Assessment/Clinical Manifestations. Because cirrhosis has a slow onset, many of the *early* manifestations are vague and nonspecific. Assess for:

- Fatigue
- Significant change in weight
- GI symptoms, such as anorexia and vomiting
- Abdominal PAIN and liver tenderness (both of which may be ignored by the patient)

Liver function problems are often found during a routine physical examination or when laboratory tests are completed for an unrelated illness or problem. The patient with *compensated cirrhosis* may be completely unaware that there is a liver problem. The first sign may present before the onset of symptoms when routine laboratory tests, presurgical evaluations, or life and health insurance assessments show abnormalities. These tests could indicate abnormal liver function or thrombocytopenia, requiring a more thorough diagnostic workup.

The development of late signs of *advanced cirrhosis* (also called "end-stage liver failure") usually cause the patient to seek medical treatment. GI bleeding, jaundice, ascites, and spontaneous bruising indicate poor liver function and complications of cirrhosis.

Thoroughly assess the patient with liver dysfunction or failure because it affects every body system. The clinical picture and course vary from patient to patient depending on the severity of the disease. Assess for:

- Obvious yellowing of the skin (jaundice) and sclerae (icterus)
- Dry skin
- Rashes
- Purpuric lesions, such as **petechiae** (round, pinpoint, red-purple lesions) or **ecchymoses** (large purple, blue, or yellow bruises)
- Warm and bright red palms of the hands (palmar erythema)
- Vascular lesions with a red center and radiating branches, known as "**spider angiomas**" (telangiectases, spider nevi, or vascular spiders), on the nose, cheeks, upper thorax, and shoulders
- Ascites (abdominal fluid)
- Peripheral dependent edema of the extremities and sacrum

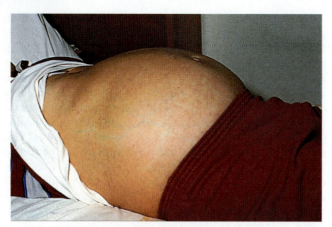

FIG. 58-2 Patient with abdominal ascites in late-stage cirrhosis.

- Vitamin deficiency (especially fat-soluble vitamins A, D, E, and K)

Abdominal Assessment. *Massive* ascites can be detected as a distended abdomen with bulging flanks (Fig. 58-2). The umbilicus may protrude, and dilated abdominal veins (caput medusae) may radiate from the umbilicus. Ascites can cause physical problems. For example, orthopnea and dyspnea from increased abdominal distention can interfere with lung expansion. The patient may have difficulty maintaining an erect body posture, and problems with balance may affect walking. Inspect and palpate for the presence of inguinal or umbilical hernias, which are likely to develop because of increased intra-abdominal pressure. *Minimal* ascites is often more difficult to detect, especially in the obese patient.

When performing an assessment of the abdomen, keep in mind that **hepatomegaly** (liver enlargement) occurs in many cases of early cirrhosis. Splenomegaly is common in nonalcoholic causes of cirrhosis. As the liver deteriorates, it may become hard and small.

Measure the patient's abdominal girth to evaluate the progression of ascites (see Fig. 58-2). To measure abdominal girth, the patient lies flat while the nurse or other examiner pulls a tape measure around the largest diameter (usually over the umbilicus) of the abdomen. The girth is measured at the end of exhalation. Mark the abdominal skin and flanks to ensure the same tape measure placement on subsequent readings. *Taking daily weights, however, is the most reliable indicator of fluid retention.*

Other Physical Assessment. Observe vomitus and stool for blood. This may be indicated by frank blood in the excrement or by a positive fecal occult blood test (FOBT) (Hema-Check, Hematest). Gastritis, stomach ulceration, or oozing esophageal varices may be responsible for the blood in the stool. Note the presence of **fetor hepaticus,** which is the distinctive breath odor of chronic liver disease and hepatic encephalopathy and is characterized by a fruity or musty odor.

Amenorrhea (no menstrual period) may occur in women, and men may exhibit testicular atrophy, **gynecomastia** (enlarged breasts), and impotence as a result of inactive hormones. Patients with problems of the hematologic system caused by hepatic failure may have bruising and petechiae (small, purplish hemorrhagic spots on the skin).

Continually assess the patient's neurologic function. Subtle changes in mental status and personality often progress to coma—a late complication of encephalopathy. Monitor for

asterixis—a coarse tremor characterized by rapid, non-rhythmic extensions and flexions in the wrists and fingers (hand-flapping).

Psychosocial Assessment. The patient with hepatic cirrhosis may undergo subtle or obvious personality, cognitive, and behavior changes, such as agitation. He or she may experience sleep pattern disturbances or may exhibit signs of emotional lability (fluctuations in emotions), euphoria (a very elevated mood), or depression. A psychosocial assessment identifies needs and helps guide care.

Repeated hospitalizations are common for patients with cirrhosis. It is a life-altering chronic disease, impacting not only the patient but also the immediate and extended family members and significant others. There are significant emotional, physical, and financial changes. Substance use may continue even as health worsens. It is important, whenever possible, to use resources available to these patients and their families. Collaborate with social workers, substance use counselors, and mental health/behavioral health care professionals as needed for patient assessment and management.

Part of the psychosocial assessment is determining if the patient is alcohol-dependent. If this is the case, observe and prepare for alcohol withdrawal (Donnelly et al., 2012). Care of the patient experiencing withdrawal can be a medical emergency. Consult mental health textbooks or references for this chapter for more information about caring for the alcohol-dependent patient.

❓ NCLEX EXAMINATION CHALLENGE

Physiological Integrity

A client previously diagnosed with liver cirrhosis visits the medical clinic. What assessment findings does the nurse expect in this client? **Select all that apply.**
A. Ecchymosis
B. Soft abdomen
C. Moist, clammy skin
D. Jaundice
E. Ankle edema
F. Fever

Laboratory Assessment. Laboratory study abnormalities are common in patients with liver disease (Table 58-3). Serum levels of *aspartate aminotransferase* (AST), *alanine aminotransferase* (ALT), and *lactate dehydrogenase* (LDH) are typically elevated because these enzymes are released into the blood during hepatic INFLAMMATION. However, as the liver deteriorates, the hepatocytes may be unable to create an inflammatory response and the AST and ALT may be normal. ALT levels are more specific to the liver, whereas AST can be found in muscle, kidney, brain, and heart. An AST/ALT ratio greater than 2 is usually found in alcoholic liver disease (Pagana & Pagana, 2014).

Increased *alkaline phosphatase* and gamma-glutamyl transpeptidase (GGT) levels are caused by biliary obstruction and therefore may increase in patients with cirrhosis. Alkaline phosphatase is a nonspecific bone, intestinal, and liver enzyme. However, alkaline phosphatase also increases when bone disease, such as osteoporosis, is present. Total serum *bilirubin* levels also rise. Indirect bilirubin levels increase in patients with cirrhosis because of the inability of the failing liver to excrete bilirubin. Therefore bilirubin is present in the urine (urobilinogen) in

TABLE 58-3   Assessment of Abnormal Laboratory Findings in Liver Disease

ABNORMAL FINDING	SIGNIFICANCE
Serum Enzymes	
Elevated serum aspartate aminotransferase (AST)	Hepatic cell destruction, hepatitis
Elevated serum alanine aminotransferase (ALT)	Hepatic cell destruction, hepatitis (most specific indicator)
Elevated lactate dehydrogenase (LDH)	Hepatic cell destruction
Elevated serum alkaline phosphatase	Obstructive jaundice, hepatic metastasis
Elevated gamma-glutamyl transpeptidase (GGT)	Biliary obstruction, cirrhosis
Bilirubin	
Elevated serum total bilirubin	Hepatic cell disease
Elevated serum direct conjugated bilirubin	Hepatitis, liver metastasis
Elevated serum indirect unconjugated bilirubin	Cirrhosis
Elevated urine bilirubin	Hepatocellular obstruction, viral or toxic liver disease
Elevated urine urobilinogen	Hepatic dysfunction
Decreased fecal urobilinogen	Obstructive liver disease
Serum Proteins	
Increased serum total protein	Acute liver disease
Decreased serum total protein	Chronic liver disease
Decreased serum albumin	Severe liver disease
Elevated serum globulin	Immune response to liver disease
Other Tests	
Elevated serum ammonia	Advanced liver disease or portal-systemic encephalopathy (PSE)
Prolonged prothrombin time (PT) or international normalized ratio (INR)	Hepatic cell damage and decreased synthesis of prothrombin

increased amounts. Fecal urobilinogen concentration is decreased in patients with biliary tract obstruction. These patients have light- or clay-colored stools.

Total serum *protein* and *albumin* levels are decreased in patients with severe or chronic liver disease as a result of decreased synthesis by the liver (Pagana & Pagana, 2014). Loss of osmotic "pull" proteins like albumin promotes the movement of intravascular fluid into the interstitial tissues (e.g., ascites). Prothrombin time/*international normalized ratio* (PT/INR) is prolonged because the liver decreases the production of prothrombin. The platelet count is low, resulting in a characteristic thrombocytopenia of cirrhosis. Anemia may be reflected by decreased red blood cell (RBC), hemoglobin, and hematocrit values. The white blood cell (WBC) count may also be decreased. *Ammonia* levels are usually elevated in patients with advanced liver disease. Serum creatinine may be elevated in patients with deteriorating kidney function. Dilutional hyponatremia (low serum sodium) may occur in patients with ascites.

Imaging Assessment. Plain x-rays of the abdomen may show hepatomegaly, splenomegaly, or massive ascites. A CT scan may be requested.

MRI is another test used to diagnose the patient with liver disease. It can reveal mass lesions, giving additional specific information. This information is helpful in determining whether the condition is malignant or benign.

Other Diagnostic Assessment. Ultrasound (US) of the liver is often the first assessment for a person with suspected liver disease to detect ascites, hepatomegaly, and splenomegaly. It can also determine the presence of biliary stones or biliary duct obstruction. Liver US is useful in detecting portal vein thrombosis and evaluating whether the direction of portal blood flow is normal.

Some patients being assessed for liver disease require biopsies to determine the exact pathology and the extent of disease progression. This procedure can be problematic because a large number of patients are at risk for bleeding. Even a **percutaneous** (through the skin) biopsy can pose a significant risk to the patient. To minimize this risk, an interventional radiologist can perform a liver biopsy using a long sheath through a jugular vein that then is threaded into the hepatic vein and liver. A tissue sample is obtained for microscopic evaluation. If a biopsy procedure is not possible, a radioisotope liver scan may be used to identify cirrhosis or other diffuse disease.

The physician may request *arteriography* if US is not conclusive in finding portal vein thrombosis. To evaluate the portal vein and its branches, a portal venogram may be performed instead, by passing a catheter into the liver and into the portal vein. This procedure is described on p. 1200 in the Transjugular Intrahepatic Portal-Systemic Shunt section.

The physician may perform an **esophagogastroduodenoscopy (EGD)** to directly visualize the upper GI tract to detect complications of liver failure. These complications may include bleeding or oozing esophageal varices, stomach irritation and ulceration, or duodenal ulceration and bleeding. EGD is performed by introducing a flexible fiberoptic endoscope into the mouth, esophagus, and stomach while the patient is under moderate sedation. A camera attached to the scope permits direct visualization of the mucosal lining of the upper GI tract. An **endoscopic retrograde cholangiopancreatography (ERCP)** uses the endoscope to inject contrast material via the sphincter of Oddi to view the biliary tract and allow for stone removals, sphincterotomies, biopsies, and stent placements if required. These procedures are described in more detail in Chapter 52.

◆ Analysis

The priority NANDA-I nursing diagnoses and collaborative problems for patients with cirrhosis include:

1. Excess Fluid Volume related to third spacing of abdominal and peripheral fluid (NANDA-I)
2. Potential for hemorrhage due to portal hypertension
3. Potential for hepatic encephalopathy due to shunting of portal venous blood and/or increased serum ammonia levels

◆ Planning and Implementation

Managing Fluid Volume

Planning: Expected Outcomes. The patient with cirrhosis is expected to have less excess fluid volume as evidenced by decreased ascites and peripheral edema and adequate circulatory volume. If ascites continues, the patient will not have respiratory distress and will manage ascites by adhering to the collaborative plan of care (see the Concept Map for liver failure due to cirrhosis on p. 1198).

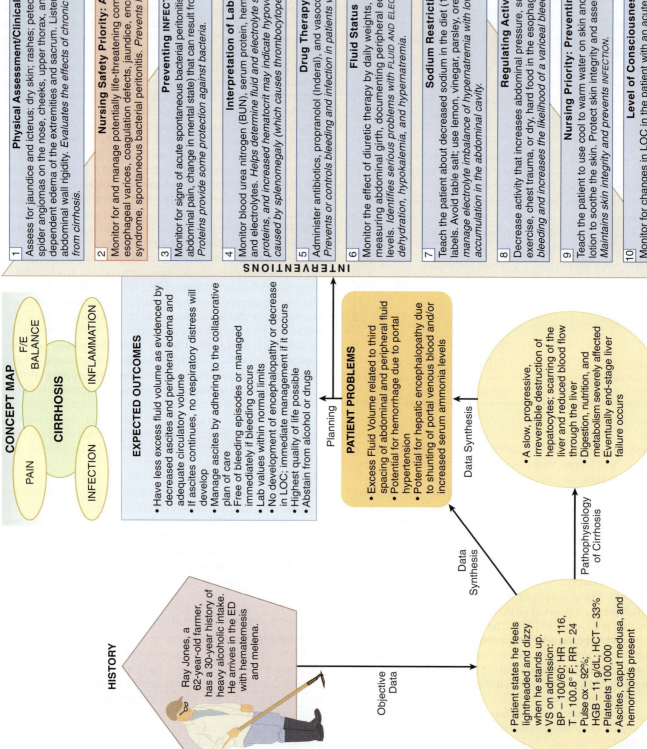

CONCEPT MAP

CIRRHOSIS
- F/E BALANCE
- INFLAMMATION
- PAIN
- INFECTION

HISTORY

Ray Jones, a 62-year-old farmer, has a 30-year history of heavy alcoholic intake. He arrives in the ED with hematemesis and melena.

Objective Data

- Patient states he feels lightheaded and dizzy when he stands up.
- VS on admission:
  BP – 100/60; HR – 116, T – 100.8° F; RR – 24
- Pulse ox – 92%;
  HGB – 11 g/dL; HCT – 33%
  Platelets 100,000
- Ascites, caput medusa, and hemorrhoids present

Pathophysiology of Cirrhosis

- A slow, progressive, irreversible destruction of hepatocytes; scarring of the liver and reduced blood flow through the liver
- Digestion, nutrition, and metabolism severely affected
- Eventually end-stage liver failure occurs

Data Synthesis

PATIENT PROBLEMS

- Excess Fluid Volume related to third spacing of abdominal and peripheral fluid
- Potential for hemorrhage due to portal hypertension
- Potential for hepatic encephalopathy due to shunting of portal venous blood and/or increased serum ammonia levels

Planning

EXPECTED OUTCOMES

- Have less excess fluid volume as evidenced by decreased ascites and peripheral edema and adequate circulatory volume
- If ascites continues, no respiratory distress will develop
- Manage ascites by adhering to the collaborative plan of care
- Free of bleeding episodes or managed immediately if bleeding occurs
- Lab values within normal limits
- No development of encephalopathy or decrease in LOC; immediate management if it occurs
- Highest quality of life possible
- Abstain from alcohol or drugs

INTERVENTIONS

1. Physical Assessment/Clinical Manifestations

Assess for jaundice and icterus: dry skin; rashes; petechiae; ecchymosis; palmar erythema; spider angiomas on the nose, cheeks, upper thorax, and shoulders; ascites; peripheral dependent edema of the extremities and sacrum. Listen to bowel sounds; assess for abdominal wall rigidity. *Evaluates the effects of chronic inflammation and necrosis resulting from cirrhosis.*

2. Nursing Safety Priority: Action Alert!

Monitor for and manage potentially life-threatening complications of cirrhosis with ascites, esophageal varices, coagulation defects, jaundice, encephalopathy, hepatic coma, hepatorenal syndrome, spontaneous bacterial peritonitis. *Prevents hemorrhage and death.*

3. Preventing INFECTION

Monitor for signs of acute spontaneous bacterial peritonitis (SBP) (low grade fever, loss of appetite, abdominal pain, change in mental state) that can result from low concentrations of proteins. *Proteins provide some protection against bacteria.*

4. Interpretation of Lab Values

Monitor blood urea nitrogen (BUN), serum protein, hemoglobin, hematocrit, platelets, and electrolytes. *Helps determine fluid and electrolyte status. Elevated BUN, decreased serum proteins, and increased hematocrit may indicate hypovolemia. Indicates destroyed platelets caused by splenomegaly (which causes thrombocytopenia and increased risk for bleeding).*

5. Drug Therapy

Administer antibiotics, propranolol (Inderal), and vasoconstrictive drugs as prescribed. *Prevents or controls bleeding and infection in patients with esophageal varices.*

6. Fluid Status

Monitor the effect of diuretic therapy by daily weights, measuring daily intake and output, documenting abdominal girth, measuring peripheral edema, and assessing electrolyte levels. *Identifies serious problems with FLUID AND ELECTROLYTE BALANCE such as dehydration, hypokalemia, and hypernatremia.*

7. Sodium Restriction

Teach the patient about decreased sodium in the diet (1 to 2 g). Review how to read nutritional labels. Avoid table salt; use lemon, vinegar, parsley, oregano, and pepper instead. *Helps to manage electrolyte imbalance of hypernatremia with low-sodium diet controlling fluid accumulation in the abdominal cavity.*

8. Regulating Activity

Decrease activity that increases abdominal pressure, such as heavy lifting or vigorous physical exercise, chest trauma, or dry, hard food in the esophagus. *Such increased activity can cause bleeding and increases the likelihood of a variceal bleed.*

9. Nursing Priority: Preventing INFECTION

Teach the patient to use cool to warm water on skin and not too much soap. Teach UAP to use lotion to soothe the skin. Protect skin integrity and assess for open areas from scratching. *Maintains skin integrity and prevents INFECTION.*

10. Level of Consciousness (LOC)

Monitor for changes in LOC in the patient with an acute bleed or with hepatic encephalopathy. *Signifies decreased perfusion to the brain.*

Concept Map by Deanne A. Blach, MSN, RN

Interventions. Fluid accumulations are minimal during the early stages of ascites. Therefore interventions are aimed at preventing the accumulation of additional fluid and moving the existing fluid collection. Nonsurgical treatment measures are used to treat ascites in most cases.

Supportive measures to control abdominal ascites include nutrition therapy, drug therapy, paracentesis, and respiratory support. The patient's FLUID AND ELECTROLYTE BALANCE is also carefully monitored. If the patient is jaundiced, he or she will likely scratch the skin because the excess bilirubin products cause irritation and pruritus (itching).

! NURSING SAFETY PRIORITY (QSEN)
Action Alert

For skin irritation and pruritus associated with jaundice, teach the patient to use cool rather than warm water on the skin and to not use an excessive amount of soap. Teach unlicensed assistive personnel to use lotion to soothe the skin. Assess for open skin areas from scratching, which could become infected.

Nutrition Therapy. The health care provider usually places the patient with abdominal ascites on a low-sodium diet as an initial means of controlling fluid accumulation in the abdominal cavity. The amount of daily sodium (Na^+) intake restriction varies, but a 1- to 2-gram (2000 mg) Na^+ restriction may be tried first. In collaboration with the dietitian, explain the purpose of the restriction and advise the patient and family to read the sodium content labels on all food and beverages. Table salt should be completely excluded. Low-sodium diets may be distasteful, so suggest alternative flavoring additives such as lemon, vinegar, parsley, oregano, and pepper. Remind the patient that seasoned and salty food is an acquired taste; in time, he or she will become used to the decrease in dietary sodium.

In general, patients with late-stage cirrhosis are malnourished and have multiple dietary deficiencies. Vitamin supplements such as thiamine (due to alcohol withdrawal), folate, and multivitamin preparations are typically added to the IV fluids because the liver cannot store vitamins. For patients with biliary cirrhosis, bile may not be available for fat-soluble vitamin transport and absorption. Oral vitamins are prescribed when IV fluid administration is discontinued.

Drug Therapy. The health care provider usually prescribes a *diuretic* to reduce fluid accumulation and to prevent cardiac and respiratory problems. Monitor the effect of diuretic therapy by weighing the patient daily, measuring daily intake and output, measuring abdominal girth, documenting peripheral edema, and assessing electrolyte levels. Serious FLUID AND ELECTROLYTE imbalances, such as dehydration, hypokalemia (decreased potassium), and hyponatremia (decreased sodium), may occur with loop diuretic therapy. Depending on the diuretic selected, the provider may prescribe an oral or IV potassium supplement. Some clinicians prescribe furosemide (Lasix) and spironolactone (Aldactone) as a combination diuretic therapy for the treatment of ascites. Because these drugs work differently, they are used for maintenance of sodium and potassium balance. For example, furosemide causes potassium loss, whereas spironolactone conserves it in the body.

All patients with ascites have the potential to develop spontaneous bacterial peritonitis (SBP) from bacteria in the collected ascitic fluid. In some patients, mild symptoms such as low-grade fever and loss of appetite occur. In others, there may be abdominal PAIN, fever, and change in mental status. When performing an abdominal assessment, listen for bowel sounds and assess for abdominal wall rigidity. Quinolones such as norfloxacin (Noroxin) are the drugs of choice for SBP. If the patient is allergic to this class of *antibiotics*, combination antibiotics like trimethoprim-sulfamethoxazole (Bactrim) are given.

Paracentesis. For some patients, abdominal paracentesis may be needed. Nursing implications associated with this procedure are described in Chart 58-1. The procedure is performed at the bedside, in an interventional radiology department, or in an ambulatory care setting. The physician inserts a trocar catheter or drain into the abdomen to remove the ascitic fluid from the peritoneal cavity. This procedure is done using ultrasound for added safety. In some situations, a short-term ascites drain catheter may be placed while the patient is awaiting surgical intervention, or tunneled ascites drains (e.g., PleurX drains) can allow a patient or family caregiver to drain ascitic fluid at home.

If SBP is suspected, a sample of fluid is withdrawn and sent for cell count and culture. If the patient has symptoms of infection, the physician may prescribe antibiotics while awaiting the culture results.

Respiratory Support. Excessive ascitic fluid volume may cause the patient to have respiratory problems. He or she may develop *hepatopulmonary syndrome*. Dyspnea develops as a result of increased intra-abdominal pressure, which limits thoracic expansion and diaphragmatic excursion. Auscultate lungs every 4 to 8 hours for crackles that could indicate pulmonary complications, depending on the patient's overall condition.

CHART 58-1 Best Practice for Patient Safety & Quality Care (QSEN)
The Patient with Paracentesis

- Explain the procedure, and answer patient questions.
- Obtain vital signs, including weight.
- *Ask the patient to void before the procedure to prevent injury to the bladder!*
- Position the patient in bed with the head of the bed elevated.
- Monitor vital signs per protocol or physician's request.
- Measure the drainage, and record accurately.
- Describe the collected fluid.
- Label and send the fluid for laboratory analysis; document in the patient record that specimens were sent.
- After the physician removes the catheter, apply a dressing to the site; assess for leakage.
- Maintain bedrest per protocol.
- Weigh the patient after the paracentesis; document in the patient record weight both before and after paracentesis.

! NURSING SAFETY PRIORITY (QSEN)
Action Alert

For the patient with hepatopulmonary syndrome, monitor his or her oxygen saturation with pulse oximetry. If needed, apply oxygen therapy to ease breathing. Elevate the head of the bed to at least 30 degrees or as high as the patient wants to improve breathing. This position, with his or her feet elevated to decrease dependent ankle edema, often relieves dyspnea. Weigh the patient daily, or delegate and supervise this activity.

FLUID AND ELECTROLYTE BALANCE problems are common as a result of the disease or treatment. Laboratory tests, such as blood urea nitrogen (BUN), serum protein, hematocrit, and electrolytes, help determine fluid and electrolyte status. An elevated BUN, decreased serum proteins, and increased hematocrit may indicate hypovolemia.

If medical management fails to control ascites, the physician may choose to divert ascites into the venous system by creating a shunt. Patients with ascites are poor surgical risks. The transjugular intrahepatic portal-systemic shunt (TIPS) is a nonsurgical procedure that is used to control long-term ascites and to reduce variceal bleeding. This procedure is described in the discussion of Interventions in the Preventing or Managing Hemorrhage section that follows.

🔘 NCLEX EXAMINATION CHALLENGE

Psychosocial Integrity

The nurse is providing teaching for a client scheduled for a paracentesis. Which statement by the client indicates the teaching has been successful?

A. "I must not use the bathroom prior to the procedure."
B. "I will lie on my stomach while the procedure is performed."
C. "I will not be allowed to eat or drink anything the night before surgery."
D. "The physician will likely remove 2 to 3 liters of fluid from my abdomen."

Preventing or Managing Hemorrhage

Planning: Expected Outcomes. The patient is expected to be free of bleeding episodes. However, if he or she has a hemorrhage, it is expected to be controlled by prompt, evidence-based interdisciplinary interventions. Esophageal variceal bleeds are the most common type of upper GI bleeding.

Interventions. All patients with cirrhosis should be screened for esophageal varices by endoscopy to detect them early *before they bleed*. If patients have varices, they are placed on preventive therapy. If acute bleeding occurs, early interventions are used to manage it. *Because massive esophageal bleeding can cause rapid blood loss, emergency interventions are needed.*

Drug Therapy. The role of early drug therapy is to *prevent* bleeding and INFECTION in patients who have varices. A nonselective *beta-blocking agent* such as propranolol (Inderal) is usually prescribed to prevent bleeding. By decreasing heart rate and the hepatic venous pressure gradient, the chance of bleeding may be reduced (Felicilda-Reynaldo, 2012b).

Up to 20% of cirrhotic patients who are admitted to the hospital due to upper GI bleeding have bacterial infections, and even more patients develop health care–associated infections, usually urinary tract infections or pneumonia (McCance et al., 2014). INFECTION is one of the most common indicators that patients will have an acute variceal bleed (AVB). Therefore cirrhotic patients with GI bleeding should receive *antibiotics* when admitted to the hospital.

If bleeding occurs, the health care team intervenes quickly to control it by combining vasoactive drugs with endoscopic therapies. *Vasoactive* drugs, such as vasopressin and octreotide acetate (Sandostatin), reduce blood flow through vasoconstriction to decrease portal pressure. Octreotide also suppresses secretion of gastrin, serotonin, and intestinal peptides, which decreases GI blood flow to help with pressure reduction within the varices (Felicilda-Reynaldo, 2012b).

Endoscopic Therapies. Endoscopic therapies include ligation of the bleeding veins or sclerotherapy. Both procedures have been very effective in controlling bleeding and improving patient survival rates. Esophageal varices may be managed with **endoscopic variceal ligation (EVL) (banding)**. This procedure involves the application of small "O" bands around the base of the varices to decrease the blood supply to the varices. The patient is unaware of the bands, and they cause no discomfort.

Endoscopic sclerotherapy (EST), also called **injection sclerotherapy**, may be done to stop bleeding. The varices are injected with a sclerosing agent via a catheter. This procedure is associated with complications such as mucosal ulceration, which could result in further bleeding.

Rescue Therapies. If rebleeding occurs, rescue therapies are used. These procedures include a second endoscopic procedure, balloon tamponade and esophageal stents, and shunting procedures. Short-term esophagogastric balloon tamponade using a Minnesota or **Sengstaken-Blakemore tube** with esophageal stents is a very effective way to control bleeding. However, the procedure can cause potentially life-threatening complications, such as aspiration, asphyxia, and esophageal perforation (Augustin et al., 2010). Similar to a nasogastric tube, the tube is placed through the nose and into the stomach. An attached balloon is inflated to apply pressure to the bleeding variceal area. Before this tamponade, the patient is usually intubated and placed on a mechanical ventilator to protect the airway. This therapy is used if the patient is not able to have a second endoscopy or TIPS procedure.

Transjugular Intrahepatic Portal-Systemic Shunt. The transjugular intrahepatic portal-systemic shunt (TIPS) is a nonsurgical procedure performed in interventional radiology departments. This procedure is used for patients who have not responded to other modalities for hemorrhage or long-term ascites. If time permits, patients have a Doppler ultrasound to assess jugular vein anatomy and patency. The patient receives heavy IV sedation or general anesthesia for this procedure. The radiologist places a large sheath through the jugular vein. A needle is guided through the sheath and pushed through the liver into the portal vein. A balloon enlarges this tract, and a stent keeps it open. Most patients also have a Doppler ultrasound study of the liver after the TIPS procedure to record the blood flow through the shunt.

Serious complications of TIPS are not common. Patients are usually discharged in 1 or 2 days and are followed up with ultrasounds for the first year after the shunt is placed. Some shunts require re-opening at least once during the first year as an ambulatory care procedure.

Other Interventions. Depending on the procedure done to control esophageal bleeding, patients usually have a nasogastric tube (NGT) inserted to detect any new bleeding episodes. Patients often receive packed red blood cells, fresh frozen plasma, dextran, albumin, and platelets through large-bore IV catheters.

Monitor vital signs every hour, and check coagulation studies, including prothrombin time (PT), partial thromboplastin time (PTT), platelet count, and international normalized ratio (INR). Additional interventions for upper GI bleeding are discussed in Chapter 55.

Preventing or Managing Hepatic Encephalopathy

Planning: Expected Outcomes. The patient is expected to be free of encephalopathy. However, if it occurs, it is expected that the interdisciplinary team will intervene early to prevent further health problems or death.

Interventions. The poorly functioning liver cannot convert ammonia and other by-products of protein metabolism to a less toxic form. They are carried by the circulatory system to the brain, where they affect cerebral function. Interventions are planned around the management of slowing or stopping the accumulation of ammonia in the body.

Because ammonia is formed in the GI tract by the action of bacteria on protein, nonsurgical treatment measures to decrease ammonia production include dietary limitations and drug therapy to reduce bacterial breakdown.

Nutrition Therapy. Patients with cirrhosis have increased nutritional requirements—high-carbohydrate, moderate-fat, and high-protein foods. However, the diet may be changed for those who have elevated serum ammonia levels with signs of encephalopathy. Patients should have a moderate amount of protein and fat foods and simple carbohydrates. Strict protein restrictions are not required because patients need protein for healing. In collaboration with the dietitian, be sure to include family members or significant others in nutrition counseling. The patient is often weak and unable to remember complicated guidelines. Brief, simple directions regarding dietary dos and don'ts are recommended. Keep in mind any financial, cultural, or personal preferences when discussing food choices, as well as the patient's food allergies.

Drug Therapy. Drugs are used sparingly because they are difficult for the failing liver to metabolize. In particular, opioid analgesics, sedatives, and barbiturates should be restricted, especially for the patient with a history of encephalopathy.

Several types of drugs, however, may eliminate or reduce ammonia levels in the body. These include lactulose (e.g., Evalose, Heptalac) or lactitol and nonabsorbable antibiotics (Felicilda-Reynaldo, 2012a). The health care provider may prescribe *lactulose* (or lactitol) to promote the excretion of ammonia in the stool. This drug is a viscous, sticky, sweet-tasting liquid that is given either orally or by NG tube. The purpose is to obtain a laxative effect. Cleansing the bowels may rid the intestinal tract of the toxins that contribute to encephalopathy. It works by increasing osmotic pressure to draw fluid into the colon and prevents absorption of ammonia in the colon. The drug may be prescribed to the patient who has manifested signs of encephalopathy, regardless of the stage. The desired effect of the drug is production of two or three soft stools per day and a decrease in patient confusion caused by this complication.

Observe for response to lactulose. The patient may report intestinal bloating and cramping. Serum ammonia levels may be monitored but do not always correlate with symptoms. Hypokalemia and dehydration may result from excessive stools. Remind unlicensed nursing personnel to help the patient with skin care if needed to prevent breakdown caused by excessive stools.

Several *nonabsorbable antibiotics* may be given if lactulose does not help the patient meet the desired outcome or if he or she cannot tolerate the drug. These drugs should not be given together. Older adults can become weak and dehydrated from having multiple stools. Neomycin sulfate (Mycifradin) or rifaximin (Xifaxan), both broad-spectrum antibiotics, may be given to act as an intestinal antiseptic (Felicilda-Reynaldo, 2012a). These drugs destroy the normal flora in the bowel, diminishing protein breakdown and decreasing the rate of ammonia production. Maintenance doses of neomycin are given orally but may also be administered as a retention enema. Long-term use has the potential for kidney toxicity and therefore is not commonly used. It cannot be used for patients with existing kidney disease.

Metronidazole (Flagyl, Novonidazol ✦) is another broad-spectrum antibiotic with similar action to neomycin, but it can cause peripheral neuropathy. Vancomycin (Vancocin) may also be given, but its long-term use can lead to resistance (Felicilda-Reynaldo, 2012a).

Frequently assess for changes in level of consciousness and orientation. Check for asterixis (liver flap) and fetor hepaticus (liver breath). These signs suggest worsening encephalopathy. Thiamine supplements and benzodiazepines may be needed if the patient is at risk for alcohol withdrawal.

💡 CLINICAL JUDGMENT CHALLENGE
Safety; Evidence-Based Practice [QSEN]

A 60-year-old man is admitted to the emergency department (ED) with a report of vomiting bright red blood. He has had liver cirrhosis for the past 10 years and states that he has been drinking heavily since his wife died last year. His blood pressure is 106/68, and his pulse rate is 94. His abdomen is distended, and he is having some difficulty breathing; his respirations are 34 per minute. You are assigned to care for this patient.

1. For what complications is this patient at risk and why? What causes these complications?
2. In what position will you place the patient and why? What evidence supports your answer? Why do you think he has tachypnea?
3. The physician suspects that he has bleeding gastroesophageal varices. What laboratory tests will he likely request and why?
4. Vasopressin is prescribed for the patient, and several large-bore IV lines are inserted. What is the purpose of this drug for this patient?
5. How will you know if the drug was effective?
6. If the drug is not effective in treating the patient, what other options are available for his management?

Community-Based Care

If the patient with late-stage cirrhosis survives life-threatening complications, he or she is usually discharged to the home or to a long-term care facility after treatment measures have managed the acute medical problems. A home care referral may be needed if the patient is discharged to the home. These chronically ill patients are often readmitted multiple times, and community-based care is aimed at optimizing comfort, promoting independence, supporting caregivers, and preventing rehospitalization. Patients with end-stage disease may benefit from hospice care. Collaborate with the case manager (CM) or other discharge planner to coordinate interdisciplinary continuing care.

Home Care Management. In collaboration with the patient, family, and case manager, assess physical adaptations needed to prepare the patient's home for recovery. Referrals for physical therapy, nutrition therapy, and transportation for physician and laboratory follow-up may be needed. The patient's rest area needs to be close to a bathroom because diuretic and/or lactulose therapy increases the frequency of urination and stools. If the patient has difficulty reaching the toilet, additional equipment (e.g., bedside commode) is necessary. Special adult-size incontinence pads or briefs may be helpful if the patient has an

---

CHART 58-2   **Patient and Family Education: Preparing for Self-Management**

Cirrhosis

Nutrition Therapy

- Consume a diet that adheres to the guidelines set by your physician, nurse, or dietitian.
- If you have excessive fluid in your abdomen, follow the low-sodium diet prescribed for you.
- Eat small, frequent meals that are nutritionally well balanced.
- Include in your diet daily supplemental liquids (e.g., Ensure or Ensure Plus) and a multivitamin.

Drug Therapy

- Take the diuretic or preventive beta blocker prescribed for you. If you experience muscle weakness, irregular heartbeat, or light-headedness, contact your health care provider right away.
- Take the medication prescribed for you that helps prevent gastrointestinal bleeding.
- Take the lactulose syrup as prescribed to maintain two or three bowel movements every day.
- Do *not* take any other medication (prescribed or over the counter) unless specifically prescribed by your health care provider.

Alcohol Abstinence

- Do not consume any alcohol.
- Seek support services for help if needed.

---

altered mental status and has incontinence. If the patient has shortness of breath from massive ascites, elevating the head of the bed and maintaining the patient in a semi-Fowler's to high-Fowler's position may help alleviate respiratory distress. Alternatively, a reclining chair with an elevated foot rest may be used.

Self-Management Education. The patient is discharged to the home setting with an individualized teaching plan (Chart 58-2) that includes nutrition therapy, drug therapy, and alcohol abstinence, if needed. The patient who has a tunneled ascites drain (e.g., PleurX drain) will need to be taught how to access the drain and remove excess fluid. *Review the home care instructions that are provided with the drainage system with both the patient and family/caregiver. Remind them to not remove more than 2000 mL from the abdomen at one time to prevent hypovolemic shock.*

The patient with encephalopathy often finds that small, frequent meals are best tolerated. If the patient's nutritional intake or albumin/pre-albumin is decreased after discharge, multivitamin supplements and supplemental liquid feedings (e.g., Ensure, Boost) are usually needed. Teach patients to avoid excessive vitamins and minerals that can be toxic to the liver, such as fat-soluble vitamins, excessive iron supplements, and niacin. Remind patients to check with their health care provider before taking any vitamin supplement.

The patient is often discharged while receiving diuretics. Provide instructions regarding the health care provider's prescription for the diuretic. Teach about side effects of therapy, such as hypokalemia. The patient may need to take a potassium supplement if he or she is taking a diuretic that is not potassium-sparing.

If the patient has had problems with bleeding from gastric ulcers, the primary care provider may prescribe an H_2-receptor antagonist agent or proton pump inhibitor to reduce acid reflux (see Chapter 55). Patients who have had episodes of spontaneous bacterial peritonitis (SBP) may be on a daily maintenance antibiotic.

Teach family members how to recognize signs of encephalopathy and to contact the health care provider if these signs develop. Reinforce that constipation, bleeding, and infections can increase the risk for encephalopathy.

Advise the patient to avoid all over-the-counter drugs, especially NSAIDs and hepatic toxic herbs, vitamins, and minerals. Reinforce the need to keep appointments for follow-up medical care. Remind the patient and family to notify the health care provider immediately if any GI bleeding (overt bleeding or melena) is noted so that re-evaluation can begin quickly.

! NURSING SAFETY PRIORITY (QSEN)

Action Alert

One of the most important aspects of ongoing care for the patient with cirrhosis is to stress the need to avoid acetaminophen (Tylenol), alcohol, and illicit drugs. By avoiding these substances, the patient may:

- Prevent further fibrosis of the liver from scarring
- Allow the liver to heal and regenerate
- Prevent gastric and esophageal irritation
- Reduce the incidence of bleeding
- Prevent other life-threatening complications

Health Care Resources. The patient with chronic cirrhosis may require a home care nurse for several visits after hospital discharge. The home care nurse can monitor the effectiveness of treatment in controlling ascites. The encephalopathic patient may need to be monitored for adherence to drug therapy and alcohol abstinence, if appropriate. Individual and group therapy sessions may be arranged to assist patients in dealing with alcohol abstinence if they are too ill to attend a formal treatment program. Because some patients may have alienated relatives over the years because of substance use, it may be necessary to help them identify a friend, neighbor, or person in their recovery group for support. If needed, refer the patient and family to self-help groups, such as Alcoholics Anonymous and Al-Anon.

The patient with cirrhosis may also desire spiritual or other psychosocial support. Finances are frequently a problem for the chronically ill patient and family; social support and community services need to be identified. The American Liver Foundation (www.liverfoundation.org) and American Gastroenterological Association (www.gastro.org) are excellent sources for more information about liver disease.

For patients who are not candidates for liver transplantation, address end-of-life issues. Discuss options such as hospice care with patients and their families (see Chapter 7). Be aware that they will go through a grieving process and will perhaps be in denial or very angry.

Evaluation: Outcomes

Evaluate the care of the patient with cirrhosis based on the identified priority patient problems. The expected outcomes include that the patient will:

- Have a decrease in or have no ascites
- Have electrolytes within normal limits (WNL)
- Not have hemorrhage or will be managed immediately if bleeding occurs
- Not develop encephalopathy or will be managed immediately if it occurs
- Have the highest quality of life possible
- Successfully abstain from alcohol or drugs (if disease is caused by these substances)

HEPATITIS

❖ PATHOPHYSIOLOGY

Hepatitis is the widespread INFLAMMATION of liver cells. *Viral* hepatitis is the most common type and can be either acute or chronic. Less common types of hepatitis are caused by chemicals, drugs, and some herbs. This section discusses hepatitis caused by a virus. Viral hepatitis results from an infection caused by one of five major categories of viruses:

- Hepatitis A virus (HAV)
- Hepatitis B virus (HBV)
- Hepatitis C virus (HCV)
- Hepatitis D virus (HDV)
- Hepatitis E virus (HEV)

Some cases of viral hepatitis are not caused by any of these viruses. These patients have non–A-E hepatitis.

Liver injury with INFLAMMATION can develop after exposure to a number of drugs and chemicals by inhalation, ingestion, or parenteral (IV) administration. Toxic and drug-induced hepatitis can result from exposure to hepatotoxins (e.g., industrial toxins, alcohol, and drugs). Hepatitis may also occur as a secondary INFECTION during the course of infections with other viruses, such as Epstein-Barr, herpes simplex, varicella-zoster, and cytomegalovirus.

After the liver has been exposed to any causative agent (e.g., a virus), it becomes enlarged and congested with inflammatory cells, lymphocytes, and fluid, resulting in right upper quadrant pain and discomfort. As the disease progresses, the liver's normal lobular pattern becomes distorted as a result of widespread inflammation, necrosis, and hepatocellular regeneration. This distortion increases pressure within the portal circulation, interfering with the blood flow into the hepatic lobules. Edema of the liver's bile channels results in obstructive jaundice (yellowing of the skin).

Classification of Hepatitis and Etiologies

The five major types of acute viral hepatitis vary by mode of transmission, manner of onset, and incubation periods. Hepatitis cases must be reported to the local public health department, which then notifies the Centers for Disease Control and Prevention (CDC).

Hepatitis A. The causative agent of hepatitis A, hepatitis A virus (HAV), is a ribonucleic acid (RNA) virus of the enterovirus family. *It is a hardy virus and survives on human hands.* The virus is resistant to detergents and acids but is destroyed by chlorine (bleach) and extremely high temperatures.

Hepatitis A usually has a mild course similar to that of a typical flu-like INFECTION and often goes unrecognized. It is spread most often by the fecal-oral route by fecal contamination either from person-to-person contact (e.g., oral-anal sexual activity) or by consuming contaminated food or water. Common sources of infection include shellfish caught in contaminated water and food contaminated by food handlers infected with HAV. The incubation period of hepatitis A is usually 15 to 50 days, with a peak of 25 to 30 days. The disease is usually not life threatening, but its course may be more severe in people older than 40 years and those with pre-existing liver disease such as hepatitis C (McCance et al., 2014).

In a small percentage of hepatitis A cases, severe illness with extrahepatic manifestations can occur. Advanced age and conditions such as chronic liver disease may cause widespread damage that requires a liver transplant. In some cases, death may occur. The incidence of hepatitis A is particularly high in non-affluent countries in which sanitation is poor. However, over 35,000 cases are diagnosed each year in the United States (American Liver Foundation, 2010). Some adults have hepatitis A and do not know it. The course is similar to that of a GI illness, and the disease and recovery are usually uneventful.

Hepatitis B. The hepatitis B virus (HBV) is not transmitted like HAV. It is a double-shelled particle containing DNA composed of a core antigen (HBcAg), a surface antigen (HBsAg), and another antigen found within the core (HBeAg) that circulates in the blood. HBV may be spread through these common modes of transmission (Lok & McMahon, 2009):

- Unprotected sexual intercourse with an infected partner
- Sharing needles
- Accidental needle sticks or injuries from sharp instruments primarily in health care workers (low incidence)
- Blood transfusions (that have not been screened for the virus, before 1992)
- Hemodialysis
- Close person-to-person contact by open cuts and sores

In addition, patients who are immunosuppressed either by disease or drug therapy are more likely to develop hepatitis B.

The clinical course of hepatitis B may be varied. Symptoms usually occur within 25 to 180 days of exposure and include (McCance et al., 2014):

- Anorexia, nausea, and vomiting
- Fever
- Fatigue
- Right upper quadrant pain
- Dark urine with light stool
- Joint PAIN
- Jaundice

Blood tests confirm the disease, although many people with hepatitis B have no symptoms.

Most adults who get hepatitis B recover, clear the virus from their body, and develop immunity. However, a small percentage of people do not develop immunity and become carriers. Hepatitis carriers can infect others even though they are not sick and have no obvious signs of hepatitis B. Chronic carriers are at high risk for cirrhosis and liver cancer. Because of the high number of newcomers from endemic areas, the incidence of hepatitis B has increased in the United States.

Hepatitis C. The causative virus of hepatitis C (HCV) is an enveloped, single-stranded RNA virus. Transmission is blood to blood. The rate of sexual transmission is very low in a single-couple relationship but increases with multiple sex partners.

HCV is spread most commonly by:

- Illicit IV drug needle sharing (highest incidence)
- Blood, blood products, or organ transplants received before 1992

- Needle stick injury with HCV-contaminated blood (health care workers at high risk)
- Unsanitary tattoo equipment
- Sharing of intranasal cocaine paraphernalia

The disease is **not** transmitted by casual contact or by intimate household contact. However, those infected are advised not to share razors, toothbrushes, or pierced earrings because microscopic blood may be on these items.

The average incubation period is 7 weeks. Acute infection and illness are not common. Most people are completely unaware that they have been infected. They are asymptomatic and not diagnosed until many months or years after the initial exposure when an abnormality is detected during a routine laboratory evaluation or when liver problems occur. Unlike with hepatitis B, most people infected with hepatitis C do not clear the virus and a chronic infection develops.

HCV usually does its damage over decades by causing a chronic inflammation in the liver that eventually causes the liver cells to scar. This scarring may progress to cirrhosis (McCance et al., 2014).

Hepatitis D. **Hepatitis D** (delta hepatitis) is caused by a defective RNA virus that needs the helper function of HBV. It occurs only with HBV to cause viral replication. This usually develops into chronic disease. The incubation period is about 14 to 56 days. As with hepatitis B, the disease is transmitted primarily by parenteral routes, especially in patients who are IV drug users. Having sexual contact with a person with HDV is also a high risk factor (McCance et al., 2014).

Hepatitis E. The **hepatitis E** virus (HEV) causes a waterborne infection associated with epidemics in the Indian subcontinent, Asia, Africa, the Middle East, Mexico, and Central and South America. Many large outbreaks have occurred after heavy rains and flooding. Like hepatitis A, hepatitis E is caused by fecal contamination of food and water.

In the United States, hepatitis E has been found only in international travelers. It is transmitted via the fecal-oral route, and the clinical course resembles that of hepatitis A. Hepatitis E has an incubation period of 15 to 64 days. There is no evidence at this time of a chronic form of the disease. The disease tends to be self-limiting and resolves on its own (McCance et al., 2014).

Complications of Hepatitis

Failure of the liver cells to regenerate, with progression of the necrotic process, results in a severe acute and often fatal form of hepatitis known as **fulminant hepatitis.** Hepatitis is considered to be chronic when liver inflammation lasts longer than 6 months. **Chronic hepatitis** usually occurs as a result of hepatitis B or hepatitis C. Superimposed infection with hepatitis D virus (HDV) in patients with chronic hepatitis B may also result in chronic hepatitis. Chronic hepatitis can lead to cirrhosis and liver cancer. Many patients have multiple infections, especially the combination of HBV with either HCV, HDV, or HIV infections (McCance et al., 2014).

Incidence and Prevalence

The incidence of hepatitis A and hepatitis B is declining as a result of CDC recommendations for vaccination. However, hepatitis B and hepatitis C are a concern because of their association with cirrhosis and liver cancer. Although exact numbers are not known, it is estimated that about 200 million people worldwide have the hepatitis C virus (HCV), making this type of hepatitis the most common type. Currently there is no vaccine for HCV. Therefore it is expected that the cases of HCV will rise over the next several decades as a result of increasing illicit drug use. This increase will require a major increase in transplantations and lead to many more deaths (Lok & McMahon, 2009).

Health Promotion and Maintenance

Hepatitis vaccines for infants, children, and adolescents have helped decrease the incidence of hepatitis A and hepatitis B. Some adults also are advised to receive these immunizations.

Measures for preventing hepatitis A in adults include:
- Proper handwashing, especially after handling shellfish
- Avoiding contaminated food or water (including tap water in countries with high incidence)
- Receiving immunoglobulin within 14 days if exposed to the virus
- Receiving the HAV vaccine before traveling to areas where the disease is common (e.g., Mexico, Caribbean)
- Receiving the vaccine if living or working in enclosed areas with others, such as college dormitories, correctional institutions, day-care centers, and long-term care facilities

Several HAV vaccines are available (e.g., Havrix and Vaqta). Both of these vaccines are made of inactivated hepatitis A virus and are given in the deltoid muscle.

Several vaccines can also provide protection against hepatitis B (HBV) infection (e.g., Engerix-B and Recombivax-HB). Twinrix is a combination HAV and HBV vaccine that is also available for adults. Examples of groups for whom immunization against HBV should be used include (Lok & McMahon, 2009):
- People who have sexual intercourse with more than one partner
- People with sexually transmitted disease (STD) or a history of STD
- Men having sex with men (MSM)
- People with any chronic liver disease (such as hepatitis C or cirrhosis)
- Patients with human immune deficiency virus (HIV) infection
- People who are exposed to blood or body fluids in the workplace, including health care workers, firefighters, and police
- People in correctional facilities
- Patients needing immunosuppressant drugs
- Family members, household members, and sexual contacts of people with HBV infection

Additional measures to prevent viral hepatitis for health care workers and others in contact with infected patients are listed in Charts 58-3 and 58-4.

❖ *PATIENT-CENTERED COLLABORATIVE CARE*

◆ *Assessment*

History. Begin by asking the patient whether he or she has had known exposure to a person with hepatitis. For the patient who presents with few or no symptoms of liver disease but has abnormal laboratory tests (e.g., elevated alanine aminotransferase [ALT] or aspartate aminotransferase [AST] level), the history may need to include additional questions regarding risk factors such as:
- Exposure to either inhaled or ingested chemical
- Use of herbal supplements

Prevention of Viral Hepatitis in Health Care Workers

- Use Standard Precautions to prevent the transmission of disease between patients or between patients and health care staff (see Chapter 23).
- Eliminate needles and other sharp instruments by substituting needleless systems. (Needle sticks are the major source of hepatitis B transmission in health care workers.)
- Take the hepatitis B vaccine (e.g., Recombivax HB), which is given in a series of three injections. This vaccine also prevents hepatitis D by preventing hepatitis B.
- For postexposure prevention of hepatitis A, seek medical attention immediately for immunoglobulin (Ig) administration.
- Report all cases of hepatitis to the local health department.

CHART 58-4 Patient and Family Education: Preparing for Self-Management

Health Practices to Prevent Viral Hepatitis

- Maintain adequate sanitation and personal hygiene. Wash your hands before eating and after using the toilet.
- Drink water treated by a water purification system.
- If traveling in underdeveloped or non-industrialized countries, drink only bottled water. Avoid food washed or prepared with tap water, such as raw vegetables, fruits, and soups. Avoid ice.
- Use adequate sanitation practices to prevent the spread of the disease among family members.
- Do not share bed linens, towels, eating utensils, or drinking glasses.
- Do not share needles for injection, body piercing, or tattooing.
- Do not share razors, nail clippers, toothbrushes, or Waterpiks.
- Use a condom during sexual intercourse, or abstain from this activity.
- Cover cuts or sores with bandages.
- If ever infected with hepatitis, never donate blood, body organs, or other body tissue.

- Use of any new prescribed drug or over-the-counter (OTC) medication
- Recent ingestion of shellfish
- Exposure to a possibly contaminated water source
- Travel to another country
- Sexual activities with men, women, or both and whether it was protected or unprotected
- Illicit drug use, IV or intranasal
- For health care workers, recent needle stick exposure
- Body piercing or tattooing
- Close living accommodations (e.g., military barracks, correctional institutions, overcrowded dormitories, long-term care facilities, day-care centers) or employment in any such setting
- Blood or blood products or organ transplants received before 1992
- Military service
- Place of birth (United States or other country) and parents' place of birth
- History of alcohol use (how many drinks each day or week)
- Human immune deficiency virus (HIV)

Physical Assessment/Clinical Manifestations. Assess whether the patient has:

- Abdominal PAIN
- Changes in skin or sclera (icterus)
- Arthralgia (joint pain) or myalgia (muscle pain)
- Diarrhea/constipation
- Changes in color of urine or stool
- Fever
- Lethargy
- Malaise
- Nausea/vomiting
- Pruritus (itching)

Lightly palpate the right upper abdominal quadrant to assess for liver tenderness. The patient may report right upper quadrant pain with jarring movements. Inspect the skin, sclerae, and mucous membranes for jaundice. He or she may present for medical treatment only after jaundice appears, believing that other vague symptoms are related to a flu-like syndrome.

Jaundice in hepatitis results from intrahepatic obstruction and is caused by edema of the liver's bile channels. Dark urine and clay-colored stools are often reported by the patient. If possible, obtain a urine and stool specimen for visual inspection and laboratory analysis. The patient may also have skin abrasions from scratching because of pruritus (itching).

Psychosocial Assessment. Viral hepatitis has various presentations, but for most infected people the initial course is mild with few or no symptoms. The long-term complications of fibrosis and cirrhosis cause the more serious problem. This is especially true for patients who have chronic HBV and HCV INFECTION.

Emotional problems for affected patients may center on their feeling sick and fatigued. General malaise, inactivity, and vague symptoms contribute to depression. Some patients often feel guilty and are remorseful about decisions made that caused the disease. These feelings are most likely to occur when the source of infection is from drug use. Family members may be angry that the patient caused the disease.

Infectious diseases such as hepatitis continue to have a social stigma. The patient may feel embarrassed by the precautions that are imposed in the hospital and continue to be necessary at home. This embarrassment may cause the patient to limit social interactions. Patients may be afraid that they will spread the virus to family and friends.

Family members are sometimes afraid of getting the disease and may distance themselves from the patient. Allow them to verbalize these feelings, and explore the reasons for these fears. Educate the patient and family members about modes of transmission, and clarify information as needed.

Patients may be unable to return to work for several weeks during the acute phases of illness. The loss of wages and the cost of hospitalization for a patient without insurance coverage may produce great anxiety and financial burden. This situation may last for months or years if hepatitis becomes chronic.

Laboratory Assessment. Hepatitis A, hepatitis B, and hepatitis C are usually confirmed by acute elevations in levels of liver enzymes, indicating liver cellular damage, and by specific serologic markers.

Levels of ALT and AST may possibly rise into the thousands in acute or fulminant cases of hepatitis. Alkaline phosphatase levels may be normal or elevated. Serum total bilirubin levels are elevated and are consistent with the clinical appearance of jaundice. Elevated levels of bilirubin are also present in the urine (Pagana & Pagana, 2014).

The presence of *hepatitis A* is established when hepatitis A virus (HAV) antibodies (anti-HAV) are found in the blood. Ongoing INFLAMMATION of the liver by HAV is indicated by the presence of immunoglobulin M (IgM) antibodies, which persist in the blood for 4 to 6 weeks. Previous infection is identified by the presence of immunoglobulin G (IgG) antibodies. These antibodies persist in the serum and provide permanent immunity to HAV.

The presence of the *hepatitis B* virus (HBV) is established when serologic testing confirms the presence of hepatitis B antigen-antibody systems in the blood and a detectable viral count (HBV polymerase chain reaction [PCR] DNA). Antigens located on the surface (shell) of the virus (HBsAg) and IgM antibodies to hepatitis B core antigen (anti-HBcAg IgM) are the most significant serologic markers. The presence of these markers establishes the diagnosis of hepatitis B. *The patient is infectious as long as hepatitis B surface antigen (HBsAg) is present in the blood.* Persistence of this serologic marker after 6 months or longer indicates a carrier state or chronic hepatitis. HBsAg levels normally decline and disappear after the acute hepatitis B episode. The presence of antibodies to HBsAb in the blood indicates recovery and immunity to hepatitis B. *People who have been vaccinated against HBV have a positive HBsAg because they also have immunity to the disease* (Pagana & Pagana, 2014).

Enzyme-linked immunosorbent assay (ELISA) is the initial screening test for patients suspected of being infected with *hepatitis C* virus (HCV). It is also the most commonly used enzyme test for HCV antibodies (anti-HCV). The antibodies can be detected within 4 weeks of the infection (Pagana & Pagana, 2014). A more specific assay called the *recombinant immunoblot assay (RIBA)* can be used as a confirmatory test. These tests show that the patient has been exposed to HCV and has developed the antibody. To identify the actual circulating virus, the HCV PCR RNA test is used. This confirms active virus and can measure the viral load. A newer diagnostic tool called the *OraQuick HCV Rapid Antibody Test* was approved by the Food and Drug Administration in the United States in 2010. It has the advantage of providing a quick diagnosis of the disease as a point-of-care test.

The presence of *hepatitis D* virus (HDV) can be confirmed by the identification of intrahepatic delta antigen or, more often, by a rise in the hepatitis D virus antibodies (anti-HDV) titer. This increase can be seen within a few days of INFECTION (Pagana & Pagana, 2014).

Hepatitis E virus (HEV) testing is usually reserved for travelers in whom hepatitis is present but the virus cannot be detected. Hepatitis E antibodies (anti-HEV) are found in people infected with the virus.

Other Diagnostic Assessment. *Liver biopsy* may be used to confirm the diagnosis of hepatitis and to establish the stage and grade of liver damage. Characteristic changes help the pathologist distinguish among a virus, drug, toxin, fatty liver, iron, and other disease. It is usually performed in an ambulatory care setting as a percutaneous procedure (through the skin) after a local anesthetic is given. If coagulation is abnormal, however, it may be done using either a CT-guided or transjugular route to reduce the risk for pneumothorax or hemothorax. *Ultrasound* also may be used.

◆ *Interventions*

The patient with viral hepatitis can be mildly or acutely ill depending on the severity of the inflammation. Most patients are not hospitalized, although older adults and those with dehydration may be admitted for a short-term stay. The plan of care for all patients with viral hepatitis is based on measures to rest the liver, promote cellular regeneration, and prevent complications, if possible.

During the acute stage of viral hepatitis, interventions are aimed at resting the inflamed liver to promote hepatic cell regeneration. *Rest* is an essential intervention to reduce the liver's metabolic demands and increase its blood supply. Collaborative care is generally supportive. The patient is usually tired and expresses feelings of general malaise. Complete bedrest is usually not required, but rest periods alternating with periods of activity are indicated and are often enough to promote hepatic healing. Individualize the patient's plan of care and change it as needed to reflect the severity of symptoms, fatigue, and the results of liver function tests and enzyme determinations. Activities such as self-care and ambulating are gradually added to the activity schedule as tolerated.

The diet should be high in carbohydrates and calories with moderate amounts of fat and protein after nausea and anorexia subside. Small, frequent meals are often preferable to three standard meals. Ask the patient about food preferences because favorite foods are tolerated better than randomly selected foods. Encourage the patient to eat foods that are appealing. High-calorie snacks may be needed. Supplemental vitamins are often prescribed.

Drugs of any kind are used sparingly for patients with hepatitis to allow the liver to rest. An antiemetic to relieve nausea

---

EVIDENCE BASED PRACTICE (QSEN)

Do Patients with Chronic Hepatitis C Use Complementary and Alternative Therapies?

Richmond, J.A., Bailey, D.E. Jr., McHutchinson, J.G., & Muir, A.J. (2010). The use of mind-body medicine and prayer among adult patients with hepatitis C. *Gastroenterology Nursing, 33*(3), 201-216.

The researchers studied the use of mind-body therapies and prayer as part of a larger, exploratory, descriptive study on the use of complementary and alternative medicine by patients with hepatitis C who were treated at one tertiary care center. According to a self-administered survey of 105 participants and semi-structured interviews of 28 participants in the study, most had used mind-body medicine in the past 12 months. The most commonly used therapies were prayer, deep breathing, and meditation to promote general well-being and relieve tension and anxiety.

Level of Evidence: 4

This study did not use an experimental design.

Commentary: Implications for Practice and Research

This exploratory descriptive study showed that patients with chronic hepatitis C use complementary and alternative medicine (CAM) in their everyday lives to promote their health and increase their quality of life. Nurses need to ensure that they ask patients about the use of CAM and which therapies are most helpful so that they can be continued as part of the patient's plan of care.

This research was the first to explore the use of CAM with this population of patients and serves as a pilot study for further research using larger sample sizes of diverse patients in multiple health care settings.

TABLE 58-4 Drug Therapy for Chronic Hepatitis B and Hepatitis C

MEDICATION	NURSING IMPLICATIONS	COMMENTS
Chronic Hepatitis B		
Tenofovir (Viread)	Monitor kidney function. Can cause bone de-mineralization. Teach risk for falls to prevent fractures.	Purpose of treatment is to achieve sustained suppression of hepatitis B virus (HBV) replication and remission of liver disease.
Adefovir (Hepsera)	Monitor kidney function.	
Lamivudine (Epivir-HBV)	Monitor kidney function. Dose is altered if co-infection with human immune deficiency virus (HIV) present.	
Entecavir (Baraclude)	Monitor kidney function.	
Chronic Hepatitis C		
Telaprevir (Incivek) Boceprevir (Victrelis) in combination with HIV medications if co-infection present PegIFN/RBV (interferon/ribavirin)	Monitor complete blood count (CBC) for anemia. Monitor chemistry panel for impaired kidney and liver function, along with electrolytes abnormalities. Peg/IFN administered subcutaneously. Instruct patients that they cannot miss a dose.	As a result of shared routes of transmission, co-infection with HIV is common.

🔆 CLINICAL JUDGMENT CHALLENGE

Patient-Centered Care; Safety `QSEN`

You are a nurse working in the emergency department (ED) of the local community hospital. You receive report from the night nurse regarding a 50-year-old man who has just returned to the United States from a month-long trip to the southern parts of Africa. For the past 2 weeks, he has been experiencing fevers on and off, malaise, anorexia, and mild abdominal discomfort. He has been taking acet-aminophen (Tylenol) for fevers and abdominal discomfort. His past medical history is significant for elevated cholesterol for which he takes only atorvastatin (Lipitor) every day. While reviewing his social history, you note that the patient reported that he is a nonsmoker, drinks 6 or 7 alcoholic drinks daily, is married, and has three children. He had his gallbladder removed when he was 43 years old.

His current vital signs are: blood pressure 126/82 mm Hg; heart rate 100 beats/min; respirations 22 breaths/min; temperature 101° F orally; pulse oximetry reading 98% on room air. The ED physician orders the following:
Diet: nothing by mouth
Laboratory studies: complete blood count and chemistry panel, uri-nalysis, blood cultures
STAT electrocardiogram (ECG) and chest x-ray
Start: 0.9% normal saline intravenously to run at 100 mL/hr
The results of his recent laboratory work are:

	LABORATORY RESULT	NORMAL RANGE
White blood cells	13,000/mm³	(4,000-12,000/mm³)
Red blood cells	7.0 million/mm³	(3.5-5.5 million/mm³)
Hemoglobin	18 g/dL	(12-16 g/dL)
Hematocrit	52%	(36-46%)
Sodium	135 mEq/L	(135-145 mEq/L)

	LABORATORY RESULT	NORMAL RANGE
Potassium	3.5 mEq/L	(3.5-4.5 mEq/L)
Magnesium	1.5 mEq/L	(1.5-2.5 mEq/L)
Serum aspartate aminotransferase (AST)	780 IU/L	(10-34 IU/L)
Serum alanine aminotransferase (ALT)	922 IU/L	(10-40 IU/L)
Blood urea nitrogen (BUN)	30 mg/dL	(8-24 mg/dL)
Creatinine	2.0 mg/dL	0.6-1.1 mg/dL
Urinalysis	Negative for blood, protein, glucose	
Blood culture	Negative for any bacterial growth	
ECG	Sinus tachycardia	
Chest x-ray	Lung fields without any noted infiltrates or masses	

1. In reviewing Mr. Goldman's laboratory values, which findings indicate abnormal liver function?
2. While reviewing Mr. Goldman's medical history, what information most likely increases his risk for abnormal liver function?
3. With further medical workup in the ED, the physician determines that Mr. Goldman is suffering from acute hepatitis A. The patient asks you how he contracted the virus. What is your best response?
4. You are educating the patient's family about receiving vaccinations against hepatitis. What information will you provide to promote their safety?

may be prescribed. However, due to the life-threatening nature of chronic hepatitis B and hepatitis C, a number of drugs are given, including antiviral and immunomodulating drugs (Table 58-4). Similar to patients with other chronic diseases, patients with hepatitis often use complementary and alternative thera-pies to promote general well-being and improve quality of life (see the Evidence-Based Practice box). Be sure to ask patients about their use of these therapies and incorporate them into the collaborative plan of care.

Community-Based Care. Home care management varies according to the type of hepatitis and whether the disease is acute or chronic. A primary focus in any case is preventing the spread of the infection. For hepatitis transmitted by the fecal-oral route, careful handwashing and sanitary disposal of feces are impor-tant. Education is therefore very important. Collaborate with the certified infection control practitioner and infectious disease specialist if needed in caring for these patients. These experts can also suggest resources for the patient and family.

CHART 58-5   **Patient and Family Education: Preparing for Self-Management**

Viral Hepatitis

- Avoid all medications, including over-the-counter drugs such as acetaminophen (Tylenol, Exdol ✚), unless prescribed by your physician.
- Avoid all alcohol.
- Rest frequently throughout the day, and get adequate sleep at night.
- Eat small, frequent meals with a high-carbohydrate, moderate-fat, and moderate-protein content.
- Avoid sexual intercourse until antibody testing results are negative.
- Follow the guidelines for preventing transmission of the disease (see Chart 58-4).

! NURSING SAFETY PRIORITY   (QSEN)

Action Alert

Teach the patient with viral hepatitis and the family to use measures to prevent infection transmission (see Chart 58-4). *In addition, instruct the patient to avoid alcohol and to check with the health care provider before taking any medication or vitamin, supplement, or herbal preparation.*

Encourage the patient to increase activity gradually to prevent fatigue. Suggest that he or she eat small, frequent meals of high-carbohydrate foods (Chart 58-5).

FATTY LIVER (STEATOSIS)

Fatty liver is caused by the accumulation of fats in and around the hepatic cells. It may be caused by alcohol use or other factors. Nonalcoholic fatty liver disease (NAFLD) and nonalcoholic steatohepatitis (NASH) are types of fatty liver disease. Causes include:

- Diabetes mellitus
- Obesity
- Elevated lipid profile

Fatty infiltration of the liver may result from faulty fat metabolism in the liver and the movement of fatty acids from adipose tissue (fat). Many patients are asymptomatic. The most common and typical finding is an elevated ALT and AST or normal ALT and elevated AST (part of a group of liver function tests [LFTs]).

MRI, ultrasound, and nuclear medicine examinations can be used to confirm excessive fat in the liver. A percutaneous biopsy can also confirm the diagnosis. Interventions are aimed at removing the underlying cause of the infiltration. Weight loss, glucose control, and aggressive treatment using lipid-lowering agents are recommended. Monitoring liver function tests is essential in disease management.

LIVER TRAUMA

The liver is one of the most common organs to be injured in patients with abdominal trauma. Damage or injury should be suspected whenever any upper abdominal or lower chest trauma is sustained. The liver is often injured by steering wheels in vehicular crashes. Common injuries include simple lacerations, multiple lacerations, avulsions (tears), and crush injuries.

The liver is a highly vascular organ and receives almost a third of the body's cardiac output. When hepatic trauma occurs, blood loss can be massive. *Observe for early signs of hypovolemic shock* (Chart 58-6).

CHART 58-6   **Key Features**

Liver Trauma

- Right upper quadrant pain with abdominal tenderness
- Abdominal distention and rigidity
- Guarding of the abdomen
- Increased abdominal pain exaggerated by deep breathing and referred to the right shoulder (Kehr's sign)
- Indicators of hemorrhage and hypovolemic shock:
  - Hypotension
  - Tachycardia
  - Tachypnea
  - Pallor
  - Diaphoresis
  - Cool, clammy skin
  - Confusion or other change in mental state

An ultrasound or CT scan of the abdomen is often done to determine the presence of a hematoma (blood clot). A decreased hematocrit may confirm suspected blood loss. Clinical manifestations include right upper quadrant PAIN with abdominal tenderness, distention, guarding, and rigidity. Abdominal pain exaggerated by deep breathing and referred to the right shoulder may indicate diaphragmatic irritation.

Liver trauma is managed in a conservative manner through new diagnostic and therapeutic modalities such as enhanced critical care monitoring and damage control surgery (Ahmed & Vernick, 2011). Patients with hepatic trauma may require multiple blood products such as packed red blood cells and fresh frozen plasma, as well as massive volume infusion to maintain adequate hydration. After surgery, the patient is admitted to a critical care unit. Monitor the patient for persistent or new bleeding. Closely monitor complete blood count and coagulation studies for trends in changes.

CANCER OF THE LIVER

❖ PATHOPHYSIOLOGY

Cancers may be *primary* tumors (hepatocellular carcinoma) starting in the liver, or they may be *metastatic* cancers that spread from another organ to the liver. They are most often seen in regions of Asia and the Mediterranean area. Worldwide, the disease kills about 1 million people each year and affects Vietnamese men more than any other group. Black and Hispanic populations have twice the rate of the disease as Euro-Americans, and older adults are affected more than other age-groups (Rossi et al., 2010). In the United States and worldwide, the incidence of liver cancer is increasing because there is an increase in cases of hepatitis C.

Chronic INFECTION with HBV and HCV frequently lead to cirrhosis, which is a risk factor for developing liver cancer. It is important to remember that cirrhosis from any cause, including alcoholic liver disease, increases the risk for cancer.

❖ PATIENT-CENTERED COLLABORATIVE CARE

● Assessment

In the early stage of cancer, most patients are without symptoms. Later in the disease, they report weight loss, anorexia, and weakness. Ask the patient if he or she has or has had recent abdominal PAIN, the most common concern. It is most often felt in the right upper quadrant before jaundice, bleeding, ascites, and edema develop. Palpation may reveal an enlarged, nodular liver.

Elevated serum *alpha-fetoprotein* (AFP) (a tumor marker for cancers of the liver, testis, and ovary) and increased *alkaline phosphatase* are also common (Pagana & Pagana, 2014). Ultrasound (US) and contrast-enhanced CT are both useful in detecting metastasis. If the primary tumor site is not known, a CT- or ultrasound-guided liver biopsy can confirm the diagnosis, although this procedure is risky because of possible bleeding and spread of the cancer cells.

◆ Interventions

Surgical resection and liver transplantation offer the only treatments for long-term survival from liver cancer. Unfortunately, most patients are not candidates for surgical removal because their tumors are unresectable. Tunneled abdominal drains, such as the PleurX drainage system, may be used at home by the patient and family to remove excess ascitic fluid. *Teach them how to empty the drain and maintain the system. Remind them not to remove more than 2000 mL of fluid at one time to prevent hypovolemic shock.*

Selective internal radiation therapy (SIRT) has been successful for some patients. Other palliative approaches include hepatic artery embolization, ablation techniques, and drug therapy. *Hepatic artery embolization* causes cell death by blocking blood supply to the tumor in the liver. It is performed under moderate sedation by an interventional radiologist who threads a catheter through the femoral artery to inject small beads into the hepatic artery to block blood flow. The patient usually stays overnight in the hospital for observation in case of bleeding. This procedure may be followed by infusing a chemotherapy agent directly into the hepatic artery (chemoembolization).

Common *ablation* procedures include radiofrequency ablation (RFA), percutaneous ethanol injection, and cryotherapy. RFA uses energy waves to heat cancer cells and kill them. It is most often performed as an ambulatory care procedure using a percutaneous laparoscopic approach. Ethanol may also be injected directly into the tumor to destroy tumor cells, although this procedure is not as commonly done as RFA (Rossi et al., 2010). Cryotherapy uses liquid nitrogen to freeze and destroy liver tumors. The general nursing care for patients having these procedures is described in Chapter 22.

Chemotherapy may be administered orally or IV. However, it is not effective in many cases. Examples of drugs used are doxorubicin (Adriamycin), 5-fluorouracil (5-FU), and cisplatin. Sorafenib (Nexavar) is a kinase inhibitor that is approved for inoperable liver cancer. Other drugs are targeted therapies that are being investigated and used with some success.

Another drug route is a catheter-directed method directly into the hepatic artery, a procedure called *hepatic arterial infusion (HAI)*. The interventional radiologist places a catheter into the artery that supplies the tumor and injects a mixture of chemotherapy and contrast agent into the tumor. This procedure has the unique effect of depositing chemotherapeutic drugs directly into the tumor without causing major systemic effects. Chapter 22 describes the general nursing care for patients receiving chemotherapy.

Patients with advanced liver cancer usually need end-of-life care and hospice services. Collaborate with the case manager to help patients and their families find the best community resources that meet their needs. Chapter 7 describes end-of-life care and hospice services in detail.

LIVER TRANSPLANTATION

❖ PATHOPHYSIOLOGY

Liver transplantation has become a common procedure worldwide. The patient with end-stage liver disease or acute liver failure who has not responded to conventional medical or surgical intervention is a potential candidate for liver transplantation. Many diseases can cause liver failure. Cirrhosis (scarring of the liver) is the most common reason for liver transplants. Other common reasons for liver transplants are chronic hepatitis B and hepatitis C, bile duct diseases, autoimmune liver disease, primary liver cancer, alcoholic liver disease, and fatty liver disease (American Liver Foundation, 2012).

Transplantation Considerations

The patient for potential transplantation has extensive physiologic and psychological assessment and evaluation by physicians and transplant coordinators. Alternative treatment should be extensively explored before committing a patient for a liver transplant. Patients who are *not* considered candidates for transplantation are those with:

- Severe cardiovascular instability with advanced cardiac disease
- Severe respiratory disease
- Metastatic tumors
- Inability to follow instructions regarding drug therapy and self-management

Liver transplantation has become the most effective treatment for an increasing number of patients with acute and chronic liver diseases. Inclusion and exclusion criteria vary among transplantation centers and are continually revised as treatment options change and surgical techniques improve.

Donor livers are obtained primarily from trauma victims who have not had liver damage. They are distributed through a nationwide program—the United Network of Organ Sharing (UNOS). This system distributes donor livers based on regional considerations and patient acuity. Candidates with the highest level of acuity receive highest priority.

The donor liver is transported to the surgery center in a solution that preserves the organ for up to 8 hours. The diseased liver is removed through an incision made in the upper abdomen. The new liver is carefully put in its place and is attached to the patient's blood vessels and bile ducts. The procedure can take many hours to complete and requires a highly specialized team and large volumes of fluid and blood replacement.

Living donors have also been used and are usually close family members or spouse. This is done on a voluntary basis after careful psychological and physiologic preparation and testing. The donor's liver is resected (usually removal of one lobe) and implanted into the recipient after removal of the diseased liver. In both the donor and the recipient, the liver regenerates and grows in size to meet the demands of the body.

Transplantation Complications

Although liver transplantations are commonly done, complications can occur. Some problems can be medically managed, whereas others require removal of the transplant. The two most common complications are acute graft rejection and infection.

The success rate for transplantations has greatly improved since the introduction many years ago of cyclosporine (cyclosporin A), an immunosuppressant drug. Today, many other anti-rejection drugs are used. (See Chapter 20 for a complete discussion of rejection and preventive drug therapy.)

Transplant rejection is treated aggressively with immunosuppressive drugs. As with all rejection treatments, the patient is at a greater risk for infection. If therapy is not effective, liver function rapidly deteriorates. Multi-system organ failure, including respiratory and renal involvement, develops along with diffuse coagulopathies and portal-systemic encephalopathy (PSE). The only alternative for treatment is emergency retransplantation.

INFECTION is another potential threat to the transplanted graft and the patient's survival. Vaccinations and prophylactic antibiotics are helpful in prevention. Immunosuppressant therapy, which must be used to prevent and treat organ rejection, significantly increases the patient's risk for infection. Other risk factors include the presence of multiple tubes and intravascular lines, immobility, and prolonged anesthesia.

In the early post-transplantation period, common INFECTIONS include pneumonia, wound infections, and urinary tract infections. Opportunistic infections usually develop after the first postoperative month and include cytomegalovirus, mycobacterial infections, and parasitic infections. Latent infections such as tuberculosis and herpes simplex may be reactivated.

The physician prescribes broad-spectrum antibiotics for prophylaxis during and after surgery. Obtain culture specimens from all lines and tubes and collect specimens for culture at predetermined time intervals as dictated by the agency's policy. If an INFECTION is detected, the physician prescribes organism-specific anti-infective agents.

The biliary anastomosis is susceptible to breakdown, obstruction, and infection. If leakage occurs or if the site becomes necrotic or obstructed, an abscess can form or peritonitis, bacteremia, and cirrhosis may develop. Observe for potential complications, which are listed in Table 58-5.

❖ PATIENT-CENTERED COLLABORATIVE CARE

Care of the patient undergoing liver transplantation requires an interdisciplinary team approach. Receiving a transplant has a major psychosocial impact. Transplant complications cause patients to be very anxious. In collaboration with the members of the health care team, assure them and their families that these problems are common and usually successfully treated.

After the patient is identified as a candidate and a donor organ is procured, the actual liver transplantation surgical procedure usually takes many hours. The length of the procedure can vary greatly.

In the immediate postoperative period, the patient is managed in the critical care unit and requires aggressive

TABLE 58-5 **Assessment and Prevention of Common Postoperative Complications Associated with Liver Transplantation**

ASSESSMENT	PREVENTION
Acute Graft Rejection	
Occurs from the 4th to 10th postoperative day	Prophylaxis with immunosuppressant agents, such as cyclosporine
Manifested by tachycardia, fever, right upper quadrant (RUQ) or flank pain, diminished bile drainage or change in bile color, or increased jaundice	Early diagnosis to treat with more potent anti-rejection drugs
Laboratory changes: (1) increased levels of serum bilirubin, transaminases, and alkaline phosphatase; (2) prolonged prothrombin time	
Infection	
Can occur at any time during recovery	Antibiotic prophylaxis; vaccinations
Manifested by fever or excessive, foul-smelling drainage (urine, wound, or bile); other indicators depend on location and type of infection	Frequent cultures of tubes, lines, and drainage
	Early removal of invasive lines
	Good handwashing
	Early diagnosis and treatment with organism-specific anti-infective agents
Hepatic Complications (Bile Leakage, Abscess Formation, Hepatic Thrombosis)	
Manifested by decreased bile drainage, increased RUQ abdominal pain with distention and guarding, nausea or vomiting, increased jaundice, and clay-colored stools	If present, keep T-tube in dependent position and secure to patient; empty frequently, recording quality and quantity of drainage
Laboratory changes: increased levels of serum bilirubin and transaminases	Report manifestations to physician immediately
	May necessitate surgical intervention
Acute Renal Failure	
Caused by hypotension, antibiotics, cyclosporine, acute liver failure, or hypothermia	Monitor all drug levels with nephrotoxic side effects
Indicators of hypothermia: shivering, hyperventilation, increased cardiac output, vasoconstriction, and alkalemia	Prevent hypotension
Early indicators of renal failure: changes in urine output, increased blood urea nitrogen (BUN) and creatinine levels, and electrolyte imbalance	Observe for early signs of renal failure, and report them immediately to the physician

monitoring and care. Assess for signs and symptoms of complications of surgery, and immediately report them to the surgeon (see Table 58-5).

Post–liver transplant patients are living longer today than ever. Teach patients to be aware of side effects of immunosuppressive drugs, such as hypertension, nephrotoxicity, and gastrointestinal disturbances. Remind them that long-term management of care includes surveillance for malignancy, metabolic syndrome, and diabetes. Teaching the patient self-examination for skin, breast, and testicular malignancies is important as well as reminders for annual Papanicolaou (Pap) smears and other cancer screening tests. Post-transplant patients need to maintain lifestyle changes to increase their longevity after surgery (Clayton, 2011; Lucey et al., 2013).

What might you NOTICE if the patient is experiencing inadequate digestion, nutrition, and metabolism as a result of impaired liver function?
- Jaundice
- Icterus
- Report of nausea and anorexia
- Vomiting
- Weight loss
- Bruising or bleeding
- Ascites

What should you INTERPRET and how should you RESPOND to a patient experiencing inadequate digestion, nutrition, and metabolism as a result of impaired liver function?

Perform and interpret physical assessment findings, including:
- Assessing respiratory status to check for dyspnea or shallow breathing
- Checking level of consciousness and cognition
- Taking vital signs (looking for fever or decreased BP) and oxygen saturation
- Checking for blood in the vomitus
- Performing an abdominal assessment, including measuring girth

- Checking urine for dark color and stool for clay-colored appearance
- Taking current weight, and comparing with previous weight
- Assessing skin for open areas
- Checking most recent laboratory values for coagulation studies and LFTs

Respond by:
- Applying oxygen to assist in ease of breathing
- Keeping head of bed elevated to at least 30 degrees
- Maintaining rest
- Collaborating with dietitian and pharmacist as needed
- Prioritizing and pacing activities to prevent fatigue
- Monitoring patient closely for complications, such as bleeding; calling the Rapid Response Team if bleeding occurs

On what should you REFLECT?
- Monitor the patient for restored digestion and nutrition, such as increased appetite.
- Think about what may have caused the liver problem.
- Consider for what complications the patient is at risk.
- Think about what members of the health care team need to provide care for this patient.

GET READY FOR THE NCLEX® EXAMINATION!

KEY POINTS

Review these Key Points for each NCLEX Examination Client Needs Category.

Safe and Effective Care Environment
- When caring for patients with cirrhosis, collaborate with the dietitian, physician, and pharmacist. **Teamwork and Collaboration** QSEN
- Refer patients with liver disorders to the American Liver Foundation; refer dying patients to hospice and other community resources as needed. **Patient-Centered Care** QSEN

Health Promotion and Maintenance
- Follow the guidelines listed in Chart 58-3 to prevent viral hepatitis in the workplace. **Evidence-Based Practice** QSEN
- Teach patients to take precautions to prevent viral hepatitis in the community as described in Chart 58-4. **Evidence-Based Practice** QSEN
- For patients with viral hepatitis, instruct them to follow the guidelines listed in Chart 58-5. **Safety** QSEN
- Teach patients to avoid alcohol and illicit drugs to prevent or slow the progression of alcohol-induced cirrhosis; remind them not to take any medication (including over-the-counter drugs) without checking with their health care provider. **Safety** QSEN

Psychosocial Integrity
- Recognize that patients with cirrhosis have mental and emotional changes due to hepatic encephalopathy. **Patient-Centered Care** QSEN
- Be aware that patients with cirrhosis and/or chronic hepatitis may feel guilty about their disease because of past habits such as drug and alcohol use. **Patient-Centered Care** QSEN
- Be aware that family members and friends may fear getting hepatitis from the patient. **Patient-Centered Care** QSEN
- Be aware that patients having liver transplantation have major concerns about the possibility of complications, such as organ rejection. **Patient-Centered Care** QSEN

Physiological Integrity
- Be aware that cirrhosis has many causes other than alcohol use (see Table 58-1). **Patient-Centered Care** QSEN

- Observe for clinical manifestations of hepatic encephalopathy (PSE) as listed in Table 58-2. **Safety** QSEN
- Monitor laboratory values of patients suspected of or diagnosed with cirrhosis of the liver as listed in Table 58-3. **Informatics** QSEN
- Monitor the patient with cirrhosis for bleeding and neurologic changes. **Safety** QSEN
- Provide care for the patient having a paracentesis as described in Chart 58-1. **Safety** QSEN
- Administer drug therapy to decrease ammonia levels (which cause PSE) in patients with cirrhosis, such as lactulose and nonabsorbable antibiotics. **Safety** QSEN
- Differentiate the five major types of hepatitis: A, B, C, D, and E. Hepatitis D occurs only with Hepatitis B and is transmitted most commonly by blood and body fluid exposure. Hepatitis A is transmitted via the fecal-oral route. Hepatitis C is the most common type and is also transmitted via blood and body fluids. **Evidence-Based Practice** QSEN

- Be aware that patients with chronic viral hepatitis often develop cirrhosis and cancer of the liver. **Evidence-Based Practice** QSEN
- Recognize that potent immunomodulators and antivirals are given to treat hepatitis B and hepatitis C; teach patients on immunomodulators to avoid large crowds and people who have INFECTIONS. **Safety** QSEN
- Monitor for bleeding in the patient with liver trauma; assume that any abdominal trauma has damaged the liver. **Safety** QSEN
- Monitor the patient having a liver transplantation for complications, such as those described in Table 58-5. **Safety** QSEN
- Report and document elevated temperature, increased abdominal PAIN and rigidity, bleeding, and/or neurologic status changes as possible indicators of liver transplantation complications. **Evidence-Based Practice** QSEN

CHAPTER 59

Care of Patients with Problems of the Biliary System and Pancreas

Lara Carver and Jennifer Powers

 http://evolve.elsevier.com/Iggy/

PRIORITY CONCEPTS

- PAIN
- NUTRITION

- INFLAMMATION

LEARNING OUTCOMES

Safe and Effective Care Environment

1. Collaborate with health care team members to provide care for patients with pancreatic disorders.
2. Identify community-based resources for patients with pancreatic disorders.

Health Promotion and Maintenance

3. Teach people about health promotion practices to prevent gallbladder disease.
4. Teach people about evidence-based health promotion practices to prevent pancreatitis.

Psychosocial Integrity

5. Describe the psychosocial needs of patients with pancreatic cancer and their families.

Physiological Integrity

6. Identify risk factors for gallbladder disease.

7. Interpret diagnostic test results associated with gallbladder disease.
8. Compare postoperative care of patients undergoing a traditional cholecystectomy with that of patients having laparoscopic cholecystectomy.
9. Compare and contrast the pathophysiology of acute and chronic pancreatitis.
10. Interpret laboratory test results associated with acute pancreatitis.
11. Interpret common assessment findings associated with acute and chronic pancreatitis.
12. Prioritize nursing care for patients with acute pancreatitis and patients with chronic pancreatitis.
13. Explain the use and precautions associated with enzyme replacement for chronic pancreatitis.
14. Develop a postoperative plan of care for patients having a Whipple procedure.

The biliary system (liver and gallbladder) and pancreas secrete enzymes and other substances that promote food digestion in the stomach and small intestine. When these organs do not work properly, the person has impaired *digestion,* which may result in inadequate NUTRITION. Collaborative care for patients with problems of the biliary system and pancreas includes the need to promote nutrition for healthy cellular function. This chapter focuses on problems of the gallbladder and pancreas. Liver disorders are described in Chapter 58.

Because of the close anatomic location of these organs, disorders of the gallbladder and pancreas may extend to other organs if the primary health problem is not treated early. INFLAMMATION is caused by obstruction (blockage) in the biliary system from gallstones, edema, stricture, or tumors. For example, gallstones in the cystic duct cause cholecystitis. Gallstones lodged in the ampulla of Vater block the flow of bile and pancreatic secretions, which can result in pancreatitis. These problems frequently cause the patient to have moderate to severe abdominal PAIN.

CHOLECYSTITIS

❖ PATHOPHYSIOLOGY

Cholecystitis is an INFLAMMATION of the gallbladder that affects many people, most commonly in affluent countries. It may be either acute or chronic, although most patients have the acute type.

Acute Cholecystitis

Two types of acute cholecystitis can occur: calculous and acalculous cholecystitis. The most common type is calculous cholecystitis, in which chemical irritation and INFLAMMATION result from gallstones (cholelithiasis) that obstruct the cystic duct (most often), gallbladder neck, or common bile duct (choledocholithiasis) (Fig. 59-1). When the gallbladder is inflamed, trapped bile is reabsorbed and acts as a chemical irritant to the gallbladder wall. Reabsorbed bile, in combination with impaired circulation, edema, and distention of the gallbladder, causes ischemia and infection. The result is tissue sloughing with

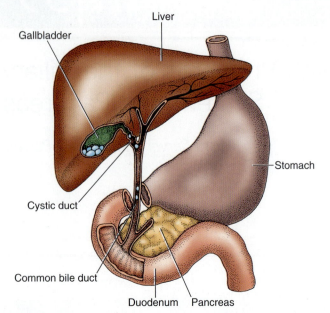

FIG. 59-1 Gallstones within the gallbladder and obstructing the common bile and cystic ducts.

necrosis and gangrene within the gallbladder itself. The gallbladder wall may eventually perforate (rupture). If the perforation is small and localized, an abscess may form. Peritonitis, infection of the peritoneum, may result if the perforation is large.

The exact pathophysiology of gallstone formation is not clearly understood, but abnormal metabolism of cholesterol and bile salts plays an important role in their formation. The gallbladder provides an excellent environment for the production of stones because it only occasionally mixes its normally abundant mucus with its highly viscous, concentrated bile. Impaired gallbladder motility can lead to stone formation by delaying bile emptying and causing biliary stasis.

Gallstones are composed of substances normally found in bile, such as cholesterol, bilirubin, bile salts, calcium, and various proteins. They are classified as either cholesterol stones or pigment stones. Cholesterol calculi form as a result of metabolic imbalances of cholesterol and bile salts. They are the most common type found in people in the United States (McCance et al., 2014).

Bacteria can collect around the stones in the biliary system. Severe bacterial invasion can lead to life-threatening *suppurative* cholangitis when symptoms are not recognized quickly and pus accumulates in the ductal system.

Acalculous cholecystitis (INFLAMMATION occurring without gallstones) is typically associated with biliary stasis caused by any condition that affects the regular filling or emptying of the gallbladder. For example, a decrease in blood flow to the gallbladder or anatomic problems such as twisting or kinking of the gallbladder neck or cystic duct can result in pancreatic enzyme reflux into the gallbladder, causing inflammation. Sphincter of Oddi dysfunction (SOD) can also occur to cause reflux and inflammation (Pfadt & Carlson, 2011). Most cases of this type of cholecystitis occur in patients with:

- Sepsis
- Severe trauma or burns
- Long-term total parenteral nutrition
- Multi-system organ failure
- Major surgery
- Hypovolemia

Chronic Cholecystitis

Chronic cholecystitis results when repeated episodes of cystic duct obstruction cause chronic INFLAMMATION. Calculi are almost always present. In chronic cholecystitis, the gallbladder becomes fibrotic and contracted, which results in decreased motility and deficient absorption.

Pancreatitis and cholangitis (bile duct INFLAMMATION) can occur as chronic complications of cholecystitis. These problems result from the backup of bile throughout the biliary tract. Bile obstruction leads to jaundice.

Jaundice (yellow discoloration of the skin and mucous membranes) and icterus (yellow discoloration of the sclera) can occur in patients with acute cholecystitis but are most commonly seen in those with the *chronic* form of the disease. Obstructed bile flow caused by edema of the ducts or gallstones contributes to *extrahepatic* obstructive jaundice. Jaundice in cholecystitis may also be caused by direct liver involvement. Inflammation of the liver's bile channels or bile ducts may cause *intrahepatic* obstructive jaundice, resulting in an increase in circulating levels of bilirubin, the major pigment of bile.

In a person with obstructive jaundice, the normal flow of bile into the duodenum is blocked, allowing excessive bile salts to accumulate in the skin. This accumulation of bile salts leads to pruritus (itching) or a burning sensation. The bile flow blockage also prevents bilirubin from reaching the large intestine, where it is converted to urobilinogen. Because urobilinogen accounts for the normal brown color of feces, clay-colored stools result. Water-soluble bilirubin is normally excreted by the kidneys in the urine. When an excess of circulating bilirubin occurs, the urine becomes dark and foamy because of the kidneys' effort to clear the bilirubin.

Etiology and Genetic Risk

A familial or genetic tendency appears to play a role in the development of cholelithiasis, but this may be partially related to familial nutrition habits (excessive dietary cholesterol intake) and sedentary lifestyles. Genetic-environment interactions may contribute to gallstone production. For example, current studies are investigating DNA expression sequences that program some people to make and secrete more cholesterol into bile, leading to the increase in cholesterol-containing gallstones. The main risk factors for developing gallstones are obesity, type 2 diabetes, dyslipidemia, and insulin resistance. Independent risk factors for developing gallstones are increase in age, female gender, and family history (Agostino et al., 2013). Also, people who experience rapid weight loss and certain intestinal diseases affecting the normal absorption of nutrients, such as Crohn's disease, are at risk for gallstones. The highest frequency of gallstone production lies among the American-Indian and Mexican-American populations (McCance, et al., 2014). Risk factors for cholecystitis are listed in Table 59-1.

The incidence of chronic cholecystitis is increased in young, thin women, especially those who are athletic (e.g., ballerinas and gymnasts). These women have chronic pain that is often misdiagnosed as gastritis.

TABLE 59-1   Risk Factors for Cholecystitis

- Women
- Aging
- American Indian, Mexican American, or Caucasian
- Obesity
- Rapid weight loss or prolonged fasting
- Increased serum cholesterol
- Women on hormone replacement therapy (HRT)

- Cholesterol-lowering drugs
- Family history of gallstones
- Prolonged total parenteral nutrition
- Crohn's disease
- Gastric bypass surgery
- Sickle cell disease
- Glucose intolerance/diabetes mellitus
- Pregnancy
- Genetic factors

CHART 59-1   Key Features

Cholecystitis

- Episodic or vague upper abdominal pain or discomfort that can radiate to the right shoulder
- Pain triggered by a high-fat or high-volume meal
- Anorexia
- Nausea and/or vomiting
- Dyspepsia (indigestion)
- Eructation (belching)
- Flatulence (gas)
- Feeling of abdominal fullness
- Rebound tenderness (Blumberg's sign)
- Fever
- Jaundice, clay-colored stools, dark urine, steatorrhea (most common with chronic cholecystitis)

GENDER HEALTH CONSIDERATIONS

Patient-Centered Care QSEN

Women who are between 20 and 60 years of age are twice as likely to develop gallstones as are men. Obesity is a major risk factor for gallstone formation, especially in women. Pregnancy and drugs such as hormone replacements and birth control pills alter hormone levels and delay muscular contraction of the gallbladder, decreasing the rate of bile emptying. The incidence of gallstones is higher in women who have had multiple pregnancies. Combinations of causative factors increase the incidence of stone formation, especially in women. Therefore some clinicians refer to the patient most at risk for acute cholecystitis and gallstones by the four **F**s:
- **F**emale
- **F**orty
- **F**at
- **F**ertile

CONSIDERATIONS FOR OLDER ADULTS

Patient-Centered Care QSEN

Older adults and patients with diabetes mellitus may have atypical manifestations of cholecystitis, including the absence of pain and fever. Localized tenderness may be the only presenting sign. The older patient may become acutely confused (delirium) as the first manifestation of gallbladder disease.

! NURSING SAFETY PRIORITY QSEN

Critical Rescue

Biliary colic may be so severe that it occurs with tachycardia, pallor, diaphoresis, and prostration (extreme exhaustion). Assess the patient for possible shock caused by biliary colic. Notify the health care provider or Rapid Response Team if these manifestations occur. Stay with the patient, and keep the head of the bed flat.

❖ PATIENT-CENTERED COLLABORATIVE CARE

◆ Assessment

Physical Assessment/Clinical Manifestations. Obtain the patient's height, weight, and vital signs, or delegate these activities to unlicensed assistive personnel (UAP). Ask about food preferences, and determine whether excessive fat and cholesterol are part of the diet. Typically, diets high in fat, high in calories, low in fiber, and high in refined white carbohydrates place patients at higher risk for developing gallstones. Inquire if any foods cause pain. Question whether any GI symptoms occur when fatty food is eaten: flatulence (gas), dyspepsia (indigestion), eructation (belching), anorexia, nausea, vomiting, and abdominal PAIN or discomfort.

Patients with cholecystitis present with abdominal PAIN, although clinical manifestations vary in intensity and frequency (Chart 59-1). Ask the patient to describe the PAIN, including its intensity and duration, precipitating factors, and any measures that relieve it. Pain may be described as indigestion of varying intensity, ranging from a mild, persistent ache to a steady, constant pain in the right upper abdominal quadrant. It may radiate to the right shoulder or scapula. In some cases the abdominal pain of chronic cholecystitis may be vague and nonspecific. The usual pattern is episodic. Patients often refer to acute pain episodes as "gallbladder attacks."

The severe PAIN of biliary colic is produced by obstruction of the cystic duct of the gallbladder or movement of one or more stones. When a stone is moving through or is lodged within the duct, tissue spasm occurs in an effort to get the stone through the small duct.

Ask patients to describe their daily activity or exercise routines to determine whether they are sedentary. Sedentary lifestyle, rapid weight loss, prolonged fasting, and pregnancy are risk factors for developing gallstones. Question whether there is a family history of gallbladder disease. Ask the patient about taking current or previous hormone replacement therapy (HRT). If the patient is female, ask if she is taking or has recently been on oral contraceptives (birth control pills).

Assessment for rebound tenderness (Blumberg's sign) and deep palpation are performed only by physicians and advanced practice nurses. To elicit rebound tenderness, the health care provider pushes his or her fingers deeply and steadily into the patient's abdomen and then quickly releases the pressure. PAIN that results from the rebound of the palpated tissue may indicate peritoneal inflammation. Deep palpation below the liver border in the right upper quadrant may reveal a sausage-shaped mass, representing the distended, inflamed gallbladder. Percussion over the posterior rib cage worsens localized abdominal pain.

In *chronic* cholecystitis, patients may have slowly developing symptoms and may not seek medical treatment until late symptoms such as jaundice (yellowing of the skin), clay-colored stools, and dark urine occur from biliary obstruction. Yellowing of the sclera (icterus) and oral mucous membranes may also be present. **Steatorrhea** (fatty stools) occurs because fat absorption is decreased because of the lack of bile. Bile is needed for the absorption of fats and fat-soluble vitamins in the intestine. As with any inflammatory process, the patient may have an elevated temperature of 99° to 102° F (37.2° to 38.9°C), tachycardia, and dehydration from fever and vomiting.

CONSIDERATIONS FOR OLDER ADULTS
Patient-Centered Care QSEN

Older adults become dehydrated much quicker than other age-groups, and they may not present with a fever. Monitor for a new onset of disorientation or acute confusion due to decreased blood volume available to oxygenate the cells of the brain (hypoxia).

Diagnostic Assessment. A differential diagnosis rules out other diseases that may cause similar symptoms, such as peptic ulcer disease, hepatitis, and pancreatitis. An increased *white blood cell* (WBC) count indicates INFLAMMATION. Serum levels of *alkaline phosphatase, aspartate aminotransferase (AST),* and *lactate dehydrogenase (LDH)* may be elevated, indicating abnormalities in liver function in patients with severe biliary obstruction. The direct (conjugated) and indirect (unconjugated) *serum bilirubin levels* are also elevated. If the pancreas is involved, serum amylase and lipase levels are elevated.

Calcified gallstones are easily viewed on abdominal x-ray. Stones that are not calcified cannot be seen. *Ultrasonography (US) of the right upper quadrant is the best initial diagnostic test for cholecystitis.* It is safe, accurate, and painless. Acute cholecystitis is seen as edema of the gallbladder wall and pericholecystic fluid.

A hepatobiliary scan (sometimes called a HIDA scan) can be performed to visualize the gallbladder and determine patency of the biliary system. In this nuclear medicine test, a radioactive tracer or chemical is injected intravenously. About 20 minutes after the injection, a gamma camera tracks the flow of the tracer from the gallbladder to determine the ejection rate of bile into the biliary duct. A decreased bile flow indicates gallbladder disease with obstruction. Teach patients having this test to have nothing by mouth before the procedure. Remind the patient that the camera is large and close to the body for most of the procedure.

When the cause of cholecystitis or cholelithiasis is not known or the patient has manifestations of biliary obstruction (e.g., jaundice), an *endoscopic retrograde cholangiopancreatography* (ERCP) may be performed. Some patients have the less invasive and safer *magnetic resonance cholangiopancreatography* (MRCP), which can be performed by an interventional radiologist. For this procedure, the patient is given oral or IV contrast material (gadolinium) before having an MRI scan (Griffin et al., 2011). Before the test, ask the patient about any history of urticaria (hives) or other allergy. MRI is also contraindicated in patients with pacemaker or other incompatible devices. Gadolinium does not contain iodine, which decreases the risk for an allergic response. Chapter 52 discusses these tests in more detail.

◆ Interventions
Acute cholecystitis is diagnosed on the basis of clinical findings, laboratory tests, and abdominal imaging. If acute infection of the gallbladder is diagnosed, emergency cholecystectomy is usually performed the same or the following day. Laparoscopic cholecystectomy is the treatment of choice for patients with acute and long-term chronic cholecystitis. This minimally invasive procedure achieves the desired outcomes of shorter recovery time, decreased expense, less postoperative pain, and minimal scarring after surgery.

Nonsurgical Management. Many people with gallstones have no symptoms. Acute PAIN is present when gallstones partially or totally obstruct the cystic or common bile duct. Most patients find that they need to avoid fatty foods to prevent further episodes of biliary colic. Withhold food and fluids if nausea and vomiting occur. IV therapy is used for hydration.

Drug Therapy. Acute biliary pain requires opioid analgesia, such as morphine or hydromorphone (Dilaudid). All opioids may cause some degree of sphincter of Oddi spasm.

Ketorolac (Toradol, Acular), an NSAID, may be used for mild to moderate pain. Be sure to monitor the patient for signs and symptoms of GI distress and pain because the drug can cause GI bleeding. The health care provider prescribes antiemetics to control nausea and vomiting. IV antibiotic therapy may also be given, depending on the cause of cholecystitis or as a one-time dose for surgery.

An option for a small number of patients with cholelithiasis (gallstones) is the use of oral bile acid dissolution or gallstone stabilizing agents. Drugs such as ursodiol (Actigall) and chenodiol (Chenodal) may be given for up to 2 years to dissolve or stabilize gallstones. A gallbladder ultrasound is required every 6 months for the first year of therapy to determine the effectiveness of the drug. Teach patients on this type of drug therapy to report diarrhea, vomiting, or severe abdominal PAIN, especially if it radiates to the shoulders, to their health care provider immediately. Remind them to take the medication with food and milk (Felicilda-Reynaldo, 2012).

Other Nonsurgical Interventions. For some patients with small stones or for those who are not good surgical candidates, a treatment that is commonly used for kidney stones can be used to break up gallstones—*extracorporeal shock wave lithotripsy (ESWL).* This procedure can be used only for patients who have a normal weight, cholesterol-based stones, and good gallbladder function. The patient lies on a water-filled pad, and shock waves break up the large stones into smaller ones that can be passed through the digestive system. During the procedure, he or she may have PAIN from the movement of the stones or duct or gallbladder spasms. A therapeutic bile acid, such as ursodeoxycholic acid (UDCA), may be used after the procedure to help dissolve the remaining stone fragments.

Another treatment option in people who cannot have surgery is the insertion of a percutaneous transhepatic biliary catheter (drain) using CT or ultrasound guidance to open the blocked duct(s) so that bile can flow (cholecystostomy). Catheters can be placed several ways, depending on the condition of the biliary ducts, in an internal, external, or internal/external drain. Biliary catheters usually divert bile from the liver into the duodenum to bypass a stricture. When all of the bile enters the duodenum, it is called an *internal* drain. However, in some cases a patient has an *internal/external* drain in which part of the bile empties into a drainage bag. Patients who need this drain for an extended period may have the external drain capped. If jaundice or leakage around the catheter site occurs, teach the patient to reconnect the catheter to a drainage bag and have a follow-up cholangiogram injection done by an interventional radiologist. An *external* only catheter is connected either temporarily or permanently to a drainage bag. A reduction in bile drainage indicates that the drain is no longer working.

Surgical Management. Cholecystectomy is a surgical removal of the gallbladder. One of two procedures is performed: the laparoscopic cholecystectomy and, far less often, the traditional open approach cholecystectomy.

Laparoscopic Cholecystectomy. Laparoscopic cholecystectomy, a minimally invasive surgery (MIS), is the "gold standard" and is performed far more often than the traditional open approach. The advantages of MIS when compared with the open approach include:

- Complications are not common.
- The death rate is very low.
- Bile duct injuries are rare.
- Patient recovery is quicker.
- Postoperative PAIN is less severe.

The laparoscopic procedure (often called a "lap chole") is commonly done on an ambulatory care basis in a same-day surgery suite. The surgeon explains the procedure, and the nurse answers questions and reinforces the instructions. Reinforce what to expect after surgery, and review pain management, deep-breathing exercises, incisional care, and leg exercises to prevent deep vein thrombosis. There is no special preoperative preparation other than the routine preparation for surgery under general anesthesia described in Chapter 14. An IV antibiotic is usually given immediately before or during surgery (Society of American Gastrointestinal and Endoscopic Surgeons [SAGES], 2013).

During the surgery the surgeon makes a very small midline puncture at the umbilicus. Additional small incisions may be needed, although single-incision laparoscopic cholecystectomy (SILC) using a flexible endoscope is often done (Salam, 2010). The abdominal cavity is insufflated with 3 to 4 liters of carbon dioxide. Gasless laparoscopic cholecystectomy using abdominal wall lifting devices is a more recent innovation in some centers. This technique results in improved pulmonary and cardiac function. A trocar catheter is inserted, through which a laparoscope is introduced. The laparoscope is attached to a video camera, and the abdominal organs are viewed on a monitor. The gallbladder is dissected from the liver bed, and the cystic artery and duct are closed. The surgeon aspirates the bile and crushes any large stones, if present, and then extracts the gallbladder through the umbilical port.

Removing the gallbladder with the laparoscopic technique reduces the risk for wound complications. Some patients have mild to severe discomfort from carbon dioxide retention in the abdomen, which may be felt throughout the thorax and shoulders.

! NURSING SAFETY PRIORITY (QSEN)

Action Alert

After a laparoscopic cholecystectomy, assess the patient's oxygen saturation level frequently until the effects of the anesthesia have passed. Remind the patient to perform deep-breathing exercises every hour.

Other postoperative care for the patient after a laparoscopic procedure is similar to that for any patient having minimally invasive endoscopic surgery (see Chapter 16). Offer the patient food and water when fully awake, and monitor for the nausea and/or vomiting that often results from anesthesia. If needed,

administer an antiemetic drug, such as ondansetron hydrochloride (Zofran), either IV push or as a disintegrating tablet. Several drug doses may be needed. Maintain an IV line to administer fluids until nausea and/or vomiting subside. Be sure to have the head of the bed elevated in the same-day surgery unit to prevent aspiration from vomiting. After nausea subsides, assist the patient to the bathroom to void. Early ambulation also promotes absorption of the carbon dioxide, which can decrease postoperative discomfort.

Administer an oral or IV push opioid as needed immediately after surgery. Continuous IV pain control is usually not required because there is only one or a few small incisions, which are covered with Steri-Strips and small adhesive bandages (e.g., Band-Aids) or are surgically glued. The glue or Steri-Strips lose their adhesiveness in about a week to 10 days and can be removed or fall off as the incision heals.

The patient is usually discharged from the hospital or surgery center the same day, although older and obese patients may stay overnight. Provide postoperative teaching regarding pain management, incision care, and follow-up appointments. Teach the patient to use ice and oral opioids for incisional pain, if needed, for a few days. For abdominal or thoracic discomfort from carbon dioxide retention, many patients report that heat application is helpful. The patient is typically allowed to bathe or shower the day after surgery.

After laparoscopic surgery, the patient can return to usual activities much sooner than those having an open cholecystectomy. Instruct the patient to rest for the first 24 hours and then begin to resume usual activities Most patients are able to resume usual activities within a week.

Some patients are able to return to their usual diet after surgery, while others must carefully monitor their diet to avoid high-fat foods. A large intake of fatty foods may result in abdominal pain and diarrhea, which could result in a mild post-cholecystectomy syndrome (PCS) (see later discussion of PCS on p. 1218). Teach patients to introduce foods high in fat one at a time to determine which foods are best tolerated.

A new minimally invasive surgical procedure is *natural orifice transluminal endoscopic surgery* (NOTES) for removal of or repair of organs. Surgery can be performed on many body organs through the mouth, vagina, and rectum. For removal of the gallbladder, the vagina is used most often in women because it can be easily decontaminated with Betadine or other antiseptic and allows easy access into the peritoneal cavity. The surgeon makes a small internal incision through the cul-de-sac of Douglas between the rectum and uterine wall to access the gallbladder. The main advantages of this procedure are the lack of visible incisions and minimal, if any, postoperative complications (Navarra et al., 2010).

Traditional Cholecystectomy. Use of the open surgical approach (abdominal laparotomy) has greatly declined during the past 25 years. Patients who have this type of surgery usually have severe biliary obstruction and the ducts are explored to ensure patency.

The surgical nurse provides the usual preoperative care and teaching in the operating suite on the day of surgery (see Chapter 14). The surgeon removes the gallbladder through an incision and explores the biliary ducts for the presence of stones or other cause of obstruction. The surgeon usually inserts a drainage tube such as a Jackson-Pratt (JP) drain. This tube is placed in the gallbladder bed to prevent fluid accumulation. The drainage is usually serosanguineous (serous fluid mixed with blood) and is stained with bile in the first 24 hours after surgery. Antibiotic therapy is given to prevent infection.

Patient care for a patient who has had a traditional open cholecystectomy is similar to the care for any patient who has had abdominal surgery under general anesthesia as described in Chapter 16. Postoperative incisional PAIN after a traditional cholecystectomy is controlled with opioids using a patient-controlled analgesia (PCA) pump. Encourage the patient to use coughing and deep-breathing exercises when pain is controlled and the incision is splinted.

Antiemetics may be necessary for episodes of postoperative nausea and vomiting. Administer the antiemetic early, as prescribed, to prevent retching associated with vomiting and thus to decrease pain related to muscle straining.

Provide care for the incision and the surgical drain. The surgeon typically removes the surgical dressing and drain within 24 hours after surgery.

The patient is NPO until fully awake postoperatively. Document the patient's level of consciousness, vital signs, and pain level. Assess the surgical incision for signs of infection, such as excessive redness or purulent drainage. Report changes to the surgeon immediately. Begin ambulation as soon as possible to prevent deep vein thrombosis and promote peristalsis.

Advance the diet from clear liquids to solid foods as peristalsis returns. The patient usually resumes solid foods and is discharged to home 1 to 2 days after surgery, depending on any complications and the patient's general condition. In the early postoperative period, if bile flow is reduced, a low-fat diet may reduce discomfort and prevent nausea. For most patients, a special diet is not required. Advise them to eat nutritious meals and avoid excessive intake of fatty foods, especially fried food, butter, and "fast food." If the patient is obese, recommend a weight-reduction program.

Teach the patient to keep the incision clean and report any changes that may indicate infection. Remind him or her to report repeated abdominal or epigastric pain with vomiting and/or diarrhea that may occur several weeks to months after surgery. These symptoms indicate possible **postcholecystectomy syndrome (PCS)**. There are multiple causes of PCS, some of which are related to the biliary system and others are not. Common causes of PCS are listed in Table 59-2. Not all patients experience PCS. Often the PAIN returns because of one of the underlying conditions listed in Table 59-2, not as a result of the cholecystectomy itself (Girometti et al., 2010).

Management depends on the exact cause but usually involves the use of endoscopic retrograde cholangiopancreatography (ERCP) to find the cause of the problem and repair it. This procedure and related nursing care are described in Chapter 52. Collaborative care includes pain management, antibiotics, nutrition and hydration therapy (possibly short-term parenteral nutrition), and control of nausea and vomiting.

ACUTE PANCREATITIS

❖ PATHOPHYSIOLOGY

Acute pancreatitis is a serious and, at times, life-threatening INFLAMMATION of the pancreas. This process is caused by a premature activation of excessive pancreatic enzymes that destroy ductal tissue and pancreatic cells, resulting in autodigestion and fibrosis of the pancreas. The pathologic changes occur in different degrees. The severity of pancreatitis depends on the extent of inflammation and tissue damage. Pancreatitis can range from mild involvement evidenced by edema and inflammation to **necrotizing hemorrhagic pancreatitis (NHP)**. NHP is diffusely bleeding pancreatic tissue with fibrosis and tissue death.

The pancreas is unusual in that it functions as both an exocrine gland and an endocrine gland. The primary *endocrine* disorder is diabetes mellitus and is discussed in Chapter 64. The *exocrine* function of the pancreas is responsible for secreting enzymes that assist in the breakdown of starches, proteins, and fats. These enzymes are normally secreted in the inactive form and become activated once they enter the small intestine. Early activation (i.e., activation within the pancreas rather than the intestinal lumen) results in the inflammatory process of pancreatitis. Direct toxic injury to the pancreatic cells and the production and release of pancreatic enzymes (e.g., trypsin, lipase, elastase) result from the obstructive damage. After pancreatic duct obstruction, increased pressure may contribute to ductal rupture allowing spillage of trypsin and other enzymes into the pancreatic parenchymal tissue. Autodigestion of the pancreas occurs as a result (Fig. 59-2). In *acute* pancreatitis, four major pathophysiologic processes occur: lipolysis, proteolysis, necrosis of blood vessels, and INFLAMMATION.

The hallmark of pancreatic necrosis is enzymatic fat necrosis of the endocrine and exocrine cells of the pancreas caused by the enzyme *lipase*. Fatty acids are released during this *lipolytic process* and combine with ionized calcium to form a soap-like product. The initial rapid lowering of serum calcium levels is not readily compensated for by the parathyroid gland. Because the body needs ionized calcium and cannot use bound calcium, hypocalcemia occurs (McCance et al., 2014).

Proteolysis involves the splitting of proteins by hydrolysis of the peptide bonds, resulting in the formation of smaller polypeptides. Proteolytic activity may lead to thrombosis and

TABLE 59-2 Common Causes of Postcholecystectomy Syndrome	
Biliary	**Non-Biliary**
• Pseudocyst	• Coronary artery disease
• Common bile duct (CBD) leak	• Intercostal neuritis
• CBD or pancreatic duct stricture or obstruction	• Unexplained pain syndrome
• Sphincter of Oddi dysfunction	• Psychiatric or neurologic disorder
• Retained or new CBD gallstone	
• Pancreatic or liver mass	
• Primary sclerosing cholangitis	
• Diverticular compression	

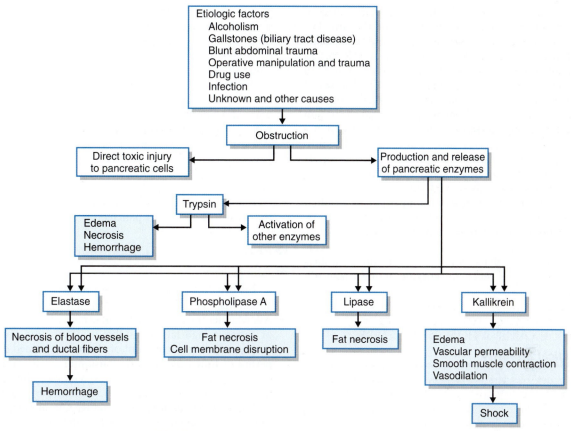

FIG. 59-2 The process of autodigestion in acute pancreatitis.

gangrene of the pancreas. Pancreatic destruction may be localized and confined to one area or may involve the entire organ.

Elastase is activated by trypsin and causes elastic fibers of the blood vessels and ducts to dissolve. The *necrosis of blood vessels* results in bleeding, ranging from minor bleeding to massive hemorrhage of pancreatic tissue. Another pancreatic enzyme, kallikrein, causes the release of vasoactive peptides, bradykinin, and a plasma kinin known as *kallidin.* These substances contribute to vasodilation and increased vascular permeability, further compounding the hemorrhagic process. This massive destruction of blood vessels by necrosis may lead to generalized hemorrhage with blood escaping into the retroperitoneal tissues. *The patient with hemorrhagic pancreatitis is critically ill, and extensive pancreatic destruction and shock may lead to death. The majority of deaths in patients with acute pancreatitis result from irreversible shock.*

The *inflammatory stage* occurs when leukocytes cluster around the hemorrhagic and necrotic areas of the pancreas. A secondary bacterial process may lead to suppuration (pus formation) of the pancreatic parenchyma or the formation of an abscess. (See discussion of Pancreatic Abscess on p. 1226.) Mild infected lesions may be absorbed. When infected lesions are severe, calcification and fibrosis occur. If the infected fluid becomes walled off by fibrous tissue, a pancreatic pseudocyst is formed. (See discussion of Pancreatic Pseudocyst on p. 1226.)

Complications of Acute Pancreatitis

Acute pancreatitis may result in severe, life-threatening complications (Table 59-3). Jaundice occurs from swelling of the head

TABLE 59-3   **Potential Complications of Acute Pancreatitis**
• Pancreatic infection (causes septic shock)
• Hemorrhage (necrotizing hemorrhagic pancreatitis [NHP])
• Acute kidney failure
• Paralytic ileus
• Hypovolemic shock
• Pleural effusion
• Acute respiratory distress syndrome (ARDS)
• Atelectasis
• Pneumonia
• Multi-organ system failure
• Disseminated intravascular coagulation (DIC)
• Type 2 diabetes mellitus

of the pancreas, which slows bile flow through the common bile duct. The bile duct may also be compressed by calculi (stones) or a pancreatic pseudocyst. The resulting total bile flow obstruction causes severe jaundice. Intermittent hyperglycemia occurs from the release of glucagon, as well as the decreased release of insulin due to damage to the pancreatic islet cells. Total destruction of the pancreas may occur, leading to type 1 diabetes mellitus (McCance et al., 2014).

Left lung pleural effusions frequently develop in the patient with acute pancreatitis. *Atelectasis and pneumonia may occur also, especially in older patients.*

Multi-system organ failure is caused by necrotizing hemorrhagic pancreatitis (NHP). The patient is at risk for acute respiratory distress syndrome (ARDS). This severe form of pulmonary edema is caused by disruption of the alveolar-capillary membrane and is a serious complication of acute pancreatitis. (See Chapter 32 for a discussion of ARDS.) In acute pancreatitis, pulmonary failure accounts for more than half of all deaths that occur in the first week of the disease.

Coagulation defects are another major potential complication and may result in death. Complex physiologic changes in the pancreas cause the release of necrotic tissue and enzymes into the bloodstream, resulting in altered coagulation. Disseminated intravascular coagulation (DIC) involves hypercoagulation of the blood, with consumption of clotting factors and the development of microthrombi.

Shock in acute pancreatitis results from peripheral vasodilation from the released vasoactive substances and the retroperitoneal loss of protein-rich fluid from proteolytic digestion. Hypovolemia may result in decreased renal perfusion and acute renal failure. Paralytic (adynamic) ileus results from peritoneal irritation and seepage of pancreatic enzymes into the abdominal cavity.

❓ NCLEX EXAMINATION CHALLENGE

Physiological Integrity

The nurse closely monitors the client with acute pancreatitis for which complication?
A. Duodenal ulcer
B. Infection
C. Pneumonia
D. Heart failure

Etiology and Genetic Risk

In many cases the cause of pancreatitis is not known, but many factors can injure the pancreas. The most common cause is biliary tract disease, with gallstones accounting for almost half of the cases of obstructive pancreatitis (McCance et al., 2014). Acute pancreatitis may occur as a result of trauma from surgical manipulation after biliary tract, pancreatic, gastric, and duodenal procedures, such as cholecystectomy, the Whipple procedure, and partial gastrectomy. The trauma may also occur as a complication of the diagnostic procedure *endoscopic retrograde cholangiopancreatography (ERCP)*, although this rarely occurs.

Other causative factors include:
- Trauma: external (blunt trauma, stab wounds, gunshot wounds [GSWs])
- Pancreatic obstruction: tumors, cysts, or abscesses; abnormal organ structure
- Metabolic disturbances: hyperlipidemia, hyperparathyroidism, or hypercalcemia
- Renal disturbances: failure or transplantation
- Familial, inherited pancreatitis
- Penetrating gastric or duodenal ulcers, resulting in peritonitis
- Viral infections, such as coxsackievirus B and human immune deficiency virus [HIV] infection
- Alcoholism
- Toxicities of drugs, including opiates, sulfonamides, thiazides, steroids, and oral contraceptives (less common)
- Cigarette smoking
- Cystic fibrosis

- Gallstones
- Abdominal surgery

Incidence and Prevalence

Pancreatic "attacks" are especially common during holidays and vacations when alcohol consumption may be high, especially in men. Women are affected most often after cholelithiasis and biliary tract problems. They are also most at risk for pancreatitis within several months after childbirth.

Death occurs in a small percentage of patients with acute pancreatitis, but with early diagnosis and treatment, mortality can be reduced. It occurs at a higher rate in *older adults* and in patients with postoperative pancreatitis. The prognosis for recovery is usually good for pancreatitis associated with biliary tract disease and poor if pancreatitis accompanies alcoholism.

❖ PATIENT-CENTERED COLLABORATIVE CARE

◆ Assessment

History. Most often the patient reports severe and constant abdominal pain. Conduct the interview *after pain is controlled.* Ask whether the abdominal PAIN occurs when drinking alcohol or eating a high-fat meal. Obtain information about alcohol usage, including the amount of alcohol consumed during what period of time (i.e., years of consumption, how much usually consumed over a particular period). Question the patient about a family or personal history of alcoholism, pancreatitis, trauma, or biliary tract disease. Ask whether any abdominal surgical interventions, such as cholecystectomy, or diagnostic procedures, such as ERCP, have been performed recently.

Ask about other medical problems known to cause pancreatitis, including peptic ulcer disease, renal failure, vascular disorders, hyperparathyroidism, and hyperlipidemia. Inquire about recent viral infections. Ask the patient or family member to list all prescription and over-the-counter (OTC) drugs taken recently, including nutritional and herbal supplements.

Physical Assessment/Clinical Manifestations. The diagnosis of pancreatitis is made based on the clinical presentation combined with the results of diagnostic studies—both laboratory and imaging assessments. Clinical manifestations of acute pancreatitis vary widely and depend on the severity of the inflammation. Typically, a patient is diagnosed after presenting with severe abdominal PAIN in the mid-epigastric area or left upper quadrant. Assess the intensity and quality of pain. The patient often states that the pain had a sudden onset and radiates to the back, left flank, or left shoulder. The pain is described as intense, **boring** (feeling that it is going through the body), and continuous and is worsened by lying in the supine position. Often the patient finds relief by assuming the fetal position (with the knees drawn up to the chest and the spine flexed) or by sitting upright and bending forward. He or she may report weight loss resulting from nausea and vomiting. Obtain the patient's weight.

When performing an abdominal assessment, inspect for:
- Generalized jaundice
- Gray-blue discoloration of the abdomen and periumbilical area
- Gray-blue discoloration of the flanks, caused by pancreatic enzyme leakage to cutaneous tissue from the peritoneal cavity

Listen for bowel sounds; absent or decreased bowel sounds usually indicate paralytic (adynamic) ileus. On light palpation, note abdominal tenderness, rigidity, and guarding as a result of peritonitis. A palpable mass may be found if a pancreatic pseudocyst is present. Pancreatic ascites creates a dull sound on percussion.

Monitor and record vital signs frequently to assess for elevated temperature, tachycardia, and decreased blood pressure, or delegate and supervise this activity. Respiratory problems, such as left lung pleural effusions, atelectasis, and pneumonia, are common in patients with acute pancreatitis. Auscultate the lung fields for adventitious sounds or diminished breath sounds, and observe for dyspnea or orthopnea.

! NURSING SAFETY PRIORITY (QSEN)

Critical Rescue

For the patient with acute pancreatitis, monitor for significant changes in vital signs that may indicate the life-threatening complication of shock. Hypotension and tachycardia may result from pancreatic hemorrhage, excessive fluid volume shifting, or the toxic effects of abdominal sepsis from enzyme damage. Observe the patient for changes in behavior and level of consciousness (LOC) that may be related to alcohol withdrawal, hypoxia, or impending sepsis with shock.

Psychosocial Assessment. If excessive alcohol is a causative factor, tactfully explore the patient's alcohol intake history. Provide patient privacy, and establish a trusting relationship. Discuss the intake of alcohol and the reasons for overindulging. Using the CAGE questionnaire to assist with determining alcohol use may be beneficial. Ask him or her when increased drinking episodes occur and, in particular, whether binges occur during holidays, vacations, or weekends or revolve around particular activities, such as television viewing. Question the patient about any recent traumatic or stressful event that may have contributed to increased alcohol consumption, such as the death of a family member or a job loss.

Laboratory Assessment. Diagnostic laboratory abnormalities are typical in patients with acute pancreatitis (Table 59-4).

TABLE 59-4   Causes of Diagnostic Laboratory Abnormalities in Acute Pancreatitis

ABNORMAL FINDING	CAUSE
Cardinal Diagnostic Tests	
Increased *serum* amylase	Pancreatic cell injury
Elevated *serum* lipase	Pancreatic cell injury
Elevated *serum* trypsin	Pancreatic cell injury
Elevated *serum* elastase	Pancreatic cell injury
Other Diagnostic Tests	
Elevated serum glucose	Pancreatic cell injury, resulting in impaired carbohydrate metabolism; decreased insulin release
Decreased serum calcium and magnesium	Fatty acids combined with calcium; seen in fat necrosis
Elevated bilirubin	Hepatobiliary obstructive process
Elevated alanine aminotransferase (ALT)	Hepatobiliary involvement
Elevated aspartate aminotransferase (AST)	Hepatobiliary involvement
Elevated leukocyte count	Inflammatory response

A variety of pancreatic and non-pancreatic disorders can cause increased serum amylase levels. In patients with pancreatitis, *amylase* levels usually increase within 12 to 24 hours and remain elevated for 2 to 3 days. Persistent elevations may be an indicator of pancreatic abscess or pseudocyst (Pagana & Pagana, 2014).

Lipase also helps determine the presence of acute pancreatitis. Serum levels may rise later than amylase and remain elevated for up to 2 weeks. Because these levels stay elevated for such a long time, the health care provider may find this test useful in diagnosing patients who are not examined until several days after the initial onset of symptoms. An increase in lipase and amylase in the urine is also expected (Pagana & Pagana, 2014).

If pancreatitis is accompanied by biliary dysfunction (biliary pancreatitis), serum *bilirubin* and *alkaline phosphatase* levels are usually elevated. A sensitive indicator of biliary obstruction in acute pancreatitis is serum *alanine aminotransferase (ALT)*. A threefold or greater rise in concentration indicates that the diagnosis of acute biliary pancreatitis is valid. Elevated *white blood cell (WBC) count and differential, erythrocyte sedimentation rate (ESR)*, and serum *glucose* levels are also common in acute pancreatitis. The levels often correlate with disease severity.

Decreased serum *calcium* and *magnesium* levels are seen with fat necrosis. Calcium levels may fall and remain decreased for 7 to 10 days. Those that consistently remain below 8 mg/dL are associated with a poor prognosis. Other tests include the basic metabolic panel (BMP), complete blood count (CBC), triglycerides, serum total protein, and albumin. The blood urea nitrogen (BUN), serum glucose, and triglycerides are usually elevated. Hemoconcentration is common as a result of third-space fluid loss. Leukocytosis (elevated WBCs) and thrombocytopenia (decreased platelets) are common (Pagana & Pagana, 2014). Albumin levels are decreased because cytokines (e.g., tumor necrosis factor [TNF]) released as part of the inflammatory response allow it to move from the bloodstream into the extravascular space. The presence of C-reactive protein suggests possible pancreatic INFLAMMATION and necrosis.

Imaging Assessment. Abdominal ultrasound is the most sensitive test to diagnose causes of pancreatitis, such as gallstones, and can be performed at the bedside. However, it is not helpful in viewing the pancreas because of overlying bowel gas. Therefore *contrast-enhanced computed tomography (CT)* provides a more reliable image and diagnosis of acute pancreatitis. This noninvasive technique may also be used to rule out pancreatic pseudocyst or ductal calculi.

An abdominal x-ray may also reveal gallstones. A chest x-ray may show elevation of the left side of the diaphragm or pleural effusion. Pancreatic stones are best diagnosed through ERCP.

◆ Analysis

The priority NANDA-I nursing diagnoses and collaborative problems for patients with acute pancreatitis include:

1. Acute Pain related to pancreatic inflammation and enzyme leakage (NANDA-I)
2. Inadequate nutrition related to the inability to ingest food and absorb nutrients

◆ Planning and Implementation

Managing Acute Pain

Planning: Expected Outcomes. The patient with acute pancreatitis is expected to state that he or she has a decrease in or absence of abdominal PAIN, as evidenced by a pain intensity scale measurement.

Interventions. The priorities for patient care are to provide supportive care by relieving symptoms, to decrease INFLAMMATION, and to anticipate or treat complications. *As for any patient, continually assess for and support the ABCs (**a**irway, **b**reathing, and **c**irculation).* In collaboration with the respiratory therapist, if available, provide oxygen and other respiratory support as needed. The collaborative plan of care depends on the severity of the illness.

Abdominal pain is the most common symptom of pancreatitis. The main focus of nursing care is aimed at controlling PAIN by interventions that decrease GI tract activity, thus decreasing pancreatic stimulation. Pain assessment to measure the effectiveness of these interventions is an essential part of nursing care.

Nonsurgical Management. *Mild* pancreatitis requires hydration with IV fluids, pain control, and drug therapy. The health care team initially attempts to relieve pain with nonsurgical interventions, which include fasting and rest, drug therapy, and comfort measures. If the patient has a life-threatening complication or requires frequent assessment, he or she is admitted to a critical care unit for invasive hemodynamic monitoring.

To rest the pancreas and reduce pancreatic enzyme secretion, withhold food and fluids (NPO) during the acute period. The health care provider prescribes IV isotonic fluid administration to maintain hydration. IV replacement of calcium and magnesium may also be needed. Measure and document intake and output. Some patients have an indwelling urinary catheter to obtain accurate measurements.

Nasogastric drainage and suction are reserved for more *severely ill* patients who have continuous vomiting or biliary obstruction. Gastric decompression using a nasogastric tube (NGT) prevents gastric juices from flowing into the duodenum.

> ⚠ **NURSING SAFETY PRIORITY** (QSEN)
>
> **Action Alert**
>
> Because paralytic (adynamic) ileus is a common complication of acute pancreatitis, prolonged nasogastric intubation may be necessary. Assess frequently for the return of peristalsis by asking the patient if he or she has passed flatus or had a stool. The return of bowel sounds is not reliable as an indicator of peristalsis return; passage of flatus or a bowel movement is the most reliable indicator. See the discussion of intestinal obstructions in Chapter 57 on p. 1157.

To decrease PAIN, the primary drug class used is opioid. Other drugs may also be prescribed. Pain management for acute pancreatitis typically begins with the administration of opioids by patient-controlled analgesia (PCA). Drugs such as morphine or hydromorphone (Dilaudid) are typically used because meperidine (Demerol) can cause seizures, especially in older adults. Other options that have been used successfully to manage acute pain include IV or transdermal fentanyl and epidural analgesia.

In *mild* pancreatitis, the pain usually subsides in 2 to 3 days. However, with *severe* acute pancreatitis, the abdominal pain and tenderness may persist for up to 2 weeks. The dosages and intervals of drug administration are individualized according to the severity of the disease and the symptoms.

Histamine receptor antagonists (e.g., ranitidine [Zantac]) and proton pump inhibitors (e.g., omeprazole [Prilosec]) help decrease gastric acid secretion. Antibiotics may be used, but they are indicated primarily for patients with acute necrotizing pancreatitis. The health care provider will prescribe appropriate antibiotics, if needed.

Helping the patient assume a side-lying position (with the legs drawn up to the chest) may decrease the abdominal PAIN of pancreatitis ("fetal position"). Sitting with the knees flexed toward the chest is also helpful.

If the patient is NPO or has an NGT, remind assistive nursing personnel to implement frequent oral and nares hygiene measures to keep mucous membranes moist and free of INFLAMMATION or crusting. Because of the drying effect of drugs and the absence of oral fluids, the mouth and oral cavity may be extremely dry, resulting in considerable discomfort and possibly parotitis (inflammation of the parotid [salivary] glands).

> ⚠ **NURSING SAFETY PRIORITY** (QSEN)
>
> **Action Alert**
>
> For the patient with acute pancreatitis, monitor his or her respiratory status every 4 to 8 hours or more often as needed, and provide oxygen to promote comfort in breathing. Respiratory complications such as pleural effusions increase patient discomfort. Fluid overload can be detected by assessing for weight gain, listening for crackles, and observing for dyspnea. Carefully monitor for signs of respiratory failure.
>
> Observe for signs and symptoms of hypocalcemia by assessing for Chvostek's and Trousseau's signs. These tests cause muscle spasms after stimulating the associated nerves. Chapter 11 discusses assessment and interventions for patients with hypocalcemia in more detail.

Lowering the patient's anxiety level may also substantially reduce pain. Explain all procedures and other aspects of patient care thoroughly. Provide reassurance, offer diversional activities such as music and reading material, and encourage visitors to direct attention away from the pain.

If pancreatitis was caused by gallstones, an ERCP with a **sphincterotomy** (opening of the sphincter of Oddi) may be performed on an urgent or emergent basis. If this procedure is not successful, surgery is required. ERCP is described in detail in Chapter 52.

Surgical Management. Surgical intervention for acute pancreatitis is usually not indicated. However, if an ERCP is not successful in removing gallstones, a laparoscopic cholecystectomy may be performed as described on p. 1217 in the discussion of Surgical Management in the Cholecystitis section.

Complications of pancreatitis, such as pancreatic pseudocyst and abscess, may also require surgical intervention. Laparoscopy (minimally invasive surgery [MIS]) may be done to drain an abscess or pseudocyst. For patients who are high surgical risks, pseudocysts or abscesses can be treated by percutaneous drainage under CT guidance.

Promoting Nutrition

Planning: Expected Outcomes. The patient with acute pancreatitis is expected to have adequate NUTRITION to meet his or her metabolic needs.

Interventions. The patient is maintained on NPO status in the early stages of pancreatitis. Antiemetics for nausea and vomiting are prescribed as needed. Patients who have severe pancreatitis and are unable to eat for 24 to 48 hours after illness onset may begin jejunal tube feeding unless paralytic ileus is present. *Early* NUTRITIONAL intervention enhances immune system functioning and may prevent complications and worsening inflammation. Enteral feeding is preferred over total parenteral nutrition (TPN) because it causes fewer episodes of glucose elevation and other complications associated with TPN. Be sure that the patient is weighed every day. Collaborate with the health care provider, dietitian, and pharmacist to plan and implement the most appropriate nutritional intervention. Chapter 60 describes collaborative care of patients receiving enteral feeding and TPN.

When food is tolerated during the healing phase, the health care provider prescribes small, frequent, moderate- to high-carbohydrate, high-protein, low-fat meals. Foods should be bland with little spice. GI stimulants such as caffeine-containing foods (tea, coffee, cola, and chocolate), as well as alcohol, should be avoided. Monitor the patient beginning to resume oral food intake for nausea, vomiting, and diarrhea. *If any of these symptoms occur, notify the health care provider immediately.*

To boost caloric intake, commercial liquid nutritional preparations supplement the diet. The health care provider may also prescribe fat-soluble and other vitamin and mineral replacement supplements. Glutamine, omega-3 fatty acids, fiber, antioxidants, and/or nucleotides may be added to the patient's nutrition plan.

Community-Based Care

Home care preparation is individualized for each patient's circumstances. Some patients may be severely weakened from their acute illness and need to confine activity to one floor, limiting stair climbing and other strenuous activities until they regain their strength. Collaborate with the case manager to plan the best place for the patient to recover and resources that may be needed.

Education needs to be started early in the hospitalization period—as soon as the acute episodes of pain have subsided. Assess the patient's and family's knowledge of the disease.

The desired outcomes for discharge planning and education are to avoid further episodes of pancreatitis and prevent progression to a chronic disease. If the patient uses alcohol, instruct him or her to abstain from drinking to prevent further pain attacks and extension of inflammation and pancreatic insufficiency. Tell the patient that if alcohol is consumed, acute PAIN will return and further autodigestion of the pancreas may lead to chronic pancreatitis.

Teach the patient to notify the health care provider after discharge to home if acute abdominal PAIN or biliary tract disease (as evidenced by jaundice, clay-colored stools, or darkened urine) occurs. These signs and symptoms are possible indicators of complications or disease progression.

Patients with acute pancreatitis may require several visits by a home care nurse if the hospital course was complicated. In these cases, home care may be needed for wound care and assistance with ADLs. The patient requires medical follow-up with the primary care physician or nurse practitioner to monitor the disease process. For those with alcoholism, provide information about groups such as Alcoholics Anonymous (AA).

Family members may attend support groups such as Al-Anon and Alateen.

◆ *Evaluation: Outcomes*

Evaluate the care of the patient with acute pancreatitis based on the identified priority patient problems. The expected outcomes include that the patient will:
- Have control of abdominal PAIN, as indicated by self-report
- Have adequate NUTRITION available to meet metabolic needs

? CLINICAL JUDGMENT CHALLENGE

Patient-Centered Care; Evidence-Based Practice; Teamwork and Collaboration; Informatics **QSEN**

A 78-year-old man is admitted from home to the medical unit with acute pancreatitis secondary to a history of gallstones, hypertension, osteoarthritis, and type 2 diabetes mellitus. He has lost 20 pounds (9 kg) in the past 2 months and reports severe boring-like abdominal pain, fatigue, and weakness. On physical assessment, he has decreased bowel sounds in all quadrants, crackles in the bases of his lungs, and signs of dehydration. Vital signs are: T, 100° F; P, 110; R, 36; and BP, 102/58.

What is the priority for this patient's care at this time? What current evidence supports your answer? Where would you look for current evidence that would help you answer this question? (Be specific in your answer.)

1. What laboratory findings would you expect him to have? Why?
2. With whom should you collaborate to meet the desired outcomes for his care?
3. What community support and health teaching is he going to require when he is discharged?

CHRONIC PANCREATITIS

❖ *PATHOPHYSIOLOGY*

Chronic pancreatitis is a progressive, destructive disease of the pancreas that has remissions and exacerbations ("flare-ups"). INFLAMMATION and fibrosis of the tissue contribute to pancreatic insufficiency and diminished function of the organ.

Chronic pancreatitis can be classified into several categories. *Alcoholism* is the primary risk factor for **chronic calcifying pancreatitis (CCP),** the most common type. In the early stages of the disease, pancreatic secretions precipitate as insoluble proteins that plug the pancreatic ducts and flow of pancreatic juices. As the protein plugs become more widespread, the cellular lining of the ducts changes and ulcerates. This inflammatory process causes fibrosis of the pancreatic tissue. Intraductal calcification and marked pancreatic tissue destruction (necrosis) develop in the late stages. The organ becomes hard and firm as a result of cell atrophy and pancreatic insufficiency.

Chronic calcifying pancreatitis is found predominantly in men, but the incidence in women is increasing. In women, chronic pancreatitis occurs more commonly among those with biliary tract disease (cholecystitis and cholelithiasis).

Chronic obstructive pancreatitis develops from INFLAMMATION, spasm, and obstruction of the sphincter of Oddi, often from cholelithiasis (gallstones). Inflammatory and sclerotic lesions occur in the head of the pancreas and around the ducts, causing an obstruction and backflow of pancreatic secretions. (See Complications of Acute Pancreatitis, p. 1219.)

Autoimmune pancreatitis is a chronic inflammatory process in which immunoglobulins invade the pancreas. Other organs may also be infiltrated, including the lungs and liver. Whereas other types of chronic pancreatitis may predispose the patient to pancreatic cancer, there is no evidence that autoimmune pancreatitis is a risk factor (Novotny et al., 2010).

Idiopathic and **hereditary chronic pancreatitis** may be associated with *SPINK1* and *CFTR* gene mutations (Midha et al., 2010). The protein encoded by the *SPINK1* gene is a trypsin inhibitor. The *CFTR* gene is associated with cystic fibrosis. Research on these gene mutations can help develop targeted drug therapy for treatment of these diseases.

Pancreatic insufficiency in any type of chronic pancreatitis causes loss of *exocrine* function. Most patients with chronic pancreatitis have decreased pancreatic secretions and bicarbonate. Pancreatic enzyme secretion must be greatly reduced to produce steatorrhea resulting from severe malabsorption of fats. These characteristic stools are pale, bulky, and frothy and have an offensive odor. The action of colonic bacteria on unabsorbed lipids and proteins is responsible for the extremely foul odor. On inspection of the stools, the fat content is visible. In severe chronic pancreatitis, stool fat output may be more than 40 g/day.

Fat malabsorption also contributes to weight loss and muscle wasting (a decrease in muscle mass) and leads to general debilitation. Protein malabsorption results in a "starvation" edema of the feet, legs, and hands caused by decreased levels of circulating albumin.

The loss of pancreatic *endocrine* function is responsible for the development of diabetes mellitus in patients with chronic pancreatic insufficiency. (See Chapter 64 for a complete discussion of diabetes mellitus.)

The patient with chronic pancreatitis may have pulmonary complications, such as pleuritic pain, pleural effusions, and pulmonary infiltrates. Pancreatic ascites may decrease diaphragmatic excursion and lung expansion, resulting in impaired ventilation. In the ill patient with chronic pancreatitis, acute respiratory distress syndrome (ARDS) may develop.

❖ PATIENT-CENTERED COLLABORATIVE CARE

◆ Assessment

Many of the clinical manifestations of chronic pancreatitis differ from those of an acute INFLAMMATION. Abdominal PAIN is the major clinical manifestation for most types of pancreatitis (Chart 59-2). For those with chronic pancreatitis, pain is typically described as a continuous burning or gnawing dullness with periods of acute exacerbation (flare-ups). The pain is very intense and relentless. The frequency of acute exacerbations may increase as the pancreatic fibrosis develops.

Perform an abdominal assessment. Abdominal tenderness is less intense in patients with chronic pancreatitis than in those with acute pancreatitis. A mass may be palpated in the left upper quadrant, which may suggest a pancreatic pseudocyst or abscess. Massive pancreatic ascites may be present, producing dullness on abdominal percussion. Because respiratory complications can occur, auscultate the lung fields for adventitious sounds or decreased aeration and observe for dyspnea or orthopnea.

Ask the patient to collect a random stool specimen if able, or ask him or her to describe the stools. The specimen may show **steatorrhea** (foul-smelling fatty stools that may increase in volume as pancreatic insufficiency progresses and lipase production decreases). Assess for unintentional weight loss, muscle wasting, jaundice, dark urine, and the manifestations of diabetes mellitus, such as polyuria (increased urinary output), polydipsia (excessive thirst), and polyphagia (increased appetite).

Diagnosis is based on the patient's clinical manifestations and laboratory and imaging assessment. *Endoscopic retrograde cholangiopancreatography* (ERCP) is done to visualize the pancreatic and common bile ducts. *Imaging studies* such as CT scanning, contrast-enhanced MRI, abdominal ultrasound (US), and endoscopic ultrasound (EUS) are also useful in making the diagnosis. In chronic pancreatitis, laboratory findings include normal or moderately elevated serum *amylase* and *lipase* levels. Obstruction of the intrahepatic bile duct can cause elevated serum *bilirubin* and *alkaline phosphatase* levels. Intermittent elevations in serum *glucose* levels are common and can be detected by blood glucose monitoring, both fasting and non-fasting.

◆ Interventions

The focus of caring for the patient with chronic pancreatitis is to manage PAIN, assist in maintaining sufficient NUTRITION, and prevent recurrence.

Nonsurgical Management. Nonsurgical interventions include primarily drug and NUTRITION therapy. The major intervention for the PAIN of chronic pancreatitis is drug therapy. Medicate the patient as prescribed according to the assessment of the intensity of pain. Evaluate the effectiveness of the drug intervention. Opioid analgesia is most frequently used initially, but dependency may occur. Non-opioid analgesics may be tried to relieve pain. (See Chapter 3 for other interventions for chronic pain.)

Pancreatic-enzyme replacement therapy (PERT) is the standard of care to prevent malnutrition, malabsorption, and excessive weight loss (Chart 59-3). Pancrelipase is usually prescribed in capsule or tablet form and contains varying amounts of amylase, lipase, and protease. Teach patients not to chew or crush pancrelipase delayed-release capsules (Creon) or enteric tablets, and teach them to take the medications with all meals and snacks.

The dosage of pancreatic enzymes depends on the severity of the malabsorption. Record the number and consistency of stools per day to monitor the effectiveness of enzyme therapy. If pancreatic enzyme treatment is effective, the stools should become less frequent and less fatty.

CHART 59-2 **Key Features**

Chronic Pancreatitis

- Intense abdominal pain (major clinical manifestation) that is continuous and burning or gnawing
- Abdominal tenderness
- Ascites
- Possible left upper quadrant mass (if pseudocyst or abscess is present)
- Respiratory compromise manifested by adventitious or diminished breath sounds, dyspnea, or orthopnea
- Steatorrhea; clay-colored stools
- Weight loss
- Jaundice
- Dark urine
- Polyuria, polydipsia, polyphagia (diabetes mellitus)

! NURSING SAFETY PRIORITY (QSEN)

Action Alert

If the patient has diabetes, the health care provider prescribes insulin or oral hypoglycemic agents for glucose control. Patients maintained on total parenteral nutrition (TPN) are particularly susceptible to elevated glucose levels and usually require regular insulin additives to the solution. Closely monitor blood glucose so that hyperglycemia is controlled. Check finger-stick blood glucose (FSBG) or sugar (FSBS) levels every 2 to 4 hours. Chapter 60 describes in detail the care associated with TPN.

The health care provider may also prescribe drug therapy to decrease gastric acid. Gastric acid destroys the lipase needed to break down fats. Controlling the acidity of the stomach with H_2 blockers or proton pump inhibitors or neutralizing stomach acid with oral sodium bicarbonate may enhance the effectiveness of PERT.

Protein and fat malabsorption result in significant weight loss and decreased muscle mass in the patient with chronic pancreatitis. Therefore the nutritional interventions for acute pancreatitis are also used for chronic pancreatitis. The patient often limits food intake to avoid increased pain. For this reason, nutrition maintenance is often difficult to achieve. Patients receive either total parenteral nutrition (TPN) or total enteral nutrition (TEN), including vitamin and mineral replacement.

Collaborate with the dietitian to teach the patient about long-term dietary management. He or she needs an increased number of calories, up to 4000 to 6000 calories/day, to maintain weight. Those foods high in carbohydrates and protein also assist in the healing process. Foods high in fat are avoided because they cause or increase diarrhea. Teach all patients to avoid alcohol. Alcohol-cessation programs may be recommended.

Surgical Management. Surgery is not a primary intervention for the treatment of chronic pancreatitis. However, it may be indicated for ongoing abdominal PAIN, incapacitating relapses of pain, or complications such as abscesses and pseudocysts.

The underlying pathologic changes determine the procedure indicated. Using laparoscopy, the surgeon incises and drains an abscess or pseudocyst. Laparoscopic cholecystectomy or choledochotomy (incision of the common bile duct) may be indicated if biliary tract disease is an underlying cause of pancreatitis. If the pancreatic duct sphincter is fibrotic, the surgeon performs a sphincterotomy (incision of the sphincter) to enlarge it. Endoscopic sphincterotomy may be used for patients who are poor surgical candidates.

In some cases laparoscopic distal pancreatectomy may be appropriate for resection of the distal pancreas or pancreas head. Endoscopic pancreatic necrosectomy and natural orifice transluminal endoscopic surgery (NOTES) are becoming more common for removing necrosed pancreatic tissue. Both procedures are performed through the GI wall without a visible skin incision. The NOTES procedure is discussed in Surgical Management on p. 1217 in the Cholecystitis section.

In a few cases, pancreas transplantation may be done. However, this procedure is performed most often for patients with severe, uncontrolled diabetes. Chapter 64 discusses pancreas transplantation.

Community-Based Care

Collaborate with the hospital-based case manager (CM) or discharge planner about home care or follow-up in another setting. A community-based CM may continue to follow the patient after hospital discharge. If the patient is discharged to home, the living area should be limited to one floor until he or she regains strength and can increase activity. Teach patients and families that toilet facilities must be easily accessible because of chronic steatorrhea and frequent defecation. If they are not easily accessible, a bedside commode is obtained for the home.

Because there is no known cure for chronic pancreatitis, patient and family education is aimed at preventing acute episodes of the disease, providing long-term care, and promoting health maintenance (Chart 59-4). Teach the patient to avoid known irritating substances, such as caffeinated beverages (stimulates the GI system) and alcohol. Collaborate with the dietitian in diet teaching, which focuses on eating bland, low-fat, frequent meals and avoiding rich, fatty foods. Stress the importance of adhering to the nutritional recommendations. Written instructions are essential, with consideration of personal and cultural food preferences.

Remind the patient and family members or significant others of the importance of adhering to pancreatic enzyme replacement. The patient must take the prescribed enzymes with meals and snacks to aid in the digestion of food and promote the absorption of fats and proteins. Teach the patient to take the enzymes before or at the beginning of the meal. Instruct him or her to report any increase in abdominal distention, cramping, and foul-smelling, frothy, fatty stools to the health care provider so that these supplements may be increased as needed. Remind the patient to report any skin breakdown so that therapeutic interventions to promote skin integrity can be started. Abdominal fistulas are common and present a difficult challenge because pancreatic secretions irritate the skin.

The frequency of defecation (whether continent or incontinent) poses challenging skin care problems. Instruct the patient to keep the skin dry and free of the abrasive fatty stools, which damage the skin. The skin should be cleaned thoroughly after each stool and a moisture barrier applied to prevent breakdown and maintain skin integrity. Many products on the market actively repel stool from the skin.

If the patient develops diabetes mellitus as a result of chronic pancreatitis, management of elevated glucose levels after discharge from the hospital may require oral antidiabetic agents or insulin injections. If this is the case, collaborate with the certified diabetic educator (CDE) to provide in-depth teaching concerning diabetes, its signs and symptoms, medical management, drug therapy, nutrition therapy, blood glucose monitoring, and general care.

Chronic illnesses are devastating for families. The high costs of medical insurance, medical treatment, and drug therapy cause serious financial problems. Often the patient with chronic pancreatitis is unable to work. Collaborate with the CM about ways to assist the patient with resources for financial help.

The patient may require several home visits by nurses, depending on the severity of the chronic health problems and home maintenance and support needs. The nurse assesses the patient for PAIN, enzyme therapy, and psychosocial adaptation to a chronic illness. Refer him or her and the family to a counselor or a self-help group, such as Alcoholics Anonymous (www.aa.org) and Al-Anon (www.al-anon.org), if appropriate.

? NCLEX EXAMINATION CHALLENGE

Physiological Integrity

Which foods will the nurse teach the client with chronic pancreatitis to avoid? **Select all that apply.**
A. Blueberries
B. Green beans
C. Bacon
D. Baked fish
E. Fried potatoes

PANCREATIC ABSCESS

Pancreatic abscesses are the most serious complication of acute necrotizing pancreatitis. If untreated, they are always fatal. After surgery, the recurrence rate is high. The abscesses form from collections of purulent liquefaction of the necrotic pancreas.

Patients with pancreatic abscesses often appear more seriously ill than those with pseudocysts. Clinical manifestations are similar. However, the temperature in patients with abscesses may spike to as high as 104°F (40°C). Drainage via the percutaneous method or laparoscopy should be performed as soon as possible to prevent sepsis. Antibiotic treatment alone does

not resolve the abscess. Death rates remain high even after surgical drainage. Many patients require multiple drainage procedures for repeated abscesses.

PANCREATIC PSEUDOCYST

❖ *PATHOPHYSIOLOGY*

Pancreatic pseudocysts, or false cysts, are so named because, unlike true cysts, they do not have an epithelial lining. They are encapsulated, saclike structures that form on or surround the pancreas. The pseudocyst wall is inflamed, vascular, and fibrotic. It may contain up to several liters of straw-colored or dark brown viscous fluid, the enzymatic exudate of the pancreas (McCance et al., 2014). Risk factors for pseudocysts are acute pancreatitis, abdominal trauma, and chronic pancreatitis.

❖ *PATIENT-CENTERED COLLABORATIVE CARE*

◆ *Assessment*

A pseudocyst can be palpated as an epigastric mass in about half of all cases. The primary presenting symptom is epigastric pain radiating to the back. Other common clinical manifestations include abdominal fullness, nausea, vomiting, and jaundice. Pseudocysts are diagnosed and their growth and resolution monitored by serial pancreatic diagnostic testing. Complications of pseudocyst formation include:
- Hemorrhage
- Infection
- Obstruction of the bowel, biliary tract, or splenic vein
- Abscess
- Fistula formation
- Pancreatic ascites

◆ *Interventions*

Pseudocysts may spontaneously resolve, or they may rupture and produce hemorrhage. Surgical intervention is necessary if the pseudocyst does not resolve within 6 to 8 weeks or if complications develop. To provide external drainage, the surgeon inserts a sump drainage tube to remove pancreatic secretions and exudate. Pancreatic fistulas are common after surgery, and skin breakdown from corrosive pancreatic enzymes in patients who have external drainage presents a major nursing care challenge.

PANCREATIC CANCER

❖ *PATHOPHYSIOLOGY*

Cancer of the pancreas is a leading cause of cancer deaths each year in the United States. It is difficult to diagnose early because the pancreas is hidden and surrounded by other organs. Treatment has limited results, and 5-year survival rates are low (American Cancer Society [ACS], 2013).

Pancreatic tumors usually originate from epithelial cells of the pancreatic ductal system. If the tumor is discovered in the early stages, the tumor cells may be localized within the glandular organ. However, this is highly unlikely. Most often, the tumor is discovered in the late stages of development and may be a well-defined mass or is diffusely spread throughout the pancreas.

The tumor may be a primary cancer, or it may result from metastasis from cancers of the lung, breast, thyroid, kidney, or skin. Primary tumors are generally adenocarcinomas and grow in well-differentiated glandular patterns. They grow rapidly and spread to surrounding organs (stomach, duodenum, gallbladder, and intestine) by direct extension and invasion of lymphatic and vascular systems. This highly metastatic lesion may eventually invade the lung, peritoneum, liver, spleen, and lymph nodes.

Clinical manifestations depend on the site of origin or metastasis. The head of the pancreas is the most common site. The tumors are usually small lesions with poorly defined margins. Jaundice results from tumor compression and obstruction of the common bile duct and from gallbladder dilation, causing the organ to enlarge.

Cancers of the body and tail of the pancreas are usually large and invade the entire tail and body. These tumors may be palpable abdominal masses, especially in the thin patient. Through metastatic spread via the splenic vein, metastasis to the liver may cause **hepatomegaly** (enlargement of the liver up to 2 to 3 times its normal size). Cancers of the body and tail spread more extensively than do pancreatic head carcinomas, with invasion of the retroperitoneum, vertebral column, spleen, adrenal glands, colon, or stomach. Regardless of where it originates, it spreads rapidly through the lymphatic and venous systems to other organs.

Venous thromboembolism is a common complication of pancreatic cancer. Necrotic products of the pancreatic tumor are believed to have thromboplastic properties resulting in the blood's hypercoagulable state. In addition, the patient is at high risk because of decreased mobility and extensive surgical manipulation.

The exact cause of pancreatic cancer is unknown. High-risk populations are those in their sixth to eighth decades of life and those with a personal history of smoking.

GENETIC/GENOMIC CONSIDERATIONS
Patient-Centered Care QSEN

A small number of those with pancreatic cancer have an inherited risk. Mutations in certain oncogenes have been identified. Mutations have also been revealed in tumor suppressor genes, such as *p16* and *BRCA2*—the same mutation that makes some women susceptible to breast and ovarian cancer. Genes responsible for hereditary nonpolyposis colorectal cancer can also increase a person's risk for pancreatic cancer (ACS, 2013).

Other risk factors associated with the disease include:
- Diabetes mellitus
- Chronic pancreatitis
- Cirrhosis
- High intake of red meat, especially processed meat like steak
- Long-term exposure to chemicals such as gasoline and pesticides
- Obesity
- Older age
- Male gender
- Cigarette smoking
- Family history
- Genetic syndromes

CHART 59-5 Key Features
Pancreatic Cancer

- Jaundice
- Clay-colored (light) stools
- Dark urine
- Abdominal pain: usually vague, dull, or nonspecific that radiates into the back
- Weight loss
- Anorexia
- Nausea or vomiting
- Glucose intolerance
- Splenomegaly (enlarged spleen)
- Flatulence
- Gastrointestinal bleeding
- Ascites (abdominal fluid)
- Leg or calf pain (from thrombophlebitis)
- Weakness and fatigue

❖ PATIENT-CENTERED COLLABORATIVE CARE
◆ Assessment

Pancreatic cancer often presents in a slow and vague manner. The presenting symptoms depend somewhat on the location of the tumor. The first sign may be jaundice, which suggests late, advanced disease (Chart 59-5). Jaundice occurs because the gallbladder and liver are commonly involved. As the tumor spreads, the yellow skin color associated with obstructive jaundice progressively worsens. Ask the patient whether the color of the stool and urine has changed. As a result of the obstructive process, the stool is clay colored and the urine is dark and frothy. Inspect the skin for dryness and scratch marks, indicating pruritus from jaundice caused by bile salt collection. Assess the sclera for icterus (yellowing) and the mucous membranes for signs of jaundice.

The enlarged gallbladder and liver may be palpable. In advanced cases of pancreatic carcinoma, the tumor may be felt as a firm, fixed mass in the left upper abdominal quadrant or epigastric region.

The most common concern is fatigue, which is described as a diminished energy level and an increased need for rest relative to the level of activity. The patient notices an inability to perform usual physical or intellectual activities.

Question the patient about abdominal PAIN, which is usually described as a vague, constant dullness in the upper abdomen and nonspecific in nature. Pain also indicates advanced stages of the disease and may be related to eating or activity. Ask whether the patient has pain in other areas of the body. Referred back pain may be caused by pressure on the nerve plexus. Some patients have leg or calf pain with swelling and redness as a result of deep vein thrombosis or thrombophlebitis.

Weigh the patient to determine the extent of weight loss and whether it has occurred rapidly. Ask about food intake and intolerances. Anorexia accompanied by early satiety, nausea, flatulence (gas), and vomiting is common. GI bleeding may develop from esophageal or gastric varices caused by the tumor pressing on the portal vein. A new diagnosis of diabetes is found in some patients.

In addition to the focused history, perform a general abdominal assessment. In particular, observe for distention and swelling, which may be **ascites** (abdominal fluid). Percussion over the ascitic abdomen elicits dullness, seen in the advanced stages of the disease process.

No specific blood tests diagnose pancreatic cancer. Serum *amylase* and *lipase* levels, as well as *alkaline phosphatase* and *bilirubin* levels, are increased. The degree of elevation depends on the acuteness or chronicity of the pancreatic and biliary damage. Elevated *carcinoembryonic antigen* (CEA) levels occur in most patients with pancreatic cancer. This test may provide early information about the presence of tumor cells. Other tumor markers such as CA 19-9 and CA 242 have been found to be useful serologic tests for monitoring a proven diagnosis and for continuing surveillance for potential spread or recurrence (Pagana & Pagana, 2014).

Abdominal *ultrasound* and *contrast-enhanced CT* are the most commonly used imaging techniques for confirming a tumor and can differentiate the tumor from a cyst. Endoscopic ultrasonography can also be performed to sample tissue for diagnosis and provide information on tumor type and size (Tonolini et al., 2012). Contrast harmonic echo-endoscopic ultrasound increases the accuracy of diagnosing solid pancreatic masses (Fusaroli et al., 2010).

Endoscopic retrograde cholangiopancreatography (ERCP) also provides visual diagnostic data. An alternative to ERCP is a percutaneous transhepatic biliary cholangiogram with placement of a percutaneous transhepatic biliary drain (PTBD). This drain decompresses the blocked biliary system by draining bile, either internally, externally, or both. Aspiration of pancreatic ascitic fluid by abdominal paracentesis may reveal cancer cells and elevated amylase levels.

◆ Interventions

Management of the patient with pancreatic cancer is geared toward preventing tumor spread and decreasing pain. These measures are not curative, only palliative. The cancers are often metastatic and recur despite treatment.

Nonsurgical Management. As in other types of cancer, chemotherapy or radiation is used to relieve pain by shrinking the tumor. It may be used before, after, or instead of surgery. *Chemotherapy* has had limited success in increasing survival time. In most cases, combining agents has been more successful than single-agent chemotherapy. 5-Fluorouracil (5-FU), a commonly used drug, may be given alone or with gemcitabine (Gemzar) for locally advanced, or unresectable, pancreatic cancers. Gemcitabine may also be given with capecitabine (Xeloda), docetaxel (Taxotere), and/or erlotinib (Tarceva), a targeted agent for unresectable or metastatic tumors. Some patients receive three or four drugs and have had more tumor shrinkage as a result. Observe for adverse drug effects, such as fatigue, rash, anorexia, and diarrhea. Chapter 22 discusses nursing implications of chemotherapy in more detail.

Other targeted therapies being investigated include growth factor inhibitors, anti-angiogenesis factors, and kinase inhibitors (also known as *tyrosine kinase inhibitors*). Kinase inhibitors are a newer group of drugs that focus on cancer cells with little or no effect on healthy cells. Chapter 22 describes general nursing interventions associated with chemotherapy.

To control pain, the patient takes high doses of opioid analgesics (usually morphine) as prescribed and uses other comfort measures before the pain escalates and peaks. Because of the poor prognosis, drug dependency is not a consideration. Chapter 3 describes in detail the care of the patient with chronic cancer PAIN.

Intensive external beam *radiation* therapy to the pancreas may offer pain relief by shrinking tumor cells, alleviating obstruction, and improving food absorption. It does not improve survival rates. Implantation of radioactive iodine (^{125}I) seeds, in combination with systemic or intra-arterial administration of floxuridine (FUDR), has also been used. The patient may experience discomfort during and after the radiation treatments. Chapter 22 describes radiation therapy in more detail.

For patients experiencing biliary obstruction who are high surgical risks, biliary stents placed percutaneously (through the skin) can ensure patency to relieve pain. These stents are devices made of plastic materials that keep the ducts of the biliary system open. Using another approach, self-expandable stents may be inserted endoscopically to relieve obstruction.

Surgical Management. Complete surgical resection of the pancreatic tumor offers the patient with pancreatic cancer the only effective treatment, but it is done only in patients with small tumors. *Partial pancreatectomy* is the preferred surgery for tumors smaller than 3 centimeters in diameter (Grützmann et al., 2011). Recent technologic advances have expanded the role of minimally invasive surgery (MIS) via laparoscopy in the staging, palliation, and removal of pancreatic cancers. The procedure selected depends on the purpose of the surgery and stage of the disease. For example, if the patient has a biliary obstruction, a laparoscopic procedure to relieve the obstruction is performed. This procedure diverts bile drainage into the jejunum.

For larger tumors, the surgeon may perform either a *radical pancreatectomy* or the *Whipple procedure (pancreaticoduodenectomy)*. These procedures have traditionally been done using an open surgical approach. Because of new advances in laparoscopic technology using a hand-assist device, this method is beginning to replace the conventional method. Some surgeons are not yet trained in how to perform this technique. Therefore the traditional open surgical approach remains the most common method of performing these surgeries.

Preoperative Care. The patient with pancreatic cancer may be a poor surgical risk because of malnutrition and debilitation. Specific care depends on the type of surgical approach being used.

Often, in the late stages of pancreatic cancer or before the Whipple procedure, the physician inserts a small catheter into the jejunum (jejunostomy) so that enteral feedings may be given. This feeding method is preferred to prevent reflux and to facilitate absorption. Feedings are started in low concentrations and volumes and are gradually increased as tolerated. Provide feedings using a pump to maintain a constant volume, and assess for diarrhea frequency to determine tolerance. Chapter 60 provides additional information about enteral feeding.

For optimal NUTRITION, TPN may be necessary in addition to tube feedings or as a single measure to provide nutrition. When central venous access is required, a peripherally inserted central catheter (PICC) or other type of IV catheter may be necessary. Meticulous IV line care is an important nursing measure to prevent catheter sepsis. Sterile dressing changes and site observation are extremely important. Additional nursing care measures for the patient receiving TPN are given in Chapter 60. Monitor nutrition indicators such as serum prealbumin and albumin.

For the laparoscopic procedure, no bowel preparation is needed. However, either approach requires that the patient have nothing by mouth (NPO) for at least 6 to 8 hours before surgery.

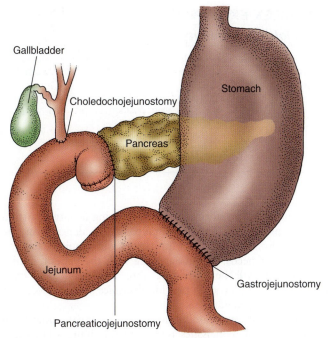

Gallbladder

Choledochojejunostomy

Stomach

Pancreas

Jejunum

Gastrojejunostomy

Pancreaticojejunostomy

FIG. 59-3 The three anastomoses that constitute the Whipple procedure: choledochojejunostomy, pancreaticojejunostomy, and gastrojejunostomy.

TABLE 59-5 Potential Complications of the Whipple Procedure	
Cardiovascular Complications • Hemorrhage at anastomosis sites with hypovolemia • Myocardial infarction • Heart failure • Thrombophlebitis **Pulmonary Complications** • Atelectasis • Pneumonia • Pulmonary embolism • Acute respiratory distress syndrome • Pulmonary edema **Metabolic Complications** • Unstable diabetes mellitus • Renal failure	**Gastrointestinal Complications** • Adynamic (paralytic) ileus • Gastric retention • Gastric ulceration • Bowel obstruction from peritonitis • Acute pancreatitis • Hepatic failure • Thrombosis to mesentery **Wound Complications** • Infection • Dehiscence • Fistulas: pancreatic, gastric, and biliary

Surgeon preference and agency policy determine the preferred protocol for preoperative preparation.

Operative Procedures. The **Whipple procedure (radical pancreaticoduodenectomy)** involves extensive surgical manipulation and is used most often to treat cancer of the head of the pancreas. The procedure entails removal of the proximal head of the pancreas, the duodenum, a portion of the jejunum, the stomach (partial or total **gastrectomy**), and the gallbladder, with anastomosis of the pancreatic duct (**pancreaticojejunostomy**), the common bile duct (**choledochojejunostomy**), and the stomach (**gastrojejunostomy**) to the jejunum (Fig. 59-3). In addition, the surgeon may remove the spleen (**splenectomy**).

Postoperative Care. In addition to routine postoperative care measures, the patient who has undergone an open radical pancreaticoduodenectomy requires intensive nursing care and is usually admitted to a surgical critical care unit. Observe for multiple potential complications of the open Whipple procedure as listed in Table 59-5.

The patient's primary benefits of MIS are a shorter postoperative recovery and less pain than with traditional open procedures. The patient having the laparoscopic Whipple surgery or radical pancreatectomy is also less at risk for severe complications. For patients having one of these procedures, observe for and implement preventive measures for these surgical complications:
- Diabetes (Check blood glucose often.)
- Hemorrhage (Monitor pulse, blood pressure, skin color, and mental status [e.g., LOC].)
- Wound infection (Monitor temperature, and assess wounds for redness and induration [hardness].)
- Bowel obstruction (Check bowel sounds and stools.)
- Intra-abdominal abscess (Monitor temperature and patient's report of severe pain.)

Immediately after surgery the patient is NPO and usually has a nasogastric tube (NGT) to decompress the stomach. Monitor

GI drainage and tube patency. In open surgical approaches, biliary drainage tubes are placed during surgery to remove drainage and secretions from the area and to prevent stress on the anastomosis sites. Assess the tubes and drainage devices for tension or kinking, and maintain them in a dependent position.

Monitor the drainage for color, consistency, and amount. The drainage should be serosanguineous. The appearance of clear, colorless, bile-tinged drainage or frank blood with an increase in output may indicate disruption or leakage of an anastomosis site. Most of the disruptions of the site occur within 7 to 10 days after surgery. Hemorrhage can occur as an early or late complication.

Place the patient in the semi-Fowler's position to reduce tension on the suture line and anastomosis site as well as to optimize lung expansion. Stress can be decreased by maintaining NGT drainage at a low or high intermittent suction level to keep the remaining stomach (if a partial gastrectomy is done) or the jejunum (if a total gastrectomy is done) free of excessive fluid buildup and pressure. The NGT also reduces stimulation of the remaining pancreatic tissue.

The development of a fistula (an abnormal passageway) is the most common and most serious postoperative complication. Biliary, pancreatic, or gastric fistulas result from partial or total breakdown of an anastomosis site. The secretions that drain from the fistula contain bile, pancreatic enzymes, or gastric secretions, depending on which site is ruptured. *These secretions, particularly pancreatic fluid, are corrosive and irritating to the skin, and internal leakage causes chemical peritonitis.* **Peritonitis** (inflammation and infection of the peritoneum causing boardlike abdominal rigidity) requires treatment with multiple antibiotics. *If you suspect any postoperative complications resulting from MIS or open surgical approaches, call the surgeon immediately and provide assessment findings that support your concerns.*

Because the *open* Whipple procedure is extensive and can take many hours to complete, maintaining fluid and electrolyte balance can be difficult. Patients often have significant intraoperative blood loss and postoperative bleeding. The intestine is exposed to air for long periods, and fluid evaporates. Significant losses of fluid and electrolytes occur from the NGT and other drainage tubes. In addition, these patients may be malnourished and have low serum levels of protein and albumin, which maintain colloid osmotic pressure within the circulating system. Reduction in the serum osmotic pressure makes the patient likely to develop third spacing of body fluids, with fluid moving from the vascular to the interstitial space, resulting in shock. These problems are less likely to occur when MIS is used. Therefore, when possible, the trained surgeon prefers to perform laparoscopic Whipple procedures to shorten operating time and prevent the many complications that can occur.

! NURSING SAFETY PRIORITY (QSEN)

Action Alert

To detect early signs of hypovolemia and prevent shock, closely monitor vital signs for decreased blood pressure and increased heart rate, decreased vascular pressures with a pulmonary artery catheter (Swan-Ganz catheter) (in ICU setting), and decreased urine output. Be alert for pitting edema of the extremities, dependent edema in the sacrum and back, and an intake that far exceeds output. Maintain sequential compression devices to prevent deep vein thrombosis.

Maintenance of prescribed IV isotonic fluid replacement with colloid replacements is important. Monitor hemoglobin and hematocrit values to assess for blood loss and the need for blood transfusions. Review electrolyte values for decreased serum levels of sodium, potassium, chloride, and calcium. IV fluid concentrations must be altered to correct these electrolyte imbalances. The physician prescribes replacement of electrolytes as needed.

Immediately after the Whipple procedure, the patient may have hyperglycemia or hypoglycemia as a result of stress and surgical manipulation of the pancreas. Most of the endocrine cells (responsible for insulin and glucagon secretion) are located in the body and tail of the pancreas. In some patients, up to half of the gland remains and diabetes does not develop. However, a large number of patients are diabetic before surgery. For patients having a radical pancreatectomy, administer insulin as prescribed because the entire pancreas is removed. Monitor glucose levels frequently during the early postoperative period, and administer insulin injections as prescribed.

Community-Based Care

The patient with pancreatic cancer is usually followed by a case manager (CM), both in the hospital and in the home or other community-based setting. Collaborate with the CM to ensure that the patient receives cost-effective treatment and that his or her needs are met.

Home Care Management. The stage of progression of pancreatic cancer and available home care resources determine whether the patient can be discharged to home or whether

---

? NCLEX EXAMINATION CHALLENGE
Physiological Integrity

A client had an open Whipple procedure yesterday for pancreatic cancer. Which nursing interventions are appropriate for this client? **Select all that apply.**
A. Monitor and document the client's nasogastric tube drainage.
B. Place the client in a side-lying position to promote wound drainage.
C. Assess the abdomen for signs of peritonitis.
D. Monitor the client's hemoglobin and hematocrit.
E. Check the client's blood glucose frequently.

---

additional care is needed in a skilled nursing facility or with a hospice provider. Home care preparations depend on the patient's physical and activity limitations and should be tailored to his or her needs. Coordinate care with the patient, family, or whoever will be providing care after discharge from the hospital—home care provider, hospice care provider, or extended-care provider.

The patient and family need compassionate emotional support to deal with issues related to this illness. The diagnosis of pancreatic cancer can frighten and overwhelm the patient and family. Assist family members in looking realistically and objectively at the amount of physical care required. Tell family members that their own physical and emotional health are at risk during this stressful period and that supportive counseling may be needed. If the family does not have a religious affiliation or a spiritual leader (e.g., a minister or a rabbi) to provide support, suggest alternative counseling options. Refer patients and families to the certified hospital chaplain if desired. It is appropriate for the nurse to make the initial contact or appointment according to the patient's or family's wishes.

Self-Management Education. When the patient is discharged to home, many interventions are palliative and aimed at managing symptoms such as pain. In many cases the diagnosis of pancreatic cancer is made a few months before death occurs. The patient needs time to adjust to the diagnosis, which is usually made too late for cure or prolonged survival. Help the patient identify what needs to be done to prepare for death, including end-of-life care. For example, he or she may want to write a will or see family members and friends whom he or she has not seen recently. The patient needs to make known to family members or others his or her specific requests for the funeral or memorial service. These actions help prepare for death in a dignified manner. Chapter 7 discusses in detail anticipatory grieving and preparation for death, as well as symptom management during the end of life.

Health Care Resources. Regular home care nursing and assistive nursing personnel visits may be scheduled to assist the patient and family by providing physical, psychological, and supportive care. Supply information about local palliative and hospice care (see Chapter 7) and cancer support groups.

NURSING CONCEPTS AND CLINICAL JUDGMENT REVIEW

What might you NOTICE if the patient is experiencing inadequate digestion and NUTRITION as a result of gallbladder and pancreatic disorders?
- Report of intense abdominal pain
- Report of nausea, especially after food
- Report of anorexia
- Vomiting
- Jaundice
- Report of weight loss
- Dark urine
- Clay-colored stools

What should you INTERPRET and how should you RESPOND to a patient experiencing inadequate digestion and NUTRITION as a result of gallbladder and pancreatic disorders?

Perform and interpret physical assessment, including:
- Taking vital signs to assess for hypovolemia and fever
- Assessing respiratory status, including breath sounds
- Conducting a complete pain assessment if possible
- Weighing the patient

- Checking laboratory values, especially enzyme levels like amylase and lipase, liver function studies, and CBC
- Assessing vomitus for quality and amount

Respond by:
- Keeping the patient's head of the bed elevated and knees flexed
- Providing pain management by comfort measures and analgesia
- Providing oxygen if the patient is having dyspnea or adventitious breath sounds
- Reassuring the patient who may be concerned about possible cancer

On what should you REFLECT?
- Observe the patient for improvement in signs and symptoms, including pain control.
- Think about what could have caused the health problem.
- Think about what else you could do to help the patient meet desired outcomes.
- Plan health teaching for patient discharge.

GET READY FOR THE NCLEX® EXAMINATION!

KEY POINTS

Review these Key Points for each NCLEX Examination Client Needs Category.

Safe and Effective Care Environment
- Collaborate with the dietitian, pharmacist, health care provider, and case manager when planning care for patients with pancreatic cancer. **Teamwork and Collaboration** QSEN
- Refer patients with end-stage pancreatic cancer for palliative and hospice care.
- Refer patients with pancreatitis who use excessive alcohol to community resources such as Alcoholics Anonymous. **Patient-Centered Care** QSEN

Health Promotion and Maintenance
- Recognize that obese, middle-aged women are most likely to have gallbladder disease. **Patient-Centered Care** QSEN
- Teach patients to avoid losing weight too quickly and to keep weight under control to help prevent gallbladder disease. **Evidence-Based Practice** QSEN
- Teach patients to avoid excessive alcohol consumption to help prevent alcohol-induced acute pancreatitis.
- Instruct patients about ways to prevent exacerbations of chronic pancreatitis as outlined in Chart 59-4.

Psychosocial Integrity
- Refer patients with pancreatic cancer for support services such as spiritual leaders and counselors for coping strategies and facilitation of the grieving process.

- Help prepare the pancreatic cancer patient and family for the death and dying process.

Physiological Integrity
- Be aware that autodigestion of the pancreas causes severe PAIN in patients with acute pancreatitis (see Fig. 59-2).
- Monitor serum laboratory values, especially amylase and lipase (both elevated), in patients with pancreatitis (see Table 59-4).
- Assess for common clinical manifestations of cholecystitis as listed in Chart 59-1.
- For patients with acute pancreatitis, provide PAIN management including opioid analgesia. **Patient-Centered Care** QSEN
- Recognize that acute PAIN relief is the first priority for patients with acute pancreatitis. **Evidence-Based Practice** QSEN
- Be aware that patients with biliary and pancreatic disorders are at high risk for biliary obstruction, a serious and painful complication.
- Assess for common clinical manifestations of chronic pancreatitis as listed in Chart 59-2.
- Document health teaching about enzyme replacement therapy as described in Chart 59-3. **Informatics** QSEN
- Assess patients with presenting clinical manifestations of pancreatic cancer as described in Chart 59-5.
- Observe for and implement interventions to prevent life-threatening complications of the Whipple procedure as outlined in Table 59-5. **Safety** QSEN

60 CHAPTER

Care of Patients with Malnutrition: Undernutrition and Obesity

Cherie R. Rebar, Nicole Heimgartner, Laura Willis

 http://evolve.elsevier.com/Iggy/

PRIORITY CONCEPTS

- NUTRITION
- FLUID AND ELECTROLYTE BALANCE

LEARNING OUTCOMES

Safe and Effective Care Environment

1. Collaborate with the health care team members when providing care for patients with malnutrition or obesity.
2. Protect bariatric patients from injury.
3. Select appropriate activities to delegate to unlicensed assistive personnel to promote a patient's NUTRITION.

Health Promotion and Maintenance

4. Provide care that meets the special nutrition needs of older adults.
5. Recall the *2010 Dietary Guidelines for Americans* recommendations.
6. Teach overweight and obese patients the importance of lifestyle changes to promote health.
7. Perform a nutrition screening for all patients to determine if they are at high risk for NUTRITION health problems.

Psychosocial Integrity

8. Assess patient responses to being obese.
9. Explain how to reduce the psychological impact for the patient who is having bariatric surgery.

Physiological Integrity

10. Interpret findings of a nutrition screening and assessment.
11. Calculate body mass index (BMI), and interpret findings.
12. Describe the risk factors for malnutrition, especially for older adults.
13. Explain why serum visceral protein levels indicate change in NUTRITION status.
14. Identify the role of supplements in restoring or maintaining nutrition.
15. Explain how to prevent complications of total parenteral nutrition (TPN).
16. Explain how to maintain enteral tube patency.
17. Describe evidence-based practices to prevent aspiration for patients with nasoenteric tubes.
18. Explain the medical complications associated with obesity.
19. Identify the role of drug therapy in the management of obesity.
20. Prioritize nursing care for patients having bariatric surgery.
21. Develop a discharge teaching plan for patients having bariatric surgery.

Carbohydrates, protein, and fat are nutrients in food that supply the body with energy. In healthy people, most of this energy undergoes digestion and is absorbed from the GI tract. Food energy is used to maintain body temperature, respiration, cardiac output, muscle function, protein synthesis, and the storage and metabolism of food sources. Therefore proper NUTRITION plays a major role in promoting and maintaining health.

Energy balance refers to the relationship between energy used and energy stored. Weight loss occurs when energy used is more than intake. If food intake is more than energy used, weight is gained. Body proteins are used for energy when calorie intake is insufficient. The body attempts to meet its calorie requirements even if it is at the expense of protein needs.

NUTRITION STANDARDS FOR HEALTH PROMOTION AND MAINTENANCE

The role of NUTRITION in disease has been a subject of interest for many years. The current focus is on health promotion and the prevention of disease by healthy eating and exercise. The Institute of Medicine of The National Academies (2014) has developed the **Dietary Reference Intakes (DRIs)** to serve as a nutrition guide that provides a scientific basis for food guidelines in the United States and Canada. Age, gender, and life stage influence the nutrient reference values of more than 40 nutrient substances (The Institute of Medicine of The National Academies, 2014). In the United States, the **Dietary Guidelines for Americans** are revised by the U.S. Department of Agriculture

(USDA) and the U.S. Department of Health and Human Services (DHHS) every 5 years. The 2010 guidelines emphasize the need to include preferences of specific racial/ethnic groups, vegetarians, and other populations when selecting foods to maintain a healthful diet that is balanced with moderation and variety. If alcohol is consumed, it should be limited to one drink per day for women and two drinks for men (U.S. Department of Agriculture [USDA], 2010). Examples of other guidelines are listed in Table 60-1.

To remind people about healthy eating habits, the USDA designed "MyPlate," a picture to demonstrate that half of each meal should consist of fruits and vegetables (Fig. 60-1). When grains are consumed, half of them should be whole grains rather than refined grain products.

Some people follow vegetarian diet patterns for health, environmental, or moral reasons. In general, vegetarians are leaner than those who consume meat. The lacto-vegetarian eats milk, cheese, and dairy foods but avoids meat, fish, poultry, and eggs. The lacto-ovo-vegetarian includes eggs in his or her diet. The vegan eats only foods of plant origin. Some people among these groups eat fish as well. Vegans can develop anemia as a result of vitamin B_{12} deficiency. Therefore they should include a daily source of vitamin B_{12} in their diets, such as a fortified breakfast cereal, fortified soy beverage, or meat substitute. All vegetarians should ensure that they get adequate amounts of calcium, iron,

zinc, and vitamins D and B_{12}. Well-planned vegetarian diets can provide adequate NUTRITION. The Academy of Nutrition and Dietetics (2013) publishes a number of credible resources regarding vegetarian health at www.eatright.org.

🌐 CULTURAL CONSIDERATIONS
Patient-Centered Care QSEN

Many people have specific food preferences based on their ethnicity or race. For example, for people of Hispanic descent, tortillas, beans, and rice *may* be desired over pasta, risotto, and potatoes. *Never assume that a person's racial or ethnic background means that he or she eats only foods associated with his or her primary ethnicity.* Health teaching about nutrition should incorporate any cultural preferences.

Some people have food allergies or intolerances. For instance, lactose intolerance (lactose is found in milk and milk products) is a common problem that occurs in a number of ethnic groups. It is found more often in Mexican Americans and black people as well as in some American Indian groups, Asian Americans, and Ashkenazi Jews. A small percentage of white people, particularly those of Mediterranean descent (e.g., Greek, Italian), are also lactose intolerant. The cause of **lactose intolerance** is an inadequate amount of the lactase enzyme, which converts lactose into absorbable glucose. Patients may benefit from learning more about the management of lactose intolerance from resources provided by organizations such as the American Dietetic Association or the Dieticians of Canada.

CONSIDERATIONS FOR OLDER ADULTS
Patient-Centered Care QSEN

The USDA recommends that older adults drink eight glasses of water a day and eat plenty of fiber to prevent or manage constipation. It also suggests daily calcium and vitamins D and B_{12} supplements and a reduction in sodium and cholesterol-containing foods.

TABLE 60-1   Examples of *2010 Dietary Guidelines for Americans*

- Control total calorie intake to manage body weight.
- Consume less than 300 mg per day of dietary cholesterol.
- Increase intake of fat-free or low-fat milk and milk products, such as milk, yogurt, cheese, or fortified soy products.
- Choose a variety of protein foods, which include seafood, lean meat and poultry, eggs, beans and peas, soy products, and unsalted nuts and seeds.
- Reduce the intake of calories from solid fats and added sugars.
- Reduce daily sodium intake to less than 2300 mg and further reduce intake to 1500 mg among persons who are 51 years of age or older and those of any age who are African American or have hypertension, diabetes, or chronic kidney disease.
- Limit the consumption of foods that contain refined grains, especially refined grains that contain solid fats, added sugars, and sodium.
- Increase vegetable and fruit intake.

Source: *Dietary Guidelines for Americans Council*. (2014). Retrieved September 2014, from http://www.fns.usda.gov/dietary-guidelines-americans-2010

One of the most recent publications from Health Canada on Nutrition is the Canada Food Guide. Compared with previous documents, it includes more culturally diverse foods, information on *trans* fats, customized individual recommendations, and exercise guidelines. Several booklets can be purchased to help people select the best foods and nutrients from the new guide, such as *Eating Well with Canada's Food Guide* (Minister of Health Canada, 2011). In addition, Canada has published a separate booklet to address the special needs of some of its indigenous people. The *Eating Well with Canada's Food Guide—First Nations, Inuit, and Métis* includes berries, wild plants, and wild game to reflect the values and traditions for aboriginal people living in Canada (Health Canada, 2011).

NUTRITION ASSESSMENT

Nutrition status reflects the balance between nutrient requirements and intake. Common factors that affect these requirements include age, gender, disease, infection, and psychological stress. Eating behavior, economic implications, emotional stability, disease, drug therapy, and cultural factors influence nutrient intake. Malnutrition (also called *undernutrition*) and obesity, discussed later in this chapter, are common nutrition health problems that may lead to many comorbidities and complications, including death.

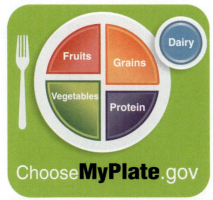

FIG. 60-1 The U.S. Department of Agriculture MyPlate.

Evaluation of nutrition status is an important part of total patient assessment and includes:

- Review of the nutrition history
- Food and fluid intake record
- Laboratory data
- Food-drug interactions
- Health history and physical assessment
- Anthropometric measurements
- Psychosocial assessment

Monitor the NUTRITION status of a patient during hospitalization as an important part of your initial assessment. Collaborate with the interdisciplinary health care team to identify patients at risk for nutrition problems.

Initial Nutrition Screening

An initial screening provides an inexpensive, quick way of determining which patients need more extensive nutrition assessment by the health care team. The Joint Commission Patient Care Standards require that a nutrition screening occur within 24 hours of the patient's hospital admission. If indicated, an in-depth nutrition assessment should be performed. When patients are in the hospital for more than a week, nutrition assessment should be part of the daily plan of care.

The initial nutrition screening includes inspection, measured height and weight, weight history, usual eating habits, ability to chew and swallow, and any recent changes in appetite or food intake. Examples of questions that help identify patients at risk for nutrition problems are part of the history and physical assessment (Chart 60-1).

The Mini Nutritional Assessment (MNA), a two-part tool that has been tested worldwide, provides a reliable, rapid assessment for patients in the community and in any health care setting. The *first* part (A-F) is a screening section that takes 3 minutes to complete and asks about food intake, mobility, and body mass index (BMI) (described on p. 1235). It also screens for weight loss, acute illness, and psychological health problems. If the patient scores 11 points or less, the *second* part (G-R) of the MNA is completed, for an additional 12 questions. The entire assessment takes only minutes to complete (Fig. 60-2). The MNA Short Form can be used as a stand-alone tool to evaluate whether the older patient is well nourished, at risk for malnutrition, or malnourished. The alternative is to take the patient's calf circumference, which can be a reliable alternative if BMI is unavailable.

Anthropometric Measurements

Anthropometric measurements are noninvasive methods of evaluating NUTRITION status. These measurements include height and weight and assessment of body mass index (BMI).

Obtain a current *height and weight* to provide a baseline. Be sure to obtain accurate measurements because patients tend to overestimate height and underestimate weight. Measurements taken days or weeks later may indicate an early change in nutrition status. *You may delegate this activity to unlicensed assistive personnel (UAP) under your supervision.*

Patients should be measured and weighed while wearing minimal clothing and no shoes. Determine the height in inches or centimeters using the measuring stick of a weight scale if the

---

CHART 60-1 **Best Practice for Patient Safety & Quality Care** QSEN
Nutrition Screening Assessment

General
- Does the patient have any conditions that cause nutrient loss, such as malabsorption syndromes, draining abscesses, wounds, fistulas, or prolonged diarrhea?
- Does the patient have any conditions that increase the need for nutrients, such as fever, burns, injury, sepsis, or antineoplastic therapies?
- Has the patient been NPO for 3 days or more?
- Is the patient receiving a modified diet or a diet restricted in one or more nutrients?
- Is the patient being enterally or parenterally fed?
- Does the patient describe food allergies, lactose intolerance, or limited food preferences?
- Has the patient experienced a recent unexplained weight loss?
- Is the patient on drug therapy—either prescription, over-the-counter, or herbal/natural products?

Gastrointestinal
- Does the patient report nausea, indigestion, vomiting, diarrhea, or constipation?
- Does the patient exhibit glossitis (tongue inflammation), stomatitis (oral inflammation), or esophagitis?
- Does the patient have difficulty chewing or swallowing?
- Does the patient have a partial or total GI obstruction?
- What is the patient's state of dentition?

Cardiovascular
- Does the patient have ascites or edema?
- Is the patient able to perform ADLs?
- Does the patient have heart failure?

Genitourinary
- Is fluid intake about equal to fluid output?
- Does the patient have an ostomy?
- Is the patient hemodialyzed or peritoneally dialyzed?

Respiratory
- Is the patient receiving mechanical ventilatory support?
- Is the patient receiving oxygen via nasal prongs?
- Does the patient have chronic obstructive pulmonary disease (COPD) or asthma?

Integumentary
- Does the patient have abnormal nail or hair changes?
- Does the patient have rashes or dermatitis?
- Does the patient have dry or pale mucous membranes or decreased skin turgor?
- Does the patient have pressure areas on the sacrum, hips, heels, or ankles?

Extremities
- Does the patient have pedal edema?
- Does the patient have cachexia?

Modified with courtesy of Ross Products Division, Abbott Laboratories, Columbus, OH.

Nestlé
NutritionInstitute

Mini Nutritional Assessment MNA®

Last name: _____ First name: _____

Sex: _____ Age: _____ Weight, kg: _____ Height, cm: _____ Date: _____

Complete the screen by filling in the boxes with the appropriate numbers. Add the numbers for the screen. If score is 11 or less, continue with the assessment to gain a Malnutrition Indicator Score.

Screening

A Has food intake declined over the past 3 months due to loss of appetite, digestive problems, chewing or swallowing difficulties?
0 = severe decrease in food intake
1 = moderate decrease in food intake
2 = no decrease in food intake ☐

B Weight loss during the last 3 months
0 = weight loss greater than 3 kg (6.6lbs)
1 = does not know
2 = weight loss between 1 and 3kg (2.2 and 6.6lbs)
3 = no weight loss ☐

C Mobility
0 = bed or chair bound
1 = able to get out of bed/chair but does not go out
2 = goes out ☐

D Has suffered psychological stress or acute disease in the past 3 months
0 = yes   2 = no ☐

E Neuropsychological problems
0 = severe dementia or depression
1 = mild dementia
2 = no psychological problems ☐

F Body Mass Index (BMI) (weight in kg) / height in m^2)
0 = BMI less than 19
1 = BMI 19 to less than 21
2 = BMI 21 to less than 23
3 = BMI 23 or greater ☐

Screening score
(subtotal max. 14 points) ☐☐

12-14 points: Normal nutritional status
8-11 points: At risk of malnutrition
0-7 points: Malnourished

For a more in-depth assessment, continue with questions G-R

Assessment

G Lives independently (not in nursing home or hospital)
1 = yes   0 = no ☐

H Takes more than 3 prescription drugs per day
0 = yes   1 = no ☐

I Pressure sores or skin ulcers
0 = yes   1 = no ☐

J How many full meals does the patient eat daily?
0 = 1 meal
1 = 2 meals
2 = 3 meals ☐

K Selected consumption markers for protein intake
• At least one serving of dairy products (milk, cheese, yoghurt) per day   yes ☐   no ☐
• Two or more servings of legumes or eggs per week   yes ☐   no ☐
• Meat, fish or poultry every day   yes ☐   no ☐
0.0 = if 0 or 1 yes
0.5 = if 2 yes
1.0 = if 3 yes ☐.☐

L Consumes two or more servings of fruit or vegetables per day?
0 = no   1 = yes ☐

M How much fluid (water, juice, coffee, tea, milk...) is consumed per day?
0.0 = less than 3 cups
0.5 = 3 to 5 cups
1.0 = more than 5 cups ☐.☐

N Mode of feeding
0 = unable to eat without assistance
1 = self-fed with some difficulty
3 = self-fed without any problem ☐

O Self view of nutritional status
0 = views self as being malnourished
1 = is uncertain of nutritional state
2 = views self as having no nutritional problem ☐

P In comparison with other people of the same age, how does the patient consider his/her health status?
0.0 = not as good
0.5 = does not know
1.0 = as good
2.0 = better ☐.☐

Q Mid-arm circumference (MAC) in cm
0.0 = MAC less than 21
0.5 = MAC 21 to 22
1.0 = MAC 22 or greater ☐.☐

R Calf circumference (CC) in cm
0 = CC less than 31
1 = CC 31 or greater ☐

Assessment (max. 16 points) ☐☐.☐

Screening score ☐☐.☐

Total Assessment (max. 30 points) ☐☐.☐

Malnutrition Indicator Score

24 to 30 points   ☐   Normal nutritional status

17 to 23.5 points   ☐   At risk of malnutrition

Ref. 1. Vellas B, Villars H, Abellan G, *et al.* Overview of MNA® - Its History and Challenges. *J Nut Health Aging.* 2006; **10:456**-465.
2. Rubenstein LZ, Harker JO, Salva A, Guigoz Y, Vellas B. Screening for Undernutrition in Geriatric Practice: Developing the Short-Form Mini Nutritional Assessment (MNA-SF). *J. Geront.* 2001; **56A**: M366-377
3. Guigoz Y. The Mini-Nutritional Assessment (MNA®) Review of the Literature – What does it tell us? *J Nutr Health Aging.* 2006; **10**: 466-487.
® Société des Produits Nestlé, S.A., Vevey, Switzerland, Trademark Owners

FIG. 60-2 The Mini Nutritional Assessment (MNA).

patient can stand. He or she should stand erect and look straight ahead, with the heels together and the arms at the sides. For patients who cannot stand or those who cannot stand erect (e.g., some older adults), use a sliding-blade **knee height caliper**, if available. This device uses the distance between the patient's patella and heel to estimate height. It is especially useful for patients who have knee or hip contractures.

Remind UAP to weigh ambulatory patients with an upright balance-beam or digital scale. Non-ambulatory patients can be weighed with a digital wheelchair or bed scale.

! NURSING SAFETY PRIORITY (QSEN)
Action Alert

For daily or sequential weights, obtain the weight at the same time each day, if possible, preferably before breakfast. Conditions such as congestive heart failure and renal disease cause weight gain; dehydration and conditions such as cancer cause weight loss. *Weight is the most reliable indicator of fluid gain or loss, so accurate weights are essential!*

Normal weights for adult men and women are available from several reference standards, such as the Metropolitan Life tables. Some health care professionals prefer these tables because they consider body-build differences by gender and body frame size.

Changes in body weight can be expressed by three different formulas:

Weight as a percentage of ideal body weight (IBW):

$$\%IBW = \frac{\text{Current weight}}{\text{Ideal body weight}} \times 100$$

Current weight as a percentage of usual body weight (UBW):

$$\%UBW = \frac{\text{Current weight}}{\text{Usual body weight}} \times 100$$

Change in weight:

$$\text{Weight change} = \frac{\text{Usual weight} - \text{Current weight}}{\text{Usual weight}} \times 100$$

An unintentional weight loss of 10% over a 6-month period at any time significantly affects nutrition status and should be evaluated. Depending on the patient's needs, weights may need to be taken daily, several times a week, or weekly for monitoring status and the effectiveness of nutrition support.

In the health care setting, *assessment of body fat* is usually calculated by the dietitian. For people who participate in a structured exercise program in the community, this assessment is typically performed by a fitness trainer or physical therapist.

The **body mass index (BMI)** is a measure of nutrition status that does not depend on frame size (Centers for Disease Control and Prevention [CDC], 2012). It indirectly estimates total fat stores within the body by the relationship of weight to height. *Therefore an accurate height is as important as an accurate weight.*

A simple calculation for estimating BMI can be programmed into handheld computers or calculators using one of these two formulas:

$$BMI = \frac{\text{Weight (lb)}}{\text{Height (in inches)}^2} \times 703$$

$$BMI = \frac{\text{Weight (kg)}}{\text{Height (in meters)}^2}$$

BMI can also be determined using a table that is linked with height and weight. The least risk for malnutrition is associated with scores between 18.5 and 25. BMIs above and below these values are associated with increased health risks (CDC, 2012a).

CONSIDERATIONS FOR OLDER ADULTS
Patient-Centered Care (QSEN)

Body weight and BMI usually increase throughout adulthood until about 60 years of age. As people get older, they often become less hungry and eat less, even if they are healthy. Ideally, older adults should have a BMI between 23 and 27.

The average daily energy intake expended by this group tends to be more than the average energy intake. This physiologic change has been called the "anorexia of aging" (Champion, 2011). Many older adults are underweight, leading to undernutrition and increased risk for illness.

? NCLEX EXAMINATION CHALLENGE
Health Promotion and Maintenance

An older adult is admitted to the hospital with pressure ulcers and septicemia. His height is 5 feet, 8 inches (1.72 meters), and he weighs 302 pounds (137 kg). His current body mass index (BMI) is _____. (Round your answer to the nearest tenth.)

Skinfold measurements estimate body fat and can be measured by either the nurse or the dietitian. The *triceps and subscapular* skinfolds are most commonly measured using a special caliper. Both are compared with standard measurements and recorded as percentiles.

The *midarm circumference (MAC) and calf circumference (CC)* can be obtained to measure muscle mass and subcutaneous fat. These measurements are needed if the Mini Nutritional Assessment tool is used. To measure MAC, place a flexible tape around the upper arm at the midpoint, taking care to hold the tape firmly but gently to avoid compressing the tissue. This measurement is usually recorded in centimeters. The midarm muscle mass (MAMM) measures the amount of muscle in the body and is a sensitive indicator of protein reserves. It can be computed from the MAC and the triceps skinfold measure. The CC is obtained using a similar procedure on the calf.

MALNUTRITION

❖ *PATHOPHYSIOLOGY*

Protein-energy malnutrition (PEM), also known as **protein-calorie malnutrition (PCM)**, may present in three forms: marasmus, kwashiorkor, and marasmic-kwashiorkor. **Marasmus** is generally a calorie malnutrition in which body fat and protein are wasted. Serum proteins are often preserved. **Kwashiorkor** is a lack of protein quantity and quality in the presence of adequate calories. Body weight is more normal, and serum proteins are low. **Marasmic-kwashiorkor** is a combined protein and energy malnutrition. This problem often presents clinically when metabolic stress is imposed on a chronically starved patient. The outcome of unrecognized or untreated PEM is often dysfunction or disability and increased morbidity and mortality.

Malnutrition (also called *undernutrition)* is a multinutrient problem because foods that are good sources of calories and protein are also good sources of other nutrients. In the malnourished patient, protein catabolism exceeds protein intake and synthesis, resulting in negative nitrogen balance, weight loss, decreased muscle mass, and weakness.

The functions of the liver, heart, lungs, GI tract, and immune system decrease in the patient with malnutrition. A decrease in serum proteins (hypoproteinemia) occurs as protein synthesis in the liver decreases. Vital capacity is also reduced as a result of respiratory muscle atrophy. Cardiac output diminishes. Malabsorption occurs because of atrophy of GI mucosa and the loss of intestinal villi.

Common complications of *severe* malnutrition in adults include:

- Leanness and cachexia (muscle wasting with prolonged malnutrition)
- Decreased activity tolerance
- Lethargy
- Intolerance to cold
- Edema
- Dry, flaking skin and various types of dermatitis
- Poor wound healing
- Infection, particularly postoperative infection and sepsis
- Possible death

Malnutrition results from inadequate nutrient intake, increased nutrient losses, and increased nutrient requirements. Inadequate nutrient intake can be linked to poverty, lack of education, substance abuse, decreased appetite, and a decline in functional ability to eat independently, particularly in older adults. Infectious diseases, such as tuberculosis and human immune deficiency virus (HIV) infection, can also cause PEM. Diseases that produce diarrhea and infections leading to anorexia result in negative calorie and protein balance. Anorexia then leads to poor food intake. Vomiting causes decreased intestinal absorption with increased nutrient losses. Medical treatments such as chemotherapy can also cause malnutrition. In addition, catabolic processes, such as that caused by prolonged immobility, increase nutrient requirements and metabolic losses.

Inadequate nutrient intake can result also when a person is admitted to the hospital or long-term care facility. For example, decreased staffing may not allow time for patients who need to be fed, especially older adults, who may eat slowly. Many diagnostic tests, surgery, trauma, and unexpected medical complications require a period of NPO or cause anorexia (loss of appetite). In a systematic integrative review, Tappenden et al. (2013) reviewed strategies needed to address the needs of hospitalized patients to prevent or treat malnutrition (see the Evidence-Based Practice box).

CULTURAL CONSIDERATIONS
Patient-Centered Care QSEN

In some cases, malnutrition results when the provided meals are different from what the patient usually eats. Be sure to identify specific food preferences that the patient can eat and enjoy that are in keeping with his or her cultural practices.

CONSIDERATIONS FOR OLDER ADULTS
Patient-Centered Care QSEN

Older adults in the community or in any health care setting are most at risk for poor nutrition, especially PEM. Risk factors include physiologic changes of aging, environmental factors, and health problems. Chart 60-2 lists some of these major factors. Chapter 2 discusses nutrition for older adults in more detail.

EVIDENCE-BASED PRACTICE QSEN
The Critical Role of Nutrition in Improving Quality of Care

Tappenden, K.A., Quatrara, B., Parkhurst, M.L., Malone, A.M., Fanjiang, G., & Ziegler, T.R. (2013). Critical role of nutrition in improving quality of care: An interdisciplinary call to action to address adult hospital malnutrition. *MEDSURG Nursing, 22*(3), 147-165.

Health care costs have increased tremendously in the United States over the past decades. With substantial changes coming in health care policy that affect the way that health care is delivered, health care facilities will need to continue searching for ways to deliver the best care at the most reasonable cost. At least one third of patients come to the hospital in a state of malnourishment, and others become malnourished after admission. Therefore ways for addressing adult hospital malnutrition are very important for both quality of care and cost containment.

The Alliance to Advance Patient Nutrition (Alliance) reflects combined efforts of the Academy of Medical-Surgical Nurses (AMSN), the Academy of Nutrition and Dietetics (AND), the American Society for Parenteral and Enteral Nutrition (ASPEN), the Society of Hospital Medicine (SHM), and Abbott Nutrition to help achieve positive patient outcomes and support improving patient nutrition. The Alliance recommends a number of strategies for meeting these outcomes, such as:

- Include nutrition as a component of all health care team member conversations and in conversation with patients and family members.
- Provide thorough explanations about the patient's nutrition status, nutrition recommendations, nutrition interventions, and post-discharge nutrition care; document these interventions in the electronic health record.

- Ensure that the patient and/or family member is given comprehensive follow-up nutrition assessment, education, and follow-up appointment recommendations at the time of discharge.
- Provide comprehensive, clear, standardized written instructions for nutrition care at home.
- Prioritize nutrition as part of self-management education, taking into consideration dietary intake, weight change, access to food, and other concerns that may affect nutrition status.

Level of Evidence: 1
The clinical evidence presented was collected and presented as a result of a systematic integrative review conducted by numerous professional health care organizations.

Commentary: Implications for Practice and Research
Quality of care, cost implications, and recovery are of primary concern for all patients who are malnourished. Collaborative efforts among the health care team members can (1) provide a more consistent and reliable approach to addressing nutrition needs for hospitalized patients, (2) avoid overlapping charges that may arise from a lack of communication, and (3) create a best practice approach for teaching the patient and family about meeting nutrition needs at the time of discharge. Nurses who work directly with patients are in a key position to provide consistent, comprehensive nutrition education; this can result in better meeting the nutrition needs of patients who are hospitalized, as well as prepare them better for self-management upon discharge.

Acute PEM may develop in patients who were adequately nourished before hospitalization but experience starvation while in a catabolic state from infection, stress, or injury. *Chronic* PEM can occur in those who have cancer, end-stage kidney or liver disease, or chronic neurologic disease.

Eating disorders such as anorexia nervosa and bulimia nervosa, which are seen most often in teens and young adults, also lead to malnutrition. Anorexia nervosa is a self-induced starvation resulting from a fear of fatness, even though the patient is underweight. Bulimia nervosa is characterized by episodes of binge eating in which the patient ingests a large amount of food in a short time. The binge eating is followed by some form of purging behavior, such as self-induced vomiting or excessive use of laxatives and diuretics. If not treated, death can result from starvation, infection, or suicide. Information about eating disorders can be found in textbooks on mental/behavioral health nursing.

❖ PATIENT-CENTERED COLLABORATIVE CARE

◆ Assessment

History. Review the medical history to determine the possibility of increased metabolic needs or NUTRITION losses, chronic disease, trauma, recent surgery of the GI tract, drug and alcohol use, and recent significant weight loss. Each of these conditions can contribute to malnutrition. For older adults, explore mental status changes and note poor eyesight, diseases affecting major organs, constipation or incontinence, and slowed reactions. Review prescription and over-the-counter (OTC) drugs, including vitamin, mineral, herbal, and other nutrition supplements.

For patients who live independently in the community, the nurse may assess their performance of instrumental activities of daily living (IADLs). Functional status can best be evaluated for institutionalized patients by assessing their ADL performance. Poor NUTRITION is a major contributing factor to decreased functional ability.

In collaboration with the dietitian, obtain information about the patient's usual daily food intake, eating behaviors, change

in appetite, and recent weight changes. If the patient is able to communicate, ask him or her to describe the usual foods eaten daily, cultural food preferences, and the times of meals and snacks. If available, ask the family these questions if the patient cannot communicate. If the patient cannot understand the questions due to language differences, locate an interpreter to assist with communication. The dietitian can more thoroughly analyze the diet, if necessary, based on your initial nutrition screening.

Ask about changes in eating habits as a result of illness, and document any change in appetite, taste, and weight loss. *A weight loss of 5% or more in 30 days, a weight loss of 10% in 6 months, or a weight that is below ideal may indicate malnutrition.*

! NURSING SAFETY PRIORITY (QSEN)

Action Alert

When assessing for malnutrition, assess for difficulty or pain in chewing or swallowing. *Unrecognized dysphagia is a common problem among nursing home residents and can cause malnutrition, dehydration, and aspiration pneumonia.* Ask the patient whether any foods are avoided and why. Ask UAP to report any choking while the patient eats. Record the occurrence of nausea, vomiting, heartburn, or any other symptoms of discomfort with eating.

Ask the patient about dental health problems, including the presence of dentures. Dentures or partial plates that do not fit well interfere with food intake. Dental caries (decay) or missing teeth may also cause discomfort while eating.

Physical Assessment/Clinical Manifestations. Assess for manifestations of various nutrient deficiencies (Table 60-2). Inspect the patient's hair, eyes, oral cavity, nails, and musculoskeletal and neurologic systems. Examine the condition of the skin, including any reddened or open areas. Anthropometric measurements may also be obtained as described on p. 1234. The nurse or UAP monitors all food and fluid intake and notes any mouth pain or difficulty in chewing or swallowing. A 3-day caloric intake may be collected and then calculated by the dietitian.

Psychosocial Assessment. The psychosocial history provides information about the patient's economic status, occupation, educational level, gender orientation, ethnicity/race, living and cooking arrangements, and mental status. Determine whether financial resources are adequate for providing the necessary food. If resources are inadequate, the social worker or case manager may refer the patient and family to available community services. Chapter 2 discusses NUTRITION in older adults in more detail.

Laboratory Assessment. Laboratory tests supply objective data that can support subjective data and identify deficiencies. Interpret laboratory data carefully with regard to the total patient; focusing on an isolated value may yield an inaccurate conclusion.

A low *hemoglobin* level may indicate anemia, recent hemorrhage, or hemodilution caused by FLUID retention. Hemoglobin may also be decreased secondary to conditions such as low serum albumin, infection, catabolism, or chronic disease. High levels may indicate hemoconcentration or dehydration or may be found secondary to liver disease.

TABLE 60-2	Manifestations of Nutrient Deficiencies		
SIGN/SYMPTOM	**POTENTIAL NUTRIENT DEFICIENCY**	**SIGN/SYMPTOM**	**POTENTIAL NUTRIENT DEFICIENCY**
Hair		**Extremities**	
Alopecia	Zinc	Subcutaneous fat loss	Calories
Easy to remove	Protein	Muscle wastage	Calories, protein
Lackluster hair	Protein	Edema	Protein
"Corkscrew" hair	Vitamin C	Osteomalacia, bone pain, rickets	Vitamin D
Decreased pigmentation	Protein		
		Hematologic	
Eyes		Anemia	Vitamin B_{12}, iron, folic acid, copper, vitamin E
Xerosis of conjunctiva	Vitamin A		
Corneal vascularization	Riboflavin	Leukopenia, neutropenia	Copper
Keratomalacia	Vitamin A	Low prothrombin time, prolonged clotting time	Vitamin K, manganese
Bitot's spots	Vitamin A		
		Neurologic	
Gastrointestinal Tract		Disorientation	Niacin, thiamine
Nausea, vomiting	Pyridoxine	Confabulation	Thiamine
Diarrhea	Zinc, niacin	Neuropathy	Thiamine, pyridoxine, chromium
Stomatitis	Pyridoxine, riboflavin, iron	Paresthesia	Thiamine, pyridoxine, vitamin B_{12}
Cheilosis	Pyridoxine, iron		
Glossitis	Pyridoxine, zinc, niacin, folic acid, vitamin B_{12}	**Cardiovascular**	
Magenta tongue	Vitamin A, riboflavin	Congestive heart failure, cardiomegaly, tachycardia	Thiamine
Swollen, bleeding gums	Vitamin C	Cardiomyopathy	Selenium
Fissured tongue	Niacin	Cardiac dysrhythmias	Magnesium
Hepatomegaly	Protein		
Skin			
Dry and scaling	Vitamin A		
Petechiae/ecchymoses	Vitamin C		
Follicular hyperkeratosis	Vitamin A		
Nasolabial seborrhea	Niacin		
Bilateral dermatitis	Niacin		

Courtesy of Ross Products Division, Abbott Laboratories, Columbus, OH.

Low *hematocrit* levels may reflect anemia, hemorrhage, excessive FLUID, renal disease, or cirrhosis. High hematocrit levels may indicate dehydration or hemoconcentration.

Serum albumin, thyroxine-binding prealbumin, and transferrin are measures of **visceral proteins**. Serum *albumin* is a plasma protein that reflects the nutrition status of the patient a few weeks before testing; therefore it is not considered to be a sensitive test. Patients who are dehydrated often have high levels of albumin, and those with fluid excess have a lowered value. The normal serum albumin level for men and women is 3.5 to 5.0 g/dL or 35 to 50 g/L (SI units) (Pagana & Pagana, 2014).

Thyroxine-binding **prealbumin (PAB)** is a plasma protein that provides a more sensitive indicator of nutrition deficiency because of its short half-life of 2 days. Depending on the laboratory test used, the normal PAB range is 15 to 36 mg/dL or 150 to 360 mg/L (SI units) (Pagana & Pagana, 2014). Although not used as commonly, serum **transferrin,** an iron-transport protein, can be measured directly or calculated as an indirect measurement of total iron-binding capacity (TIBC). It has a short half-life of 8 to 10 days and therefore is also a more sensitive indicator of protein status than albumin.

Cholesterol levels normally range between 160 and 200 mg/dL in adult men and women. Values are typically low with malabsorption, liver disease, pernicious anemia, end-stage cancer, or sepsis. A cholesterol level below 160 mg/dL has been identified as a possible indicator of malnutrition. Cholesterol testing is discussed in more detail in Chapter 36.

Total lymphocyte count (TLC) can be used to assess immune function. Malnutrition suppresses the immune system and leaves the patient more likely to get an infection. When a patient is malnourished, the TLC is usually decreased to below 1500/mm³.

◆ **Analysis**

The priority problem for the patient with malnutrition is Imbalanced Nutrition: Less Than Body Requirements related to inability to ingest or digest food or absorb nutrients (NANDA-I).

◆ **Planning and Implementation**

Improving Nutrition

Planning: Expected Outcomes. The patient with malnutrition is expected to have nutrients available to meet his or her metabolic needs as evidenced by normal serum proteins and adequate hydration.

Interventions. The preferred route for food intake is through the GI tract because it enhances the immune system and is safer, easier, less expensive, and more enjoyable.

Meal Management. The dietitian calculates the nutrients required daily and plans the patient's diet. In collaboration with the health care provider and dietitian, provide high-calorie, nutrient-rich foods (e.g., milkshakes, cheese, supplement drinks like Boost or Ensure). Assess the patient's food likes and dislikes. A feeding schedule of six small meals may be tolerated better than three large ones. A pureed or dental soft diet may be easier for those who have problems chewing or are **edentulous** (toothless).

Action Alert

Malnourished ill patients often need to be encouraged to eat. Instruct UAP who are feeding patients to keep food at the appropriate temperature and to provide mouth care before feeding. Assess for other needs, such as pain management, and provide interventions to make the patient comfortable. Pain can prevent patients from enjoying their meals. Remove bedpans, urinals, and emesis basins from sight. Provide a quiet environment, which is conducive to eating. Soft music may calm those with advanced dementia or delirium. Appropriate time should be taken so that the patient does not feel rushed through a meal.

CONSIDERATIONS FOR OLDER ADULTS
Patient-Centered Care (QSEN)

Some patients, especially older adults, may take a long time to eat even small quantities of food because they tend to be less hungry than younger adults. If available, suggest that family members bring in favorite or ethnic foods that the patient might be more likely to eat. Teach them about ways to encourage the patient to increase food intake. Chart 60-3 describes additional interventions to promote food intake in older adults.

Restorative feeding programs help nursing home residents who need special assistance. These residents often eat in a separate dining area so that time and attention can be given to them. Some nursing homes have designated food and nutrition nursing assistants and/or trained volunteers who are primarily responsible for promoting and maintaining nutrition and hydration. Delegate appropriate feeding tasks, and supervise these UAPs during resident mealtime.

Nutrition Supplements. If the patient cannot take in enough nutrients in food, fortified **medical nutrition supplements (MNSs)** (e.g., Ensure, Sustacal, Carnation Instant Breakfast [also available as lactose-free supplement]) may be given, especially to older adults. Many commercial enteral products are available. For patients with medical diagnoses such as liver and renal disease or diabetes, special products that meet those needs are available (e.g., Glucerna for diabetic patients). Nutrition supplements used in acute care, long-term care, and home care can be costly. In addition, patients may refuse them and the supplements are then wasted. In a classic study, Bender et al. (2000) found that a more successful alternative to having the MNS given by nursing assistant staff in the nursing home was to have the supplements delivered by nurses during their usual medication passes. In this study, the nurses gave 60 mL or more of the MNS at least 4 times a day with the residents' medications. As a result, the patients gained weight and had fewer pressure ulcers, thus making the program very cost-effective and providing positive clinical outcomes.

NUTRITION supplements are supplied as liquid formulas, powders, soups, coffee, and puddings in a variety of flavors. They come in different degrees of sweetness and are also available as modular supplements that provide single nutrients. Examples of modular supplements are Polycose glucose polymers for carbohydrates and Resource Beneprotein for protein, both available in liquid and powder form. Carbohydrate

CHART 60-3 Nursing Focus on the Older Adult
Promoting Nutrition Intake

- Be sure that patient is toileted and receives mouth care before mealtime.
- Be sure that patient has glasses and hearing aids in place, if appropriate, during meals.
- Be sure that bedpans, urinals, and emesis basins are removed from sight.
- Give analgesics to control pain and/or antiemetics for nausea at least 1 hour before mealtime.
- Remind unlicensed assistive personnel (UAP) to have patient sit in chair, if possible, at mealtime.
- If needed, open cartons and packages and cut up food at the patient's and/or family's request.
- Observe the patient during meals for food intake.
- Ask the patient about food likes and dislikes and ethnic food preferences.
- Encourage self-feeding, or feed the patient slowly; *delegate* this activity to UAP if desired.
- If feeding patient, sit at eye-level if culturally appropriate.
- Create an environment that is conducive to eating and socialization and relaxation, if possible.
- Decrease distractions, such as environmental noise from television, music, or other people.
- Provide adequate, nonglaring lighting.
- Keep patient away from offensive or medicinal odors.
- Keep eye contact with the patient during the meal if culturally appropriate.
- Serve snacks with activities, especially in long-term care settings; *delegate* this activity to UAP if desired.
- Document the percentage of food eaten at each meal and snack; *delegate* this activity to UAP if appropriate.
- Ensure that meals are visually appealing, appetizing, appropriately warm or cold, and properly prepared.
- Do not interrupt patients during mealtimes for nonurgent procedures or rounds.
- Assess for need for supplements between meals and at bedtime.
- Review the patient's drug profile, and discuss with the health care provider the use of drugs that might be suppressing appetite.
- If the patient is depressed, be sure that the depression is treated by the health care provider.

modulars are useful only if additional calories are needed. Protein modulars are indicated when metabolic stress causes a need for higher protein intake.

The dietitian may ask the nursing staff to keep a food and fluid intake record for at least 3 consecutive days to help assess the patient's nutrition status. Delegate this activity to UAP under your supervision. UAP also weigh the patient daily, every 3 days, or once a week, depending on the health care setting and severity of malnutrition.

Drug Therapy. Multivitamins, zinc, and an iron preparation are often prescribed to treat or prevent anemia. Monitor the patient's hemoglobin and hematocrit levels. Drug therapy can affect nutrition and elimination. For example, iron can cause constipation and zinc can cause nausea and vomiting.

If the patient still does not receive enough nutrition by mouth using the interventions just mentioned, request nutrition therapy in the form of **specialized nutrition support (SNS).** SNS consists of either total enteral nutrition (TEN) or total parenteral nutrition (TPN).

Total Enteral Nutrition. Patients often cannot meet the desired outcomes of adequate nutrition via their usual oral intake because of increased metabolic demands or a decreased ability to eat. Therefore TEN using enteral tube feeding may be necessary to supplement oral intake or to provide total nutrition.

Patients likely to receive TEN can be divided into three groups:

- Those who can eat but cannot maintain adequate NUTRITION by oral intake of food alone
- Those who have permanent neuromuscular impairment and cannot swallow
- Those who do not have permanent neuromuscular impairment but cannot eat because of their condition

Patients in the first group are often older adults or patients receiving cancer treatment who cannot meet their calorie and protein needs. In some cases, this artificial nutrition and hydration may not be desired. For example, some patients have advance directives stating that they do not want to be kept alive by artificial nutrition and hydration if certain conditions exist. *However, legal and ethical questions arise when patients are not able to make their wishes known!*

For many years it was believed that withholding food and fluids would cause discomfort. Terminally or chronically ill patients who do not eat and drink may not suffer. In fact, they may be more comfortable if food and fluids are withheld. *The decision to feed is complex, and there is no clear right or wrong answer. To compound this legal and ethical dilemma, medical complications (e.g., aspiration, pressure ulcers) are common in older adults who are tube-fed.*

Decisions about these dilemmas are aided by the advice of interdisciplinary ethics committees in health care facilities. When clinicians are making decisions about the desirability of tube feedings in these cases, the focus should be on achieving consensus by:

- Reviewing what is known about tube feedings, especially their risks and benefits
- Reviewing the medical facts about the patient
- Investigating any available evidence that would help understand the patient's wishes
- Obtaining the opinions of all stakeholders in the situation
- Delaying any action until consensus is achieved

Those in the second group of patients likely to receive TEN usually have permanent swallowing problems and require some type of feeding tube for delivery of the enteral product on a long-term basis. Examples of conditions that can cause permanent swallowing problems are strokes, severe head trauma, and advanced multiple sclerosis. Patients in the third group receive enteral NUTRITION for as long as their illness lasts. The feeding is discontinued when the patient's condition improves and he or she can eat again. TEN is contraindicated for patients in states of significant hemodynamic compromise, such as those with diffuse peritonitis, severe acute or chronic pancreatitis, intestinal obstruction, intractable vomiting or diarrhea, and paralytic ileus (Bankhead et al., 2009).

Many commercially prepared enteral products are available. A therapeutic combination of carbohydrates, fat, vitamins, minerals, and trace elements is available in liquid form. Differences among products allow the dietitian to select the right formula for each patient. A prescription from the health care provider is required for enteral nutrition, but the dietitian usually makes the recommendation and computes the amount and type of product needed for each patient.

NCLEX EXAMINATION CHALLENGE
Health Promotion and Maintenance

An older client tells the nurse that he does not have an appetite. His wife states that he refuses to eat the food she cooks. What instructions will the nurse provide for the client and wife? **Select all that apply.**
A. "Place the fork in his hand and leave the room."
B. "As long as you drink fluids, you do not need food."
C. "Let him choose what foods he might desire."
D. "Eat meals together, to make mealtime feel special."
E. "Take your time eating, and do not rush through meals."
F. "Use nutrition supplements such as Ensure throughout the day."

Methods of Administering Total Enteral Nutrition. TEN is administered as "tube feedings" through one of the available GI tubes, either through a nasoenteric or enterostomal tube. It can be used in the patient's home or any health care setting.

A **nasoenteric tube (NET)** is any feeding tube inserted nasally and then advanced into the GI tract, such as a Keofeed, Entriflex, or Dobbhoff tube. Commonly used NETs include the **nasogastric (NG) tube** and the smaller (small-bore) **nasoduodenal tube (NDT)** (Fig. 60-3, *A*). A nasojejunal tube (NJT) is also available but is used less often than the other NETs.

The NDTs are used for delivering *short-term* enteral feedings (usually less than 4 weeks) because they are easy to use and are safer for the patient at risk for aspiration *if the tip of the tube is placed below the pyloric sphincter of the stomach and into the duodenum.* Small-bore polyurethane or silicone tubes from 8 to 12 Fr external diameter are preferred. The smaller tubes are more comfortable and are less likely to cause complications such as nasal irritation, sinusitis, tissue erosion, and pulmonary compromise.

Enterostomal feeding tubes are used for patients who need *long-term* enteral feeding. The most common types are gastrostomies and jejunostomies. The surgeon directly accesses the GI tract using various surgical, endoscopic, and laparoscopic techniques.

A **gastrostomy** is a stoma created from the abdominal wall into the stomach, through which a short feeding tube is inserted by the surgeon. It may require a small abdominal incision or may be placed endoscopically. This tube is called a **percutaneous endoscopic gastrostomy (PEG)** or dual-access gastrostomy-jejunostomy (PEG/J) tube. The PEG requires monitored conscious sedation for placement and is secure and durable. An alternative to either device is the **low-profile gastrostomy device (LPGD)** (Fig. 60-3, *B* and *C*). The LPGD is available with a firm or balloon-style internal bumper or retention disk. An anti-reflux valve keeps GI contents from leaking onto the skin. This device is less irritating to the skin, longer lasting, and more cosmetically pleasing. It also allows greater patient independence. However, skin-level devices do not allow easy access for checking **residuals** (the amount of feeding that remains in the stomach).

Jejunostomies are used less often than gastrostomies. A **jejunostomy** is used for long-term feedings when it is desirable to bypass the stomach, such as with gastric disease, upper GI obstruction, and abnormal gastric or duodenal emptying.

Tube feedings are administered by bolus feeding, continuous feeding, and cyclic feeding. **Bolus feeding** is an intermittent feeding of a specified amount of enteral product at set intervals

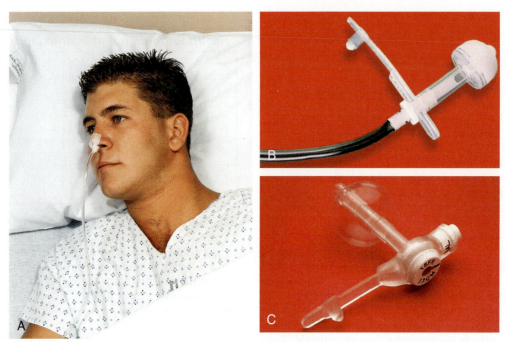

FIG. 60-3 Feeding tubes used for total enteral nutrition. **A,** Nasoduodenal tube. **B** and **C,** Gastrostomy tubes.

during a 24-hour period, typically every 4 hours. This method can be accomplished manually or by infusion through a mechanical pump or controller device. Another method of tube feeding is continuous enteral feeding. **Continuous feeding** is similar to IV therapy in that small amounts are continuously infused (by gravity drip or by a pump or controller device) over a specified time. The most commonly seen method, **cyclic feeding,** is the same as continuous feeding except the infusion is stopped for a specified time in each 24-hour period, usually 6 hours or longer ("down time"). Down time typically occurs in the morning to allow bathing, treatments, and other activities.

Infusion rates for cyclic feedings (and to some extent for intermittent bolus feeding) vary with the total amount of solution to be infused, the specific composition of the product, and the response of the patient to the feeding. The health care provider and dietitian usually decide the type, rate, and method of tube feeding, as well as the amount of additional water ("free water") needed. If the patient can swallow small amounts of food, he or she may also eat orally while the tube is in place.

The nurse is responsible for the care and maintenance of the feeding tube and the enteral feeding. Chart 60-4 lists best practices for the patient receiving TEN.

Complications of Total Enteral Nutrition. The nursing priority for care is patient safety, including preventing, assessing, and managing complications associated with tube feeding. Some complications of therapy result from the type of tube used to administer the feeding, and others result from the enteral product itself. The most common problem is the development of an obstructed ("clogged") tube. Use the tips in Chart 60-5 to maintain tube patency.

Patients receiving TEN are at risk for several other complications, including refeeding syndrome, tube misplacement and dislodgement, abdominal distention and nausea/vomiting, and FLUID AND ELECTROLYTE imbalance, often associated with diarrhea. These problems can be prevented if the patient is carefully monitored and complications are detected early.

Refeeding Syndrome. **Refeeding syndrome** is a potentially life-threatening metabolic complication that can occur when nutrition is restarted for a patient who is in a *starvation* state. When a patient is starved for nutrition, the body breaks down fat and protein, rather than carbohydrates, for energy. Protein catabolism leads to muscle and cell loss, often in major organs like the heart, liver, and lungs. The body's cells lose valuable electrolytes, including potassium and phosphate, into the plasma. Insulin secretion decreases in response to these changes. When *refeeding* begins, insulin production resumes and the cells take up glucose and electrolytes from the bloodstream, thus depleting serum levels.

> **⚠ NURSING SAFETY PRIORITY** (QSEN)
> ### *Critical Rescue*
>
> *The electrolyte shift of refeeding syndrome can cause cardiovascular, respiratory, and neurologic problems, primarily as a result of hypophosphatemia, according to a classic study by Mehanna et al. (2008). Observe for clinical manifestations of this electrolyte imbalance, including shallow respirations, weakness, acute confusion, seizures, and increased bleeding tendency. Report and document your findings immediately. More information on fluid and electrolyte imbalance can be found in Chapter 11.*

Refeeding syndrome can be prevented if patients are carefully assessed and managed for nutrition needs. Interventions to supplement or replace NUTRITION should be implemented early before the patient is in a starvation state. Patients receiving parenteral nutrition (described on pp. 1244-1245 later in this chapter) also may experience refeeding syndrome.

Tube Misplacement and Dislodgement. A serious complication is misplacement or dislodgement of the tube, *which can cause aspiration and possible death. Immediately remove any tube that you suspect is dislodged!* The Joint Commission's National Patient Safety Goals and the Centers for Medicare and Medicaid Services require all health care facilities to establish and

CHART 60-4 Best Practice for Patient Safety & Quality Care (QSEN)

Tube Feeding Care and Maintenance

- If nasogastric or nasoduodenal feeding is prescribed, use a soft, flexible, small-bore feeding tube (smaller than 12 Fr). *The initial placement of the tube should be confirmed by x-ray study.* Secure the tube with tape or a commercial attachment device after applying a skin protectant; change the tape regularly.
- Check tube placement by x-ray study when the correct position of the tube is in question; *an x-ray study is the most reliable method.*
- Per The Joint Commission's National Patient Safety Goals, if a gastrostomy or jejunostomy tube is used, assess the insertion site for signs of infection or excoriation (e.g., excessive redness, drainage). Rotate the tube 360 degrees each day, and check for in-and-out play of about $\frac{1}{4}$ inch (0.6 cm). If the tube cannot be moved, notify the health care provider immediately because the retention disk may be embedded in the tissue. Cover the site with a dry, sterile dressing, and change the dressing at least once a day.
- Check and record the residual volume every 4 to 6 hours or per facility policy by aspirating stomach contents into a syringe. If residual feeding is obtained, check with the health care provider for the appropriate intervention (usually to slow or stop the feeding for a time) or use the American Society of Parenteral and Enteral Nutrition (ASPEN) best practice recommendations.
- Check the feeding pump to ensure proper mechanical operation.
- Ensure that the enteral product is infused at the prescribed rate (mL/hr).
- Change the feeding bag and tubing every 24 to 48 hours; label the bag with the date and time of the change with your initials. Use an irrigation set for no more than 24 hours.
- For continuous or cyclic feeding, add only 4 hours of product to the bag at a time to prevent bacterial growth. *A closed system is preferred, and each set should be used no longer than 24 hours.*
- Wear clean gloves when changing or opening the feeding system or adding product; wipe the lid of the formula can with clean gauze; wear sterile gloves for critically ill or immunocompromised patients.
- Label open cans with date and time opened; cover, and keep refrigerated. Discard any unused open cans after 24 hours.
- *Do not use blue (or any color) food dye in formula because it does not assess aspiration and can cause serious complications.*
- To prevent aspiration, keep the head of the bed elevated at least 30 degrees during the feeding and for at least 1 hour after the feeding for bolus feeding; continuously maintain semi-Fowler's position for patients receiving cyclic or continuous feeding.
- Monitor laboratory values, especially blood urea nitrogen (BUN), serum electrolytes, hematocrit, prealbumin, and glucose.
- Monitor for complications of tube feeding, especially diarrhea.
- Monitor and carefully record the patient's weight and intake and output as requested by the physician or dietitian.

CHART 60-5 Best Practice for Patient Safety & Quality Care (QSEN)

Maintaining a Patent Feeding Tube

- Flush the tube with 20 to 30 mL of water (or the amount prescribed by the health care provider or dietitian):
    - At least every 4 hours during a continuous tube feeding
    - Before and after each intermittent tube feeding
    - Before and after drug administration (use warm water)
    - After checking residual volume
- If the tube becomes clogged, use 30 mL of water for flushing, applying gentle pressure with a 50-mL piston syringe.
- Avoid the use of carbonated beverage, except for existing clogs *when water is not effective.* Do not use cranberry juice.
- Whenever possible, use liquid medications instead of crushed tablets unless liquid forms cause diarrhea; make sure that the drug is compatible with the feeding solution.
- Do not mix drugs with the feeding product before giving. Crush tablets as finely as possible, and dissolve in warm water. *(Check to see which tablets are safe to crush. For example, do not crush slow-acting [SA] or slow-release [SR] drugs.)*
- Consider use of automatic flush feeding pump such as Flexiflo or Kangaroo.

implement procedures and systems to prevent patient harm from medical complications.

Several techniques should be used to confirm proper placement to prevent harm and to keep the patient safe. *An x-ray is the most accurate confirmation method and should always be done upon initial tube insertion.* After the initial placement is confirmed, check the placement before each intermittent feeding or at least every 4 to 8 hours during feeding. Also check placement before each drug administration.

The traditional auscultatory method for checking tube placement may not be reliable, especially for patients with small-bore tubes. In this method, the nurse instills 20 to 30 mL of air into the tube ("insufflation") while listening over the epigastric area (stomach) with a stethoscope. *The resulting "whooshing" sound does not guarantee correct tube placement!*

Although some patients have respiratory distress if the tube is misplaced into the lungs, others do not. Therefore better

methods for ensuring patient safety are being researched. Several safer procedures have been recommended for checking tube placement *after the initial placement has been confirmed by x-ray.* These methods include:

- Testing aspirated contents for pH, bilirubin, trypsin, or pepsin
- Assessing for carbon dioxide using capnometry

Some hospitals and nursing homes support testing the *pH of GI contents* at the bedside. To perform this procedure, aspirate a sample of the GI content, observe its color, and test its pH. When aspirating fluid, wait at least 1 hour after drug administration and then flush the tube with 20 mL of air to clear it. Collect the aspirate, and test it with pH paper. The pH of gastric fluid ranges from 0 to 4.0. If the tube has moved down into the intestines, the pH will be between 7.0 and 8.0. If the tube is in the lungs, the pH will be greater than 6.0. The pH may also be as high as 6 if the patient takes certain drugs, such as H_2 blockers (e.g., ranitidine [Zantac] and famotidine [Pepcid]). Because these drugs affect pH, bilirubin testing or capnometry may be more reliable and valid methods for predicting tube location.

Capnometry can determine if carbon dioxide is emitted from the tube (Grmec et al., 2011). A device to measure the presence of the gas is attached to the end of the tube after placement. The test is positive for carbon dioxide if the tube is placed into the lungs, rather than the stomach. *The tube should be immediately removed if the gas is detected.*

! NURSING SAFETY PRIORITY (QSEN)
Action Alert

If enteral tubes are misplaced or become dislodged, the patient is likely to aspirate. Aspiration pneumonia is a life-threatening complication associated with TEN, especially for older adults. Observe for increasing temperature and pulse, as well as for other signs of dehydration such as dry mucous membranes and decreased urinary output. Auscultate lungs every 4 to 8 hours to check for diminishing breath sounds, especially in lower lobes. Patients may become short of breath and report chest discomfort. A chest x-ray confirms this diagnosis, and treatment with antibiotics is started.

Abdominal Distention and Nausea/Vomiting. Abdominal distention, nausea, and vomiting during tube feeding are often caused by overfeeding. To *prevent* overfeeding, check gastric residual volumes every 4 to 6 hours, depending on facility policy and the needs of the patient. The American Society of Parenteral and Enteral Nutrition (ASPEN) (2011) recommends holding a feeding if the gastric residual volumes are more than 200 mL on two consecutive assessments. In some facilities, feedings are temporarily held if the gastric residual is 100 mL or more, depending on the patient. After a period of rest, the feeding can be restarted at a lower flow rate.

A problem with frequent residual assessments is that the formula may clog the tube during aspiration, even if flushed with water. If the patient's residual volumes have been low or zero and he or she has no abdominal distention, nausea, or vomiting, consider discontinuing these assessments, depending on facility policy.

FLUID AND ELECTROLYTE Imbalances. Patients receiving enteral nutrition therapy are at an increased risk for FLUID *imbalances.* They are often older or debilitated and may also have cardiac or renal problems. Fluid imbalances associated with enteral nutrition are usually related to the body's response to increased serum osmolarity, but *fluid overload* from too much tube feeding can also occur.

Osmolarity is the amount or concentration of particles dissolved in solution. This concentration exerts a specific osmotic pressure within the solution. Normal osmolarity of extracellular fluid (ECF) ranges between 270 and 300 mOsm. Enteral feeding products range in osmolarity from isotonic (about 300 mOsm) to extremely hypertonic (600 mOsm). Electrolytes (including sodium) contribute to this hypertonicity, but more of the osmolarity is determined by the concentration of proteins and sugar molecules in the enteral product. Even when the product is isotonic, the ECF can become hyperosmolar unless some hypotonic FLUIDS are also administered to the patient. This situation is most likely to develop in patients who are unconscious, unable to respond to the thirst reflex, on fluid restrictions, or receiving hyperosmotic enteral preparations.

Because increased plasma osmolarity is largely a result of extra glucose and proteins (which tend to remain in the plasma rather than move to interstitial spaces), the plasma osmotic pressure (water-pulling pressure) is increased. In this situation, intracellular and interstitial water move into and expand the plasma volume. This volume expansion results in an increased renal excretion of water (in patients with normal renal function) and leads to osmotic *dehydration.*

CONSIDERATIONS FOR OLDER ADULTS
Patient-Centered Care QSEN

If patients do *not* have normal renal and cardiac function, expansion of the plasma volume can lead to circulatory overload and pulmonary edema, especially in older adults. Therefore early identification of patients at risk for impairment of renal and/or cardiac function is important. Assess for signs and symptoms of circulatory overload, such as peripheral edema, sudden weight gain, crackles, dyspnea, increased blood pressure, and bounding pulse. Collaborate with the dietitian and health care provider to plan the correct amount of fluid to be provided.

Excessive *diarrhea* may develop when hyperosmolar enteral preparations are delivered quickly. This situation can also lead to *dehydration* through excessive water loss. Collaborate with the health care provider and dietitian for recommendations to prevent diarrhea. The dietitian usually changes the feeding to a more iso-osmolar formula. Most of these formulas can be started full strength but slowly at 15 to 20 mL/hr. The rate is gradually increased as the patient tolerates and as the expected nutrition outcome is achieved.

If diarrhea continues, especially if it has a very foul odor, evaluate the patient for *Clostridium difficile* or other infectious organisms. Contamination can occur because of repeated and often faulty handling of the feeding solution and system. *Per The Joint Commission's National Patient Safety Goals, wear clean gloves when changing systems and adding product. Sterile gloves may help prevent infection in critically ill or immunocompromised patients. A closed feeding system is preferred over an open one because the chance of contamination is lessened* (see Chart 60-4). Tubes with ports also minimize contamination by eliminating the need to open the feeding system to administer drugs.

In some cases, diarrhea may be the result of multiple liquid medications, such as elixirs and suspensions that have a very high osmolarity. Examples include acetaminophen (Tylenol), furosemide (Lasix), and phenytoin (Dilantin). Patients receiving multiple liquid drugs should be evaluated by the health care provider to determine whether their drug regimen can be changed to prevent diarrhea. Diluting these liquids may also be an option.

Depending on the patient's state of health, some electrolyte imbalances can be avoided. This is achieved by the use of enteral preparations containing lower concentrations of the electrolytes that the patient cannot handle well. For example, renal patients with high potassium levels receive a special formula that is used for this imbalance.

The two most common electrolyte imbalances associated with enteral nutrition therapy are hyperkalemia and hyponatremia. Both of these conditions may be related to hyperglycemia-induced hyperosmolarity of the plasma and the resultant osmotic diuresis. Risk for disturbances in FLUID AND ELECTROLYTE BALANCE are discussed in detail in Chapter 11.

Parenteral Nutrition. When a patient cannot effectively use the GI tract for NUTRITION, either partial or total parenteral nutrition therapy may be needed. This form of IV therapy differs from standard IV therapy in that any or all nutrients (carbohydrates, proteins, fats, vitamins, minerals, and trace elements) can be given. One liter of IV fluid containing 5% dextrose, which is often used as standard therapy, provides only 170 kcal. A hospitalized patient typically receives 3 to 4 L a day, for a total number of calories ranging between 500 and 700 a day. This calorie intake is not sufficient when the patient requires IV therapy for a prolonged period and cannot eat an adequate diet or has increased calorie needs for tissue repair and building.

Partial Parenteral Nutrition. Partial, or peripheral, parenteral nutrition (PPN) is usually given through a cannula or catheter in a large distal vein of the arm or through a peripherally inserted central catheter (PICC line). (See Chapter 13 for care of patients with PICC lines.) The alternative is used for some patients who can eat but are not able to take in enough nutrients to meet their needs. The patient must have adequate peripheral vein access and be able to tolerate large volumes of fluid to have PPN. Two types of solutions are commonly used in various combinations for PPN: IV fat (lipid) emulsions (IVFEs) and amino acid–dextrose solutions. IVFEs are usually given using a piggyback method.

! NURSING SAFETY PRIORITY (QSEN)
Critical Rescue

For patients receiving fat emulsions, monitor for manifestations of fat overload syndrome, especially in those who are critically ill. These manifestations include fever, increased triglycerides, clotting problems, and multi-system organ failure. Discontinue the IVFE infusion and report any of these changes to the health care provider immediately if this complication is suspected.

Most IVFEs (20% fat emulsion) are isotonic, but the tonicity of commercially prepared amino acid–dextrose solutions ranges from 300 mOsm to nearly 900 mOsm for PPN. Amino acid–dextrose solutions are considered more stable than IVFEs, and therefore additives (e.g., vitamins, minerals, electrolytes, trace elements) tend to be mixed with them. These solutions must be delivered through an in-line filter and are administered by an infusion pump for an accurate and constant delivery rate.

Some PPN products are a *mixture* of lipids (10% or 20% fat emulsion) and an amino acid–dextrose (usually 10%) solution. This mixture of three types of nutrients is referred to as a *3:1*, *total nutrient admixture (TNA)*, or *triple-mix solution*.

Total Parenteral Nutrition. When the patient requires intensive NUTRITION support for an extended time, the health care provider prescribes centrally administered **total parenteral nutrition (TPN)**. TPN is delivered through access to central veins, usually through a PICC line or the subclavian or internal jugular veins. Central venous catheters and associated nursing care are described in detail in Chapter 13.

Total parenteral nutrition solutions contain higher concentrations of dextrose and proteins, usually in the form of synthetic amino acids or protein hydrolysates (3% to 5%). These solutions are hyperosmotic (3 to 6 times the osmolarity of normal blood). The base solutions are available as commercially prepared solutions. The hospital or community pharmacist adds components (specific electrolytes, minerals, trace elements, and insulin) according to the patient's nutrition needs. This therapy provides needed calories and spares body proteins from catabolism for energy requirements.

The TPN solutions are administered with an infusion pump. The osmolarity of the fluid and the concentrations of the specific components make controlled delivery essential.

Patients receiving parenteral nutrition fluids are at risk for a wide variety of serious and potentially life-threatening complications. Complications may result from the solutions or from the peripheral or central venous catheter. The following discussion is limited to the complications that involve FLUID AND ELECTROLYTE BALANCE. Complications of IV cannulas and central venous catheters are discussed in Chapter 13, including infection and sepsis.

Patients receiving parenteral nutrition therapy are at high risk for fluid imbalance. Not only is fluid delivered directly into the venous system but also the extreme hyperosmolarity of the solutions stimulates fluid shifts between body fluid compartments. The hyperosmolarity is caused by their amino acid and dextrose concentrations. Increased dextrose causes hyperglycemia (increased blood glucose). As a result, some of the dextrose moves into the interstitial and intracellular spaces, where it is metabolized. However, dextrose remains in the plasma volume when the solutions are administered too rapidly, without enough insulin coverage, or in the presence of hyponatremia

and hypokalemia. The result is a shift of water from the interstitial and intracellular spaces into the plasma. Expansion of the plasma volume together with hyperglycemia can cause osmotic diuresis and lead to serious dehydration and hypovolemic shock. If the patient also has cardiac or renal dysfunction, he or she may develop fluid overload, congestive heart failure, and pulmonary edema. Monitor the infusion rate of the parenteral fluid, and give insulin as prescribed.

Monitor for these complications by taking daily weights and by documenting accurate intake and output while the patient is receiving parenteral nutrition. Serum glucose and electrolyte values are also monitored (Chart 60-6). Report any major changes or abnormalities to the health care provider, and document all assessments and interventions.

Patients receiving TPN are at an increased risk for many different disturbances of FLUID AND ELECTROLYTE BALANCE, depending on the composition of the solution and whether a fluid imbalance occurs. The health care provider usually requests frequent determinations of serum electrolyte levels to detect these imbalances. The risk for metabolic and electrolyte complications is reduced when the rate of administration is carefully controlled and patients are closely monitored for response to treatment. Potassium and sodium imbalances are common, especially when insulin is also administered as part of the therapy. Calcium imbalances, particularly hypercalcemia, are associated with TPN, although immobility may play more of a role than the actual therapy in developing this imbalance (National Institutes of Health [NIH], 2013a).

Community-Based Care

Malnourished patients can be cared for in a variety of settings, including the acute care hospital, transitional care unit, nursing home, or their own home. Malnutrition is often diagnosed when the patient is admitted to the acute care hospital or shortly after hospitalization if complications such as poor wound healing or sepsis occur. If the patient is severely compromised, he or she may require admission to a traditional nursing home for either transitional or long-term care. If adequate home support is available, he or she may be discharged to home in the care of a family member or other caregiver. Home care nurses may be needed to monitor and direct the care.

Home Care Management. The malnourished patient needs a variety of resources at home to continue aggressive NUTRITION support. If he or she can consume food by the oral route, the case manager or other discharge planner determines whether financial resources are available for the necessary nutrition supplements. If the hospital provides ambulatory nutrition counseling services, the patient is scheduled for follow-up after discharge for assessment of weight gain.

Self-Management Education. The dietitian teaches the malnourished patient and family about high-calorie, high-protein diet and NUTRITION supplements. In collaboration with the pharmacist, review specific parenteral solutions with the patient and family or significant others.

Reinforce the importance of adhering to the prescribed diet, and review any drugs the patient may be taking. If using an iron preparation, teach the importance of taking the drug immediately before or during meals. Caution the patient that iron tends to cause constipation. For the older adult already susceptible to constipation, emphasize the importance of measures for prevention, including adequate fiber intake, adequate fluids, and exercise.

Some patients are discharged to home with enteral or parenteral nutrition. Teach the family or other caregiver how to continue these therapies. Remind caregivers to consider the psychosocial aspects of these alternative methods for nutrition. For example, the caregiver can bring the enteral product and napkin to the patient on a decorative tray to make the feeding experience more elegant and "normal." Moving the feeding equipment out of view of the patient when it is not in use is also helpful.

Health Care Resources. The malnourished patient discharged to home on enteral or parenteral nutrition support needs the specialized services of a home nutrition therapy team. This team generally consists of the physician, nurse, dietitian, pharmacist, and case manager or social worker. Several commercial companies supply these services to patients at home in addition to the feeding supplies and formulas and health teaching.

◆ Evaluation: Outcomes

Evaluate the care of the malnourished patient based on the identified priority patient problem. The primary expected outcome is that he or she has available nutrients to meet the metabolic demands for maintaining weight and total protein and has adequate hydration.

OBESITY

❖ PATHOPHYSIOLOGY

Obesity is not just one disease; it includes many conditions with varying causes. The terms *obesity* and *overweight* are often used interchangeably, but they refer to different health problems. For both problems, the patient often does not consume enough

healthy nutrients and may not receive adequate nutrition. **Overweight** is an increase in body weight for height compared with a reference standard, or up to 10% greater than ideal body weight (IBW) and a body mass index (BMI) of 25 to 29. This weight may not reflect excess body fat. For example, well-developed athletes may appear overweight because of increased muscle (lean) mass, in which the proportion of muscle to fat is greater than average (NIH, 2013b).

Obesity refers to an excess amount of body fat when compared with lean body mass. The normal amount of body fat in *men* is between 15% and 20% of body weight. For *women,* the normal amount is 18% to 32%. An obese person weighs at least 20% above the upper limit of the normal range for ideal body weight and has a BMI of 30 or more. **Morbid obesity**, also called *extreme obesity,* refers to a weight that has a severely negative effect on health—usually more than 100% above IBW and a BMI over 40.

More than one third of Americans are obese (CDC, 2012b). About 10% or more of adults are morbidly obese. *This problem is the second leading cause of preventable deaths in the United States, second only to smoking, and has become a national crisis.* Obesity across the life span is considered an epidemic in the United States and Canada. Worldwide, it is recognized as a major global health problem, costing billions of dollars for health care and lost productivity.

The pathophysiology of obesity is very complex. A number of chemicals in the body, including hormones known as *adipokines,* work together to affect appetite and fat metabolism:

- **Leptin:** a hormone released by fat cells and possibly by gastric cells; it also acts on the hypothalamus to control appetite
- **Adiponectin:** an anti-inflammatory and insulin-sensitizing hormone
- **Resistin:** a hormone produced by fat cells that creates resistance to insulin activity
- **Inflammatory cytokines:** such as inflammatory interleukins and tumor necrosis factor–alpha
- **Apolipoprotein E:** one of several regulators of lipoprotein metabolism
- **Cholecystokinin:** a hormone that stimulates digestive juices and may work with leptin to increase or decrease appetite
- **Ghrelin:** the "hunger hormone" that is secreted in the stomach; increases in a fasting state and decreases after a meal

Some adipokines are neuropeptides, including orexins and anorexins, which play a role in body weight. **Orexins** are appetite stimulants; examples are ghrelin secreted by the stomach and peptide YY from the intestines. **Anorexins** decrease appetite and include leptin and insulin (McCance et al., 2014). Increased circulating plasma levels of orexins are associated with the development of obesity. However, in some people, high levels of leptin may not be effective in suppressing appetite—a condition known as *leptin resistance.* In this case, overeating and excessive weight gain can result. Hyperleptinemia also stimulates the autonomic nervous system and contributes to blood vessel inflammation and ventricular hypertrophy. These actions may help explain why obese patients are most at risk for hypertension, atherosclerosis, and heart disease (Kulie et al., 2011). Obesity is also associated with insulin resistance, which predisposes obese patients to type 2 diabetes mellitus (see Chapter 64) (NIH, 2013b).

The distribution of excess body fat rather than the degree of obesity has been used to predict increased health risks. For example, the waist circumference (WC) is a stronger predictor of coronary artery disease (CAD) than is the BMI. A WC greater than 35 inches (89 cm) in women and a WC greater than 40 inches (102 cm) in men indicate central obesity (National Institute of Diabetes and Digestive and Kidney Diseases, 2012). Central obesity is a major risk factor for CAD, stroke, type 2 diabetes, some cancers (e.g., colon, breast), sleep apnea, and early death (NIH, 2013b).

The waist-to-hip ratio (WHR) is also a predictor of CAD. This measure differentiates peripheral lower body obesity from central obesity. A WHR of 0.95 or greater in men (0.8 or greater in women) indicates android obesity with excess fat at the waist and abdomen.

Complications of Obesity

The major complications of obesity affect primarily the cardiovascular and respiratory systems. However, excess weight can also cause degeneration of the musculoskeletal system, especially the weight-bearing joints like hips and knees (osteoarthritis). Obese people are also more susceptible to infections and infectious diseases than are thinner people and tend to heal more slowly. Table 60-3 lists some of the most common complications of obesity.

Etiology and Genetic Risk

The causes of obesity involve complex interrelationships of many environmental, genetic, and behavioral factors. One of the most common causes of being overweight or obese is eating *high-fat and high-cholesterol diets*. Obesity is associated with diet when it contains a significant amount of *saturated* fat, which increases low-density lipoproteins (LDL, or LDL-C for low-density lipoproteins cholesterol). *Trans* fatty acids (TFAs), saturated fats, and cholesterol are linked to obesity and CAD (American Heart Association, 2013). By contrast, monounsaturated and polyunsaturated fats are healthy fats.

Physical inactivity has been identified as another cause of overweight and obesity. The major barriers to increasing physical activity include a lack of time, learned behaviors regarding a sedentary lifestyle, or decreased mobility associated with prolonged illness. Regular exercise is associated with lower death rates for adults of any age. It also increases lean muscle, decreases body fat, aids in weight control, and enhances psychological well-being. Although some people think that regular exercise has to include joining a fitness program or exercising for long periods, simple forms of exercise like walking 20 minutes provide the same type of benefit. Older adults can engage in this type of exercise. It does not cost money (like joining a program) and provides health benefits such as strengthening joints and improving cardiovascular health.

Another cause of obesity is *drug therapy*. Some prescribed drugs contribute to weight gain when they are taken on a long-term basis. Examples include:
- Corticosteroids
- Estrogens and certain progestins
- Nonsteroidal anti-inflammatory drugs (NSAIDs)
- Antihypertensives
- Antidepressants and other psychoactive drugs
- Antiepileptic drugs
- Certain oral antidiabetic agents

GENETIC/GENOMIC CONSIDERATIONS
Patient-Centered Care QSEN

Familial and genetic factors seem to play a very important role in obesity. When both parents are overweight, about 80% of their children will be overweight. If neither parent is overweight, fewer than 10% of the children will be overweight. In studies of identical twins, nonidentical twins, and parent-sibling relationships, about 50% of the difference in body fatness is transmitted to children and about 50% of this amount is genetically controlled (McCance et al., 2014).

Genetic composition may predispose some people but not others to obesity. Leptin, the hormone encoded by the *ob* gene, appears to send a message to the brain that the body has stored enough fat. This message serves as a signal to stop eating. In some obese people, other gene mutations have been identified, including an abnormality of the melanocortin-4 receptor that inhibits appetite in families with a history of obesity.

People who have **Prader-Willi syndrome (PWS)**, a complex neurodevelopmental genetic disorder, are typically morbidly obese. This disorder results from a hypothalamic-pituitary dysfunction that prevents appetite control (Yearwood et al., 2011).

Health Promotion and Maintenance

Obesity is a major public health problem and is associated with many complications, including death. As a result of this increasing problem, the *Healthy People 2020* agenda addresses the need to reduce the proportion of children, adolescents, and adults who are obese. *Healthy People 2020 objectives for Nutrition and Weight Status* include specific population targets related to obesity and healthy nutrition habits (Table 60-4). In

TABLE 60-3 Common Complications of Obesity

- Type 2 diabetes mellitus
- Hypertension
- Hyperlipidemia (increased serum lipids)
- Coronary artery disease (CAD)
- Stroke
- Peripheral artery disease (PAD)
- Metabolic syndrome
- Obstructive sleep apnea
- Obesity hypoventilation syndrome
- Depression and other mental health/behavioral health problems
- Urinary incontinence
- Cholelithiasis (gallstones)
- Gout
- Chronic back pain
- Early osteoarthritis
- Decreased wound healing

TABLE 60-4 Meeting *Healthy People 2020* Sample Objectives and Targets: Nutrition and Weight Status

- Reduce the proportion of adults who are obese (by 10%).
- Increase the proportion of adults who are at a healthy weight (by 10%).
- Increase the proportion of physician visits made by adult patients that include counseling about nutrition or diet (by 15.2%).
- Increase the proportion of primary care physicians who regularly assess body mass index (BMI) in their adult patients (by 10%).
- Increase the contribution of total vegetables to the diets of the population aged 2 years and older (to 1.1 cups per 1000 calories).
- Increase the contribution of fruits to the diets of the population aged 2 years and older (to 0.9 cups per 1000 calories).
- Reduce consumption of saturated fat in the population aged 2 years and older (by 9.5%).

collaboration with the dietitian, teach the importance of weight management and exercise to improve health. Even a 5% weight loss can drastically decrease the risk for coronary artery disease (CAD) and diabetes mellitus (NIH, 2013b). Nurses who practice healthful behaviors and value a healthy lifestyle are more likely to be seen by patients as credible teachers of this information (Marchiondo, 2014).

❖ PATIENT-CENTERED COLLABORATIVE CARE

◆ Assessment

History. In addition to taking a complete history regarding present and past health problems, collect this information about the patient in collaboration with the dietitian:

- Economic status
- Usual food intake
- Eating behavior
- Cultural background
- Attitude toward food
- Appetite
- Chronic diseases
- Drugs (prescribed and OTC, including herbal preparations)
- Physical activity/functional ability
- Family history of obesity
- Developmental level

A nutrition history usually includes a 24-hour recall of food intake and the frequency with which foods are consumed. The adequacy of the diet can be evaluated by comparing the amount and types of foods consumed daily with the established standards. The dietitian then provides a more detailed analysis of nutrition intake.

Physical Assessment/Clinical Manifestations. Obtain an accurate height and weight. The dietitian calculates the percentage of ideal body weight (% IBW) and the body mass index (BMI). He or she may also:

- Measure the waist circumference
- Calculate the waist-to-hip ratio
- Determine arm and calf circumferences

Examine the skin of the obese patient for reddened or open areas. Lift skinfold areas, such as pendulous breasts and abdominal aprons (**panniculus**), to observe for *Candida* (yeast) (a condition called *intertrigo*) or other infections or lesions. Infection of the panniculus is referred to as **panniculitis.**

Psychosocial Assessment. Obtain a psychosocial history to determine the patient's circumstances and emotional factors that might prevent successful therapy or that might be worsened by therapy. Interview the patient to determine his or her perception of current weight and weight reduction. Some patients do not view weight as a problem, which affects planning, treatment, and outcome. Ask the patient questions about his or her health beliefs related to being overweight, such as:

- What does food mean to you?
- Do you want to lose weight?
- What prevents you from losing weight?
- What do you think will motivate you to lose weight?
- How do you think you might benefit from losing weight?

Many patients report that they have tried multiple diets to lose weight but either the diets have not worked or they regained the weight they had initially lost. People who attempt restrictive diets become easy targets for the billion-dollar weight-loss industry, yet most dieters regain lost weight. This problem can be even more concerning for the older adult who loses weight and then regains it. Studies have shown that this cycle may contribute to loss of lean muscle mass, especially in older men (Lee et al., 2010).

The results of dieting and other efforts can lead to a sense of failure and lowered self-esteem, which often stimulates more overeating. Many overweight and obese people eat in response to environmental and emotional stressors rather than because they are hungry. Ask patients to identify their perceived stressors and what triggers their need for food.

Lifestyle changes are difficult without adequate family and community support. Assess useful coping strategies and support systems that the patient can employ during treatment for obesity.

Explore the patient's history to assess:

- Attempts at weight-reduction diets and outcomes
- Effects of obesity on lifestyle
- Effects of obesity on social interactions
- Mental health/behavioral health problems, such as depression
- Effects of obesity on intimate relationships, especially sexuality

Obese men often experience erectile dysfunction (ED), which can cause or worsen depression. Women often experience changes in their menstrual cycles and may have problems getting pregnant.

◆ Interventions

Weight is lost when energy used is greater than intake. Weight loss may be accomplished by nutrition modification with or without the aid of drugs and in combination with a regular exercise program. Patients who may be candidates for surgical treatment include those who have:

- Repeated failure of nonsurgical interventions
- A BMI equal to or greater than 40
- Weight more than 100% above IBW (i.e., morbidly obese)

Nonsurgical Management. Various nutrition approaches and drug therapy have been attempted to help obese patients achieve permanent weight loss.

Diet Programs. Diets for helping people lose weight include fasting, very-low-calorie diets, balanced and unbalanced low-energy diets, and novelty diets.

Short-term fasting programs have not been successful in treating morbidly obese patients, and prolonged fasting does not produce permanent benefits. Most patients regain the weight that was lost by this method. In addition, the risks associated with fasting (e.g., severe ketosis) require close medical supervision.

Very-low-calorie diets generally provide 200 to 800 calories/day. Two types of these diets are the *protein-sparing modified fast* and the *liquid formula diet.* The protein-sparing modified fast provides protein of high biologic value (1.5 g/kg of desirable body weight daily) within a limited number of calories. The diet produces rapid weight loss while preserving lean body mass. The liquid formula diet provides between 33 and 70 g of protein daily.

Both diets require an initial cardiac evaluation, supervision by an interdisciplinary health care team with monitoring by a physician, nutrition counseling by a dietitian, and supplementation with vitamins and minerals. These diets are only one part of a weight-reduction program. Patients who are on these diets should receive nutrition education, psychological counseling, exercise, and behavior therapy. Comparable weight losses have been achieved with both diets, but again, most patients regain the weight they lost.

Nutritionally balanced diets generally provide about 1200 calories/day with a conventional distribution of carbohydrate, protein, and fat. Vitamin and mineral supplements may be necessary if energy intakes fall below 1200 calories for women and 1800 calories for men. This diet provides conventional foods that are economical and easy to obtain. Thus the outcome of weight loss is facilitated, and it is hoped that loss is maintained. For example, Weight Watchers is an organization that provides education about nutritionally balanced diets based on a point system. They offer on-site weekly group support meetings or the option of an online community.

Unbalanced low-energy diets, such as the low-carbohydrate diet (e.g., Atkins or South Beach diet), restrict one or more nutrients. Protein and vegetables are encouraged, but certain carbohydrates and high-fat foods are not. Although they remain controversial in the medical community, these diets are extremely popular. Scientific outcome data have been conflicting.

Novelty diets, such as the grapefruit diet, the Cookie diet, and the Hollywood diet, are often nutritionally *inadequate*. This type of diet implies that a certain food or liquid increases metabolic rate or accelerates the oxidation of body fat. Weight loss is achieved because energy is restricted by food choice, but patients do not sustain weight loss after stopping the diet.

Nutrition Therapy. Nutrition recommendations for each patient are developed through close interaction among the patient, family, physician, nurse, and dietitian. The diet must meet the patient's needs, habits, and lifestyle and should be realistic.

The dietitian develops a diet plan and instructs the patient. At a minimum, the diet should:

- Have a scientific rationale
- Be nutritionally adequate for all nutrients
- Have a low risk-benefit ratio
- Be practical and conducive to long-term success

Calorie estimates are easily calculated. Resting metabolic rate is determined using a gender-specific formula that incorporates the appropriate activity factor. This figure reflects the total calories needed daily for maintaining current weight. To encourage a weight loss of 1 pound (0.45 kg) a week, the dietitian subtracts 500 calories each day. To encourage a weight loss of 2 pounds (0.9 kg) a week, 1000 calories each day are subtracted. The amount of weight lost varies with the patient's food intake, level of physical activity, and water losses. A reasonable expected outcome of 5% to 10% loss of body weight has been shown to improve glycemic control and reduce cholesterol and blood pressure. These benefits continue if the weight loss is sustained.

Exercise Program. Along with change in eating habits, a major intervention to manage obesity is to increase the type and amount of daily exercise to burn calories. For most people, adding exercise to a nutrition intervention produces more weight loss than just dieting alone. More of the weight lost is fat, which preserves lean body mass. An increase in exercise can reduce the waist circumference and the waist-to-hip ratio.

Teach patients that increasing and maintaining physical activity levels are important in maintaining weight loss. Many overweight or obese patients are so unfit that it may take several months of conditioning before they can exercise sufficiently to lose weight.

A minimum-level workout should be developed so that consistency can be achieved. The expected outcome is to maintain a lifetime of increased physical activity. The patient is likely to be less fatigued and discouraged with a low-intensity, short-duration program. Encourage sedentary (physically inactive) patients to increase their activity by walking 30 to 40 minutes at least 5 days each week. The activity may be performed all at once or divided over the course of the day. Remind the patient to exercise only under the supervision of the physician. All members of the interdisciplinary team should encourage and support any increase in physical activity. Structured national programs with support staff may be helpful for some patients. The staff typically offers diet counseling as well as cardiovascular and muscle-toning activities.

Drug Therapy. A BMI of 30 or a BMI of 27 with comorbidities is one indicator for the use of drug therapy. **Anorectic drugs** suppress appetite, which reduces food intake and, over time, may result in weight loss. The Food and Drug Administration (FDA) in the United States has pulled several drugs off the market and not approved other drugs due to concerns about cardiovascular complications associated with long-term use. Prescription drugs still available for the *long-term* treatment of obesity include orlistat (Xenical), lorcaserin (Belviq), and phentermine-topiramate (Qsymia).

Orlistat inhibits lipase and leads to partial hydrolysis of triglycerides. Because fats are only partially digested and absorbed, calorie intake is decreased. Most patients taking this drug have GI symptoms that include loose stools, abdominal cramps, and nausea unless they reduce their fat intake to less than 30% of their food intake each day. Therefore the drug should be used with caution and limited to adults between 18 and 75 years of age. Treatment is usually not extended beyond 12 months. A lower-dose 60-mg orlistat tablet (Alli) is the only *over-the-counter* weight-loss aid product that has received FDA approval for long-term use.

Lorcaserin (Belviq) works by activating the serotonin 2C receptor in the brain to help decrease appetite and create a sense of feeling full after eating small amounts of food (Mayo Clinic, 2014). Side effects may include headaches, dizziness, dry mouth, and constipation. Teach patients to report the signs of the rare but serious side effect of serotonin syndrome, including suicidal thoughts, psychiatric concerns, and problems with memory or comprehension (Mayo Clinic, 2014).

Phentermine-topiramate (Qsymia) combines a short-term weight-loss drug (phentermine) with a drug that is used to control seizures (topiramate) (Mayo Clinic, 2014). Side effects may include an increased heart rate, hand and feet tingling, insomnia, dizziness, dry mouth, and constipation. Teach patients that a rare but serious side effect that is associated with this drug is suicidal thoughts, which should immediately be reported to the prescribing health care provider (Mayo Clinic, 2014).

Other sympathomimetic drugs suppress appetite for *short-term* use along with a structured weight-management and exercise program. These drugs act on the central nervous system, including suppressing the appetite center in the hypothalamus. Examples include phentermine (Adipex-P), diethylpropion (Tenuate, Tenuate Dospan), and phendimetrazine (Bontril).

Behavioral Management. Behavioral management of obesity helps the patient change daily eating habits to lose weight. Self-monitoring techniques include keeping a record of foods eaten (food diary), exercise patterns, and emotional and situational factors. Stimulus control involves controlling the external cues that promote overeating. Reinforcement techniques are used to self-reward the behavior change. Cognitive restructuring involves modifying negative beliefs by learning positive coping self-statements. Counseling by health care professionals must continue before, during, and after treatment. The 12-step program offered by Overeaters Anonymous (www.oa.org) has helped many people lose weight, especially those who are compulsive eaters.

Complementary and Alternative Therapies. Many complementary and alternative therapies have been tested and used for obesity. These modalities aim to suppress appetite and therefore limit food intake to lose weight:

- Acupuncture
- Acupressure
- Ayurveda (a combination of holistic approaches)
- Hypnosis

Surgical Management. At any weight, some patients seek to improve their appearance by having a variety of cosmetic procedures to reduce the amount of adipose tissue in selected areas of the body. A typical example of this type of surgery is **liposuction,** which can be done in a physician's office or ambulatory surgery center. Although the patient's appearance improves, if weight gain continues, the fatty tissue will return. This procedure is not a solution for people who are morbidly obese.

Morbidly obese people who do not respond to traditional interventions may be considered for a major surgical procedure aimed at producing permanent weight loss. Patients with a body mass index (BMI) of 40 or greater or a BMI of 35 or greater along with additional risk factors are considered for surgery. Surgery has been perceived as a last resort to address weight issues, but it *is the only method that has a long-term impact on morbid obesity.*

Bariatrics. Bariatrics is a branch of medicine that manages patients with obesity and its related diseases. Surgical procedures include these three types: gastric restrictive, malabsorption, or both. *Restrictive* surgeries decrease the volume capacity of the stomach to limit the amount of food that can be eaten at one time. As the name implies, *malabsorption* procedures interfere with the absorption of food and nutrients from the GI tract.

Every year more than 200,000 people in the United States have bariatric surgical procedures (American Society for Bariatric Surgery, 2013), and that number continues to increase. The surgeon may use a conventional open approach or minimally invasive surgery (MIS). Most patients have MIS by having either the laparoscopic adjustable gastric band (LAGB) procedure or the laparoscopic sleeve gastrectomy (LSG). Both procedures are classified as restrictive surgeries (Virji, 2011). The decision of whether the patient is a candidate for the MIS is based on weight, body build, history of abdominal surgery, and co-existing medical complications. With any surgical approach, patients must agree to modify their lifestyle and follow stringent protocols to lose weight and keep the weight off. After bariatric surgery, many patients no longer have complications of obesity, such as diabetes mellitus, hypertension, depression, or sleep apnea.

Preoperative Care. Preoperative care is similar to that for any patient undergoing abdominal surgery or laparoscopy (see Chapter 14). However, obese patients are at increased surgical risks of pulmonary and thromboembolitic complications, as well as death. Some surgeons require limited weight loss before bariatric surgery to decrease these complications. Patients also have a thorough psychological assessment and testing to detect depression, substance abuse, or other mental health/behavioral health problem that could interfere with their success after surgery. Cognitive ability, coping skills, development, motivation, expectations, and support systems are also assessed. Patients who are not alert and oriented or do not have sufficient strength and mobility are not considered for bariatric surgery. *The primary role of the nurse is to reinforce health teaching in preparation for surgery.* Most bariatric surgical centers provide education sessions for groups of patients who plan to have the procedure.

Operative Procedures. *Gastric restriction* surgeries allow for normal digestion without the risk for nutrition deficiencies. In the LAGB procedure, the surgeon places an adjustable band to create a small proximal stomach pouch through a laparoscope (Fig. 60-4, *A*). The band may or may not be inflatable. For example, the REALIZE band requires that saline be injected into a balloon to control the tightness of the band. This type of procedure is considered to be restrictive; malabsorption complications usually do not occur (Virji, 2011). For the LSG, the surgeon removes the portion of the stomach where ghrelin, the "hunger hormone," is secreted. Restrictive surgeries are the easiest to perform. However, weight lost is often regained after a period of time. By contrast, patients having the malabsorption procedures maintain 60% to 70% of their weight loss even after 20 years.

The most common *malabsorption surgery* performed in the United States is the *Roux-en-Y gastric bypass (RNYGB),* which is often done as a robotic-assistive surgical procedure. This procedure results in quick weight loss, but it is more invasive with a higher risk for postoperative complications. In RNYGB, most commonly just called a **gastric bypass,** gastric resection is combined with malabsorption surgery (Virji, 2011). The patient's stomach, duodenum, and part of the jejunum are bypassed so that fewer calories can be absorbed (see Fig. 60-4, *B*).

Postoperative Care. Postoperative care depends on the type of surgery—the conventional open approach or the minimally invasive technique. Although many patients have MIS, they are

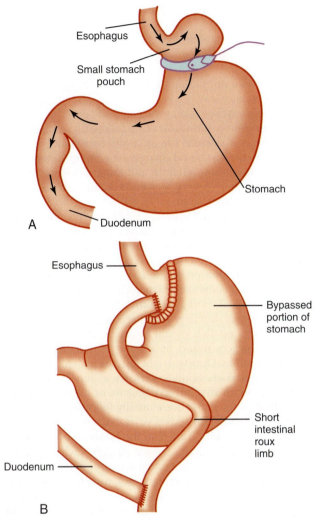

FIG. 60-4 Bariatric surgical procedures. **A,** Adjustable banded gastroplasty. **B,** Roux-en-Y gastric bypass (RNYGB).

considered as having major abdominal surgery along with all its risks and are cared for accordingly. These patients may require less than 24 hours in the hospital; some may need 1 to 2 days. Patients with open procedures may need several days to recover.

Patients having one of the MIS procedures have less pain, scarring, and blood loss. They typically have a faster recovery time and a faster return to daily activities.

The priority for immediate care of postoperative bariatric surgery patients is airway management. Patients with short and thick necks often have compromised airways and need aggressive respiratory support—possibly mechanical ventilation in the critical care unit.

All patients experience some degree of pain, but it is usually less severe when MIS is done. Patients may use patient-controlled analgesia (PCA) with morphine for up to the first 24 hours. All patients receive oral opioid analgesic agents as prescribed after the PCA is discontinued. Liquid forms of drug therapy are preferred. Acute pain management is discussed in detail in Chapter 3.

Care of the bariatric surgical patient is similar to that of any patient having abdominal or laparoscopic surgery. *A major focus is patient and staff safety.* Special bariatric equipment and accommodations, including an extra-wide bed and additional personnel for moving the patient, are needed for both the surgical suite and postoperative care units. Weight-rated beds must be wide enough to allow the patient to turn. Bed rails should not be touching the body because they can cause pressure areas. Pressure between skinfolds, as well as tubes and catheters, can also cause skin breakdown. Monitor the skin in these areas, and keep it clean and dry.

> ⚠️ **NURSING SAFETY PRIORITY** (QSEN)
> **Action Alert**
>
> Some patients who have bariatric surgery have a nasogastric (NG) tube put in place, especially after open surgical procedures. In gastroplasty procedures, the NG tube drains both the proximal pouch and the distal stomach. Closely monitor the tube for patency. *Never reposition the tube because its movement can disrupt the suture line!* The NG tube is removed on the second day if the patient is passing flatus.

Clear liquids are introduced slowly if the patient can tolerate water, and 1-ounce cups are used for each serving. Pureed foods, juice, and soups thinned with broth, water, or milk are added to the diet 24 to 48 hours after clear liquids are tolerated. Typically, the patient can increase the volume to 1 ounce over 5 minutes or until satisfied, but the diet is limited to liquids or pureed foods for 6 weeks. The patient then progresses to regular food, with an emphasis on nutrient-dense foods. Nausea, vomiting, or discomfort occurs if too much liquid is ingested.

> ⚠️ **NURSING SAFETY PRIORITY** (QSEN)
> **Critical Rescue**
>
> *Anastomotic leaks are the most common serious complication and cause of death after gastric bypass surgery. Monitor for manifestations of this life-threatening problem, including increasing back, shoulder, or abdominal pain; restlessness; and unexplained tachycardia and oliguria (scant urine). Report any of these findings to the surgeon immediately!*

In addition to the postoperative complications typically associated with abdominal and laparoscopic surgeries, bariatric patients have special needs and risks, such as the risk for anastomotic leaks (a leak of digestive juices and partially digested food through an anastomosis).

Implement these measures to prevent complications:
- Apply an abdominal binder to prevent wound dehiscence for open surgical procedures.
- Place the patient in semi-Fowler's position or use bi-level or continuous positive airway pressure (BiPAP or CPAP) ventilation at night to improve breathing and decrease risk for sleep apnea or other pulmonary complications, such as pneumonia and atelectasis.
- Monitor oxygen saturation; provide oxygen at 2 L/min as prescribed.
- Apply sequential compression stockings and administer prophylactic anticoagulant (usually heparin) therapy as prescribed to help prevent thromboembolitic complications, including pulmonary embolism (PE), a Joint Commission Core Measure intervention to prevent venous thromboembolism (VTE).

- Observe skin areas and folds for redness, excoriation, or breakdown to treat these problems early.
- Use absorbent padding between folds to prevent pressure areas and skin breakdown; make sure that tubes and catheters are not causing pressure as well.
- Remove urinary catheter within 24 hours after surgery to prevent urinary tract infection per the National Patient Safety Goals.
- Assist the patient out of bed on the day of surgery; encourage and assist with turning every 2 hours using an appropriate weight-bearing overhead trapeze. Collaborate with the physical or occupational therapist if needed for transfers or ambulation assistive devices, such as walkers.
- Ambulate patient as soon as possible to prevent postoperative complications, such as deep vein thrombosis and pulmonary embolus.
- Measure and record abdominal girth daily, as requested.
- In collaboration with the dietitian, provide six small feedings and plenty of fluids to prevent dehydration.
- Observe for signs and symptoms of **dumping syndrome** (caused by food entering the small intestine instead of the stomach) after *gastric bypass,* such as tachycardia, nausea, diarrhea, and abdominal cramping.

❓ CLINICAL JUDGMENT CHALLENGE

Patient-Centered Care; Evidence-Based Practice; Teamwork and Collaboration; Informatics QSEN

A 32-year-old morbidly obese woman had a laparoscopic sleeve gastrectomy procedure yesterday afternoon as part of a long-term plan for weight loss. She tells you that despite having had surgery, she is afraid she will not live long enough to see her children grow up. She is diaphoretic, with respirations of 32 per minute. You notice that she is wringing her hands as she talks.

1. What patient problems do you think she is having at this time? What data support your answer?
2. What priority health assessments will you perform at this time, and why?
3. How will you respond to her problems at this time, and why?
4. With which members of the health care team will you collaborate to address the patient's immediate concerns?
5. When she is ready for discharge, what health teaching will you provide related to the *Healthy People 2020 and 2010 Dietary Guidelines for Americans?* Find the complete evidence-based documents online, and develop a teaching plan for this patient.
6. To which community resources would you refer this patient, and why?

Community-Based Care

Obese patients are cared for in a variety of settings, including the acute care hospital and transitional care unit (particularly after surgery) or in their own home. Obesity is a chronic, life-long problem. Diets, drug therapy, exercise, and behavior modification can produce short-term weight losses with reasonable safety. However, most patients who do lose weight often regain the weight. Treatment of obesity should focus on the long-term reduction of health risks and medical problems associated with obesity, improving quality of life, and promoting a health-oriented lifestyle. Interdisciplinary team members need to

provide a nonjudgmental, supportive atmosphere that encourages the patient to:

- Increase physical activity
- Decrease fat intake and reliance on appetite-reducing drugs
- Establish a normal eating pattern in response to physiologic hunger
- Address psychological problems and concerns

Frequent long-term ambulatory care follow-up coordinated by a case manager is essential for successful treatment.

Teach patients that bowel changes are common after surgery, including constipation. Vitamin and mineral supplements are often needed after surgery, especially vitamin D, B-complex vitamins, iron, and calcium.

The most important features of health teaching for any obese patient and family focus on health-related behavior patterns. In collaboration with the dietitian, counsel the patient on a healthful eating pattern. The physical therapist or exercise physiologist recommends an appropriate exercise program. A psychologist may recommend cognitive restructuring approaches that help alter dysfunctional eating patterns. For patients who have surgery, additional discharge teaching is needed. Chart 60-7 lists the important areas that should be reviewed.

Bariatric surgery results in a major lifestyle change and a variety of emotions. During weight loss, the patient may become depressed or anxious. Some experience a "hibernation phase" for about a month after surgery because of physical and emotional adjustments. Patients are usually followed closely by the surgeon and dietitian for several years. Encourage them to keep all appointments and to adhere to the community-based treatment plan to ensure success. Plastic surgery, such as **panniculectomy** (removal of the abdominal apron, or **panniculus**), may be performed after weight is stabilized, usually in about 18 to 24 months.

Provide the patient with a list of available community resources, such as Overeaters Anonymous (www.oa.org) and the American Obesity Association (www.obesity.org). For surgical patients, the American Society for Metabolic and Bariatric Surgery (www.asmbs.org) may be helpful.

CHART 60-7   Patient and Family Education: Preparing for Self-Management

Discharge Teaching for the Patient After Bariatric Surgery

Nutrition: Diet progression, nutrient (including vitamin and mineral) supplements, hydration guidelines

Drug therapy: Analgesics and antiemetic drugs, if needed; drugs for other health problems

Wound care: Clean procedure for open or laparoscopic wounds; cover during shower or bath

Activity level: Restrictions, such as avoiding lifting; activity progression; return to driving and work

Signs and symptoms to report: Fever; excessive nausea or vomiting; epigastric, back, or shoulder pain; red, hot, and/or draining wound(s); pain, redness, or swelling in legs; chest pain; difficulty breathing

Follow-up care: Health care provider office or clinic visits, support groups and other community resources, counseling for patient and family

Continuing education: Nutrition and exercise classes; follow-up visits with dietitian

NURSING CONCEPTS AND CLINICAL JUDGMENT REVIEW

What might you NOTICE if the patient is experiencing inadequate NUTRITION as a result of malnutrition or obesity?

Malnutrition:
- Weight below ideal body weight or report of unexplained weight loss of 10 lbs (4.5 kg) in 6 months
- Dry, flaky skin
- Brittle nails and hair
- Leanness
- Activity intolerance
- Report of lethargy or fatigue
- Weakness
- Complications, such as infections, pressure ulcers, poor healing

Obesity:
- Weight at least 20% above ideal
- Excessive fat
- Shortness of breath during activity or at rest
- Slowed movement
- Change in gait or limping
- Complications, such as type 2 diabetes mellitus, hypertension, depression

What should you INTERPRET and how should you RESPOND to a patient experiencing inadequate NUTRITION as a result of malnutrition or obesity?

Perform and interpret assessments, including:
- Taking and recording height and weight
- Calculating BMI based on height and weight
- Checking laboratory values for hematocrit and hemoglobin and visceral proteins

- Taking complete medical history to determine associated complications and cause of nutrition problem
- Assessing impact of nutrition status on daily life, including ADLs
- Assessing coping mechanisms, especially for patients who are morbidly obese

Respond by:
- Teaching patients about their need for a healthy nutrition state
- Teaching patients how to either lose or gain weight, depending on their specific problem (e.g., nutrition supplements for malnutrition; restrictive diet and exercise for obesity)
- Teaching patients to weigh frequently
- Monitoring changes in serum visceral proteins (especially prealbumin) as an indicator of improved nutrition for malnourished patients
- Initiating total enteral or total parenteral nutrition as prescribed for malnutrition
- Informing morbidly obese patients about bariatric surgery options

On what should you REFLECT?
- Monitor patient for indicators of improved nutrition (e.g., increased prealbumin and weight for malnutrition; weight loss and decreased fat for obesity).
- Think about what may have caused these nutrition problems and how they can be prevented.
- Think about what else you can do to improve nutritional health of patients you care for.

GET READY FOR THE NCLEX® EXAMINATION!

KEY POINTS

Review these Key Points for each NCLEX Examination Client Needs Category.

Safe and Effective Care Environment
- Collaborate with the interdisciplinary health care team, especially the dietitian, health care provider, and case manager, when caring for patients with malnutrition or obesity. **Teamwork and Collaboration** `QSEN`
- Be sure that bariatric furniture and equipment are available for the obese patient in the hospital or other health care setting; avoid pressure on skinfold areas. **Safety** `QSEN`

Health Promotion and Maintenance
- Perform nutrition screening for all patients to determine if they are at risk (see Charts 60-1 and 60-2).
- Recall the recommendations included in the *2010 Dietary Guidelines for Americans* as listed in Table 60-1.
- Older patients are at increased risk for malnutrition (see Chart 60-2).

- Implement interventions to promote nutrition intake in older adults as specified in Chart 60-3. **Patient-Centered Care** `QSEN`

Psychosocial Integrity
- Be aware that some obese patients may not view their weight as a problem and are therefore unlikely to be part of a weight-reduction plan.
- Recognize that obesity can cause depression or anxiety, low self-esteem, and a disturbed body image.
- Be aware of legal and ethical issues related to tube-feeding older adults with chronic or terminal illness.

Physiological Integrity
- Review serum prealbumin, hemoglobin, and hematocrit levels to identify patients at nutrition risk.
- Assess patients with severe malnutrition for common complications, such as edema, lethargy, and dry, flaking skin.

- Provide evidence-based nursing interventions for managing total enteral nutrition as listed in Chart 60-4. **Evidence-Based Practice** QSEN
- Maintain feeding tube patency for patients receiving total enteral nutrition as described in Chart 60-5. **Safety** QSEN
- Ensure that feeding tube placement is verified by x-ray; check placement every 4 to 8 hours by aspirating gastric contents and assessing pH for nasogastric tubes. **Safety** QSEN
- Place patients receiving tube feeding in a semi-Fowler's position at all times to prevent aspiration; check residual contents every 4 hours or as designated per facility policy. **Safety** QSEN
- Use gloves when changing feeding system tubing or adding product; use sterile gloves when working with critically ill or immunocompromised patients.
- Use a feeding pump when the patient receives continuous or cyclic tube feeding.
- For patients receiving enteral or parenteral nutrition at home, teach family members or other caregivers how to provide NUTRITION while avoiding complications.
- Teach patients who are undernourished to eat high-protein, high-calorie foods and nutrition supplements.
- Provide care for patients receiving total parenteral nutrition as specified in Chart 60-6. **Evidence-Based Practice** QSEN
- Recall that normal body mass index (BMI) for adults should be between 18.5 and 25; older adults should have a BMI between 23 and 27. A BMI of 27 to 30 indicates overweight, over 30 indicates obesity, and 40 and greater indicates morbid obesity.

- Recall that obesity causes early onset of many chronic illnesses, such as osteoarthritis, diabetes mellitus, hypertension, and coronary artery disease. Pulmonary problems (e.g., obstructive sleep apnea), delayed wound healing, and infections are also common.
- Instruct obese patients about the importance of health care provider–approved exercise for weight reduction.
- Recognize that many people are following low-carbohydrate rather than low-fat diets to lose weight.
- Remember that bariatric surgery includes gastric restriction procedures or gastric bypass; a panniculectomy may be performed to remove skinfolds once weight is stabilized.
- Be alert for signs and symptoms of anastomotic leak after bariatric surgery, including severe pain, restlessness, anxiety, and unexplained tachycardia. **Safety** QSEN
- Provide postoperative care for patients having bariatric surgery to prevent complications such as wound dehiscence, respiratory distress, skin breakdown, and thromboembolitic complications, such as pulmonary embolism. Establishing and maintaining an airway is the priority for patients having bariatric surgery! **Safety** QSEN
- Observe for complications, such as dumping syndrome in patients who have a gastric bypass. Tachycardia, nausea, diarrhea, and abdominal cramping are common manifestations of dumping syndrome.
- Provide discharge teaching for patients having bariatric surgery as described in Chart 60-7.

CHAPTER **61**

Assessment of the Endocrine System

M. Linda Workman

 http://evolve.elsevier.com/Iggy/

PRIORITY CONCEPTS

- NUTRITION
- ELIMINATION

LEARNING OUTCOMES

Health Promotion and Maintenance
1. Teach all people measures to take to protect the endocrine system.

Psychosocial Integrity
2. Reduce the psychological impact for the patient and family regarding the assessment and testing of the endocrine system.

Physiological Integrity
3. Apply the principles of anatomy, physiology, and the aging process to assess the endocrine system and homeostasis.
4. Perform a focused assessment of endocrine function, incorporating information about genetic risk, age-related changes, and NUTRITION affecting endocrine function.
5. Coordinate appropriate care for patients and proper handling of specimens during testing of NUTRITION, ELIMINATION, and the endocrine system.

The tissues and organs of the endocrine system are located in many body areas (Fig. 61-1). Endocrine glands secrete hormones, which are natural chemicals that exert their effects on specific tissues known as target tissues. Target tissues are usually located some distance from the endocrine gland, with no connecting duct between the endocrine gland and its target tissue. For this reason, endocrine glands are called "ductless" glands and use the blood to transport secreted hormones to the target tissues (McCance et al., 2014). Endocrine glands include:

- Hypothalamus (a neuroendocrine gland)
- Pituitary gland
- Adrenal glands
- Thyroid gland
- Islet cells of the pancreas
- Parathyroid glands
- Gonads

The endocrine system working with the nervous system controls overall body function and regulation, including metabolism, NUTRITION, ELIMINATION, temperature, fluid and electrolyte balance, growth, and reproduction. Many interactions must occur between the endocrine system and all other body systems to ensure that each system maintains a constant normal balance (homeostasis) in response to environmental changes. For example, this regulation keeps the internal body temperature at or near 98.6° F (37° C), even when environmental temperatures vary. Other actions keep the serum sodium level between 136 and 145 mEq/L (mmol/L), regardless of whether a healthy person eats 2 g or 12 g of sodium per day.

Table 61-1 lists hormones secreted by various endocrine glands. Hormones travel through the blood to all body areas but exert their actions only on target tissues. They recognize their target tissues and exert their actions by binding to receptors on or within the target tissue cells. In general, each receptor site type is specific for only one hormone. Hormone-receptor actions work in a "lock and key" manner in that only the correct hormone (key) can bind to and activate the receptor site (lock) (Fig. 61-2). Binding a hormone to its receptor causes the target tissue to change its activity, producing specific responses.

Disorders of the endocrine system usually are related to:
- An excess of a specific hormone
- A deficiency of a specific hormone
- A receptor defect

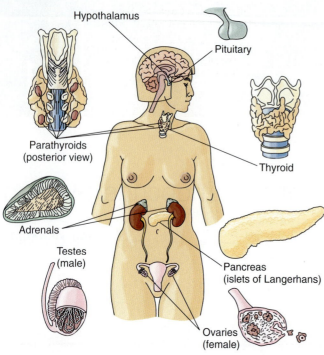

FIG. 61-1 The locations of various glands within the endocrine system.

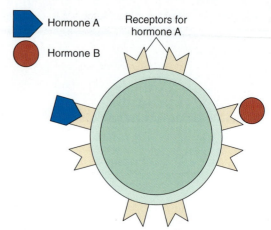

FIG. 61-2 "Lock and Key" hormone-receptor binding. *Hormone A* fits and binds to its receptors, causing a change in cell action. *Hormone B* does not fit or bind to receptors; no change in cell action results.

ANATOMY AND PHYSIOLOGY REVIEW

The control of cellular function by any hormone depends on a series of reactions working through negative feedback control mechanisms. Hormone secretion usually depends on the body's need for the final action of that hormone. When a body condition starts to move away from the normal range and a specific response is needed to correct this change, secretion of the hormone capable of starting the correcting action or response is stimulated until the need (demand) is met, and the body condition returns to the normal range. As the correction occurs, hormone secretion decreases (and may halt). This control of hormone synthesis is "negative feedback" because the hormone causes the *opposite* action of the initial condition change.

An example of a simple negative feedback hormone response is the control of insulin secretion. When blood glucose levels start to rise above normal, the hormone *insulin* is secreted. Insulin increases glucose uptake by the cells, causing a *decrease* in blood glucose levels. Thus the action of insulin (decreasing blood glucose levels) is the opposite of or negative to the condition that stimulated insulin secretion (elevated blood glucose levels).

Some hormones have more complex interactions for negative feedback. These interactions involve a series of reactions in which more than one endocrine gland, as well as the final target tissues, is stimulated. In this situation, the first hormone in the series may have another endocrine gland or glands as its target tissue. The final result of complex negative feedback for endocrine function is still opposite of the initiating condition.

An example of complex control is the interaction of the hypothalamus and the anterior pituitary with the adrenal cortex (Fig. 61-3). Low blood levels of cortisol from the adrenal cortex stimulate the secretion of corticotropin-releasing hormone (CRH) in the hypothalamus. CRH stimulates the anterior pituitary gland to secrete adrenocorticotropic hormone (ACTH). ACTH then triggers the release of cortisol from the adrenal cortex, the final endocrine gland in this series. The rising blood levels of cortisol inhibit CRH release from the hypothalamus. Without CRH, the anterior pituitary gland stops secretion of ACTH. In response, normal blood cortisol levels are maintained.

The normal blood level range of each hormone is well defined. Excesses or deficiencies of hormone secretion can lead to pathologic conditions.

TABLE 61-1	Principal Hormones of the Endocrine Glands
GLAND	**HORMONES**
Hypothalamus	Corticotropin-releasing hormone (CRH)
	Thyrotropin-releasing hormone (TRH)
	Gonadotropin-releasing hormone (GnRH)
	Growth hormone–releasing hormone (GHRH)
	Growth hormone–inhibiting hormone (somatostatin GHIH)
	Prolactin-inhibiting hormone (PIH)
	Melanocyte-inhibiting hormone (MIH)
Anterior pituitary	Thyroid-stimulating hormone (TSH), also known as *thyrotropin*
	Adrenocorticotropic hormone (ACTH, corticotropin)
	Luteinizing hormone (LH), also known as *Leydig cell–stimulating hormone (LCSH)*
	Follicle-stimulating hormone (FSH)
	Prolactin (PRL)
	Growth hormone (GH)
	Melanocyte-stimulating hormone (MSH)
Posterior pituitary	Vasopressin (antidiuretic hormone [ADH])
	Oxytocin
Thyroid	Triiodothyronine (T₃)
	Thyroxine (T₄)
	Calcitonin
Parathyroid	Parathyroid hormone (PTH)
Adrenal cortex	Glucocorticoids (cortisol)
	Mineralocorticoids (aldosterone)
Ovary	Estrogen
	Progesterone
Testes	Testosterone
Pancreas	Insulin
	Glucagon
	Somatostatin

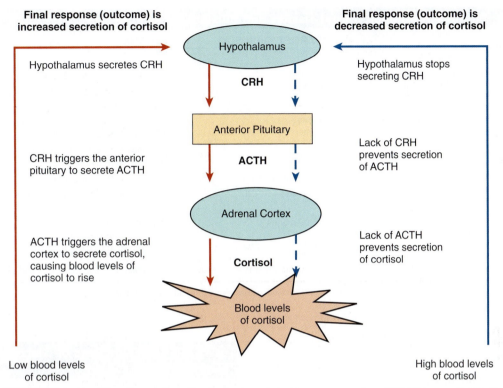

FIG. 61-3 Examples of positive and negative feedback control of hormone secretion. *ACTH,* Adrenocorticotropic hormone; *CRH,* corticotropin-releasing hormone.

Hypothalamus and Pituitary Glands

The hypothalamus is a small area of nerve and endocrine tissue located beneath the thalamus in the brain. Nerve fibers connect the hypothalamus to the rest of the central nervous system. The hypothalamus shares a small, closed circulatory system with the anterior pituitary gland, known as the *hypothalamic-hypophysial portal system.* This system allows hormones produced in the hypothalamus to travel directly to the anterior pituitary gland so that only very small amounts are wasted in systemic circulation.

The function of the hypothalamus is to produce regulatory hormones (see Table 61-1). Some of these hormones are released into the blood and travel to the anterior pituitary, where they either stimulate or inhibit the release of anterior pituitary hormones.

The pituitary gland is located at the base of the brain in a protective pocket of the sphenoid bone (see Fig. 61-1). It is divided into the anterior lobe (*adenohypophysis*) and the posterior lobe (*neurohypophysis*). Nerve fibers in the hypophysial stalk connect the hypothalamus to the posterior pituitary (Fig. 61-4).

In response to the releasing hormones of the hypothalamus, the anterior pituitary secretes some tropic hormones that stimulate other endocrine glands. Other pituitary hormones, such as prolactin, produce their effect directly on final target tissues (Table 61-2).

The hormones of the posterior pituitary—vasopressin (antidiuretic hormone [ADH]) and oxytocin—are produced in the hypothalamus and delivered to the posterior pituitary where they are stored. These hormones are released into the blood when needed.

Other factors can affect the release of hormones from the pituitary gland. Drugs, diet, lifestyle, and pathologic conditions can increase or decrease pituitary hormone secretion.

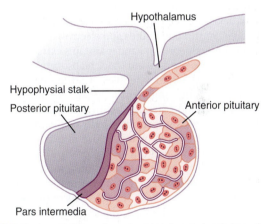

FIG. 61-4 The hypothalamus, hypophysial stalk, anterior pituitary gland, and posterior pituitary gland.

Gonads

The gonads are the male and female reproductive endocrine glands. Male gonads are the testes, and female gonads are the ovaries. Function of these glands begins at puberty when, under the influence of gonadotropic hormones secreted by the anterior pituitary, maturation of the glands and the external genitalia occurs. The testes are stimulated to produce testosterone, and the ovaries are stimulated to produce estrogen. The function of the gonads is detailed in Chapter 69.

Adrenal Glands

The adrenal glands are vascular, tent-shaped organs on the top of each kidney that have an outer cortex and an inner medulla (see Fig. 61-1). The adrenal hormones have effects throughout the body.

TABLE 61-2	Pituitary Hormones: Target Tissues and Subsequent Actions	
HORMONE	**TARGET TISSUE**	**ACTIONS**
Anterior Pituitary		
TSH (thyroid-stimulating hormone or thyrotropin)	Thyroid	Stimulates synthesis and release of thyroid hormone
ACTH (adrenocorticotropic hormone, corticotropin)	Adrenal cortex	Stimulates synthesis and release of corticosteroids and adrenocortical growth
LH (luteinizing hormone [known as *Leydig cell–stimulating hormone* in males])	Ovary / Testis	Stimulates ovulation and progesterone secretion / Stimulates testosterone secretion
FSH (follicle-stimulating hormone [known as *interstitial cell–* or *Sertoli cell–stimulating hormone* in males])	Ovary / Testis	Stimulates estrogen secretion and follicle maturation / Stimulates spermatogenesis
PRL (prolactin)	Mammary glands	Stimulates breast milk production
GH (growth hormone)	Bone and soft tissue	Promotes growth through lipolysis, protein anabolism, and insulin antagonism
MSH (melanocyte-stimulating hormone)	Melanocytes	Promotes pigmentation
Posterior Pituitary*		
Vasopressin (antidiuretic hormone [ADH])	Kidney	Promotes water reabsorption
Oxytocin	Uterus and mammary glands	Stimulates uterine contractions and ejection of breast milk

*These hormones are synthesized in the hypothalamus and are stored in the posterior pituitary gland. They are transported from the hypothalamus down the hypothalamic stalk to the posterior pituitary while bound to proteins known as *neurophysins*.

Adrenal Cortex

The adrenal cortex makes up about 90% of the adrenal gland and has cells divided into three layers. The main hormone types secreted by the cortex are the mineralocorticoids and the glucocorticoids. In addition, the cortex also secretes small amounts of sex hormones.

Mineralocorticoids are produced and secreted by the adrenal cortex to help control body fluids and electrolytes. **Aldosterone** is the major mineralocorticoid and maintains extracellular fluid volume. It promotes sodium and water reabsorption and potassium excretion in the kidney tubules. Aldosterone secretion is regulated by the renin-angiotensin system, serum potassium ion concentration, and adrenocorticotropic hormone (ACTH).

Renin is produced by specialized cells of the kidney arterioles. Its release is triggered by a decrease in extracellular fluid volume from blood loss, sodium loss, or posture changes. Renin converts renin substrate (angiotensinogen), a plasma protein, to angiotensin I. Angiotensin I is converted by a converting enzyme to form angiotensin II, the active form of angiotensin. In turn, angiotensin II stimulates the secretion of aldosterone. Chapter 11 (Fig. 11-6) further explains the renin-angiotensin system. Aldosterone causes the kidney to reabsorb sodium and water to bring the plasma volume and osmolarity back to normal.

Serum potassium level also controls aldosterone secretion. It is secreted whenever the serum potassium level increases above normal by as little as 0.1 mEq/L. Aldosterone then enhances kidney excretion of potassium to reduce the blood potassium level back to normal.

Glucocorticoids are produced by the adrenal cortex and are essential for life. The main glucocorticoid produced by the adrenal cortex is **cortisol**. Cortisol affects:

- The body's response to stress
- Carbohydrate, protein, and fat metabolism
- Emotional stability
- Immune function
- Sodium and water balance

Cortisol also influences other important body processes. For example, it must be present for catecholamine action and main-

TABLE 61-3	Functions of Glucocorticoid Hormones

- Prevent hypoglycemia by increasing liver gluconeogenesis and inhibiting peripheral glucose use
- Maintain excitability and responsiveness of cardiac muscle
- Increase lipolysis, releasing glycerol and free fatty acids
- Increase protein catabolism
- Degrade collagen and connective tissue
- Increase the number of mature neutrophils released from bone marrow
- Exert anti-inflammatory effects that decrease the migration of inflammatory cells to sites of injury
- Maintain behavior and cognitive functions

taining the normal excitability of the heart muscle cells. Glucocorticoid functions are listed in Table 61-3.

Glucocorticoid release is regulated directly by the anterior pituitary hormone *ACTH* and indirectly by the hypothalamic corticotropin-releasing hormone *(CRH)*. The release of CRH and ACTH is affected by the serum level of free cortisol, the normal sleep-wake cycle, and stress.

As described earlier and shown in Fig. 61-3, when blood cortisol levels are low, the hypothalamus secretes CRH, which triggers the pituitary to release ACTH. Then ACTH triggers the adrenal cortex to secrete cortisol. Adequate or elevated blood levels of cortisol *inhibit* the release of CRH and ACTH. This inhibitory effect is an example of a negative feedback system.

Glucocorticoid release peaks in the morning and reaches its lowest level 12 hours after each peak. Emotional, chemical, or physical stress increases the release of glucocorticoids.

Sex hormones (androgens and estrogens) are secreted in low levels by the adrenal cortex in both genders. Adrenal secretion of these hormones is usually not significant because the gonads (ovaries and testes) secrete much larger amounts of estrogens and androgens. In women, however, the adrenal gland is the major source of androgens.

💡 NCLEX EXAMINATION CHALLENGE
Physiological Integrity

What effect on circulating levels of sodium and glucose does the nurse expect in a client who has been taking an oral cortisol preparation for 2 years because of a respiratory problem?
A. Decreased sodium; decreased glucose
B. Decreased sodium; increased glucose
C. Increased sodium; decreased glucose
D. Increased sodium; increased glucose

Adrenal Medulla

The adrenal medulla is a sympathetic nerve ganglion that has secretory cells. Stimulation of the sympathetic nervous system causes the release of adrenal medullary hormones, the catecholamines (which include epinephrine and norepinephrine). These hormones travel to all areas of the body through the blood and exert their effects on target cells. The adrenal medullary hormones are not essential for life because they also are secreted by other body tissues, but they do play a role in the stress response.

The adrenal medulla secretes about 15% norepinephrine (NE) and 85% epinephrine. Hormone effects vary with the specific receptor in the cell membranes of the target tissue.

These receptors are of two types: alpha adrenergic and beta adrenergic, which are further classified as $alpha_1$ and $alpha_2$ receptors and $beta_1$, $beta_2$, and $beta_3$ receptors. NE acts mainly on alpha-adrenergic receptors, and epinephrine acts mainly on beta-adrenergic receptors.

Catecholamines exert their actions on many target organs (Table 61-4). Activation of the sympathetic nervous system, which then releases adrenal medullary catecholamines, is an important part of the stress response. Catecholamines are secreted in small amounts at all times to maintain homeostasis. Stress triggers increased secretion of these hormones, resulting in the "fight-or-flight" response, a state of heightened physical and emotional awareness.

Thyroid Gland

The thyroid gland is in the anterior neck, directly below the cricoid cartilage (Fig. 61-5). It has two lobes joined by a thin strip of tissue *(isthmus)* in front of the trachea.

The thyroid gland is composed of follicular and parafollicular cells. Follicular cells produce the thyroid hormones thyroxine (T_4) and triiodothyronine (T_3). Parafollicular cells produce thyrocalcitonin (TCT or calcitonin), which helps regulate serum calcium levels.

Control of metabolism occurs through T_3 and T_4. Both hormones increase metabolism, which causes an increase in oxygen use and heat production in all tissues. Most circulating T_4 and T_3 is bound to plasma proteins. The free hormone moves into the cell, where it binds to its receptor in the cell nucleus. Once in the cell, T_4 is converted to T_3, the most active thyroid hormone. The conversion of T_4 to T_3 is impaired by stress, starvation, dyes, and some drugs. Cold temperatures increase the conversion. Table 61-5 lists thyroid hormone functions.

Secretion of T_3 and T_4 is controlled by the hypothalamic-pituitary-thyroid gland axis negative feedback mechanism. The hypothalamus secretes thyrotropin-releasing hormone (TRH). TRH triggers the anterior pituitary gland to secrete thyroid-stimulating hormone (TSH), which then stimulates the thyroid

TABLE 61-4 Catecholamine Receptors and Effects of Adrenal Medullary Hormone Stimulation on Selected Organs and Tissues

ORGAN OR TISSUE	RECEPTORS	EFFECTS
Heart	Beta₁	Increased heart rate Increased contractility
Blood vessels	Alpha Beta₂	Vasoconstriction Vasodilation
Gastrointestinal tract	Alpha Beta	Increased sphincter tone Decreased motility
Kidneys	Beta₂	Increased renin release
Bronchioles	Beta₂	Relaxation; dilation
Bladder	Alpha Beta₂	Sphincter contractions Relaxation of detrusor muscle
Skin	Alpha	Increased sweating
Fat cells	Beta	Increased lipolysis
Liver	Alpha	Increased gluconeogenesis and glycogenolysis
Pancreas	Alpha	Decreased glucagon and insulin release
	Beta	Increased glucagon and insulin release
Eyes	Alpha	Dilation of pupils

TABLE 61-5 Functions of Thyroid Hormones in Adults

- Control metabolic rate of all cells
- Promote sufficient pituitary secretion of growth hormone and gonadotropins
- Regulate protein, carbohydrate, and fat metabolism
- Exert effects on heart rate and contractility
- Increase red blood cell production
- Affect respiratory rate and drive
- Increase bone formation and decrease bone resorption of calcium
- Act as insulin antagonists

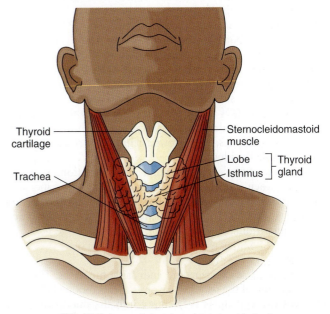

FIG. 61-5 Anatomic location of the thyroid gland.

Thyroid cartilage
Trachea
Sternocleidomastoid muscle
Lobe — Thyroid gland
Isthmus — Thyroid gland

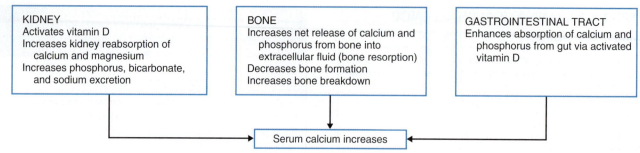

KIDNEY	BONE	GASTROINTESTINAL TRACT

Activates vitamin D
Increases kidney reabsorption of
   calcium and magnesium
Increases phosphorus, bicarbonate,
   and sodium excretion
	Increases net release of calcium and
	   phosphorus from bone into
	   extracellular fluid (bone resorption)
	Decreases bone formation
	Increases bone breakdown
		Enhances absorption of calcium and
		   phosphorus from gut via activated
		   vitamin D

Serum calcium increases

FIG. 61-6 Effects of parathyroid hormone on target tissues to maintain calcium balance.

gland to make and release thyroid hormones. If thyroid hormone levels are high, TRH and TSH release is inhibited. If thyroid hormone levels are low, release of TRH and TSH is increased. Cold and stress are two factors that cause the hypothalamus to secrete TRH, which then stimulates the anterior pituitary to secrete TSH.

Dietary intake of protein and iodine is needed to produce thyroid hormones. Iodine is absorbed from the intestinal tract as iodide. The thyroid gland withdraws iodide from the blood and concentrates it. After iodide is in the thyroid, it combines with the amino acid *tyrosine* to form T_4 and T_3. These hormones bind to thyroglobulin and are stored in the follicular cells of the thyroid gland. With stimulation, T_4 and T_3 are released into the blood. They enter many cells, where they bind to DNA receptors and turn on genes important in metabolism to regulate basal metabolic rate (BMR).

Calcium and phosphorus balance occurs partly through the actions of calcitonin (thyrocalcitonin [TCT]), which also is produced in the thyroid gland. Calcitonin lowers serum calcium and serum phosphorus levels by reducing bone resorption (breakdown). Its actions are opposite of parathyroid hormone.

The serum calcium level determines calcitonin secretion. Low serum calcium levels suppress the release of calcitonin. Elevated serum calcium levels increase its secretion.

Parathyroid Glands

The parathyroid glands consist of four small glands located close to or within the back surface of the thyroid gland (see Fig. 61-1). These cells secrete parathyroid hormone (PTH).

Parathyroid hormone regulates calcium and phosphorus metabolism by acting on bones, the kidneys, and the GI tract (Fig. 61-6). Bone is the main storage site of calcium. PTH increases **bone resorption** (bone release of calcium into the blood from bone storage sites), thus increasing serum calcium. In the kidneys, PTH activates vitamin D, which then increases the absorption of calcium and phosphorus from the intestines. In the kidney tubules, PTH allows calcium to be reabsorbed and put back into the blood.

Serum calcium levels determine PTH secretion. Secretion decreases when serum calcium levels are high, and it increases when serum calcium levels are low. PTH and calcitonin work together to maintain normal calcium levels in the blood and extracellular fluid.

Pancreas

The pancreas has exocrine and endocrine functions. The exocrine function of the pancreas involves the secretion of digestive enzymes through ducts that empty into the duodenum. The cells in the islets of Langerhans perform the pancreatic

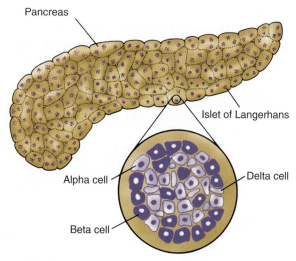

FIG. 61-7 The cells of the islets of Langerhans of the pancreas.

endocrine functions (Fig. 61-7). About one million islet cells are found throughout the pancreas.

The islets have three distinct cell types: alpha cells, which secrete glucagon; beta cells, which secrete insulin; and delta cells, which secrete somatostatin. Glucagon and insulin affect carbohydrate, protein, and fat metabolism. Somatostatin, which is secreted not only in the pancreas but also in the intestinal tract and the brain, inhibits the release of glucagon and insulin from the pancreas. It also inhibits the release of gastrin, secretin, and other GI peptides.

Glucagon is a hormone that increases blood glucose levels. It is triggered by decreased blood glucose levels and increased blood amino acid levels. This hormone helps prevent hypoglycemia. Chapter 64 discusses glucagon function in more detail.

Insulin promotes the movement and storage of carbohydrate (CHO), protein, and fat. It lowers blood glucose levels by enhancing glucose movement across cell membranes and into the cells of many tissues. Basal levels of insulin are secreted continuously to control metabolism. Insulin secretion rises in response to an increase in blood glucose levels. More information on insulin is presented in Chapter 64.

Endocrine Changes Associated with Aging

The effects of aging on the endocrine system vary. The three endocrine tissues that usually have reduced function with aging are the gonads, the thyroid gland, and the endocrine pancreas (Touhy & Jett, 2014). It is difficult to distinguish normal from abnormal endocrine activity in older adults because of chronic illness, changes in diet and activity, sleep disturbances, decreased

CHART 61-1 Nursing Focus on the Older Adult

Changes in the Endocrine System Related to Aging

CHANGES	CLINICAL FINDINGS	NURSING ACTIONS/ADAPTATIONS
Decreased antidiuretic hormone (ADH) production	Urine is more dilute and may not concentrate when fluid intake is low.	The patient is at greater risk for dehydration. Assess the older patient more frequently for dehydration. If fluids are not restricted because of another health problem, teach unlicensed assistive personnel (UAP) to offer fluids at least every 2 hours while awake.
Decreased ovarian production of estrogen	Bone density decreases.	Teach the patient to engage in regular exercise and weight-bearing activity to maintain bone density. Handle the patient carefully to avoid injury from pathologic fractures.
	Skin is thinner, drier, and at greater risk for injury.	Avoid pulling or dragging the patient. Use minimal tape on the skin. Assist patients confined to bed or chairs to change positions at least every 2 hours. Teach patients to use skin moisturizers.
	Perineal and vaginal tissues become drier, and the risk for cystitis increases.	Perform or assist the patient to perform perineal care at least twice daily. Unless another health problem requires fluid restriction, encourage all women to drink at least 2 liters of fluids daily. Teach sexually active women to urinate immediately after sexual intercourse. Teach sexually active women that using vaginal lubricants with sexual activity can reduce discomfort and the risk for tissue damage.
Decreased glucose tolerance	Weight becomes greater than ideal along with: ■ Elevated fasting blood glucose level ■ Elevated random blood glucose level ■ Slow wound healing ■ Frequent yeast infections ■ Polydipsia ■ Polyuria	Obtain a family history of obesity and type 2 diabetes. Encourage the patient to engage in regular exercise and to keep body weight within 10 lbs of ideal. Teach patients the clinical manifestations of diabetes, and instruct them to report any of these manifestations to the health care provider. Suggest diabetes testing for any patient with: ■ Persistent vaginal candidiasis ■ Failure of a foot or leg skin wound to heal in 2 weeks or less ■ Increased hunger and thirst ■ Noticeable decrease in energy level
Decreased general metabolism	Less tolerant of cold. Decreased appetite. Decreased heart rate and blood pressure (BP).	Can be difficult to distinguish from hypothyroidism. Check for additional manifestations of: ■ Lethargy ■ Constipation (as a change from usual bowel habits) ■ Decreased cognition ■ Slowed speech ■ Body temperature consistently below 97°F (36°C) ■ Heart rate below 60 beats/min Teach patients to dress warmly in cool or cold weather.

metabolism, and the use of drugs that may affect hormone function. Consider these factors when assessing the older adult with endocrine dysfunction.

Encourage the older adult to participate in regular screening examinations, including fasting and random blood glucose checks, calcium level determinations, and thyroid function testing. Chart 61-1 lists the endocrine changes that occur in the older adult.

ASSESSMENT METHODS

Patient History

Use a systems approach to obtain the history of patients with a possible endocrine problem. This approach can be difficult because of the variety and combination of clinical manifestations. Physical, psychosocial, and laboratory findings are needed for a complete assessment of endocrine function.

The age and gender of the patient provide baseline assessment data. Certain disorders are more common in older than in younger patients, such as diabetes mellitus, loss of ovarian function, and decreased thyroid function.

Manifestations of endocrine disorders can be gender related, such as the sexual effects of hyperpituitarism and hypopituitarism (see Chapter 62). Thyroid problems are more common in women (McCance et al., 2014). Assess for a history of endocrine dysfunction, manifestations that could indicate an endocrine disorder, and hospitalizations. Ask about past and current drugs, such as hydrocortisone, levothyroxine, oral contraceptives, and antihypertensive agents. The use of exogenous hormone drugs, when not needed for hormone replacement, can cause serious dysfunction in many endocrine glands. Use the opportunity to warn patients about the dangers of misusing hormone-based drugs such as androgens and thyroid hormones.

Nutrition History

NUTRITION changes or GI tract disturbances may reflect many different endocrine problems. Ask about a history of nausea, vomiting, and abdominal pain. An increase or decrease in food or fluid intake may also indicate specific disorders. For example, diabetes insipidus triggers excessive thirst and adrenal hypofunction triggers salt craving. Hunger and thirst also are associated with diabetes mellitus. Rapid changes in weight without diet changes are often associated with several endocrine disorders, including diabetes mellitus and thyroid problems.

NUTRITION deficiencies from an inadequate diet, especially of protein and iodide-containing foods (salt-water fish and seafood, iodized table salt), may be a cause of an endocrine disorder. Teach the patient about a well-balanced diet that includes at least 60 g of protein daily, less animal fat, and fewer concentrated simple sugars. Teach patients who do not eat saltwater fish on a regular basis to use iodized salt in food preparation.

Family History and Genetic Risk

Ask the patient about any family history of obesity, growth or development difficulties, diabetes mellitus, infertility, or thyroid disorders. These problems may have an autosomal dominant, recessive, or cluster pattern of inheritance.

Current Health Problems

Focus on the patient's reason for seeking health care, asking questions such as:

- Did manifestations occur gradually, or was the onset sudden?
- Have you been treated for this problem in the past?
- How have the current problems affected your activities of daily living?

These questions can provide clues to specific endocrine disorders. Also explore changes in energy levels, ELIMINATION patterns, sexual and reproductive functions, and physical features.

Energy level changes occur with many endocrine problems, especially thyroid problems (see Chapter 63) and adrenal problems (see Chapter 62). Ask the patient about any change in ability to perform ADLs, and assess his or her current energy level. For instance, has he or she been sleeping longer or are fatigue and generalized weakness present?

ELIMINATION is affected by the endocrine system. Identify the patient's past pattern of elimination to determine deviations from the normal routine. Ask about the amount and frequency of urination. Does he or she urinate frequently in large amounts? Does the patient wake during the night to urinate (**nocturia**), or is pain present with urination (**dysuria**)? Information about the frequency of bowel movements and their consistency and color may provide clues to problems in fluid balance or metabolic rate (i.e., thyroid function).

Sexual and reproductive functions are greatly affected by endocrine disturbances. Ask women about any changes in the menstrual cycle, such as increased flow, duration, and frequency of menses; pain or excessive cramping; or a change in the regularity of menses. Ask men whether they have experienced impotence. Ask men and women about a change in libido (sexual desire) or any fertility problems.

Physical appearance changes can reflect an endocrine problem. Discuss any changes that the patient perceives in physical features. Ask about changes in:

- Hair texture and distribution
- Facial contours and eye protrusion
- Voice quality
- Body proportions
- Secondary sexual characteristics

For example, ask a man whether he is shaving less often or a woman if she has noticed an increase in facial hair. These changes may be associated with pituitary, thyroid, parathyroid, or adrenal dysfunction.

Physical Assessment
Inspection

An endocrine problem can change physical features because of its effect on growth and development, sex hormone levels, fluid and electrolyte balance, and metabolism. Different clinical findings can occur with many endocrine disorders or with nonendocrine problems.

Use a head-to-toe approach for inspection. Observe the patient's general appearance, and assess height, weight, fat distribution, and muscle mass in relation to age. Heredity and age rather than a health problem may be responsible for some physical features (e.g., short stature).

When examining the head, focus on abnormalities of facial structure, features, and expression, such as:

- Prominent forehead or jaw
- Round or puffy face
- Dull or flat expression
- Exophthalmos (protruding eyeballs and retracted upper lids)

Check the lower neck for a visible enlargement of the thyroid gland. Normally the thyroid tissue cannot be observed. The isthmus may be noticeable when the patient swallows. Jugular vein distention may be seen on inspection of the neck and can indicate fluid overload.

Observe skin color, and look for areas of pigment loss (hypopigmentation) or excess (hyperpigmentation). Fungal skin infections, slow wound healing, bruising, and petechiae are often seen in patients with adrenal hyperfunction. Skin infections, foot ulcers, and slow wound healing often occur with diabetes mellitus. With some types of adrenal gland dysfunction, the skin over joints, as well as any scar tissue, may show increased pigmentation due to increased levels of adrenocorticotropic hormone (ACTH) and melanocyte-stimulating hormone.

Vitiligo (patchy areas of pigment loss) is seen with primary hypofunction of the adrenal glands and is caused by autoimmune destruction of melanocytes in the skin. This is seen most often on the face, neck, arms, and legs. Mucous membranes may have large areas of uneven pigmentation. Document the location, color, distribution, and size of skin color changes.

Inspect the fingernails for malformation, thickness, or brittleness, all of which may suggest thyroid gland problems. Examine the extremities and the base of the spine for edema, which suggests a fluid and electrolyte imbalance.

Check the trunk for any abnormalities in chest size and symmetry. Truncal obesity and the presence of a "buffalo hump" between the shoulders on the back may indicate adrenocortical excess. Hormonal imbalance may also change secondary sexual characteristics. Inspect the breasts of both men and women for size, symmetry, pigmentation, and discharge. **Striae** (reddish purple "stretch marks") on the breasts or abdomen are often seen with adrenocortical excess.

Assess the patient's hair distribution for indications of endocrine gland dysfunction. Changes can include **hirsutism** (excessive growth of body hair, especially on the face, chest, and the center abdominal line of women), excessive scalp hair loss, or changes in hair texture.

Examination of the genitalia may reveal a dysfunction in hormone secretion. Observe the size of the scrotum and penis or of the labia and clitoris in relation to standards for the patient's age. The distribution and quantity of pubic hair are often affected in hypogonadism.

Palpation

The thyroid gland and the testes can be examined by palpation. Chapters 69 and 72 discuss examination of the testes. The thyroid gland is palpated for size, symmetry, general shape, and the presence of nodules or other irregularities.

Palpate the thyroid gland by standing either behind or in front of the patient. The posterior approach may be easier (Jarvis, 2016). Having the patient swallow sips of water during the examination helps you palpate the thyroid gland, which is not easily felt when normal.

Ask the patient to sit and to lower the chin. Using the posterior approach, place both your thumbs on the back of the patient's neck, with the fingers curved around to the front of the neck on either side of the trachea. Ask the patient to swallow, and locate the thyroid as you feel it rising. To examine the right lobe, turn the patient's head to the right and gently displace the trachea to the right with your left fingers. Placing your fingers between the trachea and the neck muscles, palpate the right lobe with your right hand. Reverse this procedure to examine the left lobe.

! NURSING SAFETY PRIORITY (QSEN)
Action Alert

Always palpate the thyroid gently because vigorous palpation can stimulate a thyroid storm in a person who has or is suspected to have hyperthyroidism.

Auscultation

Auscultate the chest to assess cardiac rate and rhythm to use later as a means of assessing treatment effectiveness. Some endocrine problems induce dysrhythmias. Many endocrine problems can cause dehydration and volume depletion. Document any difference in the patient's blood pressure and pulse in the lying, standing, or sitting positions (orthostatic vital signs).

If an enlarged thyroid gland is palpated, auscultate the area of enlargement for bruits. Hypertrophy of the thyroid gland causes an increase in vascular flow, which may result in bruits.

Psychosocial Assessment

Assess the patient's coping skills, support systems, and health-related beliefs. Many endocrine problems can change a patient's behaviors, personality, and psychological responses. Ask whether the patient has noticed a change in how stress is handled, frequency of crying, or degree of patience and anger expression. The patient may not recognize these changes in himself or herself. When possible, ask the family about changes in the patient's behaviors or personality.

A number of endocrine disorders affect the patient's perception of self. For example, body features can change significantly in disorders of the pituitary, adrenal, and thyroid glands. Infertility, impotence, and other changes in sexual function may result from endocrine dysfunction. Encourage the patient to express his or her feelings and concerns about a change in appearance or in sexual function. Ask about any difficulty in coping with such changes.

Patients with endocrine problems may require lifelong drugs and follow-up care. Assess their readiness to learn and ability to carry out specific self-management skills. Patients may also face financial difficulties resulting from a prolonged medical regimen or loss of employment. A referral to social service agencies may be needed.

CHART 61-2 Best Practice for Patient Safety & Quality Care (QSEN)
Endocrine Testing

For Blood Tests:
- Check your laboratory's method of handling hormone test samples for tube type, timing, drugs to be administered as part of the test, etc. For example, blood samples drawn for catecholamines must be placed on ice and taken to the laboratory immediately.
- Explain the procedure and any restrictions to the patient.
- If you are drawing blood samples from an IV line, clear the line thoroughly. Do not use a double- or triple-lumen line to obtain samples; contamination or dilution from another port is possible.
- Emphasize the importance of taking a drug prescribed for the test on *time*. Tell the patient to set an alarm if the drug is to be taken during the night.

For Urine Tests:
- Instruct the patient to begin the urine collection (whether for 2, 4, 8, 12, or 24 hours) by first emptying his or her bladder.
- Remind the patient to *not* save the urine specimen that begins the collection. The timing for the urine collection begins *after* this specimen.
- Tell the patient to note the time of the discarded specimen and to plan to collect all urine from this time until the end of the urine collection period.
- To end the collection, instruct the patient to empty his or her bladder at the end of the timed period and *add* that urine to the collection.
- Check with the laboratory to determine any special handling of the urine specimen (e.g., Is a preservative needed? Does the container need to be kept cold?).
- If needed, make sure that the preservative has been added to the collection container at the *beginning* of the collection.
- Tell the patient about any preservative and the need to avoid splashing urine from the container, because some preservatives make the urine caustic.
- If the specimen must be kept cool or cold, instruct the patient to place the container in an inexpensive cooler with ice. The specimen container should not be kept with food or drinks.

Diagnostic Assessment
Laboratory Assessment

Laboratory tests are an essential part of the diagnostic process for possible endocrine problems. Fluids commonly used for these tests include blood, urine, and saliva (Klee, 2011). Always check with the agency's laboratory for proper collection and handling of the specimen. The specialized testing for specific disorders is described in Chapters 62 to 64. Best practices for the collection of specimens for general endocrine testing are listed in Chart 61-2.

Assays. An assay measures the level of a specific hormone in blood or other body fluid. The most common assays for endocrine testing are antibody-based immunologic assays and chromatographic assays, which include mass spectrometry. These assays are very sensitive and can detect even minute quantities of a given hormone. Many different hormone concentrations can be analyzed at the same time by the mass spectrometry method.

Stimulation/Suppression Tests. Measurement of specific hormone blood levels does not always distinguish between the normal and the abnormal. The wide normal range for some hormones makes it necessary to trigger responses by stimulation or suppression tests.

For the patient who might have an underactive endocrine gland, a stimulus may be used to determine whether the gland is capable of normal hormone production. This method is called *stimulation testing*. Measured amounts of selected hormones are given to stimulate the target gland to maximum production. Hormone levels are then measured and compared with expected normal values. Failure of the hormone level to rise with stimulation indicates hypofunction.

Suppression tests are used when hormone levels are high or in the upper range of normal. Drugs or other substances known to normally suppress hormone production are administered. Failure of suppression of hormone production during testing indicates hyperfunction.

Venous Sampling. Blood samples are taken directly from veins that drain a specific endocrine gland, and hormone levels are measured. Unexpected blood hormone levels may indicate the location of a mass, a dysfunctional gland, or a dysfunctional part of a gland.

Urine Tests. Hormone levels and their metabolites in the urine can be measured to determine endocrine function. Because many of the endocrine hormones are secreted in a pulsatile fashion, measurement of a specific hormone in a 24-hour urine collection, rather than as a single blood or urine sample, better reflects specific gland function, such as the adrenal gland. Teach the patient how to collect a 24-hour urine sample (see also Chart 61-2).

Certain hormones require additives in the container at the beginning of the collection. Instruct the patient not to discard the preservative from the container and to use caution when handling it because some are caustic. Remind him or her that this collection is timed for *exactly* 24 hours. Instruct the patient to avoid taking any unnecessary drugs during endocrine testing because some drugs can interfere with the assay.

Tests for Glucose. Tests for functions of the islet cells of the pancreas measure the *result* of pancreatic islet cell function.

Blood glucose values and the oral glucose tolerance test help diagnose diabetes mellitus. The glycosylated hemoglobin (A1C) value reveals the *average* blood glucose level over a period of 2 to 3 months. (See Chapter 64 for diabetes mellitus testing.)

Imaging Assessment

Anterior, posterior, and lateral skull x-rays may be used to view the sella turcica, the bony pocket in the skull where the pituitary gland rests. Erosion of the sella turcica indicates invasion of the wall from an abnormal growth.

MRI with contrast is the most sensitive method of imaging the pituitary gland, although CT scans can also be used to evaluate it. The thyroid, parathyroid glands, ovaries, and testes are evaluated by ultrasound. CT scans are used to evaluate the adrenal glands, ovaries, and pancreas.

Other Diagnostic Assessment

Needle biopsy is a relatively safe and quick ambulatory surgery procedure used to indicate the composition of thyroid nodules. It is used to determine whether surgical intervention is needed.

NURSING CONCEPTS AND CLINICAL JUDGMENT REVIEW

What might you NOTICE in a patient with adequate NUTRITION related to endocrine function?

Vital signs:
- Heart rate and rhythm within normal range
- Oxygen saturation of 95% or higher
- Body temperature within normal range

Physical assessment:
- Weight proportionate to height; does not appear underweight or overweight
- Muscle development even with no muscle loss or excess
- Skin color and texture normal (no jaundice, striae, waxiness, edema, excessive dryness, or severe acne)
- Body hair distribution appropriate for gender

- Scalp hair thickness similar to family members with no recent changes
- Menstrual periods regular

Psychological assessment:
- Oriented and appropriate affect
- Not confused and does not have rapid changes of emotions that are out of proportion to existing situation
- Energy level good; can engage in desired work, recreational, and personal activities
- Sleep average 6 to 8 hours, feeling rested on awakening

Laboratory assessment:
- Hormone levels and production within normal limits for age and gender
- Serum electrolyte levels within normal limits
- Blood glucose levels within normal limits

GET READY FOR THE NCLEX® EXAMINATION!

KEY POINTS

Review these Key Points for each NCLEX Examination Client Needs Category.

Health Promotion and Maintenance
- Teach all patients that misusing hormones or steroids can have an adverse effect on endocrine function. **Patient-Centered Care** QSEN

Psychosocial Integrity
- Encourage the patient to express concerns about a change in appearance, sexual function, or fertility as a result of a possible endocrine problem. **Patient-Centered Care** QSEN
- Explain all diagnostic procedures, restrictions, and follow-up care to the patient scheduled for endocrine tests. **Patient-Centered Care** QSEN
- Ask family members about changes in the patient's personality or behavior. **Patient-Centered Care** QSEN

Physiological Integrity
- Be aware that the onset of endocrine problems can be slow and insidious or abrupt and life threatening.
- Ask the patient about other family members with endocrine disorders, because some problems have a genetic component. **Evidence-Based Practice** QSEN
- Ask the patient what prescribed and over-the-counter drugs are taken on a regular basis, because some drugs can alter endocrine function. **Patient-Centered Care** QSEN
- Follow the laboratory's procedures for collecting and handling specimens for endocrine function studies. **Evidence-Based Practice** QSEN
- Differentiate normal from abnormal laboratory test findings and clinical manifestations for patients with possible endocrine problems. **Patient-Centered Care** QSEN

Care of Patients with Pituitary and Adrenal Gland Problems

M. Linda Workman

 http://evolve.elsevier.com/Iggy/

PRIORITY CONCEPTS

- FLUID AND ELECTROLYTE BALANCE
- GLUCOSE REGULATION

LEARNING OUTCOMES

Safe and Effective Care Environment

1. Protect the patient with pituitary or adrenal gland problems from injury and from problems associated with changes in FLUID AND ELECTROLYTE BALANCE.

Health Promotion and Maintenance

2. Identify the teaching priorities for the patient taking hormone replacement therapy for pituitary or adrenal hypofunction.

Psychosocial Integrity

3. Reduce the psychological impact for the patient and family experiencing pituitary or adrenal gland problems.

Physiological Integrity

4. Interpret clinical changes and laboratory data to determine the effectiveness of therapy for diabetes insipidus and for syndrome of inappropriate antidiuretic hormone (SIADH).

5. Prioritize nursing care for the patient with acute adrenal insufficiency and poor GLUCOSE REGULATION.

6. Coordinate nursing care for the patient with Cushing's disease or syndrome.

7. Coordinate care for the patient with hyperaldosteronism or pheochromocytoma.

Pituitary and adrenal gland problems alter hormone levels and change the function of many tissues and organs. When too much or too little of one or more hormones is secreted, the effects may induce physical and psychological changes. The anterior pituitary gland regulates growth, metabolism, and sexual development. The posterior pituitary gland secretes **vasopressin** (antidiuretic hormone [ADH]). Problems in this gland result in changes in FLUID AND ELECTROLYTE BALANCE. The adrenal gland secretes hormones that influence homeostasis and are life sustaining. Nursing care for the patient with pituitary or adrenal gland disorders includes assessment, patient education, evaluation of patient response to therapy, and providing support.

A complete assessment is performed to detect specific clinical findings. The patient also often undergoes many diagnostic tests and relies on the nurse for explanations. Surgical intervention may be indicated. The patient often needs lifelong hormone replacement therapy, and physical and emotional support are critical.

DISORDERS OF THE ANTERIOR PITUITARY GLAND

The anterior pituitary gland (adenohypophysis) controls growth, metabolic activity, and sexual development through the actions of these hormones:

- Growth hormone (GH; somatotropin)
- Thyrotropin (thyroid-stimulating hormone [TSH])
- Corticotropin (adrenocorticotropic hormone [ACTH])
- Follicle-stimulating hormone (FSH)
- Luteinizing hormone (LH)
- Melanocyte-stimulating hormone (MSH)
- Prolactin (PRL)

Disorders of the anterior pituitary gland can result from problems within the anterior pituitary gland itself *(primary pituitary dysfunction)*, from problems in the hypothalamus that change pituitary function *(secondary pituitary dysfunction)*, or from the influence of exogenous drugs. Regardless of the problem, one or more hormones may be undersecreted *(pituitary hypofunction)* or oversecreted *(pituitary hyperfunction)*.

HYPOPITUITARISM

❖ PATHOPHYSIOLOGY

A person with hypopituitarism has a deficiency of one or more anterior pituitary hormones. If only one hormone is affected, the condition is known as *selective hypopituitarism*. Decreased production of *all* of the anterior pituitary hormones *(panhypopituitarism)* is rare.

More often, one hormone has greatly decreased secretion and the secretion of other hormones is reduced to a lesser degree. Deficiencies of *adrenocorticotropic hormone (ACTH)* and *thyroid-stimulating hormone (TSH)* are the *most* life threatening because they cause a decrease in the secretion of vital hormones from the adrenal and thyroid glands. Adrenal gland hypofunction is discussed on pp. 1273-1276; hypothyroidism is discussed in Chapter 63.

Deficiency of the gonadotropins (luteinizing hormone [LH] and follicle-stimulating hormone [FSH]—hormones that stimulate the gonads to produce sex hormones) changes sexual function in both men and women. In men, gonadotropin deficiency results in testicular failure with decreased testosterone production that may cause sterility. In women, gonadotropin deficiency results in ovarian failure, amenorrhea, and infertility.

Growth hormone (GH) deficiency changes tissue growth patterns indirectly as a result of reduced liver production of somatomedins. These substances, especially somatomedin C, trigger growth and maintenance activities in bone, cartilage, and other tissues throughout life.

GH deficiency results from decreased GH production, failure of the liver to produce somatomedins, or a failure of tissues to respond to the somatomedins. Deficiency in children leads to short stature and general growth retardation. Deficiency in adults does not affect height but increases the rate of bone destructive activity, leading to thinner bones (osteoporosis) and an increased risk for fractures.

The cause of hypopituitarism varies. Benign or malignant pituitary tumors can compress and destroy pituitary tissue. Pituitary function can be impaired by malnutrition or rapid loss of body fat. Shock or severe hypotension reduces blood flow to the pituitary gland, leading to hypoxia and infarction. Other causes of hypopituitarism include head trauma, brain tumors or infection, radiation or surgery of the head and brain, and acquired immune deficiency syndrome (AIDS). *Idiopathic hypopituitarism* has an unknown cause.

Postpartum hemorrhage is the most common cause of pituitary infarction, which results in decreased hormone secretion. This clinical problem is known as *Sheehan's syndrome*. The pituitary gland normally enlarges during pregnancy, and when hypotension results from hemorrhage, ischemia and necrosis of the gland occur. Usually this condition develops immediately after delivery, although some cases have occurred up to several years later.

❖ PATIENT-CENTERED COLLABORATIVE CARE

◆ Assessment

Changes in physical appearance and target organ function occur with deficiencies of specific pituitary hormones (Chart 62-1). Gonadotropin (LH and FSH) deficiency results in the loss of or change in secondary sex characteristics in men and women. In male patients, look for facial and body hair loss. Ask about impotence and decreased *libido* (sex drive). Women may report amenorrhea (absence of menstrual periods), dyspareunia (painful intercourse), infertility, and decreased libido. In female patients, check for dry skin, breast atrophy, and a decrease or absence of axillary and pubic hair.

Neurologic manifestations of hypopituitarism as a result of tumor growth often first occur as changes in vision. Assess the patient's visual acuity, especially peripheral vision, for changes or loss. Headaches, diplopia (double vision), and limited eye movement are common.

CHART 62-1   Key Features

Pituitary Hypofunction

DEFICIENT HORMONE	CLINICAL MANIFESTATIONS
Anterior Pituitary Hormones	
Growth hormone (GH)	Decreased bone density Pathologic fractures Decreased muscle strength Increased serum cholesterol levels
Gonadotropins (luteinizing hormone [LH], follicle-stimulating hormone [FSH])	Women: ■ Amenorrhea ■ Anovulation ■ Low estrogen levels ■ Breast atrophy ■ Loss of bone density ■ Decreased axillary and pubic hair ■ Decreased libido Men: ■ Decreased facial hair ■ Decreased ejaculate volume ■ Reduced muscle mass ■ Loss of bone density ■ Decreased body hair ■ Decreased libido ■ Impotence
Thyroid-stimulating hormone (thyrotropin) (TSH)	Decreased thyroid hormone levels Weight gain Intolerance to cold Scalp alopecia Hirsutism Menstrual abnormalities Decreased libido Slowed cognition Lethargy
Adrenocorticotropic hormone (ACTH)	Decreased serum cortisol levels Pale, sallow complexion Malaise and lethargy Anorexia Postural hypotension Headache Hypoglycemia Hyponatremia Decreased axillary and pubic hair (women)
Posterior Pituitary Hormones	
Vasopressin (antidiuretic hormone [ADH])	Diabetes insipidus: ■ Greatly increased urine output ■ Low urine specific gravity (<1.005) ■ Hypotension ■ Dehydration ■ Increased plasma osmolarity ■ Increased thirst ■ Output does not decrease when fluid intake decreases

Laboratory findings vary widely. Some pituitary hormone levels may be measured directly. As described in Chapter 61, laboratory assessment of some pituitary hormones involves measuring the *effects* of the hormones rather than measuring the actual hormone levels. For example, blood levels of triiodothyronine (T_3) and thyroxine (T_4) from the thyroid, as well as testosterone and estradiol from the gonads, are measured easily. If levels of one or all of these hormones are low or in the low-normal range, further pituitary evaluation is necessary.

Pituitary problems may cause changes in the sella turcica (the bony nest where the pituitary gland rests) that can be seen with skull x-rays (McCance et al., 2014). Changes may include enlargement, erosion, and calcifications as a result of pituitary tumors. CT and MRI can more distinctly define bone or soft-tissue lesions. An angiogram may be used to rule out the presence of an aneurysm or other vascular problems in the area before surgery.

◆ Interventions

Management of the adult with hypopituitarism focuses on replacement of deficient hormones. Men who have gonadotropin deficiency receive sex steroid replacement therapy with androgens (testosterone). The most effective routes of androgen replacement are parenteral and transdermal. Therapy begins with high-dose testosterone and is continued until **virilization** (presence of male secondary sex characteristics) is achieved, with responses that include increases in penis size, libido, muscle mass, bone size, and bone strength. Chest, facial, pubic, and axillary hair growth also increase. Patients usually report improved self-esteem and body image after therapy is initiated. The dose may then be decreased, but therapy continues throughout life. Therapy to increase fertility requires gonadotropin-releasing hormone (GnRH) injections in addition to testosterone therapy (Melmed et al., 2011).

Androgen therapy is avoided in men with prostate cancer. Side effects of therapy include **gynecomastia** (male breast tissue development), acne, baldness, and prostate enlargement.

Women who have gonadotropin deficiency receive hormone replacement with a combination of estrogen and progesterone. The risk for hypertension or *thrombosis* (formation of blood clots in deep veins) is increased with estrogen therapy, especially among smokers. Emphasize measures to reduce risk and the need for regular health visits. For inducing pregnancy, clomiphene (Clomid) may be given to trigger ovulation. Gonadotropin-releasing hormone (GnRH) and human chorionic gonadotropin (hCG) can be used to stimulate ovulation if therapy with clomiphene fails.

Adult patients with GH deficiency may be treated with subcutaneous injections of human GH (hGH). Injections are given at night to mimic normal GH release.

? NCLEX EXAMINATION CHALLENGE

Safe and Effective Care Environment

For which client does the nurse question the prescription for androgen replacement therapy?
A. 35-year-old man who has had a vasectomy
B. 48-year-old man who takes prednisone for severe asthma
C. 62-year-old man with a history of prostate cancer
D. 70-year-old man who has hypertension and type 2 diabetes

HYPERPITUITARISM

❖ PATHOPHYSIOLOGY

Hyperpituitarism is hormone oversecretion that occurs with pituitary tumors or tissue hyperplasia (tissue overgrowth). Tumors occur most often in the anterior pituitary cells that produce growth hormone (GH), prolactin (PRL), and adrenocorticotropic hormone (ACTH). Overproduction of PRL also may occur in response to tumors that overproduce GH and ACTH. Excess ACTH may occur with increased secretion of melanocyte-stimulating hormone (MSH).

🧬 GENETIC/GENOMIC CONSIDERATIONS
Patient-Centered Care QSEN

One cause of hyperpituitarism is multiple endocrine neoplasia, type 1 (*MEN1*), in which there is inactivation of the suppressor gene *MEN1* (Manchester, 2013). This problem has an autosomal dominant inheritance pattern and is usually expressed as a benign tumor that affects the pituitary, parathyroid glands, and pancreas. In the pituitary, this problem causes excessive production of growth hormone and acromegaly. Ask a patient with acromegaly whether either parent also has this problem or has had a tumor of the pancreas or parathyroid glands.

The most common cause of hyperpituitarism is a pituitary adenoma—a benign tumor of one or more tissues within the anterior pituitary. Adenomas are classified by size, invasiveness, and the hormone secreted. As an adenoma gets larger and compresses brain tissue, neurologic changes, as well as endocrine problems, may occur. Such manifestations may include visual disturbances, headache, and increased intracranial pressure.

Prolactin (PRL)-secreting tumors are the most common type of pituitary adenoma. Excessive PRL inhibits the secretion of gonadotropins and sex hormones in men and women, resulting in *galactorrhea* (breast milk production), amenorrhea, and infertility.

Overproduction of GH in adults results in *acromegaly* (Fig. 62-1). The onset may be gradual with slow progression, and changes may remain unnoticed for years before diagnosis of the disorder. Early detection and treatment are essential to prevent irreversible changes in the soft tissues, such as those of the face, hands, feet, and skin. Other changes include increased skeletal thickness, hypertrophy of the skin, and enlargement of many organs, such as the liver and heart. Some changes may be reversible after treatment, but skeletal changes are permanent.

Bone thinning and bone cell overgrowth occur slowly. Breakdown of joint cartilage and hypertrophy of ligaments, vocal cords, and eustachian tubes are common. Nerve entrapment and poor GLUCOSE REGULATION with hyperglycemia (elevated blood glucose levels) are common.

Excess ACTH overstimulates the adrenal cortex. The result is excessive production of glucocorticoids, mineralocorticoids, and androgens, which leads to the development of Cushing's disease and problems with FLUID AND ELECTROLYTE BALANCE (see Hypercortisolism [Cushing's Disease], pp. 1276-1281).

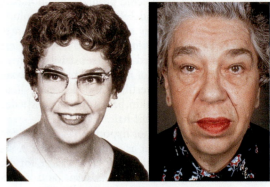

FIG. 62-1 The progression of acromegaly.

Usually, hyperpituitarism is caused by hormone-secreting benign tumors (*adenomas*) arising from one pituitary cell type. It can also be caused by hypothalamic problems that lead to excessive production of releasing hormones, which overstimulate the normal pituitary gland.

❖ PATIENT-CENTERED COLLABORATIVE CARE

◆ Assessment

The manifestations of hyperpituitarism vary with the hormone produced in excess. Obtain the patient's age, gender, and family history. Ask about any change in hat, glove, ring, or shoe size and the presence of fatigue. The patient with high GH levels may have backache and joint pain from bone changes. Ask specifically about headaches and changes in vision.

The patient with hypersecretion of PRL often reports sexual function difficulty. Ask women about menstrual changes, decreased libido, painful intercourse, and any difficulty in becoming pregnant. Ask men whether they have experienced decreased libido and impotence.

Changes in appearance and target organ function occur with excesses of specific anterior pituitary hormones (Chart 62-2). Manifestations of GH excess are increases in lip and nose sizes, a prominent brow ridge, and increases in head, hand, and foot sizes. The patient with hyperpituitarism often seeks health care because of these dramatic changes in appearance.

In a person with hyperpituitarism, usually only one hormone is produced in excess because the cell types within the pituitary gland are so individually organized. The most common hormones produced in excess with hyperpituitarism are PRL, ACTH, and GH.

Imaging assessment for hyperpituitarism is the same as for hypopituitarism. Skull x-rays are used to identify abnormalities of the sella turcica. CT scans and MRI can define soft-tissue lesions, and angiography can rule out an aneurysm or vascular malformations.

Suppression testing can help diagnose hyperpituitarism. For example, high blood glucose levels suppress the release of GH. Giving 100 g of oral glucose or 0.5 g/kg of body weight is followed by serial GH level measurements. GH levels that do not fall below 5 ng/mL indicate a positive (abnormal) result.

◆ Interventions

The expected outcomes of management for the patient who has hyperpituitarism are to return hormone levels to normal or near normal, reduce or eliminate headache and visual disturbances, prevent complications, and reverse as many of the body changes as possible.

Nonsurgical Management. Encourage the patient to express concerns about his or her altered physical appearance. Help him or her identify personal strengths and positive characteristics. Galactorrhea, gynecomastia, and reduced sexual functioning can disturb self-image and personal identity. Reassure the patient that treatment may reverse some of these problems.

Drug therapy may be used alone or in combination with surgery and radiation. The most common drugs used are the dopamine agonists *bromocriptine mesylate* (Parlodel) and *cabergoline* (Dostinex). These drugs stimulate dopamine receptors in the brain and inhibit the release of GH and PRL. In most cases, small tumors decrease until the pituitary gland is of normal size. Large pituitary tumors usually decrease to some extent.

CHART 62-2   Key Features

Anterior Pituitary Hyperfunction

Prolactin (PRL)
- Hypogonadism (loss of secondary sexual characteristics)
- Decreased gonadotropin levels
- Galactorrhea
- Increased body fat
- Increased serum prolactin levels

Growth Hormone (GH)
Acromegaly
- Thickened lips
- Coarse facial features
- Increasing head size
- Lower jaw protrusion
- Enlarged hands and feet
- Joint pain
- Barrel-shaped chest
- Hyperglycemia
- Sleep apnea
- Enlarged heart, lungs, and liver

Adrenocorticotropic Hormone (ACTH)
Cushing's Disease (Pituitary)
- Elevated plasma cortisol levels
- Weight gain
- Truncal obesity
- "Moon face"
- Extremity muscle wasting
- Loss of bone density
- Hypertension
- Hyperglycemia
- Striae and acne

Thyrotropin (Thyroid-Stimulating Hormone [TSH])
- Elevated plasma TSH and thyroid hormone levels
- Weight loss
- Tachycardia and dysrhythmias
- Heat intolerance
- Increased GI motility
- Fine tremors

Gonadotropins (Luteinizing Hormone [LH], Follicle-Stimulating Hormone [FSH])
Men:
- Elevated LH and FSH levels
- Hypogonadism or hypergonadism

Women:
- Normal LH and FSH levels

Side effects of bromocriptine include **orthostatic hypotension** (postural hypotension), gastric irritation, nausea, headaches, abdominal cramps, and constipation. Give and teach patients to take bromocriptine with a meal or a snack to reduce some of these side effects. Treatment starts with a low dose and is gradually increased until the desired level (usually 7.5 mg/day) is reached. *If pregnancy occurs, the drug is stopped immediately.*

❗ NURSING SAFETY PRIORITY (QSEN)

Drug Alert

Teach patients taking bromocriptine to seek medical care immediately if chest pain, dizziness, or watery nasal discharge occurs because of the possibility of serious side effects, including cardiac dysrhythmias, coronary artery spasms, and cerebrospinal fluid leakage.

Other agents used for acromegaly are the somatostatin analogs, especially octreotide (Sandostatin) and lanreotide (Somatuline), and a growth hormone receptor blocker, pegvisomant (Somavert). Octreotide inhibits GH release through negative feedback. Pegvisomant blocks growth hormone (GH) receptor activity and blocks production of insulin-like growth factor (IGF). Combination therapy with monthly injections of a somatostatin analog and weekly injections of pegvisomant have provided good control of the disease for some patients.

Radiation therapy does not have immediate effects in reducing pituitary hormone excesses, and several years may pass before a therapeutic effect can be seen. The use of the gamma knife and other more precise methods of delivering radiation to pituitary tumors has reduced the long-term side effects of this therapy. These side effects include hypopituitarism, optic nerve damage, and other eye and vision problems.

Surgical Management. Surgical removal of the pituitary gland and tumor (**hypophysectomy**) is the most common treatment for hyperpituitarism. Successful surgery decreases hormone levels, relieves headaches, and may reverse changes in sexual functioning.

Preoperative Care. Explain that because nasal packing is present for 2 to 3 days after surgery, it will be necessary to breathe through the mouth, and a "mustache" dressing ("drip pad") will be placed under the nose. Instruct the patient not to brush teeth, blow the nose, or bend forward after surgery. These activities can increase intracranial pressure (ICP) and delay healing, as can coughing and sneezing.

Operative Procedures. Usually a minimally invasive endoscopic transnasal approach is used instead of the more traditional transsphenoidal approach. The endoscopic approach uses smaller-diameter instruments and results in less damage to nasal structures. The procedure is performed with the patient under general anesthesia. After the gland is removed, a muscle graft is taken, often from the thigh, to support the area and prevent leakage of cerebrospinal fluid (CSF). Nasal packing is inserted after the incision is closed, and a mustache dressing is applied. If the tumor cannot be reached by either the endoscopic transnasal approach or the transsphenoidal approach, a craniotomy may be indicated (see Chapter 45).

Postoperative Care. Monitor the patient's neurologic responses, and document any changes in vision or mental status, altered level of consciousness, or decreased strength of the extremities. Observe the patient for complications such as transient diabetes insipidus (discussed on p. 1271), CSF leakage, infection, and increased ICP.

Teach the patient to report any postnasal drip or increased swallowing, which might indicate leakage of CSF. Keep the head of the bed elevated after surgery. Assess nasal drainage for quantity, quality, and the presence of glucose (which indicates that the fluid is CSF). A light yellow color at the edge of the clear drainage on the dressing is called the "halo sign" and indicates CSF. If the patient has persistent, severe headaches, CSF fluid may have leaked into the sinus area. Most CSF leaks resolve with bedrest, and surgical intervention is rarely needed.

Teach the patient to avoid coughing early after surgery because it increases pressure in the incision area and may lead to a CSF leak. Remind the patient to perform deep-breathing exercises hourly while awake to prevent pulmonary problems. Patients may have mouth dryness from mouth breathing. Instruct the patient to rinse the mouth frequently and to apply a lubricating jelly to dry lips.

CHART 62-3   Best Practice for Patient Safety & Quality Care [QSEN]

The Patient After Hypophysectomy

- Monitor the patient's neurologic status hourly for the first 24 hours and then every 4 hours.
- Monitor fluid balance, especially for output greater than intake.
- Encourage the patient to perform deep-breathing exercises.
- Instruct the patient to not cough, blow the nose, or sneeze.
- Instruct the patient to use dental floss and oral mouth rinses rather than tooth brushing until the surgeon gives permission.
- Instruct the patient to avoid bending at the waist to prevent increasing intracranial pressure.
- Monitor the nasal drip pad for the type and amount of drainage.
- Teach the patient to avoid constipation and subsequent "straining."
- Teach the patient self-administration of the prescribed hormones.

CHART 62-4   Focused Assessment

The Patient Who Has Undergone Nasal Hypophysectomy for Hyperpituitarism

Assess cardiovascular status:
- Vital signs, including apical pulse, pulse pressure, presence or absence of orthostatic hypotension, and the quality/rhythm of peripheral pulses

Assess cognition and mental status

Assess condition of operative site:
- Observe nasal area for drainage:
  If present, note color, clarity, and odor
  Test clear drainage for the presence of glucose

Assess neuromuscular status:
- Reactivity of patellar and biceps reflexes
- Oral temperature
- Handgrip strength
- Steadiness of gait
- Distant and near visual acuity
- Pupillary responses to light

Assess kidney function:
- Observe urine specimen for color, odor, cloudiness, and amount

Ask about:
- Headaches or visual disturbances
- Ease of bowel movements
- 24-hour fluid intake and output
- Over-the-counter and prescribed drugs taken

Assess patient's understanding of illness and adherence with treatment:
- Manifestations to report to health care provider
- Drug plan (correct timing and dose)

Assess for manifestations of infection, especially meningitis, such as headache, fever, and nuchal (neck) rigidity. The surgeon may prescribe antibiotics, analgesics, and antipyretics.

If the entire pituitary gland has been removed, replacement of thyroid hormones and glucocorticoids is lifelong. Best practices for care after surgery are listed in Chart 62-3.

After surgery the patient needs daily self-management regimens and frequent checkups. Chart 62-4 lists areas for focused assessment for the patient at home after a hypophysectomy. Review drug regimens and manifestations of infection and cerebral edema with the family.

After a hypophysectomy, advise the patient to avoid activities that might interfere with healing. Teach him or her to avoid bending over from the waist to pick up objects or tie shoes because this position increases ICP. Teach the patient to bend the knees and then lower the body to pick up fallen objects. ICP also increases when the patient strains to have a bowel movement. Suggest techniques to prevent constipation, such as eating high-fiber foods, drinking plenty of fluids, and using stool softeners or laxatives.

Teach the patient to avoid toothbrushing, which can disturb the operative site, for about 2 weeks after surgery. Frequent mouth care with mouthwash and daily flossing provide adequate oral hygiene. A decreased sense of smell is expected after surgery and usually lasts 3 to 4 months.

Hormone replacement with vasopressin may be needed to maintain fluid balance (see discussion of Interventions starting below in the Diabetes Insipidus section). If the anterior portion of the pituitary gland is removed, instruct the patient in cortisol, thyroid, and gonadal hormone replacement. Teach the patient to report the return of any manifestations of hyperpituitarism immediately to the primary health care provider.

DISORDERS OF THE POSTERIOR PITUITARY GLAND

Disorders of the posterior pituitary gland (**neurohypophysis**) occur with deficiency or excess of the hormone *vasopressin* (antidiuretic hormone [ADH]). ADH deficiency causes diabetes insipidus, and ADH excess causes the syndrome of inappropriate antidiuretic hormone (SIADH). Both types of problems disturb FLUID AND ELECTROLYTE BALANCE.

DIABETES INSIPIDUS

❖ PATHOPHYSIOLOGY

Diabetes insipidus (DI) is a water loss problem caused by either an ADH deficiency or an inability of the kidneys to respond to ADH. The result of DI is the excretion of large volumes of dilute urine because the distal kidney tubules and collecting ducts do not reabsorb water; this leads to **polyuria** (excessive water loss through urination), dehydration, and disturbed FLUID AND ELECTROLYTE BALANCE. Electrolyte imbalances most commonly include increased serum sodium levels.

Dehydration from this massive water loss increases plasma osmolarity, which stimulates the sensation of thirst. Thirst promotes increased fluid intake and aids in maintaining water homeostasis. *If the thirst mechanism is poor or absent or if the person is unable to obtain water, dehydration becomes more severe and can lead to death.*

> ### ❗ NURSING SAFETY PRIORITY (QSEN)
> #### Critical Rescue
> Ensure that no patient suspected of having DI is deprived of fluids for more than 4 hours, because he or she cannot reduce urine output. Continued urine output without adequate fluid intake leads to severe dehydration.

ADH deficiency is classified as nephrogenic, drug-related, primary, or secondary, depending on whether the problem is caused by insufficient production of ADH or an inability of the kidney to respond to the presence of ADH (John & Day, 2012). *Primary diabetes insipidus* is caused by a defect in the hypothalamus or posterior pituitary gland, resulting in a lack of ADH production or release. *Secondary diabetes insipidus* most often results from tumors in or near the hypothalamus or

> ### CHART 62-5 Key Features
> *Diabetes Insipidus*
>
> **Cardiovascular Manifestations**
> - Hypotension
> - Tachycardia
> - Weak peripheral pulses
> - Hemoconcentration
>
> **Kidney/Urinary Manifestations**
> - Increased urine output
> - Dilute, low specific gravity
>
> **Skin Manifestations**
> - Poor turgor
> - Dry mucous membranes
>
> **Neurologic Manifestations**
> - Decreased cognition*
> - Ataxia*
> - Increased thirst
> - Irritability*
>
> *Occurs when access to water is limited and rapid dehydration results.

> ### 🧬 GENETIC/GENOMIC CONSIDERATIONS
> #### Patient-Centered Care (QSEN)
>
> Nephrogenic diabetes insipidus is a genetic disorder in which the kidney tubules do not respond to the actions of ADH. The result is poor water reabsorption by the kidney although the actual amount of hormone produced is not deficient. This problem is most commonly inherited as an X-linked recessive disorder in which the *AVPR2* gene coding for the ADH receptor is mutated and only males are affected (Online Mendelian Inheritance in Man [OMIM], 2011). There is also an autosomal form of the disorder in which the *AQP2* gene is mutated and both males and females are affected (OMIM, 2012). When assessing a patient with DI, always ask whether anyone else in the family has ever had this disorder.

pituitary gland, head trauma, infectious processes, brain surgery, or metastatic tumors.

Drug-related diabetes insipidus is usually caused by lithium carbonate (Eskalith, Lithobid, Carbolith 🍁) and demeclocycline (Declomycin). These drugs can interfere with the response of the kidneys to ADH.

❖ PATIENT-CENTERED COLLABORATIVE CARE

◆ Assessment

Most manifestations of DI are related to dehydration (Chart 62-5). Key manifestations are an increase in urination and excessive thirst. Ask about a history of recent surgery, head trauma, or drug use (e.g., lithium). Although increased fluid intake prevents serious volume depletion, the patient who is deprived of fluids or who cannot increase oral fluid intake may develop shock from fluid loss. Manifestations of dehydration (e.g., poor skin turgor, dry or cracked mucous membranes) may be present. (See Chapter 11 for discussion of dehydration.)

Water loss produces changes in blood and urine tests. The first step in diagnosis is to measure a 24-hour fluid intake and output without restricting food or fluid intake. DI is considered if urine output is more than 4 L during this period and is greater than the volume ingested. The amount of urine excreted in 24 hours may vary from 4 to 30 L/day. Urine is dilute with a low specific gravity (less than 1.005) and low osmolarity (50 to 200 mOsm/kg).

◆ Interventions

Management focuses on controlling manifestations with drug therapy. The most preferred drug is desmopressin acetate (DDAVP), a synthetic form of vasopressin given orally or intranasally in a metered spray. The frequency of dosing varies with patient responses. Teach patients that each metered spray delivers 10 mcg and those with mild DI may need only one or two doses in 24 hours. For more severe DI, one or two metered doses 2 or 3 times daily may be needed. During severe dehydration, ADH may be given IV or IM. Ulceration of the mucous membranes, allergy, a sensation of chest tightness, and lung inhalation of the spray may occur with use of the intranasal preparations. If side effects occur or if the patient has an upper respiratory infection, oral or subcutaneous vasopressin is used rather than the intranasal form.

> ! **NURSING SAFETY PRIORITY** (QSEN)
>
> **Drug Alert**
>
> The parenteral form of desmopressin is 10 times stronger than the oral and intranasal forms, and the dosage must be reduced.

For the hospitalized patient with DI, nursing management focuses on early detection of dehydration and maintaining adequate hydration. Interventions include accurately measuring fluid intake and output, checking urine specific gravity, and recording the patient's weight daily.

Urge the patient to drink fluids in an amount equal to urine output. If fluids are given IV, ensure the patency of the access catheter and accurately monitor the amount infused hourly.

The patient with permanent DI requires lifelong drug therapy. Assess his or her ability to follow instructions and adjust dosages. Teach that polyuria and polydipsia are indications of the need for another dose.

Drugs for DI induce water retention and can cause fluid overload (see Chapter 11). *Teach all patients taking these drugs to weigh themselves daily to identify weight gain.* Stress the importance of using the same scale and weighing at the same time of day while wearing a similar amount of clothing. If a weight gain of more than 2.2 lbs (1 kg) or other signs of water toxicity occur (e.g., persistent headache, acute confusion), instruct the patient or family that the patient must go to the emergency department or call 911. Instruct him or her to wear a medical alert bracelet identifying the disorder and drugs.

SYNDROME OF INAPPROPRIATE ANTIDIURETIC HORMONE

❖ PATHOPHYSIOLOGY

The syndrome of inappropriate antidiuretic hormone (SIADH) or *Schwartz-Bartter syndrome* is a problem in which vasopressin (antidiuretic hormone [ADH]) is secreted even when plasma osmolarity is low or normal. A decrease in plasma osmolarity normally inhibits ADH production and secretion. SIADH occurs with many conditions (e.g., cancer therapy) and with specific drugs, including selective serotonin reuptake inhibitors and fluoroquinolone antibiotics (Yam & Eraly, 2012). Table 62-1 lists common causes of SIADH.

In SIADH, ADH continues to be released even when plasma is hypo-osmolar, leading to disturbances of FLUID AND ELECTROLYTE BALANCE. Water is *retained*, which results in dilutional **hyponatremia** (a decreased serum sodium level) and fluid overload. The increase in blood volume increases the kidney

TABLE 62-1	Conditions Causing the Syndrome of Inappropriate Antidiuretic Hormone
Malignancies • Small cell lung cancer • Pancreatic, duodenal, and GU carcinomas • Thymoma • Hodgkin's lymphoma • Non-Hodgkin's lymphoma	**CNS Disorders** • Trauma • Infection • Tumors (primary or metastatic) • Strokes • Porphyria • Systemic lupus erythematosus
Pulmonary Disorders • Viral and bacterial pneumonia • Lung abscesses • Active tuberculosis • Pneumothorax • Chronic lung diseases • Mycoses • Positive-pressure ventilation	**Drugs** • Exogenous ADH • Chlorpropamide • Vincristine • Cyclophosphamide • Carbamazepine • Opioids • Tricyclic antidepressants • General anesthetics • Fluoroquinolone antibiotics

ADH, Antidiuretic hormone; *CNS,* central nervous system; *GU,* genitourinary.

filtration and inhibits the release of renin and aldosterone, which increase urine sodium loss and leads to greater hyponatremia.

❖ PATIENT-CENTERED COLLABORATIVE CARE

◆ Assessment

Ask the patient about his or her medical history, which may reveal conditions that can cause SIADH. Information about these conditions should be obtained:
- Recent head trauma
- Cerebrovascular disease
- Tuberculosis or other pulmonary disease
- Cancer
- All past and current drug use

The early manifestations of SIADH are related to water retention. GI disturbances, such as loss of appetite, nausea, and vomiting, may occur first. Weigh the patient, and document any recent weight gain. Use this information to monitor responses to therapy. In SIADH, free water (not salt) is retained and dependent edema is not usually present, even though water is retained.

Water retention, hyponatremia, and fluid shifts affect central nervous system function, especially when the serum sodium level is below 115 mEq/L. The patient may have lethargy, headaches, hostility, disorientation, and a change in level of consciousness. Lethargy and headaches can progress to decreased responsiveness, seizures, and coma. Assess deep tendon reflexes, which are usually decreased.

Vital sign changes include full and bounding pulse (caused by the increased fluid volume) and hypothermia (caused by central nervous system disturbance). Chapter 11 presents other findings that occur with hyponatremia.

Water retention causes urine volume to decrease and urine osmolarity to increase. At the same time, plasma volume increases and plasma osmolarity decreases. Elevated urine sodium levels and specific gravity reflect increased urine concentration. Serum sodium levels are decreased, often as low as 110 mEq/L, because of fluid retention and sodium loss.

Radioimmunoassay of ADH along with clinical manifestations can help diagnose SIADH, but this test is usually not used for a definitive diagnosis.

◆ Interventions

Medical interventions for SIADH focus on restricting fluid intake, promoting the excretion of water, replacing lost sodium, and interfering with the action of ADH. Nursing interventions focus on monitoring response to therapy, preventing complications, teaching the patient and family about fluid restrictions and drug therapy, and preventing injury.

Fluid restriction is essential because fluid intake further dilutes plasma sodium levels. In some cases, fluid intake may be kept as low as 500 to 1000 mL/24 hr (John & Day, 2012). Dilute tube feedings with saline rather than water, and use saline to irrigate GI tubes. Mix drugs to be given by GI tube with saline.

Measure intake, output, and daily weights to assess the degree of fluid restriction needed. A weight gain of 2.2 lbs (1 kg) or more per day or a gradual increase over several days is cause for concern. A 2.2-lb (1kg) weight increase is equal to a 1000-mL fluid retention (1 kg = 1 L). Keep the mouth moist by offering frequent oral rinsing (remind the patient not to swallow the rinses).

Drug therapy with tolvaptan (Samsca) or conivaptan (Vaprisol) is used to treat SIADH when hyponatremia is present in hospitalized patients. These drugs are vasopressin antagonists that promote water excretion without causing sodium loss. Tolvaptan is an oral drug, and conivaptan is given IV. Tolvaptan has a black box warning that rapid increases in serum sodium levels (those greater than a 12 mEq/L increase in 24 hours) have been associated with central nervous system demyelination that can lead to serious complications and death. In addition, when this drug is used at higher dosages or for longer than 30 days, there is a significant risk for liver failure and death (Food and Drug Administration [FDA], 2013).

> ### ! NURSING SAFETY PRIORITY (QSEN)
> #### Drug Alert
> Administer tolvaptan or conivaptan only in the hospital setting so that serum sodium levels can be monitored closely for the development of hypernatremia.

Diuretics may be used to manage SIADH when sodium levels are near normal and heart failure is present. Be aware of the diuretic effects on sodium loss. Sodium loss can be potentiated, further contributing to the problems caused by SIADH. For milder SIADH, demeclocycline (Declomycin), an oral antibiotic, may help correct the disturbed FLUID AND ELECTROLYTE BALANCE, although it is not approved for this problem (Crawford & Harris, 2012).

Hypertonic saline (i.e., 3% sodium chloride [3% NaCl]) may be used to treat SIADH when the serum sodium level is very low (John & Day, 2012; Robinson & Verbalis, 2011). Give IV saline cautiously because it may add to existing fluid overload and promote heart failure. If the patient needs routine IV fluids, a saline solution rather than a water solution is prescribed.

Monitor the patient's response to therapy to prevent the fluid overload of SIADH from becoming worse, leading to pulmonary edema and heart failure. Any patient with SIADH, regardless of age, is at risk for these complications. The older adult or

one who also has cardiac problems, kidney problems, pulmonary problems, or liver problems is at greater risk.

Monitor for increased fluid overload (bounding pulse, increasing neck vein distention, crackles in lungs, increasing peripheral edema, reduced urine output) at least every 2 hours. *Pulmonary edema can occur very quickly and can lead to death.* Notify the health care provider of any change that indicates the fluid overload is not responding to therapy or is worse.

Providing a safe environment is critical when the serum sodium level falls below 120 mEq/L. Possible neurologic changes and the risk for seizures increase as a result of osmotic fluid shifts into brain tissue. Observe for and document changes in the patient's neurologic status. Assess for subtle changes, such as muscle twitching, before they progress to seizures or coma. Check orientation to time, place, and person every 2 hours because disorientation or confusion may be present. Reduce environmental noise and lighting to prevent overstimulation.

Flow sheets with continuing information about the level of consciousness, neurologic assessments, and laboratory data are helpful in detecting neurologic trends. The frequency of neurologic checks depends on the patient's status. For the patient with SIADH who is hyponatremic but alert, awake, and oriented, checks every 4 hours are sufficient. For the patient who has had a change in level of consciousness, perform neurologic checks at least every hour. Inspect the environment every shift, making sure that basic safety measures, such as siderails being securely in place, are observed.

> ### ? NCLEX EXAMINATION CHALLENGE
> #### Physiological Integrity
> Which urine properties indicate to the nurse that the client with syndrome of inappropriate antidiuretic hormone (SIADH) is responding to interventions?
> A. Urine output volume increased; urine specific gravity increased
> B. Urine output volume increased; urine specific gravity decreased
> C. Urine output volume decreased; urine specific gravity increased
> D. Urine output volume decreased; urine specific gravity decreased

DISORDERS OF THE ADRENAL GLAND

ADRENAL GLAND HYPOFUNCTION

❖ PATHOPHYSIOLOGY

Adrenocortical steroid production may decrease as a result of inadequate secretion of adrenocorticotropic hormone (ACTH), dysfunction of the hypothalamic-pituitary control mechanism, or direct dysfunction of adrenal gland tissue. Manifestations may develop gradually or occur quickly with stress. In acute adrenocortical insufficiency (adrenal crisis), life-threatening manifestations may appear without warning.

Insufficiency of adrenocortical steroids causes problems through the loss of aldosterone and cortisol action. Decreased cortisol levels result in poor GLUCOSE REGULATION with hypoglycemia (low blood glucose levels). Glomerular filtration and gastric acid production decrease, leading to reduced urea nitrogen excretion, which causes anorexia and weight loss.

Reduced aldosterone secretion causes disturbances of FLUID AND ELECTROLYTE BALANCE, especially of potassium, sodium, and water. Potassium excretion is decreased, causing

Emergency Care of the Patient with Acute Adrenal Insufficiency

Hormone Replacement
- Start rapid infusion of normal saline or dextrose 5% in normal saline.
- Initial dose of hydrocortisone sodium (Solu-Cortef) is 100 to 300 mg or dexamethasone 4 to 12 mg as an IV bolus.
- Administer additional 100 mg of hydrocortisone sodium by continuous IV infusion over the next 8 hours.
- Give hydrocortisone 50 mg IM concomitantly every 12 hours.
- Initiate an H_2 histamine blocker (e.g., ranitidine) IV for ulcer prevention.

Hyperkalemia Management
- Administer insulin (20 to 50 units) with dextrose (20 to 50 mg) in normal saline to shift potassium into cells.
- Administer potassium binding and excreting resin (e.g., Kayexalate).
- Give loop or thiazide diuretics.
- Avoid potassium-sparing diuretics, as prescribed.
- Initiate potassium restriction.
- Monitor intake and output.
- Monitor heart rate, rhythm, and ECG for manifestations of hyperkalemia (slow heart rate; heart block; tall, peaked T waves; fibrillation; asystole).

Hypoglycemia Management
- Administer IV glucose, as prescribed.
- Administer glucagon, as needed and prescribed.
- Maintain IV access.
- Monitor blood glucose level hourly.

ECG, Electrocardiogram.

TABLE 62-2   **Causes of Primary and Secondary Adrenal Insufficiency**

Primary Causes	Secondary Causes
• Autoimmune disease*	• Pituitary tumors
• Tuberculosis	• Postpartum pituitary necrosis
• Metastatic cancer	• Hypophysectomy
• AIDS	• High-dose pituitary or whole-brain radiation
• Hemorrhage	
• Gram-negative sepsis	
• Adrenalectomy	
• Abdominal radiation therapy	
• Drugs (mitotane) and toxins	

AIDS, Acquired immune deficiency syndrome.
*Most common cause.

Adrenal Insufficiency

Neuromuscular Manifestations
- Muscle weakness
- Fatigue
- Joint/muscle pain

Gastrointestinal Manifestations
- Anorexia
- Nausea, vomiting
- Abdominal pain
- Constipation or diarrhea
- Weight loss
- Salt craving

Skin Manifestations
- Vitiligo
- Hyperpigmentation

Cardiovascular Manifestations
- Anemia
- Hypotension
- Hyponatremia
- Hyperkalemia
- Hypercalcemia

hyperkalemia. Sodium and water excretion are increased, causing hyponatremia and hypovolemia. Potassium retention also promotes reabsorption of hydrogen ions, which can lead to acidosis.

Low adrenal androgen levels decrease the body, axillary, and pubic hair, especially in women, because the adrenals produce most of the androgens in females. The severity of manifestations is related to the degree of hormone deficiency.

Acute adrenal insufficiency, or Addisonian crisis, is a life-threatening event in which the need for cortisol and aldosterone is greater than the available supply. It often occurs in response to a stressful event (e.g., surgery, trauma, severe infection), especially when the adrenal hormone output is already reduced. The problems are the same as those of chronic insufficiency but are more severe. *Unless intervention is initiated promptly, however, sodium levels fall and potassium levels rise rapidly. Severe hypotension results from the blood volume depletion that occurs with the loss of aldosterone.* Best practices for emergency care of patients with acute adrenal insufficiency are listed in Chart 62-6.

Adrenal insufficiency (Addison's disease) is classified as primary or secondary. Causes of primary and secondary adrenal insufficiency are listed in Table 62-2. A common cause of secondary adrenal insufficiency is the sudden cessation of long-term glucocorticoid therapy. This therapy suppresses production of glucocorticoids through negative feedback by causing atrophy of the adrenal cortex. Glucocorticoid drugs must be withdrawn gradually to allow for increasing pituitary production of ACTH and activation of adrenal cells to produce cortisol.

❖ PATIENT-CENTERED COLLABORATIVE CARE

◆ Assessment

History. Ask about manifestations and factors that cause adrenal hypofunction. Ask about any change in activity level, because lethargy, fatigue, and muscle weakness are often present. Include questions about salt intake, because salt craving often occurs with hypofunction.

GI problems, such as anorexia, nausea, vomiting, diarrhea, and abdominal pain, often occur. Ask about weight loss during the past months. Women may have menstrual changes related to weight loss, and men may report impotence.

Ask whether the patient has had radiation to the abdomen or head. Document medical problems (e.g., tuberculosis or previous intracranial surgery) and all past and current drugs, especially steroids, anticoagulants, opioids, and cancer drugs.

Physical Assessment/Clinical Manifestations. The manifestations of adrenal insufficiency vary, and the severity is related to the degree of hormone deficiency (Chart 62-7). In patients with primary insufficiency, plasma ACTH and melanocyte-stimulating hormone (MSH) levels are elevated in response to the adrenal-hypothalamic-pituitary feedback system. Elevated MSH levels result in areas of increased pigmentation (Fig. 62-2). In primary autoimmune disease, patchy areas of decreased pigmentation may occur because of destruction of skin melanocytes. Body hair may also be decreased. In secondary disease, skin pigmentation is not changed.

Assess for abnormal GLUCOSE REGULATION with hypoglycemia (e.g., sweating, headaches, tachycardia, and tremors) and fluid depletion (postural hypotension and dehydration).

Hyperkalemia (elevated blood potassium levels) can cause dysrhythmias with an irregular heart rate and can result in cardiac arrest.

Psychosocial Assessment. Depending on the degree of imbalance, patients may appear lethargic, depressed, confused, and even psychotic. Assess the patient's orientation to person, place, and time. Families may report that the patient has wide mood swings and is forgetful.

Diagnostic Assessment. Laboratory findings include low serum cortisol, low fasting blood glucose, low sodium, elevated potassium, and increased blood urea nitrogen (BUN) levels (Chart 62-8). In primary disease, the eosinophil count and ACTH level are elevated. Plasma cortisol levels do not rise during provocation tests.

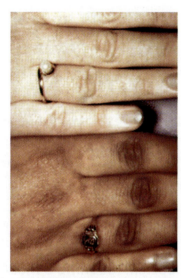

FIG. 62-2 The increased pigmentation seen in primary adrenocortical insufficiency.

Urinary 17-hydroxycorticosteroids are the glucocorticoid metabolites, and 17-ketosteroid levels reflect the adrenal androgen metabolites. Both levels are in the low or low-normal range in adrenal hypofunction.

An ACTH stimulation (provocation) test is the most definitive test for adrenal insufficiency. ACTH 0.25 to 1 mg is given IV, and plasma cortisol levels are obtained at 30-minute and 1-hour intervals. In primary insufficiency, the cortisol response is absent or very decreased. In secondary insufficiency, it is increased. When acute adrenal insufficiency is suspected, treatment is started without stimulation testing (Stewart & Krone, 2011).

Imaging Assessment. Skull x-rays, CT, MRI, and arteriography may help determine the cause of pituitary problems leading to adrenal insufficiency. CT scans may show adrenal gland atrophy.

◆ **Interventions**

Nursing interventions focus on promoting fluid balance, monitoring for fluid deficit, and preventing poor GLUCOSE REGULATION with hypoglycemia. *Because hyperkalemia can cause dysrhythmias with an irregular heart rate and result in cardiac arrest, assessing cardiac function is a nursing priority.* Assess vital signs every 1 to 4 hours, depending on the patient's condition and the presence of dysrhythmias or postural hypotension. Weigh the patient daily, and record intake and output. Monitor laboratory values to identify hemoconcentration (e.g., increased hematocrit or BUN). Chapter 11 discusses fluid volume deficit in detail.

Cortisol and aldosterone deficiencies are corrected by replacement therapy. Hydrocortisone corrects glucocorticoid deficiency (Chart 62-9). Oral cortisol replacement regimens vary. The most common drug used for this purpose is prednisone. Generally, divided doses are given, with two-thirds given in the morning and one-third in the late afternoon to mimic the normal release of this hormone. Although most patients do

CHART 62-8   Laboratory Profile

Adrenal Gland Assessment

TEST	NORMAL RANGE FOR ADULTS	SIGNIFICANCE OF ABNORMAL FINDINGS	
		HYPOFUNCTION OF THE ADRENAL GLAND	HYPERFUNCTION OF THE ADRENAL GLAND
Sodium	136-145 mEq/L	Decreased	Increased
Potassium	3.5-5.0 mEq/L	Increased	Decreased
Glucose	70-110 mg/dL (fasting) *Older adults:* slightly increased	Normal to decreased	Normal to increased
Calcium	9-10.5 mg/dL (total) 4.5-5.6 mg/dL (ionized) *Older adults:* slightly decreased	Increased	Decreased
Bicarbonate	23-30 mEq/L	Increased	Decreased
BUN	10-20 mg/dL *Older adults:* may be slightly higher	Increased	Normal
Cortisol (serum)	6 AM to 8 AM: 5-23 mcg/dL or 138-635 SI units (nmol/L) 4 PM to 6 PM: 3-13 mcg/dL or 83-359 SI units (nmol/L)	Decreased	Increased
Cortisol (salivary)	7 AM to 9 AM: 180-750 ng/dL 3 PM to 5 PM: <401 ng/dL 11 PM to midnight: <100 ng/dL		

Pagana, K., & Pagana, T. (2014). *Mosby's manual of diagnostic and laboratory tests* (5th ed.). St. Louis: Mosby.
BUN, Blood urea nitrogen; *SI,* International System of Units.

CHART 62-9 Common Examples of Drug Therapy

Hypofunction of the Adrenal Gland

DRUG AND USUAL DOSAGE	NURSING INTERVENTIONS	RATIONALES
Cortisone 25-50 mg orally daily	Instruct the patient to take the drug with meals or a snack.	GI irritation can occur.
Hydrocortisone (Cortef, Hycort ♦) 20-50 mg orally	Instruct the patient to report these signs or symptoms of excessive drug therapy: ■ Rapid weight gain ■ Round face ■ Fluid retention	Cushing's syndrome, which indicates a need for dosage adjustment, can occur.
Prednisone (Winpred ♦) 5-10 mg orally daily	Instruct the patient to report illness, such as: ■ Severe diarrhea ■ Vomiting ■ Fever	Other conditions may indicate a need for dosage change. The usual daily dosage may not be adequate during periods of illness or severe stress.
Fludrocortisone (Florinef) 0.05-0.2 mg orally daily	Monitor the patient's blood pressure. Instruct the patient to report weight gain or edema.	Hypertension is a potential side effect. Sodium-related fluid retention is possible.

NURSING SAFETY PRIORITY (QSEN)

Drug Alert

Prednisone and prednisolone are sound-alike drugs, and care is needed not to confuse them. Although they are both corticosteroids, they are not interchangeable because prednisolone is several times more potent than prednisone and dosages are not the same.

well on this regimen, some may not tolerate the dosage or may need more.

An additional mineralocorticoid hormone, such as fludrocortisone (Florinef), may be needed to maintain or restore FLUID AND ELECTROLYTE BALANCE (especially sodium and potassium). Dosage adjustment may be needed, especially in hot weather when more sodium is lost because of excessive perspiration. *Salt restriction or diuretic therapy should not be started without considering whether it might lead to an adrenal crisis.*

ADRENAL GLAND HYPERFUNCTION

The adrenal gland may oversecrete just one hormone or all adrenal hormones. Hypersecretion by the adrenal cortex results in hypercortisolism (e.g., Cushing's disease or Cushing's syndrome), hyperaldosteronism (excessive mineralocorticoid production), or excessive androgen production. Hyperstimulation of the adrenal medulla caused by a tumor (pheochromocytoma) results in excessive secretion of catecholamines (epinephrine and norepinephrine).

CLINICAL JUDGMENT CHALLENGE

Patient-Centered Care; Quality Improvement; Safety (QSEN)

The patient is a 32-year-old woman admitted to your unit after surgery for fractures of the left arm and leg resulting from a car crash. She is awake and able to verify her medical history of rheumatoid arthritis and her usual daily oral medications. These are 10 mg of prednisone, naproxen 800 mg twice daily, oral contraceptives, calcium 600 mg, and one multiple vitamin tablet. All of these are prescribed for her to receive during her hospitalization. She is concerned about pain management and how long the recovery will be for the fractures. She is friendly, somewhat anxious, asks many questions, and wants to do "her part" to ensure good recovery. Over the next 4 days, she has become quieter, mumbles that her head and stomach hurt, and now does not recognize the assistant who has been providing her daily care. When she receives her medications, she has difficulty picking them up. The nursing assistant remarks that taking her pulse is difficult because it is so slow and irregular. When you assess the patient, she is so weak that she is unable to lift her arm for a blood pressure check. Her blood pressure is 92/50, which is down from the 128/84 reading on admission. You also verify that her heart beat is slow and irregular.

1. What other assessment data should you obtain immediately and why?
2. What is the most likely cause of the changes in this patient's physical and mental status?
3. How could this problem have been avoided?
4. What specifically would be the nurse's role in preventing this problem?
5. What could be done to prevent this problem from happening again?

HYPERCORTISOLISM (CUSHING'S DISEASE)

❖ PATHOPHYSIOLOGY

Cushing's disease is the excess secretion of cortisol from the adrenal cortex, causing many problems. It is caused by either a problem in the adrenal cortex itself, a problem in the anterior pituitary gland, or a problem in the hypothalamus. In addition, glucocorticoid therapy can also lead to problems of hypercortisolism.

The presence of excess glucocorticoids, regardless of the cause, affects metabolism and all body systems. An increase in total body fat results from slow turnover of plasma fatty acids. This fat is redistributed, producing truncal obesity, "buffalo hump," and "moon face" (Fig. 62-3). Increases in the breakdown of tissue protein result in decreased muscle mass and muscle strength, thin skin, and fragile capillaries. The effects on minerals lead to bone density loss.

High levels of corticosteroids kill lymphocytes and shrink organs containing lymphocytes, such as the spleen and the lymph nodes. White blood cell cytokine production is decreased. These changes reduce the protection of the inflammatory and immune responses.

In most cases, increased androgen production also occurs and causes acne, hirsutism (increased body hair growth), and occasionally clitoral hypertrophy in women. Increased androgens disrupt the normal ovarian hormone feedback mechanism, decreasing the ovary's production of estrogens and progesterone. Oligomenorrhea (scant or infrequent menses) results.

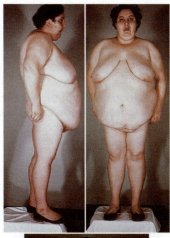
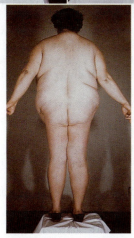

FIG. 62-3 The typical appearance of a patient with Cushing's disease or syndrome. Note truncal obesity, moon face, buffalo hump, thinner arms and legs, and abdominal striae.

Etiology

Cushing's disease or syndrome is a group of clinical problems caused by an excess of cortisol. Table 62-3 lists causes of cortisol excess. When the anterior pituitary gland oversecretes adrenocorticotropic hormone (ACTH), this hormone causes hyperplasia of the adrenal cortex in both adrenal glands and an excess of most hormones secreted by the adrenal cortex. (See Fig. 61-3 in Chapter 61.) This problem is known as **pituitary Cushing's disease** because the tissue causing the problem is the pituitary. When the excess glucocorticoids are caused by a problem in the actual adrenal cortex, usually a benign tumor (adrenal adenoma), the problem is called **adrenal Cushing's disease** and usually occurs in only one adrenal gland. When glucocorticoid excess results from drug therapy for another health problem, it is known as **Cushing's syndrome**.

Incidence and Prevalence

The most common cause of Cushing's disease is a pituitary adenoma. Women are more likely than men to develop Cushing's disease. The actual incidence of Cushing's syndrome from chronic use of exogenous corticosteroids is not known. However, because these drugs are commonly used to control serious chronic inflammatory conditions such as asthma, other respiratory problems, and rheumatoid arthritis, Cushing's syndrome is more common than Cushing's disease and affects both genders equally.

TABLE 62-3 Conditions Causing Increased Cortisol Secretion

Endogenous Secretion (Cushing's Disease)
- Bilateral adrenal hyperplasia*
- Pituitary adenoma increasing the production of ACTH (pituitary Cushing's disease)
- Malignancies: carcinomas of the lung, GI tract, pancreas
- Adrenal adenomas or carcinomas

Exogenous Administration (Cushing's Syndrome)
- Therapeutic use of ACTH or glucocorticoids—most commonly for treatment of:
  - Asthma
  - Autoimmune disorders
  - Organ transplantation
  - Cancer chemotherapy
  - Allergic responses
  - Chronic fibrosis

ACTH, Adrenocorticotropic hormone.
*Most common cause.

❖ PATIENT-CENTERED COLLABORATIVE CARE

◆ Assessment

History. Ask about the patient's other health problems and drug therapies, because glucocorticoid therapy is a common cause of hypercortisolism. Regardless of cause, the patient has many changes because of the widespread effect of excessive cortisol. The patient may report weight gain and an increased appetite. Ask about changes in activity or sleep patterns, fatigue, and muscle weakness. Ask about bone pain or a history of fractures, because osteoporosis is common in hypercortisolism. Ask about a history of frequent infections and easy bruising. Women often stop menstruating. GI problems include ulcer formation from increased hydrochloric acid secretion and decreased production of protective gastric mucus.

Physical Assessment/Clinical Manifestations. The patient with hypercortisolism has specific physical changes, although all body systems are affected (see Fig. 62-3 and Chart 62-10). Changes in fat distribution may result in fat pads on the neck, back, and shoulders ("buffalo hump"); an enlarged trunk with thin arms and legs; and a round face ("moon face"). Other changes include muscle wasting and weakness. Assess and document changes, and use these findings to prioritize patient problems.

Skin changes result from increased blood vessel fragility and include bruises, thin or translucent skin, and wounds that have not healed. Reddish purple **striae** ("stretch marks") occur on the abdomen, thighs, and upper arms because of the destructive effect of cortisol on collagen.

Acne and a fine coating of hair may occur over the face and body. In women, look for the presence of hirsutism, clitoral hypertrophy, and male pattern balding related to androgen excess.

Cardiac changes occur as a result of disturbed FLUID AND ELECTROLYTE BALANCE, especially water and mineral metabolism. Both sodium and water are reabsorbed and retained, leading to hypervolemia and edema formation. Blood pressure is elevated, and pulses are full and bounding.

Musculoskeletal changes occur as a result of nitrogen depletion and mineral loss. Muscle mass decreases, especially in arms and legs (see Fig. 62-3). Muscle weakness increases the risk for

CHART 62-10   Key Features

Hypercortisolism (Cushing's Disease/Syndrome)

General Appearance
- Moon face
- Buffalo hump
- Truncal obesity
- Weight gain

Cardiovascular Manifestations
- Hypertension
- Frequent dependent edema
- Bruising
- Petechiae

Musculoskeletal Manifestations
- Muscle atrophy (most apparent in extremities)
- Osteoporosis (bone density loss)
  - Pathologic fractures
  - Decreased height with vertebral collapse
  - Aseptic necrosis of the femur head
  - Slow or poor healing of bone fractures

Skin Manifestations
- Thinning skin
- Striae and increased pigmentation

Immune System Manifestations
- Increased risk for infection
- Decreased immune function
- Decreased inflammatory responses
- Manifestations of infection/inflammation may be masked

ACTH, Adrenocorticotropic hormone.

falls. Bone is thinner as a result of mineral loss, and osteoporosis is common, increasing the risk for pathologic fractures.

GLUCOSE REGULATION is affected by hypercortisolism. Fasting blood glucose levels are high because the liver releases glucose and the insulin receptors are less sensitive, so blood glucose does not move as easily into the tissues. Muscle mass loss also reduces glucose uptake.

Immune changes caused by excess cortisol result in immunosuppression and an increased risk for infection. Excess cortisol reduces the number of circulating lymphocytes, inhibits macrophage activity, reduces antibody synthesis, and inhibits production of cytokines and inflammatory chemicals (e.g., histamine) (McCance et al., 2014). The risk for infection is higher, and the patient may not have the expected manifestations (fever, purulent exudate, redness in the affected area) when an infection is present.

Psychosocial Assessment. Hypercortisolism can result in emotional instability, and patients often say that they do not feel like themselves. Ask about mood swings, irritability, confusion, or depression. Ask the patient whether he or she has been crying or laughing inappropriately or has had difficulty concentrating. Family members often report changes in the patient's mental or emotional status. The excess hormones stimulate the central nervous system, heightening the awareness of and responses to sensory stimulation. The patient often reports sleep difficulties and fatigue.

Laboratory Assessment. Laboratory tests include blood, salivary, and urine cortisol levels. These are high in patients with any type of hypercortisolism. Plasma ACTH levels vary,

depending on the cause of the problem. In pituitary Cushing's disease, ACTH levels are elevated. In adrenal Cushing's disease or when Cushing's syndrome results from chronic steroid use, ACTH levels are low.

Salivary cortisol levels may be used to detect hypercortisolism. Saliva is easily and painlessly collected with the use of a salivary specimen cushion placed in the cheek next to the salivary gland. A normal salivary cortisol level is lower than 2.0 ng/mL. Higher levels indicate hypercortisolism.

Urine is tested to measure levels of free cortisol and the metabolites of cortisol and androgens (17-hydroxycorticosteroids and 17-ketosteroids). In Cushing's disease, levels of urine cortisol and androgens are all elevated in a 24-hour specimen, as are urine calcium, potassium, and glucose levels.

Dexamethasone suppression testing can screen for hypercortisolism and may take place overnight or over a 3-day period. Set doses of dexamethasone are given. A 24-hour urine collection follows drug administration. When urinary 17-hydroxycorticosteroid excretion and cortisol levels are suppressed by dexamethasone, Cushing's disease is not present.

Additional laboratory findings that accompany hypercortisolism include:
- Increased blood glucose level
- Decreased lymphocyte count
- Increased sodium level
- Decreased serum calcium level

Imaging Assessment. Imaging for hypercortisolism includes x-rays, CT scans, MRI, and arteriography. These images can identify lesions of the adrenal or pituitary glands, lung, GI tract, or pancreas.

◆ Analysis

The priority NANDA-I nursing diagnoses and collaborative problems for patients with Cushing's disease or Cushing's syndrome include:
1. Fluid overload
2. Risk for Injury related to skin thinning, poor wound healing, and bone density loss (NANDA-I)
3. Risk for Infection (NANDA-I)
4. Potential for acute adrenal insufficiency

◆ Planning and Implementation

Expected outcomes of hypercortisolism management are the reduction of plasma cortisol levels, removal of tumors, and restoration of normal or acceptable body appearance. When the disorder is caused by pituitary or adrenal problems, cure is possible. When caused by drug therapy for another health problem, the focus is to prevent complications from hypercortisolism.

Restoring Fluid Volume Balance

Planning: Expected Outcomes. The patient with hypercortisolism is expected to achieve and maintain an acceptable FLUID AND ELECTROLYTE BALANCE. Indicators include that these parameters are within or close to the normal range:
- Blood pressure
- Stable body weight
- Serum electrolytes

Interventions. Interventions for patients with fluid overload from hypercortisolism focus on ensuring patient safety, restoring FLUID AND ELECTROLYTE BALANCE, and providing supportive care. Depending on the cause, surgical management may be used to reduce cortisol production.

Nonsurgical Management. Patient safety, drug therapy, nutrition therapy, and monitoring are the basis of nonsurgical interventions for hypercortisolism and fluid overload.

Patient safety includes preventing fluid overload from becoming worse, leading to pulmonary edema and heart failure. Any patient with fluid overload, regardless of age, is at risk for these complications. The older adult or one who has coexisting cardiac problems, kidney problems, pulmonary problems, or liver problems is at greater risk.

Monitor for indicators of fluid overload (bounding pulse, increasing neck vein distention, lung crackles, increasing peripheral edema, reduced urine output) at least every 2 hours. *Pulmonary edema can occur very quickly and can lead to death.* Notify the health care provider of any change that indicates fluid overload either is not responding to therapy or is worse.

The patient with fluid overload and dependent edema is at risk for skin breakdown. Use a pressure-reducing or pressure-relieving overlay on the mattress. Assess skin pressure areas, especially the coccyx, elbows, hips, and heels, daily for redness or open areas. For patients receiving oxygen by mask or nasal cannula, check the skin around the mask, nares, and ears and under the elastic band. Assist the patient to change positions every 2 hours, or ensure that others delegated to perform this intervention are diligent in this action.

Drug therapy involves the use of drugs that interfere with adrenocorticotropic hormone (ACTH) production or adrenal hormone synthesis for temporary relief. Metyrapone (Metopirone), aminoglutethimide (Elipten, Cytadren), and ketoconazole use different pathways to decrease cortisol production (Hunt, 2012). For patients with hypercortisolism resulting from increased ACTH production, cyproheptadine (Periactin) may be used because it interferes with ACTH production. Mitotane (Lysodren) is an adrenal cytotoxic agent used for inoperable tumors causing hypercortisolism. For people with increased ACTH production who have type 2 diabetes and who do not respond to other drug therapies, another drug is mifepristone (Korlym), which is a synthetic steroid that blocks glucocorticoid receptors (Aschenbrenner, 2012).

> ## ! NURSING SAFETY PRIORITY (QSEN)
> ### *Drug Alert*
>
> Mifepristone (Korlym) cannot be used during pregnancy because it also blocks progesterone receptors and would cause termination of the pregnancy.

A new drug to manage hypercortisolism resulting from a pituitary adenoma is pasireotide (Signifor). This drug binds to somatostatin receptors on the adenoma and inhibits tumor production of corticotropin. Lower levels of corticotropin lead to lower levels of cortisol production in the adrenal glands (McKeage, 2013). This subcutaneous drug does not work for people whose tumors do not have somatostatin receptors. In addition, many patients taking this drug have problems with hyperglycemia.

Monitor the patient for response to drug therapy, especially weight loss and increased urine output. Observe for manifestations of problems with FLUID AND ELECTROLYTE BALANCE, especially changes in electrocardiogram (ECG) patterns. Assess laboratory findings, especially sodium and potassium values, whenever they are drawn.

Nutrition therapy for the patient with hypercortisolism may involve restrictions of both fluid and sodium intake to control fluid volume. Review the patient's serum sodium levels whenever fluid overload is present. Often sodium restriction involves only "no added salt" to ordinary table foods when fluid overload is mild. For more pronounced fluid overload, the patient may be restricted to anywhere from 2 g/day to 4 g/day of sodium. When sodium restriction is ongoing, teach the patient and family how to check food labels for sodium content and how to keep a daily record of sodium ingested. Explain to the patient and family the reason for any fluid restriction and the importance of adhering to the prescribed restriction.

Monitoring intake and output and weight can indicate therapy effectiveness. Ensure that unlicensed assistive personnel (UAP) understand that these measurements need to be accurate, not just estimated, because treatment decisions are based on these findings. Schedule fluid offerings throughout the 24 hours. Teach UAP to check urine for color and character and to report these findings. Check the urine specific gravity (a specific gravity below 1.005 may indicate fluid overload). If IV therapy is used, infuse only the amount prescribed.

Fluid retention may not be visible. Remember that rapid weight gain is the best indicator of fluid retention and overload. Each 1 lb (about 500 g) of weight gained equates to 500 mL of retained water. Weigh the patient at the same time daily (before breakfast), using the same scale. Have the patient wear the same type of clothing for each weigh-in.

Radiation therapy is rarely used to treat hypercortisolism caused by pituitary adenomas because it is not always effective and often destroys normal tissue. Chapter 45 discusses radiation therapy to the head.

Surgical Management. The surgical treatment of adrenocortical hypersecretion depends on the cause of the disease. When adrenal hyperfunction is due to increased pituitary secretion of ACTH, removal of a pituitary adenoma using minimally invasive techniques may be attempted. Sometimes a total *hypophysectomy* (surgical removal of the pituitary gland) is needed. (See earlier discussion of hypophysectomy on pp. 1270-1271.) If hypercortisolism is caused by an adrenal tumor, an *adrenalectomy* (removal of the adrenal gland) may be needed.

Preoperative Care. Disturbances of FLUID AND ELECTROLYTE BALANCE are corrected before surgery. Continue to monitor blood potassium, sodium, and chloride levels. Dysrhythmias from potassium imbalance may occur, and cardiac monitoring is needed. Problems with GLUCOSE REGULATION and hyperglycemia are controlled before surgery.

The patient with hypercortisolism is at risk for complications of infections and fractures. Prevent infection with handwashing and aseptic technique. Decrease the risk for falls by raising top siderails and encouraging the patient to ask for assistance when getting out of bed. A high-calorie, high-protein diet is prescribed before surgery.

Glucocorticoid preparations are given before surgery. The patient continues to receive glucocorticoids during surgery to prevent adrenal crisis because the removal of the tumor results in a sudden drop in cortisol levels. Before surgery, discuss the need for long-term drug therapy.

Operative Procedures. A unilateral adrenalectomy is performed when one gland is involved. A bilateral adrenalectomy is needed when ACTH-producing tumors cannot be treated by other means or when both adrenal glands are diseased. Surgery is most often performed by laparoscopic adrenalectomy, a minimally invasive surgical approach. If necessary, an open surgery through the abdomen or the lateral flank can be performed.

Postoperative Care. After an adrenalectomy, the patient is usually sent to a critical care unit. Immediately after surgery, assess the patient every 15 minutes for shock (e.g., hypotension; a rapid, weak pulse; and a decreasing urine output) resulting from insufficient glucocorticoid replacement. Monitor vital signs, central venous pressure, pulmonary wedge pressure, intake and output, daily weights, and serum electrolyte levels.

After a bilateral adrenalectomy, patients require lifelong glucocorticoid and mineralocorticoid replacement, starting immediately after surgery. In unilateral adrenalectomy, hormone replacement continues until the remaining adrenal gland increases hormone production. This therapy may be needed for up to 2 years after surgery.

💡 NCLEX EXAMINATION CHALLENGE

Health Promotion and Maintenance

The client who is about to have a unilateral adrenalectomy for an adenoma that is causing hypercortisolism asks the nurse if she will have to continue the severe sodium restriction after surgery. What is the nurse's best response?

A. "No, once the tumor has been removed and your cortisol levels have normalized, you will not retain excess sodium anymore."

B. "No, after surgery you will have to take oral cortisol, which can be easily controlled so that your sodium levels do not rise."

C. "Yes, the fact that you are retaining sodium and have high blood pressure is related to your age and lifestyle, not the tumor."

D. "Yes, sodium is very bad for people and everyone needs to eliminate sodium completely from their diets for the rest of their lives."

Preventing Injury. The patient who has hypercortisolism is at risk for injury from skin breakdown, bone fractures, and GI bleeding. Prevention of these injuries is a major nursing care focus.

Planning: Expected Outcomes. The patient with hypercortisolism is expected to avoid injury. Indicators include:

- Skin is intact.
- Minimal or no bruising is present.
- Bones are intact.
- Stools, vomitus, and other GI secretions contain no gross or occult blood.

Interventions. Priority nursing interventions for prevention of injury focus on skin assessment and protection, coordinating care to ensure gentle handling, and patient teaching regarding drug therapy for prevention of GI ulcers.

Skin injury is a continuing risk even after surgery has corrected the cortisol excess because the changes induced in the skin and blood vessels remain for weeks to months. Assess the skin for reddened areas, excoriation, breakdown, and edema. If mobility is decreased, turn the patient every 2 hours and pad bony prominences.

Instruct the patient to avoid activities that can result in skin trauma. Teach him or her to use a soft toothbrush and an electric shaver. Instruct patients to keep the skin clean and to dry it thoroughly after washing. Excessive dryness can be prevented by using a moisturizing lotion.

Adhesive tape often causes skin breakdown. Use tape sparingly, and remove it carefully. After venipuncture, the patient may have increased bleeding because of blood vessel fragility. Exert pressure over the site for longer than normal to prevent bleeding and bruising.

Pathologic fractures from bone density loss and osteoporosis are possible for months to years after cortisol levels return to normal. Teach the patient about safety issues and dietary needs. When helping the patient move in bed, use a lift sheet instead of grasping him or her. Remind the patient to call for help when ambulating. Review the use of walkers or canes, if needed. Teach UAP to use a gait belt when walking with a patient who has bone density loss.

Coordinate with a dietitian to teach the patient about nutrition therapy. A high-calorie diet is prescribed that includes increased amounts of calcium and vitamin D. Generous amounts of milk, cheese, yogurt, and green leafy and root vegetables add calcium to promote bone density. Advise the patient to avoid caffeine and alcohol, which increase the risk for GI ulcers and may promote bone density loss.

GI bleeding is common with hypercortisolism. Cortisol (1) inhibits production of the thick, gel-like mucus that protects the stomach lining, (2) decreases blood flow to the area, and (3) triggers the release of excess hydrochloric acid. Although surgery reduces the hypercortisolism, the normal mucus and increased blood flow may take weeks to return. Interventions focus on drug therapy to reduce irritation, protect the GI mucosa, and decrease the secretion of hydrochloric acid.

Antacids buffer stomach acids and protect the GI mucosa. Teach the patient that these drugs should be taken on a regular schedule rather than on an as-needed basis.

When histamine binds to the H_2 receptors in the gastric mucosa, a series of actions release hydrochloric acid. Drugs that block the H_2-receptor site and reduce hydrochloric acid production include cimetidine (Tagamet, Peptol ♣, Novo-Cimetine ♣), ranitidine (Zantac, Apo-Ranitidine ♣), famotidine (Pepcid), and nizatidine (Axid). Omeprazole (Losec ♣, Prilosec) and esomeprazole (Nexium) inhibit the gastric proton pump and prevent the formation of hydrochloric acid.

Instruct the patient to reduce alcohol and caffeine consumption, smoking, and fasting, because these conditions cause gastric irritation. NSAIDs and drugs that contain aspirin or other salicylates can cause gastritis and intensify GI bleeding. These should be avoided or limited.

Preventing Infection. Glucocorticoids reduce both inflammation and the immune responses, increasing the risk for infection. For the patient who is taking glucocorticoid replacement therapy, the risk is ongoing. For the patient who is recovering from surgery to prevent hypercortisolism, the infection risk continues for weeks after surgery.

Planning: Expected Outcomes. The patient with hypercortisolism is expected to remain free from infection and avoid situations that increase the risk for infection. Indicators include these manifestations and behaviors:

- Does not have fever and foul-smelling or purulent drainage
- Does not have cough, chest pain, and dyspnea
- Does not have urinary frequency, urgency, or pain and burning
- Avoids crowds and large gatherings
- Obtains appropriate vaccinations
- Washes hands frequently

Interventions. Protect the patient with hypercortisolism from infection. All personnel must use extreme care during all nursing procedures. Thorough handwashing is important. Anyone with an upper respiratory tract infection who enters the patient's room must wear a mask. Observe strict aseptic technique when performing dressing changes or any invasive procedure.

Continually assess the patient for possible infection. Manifestations may not be obvious because hypercortisolism suppresses infection manifestations. Fever and the formation of pus depend on the presence of white blood cells (WBCs). The patient who is immunosuppressed may have a severe infection without pus and with only a low-grade fever.

Monitor the patient's daily complete blood count (CBC) with differential WBC count, especially neutrophils. Inspect the mouth during every shift for lesions and mucosa breakdown. Assess the lungs every 8 hours for crackles, wheezes, or reduced breath sounds. Assess all urine for odor and cloudiness. Ask about any urgency, burning, or pain on urination.

Take vital signs at least every 4 hours to assess for fever. A temperature elevation of even 1°F (or 0.5°C) above baseline is significant for a patient who is immunosuppressed and indicates infection until it has been proven otherwise.

Skin care is important for preventing infection because the skin may be the patient's only intact defense. Teach him or her about hygiene, and urge daily bathing. If the patient is immobile, turn him or her every 1 to 2 hours and apply skin lubricants.

Perform pulmonary hygiene every 2 to 4 hours. Listen to the lungs for crackles, wheezes, or reduced breath sounds. Urge the patient to deep breathe or to use an incentive spirometer every hour while awake.

Preventing Acute Adrenal Insufficiency. The patient most at risk for acute adrenal insufficiency is the one who has Cushing's syndrome as a result of glucocorticoid drug therapy. The exogenous drug inhibits the feedback control pathway (see Fig. 61-3 in Chapter 61), preventing the hypothalamus from secreting corticotropin-releasing hormone (CRH). The lack of CRH inhibits secretion of ACTH from the anterior pituitary gland. Without normal levels of ACTH, the adrenal glands atrophy and completely stop production of the corticosteroids. As a result, the patient completely depends on the exogenous drug. If the drug is stopped, even for a day or two, the atrophied adrenal glands cannot produce the glucocorticoids and the patient develops acute adrenal insufficiency, a life-threatening condition. Management of this problem is described on p. 1274.

! NURSING SAFETY PRIORITY (QSEN)

Drug Alert

Teach patients who are taking a corticosteroid for more than a week to not stop the drug suddenly. Gradual drug tapering should be done under the care of the health care provider.

Community-Based Care

Home Care Management. The patient with hypercortisolism usually has muscle weakness and fatigue for some weeks after surgery and remains at risk for falls and other injury. These problems may necessitate one-floor living for a short time, and a home health aide may be needed to assist with hygiene, meal preparation, and maintenance.

CHART 62-11   Patient and Family Education: Preparing for Self-Management

Cortisol Replacement Therapy

- Take your medication in divided doses—the first dose in the morning and the second dose between 4 PM and 6 PM.
- Take your medication with meals or snacks.
- Weigh yourself daily, and keep a record to show your health care provider.
- Increase your dosage as directed by your health care provider for increased physical stress or severe emotional stress.
- Never skip a dose of medication. If you have persistent vomiting or severe diarrhea and cannot take your medication by mouth for 24 to 36 hours, call your physician. If you cannot reach your physician, go to the nearest emergency department. You may need an injection to take the place of your usual oral medication.
- Always wear your medical alert bracelet or necklace.
- Make regular visits for health care follow-up.
- Learn how to give yourself an intramuscular injection of hydrocortisone.

Self-Management Education. The patient taking exogenous glucocorticoids who is discharged to home remains at continuing risk for problems with FLUID AND ELECTROLYTE BALANCE, especially fluid volume excess. Teach him or her and the family to monitor the patient's weight. Suggest that a record of these daily weights be kept to show the health care provider at any checkups. Also, instruct the patient to call the health care provider if more than 3 lbs are gained in a week or more than 1 to 2 lbs are gained in a 24-hour period.

Lifelong hormone replacement is needed after bilateral adrenalectomy. Teach the patient and family about adherence to the drug regimen and its side effects (Chart 62-11).

Protecting the patient from infection at home is important. Urge him or her to use proper hygiene and to avoid crowds or others with infections. Encourage the patient and all people living in the same home with him or her to have yearly influenza vaccinations. Stress that the patient should immediately notify the physician if he or she has a fever or any other indication of infection. Chart 40-10 in Chapter 40 lists guidelines for patients for infection prevention.

Health Care Resources. Immediately after returning home, the patient may need a support person to stay and provide more attention than could be given by a visiting nurse or home care aide. Contact with the health care team is needed for follow-up and identification of potential problems. The patient taking corticosteroid therapy may have manifestations of adrenal insufficiency if the dosage is inadequate. Suggest that the patient obtain and wear a medical alert bracelet listing the condition and the drug replacement therapy.

◆ Evaluation: Outcomes

Evaluate the care of the patient with hypercortisolism based on the identified priority patient problems. The expected outcomes are that the patient should:

- Maintain FLUID AND ELECTROLYTE BALANCE
- Remain free from injury
- Remain free from infection
- Not experience acute adrenal insufficiency

Specific indicators for these outcomes are listed for each priority patient problem under the Planning and Implementation section (see earlier).

HYPERALDOSTERONISM

❖ *PATHOPHYSIOLOGY*

Hyperaldosteronism is an increased secretion of aldosterone with mineralocorticoid excess. Primary hyperaldosteronism *(Conn's syndrome)* in adults results from excessive secretion of aldosterone from one or both adrenal glands, usually caused by an adrenal adenoma. In secondary hyperaldosteronism, excessive secretion of aldosterone is caused by the high levels of angiotensin II that are stimulated by high plasma renin levels. Some causes include kidney hypoxia, diabetic nephropathy, and excessive use of some diuretics. Some forms of hyperaldosterone secretion have a genetic basis and are diagnosed in childhood.

Increased aldosterone levels cause disturbances of FLUID AND ELECTROLYTE BALANCE, which then trigger the kidney tubules to retain sodium and excrete potassium and hydrogen ions. Hypernatremia, hypokalemia, and metabolic alkalosis result. Sodium retention increases blood volume, which raises blood pressure, increasing the risk for strokes, heart attacks, and kidney damage. (See Chapter 11 for discussion of electrolyte imbalances.)

❖ *PATIENT-CENTERED COLLABORATIVE CARE*

◆ *Assessment*

Hypokalemia and elevated blood pressure are the most common problems of the patient with hyperaldosteronism. He or she may have headache, fatigue, muscle weakness, dehydration, and loss of stamina. **Polydipsia** (excessive fluid intake) and **polyuria** (excessive urine output) occur less frequently. **Paresthesias** (sensations of numbness and tingling) may occur if potassium depletion is severe (Crawford, & Harris, 2011).

Hyperaldosteronism is diagnosed on the basis of laboratory studies, x-rays, and imaging with CT or MRI. Serum potassium levels are decreased, and sodium levels are elevated. Plasma renin levels are low, and aldosterone levels are high. Hydrogen ion loss leads to metabolic alkalemia (elevated blood pH). Urine has a low specific gravity and high aldosterone levels.

◆ *Interventions*

Surgery is the most common treatment for hyperaldosteronism. One or both adrenal glands may be removed. Surgery is not performed, however, until the patient's potassium levels are normal. Drugs used to increase potassium levels include spironolactone (Aldactone, Spirono, Sincomen ✤), a potassium-sparing diuretic and aldosterone antagonist. Potassium supplements may be prescribed to increase potassium levels before surgery. The patient may also benefit from a low-sodium diet before surgery.

The patient who has undergone a unilateral adrenalectomy may need temporary glucocorticoid replacement. Replacement is lifelong if both adrenal glands are removed. Glucocorticoids are given before surgery to prevent adrenal crisis. The patient receiving long-term replacement therapy should wear a medical alert bracelet. (See the discussion of adrenalectomy on pp. 1279-1280 in the Hypercortisolism [Cushing's Disease] section for more discussion of care after surgery and patient education.)

When surgery cannot be performed, spironolactone therapy is continued to control hypokalemia and hypertension. Because spironolactone is a potassium-sparing diuretic, hyperkalemia can occur in patients who have impaired kidney function or excessive potassium intake. Advise the patient to avoid potassium supplements and foods rich in potassium. Hyponatremia can occur with spironolactone therapy, and the patient may need increased dietary sodium. Instruct the patient to report manifestations of hyponatremia, such as dryness of the mouth, thirst, lethargy, or drowsiness. Teach patients to report any additional side effects of spironolactone therapy, including gynecomastia, diarrhea, drowsiness, headache, rash, **urticaria** (hives), confusion, erectile dysfunction, hirsutism, and amenorrhea. Additional drug therapy to control hypertension is often needed.

PHEOCHROMOCYTOMA

❖ *PATHOPHYSIOLOGY*

Pheochromocytoma is a catecholamine-producing tumor that arises in the adrenal medulla. These tumors usually occur as a single lesion in one adrenal gland, although they can be bilateral or in the abdomen. Pheochromocytomas are usually benign, but at least 10% are malignant.

The tumors produce, store, and release epinephrine and norepinephrine (NE). Excessive epinephrine and NE stimulate adrenergic receptors and can have wide-ranging adverse effects mimicking the action of the sympathetic division of the autonomic nervous system.

The cause is unknown, but some pheochromocytomas occur with inherited disorders such as neurofibromatosis (type 1), multiple endocrine neoplasia (MEN-2), Von Hippel-Lindau disease, and pheochromocytoma-paraganglioma syndrome (OMIM, 2014). These tumors are rare; they occur at any age but appear most commonly in patients between 30 and 50 years of age (Young, 2011).

❖ *PATIENT-CENTERED COLLABORATIVE CARE*

◆ *Assessment*

The patient often has intermittent episodes of hypertension or attacks that range from a few minutes to several hours. During these episodes, the patient has severe headaches, palpitations, profuse diaphoresis, flushing, apprehension, or a sense of impending doom. Pain in the chest or abdomen, with nausea and vomiting, can also occur. Increased abdominal pressure, defecation, and vigorous abdominal palpation can provoke a hypertensive crisis. Drugs such as tricyclic antidepressants, droperidol, glucagon, metoclopramide, phenothiazines, and naloxone can induce a hypertensive crisis in the patient with pheochromocytoma. Foods or beverages high in tyramine (e.g., aged cheese, red wine) also induce hypertension. The patient may also report heat intolerance, weight loss, and tremors.

The most common diagnostic test is blood and 24-hour urine collection for fractionated metanephrine and catecholamine levels, all of which are elevated in the presence of a pheochromocytoma. Another test that may be conducted when catecholamine levels are not consistent is the clonidine suppression test (Young, 2011). MRI or CT scans can precisely locate tumors in the adrenal gland, as well as in the chest or abdomen.

◆ *Interventions*

Surgery is the main treatment for a pheochromocytoma. One or both adrenal glands are removed (depending on whether the tumor is bilateral). After surgery, nursing interventions focus on promoting adequate tissue perfusion, nutritional needs, and comfort measures.

Hypertension is the hallmark of the disease and the most common serious complication after surgery. Monitor the blood pressure regularly, and place the cuff consistently on the same arm, with the patient in lying and standing positions. Identify stressors that may lead to a hypertensive crisis, and attempt to reduce them. Teach the patient to not smoke, drink caffeine-containing beverages, or change position suddenly. Provide a diet rich in calories, vitamins, and minerals.

> **! NURSING SAFETY PRIORITY** (QSEN)
>
> **Action Alert**
>
> Do not palpate the abdomen of a patient with a pheochromocytoma, because this action could stimulate a sudden release of catecholamines and trigger severe hypertension.

The patient often benefits from hydration before surgery because decreased blood volume increases the risk for hypotension during and after surgery. Assess the patient's hydration status, and report manifestations of dehydration or fluid overload.

The patient's blood pressure is stabilized with adrenergic blocking agents such as phenoxybenzamine (Dibenzyline) starting 7 to 10 days before surgery because of the increased risk for severe hypertension during surgery. The drug dosages are adjusted until blood pressure is controlled and hypertensive attacks do not occur. The blood volume expands, and blood pressure in the supine position returns to normal.

Anesthetic agents and touching of the tumor during surgery can cause a catecholamine release. Short-acting alpha-adrenergic blockers are given by IV bolus or continuous infusion for a hypertensive crisis.

Nursing care after surgery is similar to that for the patient who has undergone an adrenalectomy (see Hypercortisolism [Cushing's Disease], pp. 1279-1280). Monitor the patient for hypertension and for hypotension (from the sudden decrease in catecholamine levels) and for hypovolemia. Hemorrhage and shock are possible, and plasma expanders or fluids may be needed. Monitor vital signs, as well as fluid intake and output. If opioids are given, check for their effect on blood pressure.

When tumors are inoperable, management is medical, with alpha-adrenergic and beta-adrenergic blocking agents. For these patients, self-measurement of blood pressure with home monitoring equipment is essential. (See Chapter 36 for teaching priorities and community-based care of the patient with chronic hypertension.)

NURSING CONCEPTS AND CLINICAL JUDGMENT REVIEW

What might you NOTICE if the patient is experiencing disturbances of FLUID AND ELECTROLYTE BALANCE and GLUCOSE REGULATION as a result of adrenal gland hypofunction?

Assessment:
- Postural hypotension
- Irregular heart rate
- Sweating
- Headaches
- Tachycardia
- Tremors
- Muscle weakness
- Forgetfulness
- Lethargy and confusion
- Salt craving

What should you INTERPRET and how should you RESPOND to a patient experiencing disturbances of FLUID AND ELECTROLYTE IMBALANCE and GLUCOSE REGULATION as a result of adrenal gland hypofunction?

Interpret by:
- Taking vital signs
- Assessing cognition
- Assessing blood pressure in the sitting and standing positions
- Assessing muscle strength and function

Interpret laboratory values, including:
- Blood glucose levels
- Serum potassium levels
- Serum sodium levels
- Serum cortisol levels
- Blood urea nitrogen levels

Respond by:
- Ensuring fluid intake
- Providing adequate calorie and carbohydrate intake
- Monitoring for fluid deficit
- Obtaining daily weights
- Measuring intake and output
- Administering prescribed hormone replacements
- Assisting the patient with ambulation
- Monitoring electrocardiograph changes

On what should you REFLECT?
- Observe the patient for evidence of improved fluid and electrolyte balance and glucose regulation.
- Think about what patient education focus could help reduce the intensity of disturbances of fluid and electrolyte balance and glucose regulation in the future.

GET READY FOR THE NCLEX® EXAMINATION!

KEY POINTS

Review these Key Points for each NCLEX Examination Client Needs Category.

Safe and Effective Care Environment

- Handle all patients with bone density loss carefully, using lift sheets whenever possible. **Safety** QSEN
- Use good handwashing techniques before providing any care to a patient who is immunosuppressed. **Safety** QSEN
- Ensure that hormone replacement drugs are given as close to the prescribed times as possible. **Safety** QSEN

Health Promotion and Maintenance

- Instruct the patient with adrenal insufficiency to wear a medical alert bracelet and to carry simple carbohydrates with him or her at all times. **Patient-Centered Care** QSEN
- Teach the patient and family about the clinical manifestations of infection and when to seek medical advice. **Patient-Centered Care** QSEN
- Teach patients who have permanent endocrine hypofunction the proper techniques and timing of hormone replacement therapy. **Patient-Centered Care** QSEN
- Teach patients taking bromocriptine to seek medical care immediately if chest pain, dizziness, or watery nasal discharge occurs. **Safety** QSEN
- Teach patients with diabetes insipidus the proper way to self-administer desmopressin orally or by nasal spray. **Patient-Centered Care** QSEN
- Teach patients who are taking a corticosteroid for more than a week to not stop the drug suddenly. **Safety** QSEN

Psychosocial Integrity

- Encourage the patient and family to express concerns about a change in health status. **Patient-Centered Care** QSEN
- Explain all treatment procedures, restrictions, and follow-up care to the patient. **Patient-Centered Care** QSEN
- Allow patients who experience a change in physical appearance to mourn this change. **Patient-Centered Care** QSEN

Physiological Integrity

- During the immediate period after a hypophysectomy, teach the patient to avoid activities that increase intracranial pressure (e.g., bending at the waist, straining to have a bowel movement, coughing). **Patient-Centered Care** QSEN
- Measure intake and output accurately on patients who have either diabetes insipidus or syndrome of inappropriate antidiuretic hormone (SIADH). **Evidence-Based Practice** QSEN
- Teach the patient with diabetes insipidus the manifestations of dehydration. **Evidence-Based Practice** QSEN
- Ensure that no patient suspected of having DI is deprived of fluids for more than 4 hours. **Safety** QSEN
- Administer tolvaptan or conivaptan only in the hospital setting. **Safety** QSEN
- Do not confuse prednisone with prednisolone. **Safety** QSEN
- Do not palpate the abdomen of a patient who has a pheochromocytoma. **Safety** QSEN
- Work with physicians, dietitians, and pharmacists to help the patient experiencing problems of the pituitary or adrenal gland to achieve and maintain FLUID AND ELECTROLYTE BALANCE and GLUCOSE REGULATION. **Teamwork and Collaboration** QSEN

CHAPTER 63

Care of Patients with Problems of the Thyroid and Parathyroid Glands

M. Linda Workman

 http://evolve.elsevier.com/Iggy/

PRIORITY CONCEPTS

- NUTRITION
- THERMOREGULATION

LEARNING OUTCOMES

Safe and Effective Care Environment

1. Protect the patient with thyroid or adrenal parathyroid gland problems from injury and complications.

Health Promotion and Maintenance

2. Identify the teaching priorities and NUTRITION needs for the patient taking hormone replacement therapy for thyroid or parathyroid problems.

Psychosocial Integrity

3. Reduce the psychological impact for the patient and family experiencing thyroid or parathyroid gland problems.

Physiological Integrity

4. Interpret clinical changes and laboratory data to determine the effectiveness of interventions for thyroid problems.
5. Prioritize nursing care for the patient experiencing severe thyrotoxicosis (thyroid storm) and impaired THERMOREGULATION.
6. Coordinate nursing care for the patient during the first 24 hours after thyroid or parathyroid surgery.
7. Coordinate care for the patient who has hyperparathyroidism.
8. Coordinate care for the patient who has hypoparathyroidism.

The hormones secreted from the thyroid and parathyroid glands affect metabolism, THERMOREGULATION, NUTRITION, electrolyte balance, and excitable membrane activity. Problems of either gland often have many effects and manifestations. Mild disturbances produce subtle problems. More severe disturbances may produce life-threatening problems.

THYROID DISORDERS

HYPERTHYROIDISM

❖ PATHOPHYSIOLOGY

Hyperthyroidism is excessive thyroid hormone secretion from the thyroid gland. The manifestations of hyperthyroidism are called **thyrotoxicosis**, regardless of the origin of the thyroid hormones. This term is correct even when a person takes a large amount of synthetic thyroid hormones that manifests as thyrotoxicosis although he or she does not have hyperthyroidism. Thyroid hormones increase metabolism in all body organs, producing many different manifestations. Hyperthyroidism can be temporary or permanent, depending on the cause.

The excessive thyroid hormones stimulate most body systems, causing hypermetabolism and increased sympathetic nervous system activity. Manifestations are listed in Chart 63-1.

Thyroid hormones stimulate the heart, increasing both heart rate and stroke volume. These responses increase cardiac output, systolic blood pressure, and blood flow (McCance et al., 2014).

Elevated thyroid hormone levels affect protein, fat, and glucose metabolism. Protein buildup and breakdown are increased, but breakdown exceeds buildup, causing a net loss of body protein known as a **negative nitrogen balance**. Glucose tolerance is decreased, and the patient has **hyperglycemia** (elevated blood glucose levels). Fat metabolism is increased, and body fat decreases. Although the patient has an increased appetite, the increased metabolism causes weight loss and NUTRITION deficits.

Thyroid hormones are produced in response to the stimulation hormones secreted by the hypothalamus and anterior pituitary glands. Thus oversecretion of thyroid hormones changes the secretion of hormones from the hypothalamus and the anterior pituitary gland through negative feedback (see Chapter 61). Thyroid hormones also have some influence over sex hormone production. Women have menstrual problems and decreased fertility. Both men and women with hyperthyroidism have an increased **libido** (sexual interest).

Etiology and Genetic Risk

Hyperthyroidism has many causes. The most common form of the disease is Graves' disease, also called *toxic diffuse goiter.*

CHART 63-1   **Key Features**

Hyperthyroidism

Skin Manifestations
- Diaphoresis (excessive sweating)
- Fine, soft, silky body hair
- Smooth, warm, moist skin
- Thinning of scalp hair

Cardiopulmonary Manifestations
- Palpitations
- Chest pain
- Increased systolic blood pressure
- Tachycardia
- Dysrhythmias
- Rapid, shallow respirations

Gastrointestinal Manifestations
- Weight loss
- Increased appetite
- Increased stools

Neurologic Manifestations
- Blurred or double vision
- Eye fatigue
- Increased tears
- Injected (red) conjunctiva
- Photophobia
- Exophthalmos*
- Eyelid retraction, eyelid lag

- Globe lag
- Hyperactive deep tendon reflexes
- Tremors
- Insomnia

Metabolic Manifestations
- Increased basal metabolic rate
- Heat intolerance
- Low-grade fever
- Fatigue

Psychological/Emotional Manifestations
- Decreased attention span
- Restlessness and irritability
- Emotional lability
- Manic behavior

Reproductive Manifestations
- Amenorrhea
- Increased libido

Other Manifestations
- Goiter
- Wide-eyed or startled appearance (exophthalmos)*
- Enlarged spleen
- Muscle weakness and wasting

*Present in Graves' disease only.

Graves' disease is an autoimmune disorder resulting from Hashimoto's thyroiditis (HT) (Mandel et al., 2011). HT results in the production of autoantibodies to different substances and structures within the thyroid gland. In Graves' disease, these antibodies (thyroid-stimulating immunoglobulins [TSIs]) attach to the thyroid-stimulating hormone (TSH) receptors on the thyroid tissue. The thyroid gland responds by increasing the glandular cells, which enlarges the gland, forming a **goiter**, and overproduces thyroid hormones (**thyrotoxicosis**). When HT causes production of antibodies to other structures within the thyroid gland, hypothyroidism results. (See the discussion of Etiology on pp. 1291-1292) in the Hypothyroidism section.)

In Graves' disease, all the general manifestations of hyperthyroidism are present. In addition, other manifestations specific to Graves' disease may occur, including **exophthalmos** (abnormal protrusion of the eyes) and **pretibial myxedema** (dry, waxy swelling of the front surfaces of the lower legs that resembles benign tumors or keloids). *Not all patients with a goiter have hyperthyroidism.*

Hyperthyroidism caused by multiple thyroid nodules is termed **toxic multinodular goiter**. The nodules may be enlarged thyroid tissues or benign tumors (adenomas). These patients usually have had a goiter for years. The manifestations are milder than those seen in Graves' disease, and the patient does not have exophthalmos or pretibial myxedema.

Hyperthyroidism also can be caused by excessive use of thyroid replacement hormones. This type of problem is called **exogenous hyperthyroidism**.

GENETIC/GENOMIC CONSIDERATIONS
Patient-Centered Care **QSEN**

Susceptibility to Graves' disease is associated with mutations in several genes, including *GRD1*, *GRD2*, *GRDX1*, and *GRDX2*. The pattern of inheritance appears to be autosomal recessive with sex limitation to females and reduced penetrance. Graves' disease also has a strong association with other autoimmune disorders, such as diabetes mellitus, vitiligo, and rheumatoid arthritis. It often occurs in both members of identical twins (Online Mendelian Inheritance in Man [OMIM], 2014). Be sure to ask the patient with Graves' disease whether any other family members have the problem.

Incidence and Prevalence

Hyperthyroidism is a common endocrine disorder. Graves' disease can occur at any age but is diagnosed most often in women between 20 and 40 years of age (Mandel et al., 2011). Toxic multinodular goiter usually occurs after the age of 50 years and affects women 4 times more often than men (McCance et al., 2014).

❖ PATIENT-CENTERED COLLABORATIVE CARE

◆ Assessment

History. Many changes and problems occur because hyperthyroidism affects all body systems, although changes may occur over such a long period that not all patients are aware of them. Record age, gender, and usual weight. The increased metabolic rate affects NUTRITION. The patient may report a recent unplanned weight loss, an increased appetite, and an increase in the number of bowel movements per day.

A hallmark of hyperthyroidism is poor THERMOREGULATION with heat intolerance. The patient may have increased sweating even when environmental temperatures are comfortable for others. He or she often wears lighter clothing in cold weather. The patient may also report palpitations or chest pain as a result of the cardiovascular effects. Ask about changes in breathing patterns, because dyspnea (with or without exertion) is common.

Visual changes may be the earliest problem the patient or family notices, especially exophthalmos with Graves' disease (Fig. 63-1). Ask about changes in vision, such as blurring or double vision, and tiring of the eyes.

Ask whether there has been a change in energy level or in the ability to perform ADLs. Fatigue and insomnia are common. Family and friends may report that the patient has become irritable or depressed.

Ask women about changes in menses, because amenorrhea or a decreased menstrual flow is common. Initially, both men and women may have an increase in libido, but this changes as the patient becomes more fatigued.

Ask about previous thyroid surgery or radiation therapy to the neck, because some people remain hyperthyroid after surgery or are resistant to radiation therapy. Ask about past and current drugs, especially the use of thyroid hormone replacement or antithyroid drugs.

Physical Assessment/Clinical Manifestations. Exophthalmos is common in patients with Graves' disease. The wide-eyed or "startled" look is due to edema in the extraocular muscles and increased fatty tissue behind the eye, which pushes the eyeball forward and may cause problems with focusing.

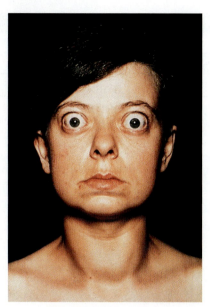

FIG. 63-1 Exophthalmos.

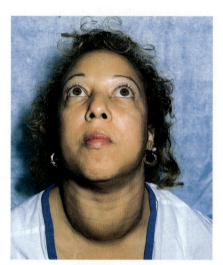

FIG. 63-2 Goiter.

Pressure on the optic nerve may impair vision. If the eyelids fail to close completely and the eyes are unprotected, they may become dry and corneal ulcers may develop. Observe the eyes for excessive tearing and a bloodshot appearance. Ask about sensitivity to light (**photophobia**).

Two other eye problems are common in all types of hyperthyroidism: eyelid retraction (eyelid lag) and globe (eyeball) lag. In eyelid lag, the upper eyelid fails to descend when the patient gazes slowly downward. In globe lag, the upper eyelid pulls back faster than the eyeball when the patient gazes upward. During assessment, ask the patient to look down and then up, and document the response.

Observe the size and symmetry of the thyroid gland. Palpate the thyroid gland to assess its size and consistency. In goiter, a generalized thyroid enlargement, the thyroid gland may increase to 4 times its normal size (Fig. 63-2). Goiters are common in Graves' disease and are classified by size (Table 63-1). Bruits (turbulence from increased blood flow) may be heard in the neck with a stethoscope. (See Chapter 61 for thyroid palpation and auscultation.)

TABLE 63-1	Goiter Classification
GOITER GRADE	**DESCRIPTION**
0	No palpable or visible goiter.
1	Mass is not visible with neck in the normal position. Goiter can be palpated and moves up when the patient swallows.
2	Mass is visible as swelling when the neck is in the normal position. Goiter is easily palpated and is usually asymmetric.

The cardiovascular problems of hyperthyroidism include increased systolic blood pressure, tachycardia, and dysrhythmias. Usually the diastolic pressure is decreased, causing a widened pulse pressure.

Inspect the hair and skin. Fine, soft, silky hair and smooth, warm, moist skin are common. Many patients notice thinning of scalp hair. Muscle weakness and hyperactive deep tendon reflexes are common. Observe motor movements of the hands for tremors. The patient may appear restless, irritable, and fatigued.

Psychosocial Assessment. The patient often has wide mood swings, irritability, decreased attention span, and manic behavior. Hyperactivity often leads to fatigue because of the inability to sleep well. Some patients describe their activity as having two modes—either "full speed ahead" or "completely stopped." Ask whether he or she cries or laughs without cause or has difficulty concentrating. Family members often report a change in the patient's mental or emotional status.

Laboratory Assessment. Testing for hyperthyroidism involves measurement of blood values for triiodothyronine (T_3), thyroxine (T_4), and thyroid-stimulating hormone (TSH). Antibodies to the TSH receptor (thyrotropin receptor [TRAbs]) are measured to diagnose Graves' disease. The most common changes in laboratory tests for hyperthyroidism are listed in Chart 63-2.

Other Diagnostic Assessment. *Thyroid scan* evaluates the position, size, and functioning of the thyroid gland. Radioactive iodine (RAI [^{123}I]) is given by mouth, and the uptake of iodine by the thyroid gland (radioactive iodine uptake [RAIU]) is measured. The half-life of ^{123}I is short, and radiation precautions are not needed. Pregnancy should be ruled out before the scan is performed. The normal thyroid gland has an uptake of 5% to 35% of the given dose at 24 hours. RAIU is increased in hyperthyroidism and can be used to identify active thyroid nodules. It is no longer the most common test for thyroid function (Mandel et al., 2011).

Ultrasonography of the thyroid gland can determine its size and the general composition of any masses or nodules. This procedure takes about 30 minutes to perform and is painless.

Electrocardiography (ECG) usually shows tachycardia. Other ECG changes with hyperthyroidism include atrial fibrillation, dysrhythmias, and changes in P and T waveforms.

◆ **Interventions**

Because Graves' disease is the most common form of hyperthyroidism, the interventions discussed in the following sections include those specific for the problems that occur with Graves' disease. The purposes of medical management are to decrease the effect of thyroid hormone on cardiac function and to reduce

CHART 63-2   Laboratory Profile

Thyroid Function

TEST	NORMAL RANGE FOR ADULTS	SIGNIFICANCE OF ABNORMAL FINDINGS	
		HYPERTHYROIDISM	HYPOTHYROIDISM
Serum T$_3$	70-205 ng/dL, or 1.2-3.4 SI units	Increased	Decreased
Serum T$_4$ (total)	4-12 mcg/dL, or 51-154 SI units	Increased	Decreased
Free T$_4$ index	0.8-2.8 ng/dL, or 10-36 SI units	Increased	Decreased
TSH stimulation test (thyroid stimulation test)	>10% in RAIU or >1.5 mcg/dL	N/A (test differentiates primary from secondary hypothyroidism)	No response in primary hypothyroidism Normal response in secondary hypothyroidism
Thyroid-stimulating immunoglobulins (TSI)	<130% of basal activity	Elevated in Graves' disease Normal in other types of hyperthyroidism	No change
Thyrotropin receptor antibodies (TRAb)	Titer: 0%	80%-95% indicates Graves' disease	No response
TSH	0.3-5.0 μU/mL or 0.3-5.0 SI units	Low in Graves' disease High in secondary or tertiary hyperthyroidism	High in primary disease Low in secondary or tertiary disease

Data from Pagana, K., & Pagana, T. (2014). *Mosby's manual of diagnostic and laboratory tests* (5th ed.). St. Louis: Mosby.
N/A, Nonapplicable; *SI,* International System of Units; *T$_3$,* triiodothyronine; *T$_4$,* thyroxine; *TSH,* thyroid-stimulating hormone.

 NCLEX EXAMINATION CHALLENGE

Physiological Integrity

Which manifestations are most often seen in general hyperthyroidism? **Select all that apply.**
A. Increased appetite
B. Cold intolerance
C. Constipation
D. Eyelid retraction
E. Insomnia
F. Palpitations
G. Tremors
H. Weight gain

thyroid hormone secretion. The priorities for nursing care focus on monitoring for complications, reducing stimulation, promoting comfort, and teaching the patient and family about therapeutic drugs and procedures.

Nonsurgical Management. *Monitoring* includes measuring the patient's apical pulse, blood pressure (BP), and temperature at least every 4 hours. Instruct the patient to report immediately any palpitations, dyspnea, vertigo, or chest pain. Increases in temperature may indicate a rapid worsening of the patient's condition and the onset of *thyroid storm,* a life-threatening event that occurs with uncontrolled hyperthyroidism and is characterized by high fever and severe hypertension. *Immediately report a temperature increase of even one degree Fahrenheit.* If this task is delegated to unlicensed assistive personnel (UAP), instruct them to report the patient's temperature to you as soon as it has been obtained. If temperature is elevated, immediately assess the patient's cardiac status. If the patient has a cardiac monitor, check for dysrhythmias.

Reducing stimulation helps prevent increasing the manifestations of hyperthyroidism and the risk for cardiac complications. Encourage the patient to rest. Keep the environment as quiet as possible by closing the door to his or her room, limiting visitors, and eliminating or postponing nonessential care or treatments.

Promoting comfort includes reducing the room temperature to decrease discomfort caused by heat intolerance. Instruct UAP to ensure the patient always has a fresh pitcher of ice water and to change the bed linen whenever it becomes damp from diaphoresis. Suggest that the patient take a cool shower or sponge bath several times each day. For patients with exophthalmos, prevent eye dryness by encouraging the use of artificial tears.

Drug therapy with antithyroid drugs is the initial treatment for hyperthyroidism. Chart 63-3 lists teaching priorities for the patient receiving drug therapy for hyperthyroidism. The preferred drugs are the thionamides, especially methimazole (Tapazole). Propylthiouracil (PTU) is used less often because of its liver toxic effects (Mandel et al., 2011). These drugs block thyroid hormone production by preventing iodide binding in the thyroid gland. The response to these drugs is delayed because the patient may have large amounts of stored thyroid hormones that continue to be released.

❗ NURSING SAFETY PRIORITY (QSEN)

Drug Alert

Although similar in action, methimazole and propylthiouracil are not interchangeable. The dosages for propylthiouracil are much higher than those for methimazole.

❗ NURSING SAFETY PRIORITY (QSEN)

Drug Alert

Methimazole can cause birth defects and should not be used during pregnancy, especially during the first trimester. Instruct women to notify their health care provider if pregnancy occurs.

Iodine preparations may be used for short-term therapy before surgery. They decrease blood flow through the thyroid gland, reducing the production and release of thyroid hormones. Improvement usually occurs within 2 weeks, but it may be weeks before metabolism returns to normal. This treatment

CHART 63-3	**Common Examples of Drug Therapy**	

Hyperthyroidism

DRUG/USUAL DOSAGE	NURSING INTERVENTION	RATIONALE
Thionamides Reduce manifestations of hyperthyroidism by preventing the new formation of thyroid hormones by inhibiting thyroid binding of iodide.		
Propylthiouracil (PTU, Propyl-Thyracil ♦) Initial dose 100-150 mg orally every 8 hr Maintenance dose 50-150 mg orally every 8 hr	Teach patient to avoid crowds and people who are ill. Teach patient to report darkening of the urine, a yellow appearance to the skin or whites of the eyes. Teach patient to check for weight gain, slow heart rate, and cold intolerance.	Drug reduces blood cell counts and the immune response, increasing the risk for infection. These manifestations may indicate liver toxicity or failure, a possible side effect of the drug. These indicate hypothyroidism and may require a lower drug dose.
Methimazole (Northyx, Tapazole) Initial dose 5-20 mg orally every 8 hr Maintenance dose 1-4 mg orally every 8 hr	Remind women to notify their health care providers if they become pregnant. Teach patient to avoid crowds and people who are ill. Teach patient to check for weight gain, slow heart rate, and cold intolerance.	This drug causes birth defects and should not be used during pregnancy. Drug reduces blood cell counts and the immune response, increasing the risk for infection. These indicate hypothyroidism and may require a lower drug dose.
Iodine and Iodine-Containing Agents The sudden excess of iodine rapidly inhibits thyroid hormone release and dramatically (but temporarily) resolves the cardiac and other manifestations of hyperthyroidism. For initial treatment of severe hyperthyroidism or thyroid storm.		
Lugol's solution Saturated solution of potassium iodide (SSKI) Dosages vary depending on the agent, how the drug is administered, and the severity of the manifestations	Administer these drugs orally 1 hour *after* a thionamide has been given. Check patient for a fever or rash, and ask about a metallic taste, mouth sores, sore throat, or GI distress.	Initially, the iodine agents can cause an increase in the production of thyroid hormones. Giving a thionamide first prevents this initial increase in thyroid hormone production. These are manifestations of *iodism*, a toxic effect of the drugs, and may require that the drug be discontinued.

can result in hypothyroidism, and the patient is monitored closely for the need to adjust the drug regimen.

Beta-adrenergic blocking drugs such as propranolol (Inderal, Detensol ♦) may be used as supportive therapy. These drugs relieve diaphoresis, anxiety, tachycardia, and palpitations but do not inhibit thyroid hormone production. See Chapters 34 and 36 for a discussion of the actions and nursing implications of these agents.

Radioactive iodine (RAI) therapy is not used in pregnant women because ^{131}I crosses the placenta and can damage the fetal thyroid gland. The patient with hyperthyroidism may receive RAI in the form of oral [131]I. The dosage depends on the thyroid gland's size and sensitivity to radiation. The thyroid gland picks up the RAI, and some of the cells that produce thyroid hormone are destroyed by the local radiation. Because the thyroid gland stores thyroid hormones to some degree, the patient may not have complete symptom relief until 6 to 8 weeks after RAI therapy. Additional drug therapy for hyperthyroidism is still needed during the first few weeks after RAI treatment.

RAI therapy is performed on an outpatient basis. One dose may be sufficient, although some patients need a second or third dose. The radiation dose is low and is usually completely eliminated within a month; however, the source is unsealed and some radioactivity is present in the patient's body fluids and stool for a few weeks after therapy. Radiation precautions are needed to prevent exposure to family members and other people. Chart 63-4 lists precautions to teach the patient during the first few weeks after receiving [131]I.

The degree of thyroid destruction varies. Some patients become hypothyroid as a result of treatment. The patient then needs lifelong thyroid hormone replacement. All patients who have undergone RAI therapy should be monitored regularly for changes in thyroid function.

Surgical Management. Surgery to remove all or part of the thyroid gland is the preferred management for Graves' disease. It is also used when a large goiter causes tracheal or esophageal compression or when hyperthyroidism does not respond to drug therapy. Removal of all (**total thyroidectomy**) or part (**subtotal thyroidectomy**) of the thyroid tissue decreases the production of thyroid hormones. After a total thyroidectomy, patients must take lifelong thyroid hormone replacement.

Preoperative Care. The patient is treated with thionamide drug therapy first to have near-normal thyroid function (**euthyroid**) before thyroid surgery. Iodine preparations also are used to decrease thyroid size and vascularity, thereby reducing the risk for hemorrhage and the potential for thyroid storm during surgery.

Hypertension, dysrhythmias, and tachycardia must be controlled before surgery. The patient with hyperthyroidism may need to follow a high-protein, high-carbohydrate diet for days or weeks before surgery.

Teach the patient to perform deep-breathing exercises. Stress the importance of supporting the neck when coughing or moving by placing both hands behind the neck to reduce strain on the incision. Explain that hoarseness may be present for a few days as a result of endotracheal tube placement during surgery.

Reassure the patient by calmly explaining the surgery and the care after surgery. Remind him or her that a drain as well as a dressing may be in place after surgery. Answer any questions the patient and family have.

Operative Procedures. Many thyroidectomies are now performed as minimally invasive surgeries or mini-incision surgeries. With these surgeries, as with the traditional open approach, the parathyroid glands and recurrent laryngeal nerves are avoided to reduce the risk for complications and injury. Usually, general anesthesia is used even for the minimally invasive techniques.

CHART 63-4   **Patient and Family Education: Preparing for Self-Management**

Safety Precautions for the Patient Receiving an Unsealed Radioactive Isotope

- Use a toilet that is not used by others for at least 2 weeks after receiving the radioactive iodine.
- Sit to urinate (males and females) to avoid splashing the seat, walls, and floor.
- Flush the toilet 3 times after each use.
- If urine is spilled on the toilet seat or floor, use paper tissues or towels to clean it up, bag them in sealable plastic bags, and take them to the hospital's radiation therapy department.
- Men with urinary incontinence should use condom catheters and a drainage bag rather than absorbent gel-filled briefs or pads.
- Women with urinary incontinence should use facial tissue layers in their clothing to catch the urine rather than absorbent gel-filled briefs or pads. These tissues should then be flushed down the toilet exclusively used by the patient.
- Using a laxative on the second and third days after receiving the radioactive drug helps you excrete the contaminated stool faster (this also decreases the exposure of your abdominal organs to radiation).
- Wear only machine-washable clothing, and wash these items separately from others in your household.
- After washing your clothing, run the washing machine for a full cycle on empty before it is used to wash the clothing of others.
- Avoid close contact with pregnant women, infants, and young children for the first week after therapy. Remain at least 3 feet (about 1 meter) away from these people, and limit your exposure to them to no more than 1 hour daily.
- Some radioactivity will be in your saliva during the first week after therapy. Precautions to avoid exposing others to this contamination (both household members and trash collectors) include:
  - Not sharing toothbrushes or toothpaste tubes
  - Using disposable tissues rather than cloth handkerchiefs, and either flushing used ones down the toilet or keeping them in a plastic bag and turning them in to the radiation department of the hospital for disposal
  - Using disposable utensils, plates, and cups
  - Selecting foods that can be eaten completely and do not result in a saliva-coated remnant (Foods to avoid are fruit with a core that can be contaminated, meat with a bone [e.g., chicken wings or legs, ribs])

Data from Al-Shakhrah, I. (2008). Radioprotection using iodine-131 for thyroid cancer and hyperthyroidism: A review. *Clinical Journal of Oncology Nursing, 12*(6), 905-912.

With a subtotal thyroidectomy, the remaining thyroid tissues are sutured to the trachea. With a total thyroidectomy, the entire thyroid gland is removed but the parathyroid glands are left with an intact blood supply to prevent causing hypoparathyroidism.

Postoperative Care. *Monitoring the patient for complications is the most important nursing action after thyroid surgery.* Monitor vital signs every 15 minutes until the patient is stable and then every 30 minutes. Increase or decrease the monitoring of vital signs based on changes in the patient's condition.

Assess the patient's level of discomfort. Use pillows to support the head and neck. Place the patient, while he or she is awake, in a semi-Fowler's position. Avoid positions that cause neck extension. Give prescribed drugs for pain control as needed.

Assist the patient to deep-breathe every 30 minutes to 1 hour. Suction oral and tracheal secretions when necessary.

Thyroid surgery can cause hemorrhage, respiratory distress, parathyroid gland injury (resulting in **hypocalcemia** [low serum calcium levels] and **tetany** [hyperexcitability of nerves and muscles]), damage to the laryngeal nerves, and thyroid storm. Remain alert to the potential for complications, and identify manifestations early.

Hemorrhage is most likely to occur during the first 24 hours after surgery. Inspect the neck dressing and behind the patient's neck for blood. A drain may be present, and a moderate amount of serosanguineous drainage is normal. Hemorrhage may be seen as bleeding at the incision site or as respiratory distress caused by tracheal compression with swelling of the site.

Respiratory distress can result from swelling, tetany, or damage to the laryngeal nerve resulting in spasms. Laryngeal **stridor** (harsh, high-pitched respiratory sounds) is heard in acute respiratory obstruction. Keep emergency tracheostomy equipment in the patient's room. Check that oxygen and suctioning equipment are nearby and in working order.

! NURSING SAFETY PRIORITY (QSEN)

Critical Rescue

When stridor, dyspnea, or other symptoms of obstruction appear after thyroid surgery, notify the Rapid Response Team.

Hypocalcemia and tetany may occur if the parathyroid glands are removed or damaged or their blood supply is impaired during thyroid surgery, resulting in decreased parathyroid hormone (PTH) levels. Ask the patient hourly about tingling around the mouth or of the toes and fingers. Assess for muscle twitching as a sign of calcium deficiency. Calcium gluconate or calcium chloride for IV use should be available in an emergency situation. (For information on the later signs of hypocalcemia, see the discussion of postoperative care on p. 1297 in the Hyperparathyroidism section and p. 1298 in the Assessment discussion in the Hypoparathyroidism section. Hypocalcemia is also discussed in Chapter 11.)

Laryngeal nerve damage may occur during surgery. This problem results in hoarseness and a weak voice. Assess the patient's voice at 2-hour intervals, and document any changes. Reassure the patient that hoarseness is usually temporary.

Thyroid storm or **thyroid crisis** is a life-threatening event that occurs in patients with uncontrolled hyperthyroidism and occurs most often with Graves' disease. Manifestations develop quickly. It is often triggered by stressors such as trauma, infection, diabetic ketoacidosis, and pregnancy. Other conditions that can lead to thyroid storm include vigorous palpation of the goiter, exposure to iodine, and radioactive iodine (RAI) therapy. Although thyroid storm after surgery is less common because of drug therapy before thyroid surgery, it can still occur.

The manifestations of thyroid storm are caused by excessive thyroid hormone release, which dramatically increases metabolic rate. *Key manifestations include fever, tachycardia, and systolic hypertension.* The patient may have abdominal pain, nausea, vomiting, and diarrhea. Often he or she is very anxious and has tremors. As the crisis progresses, the patient may become restless, confused, or psychotic and may have seizures, leading to coma. *Even with treatment, thyroid storm may lead to death.*

! NURSING SAFETY PRIORITY (QSEN)

Critical Rescue

When caring for a patient with hyperthyroidism, even after a thyroidectomy, immediately report a temperature increase of even 1°F because it may indicate an impending thyroid crisis.

CHART 63-5   Best Practice for Patient Safety & Quality Care (QSEN)

Emergency Care of the Patient During Thyroid Storm

- Maintain a patent airway and adequate ventilation.
- Give oral antithyroid drugs as prescribed: methimazole (Tapazole), up to 60 mg daily; propylthiouracil (PTU, Propyl-Thyracil ✦), 300 to 900 mg daily.
- Administer sodium iodide solution, 2 g IV daily as prescribed.
- Give propranolol (Inderal, Detensol ✦), 1 to 3 mg IV as prescribed. Give slowly over 3 minutes. The patient should be connected to a cardiac monitor, and a central venous pressure catheter should be in place.
- Give glucocorticoids as prescribed: hydrocortisone, 100 to 500 mg IV daily; prednisone, 4 to 60 mg IV daily; or dexamethasone, 2 mg IM every 6 hours.
- Monitor continually for cardiac dysrhythmias.
- Monitor vital signs every 30 minutes.
- Provide comfort measures, including a cooling blanket.
- Give non-salicylate antipyretics as prescribed.
- Correct dehydration with normal saline infusions.
- Apply cooling blanket or ice packs to reduce fever.

Emergency measures to prevent death vary with the intensity and type of manifestations. Interventions focus on maintaining airway patency, providing adequate ventilation, reducing fever, and stabilizing the hemodynamic status. Chart 63-5 outlines the best practices for emergency management of thyroid storm.

Eye and vision problems of Graves' disease are not corrected by treatment for hyperthyroidism, and management is symptomatic. Teach the patient with mild problems to elevate the head of the bed at night and to use artificial tears. If **photophobia** (sensitivity to light) is present, dark glasses may be helpful. For those who cannot close the eyelids completely, recommend gently taping the lids closed with nonallergenic tape at bedtime. These actions prevent eye irritation and injury. If pressure behind the eye continues and forces the eye forward, the blood supply to the eye can be compromised, leading to ischemia and blindness.

In severe cases, short-term steroid therapy is prescribed to reduce swelling and halt the infiltrative process. Prednisone (Deltasone, Winpred ✦) is given in high doses (often 120 mg daily) at first and then is tapered down according to the patient's response. Explain the need to reduce the prednisone gradually, and review its side effects with the patient.

Other management strategies include external radiation combined with lower-dose steroid therapy. Surgical intervention (orbital decompression) may be needed if loss of sight or damage to the eyeball is possible. Rituximab injections are an experimental approach for this problem (Mandel et al., 2011).

Health teaching includes reviewing with the patient and family the manifestations of hyperthyroidism and instructing the patient to report any increase or recurrence of these. Also teach about the manifestations of hypothyroidism (discussed in the next section) and the need for thyroid hormone replacement. Reinforce the need for regular follow-up because hypothyroidism can occur several years after radioactive iodine therapy.

The discharged patient may continue to have mood changes as a result of hyperthyroidism. Explain the reason for mood swings to the patient and family, and reassure them that these will decrease with continued treatment.

NCLEX EXAMINATION CHALLENGE
Safe and Effective Care Environment

For which assessment finding in a client who has severe hyperthyroidism does the nurse notify the Rapid Response Team?
A. An increase in premature ventricular heart contractions from 4 per minute to 5 per minute
B. An increase in or widening of pulse pressure from 40 mm Hg to 46 mm Hg
C. An increase in temperature from 99.5° F (37.5° C) to 101.3° F (38.5° C)
D. An increase of 20 mL of urine output per hour

HYPOTHYROIDISM

❖ PATHOPHYSIOLOGY

The manifestations of hypothyroidism (Chart 63-6) are the result of decreased metabolism from low levels of thyroid hormones. Thyroid cells may fail to produce sufficient levels of thyroid hormones (THs) for several reasons. Sometimes the cells themselves are damaged and no longer function normally. At other times the thyroid cells are functional but the person does not ingest enough of the substances needed to make thyroid hormones, especially iodide and tyrosine. When the production of thyroid hormones is too low or absent, the blood levels of TH are very low and the patient has a decreased metabolic rate. This lowered metabolism causes the hypothalamus and anterior pituitary gland to make stimulatory hormones, especially thyroid-stimulating hormone (TSH), in an attempt to trigger hormone release from the poorly responsive thyroid gland. The TSH binds to thyroid cells and causes the thyroid gland to enlarge, forming a goiter, although thyroid hormone production does not increase.

Most tissues and organs are affected by the low metabolic rate caused by hypothyroidism. Cellular energy is decreased, and metabolites that are compounds of proteins and sugars called *glycosaminoglycans (GAGs)* build up inside cells. This GAG buildup increases the mucus and water, forms cellular edema, and changes organ texture. The edema is mucinous and called **myxedema**, rather than edema caused by water alone. This edema changes the patient's appearance (Fig. 63-3). Non-pitting edema forms everywhere, especially around the eyes, in the hands and feet, and between the shoulder blades. The tongue thickens, and edema forms in the larynx, making the voice husky. All general physiologic function is decreased.

Myxedema coma is a rare, serious complication of untreated or poorly treated hypothyroidism. The decreased metabolism causes the heart muscle to become flabby and the chamber size to increase. The result is decreased cardiac output and decreased perfusion to the brain and other vital organs, which makes the already slowed cellular metabolism worse, resulting in tissue and organ failure. *The mortality rate for myxedema coma is extremely high, and this condition is a life-threatening emergency.* Myxedema coma can be caused by a variety of events, drugs, or conditions.

Etiology

Most cases of hypothyroidism in the United States occur as a result of thyroid surgery and radioactive iodine (RAI) treatment of hyperthyroidism. Worldwide, hypothyroidism is common in areas where the soil and water have little natural

CHART 63-6   Key Features

Hypothyroidism

Skin Manifestations
- Cool, pale or yellowish, dry, coarse, scaly skin
- Thick, brittle nails
- Dry, coarse, brittle hair
- Decreased hair growth, with loss of eyebrow hair
- Poor wound healing

Pulmonary Manifestations
- Hypoventilation
- Pleural effusion
- Dyspnea

Cardiovascular Manifestations
- Bradycardia
- Dysrhythmias
- Enlarged heart
- Decreased activity tolerance
- Hypotension

Metabolic Manifestations
- Decreased basal metabolic rate
- Decreased body temperature
- Cold intolerance

Psychological/Emotional Manifestations
- Apathy
- Depression
- Paranoia

Gastrointestinal Manifestations
- Anorexia
- Weight gain
- Constipation
- Abdominal distention

Neuromuscular Manifestations
- Slowing of intellectual functions:
  - Slowness or slurring of speech
  - Impaired memory
  - Inattentiveness
- Lethargy or somnolence
- Confusion
- Hearing loss
- Paresthesia (numbness and tingling) of the extremities
- Decreased tendon reflexes
- Muscle aches and pain

Reproductive Manifestations
Women
- Changes in menses (amenorrhea or prolonged menstrual periods)
- Anovulation
- Decreased libido

Men
- Decreased libido
- Impotence

Other Manifestations
- Periorbital edema
- Facial puffiness
- Nonpitting edema of the hands and feet
- Hoarseness
- Goiter (enlarged thyroid gland)
- Thick tongue
- Increased sensitivity to opioids and tranquilizers
- Weakness, fatigue
- Decreased urine output
- Easy bruising
- Iron deficiency anemia
- Vitamin deficiencies

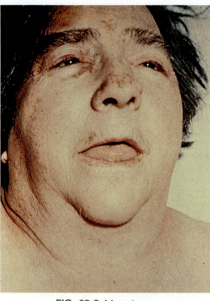

FIG. 63-3 Myxedema.

TABLE 63-2   Causes of Hypothyroidism

Primary Causes

Decreased Thyroid Tissue
- Surgical or radiation-induced thyroid destruction
- Autoimmune thyroid destruction
- Congenital poor thyroid development
- Cancer (thyroidal or metastatic)

Decreased Synthesis of Thyroid Hormone
- Endemic iodine deficiency
- Drugs:
  - Lithium
  - Propylthiouracil
  - Sodium or potassium perchlorate
  - Aminoglutethimide

Secondary Causes

Inadequate Production of Thyroid-Stimulating Hormone
- Pituitary tumors, trauma, infections, or infarcts
- Congenital pituitary defects
- Hypothalamic tumors, trauma, infections, or infarcts

iodide, causing endemic goiter. Hypothyroidism is also caused by a variety of other conditions (Table 63-2).

Incidence and Prevalence

Hypothyroidism occurs most often in women between 30 and 60 years of age. Women are affected 7 to 10 times more often than men (McCance et al., 2014).

❖ PATIENT-CENTERED COLLABORATIVE CARE

◆ Assessment

History. A decrease in thyroid hormones produces many manifestations related to decreased metabolism. However, changes may have occurred slowly and the patient may not have noticed them. Ask him or her to compare activity now with that of a year ago. The patient often reports an increase in time spent sleeping, sometimes up to 14 to 16 hours daily. Generalized weakness, anorexia, muscle aches, and paresthesias may also be present. Constipation and cold intolerance are common. Ask whether more blankets at night or extra clothing, even in warm weather, has been needed. Some changes may be subtle and are often missed, especially in older adults.

Both men and women may report a decreased libido. Women may have had difficulty becoming pregnant or have changes in menses (heavy, prolonged bleeding or amenorrhea). Men may have problems with impotence and infertility.

Ask about current or previous use of drugs, such as lithium, thiocyanates, aminoglutethimide, sodium or potassium perchlorate, or cobalt. All these drugs can impair thyroid hormone production. In particular, the cardiac drug *amiodarone* (Cordarone) often has damaging effects on the thyroid gland (Mosher, 2011). Also ask whether the patient has ever been treated for hyperthyroidism and what specific treatment was used.

Physical Assessment/Clinical Manifestations. Observe the patient's overall appearance. Fig. 63-3 shows the typical appearance of an adult with hypothyroidism. Common changes include coarse features, edema around the eyes and face, a blank expression, and a thick tongue. The patient's overall muscle movement is slow. He or she may not speak clearly and may take a longer time to respond to questions.

Cardiac and respiratory functions are decreased. Heart rate may be below 60 beats per minute, and respiratory rate may be slow. Body temperature is often lower than 97° F.

Weight gain is very common, even when the person is not overeating. Weigh the patient, and ask whether the result is the same or different from his or her weight a year ago.

Depending on the cause of hypothyroidism, the patient may have a goiter. However, some types of hypothyroidism do not induce a goiter and some types of hyperthyroidism do. The presence of a goiter suggests a thyroid problem but does not indicate whether the problem is excessive hormone secretion or too little hormone secretion.

Psychosocial Assessment. Hypothyroidism causes many problems in psychosocial functioning. Depression is the most common reason for seeking medical attention. Family members often bring the patient for the initial evaluation. The patient may be too lethargic, apathetic, or drowsy to recognize changes in his or her condition. Families may report that the patient is withdrawn and has reduced mental function. Assess his or her attention span and memory, both of which can be impaired by hypothyroidism. The mental slowness can contribute to social isolation.

Laboratory Assessment. Laboratory findings for hypothyroidism are the opposite of those for hyperthyroidism. Triiodothyronine (T_3) and thyroxine (T_4) serum levels are decreased. TSH levels are high in primary hypothyroidism but can be decreased or near normal in patients with secondary hypothyroidism (see Chart 63-2). Patients older than 80 years may have lower-than-normal levels of thyroid hormones without manifestations of hypothyroidism, and hormone replacement is not used until other manifestations are present (Touhy & Jett, 2014).

◆ **Analysis**

The priority NANDA-I nursing diagnoses and collaborative problems for patients with hypothyroidism include:

1. Impaired Gas Exchange related to decreased energy, obesity, muscle weakness, and fatigue (NANDA-I)
2. Hypotension related to altered heart rate and rhythm as a result of decreased myocardial metabolism
3. Altered cognitive functioning related to impaired brain metabolism and edema
4. Potential for myxedema coma

◆ **Planning and Implementation**

Both cardiac and respiratory problems are serious, and their management is a priority. The most common cause of death among patients with myxedema coma is respiratory failure.

Improving Gas Exchange

Planning: Expected Outcomes. The patient with hypothyroidism is expected to have improved gas exchange. Indicators include:

- Maintenance of Spo_2 of at least 90%
- Absence of cyanosis
- Maintenance of cognitive orientation

Interventions. Observe and record the rate and depth of respirations. Measure oxygen saturation by pulse oximetry, and apply oxygen if the patient has hypoxemia. Auscultate the lungs for a decrease in breath sounds. If hypothyroidism is severe, the patient may require ventilatory support. Severe respiratory distress often occurs with myxedema coma.

Sedating a patient with hypothyroidism can make gas exchange worse and is avoided if possible. When sedation is needed, the dosage is reduced because hypothyroidism increases sensitivity to these drugs. For the patient receiving sedation, assess for adequate gas exchange.

Preventing Hypotension

Planning: Expected Outcomes. The patient with hypothyroidism is expected to have adequate cardiovascular function and tissue perfusion. Indicators include that the patient:

- Maintains heart rate above 60 beats/min
- Maintains blood pressure within normal limits for his or her age and general health
- Has no dysrhythmias, peripheral edema, or neck vein distention

Interventions. The patient with hypothyroidism can have decreased blood pressure, bradycardia, and dysrhythmias. Nursing priorities are monitoring for condition changes and preventing complications. Monitor blood pressure and heart rate and rhythm, and observe for manifestations of shock (e.g., hypotension, decreased urine output, changes in mental status).

If hypothyroidism is chronic, the patient may have cardiovascular disease. *Instruct the patient to report episodes of chest pain or chest discomfort immediately.*

The patient with hypothyroidism requires lifelong thyroid hormone replacement. Synthetic hormone preparations are usually prescribed. The most common is levothyroxine sodium (Synthroid, T_4, Eltroxin ✦). Therapy is started with low doses and gradually increased over a period of weeks. *The patient with more severe symptoms of hypothyroidism is started on the lowest dose of thyroid hormone replacement.* This precaution is very important when the patient has known cardiac problems. Starting at too high a dose or increasing the dose too rapidly can cause severe hypertension, heart failure, and myocardial infarction (Brent & Davies, 2011). *Teach patients, as well as their families, who are beginning thyroid replacement hormone therapy to take the drug exactly as prescribed and not to change the dose or schedule without consulting the prescriber. Also teach them not to switch brands because the response to different drug brands can vary.*

Assess the patient for chest pain and dyspnea during initiation of therapy. The final dosage is determined by blood levels of TSH and the patient's physical responses. The dosage and time required for symptom relief vary with each patient. Monitor for and teach the patient and family about the manifestations of hyperthyroidism (see Chart 63-1), which can occur with replacement therapy.

Supporting Cognition

Planning: Expected Outcomes. The patient with hypothyroidism is expected to have cognitive function at the same level as before the thyroid problem started. Indicators include that the patient consistently:

- Demonstrates immediate memory
- Communicates clearly and appropriately for age and ability
- Is attentive during conversations

Emergency Care of the Patient During Myxedema Coma

- Maintain a patent airway.
- Replace fluids with IV normal or hypertonic saline as prescribed.
- Give levothyroxine sodium IV as prescribed.
- Give glucose IV as prescribed.
- Give corticosteroids as prescribed.
- Check the patient's temperature hourly.
- Monitor blood pressure hourly.
- Cover the patient with warm blankets.
- Monitor for changes in mental status.
- Turn every 2 hours.
- Institute Aspiration Precautions.

Interventions. Observe for and record the presence and severity of lethargy, drowsiness, memory deficit, poor attention span, and difficulty communicating. These problems should decrease with thyroid hormone treatment, and mental awareness usually returns to the patient's normal level within 2 weeks. Orient the patient to person, place, and time, and explain all procedures slowly and carefully. Provide a safe environment.

Family members may have difficulty coping with the patient's behavior. Encourage them to accept the mood changes and mental slowness as manifestations of the disease. Remind the family that these problems should improve with therapy.

Preventing Myxedema Coma. Any patient with hypothyroidism who has any other health problem or who is newly diagnosed is at risk for myxedema coma. Factors leading to myxedema coma include acute illness, surgery, chemotherapy, discontinuing thyroid replacement therapy, and the use of sedatives or opioids. Problems that often occur with this condition include:

- Coma
- Respiratory failure
- Hypotension
- Hyponatremia
- Hypothermia
- Hypoglycemia

! NURSING SAFETY PRIORITY (QSEN)

Action Alert

Myxedema coma can lead to shock, organ damage, and death. Assess the patient with hypothyroidism at least every 8 hours for changes that indicate increasing severity, especially changes in mental status, and report these promptly to the health care provider.

Treatment is instituted quickly according to the patient's manifestations and without waiting for laboratory confirmation. Best practices for emergency care of the patient with myxedema coma are listed in Chart 63-7.

Community-Based Care

Hypothyroidism is usually chronic. Patients usually live in the community and are managed on an outpatient basis. Patients in acute care settings, subacute care settings, and rehabilitation centers may have long-standing hypothyroidism in addition to other health problems. Ensure that whoever is responsible for

Thyroid Problems

Teach the patient these facts about changes in the thyroid gland related to aging:

- Thyroid hormone secretion decreases with age, but the hormone level remains stable because storage site clearance of the hormone also decreases with age.
- The basal metabolic rate decreases with age, which changes body composition from predominantly muscular to predominantly fatty.
- Older patients require lower doses of replacement thyroid hormone. Too large a dose may adversely affect the heart muscle.

overseeing the patient's daily care is aware of the condition and understands its management.

Home Care Management. The patient with hypothyroidism does not usually require changes in the home unless cognition has decreased to the point that he or she poses a danger to himself or herself. Activity intolerance and fatigue may necessitate one-floor living for a short time. If manifestations have not improved before discharge, discuss the need for extra heat or clothing because of cold intolerance. The patient may need help with the drug regimen. Discuss this issue with the family and patient, and develop a plan for drug therapy. One person should be clearly designated as responsible for drug preparation and delivery so that doses are neither missed nor duplicated.

Self-Management Education. The most important educational need for the patient with hypothyroidism is about hormone replacement therapy and its side effects. Emphasize the need for lifelong drugs, and review the manifestations of both hyperthyroidism and hypothyroidism. Teach the patient to wear a medical alert bracelet. Teach the patient and family when to seek medical interventions for dosage adjustment and the need for periodic blood tests of hormone levels. Instruct the patient to not take any over-the-counter (OTC) drugs without consulting his or her health care provider because thyroid hormone preparations interact with many other drugs. Older patients may need additional information about the effects of aging on the thyroid gland (Chart 63-8).

Advise the patient to maintain NUTRITION by eating a well-balanced diet with adequate fiber and fluid intake to prevent constipation. Caution him or her that use of fiber supplements may interfere with the absorption of thyroid hormone. Thyroid hormones should be taken on an empty stomach. Remind the patient about the importance of adequate rest.

Assist the family in understanding that the time required for resolution of hypothyroidism varies. During this time the patient may continue to have mental slowness. Teach the family to orient the patient often and to explain everything clearly, simply, and as often as needed.

Teach the patient to monitor himself or herself for therapy effectiveness. The two easiest parameters to check are need for sleep and bowel elimination. When the patient requires more sleep and is constipated, the dose of replacement hormone may need to be increased. When the patient has difficulty getting to sleep and has more bowel movements than normal for him or her, the dose may need to be decreased.

Health Care Resources. Immediately after returning home, the patient may need a support person to stay and provide day and night attention. Contact with the health care team is needed for follow-up and identification of potential problems. The patient taking thyroid drugs may have manifestations

CHART 63-9 Focused Assessment

The Patient with Thyroid Dysfunction

Assess cardiovascular status:
- Vital signs, including apical pulse, pulse pressure, presence or absence of orthostatic hypotension, and the quality and rhythm of peripheral pulses
- Presence or absence of peripheral edema
- Weight gain or loss

Assess cognition and mental status:
- Level of consciousness
- Orientation to time, place, and person
- Ability to accurately read a seven-word sentence containing no words greater than three syllables
- Ability to count backward from 100 by 3s

Assess condition of skin and mucous membranes:
- Moistness of skin, most reliable on chest and back
- Skin temperature and color

Assess neuromuscular status:
- Reactivity of patellar and biceps reflexes
- Oral temperature
- Handgrip strength
- Steadiness of gait
- Presence or absence of fine tremors in the hand

Ask about:
- Sleep in the past 24 hours
- Patient warm enough or too warm indoors
- 24-hour diet recall
- 24-hour activity recall
- Over-the-counter and prescribed drugs taken
- Last bowel movement

Assess patient's understanding of illness and adherence with therapy:
- Manifestations to report to health care provider
- Drug therapy plan (correct timing and dose)

---

of hypothyroidism if the dosage is inadequate or may have manifestations of hyperthyroidism if the dosage is too high. A home care nurse performs a focused assessment at every home visit to the patient with thyroid dysfunction (Chart 63-9).

◆ Evaluation: Outcomes

Evaluate the care of the patient with hypothyroidism based on the identified priority patient problems. The expected outcomes are that with proper management the patient should:
- Maintain normal cardiovascular function
- Maintain adequate respiratory function
- Experience improvement in thought processes

Specific indicators for these outcomes are listed for each patient problem in the Planning and Implementation section (see earlier).

THYROIDITIS

❖ PATHOPHYSIOLOGY

Thyroiditis is an inflammation of the thyroid gland. There are three types: acute, subacute, and chronic. Chronic thyroiditis (Hashimoto's disease) is the most common type.

Acute thyroiditis is caused by bacterial invasion of the thyroid gland. Manifestations include pain, neck tenderness, malaise, fever, and dysphagia (difficulty swallowing). It usually resolves with antibiotic therapy.

Subacute or granulomatous thyroiditis results from a viral infection of the thyroid gland after a cold or other upper respiratory infection. Manifestations include fever, chills,

? CLINICAL JUDGMENT CHALLENGE

Patient-Centered Care; Safety **QSEN**

The patient, a 45-year-old former school teacher, is residing in a skilled nursing facility to recover from a tibia-fibula fracture that is being managed with an external fixation system. On admission 2 weeks ago, she told you that she felt she was "getting old too fast." She explained that she had gained 54 pounds in the previous 6 months, had no energy, was often constipated, and was always cold. She teared up and said that her ability to concentrate was so bad that not only could she no longer help her high school children with their homework but also that she didn't recognize the step hazard that caused her to fall and break her ankle. Today the nursing assistant assigned to her care reports that the patient's pulse is only 42 beats per minute and that her temperature was 96°F even with two blankets. When you enter her room, she is sleeping and an untouched breakfast tray is on her table.

1. What are the priority assessment data you should obtain? Provide a rationale for your choices.
2. Should oxygen be applied? Why or why not?
3. What indications do you have that the changes in her health status are not related to complications of her fractured ankle?
4. What manifestations of hypothyroidism are in her history and present during this assessment?

---

dysphagia, and muscle and joint pain. Pain can radiate to the ears and the jaw. The thyroid gland feels hard and enlarged on palpation. Thyroid function can remain normal, although hyperthyroidism or hypothyroidism may develop.

Chronic thyroiditis (Hashimoto's disease) is a common type of hypothyroidism that affects women more often than men, usually when patients are in their 30s to 50s (Brent & Davies, 2011). Hashimoto's disease is an autoimmune disorder that is usually triggered by a bacterial or viral infection. The thyroid is invaded by antithyroid antibodies and lymphocytes, causing selective thyroid tissue destruction. When large amounts of the gland are destroyed, serum thyroid hormone levels are low and secretion of thyroid-stimulating hormone (TSH) is increased.

❖ PATIENT-CENTERED COLLABORATIVE CARE

The manifestations of Hashimoto's disease are dysphagia and painless enlargement of the gland. Diagnosis is based on circulating antithyroid antibodies and needle biopsy of the thyroid gland. Serum thyroid hormone levels and TSH levels vary with disease stage.

The patient is given thyroid hormone to prevent hypothyroidism and to suppress TSH secretion, which decreases the size of the thyroid gland. Surgery (subtotal thyroidectomy) is needed if the goiter does not respond to thyroid hormone, is disfiguring, or compresses other structures. Nursing interventions focus on promoting comfort and teaching the patient about hypothyroidism, drugs, and surgery.

THYROID CANCER

❖ PATHOPHYSIOLOGY

The four distinct types of thyroid cancer are papillary, follicular, medullary, and anaplastic (American Cancer Society, 2014). The initial manifestation of thyroid cancer is a single, painless lump or nodule in the thyroid gland. Additional manifestations depend on the presence and location of **metastasis** (spread of cancer cells).

Papillary carcinoma, the most common type of thyroid cancer, occurs most often in younger women. It is a slow-growing tumor that can be present for years before spreading to nearby lymph nodes. When the tumor is confined to the thyroid gland, the chance for cure is good with a partial or total thyroidectomy.

Follicular carcinoma occurs most often in older patients. The cancer invades blood vessels and spreads to bone and lung tissue. It can adhere to the trachea, neck muscles, great vessels, and skin, resulting in dyspnea (difficulty breathing) and dysphagia (difficulty swallowing). When the tumor involves the recurrent laryngeal nerves, the patient may have a hoarse voice.

Medullary carcinoma is most common in patients older than 50 years. This tumor often occurs as part of multiple endocrine neoplasia (MEN) type II, a familial endocrine disorder. The tumor usually secretes calcitonin, adrenocorticotropic hormone (ACTH), prostaglandins, and serotonin.

Anaplastic carcinoma is a rapid-growing, aggressive tumor that directly invades nearby structures. Manifestations include stridor (harsh, high-pitched respiratory sounds), hoarseness, and dysphagia.

A hallmark of thyroid cancer is an elevated serum thyroglobulin (Tg) level. The normal range of Tg for men is 0.5 to 53.0 ng/mL and for women is 0.5 to 43.0 ng/mL (Pagana & Pagana, 2014).

❖ PATIENT-CENTERED COLLABORATIVE CARE

Radiation therapy is used most often for anaplastic carcinoma because this cancer has usually metastasized at diagnosis. The patient is treated with ablative (enough to destroy the tissue) amounts of RAI. (See Chart 63-4 for precautions to teach the patient receiving unsealed RAI therapy.) If spread has occurred to the neck or mediastinum, external radiation is also applied. If thyroid cancer does not respond to RAI, chemotherapy is initiated.

Surgery is the treatment of choice for other types of thyroid cancer. A total thyroidectomy is usually performed with dissection of lymph nodes in the neck if regional lymph nodes are involved. (See the postoperative care discussion in the Surgical Management section for Hyperthyroidism on p. 1290.) Suppressive doses of thyroid hormone are usually taken for 3 months after surgery. Thyroglobulin levels are monitored after surgery. A rising level indicates the probable presence of cancer cells.

The patient is hypothyroid after treatment for thyroid cancer. Nursing interventions then focus on teaching the patient about the management of hypothyroidism. (See discussion of Patient-Centered Collaborative Care on pp. 1293-1294 in the Hypothyroidism section.)

PARATHYROID DISORDERS

HYPERPARATHYROIDISM

❖ PATHOPHYSIOLOGY

The parathyroid glands maintain calcium and phosphate balance (see Fig. 61-6 in Chapter 61). Serum calcium level is normally maintained within a narrow range. Increased levels of parathyroid hormone (PTH) act directly on the kidney, causing increased kidney reabsorption of calcium and increased phosphorus excretion. In hyperparathyroidism, these processes cause hypercalcemia (excessive calcium) and hypophosphatemia (inadequate blood phosphorus level).

TABLE 63-3 Causes of Parathyroid Dysfunction
Causes of Hyperparathyroidism
• Parathyroid tumor or cancer
• Congenital hyperplasia
• Neck trauma or radiation
• Vitamin D deficiency
• Chronic kidney disease with hypocalcemia
• Parathyroid hormone–secreting carcinomas of the lung, kidney, or GI tract
Causes of Hypoparathyroidism
• Surgical or radiation-induced thyroid ablation
• Parathyroidectomy
• Congenital dysgenesis
• Idiopathic (autoimmune) hypoparathyroidism
• Hypomagnesemia

In bone, excessive PTH levels increase bone *resorption* (bone loss of calcium) by decreasing *osteoblastic* (bone production) activity and increasing *osteoclastic* (bone destruction) activity. This process releases calcium and phosphorus into the blood and reduces bone density. With chronic calcium excess and hypercalcemia, calcium is deposited in soft tissues.

Although the exact triggering mechanisms are unknown, primary hyperparathyroidism results when one or more parathyroid glands do not respond to the normal feedback of serum calcium levels. The most common cause is a benign tumor in one parathyroid gland. Table 63-3 lists other causes of hyperparathyroidism.

❖ PATIENT-CENTERED COLLABORATIVE CARE

◆ Assessment

Manifestations of hyperparathyroidism may be related either to the effects of excessive PTH or to the effects of the accompanying hypercalcemia.

Ask about any bone fractures, recent weight loss, arthritis, or psychological stress. Ask whether the patient has received radiation treatment to the head or neck. The patient with chronic disease may have a waxy pallor of the skin and bone deformities in the extremities and back.

High levels of PTH cause kidney stones and deposits of calcium in the soft tissue of the kidney. Bone lesions are due to an increased rate of bone destruction and may result in pathologic fractures, bone cysts, and osteoporosis.

GI problems (e.g., anorexia, nausea, vomiting, epigastric pain, constipation, weight loss) are common when serum calcium levels are high. Elevated serum gastrin levels are caused by hypercalcemia and lead to peptic ulcer disease. Fatigue and lethargy may be present and worsen as the serum calcium levels increase. When serum calcium levels are greater than 12 mg/dL, the patient may have psychosis with mental confusion, which leads to coma and death if left untreated. (See Chapter 11 for more information about hypercalcemia.)

Serum PTH, calcium, and phosphorus levels and urine cyclic adenosine monophosphate (cAMP) levels are the laboratory tests used to detect hyperparathyroidism (Chart 63-10). X-rays may show kidney stones, calcium deposits, and bone lesions. Loss of bone density occurs in the patient with chronic hyperparathyroidism. Other diagnostic tests include arteriography, CT scans, venous sampling of the thyroid for blood PTH levels,

CHART 63-10 Laboratory Profile

Parathyroid Function

TEST	NORMAL RANGE FOR ADULTS	SIGNIFICANCE OF ABNORMAL FINDINGS	
		HYPERPARATHYROIDISM	HYPOPARATHYROIDISM
Serum calcium	Total: 9.0-10.5 mg/dL or 2.25-2.75 SI units Ionized (active): 4.64-5.28 mg/dL or 1.16-1.32 SI units	Increased in primary hyperparathyroidism	Decreased
Serum phosphorus	3.0-4.5 mg/dL or 0.97-1.45 SI units *Older adults:* May be slightly lower	Decreased	Increased
Serum magnesium	1.3-2.1 mEq/L	Increased	Decreased
Serum parathyroid hormone	C-terminal 50-330 pg/mL N-terminal 8-25 pg/mL Whole 10-65 pg/mL	Increased	Decreased
Vitamin D (calciferol)	25-80 ng/mL	Variable	Decreased
Urine cAMP	18.3-45.4 nmol/L in a 24-hour urine collection specimen	Increased	Decreased

Data from Pagana, K., & Pagana, T. (2014). *Mosby's manual of diagnostic and laboratory tests* (5th ed.). St. Louis: Mosby.
cAMP, Cyclic adenosine monophosphate; *SI,* International System of Units.

and ultrasonography. Explain the procedures and care for the patient undergoing diagnostic tests.

◆ Interventions

Surgical management is the treatment of choice for patients with hyperparathyroidism. For those who are not candidates for surgery, medication can help control the problems. Priority nursing interventions focus on monitoring and preventing injury.

Nonsurgical Management. *Diuretic and hydration therapies* are used for reducing serum calcium levels in patients who have milder disease. Usually furosemide (Lasix, Uritol ◆), a diuretic that increases kidney excretion of calcium, is used together with IV saline in large volumes to promote calcium excretion.

Drug therapy for patients who have more severe manifestations of primary or secondary hyperparathyroidism or who have hypercalcemia related to parathyroid cancer involves the use of cinacalcet (Sensipar). This drug is the first in a new class of drugs known as *calcimimetics.* When taken orally, the drug binds to calcium-sensitive receptors on parathyroid tissue. This binding reduces PTH production and release. The result is decreased serum calcium levels, stabilization of other minerals, and decreased progression of PTH-induced bone complications. The initial dose is low (30 mg orally twice daily) and is gradually increased to the maximum maintenance dose of 90 mg three times daily. The patient's serum calcium must be monitored for hypocalcemia on a regular basis for the duration of therapy.

For patients who do not respond to cinacalcet, oral phosphates are used to inhibit bone resorption and interfere with calcium absorption. IV phosphates are used only when serum calcium levels must be lowered rapidly. Calcitonin decreases the release of skeletal calcium and increases the kidney excretion of calcium. It is not effective when used alone because of its short duration of action. The therapeutic effects are greatly enhanced if calcitonin is given along with glucocorticoids.

Monitor cardiac function and intake and output every 2 hours during hydration therapy. Continuous cardiac monitoring may be needed. Compare recent ECG tracings with the patient's baseline tracings. Especially look for changes in the T waves and the QT interval, as well as changes in rate and rhythm. Monitor serum calcium levels, and immediately report any sudden drop to the health care provider. Sudden drops in calcium levels may cause tingling and numbness in the muscles.

Preventing injury is important because the patient with chronic hyperparathyroidism often has significant bone density loss and is at risk for pathologic fractures. Teach unlicensed assistive personnel (UAP) to handle the patient carefully. Use a lift sheet to reposition the patient rather than pulling him or her.

Surgical Management. Surgical management of hyperparathyroidism is a parathyroidectomy. Before surgery the patient is stabilized and calcium levels are decreased to near normal.

The operative procedure can be performed as minimally invasive surgery, mini-incision surgery, or with a traditional transverse incision in the lower neck. All four parathyroid glands are examined for enlargement. If a tumor is present on one side but the other side is normal, the surgeon removes the glands containing tumor and leaves the remaining glands on the opposite side intact. If all four glands are diseased, they are all removed.

Nursing care before and after surgical removal of the parathyroid glands is the same as that for thyroidectomy. See the Preoperative Care section on p. 1289 and the Postoperative Care section on p. 1290 for specific nursing interventions.

The remaining glands, which may have atrophied as a result of PTH overproduction, require several days to several weeks to return to normal function. A hypocalcemic crisis can occur during this critical period, and the serum calcium level is assessed frequently after surgery. Check serum calcium levels whenever they are drawn until calcium levels stabilize. Monitor for manifestations of hypocalcemia, such as tingling and twitching in the extremities and face. Check for Trousseau's and Chvostek's signs, either of which indicates potential tetany (see Chapter 11).

The recurrent laryngeal nerve can be damaged. Assess the patient for changes in voice patterns and hoarseness.

When hyperparathyroidism is due to **hyperplasia** (tissue overgrowth), three glands plus half of the fourth gland are usually removed. If all four glands are removed, a small portion of a gland may be implanted in the forearm, where it produces PTH and maintains calcium homeostasis. If all these maneuvers fail, the patient will need lifelong treatment with calcium and vitamin D because the resulting hypoparathyroidism is permanent (see next section).

HYPOPARATHYROIDISM

❖ PATHOPHYSIOLOGY

Hypoparathyroidism is a rare endocrine disorder in which parathyroid function is decreased. Problems are directly related to a lack of parathyroid hormone (PTH) secretion or to decreased effectiveness of PTH on target tissue. Whether the problem is a lack of PTH secretion or an ineffectiveness of PTH on tissues, the result is the same: *hypocalcemia*.

Iatrogenic hypoparathyroidism, the most common form, is caused by the removal of all parathyroid tissue during total thyroidectomy or by surgical removal of the parathyroid glands.

Idiopathic hypoparathyroidism can occur spontaneously. The exact cause is unknown, but an autoimmune basis is suspected. It may occur with other autoimmune disorders such as adrenal insufficiency, hypothyroidism, diabetes mellitus, pernicious anemia, and vitiligo.

Hypomagnesemia (decreased serum magnesium levels) may also cause hypoparathyroidism. Hypomagnesemia is seen in patients with malabsorption syndromes, chronic kidney disease, and malnutrition. It causes impairment of PTH secretion and may interfere with the effects of PTH on the bones, kidneys, and calcium regulation.

❖ PATIENT-CENTERED COLLABORATIVE CARE

◆ Assessment

Ask about any head or neck surgery or radiation therapy because these treatments may damage the parathyroid glands and cause hypoparathyroidism. Also ask whether the neck has ever sustained a serious injury in a car crash or by strangulation. Assess whether the patient has any manifestations of hypoparathyroidism, which may range from mild tingling and numbness to muscle tetany. Tingling and numbness around the mouth or in the hands and feet reflect mild to moderate hypocalcemia. Severe muscle cramps, spasms of the hands and feet, and seizures (with no loss of consciousness or incontinence) reflect a more severe hypocalcemia. The patient or family may notice mental changes ranging from irritability to psychosis.

The physical assessment may show excessive or inappropriate muscle contractions that cause finger, hand, and elbow flexion. This can signal an impending attack of tetany. Check for Chvostek's sign and Trousseau's sign; positive responses

indicate potential tetany (see Chapter 11). Bands or pits may encircle the crowns of the teeth, which indicate a loss of calcium from the teeth with enamel loss.

Diagnostic tests for hypoparathyroidism include electroencephalography (EEG), blood tests, and CT scans. EEG changes revert to normal with correction of hypocalcemia. Serum calcium, phosphorus, magnesium, vitamin D, and urine cyclic adenosine monophosphate (cAMP) levels may be used in the diagnostic workup for hypoparathyroidism (see Chart 63-10). The CT scan can show brain calcifications, which indicate chronic hypocalcemia.

◆ Interventions

Nonsurgical management of hypoparathyroidism focuses on correcting hypocalcemia, vitamin D deficiency, and hypomagnesemia. For patients with acute and severe hypocalcemia, IV calcium is given as a 10% solution of calcium chloride or calcium gluconate over 10 to 15 minutes. Acute vitamin D deficiency is treated with oral calcitriol (Rocaltrol), 0.5 to 2 mg daily. Acute hypomagnesemia is corrected with 50% magnesium sulfate in 2-mL doses (up to 4 g daily) IV. Long-term oral therapy for hypocalcemia involves the intake of calcium, 0.5 to 2 g daily, in divided doses.

Long-term therapy for vitamin D deficiency is 50,000 to 400,000 units of oral ergocalciferol daily. The dosage is adjusted to keep the patient's calcium level in the low-normal range (slightly hypocalcemic), enough to prevent symptoms of hypocalcemia. It must also be low enough to prevent increased urine calcium levels, which can lead to stone formation.

Nursing management includes teaching about the drug regimen and interventions to reduce anxiety. Teach the patient to eat foods high in calcium but low in phosphorus. Milk, yogurt, and processed cheeses are avoided because of their high phosphorus content. *Stress that therapy for hypocalcemia is lifelong.* Advise the patient to wear a medical alert bracelet. With adherence to the prescribed drug and diet regimen, the calcium level usually remains high enough to prevent a hypocalcemic crisis.

❓ NCLEX EXAMINATION CHALLENGE

Safe and Effective Care Environment

When taking the blood pressure of a client receiving treatment for hyperparathyroidism, the nurse observes the client's hand to undergo flexion contractions. What is the nurse's interpretation of this observation?
A. Hyperphosphatemia
B. Hypophosphatemia
C. Hypercalcemia
D. Hypocalcemia

NURSING CONCEPTS AND CLINICAL JUDGMENT REVIEW

What might you NOTICE in a patient with hyperthyroidism who demonstrates inadequate THERMOREGULATION?

Vital signs:
- Blood pressure elevated with a widened pulse pressure
- Heart rate rapid and irregular
- Temperature above 100° F

Physical assessment:
- Excessive sweating
- Smooth, warm, moist skin
- Underweight for height
- Fine hand tremors

Psychosocial assessment:
- Decreased attention span

- Restlessness and irritability
- Emotional lability

Laboratory assessment:
- Elevated T_3 and T_4 levels
- Abnormal TSH levels

What should you INTERPRET and how should you RESPOND to a patient experiencing inadequate THERMOREGULATION as a result of hyperthyroidism?

Perform and interpret physical assessment, including:
- Assessing body temperature
- Assessing cardiac effectiveness
- Checking deep tendon reflexes

Respond by:
- Maintaining a calm approach
- Cooling the environment
- Offering a sponge bath or shower
- Avoiding palpation of the neck or thyroid gland
- Maintaining a patent airway
- Administering prescribed drugs appropriately
- Notifying the health care provider of changes in cardiac or neurologic status

On what should you REFLECT?
- Think about how the environment could be made more calming.
- Think about what emergency equipment might be needed.

GET READY FOR THE NCLEX® EXAMINATION!

KEY POINTS

Review these Key Points for each NCLEX Examination Client Needs Category.

Safe and Effective Care Environment
- Keep the environment of a patient at risk for thyroid storm cool, dark, and quiet. **Safety** QSEN
- Keep emergency suctioning and tracheotomy equipment in the room of a patient who has had thyroid or parathyroid surgery. **Safety** QSEN
- Use a lift sheet to move or reposition a patient with hypocalcemia. **Safety** QSEN

Health Promotion and Maintenance
- Teach all patients to take antithyroid drugs or thyroid hormone replacement therapy as prescribed. **Patient-Centered Care** QSEN
- Teach patients to use clinical manifestations (e.g., the number of bowel movements per day, the ability to sleep) as indicators of therapy effectiveness and when the dose of thyroid hormone replacement may need to be adjusted. **Patient-Centered Care** QSEN
- Include the person who prepares the patient's meals when teaching about dietary electrolyte restrictions. **Patient-Centered Care** QSEN
- Collaborate with the registered dietitian to teach patients about diets that are restricted in calcium or phosphorus. **Teamwork and Collaboration** QSEN

Psychosocial Integrity
- Be accepting of patient behavior. **Patient-Centered Care** QSEN
- Remind patients and family members that changes in cognition and behavior related to thyroid problems are usually temporary. **Patient-Centered Care** QSEN

- Encourage the patient who has a permanent change in appearance (e.g., exophthalmia) to mourn the change. **Patient-Centered Care** QSEN

Physiological Integrity
- Be aware that:
  - The presence of a goiter indicates a problem with the thyroid gland but can accompany either hyperthyroidism or hypothyroidism.
  - Although similar in action, methimazole and propylthiouracil are not interchangeable.
  - Methimazole can cause birth defects and should not be used during pregnancy, especially during the first trimester.
- When stridor, dyspnea, or other symptoms of obstruction appear after thyroid surgery, notify the Rapid Response Team. **Safety** QSEN
- When caring for a patient with hyperthyroidism, even after a thyroidectomy, immediately report a temperature increase of even 1°F because it may indicate an impending thyroid crisis. **Evidence-Based Practice** QSEN
- Assess the cardiopulmonary status of any patient with hypothyroidism for decreased perfusion or decreased gas exchange at least every 8 hours. **Patient-Centered Care** QSEN
- Use sedating drugs or opioids sparingly with patients who have hypothyroidism. **Patient-Centered Care** QSEN
- Monitor the hydration status of patients who have hypercalcemia. **Patient-Centered Care** QSEN
- Assess the patient with hypoparathyroidism for manifestations of hypocalcemia, especially numbness or tingling around the mouth and a positive Chvostek's sign or Trousseau's sign. **Patient-Centered Care** QSEN

Care of Patients with Diabetes Mellitus

Margaret Elaine McLeod

http://evolve.elsevier.com/Iggy/

PRIORITY CONCEPTS

- GLUCOSE REGULATION
- TISSUE INTEGRITY
- SENSORY PERCEPTION
- PERFUSION

- INFECTION
- PAIN
- NUTRITION

LEARNING OUTCOMES

Safe and Effective Care Environment

1. Protect the patient who has diabetes mellitus from injury.
2. Protect the patient who has diabetes mellitus from INFECTION.

Health Promotion and Maintenance

3. Teach all people how to prevent or delay development of type 2 diabetes.
4. Teach people who have diabetes to prevent or delay long-term complications of the disorder.
5. Teach all patients with diabetes and their family members how to self-manage their disease.
6. Teach the patient with diabetes and the family the importance of foot care and good NUTRITION.
7. Work with other health care professionals to help the patient and family experiencing diabetes mellitus achieve health goals.

Psychosocial Integrity

8. Reduce the psychological impact of diabetes mellitus for the patient and family.

9. Work with other members of the health care team to ensure that patient values, preferences, and expressed needs related to diabetes mellitus are respected.

Physiological Integrity

10. Compare the risk factors, age of onset, manifestations, and pathologic mechanisms of type 1 and type 2 diabetes mellitus.
11. Apply knowledge of anatomy, physiology, and pathophysiology to assess the adequacy of GLUCOSE REGULATION for the patient with diabetes.
12. Ensure that PAIN is appropriately managed for the patient with diabetes.
13. Evaluate laboratory data and clinical manifestations to determine effectiveness of the prescribed dietary, drug, and exercise therapies for diabetes.
14. Prioritize care for the patient with diabetes experiencing hypoglycemia, ketoacidosis, or hyperglycemic-hyperosmolar state (HHS).
15. Coordinate care for the patient with diabetes in the community.

Diabetes mellitus (DM) resulting in poor GLUCOSE REGULATION is a major public health problem, and its complications, especially hypertension and **hyperlipidemia** (high blood lipid levels), cause many serious health problems. In the United States, DM is a leading cause of blindness, end-stage kidney disease, and foot or leg amputations. Many people have undiagnosed diabetes, and among those who are diagnosed, many continue to have high blood glucose levels. The complications of DM can be greatly reduced with **glycemic** (blood glucose) control along with management of hypertension and hyperlipidemia. Thus nursing priorities focus on helping the patient with diabetes achieve and maintain lifestyle changes that prevent long-term complications by keeping blood glucose levels and cholesterol levels as close to normal as possible.

Because DM is a chronic metabolic disease affecting GLUCOSE REGULATION, it requires lifelong behavioral and lifestyle changes for best management. A collaborative approach helps the patient be successful in achieving desired outcomes. As part of the team, you will plan, organize, and coordinate care with other health care team members to provide care and promote the patient's health and well-being.

❖ PATHOPHYSIOLOGY

Classification of Diabetes

For all types of diabetes mellitus (DM), the main feature is chronic **hyperglycemia** (high blood glucose level) resulting from problems with GLUCOSE REGULATION that include reduced

TABLE 64-1	**Classification of Diabetes Mellitus**

Type 1 Diabetes
- Beta-cell destruction leading to absolute insulin deficiency
- Autoimmune
- Idiopathic

Type 2 Diabetes
- Ranges from insulin resistance with relative insulin deficiency to secretory deficit with insulin resistance

Other Conditions Resulting in Hyperglycemia
- Genetic defects of beta-cell function
- Genetic defects in insulin action
- Pancreatic diseases (pancreatitis, trauma, cancer, cystic fibrosis, hemochromatosis)
- Endocrinopathies: acromegaly, Cushing's disease, glucagonoma, pheochromocytoma, hyperthyroidism, aldosteronism
- Drug- or chemical-induced hyperglycemia
- Infections: congenital rubella, cytomegalovirus, human immune deficiency virus
- Genetic syndromes associated with diabetes: Down syndrome, Klinefelter syndrome, Turner's syndrome, Huntington disease, and others

Gestational Diabetes Mellitus (GDM)
- Glucose intolerance with onset or first recognition during pregnancy

Data from American Diabetes Association (ADA). (2014d). Position statement: Diagnosis and classification of diabetes mellitus. *Diabetes Care, 37*(Suppl. 1), S81-S90.

insulin secretion or reduced insulin action (McCance et al., 2014). The disease is classified by the underlying problem causing a lack of insulin or its action and the severity of the insulin deficiency. Table 64-1 outlines the types of DM.

The Endocrine Pancreas

The pancreas has exocrine functions that are related to digestion and endocrine functions for blood GLUCOSE REGULATION. The endocrine portion of the pancreas has about 1 million small glands, the islets of Langerhans, scattered through the organ. The islet cells are only a small portion of the gland. The two types of islet cells important to glucose regulation are the *alpha* cells, which secrete glucagon, and the *beta* cells, which produce insulin and amylin. **Glucagon** is a "counterregulatory" hormone that has actions opposite those of insulin. It prevents *hypoglycemia* (low blood glucose levels) by triggering the release of glucose from cell storage sites. Insulin prevents hyperglycemia by allowing body cells to take up, use, and store carbohydrate, fat, and protein.

Active insulin is a protein made up of 51 amino acids. It is initially produced as inactive *proinsulin,* a prohormone that contains an additional amino acid chain (the C-peptide chain). Proinsulin is converted into active insulin by removal of the C-peptide (Fig. 64-1).

Insulin is secreted daily directly into liver circulation in a two-step manner. It is secreted at low levels during fasting (basal insulin secretion) and at increased levels after eating (**prandial**). An early burst of insulin secretion occurs within 10 minutes of eating. This is followed by an increasing release that lasts until the blood glucose level is normal.

Glucose Regulation and Homeostasis

Glucose is the main fuel for central nervous system (CNS) cells. Because the brain cannot produce or store much glucose, it

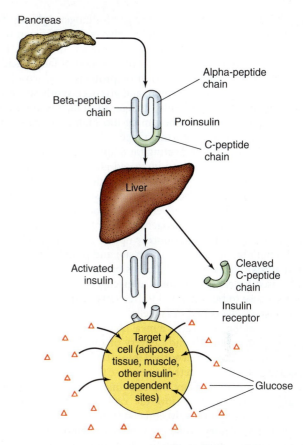

FIG. 64-1 Proinsulin, secreted by and stored in the beta cells of the islets of Langerhans in the pancreas, is transformed by the liver into active insulin. Insulin attaches to receptors on target cells, where it promotes glucose transport into the cells through the cell membranes.

needs a continuous supply from circulation to prevent neuron dysfunction and cell death. Other organs can use both glucose and fatty acids to generate energy. Glucose is stored inside cells as glycogen in the liver and muscles, and free fatty acids are stored as triglyceride in fat cells. Fat is the most efficient means of storing energy, with 9 calories of stored energy per gram. Protein and carbohydrate have only 4 calories per gram. During a prolonged fast or after illness, proteins are broken down and some of the amino acids are converted into glucose.

Several organs and hormones play a role in maintaining GLUCOSE REGULATION. During fasting, when the stomach is empty, blood glucose is maintained between 60 and 150 mg/dL (3.3 and 8.3 mmol/L) by a balance between glucose uptake by cells and glucose production by the liver. Insulin plays a pivotal role in this process.

Movement of glucose into some cells requires the presence of specific carrier proteins, known as glucose transport (GLUT) proteins, along with insulin. Insulin is like a "key" that opens "locked" membranes to glucose, allowing blood glucose to move into cells to generate energy. Insulin starts this action by binding to insulin receptors on the cell membranes, which changes membrane permeability to glucose.

Insulin exerts many effects on metabolism and cellular processes in all tissues and organs. The main metabolic effects of insulin are to stimulate glucose uptake in skeletal muscle and heart muscle and to suppress liver production of glucose and very-low-density lipoprotein (VLDL). In the liver, insulin promotes the production and storage of glycogen (**glycogenesis**) at the same time that it inhibits glycogen breakdown into glucose (**glycogenolysis**). It increases protein and lipid (fat) synthesis and inhibits **ketogenesis** (conversion of fats to acids) and **gluconeogenesis** (conversion of proteins to glucose). In muscle, insulin promotes protein and glycogen synthesis. In fat cells, it promotes triglyceride storage. Overall, insulin keeps blood glucose levels from becoming too high and helps keep blood lipid levels in the normal range.

In the *fasting state* (not eating for 8 hours), insulin secretion is suppressed, which leads to increased gluconeogenesis in the liver and kidneys, along with increased glucose generation by the breakdown of liver glycogen. In the fed state, insulin released from pancreatic beta cells reverses this process. Instead, glycogen breakdown and gluconeogenesis are inhibited. At the same time, insulin also enhances glucose uptake and use by cells and reduces both fat breakdown (**lipolysis**) and protein breakdown (**proteolysis**). When more glucose is present in liver cells than can be used for energy or stored as glycogen, insulin causes the excess glucose to be converted to free fatty acids (FFAs). These extra FFAs are deposited in fat cells.

Glucose in the blood after a meal is controlled by the emptying rate of the stomach and delivery of nutrients to the small intestine where they are absorbed into circulation. Incretin hormones (e.g., GLP-1), secreted in response to food in the stomach, have several actions. They increase insulin secretion, inhibit glucagon secretion, and slow the rate of gastric emptying, thereby preventing hyperglycemia after meals.

Counterregulatory hormones increase blood glucose by actions opposite those of insulin when more energy is needed. Glucagon is the main counterregulatory hormone. Other hormones that increase blood glucose levels are epinephrine, norepinephrine, growth hormone, and cortisol. The combined actions of insulin and counterregulatory hormones (discussed in the next section) participate in GLUCOSE REGULATION and keep blood glucose levels in the range of 60 to 100 mg/dL (3.3 to 5.6 mmol/L) to support brain function. When blood glucose levels fall, insulin secretion stops and glucagon is released. Glucagon causes glucose release from the liver. Liver glucose is made through breakdown of glycogen to glucose (glycogenolysis) and conversion of amino acids into glucose. When liver glucose is unavailable, the breakdown of fat (lipolysis) and the breakdown of proteins (proteolysis) provide fuel for energy.

? NCLEX EXAMINATION CHALLENGE

Physiological Integrity

How is hypoglycemia prevented in the healthy person who does not have diabetes even after fasting for 8 hours?

A. Metabolism is so slow when a person sleeps without eating for 8 hours that blood glucose does not enter cells to be used for energy. As a result, hypoglycemia does not occur.

B. Fasting for 8 hours triggers conversion of proteins into glycogen (glycogenesis) so that hyperglycemia develops rather than hypoglycemia.

C. Lipolysis (fat breakdown) in fat stores occurs, converting fatty acids into glucose to maintain blood glucose levels.

D. The secretion of glucagon prevents hypoglycemia by promoting glucose release from liver storage sites.

TABLE 64-2 Physiologic Response to Insufficient Insulin

- Decreased glycogenesis (conversion of glucose to glycogen)
- Increased glycogenolysis (conversion of glycogen to glucose)
- Increased gluconeogenesis (formation of glucose from noncarbohydrate sources such as amino acids and lactate)
- Increased lipolysis (breakdown of triglycerides to glycerol and free fatty acids)
- Increased ketogenesis (formation of ketones from free fatty acids)
- Proteolysis (breakdown of protein with amino acid release in muscles)

Absence of Insulin

Insulin for GLUCOSE REGULATION is needed to move glucose into many body tissues. The lack of insulin in diabetes, from either a lack of production or a problem with insulin use at its cell receptor, prevents some cells from using glucose for energy. The body then breaks down fat and protein in an attempt to provide energy and increases levels of counterregulatory hormones to make glucose from other sources. Table 64-2 outlines responses to insufficient insulin.

Without insulin, glucose builds up in the blood, causing high blood glucose levels (**hyperglycemia**). Hyperglycemia causes fluid and electrolyte imbalances, leading to the classic manifestations of diabetes: polyuria, polydipsia, and polyphagia.

Polyuria is frequent and excessive urination and results from an osmotic diuresis caused by excess glucose in the blood and urine. With diuresis, electrolytes are excreted in the urine and water loss is severe. Dehydration results, and **polydipsia** (excessive thirst) occurs. Because the cells receive no glucose, cell starvation triggers **polyphagia** (excessive eating). Despite eating, the person remains in cellular starvation until insulin is available to move glucose into the cells.

With insulin deficiency, fats break down, releasing free fatty acids. Conversion of fatty acids to **ketone bodies** (small acids) provides a backup energy source. Ketone bodies or "ketones" are abnormal breakdown products that collect in the blood when insulin is not available, leading to a type of metabolic acidosis known as ketoacidosis.

Dehydration with diabetes leads to hemoconcentration (increased blood concentration); hypovolemia (decreased blood volume); thick, concentrated blood; poor tissue PERFUSION; and hypoxia (poor tissue oxygenation), especially to the brain. Hypoxic cells do not metabolize glucose efficiently, the Krebs' cycle is blocked, and lactic acid increases, causing more acidosis.

The excess acids caused by absence of insulin increase hydrogen ion (H^+) and carbon dioxide (CO_2) levels in the blood, causing anion-gap metabolic acidosis. These products trigger the brain to increase the rate and depth of respiration in an attempt to "blow off" carbon dioxide and acid. This type of breathing is known as **Kussmaul respiration**. Acetone is exhaled, giving the breath a "rotting fruit" odor. When the lungs can no longer offset acidosis, the blood pH drops. Arterial blood gas studies show a metabolic acidosis (decreased pH with decreased arterial bicarbonate [HCO_3^-] levels) and compensatory respiratory alkalosis (decreased partial pressure of arterial carbon dioxide [$Paco_2$]).

Insulin lack initially causes potassium depletion. With the increased fluid loss from hyperglycemia, excessive potassium is excreted in the urine, leading to low serum potassium levels.

High serum potassium levels may occur in acidosis because of the shift of potassium from inside the cells to the blood. Serum potassium levels in DM, then, may be low (**hypokalemia**), high (**hyperkalemia**), or normal, depending on hydration, the severity of acidosis, and the patient's response to treatment. Chapter 12 discusses acid-base balance and acidosis in more detail.

Acute Complications of Diabetes

Three glucose-related emergencies can occur in patients with diabetes:

- Diabetic ketoacidosis (DKA) caused by lack of insulin and ketosis
- Hyperglycemic-hyperosmolar state (HHS) caused by insulin deficiency and profound dehydration
- Hypoglycemia from too much insulin or too little glucose

All three problems require emergency treatment and can be fatal if treatment is delayed or incorrect. These problems and their interventions are described later, starting on p. 1330.

Chronic Complications of Diabetes

Diabetes mellitus (DM) can lead to health problems and early death because of changes in large blood vessels (**macrovascular**) and small blood vessels (**microvascular**) in tissues and organs (McCance et al., 2014). Complications result from poor tissue PERFUSION and cell death. Macrovascular complications, including coronary heart disease, cerebrovascular disease, and peripheral vascular disease, lead to increased early death. Microvascular complications of blood vessel structure and function lead to **nephropathy** (kidney dysfunction), **neuropathy** (nerve dysfunction), and **retinopathy** (vision problems). Causes of these diabetic vascular complications include:

- Chronic hyperglycemia thickens basement membranes, which causes organ damage.
- Glucose toxicity directly or indirectly affects functional cell integrity.
- Chronic ischemia in small blood vessels causes connective tissue hypoxia and microischemia.

Chronic high blood glucose levels are the main cause of microvascular complications and allow premature development of macrovascular complications. Other risk factors contributing to poor health outcomes for people with DM include smoking, physical inactivity, obesity, hypertension, and high blood fat and cholesterol levels. Many of these factors can be modified to reduce complications related to DM.

Hyperglycemia from poor GLUCOSE REGULATION is a critical factor for long-term complications in patients with type 1 DM. Intensive therapy to maintain blood glucose levels as close to normal as possible delays the onset and progression of retinopathy, nephropathy, neuropathy, and macrovascular disease for patients with type 1 and type 2 DM. For every percentage point decrease in A1C (glycosylated hemoglobin A1C), a risk reduction of at least 25% to 30% for kidney and eye complications has been shown (American Diabetes Association [ADA], 2014b).

Macrovascular Complications

Cardiovascular Disease. Diabetes mellitus (DM) is associated with a reduced life span, largely as a result of cardiovascular disease (CVD). Most patients with DM die as a result of a thrombotic event, usually myocardial infarction (MI). Systolic and diastolic heart failure are associated with DM. Patients with DM are more likely to develop left ventricular dysfunction with heart failure and fatal cardiac dysrhythmias after MI.

Patients with diabetes, those with prediabetes, and those with metabolic syndrome are at increased risk for CVD (ADA, 2014f). This risk affects women to a greater degree than men and is influenced by the patient's ethnic group. Diabetes is now considered a "coronary heart disease risk equivalent" and a target for aggressive reduction of risk factors.

Patients with diabetes often have the traditional CVD risk factors of obesity, high blood lipid levels, hypertension, and sedentary lifestyle. Cigarette smoking and a positive family history also increase risk for CVD. Kidney disease, indicated by **albuminuria** (presence of albumin in the urine), increases the risk for coronary heart disease and mortality from MI. Patients with DM often have higher levels of C-reactive protein (CRP), an inflammatory marker associated with increased risk for cardiovascular problems and death. In addition, the presence of diabetic retinopathy is associated with an increased risk for mortality and cardiovascular events in both type 1 and type 2 DM.

Cardiovascular complication rates can be reduced through aggressive management of hyperglycemia, hypertension, and hyperlipidemia. The American Diabetes Association (ADA) recommends that blood pressure be maintained below 140/80 mm Hg and that low-density lipoprotein (LDL) cholesterol remains below 100 mg/dL (2.60 mmol/L) for patients without manifestations of CVD and below 70 mg/dL (1.8 mmol/L) for patients with manifestations of CVD (ADA, 2014f). Lifestyle modifications that focus on reducing saturated fat, *trans* fat, and cholesterol intake; increasing intake of omega-3 fatty acids, fiber, and plant sterols; weight loss (if indicated); and increasing physical activity are recommended to improve the lipid profile for patients with DM (ADA, 2013).

Priority nursing actions focus on interventions to reduce modifiable risk factors associated with CVD, such as smoking cessation, diet, exercise, blood pressure control, maintaining prescribed aspirin use, and maintaining prescribed lipid-lowering drug therapy. Many patients with DM do not have the traditional and more obvious manifestations of myocardial infarction (i.e., crushing chest pain radiating down the left arm or up the jaw). Instead the manifestations are more subtle. These include dyspnea with or without cough, extreme fatigue, and sudden onset of nausea and vomiting. Teach patients to report any of these subtle manifestations of MI to their health care provider for evaluation.

Cerebrovascular Disease. The risk for stroke is 2 to 4 times higher in people with DM compared with those who do not have the disease. Diabetes also increases the likelihood of severe carotid atherosclerosis. Hypertension, hyperlipidemia, nephropathy, peripheral vascular disease, and alcohol and tobacco use further increase the risk for stroke in people with DM.

DM also affects stroke outcomes. Patients with DM are likely to suffer irreversible brain damage with carotid emboli that produce only transient ischemic attacks in people without DM. Elevated blood glucose levels at the time of the stroke may lead to greater brain injury and higher mortality.

Microvascular Complications

Eye and Vision Complications. Legal blindness (a corrected visual acuity of 20/200 or less) is 25 times more common in patients with DM. Diabetic retinopathy (DR) is strongly related to the duration of diabetes. After 20 years of DM, nearly all patients with type 1 disease and most with type 2 disease have some degree of retinopathy. Unfortunately, DR has few manifestations until vision loss occurs.

The cause and progression of DR are related to problems that block retinal blood vessels and cause them to leak, leading to retinal hypoxia. Nonproliferative diabetic retinopathy causes structural problems in retinal vessels, including areas of poor retinal circulation, edema, hard fatty deposits in the eye, and retinal hemorrhages. Fluid and blood leak from the retinal vessels and cause retinal edema and hard exudates.

Other retinal problems include optic nerve atrophy from hypoxia and venous beading. **Venous beading** is the abnormal appearance of retinal veins in which areas of swelling and constriction along a segment of vein resemble links of sausage. It occurs in areas of retinal ischemia. Nonproliferative diabetic retinopathies develop slowly and rarely reduce vision to the point of blindness.

Proliferative diabetic retinopathy is the growth of new retinal blood vessels, also known as "neovascularization." When retinal blood flow is poor and hypoxia develops, retinal cells secrete growth factors that stimulate formation of new blood vessels in the eye. These new vessels are thin, fragile, and bleed easily, leading to eye hemorrhage and vision loss.

Visual SENSORY PERCEPTION loss from DR has several mechanisms. Central vision may be impaired by macular edema, characterized by increased blood vessel permeability and deposits of hard exudates at the center of the retina. This problem is the main cause of vision loss in the person with DM. Monthly injections of ranibizumab (Lucentis) into the vitreous can improve vision for some people with macular edema (Aschenbrenner, 2012). Vision loss also occurs from macular degeneration, corneal scarring, and changes in lens shape or clarity.

Hyperglycemia may cause blurred vision, even with eyeglasses. Hypoglycemia may cause double vision. Cataracts occur at a younger age and progress faster among patients with DM. Open-angle glaucoma also is more common in patients with DM. The management of cataracts and glaucoma is the same as for patients who do not have diabetes (see Chapter 47).

Control of blood glucose, blood pressure, and blood lipid levels is important in preventing DR. Thus patients with DM should have routine ophthalmic evaluations to detect vision problems early before vision loss occurs. The ADA recommends eye care examinations with an ophthalmologist every year after a person has been diagnosed with type 2 diabetes and yearly for a person who has had type 1 diabetes for more than 5 years (Chou et al., 2014). Not all people with DM understand the importance of these annual eye screenings (see the Evidence-Based Practice box).

EVIDENCE-BASED PRACTICE QSEN

Why Do Adults with Diabetes Forego Annual Eye Care?

Chou, C., Sherrod, C., Zhang, Z., Barker, L., Bullard, K., Crews, J., et al. (2014). Barriers to eye care among people aged 40 years and older with diagnosed diabetes, 2006-2010. *Diabetes Care, 37*(1), 180-188.

Both type 1 and type 2 diabetes mellitus (DM) are associated with major eye problems and blindness. Extensive research has shown that maintaining tight glucose control and having at least annual ophthalmologic evaluations can reduce or delay eye complications. Previous studies have indicated that vision impairment related to DM has increased by 20% in less than 10 years. The purposes of this large retrospective and descriptive study were to determine (1) about what percentage of people with diabetes mellitus were following the recommended guidelines of annual eye examinations from the time of diagnosis of type 2 DM and starting at 5 years after initial diagnosis of type 1 DM, and (2) what were the barriers to eye care for those who were not following the recommended guidelines. The researchers re-analyzed the existing data previously collected through the Behavior Risk Factor Surveillance System (BRFSS), an annual state-based random-digit-dialed telephone survey, from 22 states between the years 2006 and 2010. The defined categories of barriers to eye care were (1) cost, lack of insurance; (2) no need, have not thought of it, no reason to; (3) no eye doctor, transportation issues, couldn't get an appointment; and (4) other (everything else). More than 27,000 people who were diagnosed with DM responded to the survey.

Of the subjects with DM, 23.5% (more than 6500) reported not having had an eye examination in the previous 12 months. The barrier categories cited among these subjects were: 39.7% category **1**, 32.3% category **2**, 6.4% category **3**, and 20.5% category **4**. The majority of subjects citing barrier category **1** issues were women between the ages of 40 years and 64 years, those who have lower annual incomes, those of Hispanic or African-American ethnicity, and those who had less formal education. The majority of subjects citing barrier category **2** issues were white men, those with higher incomes, those with more formal education, and those with diagnosed visual problems. The researchers indicated that the cost issue was not surprising because Medicare does cover an annual eye examination for people older than 65 years, and the younger subjects may not have had sufficient funds or insurance to cover this cost. The surprising results were the people, especially those who already had some degree of visual problem, who said they believed there was essentially "no need" for an annual eye examination.

Level of Evidence: 4

Although very large, the study was retrospective and descriptive in nature without randomization of subject selection or assignment. The data collected relied on subject self-report and was subject to social desirability bias in that more subjects may have reported receiving annual eye examinations than actually participated in the health-seeking behavior. Also, subjects did not include people without telephones, those who had only cell phone access, those residing in institutions, and those with undiagnosed diabetes. In addition to the study size and the fact that many ethnic groups were represented, a major strength was the detailed questions asked about the barriers to eye care behaviors. The methods of statistical analysis were appropriate for the research questions posed.

Commentary: Implications for Practice and Research

The results of this study indicate that cost is a significant barrier to annual eye care for people with diabetes. Perhaps this barrier will change with the implementation of the Affordable Care Act. Nurses can help people with diabetes check their insurance policies to determine what types of eye care are covered and encourage them to make use of this benefit. Of equal concern is the subjects' beliefs that there is no compelling need for annual eye care. It is possible that some patients think that all vision issues over age 65 years are related to old age and are unavoidable. Nurses can help patients with DM understand that annual eye care can slow the progression of existing vision problems and may help prevent blindness. Other strategies for increasing adherence to annual eye care include reminders from the health care provider and nurses' asking patient's with DM during any encounter when the last eye care appointment was and reinforcing the importance of this health care behavior. More research is needed to determine specifically why patients with DM believe that annual eye care is not necessary so that more targeted interventions could be developed.

CONSIDERATIONS FOR OLDER ADULTS
Patient-Centered Care QSEN

The older patient with diabetic retinopathy also has visual changes from aging, and his or her ability to perform self-care may be seriously affected. The patient with retinopathy may have blurred vision, distorted central vision, fluctuating vision, loss of color perception, and mobility problems resulting from loss of depth perception. It is especially important to assess the patient's ability to measure and inject insulin and to monitor blood glucose levels to determine if adaptive devices are needed to assist in self-management activities.

Diabetic Peripheral Neuropathy. Diabetic peripheral neuropathy (DPN) is a progressive deterioration of nerve function that results in loss of SENSORY PERCEPTION. It is a common complication of DM and often involves all parts of the body. Damage to sensory nerve fibers results in either pain or loss of sensation. Damage to motor nerve fibers results in muscle weakness. Damage to nerve fibers in the autonomic nervous system can cause dysfunction in every part of the body. The combination of interacting factors leading to the nerve damage in DPN are:

- Hyperglycemia, long duration of DM, hyperlipidemia, low insulin levels
- Damaged blood vessels leading to reduced neuronal oxygen and other nutrients
- Autoimmune neuronal inflammation
- Increased genetic susceptibility to nerve damage
- Smoking and alcohol use

Hyperglycemia leads to DPN through blood vessel changes and reduced tissue PERFUSION that cause nerve hypoxia. Both the axon and its myelin sheath are damaged by reduced blood flow, resulting in blocked nerve impulse transmission. Excessive glucose is converted to sorbitol, which collects in nerves and impairs motor nerve conduction. Common diabetic neuropathies are listed in Table 64-3. Autonomic nervous system neuropathy leads to problems in cardiovascular, GI, and urinary function. Keeping blood glucose levels in the normal range can slow the development and progression of diabetic neuropathies.

Diabetic neuropathy can be focal or diffuse, each with different causes and rates of progression. *Diffuse neuropathies* are the most common neuropathies in DM and involve widespread nerve function loss and SENSORY PERCEPTION loss. The onset is slow, affects both sides of the body, involves motor and sensory nerves, progresses slowly, is permanent, and includes autonomic nerve dysfunction. Late complications include foot ulcers and deformities.

Focal neuropathies in DM affect a single nerve or nerve group and usually are caused by an acute ischemic event that leads to nerve damage or nerve death. Ischemic neuropathies occur when the blood supply to a nerve or nerve group is disrupted. Manifestations begin suddenly, affect only one side of the body area, and are self-limiting. The most common neuropathies affect the nerves that control the eye muscles. Manifestations begin with pain on one side of the face near the affected eye. The eye muscles become paralyzed, resulting in double vision. The problem usually resolves in 2 to 3 months.

Cardiovascular autonomic neuropathy (CAN) affects sympathetic and parasympathetic nerves to the heart and blood vessels. This problem contributes to left ventricular dysfunction, painless myocardial infarction, and exercise intolerance. Most often, CAN leads to **orthostatic hypotension** (postural hypotension) and **syncope** (brief loss of consciousness on standing). These problems result from failure of the heart and arteries to adjust to position changes by increasing heart rate and vascular tone. As a result, blood flow to the brain is interrupted briefly. Orthostatic hypotension and syncope increase the risk for falls, especially among older adults.

Autonomic neuropathy can affect the entire GI system. Common GI problems from diabetic neuropathy include gastroesophageal reflex, delayed gastric emptying and gastric retention, early satiety, heartburn, nausea, vomiting, and anorexia. Sluggish movement of the small intestine can lead to bacterial overgrowth, which causes bloating, gas, and diarrhea. Diarrhea caused by diabetes is chronic, may be severe, and often occurs at night. Constipation, the most common GI problem with DM, is intermittent and may alternate with bouts of diarrhea. **Gastroparesis** (delay in gastric emptying) is a cause of hypoglycemia.

TABLE 64-3   Features of Diabetic Neuropathy

	COMPLICATION	MANIFESTATION
Diffuse Neuropathies		
Distal symmetric polyneuropathy	Sensory alterations	Paresthesias: burning/tingling sensations, starting in toes and moving up legs Dysesthesias: burning, stinging, or stabbing pain Anesthesia: loss of sensation
	Motor alterations in intrinsic muscles of foot	Foot deformities: high arch, claw toes, hammertoes; shift of weight-bearing to metatarsal heads and tips of toes
Autonomic neuropathy	Anhidrosis	Drying, cracking of skin
	Gastrointestinal	Delayed gastric emptying, gastric retention, early satiety, bloating, nausea, vomiting, anorexia, constipation, diarrhea
	Neurogenic bladder	Atonic bladder, urinary retention
	Impotence	Erectile dysfunction
	Cardiovascular autonomic neuropathy	Early fatigue, weakness with exercise, orthostatic hypotension
	Defective counterregulation	Loss of warning signs of hypoglycemia
Focal Neuropathies		
Focal ischemia	Thoracolumbar radiculopathy with sensory and reflex loss	Pain radiating across back, side, and front of chest or abdomen
	Cranial nerve palsies, third and sixth nerves	Sudden diplopia or ptosis; eye pain
	Amyotrophy	Pain; asymmetric weakness; wasting of iliopsoas, quadriceps, and adductor muscles

Urinary problems from neuropathy result in incomplete bladder emptying and urine retention, which lead to urinary INFECTION and kidney problems. Manifestations include frequency, urgency, and incontinence.

Diabetic Nephropathy. **Nephropathy** is a pathologic change in the kidney that reduces kidney function and leads to kidney failure. Diabetes is the leading cause of chronic kidney disease (CKD) and end-stage kidney disease (ESKD) in the United States. Risk factors include a 10- to 15-year history of DM, poor blood glucose control, uncontrolled hypertension, and genetic predisposition. Patients who have a genetic predisposition appear to have higher serum uric acid levels and higher levels of tumor necrosis factor receptors. When a person has these genetic differences, the risk for progression of kidney problems to ESKD is greater even when blood glucose levels are controlled (Krolewski et al., 2014). The onset of diabetic kidney disease may be prevented and the progression to ESKD can be delayed by maintaining optimum blood GLUCOSE REGULATION, keeping blood pressure within the normal ranges, and using drug therapy to protect the kidneys (ADA, 2014b; Krolewski et al., 2014; Zitkus, 2012). Drugs that protect the kidneys are the angiotensin-converting enzyme (ACE) inhibitors and the angiotensin receptor blockers (ABRs).

Kidney disease causes progressive albumin excretion and declining glomerular filtration rate (GFR). Early manifestations of nephropathy are **microalbuminuria** (small amounts of albumin in the urine) and elevated serum uric acid levels. Annual testing for microalbuminuria is recommended for patients who have had type 1 DM for at least 5 years and in everyone with type 2 DM (ADA, 2014b).

Chronic high blood glucose levels cause hypertension in kidney blood vessels and excess kidney tissue PERFUSION. The increased pressure damages the kidney in many ways. The blood vessels become leakier, especially in the glomerulus. This leakiness allows filtration of albumin and other proteins, which then form deposits in the kidney tissue and blood vessels. Blood vessels narrow, decreasing kidney oxygenation and leading to kidney cell hypoxia and cell death. These processes worsen over time, with scarring of glomerular blood vessels and loss of urine filtration ability, leading to kidney failure.

Kidney damage is also related to hypertension for patients with DM and cardiovascular disease. Both systolic and diastolic hypertension speed the progression of diabetic nephropathy.

Male Erectile Dysfunction. Erectile dysfunction (ED) is the inability to achieve or maintain a sufficient penile erection for satisfactory sexual performance. ED occurs at a higher rate and 10 to 15 years earlier among men with DM as compared with the general population. It is related to poor blood GLUCOSE REGULATION, obesity, hypertension, heavy cigarette smoking, and the presence of other chronic vascular complications. Chapter 72 discusses erectile function problems in depth.

Cognitive Dysfunction. People age 65 years or older with diabetes are at a significantly higher risk for developing all types of dementia as compared with people who do not have the disease. Chronic hyperglycemia with microvascular disease contributes to neuron damage, brain atrophy, and cognitive impairment (Acee, 2012). These problems occur more frequently and are more severe in patients with longer-duration DM and increase the complications of neuropathy and retinopathy. Depression is highly prevalent in people with diabetes and is associated with worse outcomes.

TABLE 64-4 Differentiation of Type 1 and Type 2 Diabetes

FEATURES	TYPE 1	TYPE 2
Former names	Juvenile-onset diabetes Ketosis-prone diabetes Insulin-dependent diabetes mellitus (IDDM)	Adult-onset diabetes Ketosis-resistant diabetes Non–insulin-dependent diabetes mellitus (NIDDM)
Age at onset	Usually younger than 30 yr, occurs at any age	Peaks in 50s; may occur earlier
Symptoms	Abrupt onset, thirst, hunger, increased urine output, weight loss	Frequently none; thirst, fatigue, blurred vision, vascular or neural complications
Etiology	Viral infection	Not known
Pathology	Pancreatic beta-cell destruction	Insulin resistance Dysfunctional pancreatic beta cell
Antigen patterns	HLA-DR, HLA-DQ	None
Antibodies	ICAs present at diagnosis	None
Endogenous insulin and C-peptide	None	Low, normal, or high
Inheritance	Complex	Dominant, multifactorial
Nutritional status	Usually nonobese	60% to 80% obese
Insulin	All dependent on insulin	Required for 20% to 30%
Medical nutrition therapy	Mandatory	Mandatory

ICAs, Islet cell antibodies.

Etiology and Genetic Risk

Type 1 Diabetes. Type 1 diabetes mellitus (DM) is an autoimmune disorder in which beta cells are destroyed in a genetically susceptible person (Table 64-4). The immune system fails to recognize normal body cells as "self," and immune system cells and antibodies take destructive actions against the insulin-secreting cells in the islets. People with certain tissue types are more likely to develop autoimmune diseases, including type 1 DM. Viral infections, such as mumps and coxsackievirus infection, may trigger autoimmune destructive actions (McCance et al., 2014).

Type 2 Diabetes and Metabolic Syndrome. Type 2 DM is a progressive disorder in which the person has a combination of insulin resistance and decreased beta-cell secretion of insulin. Insulin resistance (a reduced cell response to insulin) develops

GENETIC/GENOMIC CONSIDERATIONS
Patient-Centered Care QSEN

Risk for type 1 diabetes is determined by inheritance of genes coding for the *HLA-DR* and *HLA-DQA* and *DQB* tissues types (ADA, 2014d). However, inheritance of these genes only increases the risk and most people with these genes do not develop type 1 DM. Development of DM is an interactive effect of genetic predisposition and exposure to certain environmental factors. It is unclear why some genetically susceptible people develop diabetes and others do not. Ask patients newly diagnosed with type 1 diabetes whether any other relatives have diabetes or other autoimmune disease.

from obesity and physical inactivity in a genetically susceptible person. It occurs before the onset of type 2 DM and often is accompanied by the cardiovascular risk factors of hyperlipidemia, hypertension, and increased clot formation. Most patients with type 2 DM are obese (ADA, 2014d). The specific causes of type 2 DM are not known, although insulin resistance and beta-cell failure have many genetic and nongenetic causes. Heredity plays a major role in the development of type 2 DM, although not all gene variations that increase the risk for type 2 DM are known.

Metabolic syndrome is the simultaneous presence of metabolic factors known to increase risk for developing type 2 DM and cardiovascular disease. Features of the syndrome include:

- Abdominal obesity: waist circumference of 40 inches (100 cm) or more for men and 35 inches (88 cm) or more for women
- Hyperglycemia: fasting blood glucose level of 100 mg/dL or more or on drug treatment for elevated glucose
- Abnormal A1C: between 5.5% and 6.0%
- Hypertension: systolic BP of 130 mm Hg or more or diastolic BP of 85 mm Hg or more or on drug treatment for hypertension
- Hyperlipidemia: triglyceride level of 150 mg/dL or more or on drug treatment for elevated triglycerides; high-density lipoprotein (HDL) cholesterol less than 40 mg/dL for men or less than 50 mg/dL for women

Any one of these health problems increases the rate of atherosclerosis and the risk for stroke, coronary heart disease, and early death. Teach patients about the lifestyle changes that can improve health (Bosak, 2012a). (See the Health Promotion and Maintenance section below.)

Incidence and Prevalence

More than 57 million American adults have prediabetes, defined as impaired fasting glucose (IFG) or impaired glucose tolerance (IGT) or an A1C level between 5.5% and 6.0%. IFG (fasting blood glucose levels of 100 mg/dL [5.6 mmol/L] to 125 mg/dL [6.9 mmol/L] and IGT (2-hr oral glucose tolerance values of 140 mg/dL [7.8 mmol/L] to 199 mg/dL [11.0 mmol/L]) are considered risk factors for diabetes and for cardiovascular disease. Over a 3- to 5-year period, people with prediabetes have a fivefold to fifteenfold higher risk for developing type 2 DM than do those with normal blood glucose levels. IFG and IGT are associated with obesity (especially abdominal or central obesity), dyslipidemia with high triglycerides and/or low HDL cholesterol, and hypertension (ADA, 2014d).

In the United States, nearly 26 million people are living with DM and another 79 million have prediabetes. This means

TABLE 64-5 Indications for Testing People for Type 2 Diabetes

- Testing for diabetes should be considered in people 45 years of age and older, particularly in those with a BMI greater than 25 kg/m². If normal, it should be repeated at 3-year intervals.
- Testing should be considered at a younger age or be carried out more frequently in people who are overweight (BMI >25 kg/m²) and have these additional associated factors:
  - Have a first-degree relative with diabetes
  - Are physically inactive
  - Are members of a high-risk ethnic population (e.g., African American, Hispanic American, American Indian, Asian American, or Pacific Islander)
  - Deliver a baby weighing more than 9 pounds or have been diagnosed with GDM
  - Are hypertensive (>140/90 mm Hg)
  - Have a high-density lipoprotein (HDL) cholesterol level less than 35 mg/dL (0.90 mmol/L) and/or a triglyceride level greater than 250 mg/dL (2.82 mmol/L)
  - Have polycystic ovary syndrome
  - Have IFG or IGT on previous testing
  - Have a history of vascular disease

BMI, Body mass index; *GDM,* gestational diabetes mellitus; *IFG,* impaired fasting glucose, *IGT,* impaired glucose tolerance.
Data from American Diabetes Association (ADA). (2014d). Position statement: Diagnosis and classification of diabetes mellitus. *Diabetes Care, 37*(Suppl. 1), S81-S90.

almost one third of the total U.S. population are affected by diabetes (CDC, 2011).

About 90% of people with diabetes have type 2 DM (ADA, 2014d). It is diagnosed most often among middle-aged and older adults, affecting about 9.6% of patients ages 20 to 59 years and 20.9% of patients ages 60 years and older. It is more common among men than women (National Institute of Diabetes and Digestive and Kidney Diseases [NIDDK], 2011). With the prevalence of obesity rising in North America, diabetes will become even more common.

CULTURAL CONSIDERATIONS
Patient-Centered Care QSEN

Racial and ethnic minorities have a higher prevalence and greater burden of diabetes compared with whites, and some minority groups also have higher rates of complications. The risk for diabetes is 77% higher among African Americans than non-Hispanic white Americans. At nearly 16.1%, American Indians and Alaska Indians have the highest age-adjusted prevalence of diabetes among U.S. racial and ethnic groups (Chow et al., 2012). The increase in obesity and sedentary lifestyles in the U. S. population intensifies this growing problem. The ADA has identified patients who should be tested for diabetes in Table 64-5.

The overall clinical outcomes for minority patients with diabetes are worse than for non-Hispanic whites with DM. Possible factors for these outcome differences include lack of access to health care, lifestyle issues, mistrust of the health care system, reduced financial resources, and lack of knowledge about the relationship between glucose control and complications. Be alert to the risk for diabetes whenever you are interviewing or assessing people who belong to these higher risk racial or ethnic groups.

Health Promotion and Maintenance

Diabetes causes many preventable but devastating complications and is a major public health problem. Control of diabetes and its complications is a major focus for health promotion

CHART 64-1 Laboratory Profile

Blood Glucose Values

TEST	NORMAL RANGE FOR ADULTS	SIGNIFICANCE OF ABNORMAL RESULTS
Fasting blood glucose test	<100 mg/dL (5.6 mmol/L) Older adults: Levels rise 1 mg/dL per decade of age	Levels >100 mg/dL (5.6 mmol/L) but <126 mg/dL (7.0 mmol/L) indicate impaired fasting glucose (IFG). Levels >126 mg/dL (7.0 mmol/L) obtained on at least two occasions are diagnostic of diabetes, even in older adults.
Glucose tolerance test (2-hr post-load result)	<140 mg/dL (7.8 mmol/L)	Levels >140 mg/dL (7.8 mmol/L) and <200 mg/dL (11.1 mmol/L) indicate impaired glucose tolerance (IGT). Levels >200 mg/dL (11.1 mmol/L) indicate provisional diagnosis of diabetes.
Glycosylated hemoglobin (A1C) test	4%-6%	Levels of 5.7 to 6.4% indicate increased risk for development of diabetes. Levels >8% indicate poor diabetes control and need for adherence to regimen or changes in therapy.

Data from American Diabetes Association (ADA). (2014d). Position statement: Diagnosis and classification of diabetes mellitus. *Diabetes Care, 37*(Suppl. 1), S81-S90.

activities. No interventions are successful in preventing type 1 DM, but health promotion activities focus on controlling hyperglycemia to reduce its long-term complications.

Adopting a low calorie diet that results in weight loss and increasing physical activity improve metabolic and cardiac risk factors. These improvements include reducing hypertension, increasing heart rate variability between resting rate and exercise rate, lowering triglyceride levels, increasing high-density lipoprotein cholesterol (the "good" cholesterol) levels, and reducing low-density lipoprotein cholesterol (the "bad" cholesterol) levels.

Teach all patients with DM that tight control of blood glucose levels can prevent many complications. Urge all patients with DM to regularly follow up with their health care provider or endocrinologist, to have their eyes and vision tested yearly by an ophthalmologist, and to have urine microalbumin levels assessed yearly. Early detection of changes in the eye or kidney permits adjustments in treatment regimens that can slow or halt progression of retinopathy and nephropathy. Encourage all people to maintain weight within an appropriate range for height and body build and to engage in physical activity at least 3 times per week (Bosak, 2012b).

❖ PATIENT-CENTERED COLLABORATIVE CARE

◆ Assessment

History. Ask about risk factors and manifestations related to diabetes. Age is important because type 2 diabetes mellitus (DM) is more common in older patients, especially among African Americans and Mexican Americans. Ask women how large their children were at birth, because many women who develop type 2 DM had gestational diabetes mellitus (GDM) or glucose intolerance during pregnancy (ADA, 2014d). These women often have given birth to infants weighing 9 pounds or more.

Assessing weight and weight change is important, because excess weight and obesity are risk factors for type 2 DM. The patient with type 1 DM often has weight loss with increased appetite during the weeks before diagnosis. For both types of DM, patients usually have fatigue, polyuria, and polydipsia. Ask about recent major or minor infections. In particular, ask women about frequent vaginal yeast infections. Ask all patients whether they have noticed that small skin injuries become infected more easily or take longer to heal. Also ask whether

TABLE 64-6 Criteria for the Diagnosis of Diabetes

A1C >6.5%. The test should be performed in a laboratory using a method that is NGSP certified and standardized to the DCCT assay.

Or

Fasting blood glucose greater than 126 mg/dL (7.0 mmol/L). *Fasting* is defined as no caloric intake for at least 8 hours.

Or

Two-hour blood glucose equal to or greater than 200 mg/dL (11.1 mmol/L) during oral glucose tolerance test. The test should be performed using a glucose load containing the equivalent of 75 g anhydrous glucose dissolved in water.

Or

In a patient with classic manifestations of hyperglycemia or hyperglycemic crisis, a random blood glucose concentration greater than 200 mg/dL (11.1 mmol/L). *Casual* is defined as any time of the day without regard to time since last meal. The classic symptoms of diabetes include polyuria, polydipsia, and unexplained weight loss.

NOTE: In the absence of unequivocal hyperglycemia, the first three criteria should be confirmed by repeat testing.

Data from American Diabetes Association (ADA). (2014d). Position statement: Diagnosis and classification of diabetes mellitus. *Diabetes Care, 37*(Suppl. 1), S81-S90.
DCCT, Diabetes Control and Complications Trial; *NGSP,* National Glycohemoglobin Standardization Program.

they have noticed any changes in vision or in the sense of touch.

Laboratory Assessment

Diagnosis of Diabetes. Diabetes can be diagnosed by assessing blood glucose levels. The ADA defines normal blood glucose values in Chart 64-1. A test result indicating DM should be repeated to rule out laboratory error unless manifestations of hyperglycemia or hyperglycemic crisis are also present. Table 64-6 lists criteria for the diagnosis of diabetes.

The diagnosis of diabetes mellitus includes elevated glycosylated hemoglobin levels. **Glycosylated hemoglobin (A1C)** is a standardized test that measures how much glucose permanently attaches to the hemoglobin molecule. Because glucose binds to many proteins, including hemoglobin, through a process called *glycosylation,* the higher the blood glucose level is over time, the more glycosylated hemoglobin becomes. The ADA defines A1C levels greater than 6.5% as diagnostic of DM (ADA, 2014d; Funnell, 2014).

Fasting plasma glucose (FPG) (fasting blood glucose [FBG]) is used to diagnose diabetes in nonpregnant adults. The patient should have no caloric intake for at least 8 hours (water is permitted). The blood sample needs to be obtained before insulin or oral antidiabetic agents have been taken. A diagnosis of diabetes is made with two separate test results greater than 126 mg/dL (7 mmol/L) (ADA, 2014d). *Random* or *casual* plasma (blood) glucose greater than 200 mg/dL (7.0 mmol/L) is used to diagnose diabetes in patients with severe classic hyperglycemia or hyperglycemic crisis.

Oral glucose tolerance testing (OGTT) is the most sensitive test for the diagnosis of DM. It is often used to diagnose gestational diabetes mellitus (GDM) during pregnancy and is not routinely used for general diagnosis.

Other blood tests for diabetes can help determine whether a patient has type 1 or type 2 DM. Type 1 DM results from autoimmune destruction of the beta cells of the pancreas. Markers of this destruction include islet cell autoantibodies (ICAs), autoantibodies to insulin, and autoantibodies to glutamic acid decarboxylase (GAD65). ICAs are present in 85% to 90% of people with new-onset type 1 DM.

Measurement of C-peptide levels indicates beta secretory function of the pancreas. Low to absent C-peptide levels diagnose type 1 DM, as well as late-stage type 2 DM when the ability of the pancreas to secrete insulin is severely impaired.

Screening for Diabetes. Measurement of islet cell antibodies may identify people who are at risk for developing type 1 DM. Testing to detect prediabetes and type 2 DM should be considered in patients older than 45 years and those defined as overweight (body mass index [BMI] greater than 25 kg/m²). Testing is considered for patients who are younger than 45 years and are overweight if they have additional risk factors for diabetes or have other health problems associated with diabetes. Screening for diabetes usually is done with either hemoglobin A1C levels or fasting plasma glucose levels (ADA, 2014d). The use of portable glucose meters for the diagnosis of diabetes is not recommended because of imprecise results and variance in results among the different glucose monitors (Sacks, 2011).

Ongoing Assessment. *Glycosylated hemoglobin assays* are useful because blood glucose permanently attaches to hemoglobin. The higher the blood glucose level is over time, the more glycosylated hemoglobin becomes. Thus glycosylated hemoglobin A1C (A1C) is a good indicator of the average blood glucose levels because it shows the average blood glucose level during the previous 120 days—the life span of red blood cells. A1C testing can help assess long-term glycemic control and predict the risk for complications. *Unlike the fasting blood glucose test, A1C test results are not altered by eating habits the day before the test.* This testing is performed at diagnosis and at specific intervals to evaluate the treatment plan. A1C testing is recommended at least twice yearly in patients who are meeting expected treatment outcomes and have stable blood glucose control. Quarterly assessment is recommended for patients whose therapy has changed or who are not meeting prescribed glycemic levels (ADA, 2014d). Table 64-7 shows the correlation between A1C and mean blood glucose levels.

When glucose binds to amino groups on serum proteins, especially albumin, the glycosylated protein product is called *fructosamine*. This product increases with elevated blood glucose levels in the same way as hemoglobin does but can indicate blood glucose control over a shorter period. These measures are useful for short-term follow-up of treatment changes or in patients with hemoglobin abnormalities in which A1C is not an accurate reflection of glucose control. Available tests are called

TABLE 64-7 **Correlation Between A1C Level and Mean Blood Glucose Levels**

A1C (%)	MEAN BLOOD GLUCOSE	
	Mg/dL	mmol/L
6	126	7.0
7	154	8.6
8	183	10.2
9	212	11.8
10	240	13.4
11	269	14.9
12	298	16.5

Data from American Diabetes Association (ADA). (2013). Standards of medical care in diabetes—2013. *Diabetes Care, 36*(Suppl. 1), S19.

glycosylated serum albumin (GSA), glycosylated serum protein (GSP), and *fructosamine.*

Urine Tests. *Ketone bodies* are a product of fat metabolism, and the presence of moderate to high urine ketones (hyperketonuria) indicates a severe lack of insulin. Hyperketonuria in the presence of hyperglycemia is a medical emergency that, when detected early, can be managed with insulin and careful monitoring. Urine testing for ketones should be performed during acute illness or stress, when blood glucose levels consistently exceed 300 mg/dL (16.7 mmol/L), during pregnancy, or when any manifestations of ketoacidosis are present. Ketone testing is recommended for patients with diabetes participating in a weight-loss program. Hyperketonuria without hyperglycemia suggests that weight loss is occurring without disrupting blood glucose control.

Ketone bodies appear in urine in the same proportion as they do in blood but are affected by urine volume and concentration. Thus urine ketone bodies are not used to evaluate the effectiveness of treatment for ketoacidosis.

Tests for kidney function are important in detecting kidney disease in diabetes. Persistent albuminuria in the range of 30 to 299 mg/24 hr is an indicator of early-stage diabetic nephropathy in type 1 diabetes and a marker for development of nephropathy in type 2 diabetes. Persistent albuminuria is also a marker for increased cardiovascular risk (ADA, 2014f). Screening for increased urinary albumin excretion can be performed by measurement of albumin-to-creatinine ratio in a random spot collection.

Serum creatinine is used to estimate kidney function (e.g., glomerular filtration rate) and to stage the level of chronic kidney disease. In patients with nephropathy, a rise in serum creatinine level is related to both poor blood glucose control and hypertension.

Urine glucose testing is an indirect measurement of blood glucose and is not accurate. This test is not used for monitoring DM management.

◆ *Analysis*

The priority NANDA-I nursing diagnoses and collaborative problems for patients with diabetes include:
1. Risk for Injury related to hyperglycemia (NANDA-I)
2. Potential for impaired wound healing related to endocrine and vascular effects of diabetes
3. Risk for Injury related to diabetic neuropathy (NANDA-I)

4. Acute Pain and Chronic Pain related to diabetic neuropathy (NANDA-I)
5. Risk for Injury related to diabetic retinopathy–induced reduced vision (NANDA-I)
6. Potential for kidney disease related to impaired kidney circulation
7. Potential for hypoglycemia
8. Potential for diabetic ketoacidosis
9. Potential for hyperglycemic-hyperosmolar state and coma

◆ Planning and Implementation

The management of diabetes mellitus (DM) is complex and involves extensive patient education. The Concept Map on p. 1311 highlights care issues for the patient with type 2 DM.

Preventing Injury from Hyperglycemia

Planning: Expected Outcomes. The patient with diabetes is expected to manage DM and prevent disease progression by maintaining blood glucose levels in his or her target range. Indicators are that the patient consistently demonstrates these behaviors:

- Performs treatment regimen as prescribed
- Follows recommended diet
- Monitors blood glucose using correct testing procedures
- Seeks health care if blood glucose levels fluctuate outside of recommended parameters
- Meets recommended activity levels
- Uses drugs as prescribed
- Maintains optimum weight
- Problem solves about barriers to self-management

Interventions

Nonsurgical Management. Nonsurgical management of diabetes mellitus (DM) involves nutrition interventions, blood glucose monitoring, a planned exercise program, and often, drugs to lower blood glucose levels. The nurse, together with the patient, physician, dietitian, pharmacist, case manager, and other health care professionals, plans, coordinates, and delivers care.

The American Diabetes Association (ADA) has proposed these treatment outcomes for glycosylated hemoglobin (A1C) and blood glucose levels (ADA, 2014d):

- A1C levels are maintained at 6.5% or below.
- The majority of premeal blood glucose levels are 70 to 130 mg/dL (3.9 to 7.2 mmol/L).
- Peak after-meal blood glucose levels are less than 180 mg/dL (<10.0 mmol/L).

Drug Therapy. Drug therapy is indicated when a patient with type 2 DM does not achieve blood glucose control with diet changes, regular exercise, and stress management. Several categories of drugs are available to lower blood glucose levels. Patients with type 1 DM require insulin therapy for blood glucose control.

Drugs are started at the lowest effective dose and increased every 1 to 2 weeks until the patient reaches desired blood glucose control or the maximum dosage. If the maximum dosage of one agent does not control blood glucose levels, a second agent with a different mechanism of action may be added. Insulin therapy is indicated for the patient with type 2 DM when blood glucose cannot be controlled with the use of two or three different antidiabetic agents.

Antidiabetic drugs are not a substitute for dietary modification and exercise. Teach the patient about the need for continuing

---

> **! NURSING SAFETY PRIORITY** (QSEN)
> **Drug Alert**
>
> To avoid adverse drug interactions, teach the patient who is taking an antidiabetic drug to consult with his or her primary care provider or pharmacist before using *any* over-the-counter drugs.

dietary restrictions and regular exercise while taking antidiabetic drugs.

Drug Selection. The choice of antidiabetic drug is based on cost, the patient's ability to manage multiple drug dosages, age, and response to the drugs. Shorter-acting agents (e.g., glipizide) are preferable in older patients, those with irregular eating schedules, or those with liver, kidney, or cardiac dysfunction. Longer-acting agents (e.g., glyburide, glimepiride) with once-a-day dosing are better for adherence. Beta-cell function in type 2 DM often declines over time, reducing the effectiveness of some drugs. The treatment regimen for a patient with type 2 DM may eventually require insulin therapy either alone or with other antidiabetic drugs.

Antidiabetic Drugs. Some antidiabetic drugs are oral agents, and others require subcutaneous injection. Chart 64-2 lists common antidiabetic drugs in each category.

Insulin Secretogogues. Insulin secretagogues stimulate insulin release from pancreatic beta cells and are used for patients who are still able to produce insulin.

Sulfonylurea Agents. Sulfonylurea agents lower fasting blood glucose levels by triggering the release of insulin from beta cells. Many drugs interact with sulfonylureas. Be sure to consult a drug reference book or pharmacologist when instructing patients who are prescribed a drug from this class.

Meglitinide Analogs. Meglitinide analogs are classified as insulin secretagogues and have actions and adverse effects similar to those of sulfonylureas. They tend to increase meal-related insulin secretion.

Biguanides. Metformin (Glucophage) does not increase insulin secretion. It decreases liver glucose production and decreases intestinal absorption of glucose. It also improves insulin sensitivity by increasing peripheral glucose uptake and utilization.

> **! NURSING SAFETY PRIORITY** (QSEN)
> **Drug Alert**
>
> Metformin can cause lactic acidosis in patients with renal insufficiency and should not be used by anyone with kidney disease. To prevent kidney damage, the drug should be withheld after using contrast material or any surgical procedure requiring anesthesia until adequate kidney function is established.

Insulin Sensitizers. Thiazolidinediones (TZDs) increase cellular utilization of glucose, which lowers blood glucose levels. Both of the TZDs—rosiglitazone (Avandia) and pioglitazone (Actos)—are associated with an increased risk for heart-related deaths, bone fracture, and macular edema. The Food and Drug Administration (FDA) has issued a black box warning indicating that these drugs are not to be used by patients who have symptomatic heart failure or other specific types of cardiovascular disease (Sisson et al., 2012). (A **Black Box Warning** is a government designation indicating that a drug has at least one serious side effect and must be used with caution.)

CONCEPT MAP

DIABETES MELLITUS TYPE 2

- PAIN
- PERFUSION
- SENSORY PERCEPTION
- NUTRITION
- TISSUE INTEGRITY
- INFECTION
- GLUCOSE REGULATION

INTERVENTIONS

1. Nursing Safety Priority: Critical Rescue!

Assess vital signs, provide fluids for hydration, intervene to manage BP of 160/90 mm Hg, and treat high BG level. *Treats gastroenteritis and reduces the risk of a CVA and continued vascular damage. Drug therapy may be required to achieve desired outcomes.*

2. Early Detection

Teach about tight control of BG, regular eye checkups, and urine assessment for microalbumin and ketones. *Checks for early detection of SENSORY PERCEPTION (retinopathy) and PERFUSION issues (hypertensive kidney disease, nephropathy) which permits adjustments in treatment.*

3. Interpretation of Lab Values

- Monitor K⁺ levels closely (it can be decreased, increased, or normal). *Potassium levels vary depending on hydration, the severity of any acidosis, and the patient's response to treatment.*
- Teach the patient to keep BG in the range of 60-100 mg/dL and maintain A₁c levels below 7%. *Monitors history of glucose regulation. Maintaining near normal levels delays problems with visual SENSORY PERCEPTION, INFECTION, PERFUSION, and TISSUE INTEGRITY (retinopathy, nephropathy, neuropathy, macrovascular disease).*

4. GLUCOSE REGULATION

Review with the patient the treatment regimen including nutrition, monitoring BG, when to seek medical care, recommended activity levels, using drug therapy correctly, optimum weight, and problem solving about barriers to self-management. *Prevents injury from hyperglycemia.*

5. Nursing Safety Priority: Drug Alert!

Teach the patient who is taking an antidiabetic drug to consult with the health care provider or pharmacist before using any over-the-counter drugs. *Prevents adverse drug interactions.*

6. Maintaining Nutrition

Evaluate an individualized nutritional plan in collaboration with dietitian: food intake during illness; activity level; amount of carbohydrates, fat, and fiber; consumption of alcohol; weight, and financial constraints. *Determines whether present habits are effective, need reinforcement, or require change.*

7. Preventing Complications

Teach the patient to recognize symptoms of hypoglycemia or hyperglycemia (and treatments), and when to call the health care provider. *Prevents development of diabetic ketoacidosis, prevents frequent episodes of hypoglycemia. Establishes what dietary changes are needed during illness.*

8. Health Promotion Activities – Risk Factors

Teach the patient to report decreased TISSUE PERFUSION: dyspnea, cough, extreme fatigue, and sudden onset of nausea and vomiting. *Improves CVD risk factors if the patient addresses smoking cessation, nutrition, exercise, blood pressure control, aspirin use, and adhering to prescribed lipid-lowering drug therapy.*

9. Racial and Ethnic Considerations

Explore issues related to lack of access to health care, lifestyle, mistrust of the health care system, limited financial resources, and lack of knowledge. *Racial and ethnic differences affect clinical outcomes for patients with diabetes.*

Concept Map by Deanne A. Blach, MSN, RN

EXPECTED OUTCOMES

- Manage DM and prevent progression by maintaining BG levels in expected range
- Seek care if BG levels fluctuate outside normal parameters
- Meet recommended activity level
- Use drugs as prescribed
- Maintain optimum weight
- Problem solve about barriers to self-management

Planning

PATIENT PROBLEMS

- Risk for Injury due to hyperglycemia; diabetic retinopathy; diabetic neuropathy
- Potential for impaired wound healing due to endocrine and vascular effects
- PAIN due to diabetic neuropathy
- Potential for kidney disease due to impaired kidney circulation, hypoglycemia, diabetic ketoacidosis, hyperglycemic-hyperosmolar state, and coma

Data Synthesis

LAB VALUES

- Hyperglycemia
  - BG 330 mg/dL
- Central obesity
  - waist 39 inches
  - Drug treatment for ↑ BG
- Hypertension: 160/90 mm Hg
- Triglycerides ↑ level 250 mg/dL
- HDL cholesterol 40 mg/dL

Objective Data

HISTORY

Emma Gomez is an Hispanic woman with a 20-year history of diabetes type 2. She has peripheral vascular disease and vision changes. She is admitted for gastroenteritis and a blood glucose (BG) level of 330 mg/dL.

Subjective Data

SUBJECTIVE DATA

"My vision is blurred and I have trouble with my central vision. Sometimes my vision gets a little better. I'm scared I'm going to fall when I come down the stairs because I can't tell how deep the steps are."

Data Synthesis

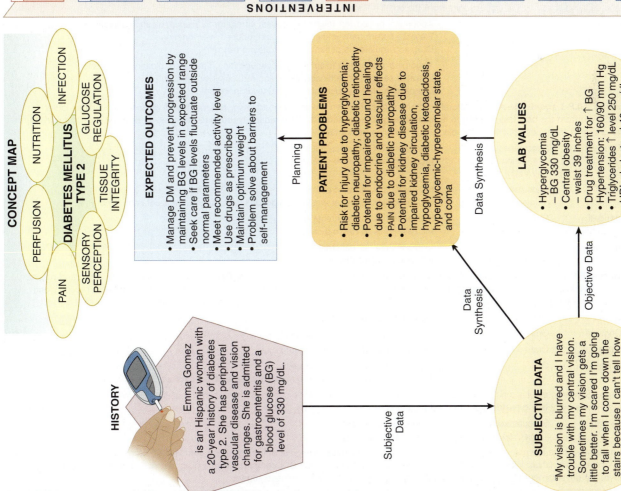

CHART 64-2   **Common Examples of Drug Therapy**

Diabetes Mellitus

DRUG/CLASS	ROUTE OF ADMINISTRATION	SIDE EFFECTS
Secretagogues—Lower fasting plasma (blood) glucose levels by triggering the release of insulin from beta cells.		
Second-Generation Sulfonylurea Agents		
Glipizide (Glucotrol)	Oral	Hypoglycemia Weight gain Interacts with many drugs
Glimepiride (Amaryl)	Oral	Hypoglycemia
Meglitinide Analogs—Lower fasting plasma (blood) glucose levels by triggering the release of insulin from beta cells.		
Repaglinide (Prandin)	Oral	Hypoglycemia
Nateglinide (Starlix)	Oral	Hypoglycemia
Biguanides		
Metformin (Glucophage)	Oral	Abdominal discomfort (diarrhea, nausea, vomiting, flatulence, indigestion) Lactic acidosis Interacts with contrast material and can induce acute kidney injury
Insulin Sensitizers—Do not increase insulin secretion. Decrease liver glucose production, reducing fasting plasma (blood) glucose release, and improve insulin receptor sensitivity. TDZs also increase cellular utilization of glucose.		
Thiazolidinediones (TZDs)		
Pioglitazone (Actos)	Oral	Increased risk for heart-related deaths; not to be used by patients with symptomatic heart failure Increased risk for bone fracture and macular edema Increased risk for liver impairment Increased risk for bladder cancer
Rosiglitazone (Avandia)	Oral	Increased risk for heart-related deaths; not to be used by patients with symptomatic heart failure Increased risk for bone fracture and macular edema Increased risk for liver impairment
Alpha-Glucosidase Inhibitors—Prevent after-meal hyperglycemia by inhibiting enzymes in the intestinal tract, reducing the rate of digestion of starches, and delaying absorption of carbohydrate from the small intestine.		
Acarbose (Precose)	Oral	Abdominal discomfort (diarrhea, nausea, vomiting, flatulence, bloating, indigestion) Elevates serum transaminase levels and reduces liver function Drug accumulates in patients with kidney impairment
Miglitol (Glyset)	Oral	Abdominal discomfort (diarrhea, nausea, vomiting, flatulence, bloating, indigestion) Elevates serum transaminase levels and reduces liver function Drug accumulates in patients with kidney impairment
Incretin Mimetics (GLP-1 agonists)—Act like natural "gut" hormones that work with insulin to lower plasma (blood) glucose levels. They lower glucagon secretion from the pancreas, leading to reduced liver glucose production. Also reduce blood glucose levels by delaying gastric emptying, slowing the rate of nutrient absorption into the blood, and reducing food intake.		
Albiglutide (Tanzeum)	Subcutaneous injection (once weekly)	Increased risk for pancreatitis Increased risk for thyroid cancer
Exenatide (Byetta)	Subcutaneous injection	Increased risk for pancreatitis Increased risk for hypersensitivity reactions, including Stevens-Johnson syndrome
Exenatide extended release (Bydureon)	Subcutaneous injection	Increased risk for pancreatitis Increased risk for thyroid cancer
Liraglutide (Victoza)	Subcutaneous injection	Increased risk for pancreatitis Increased risk for thyroid cancer
DPP-4 Inhibitors—DPP-4 is an enzyme that breaks down the natural gut hormones (GLP-1 and GIP). DPP-4 inhibitors increase the amount of natural substances that work with insulin to lower glucagon secretion from the pancreas, leading to reduced liver glucose production. Also reduce blood glucose levels by delaying gastric emptying, slowing the rate of nutrient absorption into the blood, and reducing food intake.		
Sitagliptin (Januvia)	Oral	Increased risk for acute pancreatitis
Saxagliptin (Onglyza)	Oral	Increased risk for acute pancreatitis
Linagliptin (Tradjenta)	Oral	Increased risk for acute pancreatitis
Alogliptin (Nesina)	Oral	Increased risk for acute pancreatitis Kazano (alogliptin/metformin combination) carries black box warning for lactic acidosis
Amylin Analogs—Similar to amylin, a naturally occurring hormone produced by beta cells in the pancreas that is co-secreted with insulin and lowers blood glucose levels by delaying gastric emptying and triggering satiety.		
Pramlintide (Symlin)	Subcutaneous injection	Severe hypoglycemia Nausea and vomiting
Fixed Combinations—There are many fixed combinations of oral drugs available. The side effects of these combination drugs are the same as for each component of the combination. When a drug that has the side effect of hypoglycemia is combined with a drug that does not alone produce hypoglycemia, the development of hypoglycemia is still very much a risk for the combination agent.		

Alpha-Glucosidase Inhibitors. Alpha-glucosidase inhibitors prevent after-meal hyperglycemia by delaying absorption of carbohydrate from the small intestine. These drugs inhibit enzymes in the intestinal tract, reducing the rate of digestion of starches and the absorption of glucose. This action prevents a sudden blood glucose surge after meals. These drugs do not cause hypoglycemia unless given with sulfonylureas or insulin.

Incretin Mimetics. Incretin mimetics work like the natural "gut" hormones—glucagon-like peptide-1 (GLP-1) and glucose-dependent insulinotropic polypeptide (GIP)—that are released by the intestine in response to food intake and act with insulin to perform GLUCOSE REGULATION. Drugs in this class include the GLP-1 agonists *exenatide* (Byetta), *exenatide extended-release* (Bydureon), and the glucagon-like peptide-1 (GLP-1) agonists *liraglutide* (Victoza) and *albiglutide* (Tanzeum). These drugs are used in addition to diet and exercise to improve glycemic control in adults with type 2 DM. Liraglutide carries a black box warning for thyroid tumors and is not to be used by patients with a history of medullary thyroid carcinoma.

! **NURSING SAFETY PRIORITY** (QSEN)

Drug Alert

Albiglutide (Tanzeum) is only administered once per week, not daily like other incretin mimetics.

DPP-4 Inhibitors. The natural incretins *GLP* and *GIP* are rapidly metabolized and inactivated by the enzyme *DPP-4 (dipeptidyl peptidase 4).* DPP-4 inhibitors work by reducing the inactivation of the incretin hormones so that they remain available for blood GLUCOSE REGULATION. The four DPP-4 inhibitors approved for use in patients with type 2 DM are sitagliptin (Januvia), saxagliptin (Onglyza), linagliptin (Tradjenta), and alogliptin (Nesina) (Sisson et al., 2012).

! **NURSING SAFETY PRIORITY** (QSEN)

Drug Alert

All four DPP-4 inhibitors and the incretin mimetic *liraglutide* are associated with an increased risk for pancreatitis. Warn patients taking these drugs to immediately report these manifestations to the health care provider: jaundice; sudden onset of intense abdominal pain that radiates to the back, left flank, or left shoulder; or gray-blue discoloration of the abdomen or periumbilical area.

Amylin Analogs. Amylin analogs are drugs similar to amylin, a naturally occurring hormone produced by pancreatic beta cells that works with and is co-secreted with insulin in response to blood glucose elevation. Amylin levels are deficient in patients with type 1 DM who are also deficient in insulin. Pramlintide (Symlin), an analog of amylin, is approved for patients with

---

! **NURSING SAFETY PRIORITY** (QSEN)

Drug Alert

Do not mix pramlintide and insulin in the same syringe because the pH of the two drugs is not compatible.

---

either type 1 or type 2 DM treated with insulin. It works by three mechanisms: delaying gastric emptying; reducing after-meal blood glucose levels; and triggering satiety (in the brain). (Satiety leads to decreased caloric intake and eventual weight loss.)

Sodium-Glucose Co-transport Inhibitors. Sodium-glucose co-transport inhibitors are the newest class of antidiabetic drugs. They lower blood glucose levels by preventing kidney reabsorption of the glucose that was filtered from the blood into the urine. Thus the filtered glucose is excreted in the urine rather than moved back into the blood. These oral drugs include *canagliflozin* (Invokana) and *dapagliflozin* (Farxiga).

Combination Agents. Combination agents combine drugs with different mechanisms of action. Glucovance, for example, combines glyburide with metformin. Combining drugs with different mechanisms of action may be highly effective in maintaining desired blood glucose control. Some patients may need a combination of oral agents and insulin to control blood glucose levels.

Insulin Therapy. Insulin therapy is needed for type 1 DM and also may be used for type 2 DM. The safety of insulin therapy in older patients may be affected by reduced vision, mobility and coordination problems, and decreased memory. There are many types of insulin and regimens to achieve normal blood glucose levels. Because insulin is a small protein that is quickly digested and inactivated in the GI tract, it must be administered as an injection.

Types of Insulin. Insulin is manufactured using DNA technology to produce pure human insulin. Insulin analogs are synthetic human insulins in which the structure of the insulin molecule is altered to change the rate of absorption and duration of action within the body (Dokken, 2013). An example is Lispro insulin, a rapid-acting insulin analog that is created by switching the positions of lysine and proline in one area of the insulin molecule.

Rapid-, short-, intermediate-, and long-acting forms of insulin can be injected separately, and some can be mixed in the same syringe. Insulin is available in concentrations of 100 units/mL (U-100) or 500 units/mL (U-500). U-500 is indicated only for patients with severe insulin resistance whose total daily insulin dose exceeds 200 units.

Teach the patient that the insulin types, the injection technique, the site of injection, and the patient response can all affect the absorption, onset, degree, and duration of insulin activity. Reinforce that changing insulins may affect blood glucose control and should be done only under supervision of the health care provider. Table 64-8 outlines the time activity of human insulin.

Insulin Regimens. Insulin regimens try to duplicate the normal insulin release pattern from the pancreas. The pancreas produces a constant *(basal)* amount of insulin that balances liver glucose production with glucose use and maintains normal blood glucose levels between meals. The pancreas also produces additional *(prandial)* insulin to prevent blood glucose elevation after meals. The insulin dose required for blood glucose control varies among patients. A usual starting dose is between 0.5 and 1 unit/kg of body weight per day. For multiple-dose regimens or continuous subcutaneous insulin infusion (CSII), basal insulin makes up about 40% to 50% of the total daily dosage, with the remainder divided into premeal doses of rapid-acting insulin analogs or regular insulin. Basal insulin coverage is provided by intermediate-acting insulin such as NPH insulin or by

TABLE 64-8	**Time Activity of Pharmaceutical Insulin**			
PREPARATION	**BRAND**	**ONSET (Hr)**	**PEAK (Hr)**	**DURATION (Hr)**
Rapid-Acting Insulin				
Insulin aspart	NovoLog	0.25	1-3	3-5
Insulin glulisine	Apidra	0.3	0.5-1.5	3-4
Human lispro injection	Humalog	0.25	0.5-1.5	5
Short-Acting Insulin				
Regular human insulin injection	Humulin R	0.5	2-4	5-7
	Novolin R	0.5	2.5-5	8
	ReliOn R	0.5	2.5-5	8-12
Humulin R (Concentrated U-500)	Humulin R (U-500)	1.5	4-12	24
Intermediate-Acting Insulin				
Isophane Insulin NPH injection	Humulin N	1.5	4-12	16-24+
	Novolin N	1-4	4-14	10-24+
	ReliOn N	1-4	4-14	10-24+
70% human insulin isophane suspension/30% human insulin injection	Humulin 70/30 Novolin 70/30 ReliOn 70/30	0.5	2-12	24
50% human insulin isophane suspension/50% human insulin injection	Humulin 50/50	0.5	3-5	24
70% insulin aspart protamine suspension/30% insulin aspart injection	NovoLog Mix 70/30	0.25	1-4	24
75% insulin lispro protamine suspension/25% insulin lispro injection	Humalog Mix 75/25	0.25	1-2	24
Long-Acting Insulin				
Insulin glargine injection	Lantus	2-4	None	24
Insulin detemir injection	Levemir	1	6-8	5.7-24

long-acting insulin analogs, such as insulin glargine (Lantus) or insulin detemir (Levemir). Dosages are adjusted based on the results of blood glucose monitoring.

Single daily injection protocols require insulin injection only once daily. This protocol may include one injection of intermediate- or long-acting insulin or a combination of short- and intermediate-acting insulin. Many patients with type 2 diabetes combine once-daily insulin injection with oral agent therapy.

Multiple-component insulin therapy combines short- and intermediate-acting insulin injected twice daily. Two thirds of the daily dose is given before breakfast and one third before the evening meal. Ratios of intermediate-acting and regular insulin are based on results of blood glucose monitoring.

Intensified regimens include a basal dose of intermediate- or long-acting insulin and a bolus dose of short- or rapid-acting insulin designed to bring the *next* blood glucose value into the target range. Blood glucose elevations above the target range are treated with "correction" doses of short- or rapid-acting insulin. The patient's blood glucose patterns determine insulin dosage. Frequency of blood glucose monitoring is based on the timed action of insulin and may occur as often as 8 times daily. Blood glucose testing 1 to 2 hours after meals and within 10 minutes before the next meal helps determine the adequacy of the bolus dose. The patient determines the effects of basal insulin by monitoring blood glucose levels before breakfast (fasting) and before the evening meal.

Patients on intensified insulin regimens need extensive education to achieve target blood glucose values. They need to know how to adjust insulin doses and understand NUTRITION therapy for dietary flexibility and target blood glucose values. Patients must also be able to accurately monitor blood glucose levels so that therapy decisions can be based on accurate data.

Regardless of the specific insulin regimen, adherence to insulin injection schedules is critical in achieving glycemic

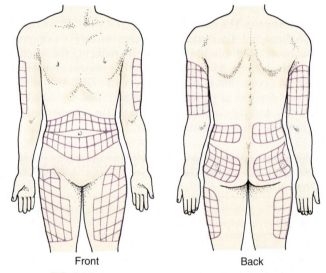

Front   Back

FIG. 64-2 Common insulin injection areas and sites.

control and maintaining A1C levels below the 6.5% needed to reduce long-term complications. At times, skipping an occasional insulin dose may be related to an unusual meal pattern for a day or a change in exercise.

Factors Influencing Insulin Absorption. Many factors affect insulin absorption and availability, including injection site; timing, type, or dose of insulin used; and physical activity.

Injection site area affects the speed of insulin absorption. Fig. 64-2 shows common insulin injection areas. Absorption is fastest in the abdomen, and except for a 2-inch radius around the navel, it is the preferred injection site area. Rotating injection site areas prevents lipohypertrophy (increased fat deposits in the skin) and lipoatrophy (loss of fatty tissue, leaving an uneven appearance). Rotation *within* one anatomic site is preferred to rotation from one area to another to prevent day-to-day changes in absorption.

Absorption rate is determined by insulin properties. The longer the duration of action, the more unpredictable is absorption. Larger doses of insulin also prolong the absorption. Factors that increase blood flow from the injection site, such as local application of heat, massage of the area, and exercise of the injected area, increase insulin absorption. Scarred sites often become favorite injection sites because they are less sensitive to pain, but these areas usually slow the rate of insulin absorption.

Injection depth changes insulin absorption. Usually, injections are made into the subcutaneous tissue. IM injection has a faster absorption and is not used for routine insulin use. Most patients lightly grasp a fold of skin and inject at a 90-degree angle; however, a 45-degree angle is advised for frail older adults and those who are cachexic. Aspiration for blood is not needed. Patients with high body mass index (BMI) levels can use 4 mm or 5 mm needles to inject insulin at a 90-degree angle without pinching a skinfold before injection. Assess the older patient's ability to inject insulin, and arrange for assistance when self-care is no longer possible.

Timing of injection affects blood glucose levels. The interval between premeal injections and eating, known as "lag time," affects blood glucose levels after meals. Insulin lispro, insulin aspart, and insulin glulisine have rapid onsets of action and should be given within 10 minutes before mealtime when blood glucose is in the target range. If hyperglycemia or hypoglycemia is not present, these insulins can be given at any time from 10 minutes before mealtime to just before eating or even immediately after eating. Regular insulin should be given at least 20 to 30 minutes before eating when glucose levels are within the target range. When blood glucose levels are above the target range, the lag time should be increased to permit insulin to begin to have an effect sooner. Rapid-acting insulin analogs can be given 15 minutes before and regular insulin 30 to 60 minutes before eating a meal. When blood glucose levels are below the target range, injection of regular insulin should be delayed until immediately before eating and injection of rapid-acting insulin should be delayed until sometime after eating the meal.

Mixing insulins can change the time of peak action. Mixtures of short- and intermediate-acting insulins produce a more normal blood glucose response in some patients than does a single dose. The patient's response to mixed insulin may differ from the response to the same insulins given separately.

! NURSING SAFETY PRIORITY (QSEN)

Drug Alert

> Do not mix any other insulin type with insulin glargine, with insulin detemir, or with any of the premixed insulin formulations, such as Humalog Mix 75/25.

Complications of Insulin Therapy. Hypoglycemia from insulin excess has many causes. Its effects and treatment are discussed on p. 1330 in the Preventing Hypoglycemia section.

Lipoatrophy is a loss of fat tissue in areas of repeated injection that results from an immune reaction to impurities in insulin. Treatment consists of injection of insulin at the edge of the atrophied area. *Lipohypertrophy* is an increased swelling of

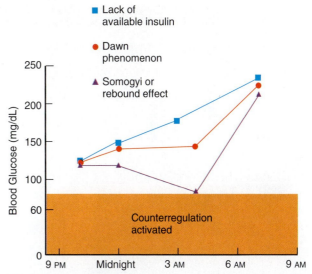

FIG. 64-3 Three blood glucose phenomena in patients with diabetes.

fat that occurs at the site of repeated insulin injections. The overlying skin has decreased sensitivity, and the area can become large and unsightly. Treatment consists of rotating the injection site among different body areas.

Two conditions of fasting hyperglycemia can occur (Fig. 64-3). *Dawn phenomenon* results from a nighttime release of growth hormone that causes release of liver glucose resulting in blood glucose elevations at about 5 to 6 AM. It is managed by providing more insulin for the overnight period (e.g., giving the evening dose of intermediate-acting insulin at 10 PM). *Somogyi phenomenon* is morning hyperglycemia from the counterregulatory response to nighttime hypoglycemia resulting in release of liver glucose. It is managed by ensuring adequate dietary intake at bedtime and evaluating the insulin dose and exercise programs to prevent conditions that lead to hypoglycemia. Both problems are diagnosed by blood glucose monitoring during the night. Help identify these problems, and teach the patient and family about management.

Alternative Methods of Insulin Administration. Many methods of insulin delivery are available in addition to traditional subcutaneous injections.

Continuous subcutaneous infusion of a basal dose of insulin (CSII) with increases in insulin at mealtimes is more effective in controlling blood glucose levels than other schedules. It allows flexibility in meal timing, because if a meal is skipped, the additional mealtime dose of insulin is not given. CSII is given by an externally worn pump containing a syringe and reservoir with rapid-acting insulin and is connected to the patient by an infusion set. Teach him or her to adjust the amount of insulin based on data from blood glucose monitoring. Rapid-acting insulin analogs are used with insulin infusion pumps (Hughes, 2012a) (Fig. 64-4).

Problems with CSII include skin infections that can occur when the infusion site is not cleaned or the needle is not changed every 2 to 3 days. CSII may lead to more episodes of ketoacidosis than other methods of insulin delivery because of inexperience in pump use, INFECTION, accidental cessation or obstruction of the infusion, or mechanical pump problems (Hughes, 2012a). Stress the importance of testing for ketones when blood glucose levels are greater than 300 mg/dL (16.7 mmol/L).

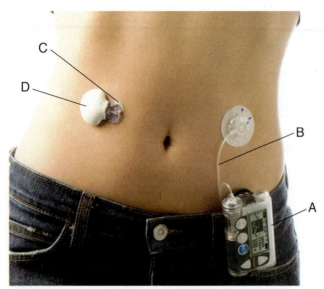

FIG. 64-4 The MiniMed Paradigm REAL-Time Insulin Pump and Continuous Glucose Monitoring System. **A,** Pump. **B,** Injection cannula. **C,** Glucose sensor. **D,** Data transmitter.

Subcutaneous Insulin Administration

- Wash your hands.
- Inspect the bottle for the type of insulin and the expiration date.
- Gently roll the bottle of intermediate-acting insulin in the palms of your hands to mix the insulin.
- Clean the rubber stopper with an alcohol swab.
- Remove the needle cover, and pull back the plunger to draw air into the syringe. The amount of air should be equal to the insulin dose. Push the needle through the rubber stopper, and inject the air into the insulin bottle.
- Turn the bottle upside down, and draw the insulin dose into the syringe.
- Remove air bubbles in the syringe by tapping on the syringe or injecting air back into the bottle. Redraw the correct amount.
- Make certain the tip of the plunger is on the line for your dose of insulin. Magnifiers are available to assist in measuring accurate doses of insulin.
- Remove the needle from the bottle. Recap the needle if the insulin is not to be given immediately.
- Select a site within your injection area that has not been used in the past month.
- Clean your skin with an alcohol swab. Lightly grasp an area of skin, and insert the needle at a 90-degree angle.
- Push the plunger all the way down. This will push the insulin into your body. Release the pinched skin.
- Pull the needle straight out quickly. Do not rub the place where you gave the shot.
- Dispose of the syringe and needle without recapping in a puncture-proof container.

Patients using CSII need intensive education. Because of the risk for hypoglycemia or hyperglycemia, he or she must be able to operate the pump, adjust the settings, and respond appropriately to alarms. Removing the pump for any length of time can result in hyperglycemia. Provide supplemental insulin schedules for times when the pump is not operational. CSII is more costly than traditional insulin injections, and not all costs are covered by insurance.

Injection devices include a needleless system and a pen-type injector in addition to traditional insulin syringes. With a needleless device, the needle is replaced by an ultrathin liquid stream of insulin forced through the skin under high pressure known as "jet injection." Insulin given by jet injection is absorbed at a faster rate and has a shorter duration of action. Cost is a drawback to this system.

Patient Education: Drugs. Provide specific instructions about insulin therapy, new drug therapies, and self-monitoring of blood glucose levels.

Insulin storage varies by use. Teach patients to refrigerate insulin that is not in use to maintain potency, prevent exposure to sunlight, and inhibit bacterial growth. Insulin in use may be kept at room temperature for up to 28 days to reduce irritation at the injection site caused by cold insulin.

To prevent loss of drug potency, teach the patient to avoid exposing insulin to temperatures below 36° F (2.2° C) or above 86° F (30° C), to avoid excessive shaking, and to protect insulin from direct heat and light. Insulin should not be allowed to freeze. Insulin glargine (Lantus) should be stored in a refrigerator (36° to 46° F [2.2° to 7.8° C]) even when in use. Teach patients to discard any unused insulin after 28 days.

Teach patients to always have a spare bottle of each type of insulin used. A slight loss in potency may occur for bottles in use for more than 30 days, even when the expiration date has not passed. Prefilled syringes are stable up to 30 days when refrigerated. Store prefilled syringes in the upright position, with the needle pointing upward, so that insulin particles do not clog it. Teach patients to roll, not shake, prefilled syringes between the hands before using.

Dose preparation is critical for insulin effectiveness and patient safety. Teach patients that the person giving the insulin needs to inspect the insulin before each use for changes (e.g., clumping, frosting, precipitation, or change in clarity or color) that may indicate loss in potency. Rapid-acting, short-acting, and glargine insulins should be clear. Preparations containing NPH insulin should be uniformly cloudy after gently rolling the vial between the hands. If potency is questionable, another vial of the same type of insulin should be used.

Syringes are the most commonly used method to administer insulin. The standard insulin syringes are marked in insulin units. They are available in 1-mL (100-U), ½-mL (50-U), and ³⁄₁₀-mL (30-U) sizes. The unit scale on the barrel of the syringe differs with the syringe size and manufacturer. Insulin syringe needles are measured in 28-, 29-, 30-, and 31-gauge and in lengths of 6 mm, 8 mm, and 12.7 mm. To ensure accurate insulin measurement, instruct the patient to always buy the same type of syringe. Chart 64-3 reviews instructions for drawing up a single insulin injection.

Disposable needles should be used only once. Reuse of an insulin syringe and needle can compromise insulin sterility. A reason not to reuse smaller (30- and 31-gauge) needles is that even with one injection, the needle tip can become bent to form a hook, which can lacerate tissue or break off to leave needle fragments in the skin (Fig. 64-5). Teach the patient to discard the syringe and needle after one use. Information on needle disposal can be obtained at www.safeneedledisposal.org.

Pen-type injectors hold small, lightweight, prefilled insulin cartridges. The injectors are easy to carry and make intensive therapy with multiple injections easier. These devices allow greater accuracy than traditional insulin syringes, especially

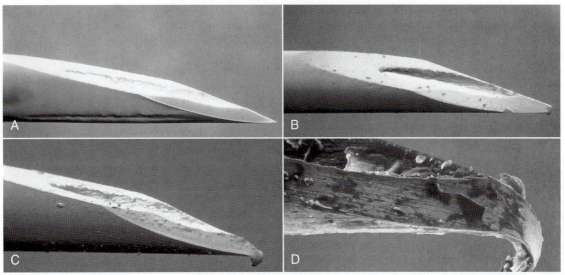

FIG. 64-5 Reuse of an insulin needle. **A,** A new needle. **B,** A needle that has been used once. **C,** A needle that has been used twice. **D,** A needle that has been used 6 times.

when measuring small doses. Discuss proper storage for pre-filled insulin pens or cartridges. Ensure that the product is appropriate to the patient's unique needs. *Pen-type injectors are not designed for independent use by visually impaired patients or by those with cognitive impairment.* Ensure that the patient has received education on its use. Each syringe or cartridge has specific requirements. Patients using the FlexPen (Novo Nordisk) must be able to attach a needle and to perform an air shot of 2 units to ensure that a dose of insulin is administered. The Institute for Safe Medication Practices (ISMP) and The Joint Commission's National Patient Safety Goals identify insulin as a *High-Alert* drug. (**High-Alert drugs** are those that have an increased risk for causing patient harm if given in error.) The ISMP cautions that digital displays on some of the newer insulin pens can be misread. If the pen is held upside down, as a left-handed person might do, a dose of 52 units actually appears to be a dose of 25 units and a dose of 12 units looks like a dose of 21 units.

Patient Education: Blood Glucose Monitoring. Self-monitoring of blood glucose (SMBG) levels provides information to assess effectiveness of the management plan. SMBG allows patients and providers to evaluate patient response to therapy and assess whether glycemic targets are being reached. Results of SMBG are useful in preventing hypoglycemia and adjusting drug

therapy, diet therapy, and physical activity. Assessment of blood glucose levels is very important for these situations:
- Manifestations of hypoglycemia/hyperglycemia
- Hypoglycemic unawareness
- Periods of illness
- Before and after exercise
- Gastroparesis
- Adjustment of diabetes drugs
- Evaluation of other drug therapies (e.g., steroids)
- Preconception planning
- Pregnancy

Technique for SMBG follows principles that are the same for most self-monitoring systems. The finger is pricked, a drop of blood flows over or is drawn into a testing strip or disc impregnated with chemicals, and the glucose value is displayed in mg/dL or mmol/L. Most meters display blood glucose results on a screen. For vision-impaired patients, "talking-meters" are available to allow independence in blood glucose monitoring.

Data obtained from SMBG are evaluated along with other measures of blood glucose (e.g., A1C values) or periodic laboratory blood glucose tests. Even when SMBG is performed correctly, the results are affected by hematocrit values (anemia falsely elevates glucose values; polycythemia falsely depresses them) and may be unreliable in the hypoglycemic or severe hyperglycemic ranges.

The performance of SMBG systems depends on accuracy of the specific blood glucose meter, operator proficiency, and test strip quality. Results are influenced by the size and quality of the blood sample; the meter's calibration to the strip in use; and environmental conditions of altitude, temperature, and moisture. Patient-specific conditions influencing results include hematocrit level, triglyceride level, high levels of substances such as ascorbic acid in blood, and the presence of hypotension or hypoxia.

Accuracy of the blood glucose monitor is ensured when the manufacturer's directions are followed. The most common source of error is related to the skill of the user rather than to errors of the instrument. Common errors involve failure to obtain a sufficient blood drop, poor storage of test strips, using expired strips, and not changing the code number on the meter to match the strip bottle code. Help the patient select a meter based on cost, ease of use, and availability of repair and servicing. Provide training, explain and demonstrate procedures, assess visual acuity, and check the patient's ability to perform the procedure using "teach-back" strategies. Glucose meters are designed to reduce user error as much as possible. Newer meters have fewer steps, include error signals for inadequate sample size, "lock out" if control solutions are not tested, and store hundreds of SMBG results. (See the *Consumer Guide* published yearly in the January edition of *Diabetes Forecast* [forecast.diabetes.org] for information to help patients determine which blood glucose meter best meets their needs.)

Accuracy and precision vary widely among capillary blood glucose monitoring devices. Teach patients to properly calibrate ("code") the machine. Instruct them to re-check the calibration and re-test if they obtain a test result that is unusual for them and whenever they are in doubt about test accuracy. Continued retraining of patients performing SMBG helps ensure accurate results because performance accuracy deteriorates over time. Laboratory glucose determinations are more accurate than SMBG.

Frequency of testing varies with the drug schedules and the patient's prescribed therapy target outcomes. The ADA recommends that patients taking multiple insulin injections or using insulin pump therapy monitor glucose levels 3 or more times daily. For patients taking less-frequent injections of insulin, non-insulin therapy, or diet therapy alone, SMBG is useful for evaluation of therapy.

Blood glucose therapy target goals are set individually for each patient. The health care team works with him or her to reach target blood glucose levels. The ADA recommends that patients with type 1 diabetes aim for A1C values less than 6.5%, premeal glucose levels of 70 to 130 mg/dL (3.9 to 7.2 mmol/L), and postmeal glucose levels less than 180 mg/dL (10.0 mmol/L) (ADA, 2013).

Infection control measures are needed for SMBG. The chance of becoming infected from blood glucose monitoring processes is reduced by handwashing before monitoring and by not reusing lancets. *Instruct patients to not share their blood glucose monitoring equipment.* Hepatitis B virus can survive in a dried state for at least 1 week. INFECTION can be spread by the lancet holder even when the lancet itself has been changed. Small particles of blood can stick to the device and infect multiple users. Regular cleaning of the meter is critical for infection control. Remind health care staff who perform blood glucose testing and family members who help with testing to wear gloves.

Many meters allow data to be downloaded by a cable or by infrared technology to a computer that has diabetes management software (Hunt et al., 2014). Some meters allow entry of additional data such as insulin dose, amounts of carbohydrate eaten, or exercise. A radio link to an insulin pump allows automatic transfer of glucose readings to a calculator that assists the patient in deciding on an appropriate insulin dose. Some patients use smart phone applications to record and trend or graph serial blood glucose levels, insulin dosages, food intake, and other data. This information can be sent to the health care provider electronically or downloaded and printed.

Once the patient learns the technical aspects of meter use, help him or her use the results of SMBG to achieve glycemic control. Post-meal glucose monitoring provides information about the effects of the size and content of their meals. SMBG allows the patient to assess effects of exercise on glucose control and provides critical information to help patients who take insulin to exercise safely. Teach patients how to use SMBG results to adjust the treatment plan. Patients should make agreed upon adjustments in the treatment plan when results are consistently out of range for a 3-day period when no change in meal plan, medications, or activity has occurred.

The U.S. Food and Drug Administration issued an Important Safety Information Notice about blood glucose measurement following use of parenteral maltose, parenteral galactose, oral xylose-containing products, and the peritoneal dialysis solution *icodextrin* (EXTRANEAL). Galactose and xylose are found in some foods, herbs, and dietary supplements; they are also used in diagnostic tests. Some meters and test strips read these substances as glucose and falsely report the blood glucose as elevated. There have been insulin overdoses with severe hypoglycemia, coma, and death when patients have used this falsely elevated glucose reading in calculating an insulin dose. The Core Measures of The Joint Commission and other agencies recommend meters and test strips that use a technology in which *only glucose* in the blood is recognized for accurate blood glucose monitoring.

> ⚠ **NURSING SAFETY PRIORITY** (QSEN)
> **Action Alert**
>
> Prevent hypoglycemia by ensuring that appropriate blood glucose testing products are used for patients receiving parenteral maltose, parenteral galactose, and oral xylose products.

It is important that staff understand the potential for hypoglycemia when patients are admitted to the hospital. In that instance, it is safest to monitor blood glucose patterns by laboratory methods. Blood glucose monitoring needs to be performed with a system in which the test strips use a different enzyme technology. The best resource for guidance in selecting a glucose monitoring system that is not reactive to maltose interference is the manufacturer of the test strip. Some manufacturers produce test strips that use more than one type of enzyme technology.

Alternate site testing allows patients to obtain blood from sites other than the fingertip and is available on many meters. However, use caution when interpreting results obtained from alternate sites. Comparison studies have shown wide variation between fingertip and alternate sites and the variation is most evident during times when blood glucose levels are rapidly changing. Teach patients that there is a lag time for blood glucose levels between the fingertip and other sites when blood glucose levels are changing rapidly and that the fingertip reading is the only safe choice at those times.

> ⚠ **NURSING SAFETY PRIORITY** (QSEN)
> **Critical Rescue**
>
> Teach patients with a history of hypoglycemic unawareness *not* to test at alternative sites.

Continuous glucose monitoring (CGM) systems monitor glucose levels in interstitial fluid to provide real-time glucose information to the user. The system consists of three parts: a disposable sensor that measures glucose levels, a transmitter that is attached to the sensor, and a receiver that displays and stores glucose information. After an initiation or warm-up period, the sensor gives glucose values every 1 to 5 minutes. Sensors may be used for 3 to 7 days, depending on the manufacturer. CGM provides information about the current blood glucose level, provides short-term feedback about results of treatment, and provides warnings when glucose readings become dangerously high or low. Most available sensors require at least two capillary glucose readings per day for calibration of the sensor. Sensor accuracy depends on these calibrations. There may be a lag time between the capillary glucose measurement and the glucose sensor value. If the blood glucose value is changing rapidly, the time between capillary and interstitial glucose values may be as long as 30 minutes. For this reason, capillary glucose readings need to be checked on all extreme values and before any corrective treatment is given.

The costs for CGM systems are substantial, starting with the cost of the device. There are additional monthly charges for disposable sensors and for the glucose test strips used to calibrate the sensors and perform FDA-required capillary glucose testing before treatment decisions are made. *Continuous glucose monitoring is meant to supplement, not replace, finger stick tests. Insulin should be given only after confirming the results of any of the continuous glucose monitoring systems.*

Nutrition Therapy. Effective self-management of diabetes requires that NUTRITION, including the meal plan, education, and counseling programs be "patientized" for each patient. A registered dietitian (RD) should be a member of the treatment team. The nurse, RD, patient, and family work together on all aspects of the meal plan, which must be realistic and as flexible as possible. Plans that consider the patient's cultural background, financial status, and lifestyle are more likely to be successful. The desired outcomes of NUTRITION and diet therapy are listed in Table 64-9.

Principles of Nutrition in Diabetes. No one meal plan is right for all patients with diabetes. Each patient's NUTRITION recommendations are based on blood glucose monitoring results, total blood lipid levels, and A1C levels. These tests help determine whether current meal and exercise patterns need adjustment or whether present habits need reinforcement. The RD individually develops a meal plan based on the patient's usual food intake, weight-management expectations, and lipid and blood glucose patterns (ADA, 2014e). Day-to-day consistency in the timing and amount of food eaten helps control blood glucose. Patients receiving insulin therapy need to eat at times that are coordinated with the timed action of insulin. Teach patients using intense insulin therapy to adjust premeal insulin to allow for timing and quantity changes in their meal plan.

Carbohydrate intake and available insulin are responsible for postmeal glucose levels, and managing carbohydrate intake is the main strategy for achieving GLUCOSE REGULATION and glycemic control. The recommendation for the patient with diabetes is a diet containing 45% of calories from carbohydrate, with a minimum intake of 130 g carbohydrate/day. However, the upper limit on daily carbohydrate intake is now considered somewhat flexible so that individual patient NUTRITION needs can be met with some variation in the carbohydrate-protein mix distribution (ADA, 2014e). The diet should include carbohydrate from fruit, vegetables, whole grains, legumes, and low-fat milk products.

The percentage of calories from carbohydrates is determined for each patient. Various starches have different blood glucose responses. The *total amount* of carbohydrate consumed each day rather than the source of the carbohydrate is still important.

Dietary fat and cholesterol intake for people with diabetes is the same as the Institute of Medicine's (IOM) recommendations for the general population to reduce the risk for cardiovascular disease. These recommendations are based on the issue that fat *quality* is more important in lipid control than is fat *quantity* (ADA, 2014e). Current recommendations are:

- Limiting total fat intake to 20% to 35% of daily calorie intake
- Choosing monounsaturated and polyunsaturated fats over saturated fats and *trans* fats
- Limiting dietary cholesterol to less than 200 mg/day
- Having two or more servings of fatty fish per week (with the exception of commercially fried fish) to provide n-3 polyunsaturated fatty acids

Trans fatty acids increase the risk for cardiovascular disease and are found in hard margarine and in foods prepared with or fried in hydrogenated and partly hydrogenated oils. Teach the patient to limit the amount of commercially fried foods and bakery goods eaten.

Further dietary fat restrictions for diabetes are determined by the RD based on specific lipid levels. Adults with diabetes should be tested annually for abnormalities of fasting serum cholesterol, triglyceride, HDL cholesterol, and calculated LDL cholesterol levels.

Protein intake of 15% to 20% of total daily calories is appropriate for patients with diabetes and normal kidney function. Some patients may need a higher percentage of calories from protein, substituted from carbohydrates, to maintain satiety and control blood glucose levels. Diets higher in protein have demonstrated improvement in insulin response but do not prevent hypoglycemia (ADA, 2014e). In patients with progressive kidney disease, reducing protein intake is needed and the level of protein reduction must be individualized.

Fiber improves carbohydrate metabolism and lowers cholesterol levels. Recommendations for the person with diabetes are the same as for the general population, which include foods

---

TABLE 64-9 Desired Outcomes of Nutrition Therapy for the Patient With Diabetes

- Achieving and maintaining blood glucose levels in the normal range or as close to normal as is safely possible
- Achieving and maintaining a blood lipid profile that reduces the risk for vascular disease
- Achieving blood pressure levels in the normal range or as close to normal as is safely possible
- Preventing or slowing the rate of development of the chronic complications of diabetes by modifying nutrient intake and lifestyle
- Addressing patient nutrition needs taking into account personal and cultural preferences and willingness to change
- Maintaining the pleasure of eating by limiting food choices only when indicated by scientific evidence
- Meeting the nutrition needs of unique times of the life cycle, particularly for pregnant and lactating women and for older adults with diabetes
- Providing self-management training for patients treated with insulin or insulin secretagogues for exercising safely, including the prevention and treatment of hypoglycemia, and managing diabetes during acute illness

containing a minimum of 25 g of fiber daily for women and 38 g daily for men (ADA, 2014e). Teach the patient to select a variety of fiber-containing foods such as legumes, fiber-rich cereals (more than 5 g fiber/serving), fruits, vegetables, and whole-grain products because they provide vitamins, minerals, and other substances important for good health.

Teach the patient that adding high-fiber foods to the diet gradually can reduce abdominal cramping, loose stools, and flatulence. An increase in fluid intake should accompany increased fiber intake. Teach the patient to pay careful attention to blood glucose levels because hypoglycemia can result when dietary fiber intake increases significantly.

Sucrose, fructose, and nonnutritive sweeteners (NNSs) are present in a variety of foods. Dietary sucrose does not increase blood glucose more than equal amounts of other starches. Intake of sucrose and sucrose-containing foods by patients with diabetes does not need to be restricted out of a concern for causing hyperglycemia. Sucrose can be included in the meal plan as long as it is adequately covered with insulin or other glucose-lowering agents; however, all people with diabetes are encouraged to avoid sugar sweetened beverages (SSBs) (ADA, 2014e). The use of nonnutritive sweeteners to enhance the taste of food while not disturbing blood glucose control is desirable. Foods sweetened with high-fructose corn syrup should be avoided by people with diabetes because this substance has been found to increase the levels of triglycerides and other lipids. Free fructose, such as that found in fruit, does not appear to alter lipid metabolism in the way that foods containing high-fructose corn syrup do (ADA, 2014e).

Alcohol consumption can affect blood glucose levels. Levels are not affected by *moderate* use of alcohol when diabetes is well controlled. Teach patients with diabetes that two alcoholic beverages for men and one for women daily can be ingested with, and in addition to, the usual meal plan. (One alcoholic beverage equals 12 ounces of beer, 5 ounces of wine, or 1.5 ounces of distilled spirits.) Because alcohol raises blood triglycerides, reducing or abstaining from alcohol is important for patients with high blood lipid levels.

> **! NURSING SAFETY PRIORITY** (QSEN)
>
> ***Action Alert***
>
> Because of the potential for alcohol-induced hypoglycemia, instruct the patient with diabetes to ingest alcohol only with or shortly after meals.

Patient Education: Prescribed Nutrition Plan. Reinforce NUTRITION information provided by the RD. The patient with DM must understand how to adjust food intake during illness, planned exercise, and social occasions (e.g., restaurant meals) when the usual time of eating may be delayed. He or she may be unable to follow the prescribed plan because of an inability to read or understand printed materials. Share dietary information with the person who prepares the meals. The RD sees each patient at least yearly to identify changes in lifestyle and make appropriate diet therapy changes. Some patients, such as those with weight-control problems or low incomes, may need more frequent evaluation and counseling.

Meal Planning Strategies. Many meal planning approaches for good NUTRITION are available. Each approach emphasizes different aspects of nutrition.

Carbohydrate (CHO) counting is a simple approach to NUTRITION and meal planning that uses label information of the nutrition content of packaged food items. Because fat and protein have little effect on after-meal blood glucose levels, CHO counting focuses on the nutrient that has the greatest impact on these levels. It uses total grams of carbohydrate, regardless of the food source. The RD determines the number of grams of carbohydrate to be eaten at each meal and snack and helps the patient make appropriate food choices. This method is effective in achieving overall blood glucose control when carbohydrate intake is consistent from day to day.

Patients using intensive insulin or pump therapies can use CHO counting to determine insulin coverage. After the amount of insulin needed to cover the usual meal is determined, insulin may be added or subtracted for changes in carbohydrate intake. An initial formula of 1 unit of rapid-acting insulin for each 15 g of carbohydrate provides flexibility to meal plans. The patient determines the grams of carbohydrate in a specific meal or snack by reading labels or weighing and measuring each item. The total grams of carbohydrate are used to calculate the bolus dose of insulin based on his or her prescribed insulin-to-carbohydrate ratio.

People at high risk for type 2 diabetes are encouraged to achieve moderate weight loss (7% total body weight), participate in regular physical activity (150 minutes per week), and reduce caloric and dietary fat intake. These at-risk people are also encouraged to increase fiber intake to at least 14 g per 1000 calories consumed and to eat foods containing whole grains.

Special considerations for type 1 diabetes include developing insulin regimens that conform to the patient's preferred meal routines, food preferences, and exercise patterns. Patients using rapid-acting insulin by injection or an insulin pump should adjust insulin doses based on the carbohydrate content of the meals and snacks. Insulin-to-carbohydrate ratios are developed and are used to provide mealtime insulin doses. Blood glucose monitoring before and 2 hours after meals determines whether the insulin-to-carbohydrate ratio is correct. For patients who are on fixed insulin regimens and do not adjust premeal insulin dosages, consistency of timing of meals and the amount of CHO eaten at each meal is important to prevent hypoglycemia.

Exercise can cause hypoglycemia if insulin is not decreased before activity. For planned exercise, reduction in insulin dosage is used for hypoglycemia prevention. For unplanned exercise, intake of additional CHO is usually needed. Moderate exercise increases glucose utilization by 2 to 3 mg/kg/min. A 70-kg (154-lb) person would need about 10 to 15 g additional CHO per hour of moderate-intensity activity. More CHO is needed for intense activity.

It is important for patients with type 1 diabetes to avoid gaining weight. Chronic high insulin levels (hyperinsulinemia) can occur with intensive management schedules and may result in weight gain. These patients may need to manage hyperglycemia by restricting calories rather than increasing insulin. Weight gain can be minimized by following the prescribed meal plan, getting regular exercise, and avoiding overtreatment of hypoglycemia.

Special considerations for type 2 diabetes focus on lifestyle changes. Many patients with type 2 diabetes are overweight and insulin resistant. NUTRITION therapy stresses lifestyle changes that reduce calories eaten and increase calories expended through physical activity. Many patients also have abnormal blood fat levels and hypertension (metabolic syndrome), making reductions of saturated fat, cholesterol, and sodium desirable. A moderate caloric restriction (250 to 500 calories less than average daily intake) and an increase in physical activity improve diabetes control and weight control. Decreases of more than 10% of body weight can result in significant improvement in A1C. Decreasing intake of cholesterol-raising fatty acids helps reduce the risk for cardiovascular disease.

When patients with type 2 diabetes need insulin, consistency in timing and carbohydrate content of meals is important. Division of the total daily calories into three meals or into smaller meals and snacks is based on patient preference.

CONSIDERATIONS FOR OLDER ADULTS
Patient-Centered Care QSEN

Older patients are at increased risk for poor nutrition, hypoglycemia, and especially dehydration, a factor in the development of hyperglycemic-hyperosmolar state (HHS). Many factors contribute to malnutrition. Nutrition needs of the older adult change as the person's taste, smell, and appetite diminish and his or her ability to obtain and prepare food decreases. Older patients who prepare their own food or have tooth loss or poorly fitting dentures may not eat enough food. Neuropathy with gastric retention or diarrhea compounds poor food intake. Impaired cognition and depression may disrupt self-care. Older patients may have a marginal food supply because of inadequate income, may have poor understanding of meal-planning needs, or may live alone and have reduced incentive to prepare or eat proper meals. They may eat in restaurants or live in situations in which they have little control over meal preparation. Regular visits by home health nurses can assist older patients in following a diabetic meal plan.

A realistic approach to nutrition therapy is essential for the older patient with diabetes. Changing the eating habits of 60 to 70 years is very difficult. The nurse, dietitian, and patient assess the patient's usual eating patterns. Teach the older patient taking antidiabetic drugs about the importance of eating meals and snacks at the same time every day, eating the same amount of food from day to day, and eating all food allowed on the diet.

Exercise Therapy. Regular exercise is an essential part of diabetic management. It has beneficial effects on carbohydrate metabolism and insulin sensitivity. Programs of increased physical activity and weight loss reduce the incidence of type 2 diabetes in patients with impaired glucose tolerance (American Association of Diabetes Educators [AADE], 2011).

Blood glucose levels remain stable in physically active patients without diabetes because of the balance between glucose use by exercising muscles and glucose production by the liver. The patient with type 1 DM cannot make the hormonal changes needed to maintain stable blood glucose levels during exercise. Without an adequate insulin supply, cells cannot use glucose. Low insulin levels trigger release of glucagon and epinephrine (counterregulatory hormones) to increase liver glucose production, further raising blood glucose levels. In the absence of insulin, free fatty acids become the source of energy. Exercise in the patient with uncontrolled diabetes results in further hyperglycemia and the formation of ketone bodies. He or she may have prolonged elevated blood glucose levels after vigorous exercise.

Exercise in the person with diabetes also can cause hypoglycemia because of increased muscle glucose uptake and inhibited glucose release from the liver. It can occur during exercise and for up to 24 hours after exercise. Replacement of muscle and liver glycogen stores, along with increased insulin sensitivity after exercise, causes insulin requirements to drop.

Benefits of Exercise. Appropriate exercise results in better blood GLUCOSE REGULATION and reduced insulin requirements for patients with type 1 DM. Exercise also increases insulin sensitivity, which enhances cell uptake of glucose and promotes weight loss.

Regular exercise decreases risk for cardiovascular disease. It decreases most blood lipid levels and increases high-density lipoproteins (HDLs). Exercise decreases blood pressure and improves cardiovascular function. Regular vigorous physical activity prevents or delays type 2 DM by reducing body weight, insulin resistance, and glucose intolerance.

Adjustments for Diabetes Complications. Exercise in the presence of long-term complications of diabetes often requires some adjustment. Vigorous aerobic or resistance exercise should be avoided in the presence of proliferative diabetic retinopathy or severe nonproliferative diabetic retinopathy. Teach the patient with retinopathy to avoid the *Valsalva maneuver* (breath holding while bearing down) and activities that increase blood pressure. Heavy lifting, rapid head motion, or jarring activities can cause vitreous hemorrhage or retinal detachment. Decreased pain sensation in the extremities increases the risk for skin breakdown and infection and for joint destruction. Teach patients with diabetic peripheral neuropathy (DPN) to wear proper footwear and to examine their feet daily for lesions. Teach anyone with a foot injury or open sore to engage in non-weight-bearing activities such as swimming, bicycling, seated yoga, or arm exercises. Those with autonomic neuropathy are at increased risk for exercise-induced injury from impaired temperature control, postural hypotension, and impaired thirst with risk for dehydration. Physical activity also can increase urine protein excretion. Encourage high-risk patients to start with short periods of low-intensity exercise and to increase the intensity and duration slowly (ADA, 2013).

Safety Assessment. Assessment before initiating an exercise program is necessary to ensure patient safety. Although current ADA guidelines do not recommend routine screening for patients with diabetes who have no manifestations of cardiovascular disease, be alert to conditions that might predispose the patient to injury or that contraindicate certain types of exercise. Regular physical activity increases the risk for both musculoskeletal injury and life-threatening cardiovascular events. Patients with diabetes often take drugs to reduce blood pressure, to normalize blood lipid concentrations, and to inhibit platelet activity. These drugs may increase fall risk, change physiologic response to exercise and physical activity, alter muscle performance, and increase bleeding risk (Sisson et al., 2012). The ADA recommends screening when any of these conditions exist:

- Chest pain or discomfort
- Abnormal electrocardiogram (ECG) suggestive of ischemia or infarction
- Peripheral or carotid occlusive disease
- Age older than 35 years with sedentary lifestyle in a patient who plans a vigorous exercise program
- Two or more risk factors in addition to diabetes, such as dyslipidemia, hypertension, tobacco use
- Family history for premature coronary artery disease, or microalbuminuria or macroalbuminuria of more than 10 years' duration
- Age older than 25 years and type 1 diabetes of more than 15 years' duration
- Severe autonomic neuropathy, severe diabetic peripheral neuropathy, history of foot lesions, and unstable proliferative retinopathy

Screening for coronary artery disease before an exercise program is started is recommended for patients with cardiovascular risk factors. Exercise treadmill testing (ETT) is used to determine if a person can exercise to 85% of his or her predicted heart rate without having ischemic changes. It also provides information about exercise capacity and functional status. Failure to achieve 85% of the predicted heart rate is associated with increased incidence of death.

Other studies to determine the risk for exercise-induced problems include medical stress tests with vasodilator therapy and stress echocardiography. Additional tests may be performed to determine the presence of obstructive lesions in coronary arteries.

Advise people with DM to perform at least 150 min/wk of moderate-intensive aerobic physical activity or 75 min/wk of vigorous aerobic physical activity or an equivalent combination of the two. In the absence of contraindications, patients with type 2 diabetes are urged to perform resistance exercise 3 times a week, targeting all major muscle groups (ADA 2013). The ADA recommends that there be no more than 2 consecutive days without aerobic physical activity.

A 5- to 10-minute warm-up period with stretching and low-intensity exercise before exercise prepares the skeletal muscles, heart, and lungs for a progressive increase in exercise intensity. After the activity session, a cool-down should be performed similarly to the warm-up. The cool-down should last 5 to 10 minutes and gradually bring the heart rate down to pre-exercise level.

Guidelines for exercise are based on blood glucose levels and urine ketone levels. Recommend that the patient test blood glucose before exercise, at intervals during exercise, and after exercise to determine if it is safe to exercise and to evaluate the effects of exercise. The absence of urine ketones indicates that enough insulin is available for glucose transport and that exercise should be effective in lowering blood glucose levels. *When urine ketones are present, the patient should **NOT** exercise.* Ketones indicate that current insulin levels are not adequate and

---

! NURSING SAFETY PRIORITY (QSEN)

Critical Rescue

Teach patients with type 1 diabetes to perform vigorous exercise only when blood glucose levels are 100 to 250 mg/dL (5.6 to 13.8 mmol/L) and no ketones are present in the urine.

CONSIDERATIONS FOR OLDER ADULTS

Patient-Centered Care (QSEN)

With age, the ability of the heart and lungs to deliver oxygen to tissues and organs declines. Muscle strength and power decline gradually. Connective tissue becomes less elastic, affecting range of motion and flexibility. Limited range of motion can alter gait, increasing risk for falls. Older adults who remain active can limit losses in muscle mass and function.

The emphasis for any activity program is on changing sedentary behavior to active behavior at any level. Encourage sedentary older adults to begin with low-intensity physical activity. Start low-intensity activities in short sessions (less than 10 minutes); include warm-up and cool-down components with active stretching. Changes in activity levels should be gradual. Formal evaluation by a physical therapist or occupational therapist may be needed. Examples of specific exercise can be found at www.geri.com.

CHART 64-4 Patient and Family Education: Preparing for Self-Management

Exercise

- Teach the patient about the relationship between regularly scheduled exercise and blood glucose levels, blood lipid levels, and complications of diabetes.
- Reinforce the level of exercise recommended for the patient based on his or her physical health.
- Instruct the patient to wear appropriate footwear designed for exercise.
- Remind the patient to examine his or her feet daily and after exercising.
- Remind the patient to stay hydrated and not to exercise in extreme heat or cold.
- Warn the patient not to exercise within 1 hour of insulin injection or near the time of peak insulin action.
- Teach patients how to prevent hypoglycemia during exercise:
  - Do not exercise unless blood glucose level is at least 80 and less than 250 mg/dL.
  - Have a carbohydrate snack before exercising if 1 hour has passed since the last meal or if the planned exercise is high intensity.
  - Carry a simple sugar to eat during exercise if symptoms of hypoglycemia occur.
  - Ensure that identification information about diabetes is carried during exercise.
- Remind the patient to check blood glucose levels more frequently on days in which exercise is performed and that extra carbohydrate and less insulin may be needed during the 24-hour period after extensive exercise.

---

that exercise would elevate blood glucose levels. Carbohydrate foods should be ingested to raise blood glucose levels above 100 mg/dL (5.6 mmol/L) before engaging in exercise. Chart 64-4 lists tips to teach the patient and family about self-management and exercise.

Blood Glucose Control in Hospitalized Patients. Hyperglycemia in hospitalized patients occurs for many reasons and is associated with poor outcomes (Kubacka, 2014). In patients without a previous diagnosis of diabetes, elevated blood glucose is often "stress hyperglycemia." Hyperglycemia may result from decline in basic level of GLUCOSE REGULATION caused by illness, decreased physical activity, withholding of antidiabetic drugs, use of drugs that cause hyperglycemia such as corticosteroids, and initiation of tube feedings or parenteral nutrition (Freeland & Funnell, 2012).

Hyperglycemia among medical-surgical patients is linked with higher infection rates, longer hospital stays, increased need for intensive care, and greater mortality. Admission glucose levels greater than 198 mg/dL (10.9 mmol/L) are associated with greater risk for mortality and complications. Hypoglycemia, defined as blood glucose values lower than 40 mg/dL (2.2 mmol/L), is an independent risk factor for mortality.

Current American Association of Clinical Endocrinologists (AACE) and ADA Core Measures recommend treatment protocols that maintain blood glucose levels between 140 and 180 mg/dL (7.8 and 10.0 mmol/L) for critically ill patients. For the majority of non–critically ill patients, premeal glucose targets should be lower than 140 mg/dL (7.8 mmol/L) with random blood glucose values less than 180 mg/dL (10.0 mmol/L). To prevent hypoglycemia, insulin regimens should be reviewed if blood glucose levels fall below 100 mg/dL (5.6 mmol/L) and should be modified when blood glucose levels are less than 70 mg/dL (3.9 mmol/L) (ADA, 2013).

Continuous IV insulin solutions are the most effective method for achieving glycemic targets in the intensive care setting. Scheduled subcutaneous injection with basal, meal, and correction elements is the preferred method for achieving and maintaining glucose control in non–critically ill patients. Using correction dose or "supplemental insulin" to correct premeal hyperglycemia in addition to scheduled prandial and basal insulin is recommended. The correction dose is determined by the patient's insulin sensitivity and current blood glucose level.

Prevention of hypoglycemia is also part of managing blood glucose levels. Causes of inpatient hypoglycemia include an inappropriate insulin type, mismatch between insulin type and/or timing of food intake, and altered eating plan without insulin dosage adjustment. The Joint Commission (TJC), together with the ADA, has established Core Measures for preventing hypoglycemia in the inpatient care of people with diabetes (The Joint Commission [TJC], 2014). These involve protocols for hypoglycemia treatment that direct staff to provide carbohydrate replacement if the patient is alert and able to swallow or to administer 50% dextrose intravenously or glucagon by subcutaneous injection if the patient cannot swallow.

There is confusion about whether to give or to hold insulin from a patient who is NPO. Administration of rapid-acting or short-acting insulin, as well as amylin and incretin mimetics, will cause hypoglycemia if a patient is not eating. Basal insulin should be administered when the patient is NPO because it controls baseline glucose levels. Insulin mixtures are not administered because they contain some short-acting or rapid-acting insulin and will cause hypoglycemia.

Surgical Management. Surgical interventions for diabetes include a pancreas transplantation. When successful, this procedure eliminates the need for insulin injections, blood glucose monitoring, and many dietary restrictions. It can eliminate the acute complications related to blood glucose control but is only partially successful in reversing long-term diabetes complications. Pancreatic transplant is successful when the patient no longer needs insulin therapy and all blood measures of glucose are normal.

Transplantation requires lifelong drug therapy to prevent graft rejection. These drug regimens have toxic side effects that restrict their use to patients who have serious progressive complications of diabetes. In addition, some anti-rejection drugs have the effect of increasing blood glucose levels. Pancreas-alone transplants are most often considered for patients with severe metabolic complications and for those with consistent failure of insulin-based therapy to prevent acute complications.

Pancreas transplantation is considered in patients with diabetes and end-stage kidney disease who have had or plan to have a kidney transplant. Normal blood glucose levels after pancreas transplantation improve kidney graft survival. Pancreas graft survival is better when performed at the time of the kidney transplant.

Whole-Pancreas Transplantation. Improved surgical techniques and newer anti-rejection drugs have improved transplantation outcomes. The 1-year survival rate for patients is above 95%, with more than 83% of patients remaining free of insulin injection and diet restrictions after 1 year. The degree of tissue-type matching affects the results.

Pancreatic transplantation is performed in one of three ways: pancreas transplant alone (PTA), pancreas after kidney (PAK)

transplant, and simultaneous pancreas and kidney (SPK) transplant. SPK transplant is the ideal procedure for patients with DM and uremia.

Operative Procedure. Most pancreatic transplants are from cadaver donors using a total pancreas still attached to the exit of the pancreatic duct. The recipient's pancreas is left in place, and the donated pancreas is placed in the pelvis. The insulin released by the pancreas graft is secreted into the bloodstream. The new pancreas also produces about 800 to 1000 mL of fluid daily, which is diverted to either the bladder or the bowel.

Excretion of pancreatic fluids can cause dehydration and electrolyte imbalance, and drainage of these fluids into the urinary bladder causes irritation. When the pancreas is attached to the bladder, the loss of fluid rich in bicarbonate may cause acidosis.

Rejection Management. A combination of drugs and antibodies is used to reverse rejection. (See Chapter 17 for a listing of agents used to prevent or manage transplant rejection.) Patients undergoing anti-rejection therapy first receive drugs to prevent viral, bacterial, and fungal infection because of the risk for opportunistic INFECTIONS. Most patients receiving high-dose steroids, as well as those on chronic long-term steroid therapy, will require dosage adjustments in insulin to achieve desired levels of glucose control.

In most episodes of rejections, kidney problems occur before pancreatic problems. An increase in serum creatinine indicates rejection of both the transplanted kidney and the pancreas. In patients with bladder drainage of pancreatic hormones, a decrease in the urine amylase level by 25% is an indication to treat rejection. High blood glucose levels are a later marker of rejection and usually indicate irreversible graft failure.

Long-Term Effects. Long-term anti-rejection therapy increases the risk for INFECTION, cancer, and atherosclerosis. When insulin drains into systemic rather than portal (liver) circulation, blood insulin levels rise (hyperinsulinemia) and increase the risk for hypertension and macrovascular disease.

Complications. Complications are common in patients taking long-term anti-rejection therapy. Monitor laboratory values, fluid and electrolyte status, physical changes, and changes in vital signs to identify possible complications. Early removal of IV and intra-arterial lines, use of sterile technique with dressing changes and catheter irrigations, strict handwashing by all health care personnel, and good pulmonary hygiene help prevent INFECTION.

Complications immediately after surgery include thrombosis, pancreatitis, anastomosis leak with INFECTION, and rejection of the transplanted pancreas. Pancreatic blood vessel thrombosis occurs in about 30% of patients after transplantation. Observe for and report any sudden drop in urine amylase levels, rapid increases in blood glucose, gross **hematuria** (bloody urine), and tenderness or pain in the graft area (iliac fossa). Pancreatitis in the transplanted organ occurs to some degree in all patients after surgery. Report elevations in serum amylase that persist after 48 to 96 hours.

The most serious complication of enteric-drained pancreas transplantation is leaking and INFECTION with intra-abdominal abscess formation. Observe for and report elevation in temperature, abdominal discomfort, and elevation in white blood cell (WBC) count. Bladder-drained pancreas transplantation has a lower rate of intra-abdominal abscess formation. However, drainage of bicarbonate-rich fluid with pancreatic enzymes into the urinary bladder can cause urinary tract infections, cystitis, urethritis, and balanitis. Metabolic acidosis occurs from the loss of large amounts of alkaline pancreatic secretions.

Assess for and document manifestations of rejection. In acute rejection, decreased kidney function is indicated by increased serum creatinine, decreased urine output, hypertension, increased weight, graft tenderness, and fever. Proteinuria is often the first indicator of chronic graft rejection. Check for increased blood amylase, lipase, or glucose; decreased urine amylase; graft tenderness; hyperglycemia; and fever. *It is especially important to assess for* INFECTION *and start appropriate therapy. Fever can indicate both infection and rejection.*

Monitor for side effects of the anti-rejection drugs. Cyclosporine (Neoral) is toxic to the kidney. Indications of toxicity are elevated creatinine and decreased urine output. Monitor WBC counts daily, because azathioprine (Imuran) can suppress bone marrow function. Common side effects of tacrolimus (Prograf) are hypertension, kidney toxicity, neurotoxicity, GI toxicity, and glucose intolerance. Prednisone has many side effects, including elevated blood glucose levels.

Islet Cell Transplantation. Islet cell transplantation eliminates the need for insulin and protects against the complications of diabetes. Wider use of this procedure is hindered by the limited supply of beta cells available for transplantation and by issues related to rejection. Islet cells from tissue-typed (HLA-matched) cadaver pancreas glands are injected into the portal vein. The new cells lodge in the liver and begin to function, secreting insulin and maintaining near-perfect blood glucose control.

Islet cell transplantation may successfully restore long-term endogenous insulin production and glycemic control in patients with type 1 diabetes and unstable baseline control. Most patients undergoing this procedure eventually have a progressive loss of islet cell function. Very few islet cell transplant recipients have remained insulin-free for more than 4 years. The reasons for this gradual loss of function are not known and make this procedure a long-term but temporary intervention. It is considered an experimental procedure.

Enhancing Surgical Recovery

Planning: Expected Outcomes. The patient with diabetes undergoing a surgical procedure is expected to recover completely without complications. Indicators include:
- Wound healing
- Absence of infection
- Maintenance of blood glucose levels within expected range

Interventions. Surgery is a physical and emotional stressor, and the patient with diabetes has a higher risk for complications. Anesthesia and surgery cause a stress response with release of counterregulatory hormones that elevate blood glucose. Stress hormones suppress insulin action, increasing the risk for ketoacidosis. Hyperglycemic-hyperosmolar state (HHS) is a common complication after major surgery and is associated with increased mortality. Diuresis from hyperglycemia can cause dehydration and increases the risk for kidney failure.

Complications of diabetes increase the risk for surgical complications. Patients with DM are at higher risk for hypertension, ischemic heart disease, cerebrovascular disease, MI, and cardiomyopathy. Heart failure is a serious risk factor and must be improved before surgery. Autonomic neuropathy may result in sudden tachycardia, bradycardia, or postural hypotension. The patient with DM is at risk for acute kidney injury and urinary retention after surgery, especially if he or she has albumin in the urine (indicator of kidney damage). Nerves to the intestinal wall

and sphincters can be impaired, leading to delayed gastric emptying and reflux of gastric acid, which increases the risk for aspiration with anesthesia. Autonomic neuropathy may cause paralytic ileus after surgery.

Preoperative Care. Patients undergoing major surgery are admitted to the hospital 2 to 3 days before surgery to optimize blood glucose control. Sulfonylureas are discontinued 1 day before surgery. Metformin (Glucophage) is stopped at least 24 hours before surgery and restarted only after kidney function is normal. All other oral drugs are stopped the day of surgery. Patients taking long-acting insulin may need to be switched to intermediate-acting insulin forms 1 to 2 days before surgery.

Preoperative blood glucose levels should be less than 200 mg/dL (11.1 mmol/L). Higher levels are associated with increased INFECTION rates and impaired wound healing.

Plan ahead for pain control after surgery. PAIN, a stressor, triggers the release of counterregulatory hormones, increasing blood glucose levels and insulin needs. Opioid analgesics slow GI motility and alter blood glucose levels. The older patient who receives opioids is more at risk for confusion, paralytic ileus, hypoventilation, hypotension, and urinary retention. Patient-controlled analgesia (PCA) systems reduce respiratory complications and confusion. (See Chapter 3 for pain interventions and Chapter 14 for general preoperative care.)

Intraoperative Care. IV infusion of insulin, glucose, and potassium is standard therapy for perioperative management of diabetes. In accordance with The Joint Commission's NPSGs, the objective is to keep the blood glucose level between 140 and 180 mg/dL (7.8 and 10.0 mmol/L) during surgery to prevent hypoglycemia and reduce risks from hyperglycemia (TJC, 2014). Insulin/glucose infusion rates are based on hourly capillary glucose tests. Higher insulin doses may be needed because stress releases glucagon and epinephrine. Patients with DM usually receive about 5 g of glucose per hour during surgery to prevent hypoglycemia, ketosis, and protein breakdown.

Monitor the patient's temperature—it may be lowered deliberately in some surgical procedures and inadvertently in others. Low operating room temperatures and large incisions also lower body temperature. Hypothermia decreases metabolic needs, depresses heart rate and contractility, causes vasoconstriction, and impairs insulin release, resulting in high blood glucose levels. Monitor arterial blood gas values for acidosis.

Postoperative Care. Hyperglycemia is associated with increased mortality after surgical procedures. Current AACE and ADA Core Measures recommend insulin protocols that maintain blood glucose between 140 and 180 mg/dL (7.8 and 10.0 mmol/L) for critically ill patients (ADA, 2013).

Protocols and computer-based programs can be used to determine the insulin infusion rate required to maintain blood glucose levels within a defined target range. Many insulin infusion algorithms are implemented by nursing staff. Continue glucose and insulin infusions as prescribed until the patient is stable and can tolerate oral feedings. Short-term insulin therapy may be needed after surgery for the patient who usually uses oral agents. For those receiving insulin therapy, dosage adjustments may be required until the stress of surgery subsides.

Monitoring. Patients with autonomic neuropathy or vascular disease need close monitoring to avoid hypotension or respiratory arrest. Those who take beta blockers for hypertension need close monitoring for hypoglycemia because these drugs mask manifestations of hypoglycemia. Patients with increased protein or nitrogen waste products in the blood may have problems with fluid management. Check central venous pressure or pulmonary artery pressure as needed.

Glucose levels are a sensitive marker of counterregulatory hormones, which are often activated before patients become febrile. Hyperglycemia often occurs before a fever.

Hyperkalemia (high blood potassium level) is common in patients with mild to moderate kidney failure and can lead to cardiac dysrhythmia. In other patients, hypokalemia (low blood potassium level) may occur and be made worse by insulin and glucose given during surgery. Monitor the cardiac rhythm and serum potassium values.

Cardiovascular monitoring by continuous electrocardiograms (ECGs) is recommended for older patients with diabetes, those with long-standing type 1 DM, and those with heart disease. Patients with diabetes are at higher risk for MI after surgery with a higher mortality rate. Changes in ECG or in potassium level may indicate a silent MI.

Kidney monitoring, especially observing fluid balance, helps detect acute kidney injury (AKI). Diagnosis of kidney impairment may require the use of x-ray studies using dyes, which may be nephrotoxic. Management of INFECTION may require the use of nephrotoxic antibiotics. Ensure adequate hydration when these drugs are used. Check for impending kidney failure by assessing fluid and electrolyte status.

Nutrition. Patients requiring clear or full liquid diets should receive about 200 g of carbohydrate daily in equally divided amounts at meals and snack times. Initial liquids should not be sugar-free. Most patients require 25 to 35 calories per kg of body weight every 24 hours. After surgery, food intake is initiated as quickly as possible with progression from clear liquids to solid foods occurring as rapidly as tolerated. Returning to a normal meal plan as soon as possible after surgery promotes healing and metabolic balance. When oral foods are tolerated, make sure the patient takes at least 150 to 200 g of carbohydrate daily to prevent hypoglycemia.

If total parenteral nutrition (TPN) is used after surgery, severe hyperglycemia may occur. Monitor blood glucose often to determine the need for supplemental insulin.

Preventing Injury from Peripheral Neuropathy

Planning: Expected Outcomes. The patient with diabetes is expected to identify factors that increase the risk for injury, practice proper foot care, and maintain skin TISSUE INTEGRITY on the feet. Indicators include that the patient consistently demonstrates these behaviors:

- Cleanses and inspects the feet daily
- Wears properly fitting shoes
- Avoids walking in bare feet
- Trims toenails properly
- Reports nonhealing breaks in the skin of the feet to the health care provider

Interventions. Patients with DM need intensive teaching about foot care. *Foot injury is the most common complication of diabetes leading to hospitalization.* Once a failure of TISSUE

INTEGRITY has occurred and an ulcer has developed, there is an increased risk for wound progression that will eventually lead to amputation. Almost all lower extremity amputations are preceded by foot ulcers. The 5-year mortality rate after leg or foot amputation ranges from 39% to 67% (National Institute of Diabetes and Digestive and Kidney Diseases [NIDDK], 2011). Neuropathy is the main factor for development of a diabetic ulcer, and an inadequate vascular supply is the main cause of poor healing (Thomas, 2013).

Motor neuropathy damages the nerves of foot muscles, resulting in foot deformities. These deformities create pressure points that gradually cause reduced TISSUE INTEGRITY with skin breakdown and ulceration. Thinning or shifting of the fat pad under the metatarsal heads decreases cushioning and increases areas of pressure. In claw toe deformity, toes are hyperextended and increase pressure on the metatarsal heads ("ball" of the foot). These changes predispose the patient to callus formation, ulceration, and INFECTION. The Charcot foot is a type of diabetic foot deformity with many abnormalities, often including a hallux valgus (turning inward of the great toe) (Fig. 64-6). The foot is warm, swollen, and painful. Walking collapses the arch, shortens the foot, and gives the sole of the foot a "rocker bottom" shape.

Autonomic neuropathy causes loss of normal sweating and skin temperature regulation, resulting in dry, thinning skin. Skin cracks and fissures increase the risk for INFECTION. Sensory neuropathy may cause PAIN, tingling, or burning (Funnell, 2014). More often it produces numbness and reduced SENSORY PERCEPTION. Without sensation, the patient does not notice injuries and loss of TISSUE INTEGRITY in the foot and does not treat them. Peripheral arterial disease reduces the blood supply to the foot, increasing the risk for ulcer formation and reducing the rate of ulcer healing (McCance et al., 2014).

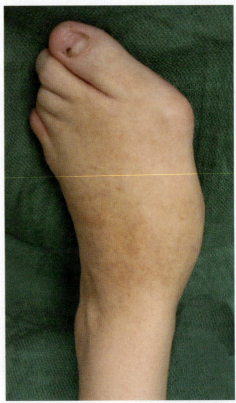

FIG. 64-6 A "Charcot foot" type of diabetic foot deformity.

Foot injuries can be caused by walking barefoot, wearing ill-fitting shoes, sustaining thermal injuries from heat (e.g., hot water bottles, heating pads, baths), or chemical burns from over-the-counter corn treatments. These injuries can lead to loss of TISSUE INTEGRITY and to amputation.

Ulcers result from continued pressure. Plantar ulcers (on the sole, usually the ball) are from standing or walking. Those on the top or sides of the foot usually are from shoes. The increased pressure causes calluses. Ulcers usually form over or around the great toe, under the metatarsal heads, and on the tops of claw toes.

Loss of TISSUE INTEGRITY with broken skin increases the risk for INFECTION. Skin tends to break in areas of pressure. Infection is common in diabetic foot ulcers and, once present, is difficult to treat. Infection also impairs GLUCOSE REGULATION, leading to higher blood glucose levels and reduced immune defenses, which further increases the risk for infection.

Prevention of High-Risk Conditions. Neuropathy of the feet and legs can be delayed by keeping blood glucose levels as near to normal as possible. Poor blood glucose control increases the risk for neuropathy and amputation. Urge smoking cessation to reduce the risk for vascular complications.

The risk for ulcers or amputation increases with duration of diabetes. Other associated factors are male gender; poor glucose control; and cardiovascular, retinal, or kidney complications. Foot-related risks include poor gait and stepping mechanics, peripheral neuropathy, increased pressure (callus, erythema, hemorrhage under a callus, limited joint mobility, foot deformities, or severe nail pathology), peripheral vascular disease, and a history of ulcers or amputation.

Peripheral Neuropathy Management. The feet should be evaluated closely at least annually. Chart 22-9 in Chapter 22 lists self-management activities for prevention of injury from peripheral neuropathy, and Table 64-10 lists foot risk categories.

Complete a full foot assessment as outlined in Chart 64-5. Sensory examination with Semmes-Weinstein monofilaments is a practical measure of the risk for foot ulcers. The nylon monofilament is mounted on a holder standardized to exert a 10-g force. A person who cannot feel the 10-g pressure at any point is at increased risk for ulcers. To perform the examination:

- Provide a quiet and relaxed setting. Ask the patient to close his or her eyes during the test.
- Test the monofilament on the patient's cheek so he or she knows what to expect.
- Test the sites noted in Fig. 64-7.
- Apply the monofilament at a right angle to the skin surface.
- Apply enough force to bend the filament using a smooth, not jabbing, motion (Fig. 64-8).

CHART 64-5   Focused Assessment

The Diabetic Foot

Assess the patient for risk for diabetic foot problems:
- History of previous ulcer
- History of previous amputation
- Assess the foot for abnormal skin and nail conditions:
- Dry, cracked, fissured skin
- Ulcers
- Toenails: thickened, long nails; ingrown nails
- Tinea pedis; onychomycosis (mycotic nails)

Assess the foot for status of circulation:
- Manifestations of claudication
- Presence or absence of dorsalis pedis or posterior tibial pulse
- Prolonged capillary filling time (greater than 25 seconds)
- Presence or absence of hair growth on the top of the foot

Assess the foot for evidence of deformity:
- Calluses, corns
- Prominent metatarsal heads (metatarsal head is easily felt under the skin)
- Toe contractures: clawed toes, hammertoes
- Hallux valgus or bunions
- Charcot foot ("rocker bottom")

Assess the foot for loss of strength:
- Limited ankle joint range of motion
- Limited motion of great toe

Assess the foot for loss of protective sensation:
- Numbness, burning, tingling
- Semmes-Weinstein monofilament testing at 10 points on each foot

---

TABLE 64-10   Foot Risk Categories

RISK CATEGORIES	MANAGEMENT CATEGORIES
Risk Category 0	**Management Category 0**
• Has protective sensation • No evidence of peripheral vascular disease • No evidence of foot deformity	• Comprehensive foot examination once a year • Patient education to include advice on appropriate footwear
Risk Category 1	**Management Category 1**
• Does not have protective sensation • May have evidence of foot deformity	• Evaluation every 3-6 months • Consider referral to a specialist to assess need for specialized treatment and follow-up • Patient education
Risk Category 2	**Management Categories 2 & 3**
• Does not have protective sensation • Evidence of peripheral vascular disease	• Evaluation every 1-3 months • Referral to a specialist • Prescription footwear • Consider vascular consultation for combined follow-up • Patient education
Risk Category 3	
• History of ulcer or amputation	

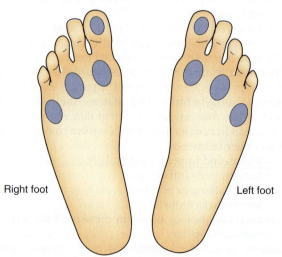

Right foot   Left foot

FIG. 64-7 Placement sites of monofilaments for testing of protective sensation.

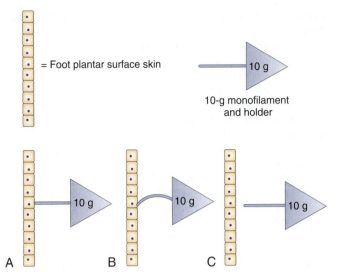

FIG. 64-8 Correct technique for sensation testing with 10-g monofilament. **A,** Apply monofilament to designated areas of the foot sole (intact skin only; see Fig. 64-7). **B,** Apply pressure to the filament either until the patient states he or she can feel the pressure or until the filament bends (see pp. 1326-1327). **C,** Quickly remove the filament without sliding it or touching other areas of the foot. *BUN,* Blood urea nitrogen; *Ca²⁺,* calcium; *HCO₃⁻,* bicarbonate; *K⁺,* potassium; *Mg²⁺,* magnesium; *Na⁺,* sodium; *PO₄,* phosphate.

- The approach, contact, and removal of the filament at each site should take 1 to 2 seconds.
- Apply the filament along the perimeter and **not** on an ulcer site, callus, scar, or necrotic tissue. Do not slide the filament across the skin or make repeated contact at the test site.

Randomize the sequence of applying the filament throughout the examination. Have the patient identify where the filament touched rather than asking "Do you feel this?"

Footwear. All patients with any degree of peripheral neuropathy are at risk for loss of TISSUE INTEGRITY and need to wear protective shoes. It is best to be fitted by an experienced shoe fitter, such as a certified podiatrist. The shoe should be ½ to ⅝ inch longer than the longest toe. Heels should be less than 2 inches high. Shoes that are too tight damage tissue. Instruct the patient to change shoes by midday and again in the evening. Socks or stockings need to fit properly and be appropriate for the planned activity. Socks should feel soft and have no thick seams, creases, or holes. They should pad the foot and absorb excess moisture. Teach patients to avoid tight stockings or those that have constricting bands. Patients with toe deformities should buy custom shoes with high, wide toe boxes and extra depth. Those with severely deformed feet, such as Charcot feet, need specially molded shoes. All new shoes need a long break-in period with frequent inspection for irritation or blistering.

Foot Care. Teach patients about preventive foot care and the need for examination of the feet and legs at each visit to a health care provider. Identify patients with high-risk foot conditions. Explain problems caused by loss of protective SENSORY PERCEPTION, the importance of monitoring the feet daily, proper care of the feet (including nail and skin care), and how to select appropriate footwear.

Assess the patient's ability to inspect all areas of the foot and to perform foot care. Teach family members how to inspect and care for the patient's feet if the patient cannot. Chart 64-6 lists foot care instructions for self-management.

CHART 64-6 **Patient and Family Education: Preparing for Self-Management**

Foot Care Instructions

- Inspect your feet daily, especially the area between the toes.
- Wash your feet daily with lukewarm water and soap. Dry thoroughly.
- Apply moisturizing cream to your feet after bathing. Do not apply to the area between your toes.
- Change into clean cotton socks every day.
- Do not wear the same pair of shoes 2 days in a row, and wear only shoes made of breathable materials, such as leather or cloth.
- Check your shoes for foreign objects (nails, pebbles) before putting them on. Check inside the shoes for cracks or tears in the lining.
- Purchase shoes that have plenty of room for your toes. Buy shoes later in the day, when feet are normally larger. Break in new shoes gradually.
- Wear socks to keep your feet warm.
- Trim your nails straight across with a nail clipper. Smooth the nails with an emery board.
- See your physician or nurse immediately if you have blisters, sores, or infections. Protect the area with a dry, sterile dressing. Do not use adhesive tape to secure dressing to the skin.
- Do not treat blisters, sores, or infections with home remedies.
- Do not smoke.
- Do not step into the bathtub without checking the temperature of the water with your wrist or thermometer. Optimal temperature is 95° F (35° C). Maximum temperature is 110° F (43° C).
- Do not use very hot or cold water. Never use hot water bottles, heating pads, or portable heaters to warm your feet.
- Do not treat corns, blisters, bunions, calluses, or ingrown toenails yourself.
- Do not go barefooted.
- Do not wear sandals with open toes or straps between the toes.
- Do not cross your legs or wear garters or tight stockings that constrict blood flow.
- Do not soak your feet.

Wound Care. The standards of care for diabetic ulcers are a moist wound environment, débridement of necrotic tissue, and elimination of pressure (offloading). Proper wound care and débridement are presented in Chapter 25.

Eliminating pressure on an infected area is essential to wound healing. Teach patients with foot ulcers to not wear a shoe on the affected foot while the ulcer is healing. Those with poor SENSORY PERCEPTION may keep walking on an ulcer because it does not hurt. This results in pressure necrosis that delays healing and increases ulcer size. Pressure is reduced by specialized orthotic devices, custom-molded shoe inserts, or shoe adjustments that redistribute weight.

Offloading redistributes force away from ulcer sites and pressure points to wider areas of the foot. Available products include total-contact casting, half shoes, removable cast walkers, wheelchairs, and crutches. Total-contact casts redistribute pressure over the bottom of the foot. Casting material is molded to the foot and leg to spread pressure along the entire surface of contact, reducing vertical force. The almost complete elimination of motion of the total-contact cast reduces plantar shear forces. The cast is removed 24 to 48 hours after application to inspect the foot and cast fit. The cast is replaced and then removed and reapplied weekly until the ulcer is healed. *Teach the patient that foot ulcers will recur unless weight is permanently redistributed.*

Managing Pain

Planning: Expected Outcomes. The patient with neuropathic pain is expected to experience relief of PAIN. Indicators include these consistent behaviors:

- Uses preventive measures
- Uses available resources to increase comfort
- Reports that pain is controlled

Interventions. Neuropathic PAIN results from damage anywhere along the nerve. Many patients with diabetes suffer from the painful neuropathy. Manifestations of diabetic neuropathy include:

- Burning
- Muscle cramps
- Piercing, stabbing, or darting pain
- Metatarsalgia (feeling as if you are walking on marbles)
- Hyperalgesia (exaggerated pain response)
- Allodynia (pain in response to normally nonpainful stimuli)
- Tingling, numbness, and loss of proprioception in lower extremities

Maintaining normal blood glucose levels and avoiding extreme fluctuations prevent neuropathy and relieve manifestations. Rapid improvement in blood glucose control may actually trigger acute peripheral neuropathy.

Several pharmacologic agents are used to manage neuropathic PAIN. The anticonvulsants *gabapentin* (Neurontin) and *pregabalin* (Lyrica) and the serotonin-norepinephrine reuptake inhibitor (SNRI) *duloxetine* (Cymbalta) are used in management of neuropathic pain. Tricyclic antidepressants such as amitriptyline hydrochloride (Elavil, Levate ✦) and nortriptyline (Pamelor) are widely used for pain but are not approved for this purpose and have some significant side effects. Their use is contraindicated for older adults and those with cardiovascular disease.

The burning of neuropathy may respond to capsaicin cream 0.075% (Axsain ✦, Zostrix-HP). Teach the patient to apply it 4 times daily for several weeks. The pain may worsen for several days after therapy is started before improving.

Unpleasant symptoms are noted with abrupt discontinuation of many of these drugs. A gradual reduction in the dose is recommended to prevent side effects.

Provide support and information on measures to reduce pain. Even having a bed cradle to lift bed clothes off hypersensitive skin can be beneficial. Assist the patient to maintain stable glucose control. *All patients with neuropathy are at increased risk for foot ulcers and require more frequent assessment and education in routine foot management.*

Preventing Injury from Reduced Vision

Planning: Expected Outcomes. The patient with diabetes is expected to be free of injury related to reduced visual SENSORY PERCEPTION and to maintain current level of vision. Indicators include:

- No further reduction of visual fields
- No double vision

Interventions

Blood Glucose Control. Poor blood GLUCOSE REGULATION (control), proteinuria, diastolic hypertension, and long duration of diabetes are risk factors for vision loss among people with diabetes (ADA, 2014a). Surgical intervention for retinal hemorrhage or new retinal blood vessel growth can reduce vision loss.

Besides regular eye examinations to evaluate retinopathy, urge the patient with impaired vision to have an optometrist or ophthalmologist assess the remaining vision and prescribe appropriate vision support. A functional vision assessment, performed by a low-vision technician, rehabilitation teacher, or diabetes educator, determines the patient's use of lighting, contrast, non-optical and low-vision devices, large-print options, and use of central or peripheral vision. Many low-vision reading aids are available as described in Chapter 47. The American Foundation for the Blind maintains a list of services for visually impaired people that is organized by type of service and geographic area. More information is available at (800) 232-5463 and www.afb.org.

Environmental Management. Not all visually impaired patients need special devices. Adjustments in lighting, contrast, color, distance, type size of printed materials, and eye movement often improve visual abilities. Chapter 47 describes general methods of enhancing vision. For the patient with diabetes and low vision, coding objects such as vials of insulin with bright colors or with felt-tipped markers helps identify the correct bottle. Bringing the blood glucose lancet or insulin syringe close to the eye makes it easier to see.

Prefilled insulin pens are not approved for use by people with severe visual impairment unless they are assisted by a person with good vision who is trained to use the pen correctly. Adaptive devices can help the patient self-administer insulin independently. Some syringes may have a magnifier attached to the syringe. Other devices include preset dose gauges (which measure the space between the end of the syringe barrel and the plunger) to help the patient draw up the correct amount of insulin by feeling this distance. The blind patient can accurately measure insulin by using products such as the Count-A-Dose Insulin Measuring Device. This device is designed to be used with the BD Lo-Dose syringe. It holds two insulin vials and has a slot to direct the syringe needle into the vials' rubber stoppers. The patient draws insulin into the syringe by turning a thumbwheel, which clicks for each unit (clicks can be both heard and felt). (See the *Consumer Guide* published yearly in the January edition of *Diabetes Forecast* [forecast.diabetes.org] for information to help patients determine which adaptive devices best meet their needs.) When teaching the patient to use an adaptive device, stress:

- Differentiating between bottles of fast-acting and slower-acting insulin by wrapping a rubber band around the fast-acting insulin bottle
- Ensuring proper placement of the device on the syringe
- Holding the insulin bottle upright when measuring insulin
- Avoiding air bubbles in the syringe by pulling a small amount of insulin into the syringe, moving the plunger in and out 3 times, and measuring insulin on the fourth draw

Design a system to determine how many doses can be drawn from a bottle so the patient does not inject air from an empty bottle instead of insulin.

Specialized adaptive equipment also is available to assist with blood glucose monitoring techniques. Assist the patient to select a blood glucose monitoring device best suited to his or her level of visual impairment. Some monitors have large display screens and easy-to-use features. Fully audio systems are available for patients who are visually impaired. The monitor uses no coding, has automatic turn-on with test strip insertion, and has a button for repeating the last message. Assess the ability of the patient to obtain an adequate blood sample and to apply it to the test strip. Commercially made blood drop guides can assist with this task.

❓ CLINICAL JUDGMENT CHALLENGE
Patient-Centered Care QSEN

During a clinic visit, you are reviewing the records of a 39-year-old patient who was diagnosed 5 years ago with type 2 diabetes. You discover that, although he has always been extremely near-sighted, he has not seen an ophthalmologist for 4 years. He has gained 12 lbs since his last visit a year ago. His laboratory values show a fasting blood glucose level of 96 mg/dL, an A1C of 8.2%, a total cholesterol of 322 mg/dL, and an LDL of 190 mg/dL. When you ask him about ophthalmology follow-up and point out his laboratory values, he replies that because he is taking prescribed antidiabetic medication, he believes that he won't have all the diabetes complications that his father had. He further tells you that he did have his eyes checked by an optometrist to make sure his prescription was accurate but that because he is younger than 40 years, he does not need intraocular pressure measurements.

1. How should you interpret his laboratory values in terms of his personal glucose regulation?
2. Should you address his weight gain? Why or why not?
3. Is he correct in thinking that an ophthalmologist visit is not necessary at this time? Explain your response.
4. Is he correct in believing that taking antidiabetic medication will prevent complications of diabetes? Explain your response.
5. How do you propose to assist this patient in managing his diabetes?

Reducing the Risk for Kidney Disease

Planning: Expected Outcomes. The patient with diabetes is expected to maintain a normal urine elimination pattern. Indicators include:

- Urine protein levels within normal limits
- 24-hour intake and output balance
- Blood urea nitrogen (BUN) and serum creatinine within the normal ranges
- Serum electrolytes within the normal ranges

Interventions

Prevention. Diabetic kidney disease is more likely to develop in patients with poor blood glucose control. Progression to end-stage kidney disease (ESKD) can be delayed or prevented by normalizing blood pressure, correcting hyperlipidemia, and restricting dietary protein. Control of hypertension is essential for the reduction of diabetic nephropathy (ADA, 2014b). Both systolic and diastolic hypertension greatly accelerate the progression of diabetic kidney disease.

Stress the need for evaluation of kidney function according to the ADA Standards of Care. Serum creatinine should be measured at least annually for an estimation of GFR in all patients with diabetes (ADA, 2013). An annual test for microalbuminuria is performed for patients who have had type 1 DM for over 5 years and in all those with type 2 DM starting at diagnosis and during pregnancy.

Persistent albuminuria in the range of 30 to 299 mg/24 hr (formerly called *microalbuminuria*) is the earliest stage of nephropathy in type 1 DM and a marker for the development of nephropathy in type 2 DM. Patients with albumin levels greater than 300 mg/24 hr (formerly called *macroalbuminuria*) are likely to progress to end-stage kidney disease (ESKD) (ADA, 2014b). Screening for increased urinary albumin excretion is performed by measurement of the albumin-creatinine ratio in a spot collection.

Aggressive control of blood glucose and hypertension in patients without microalbuminuria can avoid nephropathy. Once microalbuminuria develops, management focuses on controlling blood pressure and blood glucose, restricting dietary protein, avoiding nephrotoxic agents, promptly treating urinary tract infections, and preventing dehydration.

Control of blood pressure and blood glucose levels requires the patient's participation and effort. Prescribed drugs must be taken according to schedules, and dietary restrictions must be maintained. Teach patients about the roles of blood pressure and blood glucose levels in kidney disease. Help them maintain normal blood glucose levels and blood pressure levels below 140/80 mm Hg. Stress the need for yearly screening for microalbuminuria.

Smoking cessation is important in halting the progression of diabetic kidney disease for patients with type 1 and type 2 diabetes. Teach the patient about the risks of smoking, and refer him or her to appropriate resources for assistance in smoking cessation.

Any urinary tract INFECTION (UTI) can lead to kidney infection and further reduce kidney function. Explain the manifestations of UTI. Urge the patient to take antibiotics exactly as prescribed, completing the entire course of treatment. Reinforce the need for follow-up urine cultures to reduce the risk for kidney damage. Avoid indwelling urinary catheters when possible.

Drugs can affect kidney function either through toxic effects on the kidney or by an acute but reversible reduction in function. The most common nephrotoxic drugs are antifungal agents and aminoglycoside antibiotics. Outside the hospital, the leading nephrotoxic agents are NSAIDs such as ibuprofen (Advil) or naproxen (Aleve), when used long-term. To prevent accidental ingestion of nephrotoxic drugs, teach the patient to check with a health care provider before taking over-the-counter drugs or herbal remedies.

Radiocontrast dyes can also affect kidney function, especially in patients with preexisting kidney problems. Monitor IV hydration before and after contrast is used to prevent contrast-induced nephropathy in patients with diabetes.

Drug Therapy. Use of angiotensin-converting enzyme (ACE) inhibitors (ACEIs) or angiotensin receptor blockers (ARBs) is recommended for all patients with microalbuminuria or advanced stages of nephropathy (ADA, 2013). ACE inhibitors reduce the level of albuminuria and the rate of progression of kidney disease, although they do not appear to prevent microalbuminuria. Monitor serum potassium levels for development of hyperkalemia.

Nutrition Therapy. Patients with nephropathy should restrict protein intake to 0.8 g/kg of body weight per day. Once the glomerular filtration rate (GFR) starts falling, further reducing protein may slow the decline in kidney function. Because life-long dietary restrictions are difficult, provide ongoing teaching to encourage adherence.

Fluid and Electrolyte Management. Fluid and electrolyte management can prevent more loss of kidney function. Avoiding dehydration is important for kidney PERFUSION and function. The most common cause of dehydration in patients with diabetes is overuse of diuretics. Teach patients to report edema or symptoms of orthostatic hypotension, and provide ongoing education to promote nutrition therapy.

Dialysis for patients with DM and kidney failure is the same as for patients without diabetes (see Chapter 68). The dosage of insulin needs to be adjusted when dialysis starts.

Preventing Hypoglycemia. Hypoglycemia (low blood glucose level) induces specific manifestations and resolves when blood glucose concentration is raised. Once blood glucose levels fall below 70 mg/dL (3.88 mmol/L), a sequence of events begins with release of counterregulatory hormones, stimulation of the autonomic nervous system, and production of *neurogenic* and *neuroglycopenic* manifestations. Peripheral autonomic manifestations, including sweating, irritability, tremors, anxiety, tachycardia, and hunger, serve as an early warning system and occur before the manifestations of confusion, paralysis, seizure, and coma occur from brain glucose deprivation. *Neuroglycopenic symptoms* occur when brain glucose *gradually declines* to a low level. *Neurogenic symptoms* result from autonomic nervous activity triggered by a *rapid decline* in blood glucose (Table 64-11).

Central nervous system (CNS) function depends on a continuous supply of glucose in the blood. The brain cannot make glucose and stores only a few minutes' supply as glycogen. This needed supply is not maintained when the blood glucose level falls below critical levels.

The first defense against falling blood glucose levels in the nondiabetic person is decreased insulin secretion, decreased glucose use, and increased glucose production. Normally, insulin secretion decreases when blood glucose levels drop to about 83 mg/dL (4.5 mmol/L). Counterregulatory hormones are activated at about 67 mg/dL (3.7 mmol/L), a level well above the threshold for manifestations of hypoglycemia. The main counterregulatory hormone is glucagon. Epinephrine also becomes important in patients with DM who are deficient in glucagon. Both glucagon and epinephrine raise blood glucose levels by stimulating liver glycogen breakdown and conversion of protein to glucose. Epinephrine also limits insulin secretion.

Type 1 DM disrupts the body's response to hypoglycemia, usually within 1 to 5 years of diagnosis. Regulation of circulating insulin levels is lost because insulin comes from an injection rather than from the pancreas. As blood glucose levels fall, insulin levels do not decrease. Over time, the pancreas loses its ability to secrete glucagon in response to hypoglycemia. After a few more years of type 1 DM, the response of epinephrine to falling blood glucose levels does not occur until the blood glucose level is very low. These problems greatly increase the risk for severe hypoglycemia.

A second problem with long-standing type 1 DM is *hypoglycemic unawareness,* in which patients no longer have the warning manifestations of impending hypoglycemia that should prompt them to take preventive action (Mompoint-Williams et al., 2012). This problem occurs most often in patients who have had type 1 DM for 30 years or longer.

The blood glucose level at which manifestations of hypoglycemia occur varies among patients. Thus clinical criteria used to categorize hypoglycemia are based on manifestation severity rather than blood glucose levels. In mild hypoglycemia, the patient remains alert and able to self-manage symptoms. In severe hypoglycemia, neurologic function is so impaired that he or she needs another person's help to increase blood glucose levels.

Planning: Expected Outcomes. The patient with DM is expected to have decreased episodes of hypoglycemia and remain oriented to person, place, and time, as indicated by a Glasgow Coma Scale score above 7.

Interventions. A blood glucose level below 70 mg/dL (3.9 mmol/L) alerts you to assess for manifestations of hypoglycemia (Table 64-11; see also Table 64-12).

Blood Glucose Management. Monitor blood glucose levels before giving antidiabetic drugs, before meals, before bedtime, and when the patient is symptomatic. All patients who take insulin, those taking long-acting insulin secretagogues (glyburide [glibenclamide]), and those taking metformin in combination with glyburide (Glucovance) are at risk for hypoglycemia.

TABLE 64-11   Manifestations of Hypoglycemia

Neuroglycopenic Manifestations	Neurogenic Manifestations
• Weakness	• Adrenergic:
• Fatigue	• Shaky/tremulous
• Difficulty thinking	• Heart pounding
• Confusion	• Nervous/anxious
• Behavior changes	• Cholinergic:
• Emotional instability	• Sweaty
• Seizures	• Hungry
• Loss of consciousness	• Tingling
• Brain damage	
• Death	

TABLE 64-12   Differentiation of Hypoglycemia and Hyperglycemia

FEATURE	HYPOGLYCEMIA	HYPERGLYCEMIA
Skin	Cool, clammy	Warm, moist
Dehydration	Absent	Present
Respirations	No particular or consistent change	Rapid, deep*; Kussmaul type; acetone odor ("fruity" odor) to breath
Mental status	Anxious, nervous,* irritable, mental confusion,* seizures, coma	Varies from alert to stuporous, obtunded, or frank coma
Manifestations	Weakness,* double vision, blurred vision, hunger, tachycardia, palpitations	None specific for DKA Acidosis; hypercapnia; abdominal cramps, nausea and vomiting Dehydration: decreased neck vein filling, orthostatic hypotension, tachycardia, poor skin turgor
Glucose	<70 mg/dL (3.9 mmol/L)	>250 mg/dL (13.8 mmol/L)
Ketones	Negative	Positive

DKA, Diabetic ketoacidosis.
*Classic symptoms.

This risk is increased if they are older, have liver or kidney impairment, or are taking drugs that enhance the effects of antidiabetic drugs. Proper patient selection, drug dosage, and instructions are important factors in avoiding severe hypoglycemia. Hypoglycemia may be difficult to recognize in those who take beta-blocking drugs. Manifestations are less intense and less obvious. Manifestations of hypoglycemia in older patients may be mistaken for other conditions.

The most common causes of hypoglycemia are:
- Too much insulin compared with food intake and physical activity
- Insulin injected at the wrong time relative to food intake and physical activity
- The wrong type of insulin injected at the wrong time
- Decreased food intake resulting from missed or delayed meals
- Delayed gastric emptying from gastroparesis
- Decrease liver glucose production after alcohol ingestion
- Increased insulin sensitivity as a result of regular exercise and weight loss
- Decreased insulin clearance from progressive kidney failure

Nutrition Therapy. When the patient is hypoglycemic, start carbohydrate replacement per physician prescription or standing protocols—usually ingestion of 15 to 20 g of glucose. If the patient can swallow, give a liquid form of carbohydrate, although any carbohydrate source can be used. Ingestion of 15 to 20 g of glucose is the preferred management for blood glucose levels less than 70 mg/dL (3.9 mmol/L), repeated in about 15 minutes if manifestations have not improved or if blood glucose levels are still less than 70. The amount of carbohydrate should be increased to 30 g for glucose levels less than 50 mg/dL (2.8 mmol/L).

Ten grams (g) of oral glucose raises blood glucose levels by about 40 mg/dL over 30 minutes, and 20 g of oral glucose raises blood glucose levels by about 60 mg/dL over 45 minutes. Specific recommendations are listed in Chart 64-7.

The blood glucose level determines the form and amount of glucose used. The response should be apparent in 10 to 20 minutes; however, test blood glucose again in about 60 minutes because additional management may be needed. Fluid is absorbed much more quickly from the GI tract than are solids. Concentrated sweet fluids, such as juice with sugar added or a soft drink, may slow absorption. Management of hypoglycemia requires ingestion of glucose or glucose-containing foods. The blood glucose response correlates better with the glucose content rather than the carbohydrate content of the food. Adding protein to carbohydrate does NOT improve blood glucose response and does NOT prevent subsequent hypoglycemia. Adding fat may retard and then prolong the blood glucose response, resulting in post-treatment hyperglycemia. Commercially available products provide predictable glucose absorption.

Drug Therapy. Glucagon given subcutaneously or IM and 50% dextrose given IV are used for patients who cannot swallow. Glucagon is the main counterregulatory hormone to insulin and is used as first-line therapy for severe hypoglycemia in DM. It converts liver glycogen to glucose but is not effective in severely starved patients. Take care to prevent aspiration in patients receiving glucagon, because it often causes vomiting. Give 50% dextrose carefully to avoid extravasation because it is

hyperosmolar and can damage tissue. The effects of glucagon and dextrose are temporary. After the patient responds and is no longer nauseated, give a simple sugar followed by a small snack or meal. IV glucose is used to maintain mild hyperglycemia. Diazoxide (Proglycem) or octreotide (Sandostatin) may be required to treat sulfonylurea-induced hypoglycemia. Evaluate response by monitoring blood glucose levels for several hours because manifestations may persist. A target blood glucose level is 70 to 110 mg/dL (3.9 to 6.2 mmol/L).

CHART 64-7 Patient and Family Education: Preparing for Self-Management

Management of Hypoglycemia at Home

For *mild* hypoglycemia (hungry, irritable, shaky, weak, headache, fully conscious; blood glucose usually less than 60 mg/dL [3.4 mmol/L]):
- Treat the symptoms of hypoglycemia with 10 to 15 g of carbohydrate. You may use one of these:
  - Glucose tablets or glucose gel (dosage is printed on the package)
  - ½ cup of fruit juice
  - ½ cup of regular (nondiet) soft drink
  - 8 ounces of skim milk
  - 6 to 10 hard candies
  - 4 cubes of sugar
  - 4 teaspoons of sugar
  - 6 saltines
  - 3 graham crackers
  - 1 tablespoon of honey or syrup
- Re-test blood glucose in 15 minutes.
- Repeat this treatment if symptoms do not resolve.
- Eat a small snack of carbohydrate and protein if your next meal is more than an hour away.

For *moderate* hypoglycemia (cold, clammy skin; pale; rapid pulse; rapid, shallow respirations; marked change in mood; drowsiness; blood glucose usually less than 40 mg/dL [2.2 mmol/L]):
- Treat the symptoms of hypoglycemia with 15 to 30 g of rapidly absorbed carbohydrate.
- Take additional food, such as low-fat milk or cheese, after 10 to 15 minutes.

For *severe* hypoglycemia (unable to swallow; unconsciousness or convulsions; blood glucose usually less than 20 mg/dL [1.0 mmol/L]):
- Treatment administered by family members:
  - Administer 1 mg of glucagon as intramuscular or subcutaneous injection.
  - Administer a second dose in 10 minutes if the person remains unconscious.
  - Notify a primary care provider immediately, and follow instructions.
  - If still unconscious, transport the person to the emergency department.
  - Give a small meal when the person wakes up and is no longer nauseated.

! NURSING SAFETY PRIORITY (QSEN)

Critical Rescue

For the patient with *severe* hypoglycemia (unable to swallow, unconscious or convulsing, blood glucose usually less than 20 mg/dL [1.0 mmol/L]), treat by:
1. Giving glucagon 1 mg subcutaneously or IM
2. Repeating the dose in 10 minutes if the patient remains unconscious
3. Notifying the primary health care provider immediately, and following instructions

Prevention Strategies. Teach the patient how to prevent hypoglycemia by avoiding its four common causes: (1) excess insulin, (2) deficient intake or absorption of food, (3) exercise, and (4) alcohol intake.

Insulin excess from variable absorption of insulin can cause hypoglycemia even when insulin is injected correctly. Increased insulin sensitivity can occur with weight loss, exercise programs, and resolution of an INFECTION. Differences in insulin formulation can result in hypoglycemia. Teach the patient to not change insulin brands without medical supervision.

Deficient food intake from inadequate or incorrectly timed meals can result in hypoglycemia. Changes in gastric absorption may cause hypoglycemia in patients with delayed gastric emptying, which is more severe with solid meals, and is made worse by illness or poor glucose control. Teach the patient the importance of regularity in timing and quantity of food eaten.

Exercise often causes blood glucose levels to fall in a patient with type 1 DM. Prolonged exercise increases cellular glucose uptake for several hours after exercise. Teach the patient about blood glucose monitoring and carbohydrate consumption before and during exercise.

Alcohol inhibits liver glucose production and leads to hypoglycemia. It interferes with the counterregulatory response to hypoglycemia and impairs glycogen breakdown, making exercise-induced hypoglycemia more severe. Teach the patient to ingest alcohol only with or shortly *after* eating a meal with enough carbohydrate to prevent hypoglycemia. Warn patients to avoid excess alcohol at bedtime to prevent nighttime hypoglycemia.

Patient and Family Education. The cause of hypoglycemia may be subtle. At the onset of menses, a fall in hormone levels decreases insulin needs and contributes to hypoglycemia. When patients switch to a new bottle of insulin, hypoglycemia may occur because the fresh insulin has greater potency. Some patients have hypoglycemia when they change injection sites. Beta-blocking drugs mask manifestations that are warning signs and thus predispose patients to severe hypoglycemia. Some episodes of hypoglycemia occur without an obvious cause.

Many patients who have been treated in the emergency department for hypoglycemia do not receive adequate prevention instructions and are at continuing risk. Help each patient develop a personal treatment plan for hypoglycemia. The exact glucose rise from a set amount of carbohydrate varies; however, using the estimate that each 5 g of carbohydrate raises blood glucose about 20 mg/dL is a good starting plan. For example, the patient may be directed to take:

- 20 to 30 g of carbohydrate if the blood glucose level is 50 mg/dL (2.8 mmol/L) or less
- 10 to 15 g of carbohydrate if the blood glucose level is 51 to 70 mg/dL (2.9 to 3.9 mmol/L)

Use blood glucose monitoring results to revise or reinforce this plan.

Encourage the patient to wear a medical alert bracelet, and help him or her obtain one. This bracelet is helpful if the patient becomes hypoglycemic and is unable to provide self-care.

Teach the patient and family about the manifestations of hypoglycemia. Emphasize that delaying a meal for more than 30 minutes raises the risk for hypoglycemia when using some insulin regimens. Instruct him or her to keep a carbohydrate source nearby at all times. Teach the patient and family how to administer glucagon.

Hypoglycemia is a major risk for patients receiving intensive insulin protocols who engage in exercise programs. Explain that nightmares or headaches on days after prolonged or severe exercise may indicate hypoglycemia.

Establishing Treatment Plans. Blood glucose monitoring directs hypoglycemia management. Treatment continues until blood glucose levels reach and stay in the target range. Once blood glucose control is regained, the patient should identify the specific cause of the episode and take specific measures to prevent recurrence.

CONSIDERATIONS FOR OLDER ADULTS
Patient-Centered Care QSEN

Patients in the older age-groups are especially vulnerable to hypoglycemia. Age-related declines in kidney function and liver enzyme activity may interfere with the metabolism of sulfonylureas and insulin, thereby potentiating their hypoglycemic effects. Older patients with diabetes have impaired epinephrine release and a diminished glucagon response to falling blood glucose levels. They often have a reduced awareness of hypoglycemic manifestations. Confusion and any impairment in psychomotor performance when blood sugars are low prevent the older adult from taking appropriate steps to return the blood sugar to normal.

Instruct the older patient and family to check blood glucose values when symptoms such as unsteadiness, light-headedness, poor concentration, trembling, or sweating occur. Assess eating patterns to make sure sufficient foods are eaten at appropriate times. Encourage a patient with a poor appetite to eat a small snack at bedtime to prevent hypoglycemia during the night.

The highest rates of severe and fatal episodes of hypoglycemia are associated with the use of glyburide in patients older than 70 years. Drug regimens that require that meals be eaten on time increase the potential for hypoglycemic reactions. Complex regimens that require multiple decision points should be simplified, especially for patients with decreased functional status (Seaquist et al., 2013).

? CLINICAL JUDGMENT CHALLENGE
Safety; Quality Improvement; Teamwork and Collaboration QSEN

The patient is a 60-year-old-woman who is 1 day postoperative after a total knee replacement. She has type 2 diabetes and just recently was switched from oral antidiabetic drugs to an insulin regimen. She let her nurse know that her on-demand lunch has been ordered. The nurse tests her blood and gives her the prescribed short-acting insulin dose. An hour later the physical therapist finds her pale, confused, and clammy. Her lunch tray is on her table and appears untouched.

1. Is her condition consistent with hyperglycemia or hypoglycemia? Explain your choice.
2. What is your first action? Provide a rationale.
3. What is the most likely cause leading to this problem?
4. What could be done on this nursing care unit to prevent such an incident from happening again?

Preventing Diabetic Ketoacidosis. Diabetic ketoacidosis (DKA) is characterized by uncontrolled hyperglycemia, metabolic acidosis, and increased production of ketones. This condition results from the combination of insulin deficiency and an increase in hormone release that leads to increased liver and kidney glucose production and decreased glucose use in peripheral tissues (Fig. 64-9). Laboratory diagnosis of DKA is shown in Table 64-13. All of these changes increase ketoacid production with resultant ketonemia and metabolic acidosis.

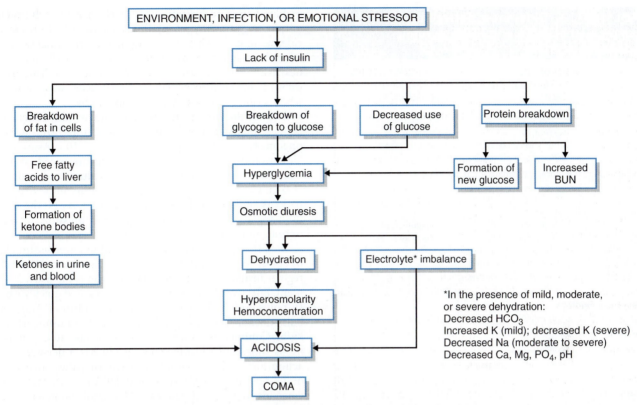

FIG. 64-9 The pathophysiologic mechanism of diabetic ketoacidosis (DKA).

DKA occurs most often in patients with type 1 DM but also can occur in those with type 2 DM who are under severe stress (e.g., trauma, surgery, infection). Some people with type 2 diabetes have a syndrome known as *ketosis-prone diabetes* or *KPD* (Palmer & Jessup, 2012). This problem is not yet fully characterized, and it is important to remember that regardless of whether the patient with DKA has type 1 or type 2 diabetes, management of the acute episode is the same. The most common precipitating factor for DKA is INFECTION. *Death occurs in up to 10% of these cases even with appropriate treatment.*

Hyperglycemia leads to osmotic diuresis with dehydration and electrolyte loss. Classic manifestations of DKA include polyuria, polydipsia, polyphagia, vomiting, abdominal pain, dehydration, weakness, confusion, shock, and coma. Mental status can vary from total alertness to profound coma. As ketone levels rise, the pH of the blood decreases and acidosis occurs. **Kussmaul respirations** (very deep and rapid respirations) cause respiratory alkalosis in an attempt to correct metabolic acidosis by exhaling carbon dioxide. Initial serum sodium levels may be low or normal. Initial potassium levels depend on how long DKA existed before treatment. After therapy starts, serum potassium levels drop quickly.

Planning: Expected Outcomes. The patient is expected to have few episodes of hyperglycemia and avoid diabetic ketoacidosis. Indicators include that the patient consistently demonstrates these behaviors:

- Maintains blood glucose levels within the prescribed target range
- Adjusts insulin doses to match eating patterns and blood glucose levels during illness
- Maintains easily digestible liquid diet containing carbohydrate and salt when nauseated

- Describes correct procedure for urine ketone testing
- Describes when to seek help from health care professional

Interventions

Blood Glucose Management. Monitor for manifestations of DKA (see Table 64-13 and Fig. 64-9). Document and use these findings to determine therapy effectiveness. *First assess the airway, level of consciousness, hydration status, electrolytes, and blood glucose level.* Check the patient's blood pressure, pulse, and respirations every 15 minutes until stable. Record urine output, temperature, and mental status every hour. When a central venous catheter is present, assess central venous pressure every 30 minutes or as prescribed. After treatment starts and these values are stable, monitor and record vital signs every 4 hours. Use blood glucose values to assess therapy and determine when to switch from saline to dextrose-containing solutions.

Fluid and Electrolyte Management. *Closely assess the patient's fluid status.* Assess for acute weight loss, thirst, decreased skin turgor, dry mucous membranes, and oliguria with a high specific gravity. Also assess for weak and rapid pulse, flattened neck veins, increased temperature, decreased central venous pressure, muscle weakness, postural hypotension, and cool, clammy, and pale skin to determine if the patient is at risk for dehydration and shock.

Manifestations of fluid volume excess include acute weight gain, full and bounding pulses, distended neck veins, pulmonary crackles, peripheral edema, and elevated central venous pressure. Acute pulmonary edema can develop quickly. Hypertension is common, especially in patients with kidney failure.

Expected manifestations of fluid balance are altered by age-related changes, by other medical conditions, and by drugs. Age-related skin changes, such as loss of elasticity and dryness, make

TABLE 64-13   Differences Between Diabetic Ketoacidosis and Hyperglycemic-Hyperosmolar State

	DIABETIC KETOACIDOSIS (DKA)	HYPERGLYCEMIC-HYPEROSMOLAR STATE (HHS)
Onset	Sudden	Gradual
Precipitating factors	Infection Other stressors Inadequate insulin dose	Infection Other stressors Poor fluid intake
Manifestations	Ketosis: Kussmaul respiration, "rotting fruit" breath, nausea, abdominal pain Dehydration or electrolyte loss: polyuria, polydipsia, weight loss, dry skin, sunken eyes, soft eyeballs, lethargy, coma	Altered central nervous system function with neurologic symptoms Dehydration or electrolyte loss: same as for DKA
Laboratory Findings		
Serum glucose	>300 mg/dL (16.7 mmol/L)	>600 mg/dL (33.3 mmol/L)
Osmolarity	Variable	>320 mOsm/L
Serum ketones	Positive at 1:2 dilutions	Negative
Serum pH	<7.35	>7.4
Serum HCO$_3^-$	<15 mEq/L	>20 mEq/L
Serum Na$^+$	Low, normal, or high	Normal or low
BUN	>30 mg/dL; elevated because of dehydration	Elevated
Creatinine	>1.5 mg/dL; elevated because of dehydration	Elevated
Urine ketones	Positive	Negative

BUN, Blood urea nitrogen; *HCO$_3^-$,* bicarbonate; *Na$^+$,* sodium.

skin turgor an unreliable indicator of dehydration. With severe hyperglycemia, the kidneys are less able to respond to changes in pH or fluid and electrolyte balance, to concentrate urine, or to regulate blood osmolarity. The risk for kidney failure rises with age, and acidosis occurs more quickly. Cardiovascular disease can cause fluid retention. In patients with poor kidney function and excess fluid volume, assess for edema around the eyes and in the limbs, increasing blood pressure, jugular venous distention, and orthostatic hypotension. Edema occurs with excess interstitial fluid and often is not apparent until interstitial volume increases by 2 to 3 L. Jugular venous pressure increases with volume overload. In severe volume depletion, the jugular venous pulsation may not be visible even with the patient lying flat.

Tachycardia is a compensatory mechanism to increase cardiac output. Older adults may not exhibit tachycardia if they are taking beta blockers or calcium channel blockers. Dry mucous membranes may be caused by anticholinergic drugs, and postural hypotension may occur with antihypertensive therapy.

The first outcome of fluid therapy is to restore volume and maintain PERFUSION to the brain, heart, and kidneys. Typically, initial infusion rates of 0.9% sodium chloride are 15 to 20 mL/kg/hr during the first hour.

The second outcome of replacing total body fluid losses is achieved more slowly. The choice for fluid replacement depends on blood pressure, hydration, serum electrolyte levels, and urine output. In general, hypotonic fluids, such as 0.45% sodium chloride, are infused at 4 to 14 mL/kg/hr after the initial fluid bolus. When blood glucose levels reach 250 mg/dL (13.8 mmol/L), 5% dextrose in 0.45% saline is usually prescribed. This solution prevents hypoglycemia and cerebral edema, which can occur when serum osmolarity declines too rapidly.

During the first 24 hours of treatment, the patient needs enough fluids to replace the actual volume lost, as well as ongoing losses. This may be as much as 6 to 10 L. Assess cardiac, kidney, and mental status to avoid fluid overload. Watch for manifestations of congestive heart failure and pulmonary edema. Central venous pressure may be monitored for older patients and those with myocardial disease. Assess the status of fluid replacement by monitoring blood pressure, intake and output, and changes in daily weight.

Drug Therapy. Insulin therapy is used to lower serum glucose by about 50 to 75 mg/dL/hr. Unless the episode of DKA is mild, regular insulin by continuous IV infusion is the usual management. Effective blood insulin levels are reached quickly when an IV bolus dose is given at the start of the infusion. An initial IV bolus dose of 0.1 unit/kg is followed by an IV infusion of 0.1 unit/kg/hr. Continuous insulin infusion is used because insulin half-life is short and subcutaneous insulin has a delayed onset of action. Subcutaneous insulin is started when the patient can take oral fluids and ketosis has stopped. DKA is considered resolved when blood glucose is less than 200 mg/mL along with a serum bicarbonate level higher than 18 mEq/L, venous pH higher than 7.3, and a calculated ion gap less than 12 mEq/L. Assess therapy effectiveness by hourly blood glucose measurements.

Acidosis Management. The key feature of DKA is elevation in blood ketone concentration (measured as serum β-hydroxybutyrate). Accumulation of ketoacids results in an increased anion gap metabolic acidosis. A normal anion gap is between 7 and 9 mEq/L; an anion gap greater than 10 to 12 mEq/L indicates metabolic acidosis.

Mild to moderate hyperkalemia is common in patients with hyperglycemia. Insulin therapy, correction of acidosis, and volume expansion decrease serum potassium concentration. To prevent hypokalemia, potassium replacement is initiated after serum levels fall below the upper limit of normal (5.0 mEq/L). *Assess for manifestations of hypokalemia, including fatigue, malaise, confusion, muscle weakness, shallow respirations, abdominal distention or paralytic ileus, hypotension, and weak pulse.* An ECG shows conduction changes related to potassium. Hypokalemia is a common cause of death in the treatment of DKA.

> **! NURSING SAFETY PRIORITY** (QSEN)
>
> **Critical Rescue**
>
> Before giving IV potassium-containing solutions, make sure the urine output is at least 30 mL/hr.

Bicarbonate is used only for severe acidosis. Sodium bicarbonate, given by slow IV infusion over several hours, is indicated when the arterial pH is 7.0 or less or the serum bicarbonate level is less than 5 mEq/L (5 mmol/L).

Patient and Family Education. Exploring the factors leading to DKA helps in planning specific educational efforts. Teach the patient and family to check blood glucose levels every 4 to 6 hours as long as manifestations such as anorexia, nausea, and vomiting are present and as long as glucose levels exceed 250 mg/dL (13.8 mmol/L). Teach them to check urine ketone levels when blood glucose levels exceed 300 mg/dL (16.7 mmol/L).

Teach the patient to prevent dehydration by maintaining food and fluid intake. Unless another health problem is present that requires fluid restriction, suggest that he or she drink at least 2 L of fluid daily and increase this amount when INFECTION is present. When nausea is present, instruct the patient to take liquids containing both glucose and electrolytes (e.g., soda pop, diluted fruit juice, and sports drinks [Gatorade]). Small amounts of fluid may be tolerated even when vomiting is present. When the blood glucose level is normal or elevated, the patient should take 8 to 12 ounces (240 to 360 mL) of calorie-free and caffeine-free liquids every hour while awake to prevent dehydration.

Liquids containing carbohydrate can be taken if the diabetic patient cannot eat solid food. Ingesting at least 150 g of carbohydrate daily reduces the risk for starvation ketosis. After consulting a primary care provider, urge the patient to take additional rapid-acting (lispro) or short-acting (regular) insulin based on blood glucose levels.

Instruct the patient and family to consult the health care provider when these problems occur:

- Blood glucose exceeds 250 mg/dL (13.8 mmol/L).
- Ketonuria lasts for more than 24 hours.
- The patient cannot take food or fluids.
- Illness lasts more than 1 to 2 days.

Also instruct them to detect hyperglycemia by monitoring blood glucose whenever the patient is ill. Illness can result in dehydration with DKA, hyperglycemic-hyperosmolar state, or both. The sooner the patient seeks treatment, the less severe the metabolic alteration. He or she should not omit insulin therapy during illness. Chart 64-8 lists guidelines for the ill patient.

❓ CLINICAL JUDGMENT CHALLENGE
Prioritization, Delegation, and Supervision

The patient, a 21-year-old college student, was brought to the emergency department (ED) by his roommate. He reports abdominal pain, polyuria for the past 2 days, vomiting several times prior to arrival, and extreme thirst. He appears flushed, and his lips and mucous membranes are dry and cracked. His skin turgor is poor. He demonstrates deep, rapid respirations; there is a rotting fruit odor to his breath. He has type 1 diabetes and "may have skipped a few doses of insulin because of cramming for final exams." He is alert and talking but is having trouble focusing on questions.

Vital signs: Blood pressure, 110/60; Pulse, 110/min; Respirations, 32/min; Temperature, 100.8° F; Fingerstick glucose, 485 mg/dL; Oxygen saturation, 99%.

1. You have completed triage assessment and history. Should you now notify his parents for permission to treat him? Why or why not?
2. Should you apply oxygen at this time? Why or why not?
3. Should you call his primary care provider? Why or why not?
4. Your work plan includes checking hourly vital signs, assessing blood glucose levels, updating the roommate about the patient's condition, and measuring the patient's emesis. Which task(s) is (are) appropriate to assign to the new nursing assistant? Provide a rationale for your choices.
5. In caring for this patient, what immediate intervention do you anticipate the ED physician will order to be performed first? Provide a rationale for your choice.
6. What IV solution do you anticipate the ED physician will order for initial fluid replacement?

CHART 64-8 Patient and Family Education: Preparing for Self-Management

Sick-Day Rules

- Notify your health care provider that you are ill.
- Monitor your blood glucose at least every 4 hours.
- Test your urine for ketones when your blood glucose level is greater than 240 mg/dL (13.8 mmol/L).
- Continue to take insulin or oral antidiabetic agents.
- To prevent dehydration, drink 8 to 12 ounces of sugar-free liquids every hour that you are awake. If your blood glucose level is below your target range, drink fluids that contain sugar.
- Continue to eat meals at regular times.
- If unable to tolerate solid food because of nausea, consume more easily tolerated foods or liquids equal to the carbohydrate content of your usual meal.
- Call your primary care provider for any of these danger signals:
  - Persistent nausea and vomiting
  - Moderate or large ketones
  - Blood glucose elevation after two supplemental doses of insulin
  - High (101.5° F [38.6° C]) temperature or increasing fever; fever for more than 24 hours
- Treat symptoms (e.g., diarrhea, nausea, vomiting, fever) as directed by your primary care provider.
- Get plenty of rest.

Preventing Hyperglycemic-Hyperosmolar State. Hyperglycemic-hyperosmolar state (HHS) is a hyperosmolar (increased blood osmolarity) state caused by hyperglycemia. The processes of HHS are outlined in Fig. 64-10. Both HHS and diabetic ketoacidosis (DKA) are caused by hyperglycemia and dehydration. HHS differs from DKA in that ketone levels are absent or low and blood glucose levels are much higher. Blood glucose levels may exceed 600 mg/dL (33.3 mmol/L), and blood osmolarity may exceed 320 mOsm/L. Table 64-13 lists the differences between DKA and HHS.

HHS results from a sustained osmotic diuresis. Kidney impairment in HHS allows for extremely high blood glucose levels. As blood concentrations of glucose exceed the renal threshold, the kidney's capacity to reabsorb glucose is exceeded.

Decreased blood volume, caused by osmotic diuresis, or underlying kidney disease, common in many older patients with diabetes, results in further deterioration of kidney function. The decreased volume further reduces glomerular filtration rate, causing the glucose level to increase. Decreased kidney PERFUSION from hypovolemia further impairs kidney function.

CONSIDERATIONS FOR OLDER ADULTS
Patient-Centered Care QSEN

HHS occurs most often in older patients with type 2 diabetes mellitus, many of whom did not know that they had diabetes. Mortality rates in older patients are as high as 40% to 70%. The onset of HHS is slow and may not be recognized. The older patient often seeks medical attention later and is sicker than the younger patient. HHS does not occur in adequately hydrated patients. Older patients are at greater risk for dehydration and HHS because of age-related changes in thirst perception, poor urine-concentrating abilities, and use of diuretics. Stress to all older adults, especially those who have diabetes, the importance of maintaining hydration.

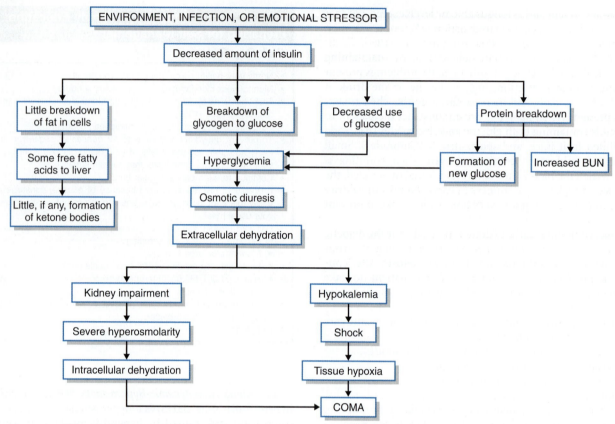

FIG. 64-10 The pathophysiologic mechanism of hyperglycemic-hyperosmolar state (HHS). *BUN*, Blood urea nitrogen.

Myocardial infarction, sepsis, pancreatitis, stroke, and some drugs (glucocorticoids, diuretics, phenytoin [Dilantin], beta blockers, and calcium channel blockers) also may cause HHS. Central nervous system (CNS) changes range from confusion to complete coma. Unlike DKA, patients with HHS may have seizures and reversible paralysis. The degree of neurologic impairment is related to serum osmolarity, with coma occurring once serum osmolarity is greater than 350 mOsm/L (350 mmol/L).

The development of HHS rather than DKA is related to residual insulin secretion. In HHS, the patient secretes just enough insulin to prevent ketosis but not enough to prevent hyperglycemia. The hyperglycemia of HHS is more severe than that of DKA, greatly increasing blood osmolarity, leading to extreme diuresis with severe dehydration and electrolyte loss.

Planning: Expected Outcomes. The patient with DM is expected to have few episodes of hyperglycemia and avoid HHS. Indicators include that the patient consistently demonstrates these behaviors:

- Maintains blood glucose levels within the target range
- Uses antidiabetic drugs appropriately
- Remains well hydrated
- Describes when to seek help from health care professionals

Interventions

Monitoring. Assess for manifestations of HHS. (See Tables 64-12 and 64-13 for manifestations of hyperglycemia.) Continually assess fluid status.

Fluid Therapy. The expected outcome of therapy is to rehydrate the patient and restore normal blood glucose levels within 36 to 72 hours. The choice of fluid replacement and the rate of infusion are critical in managing HHS. The severity of the CNS problems is related to the level of blood hyperosmolarity and cellular dehydration. Re-establishing fluid balance in brain cells is a difficult and slow process, and many patients do not recover baseline CNS function until hours after blood glucose levels have returned to normal.

The *first* priority for fluid replacement in HHS is to increase blood volume. In shock or severe hypotension, normal saline is used. Otherwise, half-normal saline (0.45% sodium chloride) is used. Infuse fluids at 1 L/hr until central venous pressure or pulmonary capillary wedge pressure begins to rise or until blood pressure and urine output are adequate. The rate is then reduced to 100 to 200 mL/hr. Half of the estimated fluid deficit is replaced in the first 12 hours, and the rest is given over the next 36 hours. Body weight, urine output, kidney function, and the presence or absence of pulmonary congestion and jugular venous distention determine the rate of fluid infusion. In patients with congestive heart failure, kidney disease, or acute kidney injury, monitor central venous pressure. *Assess the patient hourly for signs of cerebral edema—abrupt changes in mental status, abnormal neurologic signs, and coma.* Lack of

! NURSING SAFETY PRIORITY (QSEN)

Critical Rescue

For patients being managed for hyperglycemic-hyperosmolar state, immediately report changes in the level of consciousness; changes in pupil size, shape, or reaction; or seizures.

improvement in level of consciousness may indicate inadequate rates of fluid replacement or reduction in plasma (blood) osmolarity. Regression after initial improvement may indicate a too-rapid reduction in blood osmolarity. A slow but steady improvement in CNS function is the best evidence that fluid management is satisfactory.

Continuing Therapy. IV insulin is administered after adequate fluids have been replaced. The typical intervention is an initial bolus dose of 0.15 unit per kg IV followed by an infusion of 0.1 unit per kg per hour until blood glucose levels fall to 250 mg/dL (13.9 mmol/L). A reduction of blood glucose of 50 to 70 mg/dL per hour is the expected outcome. Monitor the patient closely for hypokalemia. Total body potassium depletion is often unrecognized because the blood potassium level may be normal or high as a result of dehydration. The potassium level may drop quickly when insulin therapy is started. Potassium replacement is initiated once urine output is adequate. Serum electrolytes are checked every 1 to 2 hours until stable, and the cardiac rhythm is monitored continuously for signs of hypokalemia or hyperkalemia. Patient education and interventions to minimize dehydration are similar to those for ketoacidosis.

Community-Based Care

Self-Management Education. Diabetes is a self-managed chronic disease requiring those affected to be actively involved in their own care. The concept of diabetes self-management refers to the patient's daily responsibility for almost all tasks involved in diabetes care. Education about blood glucose control for those with or at risk for diabetes occurs in a variety of health care settings. Physicians, nurses, registered dietitians, pharmacists, social workers, and psychologists all participate in the education. People with diabetes are best able to learn through educational efforts that are tailored to their individual needs.

Assessing Learning Needs and Readiness to Learn. First assess the patient's learning needs and readiness to learn. This assessment establishes what the patient already knows and what he or she needs to know. It also helps you determine the patient's ability and desire to learn. Assess the needs of both patient and family before teaching (Hughes, 2012b). Table 64-14 lists areas to include in this assessment.

Patients want information that applies directly to them. Find out what concerns the patient most about having diabetes, and ask what he or she wants to learn. Start with what the patient already knows, and build on that base. Make sure that the patient's knowledge is current and applies to his or her type of diabetes.

Your assessment may indicate that the patient is not ready to learn needed self-management behaviors. With the patient's permission, you would then teach a family member or someone close to the patient about diabetes management. You would also provide written materials on diabetes management as well as telephone numbers for the patient to call when he or she is ready to learn.

Assessing Physical, Cognitive, and Emotional Limitations. Assessing the patient's literacy is essential in developing a plan of care and providing self-management education. It is important to measure the patient's ability to read and understand written materials and conduct math calculations. Assess the patient's education and reading level to determine what level of information to present. It is important to match the literacy level of materials to the literacy level of the patient. Simplify the information you present by replacing technical terms with plain language (words people use in everyday conversation).

TABLE 64-14 **Assessment of Learning Needs for the Patient with Diabetes**
• Health and medical history
• Nutrition history and practices
• Physical activity and exercise behaviors
• Prescription and over-the-counter medications and complementary and alternative therapies and practices
• Factors that influence learning such as education and literacy levels, perceived learning needs, motivation to learn, and health beliefs
• Diabetes self-management behaviors, including experience with self-adjusting the treatment plan
• Previous diabetes self-management training, actual knowledge, and skills
• Physical factors including age, mobility, visual acuity, hearing, manual dexterity, alertness, attention span, and ability to concentrate or special needs or limitations requiring adaptive support and use of alternative skills
• Psychosocial concerns, factors, or issues including family and social support
• Current mental health status
• History of substance use including alcohol, tobacco, and recreational drugs
• Occupation, vocation, education level, financial status, and social, cultural, and religious practices
• Access to and use of health care resources

Assess the patient's ability to read printed information, insulin labels, and markings on syringes and equipment. Many with type 2 diabetes have age-related visual problems made worse by blurred vision caused by fluctuating blood glucose levels. Assess the patient's ability to reason with numbers. Determine whether the patient has the math skills needed to interpret a food label or to make adjustments in insulin doses based on glucose readings.

Assess manual dexterity for any physical limitations that may alter the teaching plan. A hand injury, tremors, or severe arthritis often leads to dosing errors with a standard syringe and may require a change in insulin preparation.

Individual learning styles vary. Visual learners think in terms of pictures and remember things best by seeing something written or by seeing visual aids. Auditory learners learn best through hearing. Kinesthetic or tactile learners learn best through touching, feeling, and experiencing what they are trying to learn. Tactile learners remember best by writing or physically manipulating the equipment. Successful diabetes self-management education uses all three learning styles by providing written handouts, discussing steps involved in a procedure such as insulin administration or self-monitoring of blood glucose, and encouraging the learner to touch and manipulate equipment. Confirm that the patient understands your instructions by having him or her "teach back" the information to you.

Tailor educational sessions to the time available and to the condition of the patient. Hospitalized people require only basic education when they are acutely ill. In these situations, it is appropriate to teach basic survival skills or focused problem-solving skills while reserving more detailed education for follow-up sessions.

Survival Skills Information. The initial phase of diabetes education involves teaching information necessary for the survival of anyone diagnosed with diabetes. Survival information includes:

- Simple information on pathophysiology of diabetes
- Learning how to prepare and administer insulin or how to take oral drugs for diabetes
- Recognition, treatment, and prevention of hypoglycemia and hyperglycemia
- Basic diet information
- Monitoring of blood glucose and ketones
- Sick-day management
- Where to buy diabetes supplies and how to store them
- When and how to notify the health care provider

In-Depth Education. In-depth education and counseling involve teaching more detailed information about survival skills and about actions for avoiding long-term complications. Educational sessions with patient and family are needed to "patientize" the diabetes regimen for *their* needs and abilities.

The person with diabetes needs to understand the pathology of diabetes. He or she should be able to discuss the action of insulin in the body and the effects of insulin deficiency. He or she should also be able to explain the effects of diet, drugs, and activity on blood glucose. The patient should be able to relate maintaining normal blood glucose levels to preventing complications. This includes relating changes in glucose level to the possible need for a change in insulin dosage.

Provide education about the manifestations of hypoglycemia along with the prescribed treatment options if the patient takes any drugs that will lower blood glucose levels. Educate patients and their families about common causes of hypoglycemia such as changes in drug regimen, increase in physical activity, and delayed or missed meals. Review manifestations of hypoglycemia at each visit. Advise patients to check their blood glucose levels before driving and make sure they have easy-to-reach snacks or fast-acting sugars with them at all times. Encourage them to always wear a medical ID tag or bracelet and to contact their health care provider if they experience low blood glucose levels more than twice a week.

Many patients require combination drug therapy to achieve GLUCOSE REGULATION in addition to aspirin and drugs to lower lipids and blood pressure. If the patient takes an oral antidiabetic drug, ask him or her to identify the drugs and describe the prescribed schedule. Determine if the patient is able to administer insulin accurately by having him or her "teach back" injection techniques. Ask the patient to discuss the onset, peak, and duration of the insulin used. The patient must be able to state when insulin is to be injected, where insulin is injected, and how insulin is stored. Review formulas for self-adjustment in insulin (when permitted by the health care provider), and explain blood glucose monitoring requirements needed to evaluate the effects of additional insulin. Stress the dangers of skipping doses. Review drug interactions, especially with older patients taking oral antidiabetic drugs.

Teach patients receiving diet therapy alone, glucose-lowering drugs, or fixed insulin doses to eat consistent amounts of carbohydrate at meals and snacks. Patients who adjust mealtime doses of insulin or those on insulin pump therapy can be taught to match their insulin dose to the carbohydrate content of their diet. The patient needs to understand what to eat, how much to eat, and when to eat. Stress the importance of eating on time, the dangers of skipping meals, and how to maintain food intake during illness. Ask the patient to describe the meal plan and explain the adjustments needed to meet diabetic diet requirements. Include the family member usually responsible for buying groceries and preparing meals in this teaching.

Regular physical activity is important for physical fitness, weight management, and blood glucose control. Assist all patients to identify activities they can do to achieve the goal of moderate-intensity activity 3 or more days a week. For patients taking insulin and/or insulin secretagogues, physical activity can cause hypoglycemia if drug dosage or carbohydrate intake is not increased. Review how to perform physical activities safely. Instruct the patient on blood glucose levels that are safe for exercise, the frequency of glucose monitoring during exercise, drug adjustments before exercise, food required before exercise, and what food to have available during exercise. He or she should be aware of the risk for injury during exercise and be able to explain the importance of protective footwear.

Self-monitoring of blood glucose provides immediate information on a person's blood glucose level and provides feedback on the effects of recent activity, drugs, and meals. The nurse's role includes teaching skills of performing the test, educating how to interpret results, and problem solving to adjust behaviors and therapy based on the information. Teach patients how to recognize when blood glucose levels are out of range, how to adjust therapy and behaviors based on self-monitoring of blood glucose (SMBG) results, and how to verify the effects of these adjustments by performing subsequent glucose testing. Also, show patients who use insulin how to use SMBG to adjust dosages to achieve glucose control while avoiding episodes of hypoglycemia.

Teach patients sick-day procedures when initially diagnosed with diabetes. Hyperglycemia often develops before INFECTION manifestations and can serve as a warning that infection is developing. Provide guidelines for the frequency of glucose testing, for ketone testing, and for insulin adjustment for those patients able to self-adjust insulin doses.

Psychosocial Preparation. The diagnosis of diabetes may represent a loss of control and flexibility. Life becomes ordered, and routines must be followed. Certain events surrounding diabetes are predictable. Taking an insulin injection and not eating for several hours causes hypoglycemia. Poorly controlled diabetes leads to complications and premature death. Tight control of blood glucose levels prevents complications.

The stress of diabetes is in addition to the demands of normal daily life. The patient must be able to integrate the demands of diabetes into daily and recreational schedules while keeping blood glucose stable.

Patients are more likely to adhere to disease management activities when the strategies make sense and seem effective. Other factors promoting adherence include the patient's belief that the activity is important, having confidence in himself or herself, and having support. Assist in healthy psychological adaptation to diabetes by providing successful educational experiences. Mastery of blood glucose monitoring helps the patient feel that he or she has control over the disease. Knowing the effects of extra activities, extra food, or extra insulin is helpful in learning to adjust the regimen.

Feeling a sense of control over the condition promotes a positive attitude about diabetes. Success in injecting insulin provides concrete evidence that he or she can master the disease. Teach by breaking a task into small, achievable units to ensure mastery. For example, a patient may begin learning how to inject insulin by first obtaining an accurate dose.

Devote as much teaching time as possible to insulin injection and blood glucose monitoring. Patients with newly diagnosed diabetes are often fearful of giving themselves injections. After

CHART 64-9 Focused Assessment

The Insulin-Dependent Patient with Diabetes During a Home or Clinic Visit

- Assess overall mental status, wakefulness, ability to converse.
- Take vital signs and weight:
  - Fever could indicate infection.
  - Are blood pressure and weight within target range? If not, why?
- Question patient regarding any change in visual acuity; check current visual acuity.
- Inspect oral mucous membranes, gums, and teeth.
- Question patient about injection areas used; inspect areas being used; assess whether patient is using areas and sites appropriately.
- Inspect skin for intactness, wounds that have not healed, new sores, ulcers, bruises, or burns; assess any previously known wounds for infection, progression of healing.
- Question patient regarding foot care.
- Assess lower extremities and feet for peripheral pulses, lack of or decreased sensation, abnormal sensations, breaks in skin integrity, condition of toes and nails.
- Question patient regarding color and consistency of stools and frequency of bowel movements; assess abdomen for bowel sounds.
- Review patient's home health diary:
  - Is blood glucose within targeted range? If not, why?
  - Is glucose monitoring being recorded often enough?
  - Is the patient's food intake adequate and appropriate? If not, why?
  - Is exercise occurring regularly? If not, why?
- Assess patient's ability to perform self-monitoring of blood glucose.
- Assess patient's procedures for obtaining and storing insulin and syringes, cleaning equipment, disposing of syringes and needles.
- Assess patient's insulin preparation and injection technique.

TABLE 64-15 Outcome Criteria for Diabetes Teaching

Before being discharged to home, the patient with diabetes or the significant other should be able to:
- Tell why insulin or an oral hypoglycemic agent is being prescribed
- Name which insulin or oral hypoglycemic agent is being prescribed, and name the dosage and frequency of administration
- Discuss the relationship between mealtime and the action of insulin or the oral hypoglycemic agent
- Discuss plans to follow diabetic diet instructions
- Prepare and administer insulin accurately
- Test blood for glucose, or state plans for having blood glucose levels monitored
- Test urine for ketones, and state when this test should be done
- Verbalize how to store insulin
- List manifestations that indicate a hypoglycemic reaction
- Tell what carbohydrate sources are used to treat hypoglycemic reactions
- Tell what manifestations indicate hyperglycemia
- Tell what dietary changes are needed during illness
- Verbalize when to call the physician or the nurse (frequent episodes of hypoglycemia, manifestations of hyperglycemia)
- Verbalize the procedures for proper foot care

this technique has been mastered, they become less anxious and are able to attend to other tasks.

Recognize that not everyone will adapt to diabetes. Some patients are unable to progress beyond the survival level. Major depression affects many patients with diabetes, having an impact on quality of life and all aspects of functioning, including self-management behaviors. Refer those who have significant problems coping with the day-to-day demands of diabetes to mental health counseling for appropriate treatment.

Home Care Management. Patients with diabetes self-manage their disease. Each day they decide what to eat, whether to exercise, and whether to take prescribed drugs. Maintaining blood glucose control depends on the accuracy of self-management skills. The nurse provides support and education to empower the patient to make informed decisions. Self-management education allows patients to identify their problems and provides techniques to help them make decisions, take appropriate actions, and alter these actions as needed.

Provide information about resources. The patient must know whom to contact in case of emergency. Older adults who live alone need to have daily telephone contact with a friend or neighbor. The patient may also need help shopping and preparing meals. He or she may have limited access to transportation and may not have sufficient supplies of food, particularly in bad weather. Because of the likelihood of visual problems in older patients, they may need assistance in preparing insulin syringes for injection or in monitoring blood glucose. Make referrals to home care or public health agencies as needed. Chart 64-9 identifies areas for assessment during a home or clinic visit.

◆ Evaluation: Outcomes

Evaluate the care of the patient with diabetes based on the identified priority patient problems. Outcome success for diabetes education is the ability of the patient to maintain blood glucose levels within their established target range. General outcome criteria are listed below and in Table 64-15. More specific outcomes are listed with each priority patient problem. The expected outcomes include that the patient should:
- Achieve blood glucose control
- Avoid acute and chronic complications of diabetes
- Avoid injury
- Experience relief of pain
- Maintain optimal visual SENSORY PERCEPTION
- Maintain a urine output in the expected range
- Have an optimal level of mental status functioning
- Have decreased episodes of hypoglycemia
- Have decreased episodes of hyperglycemia

Specific indicators for these outcomes are listed for each priority patient problem under the Planning and Implementation section (see earlier).

NURSING CONCEPTS AND CLINICAL JUDGMENT REVIEW

What might you NOTICE in a patient with diabetes mellitus who demonstrates adequate GLUCOSE REGULATION?

Vital signs:
* Blood pressure less than 140/80
* Heart rate and rhythm within the normal range
* Temperature within the normal range

Physical assessment:
* Skin intact, especially on the feet, no open wounds or sores that have failed to heal
* Weight proportionate to height; does not appear overweight or underweight
* Vision adequate for safety and participation in ADLs
* No report of pain, tingling, numbness, or burning in extremities

Psychological assessment:
* Oriented and not confused
* Willing to learn and participate in self-care
* Energy level good; can engage in desired work, recreational, and personal activities

Laboratory assessment:
* A1C levels are maintained at 6.5% or below.
* The majority of premeal blood glucose levels are 70 to 130 mg/dL (3.9 to 7.2 mmol/L).
* Peak after-meal blood glucose levels are less than 180 mg/dL (<10.0 mmol/L).
* Urine is free from ketone bodies and albumin.
* 24-hour intake and output balance.
* Blood urea nitrogen (BUN) and serum creatinine are within the normal ranges.
* Serum electrolytes are within the normal ranges.

GET READY FOR THE NCLEX® EXAMINATION!

▍KEY POINTS

Review these Key Points for each NCLEX Examination Client Needs Category.

Safe and Effective Care Environment
* Use aseptic technique during any invasive procedure when caring for a patient with diabetes. **Safety** QSEN
* Administer antidiabetic drugs and insulin in a safe manner. **Safety** QSEN
* Ensure that meals are available immediately after the patient receives an antidiabetic drug or insulin. **Safety** QSEN
* Use good handwashing techniques before providing any care to a patient who has diabetes. **Safety** QSEN

Health Promotion and Maintenance
* Encourage all patients to maintain weight within an appropriate range. **Evidence-Based Practice** QSEN
* Encourage all patients, including patients with diabetes, to participate regularly in exercise or physical activity appropriate to their health status. **Patient-Centered Care** QSEN
* Teach the patient and family about the manifestations of INFECTION and when to seek medical advice.
* Instruct patients with diabetes to wear a medical alert bracelet. **Safety** QSEN
* Instruct patients to not share blood glucose monitoring equipment. **Evidence-Based Practice** QSEN
* Reinforce to all patients with diabetes that tight control over blood glucose levels reduces the risk for the vascular complications of diabetes. **Patient-Centered Care** QSEN
* Remind patients with diabetes to have yearly eye examinations by an ophthalmologist. **Evidence-Based Practice** QSEN
* Teach patients with peripheral neuropathy to use a bath thermometer to test water for bathing, to avoid walking barefoot, and to inspect their feet daily. **Safety** QSEN
* Assess patients' visual acuity and peripheral tactile sensation to determine needed adjustments in teaching self-medication and self-monitoring of blood glucose levels.

* Instruct all patients with diabetes to avoid becoming dehydrated and to drink at least 2 L of water each day unless another medical condition requires fluid restriction. **Patient-Centered Care** QSEN
* Instruct patients who are taking sulfonylurea drugs about an increased risk for hypoglycemic reactions. **Patient-Centered Care** QSEN
* Teach patients who are taking metformin the clinical manifestations of lactic acidosis (fatigue, dizziness, difficulty breathing, stomach discomfort, irregular heartbeat). **Safety** QSEN
* Warn patients to not take over-the-counter drugs with their oral antidiabetic drugs without consulting their primary care provider.
* Teach patients to rotate insulin injection sites within one area rather than to other areas, to prevent changes in absorption. **Evidence-Based Practice** QSEN
* Use return demonstration and "teach-back" strategies when teaching the patient about drug regimen, insulin injection, blood glucose monitoring, and foot assessment. **Patient-Centered Care** QSEN
* Teach patients to administer an accurate dose of insulin using a prefilled or disposable insulin pen.
* Teach patients who experience Somogyi phenomenon (early morning hyperglycemia) to ensure an adequate dietary intake at bedtime.
* Instruct patients to always carry a glucose source.
* Teach patients who exercise to test urine for ketone bodies if blood glucose levels are greater than 250 mg/dL before engaging in strenuous exercise.
* Instruct patients in foot care as outlined in Chart 64-6.

Psychosocial Integrity
* Explore with the patient what the diagnosis of diabetes means to him or her. **Patient-Centered Care** QSEN
* Allow the patient the opportunity to express concerns about the diagnosis of diabetes or the treatment regimen.

- Explain all procedures, restrictions, drugs, and follow-up care to the patient and family.
- Instruct the patient and family on the manifestations of complications and when to seek assistance. **Safety** `QSEN`
- Pace your education sessions to match the learning needs and style of the patient. **Patient-Centered Care** `QSEN`

Physiological Integrity

- Never dilute or mix insulin glargine with any other insulin or solution. **Safety** `QSEN`
- Avoid injecting insulin within a 2-inch radius of the umbilicus.
- Avoid IM insulin injection.
- Assist patients who have PAIN from peripheral neuropathy to determine what pain-relieving drugs and techniques work best for them.
- Assess the patient's A1C level for indications of adherence to prescribed regimens and their effectiveness.
- Start carbohydrate replacement per physician prescription or standing protocols immediately on identifying a patient with hypoglycemia. **Safety** `QSEN`
- Give glucagon subcutaneously or IM and 50% dextrose IV to patients identified with hypoglycemia who cannot swallow. **Evidence-Based Practice** `QSEN`

- First assess the airway, level of consciousness, hydration status, electrolytes, and blood glucose level of any patient with diabetic ketoacidosis.
- Use blood glucose values to assess therapy effectiveness and determine when to switch from saline to dextrose-containing solutions in a patient with diabetic ketoacidosis.
- Continually assess fluid status and level of consciousness in a patient with hyperglycemic-hyperosmolar state (HHS) during the resuscitation period.
- Immediately report manifestations of cerebral edema (abrupt changes in mental status; changes in level of consciousness; changes in pupil size, shape, or reaction; seizures) in a patient with HHS to the health care provider. **Safety** `QSEN`
- Collaborate with the health care provider, diabetes nurse educator, registered dietitian, pharmacist, social worker, and case manager to individualize patient care for the person with diabetes in any care setting. **Teamwork and Collaboration** `QSEN`
- Refer patients newly diagnosed with diabetes to local resources and support groups.

CONCEPT OVERVIEW

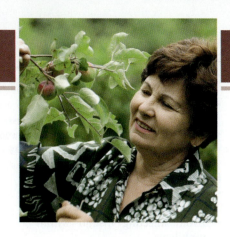

Urinary Elimination

Adequate urinary elimination is essential for body fluid homeostasis—the ability of the body to maintain its internal environment at a "steady state" and within very narrow ranges of normal, regardless of external changes. Urinary ELIMINATION alone is defined as the passage of urine through the urinary tract by means of the urinary sphincter and urethra (Giddens, 2013). However, urine cannot be eliminated unless it is first formed in the kidneys from the blood. The kidneys perform the actual work of determining which substances in body fluid will be eliminated and which will be retained. So kidney function is critical for urinary ELIMINATION to be able to maintain homeostasis of all body fluids.

The body works best when blood and other extracellular fluids maintain volumes within the normal ranges and maintain the proper ranges of electrolytes. Serious health problems and death occur when these electrolytes are much higher or lower than normal ranges. When blood volume is too high, hypertension develops and damages vital organs. When blood volume is too low, hypotension can be so severe that vital organs are not perfused with oxygen and become hypoxic. In addition, protein waste products containing nitrogen, such as urea, act as a poison and must be prevented from getting too high. Humans ingest many foods and liquids that contain water, electrolytes, and substances that will be converted to waste products. Without control mechanisms to balance the intake of these substances with their ELIMINATION, we would rapidly accumulate too much of everything and die.

As part of the renal/urinary system, the kidneys are responsible for maintaining this balance of what is taken into the body, what is allowed to remain in the body, and what is eliminated from the body. Although some products are eliminated in the stool, there is no discrimination or adjustment in bowel ELIMINATION. Urinary ELIMINATION, however, allows a person to eat and drink almost anything (except poisons and infectious organisms) in almost any amount without upsetting the homeostatic balance for body water, electrolytes, waste products, and blood pressure. For example, on one day a person may drink 2 L of fluids and eat food that contains 2 g of sodium and 5 g of potassium. The next day this same person may drink 3 L of fluids and eat food that contains 12 g of sodium and 10 g of potassium. Yet because the kidneys selectively adjust to change the amount of each substance that gets eliminated, the blood pressure, serum sodium, and serum potassium levels remain the same and within the normal ranges on both days. A "steady-state" or homeostatic balance of these substances is maintained because the kidneys adjust the output to match the intake (Fig. 1).

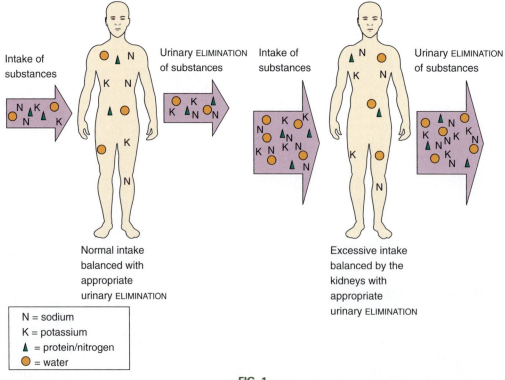

Intake of substances — Normal intake balanced with appropriate urinary ELIMINATION — Urinary ELIMINATION of substances

Intake of substances — Excessive intake balanced by the kidneys with appropriate urinary ELIMINATION — Urinary ELIMINATION of substances

N = sodium
K = potassium
▲ = protein/nitrogen
● = water

FIG. 1

When kidney function is impaired to any degree as a result of renal/urinary problems, urinary ELIMINATION is not adequate and the steady-state homeostasis of water, electrolyte, and waste products is disrupted (Fig. 2). Without intervention, this lack of steady state leads to excesses of body water, electrolytes, and nitrogenous waste products that interfere with normal organ function and can cause death.

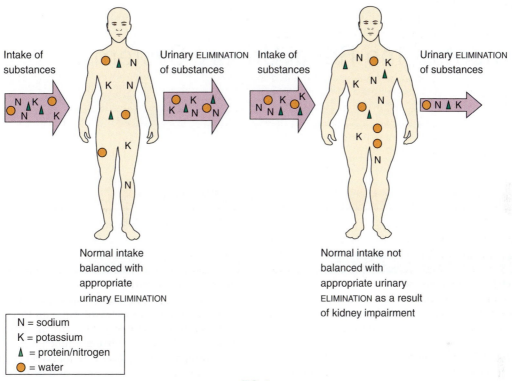

Intake of substances

Urinary ELIMINATION of substances

Intake of substances

Urinary ELIMINATION of substances

Normal intake balanced with appropriate urinary ELIMINATION

Normal intake not balanced with appropriate urinary ELIMINATION as a result of kidney impairment

N = sodium
K = potassium
▲ = protein/nitrogen
● = water

FIG. 2

65 | CHAPTER

Assessment of the Renal/Urinary System

Chris Winkelman

ⓔ http://evolve.elsevier.com/Iggy/

PRIORITY CONCEPTS

- ELIMINATION
- FLUID AND ELECTROLYTE BALANCE

- ACID-BASE BALANCE

LEARNING OUTCOMES

Safe and Effective Care Environment

1. Use principles of infection control when assessing a patient's kidney and urinary ELIMINATION for adequate FLUID AND ELECTROLYTE BALANCE and ACID-BASE BALANCE.

Health Promotion and Maintenance

2. Teach all people about the importance of maintaining an adequate oral fluid intake for FLUID AND ELECTROLYTE BALANCE.
3. Teach about or assist with cleansing of the perineum or urinary meatus after using the toilet and during daily bathing or showering.
4. Teach all people how to protect the kidneys and urinary system from toxic substances.

Psychosocial Integrity

5. Reduce the psychological impact for the patient and family regarding the assessment and testing of the renal/urinary system.

Physiological Integrity

6. Perform a focused assessment of kidney and urinary function, incorporating information from anatomy and physiology, including genetic risk and age-related changes affecting kidney and urinary function.
7. Coordinate appropriate care for patients after invasive and noninvasive testing of kidney and urinary function.
8. Use correct technique to assess the kidneys and urinary system.
9. Prioritize nursing care for the patient during the first 24 hours after invasive procedures, especially those requiring contrast material.

The renal system includes the kidneys and the entire urinary tract. The ureters, bladder, and urethra are the drainage route for the excretion of urine. Structural or functional problems in the kidneys or urinary tract may alter FLUID AND ELECTROLYTE BALANCE and ACID-BASE BALANCE.

The kidneys help maintain health in many ways. *Most important, they maintain body fluid volume and composition and filter waste products for ELIMINATION.* The kidneys also help regulate blood pressure and ACID-BASE BALANCE, produce erythropoietin for red blood cell (RBC) synthesis, and convert vitamin D to an active form.

Assessment of the patient at risk for or with actual problems of the kidneys or urinary system begins with a history and physical assessment. Understanding the anatomy, physiology, and diagnostic tests of the renal system helps you in problem solving about kidney and urinary tract function in the clinical setting. It also assists you in teaching the patient about the purpose of procedures and in physically and emotionally preparing the patient for assessment.

ANATOMY AND PHYSIOLOGY REVIEW

Kidneys

Structure

Gross Anatomy. The two kidneys are located behind the peritoneum, not in the abdominal cavity, one on either side of the spine (Fig. 65-1). The adult kidney is 4 to 5 inches (10 to 13 cm) long, 2 to 3 inches (5 to 7 cm) wide, and about 1 inch (2.5 to 3 cm) thick. The left kidney is slightly longer and narrower than the right kidney. Larger-than-usual kidneys may

indicate obstruction or polycystic disease. Smaller-than-usual kidneys may indicate chronic kidney disease (CKD).

Variation in kidney shape and number is not uncommon and does not always indicate a problem in kidney function. Some people have more than two kidneys or may have only one large, horseshoe-shaped kidney. As long as tests of kidney function are normal, these variations are of no significance.

Several layers of tissue surround the kidney, providing protection and support. The outer surface of the kidney is a layer of fibrous tissue called the **capsule** (Fig. 65-2). It covers most of the kidney except the **hilum**, which is the area where the kidney blood vessels and nerves enter and exit. It is also where the ureter exits. The capsule is surrounded by layers of fat and connective tissue.

Lying beneath the capsule are the two layers of functional kidney tissue—the cortex and the medulla. The **renal cortex** is the outer tissue layer. The **medulla** is the medullary tissue lying below the cortex in the shape of many fans. Each "fan" is called a *pyramid*. The **renal columns** are cortical tissue that dips down into the interior of the kidney and separates the pyramids.

The tip of each pyramid is called a **papilla**. The papillae drain urine into the collecting system. A cuplike structure called a **calyx** collects the urine at the end of each papilla. The calices join together to form the **renal pelvis**, which narrows to become the ureter.

The kidneys have a rich blood supply and receive a blood flow from 600 to 1300 mL/min. The blood supply to each kidney comes from the renal artery, which branches from the abdominal aorta. The renal artery divides into progressively smaller arteries, supplying all blood to areas of the kidney tissue and the nephrons. The smallest arteries (**afferent arterioles**) feed the nephrons directly to form urine.

Venous blood from the kidneys starts with the capillaries surrounding each nephron. These capillaries drain into progressively larger veins, with blood eventually returned to the inferior vena cava through the renal vein.

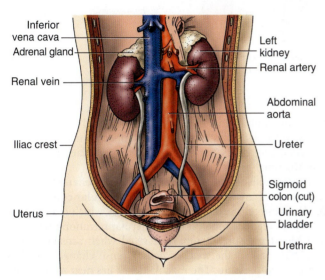

FIG. 65-1 Anatomic location of the kidneys and structures of the urinary system.

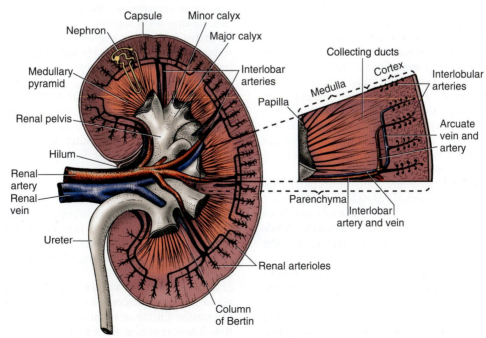

FIG. 65-2 Bisection of the kidney showing the major structures of the kidney.

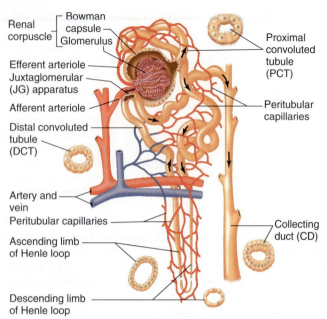

FIG. 65-3 Anatomy of the nephron—the functional unit of the kidney. The differences in appearance in tubular cells seen in a cross section reflect the differing functions of each nephron segment. Note that the particular nephron labeled here is a juxtamedullary nephron.

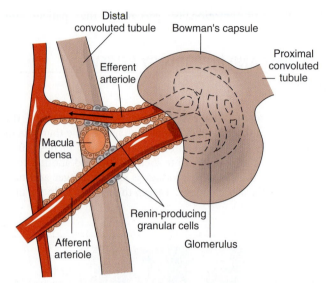

FIG. 65-4 The juxtaglomerular complex showing juxtaglomerular cells and the macula densa.

Microscopic Anatomy. The **nephron** is the functional unit of the kidney, which forms urine from blood. There are about 1 million nephrons per kidney, and each nephron separately makes urine from blood.

There are two types of nephrons: *cortical nephrons* and *juxtamedullary nephrons*. The cortical nephrons are short and lie totally within the renal cortex. The juxtamedullary nephrons (about 20% of all nephrons) are longer, and their tubes and blood vessels dip deeply into the medulla. The purpose of these longer nephrons is to concentrate urine during times of low fluid intake to allow continued excretion of body wastes with less fluid loss.

Blood supply to the nephron is delivered through the afferent arteriole—the smallest, most distal portion of the renal arterial system. From the afferent arteriole, blood flows into the **glomerulus**, which is a series of specialized capillary loops. It is through these capillaries that water and small particles are filtered from the blood to make urine. The remaining blood leaves the glomerulus through the **efferent arteriole**, which is the first vessel in the kidney's venous system. From the efferent arteriole, blood exits into either the *peritubular capillaries* around the tubular part of the cortical nephrons or the *vasa recta* around the tubular part of juxtamedullary nephrons.

Each nephron is a tubelike structure with distinct parts (Fig. 65-3). The tube begins with Bowman's capsule, a saclike structure that surrounds the glomerulus. The tubular tissue of Bowman's capsule narrows into the *proximal convoluted tubule (PCT)*. The PCT twists and turns, finally straightening into the descending limb of the *loop of Henle*. The descending loop of Henle dips in the direction of the medulla but forms a hairpin loop and comes back up into the cortex as the ascending loop of Henle.

The two segments of the ascending limb of the loop of Henle are the thin segment and the thick segment. The *distal convoluted tubule (DCT)* forms from the thick segment of the

ascending limb of the loop of Henle. The DCT ends in one of many collecting ducts located in the kidney tissue. The urine in the collecting ducts passes through the papillae and empties into the renal pelvis.

Special cells in the afferent arteriole, the efferent arteriole, and the DCT are known as the **juxtaglomerular complex** (Fig. 65-4). These cells produce and store **renin**, which is a hormone that helps regulate blood flow, glomerular filtration rate (GFR), and blood pressure. Renin is secreted when sensing cells in the DCT (called the *macula densa*) sense changes in blood volume and pressure. The macula densa lies next to the renin-producing cells. Renin is produced when the macula densa cells sense that blood volume, blood pressure, or blood sodium level is low. Renin then converts renin substrate (angiotensinogen) into angiotensin I. This leads to a series of reactions that cause secretion of the hormone *aldosterone* (Fig. 65-5). Aldosterone helps regulate FLUID AND ELECTROLYTE BALANCE by increasing kidney reabsorption of sodium and water and restoring blood pressure, blood volume, and blood sodium levels (McCance et al., 2014). It also promotes excretion of potassium (see Chapter 11).

The glomerular capillary wall has three layers (Fig. 65-6): the endothelium, the basement membrane, and the epithelium. The endothelial and epithelial cells lining these capillaries are separated by pores that filter water and small particles from the blood into Bowman's capsule. This fluid is called the "filtrate" or "early urine."

Function

The kidneys have both regulatory and hormonal functions. The regulatory functions control FLUID AND ELECTROLYTE BALANCE and ACID-BASE BALANCE. The hormonal functions control red blood cell (RBC) formation, blood pressure, and vitamin D activation.

Regulatory Functions. The kidney processes that maintain FLUID AND ELECTROLYTE BALANCE and ACID-BASE BALANCE are glomerular filtration, tubular reabsorption, and tubular secretion. These processes use filtration, diffusion, active transport, and osmosis. (See Chapter 11 for a review of these actions.)

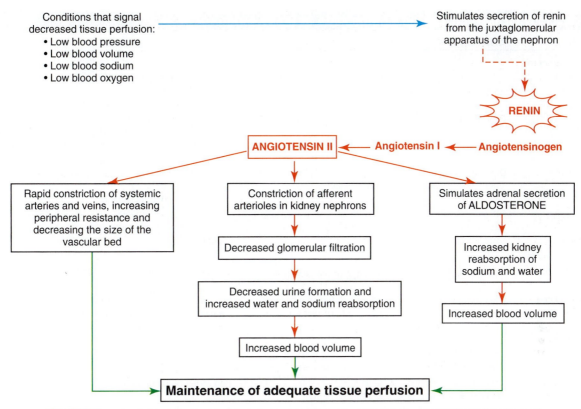

FIG. 65-5 The role of aldosterone, renin substrate (angiotensinogen), angiotensin I, and angiotensin II in the renal regulation of water and sodium.

BOWMAN'S CAPSULE

FIG. 65-6 Glomerular capillary wall.

Table 65-1 lists the functions of nephron tubules and blood vessels.

Glomerular filtration is the first process in urine formation. As blood passes from the afferent arteriole into the glomerulus, water, electrolytes, and other small particles (e.g., creatinine, urea nitrogen, glucose) are filtered across the glomerular membrane into the Bowman's capsule to form *glomerular* filtrate. As the filtrate enters the proximal convoluted tubule (PCT), it is called *tubular filtrate.*

Large particles, such as blood cells, albumin, and other proteins, are too large to filter through the glomerular capillary walls. *Therefore these substances are not normally present in the final urine.*

About 180 L of glomerular filtrate is formed from the blood each day. The rate of filtration is expressed in milliliters per minute. Normal glomerular filtration rate (GFR) averages 125 mL/min. If the entire amount of filtrate were excreted as urine, death would occur quickly from dehydration. Actually, only about 1 to 3 L is excreted each day as urine. The rest is reabsorbed back into the circulatory system (McCance et al., 2014).

GFR is controlled by blood pressure and blood flow. The kidneys self-regulate their own blood pressure and blood flow, which keeps GFR constant. GFR is controlled by selectively constricting and dilating the afferent and efferent arterioles. When the afferent arteriole is constricted or the efferent arteriole is dilated, pressure in the glomerular capillaries falls and filtration decreases. When the afferent arteriole is dilated or the efferent arteriole is constricted, pressure in the glomerular capillaries rises and filtration increases. This way the kidney maintains a constant GFR, even when systemic blood pressure changes. When systolic pressure drops below 65 to 70 mm Hg, these self-regulation processes are not effective at maintaining GFR.

Tubular reabsorption is the second process in urine formation. This reabsorption of most of the filtrate keeps normal urine output at 1 to 3 L/day and prevents dehydration. As the filtrate passes through the tubular parts of the nephron, most of the water and electrolytes is reabsorbed from the tubular lumen of the nephron and into the peritubular capillaries. This process returns most water, electrolytes, and other particles to the blood.

TABLE 65-1 Vascular and Tubular Components of the Nephron

STRUCTURE	ANATOMIC FEATURES	PHYSIOLOGIC ASPECTS
Vascular Components		
Afferent arteriole	Delivers arterial blood from the branches of the renal artery into the glomerulus	Autoregulation of renal blood flow via vasoconstriction or vasodilation Renin-producing granular cells
Glomerulus	Capillary loops with thin, semipermeable membrane	Site of glomerular filtration Glomerular filtration occurs when hydrostatic pressure (blood pressure) is greater than opposing forces (tubular filtrate and oncotic pressure)
Efferent arteriole	Delivers arterial blood from the glomerulus into the peritubular capillaries or the vasa recta	Autoregulation of renal blood flow via vasoconstriction or vasodilation Renin-producing granular cells
Peritubular capillaries (PTCs) and vasa recta (VR)	PTCs: surround tubular components of cortical nephrons VR: surround tubular components of juxtamedullary nephrons	Tubular reabsorption and tubular secretion allow movement of water and solutes to or from the tubules, interstitium, and blood
Tubular Components		
Bowman's capsule (BC)	Thin membranous sac surrounding $\frac{7}{8}$ of the glomerulus	Collects glomerular filtrate (GF) and funnels it into the tubule
Proximal convoluted tubule (PCT)	Evolves from and is continuous with Bowman's capsule Specialized cellular lining facilitates tubular reabsorption	Site for reabsorption of sodium, chloride, water, glucose, amino acids, potassium, calcium, bicarbonate, phosphate, and urea
Loop of Henle	Continues from PCT Juxtamedullary nephrons dip deep into the medulla Permeable to water, urea, and sodium chloride	Regulation of water balance
Descending limb (DL)	Continues from the loop of Henle Permeable to water, urea, and sodium chloride	Regulation of water balance
Ascending limb (AL)	Emerges from DL as it turns and is redirected up toward the renal cortex	Potassium and magnesium reabsorption in the thick segment Thin segment is impermeable to water
Distal convoluted tubule (DCT)	Evolves from AL and twists so the macula densa cells lie adjacent to the juxtaglomerular cells of afferent arteriole	Site of additional water and electrolyte reabsorption, including bicarbonate Potassium and hydrogen secretion
Collecting ducts	Collect formed urine from several tubules and deliver it into the renal pelvis	Receptor sites for antidiuretic hormone regulation of water balance

The tubules return about 99% of all filtered water back into the body (Fig. 65-7). Most water reabsorption occurs in the PCT. Water reabsorption continues as the filtrate flows down the descending loop of Henle. The thin and thick segments of the ascending loop of Henle are *not* permeable to water, and water reabsorption does not occur here.

The distal convoluted tubule (DCT) can be permeable to water, and some water reabsorption occurs as the filtrate continues to flow through the tubule. The membrane of the DCT may be made more permeable to water when *vasopressin*, also known as *antidiuretic hormone* (ADH), and aldosterone are present. Vasopressin increases tubular permeability to water, allowing water to leave the tube and be reabsorbed back into the capillaries. Vasopressin also increases arteriole constriction. Arteriole constriction alters blood pressure, which then affects the amounts of fluid and particles that exit glomerular capillaries. Aldosterone promotes the reabsorption of sodium in the DCT. Water reabsorption occurs as a result of the movement of sodium (where sodium goes, water follows).

The ability of the kidneys to vary the volume or concentration of urine helps regulate water balance regardless of fluid intake. In this way, the healthy kidney can prevent dehydration when fluid intake is low and can prevent circulatory overload when fluid intake is high.

In addition to water, some types of particles in the tubular filtrate also are returned to the blood by *tubular reabsorption*. About 50% of all urea in the filtrate is reabsorbed, although creatinine is not reabsorbed.

Most sodium, chloride, and water reabsorption occurs in the PCT. The collecting ducts are the other site of sodium, chloride, and water reabsorption. Here reabsorption is caused by aldosterone. Potassium is mostly reabsorbed in the PCT and in the thick segment of the loop of Henle.

Bicarbonate, calcium, and phosphate are mostly reabsorbed in the PCT. Bicarbonate reabsorption helps ACID-BASE BALANCE and maintains a normal blood pH. Blood levels of calcitonin and parathyroid hormone (PTH) (see Chapters 11 and 63) control calcium balance.

The kidney reabsorbs some of the glucose filtered from the blood. However, there is a limit to how much glucose the kidney can reabsorb. This limit is called the **renal threshold** or **transport maximum (tm)** for glucose reabsorption. The usual renal threshold for glucose is about 220 mg/dL. This means that at a blood glucose level of 220 mg/dL or less, all glucose is reabsorbed and returned to the blood, with no glucose present in final urine. When blood glucose levels are greater than 220 mg/dL, some glucose stays in the filtrate and is present in the urine. Normally, almost all glucose and most proteins are reabsorbed and are not present in the urine.

TABLE 65-2   Kidney Hormones and Hormones Influencing Kidney Function

	SITE	ACTION
Kidney Hormones		
Renin	Renin-producing granular cells	Raises blood pressure as result of angiotensin (local vasoconstriction) and aldosterone (volume expansion) secretion
Prostaglandins	Kidney tissues	Regulate intrarenal blood flow by vasodilation or vasoconstriction
Bradykinins	Juxtaglomerular cells of the arterioles	Increase blood flow (vasodilation) and vascular permeability
Erythropoietin	Kidney parenchyma	Stimulates bone marrow to make red blood cells
Activated vitamin D	Kidney parenchyma	Promotes absorption of calcium in the GI tract
Hormones Influencing Kidney Function		
Vasopressin (Antidiuretic hormone [ADH])	Released from posterior pituitary	Makes DCT and CD permeable to water to maximize reabsorption and produce a concentrated urine
Aldosterone	Released from adrenal cortex	Promotes sodium reabsorption and potassium secretion in DCT and CD; water and chloride follow sodium movement
Natriuretic hormones	Cardiac atria, cardiac ventricles, brain	Cause tubular secretion of sodium

CD, Collecting duct; *DCT,* distal convoluted tubule.

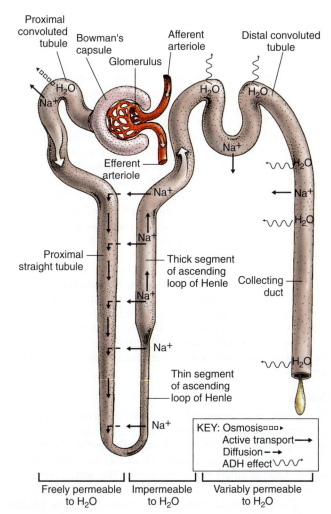

FIG. 65-7 Sodium and water reabsorption by the tubules of a cortical nephron. *ADH,* Antidiuretic hormone; *Na+,* sodium.

⚠ NURSING SAFETY PRIORITY (QSEN)

Action Alert

Report the presence of glucose or proteins in the urine of a patient undergoing a screening examination to the health care provider because this is an abnormal finding and requires further assessment.

Tubular secretion is the third process of urine formation. It allows substances to move from the blood into the early urine. During tubular secretion, substances move from the peritubular capillaries in reverse, across capillary membranes, and into the cells that line the tubules. From the cells, these substances are moved into the urine and are excreted from the body. Potassium (K^+) and hydrogen (H^+) ions are some of the substances moved in this way to maintain FLUID AND ELECTROLYTE BALANCE and ACID-BASE BALANCE (pH).

Hormonal Functions. The kidneys produce renin, prostaglandins, erythropoietin, and activated vitamin D (Table 65-2). Other kidney products, such as the kinins, change kidney blood flow and capillary permeability. The kidneys also help break down and excrete insulin.

Renin, as discussed on p. 1346 in the Microscopic Anatomy section, assists in blood pressure control. It is formed and released when there is a decrease in blood flow, blood volume, or blood pressure through the renal arterioles or when too little sodium is present in kidney blood. These conditions are detected through the receptors of the juxtaglomerular complex.

Renin release causes the production of *angiotensin II* through a series of steps (see Fig. 65-5). Angiotensin II increases systemic blood pressure through powerful blood vessel constricting effects and triggers the release of aldosterone from the adrenal glands. Aldosterone increases the reabsorption of sodium in the distal tubule of the nephron. Therefore more water is reabsorbed, which increases blood volume and blood pressure. When blood flow to the kidney is reduced, this system also prevents fluid loss and maintains circulating blood volume (see Chapter 11).

Prostaglandins are produced in the kidney and many other tissues. Those produced specifically in the kidney help regulate glomerular filtration, kidney vascular resistance, and renin production. They also increase sodium and water excretion.

Erythropoietin is produced and released in response to decreased oxygen tension in the kidney's blood supply. It triggers red blood cell (RBC) production in the bone marrow. When kidney function is poor, erythropoietin production decreases and the person develops anemia.

Vitamin D activation occurs through a series of steps. Some of these steps take place in the skin when it is exposed to sunlight, and then more processing occurs in the liver. From there, vitamin D is converted to its active form in the kidney. Activated vitamin D is needed to absorb calcium in the intestinal tract and to regulate calcium balance (McCance et al., 2014).

Ureters

Each kidney has a single ureter—a hollow tube that connects the renal pelvis with the urinary bladder. The ureter is about ½ inch (1.25 cm) in diameter and about 12 to 18 inches (30 to 45 cm) in length. The diameter of the ureter narrows in three areas:

- In the upper third of the ureter, at the point in which the renal pelvis becomes the ureter, is a narrowing known as the **ureteropelvic junction (UPJ)**.
- The ureter also narrows as it bends toward the abdominal wall (aortoiliac bend).
- Each ureter narrows at the point it enters the bladder; this point is called the **ureterovesical junction (UVJ)**.

The ureter tunnels through bladder tissue for a short distance and then opens into the bladder at the trigone (Fig. 65-8).

The ureter has three layers: an inner lining of mucous membrane (*urothelium*), a middle layer of smooth muscle fibers, and an outer layer of fibrous tissue. The middle layer of muscle fibers is controlled by several nerve pathways from the lower spinal cord.

Contractions of the smooth muscle in the ureter move urine from the kidney pelvis to the bladder. Stretch receptors in the kidney pelvis regulate this movement. For example, a large volume of urine in the kidney pelvis triggers the stretch receptors, which respond by increasing ureteral contractions and ureter peristalsis.

Urinary Bladder

Structure

The urinary bladder is a muscular sac (see Fig. 65-8) that lies directly behind the pubic bone. In men, the bladder is in front of the rectum. In women, it is in front of the vagina.

The bladder is composed of the *body* (the rounded sac portion) and the *bladder neck* (posterior urethra), which connects to the bladder body. The bladder has three linings—an inner lining of epithelial cells (*urothelium*), middle layers of smooth muscle (*detrusor muscle*), and an outer lining. The *trigone* is an area on the posterior wall between the points of ureteral entry (ureterovesical junctions [UVJs]) and the urethra.

The **internal urethral sphincter** is the smooth detrusor muscle of the bladder neck and elastic tissue. The **external urethral sphincter** is skeletal muscle that surrounds the urethra. In men, the external sphincter surrounds the urethra at the base of the prostate gland. In women, the external sphincter is at the base of the bladder. The pudendal nerve from the spinal cord controls the external sphincter.

Function

The bladder stores urine, provides continence, and enables voiding. The secretions of the urothelium lining the bladder resist bacteria.

Continence is the ability to voluntarily control bladder emptying. Continence occurs during bladder filling through the combination of detrusor muscle relaxation, internal sphincter muscle tone, and external sphincter contraction. As the bladder fills with urine, stretch sensations are transmitted to spinal sacral nerves.

Maintaining continence occurs by the interaction of the nerves that control the muscles of the bladder, bladder neck, urethra, and pelvic floor, as well as by factors that close the urethra. In the continent person, the smooth muscle of the detrusor remains relaxed during a period of urine filling and storage. Sympathetic nervous system fibers prevent detrusor muscle contraction. The control centers for voiding are located in the cerebral cortex, the brainstem, and the lower spinal cord. For urethral closure to be adequate for continence, the mucosal surfaces must be in contact and must be adhesive. Contact depends on the presence and proper function of the involved nerves and muscles. Adhesion depends on the adequate secretion of mucus-like substances.

Micturition (voiding) is a reflex of autonomic control that triggers contraction of the detrusor muscle (closing the ureter at the UVJ to prevent backflow) at the same time as relaxation of the external sphincter and the muscles of the pelvic floor. Voluntary voiding occurs as a learned response and is controlled by the cerebral cortex and the brainstem. Contraction of the external sphincter inhibits the micturition reflex and prevents voiding.

Urethra

The urethra is a narrow tube lined with mucous membranes. Its purpose is to eliminate urine from the bladder. The **urethral meatus**, or opening, is the end point of the urethra. In men, the urethra is about 6 to 8 inches (15 to 20 cm) long, with the meatus located at the tip of the penis. The male urethra has three sections:

- The prostatic urethra, which extends from the bladder through the prostate gland
- The membranous urethra, which extends from the prostate to the wall of the pelvic floor
- The cavernous urethra, which is external and extends through the length of the penis

In women, the urethra is about 1 to 1½ inches (2.5 to 3.75 cm) long and exits the bladder through the pelvic floor. The meatus lies slightly below the clitoris and directly in front of the vagina and rectum.

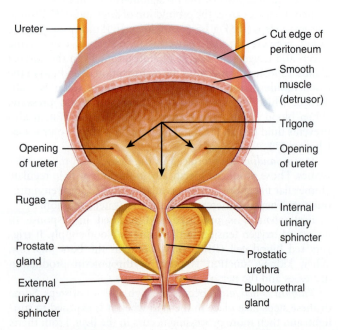

Ureter — Cut edge of peritoneum — Smooth muscle (detrusor) — Trigone — Opening of ureter — Opening of ureter — Rugae — Internal urinary sphincter — Prostate gland — Prostatic urethra — External urinary sphincter — Bulbourethral gland

FIG. 65-8 Gross anatomy of the urinary bladder.

Kidney and Urinary System Changes Associated with Aging

Kidney Changes

Changes occur in the kidney as a result of the aging process and can affect health (Chart 65-1) (Touhy & Jett, 2014). The kidney loses cortical tissue and gets smaller with age. This cortical loss is caused by reduced blood flow to the kidney. The medulla is not affected by aging, and the juxtamedullary nephron functions are preserved. The glomerular and tubular linings thicken. Both the number of glomeruli and their surface areas decrease with aging. Tubule length decreases. These changes reduce the ability of the older adult to filter blood and excrete waste products.

Blood flow to the kidney declines by about 10% per decade as blood vessels thicken. This means that blood flow to the kidney is not as adaptive in older adults, leaving nephrons more vulnerable to damage during episodes of either hypotension or hypertension.

Glomerular filtration rate (GFR) decreases with age. By age 65 years, the GFR is about 65 mL/min (half the rate of a young adult) and increases the risk for fluid overload. This decline is more rapid in patients with diabetes, hypertension, or heart failure. The combination of reduced kidney mass, reduced blood flow, and decreased GFR contributes to reduced drug clearance and a greater risk for drug reactions and kidney damage from drugs and contrast dyes in older adults.

Tubular changes with aging decrease the ability to concentrate urine, resulting in urgency (a sense of a nearly uncontrollable need to urinate) and nocturnal polyuria (increased urination at night). The regulation of sodium, acids, and bicarbonate is less efficient. Along with an age-related impairment in the thirst mechanism, these changes increase the risk for disturbances of FLUID AND ELECTROLYTE BALANCE, such as dehydration and hypernatremia (increased blood sodium levels) in the older adult. Hormonal changes include a decrease in renin secretion, aldosterone levels, and activation of vitamin D.

Urinary Changes

Changes in detrusor muscle elasticity lead to decreased bladder capacity and reduced ability to retain urine. The urge to void may cause immediate bladder emptying because the urinary sphincters lose tone and often become weaker with age. In women, weakened muscles in the pelvic floor shorten the urethra and promote incontinence. In men, an enlarged prostate gland makes starting the urine stream difficult and may cause urinary retention.

⊕ **CULTURAL CONSIDERATIONS**

Patient-Centered Care QSEN

African Americans have more rapid age-related decreases in GFR than do white people. Kidney excretion of sodium is less effective in hypertensive African Americans who have high sodium intake, and the kidneys have about 20% less blood flow as a result of anatomic changes in small blood vessels and intrarenal responses to renin. Thus African-American patients are at greater risk for kidney failure than are white patients (Jarvis, 2016). Remind African Americans that yearly health examinations should include urinalysis, checking for the presence of microalbuminuria, and evaluating serum creatinine.

CHART 65-1 Nursing Focus on the Older Adult

Changes in the Renal System Related to Aging

PHYSIOLOGIC CHANGE	NURSING INTERVENTIONS	RATIONALES
Decreased glomerular filtration rate (GFR)	Monitor hydration status.	The ability of the kidneys to regulate water balance decreases with age.
	Ensure adequate fluid intake.	The kidneys are less able to conserve water when necessary.
	Administer potentially nephrotoxic agents or drugs carefully.	Dehydration reduces kidney blood flow and increases the nephrotoxic potential of many agents. Acute or chronic kidney failure may result.
Nocturia	Ensure adequate nighttime lighting and a hazard-free environment.	Falls and injuries are common among older patients seeking bathroom facilities.
	Ensure the availability of a bedside toilet, bedpan, or urinal.	Using these items instead of getting up to the bathroom can help prevent falls.
	Discourage excessive fluid intake for 2-4 hr before the patient goes to bed.	Excessive fluid intake at night may increase nocturia.
	Evaluate drugs and timing.	Some drugs increase urine output.
Decreased bladder capacity	Encourage the patient to use the toilet, bedpan, or urinal at least every 2 hr.	Emptying the bladder on a regular basis may avoid overflow urinary incontinence.
	Respond as soon as possible to the patient's indication of the need to void.	A quick response may alleviate episodes of urinary stress incontinence.
Weakened urinary sphincters and shortened urethra in women	Provide thorough perineal care after each voiding.	The shortened urethra increases the potential for bladder infections.
		Good perineal hygiene may prevent skin irritations and urinary tract infection (UTI).
Tendency to retain urine	Observe the patient for urinary retention (e.g., bladder distention) or urinary tract infection (e.g., dysuria, foul odor, confusion).	Urinary stasis may result in a UTI, which may lead to bloodstream infections, urosepsis, or septic shock.
	Provide privacy, assistance, and voiding stimulants such as warm water over the perineum as needed.	Nursing interventions can help initiate voiding.
	Evaluate drugs for possible contribution to retention.	Anticholinergic drugs promote urinary retention.

ASSESSMENT METHODS

Patient History

Demographic information, such as age, gender, race, and ethnicity, is important to consider as nonmodifiable risk factors in the patient with any kidney or urinary problem. A sudden onset of hypertension in patients older than 50 years suggests possible kidney disease. Clinical changes with adult polycystic kidney disease typically occur in patients in their 40s or 50s. In men older than 50 years, altered urine patterns accompany prostate disease.

Anatomic gender differences make some disorders worse or more common. For example, men rarely have ascending urinary tract infections. Women have a shorter urethra and more commonly develop cystitis (bladder inflammation, most often with infection) because bacteria pass more readily into the bladder.

Ask the patient about any previous kidney or urologic problems, including tumors, infections, stones, or urologic surgery. A history of any chronic health problems, especially diabetes mellitus or hypertension, increases the risk for development of kidney disease because these disorders damage kidney blood vessels.

Exposure to certain dyes during imaging can harm the kidneys. Iodinated contrast used for CT scans is associated with both acute and chronic kidney damage. High osmolarity contrast agents can also contribute to kidney function impairment. Exposure to gadolinium-enhanced MRI can result in nephrogenic systemic fibrosis.

Ask the patient about chemical exposures at the workplace or with hobbies. Exposure to hydrocarbons (e.g., gasoline, oil), heavy metals (especially mercury and lead), and some gases (e.g., chlorine, toluene) can impair kidney function. Use this opportunity to teach patients who come into contact with chemicals at work or during leisure-time activities to avoid direct skin or mucous membrane contact with these chemicals. Use of heroin, cocaine, methamphetamine, ecstasy, and volatile solvents (inhalants) has also been associated with kidney damage.

Specifically ask the patient whether he or she has ever been told about the presence of protein or albumin in the urine. The question "Have you ever been told that your blood pressure is high?" may prompt a response different from the one to the question "Do you have high blood pressure?" Ask women about health problems during pregnancy (e.g., proteinuria, high blood pressure, gestational diabetes, urinary tract infections). Obtain information about:

- Chemical or environmental toxin exposure in occupational, diagnostic, or other settings
- Recent travel to geographic regions that pose infectious disease risks
- Recent trauma or injury, particularly to the abdomen or pelvic or genital areas
- A history of altered patterns of urinary ELIMINATION

Socioeconomic status may influence health care practices. Prevention, early detection, and treatment of kidney or urinary problems may be limited by lack of insurance or access to health care, lack of transportation, and reduced income. Low income may also result in difficulty following medical advice, having prescriptions filled, adhering to dietary instructions, and keeping follow-up appointments.

Education level may affect health-seeking practices and the patient's understanding of a disease or its manifestations.

Recurring urinary tract infections can result from not completing a course of antibiotic therapy or from not following up to ensure the infection is cleared and risks are well-managed.

The patient's health beliefs affect the approach to health and illness. Cultural background or religious affiliation may influence the belief system.

The language used by patients may be different from that used by the health care professional. When obtaining a history, listen to and explore the terms used by the patient. By using the patient's own terms, you may help him or her provide a more complete description of the problem and may decrease the patient's discomfort when discussing bodily functions.

Nutrition History

Ask the patient with known or suspected kidney or urologic disorders about his or her usual diet and any recent changes in the diet. Note any excessive intake or omission of certain food categories. Ask about food and fluid intake. Assess how much and what types of fluids the patient drinks daily, especially fluids with a high calorie or caffeine content. Use this opportunity to teach the patient the importance of drinking sufficient fluid to cause urine to be dilute (clear or very light yellow). If another medical problem does not require fluid restriction, health care providers recommend about 2 liters of fluid daily to prevent dehydration and cystitis. If the patient has followed a diet for weight reduction, the details of the diet plan are important and collaboration with a dietitian may be needed. A high-protein intake can result in temporary kidney problems. For example, a patient at risk for calculi (stone) formation who ingests large amounts of protein or has a poor fluid intake may form new stones.

Ask about any change in appetite or taste. These manifestations can occur with the buildup of nitrogenous waste products from kidney impairment. Changes in thirst or fluid intake may also cause changes in urine output. Endocrine disorders may also cause changes in thirst, fluid intake, and urine output. (See Chapter 61 for a discussion of endocrine influences on fluid balance.)

Medication History

Identify all of the patient's prescription drugs because many can impair kidney function. Ask about the duration of drug use and whether there have been any recent changes in prescribed drugs. Drugs for diabetes mellitus, hypertension, cardiac disorders, hormonal disorders, cancer, arthritis, and psychiatric disorders are potential causes of kidney problems. Antibiotics, such as gentamicin (Garamycin, Cidomycin ✦), may also cause acute kidney injury. Drug-drug interactions and drug–contrast dye interactions also may lead to kidney dysfunction.

Explore the past and current use of over-the-counter (OTC) drugs or agents, including dietary supplements, vitamins and minerals, herbal agents, laxatives, analgesics, acetaminophen, and NSAIDs. Many of these agents affect kidney function. For example, dietary supplementation with synthetic creatine, used to increase muscle mass, has been associated with compromised kidney function. High-dose or long-term use of NSAIDs or acetaminophen can seriously reduce kidney function. Some agents are associated with hypertension, hematuria, or proteinuria, which may occur before kidney dysfunction.

Family History and Genetic Risk

The family history of the patient with a suspected kidney or urologic problem is important because some disorders have a familial inheritance pattern. Ask whether his or her siblings, parents, or grandparents have had kidney problems. Past terms used for kidney disease include *Bright's disease, nephritis,* and *nephrosis.* Although nephritis is a current term describing an inflammatory process in the kidney and nephrosis is a current term describing a degenerative process in the kidney, these terms have been used by lay people for years to describe any kidney problem. Adult polycystic kidney disease, which is a genetic disorder, can occur in either gender.

Current Health Problem

The effects of severe kidney impairment are evident in all body systems. Therefore document all of the patient's current health problems. Ask him or her to describe all health concerns, because some kidney disorders cause systemic problems or problems in other body systems. Recent upper respiratory problems, achy muscles or joints, or GI problems may be related to problems of kidney function.

Assess the kidney and urologic system by asking about any changes in the appearance (color, odor, clarity) of the urine, pattern of urination, ability to initiate or control voiding, and other unusual manifestations. For example, urine that is reddish, dark brown or black, greenish, or different from the usual yellowish color usually prompts the patient to seek health care assistance. Urine typically has a mild but distinct odor of ammonia. An increase in the intensity of color, a change in odor quality, or a decrease in urine clarity may suggest infection.

Ask about changes in urination patterns, such as **incontinence** (involuntary bladder emptying), **nocturia** (urination at night), frequency, or an increase or decrease in the amount of urine. The normal urine output for adults is about 1500 to 2000 mL/day or within 500 mL of the volume of fluid ingested daily. Ask about how close the urine output is to the volume of fluid ingested. The patient usually does not know the exact amount of urine produced. A bladder diary may provide useful data. Also ask whether:

- Initiating urine flow is difficult
- A burning sensation or other discomfort occurs with urination
- The force of the urine stream is decreased (in men)
- Persistent dribbling of urine is present

The onset of pain in the flank, in the lower abdomen or pelvic region, or in the perineal area usually triggers concern and may prompt the patient to seek assistance. Ask about the onset, intensity, and duration of the pain, its location, and its association with any activity or event.

Pain associated with kidney or ureteral irritation is often severe and spasmodic. Pain that radiates into the perineal area, groin, scrotum, or labia is described as *renal colic.* This pain occurs with distention or spasm of the ureter, such as in an obstruction or the passing of a stone. Renal colic pain may be intermittent or continuous and may occur with pallor, diaphoresis, and hypotension. These general manifestations occur because of the location of the nerve tracts near or in the kidneys and ureters.

Because the kidneys are close to the GI organs and the nerve pathways are similar, GI manifestations may occur with kidney problems. These renointestinal reflexes often complicate the description of the kidney problem.

Uremia is the buildup of nitrogenous waste products in the blood as a result of some degree of kidney impairment. Manifestations include anorexia, nausea and vomiting, muscle cramps, **pruritus** (itching), fatigue, and lethargy.

Physical Assessment

The physical assessment of the patient with a known or suspected kidney or urologic disorder includes general appearance, a review of body systems, and specific structure and functions of the kidney and urinary system.

Assess the patient's general appearance, and check the skin for the presence of any rashes, bruising, or yellowish discoloration. The skin and tissues may show edema, especially in the **pedal** (foot), **pretibial** (shin), and sacral tissues and around the eyes. Use a stethoscope to listen to the lungs to determine whether fluid is present. Weigh the patient and measure blood pressure as a baseline for later comparisons.

Assess the level of consciousness and level of alertness. Record any deficits in memory, concentration, or thought processes. Family members may report subtle changes. Cognitive changes may be the result of the buildup of waste products when kidney disease is present.

Assessment of the Kidneys, Ureters, and Bladder

Assess the kidneys, ureters, and bladder during an abdominal assessment (Jarvis, 2016). Auscultate before percussion and palpation because these activities can enhance bowel sounds and obscure abdominal vascular sounds.

Inspect the abdomen and the flank regions with the patient in both the supine and the sitting positions. Observe the patient for asymmetry (e.g., swelling) or discoloration (e.g., bruising or redness) in the flank region, especially in the area of the costovertebral angle (CVA). The CVA is located between the lower portion of the twelfth rib and the vertebral column.

Listen for a bruit by placing a stethoscope over each renal artery on the midclavicular line. A **bruit** is an audible swishing sound produced when the volume of blood or the diameter of the blood vessel changes. It often occurs with blood flow through a narrowed vessel, as in renal artery stenosis.

Kidney palpation is usually performed by a physician or advanced practice nurse. It can help locate masses and areas of tenderness in or around the kidney. Lightly palpate the abdomen in all quadrants. Ask about areas of tenderness or pain, and examine nontender areas first. The outline of the bladder may be seen as high as the umbilicus in patients with severe bladder distention. *If tumor or aneurysm is suspected, palpation may harm the patient.*

Because the kidneys are located deep and posterior, palpation is easier in thin patients who have little abdominal musculature. For palpation of the right kidney, the patient is in a supine position while the examiner places one hand under the right flank and the other hand over the abdomen below the lower right part of the rib cage. The lower hand is used to raise the flank, and the upper hand depresses the abdomen as the patient takes a deep breath (Fig. 65-9) (Jarvis, 2016). The left kidney is deeper and often cannot be palpated. A transplanted kidney is readily palpated in either the lower right or left abdominal quadrant. The normal kidney is smooth, firm, and nontender.

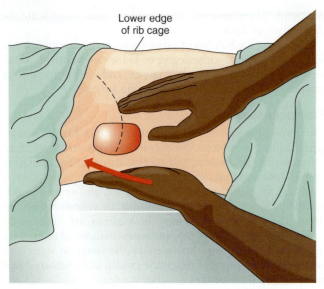

Lower edge
of rib cage

FIG. 65-9 Advanced technique for palpation of the kidney.

A distended bladder sounds dull when percussed. After gently palpating to determine the outline of the distended bladder, begin percussion on the lower abdomen and continue in the direction of the umbilicus until dull sounds are no longer produced. If you suspect bladder distention, use a portable bladder scanner to determine the amount of retained urine.

If the patient reports flank pain or tenderness, percuss the nontender flank first. Have the patient assume a sitting, side-lying, or supine position, and then form one of your hands into a clenched fist. Place your other hand flat over the CVA of the patient. Then quickly deliver a firm thump to your hand over the CVA area (Jarvis, 2016). Costovertebral tenderness often occurs with kidney infection or inflammation. Patients with inflammation or infection in the kidney or nearby structures may describe their pain as severe or as a constant, dull ache.

Assessment of the Urethra

Using a good light source and wearing gloves, inspect the urethra by examining the meatus and the tissues around it. Record any unusual discharge such as blood, mucus, or pus. Inspect the skin and mucous membranes of surrounding tissues. Record the presence of lesions, rashes, or other abnormalities of the penis or scrotum or of the labia or vaginal opening. Urethral irritation is suspected when the patient reports discomfort with urination. Use this opportunity to remind women to clean the perineum by wiping from front to back, never from back to front. Teach them that the front-to-back technique keeps organisms in stool from coming close to the urethra and decreases the risk for infection.

GENDER HEALTH CONSIDERATIONS
Patient-Centered Care (QSEN)

Women from other cultures may have undergone female circumcision. This procedure alters the anatomic appearance of the vulvar-perineal area and increases the risk for urinary tract infections. It also makes urethral inspection or catheterization difficult. Document any noted anatomic changes, and ask the patient to describe her hygiene practices for this area.

Psychosocial Assessment

Concerns about the urologic system may evoke fear, anger, embarrassment, anxiety, guilt, or sadness in the patient. Childhood learning often includes privacy with regard to toilet habits. Urologic disorders may bring up forgotten memories of difficult toilet training and bedwetting or of childhood experiences of exploring one's body. The patient may ignore manifestations or delay seeking health care because of emotional responses or cultural taboos about the urogenital area.

⍰ NCLEX EXAMINATION CHALLENGE
Health Promotion and Maintenance

The client arrives at the primary health care clinic with a problem of new abdominal pain and blood in her urine. She is afebrile. Which information is most important for the nurse to obtain from this client's history?
A. Kidney cancer in the client's family
B. Injury or trauma to the abdomen or pelvis
C. Treatment for a urinary tract infection in the past 12 months
D. Recent exposure to heavy metals, drugs, or other nephrotoxins

Diagnostic Assessment
Laboratory Assessment

Blood Tests. *Serum creatinine* is produced when muscle and other proteins are broken down. Because protein breakdown is usually constant, the serum creatinine level is a good indicator of kidney function. Serum creatinine levels are slightly higher in men than in women because men tend to have a larger muscle mass than do women. Similarly, people with greater muscle mass or muscle mass turnover (e.g., athletes) may have a slightly-higher-than-average serum creatinine level. Muscle mass and the amount of creatinine produced decrease with age. Because of decreased rates of creatinine clearance, however, the serum creatinine level remains relatively constant in older adults unless kidney disease is present.

No common pathologic condition other than kidney disease increases the serum creatinine level. The serum creatinine level does not increase until at least 50% of the kidney function is lost, and therefore *any* elevation of serum creatinine values is important and should be assessed further. Creatinine is excreted by the kidneys.

❗ NURSING SAFETY PRIORITY (QSEN)
Action Alert

A serum creatinine of 1.5 mg/dL or greater places a patient at risk for acute kidney injury (AKI) from iodinated contrast dyes and some drugs. Monitor both baseline and trend values to determine risk for and actual kidney damage, especially among patients exposed to agents that can cause kidney dysfunction. Promptly inform the health care provider of increases in serum creatinine greater than 1.5 times the baseline and urine output values of less than 0.5 mL/kg/hr for 6 or more hours.

Blood urea nitrogen (BUN) measures the effectiveness of kidney excretion of urea nitrogen, a by-product of protein breakdown in the liver. Urea nitrogen is produced mostly from liver metabolism of food sources of protein. The kidneys filter urea nitrogen from the blood and excrete the waste in urine.

CHART 65-2 Laboratory Profile

Kidney Function Blood Studies

TEST	NORMAL RANGE FOR ADULTS	SIGNIFICANCE OF ABNORMAL FINDINGS
Serum creatinine	*Males:* 0.6-1.2 mg/dL (0.053-0.106 mmol/L; 53-106 µmol/L) *Females:* 0.5-1.1 mg/dL (0.044-0.097 mmol/L; 44-97µmol/L) *Older adults:* may be decreased	An *increased level* indicates kidney impairment. A *decreased level* may be caused by a decreased muscle mass.
Blood urea nitrogen (BUN)	10-20 mg/dL (3.6-7.1 mmol/L) *Older adults:* 60-90 yr: 8-23 mg/dL (2.9-8.2 mmol/L) Older than 90 yr: 10-31 mg/dL (3.6-11.1 mmol/L)	An *increased level* may indicate liver or kidney disease, dehydration or decreased kidney perfusion, a high-protein diet, infection, stress, steroid use, GI bleeding, or other situations in which blood is in body tissues. A *decreased level* may indicate malnutrition, fluid volume excess, or severe hepatic damage.
BUN/creatinine ratio	6-25 (BUN divided by creatinine)	An *increased ratio* may indicate fluid volume deficit, obstructive uropathy, catabolic state, or a high-protein diet. A *decreased ratio* may indicate fluid volume excess.

Data from Pagana, K., & Pagana, T. (2014). *Mosby's manual of diagnostic and laboratory tests* (5th ed.). St. Louis: Mosby.

Other factors influence the BUN level, and an elevation does not always mean kidney disease is present (Chart 65-2). For example, rapid cell destruction from infection, cancer treatment, or steroid therapy may elevate BUN level. In addition, blood is a protein. Blood in the tissues rather than in the blood vessels is reabsorbed as if it were a general protein. Thus reabsorbed blood protein is processed by the liver and increases BUN levels. This means that injured tissues can result in increased BUN levels even when kidney function is normal. Also, BUN is increased by protein turnover in exercising muscle and is elevated as a result of concentration during dehydration.

The liver must function properly to produce urea nitrogen. When liver and kidney dysfunction are present, urea nitrogen levels are actually *decreased* because the liver failure limits urea production. The BUN level is not always elevated with kidney disease and is not the best indicator of kidney function. However, an elevated BUN level suggests kidney dysfunction.

Blood urea nitrogen to serum creatinine ratio can help determine whether non–kidney-related factors, such as low cardiac output or red blood cell destruction, are causing the elevated BUN level. When blood volume is deficient (e.g., dehydration) or cardiac output is low, the BUN level rises more rapidly than

the serum creatinine level. As a result, the ratio of BUN to creatinine is *increased*.

When both the BUN and serum creatinine levels increase at the same rate, the BUN/creatinine ratio remains normal. However, elevations of ***both*** serum creatinine and BUN levels suggest kidney dysfunction that is not related to dehydration or poor perfusion.

Blood osmolarity is a measure of the overall concentration of particles in the blood and is a good indicator of hydration status. The kidneys excrete or reabsorb water to keep blood osmolarity in the range of 285 to 295 mOsm/L. Osmolarity is slightly higher in older adults (285 to 301 mOsm/L). When blood osmolarity is decreased, the release of vasopressin (antidiuretic hormone [ADH]) is inhibited. Without vasopressin, the distal tubule and collecting ducts are *not* permeable to water. As a result, water is *excreted*, not reabsorbed, and blood osmolarity increases. When blood osmolarity increases, vasopressin is released. Vasopressin increases the permeability of the distal tubule to water. Then water is reabsorbed and blood osmolarity decreases.

Urine Tests

Urinalysis. Urinalysis is a part of any complete physical examination and is especially useful for patients with suspected kidney or urologic disorders (Chart 65-3). Ideally, the urine specimen is collected at the morning's first voiding. Specimens obtained at other times may be too dilute. The specimen may be collected by several techniques (Table 65-3).

Urine color comes from urochrome pigment. Color variations may result from increased levels of urochrome or other pigments, changes in the concentration or dilution of the urine, and the presence of drug metabolites in the urine. Urine smells faintly like ammonia and is normally clear without *turbidity* (cloudiness) or haziness.

Specific gravity is the concentration of particles, including electrolytes and wastes, in urine. A high specific gravity indicates concentrated urine, such as might occur from dehydration, decreased kidney blood flow, or excess vasopressin associated with stress, surgery, anesthetic agents, and certain drugs (e.g., morphine, some oral antidiabetic drugs) or syndrome of inappropriate antidiuretic hormone (SIADH) (see Chapter 62). A low specific gravity indicates dilute urine that may occur from high fluid intake, diuretic drugs, or diabetes insipidus (DI) (see Chapter 62).

Specific gravity refers to the density of urine compared with distilled water, which has a specific gravity of 1.000. The normal specific gravity of urine ranges from 1.005 to about 1.030. Kidney disease diminishes the concentrating ability of the kidney, and chronic kidney disease (CKD) may be associated with a low (dilute) specific gravity.

pH is a measure of urine acidity or alkalinity. A pH value less than 7 is acidic, and a value greater than 7 is alkaline. Urine pH is affected by diet, drugs, systemic disturbances of ACID-BASE BALANCE, and kidney tubular function. For example, a high-protein diet produces acidic urine, whereas a high intake of citrus fruit produces alkaline urine.

Urine specimens become more alkaline when left standing unrefrigerated for more than 1 hour, when bacteria are present, or when a specimen is left uncovered. Alkaline urine increases cell breakdown; thus the presence of red blood cells may be missed on analysis. In addition, alkalinity promotes bacterial overgrowth. Ensure that urine specimens are covered and delivered to the laboratory promptly or

CHART 65-3	Laboratory Profile

Urinalysis

TEST	NORMAL RANGE FOR ADULTS	SIGNIFICANCE OF ABNORMAL FINDINGS
Color	Yellow	*Dark amber* indicates concentrated urine. *Very pale yellow* indicates dilute urine. *Dark red* or *brown* indicates blood in the urine. Brown may indicate increased bilirubin level. Red also may indicate the presence of myoglobin. *Other color* changes may result from diet or drugs.
Odor	Specific aroma, similar to ammonia	*Foul smell* indicates possible infection, dehydration, or ingestion of certain foods or drugs.
Turbidity	Clear	*Cloudy urine* indicates infection, sediment, or high levels of urine protein.
Specific gravity	Usually 1.005-1.030; possible range 1.000-1.040 *Older adult:* Decreased	*Increased* in decreased kidney perfusion, inappropriate ADH secretion, or heart failure. *Decreased* in chronic kidney disease, diabetes insipidus, malignant hypertension, diuretic administration, and lithium toxicity.
pH	Average: 6; possible range: 4.6-8	*Changes* are caused by diet, drugs, infection, age of specimen, acid-base imbalance, and kidney disease.
Glucose	Fresh specimen, negative 50-300 mg/day in a 24-hour specimen	*Presence* reflects hyperglycemia or a decrease in the kidney threshold for glucose.
Ketones	None	*Presence* occurs with diabetic ketoacidosis, prolonged fasting, anorexia nervosa.
Protein	0-0.8 mg/dL 50-80 mg in a 24-hour specimen at rest <250 mg in a 24-hour specimen with exercise	*Increased* amounts may indicate stress, infection, recent strenuous exercise, or glomerular disorders.
Bilirubin (urobilinogen)	None	*Presence* suggests liver or biliary disease or obstruction.
Red blood cells (RBCs)	0-2 per high-power field	*Increased* is normal with catheterization or menses but may reflect tumor, stones, trauma, glomerular disorders, cystitis, or bleeding disorders.
White blood cells (WBCs)	0-4 per low-power field	*Increased* may indicate an infection or inflammation in the kidney and urinary tract, kidney transplant rejection, or exercise.
Casts	None	*Increased* indicates bacteria, protein, or urinary calculi.
Crystals	None	*Presence* may indicate that the specimen has been allowed to stand.
Bacteria	<1000 colonies/mL	*Increased* indicates the need for urine culture to determine the presence of urinary tract infection.
Parasites	None	*Presence* of *Trichomonas vaginalis* indicates infection, usually of the urethra, prostate, or vagina.
Leukoesterase	None	*Presence* suggests urinary tract infection.
Nitrites	None	*Presence* suggests urinary *Escherichia coli*.

Data from Pagana, K., & Pagana, T. (2014). *Mosby's manual of diagnostic and laboratory tests* (5th ed.). St. Louis: Mosby.
ADH, Antidiuretic hormone.

refrigerated. During systemic acidosis or alkalosis, the kidneys, along with blood buffers and the lungs, normally respond to keep serum pH normal. Chapter 12 discusses ACID-BASE BALANCE and imbalance.

Protein is not normally present in the urine. Levels greater than 30 mg/hr, or 200 mcg/min, are abnormal. Protein molecules are too large to pass through intact glomerular membranes. When glomerular membranes are not intact, protein molecules pass through and are excreted in the urine. Increased membrane permeability is caused by infection, inflammation, or immunologic problems. Some systemic problems cause production of abnormal proteins, such as globulin. Detection of abnormal protein types requires electrophoresis.

A random finding of **proteinuria** (usually albumin in the urine) followed by a series of negative (normal) findings does not imply kidney disease. If infection is the cause of the proteinuria, urinalyses after resolution of the infection should be negative for protein. Persistent proteinuria needs further investigation.

Microalbuminuria is the presence of albumin in the urine that is not measurable by a urine dipstick or usual urinalysis procedures. Specialized assays are used to quickly analyze a freshly voided urine specimen for microscopic levels of albumin. The normal microalbumin levels in a freshly voided specimen should range between 2.0 and 20 mg/mmol for men and between 2.8 and 28 mg/mmol for women. Higher levels indicate microalbuminuria and could mean mild or early kidney disease, especially in patients with diabetes mellitus. In 24-hour urine specimens, levels of 30 to 300 mg/24 hr, or 20 to 200 mcg/min, indicate microalbuminuria.

Glucose is filtered by the glomerulus and is reabsorbed in the proximal tubule of the nephron. When the blood glucose level rises above 220 mg/dL, the renal threshold for reabsorption is exceeded and glucose "spills over" into urine. Changes in the renal threshold for glucose occur in many patients, such as those with infection or severe stress.

Ketone bodies are formed from the incomplete metabolism of fatty acids. Three types of ketone bodies are acetone,

TABLE 65-3 Collection of Urine Specimens

NURSING INTERVENTIONS	RATIONALES
Voided Urine	
Collect the first specimen voided in the morning.	Urine is more concentrated in the early morning.
Send the specimen to the laboratory as soon as possible.	After urine is collected, cellular breakdown results in more alkaline urine.
Refrigerate the specimen if a delay is unavoidable.	Refrigeration delays the alkalinization of urine. Bacteria are more likely to multiply in an alkaline environment.
Clean-Catch Specimen	
Explain the purpose of the procedure to the patient.	Correct technique is needed to obtain a valid specimen.
Instruct the patient to self-clean before voiding:	Surface cleaning is necessary to remove secretions or bacteria from the urethral meatus.
Instruct the female patient to separate the labia and use the sponges and solution provided to wipe with three strokes over the urethra. The first two wiping strokes are over each side of the urethra; the third wiping stroke is centered over the urethra (from front to back).	
Instruct the male patient to retract the foreskin of the penis and to similarly clean the urethra, using three wiping strokes with the sponge and solution provided (from the head of the penis downward).	
Instruct the patient to initiate voiding after cleaning. The patient then stops and resumes voiding into the container. Only 1 ounce (30 mL) is needed; the remainder of the urine may be discarded into the commode.	A midstream collection further removes secretions and bacteria because urine flushes the distal portion of the internal urethra.
Ensure that the patient understands the procedure.	An improperly collected specimen may result in inappropriate or incomplete treatment.
Assist the patient as needed.	The patient's understanding and the nurse's assistance ensure proper collection.
Catheterized Specimen	
For non-indwelling (straight) catheters:	The one-time passage of a urinary catheter may be necessary to obtain an uncontaminated specimen for analysis or to measure the volume of residual urine.
Avoid routine use.	
Follow the facility's procedures for catheterization technique.	These procedures minimize bacterial entry.
For indwelling catheters:	Urine is collected from an indwelling catheter or tubing when patients have catheters for continence or long-term urinary drainage.
Apply a clamp to the drainage tubing, distal to the injection port.	Clamping allows urine to collect in the tubing at the location where the specimen is obtained.
Clean the injection port cap of the catheter drainage tubing with an appropriate antiseptic. Povidone-iodine solution or alcohol is acceptable.	Surface contamination is prevented by following the cleaning procedures.
Attach a sterile 5-mL syringe into the port, and aspirate the quantity of urine required.	A minimum of 5 mL is needed for culture and sensitivity (C&S) testing.
Inject the urine sample into a sterile specimen container.	A sterile container is used for C&S specimens.
Remove the clamp to resume drainage.	
Properly dispose of the syringe.	
24-Hour Urine Collection	
Instruct the patient thoroughly.	A 24-hr collection of urine is necessary to quantify or calculate the rate of clearance of a particular substance.
Provide written materials to assist in instruction.	Instructional materials for patients, signs, etc. remind patients and staff to ensure that the total collection is completed.
Place signs appropriately.	
Inform all personnel or family caregivers of test in progress.	
Check laboratory or procedure manual on proper technique for maintaining the collection (e.g., on ice, in a refrigerator, or with a preservative).	Proper technique prevents breakdown of elements to be measured.
On initiation of the collection, ask the patient to void, discard the urine, and note the time. If a Foley catheter is in use, empty the tubing and drainage bag at the start time and discard the urine.	Proper techniques ensure that *all* urine formed within the 24-hr period is collected.
Collect all urine of the next 24 hr.	
Twenty-four hours after initiation, ask the patient to empty the bladder and add that urine to the container.	
Do not remove urine from the collection container for other specimens.	Urine in the container is not considered a "fresh" specimen and may be mixed with preservative.

acetoacetic acid, and beta-hydroxybutyric acid. *Normally there are no ketones in urine.* Ketone bodies are produced when fat is used instead of glucose for cellular energy. Ketones present in the blood are partially excreted in the urine.

Leukoesterase is an enzyme found in some white blood cells, especially neutrophils. When the number of these cells increases in the urine or they are broken (lysed), the urine then contains leukoesterase. The presence of leukoesterase and nitrites in the urine is a sensitive screen for assessing urinary tract infections. A normal reading is no leukoesterase in the urine. A positive test (+ sign) is an indication of a urinary tract infection.

Nitrites are not usually present in urine. Many types of bacteria, when present in the urine, convert nitrates (normally found in urine) into nitrites. A positive test enhances the sensitivity of the leukoesterase test to detect urinary tract infection.

Sediment is precipitated particles in the urine. These particles include cells, casts, crystals, and bacteria. Normally, urine contains few, if any, cells. Types of cells abnormally present in the urine include tubular cells (from the tubule of the nephron), epithelial cells (from the lining of the urinary tract), red blood cells (RBCs), and white blood cells (WBCs). WBCs may indicate a urinary tract or kidney infection. RBCs may indicate *glomerulonephritis, acute tubular necrosis, pyelonephritis,* kidney trauma, or kidney cancer.

Casts are clumps of materials or cells. When cells, bacteria, or proteins are present in the urine, minerals and sticky materials clump around them and form a cast of the distal renal tubule and collecting duct. Casts are described by the type of particle they have surrounded (e.g., hyaline [protein-based] or cellular [from RBCs, WBCs, or epithelial cells]) or the stage of cast breakdown (whole cell or granular from cell breakdown). Although an isolated urinalysis with sediment from casts may be the result of strenuous exercise, repeated findings with sediment are more likely to be associated with disease.

Urine crystals come from mineral salts as a result of diet, drugs, or disease. Common salt crystals are formed from calcium, oxalate, urea, phosphate, magnesium, or other substances. Some drugs, such as the sulfates, can also form crystals.

Bacteria multiply quickly, so the urine specimen must be analyzed promptly to avoid falsely elevated counts of bacterial colonization. Normally urine is sterile, but it is easily contaminated by perineal bacteria during collection.

Recent advances in technology and molecular biology are leading to new diagnostic tests using urine, including identification of biomarkers of disease and profiling for specific proteins. Markers are being used in investigation to identify early-onset kidney dysfunction, target therapy, and predict responsiveness to intervention. Markers for angiogenesis and kidney cell adhesion, regulation, and apoptosis will likely contribute to clinical diagnostics in the future.

Urine for Culture and Sensitivity. Urine is analyzed for the number and types of organisms present. Manifestations of infection and unexplained bacteria in a urine specimen are indications for urine culture and sensitivity testing. Bacteria from urine are placed in a medium with different antibiotics. In this way we can know which antibiotics are effective in killing or stopping the growth of the organisms (organisms are "sensitive") and which are not effective (organisms are "resistant"). A clean-catch or catheter-derived specimen is best for culture and sensitivity testing.

Composite Urine Collections. Some urine collections are made for a specified number of hours (e.g., 24 hours) for more precise analysis of one or more substances. These collections are often used to measure urine levels of creatinine or urea nitrogen, sodium, chloride, calcium, catecholamines, or other components (Chart 65-4). For a composite urine specimen, *all* urine within the designated time frame must be collected (see Table 65-3). If other urine must be obtained while the collection is in progress, measure and record the amount collected but not added to the timed collection.

The urine collection may need to be refrigerated or stored on ice to prevent changes in the urine during the collection time. Follow the procedure from the laboratory for urine storage, including whether a preservative is to be added. The urine collection must be free from fecal contamination. Menstrual blood and toilet tissue also contaminate the specimen and can invalidate the results.

The collection of urine for a 24-hour period is often more difficult than it seems. With hospitalized patients, the cooperation of staff personnel, the patient, family members, and visitors is essential. Placing signs in the bathroom, instructing the patient and family, and emphasizing the need to save the urine are helpful.

Creatinine Clearance. Creatinine clearance is a calculated measure of glomerular filtration rate (GFR) and kidney function. The patient's age, gender, height, weight, diet, and activity level influence the expected amount of excreted creatinine. Thus these factors are considered when interpreting creatinine clearance test results. Decreases in the creatinine clearance rate may require reducing drug doses and often signifies the need to further explore the cause of kidney deterioration.

Commonly, creatinine clearance is calculated from serum creatinine, age, weight, urine creatinine, gender, and race. Current guidelines suggest clinical laboratories report an estimate of GFR whenever a serum creatinine is ordered, based on the modified diet in renal disease (MDRD) study equation (National Kidney Disease Education Program, 2012). The MDRD equation does not require urine to estimate GFR. The estimated GFR (eGFR) for the MDRD equation is >60 mL/min/1.73 m^2 (Pagana & Pagana, 2014). An alternate approach for calculation is the Cockcroft-Gault equation, and this equation has traditionally been used to determine the need for drug dose adjustment (Dong & Quan, 2010).

While expensive and time consuming, creatinine clearance to estimate GFR can be based on a 24-hour urine collection, although urine can be collected for shorter periods (e.g., 8 or 12 hours). The analysis compares the urine creatinine level with the blood creatinine level, and therefore a blood specimen for creatinine must also be collected. The range for normal creatinine clearance is 107 to 139 mL/min for men and 87 to 107 mL/min for women tested with a 24-hour urine collection. Values decrease 6.5 mL/min per decade of life for adults older than 40 years because of age-related decline in GFR.

Urine Electrolytes. Urine samples can be analyzed for electrolyte levels (e.g., sodium, chloride). Normally the amount of sodium excreted in the urine is nearly equal to that consumed. Urine sodium levels of less than 10 mEq/L indicate that the tubules are able to conserve (reabsorb) sodium.

Urine Osmolarity. Osmolarity measures the concentration of particles in solution. The particles in urine contributing to osmolarity include electrolytes, glucose, urea, and creatinine. Urine osmolarity can vary from 50 to 1400 mOsm/L, depending on the patient's hydration status and kidney function. With average fluid intake, the range for urine osmolarity is 300 to 900 mOsm/L. Electrolytes, acids, and other wastes of normal metabolism are continually produced. These particles are the solute load that must be excreted in the urine on a regular basis. This is referred to as *obligatory solute excretion.* If the patient loses excessive fluids, the kidney response is to save water while ridding the body of wastes by excreting small amounts of highly

CHART 65-4 Laboratory Profile

24-Hour Urine Collections

COMPONENT	NORMAL RANGE FOR ADULTS	SIGNIFICANCE OF ABNORMAL FINDINGS
Creatinine	*Males:* 1-2 g/24 hr or 14-26 mg/kg/24 hr (124-230 µmol/kg/24 hr or 7.1-17.7 mmol/24 hr) *Females:* 0.6-1.8 g/24 hr or 11-20 mg/kg/24 hr (97-177 µmol/kg/24 hr or 5.3-15.9 mmol/24 hr) *Older adults:* 10 mg/kg/24 hr (88.4 µmol/kg/24 hr) at 90 yr	*Decreased amounts* indicate a deterioration in function caused by kidney disease. *Increased amounts* occur with infections, exercise, diabetes mellitus, and meat meals.
Urea nitrogen	12-20 g/24 hr (0.43-0.71 mmol/24 hr)	*Decreased amounts* occur when kidney damage or liver disease is present. *Increased amounts* commonly result from a high-protein diet, dehydration, trauma, or sepsis.
Sodium	40-220 mEq/24 hr (40-220 mmol/24 hr)	*Decreased* in hemorrhage, shock, hyperaldosteronism, and prerenal acute kidney injury. *Increased* with diuretic therapy, excessive salt intake, hypokalemia, and acute tubular necrosis.
Chloride	110-250 mEq/24 hr (110-250 mmol/24 hr) *Older adults:* 95-195 mEq/24 hr (95-195 mmol/24 hr)	*Decreased* in certain kidney diseases, malnutrition, pyloric obstruction, prolonged nasogastric tube drainage, diarrhea, diaphoresis, heart failure, and emphysema. *Increased* with hypokalemia, adrenal insufficiency, and massive diuresis.
Calcium	100-400 mg/24 hr (2.50-7.50 mmol/kg/24 hr)	*Decreased* with hypocalcemia, hypoparathyroidism, nephrosis, and nephritis. *Increased* with calcium kidney stones, hyperparathyroidism, sarcoidosis, certain cancers, immobilization, and hypercalcemia.
*Total catecholamines	<100 mcg/24 hr (<591 mmol/24 hr)	*Increased* with pheochromocytoma, neuroblastomas, stress, or heavy exercise.
Protein	1-14 mg/dL (10-140 mg/L) or 50-80 mg/24 hr at rest	*Increased* in glomerular disease, nephrotic syndrome, diabetic nephropathy, urinary tract malignancies, and irritations.

Data from Pagana, K., & Pagana, T. (2014). *Mosby's manual of diagnostic and laboratory tests* (5th ed.). St. Louis: Mosby.
*Epinephrine and norepinephrine only; dopamine is not measured.

concentrated urine. Diet, drugs, and activity can change urine osmolarity. Thus urine with an increased osmolarity is concentrated urine with less water and more solutes. Urine with a decreased osmolarity is dilute urine with more water and fewer solutes.

❓ NCLEX EXAMINATION CHALLENGE

Physiological Integrity

The client's urinalysis shows all of these abnormal results. Which result does the nurse report to the health care provider immediately?
A. pH 7.8
B. Protein 31 mg
C. Sodium 15 mEq/L
D. Leukoesterase and nitrate positive

Bedside Sonography/Bladder Scanners. The use of portable ultrasound scanners in the hospital and rehabilitation setting by nurses is a noninvasive method of estimating bladder volume (Fig. 65-10). Bladder scanners are used to screen for post-void residual volumes and to determine the need for intermittent catheterization based on the amount of urine in the bladder

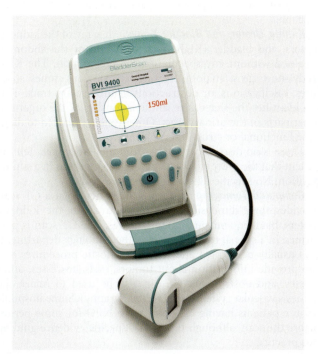

FIG. 65-10 The "BladderScan" BVI 9400, a handheld portable bladder scanner.

rather than the time between catheterizations. There is no discomfort with the scan, and no patient preparation beyond an explanation of what to expect is required.

Explain why the procedure is being done and what sensations the patient might experience during the procedure. For example, "This test will measure the amount of urine in your bladder. I will place a gel pad just above your pubic area and then place the probe, which is a little bigger and heavier than a stethoscope, on the gel."

Before scanning, select the male or female icon on the bladder scanner. Using the female icon allows the scanner software to subtract the volume of the uterus from any measurement. Use the male icon on all men and on women who have undergone a hysterectomy.

Place an ultrasound gel pad right above the symphysis pubis (pubic bone), or moisten the round dome of the scan head area with 5 mL of conducting gel to improve ultrasound conduction. Use gel on the scanner head for obese patients and those with heavy body hair in the area to be scanned. Place the probe midline over the abdomen about $1\frac{1}{2}$ inches (4 cm) above the pubic bone. Aim the scan head so the ultrasound is projected toward the expected location of the bladder, typically toward the patient's coccyx. Press and release the scan button. The scan is complete with the sound of a beep, and a volume is displayed. Two readings are recommended for best accuracy. An aiming icon on the portable bladder scanner indicates whether the bladder image is centered on the crosshairs of the scan head. If the crosshairs on the aiming icon are not centered on the bladder, the measured volume may not be accurate.

Imaging Assessment

Many imaging procedures are used to diagnose abnormalities within the urinary system (Table 65-4). Explain the procedures thoroughly to the patient, prepare him or her, and provide follow-up care. Patient education materials for many urologic tests have been developed by professional organizations such as the Society for Urologic Nurses and Associates and are freely available.

Kidney, Ureter, and Bladder X-rays. An x-ray of the kidneys, ureters, and bladder (KUB) is a plain film of the abdomen obtained without any specific patient preparation. The KUB study shows gross anatomic features and obvious stones, strictures, calcifications, or obstructions in the urinary tract. This test identifies the shape, size, and relationship of the organs to other parts of the urinary tract. Other tests are needed to diagnose functional or structural problems.

There is no discomfort or risk from this procedure. Tell the patient that the x-ray will be taken while he or she is in a supine position. No specific follow-up care is needed.

Computed Tomography. Inform the patient that a CT scan provides three-dimensional information about the kidneys, ureters, bladder, and surrounding tissues. The CT scan is performed in a special room, usually in the radiology department. It is usually performed after other diagnostic procedures and can provide information about tumors, cysts, abscesses, other masses, and obstruction. CT can also be used to image the kidney's vascular system (i.e., CT angiography). Some hospitals require patients having CT scans to be NPO for some period before the scan, although there is no specific evidence guiding this practice.

Determine whether the scan requires administration of a dye. Oral or injected contrast dye is usually given before starting

TABLE 65-4	Radiologic and Special Diagnostic Tests for Patients with Disorders of the Kidney and Urinary System
TEST	**PURPOSE**
Radiography of kidneys, ureters, and bladder (KUB) (plain film of abdomen)	To screen for the presence of two kidneys To measure kidney size To detect gross obstruction in kidneys or urinary tract
Computed tomography (CT)	To measure kidney size To evaluate contour to assess for masses or obstruction in kidneys or the urinary tract To assess renal blood flow
Magnetic resonance imaging (MRI)	Similar to CT Useful for staging of cancers
Ultrasonography (US) Can be used with a dye	To identify the size of the kidneys or obstruction (e.g., tumors, stones) in the kidneys or the lower urinary tract
(Nuclear) Renal scan	To evaluate renal perfusion To estimate glomerular filtration rate To provide functional information without exposing the patient to iodinated contrast dye
Cystoscopy	To identify abnormalities of the bladder wall and urethral and ureteral occlusions To treat small obstructions or lesions via fulguration, lithotripsy, or removal with a stone basket
Cystography and cystourethrography	To outline bladder's contour when full and examine structure during voiding To examine the structure of the urethra To detect backward urine flow
Metabolic imaging with positron emission tomography (PET)	To evaluate cysts, tumors, and other lesions, eliminating the need for biopsy in some patients

the imaging procedure. Dye use may be omitted in patients at risk for contrast-induced acute kidney injury, but the images produced are less distinct.

When a dye is used, ensure that there is sufficient oral or intravenous intake to dilute and excrete the dye. Typically, the radiologist will specify a total fluid intake of 1 liter or a variable rate to maintain urine output at 1 to 2 mL/kg/hr for up to 6 hours. When no contrast or dye is used, there is no special postprocedure care.

The contrast dye is potentially kidney-damaging (nephrotoxic). *Contrast-induced nephropathy* is the onset of *acute kidney failure* within 24 to 72 hours after the administration of iodinated contrast medium (Wood, 2012). The risk for *contrast-induced nephropathy* is greatest in patients who are older, dehydrated, have pre-existing renal insufficiency (e.g., serum creatinine levels greater than 1.5 mg/dL or estimated GFR <45 mL/min), or are also taking other nephrotoxic drugs (Davenport et al., 2014). Chart 65-5 lists assessment questions to ask before a patient undergoes testing that uses contrast material.

In addition, patients taking metformin are at risk for lactic acidosis when they receive iodinated contrast media. Metformin should be discontinued at least 24 hours before the time

Assessing the Patient About to Undergo a Kidney Test or Procedure Using Contrast Medium

Before the procedure:

- Ask the patient if he or she has ever had a reaction to contrast media. (Such a patient has the highest risk for having another reaction.)
- Ask the patient about a history of asthma. (Patients with asthma have been shown to be at greater risk for contrast reactions than the general public. When reactions do occur, they are more likely to be severe.)
- Ask the patient about known hay fever or food or drug allergies, especially to seafood, eggs, milk, or chocolate. (Contrast reactions have been reported to be as high as 15% in these patients.)
- Ask the patient to describe any specific allergic reactions (e.g., hives, facial edema, difficulty breathing, bronchospasm).
- Assess for a history of renal impairment and for conditions that have been implicated in increasing the chance of developing kidney failure after contrast media (e.g., diabetic nephropathy, class IV heart failure, dehydration, concomitant use of potentially nephrotoxic drugs such as the aminoglycosides or NSAIDs, and cirrhosis).
- Ask the patient if he or she is taking metformin (Glucophage). (Metformin must be discontinued at least 24 hours before any study using contrast media because the life-threatening complication of lactic acidosis, although rare, could occur.)
- Assess hydration status by checking blood pressure, heart and respiratory rates, mucous membranes, skin turgor, and urine concentration.
- Ask the patient when he or she last ate or drank anything.

of a procedure and for at least 48 hours after the procedure. Kidney function should be re-evaluated before the patient resumes metformin therapy.

! **NURSING SAFETY PRIORITY** QSEN

Drug Alert

Ensure that the patient who is prescribed metformin does not receive the drug after a procedure requiring IV contrast material until adequate kidney function has been determined.

All patients at risk for contrast-induced nephrotoxicity need regular assessment and collaboration with the health care provider to maintain hydration and decrease the risk for kidney damage following a dye-enhanced CT scan. Sodium bicarbonate in a liter of intravenous fluid or oral acetylcysteine (an antioxidant) may be used preprocedure to prevent contrast-induced nephrotoxic effects in radiologic procedures; however, protection provided to the kidneys is not consistent in clinical trials (Lameire & Kellum, 2013). Diuretics may be given immediately after the dye is injected to enhance dye excretion in patients who are well hydrated.

Magnetic Resonance Imaging of the Kidney. MRI provides improved contrast between normal and abnormal tissue in the renal system compared with a CT scan. As with all MRIs, the patient with metal implants (pins, pacemaker, joint replacement, aneurysmal clips, or other cosmetic or medical devices) is not eligible for this test because the magnet can move the metal implant. Gadolinium-based contrast agents have been linked with nephrogenic systemic fibrosis (Pagana & Pagana, 2014) and should not be used in patients with renal impairment, usually defined as a serum creatinine above 1.5 mg/dL or an estimated GFR less than 45 mL/min. Adults older than 60 years should be carefully evaluated for renal impairment (see the Kidney and Urinary System Changes Associated with Aging section on p. 1351).

Kidney Ultrasonography. Inform the patient that ultrasonography does not cause discomfort and is without risk. This test usually requires a full bladder. Ask the patient to drink water, if needed, to help fill the bladder. This test applies sound waves to structures of different densities to produce images of the kidneys, ureters, and bladder and surrounding tissues. Ultrasonography allows assessment of kidney size, cortical thickness, and status of the calices. The test can identify obstruction in the urinary tract, tumors, cysts, and other masses without the use of contrast dye.

The patient undergoing kidney ultrasound is usually placed in the prone position. Sonographic gel is applied to the skin over the back and flank areas to enhance sound-wave conduction. A transducer in contact with and moving across the skin delivers sound waves and measures the echoes. Images of the internal structures are produced. Skin care to remove the gel is all that is needed after ultrasonography.

Renal Scan. This imaging test is used to examine the perfusion, function, and structure of the kidneys, using the IV administration of a radioisotope. It does not use an iodinated dye and so may be used in preference to a CT scan when the patient is allergic to iodine or has impaired kidney function that places him or her at risk for kidney injury from contrast dyes.

Patient Preparation and Procedural Care. No fasting or sedation is used. A peripheral IV catheter is inserted to give the radioisotope. While the patient lies in a prone or sitting position, a camera is passed over the kidney area and records the isotope uptake on film, minutes after it is given. After initial images, the patient may be given furosemide or captopril to better visualize kidney function and blood flow. The isotope is eliminated 6 to 24 hours after the procedure. Encourage the patient to drink fluids to aid in excretion of the isotope. Because only tracer doses of radioisotopes are used, no precautions are needed related to radioactive exposure.

Renal Arteriography (Angiography). Renal arteriography allows dye to enter the renal blood vessels and generates images to determine blood vessel size and abnormalities. This test has largely been replaced by other imaging techniques (e.g., nuclear renal scans, ultrasonography, computed tomography) and is seldom used as a stand-alone diagnostic procedure. The most common use of renal arteriography is at the time of a renal angioplasty or other intervention.

Cystoscopy and Cystourethroscopy

Patient Preparation. Cystoscopy and cystourethroscopy are endoscopic procedures and require completion of a preoperative checklist and a signed informed consent statement. The urologist provides a complete description of and reasons for the procedure, and the nurse reinforces this information. Cystoscopy may be performed for diagnosis or treatment. This test is used to examine for bladder trauma (cystoscopy) or urethral trauma (cystourethroscopy) and to identify causes of urinary tract obstruction. Cystoscopy also may be used to remove bladder tumors or to plant radium seeds into a tumor, dilate the urethra and ureters with or without stent placement, stop areas of bleeding, or resect an enlarged prostate gland.

Cystoscopy may be performed under general anesthesia or under local anesthesia with sedation. The patient's age and general health and the expected duration of the procedure are considered in the decision about anesthesia. A light evening meal may be eaten. Usually the patient is NPO after midnight on the night before the cystoscopy. A bowel preparation with laxatives or enemas is performed the evening before the procedure.

Procedure. The cystoscopy is performed in a designated cystoscopic examination room. If the procedure is performed in a surgical suite under general anesthesia, the usual surgical support personnel are present (see Chapter 15). This procedure is often performed in clinics, ambulatory surgery or short-procedure units, or a urologist's office.

Assist the patient onto a table, and after sedation, place him or her in the lithotomy position. After the anesthesia is given and the area cleansed and draped, the urologist inserts a cystoscope through the urethra into the urinary bladder. This examination commonly includes the use of both the cystoscope and the urethroscope.

Follow-up Care. After this procedure with general anesthesia, the patient is returned to a postanesthesia care unit (PACU) or area. If local anesthesia and sedation were used, he or she may be returned directly to the hospital room. Ambulatory care patients undergoing cystoscopic examinations are transferred to an area for monitoring before discharge to home. Monitor for airway patency and breathing, changes in vital signs (including temperature), and changes in urine output. Also observe for the complications of bleeding and infection.

A catheter may or may not be present after cystoscopy. The patient without a catheter has urinary frequency as a result of irritation from the procedure. The urine may be pink tinged, but gross bleeding is not expected. Bleeding or the presence of clots may obstruct the catheter and decrease urine output. Monitor urine output, and notify the urologist of obvious blood clots or a decreased or absent urine output. Irrigate the Foley catheter with sterile saline, if prescribed. Notify the urologist if the patient has a fever (with or without chills) or an elevated white blood cell (WBC) count, which suggests infection. Urge the patient to take oral FLUIDS to increase urine output (which helps prevent clotting) and to reduce the burning sensation on urination.

Cystography and Cystourethrography. These tests are a series of x-rays or a continuous radiographic visualization by fluoroscopy. During the imaging, a dye fills the bladder and the bladder is emptied. Images show structure and function of the bladder and urethra. Tumors, rupture or perforation of the bladder and urethra, abnormal backflow of urine, and distortion from trauma or other pelvic masses can be seen.

Patient Preparation and Procedural Care. Explain the procedure to the patient. A urinary catheter is temporarily needed to instill contrast dye directly into the bladder for both procedures. The dye is needed to enhance x-ray visibility of the lower urinary tract and is not absorbed into the bloodstream, which reduces the risk for contrast-induced kidney injury.

After bladder filling, x-rays are taken from the front, back, and side positions. For the voiding cystourethrogram (VCUG), the patient is requested to void and x-rays are taken during the voiding. A VCUG is obtained to determine whether urine refluxes (flows backward) into the ureter. The cystogram is used in cases of trauma when urethral or bladder injury is suspected or for patients with recurrent *pyelonephritis* (kidney infection).

Monitor for infection as a result of catheter placement. In this test, the dye is not nephrotoxic because it does not enter the bloodstream and does not reach the kidney. Encourage fluid intake to dilute the urine and reduce the burning sensation from catheter irritation after removal. Monitor for changes in urine output because pelvic or urethral trauma may be present.

Retrograde Procedures. **Retrograde** means going against the normal flow of urine. A retrograde examination of the ureters and the pelvis of both kidneys (*pyelogram*), the bladder (*cystogram*), and the urethra (*urethrogram*) involves instilling dye into the lower urinary tract. Because the dye is instilled directly to obtain an outline of the structures of interest, the dye does not enter the bloodstream. Therefore the patient is not at risk for dye-induced acute kidney injury (AKI) or a systemic allergic response.

The patient is prepared for retrograde procedures (retrograde pyelography, retrograde cystography, and retrograde urethrography) in the same way as for cystoscopy. Retrograde x-rays are obtained during the cystoscopy. After placement of the cystoscope by the urologist, catheters are placed into each ureter and contrast dye is instilled into each ureter and kidney pelvis. The catheters are removed by the urologist, and x-rays are taken to outline these structures as the dye is excreted. The procedure identifies obstruction or structural abnormalities.

For patients undergoing retrograde cystoscopy or urethrography, contrast dye is instilled similarly into the bladder or urethra. Cystography and urethrography identify structural problems, such as fistulas, diverticula, and tumors.

After retrograde procedures, monitor the patient for infection caused by placing instruments in the urinary tract. Because these procedures are performed during cystoscopic examination, follow-up care is the same as that for cystoscopy.

Other Diagnostic Assessments

Urodynamic Studies. Urodynamic studies examine the processes of voiding and include:

- Tests of bladder capacity, pressure, and tone
- Studies of urethral pressure and urine flow
- Tests of perineal voluntary muscle function

These tests are often used along with voiding urographic or cystoscopic procedures to evaluate problems with urine flow and disorders of the lower urinary tract (Gray, 2011; Gray, 2012a; Gray, 2012b).

Cystometrography (CMG) can determine how well the bladder wall (detrusor) muscle functions and how sensitive it is to stretching as the bladder fills. This test provides information about bladder capacity, bladder pressure, and voiding reflexes.

Explain the procedure, and inform the patient that a urinary catheter will be needed temporarily during the procedure. Ask the patient to void normally. Record the amount and time of voiding. Insert a urinary catheter to measure the residual urine volume. The cystometer is attached to the catheter, and fluid is instilled via the catheter into the bladder. The point at which the patient first notes a feeling of the urge to void and the point at which he or she notes a strong urge to void are recorded. Bladder capacity and bladder pressure readings are recorded graphically. The patient is asked to void when the bladder instillation is complete (about 500 mL). The residual urine after voiding is recorded, and the catheter is removed.

Electromyography of the perineal muscles may be performed during this examination.

For any procedure that involves inserting instruments into the urinary tract, monitor for infection. Record the patient's temperature, the character of the urine, and urine output volume.

Urethral pressure profile (also called a *urethral pressure profilometry [UPP]*) can provide information about the nature of urinary incontinence or urinary retention.

Explain the procedure, and inform the patient that a urinary catheter will be needed temporarily during the procedure. A special catheter with pressure-sensing capabilities is inserted into the bladder. Variations in the pressure of the smooth muscle of the urethra are recorded as the catheter is slowly withdrawn.

As with any study involving inserting instruments into the urinary tract, monitor the patient for manifestations of infection.

Urine stream testing is used to evaluate pelvic muscle strength and the effectiveness of pelvic muscles in stopping the flow of urine. It is useful in assessing urinary incontinence.

Explain the procedure, and reassure the patient that efforts will be made to ensure privacy. The patient is asked to begin urinating. Three to five seconds after urination begins, the examiner gives the patient a signal to stop urine flow. The length of time required to stop the flow of urine is recorded.

Cleaning the perineal area, as after any voiding, is all that is necessary after the urine stream test.

Electromyography (EMG) of the perineal muscles tests the strength of the muscles used in voiding. This information may help identify methods of improving continence. Inform the patient that some mild, temporary discomfort may accompany placement of the electrodes. In EMG of the perineal muscles, electrodes are placed in either the rectum or the urethra to measure muscle contraction and relaxation. After the completion of EMG, administer analgesics as prescribed to promote the patient's comfort.

 NCLEX EXAMINATION CHALLENGE

Safe and Effective Care Environment

Which assessments are most important for the nurse to perform when monitoring a client who returns to the medical-surgical unit after a dye-enhanced CT scan?
A. Body temperature and urine odor
B. Kidney tenderness and flank pain
C. Urine volume and color
D. Specific gravity and pH

Kidney Biopsy

Patient Preparation. Explain that a kidney biopsy can help determine a cause of unexplained kidney problems and can help direct or change therapy. Most kidney biopsies are performed percutaneously (through skin and other tissues) using ultrasound or CT guidance. The patient signs an informed consent and is NPO for 4 to 6 hours before the procedure.

Because of the risk for bleeding after the biopsy, coagulation studies such as platelet count, activated partial thromboplastin time (aPTT), prothrombin time (PT), and bleeding time are performed before surgery. Hypertension is aggressively managed before and after the procedure because high blood pressure can make stopping the bleeding after the biopsy more difficult. Uremia also increases the risk for bleeding, and dialysis may be prescribed before a biopsy. A blood transfusion may be needed to correct anemia before biopsy.

Procedure. In a percutaneous biopsy, the nephrologist or radiologist obtains tissue samples without an incision. Patients receive sedation and are monitored throughout the procedure. The patient is placed in the prone position on the procedure table. The entry site is selected after taking preliminary images. The area is prepped and sterilely draped. A local anesthetic is injected, and the physician then inserts the biopsy device into the tissues toward the kidney. Needle depth and placement are confirmed by ultrasound or CT. While the patient holds his or her breath, the needle is advanced into the renal cortex. Samples are then taken with a spring-loaded coring biopsy needle and sent for pathologic study.

Follow-up Care. After a percutaneous biopsy, the major risk is bleeding from the biopsy site. For 24 hours after the biopsy, monitor the dressing site, vital signs (especially fluctuations in blood pressure), urine output, hemoglobin level, and hematocrit. Even if the dressing is dry and there is no hematoma, the patient could be bleeding from the site. An internal bleed is not readily visible but is suspected with flank pain, decreasing blood pressure, decreasing urine output, or other signs of hypovolemia or shock.

The patient follows a plan of strict bedrest, lying in a supine position with a back roll for additional support for 2 to 6 hours after the biopsy. The head of the bed may be elevated, and the patient may resume oral intake of food and fluids. After bedrest, the patient may have limited bathroom privileges if there is no evidence of bleeding.

Monitor for hematuria, the most common complication of kidney biopsy. Hematuria occurs microscopically in most patients, but 5% to 9% have gross hematuria. This problem usually resolves without treatment in 48 to 72 hours after the biopsy but can persist for 2 to 3 weeks. In rare cases, transfusions and surgery are required. There should be no obvious blood clots in the urine.

The patient may have some local pain after the biopsy. If aching originates at the biopsy site and begins to radiate to the flank and around the front of the abdomen, bleeding may have started or a hematoma is forming around the kidney. This pattern of discomfort with bleeding occurs because blood in the tissues around the kidney increases pressure on local nerve tracts.

If bleeding occurs, IV fluid, packed red blood cells, or both may be needed to prevent shock. In general, a small amount of bleeding creates enough pressure to compress bleeding sites. This is called a "tamponade effect." If tamponade does not occur and bleeding is extensive, surgery for hemostasis or even nephrectomy may be needed. A hematoma in, on, or around the kidney may become infected, requiring treatment with antibiotics and surgical drainage.

If no bleeding occurs, the patient can resume general activities after 24 hours. Instruct him or her to avoid lifting heavy objects, exercising, or performing other strenuous activities for 1 to 2 weeks after the biopsy procedure. Driving may also be restricted. Refer to Chapter 16 for general postoperative care for the patient who has undergone an open kidney biopsy.

♀ CLINICAL JUDGMENT CHALLENGE

Safety; Patient-Centered Care QSEN

At the start of the shift, you are assessing an 86-year-old patient who is awaiting surgery for a hip repair after a fall 12 hours ago at home. You are collecting a clean-catch urine specimen, using a bedpan, as part of the preoperative preparation. You observe that when she voids, the urine odor is foul and the urine is cloudy and full of sediment. She reports some urgency but notes that she had urgency before her fall.

1. What assessment information will you document in the chart?
2. What additional information should you ask the patient and what else should you consider?
3. Organize your thoughts into a SBAR communication (Chapter 1)
4. Who should you notify and why?

NURSING CONCEPTS AND CLINICAL JUDGMENT REVIEW

In addition to normal ranges indicating FLUID AND ELECTROLYTE BALANCE and ACID-BASE BALANCE, what might you NOTICE in a patient with adequate urinary ELIMINATION?

Vital signs:
- Body temperature is within normal range.
- Blood Pressure is within normal range.

Physical assessment:
- Daily urine output is within 500 mL of daily fluid intake.
- Skin texture is normal (no edema or superficial crystals present).
- Skin color is appropriate for ethnicity with no excessive yellowing, bruising, or petechiae.
- Urine is clear and some variation of yellow in color.
- Patient voids 300 to 500 mL per voiding.
- Patient does not report pain or burning on urination.
- Patient has no difficulty starting or stopping the stream of urine.

- Patient is continent of urine and can maintain continence without sensation of urgency.
- Patient is alert and oriented.

Psychological assessment:
- Patient is able to communicate concerns about the urinary tract system.
- Patient is aware and informed about kidney function and diagnostic tests.

Laboratory assessment:
- Hematocrit and hemoglobin are within normal limits (no anemia).
- BUN and creatinine are within normal limits.
- Serum electrolytes are within normal ranges.
- Urinalysis shows no bacteria, blood, sediment, or protein.

GET READY FOR THE NCLEX® EXAMINATION!

▌ KEY POINTS

Review these Key Points for each NCLEX Examination Client Needs Category.

Safe and Effective Care Environment
- Use sterile technique when inserting a catheter or any other instrument into the urinary system. **Safety** QSEN
- Use Contact Precautions with any patient who has drainage from the genitourinary tract. **Safety** QSEN
- Wear gloves when testing or handling urine. **Safety** QSEN
- Evaluate risk for kidney injury from diagnostic testing by asking about allergy to contrast dye or iodine and adverse reactions following the use of diagnostic agents such as gadolinium in MRI.
- Ask the patient about the use of prescribed and over-the-counter drugs that increase risk for kidney dysfunction.
- Verify that informed consent has been obtained and that the patient has a clear understanding of the potential risks before he or she undergoes invasive procedures to assess the kidneys and urinary function. **Safety** QSEN

Health Promotion and Maintenance
- Teach patients to clean the perineal area after voiding, after having a bowel movement, and after sexual intercourse. **Evidence-Based Practice** QSEN
- Urge all patients to maintain an adequate fluid intake (sufficient to dilute urine to a light yellow color). A minimum of 2 L/day may be recommended unless another health problem requires fluid restriction.
- Teach patients who come into contact with chemicals in their workplaces or for leisure-time activities to avoid direct skin or mucous membrane contact with these chemicals. **Safety** QSEN

Psychosocial Integrity
- Allow the patient the opportunity to express fear or anxiety about tests of the kidneys and urinary tract or about a potential change in kidney function. **Patient-Centered Care** QSEN
- Assess the patient's level of comfort in discussing issues related to elimination and the urogenital area.

- Explain all diagnostic procedures, restrictions, and follow-up care to the patient scheduled for tests.
- Provide as much privacy as possible for patients undergoing examination or testing of the kidney/urinary tract. **Patient-Centered Care** QSEN
- Use language and terminology that the patient can understand during discussions of kidney/urinary assessment. **Patient-Centered Care** QSEN

Physiological Integrity

- Ask the patient about kidney problems in any other members of the family, because some problems have a genetic component.
- Ask the patient about current and past drug use (prescribed, over-the-counter, and illicit), and evaluate drug use for potential nephrotoxicity.

- Use laboratory data to distinguish between dehydration and kidney impairment. **Evidence-Based Practice** QSEN
- Describe how to obtain a sterile urine specimen from a urinary catheter.
- Assess urine output closely after any procedure in which contrast dye is used IV. **Evidence-Based Practice** QSEN
- Assess the patient for bleeding or manifestations of infection after any invasive test of kidney/urinary function.
- Inform health care providers about any manifestations of complications following invasive or noninvasive tests of urinary and kidney structure or function.

Care of Patients with Urinary Problems

Chris Winkelman

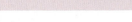 http://evolve.elsevier.com/Iggy/

The ureters, bladder, and urethra make up the urinary system. Their functions are to store the urine made by the kidney and eliminate it from the body. Problems in the urinary system can interfere with urinary ELIMINATION when the mechanics of moving urine out of the body are disrupted. Such problems can reduce control of fluids, electrolytes, nitrogenous wastes, and blood pressure.

Urinary problems affect the storage or ELIMINATION of urine. Both acute and chronic urinary problems are common and costly. More than 20 million people in the United States are treated annually for urinary tract infections, cystitis, kidney and ureter stones, or urinary incontinence (U.S. Renal Data Systems, 2012). Although life-threatening complications are rare with urinary problems, patients may have functional, physical, and psychosocial changes that reduce quality of life. Nursing interventions are directed toward prevention, detection, and management of urologic disorders.

INFECTIOUS DISORDERS

Infections of the urinary tract and kidneys are common, especially among women. Manifestations of urinary tract INFECTION (UTI) account for more than 7 million health care visits and 1 million hospital admissions annually in the United States (U.S. Renal Data Systems, 2012). Total direct and indirect costs for adult urinary tract infections are estimated at $1.6 billion each year. UTIs are the most common health care–associated INFECTION (Dudeck et al., 2013).

Urinary tract infections are described by their location in the tract. Acute infections in the lower urinary tract include *urethritis* (urethra), *cystitis* (bladder), and *prostatitis* (prostate gland). Acute *pyelonephritis* is an upper urinary tract (kidney) infection. Although the vocabulary for these infected sites reflects an inflammatory condition *(-itis),* the most common cause of INFLAMMATION in the urinary tract is INFECTION. Thus these terms are often used interchangeably to refer to either an infectious process or a noninfectious inflammatory process. Several risk factors are associated with occurrence of UTIs (Table 66-1).

The presence of bacteria in the urine is bacteriuria and can occur with any urologic infection. When bacteriuria is without manifestations of infection, it is called *colonization,* or *asymptomatic bacterial urinary tract infection or ABUTI,* and is more common in older adults. This problem may progress to acute infection or renal insufficiency when the patient has other conditions, and only then does it require treatment.

Urinary tract INFECTIONS are typically categorized as *uncomplicated* or *complicated.* An acute, uncomplicated UTI is usually cystitis or pyelonephritis in premenopausal, nonpregnant, otherwise healthy women. With an uncomplicated UTI, there

TABLE 66-1	Factors Contributing to Urinary Tract Infections
FACTOR	**MECHANISM**
Obstruction	Incomplete bladder emptying creates a continuous pool of urine in which bacteria can grow, prevents flushing out of bacteria, and allows bacteria to ascend more easily to higher structures. Bacteria have a greater chance of multiplying the longer they remain in residual urine. Overdistention of the bladder damages the mucosa and allows bacteria to invade the bladder wall.
Stones (calculi)	Large stones can obstruct urine flow. The rough surface of a stone irritates mucosal surfaces and creates a spot where bacteria can establish and grow. Bacteria can live within stones and cause re-infection.
Vesicoureteral reflux	Bacteria-laden urine is forced backward from the bladder up into the ureters and kidneys, where pyelonephritis can develop. Reflux of sterile urine can cause kidney scarring, which may promote kidney dysfunction.
Diabetes mellitus	Excess glucose in urine provides a rich medium for bacterial growth. Peripheral neuropathy affects bladder innervation and leads to a flaccid bladder and incomplete bladder emptying.
Characteristics of urine	Alkaline urine promotes bacterial growth. Concentrated urine promotes bacterial growth.
Gender	**Women** Susceptibility to periurethral colonization with coliform bacteria is increased, especially as estrogen levels fall during menopause. Use of douches, perfumed pads or toilet tissue, diaphragms, or spermicide (including spermicide-coated condoms) in women can inflame periurethral tissue and contribute to colonization. Bladder displacement during pregnancy predisposes women to cystitis and the development of pyelonephritis. A diaphragm or pessary that is too large can obstruct urine flow or traumatize the urethra. **Men** With increased age, the prostate enlarges and may obstruct the normal flow of urine, producing stasis. With increased age, prostatic secretions lose their antibacterial characteristics and predispose to bacterial proliferation in the urine. Sexually transmitted diseases may cause urethral strictures that obstruct the flow of urine and predispose to urinary stasis.
Age	Urinary stasis may be caused by incomplete bladder emptying as a result of an enlarged prostate in men and cystocele and vaginal prolapse in women. Neuromuscular conditions that cause incomplete bladder emptying, such as Parkinson disease and stroke, affect older adults more frequently. The use of drugs with intentional or unintentional anticholinergic properties in older adults contributes to delayed bladder emptying. Fecal incontinence contributes to periurethral contamination. Low estrogen in menopausal women adversely affects the cells of the vagina and urethra, making them more susceptible to infections.
Sexual activity	Sexual intercourse is the strongest risk factor for uncomplicated cystitis, particularly in young women. Irritation of the perineum and urethra during intercourse can promote migration of bacteria from the perineal area to the urinary tract in some women. Inadequate vaginal lubrication may exacerbate potential urethral irritation. Bacteria may be introduced into the man's urethra during anal intercourse or during vaginal intercourse with a woman who has a bacterial vaginitis.
Recent use of antibiotics	Antibiotics change normal protective flora, providing opportunity for pathogenic bacterial overgrowth and colonization.

is no anatomic or functional abnormality of the urinary tract. Complicated UTIs are associated with conditions that increase the risk for treatment failure or serious outcomes. These conditions or factors include obstruction, pregnancy, male gender, diabetes, neurogenic bladder, renal insufficiency, and immunosuppression (Hooton, 2012). Complicated UTIs require greater vigilance to avoid or to detect adverse events from the infection and a longer course of antimicrobial treatment. They also may require additional diagnostics to identify and manage other related health problems (comorbidities).

CYSTITIS

❖ PATHOPHYSIOLOGY

Cystitis is an inflammatory condition of the bladder. Commonly, it refers to INFLAMMATION from an INFECTION of the bladder. However, cystitis can be caused by inflammation without infection. Drugs, chemicals, or radiation, for example, cause bladder inflammation without an infecting organism. Irritants, such as feminine hygiene spray, spermicidal jellies, or

long-term use of a catheter can cause cystitis without infection. Cystitis may sometimes occur as a complication of other disorders, such as gynecologic cancers, pelvic inflammatory disorders, endometriosis, Crohn's disease, diverticulitis, lupus, or tuberculosis. Interstitial cystitis is an inflammatory disease that has no known cause.

Microbes, most commonly bacteria, move up the urinary tract from the external urethra to the bladder to cause infectious cystitis. Less commonly, spread of INFECTION through the blood and lymph fluid can occur. Mucin produced by cells lining the bladder helps maintain mucosal integrity and prevents cellular damage. Mucin may also prevent bacteria from adhering to urothelial cells. Bladder irritating factors, like concentrated urine, may interfere with the production and effectiveness of mucin.

Etiology and Genetic Risk

UTIs, like other INFECTIONS, are the result of interactions between a pathogen and the host. Usually, a high bacterial *virulence* (ability to invade and infect) is needed to overcome normal host resistance. However, a compromised host is more likely to become infected even with bacteria that have low virulence. Invading bacteria with special adhesions are more likely to cause ascending UTIs that start in the urethra or bladder and move up into the ureter and kidney. Patient-specific genetic factors such as innate inflammatory response may influence the risk for UTI.

Infectious cystitis is most commonly caused by pathogens from the bowel or, in some cases, the vagina (Hooton, 2012). About 90% of UTIs are caused by *Escherichia coli*. Less common organisms include *Staphylococcus saprophyticus, Klebsiella pneumoniae,* and organisms from the *Proteus* and *Enterobacter* species (Brusch, 2013). Other infecting microbes causing infectious cystitis are viruses, mycobacteria, parasites, and yeast (fungus), especially *Candida* species.

In most cases, organisms adhere to the perineal area and move into the urethra as a result of irritation, trauma, or instrumentation of the urinary tract. Infecting organisms then migrate to the bladder. Small urine volume or infrequent voiding, sexual intercourse, urinary tract obstruction, instrumentation, use of catheters not drained to gravity, and *vesicoureteral reflux* (backward flow of urine at the ureteral-bladder junction) are all associated with the ascending migration of infecting organisms.

Catheters are the most common factor placing patients at risk for UTIs in the hospital and long-term care settings (Mori, 2014). Within 48 hours of catheter insertion, bacterial colonization along the urethra and the catheter itself begins. About 50% of patients with indwelling catheters become infected within 1 week of catheter insertion.

How a catheter-related INFECTION occurs varies between genders. Bacteria from a woman's perineal area are more likely to ascend to the bladder by moving along the urethra. The shorter urethra in women aids in the ascending organism migration. In men, bacteria tend to gain access to the bladder from the catheter itself. Any break in the closed urinary drainage system allows bacteria to move through the lumen of the catheter. The external catheter surface also provides route for migration. Best practices to reduce the risk for catheter contamination and catheter-related UTIs are listed in Chart 66-1.

Organisms other than bacteria cause cystitis. Fungal INFECTIONS, such as those caused by *Candida*, can occur during long-term antibiotic therapy, because antibiotics change normal protective flora that reduce the adherence and virulence of pathogenic bacteria. Patients who are severely immunosuppressed, are receiving corticosteroids or other immunosuppressive agents, or have diabetes mellitus or acquired immune deficiency syndrome (AIDS) are at higher risk for fungal UTIs.

Viral and parasitic infections are rare and usually are transferred to the urinary tract from an INFECTION at another body site. For example, *Trichomonas*, a parasite found in the vagina, can also be found in the urine. Treatment of the vaginal infection also resolves the UTI.

Noninfectious cystitis may result from chemical exposure, such as to drugs (e.g., cyclophosphamide [Cytoxan, Procytox✚]); from radiation therapy; and from immunologic responses, as with systemic lupus erythematosus (SLE).

Interstitial cystitis is a rare, chronic INFLAMMATION of the entire lower urinary tract (bladder, urethra, and adjacent pelvic muscles) that is not a result of INFECTION. The condition affects women 10 times more often than men, and the diagnosis is difficult to make. Manifestations are PAIN associated with

---

CHART 66-1 Best Practice for Patient Safety & Quality Care QSEN

Minimizing Catheter-Related Infection

- Maintain good hand hygiene.
- Insert urinary catheters for appropriate use only, including:
  - Acute urinary retention or bladder obstruction
  - Accurate measurement of urine volume in critically ill patients
  - Perioperative situations that involve urologic surgery
  - Monitor urine output when large-volume infusions or diuretics are used
  - Patient requires immobilization from unstable spine or pelvic fractures
- Assess patients daily to determine the need for an indwelling catheter; the strongest predictor of a catheter-associated urinary tract infection (CAUTI) is the length of time the catheter dwells in a patient.
- Consider appropriate alternatives to an indwelling catheter such as an external device in men.
- Use sterile technique when inserting the urinary catheter.
- When emptying the urine bag, do not allow the tip of the outflow tube to touch the urine collection container. Use a dedicated container for each patient or resident.
- Select a small-size catheter, and do not overfill the balloon.
- Maintain a closed system by ensuring that catheter tubing connections are sealed securely; disconnections can introduce pathogens into the urinary tract.
- Maintain unobstructed urine flow by keeping the tubing patent and urine collection bags below the level of the bladder at all times; elevating the collection bag above the bladder causes reflux from the bag into the urinary tract.
- Monitor and report CAUTI rates, and promote ongoing best practices.
- Secure the catheter to the patient's thigh (women) or lower abdomen (men); catheter movement can cause urethral friction and irritation.
- Perform daily catheter care by washing the perineum and proximal portion of the catheter with soap and water and drying gently (removes pathogens and reduces pathogenic population).
- Consider the use of coated catheters for patients requiring indwelling catheters for more than 3 to 5 days. This coating reduces bacterial colonization along the catheter.

Application of antiseptic solutions or antibiotic ointments to the perineal area of catheterized patients has not been demonstrated to have any beneficial effect.

Adapted from Dumont, C., & Wakeman, J. (2010). Preventing catheter-associated UTIs: Survey report. *Nursing2010, 40*(12), 24-30.

---

bladder filling or voiding, usually accompanied by frequency, urgency, and nocturia (McCance et al., 2014). Pain occurs in suprapubic or pelvic areas, sometimes radiating to the groin, vulva, or rectum. Results from urinalysis and urine culture are negative for infection (Quillin & Erickson, 2012).

Although cystitis is not life threatening, infectious cystitis can lead to life-threatening complications, including pyelonephritis and sepsis. Severe kidney damage from an ascending INFECTION that began as cystitis is a rare complication unless the patient also has other predisposing factors, such as anatomic abnormalities, pregnancy, obstruction, reflux, calculi, or diabetes.

The urinary tract is the INFECTION source of severe sepsis or septic shock in about 10% to 30% of cases (Wagenlehner et al., 2013). The spread of the infection from the urinary tract to the bloodstream is termed **urosepsis**. Urosepsis is associated with complicated urinary tract infections and is more common among older adults. Sepsis is a systemic reaction to infection that can lead to overwhelming organ failure, shock, and death.

Sepsis has a high mortality and prolongs hospitalization (see Chapter 37).

Incidence and Prevalence

The incidence of UTI is second only to that of upper respiratory infections in primary care. Patients who have **frequency** (an urge to urinate frequently in small amounts), **dysuria** (PAIN or burning with urination), and **urgency** (the feeling that urination will occur immediately) account for more than 8 million health care visits annually (Foxman, 2010). About 60% of these patients will have a confirmed UTI (Lowe & Ryan-Wenger, 2012).

CONSIDERATIONS FOR OLDER ADULTS

Patient-Centered Care QSEN

The prevalence of UTIs varies with age and gender. Women of any age are more commonly affected with UTIs than are men. In men, the incidence of UTI greatly increases after 73 years of age. In women, the prevalence of UTIs increases from 20% among all women to 50% among those older than 80 years (U.S. Renal Data Systems, 2012). Skin and mucous membrane changes from a lack of estrogen appear to account for much of the increased risk in older women. Prostate disease increases risk for UTIs in men. Ask about manifestations of UTI whenever you are assessing an older adult.

Health Promotion and Maintenance

Although cystitis is common, in many cases it is preventable. In the health care setting, reducing the use and duration of indwelling urinary catheters is a major prevention strategy. When catheters must be used in institutional settings, strict attention to sterile technique during insertion is essential to reduce the risk for UTIs (see Chart 66-1). Long-term placement of urinary catheters requires aseptic technique for insertion. When *intermittent catheterization* is used in the home setting, a clean technique may be used (Newman & Willson, 2011).

! NURSING SAFETY PRIORITY QSEN

Action Alert

Ensuring that urinary catheters are used appropriately and discontinued as early as possible is everyone's responsibility. Do not allow catheters to remain in place for staff convenience.

Certain changes in fluid intake patterns, urinary ELIMINATION patterns, and hygiene patterns can help prevent or reduce cystitis in the general population. For example, a liberal water intake of 2.2 L for women and 3 L for men can promote general health. Another strategy to promote health is to have sufficient fluid intake to cause 1.5 L of clear or light yellow urine daily. Other strategies to prevent cystitis and other UTIs are listed in Chart 66-2. Although these strategies do not have consistent or high-quality evidence to support a reduced risk for UTI when followed, they are low risk and reasonable (Hooton, 2012).

❖ PATIENT-CENTERED COLLABORATIVE CARE

◆ Assessment

Physical Assessment/Clinical Manifestations. Frequency, urgency, and dysuria are the common manifestations of a urinary tract INFECTION (UTI), but other manifestations may be present (Chart 66-3). Urine may be cloudy, foul smelling, or

---

CHART 66-2 Patient and Family Education: Preparing for Self-Management

Preventing a Urinary Tract Infection

- Drink fluid liberally, as much as 2 to 3 liters daily if not contraindicated by health conditions.
- Be sure to get enough sleep, rest, and nutrition daily to maintain immunologic health.
- If spermicides are used, consider changing to another method of contraception.
- *[For women]* Clean your perineum (the area between your legs) from front to back.
- *[For women]* Avoid using or wearing irritating substances such as douches, scented lubricants for intercourse, bubble bath, tight-fitting underwear, and scented toilet tissue. Wear loose-fitting cotton underwear.
- *[For women]* Empty your bladder before and after intercourse.
- *[For both women and men]* Gently wash the perineal area before intercourse.
- Do not routinely delay urination because the flow of urine can help remove bacteria that may be colonizing the urethra or bladder.
- If you experience burning when you urinate, if you have to urinate frequently, or if you find it difficult to begin urinating, notify your physician or other health care provider right away, especially if you have a chronic medical condition (e.g., diabetes) or are pregnant.
- Consider using one or more of these therapies to reduce the risk for developing a urinary tract infection:
  - Taking cranberry substances (juice, capsules, or tablets) daily. Avoid high fructose cranberry juice to minimize calories and high glucose urine favorable to bacterial reproduction.
  - Ingesting apple cider vinegar, 2 tablespoons 3 times daily in juice.
  - Applying topical estrogen to the perineal area, if postmenopausal. Topical estrogen normalizes vaginal flora. Oral estrogens are not effective.
  - Ingesting D-mannose 500 mg tablet or 0.5-1 teaspoon of powder; D-mannose is thought to block adhesion of *E. coli* to the epithelium in the urinary tract.

Adapted from Hooton, T.M. (2012). Clinical practice: Uncomplicated urinary tract infection. *New England Journal of Medicine, 366*(11), 1028-1037.

---

blood tinged. Ask the patient about risk factors for UTI during the assessment (see Table 66-1). For noninfectious cystitis, the Pelvic Pain and Urgency/Frequency (PUF) patient symptom scale can identify patients with interstitial cystitis (Richmond, 2010).

Before performing the physical assessment, ask the patient to void so that the urine can be examined and the bladder emptied before palpation. Assess vital signs to help identify the presence of INFECTION (e.g., fever, tachycardia, and tachypnea). Inspect the lower abdomen, and palpate the bladder. Distention after voiding indicates incomplete bladder emptying.

Using Standard Precautions, record any lesions around the urethral meatus and vaginal opening. To help differentiate between a vaginal and a urinary tract INFECTION, note whether there is any vaginal discharge. Vaginal discharge and irritation are more indicative of vaginal infection. Women often report burning with urination when normal acidic urine touches labial tissues that are inflamed or ulcerated by vaginal infections or sexually transmitted diseases (STDs). Maintain privacy with drapes during the examination.

The prostate is palpated by digital rectal examination (DRE) for size, change in shape or consistency, and tenderness. The physician or advanced practice nurse performs the DRE.

Laboratory Assessment. Laboratory assessment for a UTI is a urinalysis with testing for leukocyte esterase and nitrate. The

CHART 66-3   Key Features

Urinary Tract Infection

Common Clinical Manifestations

- Frequency
- Urgency
- Dysuria
- Hesitancy or difficulty in initiating urine stream
- Low back pain
- Nocturia
- Incontinence
- Hematuria
- Pyuria
- Bacteriuria
- Retention
- Suprapubic tenderness or fullness
- Feeling of incomplete bladder emptying

Rare Clinical Manifestations

- Fever
- Chills
- Nausea or vomiting
- Malaise
- Flank pain

Clinical Manifestations that May Occur in the Older Adult

- The only manifestation may be something as vague as increasing mental confusion or frequent, unexplained falls.
- A sudden onset of incontinence or a worsening of incontinence may be the only manifestation of an early urinary tract infection (UTI).
- Fever, tachycardia, tachypnea, and hypotension, even without any urinary manifestations, may be signs of urosepsis.
- Loss of appetite, nocturia, and dysuria are common manifestations.

combination of a positive leukocyte esterase and nitrate is 68% to 88% sensitive in the diagnosis of a UTI (Lowe & Ryan-Wenger, 2012). However, when a urinalysis includes a microscopic count of bacteria, white blood cells (WBCs), and red blood cells (RBCs), the additional testing is more expensive and may not improve diagnostic accuracy. The presence of more than 20 epithelial cells/high-power field (hpf) suggests contamination. The presence of 100,000 colonies/mL or the presence of three or more WBCs (pyuria) with RBCs (hematuria) indicates INFECTION.

A urinalysis is performed on a clean-catch midstream specimen. If the patient cannot produce a clean-catch specimen, you may need to obtain the specimen with a small-diameter (6 Fr) catheter. For a routine urinalysis, 10 mL of urine is needed; smaller quantities are sufficient for culture.

A urine culture confirms the type of organism and the number of colonies. Urine culture is expensive, and initial results take at least 48 hours. It is indicated when the UTI is complicated, when it does not respond to usual therapy, or when the diagnosis is uncertain. A UTI is confirmed when more than 10^5 colony-forming units are in the urine from any patient. In patients who also have manifestations of UTI, as few as 10^3 colony-forming units may be used to confirm the infection. The presence of many different types of organisms in low colony counts usually indicates that the specimen is contaminated. Sensitivity testing follows culture results when complicating factors are present (e.g., stones or recurrent infection), when the patient is older, or to ensure the appropriate antibiotics are prescribed.

Occasionally the serum WBC count may be elevated, with the differential WBC count showing a "left shift" (see Chapter 17). This shift indicates that the number of immature

WBCs is increasing in response to the INFECTION. As a result, the number of bands, or immature WBCs, is elevated. Left shift most often occurs with urosepsis and rarely occurs with uncomplicated cystitis, which is a local rather than a systemic infection.

Other Diagnostic Assessment. The diagnosis of cystitis is based on the history, physical examination, and laboratory data. If urinary retention and obstruction of urine outflow are suspected, pelvic ultrasound or CT may be needed to locate the site of obstruction or the presence of calculi. Voiding cystourethrography (see Chapter 65) is needed when urine reflux is suspected.

Cystoscopy (see Chapter 65) may be performed when the patient has recurrent UTIs (more than three or four a year). A urine culture is performed first to ensure that no infection is present. If INFECTION is present, the urine is sterilized with antibiotic therapy before the procedure to reduce the risk for sepsis. Cystoscopy identifies abnormalities that increase the risk for cystitis. Such abnormalities include bladder calculi, bladder diverticula, urethral strictures, foreign bodies (e.g., sutures from previous surgery), and trabeculation (an abnormal thickening of the bladder wall caused by urinary retention and obstruction). Retrograde pyelography, along with the cystoscopic examination, shows outlines and images of the drainage tract.

Cystoscopy is needed to accurately diagnose interstitial cystitis. A urinalysis usually shows WBCs and RBCs but no bacteria. Common findings in interstitial cystitis are a small-capacity bladder, the presence of Hunner's ulcers (a type of bladder lesion), and small hemorrhages after bladder distention.

◆ Interventions

Nonsurgical Management. The expected outcome is to maintain an optimal urine ELIMINATION pattern. Nursing interventions for the management of cystitis focus on comfort and teaching about drug therapy, fluid intake, and prevention measures.

Drug Therapy. Drugs used to treat bacteriuria and promote patient comfort include urinary antiseptics or antibiotics, analgesics, and antispasmodics. Cure of a UTI depends on the antimicrobial levels achieved in the urine. Fluconazole is the drug of choice for treatment of *Candida* (fungal) infections. Antispasmodic drugs decrease bladder spasm and promote complete bladder emptying.

Antibiotic therapy is used for bacterial UTIs (Chart 66-4). Guidelines for uncomplicated cystitis recommend nitrofurantoin, trimethoprim/sulfamethoxazole, or fosfomycin as first-line therapy (Brusch, 2013; Hooton, 2012; Hopkins et al., 2014). Longer antibiotic treatment (7 to 21 days) and sometimes different agents are required for hospitalized patients and those with complicated UTIs (e.g., pregnant women and patients with anatomic, functional or metabolic derangements that affect the urinary tract).

! NURSING SAFETY PRIORITY   (QSEN)

Drug Alert

Two of the fluoroquinolone antibiotics, Tequin and Noroxin, are designated as sound-alike, look-alike agents with other drugs and could easily be administered in error. Take care to not confuse Tequin with Tegretol, an oral anticonvulsant, or with Ticlid, a platelet inhibitor. Take care to not confuse Noroxin with Neurontin, an oral anticonvulsant.

CHART 66-4 **Common Examples of Drug Therapy**

Urinary Tract Infections

DRUG/DOSAGE	NURSING INTERVENTIONS	RATIONALES
Antimicrobials		
Sulfonamides—Reduce Bacteria in the Urinary Tract By Direct Killing (Trimethoprim) and By Inhibiting Bacterial Reproduction (Sulfamethoxazole).		
Trimethoprim*/ sulfamethoxazole (Bactrim, Bacter-Aid, Septra, Sulfatrim, Sultrex, Roubac ♣) 160 mg trimethoprim/800 mg sulfamethoxazole orally every 12 hr	Ask patients about drug allergies, especially to sulfa drugs, before beginning drug therapy.	Allergies to sulfa drugs are common and require changing the drug therapy.
	Teach patients to drink a full glass of water with each dose and to have an overall fluid intake of 3 L daily.	Sulfamethoxazole can form crystals that precipitate in the kidney tubules. Fluid intake prevents this complication.
	Teach patients to keep out of the sun or to wear protective clothing outdoors and use a sunscreen.	This drug increases skin sensitivity to the sun and can lead to severe sunburns, even in darker-skinned patients.
	Caution patients to complete the drug regimen even if the symptoms improve or disappear sooner.	Not completing the drug regimen can lead to an infection recurrence and to bacterial drug resistance.
Fluoroquinolones—Reduce Bacteria in the Urinary Tract By Direct Killing (Bactericidal Actions) and By Inhibiting Bacterial Reproduction (Bacteriostatic Actions).		
Ciprofloxacin (Cipro, ProQuin) 250 mg orally twice daily	Teach patients taking the extended-release drugs to swallow them whole, not to crush or chew the tablets.	Crushing or chewing the tablet releases all the drug at once, ruining the extended effect.
Levofloxacin (Levaquin) 400 mg orally daily	Warn patients to not take the drug within 2 hours of taking an antacid.	Many antacids (especially those containing magnesium or aluminum) interfere with drug absorption.
	Teach patients how to take their pulse, to monitor it twice daily while on this drug, and to notify the prescriber if new-onset irregular heartbeats occur.	This class of drugs can induce serious cardiac dysrhythmias.
	Teach patients to keep out of the sun or to wear protective clothing outdoors and use a sunscreen.	Most quinolones increase skin sensitivity to the sun and can lead to severe sunburns even in darker-skinned patients.
	Caution patients to complete the drug regimen even if the symptoms improve or disappear sooner.	Not completing the drug regimen can lead to an infection recurrence and to bacterial drug resistance.
Penicillins—Reduce Bacteria in the Urinary Tract By Direct Killing (Bactericidal Actions) As a Result of Interrupting Bacterial Cell Wall Synthesis.		
Amoxicillin (Amoxil) 500 mg orally every 12 hr	Ask patients about drug allergies to penicillin before beginning drug therapy.	Allergies to penicillin are common and require changing the drug therapy.
Amoxicillin/ clavulanate (Augmentin, Clavulin ♣) 500 mg/125 mg orally every 12 hr	Teach patients to take the drug with food.	Taking it with food reduces the risk for GI upset.
	Instruct patients to call the prescriber if severe or watery diarrhea develops.	A complication of penicillin therapy is pseudomembranous colitis, which may require discontinuing the drug.
	Suggest that women who take oral contraceptives use an additional method of birth control while taking this drug.	Penicillin appears to reduce the effectiveness of estrogen-containing oral contraceptives.
	Caution patients to complete the drug regimen even if the symptoms improve or disappear sooner.	Not completing the drug regimen can lead to an infection recurrence and to bacterial drug resistance.
Cephalosporins—Reduce Bacteria in the Urinary Tract By Direct Killing (Bactericidal Actions) As a Result of Interrupting Bacterial Cell Wall Synthesis.		
Cefdinir, cefaclor, or cefpodoxime 250-500 mg orally daily	Ask about drug allergies to penicillin or cephalosporins before beginning drug therapy.	Drugs in this class are structurally similar to penicillin. Anyone with allergies to penicillin is likely to be allergic to the cephalosporins.
	Instruct patients to call the prescriber if severe or watery diarrhea develops.	A complication of penicillin therapy is pseudomembranous colitis, which may require discontinuing the drug.
	Caution patients to complete the drug regimen even if the symptoms improve or disappear sooner.	Not completing the drug regimen can lead to an infection recurrence and to bacterial drug resistance.
Other		
Fosfomycin (Monurol)—Reduces bacteria in the urinary tract by direct killing (bactericidal actions) as a result of interrupting bacterial cell wall synthesis.		
3 g orally as a one-time dose	Instruct patients to mix the contents of a package in about ½ cup of cold water, stir well, and drink all the liquid.	This oral drug is available as granules that must be dissolved before taking.
	Avoid taking this drug when also taking metoclopramide or any other drug that increases GI motility.	Drugs that increase GI motility reduce the absorption of fosfomycin.

Continued

CHART 66-4 Common Examples of Drug Therapy—cont'd

Urinary Tract Infections

DRUG/DOSAGE	NURSING INTERVENTIONS	RATIONALES
Nitrofurantoin (Furadantin, Macrobid, Macrodantin, Nephronex ♦, Urotoin)—Usually reduce bacteria in the urinary tract by inhibiting bacterial reproduction (bacteriostatic actions).		
100 mg orally every 12 hr	Teach patients to shake the bottle well before measuring the drug.	Drug is a suspension and requires shaking to ensure homogeneity.
	Suggest that patients obtain a calibrated spoon for liquid drugs and to not use household spoons.	Household spoons are not accurate for measuring drugs.
	Teach patients to drink a full glass of water with each dose and to have an overall fluid intake of at least 3 L daily.	Drug precipitates in the kidney tubules and damages the kidney. Fluid intake prevents this complication.
	Caution patients to complete the drug regimen even if the symptoms improve or disappear sooner.	Not completing the drug regimen can lead to an infection recurrence and to bacterial drug resistance.
Bladder Analgesics—*Reduce Bladder Pain and Burning on Urination by Exerting a Topical Analgesic or Local Anesthetic Effect on the Mucosa of the Urinary Tract.*		
Phenazopyridine (Azo-Dine, Prodium, Pyridiate, Pyridium, Uristat, Phenazo ♦) 200 mg orally 3 times daily, after meals	Remind patients that this drug will not treat an infection, only the symptoms.	Drug does not have any antibacterial actions.
	Teach patients to take the drug with or immediately after a meal.	Food reduces the risk for GI disturbances.
	Warn patients that urine will turn red or orange.	This expected response to the drug may stain clothing or toilets.
Antispasmodics—*Relieve Bladder Spasms by Inhibiting Nerve Stimulation to the Bladder Muscle.*		
Hyoscyamine (Anaspaz, Cystospaz, many others) 0.125-0.25 mg orally 3 to 4 times daily	Teach patients to notify the prescriber if blurred vision or other eye problems, confusion, dizziness or fainting spells, fast heartbeat, fever, or difficulty passing urine occurs.	These are manifestations of drug toxicity.
	Teach patients to wear dark glasses in sunlight or other bright-light areas.	Drug dilates the pupil and increases eye sensitivity to light.

*Trimethoprim can be given alone to patients with a sulfa allergy.

💡 NCLEX EXAMINATION CHALLENGE

Safe and Effective Care Environment

A client in the community health clinic is prescribed trimethoprim/sulfamethoxazole for cystitis. The client reports developing hives to "something called Septra." What is the nurse's best action?
A. Reassure the client that Septra is not trimethoprim/sulfamethoxazole.
B. Highlight this important information in the client's medical record.
C. Place an allergy alert band on the client's wrist.
D. Notify the prescriber immediately.

Long-term, low-dose antibiotic therapy is sometimes used for chronic, recurring INFECTION caused by structural abnormalities or stones. Trimethoprim 100 mg daily may be used for long-term management of the older patient with frequent UTIs. For women who have recurrent UTIs after intercourse, antibiotics may be prescribed to be taken after intercourse. The three most common drug treatment regimens are (1) one low-dose tablet of trimethoprim (TMP) (Proloprim, Trimpex),(2) TMP/

GENDER HEALTH CONSIDERATIONS

Patient-Centered Care QSEN

Pregnant women with a bacterial UTI require prompt and aggressive treatment because cystitis can lead to acute pyelonephritis during pregnancy. Pyelonephritis in pregnancy can cause preterm labor and adversely affect the fetus. Remind pregnant patients to contact their health care provider whenever manifestations of UTI are present.

sulfamethoxazole (half or single-strength Bactrim, Cotrim, Septra), or (3) nitrofurantoin (Macrodantin, Nephronex ♦, Novo Furantoin ♦).

Fluid Intake. Urge patients to drink enough fluid to maintain a diluted urine throughout the day and night unless fluid restriction is needed for another health problem. Some urologists recommend sufficient fluid intake to result in at least 1.5 L of urine output or 7 to 12 voidings daily. Food can provide 20% or more of fluid intake, particularly the intake of fruits and vegetables.

Drinking 50 mL of concentrated cranberry juice daily appears to decrease the ability of bacteria to adhere to the epithelial cells lining the urinary tract, decreasing the incidence of recurrent symptomatic UTIs in some patients. Cranberry juice, tablets, or capsules must be consumed for more than 4 weeks to affect the ability of *E. coli* to adhere to the urinary tract (Stapleton et al., 2012). Cranberry products have not consistently demonstrated effectiveness but are a low-cost and low-risk intervention (Hooton, 2012). It is important to note that cranberry juice is an irritant to the bladder with interstitial cystitis and should be avoided by patients with this condition. Avoiding caffeine, carbonated beverages, and tomato products may decrease bladder irritation during cystitis.

Comfort Measures. A warm sitz bath 2 or 3 times a day for 20 minutes may provide comfort and some relief of local symptoms. If burning with urination is severe or urinary retention occurs, teach the patient to sit in the sitz bath and urinate into the warm water. Urinary tract analgesics or antispasmodics may also provide comfort (see Chart 66-4).

Surgical Management. Surgery for cystitis treats the conditions that increase the risk for recurrent UTIs (e.g., removal of obstructions and repair of vesicoureteral reflux). Procedures may include cystoscopy (see Chapter 65) to identify and remove calculi or obstructions.

Community-Based Care

Assess the patient's level of understanding of the problem. His or her knowledge about factors that promote the development of cystitis determines the teaching interventions planned.

Teach the patient how to take prescribed drugs. Stress the need for correct spacing of doses throughout the day and the need to complete all of the prescribed antibiotics. If the drug will change the color of the urine, as it does with phenazopyridine (Pyridium, Urogesic, Phenazo ♣), inform the patient to expect this change.

Patients may associate discomfort with sexual activities and have feelings of guilt and embarrassment. Open and sensitive discussions with a woman who has recurrences of UTI after sexual intercourse can help her find techniques to handle the problem (see Chart 66-2). Explore with her the factors that contribute to her INFECTIONS, such as sexual penetration when the bladder is full, diaphragm use, and her general resistance to infection. Some positions during intercourse may reduce urethral irritation and subsequent cystitis. Remind the patient that vigorous cleaning of the perineum with harsh soaps and vaginal douching may irritate the perineal tissues and *increase* the risk for UTI. At the patient's request, discuss the problem with her and her partner to help them find ways of maintaining their intimate relationship.

URETHRITIS

❖ PATHOPHYSIOLOGY

Urethritis is an INFLAMMATION of the urethra. In men, manifestations include burning or difficulty urinating and a discharge from the urethral meatus. The most common cause of urethritis in men is sexually transmitted diseases (STDs). These include gonorrhea or nonspecific urethritis caused by *Ureaplasma* (a gram-negative bacterium), *Chlamydia* (a sexually transmitted gram-negative bacterium), or *Trichomonas vaginalis* (a protozoan found in both the male and female genital tract).

In women, urethritis causes manifestations similar to those of cystitis. Urethritis is known by several other terms: *pyuria-dysuria syndrome, frequency-dysuria syndrome, trigonitis syndrome,* and *urethral syndrome.* Urethritis is most common in postmenopausal women and is probably caused by tissue changes related to low estrogen levels.

❖ PATIENT-CENTERED COLLABORATIVE CARE

Ask the patient about a history of STD, painful or difficult urination, discharge from the penis or vagina, and discomfort in the lower abdomen. Urinalysis may show pyuria (white blood cells [WBCs] in the urine) without a large number of bacteria. However, results of urethral culture may indicate an STD. In women, the diagnosis may be made when urinalysis and urethral culture are negative for bacteria and there is no evidence of interstitial cystitis but manifestations persist. In such cases, pelvic examination may reveal tissue changes from low estrogen levels in the vagina. Urethroscopy may show low estrogen changes with INFLAMMATION of urethral tissues.

STDs and INFECTION are treated with antibiotic therapy. More information on STDs can be found in Chapter 74.

Postmenopausal women often have improvement in their urethral symptoms with the use of estrogen vaginal cream. Estrogen cream applied locally to the vagina increases the amount of estrogen in the urethra as well, and irritating manifestations are reduced.

█ NONINFECTIOUS DISORDERS

URETHRAL STRICTURES

Urethral strictures are narrowed areas of the urethra. These problems may be caused by complications of an STD (usually gonorrhea) and by trauma during catheterization, urologic procedures, or childbirth. About one third of urethral strictures have no obvious cause. Strictures occur more often in men than in women. They may be a factor in other urologic problems, such as recurrent UTIs, urinary incontinence, and urinary retention.

The most common manifestation of urethral stricture is obstruction of urine flow. Strictures rarely cause pain. Because urine stasis can result when flow is obstructed, the patient is at risk for developing a UTI and may have overflow incontinence. Overflow incontinence is the involuntary loss of urine when the bladder is overdistended. Assess the patient for these two problems.

A urethral stricture is treated surgically. Dilation of the urethra (using a local anesthetic) is only a temporary measure, not a curative one. Stent placement can be used in some patients. The best chance of long-term cure is with urethroplasty, which is the surgical removal of the affected area with or without grafting to create a larger opening. The recurrence rate after surgery is still high, and most patients need repeated procedures. The urethral stricture location and length are the most important factors affecting choice of interventions and recovery.

URINARY INCONTINENCE

❖ PATHOPHYSIOLOGY

Continence is the control over the time and place of urination and is unique to humans and some domestic animals. It is a learned behavior in which a person can suppress the urge to urinate until a socially appropriate location is available (e.g., a toilet). Efficient bladder emptying (i.e., coordination between bladder contraction and urethral relaxation) is needed for continence.

Incontinence is an involuntary loss of urine severe enough to cause social or hygienic problems. It is *not* a normal consequence of aging or childbirth and often is a stigmatizing and an underreported health problem. Many people suffer in silence, are socially isolated, and may be unaware that treatment is available. In addition, the cost of incontinence can be enormous.

Continence occurs when pressure in the urethra is greater than pressure in the bladder. For normal voiding to occur, the urethra must relax and the bladder must contract with enough pressure and duration to empty completely. Voiding should occur in a smooth and coordinated manner under a person's conscious control. Incontinence has several possible causes and can be either temporary or chronic (Table 66-2). Temporary causes usually do not involve a disorder of the urinary tract. The most common types of adult urinary incontinence are stress incontinence, urge incontinence, overflow incontinence, functional incontinence, and a mixed form.

TABLE 66-2   Types of Urinary Incontinence

TYPE	DEFINITION/DESCRIPTION	CAUSE	CLINICAL MANIFESTATIONS
Stress incontinence	The involuntary loss of urine during activities that increase abdominal and detrusor pressure. Patients cannot tighten the urethra sufficiently to overcome the increased detrusor pressure; leakage of urine results.	Weakening of bladder neck supports; associated with childbirth. Intrinsic sphincter deficiency caused by such congenital conditions as epispadias (abnormal location of the urethra on the dorsum of the penis) or myelomeningocele. Acquired anatomic damage to the urethral sphincter (from repeated incontinence surgeries, prostatectomy, radiation therapy, and trauma).	Urine loss with physical exertion, cough, sneeze, or exercise. Usually only small amounts of urine are lost with each exertion. Normal voiding habits (≤8 times per day, ≤2 times per night). Post-void residual usually ≤50 mL. Pelvic examination shows hypermobility of the urethra or bladder neck with Valsalva maneuvers.
Urge incontinence	The involuntary loss of urine associated with a strong desire to urinate. Patients cannot suppress the signal from the bladder muscle to the brain that it is time to urinate.	Unknown.	An abrupt and strong urge to void. May have loss of large amounts of urine with each occurrence.
Detrusor hyperreflexia (reflex incontinence)	The abnormal detrusor contractions result from neurologic abnormalities.	Central nervous system (CNS) lesions from stroke, multiple sclerosis, and parasacral spinal cord lesions. Local irritating factors such as caffeine, medications, or bladder tumor.	Post-void residual ≤50 mL.
Overflow incontinence	The involuntary loss of urine associated with overdistention of the bladder when the bladder's capacity has reached its maximum. The urethra is obstructed, so it fails to relax sufficiently to allow urine to flow, resulting in incomplete bladder emptying or complete urinary retention, causing overflow incontinence.	Diabetic neuropathy; side effects of medication; after radical pelvic surgery or spinal cord damage; outlet obstruction. Causes external to the mechanism of the urethra: an enlarged prostate (male patients) and large genital prolapse (female patients). When the cause is intrinsic to the urethra, abnormal contraction of the skeletal muscle occurs, causing obstruction. This condition, called *detrusor dyssynergia,* is seen in patients with spinal cord injuries and multiple sclerosis.	Bladder distention, often up to the level of the umbilicus. Constant dribbling of urine.
Mixed incontinence	A combination of stress, urge, and overflow incontinence.	As with each separate disorder.	As with each separate disorder.
Functional incontinence	Leakage of urine caused by factors other than disease of the lower urinary tract.		Quantity and timing of urine leakage vary; patterns are difficult to discern.
Transient causes	Transient causes improve with treatment of the underlying condition.	Loss of cognitive functioning. Loss of awareness that urination is to occur in a socially acceptable place. Abnormal openings in the urinary tract, such as a fistula or diverticulum. Drugs, such as sedatives, hypnotics, diuretics, anticholinergics, decongestants, antihypertensives, and calcium channel blockers. Diabetes insipidus or psychogenic polydipsia. Inability to get to toileting facilities. Direct bladder pressure or urethral obstruction.	Altered mental state, as in delirium, confusion, depression, dementia, sepsis, mental illness, or severe psychological stress. Urinary drainage noted from areas other than the urinary meatus. Some drugs cause altered mental state; others cause increased urine production. Increased urine output. Restraints, restricted mobility. Constipation or fecal impaction.
Permanent causes	Permanent causes are organic but may be improved with treatment.	Cognitive impairment. Traumatic or surgical effects. Those factors contributing to stress incontinence, urge incontinence, and overflow incontinence. Structural or functional defects of the bladder or the sphincters. Injuries or diseases of the spinal cord, brainstem, or cerebral cortex (neurogenic bladder). Congenital defects, including exstrophy of the bladder (bladder turned "inside out") and spina bifida.	Clinical manifestations depend on the cause.

Stress incontinence is the most common type. Its main feature is the loss of small amounts of urine during coughing, sneezing, jogging, or lifting. In the continent person, the urethra can be relaxed and tightened under conscious control because skeletal muscles of the pelvic floor surround it. When a person feels the urge to urinate, the conscious contraction of the urethra can override a bladder contraction if the urethral contraction is strong enough.

Patients with *stress incontinence* cannot tighten the urethra enough to overcome the increased bladder pressure caused by contraction of the detrusor muscle. This is common after childbirth, when the pelvic muscles are stretched and weakened. The weakened pelvic floor allows the urethra to move during exertion. If the pelvic muscles are not strengthened, this condition continues. Low estrogen levels after menopause also contribute to stress incontinence. Vaginal, urethral, and pelvic floor muscles become thin and weak without estrogen.

Urge incontinence is the perception of an urgent need to urinate as a result of bladder contractions regardless of the urine volume in the bladder. Normally when the bladder is full, contraction of the smooth muscle fibers of the bladder detrusor muscle signals the brain that it is time to urinate. Continent people override that signal and relax the detrusor muscle for the time it takes to locate a toilet. Those who suffer from urge incontinence cannot suppress the signal and have a sudden strong urge to void and often leak large amounts of urine at this time. Urge incontinence is also known as an *overactive bladder* (OAB). Overactivity may have no known cause or may be the result of abnormal detrusor contractions related to other problems. Such problems include stroke and other neurologic problems, other urinary tract problems, and irritation from concentrated urine, artificial sweeteners, caffeine, alcohol, and citric intake. Drugs, such as diuretics, and nicotine can also irritate the bladder.

Mixed incontinence is the presence of more than one type of incontinence. Often urine loss is related to both stress and urge incontinence. The manifestations mimic more than one subtype. This category is more common in older women.

Overflow incontinence occurs when the detrusor muscle fails to contract and the bladder becomes overdistended. This type of incontinence (also known as *reflex incontinence* or *underactive bladder*) occurs when the bladder has reached its maximum capacity and some urine must leak out to prevent bladder rupture. Causes for the underactive (acontractile) bladder may or may not be determined.

The urethra can be obstructed and fail to relax enough to allow urine flow. Incomplete bladder emptying or urinary retention from urethral obstruction results in overflow incontinence.

Functional incontinence is incontinence occurring as a result of factors other than the abnormal function of the bladder and urethra. A common factor is the loss of cognitive function in patients affected by dementia. To maintain continence, a person must be aware that urination needs to occur in a socially acceptable place. Patients with dementia may not have that awareness.

Etiology

Incontinence may have temporary or permanent causes. Evaluation of the incontinent patient means considering all possible causes, beginning with those that are temporary and correctable. Surgical and traumatic causes of urinary incontinence are related to procedures or surgery in the lower pelvic structures, which are areas that contain complex nerve pathways. Radical urologic, prostatic, and gynecologic procedures for treatment of pelvic cancers may result in urinary incontinence. Injury to segments S2 to S4 of the spinal cord may cause incontinence from impairment of normal nerve pathways.

Inappropriate bladder contraction may result from disorders of the brain and nervous system or from bladder irritation due to chronic INFECTION, stones, chemotherapy, or radiation therapy. Other causes of bladder contraction failure include the neuropathies associated with diabetes mellitus and syphilis. Constipation can lead to temporary urinary incontinence. Some drugs, such as anticholinergics, calcium channel blockers, diuretics, and sedatives, can cause or worsen urinary incontinence.

CONSIDERATIONS FOR OLDER ADULTS
Patient-Centered Care QSEN

Many factors contribute to urinary incontinence in older adults (Chart 66-5). An older person may have decreased mobility from many causes. In inpatient settings, mobility is limited when the older patient is placed on bedrest. Vision and hearing impairments may also prevent the patient from locating a call light to notify the nurse or assistive personnel of the need to void. Assess for these factors, and minimize them to prevent urinary incontinence. Getting out of bed to urinate is a common cause of falls among older adults.

CHART 66-5 Nursing Focus on the Older Adult
Factors Contributing to Urinary Incontinence*

Drugs
- Central nervous system depressants, such as opioid analgesics, decrease the patient's level of consciousness and the urge to void, and they contribute to constipation.
- Diuretics cause frequent voiding, often of large amounts of urine.
- Multiple drugs can contribute to changes in mental status or mobility, and they can irritate the bladder.
- Anticholinergic drugs or drugs with anticholinergic side effects are especially challenging because they affect both cognition and the ability to void. Monitor patient responses to these drugs early in treatment.

Disease
- Cerebrovascular accidents and other neurologic disorders decrease mobility, sensation, or cognition.
- Arthritis decreases mobility and causes pain.
- Parkinson disease causes muscle rigidity and an inability to initiate movement.

Depression
- Depression decreases the energy necessary to maintain continence.
- Decreased self-esteem and feelings of self-worth decrease the importance to the patient of maintaining continence.

Inadequate Resources
- Patients who need assistive devices (e.g., eyeglasses, cane, walker) may be afraid to ambulate without them or without personal assistance.
- Products that help patients manage incontinence are often costly.
- No one may be available to assist the patient to the bathroom or help with incontinence products.

*These factors are in addition to the physiologic changes of aging given in Chapter 2.

Incidence and Prevalence

Incontinence is a major health problem. As many as 25% to 45% of woman report some degree of urinary incontinence with roughly half as many men reporting this condition (Buckley et al., 2010). It is most common in older adults and in at least one half of all nursing home residents.

Increased risk for urinary incontinence occurs with pregnancy, childbirth, diabetes mellitus, and increased body mass (Buckley et al., 2010). Urinary incontinence can occur as an isolated condition or with other chronic health problems. In addition, impairments from central nervous system diseases (i.e., dementia, stroke, multiple sclerosis, Parkinson disease) and musculoskeletal disorders (i.e., osteoporosis, osteoarthritis, low back pain) contribute to reduced leg strength and mobility limitations resulting in the onset and severity of urinary incontinence (McCance et al., 2014). More than 35% of adults admitted to the hospital develop urinary incontinence (Dowling-Castronovo & Bradway, 2012). Because the problem is so common among older adults, it is recommended that all people older than 65 years be screened for urinary incontinence (DuBeau, 2013).

❖ PATIENT-CENTERED COLLABORATIVE CARE

◆ Assessment

History. Effective screening includes asking patients to respond "always," "sometimes," or "never" to these questions:

- Do you ever leak urine or water when you don't want to?
- Do you ever leak urine or water when you cough, laugh, or exercise?
- Do you ever leak urine or water on the way to the bathroom?
- Do you ever use pads, tissue, or cloth in your underwear to catch urine?

If any answer is "always" or "sometimes," proceed with a focused assessment (Chart 66-6). Incontinence may be underreported because health care professionals do not ask patients about urine loss. *Do not assume that patients will volunteer the information without specifically being asked.*

Physical Assessment/Clinical Manifestations. Assess the abdomen to estimate bladder fullness, to rule out palpable hard stool, and to evaluate bowel sounds. Urinary incontinence is confirmed by evaluating the force and character of the urine stream during voiding. Asking the patient to cough while wearing a perineal pad is useful in evaluating stress incontinence; a wet pad on forceful coughing may indicate stress incontinence.

For women, inspect the external genitalia to determine whether there is apparent urethral or uterine prolapse, cystocele (herniation of the bladder into the vagina), or rectocele. These conditions occur with pelvic floor muscle weakness. A health care provider puts on an examination glove and inserts two fingers into the vagina to assess the strength of these muscles. Strength is described as *weak, adequate,* or *strong* based on the amount of pressure felt by the health care provider as the patient tightens her vaginal muscles. Describe and document the color, consistency, and odor of any secretions from the genitourinary orifices. The urine stream interruption test (i.e., asking a patient to voluntarily start and stop urine flow during a void at least twice) is another method of determining pelvic muscle strength. For men, inspect the urethral meatus for any discharge.

CHART 66-6   Focused Assessment

The Patient with Urinary Incontinence

Note the presence of risk factors for urinary incontinence:

- Age
- If female, menopausal status
- Neurologic disease:
  - Parkinson disease
  - Dementia
  - Multiple sclerosis
  - Stroke
  - Spinal injury
- Diabetes mellitus
- Childbirth
- Urologic procedures
- Prescribed and over-the-counter drugs
- Bowel patterns
- Stress/anxiety level

Detail the symptoms of urinary incontinence:

- Leakage
- Frequency
- Urgency
- Nocturia
- Sensation of full bladder before leakage

Obtain a 24-hour intake-and-output record or a voiding diary:

- Time and amount of oral intake and continent voiding
- Time and estimated amount of incontinent leakages
- Activity around the time of leakage

Assess the patient's:

- Mobility
- Self-care ability
- Cognitive ability
- Communication patterns

Assess the environment for barriers to toileting:

- Privacy
- Restrictive clothing
- Access to toilet

A digital rectal examination (DRE) is performed by the health care provider on both male and female patients. It provides information about the nerve integrity to the bladder. The examiner determines whether there is tactile sensation in the anal area by observing whether the rectal sphincter is relaxed or contracted on digital insertion. Because nerve supply to the bladder is similar to nerve supply to the rectum, the presence of tactile sensation and a rectal sphincter that contracts suggest that the nerve supply to the bladder is intact. Impaction of stool is a cause of transient urinary incontinence and can be detected during a rectal examination. The health care provider assesses for prostate enlargement in men as a possible cause of incontinence.

Laboratory Assessment. A urinalysis is useful to rule out INFECTION. This test is the first step in the assessment of incontinent patients of any age. The presence of red blood cells (RBCs), white blood cells (WBCs), leukocyte esterase, or nitrites is an indication for culturing the urine. Any infection is treated before further assessment of incontinence.

Imaging Assessment. Determine the amount of post-void residual urine (urine remaining in the bladder immediately after voiding) by portable ultrasound. With a health care provider's order, catheterizing the patient immediately after voiding can also be used to assess residual volume. Additional imaging is rarely needed unless surgery is being considered. CT is most useful for locating abnormalities in kidneys and ureters. A voiding cystourethrogram (VCUG) or urodynamic testing may be performed to assess the size, shape, support, and function of the urinary tract system. Urodynamic testing (see Chapter 65) may take several hours and more than one visit. Electromyography (EMG) of the pelvic muscles may be a part of the urodynamic studies.

◆ *Analysis*

The priority NANDA-I nursing diagnoses and collaborative problems for patients with urinary incontinence include:

1. Stress Urinary Incontinence related to weak pelvic muscles and structural supports (NANDA-I)
2. Urge Urinary Incontinence related to decreased bladder capacity, bladder spasms, diet, and neurologic impairment (NANDA-I)
3. Reflex Urinary Incontinence related to neurologic impairment (NANDA-I)
4. Functional Urinary Incontinence related to impaired cognition or neuromuscular limitations (NANDA-I)
5. Total urinary incontinence (mixed) related to many causes

◆ *Planning and Implementation*

Several interventions are useful for each type of incontinence in addition to drugs, surgical repair, and nutrition therapy.

Reducing Stress Urinary Incontinence

Planning: Expected Outcomes. With appropriate therapy, the patient with stress urinary incontinence is expected to develop urinary continence. Indicators include that the patient rarely or never demonstrates these problems:

- Urine leakage between voidings
- Urine leakage with increased abdominal pressure (e.g., sneezing, laughing, lifting)

Interventions. Initial interventions for patients with stress incontinence include keeping a diary, behavioral interventions, and drugs. Surgery also may be an option if other interventions are not effective. Explain the purpose of a detailed diary in which the patient records times of urine leakage, activities, and foods eaten. The diary is then used by the health care provider to plan and evaluate interventions. Collection devices, absorbent pads, and undergarments may be used during the sometimes lengthy process of assessment and treatment and by those patients who elect not to pursue further interventions.

Nonsurgical Management. Drug therapy and behavioral interventions (primarily diet and exercise) for stress incontinence require the patient's active participation for success. Nursing interventions focus on teaching patients about the drugs and behavioral strategies and on providing ongoing encouragement, clarification, and support to maximize intervention effects.

Pelvic floor (Kegel) exercise therapy for women with stress incontinence strengthens the muscles of the pelvic floor (circumvaginal muscles). These muscles become strengthened, as any other skeletal muscle does, by frequent, systematic, and repeated contractions. Pelvic floor muscle training improves not only continence but also quality of life in women with urinary incontinence (Fan et al., 2013).

The most important step in teaching pelvic muscle exercises is to help the patient learn which muscle to exercise. During the pelvic examination in women and the rectal examination in men or women, instruct the patient to tighten the pelvic muscles around your fingers. Then provide feedback about the strength of the contraction. Starting and stopping the urine stream or stopping the passage of flatus indicates that the patient has correctly identified the pelvic muscles. Biofeedback devices, such as electromyography or perineometers, measure the strength of contraction. A perineometer is a tampon-shaped instrument inserted into the vagina to measure the strength of pelvic muscle contractions. The graph shows the amplitude of muscle

contraction to the patient as a method of biofeedback. Alternatively, retention of a vaginal weight also shows that the patient has identified the proper muscle (see discussion on vaginal cone therapy below).

Instructions for pelvic muscle exercises are given in Chart 66-7. Although improvement may take several months, most patients notice a positive change after 6 weeks. Teach patients to continue the exercises 10 times daily to improve and maintain pelvic muscle strength.

Nutrition therapy in the form of weight reduction is helpful for obese patients because stress incontinence is made worse by increased abdominal pressure from obesity (Wilde et al., 2014). Teach the patient to avoid bladder irritants in the diet that can contribute to urgency and frequency. For example, caffeine is a bladder irritant (Jura et al., 2011). Stress the importance of maintaining an adequate fluid intake, especially water. Refer the patient to a registered dietitian as needed.

Drug therapy can be useful for some people with stress incontinence. Because bladder pressure is greater than urethral resistance in patients with stress incontinence, drugs may be used to improve urethral resistance (Chart 66-8).

Topical estrogen to the perineal and vaginal orifice is used to treat postmenopausal women with stress incontinence, although it is not known exactly how this drug helps improve continence. Estrogen may increase the blood flow and tone of the muscles around the vagina and urethra, thus improving the patient's ability to contract those muscles during times of increased intra-abdominal stress.

Vaginal cone therapy involves using a set of five small, cone-shaped weights. They are of equal size but of varying weights and are used together with pelvic muscle exercise. The woman inserts the lightest cone, labeled *1*, into her vagina (Fig. 66-1),

CHART 66-8 Common Examples of Drug Therapy

Urinary Incontinence

DRUG/DOSAGE	NURSING INTERVENTIONS	RATIONALES
Hormones—Thought to Enhance Nerve Conduction to the Urinary Tract, Improve Blood Flow, and Reduce Tissue Deterioration of the Urinary Tract.		
*Estrogen vaginal cream daily or an estrogen-containing ring inserted monthly	Teach patients that a thin application of the cream is all that is needed. Teach patients that it takes 4-6 wks to achieve continence benefits and that benefits disappear after about 4 weeks after discontinuing regular use.	Topical use minimizes the amount of estrogen absorbed and distributed in the body. A thick application increases risk for systemic distribution. Topical administration via a cream or ring avoids systemic adverse drug effects from this hormone but also takes longer for effects.
Antispasmodics—Reduce Incontinence By Causing Bladder Muscle Relaxation.		
Oxybutynin (Ditropan) 5 mg orally 3-4 times daily; (Ditropan XL) 5-10 mg orally daily	Ask whether the patient has glaucoma before starting the drug. Suggest that patients increase fluid intake and use hard candy to moisten the mouth. Teach patients to increase fluid intake and the amount of dietary fiber. Teach patients to monitor urine output and to report an output significantly lower than intake to the health care provider. Instruct patients taking the extended-release forms of these drugs not to chew or crush the tablet/capsule.	Anticholinergics can increase intraocular pressure and make glaucoma worse. Dry mouth is a common side effect of drugs in this category. Constipation is a common side effect of drugs in this category. Drugs in this category can cause urinary retention. Crushing or chewing the tablet/capsule releases all the drug at once, ruining the extended effect and increasing the possibility of side effects.
Anticholinergics—Suppress Involuntary Bladder Contraction, Increase Urine Volume and May Increase the Bladder Capacity.		
Tolterodine (Detrol) 2 mg orally twice daily; (Detrol LA) 4 mg orally daily
Propantheline (Pro-Banthine, Propanthel ✿) 7.5-30 mg orally 3-4 times daily
Dicyclomine (Barmine, Bentyl) 10-40 mg orally 3-4 times daily
Trospium (Sanctura) 20 mg orally every 12 hr
Darifenacin (Enablex) 7.5-15 mg orally daily
Solifenacin (Vesicare) 5-10 mg orally daily
Fesoterodine (Toviaz) 4-8 mg orally daily | Ask whether the patient has glaucoma before starting the drug. Do not use these drugs if prostate hypertrophy co-exists. Teach patients to avoid dehydration and increase the amount of dietary fiber to avoid constipation. Evaluate kidney function before starting and at least annually.

Instruct the patient to avoid crushing or chewing tablets. | These drugs can increase intraocular fluid and pressure. These drugs can worsen urinary retention from prostate hypertrophy. These drugs can cause significant constipation.

These drugs may have decreased renal clearance and should either be avoided or administered in a reduced dose in patients with renal insufficiency. Most of the once-daily drugs are a long-acting formulation and should not be crushed or chewed. |
| **Alpha Adrenergic Agonists—Increase Contractile Force of the Urethral Sphincter, Increasing Resistance to Urine Outflow.** | | |
| *Midorine (ProAmatine, Orvaten) 2.5-5 mg orally every 8-12 hr
*Pseudoephedrine (Sudafed, SudoGest) 30 mg orally; also comes in an extended-release formulation | Teach the patient to monitor his or her blood pressure periodically when starting the drug. | These drugs can cause a supine hypertension; do not use with severe cardiac disease. |
| **Beta₃ Blockers—Relax the Detrusor Smooth Muscle to Increase Bladder Capacity and Urine Storage.** | | |
| Mirabegron (Myrbetriq) 25 mg orally daily | Teach the patient to periodically obtain a blood pressure and to inform the health care provider if the systolic or diastolic values increase more than 10 mm Hg or above 180/110. If the patient is taking warfarin, avoid this drug or schedule additional blood testing for potential increased risk for bleeding. | Because it is a selective beta blocker, there is some potential to increase blood pressure.

This drug may interact with warfarin due to similar metabolic pathways, resulting in prolonged international normalized ratio (INR), the test to evaluate warfarin effects. |
| **Antidepressants: Tricyclics and Serotonin-Norepinephrine Reuptake Inhibitors (SNRIs)—Increase Norepinephrine and Serotonin Levels, Which Are Thought to Strengthen the Urinary Sphincters. They Also Have Anticholinergic Actions.** | | |
| **Tricyclics**
Imipramine (Tofranil, Novo-Pramine ✿) 25-100 mg orally 4 times daily
Amitriptyline (Elavil, Levate) 10-25 mg orally daily
SNRI
*Duloxetine (Cymbalta) 20-60 mg orally daily | Warn patients not to combine these drugs with other antidepressant drugs. Instruct patients to inform their provider if they take drugs to manage hypertension. Teach patients to change positions slowly, especially in the morning. Teach patients the same interventions as for anticholinergic agents. | These drugs have significant drug-drug interactions with other antidepressants and with some antihypertensive drugs, leading to hypertensive crisis. These drugs cause dizziness and orthostatic hypotension and can increase the risk for falls. These drugs have anticholinergic activity and produce the same side effects. |

*These drugs are used off-label and do not have United States Food and Drug Administration (FDA) approval for use. However, they are commonly used to manage incontinence syndromes.

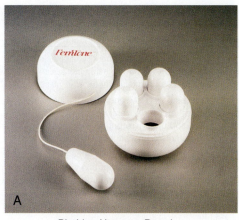

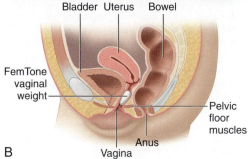

FIG. 66-1 A, FemTone vaginal weights, or cones. The number on the top of each cone represents increasing weight up to the heaviest cone, a *5*. **B,** Diagram showing the correct positioning of a vaginal weight, or cone, in place.

with the string to the outside, for a 1-minute test period. If she can hold the first cone in place without its slipping out while she walks around, she proceeds to the second cone, labeled *2*, and repeats the procedure. The patient begins her treatment with the heaviest cone she can comfortably hold in her vagina for the 1-minute test period. Treatment periods are 15 minutes twice a day. When the patient can comfortably hold the cone in her vagina for the 15-minute period, she progresses to the next heaviest weight. Treatment is completed with the cone labeled *5*.

Weighted vaginal cones can help strengthen the pelvic muscles and decrease stress incontinence but may not help pelvic prolapse. Vaginal cones do not require a prescription.

Other interventions for stress incontinence include behavior modification, psychotherapy, and electrical stimulation devices to strengthen urethral contractions. Many intravaginal and intrarectal electrical stimulation devices have been used with varying degrees of success.

A ring-shaped *pessary* inserted into the vagina may help with a prolapsed uterus or bladder when this condition is contributing to urinary incontinence. A prolapse occurs when the supportive tissue in the vagina weakens and stretches, allowing pelvic organs to protrude into the vaginal lumen. The pessary presses against the wall of the vagina to reposition pelvic organs. Generally, a pessary is removed and cleaned with soap and water on a monthly basis by the patient but can be done by the nurse for adults with cognitive or musculoskeletal impairment.

Urethral occlusion devices can be particularly helpful for activity-induced incontinence. One device, the Reliance insert, is like a tiny tampon that the patient inserts into the urethra.

After insertion, the patient inflates a tiny balloon, which rests at the bladder neck and prevents the flow of urine. To void, the patient pulls a string to deflate the balloon and removes the device. The applicator is reusable, although the tampon part is disposed of after each void.

Electrical stimulation with either an intravaginal or intrarectal electrical stimulation device is available to treat both urge and stress incontinence. Treatment consists of stimulating sensory nerves to decrease the sensation of urgency. It is done as an office-based procedure 1 to 3 times weekly for 6 to 8 weeks.

Magnetic resonance therapy involves targeted urinary tract nerves and muscles for depolarization. The patient sits on a chair containing a magnetic device, which induces depolarization and helps reduce stress-induced incontinence similar to drug-induced relaxation of muscle and nerves.

Surgical Management. Stress incontinence may be treated by a surgical sling or bladder suspension procedure (Table 66-3). A sling procedure creates a sling around the bladder neck and urethra using strips of body tissue or synthetic material (mesh). Bladder suspension procedures are more extensive, and the surgeon sutures tissue near the bladder neck to a pubic bone ligament to provide support and prevent sagging. A third surgical procedure is the injection of bulking agents into the urethral wall to provide resistance to urine outflow. Bulking agents include collagen, carbon-coated zirconium beads, and silicone implants (Shultz, 2012).

Preoperative Care. Teach the patient about the procedure, and clarify the surgeon's explanation of events surrounding the surgery. Extensive urodynamic testing (see Chapter 65) is often performed before surgery, and you must explain the need for such thorough assessment to the patient and family.

Postoperative Care. After surgery, assess for and intervene to prevent or detect complications. For prevention of movement or traction on the bladder neck, secure the urethral catheter with tape or a tube holder. If a suprapubic catheter is used instead of a urethral catheter, monitor the dressing for urine leakage and other drainage. Catheters are usually in place until the patient can urinate easily and has residual urine volume after voiding of less than 50 mL. (See Chapters 14 and 16 for a discussion of general care before and after surgery.)

Reducing Urge Urinary Incontinence

Planning: Expected Outcomes. The patient with urinary incontinence is expected to use techniques to prevent or manage urge incontinence. Indicators include that the patient often or consistently demonstrates these behaviors:

- Responds to urge in a timely manner
- Gets to toilet between urge and passage of urine
- Avoids substances that stimulate the bladder (e.g., caffeine, alcohol)

Interventions. Interventions for patients with urge incontinence or overactive bladder (OAB) include neuromodulation, drugs, and behavioral interventions. *Neuromodulation* therapy, which involves stimulation of the nerves to the bladder, can be used to manage urge incontinence. The device requires minor surgery to place the device. Other types of surgery are not the recommended treatment of this condition.

Drug Therapy. Because the hypertonic bladder contracts involuntarily in patients with urge incontinence, drugs that relax the smooth muscle and increase the bladder's capacity are prescribed (see Chart 66-8). The most effective drugs are anticholinergics, such as propantheline (Pro-Banthine, Propanthel

TABLE 66-3	Surgical Procedures for Stress Incontinence	
PROCEDURE	**PURPOSE**	**NURSING CONSIDERATIONS**
Anterior vaginal repair (colporrhaphy)	Elevates the urethral position and repairs any cystocele.	Because the operation is performed by vaginal incision, it is often done in conjunction with a vaginal hysterectomy. Recovery is usually rapid, and a urethral catheter is in place for 24-48 hr.
Retropubic suspension (Marshall-Marchetti-Krantz or Burch colposuspension)	Elevates the urethral position and provides longer-lasting results.	The operation requires a low abdominal incision and a urethral or suprapubic catheter for several days postoperatively. Recovery takes longer, and urinary retention and detrusor instability are the most frequent complications.
Needle bladder neck suspension (Pereyra or Stamey procedure)	Elevates the urethral position and provides longer-lasting results without a long operative time.	The combined vaginal approach with a needle and a small suprapubic skin incision does not allow direct vision of the operative site; however, the high complication rates may be due to the selection of patients who, because of their medical condition, are not good candidates for longer retropubic procedures.
Pubovaginal sling procedures	A sling made of synthetic or fascial material is placed under the urethrovesical junction to elevate the bladder neck.	The operation uses an abdominal, vaginal, or combined approach to treat intrinsic sphincter deficiencies. Temporary or permanent urinary retention is common postoperatively.
Midurethral sling procedures	A tensionless vaginal sling is made from polypropylene mesh (or other materials) and placed near the urethrovesical junction to increase the angle, which inhibits movement of urine into the urethra with lower intravesicular pressures.	This ambulatory surgery procedure uses a vaginal approach to improve symptoms of stress incontinence. Temporary or permanent urinary retention is common postoperatively.
Artificial sphincters	A mechanical device to open and close the urethra is placed around the anatomic urethra.	The operation is done more frequently in men. The most common complications include mechanical failure of the device, erosion of tissue, and infection.
Periurethral injection of collagen or Siloxane	Implantation of small amounts of an inert substance through several small injections provides support around the bladder neck.	The procedure can be done in an ambulatory care setting and can be repeated as often as necessary. Certain compounds may migrate after injection; an allergy test to bovine collagen must be performed before implantation.

♣), and anticholinergics with smooth muscle relaxant properties, such as oxybutynin (Ditropan and Ditropan XL), tolterodine (Detrol and Detrol LA), and dicyclomine hydrochloride (Baramine, Bentyl, Spasmoban ♣). This class of drugs has serious side effects and is used along with behavioral interventions. These drugs inhibit the nerve fibers that stimulate bladder contraction. Tricyclic antidepressants with anticholinergic and alpha-adrenergic agonist activity, such as imipramine (Tofranil, Novopramine ♣), have been used successfully. The effectiveness of other drugs, such as flavoxate (Urispas) and the antihistamines, NSAIDs, beta-adrenergic agonists, and calcium channel blockers, has yet to be determined.

Another drug therapy for urge incontinence is onabotulinumtoxinA (Botox), which received approval in 2013 from the U.S. Food and Drug Administration (FDA) for this use. The drug is injected during cystoscopy into multiple areas of the detrusor muscle of the bladder. Usually, 10 to 30 different sites are injected during one treatment session. This treatment relaxes the detrusor muscle and relieves the urge to urinate. Some patients have had relief of incontinence for as long as 6 to 9 months after injection. Side effects may include urinary

> **! NURSING SAFETY PRIORITY** (QSEN)
>
> **Drug Alert**
>
> Teach patients taking the extended-release forms of anticholinergic drugs to swallow the tablet or capsule whole without chewing it or crushing it. Chewing or crushing the tablet/capsule ruins the extended-release feature, allowing the entire dose to be absorbed quickly, which increases drug side effects.

retention, painful urination, and an increased incidence of urinary tract infections. For most patients who experience urinary retention, the condition is temporary but does require intermittent self-catheterization.

Nutrition Therapy. Teach the patient to avoid foods that irritate the bladder such as caffeine and alcohol. Spacing fluids at regular intervals throughout the day (e.g., 120 mL every hour or 240 mL every 2 hours) and limiting fluids after the dinner hour (e.g., only 120 mL at bedtime) help avoid fluid overload on the bladder and allow urine to collect at a steady pace.

Behavioral Interventions. Behavioral interventions for urge incontinence include bladder training, habit training, exercise therapy, and electrical stimulation. Interventions for urinary bladder training and urinary habit training are listed in Chart 66-9. Behavioral interventions involve a great deal of patient participation. Provide ongoing encouragement, clarification, and support to increase the effects of all interventions. Behavioral interventions are often combined with drug therapy for greatest effect.

Bladder training is an education program for the patient that begins with a thorough explanation of the problem of urge incontinence. Instead of the bladder being in control of the patient, the patient learns to control the bladder. For the program to succeed, he or she must be alert, aware, and able to resist the urge to urinate (Wilde et al., 2014).

Start a schedule for voiding, beginning with the longest interval that is comfortable for the patient, even if the interval is only 30 minutes. Instruct the patient to void every 30 minutes and to ignore any urge to urinate between the set intervals. Once he or she is comfortable with the starting schedule, increase the interval by 15 to 30 minutes. Instruct the patient

---

CHART 66-9 Best Practice for Patient Safety & Quality Care QSEN

Bladder Training and Habit Training to Reduce Urinary Incontinence

Bladder Training
- Assess patient's awareness of bladder fullness and ability to cooperate with training regimen.
- Assess the patient's 24-hour voiding pattern for 2 to 3 consecutive days.
- Base the initial interval of toileting on the voiding pattern (e.g., 45 minutes).
- Teach the patient to void every 45 minutes on the first day and to ignore or suppress the urge to urinate between the 45-minute intervals.
- Take the patient to the toilet or remind him or her to urinate at the 45-minute intervals.
- Provide privacy for toileting and run water in the sink to promote the urge to urinate at this time.
- If the patient is not consistently able to resist the urge to urinate between the intervals, reduce the intervals by 15 minutes.
- Continue this regimen for at least 24 hours or for as many days as it takes for the patient to be comfortable with this schedule and not urinate between the intervals.
- When the patient remains continent between the intervals, increase the intervals by 15 minutes daily until a 3- to 4-hour interval is comfortable for the patient.
- Praise successes. If incontinence occurs, work with the patient to re-establish an acceptable toileting interval.

Habit Training
- Assess the patient's 24-hour voiding pattern for 2 to 3 days.
- Base the initial interval of toileting on the voiding pattern (e.g., 2 hours).
- Assist the patient to the toilet or provide a bedpan/urinal every 2 hours (or whatever has been determined to be an appropriate toileting interval for the individual patient).
- During the toileting, remind the patient to void and provide cues such as running water.
- If the patient is incontinent between scheduled toileting, reduce the time interval by 30 minutes until the patient is continent between voidings.
- Assist the patient to toilet and prompt to void at prescribed intervals.
- Do not leave the patient on the toilet or bedpan for longer than 5 minutes.
- Ensure that all nursing staff members comply with the established toileting schedule and do not apply briefs or encourage the patient to "just wet the bed."
- Reduce toileting interval by 30 minutes if there are more than two incontinence episodes in 24 hours.
- If the patient remains continent at the toileting interval, attempt to increase the interval by 30 minutes until a 3- to 4-hour continence interval is reached.
- Praise the patient for successes, and spend extra time socializing with the patient.
- When incontinence occurs, ensure that the patient and bed are cleaned appropriately but do not spend extra time socializing with the patient.
- Discuss daily record of continence with staff to provide reinforcement and encourage compliance with toileting schedule.
- Include unlicensed assistive personnel in all aspects of the habit training.

---

to follow the new schedule until he or she achieves success again. As the interval increases, the bladder gradually tolerates more volume. Teach him or her relaxation and distraction techniques to maximize success in the retraining. Provide positive reinforcement for maintaining the prescribed schedule.

Habit training (scheduled toileting) is a type of bladder training that is successful in reducing incontinence in cognitively impaired patients. To use habit training, caregivers assist the patient in voiding at specific times (e.g., every 2 hours on the even hours). The goal is to get the patient to the toilet before incontinence occurs. The focus is on reducing incontinence. When that has been achieved, the focus may change to increase bladder capacity by gradually lengthening the voiding intervals, but this is only secondary.

! NURSING SAFETY PRIORITY QSEN
Action Alert

Habit training is undermined when absorbent briefs are used in place of timed toileting. Do not tell patients to "just wet the bed." A common cause of falls in health care facilities is related to patient efforts to get out of bed unassisted to use the toilet. Work with all staff members, including unlicensed assistive personnel (UAP), to implement consistently the toileting schedule for habit training.

Prompted voiding, a supplement to habit training, attempts to increase the patient's awareness of the need to void and to prompt him or her to ask for toileting assistance. Habit training otherwise relies completely on a time schedule.

Exercise therapy with pelvic muscle exercises for urge incontinence is helpful and is taught in the same way as for stress incontinence (see Chart 66-7). Improved urethral resistance helps the patient overcome abnormal detrusor contractions long enough to get to the toilet.

Reducing Reflex Urinary Incontinence

Planning: Expected Outcomes. With appropriate intervention, the patient with reflex incontinence is expected to achieve continence. Indicators include that the patient often or consistently demonstrates these behaviors:
- Recognizes the urge to void
- Maintains a predictable pattern of voiding
- Responds to urge in a timely manner
- Empties bladder completely
- Keeps urine volume in the bladder under 300 mL

Interventions. Interventions for the patient with reflex (overflow) incontinence caused by obstruction of the bladder outlet may include surgery to relieve the obstruction. The most common procedures are prostate removal (see Chapter 72) and repair of uterine prolapse (see Chapter 71).

Drug Therapy. Drugs are prescribed for short-term management of urinary retention, often after surgery. They are not used in long-term management of overflow incontinence caused by a hypotonic bladder. The most commonly used drug is bethanechol chloride (Urecholine), an agent that increases bladder pressure.

Behavioral Interventions. The most effective common behavioral interventions are bladder compression and intermittent self-catheterization.

Bladder compression uses techniques that promote bladder emptying and include the Credé method, the Valsalva maneuver, double-voiding, and splinting.

For the Credé method, teach the patient how to press over the bladder area, increasing its pressure, or to trigger nerve stimulation by tugging at pubic hair or massaging the genital area. These techniques manually assist the bladder in emptying. In the Valsalva maneuver, breathing techniques increase chest and abdominal pressure. This increased pressure is then directed toward the bladder during exhalation. With the technique of double-voiding, the patient empties the bladder and then, within a few minutes, attempts a second bladder emptying.

For women who have a large *cystocele* (prolapse of the bladder into the vagina), a technique called *splinting* both compresses the bladder and moves it into a better position. The woman inserts her fingers into her vagina, gently lifts the cystocele, and begins to urinate. A *pessary,* described earlier, can also provide relief from cystocele-related incontinence.

Intermittent self-catheterization is often used to help patients with long-term problems of incomplete bladder emptying. It is effective, can be learned fairly easily, and remains the preferred method of bladder emptying in patients who have incontinence as a result of a neurogenic bladder (Newman & Willson, 2011). These points are important in teaching the technique:

- Proper handwashing and cleaning of the catheter reduce the risk for INFECTION.
- A small lumen and good lubrication of the catheter prevent urethral trauma.
- A regular schedule for bladder emptying prevents distention and mucosal trauma.

Patients must be able to understand instructions and have the manual dexterity to manipulate the catheter. Caregivers or family members in the home can also be taught to perform straight catheterization using clean (rather than sterile) technique with good outcomes (Kannankeril et al., 2011).

Reducing Functional Urinary Incontinence

Planning: Expected Outcomes. The patient with functional urinary incontinence is expected to remain dry. Indicators include that the patient often or consistently demonstrates these behaviors:

- Uses urine containment or collection measures to ensure dryness
- Manages clothing independently

Interventions. Causes of functional (or chronic intractable) incontinence vary greatly. Some are reversible, and others are not. The focus of intervention is treatment of reversible causes. When incontinence is not reversible, urinary habit training (see Chart 66-9) is used to establish a predictable pattern of bladder emptying to prevent incontinence. A final strategy focuses on containment of the urine and protection of the patient's skin. Nonsurgical interventions include applied devices, containment, and catheterization.

Applied devices include intravaginal pessaries for women and penile clamps for men. The intravaginal pessary supports the uterus and vagina and helps maintain the correct position of the bladder. (See Chapter 71 for further discussion of pessaries.) The penile clamp is applied around the outside of the penis to compress the urethra and prevent urine leakage.

Adverse outcomes from pessaries and penile clamps include damage to the tissues from pressure and INFECTION from colonization of damaged tissues. Both devices require that the patient have either manual dexterity or a caregiver to apply and remove the device. Instruct the patient or caregivers in the use of these devices. Male patients may use an external collecting device, such as a condom catheter. Design of an effective external collecting device for women has not been as successful.

Containment is achieved with absorbent pads and briefs designed to collect urine and keep the patient's skin and clothing dry. Many types and sizes of pads are available:

- Shields or liners inserted inside a panty
- Undergarments that are full-size pads with waist straps

- Plastic-lined protective underpants
- Combination pad and pant systems
- Absorbent bed pads

A major concern with the use of protective pads is the risk for skin breakdown. Materials and costs vary. Some are reusable; others are disposable. The disposal of these products raises ecologic concerns. Avoid use of the word "diaper" when discussing these adult protective pants, however, because of the association of diapers with a baby.

Catheterization for control of incontinence may be intermittent or involve an indwelling catheter. Intermittent catheterization is preferred to an indwelling catheter because of the reduced risk for INFECTION. An indwelling urinary catheter is appropriate for patients with skin breakdown who need a dry environment for healing, for those who are terminally ill and need comfort, and for those who are critically ill and require precise measurement of urine output.

Reducing Total or Mixed Urinary Incontinence. Mixed or total urinary incontinence is a combination of two or more types of involuntary urine loss syndromes. For example, stress incontinence and urge incontinence often occur together in women during and after menopause. For the patient with mixed or total incontinence, combinations of assessment techniques (as discussed under each syndrome) are used. Interventions are also combined to promote continence. The problems and interventions for mixed incontinence are the same as for each specific type of incontinence separately. After identifying the specific types of incontinence an individual patient has, apply the appropriate priority patient problems, interventions, and expected outcomes discussed earlier with each incontinence type.

⊕ CULTURAL CONSIDERATIONS

Patient-Centered Care QSEN

Compared with white women, Asian and black women are less likely to report urinary incontinence. In addition, black women are more likely to report remission or cessation of urinary incontinence and Asian women are more likely to report improvement or a decrease of manifestations over a 2-year period when compared with white women. These cultural differences in urinary incontinence and recovery may be a result of differences in pelvic floor anatomy and function, including smaller pelvic floor area and higher urethral closure pressure in black women (Townsend et al., 2011).

🔒 CLINICAL JUDGMENT CHALLENGE

Patient-Centered Care; Evidence-Based Practice QSEN

The patient is a 52-year-old perimenopausal woman who reports a small loss of urine with coughing, laughing, and occasionally bending over. Recently she has started to leak urine just as she arrives in the bathroom but before she sits on the toilet. She states her mother has had a continuing problem with incontinence for years and seldom leaves her home. The patient wants to continue to lead an active lifestyle and wants to discuss options for preventing progression of this embarrassing condition.

1. What other information should you obtain from this patient?
2. What type or types of incontinence is she most likely to have from the information she has provided thus far?
3. Is this problem likely to be genetic? Why or why not?
4. What will you tell her regarding options for care?
5. She asks if there is anything she can do now to help reduce her urine leakage. How do you respond?

Community-Based Care

Community-based care for the patient with urinary incontinence considers his or her personal, physical, emotional, and social resources. Important personal resources for self-care include mobility, vision, and manual dexterity. When planning care, consider who will be the primary caregiver and what factors may influence the effectiveness of the plan. A recent comparative effectiveness review from the Agency for Healthcare Research and Quality (AHRQ) (2012) reports that some drugs for urinary incontinence can provide benefit but that adverse drug events, overall, lead to poor adherence. This report also provides information that nonpharmacologic and nonsurgical treatments provide significant clinical benefit with low risk for adverse effects but that these interventions are also associated with poor adherence. Ongoing relationships with health care providers may improve adherence.

Home Care Management. Assess the home environment for barriers that limit access to the bathroom. Eliminate hazards that might slow walking or lead to a fall. Such hazards include throw rugs, furniture with legs that extend into the walking area, slippery waxed or polished floors, and poor lighting.

If the patient must climb stairs to reach a bathroom, handrails should be installed and stairs kept free of obstacles. Toilet seat extenders may help provide the right level and height of seating so that maximal abdominal pressure may be applied for voiding. Portable commodes may be obtained when ambulatory access to toilets is impractical. Physical and occupational therapists are valuable resources for assisting with home care management.

Self-Management Education. Teach the patient and family about the cause of the specific type of incontinence, and discuss available treatment options for its management. The teaching plan addresses the prescribed drugs (purpose, dosage, method and route of administration, and expected and potential side effects). Instruct the patient and family about the importance of weight reduction and dietary modification to help control incontinence. Remind the patient who smokes that nicotine can contribute to bladder irritation and that coughing can cause urine leakage.

When external devices or protective pads are needed, describe the possible options and help the patient make a selection best for his or her lifestyle and resources. For patients who will use intermittent catheterization or those with artificial urinary sphincters, demonstrate the correct technique to the patient or caregiver. Evaluate return demonstrations for correct technique. Chart 66-10 also addresses teaching.

Psychosocial Preparation. The embarrassment of incontinence can be devastating to self-esteem, body image, and relationships. Sexual intimacy is often adversely affected by incontinence. The unpredictable nature of incontinence creates anxiety. Patients may be embarrassed to seek help, and even when resources are identified, they may need help to feel comfortable in using the resources. Buying supplies at a local store may threaten privacy.

Accept and acknowledge the personal concerns of the patient and caregiver. Never make their concerns seem trivial. As he or she learns the specifics of the plan that will allow control of urinary incontinence, the confidence to resume social interactions should return. Many continence supplies can be purchased online and delivered directly to the home to maintain privacy.

CHART 66-10 Patient and Family Education: Preparing for Self-Management

Urinary Incontinence

- Maintain a normal body weight to reduce the pressure on your bladder.
- Do not try to control your incontinence by limiting your fluid intake. Adequate fluid intake is necessary for kidney function and health maintenance.
- If you have a catheter in your bladder, follow the instructions given to you about maintaining the sterile drainage system.
- If you are discharged with a suprapubic catheter in your bladder, inspect the entry site for the tube daily, clean the skin around the opening gently with warm soap and water, and place a sterile gauze dressing on the skin around the tube. Report any redness, swelling, drainage, or fever to your physician.
- Do not put anything into your vagina, such as tampons, drugs, hygiene products, or exercise weights, until you check with your physician at your 6-week checkup after surgery.
- Do not have sexual intercourse until after your 6-week postoperative checkup.
- Do not lift or carry anything heavier than 5 pounds or participate in any strenuous exercise until your physician gives you postoperative clearance. In some cases, this could be as long as 3 months.
- Avoid exercises, such as running, jogging, step or dance aerobic classes, rowing, cross-country ski or stair-climber machines, and mountain biking. Brisk walking without any additional hand, leg, or body weights is allowed. Swimming is allowed after all drains and catheters have been removed and your incision is completely healed.
- If Kegel exercises are recommended, ask your nurse for specific instructions.

Health Care Resources. Referral to home care agencies for help with personal care and to continence clinics that specialize in evaluation and treatment may be helpful. In many continence clinics, nurses collaborate with physicians and other health care professionals to evaluate and manage patients. The treatment plan is specific for each patient; supplies and products are custom selected.

Patients may benefit from education and from the support of others who experience similar concerns. The National Association for Continence (NAFC) (www.nafc.org), Access to Continence Care and Treatment (www.wellweb.com/INCONT/acct/contents.htm), and the Wound, Ostomy, and Continence Nurses (www.wocn.org) publish newsletters and educational materials written with easy-to-understand explanations. The American Foundation for Urologic Disease (www.afud.com) provides information on many areas of bladder dysfunction. Local hospitals often have local NAFC-approved support groups.

❓ NCLEX EXAMINATION CHALLENGE

Safe and Effective Care Environment

For which hospitalized client does the nurse recommend the ongoing use of a urinary catheter?
A. 36-year-old woman who is blind and is receiving diuretics
B. 46-year-old man who has paraplegia and is admitted for asthma management
C. 56-year-old woman who is admitted with a vaginal-rectal fistula and has diabetes
D. 66-year-old man who has severe osteoarthritis and is a high risk for falling

◆ *Evaluation: Outcomes*

Evaluate the care of the patient with urinary incontinence based on the identified priority patient problems. The expected outcomes are that the patient will:

- Describe the type of urinary incontinence experienced
- Demonstrate knowledge of proper use of drugs and correct procedures for self-catheterization, use of the artificial sphincter, or care of an indwelling urinary catheter
- Demonstrate effective use of the selected exercise or bladder-training program
- Select and use incontinence interventions, devices, and products
- Have a reduction in the number of incontinence episodes

Specific indicators for these outcomes are listed for each priority patient problem under the Planning and Implementation section (see earlier).

UROLITHIASIS

❖ *PATHOPHYSIOLOGY*

Urolithiasis is the presence of *calculi* (stones) in the urinary tract. Stones often do not cause manifestations until they pass into the lower urinary tract, where they can cause excruciating PAIN. Nephrolithiasis is the formation of stones in the kidney. Formation of stones in the ureter is ureterolithiasis.

Urologic stones are caused by many disorders. However, the exact mechanism of stone formation is not entirely understood. Everyone excretes crystals in the urine at some time, but fewer than 10% of people form stones. Most stones contain calcium as one part of the stone complex. Struvite (15%), uric acid (8%), and cystine (3%) are more rare compositions of stones. Formation of stones involves three conditions:

- Slow urine flow, resulting in supersaturation of the urine with the particular element (e.g., calcium) that first becomes crystallized and later becomes the stone
- Damage to the lining of the urinary tract (e.g., abrasion from crystals)
- Decreased amounts of inhibitor substances in the urine that would otherwise prevent supersaturation and crystal aggregation

High urine acidity (as with uric acid and cystine stones) or alkalinity (as with calcium phosphate and struvite stones), as well as drugs (e.g., triamterene, indinavir, acetazolamide), contributes to stone formation.

One example of a metabolic problem causing stone formation begins when excessive amounts of calcium are absorbed through the intestinal tract leading to hypercalciuria. As blood circulates through the kidneys, the excess calcium is filtered into the urine, causing supersaturation of calcium in the urine. If fluid intake is poor, such as when a patient is dehydrated, supersaturation is more likely to occur and the risk for calcium combining with another compound to form a larger molecule increases. Calcium complexes often serve as a center for other deposits, and eventually a stone forms.

Stones that form in the kidney and then pass into the ureter often lodge in areas where the ureter bends or slightly changes shape. When the stone occludes the ureter and blocks the flow of urine, the ureter dilates. Enlargement of the ureter is called hydroureter.

The PAIN associated with ureteral spasm is excruciating and may cause the patient to go into shock from stimulation of

TABLE 66-4	**Metabolic Defects That Commonly Cause Kidney Stones**
METABOLIC DEFICIT	**ETIOLOGY**
Hypercalcemia	
Primary	Absorptive: increased intestinal calcium absorption Renal: decreased kidney tubular excretion of calcium
Secondary	Resorptive: hyperparathyroidism, vitamin D intoxication, kidney tubular acidosis, prolonged immobilization
Hyperoxaluria	
Primary	Genetic: autosomal recessive trait resulting in high oxalate production
Secondary	Dietary: excess oxalate from foods such as spinach, rhubarb, Swiss chard, cocoa, beets, wheat germ, pecans, peanuts, okra, chocolate, and lime peel
Hyperuricemia	
Primary	Gout is an inherited disorder of purine metabolism (20% of patients with gout have uric acid calculi)
Secondary	Increased production or decreased clearance of purine from myeloproliferative disorders, thiazide diuretics, carcinoma
Struvite	Made of magnesium ammonium phosphate and carbonate apatite; formed by urea splitting by bacteria, most commonly, *Proteus mirabilis;* needs an alkaline urine to form
Cystinuria	Autosomal recessive defect of amino acid metabolism that precipitates insoluble cystine crystals in the urine

nearby nerves. Hematuria (bloody urine) may result from damage to the urothelial lining. If the obstruction is not removed, urinary stasis can cause INFECTION and impair kidney function on the side of the blockage. As the blockage persists, hydronephrosis (enlargement of the kidney caused by blockage of urine lower in the tract and filling of the kidney with urine) and permanent kidney damage may develop.

Etiology and Genetic Risk

The cause of urolithiasis is unknown. At least 90% of patients who form stones have a metabolic risk factor. Table 66-4 lists some metabolic problems that cause stone formation. Patients who are white, older, obese, or have diabetes or gout (hyperuricemia) have increased risk for stone formation (Rodgers, 2013). Other conditions associated with stone formation and recurrence are hyperparathyroidism, urinary tract obstruction, inflammatory bowel diseases, and a history of GI problems (Fink et al., 2013).

Diet is not considered a risk for stone formation. However, calcium and vitamin D supplementation as well as high-dose

🧬 **GENETIC/GENOMIC CONSIDERATIONS**
Patient-Centered Care QSEN

Family history has a strong association with stone formation and recurrence. More than 30 genetic variations are associated with the formation of kidney stones. Single gene disorders are rare. More commonly, nephrolithiasis is a complex disease, with genetic variation in intestinal calcium absorption, kidney calcium transport, or kidney phosphate transport all associated with stone formation. Always ask a patient with a renal stone whether other family members have also had this problem.

ascorbic acid (vitamin C) intake have been implicated in stone formation (Fletcher, 2013; Rosa et al., 2013). Conversely, high intake of fluids, fruits, and vegetables, low consumption of protein, and a balanced intake of calcium, fats, and carbohydrates are prescribed to prevent and treat recurrent urolithiasis (Fink et al., 2013).

Incidence and Prevalence

The incidence of stone disease is high and varies with geographic location, race, and family history. About 12% of adults will have at least one episode of renal stone disease. The incidence is higher in men; however, struvite stones are twice as common in women. Recurrence rates vary depending on the type of treatment. The recurrence rate of untreated calcium oxalate stones is 35% to 50% in 5 to 10 years. A higher recurrence of stones occurs in patients with a family history of stone disease and in those who had their first occurrence by age 25 years.

 CULTURAL CONSIDERATIONS

Patient-Centered Care **QSEN**

The incidence of stone disease is most common in the southeastern United States, Japan, and western Europe. Calcium stone disease is more common in men than in women and tends to occur in young adults or during early middle adulthood. Kidney stone disease occurs more often in younger adults than older adults and more commonly among white people (Rodgers, 2013). For patients in these higher-risk groups, nursing care includes teaching family members, as well as patients, about the manifestations of a stone and interventions to reduce stone formation.

❖ PATIENT-CENTERED COLLABORATIVE CARE

◆ Assessment

Ask the patient about a personal or family history of urologic stones. Obtain a diet history, focusing on fluid intake patterns and supplemental vitamin or mineral intake. If he or she has a history of stone formation, ask about past treatment, whether chemical analysis of the stone was performed, and what preventive measures are followed.

The major manifestation of stones is severe PAIN, commonly called **renal colic**. Flank pain suggests that the stone is in the kidney or upper ureter. Flank pain that extends toward the abdomen or to the scrotum and testes or the vulva suggests that stones are in the ureters or bladder. Pain is most intense when the stone is moving or when the ureter is obstructed.

Renal colic begins suddenly and is often described as "unbearable." Nausea, vomiting, pallor, and diaphoresis often accompany the PAIN. A large stationary stone in the kidney (staghorn calculus), however, rarely causes much pain because it is not moving. Frequency and dysuria occur when a stone reaches the bladder. **Oliguria** (scant urine output) or **anuria** (absence of urine output) suggests obstruction, possibly at the bladder neck or urethra. *Urinary tract obstruction is an emergency and must be treated immediately to preserve kidney function.*

Assess the patient for bladder distention. He or she may appear pale, ashen, and diaphoretic and may suffer from excruciating PAIN. Vital signs may be moderately elevated with pain; body temperature and pulse are elevated with INFECTION. Blood pressure may decrease if the severe pain causes shock.

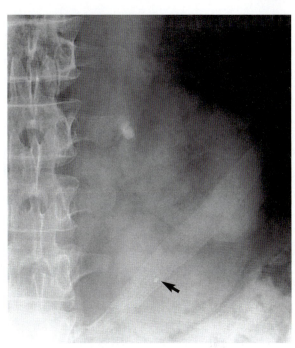

FIG. 66-2 Urinary stones on x-ray of the kidneys, ureters, and bladder (KUB).

Urinalysis is performed in patients with suspected stones. Hematuria is common, and blood may make the urine appear smoky or rusty. RBCs are usually caused by stone-induced trauma on the lining of the ureter, bladder, or urethra. WBCs and bacteria may be present as a result of urinary stasis. Increased *turbidity* (cloudiness) and odor indicate that INFECTION may also be present. Microscopic examination of the urine may identify crystals from which stones could form. Urinary pH is measured to determine acidity or alkalinity.

The serum WBC count is elevated with INFECTION. Increases in the serum calcium, serum phosphate, or serum uric acid levels indicate excess minerals are present and may contribute to stone formation.

Stones are easily seen on x-rays of the kidneys, ureters, and bladder (KUB) (Fig. 66-2), CT, and ultrasound, with ultrasound being used most commonly for screening. Noncontrast CT is the most sensitive procedure to identify urinary tract stones and can confirm the presence, shape, and location of the stones.

◆ Interventions

Nursing interventions focus on PAIN management and prevention of INFECTION and urinary obstruction. Most patients can expel the stone without invasive procedures. The most important factors regarding whether a stone will pass on its own are its composition, size, and location. The larger the stone and the higher up in the urinary tract it is, the less likely it is to be passed. When the stone is passed, it should be captured and sent to the laboratory for analysis. Other interventions are needed when the patient does not pass the stone spontaneously (Fig. 66-3).

Managing Pain. Nonsurgical and surgical approaches are used to assist the patient with a kidney stone achieve an acceptable degree of PAIN relief.

Nonsurgical Management. Nonsurgical measures to relieve pain include strategies to enhance stone passing, as well as direct pain management.

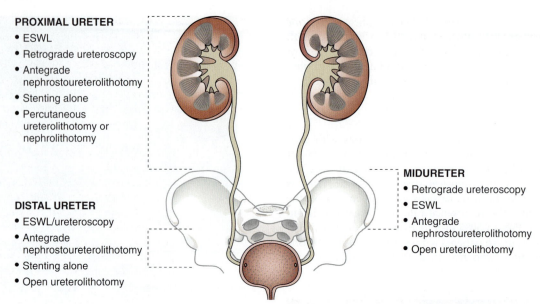

PROXIMAL URETER
- ESWL
- Retrograde ureteroscopy
- Antegrade nephrostoureterolithotomy
- Stenting alone
- Percutaneous ureterolithotomy or nephrolithotomy

MIDURETER
- Retrograde ureteroscopy
- ESWL
- Antegrade nephrostoureterolithotomy
- Open ureterolithotomy

DISTAL URETER
- ESWL/ureteroscopy
- Antegrade nephrostoureterolithotomy
- Stenting alone
- Open ureterolithotomy

FIG. 66-3 Treatment options for ureteral stones. *ESWL,* Extracorporeal shock wave lithotripsy.

Drug therapy is needed in the first 24 to 36 hours when PAIN is most severe. Opioid analgesics are used to control the severe pain caused by stones in the urinary tract and may be given IV for rapid pain relief. NSAIDs such as ketorolac (Toradol) or ketoprofen (Nexcede) in the acute phase may be quite effective. When NSAIDs are used, the risk for bleeding is increased and the use of extracorporeal shock wave lithotripsy is delayed.

Control of PAIN is more effective when drugs are given at regularly scheduled intervals or by a constant delivery system (e.g., skin patch) instead of PRN. Spasmolytic drugs, such as oxybutynin chloride (Ditropan) and propantheline bromide (Pro-Banthine, Propanthel ✦), are important for control of pain (see Chart 66-8). Give the drugs, and assess the response by asking the patient to rate the discomfort on a pain-rating scale.

Other management techniques include avoiding overhydration and underhydration in the acute phase to help make the passage of a stone less painful. Strain the urine and teach the patient to strain it to monitor for stone passage. Send any stone passed to the laboratory for analysis because preventive therapy is based on stone composition.

Two drugs may be used to aid in stone expulsion: a thiazide diuretic and allopurinol. These drugs, combined with a high fluid intake, increase urine volume or decrease urine pH and help increase the excretion of stones or stone fragments (Rosa et al., 2013). Citrate may be used to alter urine pH and interrupt intrarenal conditions that promote stone production.

Lithotripsy, also known as *shock wave lithotripsy (SWL),* is the use of sound, laser, or dry shock waves to break the stone into small fragments. The patient receives moderate sedation and lies on a flat table with the lithotriptor aimed at the stone, which is located by fluoroscopy. A local anesthetic cream is applied to the skin site over the stone 45 minutes before the procedure. During the procedure, cardiac rhythm is monitored by electrocardiography (ECG) and the shock waves are delivered in synchrony with the R wave. Shock waves at the rate of 60 to 120/min are applied over 30 to 45 minutes (Li et al., 2013). Continuous ECG monitoring for dysrhythmia and fluoroscopic observation for stone destruction are maintained.

After lithotripsy, strain the urine to monitor the passage of stone fragments. Bruising may occur on the flank of the affected side. Occasionally a stent is placed in the ureter before SWL to ease passage of the stone fragments.

Surgical Management. Minimally invasive surgical and open surgical procedures are used if urinary obstruction occurs or if the stone is too large to be passed.

Minimally Invasive Surgical Procedures. Minimally invasive surgical (MIS) procedures include stenting, ureteroscopy, percutaneous ureterolithotomy, and percutaneous nephrolithotomy.

Stenting is performed with a **stent**—a small tube that is placed in the ureter by ureteroscopy. The stent dilates the ureter and enlarges the passageway for the stone or stone fragments. This totally internal procedure prevents the passing stone from coming in contact with the ureteral mucosa, thereby reducing PAIN, bleeding, and INFECTION risk, all of which could block the ureter. A Foley catheter may be placed to facilitate passage of the stone through the urethra.

Ureteroscopy is an endoscopic procedure. The ureteroscope is passed through the urethra and bladder into the ureter. Once the stone is seen, it is removed using grasping baskets, forceps, or loops. Lithotripsy also can be performed through the ureteroscope. A Foley catheter may be placed to facilitate passage of the stone fragments through the urethra.

Percutaneous ureterolithotomy or nephrolithotomy is the removal of a stone in the ureter or kidney through the skin. The patient lies prone or on the side and receives local or general anesthesia. The physician identifies the ideal entry point with fluoroscopy and then passes a needle into the collecting system of the kidney. Once a tract has been made in the kidney, other equipment, such as an **intracorporeal** (inside the body) ultrasonic or laser lithotriptor, can be used to break up and remove the stone. An endoscope with a special attachment to grasp and extract the stone can be used. Often a nephrostomy tube is left in place at first to prevent the stone fragments from passing through the urinary tract.

Monitor the patient for complications after the procedure. Complications include bleeding at the site or through the tube, pneumothorax, and INFECTION. Monitor nephrostomy tube drainage for volume and the presence of blood in the urine, which is normal for the first 24 to 48 hours after tube placement. Provide routine nephrostomy tube care, with sterile dressing changes and tube flushing (if ordered).

Open Surgical Procedures. When other stone removal attempts have failed or when risk for a lasting injury to the ureter or kidney is possible, an *open ureterolithotomy* (into the ureter), *pyelolithotomy* (into the kidney pelvis), or *nephrolithotomy* (into the kidney) procedure may be performed. These procedures are used for a large or impacted stone.

Preoperative Care. Explain to the patient how, when, and where the procedure will be performed. Describe what he or she can expect to see, hear, and feel before and after the procedure. The patient is given nothing by mouth and also receives a bowel preparation before the procedure. (See Chapter 14 for routine care before surgery.)

Operative Procedures. The retroperitoneal area is entered through a large flank incision, as for nephrectomy (see Chapter 67), pyelolithotomy, or nephrolithotomy and through a lower abdominal incision for ureterolithotomy. The urinary tract is entered surgically, and the stone is removed. Before closure, tubes and drains may be placed (e.g., nephrostomy tube, ureteral stent, Penrose or other wound drainage device, and Foley catheter).

Postoperative Care. Follow routine procedures for assessment of the patient who has received anesthesia. (See Chapter 16 for routine care after surgery.) Monitor the amount of bleeding from incisions and in the urine. Maintain adequate fluid intake. Strain the urine to monitor the passage of stone fragments. Teach the patient how to prevent future stones through dietary changes, including consistent daily fluid intake to avoid dehydration and supersaturation.

Preventing Infection. Control of INFECTION before invasive procedures is critical for the prevention of urosepsis. Interventions include giving appropriate antibiotics, either to eliminate an existing infection or to prevent new infections, and maintaining adequate nutrition and fluid intake. Because infection always occurs with struvite stone formation, the health care team plans for long-term infection prevention.

Drug therapy involves the use of broad-spectrum antibiotics, such as the aminoglycosides (e.g., gentamicin [Garamycin]) and cephalosporins (e.g., cephalexin [Keflex, Novo-Lexin ✦]). The broad coverage is effective against gram-negative organisms. After the results of the culture and sensitivity (C&S) studies are obtained, more specific antibiotics may be prescribed. C&S studies are often done 48 hours after the start of antibiotic therapy and again 48 hours after completion of the prescribed course of therapy.

Blood levels of antibiotics may be measured to ensure that adequate levels have been reached. If the blood level of the antibiotic is not adequate, organisms may not be completely eliminated. Evidence of a new infection (e.g., chills, fever, and altered mental status) warrants the collection of a urine sample for repeat C&S tests.

For the patient with struvite stones, periodic and long-term monitoring of the urine for infection is needed. Urine cultures are checked monthly for 3 months and then quarterly for 1 year. Drugs that prevent bacteria from splitting urea, such as acetohydroxamic acid (Lithostat) and hydroxyurea (Hydrea), are often prescribed long-term for patients with struvite stones. Serum creatinine levels are monitored in patients receiving acetohydroxamic acid, and the drug is stopped if creatinine levels are above 2 mg/dL. Review interventions aimed at preventing urinary tract infection (UTI). (See Health Promotion discussion on p. 1369 in the Cystitis section.)

Nutrition therapy ideally includes adequate calorie intake with a balance of all food groups. Encourage a fluid intake sufficient to dilute urine to a light color throughout the 24-hour day (typically 2 to 3 L/day) unless another health problem requires fluid restriction.

Preventing Obstruction. Measures to prevent urinary obstruction by stones include a high intake of fluids (3 L/day or more) and accurate measures of intake and output. Fluid intake sufficient to provide diluted urine helps prevent dehydration, promotes urine flow, and decreases the chance of crystals forming a stone. Interventions also depend on the type of stone the patient has formed. Drugs, diet modification, and fluid intake are the major strategies used to prevent future stones.

Drug therapy to prevent obstruction depends on what is causing stone formation and the type of stone formed. Teach the patient the reason for the drug, and assess for side effects or adverse drug reactions. Some drugs may need to be avoided because they may contribute to stone formation.

Drugs to treat *hypercalciuria* (high levels of calcium in the urine) include thiazide diuretics (e.g., chlorothiazide [Diuril] or hydrochlorothiazide [HydroDIURIL, Urozide ✦]). These drugs promote calcium reabsorbtion from the renal tubules back into the body, thereby reducing urine calcium loads. For patients with *hyperoxaluria* (high levels of oxalic acid in the urine), allopurinol (Zyloprim) or febuxostat (Uloric) is used.

For patients with hyperuricemia or chronic gout, both allopurinol and febuxostat help prevent the formation of urate (uric acid) stones. To alkalinize the urine, drugs such as potassium citrate, 50% sodium citrate, and sodium bicarbonate are used. Lemon or orange juice may also be ingested as a daily source of citrate. The desired urine pH is 6 to 6.5. Because the normal urine pH averages 5 to 6, the desired values are termed *alkaline.*

For patients with *cystinuria* (high levels of cystine in the urine), both alpha-mercaptopropionylglycine (AMPG) and captopril (Capoten) lower urine cystine levels. They are used when hydration and urine alkalinization have not been successful.

Statins, drugs used to manage hypercholesterolemia, have also been found to reduce the incidence of stone recurrence (Sur et al., 2013). In general, with one stone, patients are advised to increase fluid intake. With two or more stones, drug therapy is advised based on the type of stone as described above (Fink et al., 2013).

Nutrition therapy depends on the type of stone formed (Table 66-5). Collaborate with the dietitian to plan for and teach the appropriate diet to the patient (Türk et al., 2011).

Other measures can help the stone pass more quickly. Urge the patient to walk as often as possible. Walking promotes passage of stones and reduces bone calcium resorption. Check the urine pH daily, and strain all urine with filter paper or a special urine sieve/strainer to collect passed stones and fragments.

Self-management education includes the key points listed in Chart 66-11. Follow-up care to evaluate effects of intervention includes a 24-hour urine collection and serum chemical analysis. The patient often has great anxiety and fear that a stone and its PAIN may recur. In addition to anxiety about the pain, the risk for repeated surgical interventions or permanent and

TABLE 66-5   Dietary Treatment for Kidney and Urinary Stones

STONE TYPE	DIETARY INTERVENTIONS	RATIONALES
Calcium oxalate	Avoid oxalate sources, such as spinach, black tea, and rhubarb. Decrease sodium intake.	Reduction of urinary oxalate content may help prevent these stones from forming. Urinary pH is not a factor. High sodium intake reduces kidney tubular calcium reabsorption.
Calcium phosphate	Limit intake of foods high in animal protein to 5-7 servings per week and never more than 2 per day. Some patients may benefit from a reduced calcium intake (milk, other dairy products). Decrease sodium intake.	Reduction of protein intake reduces acidic urine and prevents calcium precipitation. Reduction of urine calcium concentration may prevent calcium precipitation and crystallization. High sodium intake reduces kidney tubular calcium reabsorption.
Struvite (magnesium ammonium phosphate)	Limit high-phosphate foods, such as dairy products, organ meats, and whole grains.	Reduction of urinary phosphate content may help prevent these stones from forming.
Uric acid (urate)	Decrease intake of purine sources, such as organ meats, poultry, fish, gravies, red wines, and sardines.	Reduction of urinary purine content may help prevent these stones from forming.
Cystine	Limit animal protein intake (as above). Encourage oral fluid intake (500 mL every 4 hours while awake and 750 mL at night).	Reduces urinary uric acid. Increased fluid helps dilute the urine and prevents the cystine crystals from forming.

CHART 66-11   Patient and Family Education: Preparing for Self-Management

Urinary Calculi

- Finish your entire prescription of antibiotics to ensure that you will not get a urinary tract infection.
- You may resume your usual daily activities.
- Remember to balance regular exercise with sleep and rest.
- You may return to work 2 days to 6 weeks after surgery, depending on the type of intervention, your personal tolerance, and your physician's directives.
- Depending on the type of stone you had, your diet may be restricted to prevent further stone formation.
- Remember to drink at least 3 L of fluid a day to dilute potential stone-forming crystals, prevent dehydration, and promote urine flow.
- Monitor urine pH as directed (possibly up to 3 times per day).
- Expect bruising after lithotripsy. The bruising may be quite extensive and may take several weeks to resolve.
- Your urine may be bloody for several days after surgery.
- Pain in the region of the kidneys or bladder may signal the beginning of an infection or the formation of another stone. Report any pain, fever, chills, or difficulty with urination immediately to your physician or nurse.
- Keep follow-up appointments to check on infection, and have repeat cultures done.

❓ NCLEX EXAMINATION CHALLENGE

Health Promotion and Maintenance

The client passes a urinary stone that laboratory analysis indicates is composed of calcium oxalate. Based on this analysis, which instruction does the nurse specifically include for dietary prevention of the problem?
A. "Increase your intake of meat, fish, and cranberry juice."
B. "Avoid citrus fruits and citrus juices such as oranges."
C. "Avoid dark green leafy vegetables such as spinach."
D. "Decrease your intake of dairy products, especially milk."

serious kidney damage is of major concern. Psychosocial preparation is enhanced when patients know what to expect and what actions to take if problems develop. Reassure the patient that preventive and health promotion activities help prevent recurrence.

UROTHELIAL CANCER

❖ PATHOPHYSIOLOGY

Urothelial cancers are malignant tumors of the *urothelium*—the lining of transitional cells in the kidney, renal pelvis, ureters, urinary bladder, and urethra. Most urothelial cancers occur in the bladder, and the term *bladder cancer* describes this condition.

In North America, most urinary tract cancers are transitional cell carcinomas of the bladder (ACS, 2014; Canadian Cancer Society, 2014). The second most common site of urinary tract cancer is the kidney and renal pelvis. Urothelial cancers are usually low grade, have multiple points of origin (*multifocal*), and are recurrent. Once the cancer spreads beyond the transitional cell layer, it is highly invasive and can spread beyond the bladder. Because of the nature of this cancer, patients may have recurrence up to 10 years after being cancer free (ACS, 2014).

Tumors confined to the bladder mucosa are treated by simple excision, whereas those that are deeper but not into the muscle layer are treated with excision plus intravesical (inside the bladder) chemotherapy. Cancer that has spread deeper into the bladder muscle layer is treated with more extensive surgery, often a radical cystectomy (removal of the bladder and surrounding tissue) with urinary diversion. Chemotherapy and radiation therapy are used in addition to surgery. If untreated, the tumor invades surrounding tissues, spreads to distant sites (liver, lung, and bone), and ultimately leads to death.

Exposure to toxins, especially chemicals used in hair dyes and the rubber, paint, electric cable, and textile industries, increases the risk for bladder cancer. The greatest risk factor for bladder cancer is tobacco use. Other risks include *Schistosoma haematobium* (a parasite) INFECTION, excessive use of drugs containing phenacetin, and long-term use of cyclophosphamide (Cytoxan, Procytox ✚).

In the United States and Canada, about 82,690 new cases of bladder cancer are diagnosed each year, and about 17,780 deaths occur each year from the disease (ACS, 2014; Canadian Cancer Society, 2014). This cancer is rare in adults younger than 40 years and is most common after 60 years of age.

Health Promotion and Maintenance

Many people believe that tobacco use is associated with cancers only of organs that come into direct contact with it, such as the lungs. However, many compounds in tobacco enter the bloodstream and affect other organs, such as the bladder. Therefore encourage everyone who smokes to quit and nonsmokers not to start (see the Health Promotion and Maintenance section of Chapter 27 on pp. 494-496). Just as important, encourage anyone who comes into contact with dry, liquid, or gaseous chemicals to take precautions. Some people work with chemicals, and others may come into contact with them while engaging in hobbies. Many chemicals and fumes can enter the body through contact with skin and with mucous membranes in the respiratory tract. Use of personal protective equipment, such as gloves and masks, can reduce this contact. Also encourage anyone who works with chemicals to shower or bathe and change clothing as soon as contact is completed.

❓ NCLEX EXAMINATION CHALLENGE

Physiological Integrity

A 65-year-old client is seeing his primary care provider for an annual examination. Which assessment finding alerts the nurse to an increased risk for bladder cancer?
A. Smoking
B. Urine with a high specific gravity
C. Recurrent urinary tract infections
D. History of cancer in another organ or tissue

❖ PATIENT-CENTERED COLLABORATIVE CARE

◆ Assessment

Physical Assessment/Clinical Manifestations. Ask about the patient's perception of his or her general health. Document the gender and age of the patient. Ask about active and passive exposure to cigarette smoke. To detect exposure to harmful environmental agents, ask the patient to describe his or her occupation and hobbies in detail. Also ask the patient to describe any change in the color, frequency, or amount of urine and any abdominal discomfort.

Observe the patient's overall appearance, especially skin color and nutrition status. Inspect, percuss, and palpate the abdomen for asymmetry, tenderness, and bladder distention.

Examine the urine for color and clarity. Blood in the urine is often the first manifestation of bladder cancer. It may be gross or microscopic and is usually painless and intermittent. Dysuria, frequency, and urgency occur when INFECTION or obstruction is also present.

Psychosocial Assessment. Assess the patient's emotions, including his or her response to a tentative diagnosis of bladder cancer, and note anxiety, fear, sadness, anger, or guilt. Early manifestations are painless, and many patients ignore the blood in the urine because it is intermittent. They also may be reluctant to seek treatment because they suspect a sexually transmitted disease (STD). As a result, they may have guilt or anger about their own delays in seeking medical attention.

Assess the patient's coping methods and available support from family members. Social support may provide motivation and improve coping during recovery from treatment.

Diagnostic Assessment. The only significant finding on a routine urinalysis is gross or microscopic hematuria. Cytologic testing on voided urine specimens usually is not helpful. Bladder-wash specimens and bladder biopsies are the most specific tests for cancer.

Cystoscopy is usually performed to evaluate painless hematuria. A biopsy of a visible bladder tumor can be performed during cystoscopy. This is essential for staging and is usually performed in an ambulatory care surgery center. Cystoureterography may be used to identify obstructions, especially where the ureter joins the bladder. CT scans show tumor invasion of surrounding tissues. Ultrasonography shows masses but is less valuable for tumor staging. MRI may help assess deep, invasive tumors.

◆ Interventions

Therapy for the patient with bladder cancer usually begins with surgical removal of the tumor for diagnosis and staging of disease. For tumors extending beyond the mucosa, surgery is followed by intravesical chemotherapy or immunotherapy. High-grade or recurrent tumors are treated with more radical surgery plus intravesical chemotherapy, radiotherapy, or both. Systemic chemotherapy is reserved for patients with distant metastases. (See Chapter 22 for general care of the patient receiving chemotherapy or radiation therapy.)

Nonsurgical Management. Prophylactic immunotherapy with intravesical instillation of bacille Calmette-Guérin (BCG), a live virus compound, is used to prevent tumor recurrence of superficial cancers. This procedure is more effective than single-agent chemotherapy. Usually the agent is instilled in an outpatient cancer clinic and allowed to dwell in the bladder for a specified length of time, usually 2 hours. When the patient urinates, live virus is excreted with the urine.

Teach patients receiving this treatment to prevent contact of the live virus with other members of the household by not sharing a toilet with others for at least 24 hours after instillation. Instruct men to urinate while sitting down to avoid splashing the urine. After 24 hours, the toilet should be completely cleaned using a solution of 10% liquid bleach. If only one toilet is available in the household, teach the patient to flush the toilet after use and follow this by adding one cup of undiluted bleach to the bowl water. The bowl is then flushed after 15 minutes and the seat and flat surfaces of the toilet wiped with a cloth containing a solution of 10% liquid bleach. Instruct the patient to wear gloves during the cleaning and to dispose of the cloth after sealing it in a plastic bag.

Underwear or other clothing that has come into contact with the urine during the immediate 24 hours after instillation should be washed separately from other clothing in a solution of 10% liquid bleach. Sexual intercourse is avoided for 24 hours after the instillation.

Multiagent chemotherapy is successful in prolonging life after distant metastasis has occurred but rarely results in a cure. Radiation therapy is also useful in prolonging life.

Surgical Management. The type of surgery for bladder cancer depends on the type and stage of the cancer and the patient's general health. Complete bladder removal (*cystectomy*) with additional removal of surrounding muscle and tissue offers the best chance of a cure for large, invasive bladder cancers. Four alternatives for urine ELIMINATION are used after cystectomy: ileal conduit; continent pouch; bladder reconstruction, also known as *neobladder;* and ureterosigmoidostomy.

Preoperative Care. Specific patient education depends on the type and extent of the planned surgical procedure.

Coordinate education before surgery with the patient, surgeon, and enterostomal therapist (ET) or wound, ostomy, and continence nurse. Discuss the type of planned urinary diversion and the selection of a site for the stoma. Including the patient in this planning improves the chances for the patient to have a positive attitude about body image and a positive self-image. Use educational counseling to ensure understanding about self-care practices, methods of pouching, control of urine drainage, and management of odor.

The site selected for the stoma should be visible to the patient and avoid folds of skin, bones, and scar tissue. When possible, the waistline or belt area is avoided. Prepare the patient for the number and type of drains that will be present after surgery. General care before surgery is discussed in Chapter 14.

Operative Procedures. Transurethral resection of the bladder tumor (TURBT) or partial cystectomy is performed for small, early, superficial tumors. In a partial (segmental) cystectomy, a portion of the bladder is removed when there is only a single isolated bladder tumor.

When the entire bladder must be removed (complete cystectomy), the ureters are diverted into a collecting reservoir. Techniques for urinary diversion are shown in Fig. 66-4. With an ileal conduit, the ureters are surgically placed in the ileum and urine is collected in a pouch on the skin around the stoma. More often, continent reservoirs or "neobladders" are created from an intestinal graft. With cutaneous ureterostomy or ureteroureterostomy, the ureter opening is brought out onto the skin. The cutaneous ureterostomies may be located on either side of the abdomen or side by side.

Postoperative Care. After cutaneous ureterostomy, an external pouch covers the ostomy to collect urine. Work with the ET to focus care on the wound, the skin, and urinary drainage. (See Chapter 56 for ostomy care.)

The patient with a Kock's pouch, a continent reservoir, may have a Penrose drain and a plastic Medena catheter in the stoma. The drain removes lymphatic fluid or other secretions; the catheter ensures urine drainage so that incisions can heal. The patient with a neobladder usually requires 2 to 4 days in the intensive care unit (ICU) and will have a drain at first in the event the neobladder requires irrigation. Later, irrigation can be performed with intermittent catheterization. Irrigation is performed to ensure patency. There is no sensation of bladder fullness with a neobladder because sensory nerves are not attached. As a result, the patient will need to learn new cues to void, such as prescribed times or noticing a feeling of neobladder pressure. General care after surgery is discussed in Chapter 16.

Different types of drains and nephrostomy catheters are used, sometimes on a temporary basis, to drain urine from the kidney. Some are totally internal, with no drainage to the outside. Others may drain exclusively to the outside and urine is collected in a pouch or bag. For this type of drainage system, urine output remains constant. Decreased or no drainage is cause for concern and must be reported to the surgeon or nephrologist, as is leakage around the catheter. Some nephrostomy tubes are connected both to the new bladder (internal drainage) and to an external drainage system. With this type of system, urine output from the external portion of the catheter is variable. With any drainage system, intervention is needed if the external catheter is partially or completely pulled out accidentally. Immediately notify the surgeon or nephrologist. If the catheter remains partially in place, secure it from further movement. This action may result in a re-insertion process rather than a total replacement.

Community-Based Care

Self-Management Education. Teach the patient and family about drugs, diet and fluid therapy, the use of external pouching systems, and the technique for catheterizing a continent reservoir.

With some procedures, the patient may need electrolyte replacement to prevent long-term deficits. Teach him or her to avoid foods that are known to produce gas if the urinary diversion uses the intestinal tract. When intestinal production of gas is excessive, flatus can induce incontinence.

Patients who have a neobladder created often have extreme weight loss during the first few weeks after surgery. Collaborate with a dietitian to develop a diet plan specific to the patient to meet his or her caloric needs.

> ### ! NURSING SAFETY PRIORITY (QSEN)
> **Action Alert**
>
> INFECTION is common in patients who have a neobladder. Teach patients and family members the manifestations of infection and the importance of reporting them immediately to the surgeon.

Instruct the patient and family about any changes in self-care activities related to the urinary diversion. In collaboration with the enterostomal therapist, demonstrate external pouch application, local skin care, pouch care, methods of adhesion, and drainage mechanisms. If a Kock's pouch has been created, teach the patient how to use a catheter to drain the pouch. For all instruction, observe at least one return demonstration or "teach-back" session by the patient or the caregiver. Ideally, the patient assumes responsibility for self-care before discharge.

Assist the patient to prepare for the impact of urinary diversion on self-image, body image, sexual functioning, and self-esteem. Counseling provides information and support to reduce feelings of powerlessness.

Through discussions with the patient about common social situations, help him or her gain control over new toileting practices. Men with a urinary diversion into the sigmoid colon need to learn the habit of sitting to urinate. For patients of either gender, promote confidence in social situations by encouraging frequent emptying of urinary collection devices before traveling or attending social functions. Resumption of sexual activity is a major concern for many, regardless of age. Address this topic openly and with sensitivity. Cystectomy causes impotence in men, but treatment is available (see Chapter 72).

Health Care Resources. The United Ostomy Association and the American Cancer Society have educational materials that may be useful to patients. Refer patients and family members to local chapters or units of these organizations. In some areas, local support groups have meetings to assist others and to send visitors to provide peer counseling and support. Home care personnel may assist with follow-up, easing the transition from hospital to home. The Wound, Ostomy, and Continence Nurses Society has educational programs and a journal for the care of patients with ostomies.

Ureterostomies divert urine directly to the skin surface through a ureteral skin opening (stoma). After ureterostomy, the patient must wear a pouch.

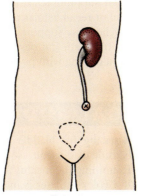

Cutaneous ureterostomy

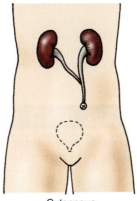

Cutaneous ureteroureterostomy

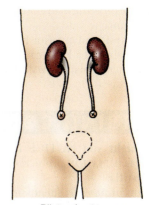

Bilateral cutaneous ureterostomy

Conduits collect urine in a portion of the intestine, which is then opened onto the skin surface as a stoma. After the creation of a conduit, the patient must wear a pouch.

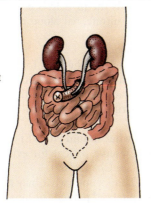

Ileal (Bricker's) conduit

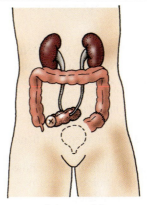

Colon conduit

Ileal reservoirs divert urine into a surgically created pouch, or pocket, that functions as a bladder. The stoma is continent, and the patient removes urine by regular self-catheterization.

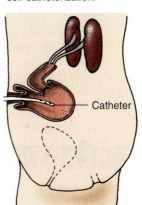

Continent internal ileal reservoir (Kock's pouch)

Sigmoidostomies divert urine to the large intestine, so no stoma is required. The patient excretes urine with bowel movements, and bowel incontinence may result.

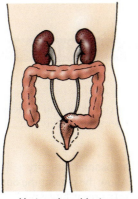

Ureterosigmoidostomy

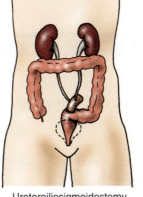

Ureteroiliosigmoidostomy

FIG. 66-4 Urinary diversion procedures used in the treatment of bladder cancer.

BLADDER TRAUMA

❖ PATHOPHYSIOLOGY

Bladder trauma can be caused by penetrating or blunt injury to the lower abdomen. Penetrating injury may occur by stabbing, gunshot wound, or other trauma in which objects pierce the abdominal wall. A fractured pelvis with puncture of the bladder by bone fragments is the most common cause of bladder trauma. Bladder trauma may also be a result of sexual assault.

Blunt trauma compresses the abdominal wall and the bladder. A seat belt may compress the bladder hard enough to cause injury, especially when the bladder is full or distended.

❖ PATIENT-CENTERED COLLABORATIVE CARE

Patients with a penetrating bladder wound often have anuria or hematuria. In the emergency department, initial assessment includes inspection of the urinary meatus for blood.

Bladder trauma, other than a simple contusion, requires surgical intervention. When bone fractures are present, they are stabilized before bladder repair to prevent further bladder damage. Surgical interventions include repairing the bladder wall and peritoneal membrane. Usually, repairs of the bladder are procedures to close the abnormal opening(s) caused by the trauma.

Patients with an anterior bladder wall injury usually have a Penrose drain and a Foley catheter in place after surgery. Those with a posterior bladder wall injury have a Penrose drain and Foley or suprapubic catheter after surgery. In some instances, vaginal or rectal fistulas may also require repair.

Psychosocial support is critical for patients who have sustained traumatic injuries. Refer them to counseling resources to assist in dealing with psychosocial issues.

NURSING CONCEPTS AND CLINICAL JUDGMENT REVIEW

What might you NOTICE if the patient is experiencing urinary ELIMINATION problems, INFLAMMATION, or INFECTION from cystitis?

- Patient urinates frequently in small amounts.
- Patient reports pain and burning on urination.
- Patient reports suprapubic pain.
- Urine is cloudy and foul-smelling.
- Urine may be darker or smoky in appearance or have obvious blood in it.

What should you INTERPRET and how should you RESPOND to a patient experiencing INFECTION, INFLAMMATION, and urinary ELIMINATION problems as a result of a UTI?

Perform and interpret physical assessment, including:
- Asking how long manifestations have been present
- Asking about low back pain (midline in men) or flank pain
- Asking whether he or she has had a UTI in the past; how long ago; how it was treated; and if antibiotics were prescribed, whether the drug course was completed
- Asking about pregnancy or the presence of any chronic health problem, especially diabetes
- Determining fluid intake and output volumes

- Assessing for bladder distention by palpation or with a bedside bladder ultrasound scanner (see Chapter 65)
- Examining the meatus for irritation
- If a Foley catheter is in place, determining why it is in use and how long it has been present
- Interpreting laboratory values:
  - Is the complete blood count within normal limits?
  - Is the urinalysis positive for bacteria, leukocyte esterase, nitrate, red blood cells, or white blood cells?

Respond by:
- Assessing the need for continuing indwelling catheter
- Teaching the patient comfort measures
- Teaching the patient the importance of completing the prescribed drug regimen

On what should you REFLECT?
- Observe patient for evidence of improved urinary output (see Chapter 65).
- Think about what may have caused this infection in a hospitalized patient (or long-term care resident) and what steps could be taken to prevent a similar episode.
- Think about what patient-teaching focus could help reduce the risk for future UTI.

GET READY FOR THE NCLEX® EXAMINATION!

KEY POINTS

Review these Key Points for each NCLEX Examination Client Needs Category.

Safe and Effective Care Environment
- Use sterile technique when inserting a catheter or any other instrument into the urinary system. **Safety** QSEN
- Use Contact Precautions with any drainage from the genitourinary tract. **Safety** QSEN
- Determine whether there is an ongoing need for an indwelling catheter. **Evidence-Based Practice** QSEN

Health Promotion and Maintenance
- Teach patients to clean the perineal area daily, after voiding, after having a bowel movement, and after sexual intercourse. **Patient-Centered Care** QSEN
- Encourage all patients to maintain an adequate fluid intake.
- Instruct women who have stress incontinence the proper way to perform pelvic floor strengthening exercises. **Patient-Centered Care** QSEN
- Urge anyone who smokes to stop smoking.
- Teach patients who come into contact with chemicals in their workplaces or with leisure-time activities to avoid direct skin and mucous membrane contact with these chemicals. **Safety** QSEN

Psychosocial Integrity
- Allow the patient the opportunity to express feelings or concerns regarding a potential chronic urinary tract disorder or a cancer diagnosis. **Patient-Centered Care** QSEN
- Use a nonjudgmental approach in caring for patients with urinary incontinence.
- Avoid referring to protective pads or pants as "diapers."
- Recognize the need for the patient undergoing cystectomy and urinary diversion to grieve about the body image change. **Patient-Centered Care** QSEN
- Assess the patient's level of comfort in discussing issues related to ELIMINATION and the urogenital area. **Patient-Centered Care** QSEN
- Use language and terminology during kidney/urinary assessment that the patient is comfortable using. **Patient-Centered Care** QSEN
- Refer patients to community resources and support groups.

Physiological Integrity

- Identify hospitalized patients at risk for bacteriuria and urosepsis.
- Report immediately any condition that obstructs urine flow.
- Instruct patients with UTI to complete all prescribed antibiotic therapy even when manifestations of INFECTION are absent.

- Evaluate daily the indications for maintaining indwelling catheters and discontinue their use as soon as possible. **Evidence-Based Practice** QSEN
- Teach patients the expected side effects and any adverse reactions to prescribed drugs.
- Assess the patient's manual dexterity and cognitive awareness before teaching a regimen of intermittent self-catheterization. **Patient-Centered Care** QSEN

Care of Patients with Kidney Disorders

Chris Winkelman

 http://evolve.elsevier.com/Iggy/

PRIORITY CONCEPTS

- ELIMINATION
- PAIN
- FLUID AND ELECTROLYTE BALANCE

- ACID-BASE BALANCE
- INFLAMMATION
- INFECTION

LEARNING OUTCOMES

Safe and Effective Care Environment

1. Collaborate with members of the health care team when providing care to patients with various types of kidney disorders.
2. Prioritize collaborative interventions for patients with kidney disorders and after nephrectomy.
3. Assess presence and extent of PAIN and suffering for patients with kidney disease.

Health Promotion and Maintenance

4. Teach patients who have other health problems that affect kidney function and ELIMINATION to manage these problems and maintain kidney health.

5. Instruct patients who are at risk for or who have kidney changes involving INFECTION or INFLAMMATION to manage kidney health appropriately.

Psychosocial Integrity

6. Reduce the psychological impact of kidney disorders for the patient and family.

Physiological Integrity

7. Identify adults at highest risk for development of an acute or chronic kidney disorder that affects FLUID AND ELECTROLYTE BALANCE.
8. Perform focused kidney/urinary assessment and re-assessment.

The role of the kidneys in urinary ELIMINATION is to filter wastes and maintain FLUID AND ELECTROLYTE BALANCE, as well as ACID-BASE BALANCE. Any problem that disrupts kidney function limits the ability to meet these roles and has the potential to impair general homeostasis (Fig. 67-1). The kidneys work together with many other organ systems. Thus kidney disorders affect systemic health and can lead to life-threatening outcomes. Kidney disorders are classified as congenital, obstructive, infectious, glomerular, and degenerative. Kidney tumors and kidney trauma are also described in this chapter. Acute kidney injury (AKI) and chronic kidney disease (CKD) are discussed in Chapter 68.

CONGENITAL DISORDERS

POLYCYSTIC KIDNEY DISEASE

❖ PATHOPHYSIOLOGY

Polycystic kidney disease (PKD) is an inherited disorder in which fluid-filled cysts develop in the nephrons (Fig. 67-2). In the dominant form, only a few nephrons have cysts until the person reaches his or her 30s. In the recessive form of the disease, nearly all nephrons have cysts from birth. Cysts develop throughout the nephron as a result of abnormal cell division.

Over time, small cysts become much larger (up to centimeters in diameter) and more widely distributed. The growing cysts damage the glomerular and tubular membranes. As the cysts fill with fluid and enlarge, the nephron and kidney function become less effective.

The kidney tissue is eventually replaced by nonfunctioning cysts, which look like clusters of grapes (see Fig. 67-2). The kidneys become very large. Each cystic kidney may enlarge to 2 or 3 times its normal size, becoming as large as a football, and may weigh 10 pounds or more each. Other abdominal organs are displaced, and the patient has PAIN. The fluid-filled cysts are also at increased risk for INFECTION, rupture, and bleeding, which increase pain.

Most patients with PKD have high blood pressure. The cause of hypertension is related to kidney ischemia from the enlarging cysts. As the vessels are compressed and blood flow to the kidneys decreases, the renin-angiotensin system is activated, raising blood pressure. Control of hypertension is a top priority because proper treatment can disrupt the process that leads to further kidney damage.

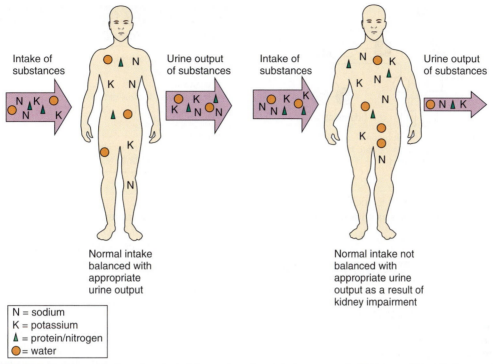

N = sodium
K = potassium
▲ = protein/nitrogen
● = water

FIG. 67-1 Unbalanced body water, electrolytes, and waste products as a result of kidney problems that prevent adjustments in urinary elimination.

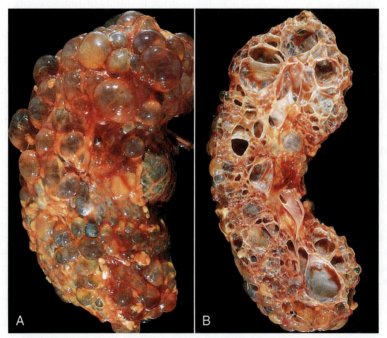

FIG. 67-2 External surface **(A)** and internal surface **(B)** of a polycystic kidney.

Cysts may occur also in other tissues, such as the liver and blood vessels. They may reduce liver function. In addition, the incidence of cerebral *aneurysms* (outpouching and thinning of an artery wall) is higher in patients with PKD. These aneurysms may rupture, causing bleeding and sudden death. For reasons as yet unknown, kidney stones occur in many patients with PKD. Heart valve problems (e.g., mitral valve prolapse), left ventricular hypertrophy, and colonic diverticula also are common in patients with PKD (McCance et al., 2014).

Etiology and Genetic Risk

PKD has several forms and can be inherited as either an autosomal dominant trait or, less commonly, as an autosomal recessive trait. People who inherit the recessive form of PKD usually

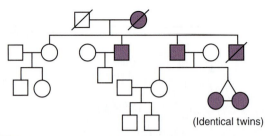

FIG. 67-3 Four-generation pedigree for autosomal dominant polycystic kidney disease (ADPKD). *Colored-in symbols* indicate family members with ADPKD. *Slashes* indicate the person has died.

die in early childhood. The 5% to 10% incidence of PKD in patients with no family history occurs as a result of a new gene mutation.

⚕ GENETIC/GENOMIC CONSIDERATIONS

Patient-Centered Care QSEN

The autosomal dominant form of PKD (ADPKD) is the most common form of polycystic disease. Children of parents who have the autosomal dominant form of PKD have a 50% chance of inheriting the gene mutation that causes the disease (*PKD1*). Fig. 67-3 shows a typical pedigree for a family with ADPKD. Presentation of ADPKD can vary for age of onset, manifestations, and illness severity, even within one family. However, it is fully penetrant, meaning that nearly 100% of people who inherit a PKD gene mutation will develop kidney cysts by age 30 (Online Mendelian Inheritance in Man [OMIM], 2014). Half of these people develop chronic kidney disease (CKD) by age 50 years. ADPKD-1 is the most common and most severe form of the autosomal dominant disease. ADPKD-2 has a slower rate of cyst formation, so manifestations occur later in life and progression to end-stage kidney disease (ESKD) and other complications is delayed.

There is no way to prevent PKD among people who have the genetic mutation, although early detection and management of hypertension may slow the progression of kidney damage. Genetic counseling may be useful for adults who have a parent with PKD. Family history analysis is a simple assessment that can be used to help identify people at risk for PKD (see Fig. 67-3).

Incidence and Prevalence

PKD is a common disorder, affecting about 600,000 people in the United States (National Kidney Foundation, 2013). It is more common in white people than in people of other races. Men and women have an equal chance of inheriting the disease because the gene responsible for PKD is not located on the sex chromosomes.

❖ PATIENT-CENTERED COLLABORATIVE CARE

◆ Assessment

History. Explore the family history of a patient with suspected or actual PKD, and ask whether either parent was known to have PKD or whether there is any family history of kidney disease. Important information to obtain is the age at which the problem was diagnosed in the parent and any related complications. Ask about constipation, abdominal discomfort, a change in urine color or frequency, high blood pressure, headaches, and a family history of sudden death from a stroke.

Polycystic Kidney Disease

- Abdominal or flank pain
- Hypertension
- Nocturia
- Increased abdominal girth
- Constipation
- Bloody or cloudy urine
- Kidney stones
- Sodium wasting and inability to concentrate urine in early stage
- Progression to kidney failure with anuria

Physical Assessment/Clinical Manifestations. Chart 67-1 lists key features of PKD. PAIN is often the first manifestation. Inspect the abdomen. A distended abdomen is common as the cystic kidneys swell and push the abdominal contents forward. Polycystic kidneys are easily palpated because of their increased size. Proceed with *gentle* abdominal palpation because the cystic kidneys and nearby tissues may be tender and palpation is uncomfortable.

The patient also may have flank PAIN as a dull ache or as sharp and intermittent discomfort. Dull, aching pain is caused by increased kidney size with distention or by INFECTION within the cyst. Sharp, intermittent pain occurs when a cyst ruptures or a stone is present. When a cyst ruptures, the patient may have bright red or cola-colored urine. Infection is suspected if the urine is cloudy or foul smelling or if there is **dysuria** (pain on urination).

Nocturia (the need to urinate excessively at night) is an early manifestation and occurs because of decreased urine concentrating ability. Patients with early PKD waste sodium and water. As kidney function further declines, the patient has increasing hypertension, edema, and uremic manifestations such as anorexia, nausea, vomiting, pruritus, and fatigue (see Chapter 68). Because berry aneurysms often occur in patients with PKD, a severe headache with or without neurologic or vision changes requires attention.

Psychosocial Assessment. As an inherited disorder, PKD may cause psychosocial responses. The patient often has seen the effects and problems of the disease in close family members. He or she may have had a parent who died or close relatives who required dialysis or transplantation. While obtaining the family history, listen carefully for spoken and unspoken feelings of anger, resentment, futility, sadness, or anxiety. Such feelings may need further exploration. The focus of the feelings may be one or both parents or the process of diagnosis and treatment. Feelings of guilt and concern for the patient's children may also complicate the issue.

Diagnostic Assessment. Urinalysis shows **proteinuria** (protein in the urine) once the glomeruli are involved. **Hematuria** (blood in the urine) may be gross or microscopic. Bacteria in the urine indicate INFECTION, usually in the cysts. Obtain a urine sample for culture and sensitivity testing when there is evidence of infection. As kidney function declines, serum creatinine and blood urea nitrogen (BUN) levels rise. With decreasing kidney function, creatinine clearance decreases. Changes in kidney handling of sodium may cause either sodium losses or sodium retention.

Diagnostic studies to detect cysts include renal ultrasound, CT, and MRI.

◆ Interventions

Interventions for the patient with PKD include PAIN management and prevention of INFECTION, constipation, hypertension, and chronic kidney disease. Newer drug therapies are being evaluated to interrupt the pathways that promote malignant cyst formation such as molecular signaling for cell division or endothelial growth (Aguiari et al., 2013). When the disease progresses and the kidneys no longer function to clear wastes, care becomes similar to that needed for the patient with end-stage kidney disease (ESKD) (see Chapter 68).

Managing Pain. PAIN management strategies include drug therapy and complementary approaches. A combination may be most effective. NSAIDs are used cautiously because they can reduce kidney blood flow. Aspirin-containing compounds are avoided to reduce the risk for bleeding.

If cyst INFECTION causes discomfort, antibiotics such as trimethoprim/sulfamethoxazole (Bactrim, Septra, Trimpex) or ciprofloxacin (Cipro) are prescribed. (See Chart 66-4 in Chapter 66.) These drugs enter the cyst wall. Monitor the serum creatinine levels because antibiotic therapy can be nephrotoxic. Apply dry heat to the abdomen or flank to promote comfort when kidney cysts are infected. When PAIN is severe, cysts can be reduced by needle aspiration and drainage; however, they usually refill.

Teach the patient methods of relaxation and comfort using deep breathing, guided imagery, or other strategies. The expected outcome is patient self-management. (See Chapter 3 for pain management.)

Preventing Constipation. Teach the patient who has adequate urine output how to prevent constipation by maintaining adequate fluid intake, increasing dietary fiber when fluid intake is more than 2500 mL/24 hr, and exercising regularly. Explain that pressure on the large intestine may occur as the polycystic kidneys increase in size. The patient should know that these recommendations for bowel management might change, particularly if ESDK also develops. Advise him or her about the use of stool softeners and bulk agents, including the careful use of laxatives, to prevent chronic constipation.

Controlling Hypertension and Preventing End-Stage Kidney Disease. Blood pressure control is necessary to reduce cardiovascular complications and slow the progression of kidney dysfunction. Nursing interventions include education to promote self-management and understanding. When kidney impairment results in decreased urine concentration with nocturia and low urine specific gravity, urge the patient to drink at least 2 L of fluid per day to prevent dehydration, which can further reduce kidney function. Restricting sodium intake may help control blood pressure. See Chapter 36 for a detailed discussion about the causes and management of hypertension.

Drug therapy for blood pressure control includes antihypertensive agents and diuretics. Antihypertensive agents include angiotensin-converting enzyme (ACE) inhibitors, calcium channel blockers, beta blockers, and vasodilators (see Chapter 36). ACE inhibitors may help control the cell growth aspects of PKD and reduce microalbuminuria.

Teach the patient and family how to measure and record blood pressure. Help the patient establish a schedule for self-administering drugs, monitoring daily weights, and keeping blood pressure records (Chart 67-2). Explain the potential side effects of the drugs. Make available written materials, such as drug teaching cards and booklets.

CHART 67-2 Patient and Family Education: Preparing for Self-Management

Polycystic Kidney Disease

- Measure and record your blood pressure daily, and notify your health care provider for consistent changes in blood pressure.
- Take your temperature if you suspect you have a fever. If a fever is present, notify your physician or nurse.
- Weigh yourself every day at the same time of day and with the same amount of clothing; notify your physician or nurse if you have a sudden weight gain.
- Limit your intake of salt to help control your blood pressure.
- Notify your physician or nurse if your urine smells foul or has blood in it.
- Notify your physician or nurse if you have a headache that does not go away or if you have visual disturbances.
- Monitor bowel movements to prevent constipation.

Many patients may have salt wasting and should not follow a sodium-restricted diet. As the disease progresses, the protein intake may be limited to slow the development of ESKD. Assist the patient and family in understanding the diet plan and why it was prescribed. Work closely with the dietitian to foster the patient's understanding. Also refer the patient for nutrition counseling.

Health Care Resources

The Polycystic Kidney Research Foundation (www.pkdcure.org) and the National Kidney & Urologic Diseases Clearinghouse (NKUDIC) of the National Institute of Diabetes and Digestive and Kidney Diseases (www2.niddk.nih.gov) conduct research and provide education about PKD. Many pamphlets are available; there is a fee for some materials. Chapters of the National Kidney Foundation (NKF) and the American Association of Kidney Patients (AAKP) also have resources for information and support.

NCLEX EXAMINATION CHALLENGE

Health Promotion and Maintenance

Which statement made by the client who is newly diagnosed with polycystic kidney disease (PKD) indicates to the nurse that additional teaching for self-management is needed?
A. "I will need to increase my daily water intake."
B. "I will restrict my sodium to less than 2 g daily."
C. "Now I will need to take a blood pressure drug daily."
D. "If I become sexually active or plan to have a family, I will seek genetic counseling."

OBSTRUCTIVE DISORDERS

HYDRONEPHROSIS, HYDROURETER, AND URETHRAL STRICTURE

❖ PATHOPHYSIOLOGY

Hydronephrosis and hydroureter are problems of urine outflow obstruction. Urethral strictures also obstruct urine outflow. Prompt recognition and treatment are crucial to prevent permanent kidney damage.

In hydronephrosis, the kidney enlarges as urine collects in the renal pelvis and kidney tissue. Because the capacity of the renal pelvis is normally 5 to 8 mL, obstruction in the renal

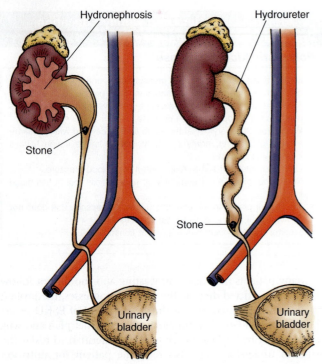

FIG. 67-4 Hydronephrosis is caused by obstruction in the upper part of the ureter. Hydroureter is caused by obstruction in the lower part of the ureter.

pelvis or at the point where the ureter joins the renal pelvis quickly distends the renal pelvis. Kidney pressure increases as the volume of urine increases. Over time, sometimes in only a matter of hours, the blood vessels and kidney tubules can be damaged extensively (Fig. 67-4).

In patients with **hydroureter** (enlargement of the ureter), the effects are similar but the obstruction is in the ureter rather than in the kidney. The ureter is most easily obstructed where the iliac vessels cross or where the ureters enter the bladder. Ureter dilation occurs above the obstruction and enlarges as urine collects (see Fig. 67-4).

In patients with a **urethral stricture**, the obstruction is very low in the urinary tract, causing bladder distention before hydroureter and hydronephrosis. The problems and kidney damage are similar without prompt treatment.

Urinary obstruction causes damage when pressure builds up directly on kidney tissue. Tubular filtrate pressure also increases in the nephron as drainage through the collecting system is impaired. With this added pressure, glomerular filtration decreases or ceases. Necrosis of the affected kidney can occur. Nitrogen waste products (urea, creatinine, and uric acid) and *electrolytes* (sodium, potassium, chloride, and phosphorus) are retained, and ACID-BASE BALANCE is impaired.

Causes of hydronephrosis or hydroureter include tumors, stones, trauma, structural defects, and fibrosis (Pengo et al., 2013). In patients with cancer, obstructed ureters may result from the tumors themselves, pelvic radiation, or surgical treatment. Early treatment of the causes can prevent hydronephrosis and hydroureter and prevent permanent kidney damage. The time needed to prevent permanent damage depends on the patient's kidney health. Permanent damage can occur in less than 48 hours in some patients and after several weeks in other patients.

❖ PATIENT-CENTERED COLLABORATIVE CARE

◆ Assessment

Obtain a history from the patient, focusing on known kidney or urologic disorders. A history of childhood urinary tract problems may indicate previously undiagnosed structural defects. Ask about his or her usual pattern of urine ELIMINATION, especially amount, frequency, color, clarity, and odor. Ask about recent flank or abdominal PAIN. Chills, fever, and malaise may be present with a urinary tract infection (UTI).

Inspect each flank to identify asymmetry, which may occur with a kidney mass, and *gently* palpate the abdomen to locate areas of tenderness. Palpate and percuss the bladder to detect distention, or use a bedside bladder scanner. Gentle pressure on the abdomen may cause urine leakage, which reflects a full bladder and possible obstruction.

Urinalysis may show bacteria or white blood cells if INFECTION is present. When urinary tract obstruction is prolonged, microscopic examination may show tubular epithelial cells. Blood chemistries are normal unless glomerular filtration has decreased. Blood creatinine and blood urea nitrogen (BUN) levels increase with a reduced glomerular filtration rate (GFR). Serum electrolyte levels may be altered with elevated blood levels of potassium, phosphorus, and calcium along with a metabolic acidosis (bicarbonate deficit).

Urinary outflow obstruction can be seen with ultrasound (US) or CT.

◆ Interventions

Urinary retention and potential for INFECTION are the primary problems. Failure to treat the cause of obstruction leads to infection and ESKD.

Urologic Interventions. If the stricture is caused by a stone, it can be located and removed using cystoscopic or retrograde urogram procedures. The urologist uses a cystoscope to guide a stone basket over the stone and removes it through the bladder. After stone removal, a plastic stent is usually left in the ureter for a few weeks to improve urine flow in the area irritated by the stone. The stent is later removed by another cystoscopic procedure.

Radiologic Interventions. When a stricture is causing hydronephrosis and cannot be corrected with urologic procedures, a **nephrostomy** is performed. Most nephrostomy drains provide only external drainage (diversion). Other styles of nephrostomy drains enter the kidney but extend to the bladder. These tubes can drain urine out to a bag or past a ureteral stricture and into the bladder, so there is both an internal and external component to the nephrostomy tubing. Externally, a fully external or an internal/external diversion drain appears the same. The urine output will fluctuate more if all urine goes to the bladder before external drainage.

Patient Preparation. If possible, the patient is kept NPO for 4 to 6 hours before the procedure. Clotting studies (e.g., international normalized ratio [INR], prothrombin time [PT], and partial thromboplastic time [PTT]) should be normal or corrected. Drugs are used to reduce hypertension. The patient receives moderate sedation for the procedure.

Procedure. The patient is placed in the prone position. The kidney is located under ultrasound or fluoroscopic guidance, and a local anesthetic is given. A needle is placed into the kidney, a soft-tipped guidewire is placed through the needle, and then a catheter is placed over the wire. The catheter tip remains in the renal pelvis, and the external end is connected to a drainage bag. The procedure immediately relieves the pressure and prevents further damage. The nephrostomy tube remains in place until the obstruction is resolved (with or without further intervention).

Follow-up Care. Assess the amount of drainage in the collection bag. The amount of drainage depends on whether a ureteral catheter is also being used (with a separate drainage bag). Patients with ureteral tubes may have all urine pass through to the bladder or may have urine drain into the collection bags. The type of urine drainage expected should be clearly communicated in the chart. If urine is expected to drain into the collection bag, assess the amount of drainage hourly for the first 24 hours. When urine drains only into the collection bag and not into the bladder, the minimum expected drainage is 30 mL/hr. If the amount of drainage decreases and the patient has back PAIN, the tube may be clogged or dislodged.

Monitor the nephrostomy site for leaking urine or blood. Urine drainage may be red-tinged for the first 12 to 24 hours after the procedure and should gradually clear. Assess the patient for manifestations of INFECTION, including fever or a change in urine character.

> **⚠ NURSING SAFETY PRIORITY** (QSEN)
>
> **Critical Rescue**
>
> After nephrostomy, notify the physician immediately when the drainage decreases or stops, drainage becomes cloudy or foul-smelling, the nephrostomy site leaks blood or urine, or the patient has back PAIN.

> **❓ NCLEX EXAMINATION CHALLENGE**
>
> **Physiological Integrity**
>
> When providing care to a client who has undergone a nephrostomy for hydronephrosis, which observation alerts the nurse to a possible complication?
> A. Urine output of 15 mL/hr
> B. Tenderness at the surgical site
> C. Blood urea nitrogen (BUN) of 23 mg/dL
> D. Pink-tinged urine draining from the nephrostomy

INFECTIOUS DISORDERS: PYELONEPHRITIS

In the healthy person, urine is normally sterile and remains sterile if there is no obstruction to urine passage in the kidney and urinary tract. When any structural abnormality is present, the risk for damage as a result of INFECTION is greatly increased. **Urinary tract infection (UTI)** is an infection in this normally sterile system. **Pyelonephritis** is a bacterial infection in the kidney and renal pelvis.

❖ PATHOPHYSIOLOGY

Pyelonephritis is either the presence of active organisms in the kidney or the effects of kidney INFECTION. **Acute pyelonephritis** is the active bacterial infection, whereas **chronic pyelonephritis** results from repeated or continued upper urinary tract infections or the effects of such infections. Chronic pyelonephritis often occurs with a urinary tract defect, with obstruction, or, most commonly, when urine refluxes from the bladder back into the ureters. **Reflux** is the reverse or upward flow of urine toward the renal pelvis and kidney.

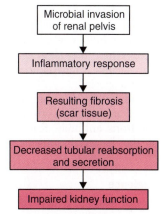

FIG. 67-5 Pathophysiology of pyelonephritis.

In pyelonephritis, organisms move up from the urinary tract into the kidney tissue. Descending infection transmitted by organisms in the blood may occur, but not often. Bacteria trigger the inflammatory response, and local edema results.

Acute pyelonephritis involves acute tissue INFLAMMATION, tubular cell necrosis, and possible abscess formation. **Abscesses**, which are pockets of INFECTION, can occur anywhere in the kidney. The infection is scattered within the kidney; healthy tissues can lie next to infected areas. Fibrosis and scar tissue develop from the inflammation. The calices thicken, and scars develop in the interstitial tissue.

Reflux of infected urine from the bladder into the ureters and kidney is responsible for most cases of chronic pyelonephritis. Reflux within the kidney can occur when some papillae in the kidney do not close properly. INFLAMMATION and fibrosis lead to deformity of the renal pelvis and calices. Repeated or continuous INFECTION creates additional scar tissue, changing blood vessel, glomerular, and tubular structure. As a result, filtration, reabsorption, and secretion are impaired and kidney function is reduced (Fig. 67-5).

Etiology and Genetic Risk

Single episodes of *acute pyelonephritis* result from bacterial INFECTION, with or without obstruction or reflux. *Chronic pyelonephritis* usually occurs with structural deformities, urinary stasis, obstruction, or reflux. Conditions that lead to urinary stasis include prolonged bedrest and paralysis. Obstruction can be caused by stones, kidney cancer, scarring from pelvic radiotherapy or surgery, recurrent infection, or injury. Reflux may occur from scarring or as a result of anatomic anomalies. Reflux also results from bladder tumor, prostate enlargement, or urinary tract stones. Reduced bladder tone from diabetic neuropathy, spinal cord injury, and neurodegenerative diseases (e.g., spina bifida, multiple sclerosis) contributes to reflux and increases the risk for pyelonephritis.

Pyelonephritis from an ascending INFECTION may follow manipulation of the urinary tract (e.g., placement of a urinary catheter), particularly in patients who are immunosuppressed or who have diabetes mellitus. In patients with chronic kidney stone disease, stones may retain organisms, resulting in ongoing infection and kidney scarring. Drug use can also contribute to pyelonephritis. In particular, high-dose or prolonged use of NSAIDs can lead to papillary necrosis and reflux.

The most common pyelonephritis-causing infecting organism is *Escherichia coli*. *Enterococcus faecalis* is common in hospitalized patients. Both organisms are in the intestinal tract. Other organisms that cause pyelonephritis in hospitalized patients include *Proteus mirabilis, Klebsiella* species, and *Pseudomonas aeruginosa.* When the INFECTION is bloodborne, common organisms include *Staphylococcus aureus* and the *Candida* and *Salmonella* species.

Other causes of kidney scarring contributing to increased risk for pyelonephritis are INFLAMMATION and inflammatory responses resulting from antibody reactions, cell-mediated immunity against the bacterial antigens, or autoimmune reactions.

Incidence and Prevalence

About 250,000 cases of acute pyelonephritis occur each year, resulting in more than 100,000 hospitalizations in the United States (U.S. Renal Data Systems, 2012). Chronic pyelonephritis is more common in women, although the exact incidence and prevalence are not known. After 65 years of age, rates of pyelonephritis for men increase greatly because of the increased incidence of prostatitis.

❖ PATIENT-CENTERED COLLABORATIVE CARE

◆ Assessment

History. Ask about a history of urinary tract INFECTIONS (UTIs), diabetes mellitus, stone disease, and defects of the genitourinary tract. Determine whether the UTIs occurred with pregnancy, and ask the patient about any previous episodes of pyelonephritis or similar problems. Ask about disease or treatment that causes immunosuppression, because they can also increase risk for pyelonephritis. Recurrences are common and may lead to a decline of kidney function. Ensure that a woman is not pregnant before radiographic imaging.

Physical Assessment/Clinical Manifestations. Ask about specific manifestations of acute pyelonephritis (Chart 67-3). Chronic pyelonephritis has a less dramatic presentation, with manifestations related to the INFECTION or reduced kidney function. Ask the patient to describe any vague urinary manifestations or abdominal discomfort. Inquire about any history of repeated low-grade fevers. Changes in urine color or odor may accompany bacteriuria. Chart 67-4 lists the kidney effects of chronic pyelonephritis.

Inspect the flanks, and gently palpate the costovertebral angle (CVA). Inspect both CVAs for enlargement, asymmetry, edema, or redness, all of which can indicate inflammation. If there is no tenderness to light palpation in either CVA, an advanced practice nurse firmly percusses each area. Tenderness or discomfort may indicate INFECTION or INFLAMMATION.

Psychosocial Assessment. The patient with any problem in the genitourinary area may have feelings of anxiety, embarrassment, or guilt. Listen carefully for signs of anxiety or specific fears, and prevent embarrassment during assessment. Feelings of guilt, often associated with sexual habits or practices, may be masked through delay in seeking treatment or through vague, nonspecific responses to specific or direct questions. Encourage patients to tell their own story in familiar, comfortable language.

Laboratory Assessment. Urinalysis shows a positive leukocyte esterase and nitrite dipstick test and the presence of white blood cells and bacteria. Occasional red blood cells, white blood cell casts, and protein may be present. The urine is cultured to determine whether gram-positive or gram-negative organisms

---

> **CHART 67-3 Key Features**
> ### Acute Pyelonephritis
>
> - Fever
> - Chills
> - Tachycardia and tachypnea
> - Flank, back, or loin pain
> - Tender costovertebral angle (CVA)
> - Abdominal, often colicky, discomfort
> - Nausea and vomiting
> - General malaise or fatigue
> - Burning, urgency, or frequency of urination
> - Nocturia
> - Recent cystitis or treatment for urinary tract infection (UTI)

> **CHART 67-4 Key Features**
> ### Chronic Pyelonephritis
>
> - Hypertension
> - Inability to conserve sodium
> - Decreased urine-concentrating ability, resulting in nocturia
> - Tendency to develop hyperkalemia and acidosis

are causing the INFECTION. The urine sample for culture and sensitivity testing, obtained by the clean-catch method, shows the bacterial species and susceptibility or resistance of the specific organism to various antibiotics. In patients with recurrent episodes of pyelonephritis or upper UTIs, more specific testing of bacterial antigens and antibodies may help determine whether the same organism is responsible for the recurrent infections.

Blood cultures are obtained for specific organisms. Other blood tests include the C-reactive protein and erythrocyte sedimentation rate to determine the presence of INFLAMMATION.

Imaging Assessment. An x-ray of the kidneys, ureters, and bladder (KUB) or CT is performed to visualize anatomy, INFLAMMATION, fluid accumulation, abscess formation, and defects in kidneys and the urinary tract. These tests also identify stones, tumors, or prostate enlargement. Urine reflux caused by incompetent bladder-ureter valve closure can be seen with a cystourethrogram. (See Chapter 65 for more information on imaging assessment.)

Other Diagnostic Assessment. Other diagnostic tests include examining antibody-coated bacteria in urine, testing for certain enzymes (e.g., lactate dehydrogenase isoenzyme 5), and radionuclide renal scan. Examining urine for antibody-coated bacteria helps identify patients who may need long-term antibiotic therapy. High-molecular-weight enzymes in urine, such as lactate dehydrogenase isoenzyme 5, are present with any kidney tissue deterioration problem and give trend data. The renal scan can identify active pyelonephritis or abscesses in or around the kidney.

◆ Analysis

The priority NANDA-I nursing diagnoses and collaborative problems for patients with pyelonephritis include:

1. Acute Pain (flank and abdominal) related to inflammation and infection (NANDA-I)
2. Potential for chronic kidney disease and end-stage kidney disease related to infectious tissue destruction

◆ *Planning and Implementation*

Managing Pain

Planning: Expected Outcomes. With proper intervention, the patient with pyelonephritis is expected to achieve an acceptable state of comfort. Indicators include that he or she often or consistently demonstrates these behaviors:

- Uses pharmacologic relief measures
- Uses NSAIDs appropriately
- Reports PAIN controlled

Interventions. Interventions may be nonsurgical or surgical. The use of several techniques that crush stones, such as lithotripsy and percutaneous ultrasonic pyelolithotomy (see Chapter 66), has decreased the need for surgery.

Nonsurgical Management. Interventions include the use of drug therapy, nutrition and fluid therapy, and teaching to ensure the patient's understanding of the treatment.

Drug therapy with antibiotics is prescribed to treat the INFECTION. At first, the antibiotics are broad spectrum. After urine and blood culture and sensitivity results are known, more specific antibiotics may be prescribed. Urinary antiseptic drugs (e.g., nitrofurantoin [Macrodantin]) may also be prescribed to provide comfort.

Nutrition therapy involves ensuring that the patient's nutrition intake has adequate calories from all food groups for healing to occur. Fluid intake is recommended at 2 L/day, sufficient to result in dilute (pale yellow) urine, unless another health problem requires fluid restriction.

Surgical Management. Surgical interventions can correct structural problems causing urine reflux or obstruction of urine outflow or can remove the source of infection.

Antibiotics are given, usually IV, to achieve adequate blood levels or sterile blood culture results. Teach the patient the nature and purpose of the proposed surgery, the expected outcome, and how he or she can participate.

The surgical procedures may be one of these: **pyelolithotomy** (stone removal from the kidney), **nephrectomy** (removal of the kidney), ureteral diversion, or reimplantation of ureter to restore proper bladder drainage.

A pyelolithotomy is needed for removal of a large stone in the kidney pelvis that blocks urine flow and causes INFECTION. Nephrectomy is a last resort when all other measures to clear the infection have failed. For patients with poor ureter valve closure or dilated ureters, **ureteroplasty** (ureter repair or revision) or ureteral reimplantation (through another site in the bladder wall) preserves kidney function and eliminates infections.

Preventing End-Stage Kidney Disease

Planning: Expected Outcomes. The patient is expected to conserve existing kidney function for as long as possible and have a slow progression to end-stage kidney disease (ESKD) once the damage has occurred. Indicators include that he or she consistently demonstrates these behaviors:

- Describes the role of antibiotics and self-administration of drugs
- Explains and offers techniques to ensure adequate nutrition and hydration
- Describes the plan for post-treatment follow-up, including knowledge of recurrent manifestations
- Modifies prescribed regimen as directed by a health care professional

Interventions. Specific antibiotics are prescribed to treat the INFECTION. Stress the importance of completing the drug therapy as directed. Discuss with the patient and family the importance of regular follow-up examinations and completing the recommended diagnostic tests.

Blood pressure control is needed to slow the progression of kidney dysfunction. When kidney impairment decreases concentrating ability, encourage the patient to drink sufficient fluid during waking hours to prevent dehydration because dehydration could further reduce kidney function. When dietary protein is restricted, refer the patient to the dietitian as needed. Other interventions related to the progression of chronic kidney disease are covered in Chapter 68.

Community-Based Care

Pyelonephritis causes fear and anxiety in the patient and family. The severity of the acute process and its potential to develop into a chronic process are frightening. The patient and the family need reassurance that treatment and preventive measures can be successful.

Home Care Management. If no surgery is performed, the patient may need help with self-care, nutrition, and drug management at home. If surgery is performed, he or she may need help with incision care, self-care, and transportation for follow-up appointments.

Self-Management Education. After assessing the patient's and family's understanding of pyelonephritis and its therapy, explain:

- Drug regimen (purpose, timing, frequency, duration, and possible side effects)
- The role of nutrition and adequate fluid intake
- The need for a balance between rest and activity, including any limitations after surgery
- The manifestations of disease recurrence
- The use of previously successful coping mechanisms

Advise the patient to complete all prescribed antibiotic regimens and to report any side effects or unusual manifestations to the health care provider rather than stopping the drugs. Refer the patient and family for nutrition counseling as needed, because many patients have special nutrition needs, such as those for diabetes or pregnancy.

Health Care Resources. The patient may also briefly need a home health care nurse to help with drug or nutrition therapy at home. Housekeeping services may be helpful while he or she is regaining strength.

◆ *Evaluation: Outcomes*

Evaluate the care of the patient with pyelonephritis based on the identified priority patient problems. Expected outcomes may include that the patient will:

- Report that PAIN is controlled
- Be knowledgeable about the disease, its treatment, and interventions to prevent or reduce disease progression

Specific indicators for these outcomes are listed for each priority patient problem in the Planning and Implementation section (see earlier).

IMMUNOLOGIC KIDNEY DISORDERS

Glomerulonephritis (GN) is the third leading cause of end-stage kidney disease (ESKD) (U.S. Renal Data Systems, 2012). Whether the disease starts in the kidney or occurs as the result of other health problems, the glomeruli are usually injured (Table 67-1). For disease that starts in the kidney, a genetic basis

TABLE 67-1 Primary Glomerular Diseases and Syndromes

- Acute glomerulonephritis
- Rapidly progressive glomerulonephritis (RPGN)
- Chronic glomerulonephritis
- Nephrotic syndrome
- Persistent, vague urinary abnormalities with few or no symptoms

TABLE 67-2 Secondary Glomerular Diseases and Syndromes

- Systemic lupus erythematosus (SLE)
- Schönlein-Henoch purpura
- Goodpasture's syndrome
- Systemic necrotizing vasculitis
- Wegener's granulomatosis
- Periarteritis nodosa (also called *polyarteritis nodosa*)
- Amyloidosis
- Diabetic glomerulopathy
- HIV-associated nephropathy
- Alport's syndrome
- Multiple myeloma
- Viral hepatitis B
- Viral hepatitis C
- Cirrhosis
- Sickle cell disease
- Nonstreptococcal postinfectious acute glomerulonephritis
- Infective endocarditis
- Hemolytic-uremic syndrome
- Thrombotic thrombocytopenic purpura

HIV, Human immune deficiency virus.

TABLE 67-3 Infectious Causes of Acute Glomerulonephritis

- Group A beta-hemolytic *Streptococcus*
- Staphylococcal or gram-negative bacteremia or sepsis
- Pneumococcal, *Mycoplasma,* or *Klebsiella* pneumonia
- Syphilis
- Visceral abscesses
- Infective endocarditis
- Hepatitis B
- Infectious mononucleosis
- Measles
- Mumps
- Rocky Mountain spotted fever
- Cytomegalovirus infection
- Histoplasmosis
- Toxoplasmosis
- Varicella
- *Chlamydia psittaci* infection
- Coxsackievirus infection
- Any bacterial, parasitic, fungal, or viral infection (potentially)

and immune-inducing INFLAMMATION problems are common. In addition, systemic diseases and INFECTIONS can have kidney effects and cause glomerular injury (Table 67-2). Conditions that lead to glomerular disease include systemic lupus erythematous and diabetic nephropathy.

Each type of disease or syndrome has a specific pathophysiology and clinical manifestations. Their *glomerular* effects are caused by injury to the glomeruli and result in proteinuria, hematuria, decreased glomerular filtration rate (GFR), edema, and hypertension. The extent and duration of kidney injury, prognosis, and specific cause vary among these syndromes.

Immunologic changes injure the glomeruli, interstitium, or tubules, and the effects may be acute or chronic. Both antibody and cellular immune responses leading to INFLAMMATION are involved. The resultant kidney disorder can be systemic or confined to the kidneys.

Most forms of INFLAMMATION-induced glomerulonephritis (GN) occur with a collection of immune complexes in the glomeruli (Fig. 20-4 in Chapter 20). An immune complex is made up of antigens (foreign substances within the body) and antibodies. The antigen can be part of any normal kidney tissue, or it can be dissolved in a body fluid (e.g., blood). Bacteria and viruses are also antigens. Exposure to bacteria, viruses, drugs, or other toxins is believed to be the trigger for glomerular injury.

Antibody reaction with antigens can cause immune complexes to form and become deposited in glomerular tissue, leading to INFLAMMATION. These complexes trigger many inflammatory mediators, such as complement, white blood cells, and blood clotting proteins, which also damage the kidney tissue. Actions that cause tissue injury include damage to cell membranes, local edema, movement of white blood cells to the site of inflammation, and platelet activation.

ACUTE GLOMERULONEPHRITIS

❖ *PATHOPHYSIOLOGY*

An INFECTION often occurs before the kidney manifestations of acute glomerulonephritis (GN). The onset of manifestations is about 10 days from the time of infection. Usually patients recover quickly and completely from acute GN. The term *acute nephritic syndrome* also describes this disorder.

Most causes of acute GN are infectious (Table 67-3) or are related to other systemic diseases (see Table 67-2). The incidence of acute GN is unknown. GN after a systemic streptococcal infection is more common in men.

❖ *PATIENT-CENTERED COLLABORATIVE CARE*

◆ *Assessment*

History. Ask about recent INFECTION, particularly of the skin or upper respiratory tract, and about recent travel or other possible exposures to viruses, bacteria, fungi, or parasites. Recent illnesses, surgery, or other invasive procedures may suggest infections. Ask about any known systemic diseases, such as systemic lupus erythematosus (SLE), which could cause acute GN.

Physical Assessment/Clinical Manifestations. Inspect the patient's skin for lesions or recent incisions, including body piercings. Assess the face, eyelids, hands, and other areas for edema because edema is present in most patients with acute GN. Assess for fluid overload and circulatory congestion that may accompany the fluid and sodium retention occurring with acute GN. Ask about any difficulty in breathing or shortness of breath. Assess for crackles in the lung fields, an S_3 heart sound (gallop rhythm), and neck vein distention.

Ask about changes in voiding patterns and any change in urine color, volume, clarity, or odor. Microscopic blood in the urine occurs, and patients often describe their urine as smoky, reddish brown, rusty, or cola colored. Ask about dysuria or oliguria. Weigh him or her to assess for fluid retention.

Take the patient's blood pressure, and compare it with the baseline blood pressure. Mild to moderate hypertension occurs with acute GN as a result of fluid and sodium retention. The patient may have fatigue, a lack of energy, anorexia, nausea, and vomiting if uremia from severe kidney impairment is present.

CONSIDERATIONS FOR OLDER ADULTS
Patient-Centered Care QSEN

The less common manifestations of acute GN are more likely to occur in older adults. Circulatory congestion often is present, causing acute GN to be easily confused with congestive heart failure (CHF). Ask any older adult with CHF about voiding patterns to determine whether the problem may be related to acute GN.

Laboratory Assessment. Urinalysis shows red blood cells (*hematuria*) and protein (*proteinuria*). An early morning specimen of urine is preferred for urinalysis because the urine is most acidic and formed elements are more intact at that time. Microscopic examination often shows red blood cell casts, as well as casts from other substances.

The glomerular filtration rate (GFR), either estimated from a single serum and urine creatinine value or measured by the 24-hour urine test for creatinine clearance, may be decreased to 50 mL/min. The older patient may have a greater decline in GFR.

A 24-hour urine collection for total protein assay is obtained. The protein excretion rate for patients with acute GN may be increased from 500 mg/24 hr to 3 g/24 hr. Serum albumin levels are decreased because of the protein lost in the urine and because of fluid retention causing dilution.

Specimens from the blood, skin, or throat are obtained for culture, if indicated. Serum creatinine and blood urea nitrogen provide information about kidney function and may be elevated, indicating impairment. Other serum tests include antistreptolysin-O titers, C3 complement levels, cryoglobulins (immunoglobulin G [IgG]), antinuclear antibodies (ANAs), and circulating immune complexes.

Antistreptolysin-O titers are increased after group A beta-hemolytic *Streptococcus* INFECTION. Complement levels are decreased when the complement system is activated. Type III cryoglobulins may be found during acute illness. ANAs suggest an autoimmune response with INFLAMMATION, and systemic lupus erythematosus (SLE) is just one possibility. Immune complexes containing IgG and C3 are often detected.

Other Diagnostic Assessment. A kidney biopsy provides a precise diagnosis of the condition, assists in determining the prognosis, and helps outline treatment (see Chapter 65). The specific tissue features are determined by light microscopy, immunofluorescent stains, and electron microscopy to identify cell type, the presence of immunoglobulins, or the type of tissue deposits.

◆ Interventions

Interventions focus on managing INFECTION, preventing complications, and providing appropriate patient education.

Managing infection as a cause of acute GN begins with appropriate antibiotic therapy. Penicillin, erythromycin, or azithromycin is prescribed for GN caused by streptococcal INFECTION. Check the patient's known allergies before giving any drug. To prevent infection spread, antibiotics for people in immediate close contact with the patient also may be prescribed. Stress personal hygiene and basic infection control principles (e.g., handwashing) to prevent spread of the organism. Teach patients the importance of completing the entire course of the prescribed antibiotic.

Preventing complications is an important nursing intervention. For patients with fluid overload, hypertension, and edema, diuretics and sodium and water restrictions are prescribed. The usual fluid allowance is equal to the 24-hour urine output plus 500 to 600 mL. Patients with oliguria usually have increased serum levels of potassium and blood urea nitrogen (BUN). Potassium and protein intake may be restricted to prevent hyperkalemia and uremia. Antihypertensive drugs may be needed to control hypertension (see Chapter 36).

Nausea, vomiting, or anorexia indicates that uremia is present. Dialysis is necessary if uremic manifestations or fluid volume excess cannot be controlled (see Chapter 68). Plasmapheresis (removal and filtering of the plasma to eliminate antibodies) also may be used (see Chapter 40).

Coordinate care to conserve patient energy. Balance activity with rest to maintain function. Relaxation techniques and participation in diversional activities can reduce emotional stress.

Preparing for self-management includes teaching the patient and family members about the purpose of prescribed drugs, the dosage and schedule, and potential adverse side effects. Ensure that they understand diet and fluid restrictions. Advise the patient to measure weight and blood pressure daily at the same time each day. Instruct him or her to notify the health care provider of any sudden increase in weight or blood pressure.

If short-term dialysis is required to control FLUID AND ELECTROLYTE BALANCE or uremic manifestations, explain peritoneal or vascular access care and dialysis schedules and routines (also see Chapter 68).

RAPIDLY PROGRESSIVE GLOMERULONEPHRITIS

Rapidly progressive glomerulonephritis (RPGN), a type of acute nephritis, is also called *crescentic glomerulonephritis* because of the presence of crescent-shaped cells in the Bowman's capsule. RPGN develops over several weeks or months and causes loss of kidney function. Patients become quite ill quickly and have manifestations of kidney impairment (hypertension, oliguria, disturbed FLUID AND ELECTROLYTE BALANCE, and uremic symptoms).

The patient may have had previous INFECTION or systemic disease, such as systemic lupus erythematosus (SLE). When associated with SLE, steroid therapy is recommended (Hahn et al., 2012). Regardless of treatment, RPGN often progresses to end-stage kidney disease (ESKD).

CHRONIC GLOMERULONEPHRITIS
❖ PATHOPHYSIOLOGY

Chronic glomerulonephritis, or *chronic nephritic syndrome,* develops over 20 to 30 years or even longer. The exact onset of the disorder is rarely identified. Often the cause of the disease is not known. Mild proteinuria and hematuria, hypertension, fatigue, and occasional edema are often the only manifestations.

Although the exact cause is not known, changes in the kidney tissue result from hypertension, INFECTION and INFLAMMATION, or poor blood flow to the kidneys. Kidney tissue atrophies, and the number of functional nephrons is greatly reduced. Biopsy in the late stages of atrophy may show glomerular changes, cell loss, protein and collagen deposits, and fibrosis of the kidney tissue. Microscopic examination shows deposits of immune complexes and inflammation.

The loss of nephrons reduces glomerular filtration. Hypertension and renal arteriolar sclerosis are often present. The glomerular damage allows proteins to enter the urine. Chronic glomerulonephritis always leads to ESKD (see Chapter 68).

❖ PATIENT-CENTERED COLLABORATIVE CARE

◆ Assessment

History. Ask about other health problems, including systemic diseases, kidney or urologic disorders, infectious diseases (e.g., streptococcal infections), and recent exposures to INFECTION. Ask about overall health status and whether increasing fatigue and lethargy have occurred.

Identify the patient's voiding pattern. Ask whether the frequency of urine ELIMINATION has increased or the quantity of urine has decreased. Ask about changes in urine color, odor, or clarity and whether dysuria or incontinence has occurred. Nocturia is a common manifestation.

Assess the patient's general comfort, and ask whether new-onset dyspnea has occurred, because fluid overload can occur with decreased urine output. Ask about and observe for changes in mental functioning (e.g., irritability, an inability to read, or incapacity during job-related functions) or disturbed concentration. Changes in memory and the ability to concentrate occur as waste products collect in the blood.

Physical Assessment/Clinical Manifestations. Assess for systemic circulatory overload. Auscultate lung fields for crackles, observe the respiratory rate and depth, and measure blood pressure and weight. Auscultate the heart for rate, rhythm, and the presence of an S_3 heart sound. Inspect the neck veins for venous engorgement, and check for edema of the feet and ankles, on the shins, and over the sacrum.

Assess for uremic manifestations, such as slurred speech, ataxia, tremors, or **asterixis** (flapping tremor of the fingers or the inability to maintain a fixed posture with the arms extended and wrists hyperextended). Inspect skin for a yellowish color, texture changes, bruises, rashes, or eruptions. Ask about itching, and document areas of dryness or any excoriation from scratching.

Diagnostic Assessment. Urine output decreases, and urinalysis shows protein, usually less than 2 g in a 24-hour collection. The specific gravity is fixed at a constant level of dilution (around 1.010) despite variable fluid intake. Red blood cells and casts may be in the urine.

The glomerular filtration rate (GFR), measured by creatinine clearance, is low. The serum creatinine level is elevated, usually greater than 6 mg/dL but may be as high as 30 mg/dL or more. The BUN is increased, often as high as 100 to 200 mg/dL.

Decreased kidney function causes disturbed FLUID AND ELECTROLYTE BALANCE. Sodium retention is common, but dilution of the plasma from excess fluid can result in a falsely normal serum sodium level (135 to 145 mEq/L) or a low sodium level (less than 135 mEq/L). When oliguria develops, potassium is not excreted and hyperkalemia occurs when levels exceed 5.4 mEq/L.

Hyperphosphatemia develops with serum levels greater than 4.7 mg/dL. Serum calcium levels are usually at the lower end of the normal range (9.0 to 10.5 mg/mL) or are slightly below normal.

Disturbances of ACID-BASE BALANCE with acidosis develop from hydrogen ion retention and loss of bicarbonate. However, there may be a decrease in serum carbon dioxide (CO_2) levels as patients breathe more rapidly to compensate for the acidosis. If respiratory compensation is present, the pH of arterial blood is between 7.35 and 7.45. A pH of less than 7.35 means that the patient's respiratory system is not completely compensating for the acidosis (see Chapter 12).

The kidneys are abnormally small on x-ray or CT. A kidney biopsy is important in the early stages of glomerulonephritis, when protein or blood is first present in the urine. Tissue changes include INFLAMMATION with a variety of cells infiltrating the glomerular tissue, deposits of immune complexes, and blood vessel sclerosis. In advanced disease, when the kidneys are small, biopsy is not usually performed.

◆ Interventions

Interventions focus on slowing the progression of the disease and preventing complications. Management consists of diet changes, fluid intake sufficient to prevent reduced blood flow to the kidneys, and drug therapy to control the problems from uremia. Eventually the patient requires dialysis or transplantation to prevent death. (Care for the patient requiring dialysis or transplantation is discussed in Chapter 68.)

NEPHROTIC SYNDROME
❖ PATHOPHYSIOLOGY

Nephrotic syndrome (NS) is a condition of increased glomerular permeability that allows larger molecules to pass through the membrane into the urine and then be excreted. This process causes massive loss of protein into the urine, edema formation, and decreased plasma albumin levels. Many agents and disorders are possible causes of NS.

The most common cause of glomerular membrane changes is an immune or inflammatory process. Defects in glomerular filtration can also occur as a result of genetic defects of the glomerular filtering system, such as Fabry disease. Altered liver activity may occur with nephrotic syndrome, resulting in increased lipid production and hyperlipidemia.

❖ PATIENT-CENTERED COLLABORATIVE CARE

The main feature of nephrotic syndrome (NS) is severe proteinuria (with more than 3.5 g of protein in a 24-hour urine sample). Patients also have low serum albumin levels of less than 3 g/dL, high serum lipid levels, fats in the urine, edema, and hypertension (Chart 67-5). Renal vein thrombosis often occurs at the same time as NS, either as a cause of the problem or as an effect. NS may progress to end-stage kidney disease (ESKD), but treatment can prevent progression in most patients.

Management varies depending on what process is causing the disorder (identified by kidney biopsy). Immunologic processes may improve with suppressive therapy using steroids and

---

CHART 67-5 Key Features

Nephrotic Syndrome

Sudden onset of these manifestations:
- Massive proteinuria
- Hypoalbuminemia
- Edema (especially facial and periorbital)
- Lipiduria
- Hyperlipidemia
- Increased coagulation
- Reduced kidney function

cytotoxic or immunosuppressive agents. Angiotensin-converting enzyme (ACE) inhibitors can decrease protein loss in the urine, and cholesterol-lowering drugs can improve blood lipid levels. Heparin may reduce vascular defects and improve kidney function. Diet changes are often prescribed. If the glomerular filtration rate (GFR) is normal, dietary intake of complete proteins is needed. If the GFR is decreased, dietary protein intake must be decreased. Mild diuretics and sodium restriction may be needed to control edema and hypertension. Assess the patient's hydration status, because vascular dehydration is common. If the plasma volume is depleted, kidney problems worsen. Acute kidney injury (AKI) may be avoided if good blood flow to the kidney is maintained.

IMMUNOLOGIC INTERSTITIAL AND TUBULOINTERSTITIAL DISORDERS

Problems can arise in the kidney tissues around the nephrons, as well as in the nephrons. These interstitial and tubulointerstitial disorders in the kidney are usually caused by immune problems and INFLAMMATION. The kidney changes may be acute or chronic. The acute effects often occur with drugs such as penicillins, cephalosporins, sulfonamides, or NSAIDs. Chronic interstitial nephritis has many causes, including NSAID use, complement activation, cyclosporin use, polycystic kidney disease, autoimmune disorders, inflammation, multiple myeloma, sickle cell disease, obstructive disorders, and radiation nephritis. Drug-induced problems often occur with a rash or an elevated eosinophil count. Fever is common in interstitial nephritis of unknown cause. Progression to ESKD occurs unless the cause is identified and removed.

DEGENERATIVE DISORDERS

Degenerative disorders that change kidney function often occur with a multisystem disorder. Many of these degenerative disorders result from changes in kidney blood vessels.

NEPHROSCLEROSIS
❖ PATHOPHYSIOLOGY

Nephrosclerosis is a problem of thickening in the nephron blood vessels, resulting in narrowing of the vessel lumens. This change decreases kidney blood flow, and the tissue is chronically hypoxic. Ischemia and fibrosis develop over time.

Nephrosclerosis occurs with hypertension, atherosclerosis, and diabetes mellitus. The more severe the hypertension, the greater the risk for severe kidney damage. Nephrosclerosis is rarely seen when blood pressure is consistently below 160/110 mm Hg. The changes caused by hypertension may be reversible or may progress to end-stage kidney disease (ESKD) within months or years. (Hypertension is the second leading cause of ESKD.)

❖ PATIENT-CENTERED COLLABORATIVE CARE

Management focuses on controlling blood pressure and reducing albuminuria to preserve kidney function. Although many antihypertensive drugs may lower blood pressure, the patient's response is important in ensuring long-term adherence to the prescribed therapy. Factors that promote adherence include once-a-day dosing, low cost, and minimal side effects.

Lack of knowledge or misinformation about hypertension poses many challenges to health care providers working with patients who have hypertension. When kidney disease occurs, adherence to therapy is even more important for preserving health.

Many drugs can control high blood pressure (see Chapter 36), and more than one agent may be needed for best control. Angiotensin-converting enzyme (ACE) inhibitors are very useful in reducing hypertension and preserving kidney function. Diuretics can maintain fluid and electrolyte balance in the presence of kidney function insufficiency. Hyperkalemia needs to be prevented when potassium-sparing diuretics, alone or in combination with other diuretics, are used to treat hypertensive patients with known kidney disease.

RENOVASCULAR DISEASE
❖ PATHOPHYSIOLOGY

Processes affecting the renal arteries may severely narrow the lumen and greatly reduce blood flow to the kidney tissues. Uncorrected renovascular disease, such as renal artery stenosis, atherosclerosis, or thrombosis, causes ischemia and atrophy of kidney tissue.

Patients with renovascular disease often have a sudden onset of hypertension, particularly in those older than 50 years. Patients with high blood pressure but with no family history of hypertension also may potentially have renal artery stenosis (RAS). RAS from atherosclerosis or blood vessel hyperplasia is the main cause of renovascular disease. Other causes include thrombosis and renal vessel aneurysms.

Atherosclerotic changes in the renal artery often occur along with sclerosis in the aorta and other vessels. Changes in the renal artery are often located where the renal artery and aorta meet. Fibrotic changes of the blood vessel wall occur throughout the length of the renal artery.

❖ PATIENT-CENTERED COLLABORATIVE CARE
◆ Assessment

Key features of renovascular disease are listed in Chart 67-6. Hypertension usually first occurs after 40 to 50 years of age, and

---

🌐 CULTURAL CONSIDERATIONS
Patient-Centered Care QSEN

Hypertension is more common in African Americans and American Indians, and the risks for ESKD from hypertension are also greater for these ethnic groups (U.S. Renal Data Systems, 2012). Between 25 and 45 years of age, the ratio of African Americans to Caucasians at risk for ESKD from hypertension is nearly 20:1. At any health care encounter with an African-American patient or an American-Indian patient, blood pressure should always be assessed. If hypertension is present, treatment and patient education can help reduce the risk for development of ESKD.

CHART 67-6 Key Features
Renovascular Disease

- Significant, difficult-to-control high blood pressure
- Poorly controlled diabetes or sustained hyperglycemia
- Elevated serum creatinine
- Decreased creatinine clearance

often the patient does not have a family history of hypertension. Diagnosis is made by magnetic resonance angiography (MRA), renal ultrasound, radionuclide imaging, or renal arteriography. MRA provides an excellent image of the renal vasculature and kidney anatomy. Radionuclide imaging is a noninvasive way of evaluating kidney blood flow and excretory function. Combining radionuclide imaging with ingestion of an angiotensin-converting enzyme (ACE) inhibitor, such as captopril, improves the accuracy of the test. A renal arteriogram makes the features of the renal blood vessels visible.

◆ Interventions

Identifying the type of defect, extent of narrowing, and condition of the surrounding blood vessels is critical for treatment choice. The patient's overall health and the size of the atrophied kidney also affect management decisions. Many patients with renovascular disease also have cardiovascular disease, and both conditions require treatment.

RAS may be managed by drugs to control blood pressure and by procedures to restore the blood supply to the kidney. Drugs may control high blood pressure but may not lead to long-term preservation of kidney function. In young and middle-aged adults, a lifetime of treatment with many drugs for high blood pressure makes treatment difficult and the outcomes uncertain.

Endovascular techniques are nonsurgical approaches to repair RAS. Stent placement with or without balloon angioplasty is an example of an endovascular intervention (see Chapter 36). After the procedure, the patient usually remains under close observation for 24 hours to monitor for sudden blood pressure fluctuations as the kidneys adjust to increased blood flow. Endovascular techniques are less risky and require less time for recovery than does renal artery bypass surgery (Escobar & Campbell, 2012).

Renal artery bypass surgery is a major procedure and requires 2 or more months for recovery. A bypass may be performed for either one or both renal arteries. A synthetic blood vessel graft is inserted to redirect blood flow from the abdominal aorta into the renal artery, beyond the area of narrowing. A splenorenal bypass can also restore blood flow to the kidney. The process is similar to other arterial bypass procedures (see Chapter 38).

DIABETIC NEPHROPATHY

❖ PATHOPHYSIOLOGY

Diabetes mellitus (DM) is the leading cause of end-stage kidney disease (ESKD) in North America (U.S. Renal Data Systems, 2012). About 36% of patients requiring dialysis or kidney transplantation have DM (U.S. Renal Data Systems, 2012). Diabetic nephropathy occurs with either type 1 or type 2 DM. Severity of diabetic kidney disease is related to the degree of hyperglycemia the patient generally experiences. With poor control of hyperglycemia, the complicating problems of atherosclerosis, hypertension, and neuropathy (which promotes loss of bladder tone, urinary stasis, and urinary tract infection) are more severe and more likely to cause kidney damage.

❖ PATIENT-CENTERED COLLABORATIVE CARE

Diabetic nephropathy is a vascular complication of diabetes. Its first manifestation is microalbuminuria, and screening for small amounts of protein in the urine should begin 5 years after the diagnosis of type 1 DM and annually after type 2 DM is diagnosed. Diabetic kidney disease is progressive.

Structural and functional changes occur in the kidneys of patients with diabetes. Initially, kidney size is slightly increased and glomerular filtration rates (GFRs) are higher than normal. Any proteinuria (albuminuria) indicates the need for aggressive treatment and a thorough diagnostic workup for comorbidities. See Chapter 64 for a detailed discussion of kidney issues in patients with diabetes.

Patients with diabetes are always considered to be at risk for ESKD. If possible, nephrotoxic agents (e.g., iodinated contrast media, aminoglycosides) and dehydration are avoided. Patients with worsening kidney function may begin to have frequent hypoglycemic episodes and a reduced need for insulin or antidiabetic agents. Explain that the kidneys metabolize and excrete insulin. When kidney function is reduced, the insulin is available for a longer time and thus less of it is needed. Some patients may believe this means their diabetes is improving with reduced insulin needs, but that is not accurate. Instead, it is an indication of worsening complications.

Desired outcomes of care to prevent the development of microalbuminuria and delay the progression to ESKD in patients with DM include:

- Achieving glycemic control (e.g., A1C <6.5%)
- Normalizing blood pressure (goal of 130/80 mm Hg or 125/75 mm Hg if proteinuria is greater than 1.0 g/24 hr and serum creatinine is greater than 1.5 mg/dL)
- Using drugs that block renin-angiotensin-aldosterone system (e.g. aldosterone)
- Treating dyslipidemia (so that the low-density lipoprotein [LDL] cholesterol is less than 100 mg/dL)

(See Chapter 64 for specific information on diabetic nephropathy.)

RENAL CELL CARCINOMA

❖ PATHOPHYSIOLOGY

Renal cell carcinoma (RCC) is the most common type of kidney cancer and is also known as *adenocarcinoma of the kidney*. As with other cancers, the healthy tissue of the kidney is damaged and replaced by cancer cells.

Systemic effects occurring with this cancer type are called *paraneoplastic syndromes* and include anemia, erythrocytosis, hypercalcemia, liver dysfunction with elevated liver enzymes, hormonal effects, increased sedimentation rate, and hypertension.

Anemia and erythrocytosis may seem confusing; however, most patients with this cancer have *either* anemia *or* erythrocytosis, not both at the same time. There is some blood loss from

TABLE 67-4	**Staging Kidney Tumors**

Stage I. Tumors up to 2.5 cm are situated within the capsule of the kidney. The renal vein, perinephric fat, and adjacent lymph nodes have no tumor.
Stage II. Tumors are larger than 2.5 cm and extend beyond the capsule but are within Gerota's fascia. The renal vein and lymph nodes are not involved.
Stage III. Tumors extend into the renal vein, lymph nodes, or both.
Stage IV. Tumors include invasion of adjacent organs beyond Gerota's fascia or metastasize to distant tissues.

Data from American Cancer Society. (2014). *Cancer facts and figures 2014.* Report No. 00-300M–No. 500814. Atlanta: Author.

hematuria, but the small amount lost does not cause anemia. The cause of the anemia and the erythrocytosis is related to kidney cell production of erythropoietin. At times, the tumor cells produce large amounts of erythropoietin, causing erythrocytosis. At other times, the tumor cells destroy the erythropoietin-producing kidney cells and anemia results.

Parathyroid hormone produced by tumor cells can cause hypercalcemia. Other hormone changes include increased renin levels (causing hypertension) and increased human chorionic gonadotropin (hCG) levels, which decrease libido and change secondary sex features.

RCC has five distinct carcinoma cell types: clear cell, papillary cell, chromophobe cell, collecting duct carcinoma, and unclassified type (Patel et al., 2012). A few RCCs are hereditary. The most well-known genetic syndrome that includes kidney cancer is von Hippel-Lindau syndrome. These cancers are highly vascular and may occur with cancers of the pancreas, central nervous system, and adrenal glands.

Kidney tumors are classified into four stages (Table 67-4). Complications include metastasis and urinary tract obstruction. The cancer usually spreads to the adrenal gland, liver, lungs, long bones, or the other kidney. When the cancer surrounds a ureter, hydroureter and obstruction may result.

The causes of nonhereditary RCC are unknown, but the risk is slightly higher for people who use tobacco or are exposed to cadmium and other heavy metals, asbestos, benzene, and trichloroethylene. Men are slightly more likely to acquire RCC, as are obese, African-American, or hypertensive people.

Kidney cancers account for about 64,000 new cases and 13,860 deaths annually in the United States (American Cancer Society [ACS], 2014). In Canada, 6000 new cases and 1750

CLINICAL JUDGMENT CHALLENGE

Safety; Patient-Centered Care QSEN

The 56-year-old African-American woman is admitted for treatment of newly diagnosed renal cell carcinoma. You find her daughter in the hallway crying. She has heard that her mother has undergone genetic testing related to her cancer diagnosis and wonders if she is at increased risk for the same condition. She was with her mother during the renal scan before admission and is also worried that this exposure to a radioactive isotope will cause cancer in her.
1. Is renal cell carcinoma commonly inherited, and why is genetic testing done?
2. Do renal scan radioisotopes require radiation precautions? Why or why not?
3. What risk factors are associated with renal cell carcinoma?
4. How can you evaluate whether your information was understood by the daughter and if follow-up is needed?

deaths from kidney cancers occur each year (Canadian Cancer Society, 2014). The 5-year survival rate is 60% in the United States. Renal cell carcinoma occurs most often in patients between 55 and 60 years of age (Patel et al., 2012).

❖ PATIENT-CENTERED COLLABORATIVE CARE

◆ Assessment

History. Ask the patient about age, known risk factors (e.g., smoking or chemical exposures), weight loss, changes in urine color, abdominal or flank discomfort, and fever. Also ask whether any other family member has ever been diagnosed with cancer of the kidney, bladder, ureter, prostate gland, uterus, ovary, or appendix.

Physical Assessment/Clinical Manifestations. Few patients with renal cell cancer have flank PAIN, obvious blood in the urine, and a kidney mass that can be palpated. Ask about the nature of the flank or abdominal discomfort. Patients often describe the pain as dull and aching. The pain may be more intense if bleeding into the tumor or kidney occurs. Inspect the flank area, checking for asymmetry or an obvious bulge. An abdominal mass may be felt through *gentle* palpation. A renal bruit may be heard on auscultation.

Bloody urine is a *late* common manifestation. Blood may be visible as bright red flecks or clots, or the urine may appear smoky or cola colored. Without gross hematuria, microscopic examination may or may not reveal red blood cells.

Inspect the skin for pallor, darkening of the nipples, and, in men, breast enlargement *(gynecomastia)* caused by changing hormone levels. Other findings may include muscle wasting, weakness, poor nutrition status, and weight loss. All tend to occur late in the disease.

Diagnostic Assessment. Urinalysis may show red blood cells. Hematologic studies show decreased hemoglobin and hematocrit values, hypercalcemia, increased erythrocyte sedimentation rate, and increased levels of adrenocorticotropic hormone (ACTH), human chorionic gonadotropin (hCG), cortisol, renin, and parathyroid hormone. Elevated serum creatinine and blood urea nitrogen (BUN) levels indicate impaired kidney function.

Kidney masses may be detected by CT scan or MRI. Ultrasound is also used to detect masses or for initial screening. Kidney biopsy may be considered to help target therapy.

◆ Interventions

Interventions focus on controlling the cancer and preventing metastasis (ACS, 2014).

Nonsurgical Management. Radiofrequency or cryo-ablation can slow tumor growth. It is a minimally invasive procedure carried out after MRI has precisely located the tumor. The procedure is used most commonly for patients who have only one kidney or who are not surgical candidates.

Chemotherapy has limited effectiveness against this cancer type. Use of biological response modifiers (BRMs) such as interleukin-2 (IL-2), interferon (INF), and tumor necrosis factor (TNF) has lengthened survival time (see Chapters 17 and 22). Newer targeted therapy agents, sorafenib (Nexavar) and temsirolimus (Torisel), were approved as treatment for patients with advanced renal cell carcinoma. Sorafenib, an oral drug taken daily, is a multikinase inhibitor that slows cancer cell division and inhibits blood vessel growth in the tumor. Temsirolimus is a weekly IV infusion that blocks a protein that is needed for cell division, inhibiting cell cycle progression. Other targeted drugs used to treat RCC are sunitinib (Sutent), everolimus (Afinitor), and pazopanib (Votrient) (Patel et al., 2012). These drugs have increased survival time of patients with advanced RCC.

Surgical Management. Renal cell carcinoma is usually treated surgically by *nephrectomy* (kidney removal). Renal cell tumors are highly vascular, and blood loss during surgery is a major concern. Before surgery, the arteries supplying the kidney may be occluded (embolized) by the interventional radiologist to reduce bleeding during nephrectomy.

Preoperative Care. Instruct the patient about surgical routines (see Chapters 14, 15, and 16). Explain the probable site of incision and the presence of dressings, drains, or other equipment after surgery. Reassure the patient about PAIN relief. Care before surgery may include giving blood and fluids IV to prevent shock.

Operative Procedures. The patient is placed on his or her side with the kidney to be removed uppermost. The trunk area is flexed to increase exposure of the kidney area. Removal of the eleventh or twelfth rib may be needed to provide better access to the kidney. The surgeon removes either part or all of the kidney and all visible tumor. The renal artery, renal vein, and fascia also may be removed after tying off the ureter. A drain may be placed in the wound before closure. The adrenal gland may be removed when the tumor is near this organ.

When a *radical* nephrectomy is performed, local and regional lymph nodes are also removed. The surgical approach may be transthoracic (as discussed in the previous paragraph), lumbar, or through the abdomen, depending on the size and location of the tumor. Radiation therapy may follow a radical nephrectomy.

Postoperative Care. Refer to Chapter 16 for care of the patient after surgery. Nursing priorities are focused on assessing kidney function to determine effectiveness of the remaining kidney, PAIN management, and preventing complications.

Monitoring includes assessing for hemorrhage and adrenal insufficiency. Inspect the patient's abdomen for distention from bleeding. Check the bed linens under the patient, because blood may pool there. Hemorrhage or adrenal insufficiency causes hypotension, decreased urine output, and an altered level of consciousness.

A decrease in blood pressure is an early indication of both hemorrhage and adrenal insufficiency. With hypotension, urine output also decreases immediately. Large water and sodium losses in the urine occur in patients with adrenal insufficiency. As a result, a large urine output is followed by hypotension and oliguria (less than 400 mL/24 hr or less than 25 mL/hr). IV replacement of fluids and packed red blood cells may be needed.

The second kidney is expected to provide adequate function, but this may take days or weeks. Assess urine output hourly for the first 24 hours after surgery (urine output of 0.5 mL/kg/hr or about 30 to 50 mL/hr is acceptable). A low urine output of less than 25 to 30 mL/hr suggests decreased blood flow to the remaining kidney and potential for acute kidney injury (AKI). The hemoglobin level, hematocrit values, and white blood cell count may be measured every 6 to 12 hours for the first day or two after surgery.

Monitor the patient's temperature, pulse rate, and respiratory rate at least every 4 hours. Accurately measure and record fluid intake and output. Weigh the patient daily.

The patient may be in a special care unit for 24 to 48 hours after surgery for monitoring of bleeding and adrenal insufficiency. A drain placed near the site of incision removes residual fluid. Because of the discomfort of deep breathing, the patient is at risk for atelectasis. Fever, chills, thick sputum, or decreased breath sounds suggest pneumonia.

Managing PAIN after surgery usually requires opioid analgesics (e.g., hydromorphone [Dilaudid] and morphine [Statex ✚]) given intravenously. The incision was made through major muscle groups used with breathing and movement. Liberal use of analgesics is needed for 3 to 5 days after surgery to manage pain. Oral agents may be tried when the patient can eat and drink.

Preventing complications focuses on INFECTION and management of adrenal insufficiency. Antibiotics may be prescribed during and after surgery to prevent infection. The need for additional antibiotics is based on evidence of infection. Assess the patient at least every 8 hours for manifestations of systemic infection or local wound infection.

Adrenal insufficiency is possible as a complication of kidney and adrenal gland removal. Although only one adrenal gland may be affected, the remaining gland may not be able to secrete sufficient glucocorticoids immediately after surgery. Steroid replacements may be needed in some patients. Chapter 62 discusses the manifestations of acute adrenal insufficiency in detail along with specific nursing interventions.

KIDNEY TRAUMA

❖ PATHOPHYSIOLOGY

Trauma to one or both kidneys is a concern in penetrating wounds or blunt injuries to the back, flank, or abdomen. Another cause of kidney trauma is iatrogenic from urologic procedures, extracorporeal shock wave lithotripsy, kidney biopsy, or percutaneous renal procedures. Blunt trauma accounts for most kidney injuries. Kidney injury has been classified into five grades based on the severity of the injury. Grade one consists of low-grade injury in the form of kidney bruising, and grade five represents the most severe trauma associated with shattering of the kidney and tearing its blood supply. Anyone can suffer kidney trauma. Strategies to prevent trauma are reviewed in Chart 67-7.

❖ PATIENT-CENTERED COLLABORATIVE CARE

◆ Assessment

Obtain a history of the patient's usual health and the events involved in the trauma from the patient, a witness, or

---

CHART 67-7   **Patient and Family Education: Preparing for Self-Management**
Preventing Kidney and Genitourinary Trauma
• Wear a seat belt.   • Practice safe walking habits.   • Use caution when riding bicycles and motorcycles.   • Wear appropriate protective clothing when participating in contact sports.   • Avoid all contact sports and high-risk activities if you have only one kidney.

emergency personnel. Documenting the mechanism of injury can help the provider determine the severity of the injury. For example, most blunt trauma from car crashes has low severity. Critical information to acquire is a history of kidney or urologic disease, surgical intervention, or health problems such as diabetes mellitus or hypertension.

Ureteral or renal pelvic injury often causes diffuse abdominal PAIN. Urine outside of the urinary tract may be visible. Ask the patient about pain in the flank or abdomen. Is the pain dull? Sharp? Constant? Intermittent? Made worse by coughing?

Patients with kidney injuries should be assessed with initial attention to the basic ABCDEs outlined in Advanced Trauma Life Support protocols. Take the patient's blood pressure, apical and peripheral pulses, respiratory rate, and temperature. Inspect both flanks for bruising, asymmetry or penetrating injuries. Also inspect the abdomen, chest, and lower back for bruising or penetrating wounds. Percuss the abdomen for distention. Inspect the urethra for blood.

Urinalysis shows hemoglobin or red blood cells from tissue damage or kidney blood vessel rupture. Microscopic examination may also show red blood cell casts, which suggest tubular damage. Hemoglobin and hematocrit values decrease with blood loss (see discussion of shock in Chapter 37).

Diagnostic procedures include ultrasound and CT. CT scan shows greater detail about blood vessel and tissue integrity. Hematomas within or through the kidney capsule can be seen, along with the integrity and patency of the urinary tract. If the patient is being taken to the operating room emergently, a one-shot high dose of ionic or nonionic IV contrast dye can be given, followed by an abdominal x-ray (KUB) to visualize the traumatic injury and any organ damage.

◆ Interventions

Nonsurgical Management. *Drug therapy* is used for bleeding prevention or control. The need for clotting factors, vitamin K, and platelets is assessed, and they are given as needed.

Fluid therapy is given to restore circulating blood volume and ensure adequate blood flow to the kidneys. Crystalloid solutions replace water and some electrolytes and include 0.9% sodium chloride (normal saline solution [NSS]), 5% dextrose in 0.45% sodium chloride, and lactated Ringer's solution. When bleeding is extensive, packed red blood cell replacement restores hemoglobin and promotes oxygenation. Fresh frozen plasma or clotting factors may help with uncontrolled bleeding. Plasma volume expanders, such as dextran or albumin, help restore plasma oncotic pressure and reduce the onset or severity of shock or fluid displacement to interstitial tissues.

During fluid restoration, give fluids at the prescribed rate and monitor the patient for indications of shock. Take vital signs as often as every 5 to 15 minutes. Measure and record urine output hourly. Output should be greater than 0.5 mL/kg/hr.

The interventional radiologist may use percutaneous or other instrumentation to drain collections of fluid or to embolize (clot) an artery or artery segment or place a stent to repair the urethra or ureters.

! NURSING SAFETY PRIORITY (QSEN)
Action Alert

If the urethral opening is bleeding, consult with the physician before attempting urinary catheterization.

Surgical Management. Most kidney injuries are managed without surgery. Many serious injuries can be treated with minimally invasive techniques such as angiographic embolization, which accesses the arteries of the kidneys through large blood vessels in the groin, similar to a cardiac catheterization. Surgery to explore the injured kidney occurs when the patient is hemodynamically unstable and appears to be losing a lot of blood from the kidney. Patients with other significant abdominal injuries, such as injuries to the bowel, spleen, or liver, who require a laparotomy may also undergo inspection and repair of the injured kidney at the same time. The aim of surgical management is to repair the injured kidney. However, if the kidney is severely injured (usually Grade 5 injury), the surgeon performs a nephrectomy.

Community-Based Care

Teach the patient and family how to assess for INFECTION and other complications following kidney trauma. The most common complications are urine leakage and delayed bleeding. Instruct the patient to check the pattern and frequency of urine ELIMINATION and to note whether the color, clarity, and amount appear normal. The development of an abscess surrounding the kidney also can occur. Instruct the patient to seek medical attention for worsening hematuria, a worrisome change, or PAIN with voiding. Chills, fever, lethargy, and cloudy, foul-smelling urine indicate a urinary tract INFECTION or abscess formation. Traumatic kidney injury can also cause hypertension from changes in perfusion and activation of the renin-angiotensin-aldosterone system (see Chapter 65 and Fig. 65-5). Advise the patient to seek medical care promptly for all new and concerning manifestations.

NURSING CONCEPTS AND CLINICAL JUDGMENT REVIEW

What might you NOTICE if the patient is experiencing problems with urinary ELIMINATION as a result of acute pyelonephritis?

- Patient urinates frequently in small amounts.
- Patient reports pain and burning on urination.
- Patient reports back or flank pain.
- Urine is cloudy and foul-smelling
- Urine may be darker or smoky or have obvious blood in it.

What should you INTERPRET and how should you RESPOND to a patient experiencing problems with urinary ELIMINATION as a result of acute pyelonephritis?

Perform and interpret physical assessment, including:

- Asking how long manifestations have been present
- Asking about low back (midline in men) or flank pain

- Asking whether he or she has had a UTI in the past; how long ago; how it was treated; and if, antibiotics were prescribed, whether the drug course was completed
- Asking about the presence of pregnancy or any chronic health problem, especially diabetes
- Asking about any nausea or vomiting and its duration
- Determining fluid intake and output volumes
- Assessing for pain over the right and left kidneys
- Weighing the patient, and asking whether this weight is more or less than his or her usual weight
- Assessing for fever and chills
- Assessing for tachycardia
- Interpreting laboratory values:
  - Is the complete blood count with differential elevated?
  - Are the BUN and serum creatinine levels elevated?

- Is the urinalysis positive for bacteria, leukocyte esterase, nitrate, red blood cells, white blood cells, or casts?

Respond by:
- Providing for pain control
- Teaching the patient the importance of completing the prescribed antibiotic drug regimen

On what should you REFLECT?
- Observe patient for evidence of improved urinary output (see Chapter 65).
- Think about what may have caused this infection and what steps could be taken to prevent a similar episode.
- Think about what patient teaching focus could help reduce the risk for future pyelonephritis and its complications.

GET READY FOR THE NCLEX® EXAMINATION!

KEY POINTS

Review these Key Points for each NCLEX Examination Client Needs Category.

Safe and Effective Care Environment
- Report immediately any condition that obstructs urine flow. **Safety** QSEN
- Check the blood pressure and urine output frequently in patients who have any type of kidney problem.
- Report immediately to the health care provider any sudden decrease of urine output in a patient with kidney disease or kidney trauma. In general, adult urine output expectations are 0.5-1 mL/kg/hr. **Safety** QSEN

Health Promotion and Maintenance
- Encourage patients with diabetes to achieve tight glycemic control.
- Encourage patients with hypertension to follow their treatment regimens to maintain blood pressure within the target range.
- Teach patients at risk for urinary tract INFECTION (UTI) to maintain a daily fluid intake of 2 L unless another health problem requires fluid restriction.
- Teach patients on antibiotic therapy for a UTI to complete the drug regimen. **Evidence-Based Practice** QSEN
- Teach all people strategies to prevent kidney trauma.

Psychosocial Integrity
- Allow the patient the opportunity to express fear or anxiety regarding the potential for chronic kidney disease and end-stage kidney disease. **Patient-Centered Care** QSEN

- Assess the patient's level of comfort in discussing issues related to ELIMINATION and the genitourinary area.
- Use language the patient is comfortable with during assessment of the kidney and urinary system. **Patient-Centered Care** QSEN
- Explain treatment procedures to patients and families.
- Refer patients with polycystic kidney disease to a geneticist or a genetic counselor.
- Refer patients to community resources, support groups, and information organizations such as the National Kidney Foundation, the Polycystic Kidney Disease Foundation, and the American Association of Kidney Patients.

Physiological Integrity
- Instruct patients with any type of kidney problem to weigh daily and to notify their health care provider if there is a sudden weight gain. **Patient-Centered Care** QSEN
- Teach patients the expected side effects and any adverse reactions to prescribed drugs, especially as they relate to kidney function.
- Teach patients the manifestations of disease recurrence and when to seek medical help.
- Explain the genetics of autosomal dominant polycystic kidney disease.
- Use laboratory data and clinical manifestations to determine the effectiveness of therapy for pyelonephritis.
- Be aware of the clinical manifestations of hydronephrosis.
- Be aware of the relationship between hypertension and kidney disease.

CHAPTER 68

Care of Patients with Acute Kidney Injury and Chronic Kidney Disease

Chris Winkelman

 http://evolve.elsevier.com/Iggy/

PRIORITY CONCEPTS

- ELIMINATION
- ACID-BASE BALANCE
- FLUID AND ELECTROLYTE BALANCE

- INFECTION
- INFLAMMATION
- PERFUSION

LEARNING OUTCOMES

Safe and Effective Care Environment

1. Collaborate with members of the health care team to reduce patient risk for kidney INFLAMMATION, kidney INFECTION, and acute kidney injury (AKI).
2. Implement interventions to protect patients with chronic kidney disease (CKD) from related systemic complications that affect ELIMINATION, FLUID AND ELECTROLYTE BALANCE, and ACID-BASE BALANCE.
3. Implement interventions to maintain patency of hemodialysis or peritoneal access when this renal replacement therapy occurs.

Health Promotion and Maintenance

4. Assess risk for AKI in patients with hemodynamic instability.
5. Collaborate with the patient and health care team to promote adequate nutrition and FLUID AND ELECTROLYTE BALANCE when AKI or CKD is diagnosed.
6. Teach transplant recipients and their families about the importance of adhering to anti-rejection therapy.

Psychosocial Integrity

7. Promote communication about patient preferences and values to plan care related to treatment for kidney failure.
8. Teach patients to use *high-quality* community resources for self-management.

Physiological Integrity

9. Compare the pathophysiology and causes of AKI with those of CKD.
10. Establish priorities in the care of patients with AKI and CKD.
11. Discuss interventions to prevent AKI.
12. Discuss the mechanisms of peritoneal dialysis (PD) and hemodialysis (HD) as renal replacement therapies.
13. Coordinate nursing care for the patient with CKD or end-stage kidney disease (ESKD).
14. Prioritize nursing care for the patient who receives a kidney transplant.

The loss of kidney function affects the ability to maintain normal processes of urinary ELIMINATION, FLUID AND ELEC-TROLYTE BALANCE, and ACID-BASE BALANCE. Kidney function loss also interrupts the activity of every organ system, particularly the immune, endocrine, skeletal, and cardiovascular systems. Acute kidney injury (AKI) is most common in the acute care setting, whereas chronic kidney disease (CKD) is more likely to be seen in community settings or as a co-existing condition in acute care settings. The characteristics of AKI and CKD are described in Table 68-1.

Both types of kidney dysfunction can result in end-stage kidney disease (ESKD), requiring renal replacement therapy (e.g., dialysis) or kidney transplant. ESKD reduces independence, shortens life, and decreases quality of life. Many diseases and conditions are associated with the onset and severity of kidney function loss.

As described in Chapter 65, kidney functions include excretion of waste, FLUID AND ELECTROLYTE BALANCE, regulation of ACID-BASE BALANCE, and hormone secretion. When kidney function declines gradually, it is diagnosed as CKD, also known as *chronic renal failure (CRF)*. The patient may have many years of abnormal serum blood urea nitrogen and creatinine values, sometimes called *renal insufficiency,* before the uremia of ESKD develops. During this time of decreased kidney function, the patient may also experience acute kidney injury (AKI). The combination of AKI and CKD, called *acute-on-chronic kidney injury,* can accelerate loss of kidney function. Low nephron numbers from CKD contribute to the progression of kidney disease (Taal et al., 2012).

When kidney decline is sudden, the functioning nephrons are overworked and kidney failure may develop with the loss of only 50% of functioning nephrons. Acute kidney injury affects

TABLE 68-1   Characteristics of Acute Kidney Injury and Chronic Kidney Disease

CHARACTERISTIC	ACUTE KIDNEY INJURY	CHRONIC KIDNEY DISEASE
Onset	Sudden (hours to days)	Gradual (months to years)
% of nephron involvement	50%-95%	Varies by stage; generally symptomatic with 75% loss and dialysis with 90%-95% loss
Duration	May not progress; full recovery (return to baseline) possible ESKD occurs in 10%-20% with lifetime reliance on dialysis or kidney transplant	Progressive and permanent Treatment and lifestyle can slow progression and delay onset of ESKD
Prognosis	Good when kidney function is maintained or returns High mortality associated with renal replacement therapy requirements of prolonged illness	Fatal without a renal replacement therapy (dialysis or transplantation) Reduced life span and potential for complex medical regimen even with optimal treatment

ESKD, End-stage kidney disease.

TABLE 68-2   The RIFLE and KDIGO Classification Systems for Severity and Outcomes of Acute Kidney Injury

	GLOMERULAR FILTRATION RATE (GFR)* CRITERIA	URINE OUTPUT CRITERIA
RIFLE Classification		
Risk stage	Serum creatinine increased × 1.5 or GFR decrease >25%	<0.5 mL/kg/hr for ≥6 hr
Injury stage	Serum creatinine increased × 2 or GFR decrease >50%	<0.5 mL/kg/hr for ≥12 hr
Failure stage	Serum creatinine increased × 3 or GFR decrease ≥75% or an absolute serum creatinine ≥354 µmol/L with an acute rise ≥4 µmol/L	<0.3 mL/kg/hr for ≥24 hr or anuria for ≥12 hr
Outcome: **L**oss	Persistent acute kidney injury (AKI), requiring renal replacement therapy for >4 wk	
Outcome: **E**nd-stage kidney disease	Requiring dialysis >3 mo	
KDIGO Classification		
Stage 1	Serum creatinine increased × 1.5-1.9 baseline or by ≥26.2 µmol/L	<0.5 mL/kg/hr for 6-12 hr
Stage 2	Serum creatinine increased × 2-2.9 baseline	<0.5 mL/kg/hr for ≥12 hr
Stage 3	Serum creatinine increased × 3 baseline or serum creatinine ≥354 µmol/L with an acute rise ≥44 µmol/L or initiation of renal replacement therapy	<0.3 mL/kg/hr for ≥24 hr or anuria for ≥12 hr

RIFLE, **R**isk, **I**njury, **F**ailure, **L**oss, **E**nd-Stage Kidney Failure; *KDIGO*, **K**idney **D**isease: **I**mproving **G**lobal **O**utcomes
*GFR must be directly measured, not estimated (Chapter 65 describes serum and urine measurement of GFR).

many body systems. Chronic kidney disease affects *every* body system. The problems that occur with kidney function loss are related to disturbances of FLUID AND ELECTROLYTE BALANCE, disturbances of ACID-BASE BALANCE, buildup of nitrogen-based wastes, and loss of kidney hormone function.

When kidney function declines to the point that the kidneys can no longer maintain homeostasis by urine ELIMINATION, renal replacement therapy is needed to prevent death from life-threatening consequences.

ACUTE KIDNEY INJURY

Pathophysiology

Acute kidney injury (AKI) has now replaced the older terminology of *acute renal failure*. AKI is a rapid reduction in kidney function resulting in a failure to maintain FLUID AND ELECTROLYTE BALANCE and ACID-BASE BALANCE. AKI occurs over a few hours or days. Most experts described AKI as one of three classes (risk, injury, and failure or Stages 1, 2, and 3 [Table 68-2]). One expert group also describes two outcomes (loss of function and end-stage kidney disease [ESKD]) following AKI. Severity of AKI is based on increases in serum creatinine and decreased urine output. Although glomerular filtration rate (GFR) is accepted as the best overall indicator of kidney function, it is not measured during acute and critical illness (Puzantian & Townsend, 2013). GFR represents the sum filtration rate of all functional nephrons. Estimations of GFR from serum creatinine are not considered accurate during critical illness. Values from direct measurements can be altered during acute and critical illness when diuretics or IV fluids are used (Moore et al., 2012; Puzantian & Townsend, 2013). Direct

measurement of GFR uses a 24-hour urinary creatinine analysis or the clearance of IV-administered markers like inulin, nonradioactive contrast agents or radioisotope compounds.

AKI not only affects kidney function but also causes systemic effects and complications described in Table 68-3. These complications increase discomfort and risk for death in the patient with new AKI. Duration of oliguria or anuria is closely correlated with lack of recovery of kidney function; the longer the duration of oliguria or anuria, the less likely the patient will return to full or baseline kidney function (Davies & Leslie, 2012).

Etiology

The causes of AKI are reduced PERFUSION to the kidneys, damage to kidney tissue, and obstruction. Diseases and conditions associated with reduced kidney PERFUSION, kidney damage, and urinary obstruction are listed in Table 68-4. (The diseases in Table 68-3 are described elsewhere in this text.) Notice that several conditions resulting in AKI are listed more than once in Table 68-4. For example, coagulopathy (disorders of bleeding and clotting; see Chapter 40) reduces perfusion, causes INFLAMMATION and direct tissue damage, and creates obstruction of urinary flow. Coagulopathy causes prerenal, intrarenal, and postrenal AKI.

TABLE 68-3 **Complications from Acute Kidney Injury**	
Metabolic	**Gastrointestinal**
• Metabolic acidosis	• Nausea
• Hyperkalemia	• Vomiting
• Hyponatremia	• Decreased peristalsis
• Hypocalcemia	• Enteral nutrition intolerance
• Hypophosphatemia	• Malnutrition
	• Ulcer formation
	• Bleeding
Cardiopulmonary	
• Peripheral and pulmonary edema	**Hematologic**
• Heart failure	• Bleeding
• Pulmonary embolism	• Thrombosis
• Pericarditis	• Anemia
• Pericardial effusion	
• Hypertension	**Renal**
• Myocardial infarction	• Permanent kidney damage
	• Chronic kidney disease (CKD)
Neurologic	• End-stage kidney disease (ESKD)
• Neuromuscular irritability or weakness	
• Asterixis	**Other**
• Seizures	• Hiccups
• Mental status changes	• Elevated parathyroid hormone
	• Low thyroid hormone
Immune/Infectious	
• Pneumonia	
• Sepsis	

TABLE 68-4 Diseases and Conditions that Contribute to Acute Kidney Injury

Perfusion Reduction (Prerenal Causes)
- Blood or fluid loss (e.g., surgery or trauma; hemorrhagic or hypovolemic shock)
- Blood pressure drugs resulting in hypotension
- Heart attack or heart failure resulting in low ejection fraction and low cardiac output
- Infection (e.g., sepsis, septic shock)
- Liver failure
- Use of aspirin, ibuprofen (e.g., Advil, Motrin IB), naproxen (e.g., Aleve), or NSAIDs
- Severe allergic reaction (anaphylaxis)
- Severe burns
- Severe dehydration
- Renal artery stenosis
- Bleeding or clotting in the kidney blood vessels (coagulopathy)
- Atherosclerosis or cholesterol deposits that block blood flow in the kidneys

Kidney Damage (Intrinsic or Intrarenal Causes)
- Glomerulonephritis or inflammation of the glomeruli
- Bleeding in the kidney
- Thrombi or emboli in the kidney blood vessels
- Hemolytic uremic syndrome, a condition of premature destruction of red blood cells caused by infection
- Systemic infection (sepsis)
- Local infection (pyelonephritis)
- Lupus, an immune system disorder causing glomerulonephritis
- Drugs, such as certain chemotherapy agents, antibiotics, dyes used during imaging tests (contrast-induced nephropathy), many antibiotics, and zoledronic acid (Reclast, Zometa), used to treat osteoporosis and high blood calcium levels (hypercalcemia)
- Multiple myeloma, a cancer of the plasma cells
- Scleroderma, a group of rare diseases affecting the skin and connective tissues
- Thrombotic thrombocytopenic purpura (TTP), a rare platelet disorder that increases clotting
- Ingested toxins, such as alcohol, heavy metals, and cocaine
- Vasculitis, an inflammation of blood vessels
- Ischemia in kidney tissue, including hypoxemia from respiratory and cardiac arrest

Urine Flow Obstruction (Postrenal Causes)
- Bladder cancer
- Cervical cancer
- Colon cancer
- Prostate cancer
- Enlarged prostate (prostate hypertrophy)
- Kidney stones (nephrolithiasis and ureterolithiasis)
- Nerve damage involving the nerves that control the bladder (neurogenic bladder)
- Blood clots in the urinary tract

AKI is more likely to occur in hospitalized adults who are older or who have pre-existing hypertension, diabetes, peripheral vascular disease, liver disease, or chronic kidney disease (CKD). Prolonged mechanical ventilation (see Chapter 32) also is an independent risk factor for the development of AKI (Akker et al., 2013).

Traditionally, AKI caused by reduced PERFUSION is classed as **prerenal failure**. It is the most common cause of AKI in acute care. Damage to kidney tissue is classed as **intrarenal** or **intrinsic renal failure** and reflects injury to the glomeruli, nephrons, or tubules. Obstruction of urine flow is also called **postrenal failure**. Although the usefulness of this classification system is a source of controversy, it does provide a framework to guide care for both prevention and treatment of AKI (Fournir, 2013). When AKI occurs in patients who already have CKD, it is called **acute-on-chronic kidney disease**. Any of these conditions can occur together such as acute prerenal and intrarenal failure occurring in someone who already has CKD. Multiple pathologies are more likely to result in end-stage kidney disease (ESKD).

With prerenal or postrenal pathology, the kidney compensates by the three responses of constricting kidney blood vessels, activating the renin-angiotensin-aldosterone pathway, and releasing antidiuretic hormone (ADH). These responses increase blood volume and improve kidney PERFUSION. However, these same responses reduce urine volume, resulting in **oliguria** (urine output less than 400 mL/day) and **azotemia** (the retention and buildup of nitrogenous wastes in the blood). Toxins can also cause blood vessel constriction in the kidney, leading to reduced kidney blood flow, oliguria, and azotemia.

INFLAMMATION, INFECTION, and damage from toxins (Table 68-5) cause intracellular changes of the tubular system in kidney tissue. Immune-mediated complexes can also damage nephrons. With extensive tubular damage, tubular cells slough and

nephrons lose the ability to repair themselves. The presence of tubular debris and sediment in urine from kidney tissue damage (intrarenal failure) is sometimes termed *acute tubular necrosis*. This term is no longer favored because supportive evidence is limited for the pathologic processes and clinical diagnosis (Moore et al., 2012).

Even with severe AKI, categorized as loss of function ("L" in *RIFLE* or stage 2 in *KDIGO* in Table 68-2), some people have return of kidney function. It is the responsibility of all health care professionals to be alert to the possibility of AKI and implement prevention strategies when risk factors are present. *Timely implementation of interventions to remove the cause of AKI may*

TABLE 68-5   Examples of Potentially Nephrotoxic Substances

Drugs

Antibiotics/Antimicrobials
- Amphotericin B
- Colistimethate
- Methicillin
- Polymyxin B
- Rifampin
- Sulfonamides
- Tetracycline hydrochloride
- Vancomycin

Aminoglycoside Antibiotics
- Gentamicin
- Kanamycin
- Neomycin
- Netilmicin sulfate
- Tobramycin

Chemotherapy agents
- Cisplatin
- Cyclophosphamide
- Methotrexate

Nonsteroidal Anti-inflammatory Drugs (NSAIDs)
- Celecoxib
- Flurbiprofen
- Ibuprofen
- Indomethacin
- Ketorolac
- Meclofenamate
- Meloxicam
- Nabumetone
- Naproxen
- Oxaprozin
- Rofecoxib
- Tolmetin

Other Drugs
- Acetaminophen
- Captopril
- Cyclosporine
- Fluorinate anesthetics
- Metformin
- D-Penicillamine
- Phenazopyridine hydrochloride
- Quinine

Other Substances

Organic Solvents
- Carbon tetrachloride
- Ethylene glycol

Non-drug Chemical Agents
- Radiographic contrast dye (e.g., iodinated dyes, high-osmolar dyes, and gadolinium)
- Pesticides
- Fungicides
- Myoglobin (from breakdown of skeletal muscle)

Heavy Metals and Ions
- Arsenic
- Bismuth
- Copper sulfate
- Gold salts
- Lead
- Mercuric chloride

and correction of problems causing reduced kidney blood flow often restore function before tissue damage can occur. Evaluate the patient's fluid status. Accurately measure intake and output and check body weight to identify changes in fluid balance. Note the characteristics of the urine, and report new sediment, hematuria (smoky or red color), foul odor, or other worrisome changes. It is important to immediately report to the health care provider a urine output of less than 0.5 mL/kg/hr that persists for more than 2 hours. Some experts suggest that 0.3 mL/kg/hr for more than 2 hours should be reported (Ralib et al., 2013). Waiting for 6 hours of oliguria to meet RIFLE criteria may promote kidney damage—act early!

! NURSING SAFETY PRIORITY (QSEN)
Critical Rescue

In any acute care setting, preventing volume depletion and providing intervention early when volume depletion occurs are nursing priorities. Reduced PERFUSION from volume depletion is a common cause of AKI. Recognize the manifestations of volume depletion (low urine output, decreased systolic blood pressure, decreased pulse pressure, orthostatic hypotension, thirst, rising blood osmolarity). Intervene early with oral fluids, or in the patient who is unable to take or tolerate oral fluid, request an increase in IV fluid rate from the health care provider to prevent permanent kidney damage.

Monitor laboratory values for any changes that reflect poor kidney function. A clinically significant increase in creatinine, especially when the increase occurs over hours or a few days, is a concern and should be reported urgently to the health care providers. Other laboratory values that help monitor kidney function include serum blood urea nitrogen (BUN); serum potassium, sodium, and osmolarity; and urine specific gravity and electrolytes.

Be aware of nephrotoxic substances that the patient may ingest or be exposed to (see Table 68-5). Question any prescription for potentially nephrotoxic drugs, and validate the dose before the patient receives the drug. Many antibiotics have nephrotoxic side effects. NSAIDs can cause or increase the risk for AKI. Combining two or more nephrotoxic drugs dramatically increases the risk for AKI. If a patient must receive a known nephrotoxic drug, closely monitor laboratory values, including BUN, creatinine, and drug peak and trough levels, for indications of reduced kidney function. When nephrotoxic agents are used, nephrons may be protected by administering a pretreatment oral or IV bolus of fluid volume.

prevent ESKD and need for lifelong renal replacement therapy or a renal transplant.

Incidence and Prevalence

The reported prevalence of AKI from United States data ranges from 1% (community-acquired) up to 7.1% (hospital-acquired) of all hospital admissions. As many as 30% of patients admitted to an ICU experience an episode of AKI (Fournir, 2013). Transient azotemia and oliguria occur in as many as 40% of all inpatients (Uchino et al., 2010). AKI is associated with an in-hospital and 1-year mortality rate of up to 60% (Ralib et al., 2013).

Health Promotion and Maintenance

Keep in mind that severe blood volume depletion can lead to kidney injury even in people who have no known kidney problems. Urge all healthy people to avoid dehydration by drinking 2 to 3 L of water daily. This is especially important for athletes or any person who performs strenuous exercise or work and sweats heavily.

Nurses have an essential role in the prevention of AKI in hospitalized patients. Always be on the lookout for signs of impending kidney dysfunction through physical assessment and close monitoring of laboratory values. Early recognition

❖ PATIENT-CENTERED COLLABORATIVE CARE
◆ Assessment

History. The accurate diagnosis of AKI, including its cause, depends on a detailed history. Ask the patient about recent surgery or trauma, transfusions, or other factors that might lead to reduced kidney blood flow. Obtain a drug history, especially treatment with antibiotics and NSAIDs. Ask about recent imaging procedures requiring injection of a contrast dye. Coexisting conditions of advanced age, diabetes mellitus, long-term hypertension, systemic lupus erythematosus, major or systemic INFECTION (sepsis), systemic INFLAMMATION from any cause, and coagulopathy or treatment for bleeding or clotting disorders increase the risk for AKI.

CHART 68-1 Laboratory Profile		

Kidney Disease

TEST	NORMAL RANGE FOR ADULTS	VALUES IN KIDNEY DISEASE
Serum creatinine	*Male:* 0.6-1.2 mg/dL *Female:* 0.5-1.1 mg/dL *Older adults:* Decreased	**In Chronic Kidney Disease** May increase by 0.5-1.0 mg/dL every 1-2 yr May be as high as 15-30 mg/dL *before* manifestations of severe CKD are present **In Acute Kidney Injury** Increase of 1-2 mg/dL every 24-48 hr May increase 1-6 mg/dL in 1 wk or less
Blood urea nitrogen	10-20 mg/dL *Older adults:* May be slightly increased	**In Chronic Kidney Disease** May reach 180-200 mg/dL *before* manifestations develop **In Acute Kidney Injury** Often increases by 10-20 mg/dL at same pace as serum creatinine level May reach 80-100 mg/dL within 1 wk
Serum sodium	136-145 mEq/L; 136-145 mmol/L (SI units)	Normal, increased, or decreased
Serum potassium	3.5-5.0 mEq/L; 3.5-5.0 mmol/L (SI units)	Increased
Serum phosphorus (phosphate)	3.0-4.5 mg/dL; 0.97-1.45 mmol/L (SI units) *Older adults:* May be slightly decreased	Increased
Serum calcium	Total calcium: 9.0-10.5 mg/dL; 2.25-2.75 mmol/L (SI units) Ionized calcium: 4.5-5.6 mg/dL; 1.05-1.3 mmol/L (SI units) *Older adults:* Slightly decreased	Decreased
Serum magnesium	1.3-2.1 mEq/L; 0.65-1.05 mmol/L	Increased
Serum carbon dioxide combining power (bicarbonate)	23-30 mEq/L (venous); 23-30 mmol/L (SI units)	Decreased
Arterial blood pH	7.35-7.45	Decreased (in metabolic acidosis) or normal
Arterial blood bicarbonate (HCO_3^-)	21-28 mEq/L	Decreased
Arterial blood $PaCO_2$	35-45 mm Hg	Decreased
Hemoglobin	*Female:* 12-16 g/dL; 7.4-9.9 mmol/L (SI units) *Male:* 14-18 g/dL; 8.7-11.2 mmol/L (SI units) *Older adults:* Slightly decreased	Decreased
Hematocrit	*Female:* 37%-47% *Male:* 42%-52% *Older adults:* May be slightly decreased	Decreased to 20%
Blood osmolarity	285-295 mOsm/kg or mmol/kg (SI)	Elevated in volume-depleted states, increasing the risk for acute kidney injury

Data from Pagana, K., & Pagana, T. (2014). *Mosby's manual of diagnostic and laboratory tests* (5th ed.). St. Louis: Mosby.
CKD, Chronic kidney disease; *SI,* International System of Units.

To identify immune-mediated acute glomerulonephritis, ask about acute illnesses such as influenza, colds, gastroenteritis, and sore throats. Ask whether urine color is darker or appears smoky.

Anticipate AKI following any episode of hypotension, shock, burns, or heart failure exacerbation. Any problem in which the blood volume is depleted can contribute to AKI such as extensive bowel preparations, being NPO before surgery, or dehydration from exercise.

Consider whether there is a history of urinary obstructive problems. Ask the patient about any difficulty in starting the urine stream, changes in the amount or appearance of the urine, narrowing of the urine stream, nocturia, urgency, or manifestations of kidney stones. Also ask about any cancer history that may cause urinary obstruction.

Physical Assessment/Clinical Manifestations. The manifestations of AKI are related to the buildup of nitrogenous wastes (azotemia), decreased urine output (oliguria), as well as to the underlying cause. As AKI progresses in severity, the patient may have manifestations of fluid overload (because in AKI, fluid is not eliminated) including pulmonary crackles, dependent and generalized edema, decreased oxygenation (low peripheral oxygenation or Spo_2), increased respiratory rate, and dyspnea. See Chapter 11 for further assessment related to fluid overload.

Laboratory Assessment. The many changes in laboratory values in the patient with AKI are similar to those occurring in chronic kidney disease (CKD) (Chart 68-1). A rising serum creatinine is more likely to indicate prolonged or permanent kidney damage. Expect to see rising BUN levels and abnormal blood electrolytes values. Patients with AKI, however, usually do *not* have the anemia associated with CKD unless there is blood loss from another condition (e.g., surgery, trauma) or when BUN levels are high enough to break (lyse) red blood cells.

In early AKI, urine tests provide important information. Urine sodium levels may reflect an inability to concentrate urine. Urine may be dilute with a specific gravity near 1.000 or concentrated with a specific gravity greater than 1.030. The presence of urine sediment (e.g., red blood cells [RBCs], RBC casts, and tubular cells), myoglobin, or hemoglobin may contribute to nephron damage.

Imaging Assessment. Ultrasonography is useful in the diagnosis of kidney and urinary tract obstruction. Dilation of the renal calyces and collecting ducts, as well as stones, can be detected. Ultrasonography can show kidney size and patency of the ureters.

CT scans without contrast dye can determine adequacy of kidney blood flow and identify obstruction or tumors. Contrast dyes are usually avoided to prevent further kidney damage. An MRI may be used in place of CT scan at some medical centers.

X-rays of the pelvis or kidneys, ureters, and bladder (KUB) may be used to provide an initial screening view of kidneys and the urinary tract to determine the cause of AKI. Enlarged kidneys with obstruction may show hydronephrosis. X-rays can show stones obstructing the renal pelvis, ureters, or bladder. More commonly, ultrasound is used to screen for hydronephrosis.

A nuclear medicine study called *MAG3* may be used to determine the nature of the kidney failure and measure GFR. A renal scan can determine whether blood flow to the kidneys is sufficient. Cystoscopy or retrograde pyelography may be needed to identify obstructions of the lower urinary tract.

Other Diagnostic Assessments. Kidney biopsy is performed if the cause of AKI is uncertain and manifestations persist or an immunologic disease is suspected. Prepare the patient before the test, particularly managing both hypotension and hypertension. Hypertension can contribute to intrarenal hemorrhage following needle biopsy. Provide follow-up care. Be aware of all test results, and understand how they might affect the treatment regimen. (See Chapter 65 for a detailed discussion of diagnostic tests related to the kidney.)

? NCLEX EXAMINATION CHALLENGE

Safe and Effective Care Environment

An 84-year-old male client is being admitted after surgery to remove a section of his bowel (colectomy) following a diagnosis of colon cancer. His urine output from an indwelling urinary catheter after 3 hours in the postanesthesia care unit plus the amount in the bag on admission to the medical-surgical unit totals 100 mL. The urine is cloudy and dark yellow. He also has a history of hypertension. After evaluating the patency of the collection device, what is the most appropriate action for the nurse to perform?
A. Notify the health care provider of the low urine output.
B. Increase the rate of IV fluids until urine output is 0.5mL/kg/hr.
C. Continue to assess the client and re-evaluate urine output in 4 hours.
D. Ask about his typical voiding patterns and about any previous episodes of urinary problems.

◆ Interventions

A reduction in blood flow to the kidneys may initially not be recognized when there is no associated drop in systemic blood pressure (Davies & Leslie, 2012). Autoregulation and the renin-angiotensin-aldosterone system effectively maintain normal kidney blood flow and glomerular filtration rate. However, these mechanisms may not be working well in the critically ill patient. Thus current guidelines suggest that a mean arterial pressure (MAP) of 65 mm Hg be maintained to promote kidney PERFUSION. The calculation of MAP is illustrated in Table 68-6.

TABLE 68-6 Calculation of Mean Arterial Pressure (MAP)

$$MAP = (SBP + [2 \times DBP]) \div 3$$

Example:
Blood pressure 130/80; SBP = 130; DBP = 80
$(130 + [2 \times 80]) \div 3 =$
$(130 + 160) \div 3 =$
$290 \div 3 =$
$96.666 = 97$ mm Hg. **NOTE:** this value of 97 mm Hg is safe in relation to kidney perfusion and reduces risk for acute kidney injury (AKI) and progression of chronic kidney disease (CKD). A normal range for MAP is 70-110 mm Hg for healthy adults.

Abbreviations: SBP = systolic blood pressure; DBP = diastolic blood pressure

---

MAP is often displayed as a component of automated blood pressure measurement devices and during intra-arterial blood pressure measurement at the ICU bedside. Observations about peripheral edema, increased daily weight, and reduced urine output can identify patients with a positive fluid balance from AKI. Blood sampling of patients at risk for AKI allows monitoring of kidney function and early recognition of elevated serum creatinine. Communicate these observations early and often to the provider so that interventions can promote kidney health and interrupt the progression of AKI when it occurs. Surviving kidney tubule cells possess a remarkable ability to regenerate and proliferate, and early identification can both stop progression of AKI and aid in recovery of kidney function.

Not all patients with AKI experience oliguria. Inflammatory causes of AKI may allow proteins to enter the glomerulus, and these proteins can hold fluid in the filtrate, causing a *polyuria* (excess urine output). During AKI with high-volume urine output, hypovolemia and electrolyte *loss* are the main problems. The patient in the diuretic phase of AKI needs a plan of care that focuses on fluid and electrolyte *replacement* and monitoring. Onset of polyuria can be the start of recovery from AKI.

Base the desired outcomes of care on collaboration and communication with health care team members. Update the plan of care for either restriction or liberal administration of fluid based on timely and accurate health care team communication.

Frequent serum monitoring, close surveillance of intake and output, drug therapy, nutrition, careful administration of fluids and minerals, and renal replacement therapy are commonly used to manage AKI.

Drug Therapy. The health care team should consult the inpatient pharmacist for drug adjustment based on kidney function. As kidney function changes, drug dosages are changed. It is important to be knowledgeable about the site of drug metabolism and especially careful when giving drugs. Continuously monitor the patient with AKI for adverse drug events and interactions of the drugs that he or she is receiving. Diuretics may be used to increase urine output in AKI. Diuretic-induced urine output does not preserve kidney function or stop AKI, but diuretics do rid the body of retained fluid and electrolytes in the patient with AKI that has not progressed to ESKD.

Fluid challenges are often used to promote kidney PERFUSION. In patients without fluid overload, 500 to 1000 mL of normal saline may be infused over 1 hour. Patients with AKI often require central venous pressure (CVP) monitoring. When cardiac disease is also present and worsening, measurement of pulmonary arterial pressure by means of a pulmonary artery catheter for accurate evaluation of hemodynamic status may be needed. During fluid challenges, closely assess the response to fluid and slow the infusion if indications of fluid overload, particularly respiratory distress, occur.

Calcium channel blockers may be used to treat AKI resulting from nephrotoxins. These drugs prevent the movement of calcium into the kidney cells, maintain kidney cell integrity, and improve kidney blood flow. If they do not improve GFR as estimated by serum creatinine (described in Chapter 65), calcium channel blockers are stopped.

Investigation is ongoing to identify biomarkers that can indicate kidney injury early. Neutrophil gelatinase-associated lipocalin (NGAL) and kidney injury molecule-1 (KIM-1) are promising new biomarkers to identify AKI and guide treatment (Obermüller et al., 2014; Vanmassenhove et al., 2013).

Nutrition Therapy. Patients who have AKI often have a high rate of *catabolism* (protein breakdown). Increases in metabolism and protein breakdown may be related to the stress of illness and the increase in blood levels of catecholamines, cortisol, and glucagon. The rate of protein breakdown correlates with the severity of uremia and azotemia. Catabolism causes the breakdown of muscle for protein and increases azotemia.

A registered dietitian will calculate the patient's protein and caloric needs. Whereas this occurs for all patients admitted to an ICU, a consult may need to be requested for inpatients outside of the ICU or for those in the community settings. Work with the dietitian to establish a diet with specified amounts of protein, sodium, and fluids. For the patient who does not require dialysis, 0.6 g/kg of body weight or 40 g/day of protein is usually prescribed. For patients who do require dialysis, the protein level needed will range from 1 to 1.5 g/kg. The amount of dietary sodium ranges from 60 to 90 mEq/kg. If high blood potassium levels are present, dietary potassium is restricted to 60 to 70 mEq/kg. The daily amount of fluid permitted is calculated to be equal to the urine volume plus 500 mL. Assess food intake every shift to ensure that caloric intake is adequate.

Many patients with AKI are too ill or their appetite is too poor to meet caloric goals. For these patients, nutrition support is needed. Nutrition support can include oral supplements, enteral nutrition, or parenteral nutrition (hyperalimentation). The purposes of nutrition support in AKI are to provide sufficient nutrients to maintain or improve nutrition status, to preserve lean body mass, to restore or maintain fluid balance, and to preserve kidney function.

There are several kidney-specific formulations of oral supplements and enteral solutions (e.g., Nepro, Suplena Renalcal, and NovaSource Renal). As a rule, specialty tube feedings for kidney patients are lower in sodium, potassium, and phosphorus and higher in calories than are standard feedings. Enteral nutrition, delivered with a nasogastric or nasojejunal tube (these tubes can also be placed orally), is an effective route to deliver nutrition support. If TPN is used, the IV solutions are mixed to meet the patient's specific needs. Because kidney function is unstable in AKI, continuously monitor fluid balance (intake and output) and serum electrolyte levels to indicate how the supplementation affects FLUID AND ELECTROLYTE BALANCE. IV fat emulsion (Intralipid) infusions can provide a nonprotein source of calories. In uremic patients, fat emulsions are used in place of glucose to avoid the problems of excessive sugars.

Renal Replacement Therapy. Renal replacement therapy (RRT), also called *dialysis,* is used for patients with loss of kidney function. Indications for dialysis use include symptomatic uremia (pericarditis, neuropathy, or unexplained decline in cognition), persistent or rapidly rising high potassium levels (i.e., greater than 6.5 mEq/L), severe metabolic acidosis (pH less than 7.1), or fluid overload that compromises tissue PERFUSION. When AKI is associated with drug or alcohol intoxication, RRT also can remove toxins.

Immediate vascular access for RRT in patients with AKI is made by placement of a catheter specific for dialysis (Fig. 68-1). The catheter is placed in a central vein using best practices to avoid catheter-associated bloodstream infections (see Chapter 13, pp. 193-196). Placement of a dialysis catheter requires informed consent and a "time-out" similar to other surgical procedures (see Chapter 14, Care of Preoperative Patients). The catheter is not used to acquire blood samples, give drugs or fluid, or monitor central venous pressure. Provide site care in accordance with institutional policy and best practices to avoid catheter-related bloodstream INFECTION (CR-BSI).

A long-term dialysis catheter may be placed in the radiology department using a tunneling technique. The patient receives moderate sedation. Under ultrasound or fluoroscopic guidance, the physician makes a small incision where the internal jugular vein passes behind the clavicle. A 6- to 8-cm tunnel is created away from the site of the incision. A long-term hemodialysis catheter is inserted through the tunnel and into the jugular vein. Keeping a segment of the catheter within the subcutaneous tissues before entering the jugular vein reduces the risk for INFECTION. These centrally placed catheters are dedicated to dialysis alone and require aseptic dressing changes as for all central venous catheters.

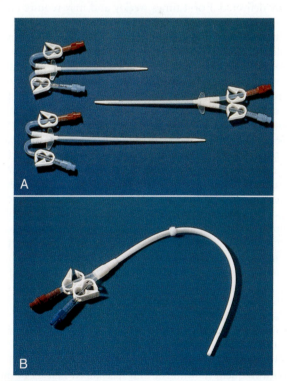

FIG. 68-1 Subclavian dialysis catheters. These catheters are radiopaque tubes that can be used for hemodialysis access. The Y-shaped tubing allows arterial outflow and venous return through a single catheter. **A,** Mahurkar catheters, made of polyurethane and used for short-term access. **B,** A PermCath catheter, made of silicone and used for long-term access.

Dialysis catheters have two lumens—one for outflow and one for inflow. This allows the patient's blood to flow out and, once dialyzed, to be returned through the inflow lumen. Some catheters have a third lumen for the dialysis nurse to sample venous blood or give drugs and fluid during dialysis.

Intermittent Versus Continuous Renal Replacement Therapy.
Renal replacement therapy (RRT) is a supportive strategy to purify blood, substituting for the normal function of the kidney. Particles are separated from blood based on the different ability of particles to pass through (diffuse) a membrane. RRT can be delivered intermittently, continuously, or as a hybrid of these treatment approaches to hospitalized patients. There is no difference in the number of patients who go on to recover kidney function based on the type of RRT administered during AKI. Mortality is significant, regardless of modality, among patients with AKI who require RRT, and this mortality is around 50% while in the hospital (Elseviers et al., 2010).

Intermittent RRT, sometimes called *hemodialysis*, is delivered over 3 to 6 hours. Generally a technician or nurse with specialized training brings the dialysis machine to the bedside of a critically ill patient. Patients who do not need intensive care may be transported to an inpatient dialysis unit for the duration of the RRT treatment.

Intermittent RRT uses a dialysis machine to mix and monitor the dialysate. Dialysate is the fluid that helps remove the unwanted particles and waste products from blood. Dialysate is prescribed by the health care provider as an admixture to restore electrolytes and minerals to normal levels in the blood. The machine also monitors the flow of blood while it is outside of the body. Alarms are set and monitored by the dialysis technician or nurse to ensure safe and effective flow. This type of RRT has a long history of safety and effectiveness in ESKD. It is usually delivered 3 or 4 times weekly and may require anticoagulation in the dialysis circuit. However, this high-intensity treatment creates shifts of fluid and electrolytes that may not be tolerated in acutely and critically ill patients.

Continuous renal replacement therapies (RRTs), also known as *hemofiltration*, are alternative methods for removing wastes and restoring FLUID AND ELECTROLYTE BALANCE in hospitalized adults with AKI who are too unstable to tolerate the changes in blood pressure that occur with intermittent conventional hemodialysis. In all hemodialysis, blood is passed through a filter to remove waste and undesired particles. Unlike intermittent hemodialysis, continuous RRT removes and returns blood over 12 to 24 hours each day. Another difference between continuous RRT and intermittent hemodialysis is the approach used to remove particles from blood. Hemofiltration uses ultrafiltration, whereas diffusion is used in intermittent dialysis to remove toxins and other particles. *Ultrafiltration* is the separation of particles from a suspension by passage through a filter with very fine pores. In ultrafiltration, the separation is performed by convective transport. During intermittent hemodialysis, separation depends on differential diffusion. Some approaches to continuous RRT combine ultrafiltration with diffusion (combined hemofiltration and hemodialysis).

Continuous RRT occurs only in the ICU because of (1) the need for frequent monitoring and specialized skill set to maintain safety during *extracorporeal circulation* (blood flow outside the body) and (2) the need for ongoing replacement of fluid and electrolytes. Many agencies require nurses who deliver continuous RRT to attend classes and demonstrate competency in

care annually. The American Nephrology Nurses Association provides resources for RRT policies and procedures.

There are several strategies to provide hemofiltration to critically ill patients. Continuous venovenous hemofiltration (CVVH) is more commonly used. CVVH is powered by a pump that drives blood from the patient catheter into the dialyzer (filter). The ultrafiltrate fluid is then collected into a bag for disposal. There may be a second pump that acts on the ultrafiltrate tubing to create negative pressure and increase fluid removal. Replacement fluid is infused via the inflow circuit in some systems. The pump increases the risk for an air embolus, but RRT systems should have alarms that detect air. These systems may also use anticoagulants but at lower doses than needed for systems using arterial access. CVVH can also be combined with dialysis (continuous venovenous hemofiltration and dialysis [CVVHD]). CVVHD is similar to intermittent RRT except that the rates of blood circulation and waste formation are much slower with CVVHD, thus the need for continuous therapy (Golestaneh et al., 2012).

Another modality for RRT is a hybrid of continuous and intermittent approaches. Slow continuous ultrafiltration (SCUF) provides slow removal of fluid over 12 to 24 hours. It can be useful when azotemia or uremia is not a concern (Streets & Vickers, 2012). Sustained low-efficiency dialysis (SLED) uses the dialysis machine to deliver prolonged dialysis for 12 to 24 hours. Lower blood flow and dialysate flow rates remove both particles and water and may be better tolerated by the unstable or critically ill patient, with fewer episodes of hypotension.

Continuous RRT is expensive and resource intensive (Allegretti et al., 2013; Golestaneh et al., 2012). It requires consultation and collaboration with the nephrologist and, often, with nurses specialized in dialysis delivery. Clear evidence about when to start or stop RRT when AKI occurs does not yet exist. Conservative management of FLUID AND ELECTROLYTE BALANCE, ACID-BASE BALANCE, and drug therapy is an acceptable and reasonable approach to manage AKI. This approach may be associated with less mortality up to 2 years following RRT for AKI.

Posthospital Care.
The care for a patient with AKI after discharge from the hospital varies, depending on the status of the kidney function when the patient is discharged. The course of AKI varies, with recovery lasting up to several months. If the kidney injury is resolving, follow-up care may be provided by a nephrologist or by the family physician in consultation with the

---

❓ NCLEX EXAMINATION CHALLENGE

Physiological Integrity

The nurse is completing documentation for a client with acute kidney injury who is being discharged today. The nurse notices that the client has a serum potassium level of 5.8 mEq/L. Which is the priority nursing action?

A. Asking the client to drink an extra 500 mL of water to dilute the electrolyte concentration and then re-checking the serum potassium level.

B. Encouraging the client to eat potassium-binding foods and to contact his or her primary care provider within 24 hours.

C. Checking the remaining values on the electrolyte panel and informing the primary care provider of all results before the client is discharged.

D. Applying a cardiac monitor and evaluating the client's muscle strength and muscle irritability.

nephrologist. Frequent medical visits are necessary, as are scheduled laboratory blood and urine tests to monitor kidney function. A dietitian can plan modifications to the patient's diet according to the degree of kidney function and ongoing nutrition needs. Fluid restrictions and daily weights may be advised to avoid fluid overload while kidneys are recovering.

About 10% of patients who receive RRT for AKI in the hospital experience ESKD and require chronic intermittent dialysis or renal transplantation (Allegretti et al., 2013). In patients who require dialysis at discharge following AKI, follow-up care is similar to that needed for patients with ESKD from CKD (see Community-Based Care, pp. 1444-1446). Depending on their level of independence and family support, patients may also need home care nursing or social work assistance.

CHRONIC KIDNEY DISEASE

❖ PATHOPHYSIOLOGY

Unlike acute kidney injury (AKI), **chronic kidney disease (CKD)** is a progressive, irreversible disorder and kidney function does *not* recover (Taal et al., 2012). When kidney function is too poor to sustain life, CKD becomes **end-stage kidney disease (ESKD)**. Terms used with CKD include **azotemia** (buildup of nitrogen-based wastes in the blood), **uremia** (azotemia with clinical manifestations [Chart 68-2]), and **uremic syndrome**. See Table 68-1 for a comparison of AKI and CKD.

Stages of Chronic Kidney Disease

The kidneys fail in an organized fashion involving five stages based on estimated glomerular filtration rate (GFR). Direct measurement (described in Chapter 65, using a 3-hour or 24-hour urine collection) is advised for the most accurate estimation of GFR. The five stages of CKD are described in Table 68-7. CKD starts with a normal GFR but increased risk for kidney damage. In the first stage, the person may have a normal GFR (greater than 90 mL/min) but urine findings or structural abnormalities or genetic trait point to kidney disease. The patient is at increased risk for kidney damage from INFECTION, INFLAMMATION, pregnancy, dehydration, and hypotension or hypertension. Careful management of conditions like diabetes, hypertension, and heart failure can slow the progression of CKD even before GFR changes and manifestations of CKD occur (Wynne et al., 2012).

In the next stage, *mild CKD*, GFR is reduced, ranging between 60 and 89 mL/min. Kidney nephron damage has occurred, and there may be slight elevations of metabolic wastes in the blood because of nephron loss. Levels of blood urea nitrogen (BUN), serum creatinine, uric acid, and phosphorus are not sensitive enough to define this stage. Increased output of dilute urine may occur at this stage of CKD and contribute to severe dehydration.

CHART 68-2 Key Features

Uremia

- Metallic taste in the mouth
- Anorexia
- Nausea
- Vomiting
- Muscle cramps
- Uremic "frost" on skin
- Itching
- Fatigue and lethargy
- Hiccups
- Edema
- Dyspnea
- Paresthesias

> **! NURSING SAFETY PRIORITY (QSEN)**
> **Action Alert**
>
> Teach patients with mild CKD that carefully managing fluid volume, blood pressure, electrolytes, and other kidney-damaging diseases by following prescribed drug and nutrition therapies can prevent damage and slow the progression to ESKD.

In *moderate CKD*, GRF reduction continues and ranges between 30 and 59 mL/min. Nephron damage is greater, and azotemia is present. Ongoing management of the underlying conditions that cause nephron damage is essential, especially glycemic and blood pressure control. Restriction of fluids, proteins, and electrolytes is needed.

Over time, patients progress to *severe CKD* (the fourth stage) and *end-stage kidney disease* (ESKD) (the fifth stage). Excessive amounts of urea and creatinine build up in the blood, and the kidneys cannot maintain homeostasis. Severe impairments of FLUID AND ELECTROLYTE BALANCE and ACID-BASE BALANCE occur. Without renal replacement therapy, death results from ESKD.

TABLE 68-7 Stages of Chronic Kidney Disease

STAGE	ESTIMATED GLOMERULAR FILTRATION RATE	INTERVENTION
Stage 1 At risk; normal kidney function but urine findings or structural abnormalities or genetic trait point to kidney disease	>90 mL/min	Screen for risk factors and manage care to reduce risk: • Uncontrolled hypertension • Diabetes mellitus • Chronic kidney or urinary tract infection • Family history of genetic kidney diseases • Exposure to nephrotoxic substances
Stage 2 Mild chronic kidney disease (CKD); reduced kidney function; laboratory values and other findings (e.g. structural changes) point to kidney disease	60-89 mL/min	Focus on reduction of risk factors
Stage 3 Moderate CKD	30-59 mL/min	Implement strategies to slow disease progression
Stage 4 Severe CKD	15-29 mL/min	Manage complications Discuss patient preferences and values Educate about options and prepare for renal replacement therapy
Stage 5 End-stage kidney disease (ESKD)	<15 mL/min	Implement renal replacement therapy or kidney transplantation

Kidney Changes

CKD with greatly reduced GFR causes many problems, including abnormal urine production, severe disruption of FLUID AND ELECTROLYTE BALANCE, and metabolic abnormalities. Because healthy nephrons become larger and work harder, urine production and water ELIMINATION are sufficient to maintain essential homeostasis until about three fourths of kidney function is lost. As the disease progresses, the ability to produce diluted urine is reduced, resulting in urine with a fixed osmolarity (*isosthenuria*). As kidney function continues to decline, the BUN increases and urine output decreases. At this point, the patient is at risk for fluid overload.

Metabolic Changes

Urea and creatinine excretion are disrupted by CKD. Creatinine comes from proteins present in skeletal muscle. The rate of creatinine excretion depends on muscle mass, physical activity, and diet. Without major changes in diet or physical activity, the serum creatinine level is constant. Creatinine is partially excreted by the kidney tubules, and a decrease in kidney function leads to a buildup of serum creatinine. Urea is made from protein metabolism and is excreted by the kidneys. The BUN level normally varies directly with protein intake.

Sodium excretion changes are common. Early in CKD, the patient is at risk for *hyponatremia* (sodium depletion) because there are fewer healthy nephrons to reabsorb sodium. Thus sodium is lost in the urine. Polyuria of mild to moderate CKD also causes sodium loss.

In the later stages of CKD, kidney excretion of sodium is reduced as urine production decreases. Then sodium retention and high serum sodium levels (*hypernatremia*) can occur with only modest increases in dietary sodium intake. This problem leads to severe disruption of FLUID AND ELECTROLYTE BALANCE (see Chapter 11). Sodium retention causes hypertension and edema.

Even with sodium retention, the serum sodium level may appear normal because plasma water is retained at the same time. If fluid retention occurs at a greater rate than sodium retention, the serum sodium level is falsely low because of dilution (see Chart 68-1).

Potassium excretion occurs mainly through the kidney. Any increase in potassium load during the later stages of CKD can lead to **hyperkalemia** (high serum potassium levels). Normal serum potassium levels of 3.5 to 5 mEq/L are maintained until the 24-hour urine output falls below 500 mL. High potassium levels then develop quickly, reaching 7 to 8 mEq/L or greater. Life-threatening changes in cardiac rate and rhythm result from this elevation due to abnormal depolarization and repolarization. Other factors contribute to high potassium levels in CKD, including the ingestion of potassium in drugs, failure to restrict dietary potassium, tissue breakdown, blood transfusions, and bleeding or hemorrhage. (See Chapter 11 for discussion of potassium problems.)

ACID-BASE BALANCE is affected by CKD. In the early stages, blood pH changes little because the remaining healthy nephrons increase their rate of acid excretion. As more nephrons are lost, acid excretion is reduced and metabolic acidosis results (see Chapter 12).

Many factors lead to acidosis in CKD. First, the kidneys cannot excrete excessive hydrogen ions (acids). Normally, tubular cells move hydrogen ions into the urine for excretion, but ammonium and bicarbonate are needed for this movement

to occur. In patients with CKD, ammonium production is decreased and reabsorption of bicarbonate does not occur. This process leads to a buildup of hydrogen ions and reduced levels of bicarbonate (*base deficit*). High potassium levels further reduce kidney ammonium production and excretion.

As CKD worsens and acid retention increases, increased respiratory action is needed to keep blood pH normal. The respiratory system adjusts or compensates for the increased blood hydrogen ion levels (acidosis or decreased pH) by increasing the rate and depth of breathing to excrete carbon dioxide through the lungs. This breathing pattern, called **Kussmaul respiration**, increases with worsening kidney disease. Serum bicarbonate measures the extent of metabolic acidosis (bicarbonate deficit). Patients with CKD usually need alkali replacement to counteract acidosis.

Calcium and phosphorus balance is disrupted by CKD. A complex, balanced normal reciprocal relationship exists between calcium and phosphorus (used interchangeably with phosphate) and is influenced by vitamin D (see Chapter 11). The kidney produces a hormone needed to activate vitamin D, which then enhances intestinal absorption of calcium.

Normally, excess dietary phosphorus is excreted by the kidneys in the urine. In CKD, phosphorus overload leads to secretion of a phosphaturic hormone from bone (Fukagawa et al., 2013). This hormone, fibroblast growth factor 3 (GG3), contributes to mineral imbalance.

Parathyroid hormone (PTH) controls the amount of phosphorus in the blood by causing tubular excretion of phosphorus when there is an excess. An early effect of CKD is reduced phosphorus excretion (Fig. 68-2). As plasma phosphorus levels increase (*hyperphosphatemia*), calcium levels decrease (*hypocalcemia*). Chronic low blood calcium levels stimulate the parathyroid glands to release more PTH. Under the influence of additional PTH, calcium is released from storage areas in bones

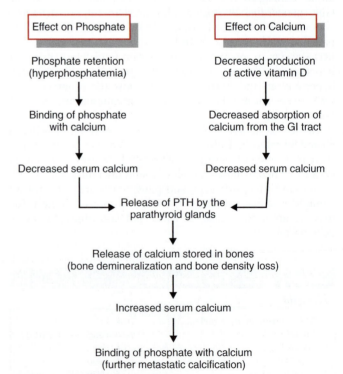

FIG. 68-2 The effects of kidney dysfunction on phosphorus and calcium balance. *PTH*, Parathyroid hormone.

(bone resorption), which results in bone density loss. The extra calcium from the bone is needed to balance the excess plasma phosphorus level. The problem of low blood calcium levels is made worse with severe CKD because kidney cell damage also reduces production of active vitamin D. Thus less calcium is absorbed through the intestinal tract in the absence of sufficient vitamin D.

The problems in bone metabolism and structure caused by CKD-induced low calcium levels and high phosphorus levels are called renal osteodystrophy. Bone mineral loss causes bone pain, spinal sclerosis, fractures, bone density loss, osteomalacia, and tooth calcium loss.

Crystals formed from excessive calcium phosphorus are called *metastatic calcifications* and may precipitate in many body areas. When the plasma level of the calcium-phosphorus product (serum calcium level multiplied by the serum phosphorus level) exceeds 70 mg/dL, the crystals may lodge in the kidneys, heart, lungs, major blood vessels, joints, eyes (causing conjunctivitis), and brain. Skin itching increases with calcium-phosphorus imbalances.

Calcium is also deposited in atherosclerotic plaques and in the intima of blood vessels. Vascular calcium deposits are a marker of significant risk for cardiovascular disease.

Cardiac Changes

Hypertension is common in most patients with CKD. This problem may be either the cause or the result of CKD. In patients who have other causes of hypertension such as atherosclerosis, the increased blood pressure damages the glomerular capillaries and eventually ESKD results.

CKD itself elevates blood pressure by causing fluid and sodium overload and dysfunction of the renin-angiotensin-aldosterone system. Hypertension alone can damage kidney arterioles, reducing PERFUSION. A decrease in kidney blood flow results in the production and release of a number of signaling chemicals, including renin, to improve blood flow to the kidney. The release of renin triggers the production of angiotensin and aldosterone. Angiotensin causes blood vessel constriction and increases blood pressure. Aldosterone, a hormone released by the adrenal glands, stimulates kidney tubules to reabsorb sodium and water. These actions increase plasma volume and raise blood pressure. However, in the presence of CKD, an increase in blood pressure may not result in increased blood flow, and the production of renin continues, which creates a cycle of vasoconstriction in kidney arterioles and peripheral arterioles. The result is severe hypertension that worsens kidney function. Hypertension with CKD is difficult to manage. Many patients with CKD have heart damage and heart enlargement from the long-term hypertension that results in coronary artery damage and poor coronary artery perfusion.

Hyperlipidemia occurs in CKD from changes in fat metabolism that increase triglyceride, total cholesterol, and low-density lipoprotein (LDL) levels. These changes increase the patient's risk for coronary artery disease and acute cardiac events. Problems with lipids and atherosclerosis are significantly increased for the patient with both CKD and diabetes.

Heart failure may occur in CKD because it increases the workload on the heart as a result of anemia, hypertension, and fluid overload. Left ventricular enlargement and heart failure are common in ESKD. Uremia may cause *uremic cardiomyopathy,* the uremic toxin effect on the myocardium. Heart failure also may occur in these patients because of hypertension and

coronary artery disease. Cardiac disease is a leading cause of death in patients with ESKD.

Pericarditis also occurs in patients with CKD. The pericardial sac becomes inflamed by uremic toxins or INFECTION. If it is not treated, this problem leads to pericardial effusion, cardiac tamponade, and death. Manifestations include shortness of breath from low cardiac output, severe chest pain, tachycardia, narrow *pulse pressure* (close values for systolic and diastolic blood pressure), low-grade fever, and a pericardial friction rub that can be heard with a stethoscope placed over the left sternal border. Dysrhythmias may occur with uremia and uremic pericarditis. Treatment of tamponade requires removal of pericardial fluid by placement of a needle, catheter, or drainage tube into the pericardium.

Hematologic Changes

Anemia is a common problem in patients in the later stages of CKD, and it worsens the CKD manifestations. The causes of anemia include a decreased erythropoietin level that decreases red blood cell (RBC) production, decreased RBC survival time resulting from uremia, iron and folic acid deficiencies, and increased bleeding as a result of impaired platelet function.

Gastrointestinal Changes

Uremia affects the entire GI system. The flora of the mouth change with uremia. The mouth contains the enzyme *urease,* which breaks down urea into ammonia. The ammonia generated then causes *halitosis* (bad breath) and *stomatitis* (mouth INFLAMMATION).

Anorexia, nausea, vomiting, and hiccups are common in patients with uremia. The specific cause of these problems is unknown but may be related to high BUN and creatinine levels as well as acidosis.

Peptic ulcer disease is common in patients with uremia, but the exact cause is unclear. Uremic colitis with watery diarrhea or constipation may also be present with uremia. Ulcers may occur in the stomach or intestine, causing erosion of blood vessels. The blood loss caused by these erosions may lead to hemorrhagic shock from severe GI bleeding.

Etiology and Genetic Risk

The causes of CKD are complex (Table 68-8). More than 100 different disease processes can result in progressive loss of kidney function (see also Chapter 67). Two main causes of CKD leading to dialysis are hypertension and diabetes mellitus. African-American patients are much more likely to develop ESKD and to have hypertensive ESKD.

Incidence and Prevalence

The number of patients being treated for CKD is increasing, particularly among people older than 65 years. Over 871,000 people in the United States are being treated for ESKD (U.S. Renal Data Systems [USRDS], 2014). As many as 25% of patients receiving treatment for ESKD die in the first year of dialysis. Chart 68-3 addresses the prevention of kidney and urinary problems.

Health Promotion and Maintenance

The health-promotion activities to prevent or delay the onset of CKD focus on controlling the diseases that lead to its development, such as diabetes mellitus and hypertension. Educating and encouraging the patient to accept lifestyle modifications

TABLE 68-8 Selected Causes of Chronic Kidney Disease

Glomerular Disease
- Glomerulonephritis
- Basement membrane disease
- Goodpasture's syndrome
- Intercapillary glomerulosclerosis

Tubular Disease
- Chronic hypercalcemia
- Chronic potassium depletion
- Fanconi's syndrome
- Heavy metal (lead) poisoning

Vascular Disease of the Kidney
- Ischemic disease of the kidney
- Bilateral renal artery stenosis
- Nephrosclerosis
- Hyperparathyroidism

Inherited or Genetic Conditions
- Hypoplastic kidneys
- Medullary cystic disease
- Polycystic kidney disease

Infection
- Pyelonephritis
- Tuberculosis

Systemic Vascular Disease
- Intrarenal renovascular hypertension
- Extrarenal renovascular hypertension

Metabolic Kidney Disease
- Diabetes
- Amyloidosis
- Gout (hyperuricemic nephropathy)
- Milk-alkali syndrome
- Sarcoidosis

Connective Tissue Disease
- Progressive systemic sclerosis
- Systemic lupus erythematosus
- Polyarteritis

Urinary Tract Disease
- Obstructive uropathy

NOTE: List is not all-inclusive.

CHART 68-3 Patient and Family Education: Preparing for Self-Management

Prevention of Kidney and Urinary Problems

- Be alert to the general appearance of your urine. Note any changes in its color, clarity, or odor.
- Changes in the frequency or volume of urine passage occur with changes in fluid intake. More frequent or infrequent voiding not associated with changes in fluid intake may signal health problems.
- Any discomfort or distress with the passage of urine is not normal. Pain, burning, urgency, aching, or difficulty with initiating urine flow or complete bladder emptying is of some concern.
- The kidneys need 1 to 2 liters of fluid a day to flush out your body wastes. Water is the ideal flushing agent.
- Avoid sugary, high-calorie drinks; they provide low-quality calories that contribute to weight gain and hyperglycemia-induced diuresis.
- Changes in kidney function are often silent for many years. Periodically ask your health care provider to measure your kidney function with a blood test (serum creatinine) and a urinalysis.
- If you have a history of kidney disease, diabetes mellitus, hypertension (high blood pressure), or a family history of kidney disease, you should know your serum creatinine level and your glomerular filtration rate (either estimated from serum creatinine or measured with a 24-hour creatinine urine collection). At least one checkup per year that includes laboratory blood and urine testing of kidney function is recommended.
- If you are identified as having decreased kidney function, ask about whether any prescribed drug, diagnostic test, or therapeutic procedure will present a risk to your current kidney function. Evaluate the contribution of diet to risk for kidney disease with your health care provider or a dietitian. Check out all nonprescription drugs with your physician or pharmacist before using them.

and how to implement them are incorporated into the plan of care in an ongoing manner. Diet adjustments (e.g., sodium, protein, and cholesterol restriction), weight maintenance (i.e., achieve body mass index of 22-25 kg/m^2), cessation of smoking, participation in 30 to 60 minutes of moderate-intensity exercise daily, and limitation of alcohol to 1 or 2 drinks daily are examples of lifestyle recommendations for the patient with CKD (Saccomano & DeLuca, 2012). Identifying patients who have diabetes or hypertension at an early stage is critical to CKD prevention. Teach patients to adhere to drug and diet regimens and to engage in regular physical activity to prevent the blood vessel changes and cascade of kidney cell damage that lead to CKD. Instruct patients with diabetes to keep their blood glucose levels within the prescribed range. Teach patients with hypertension that drug therapy reduces vessel damage. Lifestyle changes in diet and activity promote health and healthy kidneys. Urge patients with diabetes or hypertension to have yearly testing for microalbuminuria along with serum creatinine and BUN.

Teach everyone treated for an INFECTION anywhere in the kidney/urinary system to take all antibiotics as prescribed. Urge everyone to drink at least 2 L of water daily unless a health problem requires fluid restriction. Caution people who use NSAIDs to use the lowest dose for the briefest time period because these drugs interfere with blood flow to the kidney. High-dose and long-term NSAID use reduces kidney function.

❖ PATIENT-CENTERED COLLABORATIVE CARE

◆ Assessment

History. When taking a history from a patient with risk for or actual chronic kidney disease (CKD), document the patient's age and gender. Accurately measure weight and height, and ask about usual weight and recent weight gain or loss. Weight gain may indicate fluid retention from poor kidney function. Weight loss may be the result of anorexia from high blood urea levels.

Obtain a complete history of kidney and urologic disorders, long-term health problems, and drug use. Long-term health problems such as hypertension, diabetes, systemic lupus erythematosus, arthritis, cancer, and tuberculosis can cause decreased kidney function. Ask the patient about family members' kidney disease that might indicate a genetic problem.

Document the use of current and past prescription and over-the-counter drugs because many drugs are nephrotoxic and can cause kidney damage (see Table 68-5). Inquire about contrast-induced nephropathy by asking if the patient has had x-rays or CT scan with dye.

Examine the patient's dietary habits, and discuss any present GI problems. A change in the taste of foods often occurs with CKD. Patients may report that sweet foods are not as appealing or that meats have a metallic taste. Ask about the presence of nausea, vomiting, anorexia, hiccups, diarrhea, or constipation. These manifestations may be the result of excess wastes that the body cannot excrete because of kidney disease.

Ask about the patient's energy level and any recent injuries or bleeding. Explore changes in his or her daily routine as a possible *result* of fatigue. Fatigue is a common and often profound problem among patients with CKD, particularly among patients receiving dialysis (Horigan et al., 2012). Weakness, drowsiness, and shortness of breath suggest impending pulmonary edema or neurologic degeneration. Ask about bruising or bleeding, which can be caused by hematologic changes from uremia.

Discuss urine ELIMINATION in detail, including frequency of urination, appearance of the urine, and any difficulty starting or controlling urination. These data can help identify urologic problems that may influence existing kidney function.

❓ NCLEX EXAMINATION CHALLENGE

Health Promotion and Maintenance

A 60-year-old African-American client is newly diagnosed with mild chronic kidney disease (stage 2 CKD). She has a history of diabetes, and her current A1C is 8.0%. She asks the nurse whether any of the following factors could have caused this problem. Which factor should the nurse indicate may have influenced the development of CKD?

A. She heavily salted her food as a child and teenager but added no extra salt to her food as an adult.
B. Her chronic hyperglycemia causes blood vessel changes in the kidney that can damage kidney tissue.
C. Her paternal grandparents had type 2 diabetes and hypertension.
D. She drinks 2 cups of coffee with cream daily.

Physical Assessment/Clinical Manifestations. CKD causes changes in all body systems (Chart 68-4). Most manifestations are related to changes in FLUID AND ELECTROLYTE BALANCE, ACID-BASE BALANCE, and buildup of nitrogenous wastes.

Neurologic manifestations of CKD and uremic syndrome vary (see Chart 68-4). Observe for problems ranging from lethargy to seizures or coma, which may indicate uremic encephalopathy. Assess for sensory changes that appear in a glove-and-stocking pattern over the hands and feet (peripheral neuropathy). Check for weakness in the upper and lower extremities (e.g., uremic neuropathy).

If untreated, encephalopathy can lead to seizures and coma. Dialysis is used for CKD when neurologic problems result. The manifestations of encephalopathy may resolve with dialysis. However, improvement in neuropathy is limited if it is severe and motor function is impaired.

Cardiovascular manifestations of CKD and uremia result from fluid overload, hypertension, heart failure (HF), pericarditis, potassium-induced dysrhythmias, and cholesterol/calcium (plaque) deposits in blood vessels. Assess for manifestations of reduced sodium and water excretion. Circulatory overload, if untreated, leads to hypertension, pulmonary edema, peripheral edema, and HF.

Assess heart rate and rhythm, listening for extra sounds (particularly an S_3), irregular patterns, or a pericardial friction rub. Unless a dialysis vascular access has been created, measure blood pressure in each arm. Assess the jugular veins for distention, and assess for edema of the feet, shins, and sacrum and around the eyes. Crackles during lung auscultation and shortness of breath with exertion and at night suggest fluid overload.

Respiratory manifestations of CKD also vary (e.g., breath that smells like urine [*uremic fetor* or uremic halitosis], deep sighing, yawning, shortness of breath). Observe the rhythm, rate, and depth of breathing. Tachypnea and hyperpnea (increased depth of breathing) occur with metabolic acidosis.

With severe metabolic acidosis, extreme increases in rate and depth of ventilation (Kussmaul respirations) occur. A few patients have pneumonitis, or *uremic lung*. In these patients, assess for thick sputum, reduced coughing, tachypnea, and

---

CHART 68-4 Key Features

Severe Chronic and End-Stage Kidney Disease

Neurologic Manifestations
- Lethargy and daytime drowsiness
- Inability to concentrate or decreased attention span
- Seizures
- Coma
- Slurred speech
- Asterixis (jerky movements or "flapping" of the hands)
- Tremors, twitching, or jerky movements
- Myoclonus
- Ataxia (alteration in gait)
- Paresthesias

Cardiovascular Manifestations
- Cardiomyopathy
- Hypertension
- Peripheral edema
- Heart failure
- Uremic pericarditis
- Pericardial effusion
- Pericardial friction rub
- Cardiac tamponade
- Cardiorenal syndrome

Respiratory Manifestations
- Uremic halitosis
- Tachypnea
- Deep sighing, yawning
- Kussmaul respirations
- Uremic pneumonitis
- Shortness of breath
- Pulmonary edema
- Pleural effusion
- Depressed cough reflex
- Crackles

Hematologic Manifestations
- Anemia
- Abnormal bleeding and bruising

Gastrointestinal Manifestations
- Anorexia
- Nausea
- Vomiting
- Metallic taste in the mouth
- Changes in taste acuity and sensation
- Uremic colitis (diarrhea)
- Constipation
- Uremic gastritis (possible GI bleeding)
- Uremic fetor (breath odor)
- Stomatitis

Urinary Manifestations
- Polyuria, nocturia (early)
- Oliguria, anuria (later)
- Proteinuria
- Hematuria
- Diluted, straw-colored urine appearance (early)
- Concentrated and cloudy urine appearance (later)

Integumentary Manifestations
- Decreased skin turgor
- Yellow-gray pallor
- Dry skin
- Pruritus
- Ecchymosis
- Purpura
- Soft-tissue calcifications
- Uremic frost (late, premorbid)

Musculoskeletal Manifestations
- Muscle weakness and cramping
- Bone pain
- Fractures
- Renal osteodystrophy

Reproductive Manifestations
- Decreased fertility
- Infrequent or absent menses
- Decreased libido
- Impotence
- Sexual dysfunction

---

fever. A pleural friction rub may be heard with a stethoscope. Patients often have pleuritic pain with breathing. Auscultate the lungs for crackles, which indicate fluid overload.

Hematologic manifestations of CKD include anemia and abnormal bleeding. Check for indicators of anemia (e.g., fatigue, pallor, lethargy, weakness, shortness of breath, dizziness). Check for abnormal bleeding by observing for bruising, petechiae, purpura, mucous membrane bleeding in the nose or gums, or intestinal bleeding (black, tarry stools [melena]).

GI manifestations of CKD include foul breath and mouth INFLAMMATION or ulceration. Document any abdominal pain, cramping, or vomiting. Test all stools for occult blood.

Skeletal manifestations of CKD are related to osteodystrophy from poor absorption of calcium and continuous bone calcium loss. Adults with osteodystrophy have thin, fragile bones that are at risk for pathologic fractures with even slight trauma. Vertebrae become more compact and may bend forward, leading to an overall loss of height. Ask about changes in height and any unexplained bone pain. Observe for spinal curvatures and any unusual bumps or protrusions in bone areas that may indicate fractures. Handle the patient carefully during examination and care.

Urine manifestations in CKD reflect the kidneys' decreasing function. At first, urine amount, frequency, and appearance change. Protein, sediment, or blood may be in the urine.

The amount and composition of the urine change as kidney function decreases. With the onset of mild to moderate CKD, the urine may be more dilute and clearer because tubular reabsorption of water is reduced. The actual urine output in a patient with CKD varies with the amount of remaining kidney function. The patient with severe CKD or ESKD usually has oliguria, but some patients continue to produce 1 L or more daily. Daily urine volume usually changes again after dialysis is started. A long duration of oliguria is an indication that recovery of kidney function is not to be expected.

Skin manifestations of CKD occur as a result of uremia. Pigment is deposited in the skin, causing a yellowish coloration, or darkening when skin is brown or bronze. The anemia of CKD causes a sallowness, appearing as a faded suntan on lighter-skinned patients.

Skin oils and turgor are decreased in patients with uremia. A distressing problem of uremia is severe *pruritus* (itching). Uremic frost, a layer of urea crystals from evaporated sweat, may appear on the face, eyebrows, axillae, and groin in patients with advanced uremic syndrome. Assess for bruises (*ecchymosis*), purple patches (*purpura*), and rashes.

Psychosocial Assessment. Chronic kidney disease (CKD) and its treatment disrupt many aspects of a patient's life. Psychosocial assessment and support are part of the nurse's role from the time that CKD is first diagnosed. Ask about the patient's understanding of the diagnosis and what the treatment regimen means to him or her (e.g., diet, drugs, dialysis). Assess for anxiety and for the coping styles used by the patient or family members. Issues affected by CKD include family relations, social activity, work patterns, body image, and sexual activity. The long-term nature of severe CKD and ESKD, the many treatment options, and the uncertainties about the course of the disease and its treatment require ongoing psychosocial assessment.

Laboratory Assessment. CKD causes extreme changes in many laboratory values (see Chart 68-1). Monitor these blood values: creatinine, blood urea nitrogen (BUN), sodium, potassium, calcium, phosphorus, bicarbonate, hemoglobin, and hematocrit. Also monitor GFR for trends.

A urinalysis is performed. In the early stages of CKD, urinalysis may show excessive protein, glucose, red blood cells (RBCs) and white blood cells (WBCs), and decreased or fixed specific gravity. Urine osmolarity is usually decreased. As CKD progresses, urine output decreases dramatically and osmolarity increases.

Glomerular filtration rate (GFR) can be estimated from serum creatinine levels, age, gender, race, and body size. But this type of estimation is generally considered for screening rather than for staging of CKD. Estimation of GFR based on serum creatinine is also useful to calculate drug dose or drug frequency when reduced renal function is a concern. However, to determine stage of CKD, a urine collection of 3 hours to 24 hours is usually done.

In severe CKD, measurements of the serum creatinine and BUN levels may be used to determine the presence and degree of uremia. Serum creatinine levels may increase gradually over a period of years, reaching levels of 15 to 30 mg/dL or more, depending on the patient's muscle mass. BUN levels are directly related to dietary protein intake. Without protein restriction, BUN levels may rise to 10 to 20 times the value of the serum creatinine level. With dietary protein restriction, BUN levels are elevated but less than those of non–protein-restricted patients. Fluid balance also affects BUN.

Imaging Assessment. Few x-ray findings are abnormal with CKD. Bone x-rays of the hand can show renal osteodystrophy. With long-term ESKD, the kidneys shrink (except for ESKD caused by polycystic kidney disease) and may be 8 to 9 cm or smaller. This small size results from atrophy and fibrosis. If CKD progresses suddenly, a kidney ultrasound or CT scan without contrast medium may be used to rule out an obstruction. (See Chapter 65 for a complete description of diagnostic tests for kidney function.)

◆ Analysis

The patient with CKD usually has had a progressive reduction of kidney function and is often hospitalized for adjustment of the treatment plan. The focus of care is to manage problems and prevent complications. The priority NANDA-I nursing diagnoses and collaborative problems for patients with CKD include:

1. Excess Fluid Volume related to the inability of diseased kidneys to maintain body fluid balance (NANDA-I)
2. Potential for pulmonary edema related to fluid overload
3. Decreased Cardiac Output related to reduced stroke volume, dysrhythmias, fluid overload, and increased peripheral vascular resistance (NANDA-I)
4. Inadequate nutrition related to inability to ingest, digest, or absorb food and nutrients as a result of physiologic factors
5. Risk for Infection related to skin breakdown, immune-related kidney dysfunction, or malnutrition (NANDA-I)
6. Risk for Injury related to effects of kidney disease on bone density, blood clotting, and drug elimination (NANDA-I)
7. Fatigue related to kidney disease, anemia, and reduced energy production (NANDA-I)
8. Anxiety related to threat to or change in health status, economic status, relationships, role function, systems, or self-concept; situational crisis; threat of death; lack of knowledge about diagnostic tests, disease process, treatment; loss of control; or disrupted family life (NANDA-I)

◆ Planning and Implementation

The Concept Map on p. 1425 discusses nursing care issues related to patients who have end-stage kidney disease (ESKD).

Managing Fluid Volume

Planning: Expected Outcomes. The patient with CKD is expected to achieve and maintain an acceptable FLUID AND ELECTROLYTE BALANCE. Indicators include that blood pressure, central venous pressure, and electrolytes are normal or nearly normal. Body weight is stable (±2 lbs overnight and 5 lbs weekly) and does not increase more than 3 pounds between dialysis sessions.

CONCEPT MAP

PERFUSION

ACID-BASE BALANCE

INFECTION

END-STAGE KIDNEY DISEASE

ELIMINATION

INFLAMMATION

FLUID AND ELECTROLYTE BALANCE

History

Joe Brown is a 55-year-old African-American man who has a lengthy history of type 2 diabetes, coronary artery disease, and hyperlipidemia. He has had complete loss of kidney function for 4 months. His vital signs are T – 100° F; P – 104 and irregular; R – 32; BP – 160/100 mm Hg.

Data Synthesis →

- Age 55, male, height 5'9" 225 lbs, recent weight gain of 8 lbs.
- History of kidney stones, uncontrolled DM type 2, drug use, hypertension, and hyperlipidemia. Family history of polycystic kidney disease.
- Chronic use of NSAIDs for arthritis pain.
- Reports that desserts "don't taste sweet like before" and meat leaves a metallic taste. Some nausea and anorexia.
- Reports feeling weak and tired and is often short of breath. He has several bruises on his arms and legs at different stages.
- States he urinates dark-colored urine in small amounts a few times a day.

Data Synthesis →

PATIENT PROBLEMS

- Excess Fluid Volume due to inability of kidneys to maintain body fluid balance
- Potential for pulmonary edema due to fluid overload
- Decreased Cardiac Output due to reduced stroke volume, dysrhythmias, fluid overload, and increased peripheral vascular resistance
- Inadequate nutrition due to inability to ingest, digest, or absorb food and nutrients as a result of physiologic factors
- Risk for Infection related to skin breakdown, immune-related kidney dysfunction, or malnutrition
- Risk for Injury due to effects of kidney disease on bone density, blood clotting, and drug elimination
- Fatigue related to kidney disease, anemia, and reduced energy production
- Anxiety due to threat to or change in health status, economic status, relationships, role function, systems, or self-concept; situational crisis; threat of death; lack of knowledge about diagnostic tests, disease process, treatment; loss of control; or disrupted family life

← Planning

EXPECTED OUTCOMES

- Achieve an acceptable fluid balance
- Maintain a stable body weight
- No exhibiting signs of pulmonary edema
- Maintain adequate cardiac output
- Maintain adequate nutrition
- Remain free of infection
- Remain free of injury
- Decreased fatigue

INTERVENTIONS

1 Physical Assessment

Assess for presence of S$_3$ or pericardial friction rub, chest pain, jugular vein distention, edema, fatigue, dyspnea, crackles, weight change, skin integrity, pruritus, skin discoloration, mental status, seizure activity, sensory changes, LE weakness, anorexia, nausea, vomiting, stomatitis, melena, urine amount/frequency/appearance, bone pain, presence of hyperglycemia secondary to diabetes, signs of bleeding disorders (petechiae, purpura, ecchymosis). *Guides patient care; assesses for signs of kidney failure.*

2 Fluid Management

Monitor vital signs, intake and output, weight, hydration status, treat hypertension with drug therapy. *Monitors for fluid overload; sodium retention causes hypertension and edema.*

3 Monitoring for Pulmonary Edema

- Assess for restlessness, anxiety, tachycardia, shortness of breath, crackles, decreased breath sounds, frothy, blood-tinged sputum, and diaphoresis. *Indicates pulmonary edema; uremic injury to lung blood vessels causes inflammation.*
- Position the patient in high Fowler's; give oxygen, loop diuretics, and measure urine output every 15-30 minutes. *Decreases fluid volume, improves gas exchange and PERFUSION.*
- Monitor vital signs and assess breath sounds at least every 2 hours. *Evaluates the patient's response to treatment.*

4 Maintaining Acid-Base Balance

Ensure participation in renal replacement therapies, either peritoneal dialysis (PD) or hemodialysis (HD). *Improves fluid, electrolyte, and acid-base balance; removes nitrogenous wastes.*

5 Interpretation of Lab Values

Monitor lab values – Blood urea nitrogen (BUN), serum creatinine, creatinine clearance, complete blood count, electrolytes. *Determines the effectiveness of therapy for kidney failure.*

6 Monitoring Cardiac Output

Assess for signs of heart failure. Administer calcium channel blockers, ACE inhibitors, alpha-adrenergic and beta-adrenergic blockers, and vasodilators. *Controls blood pressure, which is essential to preserve kidney function.*

7 Enhancing Nutrition

Collaborate with the dietitian to determine calories; protein, fluid, potassium, sodium, and phosphorus restrictions; vitamin and mineral supplements. *Provides a balance of food and fluids to prevent malnutrition and avoid complications.*

8 Preventing Infection

Provide meticulous skin care; inspect vascular access site or peritoneal dialysis catheter site for redness, swelling, pain, and drainage. Monitor vital signs for fever and tachycardia. *Prevents and detects early signs of infection.*

9 Health Promotion and Maintenance

Teach the patient and family the importance of adhering to prescribed fluid and dietary restrictions, medications, and dialysis as scheduled. *Promotes health and reduces complications.*

10 Psychosocial Integrity

Encourage the expression of concerns about risks for death and lifestyle disruption; determine the presence of anxiety or maladaptive behavior. Refer to community health or support groups. *Minimizes the impact that depression, anxiety, and nonacceptance have on mental well-being.*

Concept Map by Deanne A. Blach, MSN, RN

CHART 68-5 Best Practice for Patient Safety & Quality Care (QSEN)

Managing Fluid Volume

- Weigh the patient daily at the same time each day, using the same scale, with the patient wearing the same amount and type of clothing, and graph the results.
- Observe the weight graph for trends (1 L of water weighs 1 kg).
- Accurately measure all fluid intake and output.
- Teach the patient and family about the need to keep fluid intake within prescribed restricted amounts and to ensure that the prescribed daily amount is evenly distributed throughout the 24 hours.
- Monitor for these manifestations of fluid overload at least every 4 hours:
  - Decreased urine output
  - Rapid, bounding pulse
  - Rapid, shallow respirations
  - Presence of dependent edema
  - Auscultation of crackles or wheezes
  - Presence of distended neck veins in a sitting position
  - Decreased oxygen saturation
  - Elevated blood pressure
  - Narrowed pulse pressure
- Assess level of consciousness and degree of cognition.
- Ask about the presence of headache or blurred vision.

Interventions. Management of the patient with CKD includes drug therapy, nutrition therapy, fluid restriction, and dialysis. Dialysis using extracorporeal blood circulation (hemodialysis) is done intermittently for 3 to 4 hours, typically 3 days per week. Alternatively, some patients with ESKD receive peritoneal dialysis. PD uses the peritoneum as the dialyzing membrane. The dialysate is infused through a catheter implanted in the peritoneum. Dialysis for ESKD is described on pp. 1431-1437 in this chapter.

The purpose of fluid management is to attain fluid balance and prevent complications of fluid overload (Chart 68-5). Monitor the patient's intake and output and hydration status. Assess for manifestations of fluid overload (e.g., lung crackles, edema, distended neck veins).

Drug therapy with diuretics is prescribed for patients with mild to severe CKD to increase urinary ELIMINATION of fluid. The increased urine output produced from these drugs helps reduce fluid overload and hypertension in patients who still have some urine output. Diuretics are seldom used in ESKD after dialysis is started because, as kidney function is reduced, these drugs can have harmful side effects on the remaining kidney cells and on a patient's hearing.

Assess fluid status by obtaining daily weights and reviewing intake and output. Daily weight gain in these patients indicates fluid retention rather than true body weight gain. Estimate the amount of fluid retained: 1 kg of weight equals about 1 L of fluid retained. Weigh the patient daily at the same time each day, on the same scale, wearing the same amount of clothing, and after voiding (if the patient is not anuric). Monitor weight for changes before and after dialysis.

Fluid restriction is often needed. Consider all forms of fluid intake, including oral, IV, and enteral sources, when calculating fluid intake. Assist the patient in spreading oral fluid intake over a 24-hour period. Monitor his or her response to fluid restriction, and notify the health care provider if manifestations of fluid overload persist or worsen.

Preventing Pulmonary Edema

Planning: Expected Outcomes. The patient with CKD is expected to remain free of pulmonary edema by maintaining optimal fluid balance. Indicators include that the patient has no breathing difficulty and no adventitious lung sounds (e.g., crackles, wheezes) with auscultation and that oxygen saturation remains greater than 92%.

Interventions. In the patient with CKD, pulmonary edema can result from left-sided heart failure related to fluid overload or from blood vessel injury. In left-sided heart failure, the heart is unable to eject blood adequately from the left ventricle, leading to an increased pressure in the left atrium and in the pulmonary blood vessels. The increased pressure causes fluid to cross the capillaries into the pulmonary tissue, forming edema (McCance et al., 2014). Pulmonary edema can also occur from injury to the lung blood vessels as a result of uremia. This condition causes INFLAMMATION and capillary leak. Fluid then leaks from pulmonary circulation into the lung tissue and the alveoli. It may also leak into the pleural space, causing a *pleural effusion.*

Assess the patient for early indicators of pulmonary edema, such as restlessness, anxiety, rapid heart rate, shortness of breath, and crackles that begin at the base of the lungs. As pulmonary edema worsens, the level of fluid in the lungs rises. Auscultation reveals increased crackles and decreased breath sounds. The patient may have frothy, blood-tinged sputum. As cardiac and pulmonary function decrease further, the patient becomes diaphoretic and cyanotic.

The patient with pulmonary edema usually is admitted to the hospital for aggressive treatment and continuous cardiac monitoring. Place the patient in a high-Fowler's position and give oxygen to improve gas exchange. Drug therapy with kidney failure and pulmonary edema is difficult because of potential adverse drug effects on the kidneys. Loop diuretics such as IV furosemide (Lasix) are used to manage pulmonary edema. Kidney impairment increases the risk for *ototoxicity* (ear damage with hearing loss) with furosemide; thus IV doses are given cautiously. Diuresis usually begins within 5 minutes of giving IV furosemide. Measure urine output every 15 to 30 minutes during the acute episode and every hour thereafter until the patient is stabilized. Monitor vital signs and assess breath sounds at least every 2 hours to evaluate the patient's response to this treatment.

IV morphine sulfate (1 to 2 mg) can be prescribed to reduce myocardial oxygen demand by triggering blood vessel dilation and to provide sedation. Dosage adjustments are needed to achieve the desired response and avoid respiratory depression. Monitor the patient's respiratory rate, oxygen saturation, and blood pressure hourly during this therapy. Other drugs that dilate blood vessels, such as nitroglycerin, may be given as a continuous infusion to reduce pulmonary pressure from left heart failure. Monitor vital signs at least hourly because this drug combination may cause severe hypotension.

Monitor serum electrolyte levels daily, and report abnormalities to the health care provider so that imbalances can be corrected quickly. If using electrocardiogram (ECG) monitoring, identify dysrhythmias as they occur and report changes in rhythm that affect consciousness or blood pressure immediately to the health care provider. Monitor oxygen saturation levels by pulse oximetry, and consult with the respiratory therapist for the optimal method to deliver oxygen (e.g., facemask, nasal cannula, or noninvasive mechanical support [see Chapter 28]). Monitor the patient for worsening of the condition, manifested as increasing hypoxemia. He or she may require temporary intubation and mechanical ventilation if respiratory failure occurs.

Patients with CKD who have existing cardiac problems, high blood pressure, or chronic fluid retention are at increased risk for developing pulmonary edema. They are less likely to respond quickly to treatment and are more likely to develop problems related to drug therapy. Ultrafiltration may be used with these patients to reduce fluid volume.

Increasing Cardiac Output

Planning: Expected Outcomes. The patient with CKD is expected to attain and maintain adequate cardiac output. Indicators include that systolic and diastolic blood pressures, ejection fraction, peripheral pulses, and cognitive status are either normal or nearly normal.

Interventions. Many patients with long-standing hypertension are at risk for CKD and accelerated progression of kidney failure once CKD occurs. *Therefore blood pressure control is essential in preserving kidney function.* To control blood pressure, calcium channel blockers, angiotensin-converting enzyme (ACE) inhibitors, alpha-adrenergic and beta-adrenergic blockers, and vasodilators may be prescribed. ACE inhibitors are the most effective drugs to slow the progression of CKD in patients with hypertension. Calcium channel blockers can improve the GFR and blood flow within the kidney.

More information on the specific drugs for blood pressure control can be found in Chapter 36. Indications vary depending on the patient, and these drugs are used carefully to avoid complications. Different dosages and combinations may be tried until blood pressure control is adequate and side effects are minimized.

Teach the patient and family to measure blood pressure daily. Evaluate their ability to measure and record blood pressure accurately using their own equipment. Re-check measurement accuracy on a regular basis. Teach the patient and family about the relationship of blood pressure control to diet and drug therapy. Instruct the patient to weigh daily and to bring records of blood pressure measurements, drug administration times, and weights for discussion with the physician, nurse, or registered dietitian.

Assess the patient on an ongoing basis for manifestations of reduced cardiac output, heart failure, and dysrhythmias. These topics are discussed in Chapters 35 through 38.

Enhancing Nutrition

Planning: Expected Outcomes. The patient with CKD is expected to maintain adequate nutrition. The patient should have a protein-caloric intake appropriate for his or her weight-to-height ratio, muscle tone, and laboratory values (serum albumin, hematocrit, hemoglobin).

Interventions. The nutrition needs and diet restrictions for the patient with CKD vary according to the degree of kidney function and the type of renal replacement therapy used (Table 68-9). The purpose of nutrition therapy is to provide the food and fluids needed to prevent malnutrition and avoid complications from CKD.

The patient is referred to a dietitian for dietary teaching and planning. Work with the dietitian to teach the patient about diet changes that are needed as a result of CKD. Common changes include control of protein intake; fluid intake limitation; restriction of potassium, sodium, and phosphorus intake; taking vitamin and mineral supplements; and eating enough calories to meet metabolic need.

Protein restriction early in the course of the disease prevents some of the problems of CKD and may preserve kidney function. Protein is restricted on the basis of the degree of kidney impairment (reduced GFR) and the severity of the manifestations. Buildup of waste products from protein breakdown is the main cause of uremia.

The glomerular filtration rate (GFR) and treatment of CKD is used to guide safe levels of protein intake. A patient with a severely reduced GFR who is *not* undergoing dialysis is usually permitted 0.55 to 0.60 g of protein per kilogram of body weight (e.g., 40 g of protein daily for a 150-lb [70-kg] adult). If protein is lost in the urine, protein is added to the diet in amounts equal to that lost in the urine. Protein requirements are calculated based on actual body weight (corrected for edema), not ideal body weight.

The patient with ESKD receiving dialysis needs more protein because some protein is lost through dialysis. Protein requirements are tailored according to the patient's post-dialysis, or "dry," weight. Generally, patients receiving dialysis are allowed about 1 to 1.5 g of protein/kg/day. Peritoneal dialysis (PD) patients are allowed 1.2 to 1.5 g of protein/kg/day because protein is lost with each exchange. Suggested protein-containing foods are milk, meat, or eggs. If protein intake is not adequate, significant muscle wasting can occur. BUN and serum prealbumin and albumin levels are used to monitor the adequacy of protein intake. Decreased serum prealbumin or albumin levels indicate poor protein intake.

Sodium restriction is needed in patients with little or no urine output. Both fluid and sodium retention cause edema, hypertension, and heart failure (HF). Most patients with CKD retain sodium; a few cannot conserve sodium.

Estimate fluid and sodium retention status by monitoring the patient's body weight and blood pressure. In uremic patients not receiving dialysis, sodium is limited to 1 to 3 g daily and fluid intake depends on urine output. In patients receiving dialysis, the sodium restriction is 2 to 4 g daily and fluid intake

TABLE 68-9	**Dietary Restrictions Needed for Severe Kidney Disease**		
DIETARY COMPONENT	**WITH CHRONIC UREMIA**	**WITH HEMODIALYSIS**	**WITH PERITONEAL DIALYSIS**
Protein	0.55-0.60 g/kg/day	1.0-1.5 g/kg/day	1.2-1.5 g/kg/day
Fluid	Depends on urine output but may be as high as 1500-3000 mL/day	500-700 mL/day plus amount of urine output	Restriction based on fluid weight gain and blood pressure
Potassium	60-70 mEq/day	70 mEq/day	Usually no restriction
Sodium	1-3 g/day	2-4 g/day	Restriction based on fluid weight gain and blood pressure
Phosphorus	700 mg/day	700 mg/day	800 mg/day

is limited to 500 to 700 mL plus the amount of any urine output. Instruct the patient not to add salt at the table or during cooking. Many foods are significant sources of sodium (e.g., processed foods, fast foods, potato chips, pretzels, pickles, ham, bacon, sausage) and difficult to moderate or remove from one's diet. Inattention to sodium intake can increase the duration or number of dialysis treatments and contribute to *disequilibrium syndrome* (feeling "zonked") following dialysis.

Potassium restriction may be needed because high blood potassium levels can cause dangerous cardiac dysrhythmias. Monitor the ECG for tall, peaked T waves caused by hyperkalemia. Document serum potassium levels. Instruct the patient with ESKD to limit potassium intake to 60 to 70 mEq/day. Teach him or her to read labels of seasoning agents carefully for sodium and potassium content. Chart 11-6 in Chapter 11 lists common foods that are low in potassium and are permitted, along with foods that are high in potassium and should be avoided. Instruct patients to avoid salt substitutes composed of potassium chloride. Those receiving peritoneal dialysis or who are producing urine may not need potassium restriction.

Phosphorus restriction for control of phosphorus levels is started early in CKD to avoid renal osteodystrophy (bone defects). Monitor serum phosphorus levels. Dietary phosphorus restrictions and drugs to assist with phosphorus control may be prescribed. Phosphate binders must be taken at mealtimes. Most patients with CKD already restrict their protein intake, and because high-protein foods are also high in phosphorus, this reduces phosphorus intake. Chapter 11 lists foods high in potassium, sodium, and phosphorus. Cinacalcet (Sensipar), a drug to control parathyroid hormone excess, is also used to manage hyperphosphatemia and hypocalcemia.

Vitamin and mineral supplementation is needed daily for most patients with CKD. Low-protein diets are also low in vitamins, and water-soluble vitamins are removed from the blood during dialysis. Anemia also is a problem in patients with CKD because of the limited iron content of low-protein diets and decreased kidney production of erythropoietin. Thus supplemental iron is needed. Calcium and vitamin D supplements may be needed, depending on the patient's serum calcium levels and bone status.

Nutrition needs for patients undergoing peritoneal dialysis (PD) are slightly different from those for patients undergoing dialysis. Because protein is lost with the dialysate in PD, replacing lost protein is needed. Often 1.2 to 1.5 g of protein per kilogram of body weight per day is recommended. Patients may have anorexia and have difficulty eating enough protein. High-calorie oral supplements may also be needed (e.g., Magnacal Renal, Ensure Plus). Sodium restriction varies with fluid weight gain and blood pressure. Usually dietary potassium does not need to be restricted because the dialysate is potassium-free. Any potassium restriction is determined by serum potassium levels.

Collaborate with the dietitian to assess each patient's nutrition needs. Teach the patient the dietary regimen, and evaluate his or her understanding of and adherence to it. Give the patient and family written examples of the diet to promote adherence. Help patients adapt diet restrictions to their budget, ethnic background, and food preferences.

Preventing Infection

Planning: Expected Outcomes. The patient with CKD is expected to remain free of INFECTION. Indicators include that the patient will have only mild or no fever, no lymph node enlargement, negative urine culture, negative dialysis access site culture, and white blood cell count either within the normal range or only slightly elevated.

Interventions. Provide meticulous care to any areas where skin is not intact (e.g., incisions, site of drains, puncture sites, cracked or excoriated skin, pressure ulcers), and provide preventive skin care to intact areas. For patients with ESKD undergoing dialysis, inspect the vascular access site or peritoneal dialysis catheter insertion site every shift for redness, swelling, pain, and drainage. Monitor vital signs for manifestations of INFECTION (e.g., fever, tachycardia).

Preventing Injury

Planning: Expected Outcomes. The patient with CKD is expected to remain free of injury. Indicators include that the patient should not have any of these problems:

- Pathologic fractures
- Toxic side effects from drug therapy
- Bleeding

Interventions. *Injury prevention strategies* are needed because the patient with long-standing CKD may have brittle, fragile bones that fracture easily and cause little pain. When lifting or moving a patient with fragile bones, use a lift sheet rather than pulling the patient. Teach unlicensed assistive personnel (UAP) the correct use of lift sheets. Observe for normal range of joint motion and for any unusual surface bumps or depressions over bony areas.

Managing drug therapy in patients with CKD is a complex clinical problem. Many over-the-counter drugs contain agents that alter kidney function. Therefore it is important to obtain a detailed drug history. Know the use of each drug, its side effects, and its site of metabolism.

Certain drugs must be avoided, and the dosages of others must be adjusted according to the degree of remaining kidney function. As the patient's kidney function decreases, repeated dosage adjustments are necessary. Assess for side effects and indications of drug toxicity, and notify the prescriber as appropriate.

! NURSING SAFETY PRIORITY (QSEN)

Drug Alert

Monitor the patient with severe CKD or ESKD closely for drug-related complications, and ensure that dosages are adjusted as needed. Consult with the pharmacist to determine safe effective doses.

Many drugs are routinely given to patients with CKD, and some of the common drugs are detailed in Chart 68-6. Know the rationale for these drugs and the indicated nursing interventions. Many patients also have cardiac disease and may require cardiac drugs such as digoxin. Patients with severe CKD and ESKD are particularly at risk for digoxin toxicity because the drug is excreted by the kidneys. When caring for patients with CKD who are receiving digoxin, monitor for indications of

---

! NURSING SAFETY PRIORITY (QSEN)

Drug Alert

Doses of digoxin are much lower than for most drugs. When digoxin is administered to older adults with kidney disease, the prescribed daily dose may be even lower (0.0625 mg). Check and recheck the dosage before administering digoxin to a patient with kidney disease.

toxicity, such as nausea, vomiting, anorexia, visual changes, restlessness, headache, fatigue, confusion, bradycardia, and tachycardia. Monitor the serum drug levels to be certain they are in the therapeutic range (0.8-2 ng/mL). Also closely monitor the serum potassium levels of any patient receiving digoxin.

Drugs to control an excessively high phosphorus level include phosphate-binding agents. Non-calcium binders may be preferred to reduce the risk for extraskeletal deposition of calcium and subsequent vessel disease or stone formation (Lewis, 2012). These drugs help prevent renal osteodystrophy and related

CHART 68-6 Common Examples of Drug Therapy

Chronic Kidney Disease

DRUG/DOSAGE	ACTION/PURPOSE	NURSING INTERVENTIONS	RATIONALES
Loop Diuretics			
Furosemide (Lasix) Bumetanide (Bumex, Burinex) Dose varies with severity of kidney damage; not effective in ESKD	Manage volume overload when urinary elimination is still present.	Monitor intake and output. Monitor electrolytes.	Generally the expected outcome is for output to be greater than intake by 500-1000 mL per 24 hr. Loop diuretics result in loss of potassium; this can be a desired effect in patients with hyperkalemia
Vitamins and Minerals			
Phosphate Binders: Calcium acetate (PhosLo) 2-4 capsules with each meal Calcium carbonate (Caltrate, Oystercal, others) 2-4 capsules with each meal Lanthanum carbonate (Fosrenol) 500-1000 mg tablets Sevelamer (Renagel, Renvela) 400-800 mg Taken just before or with meals	High blood phosphorus levels cause hypocalcemia and osteodystrophy. These drugs bind to dietary phosphorous and phosphate, typically by using calcium to form an insoluble calcium phosphate such that neither mineral is absorbed from the gastrointestinal tract. These are non-calcium, non-aluminum phosphate binders.	Teach patients to take drugs with meals. Teach patients not to take these drugs within 2 hours of other schedule drugs. Teach patients to separate administration of phosphate binders from other scheduled drugs by 2 or more hours. Monitor both serum phosphorus and calcium levels. Monitor for constipation. Teach patients to report muscle weakness, slow or irregular pulse, or confusion to the prescriber.	Oral phosphate binders reduce hyperphosphatemia common in severe CKD and ESKD. Many of these drugs can bind with other oral drugs—notably cardiovascular drugs and antibiotics. Drugs that use calcium to bind phosphorus can cause hypercalcemia. Bound phosphorus is excreted in feces. These drugs can cause significant constipation leading to fecal impaction or ileus. Manage constipation with stool softeners like docusate or bowel stimulants such as senna. These are manifestations of hypophosphatemia, which require dosage adjustment.
Multivitamins and vitamin B supplements: Folic acid (vitamin B₉, Folvite, Novo-Folacid ♦) 1 mg orally daily	When the patient is receiving dialysis, many essential vitamins and minerals are removed from the blood. Replacement is needed to prevent severe deficiencies.	Teach patients to take the drugs after dialysis. Teach patients to take iron supplements (ferrous sulfate) with meals.	Dialysis removes the drug from the blood. Food reduces nausea and abdominal discomfort.
Iron Salts: Ferrous sulfate (Feosol, Novoferrosulfa ♦) 325 mg orally three or four times daily Iron sucrose (Venofer) 20 mg/mL; 100 mg per dialysis session		Teach patients to take stool softeners daily while taking iron supplements. Remind patients that iron supplements change the color of the stool.	Oral iron preparations cause constipation, and most patients with kidney disease must reduce their fluid intake, further increasing the risk for constipation. Knowing the expected side effects decreases anxiety when they appear.
Vitamin D: Calcitriol (Rocaltrol, Calcijex, Vectical) 0.25-0.5 mcg capsules or 1 mcg/mL solution Paricalcitol (Zemplar) 1-4 mcg capsules or injectable solution	This is the active form of vitamin D. It is used to suppress parathyroid production and secretion and to treat hypocalcemia.	Monitor serum levels of vitamin D and calcium.	Monitor for hypocalcemia or evidence of vitamin D toxicity.
Doxercalciferol (Hectorol) 0.25-2.5 mg, given 3 times/weekly at dialysis	This is a vitamin D analog that does not require activation by the kidneys.		

Continued

CHART 68-6   Common Examples of Drug Therapy—cont'd

Chronic Kidney Disease

DRUG/DOSAGE	ACTION/PURPOSE	NURSING INTERVENTIONS	RATIONALES
Erythropoietin-Stimulating Agents (ESAs)			
Epoetin alfa (Epogen, Procrit, generic) 50-100 units/kg subcutaneously or IV three times a week for patients on dialysis Darbepoetin alfa (Aranesp) 0.45 mcg/kg subcutaneously or IV once weekly for patients on dialysis	Drug prevents anemia by stimulating red blood cell growth and maturation in the bone marrow.	Monitor hemoglobin values. Start when hemoglobin is less than 10 g/dL and the rate of decline indicates the likelihood of requiring a red blood cell transfusion. Once the hemoglobin level is greater than 11 g/dL, reduce or interrupt dose. Teach patients to report any of these side effects to the prescriber as soon as possible: chest pain, difficulty breathing, high blood pressure, rapid weight gain, seizures, skin rash or hives, swelling of feet or ankles.	Drug can induce serious cardiovascular problems, such as myocardial infarction (MI).
Parathyroid Hormone Modulator			
Cinacalcet (Sensipar) 30-180 mg daily	Reduce parathyroid hormone levels. This drug increases the sensitivity to calcium on the chief cell receptors in the parathyroid gland.	Monitor levels of serum calcium. Teach the patient to monitor for diarrhea and muscle pain (myalgia).	This drug should not be used in severe hypocalcemia (levels less than 8.4 mg/dL).

CKD, Chronic kidney disease; *ESKD*, end-stage kidney disease.

injuries. Stress the importance of taking these agents and all prescribed drugs.

Hypophosphatemia (low serum phosphorus levels) is a complication of phosphate binding, especially in patients who are not eating adequately but who are continuing to take phosphate-binding drugs. *Hypercalcemia* (high serum calcium levels) also is a possible complication for patients taking calcium-containing compounds to control phosphorus excess. In patients taking aluminum-based phosphate binders for prolonged periods, aluminum deposits may cause bone disease or permanent neurologic problems. Monitor the patient for muscle weakness, anorexia, malaise, tremors, and bone pain.

Teach patients with kidney disease to avoid antacids containing magnesium. These patients cannot excrete magnesium and thus should avoid additional intake.

Some drugs, in addition to those used to treat kidney failure, require special attention. These drugs include antibiotics, opioids, antihypertensives, diuretics, insulin, and heparin.

Many antibiotics are safe for patients with CKD, but those excreted by the kidney require dose adjustment. To prevent complications of bloodstream INFECTION from mouth bacteria, prophylactic antibiotic treatment is given to patients with CKD before any dental procedures. The antibiotic used varies with the patient's needs and the health care provider's preference.

Give opioid analgesics cautiously in patients with severe CKD or ESKD because the effects often last longer. Patients with uremia are sensitive to the respiratory depressant effects of these drugs. Because opioids are broken down by the liver and not the kidneys, the dosages are often the same regardless of the level of kidney function. Monitor the patient's reactions closely after opioids are given to determine whether adjustments are needed.

As CKD progresses, the patient with diabetes often requires reduced doses of insulin or antidiabetic drugs because the failing kidneys do not excrete or metabolize these drugs well. Thus the drugs are effective longer, increasing the risk for

hypoglycemia. Monitor blood glucose levels at least 4 times daily to assess whether a dosage change is needed.

Poor platelet function and capillary fragility in CKD make anticoagulant therapy risky. Monitor patients receiving heparin, warfarin, or any anticoagulant every shift for bleeding. See Chapter 40 for more information on caring for patients at increased risk for bleeding.

Minimizing Fatigue

Planning: Expected Outcomes. The patient with chronic kidney disease (CKD) is expected to conserve energy by balancing activity and rest. Indicators include that the patient will be able to participate in self-care activities, have interest in surroundings, and demonstrate mental concentration.

Interventions. Some causes of fatigue in the patient with CKD include vitamin deficiency, anemia, and buildup of urea. All patients are given vitamin and mineral supplements because of diet restrictions and vitamin losses from dialysis. Avoid giving these supplements before hemodialysis (HD) treatment because they will be dialyzed out of the body and the patient will receive no benefit.

The anemic patient with CKD is treated with agents to stimulate red blood cell production (Dutka, 2012). The outcome of this therapy is to maintain a hemoglobin level around 10 g/dL. This therapy is effective in triggering bone marrow production of red blood cells if the patient has adequate iron stores. Iron supplements may be needed if patients are iron deficient. Many who receive these drugs report improved appetite and sexual function along with decreased fatigue. The increased production of all blood cells from this therapy may increase blood pressure. The improved appetite challenges patients in their attempts to maintain protein, potassium, and fluid restrictions and requires additional education.

Reducing Anxiety

Planning: Expected Outcomes. The patient with CKD is expected to have reduced tension and apprehension. Indicators include that the patient consistently demonstrates these behaviors:

- Seeks information to reduce anxiety
- Uses effective coping strategies
- Reports an absence of anxiety manifestations

Interventions. The nurse coordinates a team of health care professionals to support and counsel the patient and family, often over many years of treatment. The nurse has the most contact with the patient when he or she is hospitalized or undergoing in-center dialysis treatments. Perform an ongoing assessment of the patient's anxiety level. Observe behavior for cues indicating anxiety (e.g., anxious facial expressions, clenching of hands, tapping of feet, withdrawn posture, absence of eye contact, an increased pulse rate). Evaluate the support systems, such as the involvement of family and friends with the patient's care.

Unfamiliar settings and lack of knowledge about treatments and tests can increase the patient's anxiety level. Explain all procedures, tests, and treatments. Identify the patient's knowledge needs about kidney disease. Provide instruction at a level he or she can understand using a variety of written and visual materials.

Provide continuity of care, whenever possible, by using a consistent nurse-patient relationship to decrease anxiety and promote discussions of concerns. As you develop the nurse-patient relationship, encourage the patient to discuss current problems or concerns.

Encourage the patient to ask questions and discuss fears about the diagnosis. An open atmosphere that allows for discussion can decrease anxiety. Facilitate discussions with family members about the prognosis and the impact on lifestyle.

Renal Replacement Therapies

Renal replacement therapy (RRT) is needed when the pathologic changes of stage 4 and stage 5 CKD are life threatening or pose continuing discomfort. When the patient can no longer be managed with conservative therapies, such as diet, drugs, and fluid restriction, dialysis is indicated. Transplantation may be discussed at any time.

Hemodialysis

Intermittent hemodialysis (HD) is the most common RRT used with ESKD (Table 68-10). Dialysis removes excess fluids and waste products and restores chemical and electrolyte balance. HD involves passing the patient's blood through an artificial semipermeable membrane to perform the filtering and excretion functions of the kidney. This therapy usually requires technicians to provide meticulous care to the machines delivering HD and nurses to implement and supervise direct care. Such measures are essential to safe HD. Technical or human error can lead to avoidable complications (e.g., hemolysis, air embolism, dialysate error, contamination).

Patient Selection. Any patient may be considered for intermittent HD therapy. Starting HD depends on manifestations from disruptions of FLUID AND ELECTROLYTE BALANCE and waste and toxin accumulation, not the GFR alone (Yeun et al., 2012). Dialysis is started immediately for patients who have:

- Fluid overload that does not respond to diuretics (including fluid overload with **pericarditis**)
- Symptomatic **hyperkalemia**
- **Calciphylaxis** (a condition of thrombosis and skin necrosis that can occur in stage 5 CKD)

TABLE 68-10	**Comparison of Hemodialysis and Peritoneal Dialysis**
HEMODIALYSIS	**PERITONEAL DIALYSIS**
Advantages	
More efficient clearance of wastes	Flexible schedule for exchanges
Short time needed for treatment	Few hemodynamic changes during and following exchanges
	Less dietary and fluid restrictions
Complications	
Disequilibrium syndrome	Protein loss
Muscle cramps and back pain	Peritonitis
Headache	Hyperglycemia from dialysate
Itching	Respiratory distress
Hemodynamic and cardiac adverse events (hypotension, cell lysis contributing to anemia, cardiac dysrhythmias)	Bowel perforation
	Infection
Infection	Weight gain; discomfort from "carrying" 1-2 liters in abdomen during dwell time; potential for back pain or development of hernia
Increased risk for subdural and intracranial hemorrhage from anticoagulation and changes in blood pressure during dialysis	
Contraindications	
Hemodynamic instability or severe cardiac disease	Extensive peritoneal adhesions, fibrosis, or active inflammatory gastrointestinal disease (e.g., diverticulitis, inflammatory bowel conditions)
Severe vascular disease that prevents vascular access	
Serious bleeding disorders	Ascites or massive central obesity
Uncontrolled diabetes	Recent abdominal surgery
Access	
Vascular access route	Intra-abdominal catheter
Procedure	
Complex; requires a second person trained in the technique whether completed at home or at a dialysis unit/center	Simple, easier to complete at home compared with at-home hemodialysis
Special training for center personnel and in-home use; requires at least two people to manage process	Less complex training; typically managed by patient; can be managed by one person

- Symptomatic toxin ingestion such as drug overdose or poisoning that is dialyzable (see Table 68-13)

Most commonly, hemodialysis for CKD is started when uremic manifestations (e.g., nausea and vomiting, decreased attention span, decreased cognition, and pruritus) are present.

Many patients survive for years with HD therapy, and others may live only a few months. How long the patient survives using HD therapy depends on his or her age, the cause of CKD, and the presence of other diseases, such as cardiovascular disease or diabetes. General patient selection criteria are:

- Irreversible kidney failure when other therapies are unacceptable or ineffective
- No disorders that would seriously complicate HD
- Patient values and preferences
- Expected ability to continue or resume roles at home, work, or school

Dialysis Settings. Patients with CKD may receive HD treatments in many settings, depending on specific needs. Regardless of the setting for therapy, they need ongoing nursing support to maintain this complex and lifesaving treatment.

Patients may be dialyzed in a hospital-based center if they have recently started treatment or have complicated conditions that require close supervision. Stable patients not requiring intense supervision may be dialyzed in a community or free-standing dialysis center. Selected patients may participate in complete or partial self-care in an ambulatory care center or with in-home HD.

In-home HD is the least disruptive and allows the patient to adapt the regimen to his or her lifestyle. Many cannot participate in in-home dialysis because they lack a skilled partner to assist with the therapy and manage the dialysis machine. Some patients and partners find the use of in-home dialysis to be too stressful. In addition, a water treatment system must be installed in the home to provide a safe, clean water supply for the dialysis process. More compact and more easily managed systems have contributed to the growth of in-home HD (Yeun et al., 2012).

Procedure. Dialysis works using the passive transfer of toxins by diffusion. **Diffusion** is the movement of molecules from an area of higher concentration to an area of lower concentration. The rate of diffusion during dialysis is most dependent on the difference in the solute concentrations between the patient's blood and the dialysate. Large molecules, such as RBCs and most plasma proteins, cannot pass through the membrane.

When HD is started, blood and **dialysate** (dialyzing solution) flow in opposite directions across an enclosed semipermeable membrane. The dialysate contains a balanced mix of electrolytes and water that closely resembles human plasma. On the other side of the membrane is the patient's blood, which contains nitrogen waste products, excess water, and excess electrolytes. During HD, the waste products move from the blood into the dialysate because of the difference in their concentrations (diffusion). Some water is also removed from the blood into the dialysate by *osmosis.* Electrolytes can move in either direction, as needed, and take some fluid with them. Potassium and sodium typically move out of the plasma into the dialysate. Bicarbonate and calcium generally move from the dialysate into the plasma. This circulating process continues for a preset length of time, removing nitrogenous wastes and reestablishing FLUID AND ELECTROLYTE BALANCE, as well as restoring ACID-BASE BALANCE. Water volume may be removed from the plasma by applying positive or negative pressure to the system.

The HD system includes a dialyzer, dialysate, vascular access routes, and an HD machine. The artificial kidney, or **dialyzer** (Fig. 68-3), has four parts: a blood compartment, a dialysate compartment, a semipermeable membrane, and an enclosed support structure.

Dialysate is made from water and chemicals and is free of any waste products or drugs. Often dialysate is made in the pharmacy in an acute care setting. It may be made by technicians in dialysis centers. Because bacteria and other organisms are too large to pass through the membrane, dialysate is not sterile. The water used in dialysate must meet specific standards and usually requires special treatment before mixing the dialysate. The dialysate composition may be altered according to the patient's needs for management of electrolyte imbalances. During HD, the dialysate is warmed to 100°F (37.8°C) to increase the diffusion rate and to prevent hypothermia.

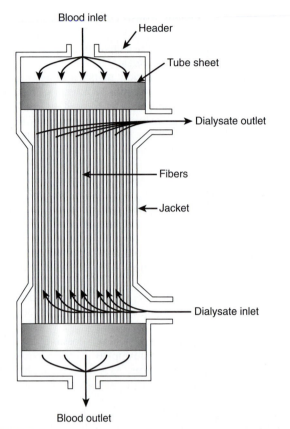

FIG. 68-3 Hollow fiber dialyzer (artificial kidney) used in hemodialysis.

The HD machine has built-in safety features such as the ability to record patient vital signs, blood and dialysate flows, arterial and venous pressures, delivered dialysis dose, plasma volume changes and thermal changes. If any of these problems are detected, an alarm sounds to protect the patient from life-threatening complications.

All dialyzers function in a similar manner. Fig. 68-4 shows a comparison of fluid and particle movement across the dialyzer membranes, comparing intermittent HD with continuous renal replacement circuits. For intermittent HD, the number and length of treatments depend on the amount of wastes and fluid to be removed, the clearance capacity of the dialyzer, and the blood flow rate to and from the machine. Fig. 68-5 shows a typical intermittent dialysis machine. Most patients receive three 4-hour treatments over the course of a week. For those with some ongoing urine production, two 5- to 6-hour treatments a week may be adequate. If the patient gains large amounts of fluid, a longer HD treatment time may be needed to remove the fluid without hypotension or severe side effects.

Anticoagulation. Blood clotting can occur during dialysis. Anticoagulation, usually with heparin, is most often delivered into the blood circuit via a pump. In patients with high risk for bleeding, a reduced dose, regional anticoagulation (using citrate rather than heparin for anticoagulation or reversing heparin actions by administering protamine before returning blood to the patient), or no anticoagulation may be used. Patient response to heparin varies, and the dose is adjusted on the basis of each patient's need.

Heparin remains active in the body for 4 to 6 hours after dialysis, increasing the patient's risk for hemorrhage during and immediately after HD treatments. Invasive procedures must be

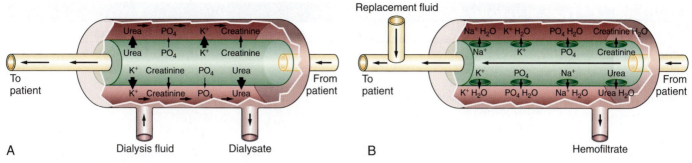

FIG. 68-4 Comparison of hemodialysis and hemofiltration fluid and solute movements across the membrane. Demonstrates this movement in hemodialysis **(A)** and in hemofiltration **(B)**. The *arrows* that cross the membrane indicate the predominant direction of movement of each solute through the membrane; the relative size of the *arrows* indicates the net amounts of the solute transferred. Other *arrows* indicate the direction of flow.

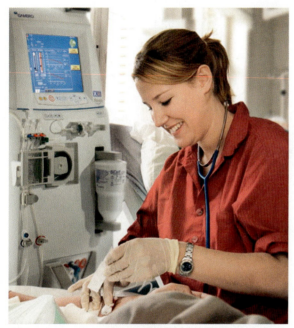

FIG. 68-5 Renal replacement therapy with an intermittent hemodialysis machine.

avoided during that time. Monitor him or her closely for any manifestations of bleeding or hemorrhage. Protamine sulfate is an antidote to heparin and always should be available in the dialysis setting.

Vascular Access. Vascular access is required for hemodialysis (Table 68-11 and Fig. 68-6). The procedure requires the easy availability of a large amount of blood flow: at least 250 to 300 mL/min, usually for a period of 3 to 4 hours. Normal venous cannulation does not provide this high rate of blood flow.

Long-term vascular access is internal for most patients having long-term HD (see Table 68-11). The two common choices are an internal arteriovenous (AV) fistula or an AV graft (see Fig. 68-6 A, B, and C). *AV fistulas* are formed by surgically connecting an artery to a vein. The vessels used most often are the radial or brachial artery and the cephalic vein of the nondominant arm. Fistulas increase venous blood flow to 250 to 400 mL/min, the amount needed for effective dialysis.

Time is needed after anastomosis for the AV fistula to develop. As the AV fistula "matures," the increased pressure of the arterial blood flow into the vein causes the vessel walls to

thicken. This thickening increases their strength and durability for repeated cannulation. Patients differ in the amount of time needed for the fistula to mature. Some fistulas may not be ready for use for as long as 4 months after the surgery, and a temporary vascular access (AV shunt or HD catheter) is used during this time. Fig. 68-7 shows a mature fistula.

To access a fistula, cannulate it by inserting two needles—one toward the venous blood flow and one toward the arterial blood flow. This procedure allows the HD machine to draw the blood out through the arterial needle and return it through the venous needle.

Arteriovenous grafts are used when the AV fistula does not develop or when complications limit its use. The polytetrafluoroethylene (PTFE) graft is a synthetic material (GORE-TEX). This type of graft is commonly used for older patients using HD. Figs. 68-6, *A*, and 68-7 show a patient's fistula.

Precautions. Some precautions are needed to ensure the functioning of an internal AV fistula or AV graft. First assess for adequate circulation in the fistula or graft as well as in the lower portion of the arm. Check distal pulses and capillary refill in the arm with the fistula or graft. Then check for a bruit or a thrill by auscultation or palpation over the access site. Chart 68-7 lists best practices for care of the patient with an HD access.

> **! NURSING SAFETY PRIORITY** (QSEN)
> **Action Alert**
>
> Because repeated compression can result in the loss of the vascular access, avoid taking the blood pressure or performing venipunctures in the arm with the vascular access. Do not use an AV fistula or graft for delivery of IV fluids.

Complications. Complications can occur with any type of access. The most common problems are thrombosis or stenosis, INFECTION, aneurysm formation, ischemia, and heart failure. Table 68-12 lists strategies to prevent access complications.

Thrombosis, or clotting of the AV access, is the most frequent complication. Most grafts fail because of high-pressure arterial flow entering the venous system. The muscle layers of the veins react to this increased pressure by thickening. The venous thickening reduces or occludes blood flow. An interventional radiologist can re-open failing grafts with the injection of a thrombolytic drug (e.g., tPA) to dissolve the clot. The clot usually dissolves within minutes, and often a stricture is revealed

TABLE 68-11	**Types of Vascular Access for Hemodialysis**		
ACCESS TYPE	**DESCRIPTION**	**LOCATION**	**TIME TO INITIAL USE**
Permanent			
AV fistula	An internal anastomosis of an artery to a vein	Forearm Upper arm	2-4 mo or longer
AV graft	Synthetic vessel tubing tunneled beneath the skin, connecting an artery and a vein	Forearm Upper arm Inner thigh	1-2 wk
Temporary			
Dialysis catheter	A specially designed catheter with separate lumens for blood outflow and inflow	Subclavian, internal jugular, or femoral vein	Immediately after insertion and x-ray confirmation of placement
Subcutaneous device	An internal device with two metallic access ports and two catheters inserted into large central veins	Subclavian	

AV, Arteriovenous.

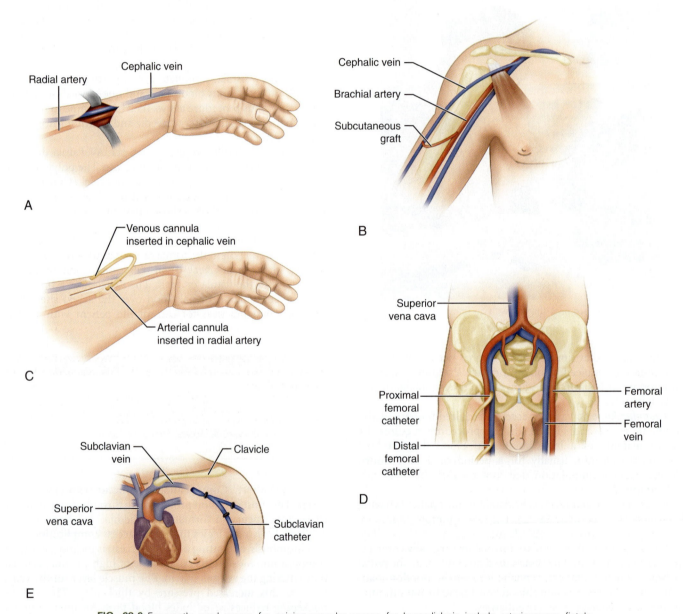

FIG. 68-6 Frequently used means for gaining vascular access for hemodialysis include arteriovenous fistula **(A)**, arteriovenous graft **(B)**, external arteriovenous shunt **(C)**, femoral vein catheterization **(D)**, and subclavian vein catheterization **(E)**. **A** and **B** are options for long-term vascular access for hemodialysis. **C, D,** and **E** are used for short-term access for intermittent hemodialysis or for continuous renal replacement therapy in acute care.

TABLE 68-12	Interventions for Preventing Complications in Hemodialysis Vascular Access		
ACCESS TYPE	**BLEEDING**	**INFECTION**	**CLOTTING**
AV fistula or AV graft	Apply pressure to the needle puncture sites.	Prepare skin using best practices before cannulation. Typically 2% chlorhexidine is used, similar to central line skin preparation. Between hemodialysis sessions, the patient should wash the area with antibacterial soap and rinse with water.	Avoid constrictive devices. Rotate needle insertion sites with each hemodialysis treatment. Assess for thrill and bruit.
Hemodialysis catheters (temporary and permanent)	Monitor the access site.	Use aseptic technique to dress site and access catheter.	Place a heparin or heparin/saline dwell solution after hemodialysis treatment. Do not use access except for dialysis treatments.

AV, Arteriovenous.

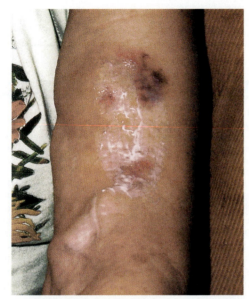

FIG. 68-7 A mature fistula for hemodialysis access. The increased pressure from the anastomosed artery forced blood into the vein. This process caused the vein to dilate enough for fistula needles to be placed for hemodialysis. When the vein is sufficiently dilated, a process that takes 8 to 12 weeks, the fistula is said to be "developed" or "mature."

at the point where the graft and the vein connect. The stricture can be corrected by balloon angioplasty.

Most infections of the vascular access are caused by *Staphylococcus aureus* introduced during cannulation. Prepare the skin with an antibacterial agent according to agency policy before cannulation to prevent INFECTION.

Aneurysms can form in the fistula and are caused by repeated needle punctures at the same site. Large aneurysms may cause loss of the fistula's function and require surgical repair.

Ischemia occurs in a few patients with vascular access when the fistula decreases arterial blood flow to areas below the fistula (*steal syndrome*). Manifestations vary from cold or numb fingers to gangrene. If the collateral circulation is poor, the fistula may need to be surgically tied off and a new one created in another area to preserve extremity circulation.

Shunting of blood directly from the arterial system to the venous system, through the fistula, can cause heart failure in patients with limited cardiac function. This complication is rare, but if it does occur, the fistula may need to be revised to reduce arterial blood flow.

Temporary Vascular Access. Temporary access with special catheters can be used for patients requiring immediate HD. A catheter designed for HD may be inserted into the subclavian,

---

CHART 68-7 Best Practice for Patient Safety & Quality Care QSEN

Caring for the Patient with an Arteriovenous Fistula or Arteriovenous Graft

- Do not take blood pressure readings using the extremity in which the vascular access is placed.
- Do not perform venipunctures or start an IV line in the extremity in which the vascular access is placed.
- Palpate for thrills and auscultate for bruits over the vascular access site every 4 hours while the patient is awake.
- Assess the patient's distal pulses and circulation in the arm with the access.
- Elevate the affected extremity postoperatively.
- Encourage routine range-of-motion exercises.
- Check for bleeding at needle insertion sites.
- Assess for manifestations of infection at needle sites.
- Instruct the patient not to carry heavy objects or anything that compresses the extremity in which the vascular access is placed.
- Instruct the patient not to sleep with his or her body weight on top of the extremity in which the vascular access is placed.

AV, Arteriovenous.

internal jugular, or femoral vein. The lumens of these devices are much smaller than the permanent accesses, and more time (4 to 8 hours) is required to complete a dialysis session.

Subcutaneous devices may also be surgically inserted to provide temporary access for HD. Implanted beneath the skin, these devices are composed of two small metallic ports with attached catheters that are inserted into large central veins. The ports of subcutaneous devices have internal mechanisms that open when needles are inserted and close when needles are removed. Blood from one port flows from the body to the HD machine and returns to the body via the other port. These devices may be ideal for patients waiting for permanent access placement or a kidney transplant.

? CLINICAL JUDGMENT CHALLENGE

Evidence-Based Practice; Patient-Centered Care QSEN

The patient just completed a vascular "mapping" procedure with an angiogram to plan the site of an AV fistula for hemodialysis. You are considering the care priorities for the patient's return when the AV fistula is formed.
1. What are important teaching points for the period immediately following AV fistula formation?
2. The patient asks if there is anything she can do to make this AV fistula last a long time. How should you respond to promote best practices in AV fistula self-management?
3. What else should this patient know about AV fistula care?

TABLE 68-13 Examples of Dialyzable Drugs

Consult the pharmacist, nephrologist, or dialysis nurse to plan the best time to administer a drug based on the dialysis schedule.

Aminoglycosides
- Amikacin
- Gentamicin
- Tobramycin

Antituberculosis Agents
- Ethambutol
- Isoniazid

Antiviral and Antifungal Agents
- Acyclovir
- Ganciclovir
- Fluconazole

Cephalosporins
- Cefaclor
- Cefazolin
- Cefoxitin
- Ceftizoxime
- Ceftriaxone
- Cefuroxime
- Cefepime

Anticonvulsants
- Ethosuximide
- Gabapentin
- Phenobarbital

Penicillins
- Amoxicillin
- Ampicillin
- Cloxacillin
- Dicloxacillin
- Mezlocillin
- Penicillin G
- Ticarcillin

Miscellaneous
- Aztreonam
- Cimetidine
- Vitamins
- Clavulanic acid
- Allopurinol
- Enalapril
- Aspirin

Hemodialysis Nursing Care. Many drugs are dialyzable (i.e., can be partially removed from the blood during dialysis). Coordinate with the health care provider to assess the patient's drug regimen and determine which drugs should be held until after HD treatment. Table 68-13 lists common dialyzable drugs that should be given *after* rather than before HD. Consult the dialysis nurse or nephrologists to determine if antihypertensive drugs should be given before a scheduled dialysis treatment; some short-acting antihypertensives can contribute to hypotension during dialysis (Ryan, 2012).

The time required to complete an HD treatment usually is at least 4 hours. During this time patients may use various distraction techniques to prevent boredom. This time can be used also for brief health teaching opportunities (see the Quality Improvement box).

Post-Dialysis Care. Closely monitor the patient immediately and for several hours after dialysis for any side effects from the treatment. Common problems include hypotension, headache, nausea, vomiting, dizziness, and muscle cramps.

Obtain vital signs and weight for comparison with pre-dialysis measurements. Blood pressure and weight are expected to be reduced as a result of fluid removal. Hypotension may require rehydration with IV fluids, such as normal saline. The patient's temperature may also be elevated because the dialysis machine warms the blood slightly. If he or she has a fever, sepsis may be present and a blood sample is needed for culture and sensitivity.

The heparin required during HD increases the risk for excessive bleeding. All invasive procedures must be avoided for 4 to 6 hours after dialysis. Continually monitor the patient for hemorrhage during and for at least 1 hour after dialysis (Chart 68-8).

Complications of Hemodialysis. Few adverse events occur during a 3- to 4-hour HD treatment under current practice protocols. Improved water treatment, more physiologic solutions, and improvements in HD equipment and procedures

CHART 68-8 Best Practice for Patient Safety & Quality Care (QSEN)

Caring for the Patient Undergoing Hemodialysis

- Weigh the patient before and after dialysis.
- Know the patient's dry weight.
- Discuss with the health care provider whether any of the patient's drugs should be withheld until after dialysis.
- Be aware of events that occurred during previous dialysis treatments.
- Measure blood pressure, pulse, respirations, and temperature.
- Assess for manifestations of orthostatic hypotension.
- Assess the vascular access site.
- Observe for bleeding.
- Assess the patient's level of consciousness.
- Assess for headache, nausea, and vomiting.

QUALITY IMPROVEMENT (QSEN)

Using Hemodialysis Time as a Teachable Moment

Wilson, B., & Lawrence, J. (2013). Implementation of a foot assessment program in a regional satellite hemodialysis setting. *Canadian Association of Nephrology Nurses and Technologists Journal, 23*(2), 41-47.

Because many patients receiving hemodialysis (HD) also have diabetes, the authors designed a quality improvement project to implement guidelines for foot care among their patients in an ambulatory care HD setting. The program included a one-time full assessment of risk for all patients followed by a monthly foot check for all patients with diabetes. Results included early identification of patients with a foot problem, timelier referral for treatment of foot problems, and a high degree of staff and patient satisfaction with the program.

Commentary: Implications for Practice and Research

This is an example of translating guidelines into practice and using guidelines in an uncommon setting to provide consistent assessment for diabetic patients at high risk for impaired self-management. Although the guidelines were Canadian and the implementation occurred in a single site, the steps to translating a guideline into practice and evaluating adherence to practice can be followed by other sites interested in delivering high-quality care to high-risk patients who receive hemodialysis.

! NURSING SAFETY PRIORITY (QSEN)

Critical Rescue

Hypotension can occur in up to 50% of HD treatments (Yeun et al., 2012). Heat transfer from warmed solutions can result in vasodilation and a drop in blood pressure. When this occurs, consider reducing the temperature of the dialysate to 35°C (95°F). A shift of fluid from the intravascular to extravascular space related to the difference in electrolytes concentrations between HD solutions and blood also contributes to low blood pressure. Whereas modest declines in blood pressure can be addressed by adjusting the rate of extracorporeal blood flow and placing the patient in a legs-up (Trendelenburg) position, sustained or symptomatic hypotension is treated with a fluid bolus of 100 to 250 mL of normal saline or sometimes albumin or mannitol. A second bolus may be needed. If hypotension persists, consider that new-onset myocardial injury or pericardial disease may be a contributing factor and administer oxygen, reduce the blood flow, and notify the health care provider urgently. Discontinue HD when hypotension continues despite cooling dialysate or providing up to two bolus infusions.

have significantly improved safe care for patients receiving this treatment. Complications during HD include hypotension, dialysis disequilibrium syndrome, cardiac events, and reactions to dialyzers.

Dialysis disequilibrium syndrome may develop during HD or after HD has been completed. It is characterized by mental status changes and can include seizures or coma; it is uncommon to observe this severity of disequilibrium syndrome with today's HD practice. A mild form of disequilibrium syndrome includes manifestations of nausea, vomiting, headaches, fatigue, and restlessness. It is thought to be the result of a rapid reduction in electrolytes and other particles (**solutes**) in a short time frame. Maintaining a low blood flow or reducing blood flow with the onset of manifestations can prevent this syndrome.

Cardiac events during HD are associated with underlying cardiovascular disease, especially left ventricular hypertrophy, coronary vascular disease, and a history of cardiac dysrhythmias. These conditions are described in Chapters 35, 36, and 38. Cardiac events leading to a full cardiac arrest are most concerning in an ambulatory care or in-home HD setting. Although cardiac arrest is a rare event, the setting should be equipped with an automatic defibrillator and staff or family trained in cardiopulmonary resuscitation. Often cardiac arrest is related to new-onset cardiac ischemia. The patient then needs to be managed in an acute care setting in which the presence of myocardial disease can be evaluated and cardiac treatment optimized.

Pericardial disease is a complication of patients with ESKD. Assess the patient's heart sounds for the presence of a pericardial rub prior to dialysis. Intensification of dialysis may be used to treat this complication. Other treatment might include NSAID use or surgery as described on p. 1421.

Reactions to dialyzers still occur, although more biocompatible membranes and careful attention to rinsing the dialyzer before use (to eliminate sterilizing agents) have reduced this type of adverse event during HD. Reactions occur during a "first-time" use of the filter and resemble an anaphylactic episode early during HD, with profound hypotension (Chapter 20 describes anaphylactic reactions). With suspected dialyzer reactions, the nurse does not return the blood to the patient and discontinues HD. Corticosteroids may be used to treat the immune reaction.

Other potential complications of recurrent HD require the nurse to monitor the level of consciousness and vital signs frequently during treatment and to slow or stop HD when manifestations occur. Hypoglycemia is a rare adverse HD event and more likely to occur when the patient has diabetes. Hypoglycemia is managed by providing glucose and increasing dialysis glucose concentration in subsequent treatments. Hemorrhage can occur when needle dislodgement or circuit connections become loose and is amplified by the anticoagulation treatment to maintain circuit patency. Some hemolysis will occur because of mechanical trauma to red blood cells, contributing to the anemia of CKD and, perhaps, sensations of dyspnea or chest tightness.

Infectious diseases transmitted by blood transfusion are a serious complication of long-term HD. Two of the most serious blood-transmitted infections are hepatitis and human immune deficiency virus (HIV) infection. *Hepatitis B infection* and *hepatitis C infection* in patients with CKD have decreased because the use of erythropoietin-stimulating agents (ESAs) has reduced the need for blood transfusions to maintain red blood cell counts. Hepatitis is a problem because of the blood access and the risk for contamination during HD. The viruses can be transmitted through the use of contaminated needles or instruments, by entry of contaminated blood through open wounds in the skin or mucous membranes, or through transfusions with contaminated blood. Monitor all patients receiving HD for manifestations of hepatitis (see Chapter 58).

HIV is a bloodborne virus that poses some risk for patients undergoing HD. Fortunately, the risks for HIV transmission are reduced by the consistent practice of Standard Precautions, routine screening of donated blood for HIV, and decreased need for blood transfusions with CKD and ESKD. Patients who have been undergoing HD or who received frequent transfusions during the early to middle 1980s are at risk for acquired immune deficiency syndrome (AIDS) (see Chapter 19).

CONSIDERATIONS FOR OLDER ADULTS

Patient-Centered Care QSEN

Between the years 2000 and 2010, a threefold increase in the number of older adults diagnosed with CKD occurred (Elliott, 2012). In 2010, the number of patients ages 60 years and older increased to more than 25% of patients beginning ESKD therapy (USRDS, 2014). The overall mean age for new patients requiring dialysis is 64.6. Patients older than 65 years who are receiving HD are more at risk for dialysis-induced hypotension. These patients require more frequent monitoring during and after dialysis.

Peritoneal Dialysis

Peritoneal dialysis (PD) allows exchanges of wastes, fluid, and electrolytes to occur in the peritoneal cavity. PD is slower than hemodialysis (HD), however, and more time is needed to achieve the same effect. Other disadvantages of PD are the protein loss in outflow fluid, risk for peritoneal injury, and potential discomfort from indwelling fluid. Advantages and complications are listed in Table 68-10. The use of PD has deceased and currently accounts for less than 10% of dialysis (USRDS, 2014).

Patient Selection. Most patients with CKD can select either HD or PD. For those who are unstable and those who cannot tolerate anticoagulation, PD is less hazardous than HD. For some patients, vascular access problems may eliminate HD as an option. At times a patient may use PD until a new arteriovenous (AV) fistula matures. PD is often the treatment of choice for older adults because it offers more flexibility if his or her status changes frequently.

Peritoneal dialysis *cannot* be performed if peritoneal adhesions are present or if extensive intra-abdominal surgery has been performed. In these cases, the surface area of the peritoneal membrane is not sufficient for adequate dialysis exchange. Peritoneal membrane fibrosis may occur after repeated INFECTION, which decreases membrane permeability.

Procedure. A siliconized rubber (Silastic) catheter is surgically placed into the abdominal cavity for infusion of dialysate (Fig. 68-8). Usually 1 to 2 L of dialysate is infused by gravity (*fill*) into the peritoneal space over a 10- to 20-minute period, according to the patient's tolerance. The fluid stays (*dwells*) in the cavity for a specified time prescribed by the physician. The fluid then flows out of the body (*drains*) by gravity into a drainage bag. The peritoneal outflow contains the dialysate and the excess water, electrolytes, and nitrogen-based waste products. The dialyzing fluid is called peritoneal *effluent* on outflow. The three phases of the process (infusion, or "fill"; dwell; and outflow, or drain) make up one PD exchange. The number and frequency of PD exchanges are prescribed by the physician, depending on manifestations and laboratory data.

Process. Peritoneal dialysis occurs through diffusion and osmosis across the semipermeable peritoneal membrane and capillaries. The peritoneal membrane is large and porous. It allows solutes (particles) and water to move from an area of higher concentration in the blood to an area of lower concentration in the dialyzing fluid (diffusion).

The peritoneal cavity is rich in capillaries and is a ready access to the blood supply. The fluid and waste products dialyzed from the patient move through the blood vessel walls, the interstitial tissues, and the peritoneal membrane and are removed when the dialyzing fluid is drained from the body.

PD efficiency is affected by many factors. INFECTION can cause scarring and reduce capillary blood flow. Vascular disease and decreased PERFUSION of the peritoneum reduce PD diffusion. For PD, water removal depends on the concentration of the dialysate. PD efficiency can be altered by the *tonicity* (i.e., number of particles per liter of fluid) of the dialysate. Increasing the dialysate glucose concentration makes the solution more hypertonic. The more hypertonic the solution, the greater the osmotic pressure for water filtration and fluid removal from the patient during an exchange. The dialysate concentration is prescribed on the basis of the patient's fluid status.

Dialysate Additives. Heparin may be added to the dialysate to prevent clotting of the catheter or tubing. Usually intraperitoneal (IP) heparin is needed only after new catheter placement or if peritonitis occurs. IP heparin is not absorbed systemically and does not affect blood clotting.

Other agents that may be given in the dialysate include potassium and antibiotics. Commercially prepared dialysate does not contain potassium. Some patients need potassium added to the dialysate to prevent hypokalemia. Antibiotics may be given by the IP route when peritonitis is present or suspected. Potassium and antibiotics are not mixed in the same dialysate bag because interactions may reduce the antibiotic effect.

Types of Peritoneal Dialysis. Many types of PD are available, including continuous ambulatory PD, multiple-bag continuous ambulatory PD, automated PD, intermittent PD, and continuous-cycle PD. The type selected depends on the patient's ability and lifestyle. The two most commonly used types of PD are continuous ambulatory peritoneal dialysis and continuous cycling peritoneal dialysis.

Continuous ambulatory peritoneal dialysis (CAPD) is performed by the patient with the infusion of four 2-L exchanges of dialysate into the peritoneal cavity. Each time, the dialysate remains for 4 to 8 hours, and these exchanges occur 7 days a week (Figs. 68-9 through 68-11). During the dwell period, the patient can use a continuous connect system or disconnect and

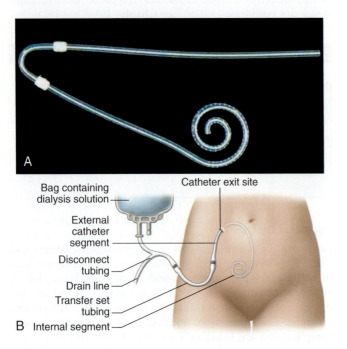

FIG. 68-8 Peritoneal dialysis catheter. **A,** The actual Silastic peritoneal dialysis catheter. **B,** Positioning of the Silastic catheter within the abdominal cavity.

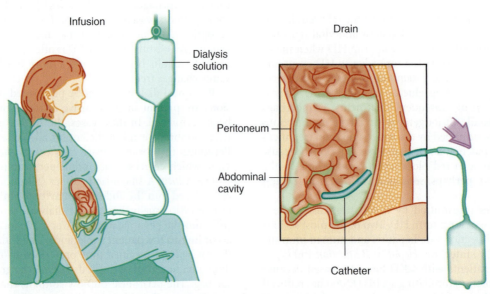

FIG. 68-9 Peritoneal dialysis exchange for control of fluids, electrolytes, nitrogenous wastes, blood pressure, and acid-base balance. The peritoneal membrane acts as the dialyzing membrane.

reconnect at a later time. Most long-term patients with PD prefer to complete exchanges overnight with an automated cycler (automatic peritoneal dialysis [APD], described below).

With the continuous *connect* system (straight transfer set), the dialysate bag is attached to the catheter by 48-inch tubing. The empty bag and tubing are folded and worn beneath the clothing until they are used for outflow. After draining, the

patient removes the bag and connects a new bag to repeat the process.

With the *disconnect system* (Y–transfer set), the patient removes the connecting tubing and empties the dialysate bag after inflow and attaches a cap to the PD catheter. The disconnect system eliminates the need to wear the tubing and bag but requires opening the system 2 extra times with each exchange. The extra opening of the system increases the risk for INFECTION.

With CAPD, no machine is necessary and no partner is required. However, it is best for a partner also trained in CAPD to be available as a support for the patient if illness occurs. Devices to assist in the safe, sterile connection of the tubing spike into the dialysate bag are available. These are useful for patients with poor vision, limited manual dexterity, or reduced hand and arm strength. CAPD allows constant removal of fluid and wastes and more closely resembles kidney action than HD. Some patients even perform their own exchanges while hospitalized.

Continuous-cycle peritoneal dialysis (CCPD) is a form of automated dialysis that uses an automated cycling machine. Exchanges occur at night while the patient sleeps. The final exchange of the night is left to dwell through the day and is drained the next evening as the process is repeated. CCPD offers the advantage of 24-hour dialysis, as in CAPD, but the sterile catheter system is opened less often.

Automated peritoneal dialysis (APD) may be used in the acute care setting, the ambulatory care dialysis center, or the patient's home. APD uses a cycling machine for dialysate inflow, dwell, and outflow according to preset times and volumes. A warming chamber for dialysate is part of the machine (Fig. 68-12). The functions are programmed for the patient's specific needs. A typical prescription calls for 30-minute exchanges (10/10/10 for inflow, dwell, and outflow) for a period of 8 to 10 hours. The machines have many safety monitors and alarms and are relatively simple to learn to use.

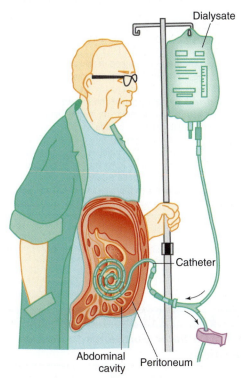

FIG. 68-10 A patient performing continuous ambulatory peritoneal dialysis (CAPD). Note that the patient can walk with this setup.

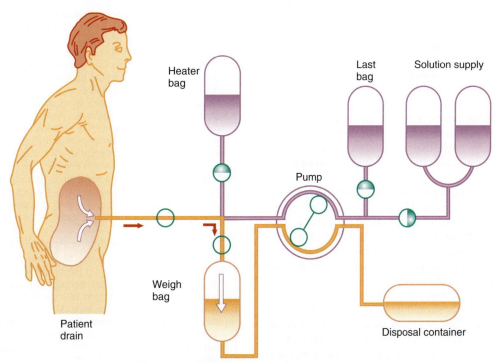

FIG. 68-11 Peritoneal dialysis machine circuit in automated peritoneal dialysis (APD).

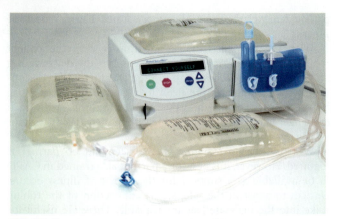

FIG. 68-12 A cycler machine for automated peritoneal dialysis at home.

Automated peritoneal dialysis has several advantages. It permits in-home dialysis while the patient sleeps, allowing him or her to be dialysis-free during waking hours. The incidence of peritonitis is reduced with APD because fewer connections and disconnections are needed. Also, APD can be used to deliver larger volumes of dialysis solution for patients who need higher clearances.

Intermittent peritoneal dialysis (IPD) combines osmotic pressure gradients with true dialysis. The patient usually requires exchanges of 2 L of dialysate at 30- to 60-minute intervals, allowing 15 to 20 minutes of drain time. For most patients, 30 to 40 exchanges of 2 L three times weekly are needed. IPD treatments can be automated or manual.

Complications. Complications are possible with PD, but many can be prevented with meticulous care and appropriate patient education for self-management. Problems and complications are more common when evidence-based guidelines for catheter care are not followed (see the Quality Improvement box regarding PD catheters).

Peritonitis is the major complication of PD, most commonly caused by connection site contamination. To prevent peritonitis, use meticulous sterile technique when caring for the PD catheter and when hooking up or clamping off dialysate bags (Chart 68-9).

Manifestations of peritonitis include cloudy dialysate outflow (effluent), fever, abdominal tenderness, abdominal pain, general malaise, nausea, and vomiting. *Cloudy or opaque effluent is the earliest indication of peritonitis.* Examine all effluent for color and clarity to detect peritonitis early. When peritonitis is suspected, send a specimen of the dialysate outflow for culture and sensitivity study, Gram stain, and cell count to identify the infecting organism.

Pain during the inflow of dialysate is common when patients are first started on PD therapy. Usually this pain no longer occurs after a week or two of PD. Cold dialysate increases discomfort. Warm the dialysate bags before instillation by using a heating pad to wrap the bag or by using the warming chamber of the automated cycling machine. *Microwave ovens are not recommended for the warming of dialysate.*

Exit site and tunnel infections are serious complications. The exit site from a PD catheter should be clean, dry, and without pain or INFLAMMATION. Exit-site INFECTIONS (ESIs) can occur with any type of PD catheter. These infections are difficult to treat and can become chronic. They can lead to peritonitis, catheter failure, and hospitalization. Dialysate leakage and

---

CHART 68-9 **Best Practice for Patient Safety & Quality Care** (QSEN)

Caring for the Patient with a Peritoneal Dialysis Catheter

- Mask yourself and your patient. Wash your hands.
- Put on sterile gloves. Remove the old dressing. Remove the contaminated gloves.
- Assess the area for signs of infection, such as swelling, redness, or discharge around the catheter site.
- Use aseptic technique:
  - Open the sterile field on a flat surface, and place two precut 4 × 4–inch gauze pads on the field.
  - Place three cotton swabs soaked in povidone-iodine or other solution prescribed by your health care provider on the field. Put on sterile gloves.
- Use cotton swabs to clean around the catheter site. Use a circular motion starting from the insertion site and moving away toward the abdomen. Repeat with all three swabs.
- As an alternative (if recommended by your health care provider or clinic), cleanse the area with sterile gauze pads using soap and water. Use a circular motion starting from the insertion site and moving away toward the abdomen. Rinse thoroughly.
- Apply precut gauze pads over the catheter site. Tape only the edges of the gauze pads.

QUALITY IMPROVEMENT (QSEN)

Follow PD Catheter Guidelines to Reduce Complications

Wong, L.P., Yamamoto, K.T., Reddy, V., Cobb, D., Chamberlin, A., Pham, H., et al. (2014). Patient education and care for peritoneal dialysis catheter placement: A quality improvement study. *Peritoneal Dialysis International, 34*(1), 12-23.

Although there are practice guidelines for placement of a peritoneal dialysis (PD) catheter, it is unknown if these recommendations are followed. The authors observed the care of 46 new patients at a single site—a regional PD center in the United States Northwest. Patients completed a questionnaire derived from the International Society for Peritoneal Dialysis (ISPD) catheter guidelines and were followed for early complications.

Results indicated that there were many and serious deviations from the ISPD catheter guidelines and that these deviations were linked to adverse outcomes. For example, after insertion, 20% of patients reported not being given instructions for follow-up care and 46% reported not being taught the warning signs of PD catheter infection. In 41% of patients, a complication developed, with 30% of patients experiencing a catheter or exit-site problem and 11% developing infection. Improving patient education and care coordination for PD catheter placement were identified as the next steps in the quality improvement (QI) cycle.

Commentary: Implications for Practice and Research

This study shows the initial steps of gathering information in a Plan-Do-Study-Act cycle of QI. First the guidelines for care were identified, and then they were operationalized as a patient questionnaire with a focus on education and as a provider checklist to observe components of high-quality care. The data were then linked to patient outcomes. The association of less-than-optimal education and care to serious and recurrent adverse patient outcomes is a powerful approach to develop essential interventions with the next cycle in order to provide safe, effective care.

pulling or twisting of the catheter increase the risk for ESIs. A Gram stain and culture should be performed when exit sites have purulent drainage.

Tunnel infections occur in the path of the catheter from the skin to the cuff. Manifestations include redness, tenderness, and pain. ESIs are treated with antimicrobials. Deep cuff infections may require catheter removal.

Poor dialysate flow is usually related to constipation. To prevent constipation, a bowel preparation is prescribed before placement of the PD. An enema before starting PD may also prevent flow problems. Teach patients to eat a high-fiber diet and to use stool softeners to prevent constipation. Other causes of flow difficulty include kinked or clamped connection tubing, the patient's position, fibrin clot formation, and catheter displacement.

Ensure that the drainage bag is lower than the patient's abdomen to enhance gravity drainage. Inspect the connection tubing and PD system for kinking or twisting. Ensure that clamps are open. If inflow or outflow drainage is still inadequate, reposition the patient to stimulate inflow or outflow. Turning the patient to the other side or ensuring that he or she is in good body alignment may help. Having the patient in a supine low-Fowler's position reduces abdominal pressure. Increased abdominal pressure from sitting or standing or from coughing contributes to leakage at the PD catheter site.

Fibrin clot formation may occur after PD catheter placement or with peritonitis. Milking the tubing may dislodge the fibrin clot and improve flow. An x-ray is needed to identify PD catheter placement. If displacement has occurred, the physician repositions the PD catheter.

Dialysate leakage is seen as clear fluid coming from the catheter exit site. When dialysis is first started, small volumes of dialysate are used. It may take patients 1 to 2 weeks to tolerate a full 2-L exchange without leakage around the catheter site. Leakage occurs more often in obese patients, those with diabetes, older adults, and those on long-term steroid therapy. During periods of catheter leak, patients may require hemodialysis (HD) support.

Other complications of PD include bleeding, which is expected when the catheter is first placed, and bowel perforation, which is serious. When PD is first started, the outflow may be bloody or blood tinged. This condition normally clears within a week or two. After PD is well-established, the effluent should be clear and light yellow. Observe for and document any change in the color of the outflow. Brown-colored effluent occurs with a bowel perforation. If the outflow is the same color as urine and has the same glucose level, a bladder perforation is probable. Cloudy or opaque effluent indicates INFECTION.

Nursing Care During Peritoneal Dialysis. In the hospital setting, PD is routinely started and monitored by the nurse. Before the treatment, assess baseline vital signs, including blood pressure, apical and radial pulse rates, temperature, quality of respirations, and breath sounds. Weigh the patient, always on the same scale, before the procedure and at least every 24 hours while receiving treatment. Weight should be checked after a drain and before the next fill to monitor the patient's "dry weight." Baseline laboratory tests, such as electrolyte and glucose levels, are obtained before starting PD and are repeated at least daily during the PD treatment.

Continually monitor the patient during PD. Take and record vital signs every 15 to 30 minutes. Assess for respiratory distress, pain, or discomfort. Check the dressing around the catheter exit site every 30 minutes for wetness during the procedure. Monitor the prescribed dwell time, and initiate outflow. Assess blood glucose levels in patients who absorb glucose.

Observe the outflow pattern (outflow should be a continuous stream after the clamp is completely open). Measure and record the total amount of outflow after each exchange. Maintain accurate inflow and outflow records when hourly PD exchanges are performed. When outflow is less than inflow, the difference is retained by the patient during dialysis and is counted as fluid intake. Weigh the patient daily to monitor fluid status.

Kidney Transplantation

Dialysis and kidney transplant are life-sustaining *treatments* for end-stage kidney disease (ESKD). Kidney transplant is not considered a "cure." Each patient, in consultation with a nephrologist, determines which type of therapy is best suited to his or her physical condition and lifestyle. About 17,000 to 18,000 kidney transplants are performed yearly in the United States. Currently about 159,000 people are awaiting kidney transplant in North America. The median time on the waiting list is 678 days (USRDS, 2014).

Candidate Selection Criteria. Candidates for transplantation must be free of medical problems that might increase the risks from the procedure. The usual age-range for kidney transplant is 2 to 70 years. Patients older than 70 years are considered for transplant on an individual basis because complications are more common in the older adult.

The patient is thoroughly assessed before he or she is considered for a kidney transplant. Patients who have advanced, uncorrectable cardiac disease are excluded from the procedure because these problems are made worse by transplantation. Other conditions that preclude kidney transplant include metastatic cancer, chronic INFECTION, and severe psychosocial problems such as alcoholism or chemical dependency. Long-standing pulmonary disease increases the risk for complications and death from respiratory infection. Patients with diseases of the GI system, such as peptic ulcers and diverticulosis, require treatment before consideration for transplantation because some diseases are made worse by the large doses of steroids used after surgery.

The urinary system is completely evaluated to ensure normal urine flow. Many patients with ESKD have not used their lower urinary tract for years, and ureteral or bladder problems may require surgical correction before a kidney is transplanted.

Patients with a recent history of cancer are treated with dialysis because of the shortage of donor organs and the uncertain life expectancy of these patients. In addition, the drugs used after the procedure increase the risk for cancer recurrence. If more than 2 to 5 years have passed since cancer eradication, the patient can be considered for a transplant.

Diabetes mellitus and other endocrine problems cause great risks. Patients with these problems can have a kidney transplant but require intense observation and management to limit complications. Other pre-existing conditions are considered on an individual basis, depending on the patient's health status. Kidney transplantation is considered for most patients with ESKD and is the optimal therapy for many people.

Donors. Kidney donors may be living donors (related or unrelated to the patient), non-heart-beating donors (NHBDs), and cadaveric donors. The available kidneys are matched on the basis of tissue type similarity between the donor and the recipient. NHBDs are persons declared dead by cardiopulmonary criteria. Kidneys from NHBDs are removed (harvested) immediately after death in cases in which patients have previously given consent for organ donation. If immediate removal must be delayed, the organ is preserved by infusing a cool preservation solution into the abdominal aorta after death is declared and until surgery can be performed. Cadaveric donors are usually people who suffered irreversible brain injury, most often as a result of trauma. These donors are maintained with mechanical ventilation and must have sufficient PERFUSION for the kidneys to remain viable.

The size of the kidney is seldom a problem in adults. Kidneys transplanted from children become larger to meet adult needs within a few months.

Organs from living *related* donors (LRDs) have the highest rates of kidney graft survival (90%). A living donor is one who is medically compatible with the recipient (Ficorelli et al., 2013). LRDs are usually at least 18 years old and are seldom older than 65 years, although there are reports of donors age 70 years with good outcomes for both the donor and recipient (Berger et al., 2011). Physical criteria for donors include:
* Absence of systemic disease and INFECTION
* No history of cancer
* No hypertension or kidney disease
* Adequate kidney function as determined by diagnostic studies

LRDs must express a clear understanding of the surgery and a willingness to give up a kidney. Some transplant centers require a psychiatric evaluation to assess the donor's motivation.

A paired or chain exchange donation can be done when two kidney donor/recipient pairs have blood types that are not compatible (Gentry et al., 2011). The recipients trade donors so that each recipient can receive a kidney with a compatible blood type and tissue type (Fig. 68-13). Once the evaluations of all

donors and recipients are completed, the series of kidney transplant operations are scheduled to occur consecutively (www.paireddonaton.org).

Because of advances in immunosuppressant therapy and medical management, the United Network for Organ Sharing (UNOS) reported 1-year kidney transplant graft survival to be almost 95% for all centers in the United States during 2012 (UNOS, 2014).

Preoperative Care. Many issues related to patient health and the actual transplant procedure must be addressed before surgery. The *Clinical Pathway* on the *Evolve* website highlights care needs for the patient undergoing kidney transplantation.

Immunologic studies are needed because the major barrier to transplant success after a suitable donor kidney is available is the body's ability to reject "foreign" tissue. This immunologic process can attack the transplanted kidney and destroy it. For immunologic problems to be overcome, tissue typing is performed on all candidates. These studies include simple blood typing and human leukocyte antigen (HLA) studies, as well as other tests. A donated kidney *must* come from a donor who is the same blood type as the recipient. The HLAs are the main immunologic feature used to match transplant recipients with compatible donors. The more similar the antigens of the donor are to those of the recipient, the more likely the transplant will be successful and rejection will be avoided (see Chapter 17).

Nursing actions before surgery include teaching about the procedure and care after surgery, in-depth patient assessment, coordination of diagnostic tests, and development of treatment plans. See Chapter 14 for more discussion of standard preoperative nursing care.

The patient usually requires dialysis within 24 hours of the surgery and often receives a blood transfusion before surgery. Usually blood from the kidney donor is transfused into the recipient. This procedure increases graft survival of organs from living related donors (LRDs).

Operative Procedures. The donor nephrectomy procedure varies depending on whether the donor is a non-heart-beating donor (NHBD), cadaveric donor, or living donor (Beach et al., 2011). The NHBD or cadaveric donor nephrectomy is a sterile autopsy procedure performed in the operating room. All arterial and venous vessels and a long piece of ureter are preserved. After removal, the kidneys are preserved until time for implantation into the recipient. The technique for kidney removal from living donors is a laparoscopic procedure. Donors need postoperative nursing care and support for the psychological adjustment to loss of a body part.

Transplantation surgery usually takes several hours. The new kidney is usually placed in the right or left anterior iliac fossa (Fig. 68-14) instead of the usual kidney position. This placement allows easier connection of the ureter and the renal artery and vein. It also allows for easier kidney palpation. The recipient's own failed kidneys are not removed unless chronic kidney INFECTION is present or, as in the case of polycystic kidney disease, the nonfunctioning, enlarged kidneys cause pain. After surgery, the patient is taken to the postanesthesia care unit and then, when stable, to a designated unit in the transplant center or to a critical care unit.

Postoperative Care. Care of the recipient after surgery requires that nurses be knowledgeable about the expected clinical findings and potential complications. Nursing care includes ongoing physical assessment, especially evaluation of kidney function. The most common complications occurring in

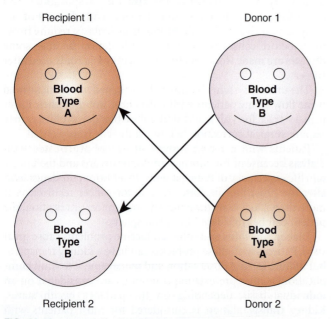

FIG. 68-13 An example of a paired exchange kidney donation. *Donor 1* is related to or acquainted with *recipient 1* and has agreed to donate a kidney but is not a blood type or tissue type match with *recipient 1*. *Donor 1* is compatible with *recipient 2* and agrees to donate a kidney to *recipient 2* if *donor 2* agrees to donate a kidney to *recipient 1* with confirmed compatibility to *recipient 1*.

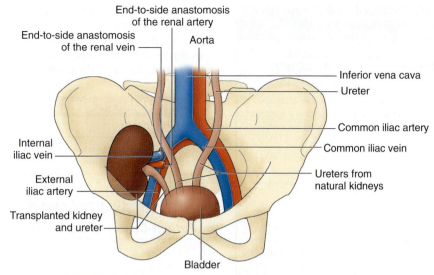

End-to-side anastomosis
of the renal artery

End-to-side anastomosis
of the renal vein

Aorta

Inferior vena cava

Ureter

Common iliac artery

Common iliac vein

Internal
iliac vein

External
iliac artery

Ureters from
natural kidneys

Transplanted kidney
and ureter

Bladder

FIG. 68-14 Placement of a transplanted kidney in the right iliac fossa.

patients after renal transplant are rejection and INFECTION. Immunosuppressive drug therapy used to prevent tissue rejection impairs healing and increases the risk for INFECTION.

Urologic management is essential to graft success. A urinary catheter is placed for accurate measurements of urine output and decompression of the bladder. Decompression prevents stretch on sutures and ureter attachment sites on the bladder.

Assess urine output at least hourly during the first 48 hours. An abrupt decrease in urine output may indicate complications such as rejection, acute kidney injury (AKI), thrombosis, or obstruction. Examine the urine color. The urine is pink and bloody right after surgery and gradually returns to normal over several days to several weeks, depending on kidney function. Obtain daily urine specimens for urinalysis, glucose measurement, the presence of acetone, specific gravity measurement, and culture (if needed).

Occasionally, continuous bladder irrigation is prescribed to decrease blood clot formation, which could increase pressure in the bladder and endanger the graft. Perform routine catheter care, according to agency policy, to reduce catheter-associated urinary tract infection (CAUTI). The catheter is removed as soon as possible to avoid INFECTION—usually 3 to 5 days after surgery. After surgery, the function of the transplanted kidney (graft) can result in either oliguria or diuresis. Oliguria may occur as a result of ischemia and AKI, rejection, or other complications. To increase urine output, the health care provider may prescribe diuretics and osmotic agents. Closely monitor the patient's fluid status because fluid overload can cause hypertension, heart failure, and pulmonary edema. Evaluate his or her fluid status by weighing daily, measuring blood pressure every 2 to 4 hours, and measuring intake and output.

Instead of oliguria, the patient may have diuresis, especially with a kidney from a living related donor (LRD). Monitor intake and output, and observe for disruptions of FLUID AND ELECTROLYTE BALANCE, such as low potassium and sodium levels. Excessive diuresis may cause hypotension.

Complications. Many complications are possible after kidney transplantation. Early detection and intervention improve the chances for graft survival.

> **! NURSING SAFETY PRIORITY (QSEN)**
> *Critical Rescue*
>
> Notify the physician immediately about hypotension or excessive diuresis (e.g., unanticipated urine output 500-1000 mL greater than intake over 12-24 hours or other goal for intake and output (I&O)) because hypotension reduces blood flow and oxygen to the new kidney, threatening graft survival.

Rejection is the most serious complication of transplantation and is the leading cause of graft loss. A reaction occurs between the tissues of the transplanted kidney and the antibodies and cytotoxic T-cells in the recipient's blood. These substances treat the new kidney as a foreign invader and cause tissue destruction, thrombosis, and eventual kidney necrosis.

The three types of rejection are hyperacute, acute, and chronic. Acute rejection is the most common type with kidney transplants. It is treated with increased immunosuppressive therapy and often can be reversed. Rejection is diagnosed by manifestations, a CT or renal scan, and kidney biopsy. Table 68-14 lists the features of the three types of rejection. Chapter 17 discusses their causes and treatment.

Ischemia from delayed transplantation following harvesting can contribute to AKI. Newly transplanted patients with AKI may need dialysis until adequate urine output returns and the blood urea nitrogen (BUN) and creatinine levels normalize. Biopsy can be used to determine if oliguria is the result of AKI or rejection.

Thrombosis of the major renal blood vessels may occur during the first 2 to 3 days after the transplant. A sudden decrease in urine output may signal impaired PERFUSION resulting from thrombosis. Ultrasound of the kidney may show decreased or absent blood supply. Emergency surgery is required to prevent ischemic damage or graft loss.

Renal artery stenosis may result in hypertension. Other manifestations include a bruit over the artery anastomosis site and decreased kidney function. A CT or renal scan can quantify the blood flow to the kidney. The involved artery may be repaired surgically or by balloon angioplasty in the radiology

TABLE 68-14   **Comparison of Hyperacute, Acute, and Chronic Post-Transplant Rejection**

HYPERACUTE REJECTION	ACUTE REJECTION	CHRONIC REJECTION
Onset		
Within 48 hours after surgery	1 week to any time postoperatively; occurs over days to weeks	Occurs gradually during a period of months to years
Clinical Manifestations		
Increased temperature	Oliguria or anuria	Gradual increase in BUN and serum creatinine levels
Increased blood pressure	Temperature over 100° F (37.8° C)	
Pain at transplant site	Increased blood pressure	Fluid retention
	Enlarged, tender kidney	Changes in serum electrolyte levels
	Lethargy	
	Elevated serum creatinine, BUN, potassium levels	Fatigue
	Fluid retention	
Treatment		
Immediate removal of the transplanted kidney	Increased doses of immunosuppressive drugs	Conservative management until dialysis is required

BUN, Blood urea nitrogen.

department. The decision to perform a balloon repair is determined by the amount of healing time after the surgery.

Other vascular problems include vascular leakage or thrombosis, both of which require an emergency transplant nephrectomy.

Other complications may involve the surgical wound or urinary tract. Wound problems, such as hematomas, abscesses, and lymphoceles (cysts containing lymph fluid), increase the risk for infection and exert pressure on the new kidney. INFECTION is a major cause of death in the transplant recipient. Prevention of infection is essential. Strict aseptic technique and handwashing must be rigorously enforced. Transplant recipients may not have the usual manifestations of infection because of the immunosuppressive therapy. Low-grade fevers, mental status changes, and vague reports of discomfort may be the only manifestations before sepsis. Always consider the possibility of infection with any patient after a kidney transplant. Urinary tract complications include ureteral leakage, fistula, or obstruction; stone formation; bladder neck contracture; and graft rupture. Surgical intervention may be required.

Immunosuppressive Drug Therapy. The success of kidney transplantation depends on changing the patient's immunologic response so that the new kidney is not rejected as a foreign organ. Immunosuppressive drugs protect the transplanted organ. These drugs include corticosteroids, inhibitors of T-cell proliferation and activity (azathioprine, mycophenolic acid, cyclosporine, and tacrolimus), mTOR inhibitors (to disrupt stimulatory T-cell signals), and monoclonal antibodies. Chapter 17 discusses the mechanisms of action for these agents and the associated patient responses. Patients taking these drugs are at an increased risk for death from INFECTION.

Some patients do not follow the regimen correctly and are at high risk for losing the transplanted kidney. Work with the patient to ensure adherence to the drug regimen.

Despite the complexity of drug regimens following kidney transplantation, 85.5% of patients are living 5 years after transplantation compared with 35.8% of patients who receive dialysis for 5 years. The costs of HD are 3 times the cost of kidney transplantation over the same 5 years (USRDS, 2014).

> **! NURSING SAFETY PRIORITY** (QSEN)
> **Action Alert**
>
> Teach patients and families about the importance of adhering to the anti-rejection drug regimen to prevent transplant rejection.

> **? CLINICAL JUDGMENT CHALLENGE**
> **Patient-Centered Care** (QSEN)
>
> The patient is a 64-year-old man with ESKD who has been on hemodialysis for 3 years while waiting for a kidney transplant. He expresses frustration with the wait from time to time and has told you that he fears that he will be considered too old to receive a kidney if much more time goes by. He states that he feels "chained" to the dialysis center.
> 1. How should you respond to his concern about age possibly affecting his ability to be a transplant recipient?
> 2. How do you respond to his feeling about being chained to the dialysis center?
> 3. What other resources can you offer to help him be informed and deal with the emotional aspects of dialysis?

Community-Based Care

Home Care Management. Because of the complex nature of CKD, its progressive course, and many treatment options, a case manager is helpful in planning, coordinating, and evaluating care. As kidney disease progresses, the patient is seen by a physician or nurse practitioner regularly. Together with the dietitian and social worker, evaluate the home environment and determine equipment needs before discharge. Once the patient is discharged, home care nurses direct care and monitor progress.

Provide health teaching about the diet in kidney disease and the progression of disease. As CKD approaches end-stage kidney disease (ESKD), one of these treatment methods is chosen: hemodialysis (HD), peritoneal dialysis (PD), or transplantation. For each form of treatment, the patient and partner must learn about the procedures and consider his or her personal lifestyle, support systems, and methods of coping. Decision making about treatment type or even whether to pursue treatment is difficult for patients and families. Provide information and emotional support to assist patients with these decisions.

Teach patients who select hemodialysis (HD) about the machine and vascular access care. If in-home HD is selected, preparations are needed for the appropriate equipment, including a water treatment system. Referral to a home health care agency is essential for a successful transition to at-home HD. A home care visit occurs before discharge to coordinate equipment setup. Family members or agency staff must be available to respond to alarms during treatment. Because nocturnal HD is a growing modality, additional safety considerations must be addressed, including a plan for treatment discontinuation or generator backup during power outages. Regardless of whether the treatment occurs at home or in a center, promote independence through teaching and best practices in self-management.

The patient receiving PD needs extensive training in the procedure. He or she also needs help in obtaining equipment and the many supplies needed. Home care nurses assess patients, monitor vital signs, assess adherence with drug and diet regimens, and monitor for manifestations of peritonitis.

The nurse plays a vital role in the long-term care of the patient with a kidney transplant. Facilitate acceptance and understanding of the anti-rejection drug regimen as a part of daily life. Carefully monitor for indications of graft rejection and for complications, such as INFECTION. Chart 68-10 describes the focused assessment for the patient following kidney transplant.

Self-Management Education. Instruct patients and family members in all aspects of nutrition therapy, drug therapy, and complications. Teach them to report complications, such as fluid overload and INFECTION. When a patient has a specific form of therapy, such as dialysis or transplantation, focus teaching on the chosen type of intervention. Assess the need for immunizations, and request a prescription to administer needed ones before transplantation.

CHART 68-10 Focused Assessment

The Patient Following Kidney Transplant

Assess cardiovascular and respiratory status, including:
- Vital signs, with special attention to blood pressure
- Presence of S_3 or pericardial friction rub
- Presence of chest pain
- Presence of edema (periorbital, pretibial, sacral)
- Jugular vein distention
- Presence of dyspnea
- Presence of crackles, beginning at the lung bases and extending upward

Assess nutritional status, including:
- Weight gain or loss
- Presence of anorexia, nausea, or vomiting

Assess kidney status, including:
- Amount, frequency, and appearance of urine (in non-anuric patients)
- Presence of bone pain
- Presence of hyperglycemia secondary to diabetes

Assess hematologic status, including:
- Presence of petechiae, purpura, ecchymoses
- Presence of fatigue or shortness of breath

Assess gastrointestinal status, including:
- Presence of stomatitis
- Presence of melena

Assess integumentary status, including:
- Skin integrity
- Presence of pruritus
- Presence of skin discoloration

Assess neurologic status, including:
- Changes in mental status
- Presence of seizure activity
- Presence of sensory changes
- Presence of lower extremity weakness

Assess laboratory data, including:
- BUN
- Serum creatinine
- Creatinine clearance
- CBC
- Electrolytes

Assess psychosocial status, including:
- Presence of anxiety
- Presence of maladaptive behavior

BUN, Blood urea nitrogen; *CBC,* complete blood count.

Hemodialysis (HD) is the most complex form of therapy for the patient and family to understand. Even if patients receive HD in a dialysis center instead of at home, they are expected to have some knowledge of the process. Teach the patient or a family member to care for the vascular access and to report signs of INFECTION and stenosis. Those who plan to have in-home HD will need a partner. Both the patient and the partner must be taught the entire process of HD and must be able to perform it independently before the patient is discharged.

Peritoneal dialysis (PD) involves extensive health teaching for the patient and family. Emphasize sterile technique because peritonitis is the most common complication of PD. Instruct patients to report any manifestation of peritonitis, especially cloudy effluent and abdominal pain. If peritonitis develops, teach patients how to give themselves antibiotics by the intraperitoneal (IP) route. Stress the importance of completing the antibiotic regimen. Remind patients that repeated episodes of peritonitis can reduce the effectiveness of PD, which may require the transfer to HD.

The patient receiving a kidney transplant also needs extensive health teaching. Provide instruction about drug regimens, home monitoring, immunosuppression, manifestations of rejection, INFECTION, and prescribed changes in the diet and activity level.

Psychosocial Preparation. Provide psychological support for the patient and family. Help the patient adjust to the diagnosis of kidney failure and eventually accept the treatment regimens.

Many patients view dialysis as a cure instead of lifelong management. For many patients, reduction of uremic manifestations in the first weeks after starting dialysis treatment creates a sense of well-being (the "honeymoon" period). They feel better physically, and their mood may be happy and hopeful. At this time they tend to overlook the discomfort and inconvenience of dialysis. Use this time to begin health teaching. Stress that although manifestations are reduced, not to expect a complete return to the previous state of well-being before ESKD.

Many patients become discouraged during the first year of treatment. This mood state may last a few months to a year or longer. The difficulties of incorporating dialysis into daily life are staggering, and patients may become depressed as problems occur. They may struggle with the idea of having to be permanently dependent on a disruptive therapy. Patients may feel helpless and dependent. Some people may deny the need for dialysis or may not adhere to drug therapy and diet restrictions. Monitor any behaviors that may contribute to nonadherence, and suggest psychiatric referrals. Help the patient and family focus on the positive aspects of the treatments. Continue health education with patients as active participants and decision makers.

Most patients with CKD eventually enter a phase of acceptance or resignation. Each person reacts differently. To make this long-term adaptation, the patient must adjust to continuous change. Concerns depend on the patient's health and specific treatment method.

After patients have accepted or become resigned to the chronic aspect of their disease, they usually attempt to return to their previous activities. Resuming the previous level of activity, however, may not be possible. Help patients develop realistic expectations that allow them to lead active, productive lives.

Health Care Resources. Professionals from many disciplines are resources for the patient with ESKD. Home care nurses monitor the patient's status and evaluate maintenance of the prescribed treatment regimen (HD or PD). Social services are often involved because of the complex process of applying for financial aid to pay for the required medical care. A physical therapist may be beneficial in helping to improve the patient's functional health. A dietitian can assist the patient and family members in understanding special dietary needs. A psychiatric evaluation may be needed if depressive symptoms are present. Pharmacists provide invaluable insight and teaching about drug therapy and adjustments to meet outcomes. Clergy and pastoral care specialists offer spiritual support.

Patients with CKD are routinely followed by a physician, usually a nephrologist. Organizations such as the National Kidney Foundation (NKF), the American Kidney Fund, and the National Association of Patients on Hemodialysis and Transplantation (NAPHT) may be helpful to patients and families.

◆ Evaluation: Outcomes

Evaluate the care of the patient with CKD based on the identified priority problems. The expected outcomes are that with appropriate management the patient should:

- Achieve and maintain appropriate FLUID AND ELECTROLYTE BALANCE
- Maintain an adequate nutrition status
- Avoid INFECTION at the vascular access site
- Use effective coping strategies
- Report an absence of physical manifestations of anxiety
- Prevent or slow systemic complications of CKD, including osteodystrophy

Specific indicators for these outcomes are listed for each priority problem under the Planning and Implementation section (see earlier).

NURSING CONCEPTS AND CLINICAL JUDGMENT REVIEW

What might you NOTICE if the patient is experiencing reduced PERFUSION and altered urinary ELIMINATION related to acute kidney injury?

- Hemodynamic instability, especially hypotension and tachycardia that persist or recur
- Urine output (elimination) of less than 0.5 mL/kg/hr for more than 2 hours; some experts suggest reporting urine output of less than 0.3 mL/kg/hr for more than 2 hours.
- Serum creatinine increased above baseline or admission values
- Patient reports of back or flank pain
- Urine that has sediment or is dark or smoky or has obvious blood in it
- Signs of abnormalities in fluid and electrolytes including dehydration and abnormal serum and urine potassium and sodium values

How should you INTERPRET and how should you RESPOND to a patient experiencing complications from INFECTION, INFLAMMATION, disturbances in FLUID AND ELECTROLYTE BALANCE, and altered ACID-BASE BALANCE as a result of chronic kidney disease?

Perform and interpret physical assessment, including:
- Asking how long manifestations have been present
- Determining fluid intake and output volumes
- Weighing the patient, and asking whether this weight is more or less than the usual weight
- Assessing for tachycardia, hypertension, and hypotension
- Assessing for pulmonary congestion
- Assessing for skin tissue integrity related to risk for injury from uremia and edema
- Interpreting laboratory values:
  - BUN and serum creatinine levels elevated with altered cognition
  - Serum potassium level elevated with potential for cardiac dysrhythmias
  - Low serum calcium indicating risk for renal osteodystrophy
  - Arterial pH or venous base deficit

Respond by:
- Ensuring hemodynamic stability
- Monitoring urine output
- Monitoring for fluid overload and, after dialysis, dehydration
- Evaluating laboratory results regularly with physical assessment
- Evaluating patient risk for falls or other unsafe situations
- Promoting best practices related to care of the patient with vascular access for hemodialysis
- Providing education about drugs used to manage CKD and kidney transplant

On what should you REFLECT?
- Observe patient for evidence of improved urine output after implementing the plan of care for AKI.
- Plan care to avoid periods of inadequate kidney perfusion from hypotension and dehydration.
- Identify and evaluate the effect of interventions to minimize the risk for infection, including appropriate administration of immunizations, particularly in patients with CKD and altered immunity from kidney transplant.
- Think about topics for patient teaching that could help prevent complications from AKI or progressive CKD.
- Explore how patient preferences and values affect patient decisions about self-management in CKD.
- Explain how immunosuppression in kidney transplant patients and patients with ESKD alters immune responses, including inflammation.
- Consider how timeliness (routine versus urgent versus immediate) and accuracy (e.g., isolated versus trend, and complete versus focused data) of communication to the health care provider or other health care team members can avoid or reduce complications, worsening CKD, transplant rejection, and severity of AKI.
- Inform health care providers about signs of local or systemic infection, vital signs that are not within normal ranges or ranges that are not acceptable for the patient, abnormal laboratory results, or other changes in patient status that require urgent assessment and intervention.

GET READY FOR THE NCLEX® EXAMINATION!

KEY POINTS

Review these Key Points for each NCLEX Examination Client Needs Category.

Safe and Effective Care Environment

- Use sterile technique when initiating and providing renal replacement therapy. **Safety** **QSEN**
- Implement fall precautions and consider physical therapy referral for patients with CKD osteodystrophy to prevent fractures. **Safety** **QSEN**
- Use skin protective measures to reduce injury and pressure ulcer formation in patients with CKD. **Safety** **QSEN**
- Communicate to health care providers patient assessments that indicate dehydration or hypovolemia to avoid inadequate kidney PERFUSION. **Teamwork and Collaboration** **QSEN**
- Avoid taking blood pressure measurements or drawing blood from an arm with a vascular access (AV fistula or graft). **Safety** **QSEN**
- Do not use a renal replacement vascular access device (the AV fistula or graft site) to give IV fluids. **Safety** **QSEN**

Health Promotion and Maintenance

- Encourage patients with AKI, CKD, or end-stage kidney disease (ESKD) to follow fluid and dietary restrictions regarding sodium, potassium, and protein.
- Teach patients the expected side effects, any adverse reactions to prescribed drugs, and when to contact the prescriber. **Safety** **QSEN**
- Teach patients using peritoneal dialysis the manifestations of peritonitis. **Patient-Centered Care** **QSEN**
- Teach patients receiving immunosuppressive therapy for kidney transplantation to assess themselves daily for fever, general malaise, and nausea or vomiting, as well as weight gain, indicating new fluid retention. **Patient-Centered Care** **QSEN**

Psychosocial Integrity

- Allow patients the opportunity to express concerns about the disruption of lifestyle and considerations for end-of-life care as a result of kidney failure. **Patient-Centered Care** **QSEN**
- Use language and terminology that are comfortable for the patient. **Patient-Centered Care** **QSEN**
- Assess the patient for depression and nonacceptance of the diagnosis or treatment plan. **Patient-Centered Care** **QSEN**
- Refer patients to community resources and support groups. **Informatics** **QSEN**

Physiological Integrity

- Report immediately any condition that obstructs urine flow. **Safety** **QSEN**
- Collaborate with the dietitian to teach patients about needed fluid, sodium, potassium, or dietary protein restriction. **Teamwork and Collaboration** **QSEN**
- Inform the health care provider urgently or immediately about hemodynamic instability, change in cognition, manifestations of INFECTION, newly abnormal serum electrolytes, and urine output less than 0.5mL/kg/hr for more than 2-4 hours (unless the patient is oliguric or anuric from ESKD). **Teamwork and Collaboration** **QSEN**
- Teach patients in the early stages of CKD the manifestations of dehydration. **Patient-Centered Care** **QSEN**
- Teach patients in the later stages of CKD the manifestations of fluid overload and hyperkalemia. **Patient-Centered Care** **QSEN**
- Avoid all invasive procedures in the 4 to 6 hours following hemodialysis. **Evidence-Based Practice** **QSEN**

CONCEPT OVERVIEW

Sexuality

Unlike the physiologic human needs introduced in other section openers of this text, *sexuality* is a complex integration of many physiologic, emotional, social, and cultural aspects of well-being. It is closely associated with self-concept, self-esteem, role relationships, sexual response, gender identity, and reproduction. Sexuality comprises other related human needs, such as belonging, intimacy (e.g., touching, kissing), sharing, and caring. When these needs are met, a person is sexually healthy (Fig. 1).

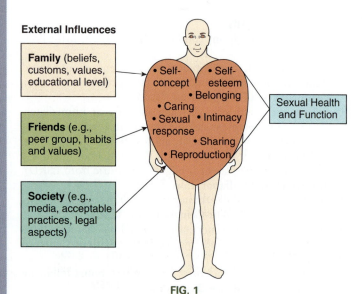

External Influences

Family (beliefs, customs, values, educational level)

Friends (e.g., peer group, habits and values)

Society (e.g., media, acceptable practices, legal aspects)

• Self-concept • Self-esteem • Belonging • Caring • Intimacy • Sexual response • Sharing • Reproduction

Sexual Health and Function

FIG. 1

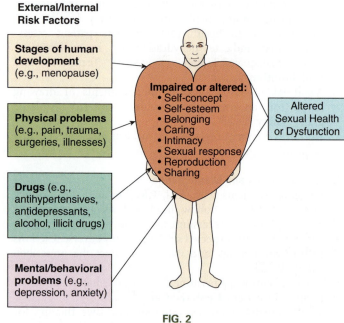

External/Internal Risk Factors

Stages of human development (e.g., menopause)

Physical problems (e.g., pain, trauma, surgeries, illnesses)

Drugs (e.g., antihypertensives, antidepressants, alcohol, illicit drugs)

Mental/behavioral problems (e.g., depression, anxiety)

Impaired or altered: • Self-concept • Self-esteem • Belonging • Caring • Intimacy • Sexual response • Reproduction • Sharing

Altered Sexual Health or Dysfunction

FIG. 2

Sexuality, therefore, is a vital part of one's holistic being from birth to death. During the stages of human development, a person's attitudes, beliefs, and values related to sexuality are influenced and shaped by the environment, including family, friends, and society. For example, cultural beliefs affect the nature of physical sexual pleasure. The media also play a large role in developing one's views on sexuality. Some societies, such as the United States, tend to value youth and beauty more than aging and wisdom. As a result, people in these societies may feel less physically attractive and desirable for intimacy and belonging as they age.

Various external and internal risk factors can alter or impair sexual health. In many cases, they cause physical sexual dysfunction, which then affects emotional needs such as self-esteem (Fig. 2). These factors include:

- Stages of human development
- Physical health problems
- Drugs
- Mental/behavioral health problems

The *stages of human development* typically influence human sexuality, especially when menopause occurs in middle adulthood. Although each woman's response is different, menopause may result in a decreased libido (desire for sexual contact or intercourse). Relationships with her sexual partner(s) are altered, and interpersonal conflict can occur.

Physical health problems also can negatively affect sexual health. For example, chronic pain may cause decreased physical contact and a lowered self-concept along with chronic fatigue and decreased energy. Sexual dysfunction commonly occurs in people with chronic diseases such as diabetes and hypertension. Reproductive diseases (e.g., sexually transmitted diseases, testicular cancer) and their treatments (e.g., radiation therapy, surgery) can also affect sexuality, both physically and emotionally. Physical trauma such as spinal cord injury may prevent a person from having sexual intercourse.

Certain prescription or recreational *drugs* can cause impotence (inability to have an erection) or infertility. Alcohol and many antihypertensive agents, antidepressants, and illicit drugs interfere with sexual function in men.

Mental/behavioral health problems can also result in altered sexual health. Common examples include depression and severe anxiety states. In some cases, concern about physical performance can lead to sexual dysfunction.

Assessment of the Reproductive System

Donna D. Ignatavicius

ℯ http://evolve.elsevier.com/Iggy/

PRIORITY CONCEPTS

- PAIN
- SEXUALITY

- INFECTION

LEARNING OUTCOMES

Health Promotion and Maintenance
1. Teach patients about recommended guidelines for selected reproductive screening tests.

Psychosocial Integrity
2. Identify general psychological responses to reproductive health problems that affect SEXUALITY.

Physiological Integrity
3. Review the anatomy and physiology of the male and the female reproductive systems.

4. Identify reproductive changes associated with aging and their implications for nursing care.
5. Perform a focused physical assessment of the patient with male or female reproductive system problems.
6. Explain the use of laboratory testing for patients with suspected or actual reproductive health problems.
7. Develop an evidence-based teaching plan for a patient undergoing endoscopic studies for reproductive health problems.

The first health care professional to assess the patient with a reproductive system health problem or hear a patient's concern about a reproductive problem is often the nurse. These problems typically affect the need for SEXUALITY, both its physical and psychosocial aspects, and are difficult for many people to discuss. Assessment of the male and the female reproductive systems should be part of every complete physical assessment. *Be aware of and sensitive to differences in sexual orientation and practices.*

This chapter reviews the focused reproductive system assessment that a nurse generalist performs. An advanced practice nurse or other health care provider performs the comprehensive reproductive examination. A more detailed discussion of human SEXUALITY is found in a fundamentals or basic nursing text.

ANATOMY AND PHYSIOLOGY REVIEW

Structure and Function of the Female Reproductive System

The female reproductive system is located both outside (external) and inside (internal) the body.

External Genitalia

The external female genitalia, or **vulva,** extend from the mons pubis to the anal opening. The mons pubis is a fat pad that covers the symphysis pubis and protects it during coitus (sexual intercourse).

The labia majora are two vertical folds of adipose tissue that extend posteriorly from the mons pubis to the perineum. The size of the labia majora varies depending on the amount of fatty tissue present. The skin over the labia majora is usually darker than the surrounding skin and is highly vascular. It protects inner vulval structures and enhances sexual arousal.

The labia majora surround two thinner, vertical folds of reddish epithelium called the *labia minora.* The labia minora are highly vascular and have a rich nerve supply. Emotional or physical stimulation produces marked swelling and sensitivity. Numerous sebaceous glands in the labia minora lubricate the entrance to the vagina. The clitoris is a small, cylindric organ that is composed of erectile tissue with a high concentration of sensory nerve endings. During sexual arousal, the clitoris becomes larger and increases sexual sensation.

The vestibule is a longitudinal area between the labia minora, the clitoris, and the vagina that contains Bartholin glands and the openings of the urethra, Skene's glands (paraurethral glands), and vagina. The two Bartholin glands, located deeply toward the back on both sides of the vaginal opening, secrete lubrication fluid during sexual excitement. Their ductal openings are usually not visible.

The area between the vaginal opening and the anus is the perineum. The skin of the perineum covers the muscles, fascia, and ligaments that support the pelvic structures.

Internal Genitalia

The internal female genitalia are shown in Fig. 69-1. The vagina is a hollow tube that extends from the vestibule to the uterus. Ovarian hormones (primarily *estrogen*) influence the amounts of glycogen and lubricating fluid secreted by the vaginal cells. The normal vaginal bacteria (flora) interact with the secretions to produce lactic acid and maintain an acidic pH (3.5 to 5) in the vagina. This acidity helps prevent infection in the vagina.

At the upper end of the vagina, the uterine cervix projects into a cup-shaped vault of thin vaginal tissue. The recessed pockets around the cervix permit palpation of the internal pelvic organs. The posterior area provides access into the peritoneal cavity for diagnostic or surgical purposes.

The uterus (or "womb") is a thick-walled, muscular organ attached to the upper end of the vagina. This inverted pear–shaped organ is located within the true pelvis, between the bladder and the rectum. The uterus is made up of the body and the cervix.

The cervix is a short (1 inch [2.5 cm]), narrowed portion of the uterus and extends into the vagina. The surfaces of the cervix and the canal are the sites for Papanicolaou (Pap) testing. (See discussion on p. 1454.)

The fallopian tubes (uterine tubes) insert into the fundus of the uterus and extend laterally close to the ovaries. They provide a duct between the ovaries and the uterus for the passage of ova and sperm. In most cases, the ovum is fertilized in these tubes.

The ovaries are a pair of almond-shaped organs located near the lateral walls of the upper pelvic cavity. After menopause, they become smaller. These small organs develop and release ova and produce the sex steroid hormones (estrogen, progesterone, androgen, and relaxin). Adequate amounts of these hormones are needed for normal female growth and development and to maintain a pregnancy.

Breasts

The female breasts are a pair of mammary glands that develop in response to secretions from the hypothalamus, pituitary gland, and ovaries. The breasts are an accessory of the reproductive system that nourish the infant after birth.

Breast tissue is composed of a network of glandular and ductal tissue, fibrous tissue, and fat. The proportion of each component of breast tissue depends on genetic factors, nutrition, age, and obstetric history. The breasts are supported by

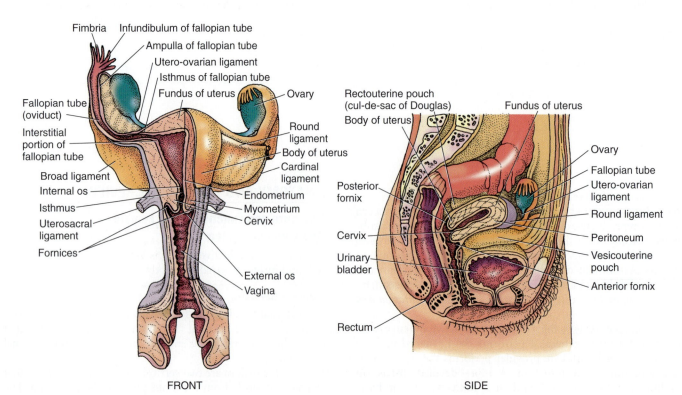

FRONT   SIDE

FIG. 69-1 Internal female genitalia.

ligaments that are attached to underlying muscles. They have abundant blood supply and lymph flow that drain from an extensive network toward the axillae (Fig. 69-2).

Structure and Function of the Male Reproductive System

The male reproductive system also consists of external and internal genitalia. The primary male hormone for sexual development and function is *testosterone*. Testosterone production is fairly constant in the adult male. Only a slight and gradual reduction of testosterone production occurs in the older adult male until he is in his 80s. Low testosterone levels decrease muscle mass, reduce skin elasticity, and lead to changes in sexual performance.

The penis is an organ for urination and intercourse consisting of the body or shaft and the glans penis (the distal end of the penis). The glans is the smooth end of the penis and contains the opening of the urethral meatus. The urethra is the pathway for the exit of both urine and semen. A continuation of skin covers the glans and folds to form the prepuce (foreskin). Surgical removal of the foreskin (circumcision) for religious or cultural reasons is a common procedure in the United States and other Western countries.

The scrotum is a thin-walled, fibromuscular pouch that is behind the penis and suspended below the pubic bone. This pouch protects the testes, epididymis, and vas deferens in a space that is slightly cooler than inside the abdominal cavity. The scrotal skin is darkly pigmented and contains sweat glands, sebaceous glands, and few hair follicles. It contracts with cold, exercise, tactile stimulation, and sexual excitement.

The internal male genitalia are shown in Fig. 69-3. The major organs are the testes and prostate gland. The testes are a pair of oval organs in the scrotum that produce sperm and testosterone. Each testis is suspended in the scrotum by the spermatic cord, which provides blood, lymphatic, and nerve supply to the testis. Sympathetic nerve fibers are located on the arteries in the cord, and sympathetic and parasympathetic fibers are on the vas deferens. When the testes are damaged, these autonomic nerve fibers transmit excruciating PAIN and a sensation of nausea.

The epididymis is the first portion of a ductal system that transports sperm from the testes to the urethra and is a site of sperm maturation. The vas deferens, or ductus deferens, is a firm, muscular tube that continues from the tail of each epididymis. The end of each vas deferens is a reservoir for sperm and tubular fluids. They merge with ducts from the seminal vesicle to form the ejaculatory ducts at the base of the prostate

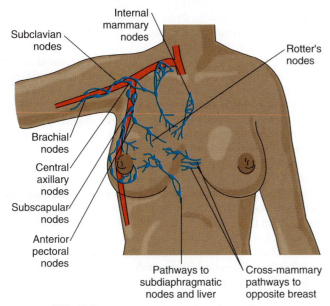

FIG. 69-2 Lymphatic drainage of the female breast.

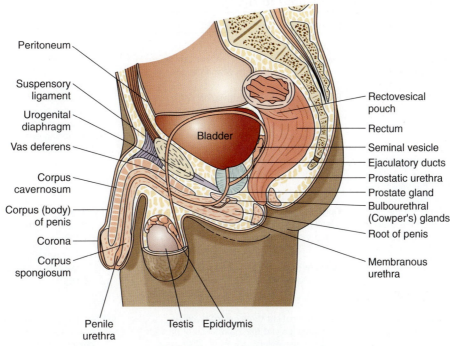

FIG. 69-3 Internal male genitalia.

gland. Sperm from the vas deferens and secretions from the seminal vesicles move through the ejaculatory duct to mix with prostatic fluids in the prostatic urethra.

The prostate gland is a large accessory gland of the male reproductive system that can be palpated via the rectum. The gland secretes a milky alkaline fluid that adds bulk to the semen, enhances sperm movement, and neutralizes acidic vaginal secretions. Men older than 50 years commonly have an enlarged prostate (benign prostatic hyperplasia [BPH]), which can cause problems such as overflow incontinence and nocturia (nighttime urination). Prostate function depends on adequate levels of testosterone.

REPRODUCTIVE CHANGES ASSOCIATED WITH AGING

Age affects the function of both the male and the female reproductive systems. Many changes in the reproductive system occur as people age (Chart 69-1).

ASSESSMENT METHODS

Patient History

Establish a trusting relationship with the patient. Many patients are hesitant to share their reproductive history or concerns about SEXUALITY. Respect their choice to refuse to answer questions about their reproductive problems or sexual practices. Assess the patient's health habits, such as diet, sleep, and exercise patterns. Low levels of body fat may be related to ovarian dysfunction. Assess for alcohol, tobacco, and drug use (prescribed, over-the-counter [OTC], and illicit drugs), because libido (sex drive), sperm production, and the ability to have or sustain an erection can be affected by these substances.

Ask female patients about the date and result of their most recent Pap test, breast self-examination, and vulvar self-examination. Determine when male patients older than 50 years had their last prostate examination and prostate-specific antigen test.

Ask about childhood illnesses that could have an effect on the reproductive system. For example, mumps in men may cause orchitis (painful inflammation and swelling of the testes) and can lead to testicular atrophy and sterility. Also ask whether the patient has had any infections. Pelvic inflammatory disease or a ruptured appendix followed by peritonitis can cause pelvic scarring and strictures or adhesions in the fallopian tubes. Salpingitis (uterine tube INFECTION) is often caused by chlamydia and can result in female infertility. A history of infections or prolonged fever in males may have damaged sperm production or caused obstruction of the seminal tract, which can cause infertility.

Assess for chronic illnesses or surgeries that could affect reproductive function. Disorders that affect a woman's metabolism or nutrition can depress ovarian function and cause amenorrhea (absence of menses). Patients with diabetes mellitus may experience physiologic changes such as vaginal dryness or impotence. Chronic disorders of the nervous system, respiratory system, or cardiovascular system can alter the sexual response.

Ask whether the patient has been treated with radiation therapy. Inquire about the prolonged use of corticosteroids, internal or external estrogen, testosterone, or chemotherapy drugs, which can lead to reproductive system dysfunction.

Data about sexual activity are vital parts of the patient's history. Sexual orientation should not be assumed. Patients who are lesbian, gay, bisexual, transgender, and queer/questioning (LGBTQ) are often not fully assessed by health care

---

CHART 69-1 Nursing Focus on the Older Adult

Changes in the Reproductive System Related to Aging

PHYSIOLOGIC CHANGE	NURSING INTERVENTIONS	RATIONALES
Women		
Graying and thinning of the pubic hair	Discuss changes with the patient (applies to all structures for both women and men).	Education helps prevent problems with body image (applies to all structures for both women and men).
Decreased size of the labia majora and clitoris		
Drying, smoothing, and thinning of the vaginal walls	Provide information about vaginal estrogen therapy and water-soluble lubricants.	Education enables the patient to make informed decisions about the treatment of vaginal dryness, which can cause painful intercourse.
Decreased size of the uterus	Provide information about Kegel exercises to strengthen pelvic muscles. Urinary incontinence can be a major problem.	Strengthening exercises may prevent or reduce pelvic relaxation and urinary incontinence.
Atrophy of the endometrium		
Decreased size and marked convolution of the ovaries		
Loss of tone and elasticity of the pelvic ligaments and connective tissue		
Increased flabbiness and fibrosis of the breasts, which hang lower on the chest wall; decreased erection of the nipples	Teach or reinforce the importance of breast self-awareness, clinical breast examinations, and mammography.	These methods can detect masses or other changes that may indicate the presence of cancer.
Men		
Graying and thinning of the pubic hair	Teach or reinforce the importance of testicular self-examination (TSE).	TSE may detect changes that may indicate cancer.
Increased drooping of the scrotum and loss of rugae		
Prostate enlargement, with an increased likelihood of urethral obstruction	Teach the patient the signs of urethral obstruction and the importance of prostate cancer screening.	Education helps the patient detect enlargement or obstruction, which may indicate the presence of cancer.

professionals. These patients feel more comfortable sharing this information about their reproductive health and sexual activity when approached in a caring, nonjudgmental way. Chapter 1 describes sensitive interviewing techniques that are appropriate for LGBTQ patients. Chapter 73 in this unit discusses assessment and care of transgender patients in detail.

🌐 CULTURAL CONSIDERATIONS
Patient-Centered Care QSEN

Other cultural beliefs and practices influence lifestyle and sexual activity. A person's religious beliefs often influence specific sexual practices, the acceptable number of sexual partners, and contraceptive use. Be sensitive to these differences by being nonjudgmental and showing acceptance.

Nutrition History

A nutrition history is important when assessing the reproductive system. Fatigue and low libido may occur as a result of poor diet and anemia. The World Cancer Research Fund estimates that about one quarter to one third of the new *preventable* cancer cases expected to occur in the United States in 2014 will be related to overweight or obesity, physical inactivity, and poor nutrition (American Cancer Society [ACS], 2014a). Ask the patient to recall his or her dietary intake for a recent 24-hour period to assess nutritional quality.

Assess the patient's height, weight, and body mass index. The patient may be hesitant to discuss practices such as bingeing, purging, anorexic behaviors, or excessive exercise. A certain level of body fat and weight is necessary for the onset of menses and the maintenance of regular menstrual cycles. Decreased body fat results in insufficient estrogen levels.

GENDER HEALTH CONSIDERATIONS
Patient-Centered Care QSEN

Women have special nutrition needs. Heavy menstrual bleeding, particularly in women who have intrauterine devices, may require iron supplements. Teach all women about their body's need for calcium. Although adequate calcium intake throughout life is needed, it is especially important during and after menopause to help prevent osteoporosis due to decreased estrogen production (see Chapter 50).

Family History and Genetic Risk

The family history helps determine the patient's risk for conditions that affect reproductive functioning. A delayed or early development of secondary sex characteristics may be a familial pattern.

The current age and health status of family members are important. Evidence of medical diseases or reproductive problems in family members (e.g., diabetes, endometriosis, reproductive cancer) provides a fuller understanding of the patient's current symptoms. For example, daughters of women who were given diethylstilbestrol (DES) to control bleeding during pregnancy are at increased risk for infertility and reproductive tract cancer.

Specific *BRCA1* and *BRCA2* gene mutations increase the overall risk for breast or ovarian cancer (ACS, 2014c). Men with first-degree relatives (e.g., father, brother) with prostate cancer

---

CHART 69-2 Best Practice for Patient Safety & Quality Care QSEN

Assessing the Patient with Reproductive Health Problems

PATIENT CONCERN	NURSING ASSESSMENT
Pain	Type and intensity of pain Location and duration of pain Factors that relieve or worsen pain Relationship to menstrual, sexual, urinary, or GI function Medications
Bleeding	Presence or absence of bleeding Character and amount of bleeding Relationship of bleeding to events or other factors (e.g., menstrual cycle) Onset and duration of bleeding Presence of associated symptoms, such as pain
Discharge	Amount and character of discharge Presence of genital lesions, bleeding, itching, or pain Presence of symptoms or discharge in sexual partner
Masses	Location and characteristics of mass Presence of associated symptoms, such as pain Relationship to menstrual cycle

---

are at greater risk for the disease than are men in the general population.

Current Health Problems

Patients often seek medical attention as a result of PAIN, bleeding, discharge, and masses (Chart 69-2). Pain related to reproductive system disorders may be confused with symptoms usually associated with GI or urinary health problems (e.g., urinary frequency). Ask the patient to describe the nature of the pain, including its type, intensity, timing and location, duration, and relationship to menstrual, sexual, urinary, or GI function. Assess the factors that exacerbate (worsen) or relieve the pain. Ask about sleeping patterns and if pain or other symptoms affect the ability to get adequate rest (Ruhl, 2010).

Heavy *bleeding* or a lack of bleeding may concern the patient. The possibility of pregnancy in any sexually active woman with amenorrhea must be considered. Postmenopausal bleeding needs to be evaluated. Ask the patient to describe the amount and characteristics of abnormal vaginal bleeding. Assess whether the bleeding occurs in relation to the menstrual cycle or menopause, intercourse, trauma, or strenuous exercise. For male patients, ask about the presence of penile bleeding. Ask any patient who has abnormal bleeding about associated symptoms, such as PAIN, cramping or abdominal fullness, a change in bowel habits, urinary difficulties, and weight changes.

Discharge from the male or female reproductive tract can cause irritation of the surrounding tissues, itching, PAIN, embarrassment, and anxiety. Ask about the amount, color, consistency, odor, and chronicity of discharge that may be present from orifices used during sexual activity. Drugs (e.g., antibiotics) and clothing (e.g., tight jeans, synthetic underwear fabric) may cause or worsen genital discharge. Many types of discharge are caused by sexually transmitted diseases (STDs) or other INFECTION (see Chapter 74).

Masses in the breasts, testes, or inguinal area must be evaluated. Patients can sometimes relate changes in character or size of masses to menstrual cycles, heavy lifting, straining, or trauma. Ask about associated symptoms such as tenderness, heaviness, PAIN, dimpling, and tender lymph nodes.

Physical Assessment

Assessment of the Female Reproductive System

The nurse generalist does not perform a comprehensive female or male reproductive examination. However, you should perform a focused assessment related to specific concerns of the patient. The primary care provider conducts a more detailed gynecologic assessment as described below; the generalist nurse often assists with the examination.

Immediately before the pelvic and breast examinations, ask the patient to empty her bladder and undress completely. Drape the patient adequately to provide modesty throughout the examination. Remove drapes only over the region being examined, and replace them after that area has been assessed. Mirrors can be used to facilitate teaching if the patient so desires. The examination should be performed in a room that has adequate lighting for body inspection, that has comfortable temperature, and that ensures privacy.

The physical examination of the female reproductive system includes the breasts (see Chapter 70), cardiovascular system, and abdomen. The patient's arms should be at her sides or over her chest to allow better relaxation of the abdominal muscles. During the gynecologic examination, the primary care provider palpates for symptomatic and asymptomatic abdominopelvic masses, which can be of reproductive, intestinal, or urinary tract origin. Gynecologic masses, such as ovarian masses, may be further differentiated from lesions on the body of the uterus during the bimanual portion of the pelvic examination.

Inspection of the female genitalia and the pelvic examination are usually performed at the end of a head-to-toe physical assessment. The patient is often more apprehensive about these portions of the examination than about any other part. PAIN or lack of privacy during previous pelvic or breast examinations may prevent the patient from relaxing.

Other than determining pregnancy or infertility, a pelvic examination is indicated to assess for:

- Menstrual irregularities
- Unexplained abdominal or vaginal PAIN
- Vaginal discharge, itching, sores, or INFECTION
- Rape trauma or other pelvic injury
- Physical changes in the vagina, cervix, and uterus

Assessment of the Male Reproductive System

Unless a male patient seeks health care for a specific problem, the health care provider may not perform a reproductive assessment, depending on the setting and the age of the patient. Men are often embarrassed and anxious when the reproductive system is assessed. The patient may be concerned about discomfort, the developmental stage of his genitalia, or the possibility of an erection during the examination. If he does have an erection, the examiner should assure him that this is a normal response to a tactile stimulus (touch) and should continue the examination.

Explain each step of the assessment procedure before it is performed. The patient needs to be reassured that the health care provider will stop and change the assessment plan or technique if the patient experiences pain during the examination. Teach relaxation techniques and provide nonjudgmental support during the examination to increase comfort.

Psychosocial Assessment

The psychosocial assessment may provide information about factors that affect the patient's health status. During the social history, ask about sources of support, strengths, and coping reactions to illness or dysfunction.

A patient's personal experiences, culture, and/or spiritual beliefs may influence his or her ability to enjoy a satisfactory sexual life. These factors may include:

- Sexual trauma or abuse inflicted during childhood or adulthood
- Punishment for masturbation
- Psychological trauma
- Cultural influences, such as the idea of female passivity during intercourse
- Concerns about sexual partners or sexual lifestyle
- Use of alcohol or street drugs

Fears may affect the patient's satisfaction with SEXUALITY or body image. He or she may also be concerned about the potential or actual reaction of family members to reproductive health problems (see Chart 69-2). Use nonjudgmental listening to continue development of trust between yourself and the patient, allowing the patient to openly express feelings or concerns.

Diagnostic Assessment

Laboratory Assessment

Chart 69-3 summarizes important laboratory tests associated with reproductive function. The **Papanicolaou test (Pap test)**, or **Pap smear**, is a cytologic study that is effective in detecting precancerous and cancerous cells within the female patient's cervix. It is done immediately before the pelvic examination. A speculum is inserted into the vagina, and several samples of cells from the cervix are obtained with a small brush or spatula. The specimens are placed on a glass slide and sent to the laboratory for examination.

The Pap test should be scheduled between the patient's menstrual periods so that the menstrual flow does not interfere with laboratory analysis. Teach women not to douche, use vaginal medications or deodorants, or have sexual intercourse for at least 24 hours before the test, because these may interfere with test interpretation.

The American Cancer Society (ACS) advises all women to begin having an annual Pap test at 21 years of age. Women younger than 21 years should not be tested (ACS, 2014a). Between ages 21 and 29 years, women should have a Pap test every 3 years; women between ages 30 and 65 years should have a Pap test plus a human papilloma virus (HPV) test ("co-testing") every 5 years. More information on the HPV test is found later in this chapter. In the absence of co-testing, this population should still have a Pap test every 3 years. According to the ACS, women older than 65 years who have had regular cervical cancer testing with normal results should not receive Pap tests (ACS, 2014a). Recommended guidelines from other health care organizations suggest a Pap test every 3 years for women older than 60 years. Those who have had a history of a serious cervical precancerous lesion should be tested annually for at least 20 years after that diagnosis, regardless of age (ACS, 2014a).

Other types of laboratory testing include cytologic vaginal *cultures*, which can detect bacterial, viral, fungal, and parasitic disorders. Examination of cells from the vaginal walls can evaluate estrogen balance.

The **human papilloma virus (HPV) test** can identify many high-risk types of HPV INFECTION associated with the

CHART 69-3 Laboratory Profile

Reproductive Assessment

TEST	NORMAL RANGE FOR ADULTS	SIGNIFICANCE OF ABNORMAL FINDINGS
Serum Studies		
Follicle-stimulating hormone (FSH) (Follitropin)	*Men:* 1.42-15.4 IU/L *Women:* follicular phase, 1.37-9.9 IU/L; midcycle, 6.17-17.2 IU/L; luteal phase, 1.09-9.2 IU/L; postmenopause, 19.3-100.6 IU/L	Decreased levels indicate possible infertility, anorexia nervosa, neoplasm. Elevations indicate possible Turner's syndrome.
Luteinizing hormone (LH) (Lutropin)	*Men:* 1.24-7.8 IU/L *Women:* follicular phase, 1.68-15 IU/L; midcycle, 21.9-56.6 IU/L; luteal phase, 0.61-16.3 IU/L; postmenopause, 14.2-52.3 IU/L	Decreased levels indicate possible infertility, anovulation. Elevations indicate possible ovarian failure, Turner's syndrome.
Prolactin	*Men:* 3-13 ng/mL *Women:* 3-27 ng/mL Pregnant women: 20-400 ng/mL	Elevations indicate possible galactorrhea (breast discharge), pituitary tumor, disease of hypothalamus or pituitary gland, hypothyroidism.
Estradiol	*Men:* 10-50 pg/mL *Women:* follicular phase, 20-350 pg/mL; midcycle, 150-750 pg/mL; luteal phase, 30-450 pg/mL; postmenopause, ≤20 pg/mL	Elevations of estradiol, total estrogens, and estriol in men indicate possible gynecomastia, decreased body hair, increased fat deposits, feminization, testicular tumor; in women, ovarian tumor.
Estriol	Men and nonpregnant women: N/A	Decreased levels of estradiol, total estrogens, and estriol in women indicate possible amenorrhea, climacteric, impending miscarriage, hypothalamic disorders.
Progesterone	*Men:* 10-50 ng/dL *Women:* follicular phase, <50 ng/dL; luteal phase, 300-2500 ng/dL; postmenopausal, <40 ng/dL	Decreased levels in women indicate possible inadequate luteal phase, amenorrhea. Elevations in women indicate possible ovarian luteal cysts. Decreased levels may indicate ovarian neoplasm, ovarian dysfunction.
Testosterone	*Men:* 280-1080 ng/dL *Women:* <70 ng/dL	Increased levels in men indicate possible testicular tumor, hyperthyroidism. Decreased levels in men indicate possible hypogonadism. Elevations in women indicate possible adrenal neoplasm, ovarian neoplasm, polycystic ovary syndrome.
Prostate-specific antigen	*Men:* 0-2.5 ng/mL	Increased levels may indicate prostatitis, benign prostatic hyperplasia, prostate cancer.
Urine Studies		
Total estrogens	*Men:* 4-25 mcg/24 hr *Women:* 4-60 mcg/24 hr	Elevations indicate possible testicular tumors. Decreased levels indicate possible ovarian dysfunction.
Pregnanediol	*Men:* 0-1.9 mg/24 hr *Women:* follicular phase, <2.6 mg/24 hr; luteal phase, 2.6-10.6 mg/24 hr	Elevations indicate possible luteal ovarian cysts, ovarian neoplasms, adrenal disorders. Decreased levels indicate possible amenorrhea.
17-Ketosteroids	Men (20-50 yr): 6-20 mg/24 hr Women (20-50 yr): 6-17 mg/24 hr Values decrease with age	Elevations indicate possible Cushing's syndrome, increased androgen or cortisol production, severe stress. Decreased levels indicate possible Addison's disease, hypopituitarism.

Data from Pagana, K.D., & Pagana, T.J. (2014). *Mosby's manual of diagnostic and laboratory tests* (12th ed.). St. Louis: Mosby.
1 mcg, 1 microgram or 1 millionth of a gram; *1 ng,* 1 nanogram or 1 billionth of a gram; *1 pg,* 1 picogram or 1 trillionth of a gram.

development of cervical cancer. This test can be done at the same time as the Pap test for women older than 30 years and for women of any age who have had an abnormal Pap test result (ACS, 2014a). It does not take the place of the Pap test because it tests for viruses that can cause cell changes in the cervix that, if not treated, could lead to cancer. Cells are collected from the cervix and sent to a laboratory for analysis. Women who have normal Pap test results and no HPV infection are at very low risk for developing cervical cancer. Conversely, women with an abnormal Pap test result and a positive HPV test are at higher risk if not treated.

Serum levels of follicle-stimulating hormone (FSH), luteinizing hormone (LH), and prolactin are helpful in the diagnosis of male and female reproductive tract disorders. No nutrition restrictions are necessary before the test. Serum testing can also detect estrogen, progesterone, and testosterone levels in men and women. See Chart 69-3 for normal values and the significance of abnormal findings.

Serologic studies detect antigen-antibody reactions that occur in response to foreign organisms. This form of diagnostic testing is helpful only after an infection has become well established. Serologic testing can be used in the evaluation of exposure to organisms causing syphilis, rubella, and herpes simplex virus type 2 (HSV2). Results may be read as *nonreactive, weakly reactive,* or *reactive.* A single titer is not as revealing as serial titers, which can detect the rise in antibody reactions as the body continues to fight the infection (see Chapter 74).

The *prostate-specific antigen (PSA)* test is used to screen for prostate cancer and to monitor the disease after treatment. PSA levels less than 2.5 ng/mL may be considered normal, although there is no agreement on that value and how it is affected by age. Elevated PSA levels may be associated with prostate cancer. Older men, particularly African-American men, often have a higher normal PSA, especially as they age (Pagana & Pagana, 2014). Chapter 72 discusses this test in more detail.

Imaging Assessment

Computed Tomography. CT scans for reproductive system disorders involve the abdomen and the pelvis. Health care providers can detect and evaluate masses and identify lymphatic enlargement from metastasis. This scan can differentiate solid tissue masses from cystic or hemorrhagic structures.

Hysterosalpingography. A hysterosalpingogram is an x-ray that uses an injection of a contrast medium to visualize the cervix, uterus, and fallopian tubes (American Congress of Obstetricians and Gynecologists [ACOG], 2011). This test is used to evaluate tubal anatomy and patency and uterine problems such as fibroids, tumors, and fistulas. The study should not be attempted for at least 6 weeks after abortion, delivery, or dilation and curettage. Other contraindications include reproductive tract infection and uterine bleeding.

The examination is best performed in the first half (days 1-14) of the patient's menstrual cycle, which reduces the chance that the patient may be pregnant (ACOG, 2011). Patients preparing to have a hysterosalpingogram should be instructed to follow the recommendations of their health care provider, which may include taking an over-the-counter pain reliever before the procedure (ACOG, 2011).

On the day of the examination, confirm the date of the patient's last menstrual period. Ask about allergies to iodine dye or shellfish. The health care provider will share benefits and risks of the procedure with the patient. You, as the nurse, may witness the signed informed consent. Be aware that the patient may experience some nausea and vomiting, abdominal cramping, or faintness during the procedure. Provide support and assistance with relaxation techniques as needed.

After the patient is placed in lithotomy position, the health care provider will insert a speculum to view the cervix. Dye is injected through the cervix to fill and highlight the interior of the cervix, uterus, and fallopian tubes. If the fallopian tubes are patent, the contrast material spills into the peritoneal cavity. Usually, only two or three views are obtained to show the path and distribution of the contrast medium.

The patient may experience pelvic PAIN after the study and should receive analgesic medications as ordered. Inform her that she may also have referred PAIN to the shoulder because of irritation of the phrenic nerve. Provide a perineal pad after the test to prevent soiling of clothes as the dye drains from the cervix. Instruct the patient to contact her health care provider if bloody discharge continues for 4 days or longer and to immediately report any signs of infection, such as lower quadrant PAIN, fever, malodorous discharge, or tachycardia.

Mammography. Mammography is an x-ray of the soft tissue of the breast. Mammograms assess differences in the density of breast tissue. They are especially helpful in evaluating poorly defined masses, multiple masses or nodules, nipple changes or discharge, skin changes, and PAIN. Mammography can detect about 78% of cancers that are not palpable by physical examination in women younger than 50 years and 83% in women older than 50 years (Susan G. Komen, 2013). However, some actual cancers may not appear on mammography or may appear as benign (ACS, 2014b).

In young women's breasts, there is little difference in the density between normal glandular tissue and malignant tumors, which makes the mammogram less useful for evaluation of breast masses in these women. For this reason, annual screening mammograms are not recommended for women younger than 40 years (ACS, 2014b). In older women, the amount of fatty tissue is higher and the fatty tissue appears lighter than cancers. Cancer and cysts may have the same density. Cysts usually have smooth borders, and cancers often have starburst-shaped margins.

No dietary restrictions are necessary before the mammogram. Remind the patient not to use creams, lotions, powders, or deodorant on the breasts or underarms before the study because these products may be visible on the mammogram and lead to misdiagnosis. If there is any possibility that the patient is pregnant, the test should be rescheduled. Explain the purpose of the study and its anticipated discomforts. Provide a gown and privacy to undress above the waist. Allow the patient to express concerns about the mammogram and the presence of any lumps.

When performing a standard mammogram, a technician positions the patient next to the x-ray machine with one breast exposed. A film plate and the platform of the machine are placed on opposite sides of the breast to be examined. The technician includes as much breast tissue as possible between the plates. The woman may experience some temporary discomfort when the breast is compressed (for about a minute for each of four positions). The entire test takes about 15 minutes. The patient usually is asked to wait until the films are reviewed in case a view needs to be repeated. If a digital mammogram is performed, the images are recorded and saved as computer files (ACS, 2014b).

Inform the patient when to expect the report of the results. Because this is a time when the patient is anxious about the health of her breasts, teach or reinforce the importance of breast self-awareness and provide instructions as needed.

Other Diagnostic Assessment

Ultrasonography. Ultrasonography (US) is a technique that is used to assess fibroids, cysts, and masses. It can be used to monitor the progress of tumor regression after medical treatment. US is also helpful in differentiating solid tumors from cysts in breast examinations. In men, ultrasound can test for varicoceles, scrotal abnormalities, and problems of the ejaculatory ducts and seminal vesicles and the vas deferens (Pagana & Pagana, 2014).

For an abdominal, breast, or scrotal scan, the technician exposes the area and applies gel to the area to be scanned, which provides better transmission of sound waves from the transducer through the patient's skin. The transducer is moved in a linear pattern across the area being tested to outline and define soft-tissue masses and to differentiate tumor type, ascites, and encapsulated fluid.

For a *transvaginal* or *transrectal* scan, the transducer is covered with a condom onto which transmission gel has been placed. The transducer is then inserted into the vagina or rectum as indicated. Women should have an empty or only partially filled bladder if they are having a transvaginal ultrasound. Patients having an internal ultrasound should be informed that they might feel some mild discomfort associated with pressure of the probe (Levin, 2012).

Magnetic Resonance Imaging. MRI uses a magnetic field and radiofrequency energy to scan for pelvic tumors. This scan distinguishes between normal and malignant tissues. MRIs are used in addition to mammograms to assess for breast cancer in women who have a genetic risk (ACS, 2014c). The use of MRI in evaluating patients with dense breast tissue may reduce the need for biopsy.

Endoscopic Studies

Colposcopy. A colposcope allows three-dimensional magnification and intense illumination of epithelium with suspected disease. Colposcopy is suited for inspection of a female patient's cervical epithelium, vagina, and vulvar epithelium. Because it provides accurate site selection, this procedure can locate the exact site of precancerous and malignant lesions for biopsy.

Inform the patient that she should not douche or use vaginal preparations for 24 to 48 hours before the test. This nearly painless procedure is better tolerated if it is explained in advance and if the actual colposcope instrument is shown to the patient. Explain that the health care provider may take a biopsy while performing colposcopy.

Provide the patient with a gown and privacy, and instruct her to undress from the waist down. Assist the patient to the lithotomy position. The health care provider locates the cervix or vaginal site through a speculum examination. Lubricants other than water should not be used. Cells in the area may be stained or left unstained to enhance visibility. The cervix will be cleaned and moistened with normal saline to increase the visibility of vascular patterns and the junction between the columnar epithelium and the squamous epithelium. Acetic acid is applied to the cervix to draw moisture from the tissue and to accentuate important features. The health care provider then uses a colposcope or colpomicroscope to inspect the area in question, and a biopsy specimen can be taken if abnormal cells are seen. (See Cervical Biopsy section on p. 1458.)

After the procedure, allow the patient to rest for a few minutes, especially if she had a biopsy performed. Provide privacy and supplies to clean the perineum and a perineal pad to absorb any dye or discharge. Inform the patient that she may wish to wear a sanitary pad, as mild cramping, spotting, or dark or black-colored discharge (from medication applied to the cervix to reduce bleeding) may occur for several days (Johns Hopkins Medicine, 2014). Remind the patient to take pain relievers as recommended by her health care provider but to avoid aspirin to decrease the chance of bleeding. The patient should be instructed to refrain from douching, using tampons, and having sexual intercourse for 1 week (or as instructed by the health care provider) (Johns Hopkins Medicine, 2014).

Laparoscopy. Laparoscopy is a direct examination of the pelvic cavity through an endoscope. This procedure can rule out an ectopic pregnancy, evaluate ovarian disorders and pelvic masses, and aid in the diagnosis of infertility and unexplained pelvic PAIN. Laparoscopy is also used during surgical procedures such as:

- Tubal sterilization
- Ovarian biopsy
- Cyst aspiration
- Removal of endometriosis tissue
- Lysis of adhesions around the fallopian tubes
- Retrieval of "lost" intrauterine devices

A laparoscopy may be used instead of a laparotomy for minor surgical procedures because it uses small incisions, involves less discomfort, and does not require overnight hospitalization.

The surgeon describes benefits and risks of the procedure to the patient. Risks include complications associated with the use of general anesthesia, postoperative shoulder pain from irritation of the phrenic nerve, effects of carbon dioxide gas and/or peritoneal stretching (Taş et al., 2013), irritation at the incision site, and the rare occurrence of infection or electrical burns. As the nurse, you may witness the patient signing the informed consent. A laparoscopy can be performed with a regional or general anesthetic.

After the patient is anesthetized and placed in the lithotomy position, a urinary catheter is inserted to drain the bladder. The operating table is placed in slight Trendelenburg position to allow the intestines to fall away from the pelvis. The cervix is held with a cannula to allow movement of the uterus during laparoscopy (Fig. 69-4). The surgeon inserts a needle below the umbilicus to infuse carbon dioxide (CO_2) into the pelvic cavity, which distends the abdomen and permits better visualization of the organs. After the trocar and cannula are in place in the abdominal cavity, the surgeon removes the trocar and inserts the laparoscope. The surgeon can then visualize the pelvic cavity and reproductive organs. Further instrumentation is possible through one or more small incisions. The laparoscope is removed at the end of the procedure, and the abdomen is deflated. The small incision is closed with absorbable sutures and dressed with an adhesive bandage.

The patient is usually discharged on the day of the procedure. Discomfort from the incision is managed by oral analgesics. The greatest discomfort is due to referred shoulder PAIN. Most of these sensations disappear within 48 hours. Instruct the patient to change the small adhesive bandage as needed and to observe the incision for signs of infection or hematoma. Remind

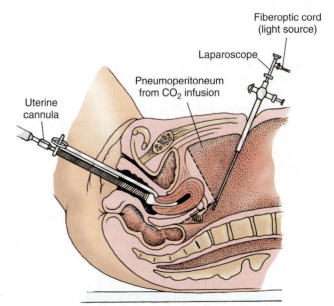

FIG. 69-4 Laparoscopy. *CO_2*, Carbon dioxide.

her also to avoid strenuous activity for the first week after the procedure.

Hysteroscopy. Hysteroscopy is a procedure that uses a fiber-optic camera to visualize the uterus to diagnose and treat causes of abnormal bleeding (Cleveland Clinic, 2013). The hysteroscope includes a fiberoptic camera that is inserted into the vagina to examine the cervix and uterus. Diagnostic hysteroscopy is used to diagnose new problems with the uterus or to confirm results from other tests (Cleveland Clinic, 2013). Hysteroscopy can also be used before or during other procedures (e.g., laparoscopy) for infertility and unexplained bleeding. The procedure is best performed 5 days after menses has ceased to reduce the possibility of pregnancy.

The physician informs the patient of benefits and risks associated with the procedure and obtains consent. You may witness the patient signing the informed consent. The preparation is the same as for a pelvic examination. After the patient is placed in lithotomy position, she is usually anesthetized with a paracervical or other regional block before the cervix is dilated. The physician inserts the hysteroscope through the cervix. Because this distends the uterus, cells can be pushed through the fallopian tubes and into the pelvic cavity. Therefore hysteroscopy is contraindicated in patients with suspected cervical or endometrial cancer, in those with infection of the reproductive tract, and in pregnant patients.

Care is the same as that after a pelvic examination. Analgesics may be prescribed if the patient has cramping or shoulder PAIN.

Biopsy Studies

Cervical Biopsy. In a cervical biopsy, cervical tissue is removed for cytologic study. A biopsy is indicated for an identifiable cervical lesion, regardless of the cytologic findings. The health care provider usually performs a biopsy in conjunction with colposcopy as a follow-up to a suspicious Pap test finding. The procedure may be performed in a clinic or office setting.

Several techniques can be used for a cervical biopsy. If a lesion is clearly visible, an endocervical curettage can be performed as an ambulatory care procedure and with little or no anesthetic. Conization (removal of a cone-shaped sample of tissue) and loop electrosurgical excision procedures (LEEPs) are usually not done unless the cervical biopsy findings are positive or the results of the colposcopy are unsatisfactory (Lowdermilk & Perry, 2014). Conization can be done as a cold-knife procedure, a laser excision, or an electrosurgical incision.

The biopsy is usually scheduled when the woman is in the early proliferative phase of the menstrual cycle, when the cervix is least vascular. Because a biopsy evaluates potentially cancerous cells, your patient may be anxious and need time to discuss her feelings and fears. The use of relaxation techniques may assist comfort. Assist her into the lithotomy position, recognizing that further preparation depends on the type of procedure to be performed.

The physician may anesthetize the patient according to the needs of the chosen procedure. He or she visualizes the cervix and obtains the tissue sample, which is immediately placed into a formalin solution. The type of anesthetic used for the procedure determines the type of immediate care that is needed after the procedure. Discharge instructions can be found in Chart 69-4.

Endometrial Biopsy. Both endometrial biopsy and aspiration are used to obtain cells directly from the lining of the uterus to assess for cancer of the endometrium. Biopsy helps assess

---

> **CHART 69-4** **Patient and Family Education:**
> **Preparing for Self-Management**
>
> ### The Patient Recovering from Cervical Biopsy
>
> * Do not lift any heavy objects until the site is healed (about 2 weeks).
> * Rest for 24 hours after the procedure.
> * Report any excessive bleeding (more than that of a normal menstrual period) to your health care provider.
> * Report signs of infection (fever, increased pain, foul-smelling drainage) to your health care provider.
> * Do not douche, use tampons, or have vaginal intercourse until the site is healed (about 2 weeks).
> * Keep the perineum clean and dry by using antiseptic solution rinses (as directed by your health care provider) and changing pads frequently.

menstrual disturbances (especially heavy bleeding) and infertility (corpus luteum dysfunction).

When menstrual disturbances are being evaluated, the biopsy is generally done in the immediate premenstrual period to provide an index of progesterone influence and ovulation. A biopsy performed in the second half of the menstrual cycle (about days 21 and 22) evaluates corpus luteum function and the presence or absence of a persistent secretory endometrium. Postmenopausal women may undergo biopsies at any time.

Menstrual data should be obtained from the patient and are included on the specimen request for the pathologist. Prepare the patient in the same way as you would for a pelvic examination. Advise her that she may experience some cramping when the cervix is dilated. Analgesia before the procedure and relaxation and breathing techniques during the procedure may be helpful to make her more comfortable.

An endometrial biopsy is usually done as an office procedure with or without anesthesia. After the uterus is measured and the cervix dilated, the physician inserts the curette or intrauterine cannula into the uterus. A portion of the endometrium is withdrawn using either the cuplike end of the curette or suction equipment and is placed into a formalin solution to be sent for histologic examination. The patient will likely have moderate cramping. Allow her to rest on the examining table until the cramping has subsided. Provide a perineal pad and a wipe to clean the perineum. Teach her that spotting may be present for 1 to 2 days but any signs of infection or excessive bleeding should be reported to the physician. Instruct the patient to avoid intercourse or douching until all discharge has ceased.

Breast Biopsy. All breast masses should be evaluated for the possibility of cancer. It is important to recognize that breast cancer can occur in men as well as women (National Cancer Institute, 2014). Fibrocystic lesions, fibroadenomas, and intraductal papillomas can be differentiated by biopsy. Any discharge from the breasts is examined histologically.

Provide instructions to the patient depending on the type of biopsy performed and the type of anesthesia used. The patient usually receives a local anesthetic, and the tissue either is aspirated through a large-bore needle (core-needle biopsy) or is removed using a small incision to extract multiple samples of tissue.

Aspirated fluid from benign cysts may appear clear to dark green–brown. Bloody fluid suggests cancer. These specimens undergo histologic evaluation. If cancer is found, the tissue is evaluated for estrogen receptor analysis. Chapter 70 discusses types of breast cancer and their relationship to estrogen receptors.

Teach that discomfort after the procedure is usually mild and can be controlled with analgesics or the use of ice or heat, depending on the type and extent of the biopsy. Educate the patient about how to assess the area or incision for bleeding and edema. Tell women to wear a properly supportive bra continuously for 1 week after surgery or as recommended by their surgeon. Remind the patient that numbness around the biopsy site may last several weeks. If cancer is identified, provide emotional support and reinforce information about follow-up treatment options.

Prostate Biopsy. When prostate cancer is suspected, a biopsy must be performed. This can be done by transurethral biopsy, by inserting a needle through the area of skin between the anus and scrotum, or, most commonly, by transrectal biopsy (Mayo Clinic, 2013). Preparation for the procedure depends on the technique used to puncture the gland.

Explain to the patient that he may experience some discomfort. Teach him about breathing and relaxation techniques that may be helpful to use during the procedure. Because the purpose of this procedure is to evaluate prostate cells for cancer, allow him time to discuss his anxieties and fears.

Assist the patient who is undergoing transrectal biopsy into the side-lying position with his knees pulled up toward his chest (Mayo Clinic, 2013). The physician will cleanse the area, apply gel, and then insert a thin ultrasound probe into the patient's rectum to anesthetize (if needed) and guide the biopsy needle into place. The biopsy is collected over a 5- to 10-minute period. The patient may experience a brief, uncomfortable feeling each time the needle collects a sample.

After prostate biopsy, educate the patient to take the entire prescribed antibiotic. Remind him that he may experience slight soreness, light rectal bleeding, and blood in the urine or stools for a few days. Semen may be red or rust-colored for several weeks. Teach the patient to contact his health care provider if he has prolonged or heavy bleeding, worsening pain, swelling in the area of biopsy, and/or difficulty urinating (Mayo Clinic, 2013). Rarely, sepsis can develop after a prostate biopsy. Teach the patient to contact his health care provider immediately if he experiences fever, pain when urinating, or penile discharge.

💡 NCLEX EXAMINATION CHALLENGE

Physiological Integrity

A client has undergone a transrectal biopsy for suspected prostate cancer. The nurse teaches which postoperative condition should immediately be reported to the health care provider?
A. Fever the next morning
B. Blood in urine 1 day postprocedure
C. Scant rectal bleeding for 2 days
D. Reddish-tinted semen 3 weeks after biopsy

NURSING CONCEPTS AND CLINICAL JUDGMENT REVIEW

What might you EXPECT to see in a patient without reproductive health problems that affect SEXUALITY?

Physical assessment:
• No vaginal bleeding other than normal menstruation
• No unusual vaginal discharge
• No penile bleeding or discharge
• No masses or lesions on internal or external genitalia
• Reports ability to have intercourse without pain

Psychosocial assessment:
• Reports satisfaction with sexual activity
• Reports satisfaction with body image

Laboratory assessment:
• Sex hormones within normal limits for age and gender
• Prostate-specific antigen within normal limits for age

GET READY FOR THE NCLEX® EXAMINATION!

KEY POINTS

Review these Key Points for each NCLEX Examination Client Needs Category.

Health Promotion and Maintenance
• Encourage women to follow recommended Pap screening guidelines for early detection of precancerous and cancerous cells from the cervix. **Evidence-Based Practice** QSEN
• Assess and respect cultural preferences when identifying risks for certain reproductive problems and when evaluating health promotion practices. **Patient-Centered Care** QSEN

Psychosocial Integrity
• Allow the patient to express fear or anxiety regarding potential changes in sexual or reproductive function.

• Assess the patient's level of comfort in discussing issues related to reproductive health and SEXUALITY. **Patient-Centered Care** QSEN
• Encourage patients to express feelings of anxiety or discomfort related to genital examinations and testing of the reproductive system.

Physiological Integrity
• Urge patients with PAIN, bleeding, discharge, masses, or changes in reproductive function to see their health care provider. **Safety** QSEN
• Provide privacy for patients undergoing examination or testing of the reproductive system.

- Recognize that reproductive changes occur with aging, as described in Chart 69-1.
- Recall the selected laboratory tests used for diagnosing reproductive health problems as outlined in Chart 69-3.
- Explain all diagnostic procedures, restrictions, and follow-up care to the patient scheduled for tests.

- Teach women to report symptoms of infection to their health care provider after endoscopic procedures and biopsies of the breast, cervix, and endometrium. **Safety** QSEN
- Instruct men to report symptoms of infection to their health care provider after a transrectal biopsy of the prostate. **Safety** QSEN

CHAPTER 70

Care of Patients with Breast Disorders

Mary Justice

http://evolve.elsevier.com/Iggy/

PRIORITY CONCEPTS

- INFECTION
- PAIN
- SEXUALITY

LEARNING OUTCOMES

Safe and Effective Care Environment

1. Collaborate with health care team members to identify community resources for patients with breast cancer.

Health Promotion and Maintenance

2. Describe the three-pronged approach to early detection of breast masses: mammography, clinical breast examination (CBE), and breast self-awareness.
3. Teach patients who choose breast self-examination (BSE) as an option to use correct technique.
4. Explain the options available to a person at high genetic risk for breast cancer.
5. Evaluate patient risk factors for breast cancer.

Psychosocial Integrity

6. Reduce the psychosocial impact for the patient and family who have received a diagnosis of breast cancer.
7. Discuss SEXUALITY issues with the patient having breast surgery.

8. Describe body image changes that can result from breast cancer surgery.

Physiological Integrity

9. Compare assessment findings associated with benign breast lesions with those of malignant breast lesions.
10. Explain implications of breast reduction and breast augmentation.
11. Discuss treatment options for breast cancer.
12. Develop a personalized postoperative collaborative plan of care for a patient with breast cancer, including PAIN management.
13. Describe the role of radiation and drug therapy in the care of patients with breast cancer.
14. Identify the role of complementary and alternative therapies in breast cancer management.
15. Explain evidence-based options that are available to a woman considering breast reconstruction.

Breast disorders may be benign or cancerous. Changes in the breast can cause a great deal of anxiety for women. An ever-increasing amount of health information is communicated through various types of media that often leads to anxiety and confusion about one's risk for breast cancer (Justice et al., 2012). As a result, many women seek advice for breast changes that they perceive to be abnormal. Nurses are often in the position of assisting patients by providing accurate information about benign breast disorders and breast cancer.

BENIGN BREAST DISORDERS

Benign breast conditions are very common. Noncancerous changes to breast tissue can present as breast lumps, discomfort or PAIN, and nipple changes (Amin et al., 2013). Most breast lumps are benign. Because the incidence of breast disease is related to age, breast disorders are described below in an age-related order (Table 70-1).

FIBROADENOMA

Fibroadenomas are the most common benign tumor in women during the reproductive years. However, they also may occur in a few postmenopausal women. A fibroadenoma is a mass of connective tissue that is unattached to the surrounding breast tissue and is usually discovered by the woman herself or during mammography. Although the immediate fear is that of breast cancer, the risk for cancer occurring within a fibroadenoma is very small. On clinical examination, the tumors are oval, freely mobile, and rubbery. Their size varies from smaller than 0.4 inch (1 cm) in diameter to as large as 6 inches (15 cm) in diameter.

Fibroadenomas may occur anywhere in the breast. The health care provider may request a breast ultrasound examination or may perform a needle aspiration to establish whether the lump is cystic (fluid-filled) or solid. If the lesion is solid, excision in an ambulatory care setting using local anesthesia is sometimes the treatment of choice.

TABLE 70-1 Typical Presentation of Benign Breast Disorders

BREAST DISORDER	DESCRIPTION	INCIDENCE
Fibroadenoma	Most common benign lesion; solid mass of connective tissue that is unattached to the surrounding tissue	During teenage years into the 30s (most commonly)
Fibrocystic breast condition	Breast PAIN and tender lumps; the lumps are rubbery, ill defined, and commonly found in the upper outer quadrant of the breast	Onset late teens and 20s; usually subsides after menopause
Ductal ectasia	Hard, irregular mass or masses with nipple discharge, enlarged axillary nodes, redness, and edema; difficult to distinguish from cancer	Women approaching menopause
Intraductal papilloma	Mass in duct that results in nipple discharge; mass is usually not palpable	Women 40 to 55 yr of age

FIBROCYSTIC BREAST CONDITION

❖ PATHOPHYSIOLOGY

Fibrocystic changes of the breast include a range of changes involving the lobules, ducts, and stromal tissues of the breast. Because these changes affect at least half of women over the life span, they are referred to as **fibrocystic breast condition (FBC)** rather than *fibrocystic disease*. This condition most often occurs in premenopausal women between 20 and 50 years of age and is thought to be caused by an imbalance in the normal estrogen-to-progesterone ratio. Typical symptoms include breast PAIN and tender lumps or swelling in the breasts. The symptoms are more noticeable before a woman's menstrual period (American Cancer Society [ACS], 2013a).

The two main features of FBC are fibrosis and cysts. Areas of fibrosis are made up of fibrous connective tissue and are firm or hard. Cysts are spaces filled with fluid lined by breast glandular cells. Microcysts are small, nonpalpable cysts inside the breast glands. Macrocysts occur when fluid continues to build up. They often enlarge in response to monthly hormonal changes, stretching the surrounding breast tissue, and become PAINful. Symptoms usually resolve after menstruation and then recur before the next menstrual period in a cyclic fashion. Breast ultrasound is used to confirm the presence of a cyst.

Postmenopausal women taking hormone replacement therapy (HRT) may develop FBC or experience worsening of symptoms. Having cysts or fibrosis does not increase a woman's chance of developing breast cancer. However, if a lump is very firm or has other features raising the concern about cancer, mammography is indicated. A needle biopsy or a surgical biopsy may be needed to make sure cancer is not present. Biopsy may be indicated in these situations:

- No fluid is aspirated.
- The mammogram shows suspicious findings.
- A mass remains palpable after aspiration.
- The aspirated fluid reveals cancer cells.

Symptoms often resolve after menopause when estrogen decreases.

❖ PATIENT-CENTERED COLLABORATIVE CARE

Management of FBC focuses on the symptoms of the condition. Suggest supportive measures for women with mild discomfort. The use of analgesics or limiting salt intake before menses to help decrease swelling may be helpful. Teach patients that wearing a supportive bra, even to bed, can reduce PAIN by decreasing tension on the ligaments. Local application of ice or heat may provide temporary relief of pain. For a small number of women, draining the cysts by needle aspiration can help relieve painful symptoms. Many women find relief with the reduction of dietary caffeine and other stimulants, although research has not found stimulants to have a significant impact on FBC (ACS, 2013a).

In women with severe symptoms of FBC, hormonal drugs such as oral contraceptives or selective estrogen receptor modulators (SERMs) may be prescribed to suppress oversecretion of estrogen and correct luteal insufficiency. Vitamin supplements have also been suggested to relieve symptoms, but research has not consistently shown these to be effective; some may have dangerous side effects if taken in large doses. Diuretics may be prescribed to decrease premenstrual breast engorgement.

⚠ NURSING SAFETY PRIORITY (QSEN)

Drug Alert

Explain to women the benefits and risks associated with hormonal drug therapy for FBC, such as stroke, liver disease, and increased intracranial pressure. Teach them to seek medical attention immediately if any signs or symptoms of these complications occur.

Encourage the patient to continue prescribed drug therapy, and monitor the effectiveness of these interventions. Teach the patient to become familiar with the normal feel and texture of her breasts so she is aware of any changes.

DUCTAL ECTASIA

Ductal ectasia is a benign breast problem that is usually seen in women approaching menopause. It occurs when a breast duct dilates and its walls thicken, causing the duct to become blocked. The ducts in the subareolar area are most often affected. These ducts become distended and filled with cellular debris, which activates an inflammatory response. Two manifestations result from these changes:

- A mass develops that feels hard, has irregular borders, and may be tender.
- A greenish brown nipple discharge, enlarged axillary nodes, and redness and edema over the site of the mass are noted.

Ductal ectasia does not affect a woman's breast cancer risk. However, if a mass is present, it may be difficult to distinguish it from breast cancer. Because the risk for breast cancer is increased among women in the menopause age-group, accurate diagnosis is vital. A microscopic examination of the nipple discharge is performed to detect any atypical or malignant cells, and the affected area is excised. Nursing care is directed at reducing the anxiety associated with the threat of breast cancer and at supporting the woman through the diagnostic and treatment procedures. Ductal ectasia may improve without treatment. Warm compresses and antibiotics may be helpful. If symptoms do not improve, the abnormal duct may be surgically removed.

INTRADUCTAL PAPILLOMA

Intraductal papilloma occurs most often in women 40 to 55 years of age. A benign process in the epithelial lining of the duct forms a papilloma (pedunculated outgrowth of tissue). As it grows, trauma and erosion within the duct result in a bloody or serous nipple discharge. A mass is rarely palpable.

Diagnosis is aimed first at ruling out breast cancer. Microscopic examination of the nipple discharge and surgical excision of the mass and ductal area are usually indicated.

ISSUES OF LARGE-BREASTED WOMEN

Although Western society emphasizes large breasts as a positive attribute, women with excessive breast tissue often have health problems and discomfort. For instance, a woman with large breasts may have difficulty finding clothes that fit well and in which she feels attractive. The breast size may be out of proportion to the rest of the body, which adds to the problem of finding clothes that fit. Larger bras are expensive and may need to be specially ordered. The woman may have large dents in the shoulders from bra straps. In addition, many large-breasted women develop fungal INFECTIONS under the breasts, especially in hot weather, because it is difficult to keep this area dry and exposed to air.

Backaches from the added weight are also common. If well-fitting bras do not help and obesity is not part of the problem, the only alternative for this condition may be breast reduction surgery. The surgeon removes excess breast tissue and then repositions the nipple and remaining skin flaps to produce the best cosmetic effect. This operation is a major surgical procedure and is called a reduction mammoplasty.

The decision to have the procedure is usually made after years of living with the discomfort of excessive breast size. Listen to the woman verbalize her feelings, and reinforce information as appropriate. The nursing care after surgery is similar to that for the woman having reconstructive surgery. (See discussion of Breast Reconstruction, p. 1476, in the Surgical Management section.)

ISSUES OF SMALL-BREASTED WOMEN

Some women choose to have breast augmentation surgery to increase or improve the size, shape, or symmetry of their breasts. Most health insurers do not pay for this procedure. Most surgeries involve the implantation of saline-filled or silicon prostheses. Some are constructed from the women's own tissue in much the same way as for reconstruction after mastectomy. *Saline* implants are filled with sterile saline and can be filled with the amount needed to get the shape and firmness the woman wants. If the implant shell leaks, the saline will be safely absorbed by the body. *Silicone* implants are filled with an elastic gel, which can leak into the breast and will not be absorbed. The plastic surgeon reviews the advantages and disadvantages of each implant or natural procedure.

After surgery, the patient can be discharged to home the same day or the day after. Remind the family or significant other that someone should stay with her for at least 24 hours after surgery. The incisions may or may not have dressings depending on the surgeon and type of surgery.

> **! NURSING SAFETY PRIORITY** (QSEN)
> **Action Alert**
>
> Before breast augmentation surgery, teach the patient to stop smoking (to promote healing), avoid aspirin and other NSAIDs, and avoid herbs that can cause bleeding during the procedure, such as garlic, *Ginkgo biloba*, and ginseng. Tell her that the incisions will be hidden as much as possible, either under the pectoral muscle or directly behind the breast tissue as a submammary placement. One or more wound drains will be inserted during surgery, and she will need to know how to care for those drains at home. Review possible postoperative complications, including INFECTION and implant leakage, which can cause severe PAIN and possible fever.

> **! NURSING SAFETY PRIORITY** (QSEN)
> **Action Alert**
>
> Remind the patient after breast augmentation that for the first few days she should expect soreness in her chest and arms. Her breasts will feel tight and sensitive, and the skin over her breasts may feel warm or may itch. Teach the patient that she will have difficulty raising her arms over her head and should not lift, push, or pull anything until the surgeon permits. Teach her to also avoid strenuous activity or twisting above her waist. Remind the patient to walk every few hours to prevent deep vein thrombi. Tell her to expect some swelling of the breasts for 3 to 4 weeks after surgery.

An important issue for patients who have breast augmentation surgery is breast cancer surveillance. Breast self-examination (BSE) and clinical breast examination (CBE) can still be performed because the prosthesis is placed behind the woman's normal breast tissue, actually pushing it forward. However, screening mammography may not be as sensitive because the amount of visualized breast tissue is decreased. Additional x-rays, called *implant displacement views,* may be used to examine the breast tissue more completely (ACS, 2013a). Although there is no conclusive evidence that breast augmentation increases breast cancer risk, further research is needed regarding diagnosis and prognosis of breast cancer among women with cosmetic breast implants (Lavigne et al., 2013). Teach women desiring cosmetic breast augmentation about the differences in breast cancer screening.

GYNECOMASTIA

Gynecomastia literally means "female breasts" and is a symptom rather than a disease. It is usually a benign condition of breast enlargement in *men* (Fig. 70-1). However, gynecomastia can be a result of a primary cancer such as lung or testicular cancer. The enlargement is usually bilateral but may be asymmetric in a few cases. The condition is caused by abnormal growth of the glandular tissue, including the mammary ducts and ductal tissue. In many instances it is difficult to determine gynecomastia from breast enlargement related to excess adipose tissue. Other causes of gynecomastia include:

- Drugs, such as anti-androgen agents and corticosteroids
- Aging
- Obesity
- Underlying disease causing estrogen excess, such as malnutrition, liver disease, or hyperthyroidism
- Androgen-deficiency states, such as age, chronic kidney disease, or alcoholism

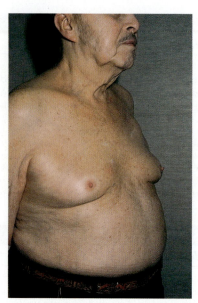

FIG. 70-1 Gynecomastia.

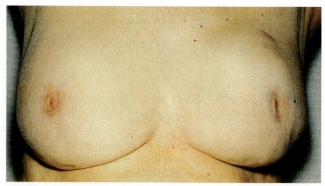

FIG. 70-2 Skin dimpling on a breast as a result of fibrosis or breast cancer.

Although gynecomastia is not common, men with abnormal breast findings, especially a breast mass, should be carefully evaluated for breast cancer.

BREAST CANCER

❖ PATHOPHYSIOLOGY

Excluding skin cancers, breast cancer is the most commonly diagnosed cancer in women and is second only to lung cancer as a cause of female cancer deaths (ACS, 2013b). Therefore most references in this section are to women with breast cancer. Because of the high incidence of the disease, almost every woman knows of someone with the disease. Thus most women have strong reactions to the threat of breast cancer. These reactions greatly influence health habits, including breast self-examination (BSE) and the patient's readiness to seek care when a suspicious area is discovered. Nurses play a key role in early detection by educating women about screening guidelines, risk factors for breast cancer, and BSE. Men should also be taught about this disease.

Early detection is the key to effective treatment and survival. The 5-year relative survival rate is lower for women who are diagnosed with an advanced stage of breast cancer. The 5-year survival rate for localized breast cancer is 98.6%, whereas the rate drops to 83.8% when the cancer has spread to the regional lymph nodes (ACS, 2013b). Survival drops dramatically when breast cancer is metastatic (spread to distant sites).

Cancer of the breast begins as a single transformed cell that grows and multiplies in the epithelial cells lining one or more of the mammary ducts or lobules. It is a heterogeneous disease, having many forms with different clinical presentations and responses to therapy (Weigelt et al., 2010). Some breast cancers will present as a palpable lump in the breast, whereas others show up only on a mammogram.

There are two broad categories of breast cancer: noninvasive and invasive. About 20% are *noninvasive;* the remaining 80% are invasive. As long as the cancer remains within the duct, it is noninvasive. The cancer is classified as *invasive* when it penetrates the tissue surrounding the duct. Most of these cancers arise from the intermediate ducts. Metastasis occurs when cancer cells leave the breast via the blood and lymph systems, which permits spread of these cells to distant sites. The most common sites of metastasis are bone, lung, brain, and liver. The course of metastatic breast cancer is related to the site affected and to the function impaired. The processes involved in cancer development are described in Chapter 21.

Noninvasive Breast Cancers

Ductal carcinoma in situ (DCIS) is an early *noninvasive* form of breast cancer. In DCIS, cancer cells are located within the duct and have not invaded the surrounding fatty breast tissue. Because of mammography screening and earlier detection, the number of women diagnosed with DCIS has increased. If left untreated, it is estimated that 14% to 53% of DCIS would become invasive and spread into the breast tissue surrounding the ducts over a period of 10 years (Morgan et al., 2011). Currently there is no way to determine which DCIS lesions will progress to invasive cancer and which ones will remain unchanged. This uncertainty causes anxiety and decisional conflict in many women diagnosed with DCIS. It is important to convey to patients the ways in which DCIS differs from invasive cancer and that DCIS cells lack the biologic capacity to metastasize.

Another type of noninvasive cancer is **lobular carcinoma in situ (LCIS).** This cancer is rare and occurs as an abnormal cell growth in the lobules (milk-producing glands) of the breast. It is not a true cancer, but having LCIS increases one's risk for developing a separate breast cancer later. It is usually diagnosed before menopause in women 40 to 50 years of age. Traditionally, LCIS is treated with close observation only. Women with LCIS and other breast cancer risk factors may want to consider prophylactic treatment options such as tamoxifen, raloxifene, or prophylactic mastectomy (ACS, 2013a).

Invasive Breast Cancers

The most common type of invasive breast cancer is **infiltrating ductal carcinoma.** As the name implies, the disease originates in the mammary ducts and grows in the epithelial cells lining these ducts. Once invasive, the cancer grows into the tissue around it in an irregular pattern. If a lump is present, it is felt as an irregular, poorly defined mass. As the tumor continues to grow, **fibrosis** (replacement of normal cells with connective tissue and collagen) develops around the cancer. This fibrosis may cause shortening of Cooper's ligaments and the resulting typical skin dimpling that is seen with more advanced disease (Fig. 70-2). Another sign, sometimes indicating late-stage breast

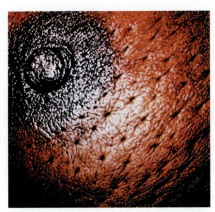

FIG. 70-3 Breast edema giving the skin an "orange peel" *(peau d'orange)* appearance.

cancer, is an edematous thickening and pitting of breast skin called *peau d'orange* (orange peel skin) (Fig. 70-3).

A rare but highly aggressive form of invasive breast cancer is **inflammatory breast cancer** (IBC). Symptoms include swelling, skin redness, and PAIN in the breasts. IBC seldom presents as a palpable lump and may not show up on a mammogram. Because it is usually diagnosed at a later stage than other types of breast cancer, it is often harder to treat successfully (ACS, 2013a).

Breast Cancer in Men

Male breast cancer is rare, occurring in fewer than 1% of all cases. The average age of onset is 68 years (Mattarella, 2010). Causes are not completely understood, but there is a strong association between male breast cancer, family history, and genetic factors. (See discussion of genetic risk below.)

Men usually present with a hard, painless, subareolar mass; gynecomastia may be present. Occasionally the man may have nipple discharge, retraction, erosion, or ulceration. Because *men* usually do not suspect breast cancer when they feel a lump, diagnosis frequently is delayed (Mattarella, 2010). Thus men have a slightly lower overall survival than do women. However, there are more similarities than differences between male and female breast cancer (Greif et al., 2012). Treatment of breast cancer in men is the same as in women at a similar stage of disease.

Breast Cancer in Young Women

Media coverage and accounts of women with breast cancer often portray women younger than 60 years, misleading many to overestimate the incidence of breast cancer in younger women (National Breast Cancer Coalition [NBCC], 2012). Nevertheless, about 4.6% of breast cancer cases occur in women younger than 40 years (ACS, 2013b). Genetic predisposition is a stronger risk factor for younger women than older women (Pollán, 2010). Younger women frequently present with more aggressive forms of the disease, and the number of cases of advanced breast cancer in younger women is increasing (Johnson et al., 2013). Screening tools can be less effective for this group because the breasts are denser; therefore regular screening mammograms before the age of 40 years are not recommended for average-risk women (ACS, 2013a). Nurses should encourage women who have symptoms to seek evaluation and not watch and wait. Younger women with breast cancer face unique issues associated with treatment. These include surgical menopause, infertility after treatment, and sexual dysfunction (Kedde et al., 2013).

Etiology and Genetic Risk

There is no single known cause for breast cancer. *Being an older woman or man is the primary risk factor, although some people are at higher risk than others.* Several breast cancer risk factors have been identified; some are modifiable, whereas others are not (ACS, 2013b). Risk factors have varying degrees of influence on breast cancer development. Having several risk factors increases one's risk more than having a single risk factor. Table 70-2 lists major breast cancer risk factors according to the varying degree of risk. Assist women to clarify that not all risk factors are the same.

⚕ GENETIC/GENOMIC CONSIDERATIONS
Patient-Centered Care QSEN

Mutations in several genes, such as *BRCA1* and *BRCA2,* are related to hereditary breast cancer. People who have specific mutations in either one of these genes are at a high risk for developing breast cancer as well as ovarian cancer. However, only 5% to 10% of all breast cancers are hereditary. Only women with a strong family history and a reasonable suspicion that a mutation is present have genetic testing for *BRCA* mutations (ACS, 2013a). Encourage women to talk with a genetics counselor to carefully consider the benefits and potential harmful consequences of genetic testing before these tests are done.

Knowledge of modifiable risk factors can help women develop strategies for prevention of breast cancer. These include avoiding weight gain and obesity, engaging in regular physical activity, and minimizing alcohol intake. Breast-feeding for a year or more has been shown to have a protective influence on breast cancer as does avoidance of hormone replacement therapy (HRT) for menopausal symptoms. Encourage women seeking help for menopausal symptoms to discuss the benefits and risks of hormonal therapy with their health care provider. Environmental causes of breast cancer are the subject of increasing research and concern for many women. Environmental estrogens found to influence breast cancer development in animals include DDT found in pesticides, perfluorooctanoic acid (PFOA) found in nonstick cookware, and bisphenol A (BPA) found in plastic food containers. More research is needed to discover the effect of these chemicals on human breast cancer (Schmidt, 2012), but many women are choosing to avoid them as a precaution. (See the Evidence-Based Practice box.)

Incidence and Prevalence

The American Cancer Society estimated the incidence of breast cancer in the United States to be 232,340 in 2013. Breast cancer is the second leading cause of cancer death in women, exceeded only by lung cancer, and 39,629 are likely to die of the disease (ACS, 2013b).

Health Promotion and Maintenance

The American Cancer Society (ACS) establishes evidence-based guidelines for breast cancer screening in women. Guidelines have not been recommended for screening men in the general population because breast cancer in men is so uncommon (ACS, 2013a). Encourage men with a strong family history or known genetic mutations to discuss screening with their health care provider.

TABLE 70-2   Risk Factors for Breast Cancer

FACTORS	COMMENTS
High Increased Risk (Relative Risk >4.0)	
Female gender	Ninety-nine percent of all breast cancers occur in women.
Age >65 years	Risk increases across all ages until age 80 years.
Genetic factors	Inherited mutations of *BRCA1* and/or *BRCA2* increase risk.
History of a previous breast cancer	The risk for developing a cancer in the opposite breast is 5 times greater than for the average population at risk.
Breast density	Dense breasts contain more glandular and connective tissue, which increases the risk for developing breast cancer.
Atypical hyperplasia	Biopsy-confirmed atypical hyperplasia is a high relative risk.
Moderate Increased Risk (Relative Risk 2.1–4.0)	
Family history	Two first-degree relatives with breast cancer increases risk.
Ionizing radiation	Women who received frequent low-level radiation exposure to the thorax had an increased risk, especially if the exposure occurred during periods of rapid breast formation.
High postmenopausal bone density	High estrogen levels over time both strengthen bone and increase breast cancer risk.
Low Increased Risk (Relative Risk 1.1–2.0)	

Reproductive history
    Nulliparity OR
    First child born after age 30 years
	Childless women have an increased risk, as do women who bear their first child near or after age 30.

Menstrual history
    Early menstruation OR
    Late menopause OR
    Both
	The risk for breast cancer rises as the interval between menarche and menopause increases. Women who undergo bilateral oophorectomy before age 35 years have less risk for breast cancer than women who undergo natural menopause.

Recent oral contraceptive use	There is a slight increase in breast cancer risk in women taking oral contraceptives. The risk returns to normal after 10 years of stopping the pill.
Recent hormone replacement therapy (HRT)	Use of HRT containing both estrogen and progestin increases risk; risk diminishes after 5 years of discontinuation.
Obesity	Postmenopausal obesity (especially increased abdominal fat), increased body mass, insulin resistance, and hyperglycemia have been reported to be associated with an increased risk for breast cancer.
Other Risk Factors	
Alcohol	Risk is dose-dependent; consumption of 3 to 14 drinks per week is associated with a slight increase in risk; risk increases with increased consumption.
High socioeconomic status	Breast cancer incidence is greater in women of higher education and socioeconomic background. This relationship is possibly related to lifestyle differences, such as later age at first birth.
Jewish heritage	Women of Ashkenazi Jewish heritage have higher incidences of *BRCA1* and *BRCA2* genetic mutations.

Modified from American Cancer Society. (2013). *Breast cancer facts & figures 2011-2012.* Atlanta: Author.

EVIDENCE-BASED PRACTICE (QSEN)

Does Night-Shift Work Increase the Risk for Breast Cancer?

Kamdar, B., Tergas, A., Mateen, F., Bhayani, N., & Oh, J. (2013). Night-shift work and risk of breast cancer: A systematic review and meta-analysis. *Breast Cancer Research and Treatment, 138*(1), 291-301.

Researchers conducted a systematic review and meta-analysis of studies examining night-shift work and its relationship with breast cancer. Previous studies have suggested that night-shift workers, such as flight attendants and nurses, may lack adequate melatonin, which may contribute to an increase in breast cancer risk. Fifteen studies were included in the analysis. The researchers determined that the findings of these studies were limited due to unmeasured confounding and substantial heterogeneity observed among the studies. They concluded there is weak evidence to support previous findings that night-shift work is associated with an increased breast cancer risk.

Level of Evidence: 1
The study utilized a systematic review of the literature and meta-analysis of multiple studies to make conclusions.

Commentary: Implications for Practice and Research
Nurses should be aware of the validity of publicized studies as well as ongoing research in this area. This meta-analysis found lack of consistencies among studies about shift work and breast cancer risk. Future studies involving large sample sizes and diverse occupational and geographic populations are necessary. The increasing number of around-the-clock workers raises important public health and policy issues.

🌐 CULTURAL CONSIDERATIONS

Patient-Centered Care (QSEN)

One of every 8 women in the United States will develop breast cancer by age 70 years. Euro-American women older than 40 years are at a greater risk than other racial/ethnic groups, but the rate of breast cancer in African-American women *younger than 40 years* is higher than for others in that age-group. African-American women have a higher death rate at any age when compared with other women with the disease (ACS, 2013b). Cultural disparities with regard to breast cancer stage and mortality are persistent. Ooi et al. (2011) found that non-Hispanic white women are more likely to present with an earlier-stage breast cancer than American-Indian/Alaska-Native, Asian-Indian/Pakistani, Black, Filipino, Hawaiian, Mexican,

Puerto Rican, and Samoan women. These groups are also more likely to present with more aggressive breast cancer that is harder to treat, such as *triple negative breast cancer*. In this type of breast cancer, cells lack receptors for estrogen, progesterone, and the protein *HER2*. African-American and Puerto Rican women have the highest risk for triple negative breast cancer. Breast cancer death rates are highest in African-American, Hawaiian, Puerto Rican, and Samoan women. Cultural disparities should be addressed with targeted interventions that are appropriate for specific cultural and ethnic groups. Nurses need to be culturally competent to assist women to overcome barriers to care.

The ACS recommendation for early detection by screening for breast masses is a screening mammogram for women ages 40 years and older and a clinical breast examination (CBE) by a health care professional at least every 3 years for women 20 to 40 years old. Monthly breast self-examination (BSE) is less emphasized today than in the past several decades. It is recommended as an option to women to increase breast self-awareness beginning at age 20.

Mammography

The use of mammography (x-ray of the breasts) screening for healthy, average-risk women continues to be studied for its effectiveness. In 2009, the U.S. Preventive Services Task Force (USPSTF) recommended raising the screening age for average-risk women from 40 to 50 years (USPSTF, 2009). Scientific evidence shows there are benefits as well as risks associated with mammography, and disagreement exists about the emphasis that should be placed on each one. However, the ACS and The American College of Obstetricians and Gynecologists (ACOG) continue to recommend that all women ages 40 years and older have a screening mammogram annually (ACOG, 2011). Educate women on the advantages and disadvantages of breast screening techniques so that they can make informed decisions about the screening methods best suited to their individual situations (Association of Women's Health, Obstetric, and Neonatal Nursing [AWHONN], 2010).

According to guidelines of the American Society of Clinical Oncology, women who are asymptomatic following breast cancer treatment should be screened with annual mammograms, without additional tests (Khatcheressian et al., 2013). A small number of women who have known genetic mutations and/or other high risk factors for breast cancer should have screening with MRI in addition to annual mammography (ACS, 2013a). Encourage women with moderate risk factors to discuss with their health care provider the benefits and limitations of adding MRI screening to their annual mammograms. MRI screening is not recommended for women with low breast cancer risk factors.

Breast ultrasound is sometimes used in addition to mammography when problems are found during routine screening and for some women with dense breast tissue. Although the use of ultrasound has added benefits over mammography alone, it is not recommended as part of routine breast cancer screening for women who are average risk for breast cancer (ACS, 2013a).

Breast Self-Awareness/Self-Examination

Nurses working with women should teach them the importance of becoming familiar with the appearance and feel of their breasts. Any changes detected by the woman should be reported to her health care provider. Teach a woman that lumps are not necessarily abnormal. For premenopausal women, lumps can come and go with the menstrual cycle. Most lumps that are detected and tested are not cancerous.

Some women may want to practice regular breast self-examination (BSE) as a method for breast self-awareness. Evidence shows that monthly BSE is no more beneficial than women simply being aware of what is normal for their own breasts and women are just as likely to find a lump by chance (ACS, 2013a). However, BSE should be presented as an option to women beginning in their early 20s. In addition to breast self-awareness, emphasis should be placed on mammography and clinical breast examination for early detection of breast cancer. The combined approach is better than any single test (ACS, 2013a). A woman who chooses to perform BSE should be taught the correct technique and have it reviewed by a health care professional during her clinical breast examination.

The BSE technique is similar for women and men. Use teaching models of normal and abnormal breasts when teaching BSE. Discuss the proper timing for BSE. Instruct premenopausal women to examine their breasts 1 week after the menstrual period. At this time, hormonal influence on breast tissue is decreased, so fluid retention and tenderness are reduced. Teach women whose breast tissue is no longer influenced by hormonal fluctuations, such as after a total hysterectomy or menopause, to pick a day each month to do BSE, such as the first day of the month. Chart 70-1 describes the procedure for breast self-examination and may be used as a patient resource.

Clinical Breast Examination

Clinical breast examination (CBE) is typically performed by advanced practice nurses and other health care providers. Clinicians who perform CBE ideally go through simulation training and exposure to patients to become proficient at the technique

CHART 70-1   Best Practice for Patient Safety & Quality Care   QSEN

Performing Breast Self-Examination

1. Lie down on your back, and place your right arm behind your head. Lying down spreads the breast tissue evenly over the chest wall, making it easier to feel all the breast tissue.
2. Use the finger pads of the three middle fingers on your left hand to feel for lumps in the right breast. Use overlapping dime-size circular motions of the finger pads to feel the breast tissue.
3. Use three different levels of pressure to feel all the breast tissue. Light pressure is needed to feel the tissue closest to the skin; medium pressure to feel a little deeper; and firm pressure to feel the tissue closest to the chest and ribs. It is normal to feel a firm ridge in the lower curve of each breast.
4. Move around the breast in an up-and-down pattern starting at an imaginary line drawn straight down your side from the underarm and moving across the breast to the middle of the chest bone (sternum or

breastbone). Be sure to check the entire breast area going down until you feel only ribs, and up to the neck.
5. Repeat the exam on your left breast, putting your left arm behind your head and using the finger pads of your right hand to do the exam.
6. While standing in front of a mirror with your hands pressing firmly down on your hips, look at your breasts for any changes of size, shape, contour, or dimpling and look at your nipples and breast skin for redness or scaling. (The pressing-down-on-the-hips position contracts the chest wall muscles and enhances any breast changes.)
7. Examine each underarm while sitting up or standing and with your arm only slightly raised so you can easily feel in this area. Raising your arm straight up tightens the tissue in this area and makes it harder to examine.

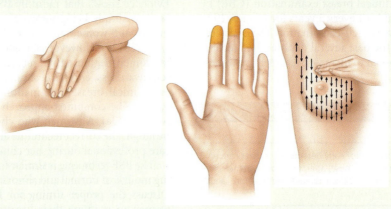

Adapted from the American Cancer Society. (2013). *Detailed guide: How to examine your breasts.* Atlanta: Author. Available from www.cancer.org.

(Bryan & Snyder, 2013). It is recommended that the CBE be part of a periodic health assessment, at least every 3 years for women in their 20s and 30s, and every year for asymptomatic women at least 40 years of age (ACS, 2013a). Teach patients what to expect during this examination. First, they will be asked to undress from the waist up. The examiner inspects the breasts for abnormalities in size and shape and for skin and nipple changes. Then, using the pads of the fingers, the examiner palpates the breasts for any lumps and, if present, whether such lumps are attached to the skin or deeper tissues. The area under both arms is also examined.

Options for High-Risk Women

Women with a personal history of breast cancer are at risk for developing a recurrence or a new breast cancer. Those with known *BRCA1* and *BRCA2* genetic mutations, strong family history, or other high-risk factors are also considered high-risk. Women in this category usually practice *close surveillance* as a prevention option. It is referred to as "secondary prevention" and is used to detect cancer early in the initial stages. In addition to annual mammography and clinical breast examination, high-risk women are recommended to have an annual breast MRI screening (ACS, 2013a). Close surveillance may begin as early as age 30 years, but evidence is limited regarding the best age at which to start screening. Encourage high-risk women to discuss their personal preferences for close surveillance with their health care providers.

Options currently available for reducing a woman's breast cancer risk are **prophylactic mastectomy** (preventive surgical removal of one or both breasts), prophylactic **oophorectomy** (removal of the ovaries), and anti-estrogen chemopreventive drugs. Although each option significantly reduces the risk for breast cancer, no option completely eliminates it. Each option has its own risks and potentially serious complications.

Even though a woman may decide to have a *prophylactic mastectomy,* there is a small risk that breast cancer will develop in residual breast glandular tissue because no mastectomy reliably removes all mammary tissue. Women must also understand that breast reconstruction after a prophylactic mastectomy is very different from breast augmentation. It is a more complex surgical procedure with a greater potential for complications. The decision to have this type of surgery can be a very difficult one to make. Women may find it helpful to reach out to a breast cancer support organization and talk to someone who has been through a prophylactic mastectomy. The majority of patients express long-term satisfaction with this surgical procedure (Soran et al., 2013).

Women undergoing *oophorectomy* will likely experience menopausal symptoms, although some estrogen remains in body fat tissue. *Anti-estrogen drugs* reduce breast cancer recurrence but carry other risks such as blood clots and endometrial cancer. Encourage women to carefully consider the benefits and risks of breast cancer–risk-reducing options and to discuss them with their health care provider.

❖ PATIENT-CENTERED COLLABORATIVE CARE

◆ Assessment

History. Often the history is taken after a mass has been discovered but before a diagnosis has been made for a woman or man with breast cancer. For some patients, the history may be obtained at the time they are seen for treatment of an identified cancer. The interview should focus on three major areas: risk factors, the breast mass, and health maintenance practices.

Record age, gender, marital status, weight, and height. Marital status and identifying the patient's primary support person provide information about who should be included in the patient's care, teaching, and support.

🌐 CULTURAL CONSIDERATIONS

Patient-Centered Care QSEN

Remember that some cultures do not allow the man to be part of a woman's care or only women are allowed to care for her (e.g., Arab Muslim women). Other cultures are male-predominant and all decisions about female care are made by the man (e.g., Nigerian women).

Ask specific information on personal and family histories of breast cancer. In addition to increasing the woman's own risk, these factors also affect any sisters' or daughters' risk and should be part of later counseling.

Ask about the woman's gynecologic and obstetric history, including:

- Age at menarche
- Age at menopause
- Symptoms of menopause
- Age at first child's birth
- Number of children/pregnancies

Prolonged hormonal stimulation (e.g., early menses, late menopause) increases a woman's risk, as do birth of the first child after 30 years of age and nulliparity (having no children).

A history of the breast mass or lump reveals not only the course of the disease but also information related to health care–seeking practices and health-promoting behaviors. Ask the patient about how, when, and by whom the mass was discovered and the time between discovery and seeking care. If the patient found the mass, ask how it was discovered. The answer to this question reveals the need for discussion and teaching about health promotion practices, regardless of whether the mass proves to be cancerous. If there was a delay between discovery and seeing the health care provider, ask what caused the delay. These questions are linked to the psychosocial assessment but also reveal the length of time that the tumor has been present. Ask what procedures have been performed to diagnose the problem. Also, ask patients if they have noticed any other changes in their body within the past year. This information can help determine whether there has been obvious cancer spread. Ask especially about the presence of joint or bone PAIN.

Ask about the use of alcohol intake, because this is a factor that may increase breast cancer risk. Ask what prescribed and over-the-counter (OTC) drugs are used—specifically, hormonal supplements such as estrogen and natural or herbal substances that stimulate hormones. Estrogen can be taken orally, intravaginally, or via a transdermal patch. Document the type and

---

CHART 70-2 Best Practice for Patient Safety & Quality Care QSEN

Assessing a Breast Mass

- Identify the location of the mass by using the "face of the clock" method.
- Describe the shape, size, and consistency of the mass.
- Assess whether the mass is fixed or movable.
- Note any skin changes around the mass, such as dimpling (peau d'orange), increased vascularity, nipple retraction, and ulceration.
- Assess the adjacent lymph nodes—both axillary and supraclavicular nodes.
- Ask patients if they experience pain or soreness in the area around the mass.

---

form of hormones (birth control pills or patches, supplements) and length of use.

Physical Assessment/Clinical Manifestations. Document in the electronic medical record any abnormal findings from the clinical breast examination. Describe specific information about a breast mass (Chart 70-2) such as location, using the "face of the clock" method; shape; size; consistency; and whether the mass is mobile or fixed to the surrounding tissue. Note any skin change, such as *peau d'orange* (dimpling, orange peel appearance), redness and warmth, nipple retraction, or ulceration, which can indicate advanced disease. Document the location of any enlargements of axillary and supraclavicular lymph nodes. Evaluate the presence of PAIN or soreness in the affected breast.

Psychosocial Assessment. A breast cancer diagnosis is usually an unanticipated event in the life of a woman who feels physically well. It initiates a sudden and distressing transition into a potentially life-threatening illness. Feelings of fear, shock, and disbelief are predominant as a woman learns about her disease and faces numerous treatment decisions. Psychological distress is common at cancer diagnosis and at the end of treatment. A previous history of mental illness, age, and life circumstances can contribute to increased psychological distress (Williams, 2012). Encourage expression of feelings, and determine if a referral to a breast cancer support group would be helpful. Talking with someone who has been through the experience is particularly helpful in dealing with the emotional aspects of the disease.

Assess the patient's need for information. Some people may not be ready for a lot of information at first. Most want to know how advanced the disease is, the likelihood of cure, treatment options and side effects, how treatment will affect their life and self-image, how family or partners will be affected, and what is required for home self-management. A previous experience with cancer, especially with other people who had breast cancer, influences the reactions to the disease. Ask patients and family members whether they have known anyone with breast cancer, and explore their feelings about the disease. The Internet is a primary source of information through which breast cancer information is sought and shared. Increasingly, the information on the Internet is provided by patients themselves (Quinn et al., 2013). Clarify health information the patient has received on the Internet, and provide current information about the stage of the disease and treatment options.

Assess the patient for problems related to SEXUALITY. Sexual dysfunction affects most breast cancer survivors in some way.

Sometimes the sexual dysfunction is related to the loss of a breast and the threat to one's femininity, but many women also equate a breast cancer diagnosis and treatment effects with the aging process (Klaeson et al., 2011). Lack of libido (sexual desire) related to hormonal changes, psychological distress, and severe anxiety is commonly experienced by women with breast cancer. If the patient does not discuss sexual concerns voluntarily, ask about the frequency of and satisfaction with sexual relations with her partner. Use resources that provide education about alternative expressions of intimacy and a focus on pleasure rather than performance. Refer the patient and her partner to counseling if appropriate.

GENDER HEALTH CONSIDERATIONS

Patient-Centered Care QSEN

Research is limited about breast cancer and women who identify as lesbian, but it is thought that breast cancer is more common in this group (Beredjick, 2012). A possible explanation is that risk factors for breast cancer, such as smoking, alcohol use, obesity, and infrequent pregnancy, are more common in this group (ACS, 2013a). Lesbian and bisexual women are less likely to have health insurance and get regular cancer screenings (see Chapter 73). Factors include fear and distrust of culturally incompetent health care providers. They may also be less focused on their breasts and breast cancer risk. Nurses' awareness and sensitivity to these issues help establish trust. Emphasize the importance of screening and early detection. Assess the need for referrals to support organizations such as the National LGBT Cancer Network (2013).

Laboratory Assessment. The diagnosis of breast cancer relies on pathologic examination of tissue from the breast mass. After the diagnosis of cancer is established, laboratory tests, including pathologic study of the lymph nodes, help detect possible metastases. Elevated liver enzyme levels indicate possible liver metastases, and increased serum calcium and alkaline phosphatase levels suggest bone metastases.

Imaging Assessment. Mammography is a sensitive screening tool for breast cancer. The uniqueness of this test results from its ability to reveal preclinical lesions (masses too small to be palpated manually). Most breast centers now use *digital mammography*—a system that is able to read, file, and transmit mammograms electronically. Women should be screened with mammography annually beginning at age 40 years (ACS, 2013a). Patient preparation and the procedure for mammography are discussed in Chapter 69. Some women may voice concern about radiation exposure with mammograms. Reassure them the dose is very small and the risk for harm from radiation is minimal (ACS, 2013b). Breast *tomosynthesis* is an emerging technology that is similar to mammography but uses three-dimensional images. It has the potential to improve detection of breast cancer by better differentiating suspicious from normal tissue (Alakhras et al., 2013). Although tomosynthesis has been approved by the Food and Drug Administration (FDA), its role in breast cancer screening and diagnosis has not yet been established (ACS, 2013a).

Ultrasonography of the breast is an additional diagnostic tool used to clarify findings on mammography. If the mammogram reveals a lesion, ultrasonography is helpful in differentiating a fluid-filled cyst from a solid mass. Mammography screening combined with ultrasound may be effective for detecting cancers in women with dense breasts, but currently it is not recommended for routine breast cancer screening (ACS, 2013a).

MRI is used for screening high-risk women and better examination of suspicious areas found by a mammogram (ACS, 2013b). MRI is more expensive than mammography. Most insurance companies will cover a portion of the cost if the woman is shown to be high risk. Although higher-quality images are produced, there is concern about high costs and access to quality breast MRI services for high-risk women (ACS, 2013b).

If the patient has an invasive breast cancer, other imaging tests may be done to rule out metastases. A chest x-ray is done to screen for lung metastases. Bone, liver, and brain scans and CT scans of the chest and abdomen can reveal distant metastases.

Other Diagnostic Assessment. Whereas imaging techniques serve as tools for screening and more precise visualization of potential breast cancers, *breast biopsy (pathologic examination of the breast tissue) is the only definitive way to diagnose breast cancer*. Breast tissue is obtained by one of several types of biopsies (see Chapter 69). Tissue samples are analyzed by a pathologist to determine the presence of breast cancer. If breast cancer is identified, it is classified according to the size and type of breast cancer, the histologic grade, and the type of receptors on the cells. These characteristics are used to guide treatment. For example, a small, noninvasive breast cancer may be treated only with lumpectomy and radiation, whereas a larger, aggressive tumor (one with a high histologic grade) may be treated with a mastectomy and chemotherapy, followed by radiation. Cancer cells that contain estrogen receptors (*ER positive*) or progesterone receptors (*PR positive)* have a better prognosis and usually respond to hormonal therapy. If the type of breast cancer is *HER2,* or one in which the *neu* gene product is overexpressed, it may be treated successfully with trastuzumab (Herceptin), which is a breast cancer *targeted therapy* for this specific type.

Most women, even those with very small tumors, receive some sort of treatment in addition to surgery for breast cancer. Research has focused on ways to predict clinical outcomes so that low-risk women may avoid unnecessary treatments. Gene expression profiling systems, such as Oncotype DX and MammaPrint, have been developed to help predict clinical outcomes by analyzing genes in breast cancer tissue. Some clinicians use this information in addition to the pathologic analysis for guiding treatment decisions. These multi-gene tests have been shown to be accurate predictors of patient prognosis and response to therapy in breast cancer (Jankowitz & Lee, 2013). Their role in clinical practice continues to evolve.

◆ Analysis

The priority NANDA-I nursing diagnoses and collaborative problems for patients with breast cancer include:

1. Ineffective Coping related to unanticipated breast cancer diagnosis (NANDA-I)
2. Potential for metastasis of cancer to other parts of the body

◆ Planning and Implementation

Developing Coping Strategies

Planning: Expected Outcomes. The patient with breast cancer is expected to report the use of methods to help increase coping ability and reduce anxiety. The patient will maintain relationships and participate as an active partner in management of her disease.

Interventions. The anxiety and uncertainty for the patient with breast cancer begin the moment a lump is discovered or when a mammogram reveals an abnormality. These feelings may be related to past experiences and personal associations with the disease. Assess the patient's perceptions of his or her own situation. Allow the patient to ventilate these feelings even if a diagnosis has not been established.

If the mass has been diagnosed as cancer, many people feel a partial sense of relief to be dealing with a known entity. A feeling of shock or disbelief usually occurs. It is difficult to accept a diagnosis of cancer when one feels basically well. Patients and their families or significant others deal in individual ways with the mix of feelings. Flexibility is the key to nursing care. Adjust your approach to care as the patient's emotional state changes. Those who have an interval between the diagnosis and treatment during which they actively participate in the choice of treatment cope more effectively after surgery, no matter which treatment is chosen.

An integral part of the plan to meet these emotional needs is the use of outside resources. Health care providers working with breast cancer may know other patients willing to make a preoperative visit. For example, the patient who is worried in particular about the side effects of radiation therapy may benefit more from talking to someone who has undergone radiation than from talking to the nurse or health care provider. Be sure to assess his or her preference.

Assess the patient's need for knowledge. Some may want to read and discuss any available information. Provide accurate information, and clarify any misinformation the patient may have received by the media, on the Internet, or from family and friends. The American Cancer Society (www.cancer.org) and Breastcancer.org (www.breastcancer.org) are two Internet sources that provide evidence-based information in language a lay person can understand.

> **! NURSING SAFETY PRIORITY** (QSEN)
>
> *Action Alert*
>
> Women are exposed to many misconceptions and much misinformation about breast cancer through various media. Clarify misconceptions and provide current information regarding risk factors, screening recommendations, and treatment for breast cancer.

Decreasing the Risk for Metastasis

Planning: Expected Outcomes. The patient with breast cancer is expected to remain free of metastases or recurrence of disease, if possible. If cancer recurs, the patient will experience optimal health outcomes, including potential palliation and end-of-life care.

Interventions. There are many surgical and nonsurgical options for breast cancer treatment. Because of the various options, the patient with breast cancer often faces difficult decisions. Although patients are living longer with metastatic disease, the 5-year survival rate remains low. Once cancer is diagnosed, the extent and location of metastases determine the overall therapeutic strategy. The emphasis of breast cancer treatment is on preventing or stopping the spread of tumor cells that leads to distant metastasis. Treatment is tailored specifically

to each patient, taking into account other health problems and the patient's ability to tolerate a particular therapy.

Nonsurgical Management. For patients with breast cancer at a stage for which surgery is the main treatment, follow-up with adjuvant (in addition to surgery) radiation, chemotherapy, hormone therapy, or targeted therapy is commonly prescribed. For those who cannot have surgery or whose cancer is too advanced, these therapies are used to promote comfort (palliation). These options are discussed in the Adjuvant Therapy section on p. 1476.

Complementary and Alternative Therapies. Women with breast cancer often cope with distressing symptoms related to the disease itself or the side effects of chemotherapy, radiation, and hormonal therapy. Common symptoms associated with these therapies include PAIN, nausea, hot flashes, anxiety, depression, and fatigue. Physical and emotional symptoms associated with breast cancer may be eased with the use of complementary and alternative medicine (CAM). Up to 80% of women use some form of CAM during breast cancer treatment (Wyatt et al., 2010). The most frequently used types of CAM are biologically based therapies such as vitamins, special cancer diets, and herbal therapy. Prayer is also widely used. Other types of CAM are mind-body or body-based such as guided imagery and massage. Encourage women to seek a practitioner with a certification or license for the specific type of CAM therapy. In some states, a certification or license is required for acupuncture, chiropractic therapy, massage, and shiatsu. Some types of CAM can be self-taught or done alone after a few sessions of instruction. Table 70-3 lists complementary therapies for specific symptoms associated with breast cancer and its treatments.

Although the use of CAM can improve quality of life, its use does not alter the outcome of breast cancer and should not be used in place of standard treatment (Saquib et al., 2012). Encourage patients who are interested in trying CAM therapies to check with their health care provider before using them. Refer patients to reliable resources for information about CAM. The website *breastcancer.org* provides accurate information about complementary therapies and the extent to which they have been researched in breast cancer patients. Cost may be a factor in decision making since not all insurances provide

TABLE 70-3	**Complementary and Alternative Medicine (CAM) for Breast Cancer**
SYMPTOM	**CAM**
Physical	
Pain	Acupuncture, chiropractic therapy, hypnosis, massage, music, reiki, shiatsu
Nausea/vomiting	Acupuncture, aromatherapy, ginger, hypnosis, progressive muscle relaxation, shiatsu
Fatigue	Acupuncture, massage, meditation, reiki, tai chi, yoga
Hot flashes	Acupuncture, black cohosh, flaxseed
Muscle tension	Aromatherapy, massage, shiatsu
Emotional	
Anxiety/stress/fear	Aromatherapy, guided imagery, hypnosis, journaling, massage, meditation, music therapy, progressive muscle relaxation, prayer, support groups, tai chi, yoga
Depression	Aromatherapy, yoga, journaling, progressive muscle relaxation

coverage for CAMs. Teach the patient that all ingested CAM agents potentially risk interaction with conventional drugs.

Surgical Management. The most common types of breast surgeries are shown in Fig. 70-4. Although controversy exists concerning the best treatment for breast cancer, experts agree that the mass itself should be removed to reduce the risk for local recurrence. A large tumor is sometimes treated with chemotherapy, called **neoadjuvant therapy,** to shrink the tumor before it is surgically removed. An advantage of this therapy is that cancers can be removed by lumpectomy rather than mastectomy.

Axillary lymph nodes are analyzed for the presence of cancer and staging purposes. Axillary lymph node dissection (ALND) is usually done when there are palpable axillary lymph nodes or when cancer is suspected to be at a later stage. Sentinel lymph node biopsy (SLNB) is a much less invasive approach now preferred by most surgeons for analyzing lymph nodes in early-stage breast cancers with low to moderate risk for lymph node involvement. SLNB is shown in Fig. 70-5. In this method, the sentinel lymph node is identified during breast surgery by injecting the breast with radioisotope and/or dye that travels via lymphatic pathways to the sentinel lymph node. The nodes that take up the dye (or give off a certain level of radiation picked up by a handheld counter) are removed and examined for the presence of cancer cells. It is believed that if cancer cells have traveled through the lymph channels, the cells will lodge in the sentinel nodes. Travel beyond these nodes to higher-level nodes may occur as a secondary event. Therefore the absence of cancer cells in the sentinel nodes is an indicator that no other nodes in the regional area are involved.

Preoperative Care. Care of the patient facing surgery for breast cancer focuses on psychological preparation and preoperative teaching. Priority nursing interventions are directed toward relieving anxiety and providing information to increase patient knowledge. *Include the spouse or partner, who may be experiencing similar stress and confusion, in the health teaching unless the patient's culture does not permit this approach.*

Review the type of procedure planned. Use open-ended questions (e.g., "What type of surgery are you having? Can you explain what will happen?") to assess the current level of knowledge. Provide postoperative information, including:

- The need for a drainage tube
- The location of the incision
- Mobility restrictions
- The length of the hospital stay (if any)
- The possibility of adjuvant therapy
- General preoperative and postoperative information needed by any surgical patient (see Chapters 14 and 16)

Supplement teaching with written or electronic materials for the patient and family to take home as references. This information should include whom to call in case there are any

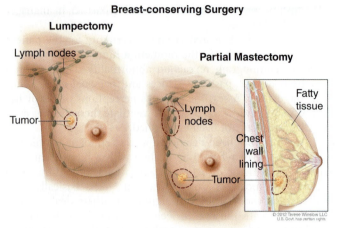

Breast-conserving Surgery

Breast-conserving surgery. Dotted lines show the area containing the tumor that is removed and some of the lymph nodes that may be removed.

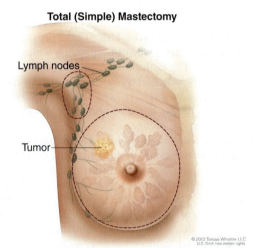

Total (Simple) Mastectomy

Total (simple) mastectomy. The dotted line shows where the entire breast is removed. Some lymph nodes under the arm may also be removed.

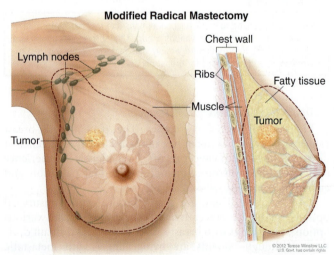

Modified Radical Mastectomy

Modified radical mastectomy. The dotted line shows where the entire breast and some lymph nodes are removed. Part of the chest wall muscle may also be removed.

FIG. 70-4 Surgical treatment for breast cancer.

Sentinel Lymph Node Biopsy

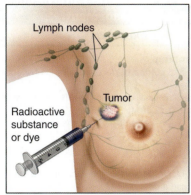
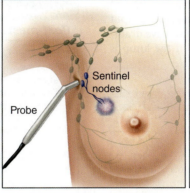
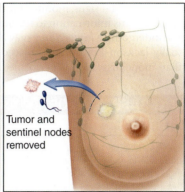

© 2010 Terese Winslow
U.S. Govt. has certain rights

Sentinel lymph node biopsy of the breast. A radioactive substance and/or blue dye is injected near the tumor (first panel). The injected material is detected visually and/or with a probe that detects radioactivity (middle panel). The sentinel nodes (the first lymph nodes to take up the material) are removed and checked for cancer cells (last panel).

FIG. 70-5 Sentinel lymph node biopsy of the breast.

complications. Address body image issues before surgery to correct misconceptions about appearance after surgery. If available, suggest that patients and their caregivers attend classes before surgery in an ambulatory care setting, such as a breast cancer center, to promote successful early discharge from the hospital. Programs that provide emotional support, information, and opportunities for discussion related to SEXUALITY, body image, and preoperative and postoperative care enhance the recovery of the short-stay mastectomy patient.

Operative Procedures. Types of breast surgeries are shown in Fig. 70-5. During **breast-conserving surgery,** such as a *lumpectomy,* the surgeon removes the tumor and a small amount of tissue rather than the entire breast. A partial mastectomy is surgery to remove part of the breast that contains cancer and some normal tissue around it. *Margins* refer to the distance between the tumor and the edge of the surrounding tissue. The desired outcome of breast-conserving surgery is to obtain negative *margins* in which no cancer cells extend to the edge of the tissue. Typically, radiation therapy follows to kill any residual tumor cells.

Breast-conserving procedures are usually performed in same-day surgical settings. The cosmetic results of these surgeries are good to excellent, and the psychological benefits of avoiding breast removal are significant for patients who choose this option.

Despite advances in breast-conserving surgery, mastectomy remains a popular option for breast cancer treatment and women are increasingly choosing it for prophylactic treatment (McLaughlin, 2013). Typically, indications for a mastectomy include multi-centric disease (tumor is present in different quadrants of the breast), inability to have radiation therapy, presence of a large tumor in a small breast, and patient preference. Mastectomy does not conserve the breast; the affected breast is completely removed. A total (simple) mastectomy is surgery to remove the whole breast that has cancer. A modified radical mastectomy removes the breast tissue, lymph nodes, and sometimes, part of the underlying chest wall muscle. If reconstruction is to be performed at the same time as the mastectomy, less-invasive techniques, such as incising a ½-inch flap of skin around the nipple (excising the same amount of breast tissue as with conventional mastectomy), may be performed.

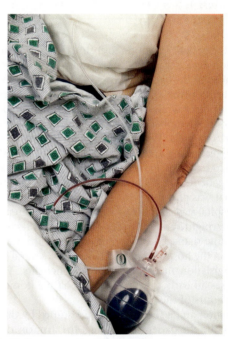

FIG. 70-6 Jackson-Pratt drain in place after a mastectomy.

Skin flaps or expanders may be used to create a breast mound at the time of the original procedure.

Postoperative Care. Before the patient returns from surgery, inform the staff to avoid using the affected arm for measuring blood pressure, giving injections, or drawing blood. He or she returns from the postanesthesia care unit (PACU) as soon as vital signs return to baseline levels and if no complications have occurred. Assess vital signs on a schedule of decreasing frequency, such as every 30 minutes for 2 times, every hour for 2 times, and then every 4 hours. During these checks, assess the dressing for bleeding.

During a *modified radical mastectomy,* the surgeon places one or two drainage tubes, usually Jackson-Pratt drains, under the skin flaps and attaches the tubes to a small collection chamber (Fig. 70-6). Gentle suction is exerted, and fluid that would accumulate under the flaps and delay healing is collected. Various drains are available, but all allow the drainage to be seen and measured. When taking vital signs, monitor for the amount and color of drainage. Add this information to the intake and output record. Patients undergoing a *lumpectomy* may also have drainage tubes (usually Jackson-Pratt drains) placed if the lump is large or if axillary node dissection is performed.

! NURSING SAFETY PRIORITY (QSEN)
Action Alert

Per TJC National Patient Safety Goal recommendations, to decrease the chance of surgical site infection, carefully observe the surgical wound after breast surgery for signs of swelling and infection throughout recovery. Assess the incision and flap of the post-mastectomy patient for signs of bleeding, infection, and poor tissue perfusion. With short hospital stays, drainage tubes are usually removed about 1 to 3 weeks after hospital discharge when the patient returns for an office visit. The drainage amount should be less than 25 mL in a 24-hour period. Inform the patient that tube removal may be uncomfortable although these tubes lie just under the skin. Provide or suggest analgesia before they are removed. Document all findings, and report any abnormalities to the surgeon immediately.

Assess the patient's position to ensure that the drainage tubes or collection device is not pulled or kinked. The patient should have the head of the bed up at least 30 degrees with the affected arm (the arm on the same side as the axillary dissection) elevated on a pillow while awake. Keeping the affected arm elevated promotes lymphatic fluid return after removal of lymph nodes and channels. Provide other basic comfort measures, such as repositioning and analgesics as prescribed on a regular basis until PAIN ceases. Patient-controlled analgesia may be used for some patients for a short time depending on the type of surgery that was performed.

The hospital stay after breast surgery is short, often same-day or just overnight, and recovery is usually not complicated. Because some managed care plans will not authorize an overnight stay in the hospital after a mastectomy, several states have enacted legislation mandating inpatient benefits. The patient who chooses an early discharge should have a home care visit within 24 hours of the discharge.

Ambulation and a regular diet are resumed by the day after surgery. While the patient is walking, the arm on the affected side may need to be supported at first. Gradually, the arm should be allowed to hang straight by the side. Instruct the patient to avoid the hunched-back position with the arm flexed because of the risk for elbow contracture. Beginning exercises that do not stress the incision can usually be started on the first day after surgery. These exercises include squeezing the affected hand around a soft, round object (a ball or rolled washcloth) and flexion/extension of the elbow. The progression to more strenuous exercises depends on the subsequent procedures planned (e.g., reconstruction) and the surgeon's prescription.

As soon as the patient is ambulatory and surgical PAIN is under control, he or she is discharged to home. Common instructions for exercises after mastectomy are listed in Chart 70-3.

Breast Reconstruction. Breast reconstruction after or during mastectomy for women is common with few complications. Patients consult with the plastic surgeon to discuss the type of reconstruction, timing of the procedure, and technique desired. Many women prefer reconstruction immediately after

---

CHART 70-3   Patient and Family Education: Preparing for Self-Management
Post-mastectomy Exercises

Hand Wall Climbing
- Face the wall, and put the palms of your hands flat against the wall at shoulder level.
- Flex your fingers so that your hands slowly "walk" up the wall.
- Stop when your arms are fully extended.
- Slowly "walk" your hands back down the wall until they return to shoulder level.

Pulley Exercise
- Drape a 6-foot-long rope over a shower curtain rod or over the top of a door. If you use a door for this exercise, have someone put a nail or hook at the top of the door so that the rope does not slip off.
- Grab the ends of the rope, one in each hand, and extend your arms out to your sides until they are straight.
- Keeping your arms straight, pull down with your left arm to raise your right arm as high as you can.
- Pull down with your right arm to raise your left arm as high as you can.

Rope Turning
- Tie a rope to the knob of a closed door.
- Hold the other end of the rope and step back from the door until your arm is almost straight out in front of you.
- Swing the rope in a circle. Start with small circles, and gradually increase to larger circles as you become more flexible.

? NCLEX EXAMINATION CHALLENGE
Physiological Integrity

The nurse is assigned to care for a client who has undergone a modified radical left mastectomy for breast cancer. When delegating care, which statement by the nursing assistant would require further teaching by the nurse?
A. "I will report urine intake and output to you."
B. "If the client appears to be in pain, I will tell you right away."
C. "It is important for me to take blood pressure on the client's left arm."
D. "When ambulating, I will assist the client to stand straight with arms hanging at the side."

---

mastectomy using their own tissue (autogenous reconstruction). Breast reconstruction at the time of mastectomy, both autogenous and prosthetic, may lessen the psychological strain associated with undergoing a mastectomy.

The surgeon should offer the option of breast reconstruction before surgery is performed. If the woman does not choose immediate reconstructive surgery, a temporary prosthesis can be used. Refer the patient to the American Cancer Society's *Reach to Recovery* program (www.cancer.org). In this program, a volunteer who has had breast cancer surgery visits the woman at home, offering information on breast forms, clothing, coping with breast cancer, and possible reconstructive options. For this intervention to be as helpful as possible, the volunteer should be about the same age as the patient and have experienced the same surgical procedure.

Evaluate the woman's level of satisfaction with her prosthesis several weeks after surgery. Assess her attitude by asking about future plans for restoring appearance. Although reconstruction is not appropriate for some women and others may not be

TABLE 70-4	**Examples of Breast Reconstruction Procedures**		
PROCEDURE	**DESCRIPTION**	**PROCEDURE**	**DESCRIPTION**
Implantation	An implant matching the size of the other breast is placed under the muscle on the operative side to create a breast mound.	Myocutaneous flaps	A flap of skin, fat, and muscle is transferred from the donor site to the operative area. The flap contains an appropriate amount of fat to match the other breast and is similar in appearance to breast tissue. A blood supply is established by reanastomosis of vessels from the operative area to those with the flap when possible. A new nipple may be created with tissue from areas such as the labia or upper, inner thigh. Nipples can also be created by tattooing.

Latissimus dorsi musculocutaneous flap

Abdominal myocutaneous flap

Tissue expansion	A tissue expander is placed under the muscle and gradually expanded with saline to stretch the overlying skin and create a pocket. After several weeks, the tissue expander is exchanged for an implant.		

interested in it, the surgeon should discuss the indications and contraindications, advantages and disadvantages, and typical recovery. If immediate reconstruction is chosen, the surgeon should be aware of this before surgery so that plans can be coordinated with those of the plastic surgeon.

Several procedures are available for restoring the appearance of the breast (Table 70-4). Reconstruction may begin during the original operative procedure or later in one to several stages. Common types of breast reconstruction are:

- Breast expanders (saline or gel)
- Autologous reconstruction using the patient's own skin, fat, and muscle

Breast expanders are the most common method of breast reconstruction used today in the United States. A tissue expander

is a balloon-like device with a resealable metal port that is placed under the pectoralis muscle. A small amount of normal saline is injected intraoperatively into the expander to partially inflate it. The patient then receives additional weekly saline injections for about 6 to 8 weeks until the expander is fully inflated. When full expansion is achieved, the tissue expander is then exchanged for a permanent implant during surgery in an ambulatory care center. The permanent implant is filled with either saline or silicone gel. Despite earlier claims that silicone gel caused autoimmune diseases like lupus and arthritis, silicone implants have been safely used in the majority of women who choose this type of breast implant.

Autologous reconstruction using the patient's own skin, fat, and muscle is advantageous because the donor site tissue is similar in consistency to the natural breast. Therefore the results more closely resemble a real breast as compared with implant reconstruction. Flap donor sites include the latissimus dorsi flap (back muscle); transverse rectus abdominis myocutaneous flap, known as the *TRAM flap* (abdominal muscle); and the gluteal flap (buttock muscle). Reconstruction of the nipple-areola complex is the last stage in the reconstruction of the breast. If necessary, a new nipple may be created with other body tissue, such as from the labia, abdomen, or inner thigh.

Women who have had a mastectomy and breast reconstruction in one breast should have close surveillance breast cancer screening in the contralateral (opposite) breast, including imaging with mammography or mammography and MRI. Mammography and MRI are not recommended to be routinely done in reconstructed breasts because most local recurrences of breast cancer in the residual tissue are palpable during clinical breast examination (Zakhireh et al., 2010). Nursing care of the woman who has undergone breast reconstruction is outlined in Chart 70-4.

Adjuvant Therapy. The decision to follow the original surgical procedure with **adjuvant therapy** (in addition to surgery) for breast cancer is based on:

- The stage of the disease
- The patient's age and menopausal status
- Patient preferences
- Pathologic examination
- Hormone receptor status
- Presence of a known genetic predisposition

Adjuvant therapy for breast cancer consists of radiation therapy and drug therapy. The purpose of radiation therapy is to reduce

the risk for local recurrence of breast cancer. Drug therapy includes chemotherapy, targeted therapy, and/or hormonal therapy. These drugs destroy breast cancer cells that may be present anywhere in the body. They are typically delivered after surgery for breast cancer, although **neoadjuvant** chemotherapy may be given to reduce the size of a tumor before surgery. Hormonal therapy is a chemoprevention option for high-risk women with a personal history of breast cancer.

Radiation Therapy. Radiation therapy is administered after breast-conserving surgery to kill breast cancer cells that may remain near the site of the original tumor. This therapy can be delivered to the whole breast or to only part of the breast. Whole-breast irradiation is delivered by external beam radiation over a period of 5 to 6 weeks. Partial breast irradiation (PBI) has become a newer option for women with early-stage breast cancer. PBI is a convenient alternative to whole breast radiation. Less time is needed for completion, and outcomes are comparable to whole breast radiation (Edwards et al., 2013). The advantage of this type of radiation is that it is delivered over a much shorter time interval, eliminating the need for daily trips for treatment. The types of methods available for delivering *partial-breast irradiation* include:

- Interstitial brachytherapy, in which several catheters loaded with a radioactive source are inserted at the lumpectomy cavity and surrounding margin, is given over a period of 4 to 5 days.
- Balloon brachytherapy, also known as *MammoSite*, involves the use of a single balloon-tipped catheter that is surgically placed near the tumor bed. The catheter is loaded with a radiation source and inflated to conform to the total cavity. Ten total treatments are given, with at least 6 hours between each treatment.
- Intraoperative radiation therapy is the most accelerated form of partial breast irradiation. It utilizes a high single dose of radiation delivered during the lumpectomy surgery.

Nursing care for the patient undergoing radiation therapy includes patient education and side effect management. Skin changes are a major side effect during this therapy (see Chapter 22). If brachytherapy is planned, instruct patients about the procedure. Assure them that they will be radioactive only while the radiation source is dwelling inside the breast tissue.

CHART 70-4 Best Practice for Patient Safety & Quality Care (QSEN)

Postoperative Care of the Patient After Breast Reconstruction

- Assess the incision and flap for signs of infection (excessive redness, drainage, odor) during dressing changes.
- Assess the incision and flap for signs of poor tissue perfusion (duskiness, decreased capillary refill) during dressing changes.
- Avoid pressure on the flap and suture lines by positioning the patient on her nonoperative side and avoiding tight clothing.
- Monitor and measure drainage in collection devices, such as for Jackson-Pratt drains.
- Teach the patient to return to her usual activity level gradually and to avoid heavy lifting.
- Remind the patient to avoid sleeping in the prone position.
- Teach the patient to avoid participation in contact sports or other activities that could cause trauma to the chest.
- Teach the patient to minimize pressure on the breast during sexual activity.
- Remind the patient to refrain from driving until advised by the physician.
- Remind the patient to ask at the 6-week postoperative visit when full activity can be resumed.
- Reassure the patient that optimal appearance may not occur for 3 to 6 months postoperatively.
- If implants have been inserted, teach the proper method of breast massage to enhance expansion and prevent capsule formation (consult with the physician).
- Emphasize breast self-awareness; if the patient performs breast self-examination (BSE), review her technique.
- Remind the patient of the importance of clinical breast examination and follow-up surveillance by her physician.

! NURSING SAFETY PRIORITY (QSEN)

Action Alert

Teach women undergoing brachytherapy for breast cancer that radiation is contained in the temporary implant. The risk for others to be exposed to radiation is very small. Body fluids and items contacted by patients with brachytherapy are not radioactive. However, during the time the radiation is delivered, it is recommended they limit visitors, including pregnant women and children.

Chemotherapy. Chemotherapy for breast cancer is delivered systemically via the central IV route, such as an implantable venous access device (Port-a-Cath). Its purpose is to kill undetected breast cancer cells that may have left the original tumor and moved to more distant sites. Chemotherapy is recommended for treatment of invasive breast cancer after surgery (adjuvant chemotherapy). It may also be given before surgery to reduce the size of the tumor (neoadjuvant chemotherapy). Chemotherapy is most effective when combinations of more than one drug are used. Table 70-5 lists common chemotherapy agents used in breast cancer and their mechanism of action. Chemotherapy drugs are usually delivered in four to six cycles, with each period of treatment followed by a rest period to give the body time to recover from the effects of the drugs. Each cycle is 2 to 3 weeks long. The total treatment time is 3 to 6 months, although treatment may be longer for advanced breast cancer. Many combinations of drugs are used, and no one combination has been proven to be superior over others (ACS, 2013a). A common chemotherapy regimen for breast cancer treatment is Cytoxan, Adriamycin, and fluorouracil, which is also known as 5-FU (CAF). In early-stage breast cancer, chemotherapy regimens lower the risk for breast cancer recurrence. In advanced breast cancer, chemotherapy regimens reduce cancer size in many patients.

Nurses must be very proficient in the preparation and administration of chemotherapy drugs and knowledgeable about various venous access devices. They must also be able to manage the distressing symptoms associated with side effects of chemotherapy. Chapter 22 discusses general nursing management of alopecia, nausea and vomiting, mucositis, and bone marrow suppression. Fatigue and sleep disturbance are often major concerns as side effects of chemotherapy.

! NURSING SAFETY PRIORITY (QSEN)

Action Alert

Teach patients undergoing chemotherapy with anthracyclines such as doxorubicin (Adriamycin) to be aware of cardiotoxic effects. Instruct them to report excessive fatigue, shortness of breath, chronic cough, and edema to the health care provider.

Chemotherapy is unpleasant and expensive and can have life-threatening short-term and long-term side effects. Because more women are living longer with breast cancer, long-term effects are increasingly emerging. Although targeted therapy is effective with fewer side effects, some side effects are nevertheless life threatening. For example, cardiac toxicity is a risk associated with the use of Herceptin, particularly when it is combined with other chemotherapy. Chemotherapy and ovarian suppression can result in infertility, a devastating effect for women of childbearing age. Hormonal therapy can result in long-term ill effects from bone loss. Discuss patient concerns, provide accurate information, and assist him or her in decision making.

Targeted Therapy. Targeted cancer therapies are drugs that target specific characteristics of cancer cells, such as a protein, an enzyme, or the formation of new blood vessels. The advantage of targeted therapy over traditional chemotherapy is that targeted therapy is less likely to harm normal, healthy cells and therefore it has fewer side effects. Table 70-5 lists targeted chemotherapy drugs used in breast cancer. One of the first targeted therapies developed for breast cancer is the monoclonal antibody *trastuzumab* (Herceptin). This drug targets the *HER2/neu* gene product in breast cancer cells. Several other targeted therapies have been developed since Herceptin.

Hormonal Therapy. Table 70-5 lists hormonal therapy drugs used in breast cancer prevention and treatment. The purpose of hormonal therapy is to reduce the estrogen available to breast tumors to stop or prevent their growth. *Premenopausal* women whose main estrogen source is the ovaries may benefit from

TABLE 70-5	Drug Therapy for Breast Cancer	
CATEGORY	**MECHANISM OF ACTION**	**AGENTS**
Chemotherapy		
Anthracyclines	Inhibit DNA synthesis in susceptible cells	doxorubicin (Adriamycin) (A) epirubicin (Ellence) (E) daunorubicin (Cerubidine) mitoxantrone (Novantrone)
Taxanes	Inhibit microtubule network in rapidly dividing cells	docetaxel (Taxotere) (D) paclitaxel (Taxol) (P) paclitaxel, protein-bound (Abraxane)
Alkylating agents	Interfere with the replication of susceptible cells	cyclophosphamide (Cytoxan) (C) thiotepa (Thioplex)
Antimetabolites	Inhibit DNA synthesis and cellular replication in rapidly dividing cells	methotrexate (Mexate) (M) fluorouracil (5-FU) (F) capecitabine (Xeloda) gemcitabine (Gemzar)
Additional Chemotherapy Drugs Used in Advanced Breast Cancer		
Vinca alkaloids	Interfere with genes, stopping cells from reproducing	vinorelbine (Navelbine) vincristine (Oncovin)
Platinum-based	Weakens or destroys breast cancer cells by damaging genetic material	carboplatin (Paraplatin)
Microtubule inhibitor	Disrupts cells division by interfering with microtubulin	eribulin (Halaven)
Epothilone	Interferes with cancer cell division	ixabepilone (Ixempra)
Antitumor antibiotic	Damages genes, interfering with reproduction	mitomycin (Mutamycin)
Targeted Therapy	Selectively targets critical steps in the processes required for tumor growth, viability, or invasion	trastuzumab (Herceptin) lapatinib (Tykerb) pertuzumab (Perjeta) everolimus (Afinitor) T-DM1 (Kadcyla)
Hormonal Therapy		
LH-RH agonists	Block release of LH and FSH, thereby preventing ovarian production of estrogen	goserelin (Zoladex) leuprolide (Lupron)
Selective estrogen receptor modulators (SERMs)	Bind to estrogen receptors; have both agonist and antagonist properties (selectively block action of estrogen in the breast but not in other organs)	tamoxifen (Nolvadex) raloxifene (Evista) toremifene (Fareston)
Aromatase inhibitors	Prevent conversion of adrenal and ovarian androgens to estrogens by inhibiting the aromatase enzyme	anastrozole (Arimidex) letrozole (Femara) exemestane (Aromasin)
Estrogen receptor down-regulators	Induce degradation of estrogen receptor	fulvestrant (Faslodex)

FSH, Follicle-stimulating hormone; *LH,* luteinizing hormone; *LH-RH,* luteinizing hormone–releasing hormone.

LH-RH agonists that inhibit estrogen synthesis. These drugs include leuprolide (Lupron) and goserelin (Zoladex), which suppress the hypothalamus from making luteinizing hormone–releasing hormone (LH-RH). When LH-RH is inhibited, the ovaries do not produce estrogen. Although the suppression of ovarian function decreases breast cancer risk, the drastic drop in estrogen causes significant menopausal symptoms. Therefore the decision to use these drugs is not made lightly.

Selective estrogen receptor modulators (SERMs), on the other hand, do not affect ovarian function. Rather, they block the effect of estrogen in women who have estrogen receptor (ER)–positive breast cancer. SERMs are also used as chemoprevention in women at high risk for breast cancer and in women with advanced breast cancer. For women with hormone receptor–positive breast cancer, tamoxifen reduces the chances of the cancer coming back by about half (ACS, 2013a). A recent study demonstrated that taking tamoxifen for 10 years, rather than 5 years, achieves the best benefit for risk reduction (Davies et al., 2013). Common side effects of SERMs include hot flashes and weight gain. Rare but serious side effects of these drugs include endometrial cancer and thromboembolic events.

Aromatase inhibitors (AIs) are used in *postmenopausal* women whose main source of estrogen is not the ovaries but, rather, body fat. AIs reduce estrogen levels by inhibiting the conversion of androgen to estrogen through the action of the enzyme *aromatase*. AIs are beneficial when given to postmenopausal women for up to 5 years. Treatment with AIs usually follows treatment with tamoxifen. Studies are underway to determine whether it is beneficial to take AIs longer than 5 years (ACS, 2013a). A side effect of AIs, not seen with tamoxifen, is loss of bone density. Women taking AIs are candidates for bone-strengthening drugs and must be closely monitored for osteoporosis. Fulvestrant (Faslodex), a second-line hormonal therapy for postmenopausal women with advanced breast cancer, is used after other hormonal treatments have stopped working.

Stem Cell Transplantation. Autologous or allogeneic stem cell transplantation is an option for patients with a high risk for recurrence or who have advanced disease. **Autologous bone marrow transplantation** (taken from the patient's bone marrow), peripheral blood stem cell transplantation (taken from circulating blood), or **allogeneic bone marrow transplantation** (taken from a healthy donor's bone marrow or peripheral blood) is performed as a means of rescue therapy after very high doses of chemotherapy. The general care of the patient undergoing bone marrow or stem cell transplantation is discussed in Chapter 22.

Community-Based Care

Home Care Management. In collaboration with the case manager and members of the interdisciplinary health care team, make the appropriate referrals for care after discharge. Preoperative teaching and arrangements for home care management and referrals (*Reach to Recovery*, social services, home care) can be started before surgery or other treatment.

The patient who has undergone breast surgery can be discharged to the home setting unless other physical disabilities exist. Some are discharged the day after surgery with Jackson-Pratt or other types of drains in place. Many patients are discharged to home on the day of surgery. Older adults should not be sent home without a family member or friend who can stay with them for 1 to 2 days. These patients may need some assistance at home with drain care, dressings, and ADLs because of

---

> ### CHART 70-5 Patient and Family Education: Preparing for Self-Management
> #### *Recovery from Breast Cancer Surgery*
>
> - There may be a dry gauze dressing over the incision when you leave the hospital. You may change this dressing if it becomes soiled.
> - A small, dry dressing will be around the site where a drain is placed. Often there is some leakage of fluid around the drain. Check the gauze dressing for drainage, and change it if it becomes soiled. Some leakage is normal, but if the dressing becomes soaked more than once a day, call your health care provider.
> - You have been taught how to empty the reservoir from your drain and how to measure the volume of drainage. You should empty the reservoir twice a day and record the measurements.
> - Drains are generally removed when drainage is less than 25 mL in 24 hours.
> - Drains are often removed at the same time as the stitches or staples, generally 7 to 10 days (could be as long as 3 weeks if needed) after surgery.
> - You may take sponge baths or tub baths, making certain that the area of the drain and incision stays dry. You may shower after the stitches, staples, and drains are removed.
> - You can begin using your arm for normal activities, such as eating or combing your hair. Exercises involving the wrist, hand, and elbow, such as flexing your fingers, circular wrist motions, and touching your hand to your shoulder, are very good. You can usually resume more strenuous exercises after the drains have been removed.
> - You can expect some discomfort or mild pain after surgery, but within 4 to 5 days, most women have no need for pain medication or require medication only at bedtime.
> - Numbness in the area of the surgery and along the inner side of the arm from the armpit to the elbow occurs in almost all women. It is the injury to the nerves that causes sensation to the skin in those areas. Women have described sensations of heaviness, pain, tingling, burning, and "pins and needles." Neuropathic pain is sometimes relieved by gabapentin (Neurontin). These sensations change over the months and usually resolve by 1 year.
> - Pamphlets on exercises, hand and arm care, and general facts about breast cancer are available from us or from a volunteer visitor. The American Cancer Society has volunteers who have had surgery similar to yours and are available to visit you.

PAIN and impaired range of motion of the affected arm. Summaries of continuing care instructions are given in Charts 70-5 and 70-6.

Teach patients that activities involving stretching or reaching for heavy objects should be avoided temporarily. This restriction can be discussed with a family member or significant other who can perform these tasks or place the objects within easy reach.

Self-Management Education. The teaching plan for the patient after surgery includes:
- Measures to improve body image
- Information about interpersonal relationships and roles
- Exercises to regain full range of motion
- Measures to prevent INFECTION of the incision (per The Joint Commission's National Patient Safety Goals)
- Measures to avoid lymphedema
- Measures to avoid injury, INFECTION, and swelling of the affected arm (per The Joint Commission's National Patient Safety Goals)
- Care of the incision and drainage device

Teach incisional care to the patient, family, and/or other caregiver. The patient may wear a light dressing to prevent irritation. Explain that no lotions or ointments should be used on the area

CHART 70-6 Home Care Assessment

Patients Recovering from Breast Cancer Surgery

Assess cardiovascular, respiratory, and urinary status:
- Vital signs
- Lung sounds
- Urine output patterns

Assess for pain and effectiveness of analgesics.

Assess dressing and incision site:
- Excess drainage
- Manifestations of infection
- Wound healing
- Intact staples

Assess drain and site:
- Drainage around drain site and in drain reservoir
- Color and amount of drainage
- Manifestations of infection

Review patient's recordings of drainage.

Evaluate patient's ability to care for and empty drain reservoir.

Assess status of affected extremity:
- Range of motion
- Ability to perform exercise regimen
- Lymphedema

Assess nutritional status:
- Food and fluid intake
- Presence of nausea and vomiting
- Bowel sounds

Assess functional ability:
- Activities of daily living
- Mobility and ambulation

Assess home environment:
- Safety
- Structural barriers

Assess patient's compliance and knowledge of illness and treatment plan:
- Follow-up appointment with surgeon
- Manifestations to report to health care provider
- Hand and arm care guidelines
- Referral to *Reach to Recovery*

Assess patient and caregiver coping skills:
- Whether patient and/or caregiver has looked at incision site
- Patient's and/or caregiver's reaction to incision site

---

beyond that. Some YWCA locations have a free program called *ENCORE,* which supports women and men following breast cancer surgery. The program includes exercise to music, exercise in water, and peer psychological support. Patients may participate as early as 3 weeks after surgery. Before discharge, the surgeon may prescribe precautions or limitations specific to plans for future procedures, such as reconstruction.

Lymphedema, an abnormal accumulation of protein fluid in the subcutaneous tissue of the affected limb after a mastectomy, is a commonly overlooked topic in health teaching. Risk factors include injury or INFECTION of the extremity, obesity, presence of extensive axillary disease, and radiation treatment. Once it develops, it can be very difficult to manage, and *lifelong measures must be taken to prevent it.* Nurses play a vital role in educating patients about this complication. Teach your patient to immediately report symptoms of lymphedema such as sensations of heaviness, aching, fatigue, numbness, tingling, and/or swelling in the affected arm, as well as swelling in the upper chest (Mohler & Mondry, 2013).

! NURSING SAFETY PRIORITY (QSEN)

Action Alert

Provide information needed to help the patient avoid INFECTION and subsequent lymphedema of the affected arm after the mastectomy. Teach the importance of avoiding having blood pressure measurements taken on, having injections in, or having blood drawn from the arm on the side of the mastectomy. Instruct the patient to wear a mitt when using the oven, wear gloves when gardening, and treat cuts and scrapes appropriately. If lymphedema occurs, early intervention provides the best chance for control. Nurses should not assume that women with lymphedema are disabled; they are able to live full lives within this limitation (Ridner et al., 2012). A referral to a lymphedema specialist may be necessary for the patient to be fitted for a compression sleeve and/or glove, to be taught exercises and manual lymph drainage, and to discuss ways to modify daily activities to avoid worsening the problem. Management is directed toward measures that promote drainage of the affected arm. Teach patients, especially those who have had axillary lymph nodes removed, that measures to prevent lymphedema are lifelong and include avoiding trauma to the arm on the side of the mastectomy.

---

and that the use of deodorant under the affected arm should be avoided until healing is complete. Although swelling and redness of the scar itself are normal for the first few weeks, swelling, redness, increased heat, and tenderness of the surrounding area indicate INFECTION and should be reported to the surgeon immediately. If a lymph node dissection was performed, instruct the patient to elevate the affected arm on a pillow for at least 30 minutes a day for the first 6 months. Ask the patient to have someone bring a loose-fitting, non-wire bra or camisole for her to try before discharge with a soft, cotton-filled or polyester fiber–filled form supplied by the hospital or by *Reach to Recovery.* The patient wears this form until the incision is completely healed and the health care provider approves the fitting of a more sophisticated prosthesis, usually 6 to 8 weeks after discharge. Encourage the patient to dress in loose-fitting street clothes at home, not pajamas, to further enhance a positive self-image.

Teach the patient to continue performing the exercises that began in the hospital. Active range-of-motion exercises should begin 1 week after surgery or when sutures and drains are removed. Emphasize that reaching and stretching exercises should continue only to the point of PAIN or pulling, never

Psychosocial Preparation. Concerns about appearance after surgery are common and are often a threat to the patient's self-concept as a woman. Before breast surgery, the woman and her partner can benefit from an explanation of the expected post-operative appearance. After a modified radical mastectomy, the chest wall is fairly smooth and has a horizontal incision from the axilla to the midchest area. After breast-conserving surgery, scars vary according to the amount of breast tissue removed. Women are sometimes shown pictures of post-mastectomy reconstruction but are disappointed with their own results. Emphasize that scars will fade and edema will lessen with time. Scars may be red and raised at first, but these features lessen in the first few months. After surgery, encourage the woman to look at her incision when she is ready. Do not push her to accept this body image change immediately.

Much of one's body image is a reflection of how others respond. Therefore the response of the patient's family or partner to the surgery is crucial in determining the effect on self-concept. These people may also need the support of the nurse. They may have concerns about their ability to accept the changes and need to discuss these feelings with an objective listener. They may also need help with communicating their feelings, both negative and positive, with their loved one. Involving them in teaching may also help reinforce learning and increase retention.

Discuss sexual concerns before discharge. Most surgeons recommend avoiding sexual intercourse for 4 to 6 weeks. Patients may prefer to lay a pillow over the surgical site or to wear a bra, camisole, or T-shirt to prevent contact with the surgical site during intercourse. He or she may be embarrassed to discuss the topic of SEXUALITY. Be sensitive to possible concerns, and approach the subject first.

For young women, issues related to childbearing may be a concern. Chemotherapy and radiation are considered serious teratogenic (birth defect–causing) agents. Advise sexually active patients receiving chemotherapy or radiotherapy to use birth control during therapy. The method and length of birth control should be discussed with the health care provider.

Health Care Resources. Resources available to the patient after discharge include personal support and community programs. After discharge, the spouse or partner may need help in planning support for home responsibilities. For example, a partner who may be assuming additional duties at home and work may feel stressed. Discussing the need for ongoing emotional support is also beneficial to both the patient and partner. Leaving the hospital and appearing normal do not end the anxiety and fear. Identifying a support person with whom the patient or couple can explore these feelings and discussing the need to ventilate feelings enhance personal and family recovery.

Numerous support and educational resources are available to those diagnosed with breast cancer. Nurses must provide accurate and current information to patients who may have obtained inaccurate information from various media. There are over 2 million breast cancer survivors in the United States, and many men and women are active in breast cancer support and advocacy organizations. National breast cancer organizations are accessible online, and many of them have local affiliates. Examples of such organizations are Susan G. Komen for the Cure, the National Breast Cancer Coalition, Y-Me, Sisters Network, Young Survival Coalition, and Pink Ribbon Girls. Local support organizations can be accessed through the health care provider, the local hospital, wellness centers, home care agencies, or by word of mouth. The American Cancer Society (ACS) (www.cancer.org) is a comprehensive resource for information and support.

💡 CLINICAL JUDGMENT CHALLENGE

Patient-Centered Care; Safety; Evidence-Based Practice QSEN

A 46-year-old Caucasian lesbian woman is diagnosed with breast cancer and scheduled for a radical right mastectomy and chemotherapy. She tells you that she often feared developing cancer because her mother and aunt were both diagnosed with breast cancer in their 40s. She says she is fearful because her employer does not offer insurance and she is not eligible to be covered under her partner's insurance plan. She also shares that she feels sad because she has been attempting to get pregnant for the first time and she now realizes that this will not be possible for the foreseeable future.

1. What evidence-based risk factors does this patient have?
2. What discharge instructions will you provide for her and why?
3. What will you teach the patient about chemotherapy to maintain her safety?
4. How might you help address the patient's emotional concerns?

NURSING CONCEPTS AND CLINICAL JUDGMENT REVIEW

What might you NOTICE if a patient is experiencing impaired SEXUALITY as a result of breast cancer or other disorder?
- Breast swelling or lump (with or without pain)
- Discharge from nipple(s)
- Skin dimpling or orange peel appearance
- Asymmetric breast tissue
- Very large or very small breasts
- Skin redness and warmth

What should you INTERPRET and how should you RESPOND to a patient having impaired SEXUALITY as a result of breast cancer or other disorder?

Perform and interpret physical assessment, including:
- Taking a thorough patient and family history
- Examining each breast, comparing sides, and documenting
- Assessing pain and documenting
- Assessing psychosocial reaction to the breast changes

Respond by:
- Checking recent mammogram test or other imaging assessment results
- Acknowledging patient's concerns about body image and sexuality changes
- Asking the patient about resources for support that have been used in the past for coping with crisis
- Preparing the patient for testing and possible biopsy
- Listening to the patient's concerns in a nonjudgmental manner

On what should you REFLECT?
- Consider what health care resources (team members) the patient and family will need throughout disease management.
- Think about what other community resources the patient and family will need.
- Observe the patient's progress in adapting to body image changes.

GET READY FOR THE NCLEX® EXAMINATION!

KEY POINTS

Review these Key Points for each NCLEX Examination Client Needs Category.

Safe and Effective Care Environment
- In collaboration with the health care team, identify community resources for patients with breast cancer, including *Reach to Recovery* of the American Cancer Society. **Teamwork and Collaboration** QSEN

Health Promotion and Maintenance
- Identify patients at high risk for breast cancer, especially women with family history of breast cancer at a young age; those who have had early menarche, late menopause, or first pregnancy after 30 years of age; or those who are nullipara.
- Discuss benefits and risks of options available to women who are high risk for breast cancer, including close surveillance and prophylactic surgery.
- Teach women to become self-aware of breasts and any breast changes; teach breast self-examination (BSE) to women who choose this method of breast self-awareness. **Patient-Centered Care** QSEN
- Encourage women to have screening mammography according to recommended guidelines. Baseline screening should begin at 40 years of age and continue yearly. In high-risk women, screening should be started earlier. **Evidence-Based Practice** QSEN
- Encourage women to have a clinical breast examination (CBE) according to recommended guidelines. **Evidence-Based Practice** QSEN

Psychosocial Integrity
- Assess patients' reactions to the diagnosis of breast cancer and the effect of breast cancer treatment on their body image and SEXUALITY. **Patient-Centered Care** QSEN
- Identify resources that facilitate patients' grief work and coping skills.

- Allow patients opportunities to express feelings of grief, fear, and anxiety.
- Teach women ways to minimize surgical area deformity and enhance body image, such as use of a breast implant (prosthesis) or the option of breast reconstruction.
- Address the reactions of family and significant others to the diagnosis of breast cancer; provide support and education.

Physiological Integrity
- Assess benign lumps as mobile and round or oval; assess possible malignant lumps as fixed and irregularly shaped, often in the upper outer breast quadrant.
- A breast reduction is an option to promote comfort for women with very large, heavy breasts.
- A breast augmentation is an elective procedure for women with small breasts or for women who desire reconstruction after breast removal.
- After breast cancer surgery, assess vital signs, dressings, drainage tubes, and amount of drainage.
- Notify the health care team that the arm of the surgical mastectomy side should not be used for blood pressures, blood drawing, or injections. **Safety** QSEN
- Assess the return of arm and shoulder mobility after breast surgery and axillary dissection.
- Assess for the presence of lymphedema, and assist the patient to perform therapeutic measures to reduce lymphedema in the affected arm. **Safety** QSEN
- Teach the patient measures to prevent lymphedema after axillary node dissection.
- Observe for and report other complications of breast cancer surgery or breast reconstruction, especially infection and inadequate vascular perfusion. **Safety** QSEN
- After an axillary lymph node dissection, elevate the affected arm on a pillow.
- Radiation and drug therapy are used most often as adjuvant therapy after breast surgery but may be used before surgery to shrink the tumor.

71 | CHAPTER

Care of Patients with Gynecologic Problems

Donna D. Ignatavicius

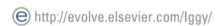 http://evolve.elsevier.com/Iggy/

PRIORITY CONCEPTS

- INFECTION
- PAIN
- SEXUALITY
- ELIMINATION

LEARNING OUTCOMES

Safe and Effective Care Environment
1. Collaborate with members of the health care team when providing care for patients with gynecologic cancers.
2. Teach patients about community-based resources for patients with gynecologic health problems.
3. Develop a community-based plan of care for patients with gynecologic cancers.

Health Promotion and Maintenance
4. Identify risk factors for gynecologic cancers.
5. Describe evidence-based health promotion and maintenance measures to help prevent or early-detect gynecologic cancers.

Psychosocial Integrity
6. Reduce the psychological impact for the patient who has received a diagnosis of a gynecologic health problem.

7. Discuss ways to help patients adapt to physical changes, including impaired SEXUALITY, caused by gynecologic problems and their treatment.

Physiological Integrity
8. Describe the mechanisms of action, side effects, and nursing implications of drug therapy for endometriosis.
9. Develop a teaching plan for a patient with a vaginal inflammation or INFECTION.
10. Prioritize care after surgery for the woman undergoing an anterior and/or posterior repair.
11. Develop a plan of care for a patient undergoing a hysterectomy.
12. Explain the purpose and side effects of radiation and chemotherapy for patients with gynecologic cancers.
13. Teach patients about complementary and alternative therapies that they may wish to explore.

Common gynecologic symptoms that women experience are PAIN, vaginal discharge, and bleeding. Some patients also have urinary ELIMINATION symptoms associated with their gynecologic problem. Women are often hesitant to seek medical attention for these problems because of fear of a life-threatening disease diagnosis or concern about privacy and dignity. Be sensitive to the woman's concerns and encourage discussion about menstrual or other reproductive problems. Teach women about their bodies, and help them recognize when professional help should be sought. Teach them how to make informed decisions about treatments. Assess the effects of gynecologic disorders on SEXUALITY in any setting. These health problems often impair sexual function and therefore can affect the woman's relationship with her partner. Remember that SEXUALITY affects a woman's sense of being, self-esteem, and body image.

ENDOMETRIOSIS

❖ PATHOPHYSIOLOGY

Endometriosis is endometrial (inner uterine) tissue implantation *outside* the uterine cavity. The tissue typically appears on

the ovaries and the cul-de-sac (posterior rectovaginal wall) and less commonly on other pelvic organs and structures (Fig. 71-1). A "chocolate" cyst, also called an *endometrioma,* is an area of endometriosis on an ovary. The disease affects millions of women in their 30s and 40s. Endometriosis responds to cyclic hormonal stimulation just as if it were in the uterus. Monthly cyclic bleeding occurs at the ectopic (out of place) site of implantation, which irritates and scars the surrounding tissue. Scarring can lead to adhesions, causing infertility (inability to become pregnant). Endometriosis progresses slowly and regresses during pregnancy and at menopause. The most common site for endometriosis is the ovaries (Saul, 2013). Although cancer of the endometrium is possible, simply having endometriosis does not mean that a patient is at high risk. Estrogen, tamoxifen, hereditary conditions, and amount of body fat are more strongly linked to development of endometrial cancer (National Cancer Institute [NCI], 2013a).

The cause of endometriosis is unknown. Retrograde menstruation, a condition in which the menstrual blood (which contains endometrial cells) may flow back through the fallopian tube, emptying into the pelvic cavity (instead of outside the

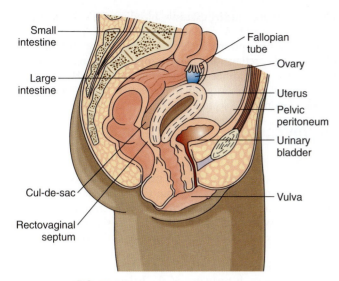

Small intestine

Large intestine

Cul-de-sac

Rectovaginal septum

Fallopian tube

Ovary

Uterus

Pelvic peritoneum

Urinary bladder

Vulva

FIG. 71-1 Common sites of endometriosis.

body), is thought to be a cause. The displaced cells stick to surfaces within the pelvic cavity and grow, thicken, and bleed during each menstrual cycle. Embryonic cell growth, surgical scar implantation, endometrial cell transport (via the lymphatic system), and immune system disorders are also thought to be possible causes for endometriosis (Mayo Clinic, 2013).

❖ PATIENT-CENTERED COLLABORATIVE CARE

◆ Assessment

Take a detailed history, including the woman's menstrual history, sexual history (including any patient concerns regarding history of abuse), and bleeding characteristics. A thorough menstrual history includes onset, duration, flow type and characteristics, and regularity. *PAIN is the most common symptom of endometriosis.* The pain usually peaks just before the menstrual flow. It is usually located in the lower abdomen, causing many women to feel a sense of rectal pressure. The degree of pain is not related to the extent of the endometriosis but, instead, to the site. Often, women with minimal disease have more severe pain than do women with extensive disease. Other manifestations include **dyspareunia** (painful sexual intercourse), painful defecation, low backache, and infertility. GI disturbances such as nausea and diarrhea are also common.

A pelvic examination performed by the health care provider may reveal pelvic tenderness, tender nodules in the posterior vagina, and limited movement of the uterus. A psychosocial assessment may reveal anxiety because of uncertainty about the diagnosis or frustration because of PAIN. The woman may also have concerns about her self-concept if she is infertile but wants to become pregnant.

Diagnostic tests may rule out pelvic inflammatory disease caused by chlamydia or gonorrhea. Serum cancer antigen *CA-125* may be positive in women with endometriosis (Mayo Clinic, 2011). Transvaginal ultrasound is used to determine whether pelvic masses are endometriosis or malignant.

◆ Interventions

Hormonal and surgical management may be used, depending on the symptoms, the extent of disease, the woman's desire for

childbearing, and her treatment option preferences. Collaborative care consists of interventions that:

- Reduce PAIN
- Restore sexual function
- Alleviate anxiety related to the disease and the uncertainty of the diagnosis
- Educate the patient about the disease and its treatment
- Alleviate fear related to the possibility of laparoscopy or surgery
- Prevent self-concept disturbance related to infertility

Nonsurgical Management. Several resources, such as the Endometriosis Association (www.endometriosisassn.org) and RESOLVE (an organization for infertile couples) (www.resolve.org), offer information on endometriosis that is helpful for patients and caregivers.

Menstrual cycle control using oral contraceptives or progestins, such as oral medroxyprogesterone acetate (Provera, Alti-MPA✤ Novo-Medrone❦) and norethindrone acetate (Aygestin, Norlutate❦), may be prescribed. Injectable forms of progestins, such as medroxyprogesterone acetate (Depo-Provera), may be more convenient because these drugs are given less frequently.

Continuous low-level heat using wearable heat packs may provide temporary PAIN relief. Relaxation techniques, yoga, massage, and biofeedback may decrease muscle tissue hypoxia and hypertonicity and relieve ischemia by increasing blood flow to the affected areas. Calcium and magnesium may also relieve muscle cramping for some patients.

Surgical Management. Surgical management of endometriosis for a woman who wants to remain fertile involves ablation, a laparoscopic removal of endometrial implants and adhesions, in a same-day surgical setting. Chapter 16 describes the general postoperative care for patients having surgery. The surgeon may use a laser to treat endometriosis by vaporizing adhesions and endometrial implants. Teach patients that temporary postoperative PAIN from carbon dioxide, used during laparoscopy to better visualize internal organs, can occur in the shoulders and chest.

DYSFUNCTIONAL UTERINE BLEEDING

❖ PATHOPHYSIOLOGY

Dysfunctional uterine bleeding (DUB) is excessive and frequent bleeding (more than every 21 days). It is a diagnosis of exclusion, made after ruling out anatomic or systemic conditions such as drug therapy or disease. DUB occurs most often at the beginning or end of a woman's reproductive years—when ovulation is becoming established or when it is becoming irregular at or after menopause.

Normally the menstrual cycle is a series of delicately timed hormonal events regulated by hypothalamic, pituitary, ovarian, and uterine functions. **Menses,** the sloughing of the endometrial lining, is an expected result. DUB occurs when there is a hormonal imbalance, generally when the ovaries fail to ovulate. This decreases progesterone production, which is needed to mature the uterine lining and prevent overgrowth. Without progesterone, prolonged estrogen stimulation causes the endometrium to grow past its hormonal support, causing disordered shedding of uterine lining. Most cases of DUB are classified into two types: anovulatory DUB (most common) and ovulatory DUB. Common risk factors for DUB during the reproductive years are listed in Table 71-1.

TABLE 71-1   **Risk Factors for Dysfunctional Uterine Bleeding**

- Obesity
- Extreme weight loss or gain
- Age older than 40 years
- High stress levels
- Polycystic ovary disease
- Long-term drug use (e.g., oral contraceptives)
- Excessive exercise

❖ PATIENT-CENTERED COLLABORATIVE CARE

◆ Assessment

Take a complete menstrual history. Ask about illnesses, changes in weight or nutritional intake, exercise, drug ingestion, and whether the woman experiences PAIN.

Assess for symptoms of anemia or systemic disease, such as:

- Renal or hepatic disease
- Abnormal weight
- Signs of hormonal dysfunction, such as thyroid enlargement or male hair pattern
- Evidence of abdominal PAIN or masses

The health care provider inspects the external genitalia, does a bimanual pelvic examination, performs a Papanicolaou (Pap) test to assess for the presence of cervical cancer, and does a rectal examination to identify INFECTIONS, lesions, or tenderness. Vaginal specimens are also tested for sexually transmitted diseases (STDs) such as chlamydia. Women at high risk for endometrial cancer should also have an endometrial biopsy. Risk factors are described later in this chapter.

A complete blood count may be taken to determine whether the patient is anemic. Thyroid-stimulating hormone and reproductive hormone levels may also be evaluated.

Transvaginal ultrasound may reveal leiomyomas (fibroids) and measure an excessively thick endometrium. *Sonohysterography* uses vaginal ultrasound to visualize the uterus after sterile saline is infused through the cervix, thus outlining the inner uterine cavity (American Congress of Obstetricians and Gynecologists [ACOG], 2011).

◆ Interventions

Nonsurgical Management. As with endometriosis, hormone manipulation is usually the treatment of choice for women with anovulatory DUB. The drugs used depend on the severity of bleeding and age of the patient. Progestin or combination hormone therapy (estrogen and progestin) may be given when bleeding is heavy and acute. For nonemergent bleeding, contraceptives (oral or patch) provide the progestin (artificial progesterone) needed to stabilize the endometrial lining. Progestin-only pills (e.g., norethindrone [Aygestin, Norlutate ◆]) or long-acting progestins (e.g., injectable medroxyprogesterone acetate [Depo-Provera]) are preferable for women older than 35 years who smoke or are at risk for thrombophlebitis.

Explain the desired outcomes and the side effects of these drugs, and evaluate the woman's knowledge of the effects, dosage, and schedule. Remind her to take the drug exactly as prescribed and not to skip a dose or run out of it. If bleeding worsens, teach her to call her health care provider immediately.

Surgical Management. Removal of the built-up uterine lining, called endometrial ablation, stops the blood flow to fibroids that are causing excessive bleeding. This is a safe alternative for women who do not respond to medical management. Other invasive options include uterine artery embolization, dilation and curettage, and hysterectomy. A hysterectomy is performed only after other treatments have failed. (Hysterectomy is discussed under Surgical Management on p. 1489 of the Uterine Leiomyoma section.)

VULVOVAGINITIS

❖ PATHOPHYSIOLOGY

Vaginal discharge and itching are two common problems experienced by most women at some time in their lives. Vaginal INFECTIONS may be transmitted sexually and non-sexually. Gonorrhea, syphilis, chlamydia, and herpes simplex virus infections are sexually transmitted diseases (STDs) discussed in Chapter 74.

Vulvovaginitis is inflammation of the lower genital tract resulting from a disturbance of the balance of hormones and flora in the vagina and vulva. It may be characterized by itching, change in vaginal discharge, odor, or lesions. The most common causes include:

- Fungal (yeast) INFECTIONS (*Candida albicans*)
- Bacterial vaginosis
- STDs (*Trichomonas vaginalis*)
- Postmenopausal vaginal atrophy
- Changes in the normal flora or pH (from douching)
- Chemical irritant or allergens (vaginal spray, fabric dyes, detergent) or foreign body (tampon)
- Drugs, especially antibiotics
- Immunosuppression from diabetes or human immune deficiency virus (HIV)

Primary INFECTIONS that affect the vulva include *herpes genitalis* and *condylomata acuminata* (human papilloma virus, venereal warts) (see Chapter 74). Secondary infections of the vulva are caused by organisms responsible for the many types of vaginitis, including *candidiasis*. Pediculosis pubis (crab lice, or "crabs") and scabies (itch mite) are common parasitic infestations of the skin of the vulva. Other causes of vulvitis include:

- Atrophic vaginitis
- Lichen planus (thickened, leathery skin from scratching)
- Vulvar leukoplakia (postmenopausal atrophy and thickening of vulvar tissues)
- Vulvar cancer
- Urinary incontinence

Some women may have an *itch-scratch-itch cycle,* in which the itching leads to scratching, which causes excoriation that then must heal. As healing takes place, itching occurs again. If the cycle is not interrupted, the chronic scratching may lead to the white, thickened skin of lichen planus. This dry, leathery skin cracks easily, increasing the risk for infection.

❖ PATIENT-CENTERED COLLABORATIVE CARE

Assess for vulvovaginitis by asking questions about the symptoms, assisting with a pelvic examination, and obtaining vaginal smears for laboratory testing. Ask if the patient is experiencing an itching or burning sensation, erythema (redness), edema, and/or superficial skin ulcers. Use a nonjudgmental approach and provide reassurance during the assessment because the patient may be embarrassed or afraid to discuss her symptoms.

CHART 71-1 Patient and Family Education: Preparing for Self-Management
Vaginal Infections

- Your risk for getting vaginal infections increases if you have sex with more than one person.
- When you have a vaginal infection, do not have sexual intercourse, if possible, or at least make sure that your partner wears a condom.
- All sexual partners may need to be treated for infection.
- The only way to identify what infection you have is to be examined by a health care provider and to follow up to get the results of laboratory tests.
- Take all of your medicine as prescribed, not just until your symptoms go away.

CHART 71-2 Patient and Family Education: Preparing for Self-Management
Prevention of Vulvovaginitis

- Wear cotton underwear.
- Avoid wearing tight clothing, such as pantyhose or tight jeans, because they can cause chafing. You can also get hot and sweaty, which can increase the risk for infection.
- Always wipe front to back after having a bowel movement or urinating.
- During bath or shower, cleanse inner labial mucosa with water, not soap.
- Do not douche or use feminine hygiene sprays.
- If your sexual partner has an infection of the sex organs, do not have intercourse with him or her until he or she has been treated.
- You are more likely to get an infection if you are pregnant, have diabetes, take oral contraceptive drugs, or are menopausal.
- Practice vulvar self-examination monthly.

Encourage her to talk about her problem and its effect on her sexual health.

Interventions for vulvovaginitis depend on the specific vaginal INFECTION. Proper health habits can benefit treatment. Instruct the patient to get enough rest and sleep, observe good dietary habits, exercise regularly, and use good personal hygiene. Teach her about how to manage her infection (Chart 71-1) and how to prevent further infections (Chart 71-2).

Wet compresses, warm or tepid sitz baths for 30 minutes several times a day, and topical drugs such as estrogens and lidocaine can help relieve itching. Encourage the patient to wear breathable fabrics such as cotton and to avoid irritants or allergens in products such as laundry detergents or bath products.

Treatment of pediculosis and scabies is used if needed and includes:

- Applying lindane (Kwell, Kwellada ✦) lotion, shampoo, or cream to the affected area as directed
- Cleaning affected clothes, bedding, and towels
- Disinfecting the home environment (lice cannot live for more than 24 hours away from the body)

CHART 71-3 Patient and Family Education: Preparing for Self-Management
Prevention of Toxic Shock Syndrome

- Wash your hands before inserting a tampon.
- Do not use a tampon if it is dirty.
- Insert the tampon carefully to avoid injuring the delicate tissue in your vagina.
- Change your tampon every 3 to 6 hours.
- Do not use superabsorbent tampons.
- Use sanitary napkins (instead of tampons) at night.
- Call your health care provider if you suddenly experience a high temperature, vomiting, or diarrhea.
- Do not use tampons at all if you have had toxic shock syndrome.
- Not using tampons almost guarantees that you will not get toxic shock syndrome.

❓ NCLEX EXAMINATION CHALLENGE
Health Promotion and Maintenance

A client tells the nurse that she has vaginal itching. Which client statement would cause the nurse to further assess for symptoms of vaginitis? **Select all that apply.**
A. "I always use the same detergent when washing clothes."
B. "All of my immunizations, including Gardasil, are up to date."
C. "I've scratched so hard that it gets raw, but then it feels better for awhile."
D. "My boyfriend and I broke up last month, but we are together again now."
E. "My health care provider prescribed antibiotics for my sinus infection last week."

TOXIC SHOCK SYNDROME

❖ *PATHOPHYSIOLOGY*

Toxic shock syndrome (TSS) can result from menstruation and tampon use. Other conditions associated with TSS include surgical wound INFECTION, nonsurgical infections, gynecologic surgeries, and use of internal contraceptives.

In INFECTION related to menstruation, menstrual blood provides a growth medium for *Staphylococcus aureus* (or, less frequently, Group A *Streptococcus* [GAS], also known as *Streptococcus pyogenes*). Exotoxins produced from the bacteria cross the vaginal mucosa to the bloodstream via microabrasions from tampon insertion or prolonged use. TSS can be fatal. Extensive public education has led to a decreased number of women developing the infection.

❖ *PATIENT-CENTERED COLLABORATIVE CARE*

TSS usually develops within 5 days after the onset of menstruation. Most common symptoms include fever, rash, myalgias, sore throat, edema, and hypotension (Low, 2013). The rash associated with TSS often looks like a sunburn, and patients often develop broken capillaries in the eyes and skin. Educate all women on prevention of TSS (Chart 71-3).

Treatment includes removal of the INFECTION source, such as a tampon; restoring fluid and electrolyte balance; administering drugs to manage hypotension; and IV antibiotics. Other measures may include transfusions to reverse low platelet counts and corticosteroids to treat skin changes.

PELVIC ORGAN PROLAPSE

❖ *PATHOPHYSIOLOGY*

The pelvic organs are supported by a sling of muscles and tendons, which sometimes become weak and no longer able to hold an organ in place. **Uterine prolapse,** the most common type of **pelvic organ prolapse (POP),** can be caused by neuromuscular damage of childbirth; increased intra-abdominal

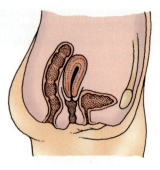

In **grade I uterine prolapse**, the uterus bulges into the vagina, but the cervix does not protrude through the entrance to the vagina.

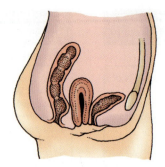

In **grade II uterine prolapse**, the uterus bulges farther into the vagina, and the cervix protrudes through the entrance to the vagina.

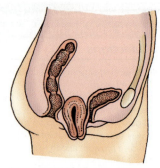

In **grade III uterine prolapse**, the body of the uterus and the cervix protrude through the entrance to the vagina. The vagina is turned inside out.

FIG. 71-2 Types of uterine prolapse.

Cystocele

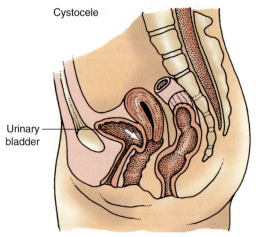

Urinary bladder

Rectocele

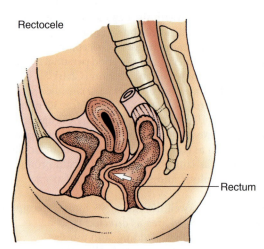

Rectum

FIG. 71-3 In cystocele, the urinary bladder is displaced downward, causing bulging of the anterior vaginal wall. In rectocele, the rectum is displaced, causing bulging of the posterior vaginal wall.

pressure related to pregnancy, obesity, or physical exertion; or weakening of pelvic support due to decreased estrogen. The stages of uterine prolapse are described by the degree of descent of the uterus (Fig. 71-2) through the pelvic floor.

Whenever the uterus is displaced, other structures such as the bladder, rectum, and small intestine can protrude through the vaginal walls (Fig. 71-3). A **cystocele** is a protrusion of the bladder through the vaginal wall (urinary bladder prolapse), which can lead to stress urinary incontinence (SUI) and urinary tract infections (UTIs). A **rectocele** is a protrusion of the rectum through a weakened vaginal wall (rectal prolapse).

❖ PATIENT-CENTERED COLLABORATIVE CARE

◆ Assessment

Patients with suspected uterine prolapse may report a feeling of "something falling out," dyspareunia (painful intercourse), backache, and heaviness or pressure in the pelvis. A pelvic examination may reveal a protrusion of the cervix or anterior vaginal wall when the woman is asked to bear down. Listen to her concerns, and note signs of anxiety or depression from having long-term symptoms.

Ask the patient whether she has urinary ELIMINATION problems, such as difficulty emptying her bladder, urinary frequency

and urgency, a urinary tract infection, or **stress urinary incontinence (SUI)** (loss of urine during activities that increase intra-abdominal pressure, such as laughing, coughing, sneezing, or lifting heavy objects). These symptoms may be associated with a *cystocele* (bladder prolapse).

Diagnostic tests include cystography (to show the presence of bladder herniation), measurement of residual urine by bladder ultrasound, and urine culture and sensitivity testing. Radiographic imaging of urinary anatomy and voiding function is useful in determining the degree of *cystocele* (prolapse).

Rectocele assessment usually includes symptoms of constipation, hemorrhoids, fecal impaction, and feelings of rectal or vaginal fullness. A vaginal and rectal examination may show a bulge of the posterior vaginal wall when the woman is asked to bear down.

◆ Interventions

Interventions are based on the degree of the POP. Conservative treatment is preferred over surgical treatment when possible.

Nonsurgical Management. Teach women to improve pelvic support and tone by doing pelvic floor muscle exercises (PFMEs, or Kegel exercises). Space-filling devices such as pessaries or spheres can be worn in the vagina to elevate the uterine prolapse. Intravaginal estrogen therapy may be prescribed for the postmenopausal woman to prevent atrophy and weakening of vaginal walls. Women with bladder symptoms may benefit from bladder training and attention to complete emptying. Management of a rectocele focuses on promoting bowel elimination. The health care provider usually prescribes a high-fiber diet, stool softeners, and laxatives.

Surgical Management. Surgery may be recommended for severe symptoms of POP, with preference given to the least invasive approach. Address the fears and concerns of the patient and her family.

Transvaginal repair for pelvic organ prolapse (POP) using surgical vaginal mesh or tape is a commonly performed minimally invasive technique. It is particularly useful for women who are very obese. Depending on the procedure that is planned, the patient has either local or general anesthesia. The surgeon creates a sling with the mesh or tape, and the woman is discharged the same day. Procedures done under local anesthesia can be done in the surgeon's office. Since 2008, patient report of complications associated with the use of transvaginal mesh has required the U.S. Food and Drug Administration (2011) to release an initial report and update advising about the safety and effectiveness of the use of this product for POP. Complications associated with the use of transvaginal mesh for POP include vaginal mesh erosion, painful sexual intercourse, infection, urinary ELIMINATION problems, bleeding, and organ perforation (U.S. Food and Drug Administration [USFDA], 2011). Three deaths associated with this procedure (two bowel perforations and one hemorrhage) were also reported between 2008 and 2010 (USFDA, 2011).

! NURSING SAFETY PRIORITY (QSEN)

Action Alert

To help the patient decide if she should have any surgical procedure using mesh or tape, be sure that she is provided with information regarding informed consent prior to surgery. Reinforce information about possible adverse events, the signs and symptoms of infection, and when she should contact her surgeon. Provide the patient with the manufacturer's labeling and written information.

Teach patients who have had the mesh or tape procedure to avoid strenuous exercise, heavy lifting, and sexual intercourse for 6 weeks. After 6 weeks, the patient may gradually begin to return to regular activities but must be educated about prevention of increasing intra-abdominal pressure (e.g., constipation, weight-lifting, cigarette smoking) for a minimum of 3 months to allow proper healing and prevent POP recurrence (Lazarou, 2012).

Alternatives to minimally invasive surgery are open surgical techniques. An **anterior colporrhaphy** (anterior repair) tightens the pelvic muscles for better *bladder* support. A vaginal surgical approach is used and may be done as a laparoscopic-assisted procedure. Nursing care for a woman undergoing an anterior repair is similar to that for a woman undergoing a vaginal hysterectomy.

After surgery, instruct the patient how to splint her abdomen to protect sutures and to limit her activities. Teach her to *avoid lifting anything heavier than 5 pounds, strenuous exercises, and sexual intercourse for 6 weeks.* For discomfort, she may use heat either as a moist heating pad or warm compresses applied to the abdomen. A hot bath may also be helpful. Sutures do not

need to be removed because some are absorbable and others will fall out as healing occurs. Tell the woman to notify her health care provider if she has signs of INFECTION, such as fever, persistent PAIN, or purulent, foul-smelling discharge. Encourage her to keep her follow-up appointment after surgery.

Posterior colporrhaphy (posterior repair) reduces *rectal* bulging. If both a cystocele and a rectocele are present, an *anterior and posterior colporrhaphy (A&P repair)* is performed.

The nursing care after a posterior repair is similar to that after any rectal surgery. After surgery, a low-residue (low-fiber) diet is usually prescribed to decrease bowel movements and allow time for the incision to heal. Instruct the patient to avoid straining when she does have a bowel movement so that she does not put pressure on the suture line. Bowel movements are often painful, and she may need pain medication before having a stool. Provide sitz baths or delegate this activity to unlicensed nursing personnel to relieve the woman's discomfort. Health teaching for the patient undergoing a posterior repair is similar to that for the patient undergoing an anterior repair. Vaginal hysterectomy may accompany any uterine prolapse repair surgery unless the woman wants to become pregnant. This procedure is described on p. 1489.

BENIGN NEOPLASMS

OVARIAN CYST

Functional ovarian cysts can occur in a woman of any age but are rare after menopause. Other cysts and tumors of the ovaries are not related to the menstrual cycle but arise from ovarian tissue. Primary assessment involves pelvic examination and transvaginal ultrasound. Further testing with CT, MRI, or laparoscopic biopsy to rule out cancer may be needed. Some ovarian cysts disappear over time, and others cause discomfort for a prolonged period. Laparoscopic surgery to remove the cyst or ovary may be needed.

UTERINE LEIOMYOMA

❖ PATHOPHYSIOLOGY

Leiomyomas, also called **fibroids** or **myomas**, are benign, slow-growing solid tumors of the uterine myometrium (muscle layer). They are classified according to their position in the layers of the uterus: intramural, submucosal, and subserosal (Fig. 71-4).

Intramural leiomyomas are contained in the uterine wall within the myometrium. *Submucosal* leiomyomas protrude into the cavity of the uterus and can cause bleeding and disrupt pregnancy. *Subserosal* leiomyomas protrude through the outer surface of the uterine wall and may extend to the broad ligament, pressing other organs (McCance et al., 2014).

Although most fibroids develop within the uterine wall, a few may appear in the cervix. Pedunculated leiomyomas are attached by a pedicle (stalk) to the outside of the uterus and occasionally break off and attach to other tissues (parasitic fibroids).

Although the cause is not known, leiomyomas develop from excessive local growth of smooth muscle cells. This may be a genetic error causing a lack of ability to halt growth. The growth of leiomyomas may be related to stimulation by estrogen, progesterone, and growth hormone. This explains why fibroids sometimes enlarge during pregnancy and diminish in size after menopause.

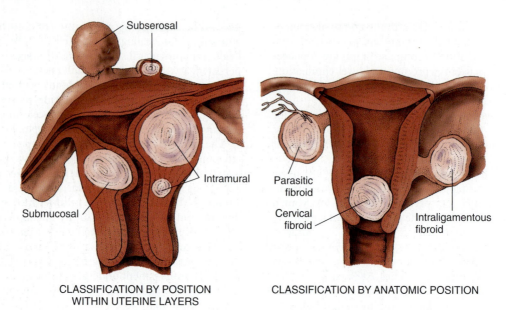

CLASSIFICATION BY POSITION
WITHIN UTERINE LAYERS

CLASSIFICATION BY ANATOMIC POSITION

FIG. 71-4 Classification of uterine leiomyomas.

The incidence of leiomyomas increases as women get older. Women who have never been pregnant also are at a high risk. Many women have asymptomatic fibroids, whereas others have severe symptoms.

❖ PATIENT-CENTERED COLLABORATIVE CARE

◆ Assessment

Women with fibroids usually do not have pain, although acute PAIN may occur with twisting of the fibroid on its stalk. *The patient often seeks medical attention because of heavy vaginal bleeding.* Ask about how many tampons or menstrual pads she uses a day. She may report a feeling of pelvic pressure, constipation, or urinary frequency or retention. These symptoms result when an enlarged fibroid presses on other organs. The patient may notice that her abdomen has increased in size. Assess the woman's abdomen for distention or enlargement. Ask if she has dyspareunia (painful intercourse) and/or infertility (inability to become pregnant).

Abdominal, vaginal, and rectal examinations usually reveal the presence of a uterine enlargement. Further diagnostic procedures are needed to differentiate benign tumors from cancerous ones.

Symptoms such as dyspareunia may significantly lower the patient's quality of life. A woman who is symptomatic may fear that she has cancer or may have anxiety about abnormal bleeding or her failure to conceive. She may also be concerned if surgery is recommended if she desires pregnancy. Assess the woman's feelings and concerns about her symptoms and fears of the unknown. If hysterectomy is recommended, explore the significance of the loss of the uterus for the woman and her partner. Discuss SEXUALITY issues with the patient based on your assessment.

A complete blood count may identify iron deficiency anemia (related to bleeding). A pregnancy test is done to determine whether pregnancy is the cause of the uterine enlargement. An endometrial biopsy may be performed to evaluate for endometrial cancer.

Transvaginal ultrasound alone or with saline infusion (saline sonogram) provides a picture of a submucosal fibroid that may

protrude into the uterine cavity. The health care provider may then choose to directly view a tumor and perform a biopsy using *laparoscopy* (for tumors on the outside of the uterus) or *hysteroscopy* (for tumors accessible inside the uterus). *MRI* can differentiate between benign and malignant lesions.

◆ Interventions

Asymptomatic fibroids do not need treatment. Management depends on the size and location of the tumor and the woman's desire for future pregnancy. Women who still desire pregnancy can take drug therapy or have magnetic resonance–guided focused ultrasound surgery or laparoscopic myomectomy to remove the tumor. Uterine artery embolization and hysterectomy are choices for women who no longer desire pregnancy.

Nonsurgical Management. If the woman is menopausal, the fibroids usually shrink and surgery may not be necessary. *Teach the patient who is receiving hormone replacement therapy for menopausal symptoms that the fibroids may continue to grow because of estrogen stimulation.*

If the woman has few symptoms or desires childbearing, the health care provider may recommend intermittent observation and examination. As with dysfunctional uterine bleeding, mild leiomyoma symptoms can be managed with oral contraception.

Magnetic resonance–guided focused ultrasound is a noninvasive, painless technique for women with few smaller fibroids who wish to preserve their fertility. The woman lies prone on an MRI scanner, which provides a three-dimensional image of the pelvis. The radiologic clinician then guides a focused pulse of ultrasound to heat the tumor to destroy it.

An alternative to surgery for the woman who does not desire pregnancy is **uterine artery embolization** (also called *uterine fibroid embolization [UFE]*) under conscious sedation. The interventional radiologist uses a percutaneous catheter inserted through the femoral artery to inject polyvinyl alcohol pellets into the uterine artery. The resulting blockage starves the tumor of circulation, allowing it (or them) to shrink.

Before discharge, tell the patient to observe for post-embolectomy syndrome—a flu-like illness that some women develop that lasts about 5 to 7 days (Northwest Radiology

! **NURSING SAFETY PRIORITY** (QSEN)

Action Alert

After uterine artery embolization, the woman may have severe cramping within the first 24 hours caused by decreased blood flow to the uterus. Cramping can last from a few days to 2 weeks. Assess her pain level, and provide analgesics as needed. If a vascular closure device is used at the arterial insertion site (most commonly), raise the head of the bed. Help the patient ambulate in about 2 hours after the procedure. If a closure device was not used, keep her on bedrest with the legs immobilized for 4 hours before ambulating to prevent bleeding. Patients generally recover quickly, returning to normal activities within 7 to 10 days after the procedure (Storck, 2012.)

Associates, 2014). Teach her to resume usual activities slowly. Most patients can return to work or daily routine within a week. She should avoid strenuous activity until the physician recommends it.

Surgical Management. When possible, minimally invasive surgical (MIS) techniques are performed, such as a myomectomy. If not, a hysterectomy is the procedure of choice.

Uterus-Sparing Surgeries. If the woman desires children, the surgeon may perform a laparoscopic or hysteroscopic **myomectomy** (the removal of leiomyomas from the uterus) (Bradley, 2013). During this procedure, a laser may be used to remove the tumors. This minimally invasive procedure is usually performed in the early phase of the menstrual cycle to minimize blood loss and to avoid the possibility of interrupting an unsuspected pregnancy. A small percentage of leiomyomas recur after surgery. Scarring makes the uterus more likely to rupture during labor, so future deliveries will be planned cesarean deliveries. Nursing care is similar to that for a woman undergoing a hysterectomy (see below).

In selected cases (e.g., submucous fibroids, menorrhagia), a *transcervical endometrial resection (TCER)* is performed via hysteroscopy. A hysteroscope (endoscope) is inserted into the uterus, and the endometrium is destroyed using diathermy (heat) or radioablation.

! **NURSING SAFETY PRIORITY** (QSEN)

Critical Rescue

Monitor for rare but potential complications of hysteroscopic surgery, which include:
- Fluid overload (fluid used to distend the uterine cavity can be absorbed)
- Embolism
- Hemorrhage
- Perforation of the uterus, bowel, or bladder and ureter injury
- Persistent increased menstrual bleeding
- Incomplete suppression of menstruation

Monitor for any indications of these problems, and report signs and symptoms, such as severe pain and heavy bleeding, to the surgeon immediately. Scarring may cause a small risk for complications in future pregnancies.

Hysterectomy. Leiomyomas are the most common reason for hysterectomies. Hysterectomies may be performed abdominally, vaginally, or with laparoscopic or robotic assistance based on the patient's clinical reason for hysterectomy and the surgeon's area of technical expertise (Falcone, 2014).

A *total abdominal hysterectomy (TAH)* is usually performed for leiomyomas larger than the size of a 16-week pregnancy. The

TABLE 71-2 Common Gynecologic Surgeries

Total Hysterectomy
All of the uterus, including the cervix, is removed. The procedure may be vaginal or abdominal, with laparoscopic or robotic assistance.

Bilateral Salpingo-Oophorectomy (BSO)
Fallopian tubes and ovaries are removed.

Panhysterectomy
Total abdominal hysterectomy and BSO: The uterus, ovaries, and fallopian tubes are removed.

Radical Hysterectomy
The uterus, cervix, adjacent lymph nodes, the upper third of the vagina, and the surrounding tissues (parametrium) are removed.

uterus and cervix are most often removed by laparoscopic-assisted minimally invasive surgery (MIS), which requires one or more very small umbilical incisions. The traditional open surgery is performed through a horizontal bikini incision. A *total vaginal hysterectomy (TVH)* requires no skin incision because the uterus is removed through the vagina.

Some surgeons use robotic technology to assist in performing a TAH, although it is much more expensive than a traditional vaginal or laparoscopic approach (ACOG, 2013). Robotic surgery is helpful when performing hysterectomies on patients who are extremely obese (Gallo et al., 2012). In both vaginal and abdominal hysterectomies, the surgeon removes the uterus from the five supporting ligaments, which are then attached to the vaginal cuff so that normal depth of the vagina is maintained (Table 71-2).

Preoperative teaching by the health care team begins in the surgeon's office. Explain procedures that routinely take place before surgery, including laboratory tests and expected drugs such as a prophylactic antibiotic. Depending on the type of surgical technique planned, teach about the need for turning, coughing, and deep-breathing exercises; incentive spirometry; early ambulation; and PAIN relief. (See Chapter 14 for a discussion of general patient care before surgery.)

Psychological assessment is essential. Assess the significance of the surgery for the woman and her partner related to SEXUALITY. If it involves loss of the uterus, she may feel a great loss if she wishes to become pregnant. Many women relate their uterus to self-image and femininity or believe that their sexual function is related to their uterus. Although surgical menopause by hysterectomy can create loss of libido and vaginal changes if the ovaries are also removed, teach the patient that vaginal estrogen cream and gentle dilation can help correct that. Reassure her regarding any misperceptions about the effects of hysterectomy, such as association with masculinization and weight gain. Assess the patient's support system. She may fear rejection by her sexual partner. Include the partner in all teaching sessions (if the patient prefers) unless this practice is not culturally acceptable.

Patients who have *uterus-sparing surgeries* usually go home the same day of surgery. They often experience less postoperative PAIN and fewer complications when compared with patients who have their uterus and cervix removed. Teach patients that they usually return to usual daily activities in 2 weeks but sexual intercourse should be avoided for at least 6 weeks.

Postoperative care of the woman who has undergone a *TAH* is similar to that of any patient who has had laparoscopic or

CHART 71-4 Focused Assessment

Postoperative Nursing Care of the Patient after Total Abdominal Hysterectomy

- Assess cardiovascular, respiratory, renal, and gastrointestinal status, including:
  - Vital signs
  - Heart, lung, and bowel sounds
  - Urine output
  - Temperature and color of the skin
  - Red blood cell, hemoglobin, and hematocrit levels
  - Activity tolerance
  - Dressing and drains for color and amount of drainage
  - Perineal pads for vaginal bleeding and clots
  - Fluid intake (IVs until peristalsis returns and patient is tolerating oral intake)
- Teach the patient to use these interventions to prevent postoperative complications:
  - Cough and deep-breathing exercises
  - Incentive spirometry
  - Sequential compression devices
  - Ambulation
  - Avoidance of heavy lifting or strenuous activity
  - Adequate hydration
- Assess the home care teaching needs of the patient related to the illness and surgery, including:
  - Physiologic effects of the surgery
  - Signs or symptoms to report
  - Side or toxic effects of medications
  - Activity limitations related to driving and use of stairs
  - Follow-up care
  - Postoperative restrictions related to sexual activity, use of tampons, and bathing
  - Care of wound and/or drains
- Assess the patient's coping skills and reaction to the diagnosis and surgical procedure.

CHART 71-5 Patient and Family Education: Preparing for Self-Management

Care after a Total Vaginal or Abdominal Hysterectomy

Expected Physical Changes
- You will no longer have a period, although you may have some vaginal discharge for a few days after you go home.
- It will not be possible for you to become pregnant, and birth control methods are no longer needed. (Condoms should still be used to decrease the chance of getting a sexually transmitted disease [STD].)
- If your ovaries were removed, you may have some menopause symptoms such as hot flushes, night sweats, and vaginal dryness.
- It is normal to tire more easily and require more sleep and rest during the first few weeks after surgery.

Activity
- Limit stair climbing to fewer than 5 times per day.
- Do not lift anything heavier than 5 to 10 lbs.
- Gradually increase walking as exercise, but stop before you become fatigued.
- Avoid the sitting position for any extended period. When you sit, do not cross your legs at the knees.
- Avoid jogging, aerobic exercise, participating in sports, and any strenuous activity for 2 to 6 weeks, depending on what type of surgical procedure was performed.
- Do not drive until your surgeon has told you it is alright.

Sexual Activity
- Do not engage in sexual intercourse for 4 to 6 weeks or as prescribed by your surgeon.
- If you had a vaginal "repair" as part of your surgery, the first time you have intercourse you may have some tenderness or pain because the vaginal walls are tighter. Careful intercourse and the use of water-based lubricants can help reduce this discomfort. This discomfort usually goes away with time and stretching of the vagina.

Complications
- Take your temperature twice each day for the first 3 days after surgery. Report fevers of over 100°F (38°C).
- Check your incision, if you have any, daily for signs of infection (increasing redness, open areas, drainage that is thick or foul-smelling, incision pain).

Symptoms to Report to Your Surgeon
- Increased vaginal drainage or change in drainage (bloodier, thicker, foul-smelling)
- Temperature over 100°F (38°C)
- Pain, tenderness, redness, or swelling in your calves
- Pain or burning on urination

traditional open abdominal surgery (see Chapter 16). Assess (Chart 71-4):
- Vaginal bleeding (there should be less than one saturated perineal pad in 4 hours)
- Abdominal bleeding at the incision site(s) (a small amount is normal)
- Intactness of the incision(s)
- Urine output per urinary catheter for 24 hours or less (for open surgery only)
- PAIN

Specific postoperative interventions for a *vaginal hysterectomy* include:
- Assessment of vaginal bleeding (there should be less than one saturated pad in 4 hours)
- Urinary catheter care
- Perineal care

❓ NCLEX EXAMINATION CHALLENGE

Physiological Integrity

A client returns from surgery after a total vaginal hysterectomy. Upon initial assessment, which finding by the nurse requires immediate intervention?
A. Clean, intact dressing
B. Excessive vaginal bleeding
C. Temperature of 99°F
D. Client statement that pain is "4" on scale of 0-10

Community-Based Care

If the patient had a hysterectomy, teach her to limit stair climbing for several weeks. If she lives alone and is not permitted to drive for several weeks, she may need to arrange for transportation for follow-up surgical visits.

Teach the woman who has undergone an abdominal hysterectomy about the expected physical changes, any activity restrictions, diet, sexual activity, wound care, complications, and the need for follow-up care. Chart 71-5 lists areas to include for health teaching.

Generally, women are more accepting of surgery if they have completed childbearing, have interests outside the home, work, have no misconceptions about the effects of hysterectomy, and have support from the family, especially their sexual partner. Psychological reactions can occur months to years after surgery, particularly if sexual functioning and libido are diminished. Women identified as being at high risk for psychological problems may need long-term follow-up care or referral. They may need to be counseled about signs of depression. Intermittent sadness is normal, but continued feelings of low self-esteem or loss of interest or pleasure in usual activities and pastimes is not expected and should be evaluated. Provide written materials, and focus on the positive aspects of the woman's life to help decrease adverse psychological reactions.

BARTHOLIN CYST

Bartholin cyst is a common disorder of the vulva. It results from obstruction of the duct of the Bartholin gland. The secretory function of the gland continues, and the fluid fills the obstructed duct. The main causes of the obstruction are INFECTION, thickened mucus near the ductal opening, or trauma, such as lacerations.

The patient may be asymptomatic if the cyst is small. Ask if she has dyspareunia (painful intercourse) or inadequate genital lubrication. Assess for swelling in the perineal area. A large cyst usually causes constant local pain and may cause difficulty walking or sitting. Assessment of the vulva reveals a unilateral swelling immediately beneath the skin in the posterior portion of the vulva. The cyst may appear brown or bloody, depending on its contents. Vaginal discharge may be present with a Bartholin *abscess* if an infection, such as one caused by a sexually transmitted organism, is present (Braun, 2014).

If the cyst is draining, a fluid sample is sent to the laboratory to culture for gonorrhea and/or other organisms. If the woman is older than 40 years, a biopsy of the cyst may be done to identify possible cancer.

If the woman is asymptomatic, no intervention is needed. An abscess usually ruptures spontaneously within 72 hours of forming. Teach the patient to take over-the-counter or prescribed analgesics and apply moist heat (sitz baths or hot wet packs) to the vulva. Cultures most often reveal *Escherichia coli* or *S. aureus,* for which antibiotics are prescribed.

Simple incision and drainage (I&D) may provide temporary relief. However, cysts tend to recur when the opening of the duct re-obstructs. Usually the surgeon establishes a permanent opening for drainage. Marsupialization (formation of a pouch that is a new duct opening) is performed using local, regional, or general anesthesia. Discomfort after surgery may be relieved with analgesics and sitz baths. Prophylactic antibiotics may be prescribed.

The Bartholin glands may be totally removed in older women when cancer is suspected or if infections with abscess formation recur. Care after surgery includes:

- Application of ice packs or sitz baths several times a day for comfort and promotion of healing
- Analgesics for PAIN
- Prophylactic antibiotics
- Assessment of the incision for signs of healing or INFECTION

CERVICAL POLYP

Cervical polyps are *pedunculated* (on stalks) tumors that arise from the mucosa and extend through the opening of the cervical os. Although the cause is not completely understood, they may result from a hyperplasia (overgrowth) of the endocervical epithelium in response to estrogen, chronic inflammation, and/or clogged blood vessels in the cervix (Storck, 2014). Polyps may also be due to inflammation or to localized vascular congestion of the cervical blood vessels. They are the most common benign growth of the cervix and occur most often in women older than 40 years who have had several children.

Some patients are asymptomatic; others may have premenstrual or postmenstrual bleeding, experience bleeding after douching or intercourse, and/or have leukorrhea (white or yellow mucus) (Storck, 2014). A speculum examination may reveal a small single polyp or multiple polyps. They are bright red, are soft and fragile, and may bleed when touched.

Polyp removal is usually accomplished as a simple office procedure. The base of the polyp is grasped with a clamp, and the polyp is gently twisted off and sent to the pathology laboratory for evaluation. Cautery usually stops any bleeding at the site of removal and is also effective when removing larger polyps (Storck, 2014). The woman does not feel any pain during the procedure. Instruct her to avoid tampon use, douches, and sexual intercourse for a week or until healing has taken place.

GYNECOLOGIC CANCERS

ENDOMETRIAL (UTERINE) CANCER

❖ *PATHOPHYSIOLOGY*

Endometrial cancer (cancer of the inner uterine lining) is the most common gynecologic malignancy (Nguyen et al., 2013). This chapter includes two other common gynecologic cancers, but the disease can affect any organ in the reproductive tract.

Endometrial cancer grows slowly in most cases, and early symptoms of vaginal bleeding generally lead to prompt evaluation and treatment. As a result, this type of cancer has a good prognosis. *Adenocarcinoma* is the most common type of tumor. It arises from the glandular part of the endometrium and usually follows endometrial hyperplasia (overgrowth).

The initial growth of the cancer is within the uterine cavity, followed by extension into the myometrium and the cervix. Stage I endometrial cancer is confined to the endometrium. Stage II cancer also involves the cervix, and stage III reaches the vagina or lymph nodes. Stage IV endometrial cancer has spread to the bowel or bladder mucosa and/or beyond the pelvis (McCance et al., 2014).

Metastasis outside the uterus occurs in these ways:

- Through lymphatic spread to the ovaries and parametrial, pelvic, inguinal, and para-aortic lymph nodes
- By blood to the lungs, liver, or bones
- By transtubal or intra-abdominal spread to the peritoneal cavity

Etiology and Genetic Risk

Endometrial cancer is strongly associated with conditions causing prolonged exposure to estrogen without the protective effects of progesterone. Risk factors for endometrial cancer are listed in Table 71-3. Although most cases of endometrial cancer do not have a genetic predisposition, it is more common in families who have gene mutations for hereditary nonpolyposis colon cancer (HNPCC) (National Cancer Institute [NCI], 2013b).

Incidence and Prevalence

In 2013, it was estimated that there will be 49,560 new cases of endometrial cancer in the United States, with 8,910 deaths associated with this condition. White women get the disease more

TABLE 71-3   Risk Factors for Endometrial (Uterine) Cancer and Cervical Cancer

ENDOMETRIAL (UTERINE) CANCER	CERVICAL CANCER
• Women in reproductive years	• Girls and young women
• Family history of endometrial cancer or HNPCC	• Infection with HPV
• Diabetes mellitus	• Multiparity (multiple births)
• Hypertension	• Smoking
• Obesity	• Younger than 18 years at first intercourse
• Uterine polyps	• Multiple sex partners
• Late menopause	• African American
• Nulliparity (no childbirths)	• Oral contraceptive use
• Smoking	• History of STDs
• Tamoxifen (Nolvadex) given for breast cancer	• Obesity or poor diet
	• Family history of cervical cancer
	• HIV/AIDS
	• Lower socioeconomic status
	• Sexual partner had a previous partner who developed cervical cancer
	• Intrauterine exposure to DES

AIDS, Acquired immune deficiency syndrome; *DES,* diethylstilbestrol; *HIV,* human immune deficiency virus; *HNPCC,* hereditary nonpolyposis colon cancer; *HPV,* human papilloma virus; *STDs,* sexually transmitted diseases.

often than African-American women, but African-American women die more often from the disease (American Cancer Society [ACS], 2013a). The causes for these differences are not known.

❖ PATIENT-CENTERED COLLABORATIVE CARE

◆ Assessment

Physical Assessment/Clinical Manifestations. *The main symptom of endometrial cancer is postmenopausal bleeding. Ask the patient how many tampons or menstrual pads she uses each day.* Some women also have a watery, bloody vaginal discharge, low back or abdominal PAIN, and low pelvic PAIN (caused by pressure of the enlarged uterus). Ask the patient to describe the exact location and intensity of her discomfort. A pelvic examination may reveal the presence of a palpable uterine mass or uterine polyp. The uterus is enlarged if the cancer is advanced.

Laboratory Assessment. Several laboratory tests are used to determine the overall condition of the woman with possible or confirmed endometrial cancer. For example, the complete blood count typically shows anemia because the patient has heavy bleeding. Serum tumor markers to assess for metastasis include CA-125 (cancer antigen–125) and alpha-fetoprotein (AFP), both of which may be elevated when ovarian cancer is present (Pagana & Pagana, 2013). A human chorionic gonadotropin (hCG) level may be taken to rule out pregnancy before treatment for cancer begins. Genetic testing may be done for the mutation causing hereditary nonpolyposis colorectal cancer (HNPCC) if there is a family history of this disease.

Other Diagnostic Assessment. *Transvaginal ultrasound* and *endometrial biopsy* are the gold standard tests to determine the presence of endometrial thickening and cancer. Saline may be infused during the ultrasound to improve the image of the uterine cavity. The clinician then collects an endometrial biopsy from inside the uterus via a thin, flexible suction curette through the cervix (Pagana & Pagana, 2013).

Other diagnostic tests to determine the patient's overall health status and the presence of metastasis (cancer spread) include:

- Chest x-ray
- Intravenous pyelography (IVP) or excretory urography to assess renal function and to assess for renal metastasis
- Abdominal ultrasound
- CT of the pelvis
- MRI of the abdomen and pelvis
- Liver and bone scans to assess for distant metastasis

Some women also have a hysteroscopic examination of the uterus and proctosigmoidoscopy depending on the stage of their cancer.

Psychosocial Assessment. Before a diagnosis is made, the woman may deny that the symptoms are related to cancer. During the diagnostic phase, the woman may express fears and concerns about having the disease. After the diagnosis is confirmed, she may express disbelief, anger, depression, anxiety, or withdrawal behaviors. Assess these emotional reactions, and encourage the patient to discuss her feelings. Ask her about how she copes with other stressful events, and assess her support systems.

◆ Analysis

The priority NANDA-I nursing diagnoses and collaborative problems for patients with endometrial cancer include:

1. Potential for disease metastasis
2. Ineffective Coping related to the diagnosis of cancer and fear of dying (NANDA-I)

◆ Planning and Implementation

Reducing the Risk for Metastasis

Planning: Expected Outcomes. The patient is expected to be free of metastatic disease if she has been diagnosed without obvious metastasis. For patients whose cancer has already spread, the expected outcomes are to have the highest quality life for as long as possible. In some cases, palliation and end-of-life care are needed.

Interventions. Surgical removal and cancer staging of the tumor with adjacent lymph nodes are the most important interventions for endometrial cancer. Cancer staging is often done using minimally invasive techniques, such as laparoscopic or robotic-assisted procedures.

Surgical Management. For stage I disease, the gynecology oncologist usually removes the uterus, fallopian tubes, and ovaries (**total hysterectomy** and **bilateral salpingo-oophorectomy [BSO]**), as well as peritoneum fluid or washings for cytologic examination. Laparoscopic surgery has fewer complications, shorter hospital stay, and less cost. A radical hysterectomy with bilateral pelvic lymph node dissection and removal of the upper third of the vagina is performed for stage II cancer. Nursing care for a radical hysterectomy is the same as that for a simple hysterectomy except that the woman's hospitalization is usually longer and her convalescence may be extended. (See p. 1489 for discussion of hysterectomy in this chapter.) Radical surgery and node dissection can also be done as a minimally invasive procedure using laparoscopic or robotic-assisted technology.

Nonsurgical Management. Nonsurgical interventions (radiation therapy and chemotherapy) are typically used postoperatively and depend on the surgical staging.

Radiation Therapy. The oncologist may prescribe radiation therapy to be delivered by external beam and/or brachytherapy for stage II and stage III cancers. Women with stage II disease may use brachytherapy (internal) radiation to prevent recurrence of vaginal cancer and improve survival.

The purpose of *brachytherapy* is to prevent disease recurrence. The radiologist places an applicator within the woman's uterus through the vagina. After the correct position of the applicator is confirmed by x-ray, the radioactive isotope is placed in the applicator and remains for several minutes. This procedure may be repeated between 2 and 5 times once or twice a week. Some patients also have external beam radiation while having brachytherapy treatment sessions. There are no restrictions for the woman to stay away from her family or the public between treatments.

While the radioactive implant is in place, radiation is emitted that can affect other people. The amount of time needed for the therapy depends on the amount of radiation emitted from the source. The radiologist calculates the time needed for a specific dose of radiation.

Inform the patient that she is restricted to bedrest during the treatment session. Excessive movement in bed is restricted to prevent dislodgment of the radioactive source. Chart 71-6 lists the health teaching for the patient having brachytherapy for gynecologic cancer. Teach patients about when to call the health care provider after each treatment session.

External beam radiation therapy (EBRT or XRT) may be used to treat any stage of endometrial cancer in combination with surgery, brachytherapy, and/or chemotherapy. Depending on the extent of the tumor, the treatment is given on an ambulatory care basis for 4 to 6 weeks. Tissue around the tumor and pelvic wall nodes also are treated. *Teach the patient to monitor for signs of skin breakdown, especially in the perineal area; to avoid sunbathing; and to avoid washing the markings outlining the treatment site.* Chapter 22 discusses nursing care of patients receiving radiation therapy in more detail.

Drug Therapy. Chemotherapy is used as palliative treatment in advanced and recurrent disease when it has spread to distant parts of the body, but it is not always effective. Although the combination can vary, three of the most common agents used for endometrial cancer are doxorubicin (Adriamycin), cisplatin (Platinol), and paclitaxel (Taxol). Chapter 22 describes chemotherapy and general nursing care during treatment.

Every woman experiences cancer differently. Many complementary therapies have evidence of benefit in decreasing the side effects of drug therapy and boosting the immune system. Provide your patient with information that will help her make informed, evidence-based decisions. Encourage her to check with her oncologist and/or pharmacist because some alternative therapies can be harmful or interfere with cancer treatment. Current evidence-based information is available at the American Cancer Society website (www.cancer.org) about mind-body therapies, healing touch, herbs, vitamins, nutrition, and biologic therapies.

Helping the Patient Develop Coping Strategies

Planning: Expected Outcomes. The patient is expected to develop coping strategies that will help her deal with the diagnosis and collaborative care for endometrial cancer.

Interventions. Women need to discuss their concerns about the presence of cancer and the potential for recurrence. Provide emotional support, and create an atmosphere that encourages them to ask questions or express their fears and concerns. Include family members or significant others in discussions when the patient desires and when this is possible.

Reactions to radiation therapy vary. Some women feel "radioactive" or "unclean" after treatments and may exhibit withdrawal behaviors. Reassure them by correcting any misconceptions. Patients who have chemotherapy may be upset if **alopecia** (hair loss) occurs. Warn them of this possibility before treatment starts. Wigs, scarves, or turbans can be worn until the hair grows back. Many women select these replacements before they lose their hair. Others shave their heads and begin wearing them immediately as the treatment begins. Tell women about these options so that they can make decisions with which they are personally comfortable.

Often patients experience emotional crises because of the physical effects of cancer treatments. Radical hysterectomy may be seen as mutilating. Both radiation and chemotherapy have side effects that change physical appearance and body image. Women may have a grief reaction to these changes. The feelings of loss depend on the visibility of the loss and the loss of function. Help the patient adapt to the body changes. Using a calm and accepting approach, encourage self-management as soon as her physical condition is stable.

Death can occur with or without treatment. The patient and family want the woman to pass the 5-year survival mark without a recurrence of disease. If there is a recurrence, they may be hostile and have manifestations of a grief reaction. Encourage patients and their families to discuss their feelings. Refer to support services such as certified hospital chaplain or other spiritual leader, social worker, or counselor. Response to loss and grieving is discussed in Chapter 7.

Community-Based Care

Home Care Management. The woman with endometrial cancer is managed at home unless surgery is indicated. After surgery, she is usually discharged to her home. Home care after surgery for endometrial cancer is the same as that after a hysterectomy. (See discussion off Hysterectomy on p. 1489 in the Uterine Leiomyoma section.) Patients who are receiving chemotherapy or radiation therapy are treated on an ambulatory care basis. Most women are surprised by the fatigue caused by radiation and chemotherapy. Help the patient and her family plan daily activities around trips to the clinic or the health care provider's office. If the tumor recurs and cure is not likely, the woman and her family need to think about hospice care and whether she can be cared for in the home.

CHART 71-6 Best Practice for Patient Safety & Quality Care QSEN

Health Teaching for the Patient Having Brachytherapy for Gynecologic Cancer

- Teach the patient to report any of these signs and symptoms to the health care provider immediately:
  - Heavy vaginal bleeding
  - Urethral burning for more than 24 hours
  - Blood in the urine
  - Extreme fatigue
  - Severe diarrhea
  - Fever over 100° F (38° C)
  - Abdominal pain
- Teach the patient that she is not radioactive between treatments and there are no restrictions on her interactions with others.

Self-Management Education. Teach the patient to report vaginal or rectal bleeding, foul-smelling discharge, abdominal PAIN or distention, and hematuria to the health care provider. These symptoms may be the result of the disease or its treatment.

The high dose of radiation causes sterility, and vaginal shrinkage can occur. Vaginal dilators can be used with water-soluble lubricants for 10 minutes each day until sexual activity resumes, generally within 4 weeks (ACS, 2013b). Reassure the woman that she is not radioactive and that her partner will not "catch" cancer by engaging in sexual intercourse.

Review all prescribed drugs, including the dosage and schedule, effects, and side effects. Emphasize the importance of keeping appointments for follow-up care.

Health Care Resources. In the United States, local American Cancer Society chapters provide written materials about endometrial cancer and information about local support groups. Each province in Canada also has a division of the Canadian Cancer Society (www.cancer.ca). If the patient is in the terminal stages of cancer, hospice care may be appropriate (see Chapter 7). If nursing care is needed at home, the hospital nurse or case manager makes referrals to a home health care agency. A referral to a social services agency may be needed if the patient cannot meet the financial demands of treatment and long-term follow-up.

CERVICAL CANCER

❖ PATHOPHYSIOLOGY

The uterine cervix is covered with squamous cells on the outer cervix and columnar (glandular) cells that line the endocervical canal. Papanicolaou (Pap) tests sample cells from both areas as a screening test for cervical cancer. The squamo-columnar junction is the *transformation zone* where most cell abnormalities occur. The adolescent has more columnar cells exposed on the outer cervix, which may be one reason she is more vulnerable to sexually transmitted diseases (STDs) and human immune deficiency virus (HIV). In contrast, in the menopausal woman, the squamo-columnar junction may be higher up in the endocervical canal, making it difficult to sample for a Pap test.

Premalignant changes are described on a continuum from *atypia* (suspicious) to *cervical intraepithelial neoplasia (CIN)* to *carcinoma in situ (CIS)*, which is the most advanced premalignant change. It generally takes years for the cervical cells to transform from normal to premalignant to invasive cancer. CIN, sometimes called *dysplasia,* is graded on a scale of 1 to 3 depending on the appearance of the cervical tissue under a microscope (ACS, 2014b). Not much tissue appears abnormal in CIN1 (mild dysplasia), which is thought to be the least serious cervical pre-cancer; more tissue appears abnormal in CIN2 (moderate dysplasia). Most tissue looks abnormal in CIN3 (severe dysplasia as well as carcinoma *in situ*), which is the most serious pre-cancer (ACS, 2014b).

Most cervical cancers arise from the squamous cells on the outside of the cervix. The other cancers arise from the mucus-secreting glandular cells (adenocarcinoma) in the endocervical canal. The disease spreads by direct extension to the vaginal mucosa, lower uterine segment, parametrium, pelvic wall, bladder, and bowel. Metastasis is usually confined to the pelvis, but distant spread can occur through lymphatic spread and the circulation to the liver, lungs, or bones.

Etiology

Human papilloma virus infection (HPV) is the most common type of STD in the United States (Centers for Disease Control and Prevention [CDC], 2014b). Almost all women will have HPV sometime in their life, but not all types lead to cancer. Most cases of cervical cancer are caused by certain types of HPV. The high-risk HPV types, especially strains 16 and 18, impair the tumor-suppressor gene and cause most of the cervical cancers. The unrestricted tissue growth can spread, becoming invasive and metastatic. Strains 6 and 11 are associated with genital warts (McCance et al., 2014). Risk factors for cervical cancer are listed in Table 71-3.

Incidence and Prevalence

Invasive cancer of the cervix is the third most common cancer of the female genital system, after ovarian and uterine cancer. The number of cases of cervical cancer (and deaths from cervical cancer) has decreased significantly over the past 40 years because more women regularly get Pap tests (CDC, 2014a).

Health Promotion and Maintenance

Girls and young women (ages 9 through 26 years) should receive one of the two currently used HPV vaccines, *Gardasil* and *Cervarix,* ideally before their first sexual contact to receive protection against the highest-risk HPV types that are responsible for most cervical cancers. It is also given for boys and young men (ages 9 through 26 years) to prevent genital warts because it protects against the 6 and 11 HPV strains and to prevent anal cancer, which is caused by HPV strains 16 and 18 (Merck Sharpe & Dohme Corporation, 2014). Cervarix protects girls and women ages 9 through 25 years against INFECTION for HPV strains 16 and 18 to prevent cervical cancer (GlaxoSmithKline, 2012).

Teach all young adults and parents of minors about the importance of receiving the vaccine and the need to have the entire series (3 injections over 6 months). Tell them that the most frequent side effects are related to local irritation from the injections (e.g., PAIN, redness). Other common side effects include nausea, vomiting, dizziness, headache, and diarrhea.

The American Cancer Society (ACS) recommends that women have periodic pelvic examinations and Pap tests to screen for cervical cancer early. Teach women that they should begin these screening precautions at the age of 21 years. Between ages 21 and 29 years, women should have a Pap test every 3 years; women between ages 30 and 65 years should have a Pap test plus a human papilloma virus (HPV) test ("co-testing") every 5 years. More information on the HPV test is found later in this chapter. In the absence of co-testing, this population should still have a Pap test every 3 years. According to the ACS, women older than 65 years who have had regular cervical cancer testing with normal results should not receive Pap tests (ACS, 2014a). Recommended guidelines from other health care organizations suggest a Pap test every 3 years for women older than 60 years. Those who have had a history of a serious cervical pre-cancerous lesion should be tested annually for at least 20 years after that diagnosis, regardless of age (ACS, 2014a).

❖ PATIENT-CENTERED COLLABORATIVE CARE

◆ Assessment

Physical Assessment/Clinical Manifestations. The patient who has preinvasive cancer is often asymptomatic. *The classic symptom of invasive cancer is painless vaginal bleeding.* Ask the patient if she has had or now has bleeding. It may start as spotting between menstrual periods or after sexual intercourse or douching. As the cancer grows, bleeding increases in frequency, duration, and amount and may become continuous.

Ask the woman if she has a watery, blood-tinged vaginal discharge that becomes dark and foul-smelling (occurs as the disease progresses). Leg pain (along the sciatic nerve) or swelling of one leg may be a late symptom or may indicate recurrent disease. Flank pain may be a late symptom of hydronephrosis, indicating advanced cancer pressing on the ureters, backing up the urine into the kidney. Ask the patient if she has had other signs of recurrence or metastasis such as:

- Unexplained weight loss
- Dysuria (painful urination)
- Pelvic PAIN (caused by pressure of the tumor on the bladder or the bowel)
- Hematuria (bloody urine)
- Rectal bleeding
- Chest PAIN
- Coughing

A physical examination may not reveal any abnormalities in early preinvasive cervical cancer. The internal pelvic examination may identify late-stage disease.

Diagnostic Assessment. If Pap results are abnormal, an *HPV-typing DNA test* of the cervical sample can determine the presence of one or more high-risk types. The health care provider may perform a colposcopic examination to view the transformation zone. Colposcopy is a procedure in which application of an acetic acid solution is applied to the cervix. The cervix is then examined under magnification with a bright filter light that enhances the visualization of the characteristics of dysplasia or cancer. If abnormal tissue is recognized, multiple biopsies of the cervical tissue are performed.

If atypical glandular cells are suspected, the health care provider may perform an *endocervical curettage* (scraping of the endocervix wall) as well. Inform her that a small amount of bleeding is expected for up to 2 weeks after the biopsies.

◆ **Interventions**

Interventions for the woman with cervical cancer are similar to those for endometrial cancer: surgery, which is possibly followed by radiation and chemotherapy for later-stage disease.

Surgical Management. Early stage I management techniques include local cervical ablation therapies of electrosurgical excision, laser therapy, or cryosurgery. Small tumors that are only microinvasive are managed with excisional conization or hysterectomy. Early-stage *invasive* cancers are managed with radical surgery and radiation. Advanced inoperable cancers are treated with radiation. Factors that influence the choice of localized treatment versus surgical intervention include patient overall health, desire for future childbearing, tumor size, stage, cancer cell type, degree of lymph node involvement, and patient preference.

Early Surgical Procedures. The loop electrosurgical excision procedure (LEEP) is short (10 to 30 minutes) and is performed in a physician's office or in an ambulatory care setting with a local anesthetic injected into the cervix. A thin loop-wire electrode that transmits a painless electrical current is used to cut away affected tissue. LEEP is both a diagnostic procedure and a treatment, because it provides a specimen that can be examined by a pathologist to ensure the lesion was completely removed. Little discomfort is associated with this procedure.

CHART 71-7 Patient and Family Education: Preparing for Self-Management

Care after Local Cervical Ablation Therapies

- Refrain from sexual intercourse.
- Do not use tampons.
- Do not douche.
- Take showers rather than tub baths.
- Avoid lifting heavy objects.
- Report any heavy vaginal bleeding, foul-smelling drainage, or fever.
  The usual time period for these restrictions is 3 weeks. Your health care provider may prescribe a different (longer or shorter) time frame for you.

Spotting after the procedure is common. Teach patients to adhere for 3 weeks to the restrictions listed in Chart 71-7.

Laser therapy is also an office procedure used for early cancers. A laser beam is directed to the abnormal tissues, where energy from the beam is absorbed by the fluid in the tissues, causing them to vaporize. A small amount of bleeding occurs with the procedure, and the woman may have a slight vaginal discharge. Healing occurs in 6 to 12 weeks. A disadvantage of this procedure is that no specimen is available for study.

Cryotherapy involves freezing of the cancer, causing subsequent necrosis. The procedure is often painless, although some women have slight cramping after the procedure. The patient has a heavy watery discharge for several weeks after the procedure. Instruct her to follow the restrictions in Chart 71-7.

In cases of microinvasive cancer, a *conization* can remove the affected tissue while still preserving fertility. This procedure is done when the lesion cannot be visualized by colposcopic examination. A cone-shaped area of cervix is removed surgically and sent to the laboratory to determine the extent of the cancer. Potential complications from this procedure include hemorrhage and uterine perforation Long-term follow-up care is needed because new cancers can develop.

Hysterectomy. A total hysterectomy may be performed as treatment of microinvasive cancer if the woman does not want children or more children. A laparoscopic approach is commonly used. A radical hysterectomy and bilateral pelvic lymph node dissection may be as effective as radiation is for treating cancer that has extended beyond the cervix but not to the pelvic wall. Care for patients undergoing hysterectomy is found in the Uterine Leiomyoma section on pp. 1489-1491.

Nonsurgical Management. Radiation therapy is reserved for invasive cervical cancer. Brachytherapy and external beam radiation therapy are used in combination, depending on the extent and location of the lesion. The procedure is similar to that described on pp. 1492-1493 for endometrial cancer.

A combination of chemotherapy with cisplatin (Platinol) and radiation may also be used. This treatment modality shows increased survival times but increased toxicity for many patients. Examples of other drugs used alone or in combination include paclitaxel (Taxol), carboplatin, fluorouracil (5-FU), and mitomycin. See Chapter 22 for more information about the general nursing care for the patient on chemotherapy and radiation.

OVARIAN CANCER

❖ *PATHOPHYSIOLOGY*

Most ovarian cancers are epithelial tumors that grow on the surface of the ovaries. These tumors grow rapidly, spread

TABLE 71-4　Risk Factors for Ovarian Cancer

- Older than 40 years
- Family history of ovarian or breast cancer or HNPCC
- Diabetes mellitus
- Nulliparity
- Older than 30 years at first pregnancy
- Breast cancer
- Colorectal cancer
- Infertility
- *BRCA1* or *BRCA2* gene mutations
- Early menarche/late menopause
- Endometriosis
- Obesity/high-fat diet

HNPCC, Hereditary nonpolyposis colon cancer.

quickly, and are often bilateral. Tumor cells spread by direct extension into nearby organs and through blood and lymph circulation to distant sites (McCance et al., 2014). Free-floating cancer cells also spread through the abdomen to seed new sites, usually accompanied by ascites (abdominal fluid).

Ovarian cancer seems to be disordered growth in response to excessive exposure to estrogen. This would explain the protective effects of pregnancies and oral contraceptive use, both of which interrupt the monthly estrogen exposure. Table 71-4 lists known and suspected risk factors for ovarian cancer.

Ovarian cancer is the leading cause of death from female reproductive cancers, but it is not the most common type of cancer (ACS, 2013a). The incidence increases in women older than 50 years, and most are diagnosed after menopause. Family history accounts for a small percentage of cases. These women carry *BCRA1* or *BCRA2* genetic mutations. Of these, some choose to have an elective **bilateral salpingo-oophorectomy (BSO)** (removal of both ovaries and fallopian tubes) to prevent ovarian cancer.

Survival rates are low because ovarian cancer is often not detected until its late stages. It is important for nurses to teach women to *"think ovarian"* if they have vague abdominal and GI symptoms.

Health Promotion and Maintenance

Health promotion measures to help prevent ovarian cancer include maintaining a normal weight and eating a well-balanced diet. Women who have had tubal ligation, used oral contraception, and breast-fed their children also have less risk for having the disease (ACS, 2014a).

❖ PATIENT-CENTERED COLLABORATIVE CARE

◆ Assessment

Most women with ovarian cancer have had mild symptoms for several months but may have thought they were due to normal perimenopausal changes or stress. They may report abdominal pain or swelling or have vague GI disturbances such as dyspepsia (indigestion) and gas. Ask the patient if she has had urinary frequency or incontinence, unexpected weight loss, and/or vaginal bleeding.

Complications of advanced metastatic cancer include:
- Pleural effusion
- Ascites
- Lymphedema
- Intestinal obstruction
- Malnutrition

On pelvic examination, an abdominal mass may not be palpable until it reaches a size of 4 to 6 inches (10 to 15 cm). Any enlarged ovary found after menopause should be evaluated as

though it were malignant. A Pap smear is of limited value for detecting ovarian cancer.

A cancer antigen test, *CA-125,* measures the presence of damaged endometrial and uterine tissue in the blood. It may be elevated if ovarian cancer is present, but it can also be elevated in patients with endometriosis, fibroids, pelvic inflammatory disease, pregnancy, and even menses (Pagana & Pagana, 2013). It is also useful for monitoring a patient's progress during and after treatment. Transvaginal ultrasonography, chest radiography, and CT are part of a complete workup to evaluate for metastasis. Complete blood work includes a liver profile if there is ascites.

The woman with ovarian cancer has concerns similar to those described for the patient with endometrial cancer (see p. 1493 of this chapter). Because the cancer is often diagnosed in an advanced stage, thoughts of death and dying, menopause, and loss of fertility come as a shock.

💡 CLINICAL JUDGMENT CHALLENGE

Patient-Centered Care; Evidence-Based Practice; Informatics; Teamwork and Collaboration QSEN

A 34-year-old woman is diagnosed with ovarian cancer today. She tells you that she "can't believe this," and that "this must be the wrong diagnosis." She states that she and her husband had planned to get pregnant later this year and that she "cannot lose" her ovaries. However, she is scheduled to have a bilateral salpingo-oophorectomy and hysterectomy in 2 days. Her oncologist told her that after she recovers from surgery, she may need to have adjuvant chemotherapy to destroy any remaining cancer cells.

1. What preoperative teaching will you provide for this patient and why?
2. How will you address this patient's statements about disbelief of the diagnosis?
3. How will you approach the patient's feelings about getting pregnant later this year?
4. Do you believe that this patient understands the implications of a bilateral salpingo-oophorectomy? If not, what would be your next nursing action?
5. What will you tell her about chemotherapy that may be necessary after surgery?
6. Where would you search for evidence about her expected quality of life and prognosis?
7. To what community resources would you refer this patient after discharge?

◆ Interventions

Nursing care of the patient with ovarian cancer is similar to that for endometrial or cervical cancer. The options for treatment depend on the extent of the cancer and usually include surgery first, followed by chemotherapy. Radiation is used for more widespread cancers.

Surgical Management. Diagnosis depends on surgical exploration. Exploratory laparotomy (abdominal surgery) is performed to diagnose, treat, and stage ovarian tumors. A total abdominal hysterectomy, bilateral salpingo-oophorectomy (removal of the ovaries and fallopian tubes), and pelvic and para-aortic lymph node dissection are usually performed. Very large tumors that cannot be removed are debulked (cytoreduction). These procedures can be performed via laparoscopic technique to decrease recovery time, minimize PAIN, and reduce postoperative complications. (See p. 1489 for discussion of laparoscopic hysterectomy in this chapter.) Ovarian cancer is staged during surgery.

Nursing care of the patient is similar to that for any patient having abdominal surgery (see Chapter 16). As for any patient after abdominal surgery, assess vital signs and PAIN and maintain catheters and drains. Teach her the importance of antiembolism stockings, incentive spirometry, and early ambulation. Infections after ovarian cancer surgery commonly affect the respiratory and urinary tracts. Assess vital signs, and monitor the quantity and quality of urine output.

Nonsurgical Management. After cytoreduction and staging of ovarian cancer, chemotherapy is the treatment that is used most often. For all stages of ovarian cancer, cisplatin (Platinol), carboplatin, and taxanes of all types are the most common postoperative *drugs* used for treating ovarian cancer. They may be given IV and/or intraperitoneally. Intraperitoneal (IP) therapy is described in Chapter 13. New drugs continue to be tested that use monoclonal antibodies, hormones, and agents that target cell growth and tumor blood supply.

Community-Based Care

Patients having surgery usually return to their home. Teach them to avoid tampons, douches, and sexual intercourse for at least 6 weeks or as instructed by the health care provider. Remind them to keep their follow-up surgical appointment and talk with the health care provider about resuming usual activities. Refer patients and their families to Gilda's Club (www.gildasclub.org) and the National Ovarian Cancer Coalition (NOCC) (www.ovarian.org) for more information and support groups. In Canada, the National Ovarian Cancer Association (www.ovariancanada.org) is available for the same purpose.

For patients with advanced metastatic disease, collaborate with the case manager, patient, and family for possible referral to hospice. Chapter 7 discusses end-of-life care and hospice in detail. The woman who is faced with the diagnosis of advanced ovarian cancer is usually very anxious about dying. Encourage her to discuss her feelings. Provide realistic assurance, as well as accurate information about treatments. Patients report their most distressing moments in the hospital were when they thought they were not getting adequate information. Encourage them to use their support systems of family members, friends, and clergy, including the hospital chaplain. Grief counseling is very appropriate. A visit from another woman who has survived a similar disease or referral to a support group may decrease fears. Refer the patient who fears passing the *BRCA1* or *BRCA2* gene to her daughter for genetic counseling and testing.

Ovarian cancer has a high recurrence rate. After recurrence, the cancer is treatable but no longer curable. If this occurs, the patient may deny symptoms at first or express feelings of anger and grief. The family is often fearful of the outcome. Provide encouragement and support during this difficult time, and help the patient and her family work through their grief and prepare for death.

NURSING CONCEPTS AND CLINICAL JUDGMENT REVIEW

What might you NOTICE if the patient is experiencing impaired SEXUALITY as a result of gynecologic problems?
- Irregular or abnormal vaginal bleeding
- Vaginal discharge
- Report of perineal itching or burning
- Report of painful intercourse
- Abdominal distention and discomfort
- Report of irritability, anxiety, or depression
- Report of decreased libido

What should you INTERPRET and how should you RESPOND to the patient experiencing impaired SEXUALITY as a result of gynecologic problems?

Perform and interpret physical assessment, including:
- Conducting an abdominal assessment
- Conducting a thorough pain assessment

- Checking for bleeding and amount (number of pads or tampons)
- Listening to patient's concerns about her sexuality

Respond by:
- Helping the patient into a sitting position
- Providing pain-relief measures, such as heat and analgesia
- Referring the patient to a sexual or intimacy counselor (including the patient's partner if desired)

On what should you REFLECT?
- Think about what else you can do to help provide psychosocial support.
- Prepare for complications, such as hemorrhage, if the patient is bleeding.
- Evaluate pain level after interventions.

GET READY FOR THE NCLEX® EXAMINATION!

KEY POINTS

Review these Key Points for each NCLEX Examination Client Needs Category.

Safe and Effective Care Environment
- Refer patients with gynecologic problems to appropriate community resources such as the American Cancer Society and the Endometriosis Association. **Teamwork and Collaboration** QSEN

- Collaborate with the case manager when planning care for patients with gynecologic cancers. **Teamwork and Collaboration** QSEN

Health Promotion and Maintenance
- Teach women to follow the American Cancer Society's screening guidelines to prevent and early-detect for gynecologic cancers.

- Teach all women to have regular Pap tests based on their risk factors.
- Teach women to practice safe sex to prevent INFECTION of the reproductive organs.
- Teach women about risk factors for gynecologic cancers as described in Tables 71-3 and 71-4.
- Teach women how to prevent toxic shock syndrome (TSS) as listed in Chart 71-3. **Safety** `QSEN`

Psychosocial Integrity

- Explain all tests, procedures, and treatments, especially if they cause PAIN during or after the procedures.
- Assess the patient's anxiety before any gynecologic surgery, and encourage the patient to discuss her feelings. **Patient-Centered Care** `QSEN`
- Encourage women who are having procedures that may interfere with fertility and/or SEXUALITY to express feelings of fear or grief. **Patient-Centered Care** `QSEN`
- Encourage women with chronic or serious health problems to consider using support groups or counseling.

Physiological Integrity

- Urge any woman who experiences postmenopausal vaginal bleeding to consult with her gynecologic health care provider as soon as possible. **Safety** `QSEN`
- Assess for symptoms of problems associated with urinary ELIMINATION.
- Assess for symptoms associated with toxic shock syndrome.
- Teach patients about specific restrictions after local cervical ablation therapy (see Chart 71-7).
- When caring for a patient who has a radioactive implant, use best practices as described in Chart 71-6. **Teamwork and Collaboration** `QSEN`
- Teach the patient who is going home after a hysterectomy how to monitor for INFECTION and other complications. **Safety** `QSEN`
- Instruct patients receiving external beam radiation to the abdomen to gently wash the area; to not apply creams or lotions (unless prescribed by the radiologist); to not wash off marking; to avoid exposing the area to sunlight or temperature extremes; and to wear soft, nonirritating clothing.

CHAPTER 72

Care of Patients with Male Reproductive Problems

Donna D. Ignatavicius

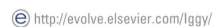
http://evolve.elsevier.com/Iggy/

PRIORITY CONCEPTS

- PAIN
- ELIMINATION
- INFECTION
- REPRODUCTION

LEARNING OUTCOMES

Safe and Effective Care Environment
1. Collaborate with health care team members to provide care for patients with male reproductive health problems.

Health Promotion and Maintenance
2. Teach men and their partners about community resources for reproductive cancers.
3. Develop a health teaching plan for men to prevent or detect early male reproductive cancers.

Psychosocial Integrity
4. Explain the psychosocial needs of men who have male reproductive problems.

Physiological Integrity
5. Identify the clinical manifestations of benign prostatic hyperplasia (BPH) as they affect urinary ELIMINATION.
6. Describe the nursing implications for pharmacologic management of BPH.
7. Develop an evidence-based postoperative plan of care for a patient undergoing surgery for benign prostatic hyperplasia.

8. Evaluate patient risk factors for male reproductive cancers.
9. Identify complementary and alternative therapies to incorporate into the patient's plan of care.
10. Discuss treatment options for prostate cancer with patients, partners, and/or families.
11. Provide preoperative teaching for patients having a radical prostatectomy.
12. Identify adverse effects of radiation therapy for male reproductive cancers.
13. Develop a community-based plan of care for a man with prostate cancer.
14. Describe the options for treating erectile dysfunction.
15. Identify cultural considerations related to male reproductive problems.
16. Develop a plan of care for a patient with testicular cancer, including fertility issues.
17. Compare the assessment and treatment for hydrocele, spermatocele, and varicocele.

Male reproductive problems can range from short-term INFECTIONS to long-term health care problems that require end-of-life care. Any health issue that affects the male reproductive system can affect the human needs for SEXUALITY and urinary ELIMINATION. For example, some patients have surgeries that damage essential nerves that are needed to have an erection. Others have disorders that psychologically prevent the patient from engaging in his usual sexual activity.

The role of the nurse and other health care team members is to be open, supportive, and nonjudgmental when caring for men with reproductive problems. Respect the man's privacy at all times.

BENIGN PROSTATIC HYPERPLASIA

❖ PATHOPHYSIOLOGY

Benign prostatic hyperplasia (BPH) is a very common health problem, but the exact cause is unclear. It is likely the result of a combination of aging and the influence of androgens that are present in prostate tissue, such as dihydrotestosterone (DHT) (McCance et al., 2014). With aging and increased DHT levels, the glandular units in the prostate undergo nodular tissue **hyperplasia** (an increase in the number of cells). This altered tissue promotes local inflammation by attracting cytokines and other substances (McCance et al., 2014).

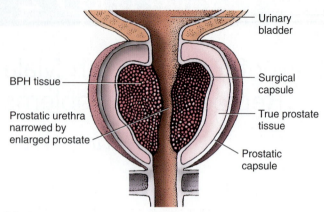

FIG. 72-1 Benign prostatic hyperplasia (BPH) grows inward, causing narrowing of the urethra.

As the prostate gland enlarges, it extends upward into the bladder and inward, causing *bladder outlet obstruction* (Fig. 72-1). In response, the urinary system is affected in several ways. First, the detrusor (bladder) muscle thickens to help urine push past the enlarged prostate gland (McCance et al., 2014). In spite of the bladder muscle change, the patient has increased residual urine (stasis) and chronic urinary retention. The increased volume of residual urine often causes **overflow urinary incontinence,** in which the urine "leaks" around the enlarged prostate causing dribbling. Urinary stasis can also result in urinary tract INFECTIONS and bladder calculi (stones).

In a few patients, the prostate becomes very large and the man cannot void (acute urinary retention [AUR]). The patient with this problem requires emergent care. In other patients, chronic urinary retention may result in a backup of urine and cause a gradual dilation of the ureters (**hydroureter**) and kidneys (**hydronephrosis**) if BPH is not treated. These urinary ELIMINATION problems can lead to chronic kidney disease as described in Chapter 68.

❖ PATIENT-CENTERED COLLABORATIVE CARE

◆ Assessment

History. When taking a history, several standardized assessment tools are used to help the health care provider determine the severity of lower urinary tract symptoms (LUTS) associated with prostatic enlargement. One of the most commonly used assessments is the International Prostate Symptom Score (I-PSS), which incorporates the American Urological Association Symptom Index (AUA-SI) (Fig. 72-2) as questions 1 through 7. The additional question included on the I-PSS is the effect of the patient's urinary symptoms on quality of life. Most patients complete the questions as a self-administered tool because it is available in many languages. If the patient is illiterate (does not read) or does not feel like reading the questions, the nurse or health care provider can ask them. Be sure that older men wear their glasses or contact lenses if needed.

Physical Assessment/Clinical Manifestations. Ask about the patient's current urinary ELIMINATION pattern. Assess for urinary frequency and urgency. Determine the number of times the patient awakens during the night to void (**nocturia**). Other symptoms of LUTS include:

- Difficulty in starting (hesitancy) and continuing urination

- Reduced force and size of the urinary stream ("weak" stream)
- Sensation of incomplete bladder emptying
- Straining to begin urination
- Post-void (after voiding) dribbling or leaking

If frequency and nocturia do not occur with restricted urinary flow, the patient may have an INFECTION or other bladder problem. Ask whether the patient has had **hematuria** (blood in the urine) when starting the urine stream or at the end of voiding. BPH is a common cause of hematuria in older men.

The health care provider examines the patient for physical changes of the prostate gland. Remind the patient to void before the physical examination. Inspect and palpate the abdomen for a distended bladder. The health care provider may percuss the bladder. If the patient has a sense of urgency when gentle pressure is applied, the bladder may be distended. Obese patients are best assessed by percussion or bedside ultrasound bladder scanner rather than by inspection or palpation.

Prepare the patient for the prostate gland examination. Tell him that he may feel the urge to urinate as the prostate is palpated. Because the prostate is close to the rectal wall, it is easily examined by digital rectal examination (DRE). If needed, help the patient bend over the examination table or assume a side-lying fetal position, whichever is the easiest position for him. The health care provider examines the prostate for size and consistency. BPH presents as a uniform, elastic, nontender enlargement, whereas cancer of the prostate gland feels like a stony-hard nodule. Advise the patient that after the prostate gland is palpated, it may be massaged to obtain a fluid sample for examination to rule out **prostatitis** (inflammation and possible INFECTION of the prostate), a common problem that can occur with BPH. If the patient has bacterial prostatitis, he is treated with broad-spectrum antibiotic therapy to prevent the spread of infection (McCance et al., 2014).

Psychosocial Assessment. Patients who have nocturia and other LUTS may be irritable or depressed as a result of interrupted sleep and annoying visits to the bathroom. Assess the effect of sleep interruptions on the patient's mood and mental status.

Post-void dribbling and overflow incontinence may cause embarrassment and prevent the patient from socializing or leaving his home. For some patients, this social isolation can affect quality of life and lead to clinical depression and/or severe anxiety. Johnson et al. (2010) found a strong correlation between depression and BPH in older men. Depressed patients were 3 times more likely to have severe symptoms.

Laboratory Assessment. A *urinalysis* and urine *culture* are typically obtained to diagnose urinary tract infection and microscopic hematuria. If INFECTION is present, the urinalysis measures the number of white blood cells (WBCs).

Other laboratory studies that may be performed include:
- A *complete blood count* (CBC) to evaluate any evidence of systemic infection (elevated WBCs) or anemia (decreased red blood cells [RBCs]) from hematuria
- *Blood urea nitrogen* (BUN) and serum creatinine levels to evaluate renal function (both are usually elevated with kidney disease)
- A *prostate-specific antigen* (PSA) and a serum acid phosphatase level if prostate cancer is suspected (both are typically elevated in patients who have prostate cancer)
- *Culture and sensitivity* of prostatic fluid (if expressed during the examination)

International Prostate Symptom Score (I-PSS)

Patient Name:_____ Date of Birth:_____ Date Completed_____

In the past month:	Not at All	Less Than 1 in 5 Times	Less Than Half the Time	About Half the Time	More Than Half the Time	Almost Always	Your Score
1. Incomplete Emptying How often have you had the sensation of not emptying your bladder?	0	1	2	3	4	5	
2. Frequency How often have you had to urinate less than every 2 hours?	0	1	2	3	4	5	
3. Intermittency How often have you found you stopped and started again several times when you urinated?	0	1	2	3	4	5	
4. Urgency How often have you found it difficult to postpone urination?	0	1	2	3	4	5	
5. Weak Stream How often have you had a weak urinary stream?	0	1	2	3	4	5	
6. Straining How often have you had to strain to start urination?	0	1	2	3	4	5	
	None	1 Time	2 Times	3 Times	4 Times	5 Times	
7. Nocturia How many times do you typically get up at night to urinate?	0	1	2	3	4	5	
Total I-PSS Score							

Score: 1-7: Mild   8-19: Moderate   20-35: Severe

Quality of Life Due to Urinary Symptoms	Delighted	Pleased	Mostly Satisfied	Mixed	Mostly Dissatisfied	Unhappy	Terrible
If you were to spend the rest of your life with your urinary condition just the way it is now, how would you feel about that?	0	1	2	3	4	5	6

FIG. 72-2 The International Prostate Symptom Score (I-PSS).

Continued

About the I-PSS

The International Prostate Symptom Score (I-PSS) is based on the answers to seven questions concerning urinary symptoms and one question concerning quality of life. Each question concerning urinary symptoms allows the patient to choose one out of six answers indicating increasing severity of the particular symptom. The answers are assigned points from 0 to 5. The total score can therefore range from 0 to 35 (asymptomatic to very symptomatic).

The questions refer to the following urinary symptoms:

Questions	Symptom
1	Incomplete emptying
2	Frequency
3	Intermittency
4	Urgency
5	Weak Stream
6	Straining
7	Nocturia

Question 8 refers to the patient's perceived quality of life.

The first seven questions of the I-PSS are identical to the questions appearing on the American Urological Association (AUA) Symptom Index, which currently categorizes symptoms as follows:

Mild (symptom score less than or equal to 7)
Moderate (symptom score range 8 to 19)
Severe (symptom score range 20 to 35)

The International Scientific Committee (SCI), under the patronage of the World Health Organization (WHO) and the International Union Against Cancer (UICC), recommends the use of only a single question to assess the quality of life. The answers to this question range from "delighted" to "terrible," or 0 to 6. Although this single question may or may not capture the global impact of benign prostatic hyperplasia (BPH) symptoms or quality of life, it may serve as a valuable starting point for a doctor-patient conversation.

The SCI has agreed to use the symptom index for BPH, which has been developed by the AUA Measurement Committee, as the official worldwide symptoms assessment tool for patients suffering from prostatism.

The SCI recommends that physicians consider the following components for a basic diagnostic workup: history; physical examination; appropriate labs such as U/A, creatinine, etc.; and DRE or other evaluation to rule out prostate cancer.

FIG. 72-2, cont'd

Other Diagnostic Assessment. Imaging studies that are typically performed are *transabdominal ultrasound* and/or *transrectal ultrasound (TRUS)*. The patient having a TRUS lies on his side while the transducer is inserted into the rectum for viewing the prostate and surrounding structures. A tissue biopsy may also be done if the health care provider is uncertain whether the prostatic problem is benign or malignant.

In some cases the physician uses a cystoscope to view the interior of the bladder, the bladder neck, and the urethra. This examination is used to study the presence and effect of bladder neck obstruction and is usually done in an ambulatory care setting. See Chapter 66 for a detailed description of *cystoscopy* and the nursing care needed for patients having this procedure.

Residual urine may be determined by *bladder ultrasound* immediately after the patient voids. As an alternative, because the patient voids before cystoscopy, residual urine may be measured when the cystoscope is inserted. *Urodynamic pressure-flow studies* may help diagnose and grade bladder outlet obstruction and detrusor muscle function.

◆ *Analysis*

The priority NANDA-I nursing diagnosis for the patient with benign prostatic hyperplasia (BPH) is Impaired

Urinary Elimination related to bladder outlet obstruction (NANDA-I).

◆ *Planning and Implementation*
Improving Urinary Elimination
Planning: Expected Outcomes. The patient with BPH is expected to have a normal urinary ELIMINATION pattern without urinary hesitancy, urgency, or infection.

Interventions. Patients with symptomatic BPH are first treated with nonsurgical interventions, such as drug therapy. The Concept Map on p. 1504 shows nursing assessment and collaborative interventions for the patient with BPH.

Nonsurgical Management. Drug therapy is a popular option for treating BPH. For patients with acute urinary retention (AUR) or for those who do not respond to or cannot tolerate drug therapy, noninvasive procedures or surgery is the treatment of choice.

Drug Therapy. Drugs from two major categories may be used alone, but most commonly they are given in combination. The health care provider usually prescribes a *5-alpha reductase inhibitor (5-ARI)* as first-line drug therapy. Examples of these drugs are finasteride (Proscar) and dutasteride (Avodart). Normally, testosterone is converted to DHT in the prostate gland by the enzyme *5-alpha reductase.* By taking an enzyme-inhibiting agent, the patient's DHT levels decrease, which results in reducing the enlarged prostate.

! NURSING SAFETY PRIORITY (QSEN)
Drug Alert

Remind patients who are being treated with a 5-ARI for BPH that they may need to take it for as long as 6 months before improvement is noticed. Teach them about possible side effects, which include erectile dysfunction (ED), decreased libido (sexual desire), and dizziness due to orthostatic hypotension. *Remind them to change positions carefully and slowly!*

The alpha-adrenergic receptors in prostatic smooth muscle enable the prostate gland to respond to *alpha-1 selective blocking agents,* such as tamsulosin (Flomax), alfuzosin (Uroxatral), doxazosin (Cardura, Cardura-1✦), and silodosin (Rapaflo). Tamsulosin is also available as an over-the-counter (OTC) drug. These drugs relax smooth muscles in the prostate gland, creating less urinary resistance and improved urinary flow. They also cause peripheral vasodilation and reduced peripheral vascular resistance.

! NURSING SAFETY PRIORITY (QSEN)
Drug Alert

If giving alpha blockers in an inpatient setting, assess for orthostatic (postural) hypotension, tachycardia, and syncope ("blackout"), especially after the first dose is given to older men. If the patient is taking the drug at home, teach him to be careful when changing position and to report any weakness, lightheadedness, or dizziness to the health care provider immediately. Bedtime dosing may decrease the risk for problems related to hypotension. Teach patients taking a 5-ARI or alpha-blocking drug to keep all appointments for follow-up laboratory testing because both drug classes can cause liver dysfunction.

The most effective drug therapy approach for many patients is a combination of a 5-ARI drug and an alpha-1 selective blocking agent. A commonly prescribed drug regimen is finasteride and doxazosin. Newer drugs, such as Jalyn, provide a combination of dutasteride and tamsulosin in a once-a-day capsule.

Other drugs may be helpful in managing specific urinary symptoms. For example, low-dose oral desmopressin, a synthetic antidiuretic analog, has been used successfully for nocturia (Wang et al., 2011). Tadalafil (Cialis), a drug usually given to treat erectile dysfunction, has also been approved for some men with BPH because it can improve lower urinary tract symptoms.

Complementary and Alternative Therapies. Although many men use *Serenoa repens* (saw palmetto extract), a plant extract, to help manage the urinary symptoms associated with BPH, studies on the effectiveness of this herb have not shown that it is effective (Barry et al., 2011). Teach patients who want to try these herbs and other natural substances that scientific evidence to prove they are useful is lacking. However, if they choose to take them, remind them to check with their health care provider before taking any OTC natural substance. Some herbs interfere with prescription drugs the patient may be taking for other health problems.

Other Nonsurgical Interventions. Other interventions that may reduce obstructive symptoms include those that cause the release of prostatic fluid such as frequent sexual intercourse. This approach is helpful for the man whose obstructive symptoms result from an enlarged prostate with a large amount of retained prostatic fluid.

Teach patients with BPH to avoid drinking large amounts of fluid in a short time; to avoid alcohol, diuretics, and caffeine; and to void as soon as they feel the urge. These measures are aimed at preventing overdistention of the bladder, which may result in loss of detrusor muscle tone. Teach patients to avoid any drugs that can cause urinary retention, especially anticholinergics, antihistamines, and decongestants. *Emphasize the importance of telling any health care provider about the diagnosis of BPH so that these drugs are not prescribed.*

If drug therapy or other measures are not helpful in relieving urinary symptoms, several noninvasive techniques are available to destroy excess prostate tissue using a variety of heat methods (**thermotherapy**). These procedures are often done in a physician's office or another ambulatory care setting. Examples include:

- **Transurethral needle ablation (TUNA)** (low radiofrequency energy shrinks the prostate)
- **Transurethral microwave therapy (TUMT)** (high temperatures heat and destroy excess tissue)
- **Interstitial laser coagulation (ILC),** also called **contact laser prostatectomy (CLP)** (laser energy coagulates excess tissue)
- **Electrovaporization of the prostate (EVAP)** (high-frequency electrical current cuts and vaporizes excess tissue)

Prostatic stents may be placed into the urethra to maintain permanent patency after a procedure for destroying or removing prostatic tissue. All of these highly technical treatments use local or regional anesthesia and do not require an indwelling urinary catheter. They are also associated with less risk for complications such as intraoperative bleeding and erectile dysfunction when compared with traditional surgical approaches. Patients can return to their usual activities in a day or two.

CONCEPT MAP

BENIGN PROSTATIC HYPERPLASIA (BPH)

- PAIN
- ELIMINATION
- SEXUALITY

INTERVENTIONS

1 Nonjudgment

Respect privacy at all times. *Being open, supportive, and nonjudgmental when caring for the patient with SEXUALITY issues facilitates trust.*

2 Physical Assessment of Elimination

Perform focused assessment of urinary pattern: frequency, hesitancy, urgency, presence of weak stream, nocturia, sensation of incomplete emptying, straining, hematuria, and post-void dribbling. *Evaluates whether BPH is causing hematuria. If frequency and nocturia do not occur with this elimination problem of restricted urinary flow, it may be infection or other bladder problem.*

3 Drug Therapy

Explain the mechanisms of action, side effects, and implications for drug therapy for BPH. *Minimizes side effects and the potential for injury.*

4 Nursing Safety Priority: Drug Alert!

- Assess for orthostatic hypotension, tachycardia, and syncope from alpha blockers. *Minimizes potential for injury from falls from orthostatic hypotension.*
- Instruct the patient to report weakness, lightheadedness, or dizziness; monitor liver function, and side effects, including erectile dysfunction, and decreased libido. *Providing accurate discharge information prevents serious complications.*

5 Interpretation of Lab Values

- Obtain urinalysis (U/A) and culture, and complete blood count. *U/A and culture detects UTI and hematuria; ↑ WBC is sign of infection, ↓ RBC indicates anemia from hematuria.*
- Obtain blood urea nitrogen (BUN) and serum creatinine, prostate-specific antigen (PSA), and serum acid phosphatase level. *BUN and serum creatinine increase detects renal dysfunction; increased PSA and serum phosphatase detects prostate cancer.*
- Obtain culture and sensitivity of prostatic fluid if expressed during the exam. *Rules out prostatitis.*

6 Reducing Obstructive Symptoms

- Instruct the patient to avoid large amounts of fluid, alcohol, diuretics, caffeine; void as soon as the urge is felt. *Promotes ELIMINATION and prevents bladder overdistention.*
- Inform the patient that frequent sexual intercourse can reduce obstructive symptoms. *Relieves symptoms in the patient who has a large amount of retained prostatic fluid.*
- Teach to avoid anticholinergics, antihistamines, and decongestants. *These medications cause urinary retention.*

7 Psychosocial Integrity and Sexuality

Assess the patient's acceptance of body image related to BPH and its impact on sleep and sexual function that affects mood and mental status. *Evaluates irritability or depression that may occur with nocturia. Evaluates embarrassment of postvoid incontinence that can prevent socialization. Evaluates effect on SEXUALITY.*

8 Herbal Remedies

Remind the patient to check with the provider before taking complementary therapies. *Teaches patients that scientific evidence is lacking. Some herbs such as saw palmetto used for urinary symptoms can interfere with prescription drugs.*

9 Treatment Options – TURP

If surgery is a chosen treatment option, consider the patient's general physical condition, size of prostate, patient preferences, anxiety, and misconceptions. *Assists with options for treatment of BPH and prevents postoperative complications.*

Concept Map by Deanne A. Blach, MSN, RN

EXPECTED OUTCOMES

Normal urinary elimination pattern without urinary hesitancy, urgency, or infection

Planning

PRIORITY PATIENT PROBLEMS

Impaired Urinary Elimination related to bladder outlet obstruction

Data Synthesis

HISTORY

Davey Smitt, a 64-year-old with BPH, is admitted with a urinary tract infection (UTI), hematuria, and hydronephrosis. His wife says their sexual relationship has been nonexistent due to her husband's BPH. He has used saw palmetto extract for his urinary symptoms with some relief.

Pathophysiology

As the prostate gland enlarges, bladder outlet obstruction occurs and the patient develops urinary stasis and retention.

- Increased volume of residual → overflow incontinence → urine "leaks" around enlarged prostate → dribbling
- Urinary stasis → UTI and bladder calculi
- Chronic retention → backup of urine causes gradual dilation of ureters, hydronephrosis if not treated

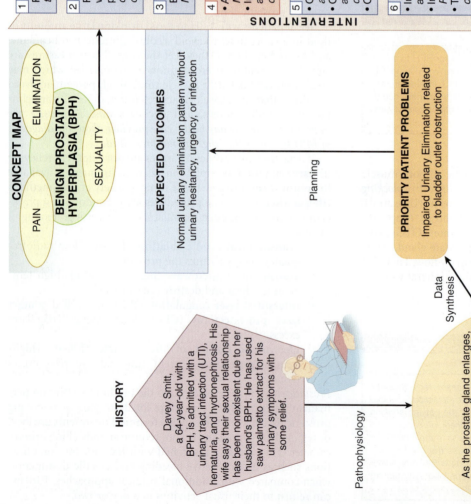

Surgical Management. For patients who are not candidates for nonsurgical management or do not want to take drugs or have other treatment options, surgery may be performed. The gold standard continues to be a **transurethral resection of the prostate (TURP)** in which the enlarged portion of the prostate is removed through an endoscopic instrument. The newer holmium laser enucleation of the prostate (HoLEP) procedure is a minimally invasive surgical technique that is gaining popularity. For a few men, an open prostatectomy (entire prostate removal) may be performed. (See discussion of Surgical Management on p. 1509 in the Prostate Cancer section.) Some or all of these criteria indicate the need for surgery:

- Acute urinary retention (AUR)
- Chronic urinary tract infections secondary to residual urine in the bladder
- Hematuria
- Hydronephrosis

Preoperative Care. When planning surgical interventions, the patient's general physical condition, the size of the prostate gland, and the man's preferences are considered. The patient may have many fears and misconceptions about prostate surgery, such as believing that automatic loss of sexual functioning or permanent incontinence will occur. Assess the patient's anxiety, correct any misconceptions about the surgery, and provide accurate information to him and his family. Regardless of the type of surgery to be performed, reinforce information about anesthesia (see Chapter 15). Remind patients taking anticoagulants that the drugs will be discontinued prior to a TURP or open prostate surgery to prevent postoperative bleeding. Other general preoperative care is described in Chapter 14.

The patient may have other medical problems that increase the risk for complications of general anesthesia and may be advised to have regional anesthesia. Epidural and spinal anesthesia are the most common types of anesthesia used for a TURP. Because the patient is awake, it is easier to assess for hyponatremia (low serum sodium), fluid overload, and water intoxication, which can result from large-volume bladder irrigations.

After a TURP, all patients have an indwelling urethral catheter. *Be sure that they know that they will feel the urge to void while the catheter is in place.* Tell the patient that he will likely have traction on the catheter that may cause discomfort. However, reassure him that analgesics will be prescribed to relieve his pain. Explain that it is normal for the urine to be blood-tinged after surgery. Small blood clots and tissue debris may pass while the catheter is in place and immediately after it is removed. Some patients also have a continuous bladder irrigation (CBI) depending on the procedure performed.

Operative Procedures. The traditional TURP is a "closed" surgery. To perform the procedure, the surgeon inserts a resectoscope (an instrument similar to a cystoscope, but with a cutting and cauterizing loop) through the urethra. The enlarged portion of the prostate gland is then removed in small pieces (prostate chips). A similar procedure is the transurethral incision of the prostate (TUIP) in which small cuts are made into the prostate to relieve pressure on the urethra. This alternate technique is used for smaller prostates. To prevent bleeding and excess clotting, a fibrinolytic inhibitor like tranexamic acid (Cyklokapron) may be used during surgery.

The disadvantage of a TURP is that, because only small pieces of the gland are removed, remaining prostate tissue may continue to grow and cause urinary obstruction, requiring additional TURPs. Also, urethral trauma from the resectoscope with resulting urethral strictures is possible.

In many large medical centers around the world, specialists can perform newer surgical treatments, such as the *holmium laser enucleation of the prostate (HoLEP)* (Eltabey et al., 2010). For this procedure, the surgeon uses the laser to remove the obstructive prostatic tissue and then pushes the tissue into the bladder for removal. Very little blood is lost during the short procedure and is therefore safe for patients taking anticoagulants.

Postoperative Care. After both the TURP and HoLEP procedures, a urinary catheter is placed into the bladder. Traction is often applied on the catheter for the patient having a TURP by pulling it taut and taping it to the patient's abdomen or thigh. If the catheter is taped to the patient's thigh, instruct him to keep his leg straight. The patient having the HoLEP procedure has a urinary catheter overnight, but the patient with a TURP may have a catheter and continuous bladder irrigation (CBI) in place for several days. In some cases the patient is discharged with the catheter in place.

For patients with a CBI, a 3-way urinary catheter is used to allow drainage of urine and inflow of a bladder irrigating solution. Be sure to maintain the flow of the irrigant to keep the urine clear. When measuring the fluid in the urinary drainage bag, be sure to subtract the amount of irrigating solution that was used to determine actual urinary output.

❓ NCLEX EXAMINATION CHALLENGE

Physiological Integrity

A client has a urinary catheter and continuous bladder irrigation after a transurethral resection of the prostate this morning. The amount of bladder irrigating solution that has infused over the past 12 hours is 1000 mL. The amount of fluid in the urinary drainage bag is 1725 mL. The nurse records that the client had ____ mL urinary output in the past 12 hours.

CONSIDERATIONS FOR OLDER ADULTS

Patient-Centered Care **QSEN**

When caring for older men who may become confused after surgery, reorient them frequently and remind them not to pull on the catheter. If the patient is restless or "picks" at tubes, provide a familiar object such as a family picture for him to hold for distraction and a feeling of security. Do not restrain the patient unless all other alternatives have failed.

Remind the patient that because of the urinary catheter's large diameter and the pressure of the retention balloon on the internal sphincter of the bladder, he will feel the urge to void continuously. This is a normal sensation, not a surgical complication. Advise the patient not to try to void around the catheter, which causes the bladder muscles to contract and may result in painful spasms. Chart 72-1 summarizes the nursing care for patients having a TURP.

If the bleeding is *venous,* the urine output is burgundy, with or without any change in vital signs. *Inform the surgeon of any bleeding.* Closely monitor the patient's hemoglobin (Hgb) and hematocrit (Hct) levels for anemia as a result of blood loss.

When the urinary catheter is removed, the patient may experience burning on urination and some urinary frequency,

CHART 72-1   Best Practice for Patient Safety & Quality Care (QSEN)

Care of the Patient After Transurethral Resection of the Prostate

- Monitor the patient closely for signs of infection. Older men undergoing prostate surgery often also have underlying chronic diseases (e.g., cardiovascular disease, chronic lung disease, diabetes).
- Help the patient out of the bed to the chair as soon as permitted to prevent complications of immobility. Older men may need assistance because of underlying changes in the musculoskeletal system (e.g., decreased range of motion, stiffness in joints). These patients are at *high risk* for falls.
- Assess the patient's pain every 2 to 4 hours, and intervene as needed to control pain.
- Provide a safe environment for the patient. Anticipate a temporary change in mental status for the older patient in the immediate postoperative period as a result of anesthetics and unfamiliar surroundings. Reorient the patient frequently. Keep catheter tubes secure.
- Maintain the rate of the continuous bladder irrigation to ensure clear urine without clots and bleeding.
- Use normal saline solution for the intermittent bladder irrigant unless otherwise prescribed. Normal saline solution is isotonic.
- Monitor the color, consistency, and amount of urine output.
- Check the drainage tubing frequently for external obstructions (e.g., kinks) and internal obstructions (e.g., blood clots, decreased output).
- Assess the patient for reports of severe bladder spasms with decreased urinary output, which may indicate obstruction.
- If the urinary catheter is obstructed, irrigate the catheter per agency or surgeon protocol.
- Notify the physician immediately if the obstruction does not resolve by hand irrigation or if the urinary return becomes ketchup-like.

! NURSING SAFETY PRIORITY (QSEN)

Critical Rescue

After a TURP, monitor the patient's urine output every 2 hours and vital signs, including pain assessment, every 4 hours for the first postoperative day. Assess for postoperative bleeding. *Patients who undergo a TURP or open prostatectomy are at risk for severe bleeding or hemorrhage after surgery. Although rare, bleeding is most likely within the first 24 hours.* Blood transfusions may be given after a TURP surgery but are not needed after the HoLEP procedure. Bladder spasms or movement may trigger fresh bleeding from previously controlled vessels. This bleeding may be arterial or venous, but venous bleeding is more common.

If arterial bleeding occurs, the urinary drainage is bright red or ketchup-like with numerous clots. Notify the surgeon immediately, and irrigate the catheter with normal saline solution per physician or hospital protocol. In rare instances the surgeon may prescribe aminocaproic acid (Amicar) to control bleeding. If this drug does not work, surgical intervention may be needed to clear the bladder of clots and to stop bleeding.

dribbling, and leakage. Reassure him that these symptoms are normal and will decrease. The patient may also pass small clots and tissue debris for several days after the TURP. *Instruct him to increase fluid intake to at least 2000 to 2500 mL daily, which helps decrease dysuria and keep the urine clear.* An older patient who has renal disease or who is at risk for heart failure may not be able to tolerate this much fluid. By the time of discharge (usually 2 to 3 days after surgery depending on age and progress), he should be voiding 150 to 200 mL of clear yellow urine every 3 to 4 hours. By discharge, pain is minimal and analgesics may not be required.

Observe for other possible but uncommon complications of TURP, such as INFECTION and incontinence. Teach the patient that sexual function should not be affected after surgery but that retrograde ejaculation is possible. In this case, most of the semen flows backwards into the bladder so only a small amount will be ejaculated from the penis.

Community-Based Care

The patient with benign prostatic hyperplasia (BPH) is typically managed at home. Patients who have surgery are also discharged to their home or other setting from where they were admitted. Some patients, especially those who have had a TURP, may have temporary loss of control of urination or a dribbling of the urine. Reassure the patient that these symptoms are almost always temporary and will resolve. Also remind him that REPRODUCTION ability should not be affected by surgery.

Assist the patient and his family in finding ways to keep his clothing dry until sphincter control returns. Instruct him to contract and relax his sphincter frequently to re-establish urinary ELIMINATION control (Kegel exercises). External urinary (condom) catheters are not used except in extreme cases because they may give the patient a false sense of security and delay urinary control.

Patients having the HoLEP procedure typically stay in the hospital overnight and usually have no urinary symptoms after surgery. This procedure may soon replace the TURP as the gold standard for surgical management of the patient with BPH.

? NCLEX EXAMINATION CHALLENGE

Physiological Integrity

A client had a transurethral resection of the prostate (TURP) with continuous bladder irrigation yesterday. The staff nurse notes that the urinary drainage is bright red and thick. What is the nurse's best action?
A. Notify the charge nurse as soon as possible.
B. Increase the rate of the bladder irrigation.
C. Document the assessment in the medical record.
D. Prepare the patient for a blood transfusion.

PROSTATE CANCER

❖ PATHOPHYSIOLOGY

Prostate cancer is the second most common type of cancer in men in the world and if found early has a nearly 100% cure rate. Men older than 65 years have the greatest risk for the disease. In the United States, it affects African-American men more commonly than Euro-American men and at an earlier age. The exact cause for this difference is not known (Hegarty & Bailey, 2011).

Testosterone and dihydrotestosterone (DHT) are the major androgens (male hormones) in the adult male. Testosterone is produced by the testis and circulates in the blood. DHT is a testosterone derivative in the prostate gland. In some patients the prostate grows very rapidly, leading to noncancerous high-grade prostatic intraepithelial neoplasia (PIN). Patients with PIN are at a higher risk for developing prostate cancer than are men who do not have that growth pattern.

Many prostate tumors are androgen-sensitive (McCance et al., 2014). Most are adenocarcinomas and arise from

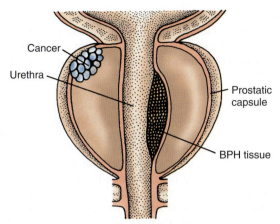

FIG. 72-3 The prostate gland with cancer and benign prostatic hyperplasia (BPH). Note that cancer normally arises in the periphery of the gland, whereas BPH occurs in the center of the gland.

epithelial cells located in the posterior lobe or outer portion of the gland (Fig. 72-3).

Of all malignancies, prostate cancer is one of the slowest growing, and it metastasizes (spreads) in a predictable pattern. Common sites of metastasis are the nearby lymph nodes, bones, lungs, and liver (McCance et al., 2014). The bones of the pelvis, sacrum, and lumbar spine are most often affected. Chapter 21 describes staging categories of localized and advanced cancers.

Prostate cancer is caused by a number of factors. Advanced age is the leading risk factor. Race is the second most common risk factor, and family history of prostate cancer is the third most common risk factor for this malignancy. The risk increases twofold for men who have a first-degree relative (brother, father) with the disease.

🌐 CULTURAL CONSIDERATIONS
Patient-Centered Care QSEN

Race is the second most common risk factor for prostate cancer because the disease affects African Americans more often than other ethnic/racial groups, followed by Caucasians (Euro-Americans) and Hispanic-American men. The reasons for these differences are not known but may be related to socioeconomic factors, health care access, health insurance, education, and diet (Dunn & Kazer, 2011).

Other risk factors that may play a role are eating a diet high in animal fat (e.g., red meat) and complex carbohydrates or having a low-fiber intake. Men who have had a vasectomy or those who were exposed to environmental toxins, such as arsenic, may also be at increased risk for the disease (McCance

🧬 GENETIC/GENOMIC CONSIDERATIONS
Patient-Centered Care QSEN

Many gene mutations play a role in various types of prostate cancer. Some men with the most aggressive prostate cancers have *BRCA2* mutations similar to those women who have *BRCA2*-associated breast and ovarian cancers. The most common genetic factor that increases the risk for prostate cancer is a mutation in the glutathione S-transferase *(GST P1)* gene. This gene is normally part of the pathway that helps prevent cancer (McCance et al., 2014).

EVIDENCE-BASED PRACTICE QSEN
What Are the Evidence-Based Recommendations for Prostate-Specific Antigen Screening for Prostate Cancer?

O'Rourke, M.E. (2011). The prostate-specific antigen screening conundrum: Examining the evidence. *Seminars in Oncology Nursing, 27*(4), 251-259.

The researchers reviewed the current guidelines and recommendations for prostate-specific antigen (PSA) screening from a variety of nursing and medical literature. They found multiple recommendations from randomized controlled trials (RCTs) and various national and international organizations, including the National Comprehensive Cancer Network, The American College of Preventive Medicine, and the Advisory Committee on Cancer Prevention of the European Union. However, there was no consensus regarding the normal values of PSA for age-groups or when PSA screening is needed. Most guidelines made adjustments for age and race because the PSA normal value is likely to increase as a man ages and African-American men tend to have higher normal PSA values than other groups.

Level of Evidence: 1
The researchers used a systematic literature review of RCTs and guidelines from various professional international and national organizations.

Commentary: Implications for Practice and Research
Nurses need to explain to men that there is no consensus regarding PSA screening. Instead, men should talk with their primary health care provider and identify risk factors that may influence the decision for PSA screening. More RCTs are needed to establish guidelines for prostate screening to assist health care providers as they counsel their patients.

et al., 2014). Although controversial, some researchers believe that excessive intake of vitamin E and omega-3 fish oil supplements may increase the risk for prostate cancer (American Cancer Society [ACS], 2014a).

Health Promotion and Maintenance
Teach men about the most recent American Cancer Society (ACS) guidelines for prostate cancer screening and early detection (ACS, 2014a). The current recommendations are that men should make an informed decision about whether to have prostate cancer screening. Although not agreed upon by all authoritative sources, starting at the age of 50 years, men should discuss the options of having prostate-specific antigen testing with their health care provider (see the Evidence-Based Practice box). Men at a higher risk for prostate cancer, including African Americans or men who have a first-degree relative with prostate cancer before the age of 65 years, should have this discussion at age 45 years. Men who have multiple first-degree relatives with prostate cancer at an early age should discuss screening at age 40 years (O'Rourke, 2011).

Although a family history of prostate cancer cannot be changed, certain nutritional habits can be altered to possibly decrease the risk for the disease. First, teach men to eat a healthy, balanced diet, including decreasing animal fat (e.g., red meat). Instead of red meat, remind them to eat more fish and other foods high in *omega-3 fatty acids* because they are thought to be helpful in preventing cancer. Also reinforce the need to increase fruits, vegetables, and high-fiber foods (Carmody et al., 2012).

❖ PATIENT-CENTERED COLLABORATIVE CARE

◆ Assessment

History. Assess the patient's age, race/ethnicity, and family history of prostate cancer. Ask about his nutritional habits, especially focusing on the intake of red meat, fish, and fruits and vegetables. Assess whether the patient has any problems with urinary ELIMINATION. Take a drug history to determine if he is taking any medication that could affect voiding. The first symptoms that the man may report are related to bladder outlet obstruction, such as difficulty in starting urination, frequent bladder INFECTIONS, and urinary retention. Ask about urinary frequency, **hematuria** (blood in the urine), and **nocturia** (voiding during the night). Ask if he has had any PAIN during intercourse, especially when ejaculating. Inquire if the patient has had or currently has any other pain (particularly bone pain), a symptom associated with advanced prostate cancer. Ask him if he has had any recent unexpected weight loss.

Take a sexual history for recent changes in desire or function. Ask about current or previous sexually transmitted diseases, penile discharge, or scrotal pain or swelling.

Physical Assessment/Clinical Manifestations. Most *early* cancers are diagnosed while the patient is having a routine physical examination or is being treated for benign prostatic hyperplasia (BPH). Gross blood in the urine (hematuria) is a common clinical manifestation of *late* prostate cancer. Assess for PAIN in the pelvis, spine, hips, or ribs. Complete a thorough pain assessment. Palpate for swollen lymph nodes, especially in the groin areas. Pain and swollen nodes also indicate advanced disease that has spread. Take and record the patient's weight because unexpected weight loss is also common when the disease is advanced.

Prepare the patient for a digital rectal examination (DRE). On rectal examination, a prostate that is found to be stony hard and with palpable irregularities or indurations is suspected to be malignant.

Psychosocial Assessment. A diagnosis of any type of cancer causes fear and anxiety for most people. Some men, particularly African Americans, develop the disease in their 40s and 50s when they are perhaps planning their retirements, putting their children through college, and/or enjoying their middle years. Assess the reaction of the patient to the diagnosis, and observe how his family reacts to the illness. Men may describe their feelings as shock, fear, anger, and "roller coaster." Expect that patients usually go through the grieving process and may be in denial or depressed. Determine what support systems they have, such as spiritual leaders or community group support, to help them through diagnosis, treatment, and recovery.

One of the biggest concerns for the man may be his ability for sexual function after cancer treatment. Tell him that function will depend on the type of treatment he has. Common surgical techniques used today do not involve cutting the perineal nerves that are needed for an erection. A dry climax may occur if the prostate is removed because it produces most of the fluid in the ejaculate. Refer the patient to his surgeon (urologist), sex therapist, or intimacy counselor if available.

Laboratory Assessment. **Prostate-specific antigen (PSA)** is a glycoprotein produced by the prostate. *PSA analysis is used as a screening test for prostate cancer.* If the test is performed, it should be drawn before the DRE because the examination can cause an increase in PSA due to prostate irritation.

Most authoritative sources agree that the normal blood level of PSA in men younger than 50 years is less than 2.5 ng/mL. PSA levels increase to as high as 6.5 ng/mL when men reach their 70s. *African-American men have a slighter higher normal value, but the reason for this difference is not known. Because other prostate problems also increase the PSA level, it is not specifically diagnostic for cancer.* The level associated with prostate cancer, however, is usually much higher than those occurring with problems such as prostatitis and benign prostatic hyperplasia (Pagana & Pagana, 2014).

An elevated PSA level should decrease a few days after a prostatectomy for cancer. An increase in the PSA level several weeks after surgery may indicate that the disease has recurred.

Because PSA is not absolutely specific to prostate cancer, another test, *early prostate cancer antigen (EPCA-2)*, may be a serum marker for prostate cancer. It can detect changes in the prostate gland early and is a very sensitive test. EPCA-2 may also eliminate the need to perform a biopsy of prostate tissue (Pagana & Pagana, 2014).

Other Diagnostic Assessment. After assessments by DRE and PSA, most patients have a *transrectal ultrasound (TRUS)* of the prostate in an ambulatory care or imaging setting. The technician inserts a small probe into the rectum and obtains a view of the prostate using sound waves. If prostate cancer is suspected, a *biopsy* is usually performed in the physician's office to obtain an accurate diagnosis. Prior to the procedure, the physician uses lidocaine jelly on the ultrasound probe and/or injects lidocaine into the prostate gland to promote patient comfort (Dunn & Kazer, 2011).

> ❗ **NURSING SAFETY PRIORITY** (QSEN)
>
> ### Action Alert
>
> After a *transrectal ultrasound with biopsy*, instruct the patient about possible complications, although rare, including hematuria with clots, signs of infection, and perineal pain. Teach him to report fever, chills, bloody urine, and any difficulty voiding. Advise him to avoid strenuous physical activity and to drink plenty of fluids, especially in the first 24 hours after the procedure. Teach him that a small amount of bleeding turning the urine pink is expected during this time. However, bright red bleeding should be reported to the health care provider immediately.

After prostate cancer is diagnosed, the patient has additional imaging and blood studies to determine the extent of the disease. Common tests include lymph node biopsy, CT of the pelvis and abdomen, and MRI to assess the status of the pelvic and para-aortic lymph nodes. A radionuclide bone scan may be performed to detect metastatic bone disease. An enlarged liver or abnormal liver function study results indicate possible liver metastasis.

Patients with advanced prostate cancer often have *elevated* levels of *serum acid phosphatase*. Most men with bone metastasis have *elevated serum alkaline phosphatase* levels and severe PAIN.

◆ Interventions

As with any cancer, accurate staging and grading of prostate tumors guide treatment planning and monitoring during the course of the disease. Patients are faced with several treatment options. A urologist and oncologist are needed to help patients make the best decision. Because prostate cancer is slow growing with late metastasis, older men who are asymptomatic and have other illnesses may choose observation without immediate active treatment, especially if the cancer is early stage. This option is known as active surveillance (AS). This form of treatment involves initial surveillance with active treatment only if the symptoms become bothersome. The average time from diagnosis to start of treatment is up to 10 years. During the AS period, men are monitored at regular intervals through DRE and PSA testing. Factors that are considered in choosing AS include potential side effects of treatment (e.g., urinary incontinence, erectile dysfunction), estimated life expectancy, and the risk for increased morbidity and mortality from not seeking active treatment (Hegarty & Bailey, 2011).

Patients who have very early–stage cancer of the prostate who choose AS require close follow-up by their health care provider. If obstruction occurs, a transurethral resection of the prostate (TURP) may be done. The care of patients having this procedure is described in the discussion of Surgical Management on p. 1505 in the Benign Prostatic Hyperplasia section.

Specific management is based on the extent of the disease and the patient's physical condition. The patient may undergo surgery for a biopsy, staging and removal of the tumor, or palliation to control the spread of disease or relieve distressing symptoms. As with AS, the health care provider and patient must weigh the benefits of treatment against potential adverse effects such as incontinence and erectile dysfunction (ED).

Surgical Management. Surgery is the most common intervention for a cure. Minimally invasive surgery (MIS) or, less commonly, an open surgical technique for radical prostatectomy (prostate removal) is usually performed. A bilateral orchiectomy (removal of both testicles) is another palliative surgery that slows the spread of cancer by removing the main source of testosterone.

Preoperative Care. Preoperative care depends on the type of surgery that will be done. Minimally invasive surgery (MIS) is most appropriate for localized prostate cancer and is used as a curative intervention. The most common procedure is the *laparoscopic radical prostatectomy (LRP)*, most often with robotic assistance (Chitlik, 2011). Other newer procedures include transrectal high-intensity focused ultrasound (HIFU) and cryosurgery. Patients who qualify for LRP must have a PSA less than 10 ng/mL and have no previous hormone therapy or abdominal surgeries. Remind the patient that the advantages of this procedure over open surgery are (Dunn & Kazer, 2011):

* Decreased hospital stay (1 to 2 days)
* Minimal bleeding
* Smaller or no incisions and less scarring
* Less postoperative discomfort
* Decreased time for urinary catheter placement
* Fewer complications
* Faster recovery and return to usual activities
* Nerve-sparing advantages

For the patient undergoing an *open* radical prostatectomy, provide preoperative care as for any patient having surgery (see Chapter 14).

Operative Procedures. For the *LRP procedure*, the patient is placed in lithotomy positioning with steep Trendelenburg. Nurses in the OR ensure that the patient maintains a balanced body temperature and positions the patient to prevent injury (Chitlik, 2011). The urologist makes one or more small punctures or incisions into the abdomen. A laparoscope with a camera on the end is inserted through one of the incisions while other instruments are inserted into the other incisions. The robotic system may be used to control the movement of the instruments by a remote device. The prostate is removed along with nearby lymph nodes, but perineal nerves are not affected.

The *open* radical prostatectomy can be performed via several surgical approaches, depending on the patient's desired outcomes and the staging of the disease. The transperineal and retropubic (nerve-sparing) approaches are most commonly used. The surgeon removes the entire prostate gland along with the prostatic capsule, the cuff at the bladder neck, the seminal vesicles, and the regional lymph nodes. The remaining urethra is connected to the bladder neck. The removal of tissue at the bladder neck allows the seminal fluid to travel upward into the bladder rather than down the urethral tract, resulting in retrograde ejaculations.

Postoperative Care. Provide postoperative care of the patient after *open* radical prostatectomy as summarized in Chart 72-2. Nursing interventions include all the typical care for a patient undergoing major surgery. Maintaining hydration, caring for wound drains (open procedure), managing PAIN, and preventing pulmonary complications are important aspects of nursing care. (See general postoperative care in Chapter 16.)

Assess the patient's pain level, and monitor the effectiveness of PAIN management with opioids given as patient-controlled analgesia (PCA), a common method of delivery during the first 24 hours after surgery. Administer a stool softener if needed to prevent possible constipation from the drugs. Patients having the minimally invasive surgery have much less pain and fewer complications.

The patient has an indwelling urinary catheter to straight drainage to promote urinary ELIMINATION. Monitor intake and output every shift and record, or delegate this activity to and supervise unlicensed assistive personnel (UAP). An antispasmodic may be prescribed to decrease bladder spasm induced by the indwelling urinary catheter. The time for catheter removal depends on the type of procedure that is performed and overall patient condition. Those with open surgical procedures use the catheter for 7 to 10 days or longer.

CHART 72-2 **Best Practice for Patient Safety & Quality Care** QSEN

Care of the Patient After an Open Radical Prostatectomy

* Encourage the patient to use patient-controlled analgesia (PCA) as needed.
* Help the patient get out of bed into a chair on the night of surgery and ambulate by the next day.
* Maintain the sequential compression device until the patient begins to ambulate.
* Monitor the patient for deep vein thrombosis and pulmonary embolus.
* Keep an accurate record of intake and output, including Jackson-Pratt or other drainage device drainage.
* Keep the urinary meatus clean using soap and water.
* Avoid rectal procedures or treatments.
* Teach the patient how to care for the urinary catheter because he may be discharged with the catheter in place.
* Teach the patient how to use a leg bag.
* Emphasize the importance of not straining during bowel movement. Advise the patient to avoid suppositories or enemas.
* Remind the patient about the importance of follow-up appointments with the physician to monitor progress.

Ambulation should begin no later than the day after surgery. Provide assistance in walking the patient when he first gets out of bed. Assess for scrotal or penile swelling from the disrupted pelvic lymph flow. If this occurs, elevate the scrotum and penis and apply ice to the area intermittently for the first 24 to 48 hours.

Many patients who have the minimally invasive techniques are discharged in 1 to 3 days after surgery and can resume usual activities in about a week or two. Those who have open procedures are discharged in 2 to 3 days or longer, depending on their progress.

Remind patients that common potential long-term complications of open radical prostatectomy are erectile dysfunction (ED) and urinary incontinence. For ED, drugs such as sildenafil (Viagra) may be effective. *Urge incontinence* may occur because the internal and external sphincters of the bladder lie close to the prostate gland and are often damaged during the surgery. Kegel perineal exercises may reduce the severity of urinary incontinence after radical prostatectomy. Teach the patient to contract and relax the perineal and gluteal muscles in several ways. For one of the exercises, teach him to:

1. Tighten the perineal muscles for 3 to 5 seconds as if to prevent voiding, and then relax.
2. Bear down as if having a bowel movement.
3. Relax and repeat the exercise.

Show him how to inhale through pursed lips while tightening the perineal muscles and how to exhale when he relaxes. To regain urinary control, teach the patient to practice holding an object, such as a pencil, in the fold between the buttock and the thigh. He may also sit on the toilet with the knees apart while voiding and start and stop the stream several times.

Nonsurgical Management. Nonsurgical management may be an adjunct to surgery or alternative intervention if the cancer is widespread or the patient's condition or age prevents surgery. Available modalities include radiation therapy, hormone therapy, and chemotherapy (less often).

Radiation Therapy. External or internal radiation therapy may be used in the treatment of prostate cancer or as "salvage" treatments when cancer recurs. It may also be done for palliation of the patient's symptoms.

External beam radiation therapy (EBRT or XRT) comes from a source outside the body. Patients are usually treated 5 days a week for 4 to 6 weeks (Dunn & Kazer, 2011). Three-dimensional conformal radiation therapy (3D-CRT) can more accurately target prostate tissue and can reduce side effects such as damage to the rectum. An advanced type of this radiation called *intensity-modulated radiation therapy* provides very high doses to the prostate. EBRT can also be used to relieve pain from bone metastasis or given following radical prostatectomy. Teach patients that external beam radiation causes ED in many men well after the treatment is completed.

Teach patients that other complications from EBRT include urinary frequency, diarrhea, and *acute radiation cystitis,* which causes persistent pain and hematuria. Symptoms are usually mild to moderate and subside in 6 weeks after treatment. Drugs to prevent urinary urgency such as tolterodine (Detrol LA) may be prescribed. Teach the patient to avoid caffeine and continue drinking plenty of water and other fluids.

Radiation proctitis (rectal mucosa inflammation) may also develop but is less likely with 3D-CRT. The man reports rectal urgency and cramping and passes mucus and blood. Teach him to report these symptoms to the health care provider. Like

cystitis, this problem usually resolves in 4 to 6 weeks after the treatment stops. If proctitis occurs, teach patients to limit spicy or fatty foods, caffeine, and dairy products.

Low-dose brachytherapy (internal radiation) can be delivered by implanting low-dose radiation seeds, needles, or wires directly into and around the prostate gland. This treatment includes ultrasonically guided interstitial or radioactive implantation. These procedures are done on an ambulatory care basis and are the most cost-effective treatment for early-stage prostate cancer. Reassure the patient that the dose of radiation is low and that the radiation will not pose a hazard to him or others. Teach him that ED, urinary incontinence, and rectal problems do occur in a small percentage of cases. Fatigue is also common and may last for several months after the treatment stops. Chapter 22 describes general nursing care for patients having radiation therapy.

Drug Therapy. Drug therapy may consist of either hormone therapy (androgen deprivation therapy [ADT]) or chemotherapy.

Hormone Therapy. Because most prostate tumors are hormone dependent, patients with extensive tumors or those with metastatic disease may be managed by androgen deprivation. Luteinizing hormone–releasing hormone (LH-RH) agonists or anti-androgens can be used.

Examples of *LH-RH agonists* are leuprolide (Lupron), goserelin (Zoladex), and triptorelin (Trelstar). These drugs first stimulate the pituitary gland to release the luteinizing hormone (LH). After about 3 weeks, the pituitary gland "runs out" of LH, which reduces testosterone production by the testes.

! NURSING SAFETY PRIORITY (QSEN)

Drug Alert

Teach patients taking LH-RH agonists that side effects include "hot flashes," erectile dysfunction, and decreased **libido** (desire to have sex). Some men also have **gynecomastia** (breast tenderness and growth). These drugs can also cause osteoporosis. Bisphosphonates like pamidronate (Aredia) are prescribed to prevent bone fractures. They can also be used to slow the damage caused by bone metastasis.

Anti-androgen drugs, also known as *androgen deprivation therapy (ADT),* work differently in that they block the body's ability to use the available androgens (Dunn & Kazer, 2011). These drugs are the major treatment for metastatic disease. Examples include flutamide (Eulexin, Euflex ✦), bicalutamide (Casodex), and nilutamide (Nilandron). These drugs inhibit tumor progression by blocking the uptake of testicular and adrenal androgens at the prostate tumor site.

Anti-androgens may be used alone or in combination with LH-RH agonists for a total or maximal androgen blockade (hormone ablation). Patients who have this drug combination often have "hot flashes" similar to those experienced by menopausal women, and they can decrease the patient's perceived quality of life. Ask the patient if he has been experiencing this problem. Megestrol acetate may be prescribed for this uncomfortable condition.

Chemotherapy. Systemic chemotherapy may be an option for patients whose cancer has spread and for whom other therapies have not worked. For example, small cell prostate cancer is rare and is more responsive to chemotherapy than to hormone therapy. Docetaxel (Taxotere) plus prednisone given every 3 weeks is the preferred treatment. A combination of cisplatin (Platinol) and etoposide (VP-16, VePesid) may also be effective for this type of cancer. Chapter 22 describes general nursing care for patients receiving chemotherapy.

Community-Based Care

Patient-centered collaborative care of the man with prostate cancer should include his partner, if any, and family. The diagnosis and treatment of cancer greatly affect couples who survive the disease. Recognize that the patient and partner have specific physical and psychosocial needs that should be addressed before hospital discharge and management should continue in the community setting.

Patients with prostate cancer may require care in a wide variety of settings: at the hospital, the radiation therapy department, the oncologist's office, or home at any stage of the disease process. Specific interventions depend on which treatment the patient had or if he had a combination of treatments. This section focuses on the needs of those who had a radical prostatectomy.

Home Care Management. Discharge planning and health teaching start early, even before surgery. A patient can better plan home care management when he knows what to expect. Collaborate with the case manager to coordinate the efforts of various health care providers, surgical unit nursing staff, and possibly a home care nurse. As specified by The Joint Commission and other accrediting agencies, continuity of care is essential when caring for this patient because he may need weeks or months of therapies.

Self-Management Education. An important area of teaching for the patient going home after an *open* radical prostatectomy may be urinary catheter care. An indwelling urinary catheter may be in place for up to several weeks, depending on the surgical technique that was used. Teach him and his family how to care for the catheter, use a leg bag, and identify manifestations of INFECTION and other complications. See Chart 72-3 for patient and family education.

Encourage the patient to walk short distances. Lifting may be restricted to no more than 15 pounds for up to 6 weeks if an open procedure was done. Remind him to maintain an upright position and not walk bent or flexed. Vigorous exercise such as running or jumping should be avoided for at least 12 weeks and then gradually introduced. By contrast, patients having the minimally invasive laparoscopic surgery can usually return to work or usual activities in about a week.

Teach the patient to not strain to defecate. A stool softener may be prescribed to reduce the need for straining. If an opioid is prescribed for PAIN management, encourage the patient to drink adequate water to prevent constipation.

If the patient had an *open* radical prostatectomy, teach him to shower for the first 2 to 3 weeks rather than soak in a bathtub. Patients who had a laparoscopic procedure can usually shower in 1 to 2 days. Teach them to remove the small bandage but leave the Steri-Strips in place (they should fall off in about a week). Show patients how to inspect the incision or puncture site(s) daily for signs of INFECTION. Remind them to keep all follow-up appointments. PSA blood tests are taken 6 weeks after surgery and then every 4 to 6 months to monitor progress.

Health Care Resources. Refer the patient and partner to agencies or support groups such as the American Cancer Society's *Man to Man* program to help cope with prostate cancer. This program provides one-on-one education, personal visits, educational presentations, and the opportunity to engage in open and candid discussions. Another prostate cancer support group is *Us TOO International* (www.ustoo.com) sponsored by the Prostate Cancer Education and Support Network. This group provides education and support with national and international chapters. Information can also be obtained from the Prostate Cancer Foundation (www.prostatecancerfoundation.org) or the National Prostate Cancer Coalition (www.fightprostatecancer.org). Other personal and community support services such as spiritual leaders or churches and synagogues are also important to many patients.

For same-sex couples surviving prostate cancer, *Malecare* (http://malecare.org) is an excellent resource. This nonprofit organization provides support groups for gay and bisexual men and their partners (Galbraith et al., 2011). Another resource is *A Gay Man's Guide to Prostate Cancer*, which was updated in 2011.

Some men have erectile dysfunction (ED) for the first 3 to 18 months after a prostatectomy. Refer them to a specialist who can help with this problem. (ED is discussed briefly in the Erectile Dysfunction section, p. 1512.) Refer patients with urinary incontinence to a urologist who specializes in this area. Drug therapy and other strategies may be used. Chapter 66 discusses incontinence management in detail.

CHART 72-3 Patient and Family Education: Preparing for Self-Management

Urinary Catheter Care at Home

- Once a day, gently wash the first few inches of the catheter starting at the penis and washing outward with mild soap and water.
- Rinse and dry the catheter well.
- If you have not been circumcised, push the foreskin back to clean the catheter site; when finished, push the foreskin forward.
- Change the drainage bag at least once a week as needed:
  - Hold the catheter with one hand and the tubing with the other hand, and twist in opposite directions to disconnect.
  - Place the end of the catheter in a clean container to catch leakage of urine.
  - Remove the rubber cap from the tubing of the leg bag or clean drainage bag.
  - Clean the end of the new tubing with alcohol swabs.
  - Insert the end of the new tubing into the catheter, and twist to connect securely.
- Clean the drainage bag just removed by pouring a solution of one part vinegar to two parts water through the tubing and bag. Rinse well with water, and allow the bag to dry.

💡 CLINICAL JUDGMENT CHALLENGE

Patient-Centered Care (QSEN)

A urologist tells a 70-year-old man that his biopsy revealed stage 2 prostate cancer. The patient has lived with his male life partner for 20 years; they are both very upset about his diagnosis and prognosis. The urologist states that the patient is a candidate for laparoscopic prostatectomy.

1. As the office nurse, what is your best response to the patient and his partner at this time?
2. How would you describe his likely prognosis?
3. What health teaching will the patient and partner need?
4. What community resources will you recommend and why?

PROSTATITIS

❖ PATHOPHYSIOLOGY

Prostatitis is an inflammation of the prostate gland. Duration of symptoms, presence or absence of WBCs in the urine, and urinary culture results determine the classification.

Bacterial prostatitis often occurs with urethritis or an INFEC- TION of the lower urinary tract. Organisms may reach the pros- tate via the bloodstream or the urethra. The most common organisms are *Escherichia coli, Enterobacter, Proteus,* and group D streptococci. Acute bacterial prostatitis may be manifested by fever, chills, **dysuria** (painful urination), urethral discharge, and a boggy, tender prostate. Gentle palpation of the prostate usually results in a urethral discharge, which has WBCs in the prostatic secretions.

Chronic bacterial prostatitis generally occurs in older men and has a less dramatic presentation than acute bacterial pros- tatitis and without the systemic manifestations. The patient reports experiencing hesitancy, urgency, dysuria, difficulty ini- tiating and terminating the flow of urine, and decreased strength and volume of urine. Also, there may be discomfort in the perineum, scrotum, and penis.

❖ PATIENT-CENTERED COLLABORATIVE CARE

The patient with chronic prostatitis usually reports backache, perineal PAIN, mild dysuria, and urinary frequency. Hematuria may be present. The prostate may feel irregularly enlarged, firm, and slightly tender when palpated. The patient often has an elevated serum WBC count and prostate-specific antigen (PSA) level.

Complications of prostatitis are **epididymitis** (inflamma- tion of the epididymis) and **cystitis** (inflammation of the bladder). The patient with either acute or chronic bacterial prostatitis is likely to develop urinary tract INFECTIONS. Sexual functioning may be impaired because of discomfort.

Early diagnosis and treatment of prostatitis with antimicro- bials are important. Treatment may last from weeks to many months because there is poor penetration of antibiotics into prostatic tissue. Acute bacterial prostatitis may require hospital- ization with aggressive IV antibiotics.

Emphasize the importance of comfort measures, such as sitz baths, muscle relaxants, and NSAIDs. Stool softeners are pre- scribed to prevent straining and rectal irritation of the prostate during a bowel movement. Alpha blockers such as tamsulosin (Flomax) may be given to promote voiding. Teach patients to avoid alcohol, coffee, tea, and spicy foods that irritate symp- toms. Instruct them to avoid over-the-counter cold prepara- tions containing decongestants or antihistamines that may cause urinary retention.

Teach the patient with chronic prostatitis about the long- term nature of the problem. Because prostatitis can cause other urinary tract INFECTIONS, explain the importance of long- term antibiotic therapy and increasing fluid intake. Remind him to take the prescribed antibiotics on schedule. Because sulfamethoxazole-trimethoprim (Bactrim, Septra) diffuses into the prostatic fluid, it is often the antibiotic of choice. *Before drug administration, be sure that the patient does not have any allergy to sulfa drugs.*

Teach the patient about activities that drain the prostate (sexual intercourse, masturbation), which may help in the man- agement of chronic prostatitis. Inform him that prostatitis is not infectious or contagious.

ERECTILE DYSFUNCTION

❖ PATHOPHYSIOLOGY

Erectile dysfunction (ED), also known as *impotence,* is the inability to achieve or maintain an erection for sexual inter- course. It affects millions of men in the United States. There are two major types of ED: organic and functional.

Organic ED is a gradual deterioration of function. The man first notices diminishing firmness and a decrease in frequency of erections. Causes include (McCance, et al., 2014):

- Inflammation of the prostate, urethra, or seminal vesicles
- Surgical procedures such as prostatectomy
- Pelvic fractures
- Lumbosacral injuries
- Vascular disease, including hypertension
- Chronic neurologic conditions, such as Parkinson disease or multiple sclerosis
- Endocrine disorders, such as diabetes mellitus (a major cause) or thyroid disorders
- Smoking and alcohol consumption
- Drugs, such as antihypertensives
- Poor overall health that prevents sexual intercourse

If the patient has episodes of ED, it usually has a *functional* (psychological) cause. Men with functional ED usually have normal nocturnal (nighttime) and morning erections. Onset is usually sudden and follows a period of high stress.

❖ PATIENT-CENTERED COLLABORATIVE CARE

If possible, the physician determines the cause of the ED through a variety of diagnostic testing, including measuring serum hormone levels and using Doppler ultrasonography to determine blood flow to the penis. The most common interven- tion for ED is drug therapy. Other interventions include vacuum devices, intracorporal injections, intraurethral applications, and prostheses (implants).

First-line oral drugs used to manage ED, phosphodiesterace-5 (PDE-5) inhibitors, work by relaxing the smooth muscles in the corpora cavernosa so blood flow to the penis is increased. The veins exiting the corpora are compressed, limiting outward blood flow and resulting in penile **tumescence** (swelling). Teach patients to take the pill 1 hour before sexual intercourse. For some drugs, such as sildenafil (Viagra) and vardenafil (Levitra), sexual stimulation is needed within $\frac{1}{2}$ to 1 hour to promote the erection. With other drugs, such as tadalafil (Cialis), erec- tion can be stimulated over a longer period. Because the erec- tion occurs more naturally compared with other treatment options, most men and their partners prefer this option.

> ❗ **NURSING SAFETY PRIORITY** (QSEN)
> *Drug Alert*
>
> Instruct patients taking PDE-5 inhibitors to abstain from alcohol before sexual intercourse because it may impair the ability to have an erection. Common side effects of these drugs include dyspepsia (heartburn), headaches, facial flushing, and stuffy nose. If more than one pill a day is being taken, leg and back cramps, nausea, and vomiting also may occur. *Teach men who take nitrates to avoid PDE-5 inhibitors because the vasodilation effects can cause a profound hypotension and reduce blood flow to vital organs.* For patients who cannot take these drugs or do not respond to them, other methods are available to achieve an erection.

The basic design of a *vacuum constriction device (VCD)* is a cylinder that fits over the penis and sits firmly against the body. Using a pump, a vacuum is created to draw blood into the penis to maintain an erection. A rubber ring (tension band) is placed around the base of the penis to maintain the erection, and the cylinder is removed.

Injecting the penis with vasodilating drugs can make the penis erect by engorging it with blood. The most common agents used for this purpose include (Lilley et al., 2014):

- Alprostadil (Caverject), a synthetic vasodilator identical to prostaglandin E_1 produced in the body
- Paverine, also a vasodilator
- Phentolamine (Regitine), an alpha-1, alpha-2 selective adrenergic receptor antagonist
- A combination of any or all of these drugs

Adverse drug effects include priapism (prolonged erection), penile scarring, fibrosis, bleeding, bruising at the injection site, pain, infection, and vasovagal responses.

Penile implants (prostheses) are used when other modalities fail. Devices include semirigid, flexible, or hydraulic inflatable and multi-component or one-piece instruments. The three-piece inflatable device is the most commonly implanted prosthesis. A reservoir is placed in the scrotum. Tubes carry the fluid into the inflatable pieces that are placed in the penis. To inflate the prosthesis, the man squeezes the pump located in the scrotum. To deflate the prosthesis, a release button is activated. Advantages include the man's ability to control his erections. The major disadvantages include device failure and infection. The device is implanted as an ambulatory care surgical procedure. *Teach the patient to observe the surgical site for bleeding and* INFECTION.

? NCLEX EXAMINATION CHALLENGE

Health Promotion and Maintenance

The nurse is teaching a client about taking sildenafil (Viagra) for erectile dysfunction. Which statement by the client indicates a need for further teaching?
A. "I should have sex within an hour after taking the drug."
B. "I should avoid alcohol when on the drug or it might not work well."
C. "I can expect to maybe get a stuffy nose or headache when I take the drug."
D. "If I have chest pain during sex, I should take a nitroglycerin tablet."

TESTICULAR CANCER

❖ PATHOPHYSIOLOGY

Testicular cancer is a rare cancer that most often affects men between 20 and 35 years of age but can affect men of any age (American Cancer Society [ACS], 2014b). It usually strikes men at a productive time of life and thus has significant economic, social, and psychological impact on the patient and his family and/or partner. With early detection by testicular self-examination (TSE) (Chart 72-4) and treatment, testicular cancer has a 95% cure rate (Viatori, 2012). It can occur in one testicle or both.

Primary testicular cancers fall into two major groups:

- Germ cell tumors arising from the sperm-producing cells (account for most testicular cancers)

CHART 72-4   Patient and Family Education: Preparing for Self-Management

Testicular Self-Examination

- Examine your testicles monthly immediately after a bath or a shower, when your scrotal skin is relaxed.
- Examine each testicle by gently rolling it between your thumbs and fingers. Testicular tumors tend to appear deep in the center of the testicle.
- Look and feel for any lumps; smooth, rounded masses; or any change in the size, shape, or consistency of the testes.
- Report any lump or swelling to your doctor as soon as possible.

TABLE 72-1   Classification of Testicular Tumors

GERM CELL (GERMINAL) TUMORS	NON–GERM CELL (NONGERMINAL) TUMORS

• Seminoma
• Nonseminoma:
  • Embryonal carcinoma
  • Teratoma
  • Choriocarcinoma
	• Interstitial cell tumor
	• Androblastoma

- Non–germ cell tumors arising from the stromal, interstitial, or Leydig cells that produce testosterone (account for a very small percentage of testicular cancers)

Testicular germ cell tumors are classified into two broad categories: seminomas and nonseminomas (Table 72-1). The most common type of testicular tumor is *seminoma*. Patients with seminomas have the most favorable prognoses because the tumors are usually localized, metastasize late, and respond to treatment (Viatori, 2012). They often are diagnosed when they are still confined to the testicles and retroperitoneal lymph nodes.

Non–germ cell tumors are classified as either *interstitial cell tumors* or *androblastomas* (testicular adenomas). Most of these tumors do not metastasize. Interstitial cell tumors arise from the Leydig cells, which secrete testosterone into the bloodstream. Androblastomas sometimes secrete estrogen, which accounts for the feminization and gynecomastia (breast enlargement) occasionally seen in these men.

The risk for testicular tumors is higher in males who have an undescended testis (cryptorchidism) or have human immune deficiency virus (HIV) infection (McCance, et al., 2014).

🧬 GENETIC/GENOMIC CONSIDERATIONS

Patient-Centered Care QSEN

Men are at a higher risk for testicular cancer if they have a family history of the disease (Viatori, 2012). The incidence is higher among identical twins, brothers, and other close male relatives. Euro-American men are at a higher risk for testicular cancer than men of other races or ethnicities (Viatori, 2012). The reason for these differences is not known.

Primary testicular cancer is rarely bilateral. Other cancers such as leukemia, lymphoma, and metastatic carcinomas may invade the testes. A man with bilateral testicular tumors is more likely to have metastatic disease to the testes than primary cancer.

❖ PATIENT-CENTERED COLLABORATIVE CARE

◆ Assessment

Physical Assessment/Clinical Manifestations. When taking a history from a patient with a suspected testicular tumor, consider the risk factors. Assess for other risk factors, including a history or presence of an undescended testis and a family history of testicular cancer.

The most common manifestation is a painless, hard swelling or enlargement of the testicle. Patients with discomfort such as heaviness or aching in the lower abdomen or the scrotum may have metastatic disease. Determine how long any manifestations have been present.

Assess the patient's family situation. Is the patient sexually active? If so, what is his sexual preference? Does he have children? Does he want children in the future? Depending on the treatment plan chosen, would he be interested in sperm storage in a sperm bank?

If the man has one healthy testis, he can function sexually and may not have any problem with REPRODUCTION. If he has a retroperitoneal lymph node dissection or chemotherapy, he may become sterile because of treatment effects on the sperm-producing cells or surgical trauma to the sympathetic nervous system resulting in retrograde ejaculations.

The testes, lymph nodes, and abdomen should be thoroughly examined. Patients may feel embarrassed about having this examination. Provide privacy, and explain the procedure to the patient. Inspect the testicles for swelling or a lump that the patient reports is painless. An advanced practice nurse or other health care provider palpates the testes for lumps and swelling that are not visible (Chart 72-5). The presence of any testicular PAIN, lymph node swelling, bone pain, abdominal masses, sudden hydrocele (fluid in the scrotum), or gynecomastia often indicates metastatic disease.

Psychosocial Assessment. Because testicular cancer and its treatment often lead to sexual dysfunction, pay close attention to the psychosocial aspects of the disease. Sexuality is an issue for men of any age, but it may be even more of an issue for younger men. Even if the cancer is detected at an early stage and the patient is cured after surgery, he may be afraid that he will be sexually deficient. He may also think of himself as "less than a whole person." These fears can disrupt the psychosocial and sexual development of young males and can threaten their identity. The patient may be afraid that he will be unable to perform sexually, will no longer be sexually attractive or desirable, and will face rejection. Feelings of sexual inadequacy may be denied, repressed, or displaced, causing increased stress on the man's personal and work relationships.

Assess the man's support systems, including his partner, family members, and friends. Ask him where he feels that he can be supported, such as a religious or spiritual group, community club, or social group. Friends are often very helpful during this difficult time.

Laboratory Assessment. Common serum tumor markers that confirm a diagnosis of testicular cancer are:

- Alpha-fetoprotein (AFP)
- Beta human chorionic gonadotropin (hCG)
- Lactate dehydrogenase (LDH)

Serum testosterone levels are increased when the tumor affects the Leydig cells, which produce this hormone. Drugs such as alcohol and antiepileptic drugs can also cause an increase in testosterone (Pagana & Pagana, 2014).

Other Diagnostic Assessment. When a patient has a change in testis size, shape, or texture, *ultrasonography* can determine whether the mass is solid or fluid filled. It also can help differentiate benign masses from malignant ones.

After the diagnosis of testicular cancer, the patient should have a *CT* scan of the abdomen and the chest to identify small metastatic lesions. *Lymphangiography* shows a view of the body's lymph system to look for spread to other areas.

MRI is used to detect enlarged lymph nodes and abnormal nodules in certain organs that may indicate metastasis from the testicles. Chest x-rays and bone scans may also be performed if metastasis is suspected.

◆ Interventions

At diagnosis, the incidence of **oligospermia** (low sperm count) and **azoospermia** (absence of living sperm) is common in patients with testicular cancer. This problem is thought to be related to higher testicular temperatures created by cancer cell metabolism. The man may not discover that he has reduced sperm count until he has a sperm count performed before surgery.

Health teaching about REPRODUCTION, fertility, and sexuality is started in the pretreatment phase. Review the normal reproductive function, as well as the possible effects of cancer and its treatment on reproductive function. Explore with the patient various reproductive options if desired (Chart 72-6). A sperm bank facility provides comprehensive information on

---

CHART 72-5   Focused Assessment

The Patient with a Testicular Lump

- Obtain a medical history from the patient:
  - When was the lump discovered?
  - Are there any other symptoms (sensation of heaviness, dragging in testicle, pain, discharge from penis)?
  - Is there a history of cryptorchidism?
- An advanced practice nurse or other health care provider will assess the genital system. They will:
  - Inspect and palpate the scrotal contents, have the patient perform a Valsalva maneuver, and palpate for a varicocele.
  - Any lump or enlargement that does not transilluminate should be suspected as malignant.
- Palpate for any enlarged lymph nodes. Always wear gloves during the examination of the male genitalia. The most common areas for lymphadenopathy are in the inguinal or supraclavicular regions.
- Assess the abdomen for a possible mass or hepatomegaly.

CHART 72-6   Patient and Family Education: Preparing for Self-Management

Sperm Banking

- You may want to investigate sperm storage in a sperm bank as a way to preserve your sperm for future use.
- No one knows how long sperm can be stored successfully, but pregnancies have resulted from sperm stored for longer than 10 years.
- Check with the sperm bank to see how much it charges to process and store your sperm and to see whether you must pay when the service is provided.
- Investigate whether your health insurance company will reimburse you for sperm collection and storage.

semen collection, storage of semen, the storage contract, costs, and the insemination process.

When preparing the patient for the collection and storage of sperm, assume the role of patient advocate and keep in mind the effect of the cancer diagnosis. The psychological benefit of having stored sperm may be important for the man and may influence his response to treatment. For some men, knowing that the potential for being a father still exists may help them cope with other fears, such as alopecia or erectile dysfunction (ED).

Suggest that the patient arrange for semen storage, if desired, as soon as possible after diagnosis. Sperm collection should be completed before he begins radiation therapy or chemotherapy or undergoes a radical lymph node dissection. After radiation therapy or chemotherapy has been started, the patient is at increased risk for producing mutagenic sperm, which may not be viable or may result in fetal abnormalities.

The patient's diagnosis and his physical condition may not allow treatment to be postponed, thus making sperm storage impossible. Also, some men may have personal or religious beliefs that do not allow sperm storage. For those who are not candidates for sperm storage in a sperm bank and for those who choose not to bank, discuss other options for REPRODUCTION such as donor insemination or adoption.

Surgical Management. Surgery is the main treatment for testicular cancer. For stage 0 or 1 (localized disease), the surgeon performs a unilateral **orchiectomy** to remove the affected testicle. Every effort is made to remove the cancerous testis as an intact organ to prevent releasing cancer cells into the surgical site. Depending on the type and stage of the cancer, radical retroperitoneal lymph node dissection (RPLND) may also be done.

Preoperative Care. Like most patients with cancer, the man with testicular cancer is very apprehensive. Offer support, and reinforce the teaching provided by the surgeon. Teach the patient and his family or partner about what to expect after surgery. For patients with very early disease, minimally invasive surgery (MIS) using a laparoscope is performed rather than using an open incision. For patients having MIS, teach them that carbon dioxide may be used as part of the surgery. Carbon dioxide can cause chest or shoulder pain from diaphragmatic irritation after the procedure.

Operative Procedures. Most patients with seminoma have only one surgery to remove the diseased testicle through the groin (inguinal) for a cure. A frozen section of the tumor is examined to confirm the type and stage of the cancer. A gel-filled silicone prosthesis may be surgically implanted into the scrotum at the time of the orchiectomy or later if the patient desires. Reassure the patient that this procedure does not impair fertility or sexual function. He cosmetically appears to have two testes (reconstructive surgery).

Some men have more advanced disease or tumor types that are more aggressive. Two options are available for the lymph node dissection: a traditional open approach and minimally invasive surgery (MIS) using a laparoscope. To perform the *open* approach, the surgeon removes the retroperitoneal nodes in the iliac and lumbar regions. Because the blood supply and the lymphatic vessels of the testes and kidneys are directly related, an extensive midline incision from the xiphoid process to the pubis is necessary. Removal of the sympathetic ganglia eliminates peristalsis in the vas deferens and contractions of the seminal vesicles. This disruption results in sterility because the

man's ejaculate no longer contains sperm. However, having a normal erection and experiencing orgasm usually are not affected.

The MIS procedure involves using a laparoscope through several small "keyhole" incisions through which the nodes are dissected for examination. This technique shortens the time the patient is in the operating suite, minimizes bleeding, and causes less pain after surgery. The patient has fewer postoperative complications and a shorter hospital stay.

Postoperative Care. Nursing care for the patient after surgery depends on the type of surgical procedure that was performed and the extent of the disease process.

> **! NURSING SAFETY PRIORITY** (QSEN)
>
> **Action Alert**
>
> Because of the length of the *open* orchiectomy and lymph node dissection approach, manipulation of the abdominal and retroperitoneal viscera, and the loss of lymphatic fluid, observe, assess, and report any complications of this major abdominal surgery (e.g., paralytic ileus) (see Chapter 16). Monitor vital signs (including pain), hydration, and pulmonary function carefully for the first 24 to 48 hours. Ambulate the patient as soon as possible, and teach him how to use the incentive spirometer. Assess the patency of the urinary catheter. Be sure the patient wears antiembolism stockings or devices, and provide care for surgical incisions and wound drains.
>
> The patient having the *laparoscopic* procedure may have a urinary catheter in place for 1 to 2 days. The other advantages of the MIS procedure are that patients have less pain and fewer complications than those who had the open surgery. Chapter 15 describes laparoscopic surgery in detail.

> **? NCLEX EXAMINATION CHALLENGE**
>
> **Physiological Integrity**
>
> A client had an orchiectomy and laparoscopic radical retroperitoneal lymph node dissection this morning. What is the nurse's priority for care?
> A. Assess the client's pain level and provide pain management.
> B. Ensure that the client's urinary catheter is draining clear yellow urine.
> C. Observe the client's incision for redness, swelling, and drainage.
> D. Apply oxygen therapy via nasal cannula at 2 L/min.

Nonsurgical Management. Combination *chemotherapy* may be used as adjuvant therapy for nonseminomatous testicular tumors or as primary treatment when there is evidence of metastatic disease. Many drug regimens are used, including varying combinations of bleomycin, etoposide, and cisplatin (BEP). The specific combination of drugs and the frequency, cycling, and duration of treatment vary from patient to patient, depending on the extent of the disease and the protocol being followed. Chapter 22 discusses the general nursing care for the patient receiving chemotherapy.

Patients having chemotherapy are at risk for certain health problems that are associated with these drugs. Examples of these problems include hypertension, hyperlipidemia, lung toxicity, anemia, and leukemia (Viatori, 2012). Teach patients taking these drugs about the long-term effects for which they should be continually and carefully monitored by their health care providers.

After orchiectomy for localized disease, *external beam radiation therapy* (EBRT) may be used. The remaining testis is shielded with a lead cup to preserve reproductive function. Even with these precautions, the patient may have a temporary decreased sperm count as a result of radiation scatter. Normally the sperm count returns to the pretreatment level within 24 to 30 months after the radiation treatment is completed. If metastases develop outside the lymphatic system, the man may still be cured with radiation therapy if the area of involvement is limited. If lymphatic involvement is extensive or if the visceral organs are involved, combination chemotherapy is used.

Community-Based Care

The patient is usually hospitalized for multiple days after an *open* radical retroperitoneal lymph node dissection but for just 1 to 2 days for the *MIS* laparoscopic procedure.

After an open *orchiectomy,* unless the patient has a wound complication, he is discharged without a dressing on the inguinal incision. A scrotal support may be needed for several days. He may want to wear a dry dressing to prevent clothing from rubbing on the sutures and causing irritation. Tell him that the sutures will be removed in the physician's office 7 to 10 days after surgery.

> ⚠ **NURSING SAFETY PRIORITY** (QSEN)
>
> *Action Alert*
>
> For the patient who has undergone testicular surgery, emphasize the importance of scheduling a follow-up visit with the surgeon to examine the incision for healing and complications. Instruct him to notify the surgeon if chills, fever, increasing tenderness or pain around the incision, drainage, or dehiscence of the incision occurs. These manifestations may indicate INFECTION for which antibiotics are needed. Instruct the patient who had a laparoscopic orchiectomy that he will be able to resume most of his usual activities within 1 week after discharge. He can take a shower in 1 or 2 days after surgery, but be sure he does not remove the Steri-Strips. These strips will loosen and fall off in about a week after surgery.

Patients who also had an *open retroperitoneal lymph node dissection* recover more slowly. They should not lift anything over 15 pounds, should avoid stair climbing, and should not drive a car for several weeks. Be sure that bathroom facilities are on the first floor of the house where he can easily access them.

Explain the importance of performing monthly testicular self-examination (TSE) on the remaining testis and scheduling follow-up examinations with the physician. The patient who has had testicular cancer should schedule tests for urinary and serum levels of tumor markers and CT or MRI studies as part of his routine follow-up for at least 3 years.

Depending on the pathologic findings and the stage of the cancer, the patient may need further treatment. This information may not be known at the time of discharge. If it is known that the patient needs further surgery, he and his family need information about the future surgery. If it is known that he must undergo radiation therapy or chemotherapy, he needs education about these treatments as soon as possible.

The man who has testicular cancer needs emotional support. If permanent sterility occurs and sperm storage has not been feasible, he may desire counseling about other reproductive options. Refer the patient to agencies or support groups, such as the American Fertility Society (www.theafa.org) or RESOLVE: The National Infertility Association (www.resolve.org) (organizations for infertile couples).

OTHER PROBLEMS AFFECTING THE TESTES AND ADJACENT STRUCTURES

Problems that develop inside the scrotum usually occur as a mass or as scrotal edema. Some problems produce pain, but others do not. Fig. 72-4 shows some of the most common conditions found in adult men, including hydrocele, spermatocele, and varicocele. In addition to local comfort measures, these masses are either drained or removed surgically. Scrotal support, heat, and analgesics are needed after surgery. Teach patients to follow up with their health care provider.

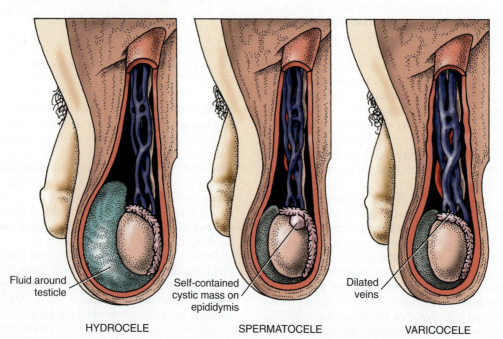

Fluid around testicle — HYDROCELE
Self-contained cystic mass on epididymis — SPERMATOCELE
Dilated veins — VARICOCELE

FIG. 72-4 Common problems affecting the testes and adjacent structures.

NURSING CONCEPTS AND CLINICAL JUDGMENT REVIEW

What might you NOTICE if the patient is experiencing impaired SEXUALITY as a result of male reproductive problems?
- Lump or swelling in prostate or scrotum
- Report of pain in scrotum or during ejaculation
- Report of difficulty voiding (e.g., starting urine stream)
- Hematuria
- Report of dribbling of urine (incontinence)
- Report of inability to have a penile erection
- Report of decreased libido

What should you INTERPRET and how should you RESPOND to a patient experiencing impaired SEXUALITY as a result of male reproductive problems?

Perform and interpret physical assessment, including:
- Conducting a complete pain assessment
- Inspecting and palpating bladder for distention
- Inspecting and palpating scrotum for swelling or masses
- Palpating lymph nodes for swelling, especially in the inguinal areas
- Sending urine sample for urinalysis and culture
- Checking most recent laboratory values for PSA, CBC, and serum tumor markers

Respond by:
- Catheterizing patient if retaining urine
- Providing pain-relief measures, such as ice or medication as prescribed
- Elevating scrotum if swollen
- Arranging for consultation with sex or intimacy therapist if patient desires

On what should you REFLECT?
- Evaluate patient for need for indwelling urinary catheter.
- Evaluate effectiveness of actions to control pain and swelling.
- Think about what additional resources the patient will need to cope with his problem.

GET READY FOR THE NCLEX® EXAMINATION!

KEY POINTS

Review these Key Points for each NCLEX Examination Client Needs Category.

Safe and Effective Care Environment
- Teach patients with prostate cancer about American Cancer Society's *Man to Man* program and the American Foundation for Urologic Disease's *Us TOO International* program to help men and their partners cope with prostate cancer.
- Teach patients to report signs of INFECTION when caring for a urinary catheter in the home. **Safety** QSEN

Health Promotion and Maintenance
- Teach men at risk for prostate cancer to follow the current American Cancer Society's screening and early detection guidelines. **Evidence-Based Practice** QSEN
- Teach men how to perform testicular self-examination as described in Chart 72-4.
- Teach uncircumcised men the importance of keeping the penis clean to prevent penile cancer.

Psychosocial Integrity
- Because most patients with testicular cancer are young and middle-aged adults, assess their reaction to the possible loss of REPRODUCTION ability.
- Because of the high incidence of erectile dysfunction after radical prostatectomy, assess the patient's adjustment to these changes in body function. **Patient-Centered Care** QSEN
- Assess the patient's anxiety before prostate surgery, and allow him to express feelings of fear or grief. **Patient-Centered Care** QSEN

Physiological Integrity
- Perform a focused physical assessment for patients reporting lumps or swelling in their genital area; inspect and palpate bladder and scrotum.
- Observe for and report complications after radical prostatectomy, including infection, severe PAIN, urinary infection, urinary ELIMINATION problems, and erectile dysfunction. **Safety** QSEN
- Observe for and report bloody urine with clots after TURP; increase continuous bladder irrigation or irrigate the bladder per agency or surgeon protocol. **Safety** QSEN
- Maintain traction on the urinary catheter and continuous bladder irrigation after a TURP. **Safety**
- Teach patients about drug therapies (5-ARIs and alpha blocking agents) used to treat BPH, including side effects such as orthostatic hypotension, erectile dysfunction, decreased libido, dizziness, and liver dysfunction. **Safety** QSEN
- Teach patients to avoid any drugs that can cause urinary retention, especially anticholinergics, antihistamines, and decongestants if BPH is present. **Evidence-Based Practice** QSEN
- Remind patients wanting to use complementary and alternative therapies to check with their health care providers before using them.
- Eating a well-balanced diet with plenty of fish and fruits and vegetables may help prevent prostate cancer.
- Reinforce the man's option for managing prostate cancer; some procedures and drugs cause erectile dysfunction and incontinence either temporarily or permanently.
- Use the information listed in Chart 72-3 to teach patients urinary catheter care after prostate cancer surgery.

- Teach patients about not lifting more than 15 lb (6.8 kg) after open prostate surgery. **Safety** **QSEN**
- Options for erectile dysfunction (ED) include drug therapy (most common), vacuum assist devices, penile injections, transurethral suppositories, or penile implants.
- Be aware that African-American middle-aged men are the most at risk for prostate cancer; Euro-American young men are the most at risk for testicular cancer.
- Teach patients to report symptoms of radiation cystitis or proctitis to their health care provider as soon as possible;

these complications resolve in 4 to 6 weeks after the end of radiation therapy.
- Teach patients and their partners about hormone therapy used to manage prostate cancer: LH-RH agonists and anti-androgen drugs.
- Be aware that sexually transmitted diseases (STDs) are a major cause of male reproductive system INFECTIONS.

CHAPTER 73

Care of Transgender Patients

Donna D. Ignatavicius and Stephanie M. Ignatavicius

ⓔ http://evolve.elsevier.com/Iggy/

PRIORITY CONCEPTS

- SEXUALITY
- REPRODUCTION

LEARNING OUTCOMES

Safe and Effective Care Environment
1. Describe the need to collaborate with members of the health care team to provide high-quality care for transgender patients.
2. Explain the role of the nurse as a leader to promote advocacy for transgender people.

Health Promotion and Maintenance
3. Develop a health teaching plan for transgender patients who take hormone therapy and/or have gender reassignment surgery.
4. Identify appropriate resources for accurate trans-health information and ongoing preventive health care.

Psychosocial Integrity
5. Discuss how to use culturally sensitive terminology when providing care for transgender patients.

6. Identify the major sources of stress that contribute to transgender health issues.
7. Explain the major challenges for transgender patients in obtaining health care.

Physiological Integrity
8. Describe the side effects and adverse effects of feminizing and masculinizing hormone therapy, including effects of SEXUALITY and REPRODUCTION.
9. Identify laboratory test values that require monitoring for patients taking hormone therapy.
10. Describe the preoperative care needed for male-to-female or female-to-male patients having genital surgery.
11. Prioritize postoperative nursing care for patients having feminizing or masculinizing genital surgery.

The American Nurses Association (ANA) *Code of Ethics* states that the nurse practices with compassion and respect for the dignity and worth of every patient (ANA, 2001). The Institute of Medicine and the Quality and Safety Education for Nurses (QSEN) Institute further identified the need for nurses to be competent in patient-centered care (see Chapter 1). This competency ensures that nurses provide care with sensitivity and respect for diverse patients, even if those patients have values and preferences different from their own (ANA, 2001). Diversity is often discussed as ethnicity and race, but other cultural aspects such as sexual orientation and gender identity are part of the diverse human experience. An estimated 9 million people in the United States identify themselves as sexual and gender minorities (Gates, 2011).

People of minority sexual and gender identities are often grouped under one population category described by the acronym **LGBTQ**—lesbian, gay, bisexual, transgender, and queer/questioning (people who do not feel they belong in any other subgroup) (Table 73-1) (Eliason et al., 2013; Pettinato, 2012). Some literature includes only "LGBT." These evolving labels are misleading regarding people who identify as transgender. The grouping of SEXUALITY (sexual attraction and behavior) and gender identity (sense of maleness or femaleness) suggests that these two concepts are related or dependent upon one another, but they are different. *LGB* refers to specific sexual orientation. However, transgender people may identify as heterosexual, homosexual, both, or neither. Nurses and other health care professionals should not assume that transgender patients have the same experiences or health care needs as those who identify as lesbian, gay, or bisexual.

PATIENT-CENTERED TERMINOLOGY

Commonly, gender is categorized as one of two terms: *male* and *female.* For the majority of people, these descriptors are accurate. However, some people do not clearly fit into either category and may define themselves as *transgender.* Identifying oneself as transgender is not a choice or lifestyle but, rather, an inner sense of being born in the wrong body. When transgender people pursue ways of affirming their physical body and

TABLE 73-1 **Appropriate Terminology Associated with Transgender Health**

TERM	DEFINITION
Coming out	A lesbian, gay, bisexual, transgender, and queer/questioning (LGBTQ) person's public disclosure regarding sexual orientation or gender identity
Female-to-male	An adjective to describe people who were female at birth and are changing (or have changed) to a more masculine body or male
Gender dysphoria	Emotional or psychological distress caused by an incongruence between one's natal (birth) sex and gender identity
Gender identity	A person's inner sense of being a male, a female, or an alternative gender (e.g., genderqueer)
Genderqueer	An identity label used by some people whose gender identity does not conform to one of the two categories of male or female
Male-to-female	An adjective to describe people who were male at birth and are changing (or have changed) to a more feminine body or female
Sex (also called *natal sex*)	The gender assigned at one's birth
Sex reassignment surgery (SRS) (also called *gender reassignment surgery* or *gender affirmation surgery*)	A group of surgical procedures that change primary and/or secondary sex characteristics to affirm a person's gender identity
Transgender	An adjective to describe a person who crosses or transcends culturally defined categories of gender
Transition	The period of time when transgender people change from the gender role associated with their sex to a different gender role
Transsexual	Term often used by health care professionals to describe people who want to change or have changed their primary and/or secondary sex characteristics

as age 2 years and is usually present in most children during the early elementary years. Transgender people feel a mismatch between their gender identity and natal sex, often extending back into early childhood. When this incongruence occurs, they can experience gender dysphoria, or discomfort with one's natal sex (APA, 2013; Edwards-Leeper & Spack, 2013). Some people who have gender dysphoria may seek interventions for sex reassignment to transition to the preferred gender.

The term "transgender" is often used as an umbrella description for all people whose gender identity and presentation do not conform to social expectations (Aramburu Alegria, 2011). In this text, transgender describes patients who self-identify as the opposite gender or a gender that does not match their natal sex (APA, 2013; Jenner, 2010). For proper usage, transgender should be used only in adjective form. For example, a patient "is transgender," "identifies as transgender," or "is a transgender patient." Note that "transgender" never ends in "-ed." The term "transgender" should not be used as a noun, and a patient should never be described as "*a transgender*."

According to *The Diagnostic and Statistical Manual of Mental Disorders* (APA, 2013), prevalence of gender dysphoria ranges from 5 to 14 in 1000 natal males and from 2 to 3 in 1000 natal females. However, these data describe the number of people who experience discontent with the gender they were assigned at birth and do not give an accurate estimate of the number of people who identify as transgender. Other studies have shown that the prevalence of transgender people is between 1 in 11,900 and 1 in 200,000 people (Coleman et al., 2011). Most scholars suggest that the prevalence is much higher, and more research is needed to collect more accurate demographic data for this population.

Another common term is transsexual, which generally describes a person who has modified his or her natal body to match the appropriate gender identity, either through cosmetic, hormonal, or surgical means (APA, 2013; Jenner, 2010). "Transsexual" can be used as both an adjective and a noun, such that a patient can be described "as transsexual" or "as a transsexual." People who were born with anatomically male parts but identify as and/or live as female are known as "male-to-female" or "MtF." Male-to-female people are also known as "transwomen," with the gender descriptor indicating the current-lived gender identity. Conversely, "transmen" are natal females who identify as and/or live as men. They are described as "female-to-male" or "FtM."

Transgender people are sometimes described as "transvestites" or "cross-dressers," often in a judgmental or negative manner. These terms should not be used unless the patient identifies as such. Other terms, such as "tranny," "he-she," or "shemale," are offensive and hurtful. These terms and other negative comments should never be used.

A patient may self-identify with any of the above terms or choose not to be defined at all. Become familiar with appropriate terms and concepts, but do not force definitions on your patients. Instead, if you are unsure how to address patients, during your nursing assessment ask them how they define their gender identity.

appearance with their gender identity, their interaction with the health care system requires knowledge, respect, compassion, and specialized nursing care.

Using appropriate terminology is essential to demonstrating respect (see Table 73-1). Of utmost importance is the distinction between gender and sex. Gender, also known as gender identity, describes a person's inner sense of maleness or femaleness and is not related to reproductive anatomy. Gender identity describes one's social role as a man or a woman (American Psychiatric Association [APA], 2013). Sex, also known as *biological* or natal sex, refers to a person's genital anatomy present at birth (Edwards-Leeper & Spack, 2013).

When babies are born, the gender of the child is determined by the genitalia present, but there is no way of knowing the child's true sense of gender. The sense of gender and feelings toward maleness or femaleness can develop in children as early

TRANSGENDER HEALTH ISSUES

Transgender people (also referred to as *trans-people*) encounter frequent discrimination and are faced with numerous stressful situations related to their identity. Sources of stress such as job discrimination and bias-related harassment can have an impact on patients' physical and psychological health. In a 2011 national survey on discrimination, the majority of transgender people had experienced mistreatment in the workplace. Also, almost half of transgender respondents reported loss of job or denial of promotion due to their transgender identity (Grant et al., 2011). As a result, they may be homeless, use alcohol or drugs as coping mechanisms, and ignore their health needs (Grant et al., 2011). In some cases they may turn to sex work (prostitution) as a mechanism for survival (Chestnut et al., 2013; Grant et al., 2011). Only a small subset of primarily MtF transgender people engage in sex work, which can expose them to human immune deficiency virus (HIV) and sexually transmitted disease (STD).

Transgender people are also vulnerable to bias-related violence and verbal harassment, including threats and intimidation (Chestnut et al., 2013; Shipherd et al., 2011). MtF people are more than 2 times more likely to experience physical violence and discrimination than non-transwomen; the likelihood of harassment is even greater for transwomen of color (Chestnut et al., 2013). A recent report indicated that half of LGBTQ-related hate crime homicides in the United States were committed against transwomen (Chestnut et al., 2013). Factors that increase this risk for violence include poverty, homelessness, and sex work.

Having an identity that puts a person at risk for violence and mistreatment can lead to emotional distress, particularly if the person has been directly victimized. Transgender people who have experienced traumatic situations may demonstrate manifestations of posttraumatic stress disorder (PTSD) and/or depression (Shipherd et al., 2011). They may turn to a variety of coping strategies to deal with distress, some of which can negatively impact physical health. In a 2010 national survey, 26% of transgender people reported current or previous alcohol or drug use to cope with discrimination and mistreatment; however, the number of people who use substances recreationally may be higher (Grant et al., 2010). Rates of smoking in the transgender community are higher than the rates in the LGB community and general population of U.S. adults. Most important, major life stressors, emotional distress, and lack of resources can lead to suicidal ideation or suicide attempt when all other methods of coping have failed. In a sample of over 7000 transgender adults, 41% reported at least one suicide attempt in their lifetime (Grant et al., 2010).

STRESS AND TRANSGENDER HEALTH

Transgender people have additional sources of stress when attempting to access health care, such as lack of health insurance due to unemployment. This barrier to health care causes them to postpone both acute and preventive medical care. For those people who are insured, coverage for health care related to gender transition (gender reassignment), such as hormone use and surgery, is often denied (Grant et al., 2010; Lombardi, 2010).

When transgender people gain access to health care, they are often fearful and anxious about the providers and setting. In particular, they may be hesitant to disclose their transgender status due to fear of discrimination or ridicule (Aramburu Alegria, 2011; Lombardi, 2010). They may also fear that this information will be documented in health records and shared with family members. This reluctance is increased if they have had previous negative experiences with health care providers. One national survey found that 19% of transgender adults were refused health care services due to their gender identity, while 28% reported receiving verbal harassment in a health care setting. Male-to-female transgender people were more likely to encounter discrimination and avoid health care due to these experiences (Grant et al., 2010). Even with providers who seem tolerant and caring with transgender patients, there is still a risk for patients overhearing jokes in the hallway and defamatory comments (Rounds et al., 2013).

Another source of stress faced by many transgender people is lack of health care–professional knowledge regarding health care needs (Aramburu Alegria, 2011; Jenner, 2010). When this situation occurs, transgender patients are put in a position of acting as health care experts, which can limit the quality of their care. While most transgender patients generally expect their providers to have some level of knowledge or know where to seek answers (Rounds et al., 2013), at least half of them find they have to teach their providers. When they encounter providers who are unfamiliar with the specific health care needs of their population, patient confidence is likely to diminish drastically and affect desire for future health care.

Whereas transgender patients may encounter providers who do not understand or who overlook their gender identity, some may encounter health care professionals who over-focus on it. Although it is important to be generally knowledgeable about a patient's gender status and understand how it may affect health care needs, this factor is not always relevant for every health problem. For example, transgender patients with fractures or influenza do not need to be extensively questioned about their gender identity. Whereas there are instances in which the presenting manifestations require transgender-specific care, there are also many other instances that require the same health care that all patients receive. At these times, most transgender patients prefer to be treated as any other patient (Rounds et al., 2013). Therefore use sound clinical judgment to decide if one's gender identity impacts patient assessment and care.

NEED TO IMPROVE TRANSGENDER HEALTH CARE

During the past few years, several national documents were published by the U.S. Department of Health and Human Services and private health care organizations that call for improvement in LGBTQ health care. These important publications include:

- *Healthy People 2020*
- The Institute of Medicine's (IOM) report on LGBT health
- The Joint Commission field guide for care of LGBT patients
- World Professional Association for Transgender Health standards of care

The U.S. Department of Health and Human Services' *Healthy People 2010* publication did *not* include the need to improve health care for LGBT people. As a result of this omission, a companion document was developed by the Gay and Lesbian Medical Association (GLMA) to address special health care needs of this population across the life span. Ten common health problems affecting the LGBT group were identified, including cancer, nutrition and weight, and sexually transmitted disease.

The *Healthy People 2020* agenda added objectives for improving the health of LGBT people, including the need to recognize and address the special health needs of transgender patients of all ages.

One major objective is to develop a system to identify patients who identify as LGBTQ. This objective is similar to the recommendation in the Institute of Medicine's (IOM) publication entitled *The Health of LGBT People: Building a Foundation for Better Understanding* (IOM, 2011).

The IOM LGBT health report calls for the need for more research to identify the special health care concerns of LGBT people of all ages. To help meet this outcome, the document outlined the need to collect more demographic data to better identify this population. LGBTQ people need to feel safe when disclosing this very personal information.

In 2011, The Joint Commission (TJC) published a similar document that recommends ways for health care agencies to create a welcoming and safe environment for LGBT patients. In response to growing attention to the need for cultural competence for all health care professionals and to provide quality health care for sexual and gender minority patients, TJC published a field guide for health care agencies to improve LGBT patient care (TJC, 2011). Chart 73-1 lists the recommendations for health care agencies in designing a safe environment for LGBT patient care. Fig. 73-1 shows an example of a "safe zone" image that should be used to reassure these patients that they are in a safe place where they can receive respectful and knowledgeable quality care.

Also in 2011, the World Professional Association for Transgender Health (WPATH) updated its standards of care (Coleman et al., 2011). This document outlines core principles that nurses and other health care professionals should follow when caring for transgender patients (Table 73-2).

❖ *PATIENT-CENTERED COLLABORATIVE CARE*

◆ *Assessment*

As with any patient, it is best to ask during the nursing history and physical assessment how he or she prefers to be addressed. For example, for non-transgender patients, some people may go by a nickname or by their middle name and prefer to be addressed as such. For transgender patients, it is not uncommon for driver's licenses, insurance cards, and other forms of identification to retain their birth names (and by extension, birth sex) because it can be difficult to change this information,

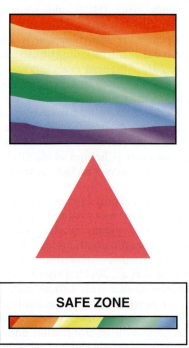

FIG. 73-1 The Safe Zone—rainbow or pink triangle signs welcome LGBTQ patients in a health care agency.

CHART 73-1   Best Practice for Patient Safety & Quality Care QSEN

The Joint Commission Recommendations for Creating a Safe, Welcoming Environment for LGBTQ Patients

- Post the *Patients' Bill of Rights* and nondiscrimination policies in a visible place.
- Make waiting rooms inclusive of LGBTQ patients and families, such as posting *Safe Zone*, rainbow, or pink triangle signs.
- Designate unisex or single-stall restrooms.
- Ensure that visitation policies are equitable for families of LGBTQ patients.
- Avoid assumptions about any patient's sexual orientation and gender identity.
- Include gender-neutral language on all medical forms and documents; e.g., "partnered" in addition to married, single, or divorced categories.
- Reflect the patient's choice of terminology in communication and documentation.
- Provide information on special health concerns for LGBTQ patients.
- Become knowledgeable about LGBTQ health needs and care.
- Refer LGBTQ patients to qualified health care professionals as needed.
- Provide community resources for LGBTQ information and support as needed.

Adapted from The Joint Commission (TJC). (2011). *Advancing effective communication, cultural competence, and patient- and family-centered care for the lesbian, gay, bisexual, and transgender community.* Retrieved September 2013, from www.jointcommission.org/lgbt.

TABLE 73-2   Core Principles for Health Care Professionals Who Care for Transgender Patients

- Become knowledgeable about the health care needs of transgender and other gender-nonconforming people.
- Become knowledgeable about the treatment options for transgender patients and required follow-up care.
- Do not assume that all transgender patients are the same; treat each one as an individual and develop an individualized plan of care.
- Demonstrate respect for patients with nonconforming gender identities.
- Provide culturally sensitive care and use appropriate terminology that affirms the patient's gender identity.
- Facilitate patient access to appropriate and knowledgeable health care providers.
- Seek informed consent before providing treatment.
- Offer continuity of care or refer patients for ongoing quality health care.
- Advocate for patients within their families and communities.

Adapted from Coleman, E., Bockting, W., Botzer, M., Cohen-Kettenis, P., DeCuypere, G., Fladman, J., et al., (2011). Standards of care for the health of transsexual, transgender, and gender-nonconforming people (Version 7). *International Journal of Transgenderism, 13*, 165-232; Rounds, K.E., McGrath, B.B., & Walsh, E. (2013). Perspectives on provider behaviors: A qualitative study of sexual and gender minorities regarding quality of care. *Contemporary Nurse, 44*(1), 99-110.

particularly if a person is in the process of transitioning. Therefore nurses may receive patient documentation with misleading patient data. For example, a nurse may receive a health care record listing a male name and birth sex yet encounter a patient presenting as female in appearance. It can be offensive and embarrassing for the patient who clearly identifies as female to be called "Mister," "sir," or the male birth name. Not only does it communicate disrespect, it also signals to the patient that she may receive inadequate care or that the environment is unsafe.

In addition to preferred names, correct pronoun usage is also important. Each patient has his or her own preference. For example, an MtF patient may visit a clinic during lunch hour at work. Because the patient has not disclosed the transgender identity at work, this patient maintains male dress and demeanor at the office. Though the patient may identify as female and live as female at home, the patient may request the nurse to use male pronouns (he, him, his) to match the patient's current presentation and may not disclose the transgender identity to the nurse. Conversely, even though the patient presents at the time as male, the patient may request the nurse to use female pronouns (she, her, hers) because the patient identifies with a female gender identity.

In general, use pronouns that match the patient's physical presentation and dress. Even though the biological sex may not match, patients presenting as female should be addressed as female and patients presenting as male should be addressed as male. With changing styles and trends, it can sometimes be difficult to assess by clothing alone. However, with a patient whose birth sex is listed as female yet presents in traditionally male attire, facial hair, and a men's hairstyle, it is most appropriate to address this patient as male. Understandably, the clinical setting can be fast-paced and nurses may encounter multiple patients at a time; however, taking time to use clinical judgment is important. Appropriately interacting with a transgender patient can sometimes mean the difference between the patient continuing to seek health care or not.

In a few cases, patients may not identify as male or female and prefer to not use male or female pronouns. These patients often feel that the binary gender system in which a person must fit clearly into one category or the other is too limiting. Though this is a small subset of the transgender population, it is important to be aware of this subculture in case you encounter a patient who refuses to identify with a specific gender or instead identifies as genderqueer (the Q in LGBTQ). Genderqueer patients may request the use of gender neutral pronouns, or they may use these pronouns in the nurse's presence. For many genderqueer people, the pronoun "they" is preferred instead of "he" or "she."

Getting used to using the correct name or pronoun can take some time. Occasionally, nurses will know their patient's preferred name or pronoun but accidentally say the wrong one. Transgender patients encounter this situation often and typically anticipate an error at times. When this error occurs, it is best to self-correct and continue with care rather than make a prolonged apology. Focusing too much on the error may make the patient more uncomfortable because more attention has been drawn to the situation. Most transgender patients, particularly those who live full time in their gender-affirming role, wish to be treated like any other patient.

History. Interventions for transgender people who experience gender dysphoria (discomfort with one's natal sex) include one or more of these options (Coleman et al., 2011):

- Changes in gender expression that may involve living part time or full time in another gender role
- Psychotherapy to explore gender identity and expression, improve body image, or strengthen coping mechanisms
- Hormone therapy to feminize or masculinize the body
- Surgery to change primary and/or secondary sex characteristics (e.g., the breasts/chest, facial features, internal and/or external genitalia)

During the health history, inquire about which interventions the patient has had, if any, or if there are plans to have them in the future. Ask about current use of *drug therapy*, including hormones and other feminizing or masculinizing agents, including silicone injections. These medications are usually prescribed by endocrinologists or other specialists in transgender health care, but some patients may obtain them from nonmedical sources, including the Internet.

Exogenous hormone therapy can cause adverse health problems and requires careful patient monitoring, including laboratory testing. For example, estrogen therapy can cause increased health risks such as increased blood clotting causing venous thromboembolism (VTE), elevated blood glucose, hypertension, estrogen-dependent cancers, and fluid retention (Brennan et al., 2012). Smoking and obesity increase these risks. The risks also increase with higher doses of the medication. Ask the patient about a history of these problems.

Inquire about the patient's *surgical history*. For the MtF patient, ask about breast surgery and any surgical changes to the genitalia, such as a penectomy (removal of the penis) and vaginoplasty (creation of a vagina). The MtF patient still has the prostate gland. For older patients, ask about any problems with prostate health problems, such as urinary dribbling and retention. For the FtM patient, ask whether a hysterectomy, bilateral salpingo-oophorectomy (BSO), mastectomy, phalloplasty (creation of a penis), and/or scrotoplasty (creation of a scrotum) was performed.

Keep in mind that health insurance usually does not cover the cost of the transition process and patients may seek alternative care. For example, hormones may be obtained illegally or from countries that do not have quality controls for medication. MtF patients may seek silicone for creating breasts from nonmedical people, causing a high risk for hepatitis C and silicone complications (Brennan et al., 2012). Ask patients about the use of these alternatives as a part of their transition process.

Physical Assessment. Be sure to review the transgender patient's health record carefully before performing a physical assessment. Be culturally sensitive, nonjudgmental, and respectful during the assessment. Be aware that transgender patients may be young, middle-aged, or older adults.

CONSIDERATIONS FOR OLDER ADULTS
Patient-Centered Care QSEN

Transgender patients who are older than 65 years lived in an era when most of them concealed their sexual orientation and true gender identity due to social stigma. These people have not been well studied as a group, but research indicates that those who lived with a partner have fewer mental health problems and better self-esteem compared with those who lived alone (Brennan et al., 2012).

When assessing transgender patients, be aware that they will be in varying stages of transition. Some patients present with no obvious physical signs that they are in the process of transitioning. Others have had gender reassignment surgery such that their new appearance matches their gender identity. Realize a transgender patient's genitalia may not match his or her physical appearance.

Psychosocial Assessment. If gender and SEXUALITY are relevant to the patient's presenting health problem, ask specific questions to determine how these factors may impact care. Reassure patients that their responses are confidential and will not be shared with any family, friends, or significant others without the patient's permission. However, evidence of abuse must be reported as mandated by law. Appropriate screening questions about gender and sexuality include (Coleman et al., 2011):

- Are you experiencing any challenges, concerns, or anxiety related to your sexuality?
- Related to your gender, how do you identify?
- Are you experiencing any sadness, depression, or thoughts of hurting yourself?
- Have you experienced any violence or discrimination in your personal or work life?
- Are you currently being seen by a counselor or psychologist related to your sexuality and gender identity? If so, why?

If the responses to these questions indicate that the patient has potential or actual mental health problems, consult with the health care provider for further evaluation by a qualified mental health care professional, such as a clinical psychologist.

◆ **Interventions**

Nurses care for transgender patients who are transitioning or have completed gender reassignment. They may care for them for health problems related to their transition process or for problems that are unrelated to the patient's SEXUALITY or gender identity. In general, care for transgender patients with most health problems is the same as for any other patient. However, some interventions such as hormone therapy may affect nursing assessment and care. As a leader in health care, advocate for transgender patients and provide health teaching to promote their health. Encourage them to include their sexual partner, if any, in discussions about the transition process.

Nonsurgical Management. The primary nonsurgical interventions for transgender patients include drug (hormone) therapy, counseling about REPRODUCTION and reproductive health, and vocal therapy. The type of intervention depends on whether the patient is transitioning from MtF or FtM.

Drug Therapy. Drug therapy may be started after a psychosocial assessment by a qualified mental health care professional and informed consent has been obtained. According to WPATH's most recent standards of care, the criteria for hormone therapy include:

- Continuing and well-documented gender dysphoria
- Patient ability to make a fully informed decision and give consent to treatment
- Patient older than 18 years
- Well-controlled existing medical or mental health problems, if any

Drugs for MtF Patients. Patients transitioning from male to female (MtF) typically take a combination of estrogen therapy and androgen-reducing medications to achieve feminizing effects. Expected physical changes from *estrogen therapy* are breast enlargement, thinning hair, decreased testicular size, decreased erectile function, and increased body fat compared

---

TABLE 73-3   Feminizing Drug Therapy for MtF Patients: Expected Changes and Monitoring

Expected Physical Changes
- Enlargement of breast tissue (gynecomastia)
- Decreased testicular size
- Decreased erectile function
- Decreased libido (sex drive)
- Decreased body hair growth
- Decreased male pattern baldness
- Increased fat compared with muscle
- Softening of skin

Laboratory/Imaging Studies
- Chemistry panel (including glucose and electrolytes)
- Liver function tests
- Lipid profile
- Complete blood count
- Prostate-specific antigen (PSA) if recommended for age-group
- Mammogram (when breast tissue develops)
- Papanicolaou (Pap) smear (if vagina present)

---

with muscle mass (Table 73-3). Because oral estrogen (ethinyl estradiol) can increase the risk for venous thromboembolism, transdermal estrogen (Climara) or injectable estradiol is preferred for use in transgender patients. The typical dosing is two 0.1-mg patches changed twice weekly (Aramburu Alegria, 2011). Injectable estradiol is usually prescribed in a dose between 5 and 20 mg IM every 2 weeks. Progesterone may also be prescribed for 10 days each month.

Before the first dose of transdermal estrogen, teach the patient to apply the patch to an area that is hairless to ensure good contact with the skin. When changing to a new patch, wash any excess drug from the skin where the previous patch was applied.

Teach patients taking any form of estrogen about side effects such as headache, breast tenderness, nausea/vomiting, and weight gain (often due to fluid retention) or loss. Tell them to report increased feelings of anxiety or depression to their health care provider. Estrogens can also cause estrogen-dependent cancers, hypertension (due to fluid retention), venous thromboembolism (VTE) such as deep vein thrombosis (DVT), and gallbladder disease (Brennan et al., 2012). Teach patients to follow up with their health care provider to monitor for these potential adverse drug effects. Diagnostic testing is part of follow-up and monitoring, as listed in Table 73-3.

❓ NCLEX EXAMINATION CHALLENGE

Physiological Integrity

The nurse provides health teaching for a client receiving estrogen therapy. Which statement by the client indicates a need for further teaching?

A. "I need to check my blood pressure frequently when taking this drug."

B. "I will call my doctor if I have any redness or swelling in my legs."

C. "I will drink extra fluids because this drug will cause me to urinate a lot."

D. "I will eat more oranges and bananas to replace the potassium I lose."

In addition to estrogen therapy, androgen-reducing agents (anti-androgens) are often given to block the effects of testosterone, including (Coleman et al., 2011):

- Spironolactone (Aldactone), a low-cost diuretic that also inhibits testosterone secretion and androgen binding to androgen receptors.
- 5-alpha reductase inhibitors (e.g., finasteride [Proscar]), drugs typically used to treat benign prostatic hyperplasia (BPH). These drugs block the conversion of testosterone to a more active ingredient to decrease the hair loss associated with estrogen therapy and shrink prostate tissue.
- GnRH agonists (e.g., goserelin [Zoladex]), neurohormones that block the gonadotropin-releasing hormone receptor, thus inhibiting the release of the follicle-stimulating hormone (FSH) and luteinizing hormone (LH). These drugs are more expensive and are available only as implants and parenteral preparations.

TABLE 73-4	Masculinizing Drug Therapy for FtM Patients: Expected Changes and Monitoring
Expected Changes	**Laboratory/Imaging Studies**
• Voice deepening • Body hair growth (hirsutism) • Breast atrophy • Increased libido • Increased aggression • Clitoral growth • Redistribution of fat • Laryngeal prominence	• Lipid profile • Liver function tests • Complete blood count • Papanicolaou (Pap) smear (if vagina present) • Mammogram (if breast tissue present)

! NURSING SAFETY PRIORITY (QSEN)

Drug Alert

Teach patients taking *spironolactone* to monitor their blood pressure and have periodic laboratory tests to assess for hyperkalemia if the health care provider determines them to be at risk for these drug effects. Remind them that increased serum potassium can cause cardiac dysrhythmias and skeletal muscle spasticity.

Common side effects of finasteride and other *5-alpha reductase inhibitors* include dizziness, cold sweats, and chills. These manifestations typically decrease over time. If patients continue to have these side effects, instruct them to contact their health care provider.

Teach patients receiving *GnRH agonists* how to self-administer subcutaneous injections. Major side effects of these drugs are tachycardia and other cardiac dysrhythmias. Remind patients to follow up with their health care provider to monitor heart rate and rhythm. Teach them to call 911 if they experience chest pain.

Drugs for FtM Patients. Testosterone is the major drug used for achieving masculinizing effects in transgender people transitioning from female to male; however, much of the available drug converts to estrogen in the body (Coleman et al., 2011). This drug can be taken orally, transdermally, or parenterally (IM). Buccal and implantable forms of testosterone are also available. Oral testosterone (Andriol) is the least effective form of the drug. Depo-Testosterone, the most common IM preparation, is usually started in a low dose and increased to 100 to 200 mg every 1 to 2 weeks (Lilley et al., 2014). Teach patients the importance of not sharing needles to prevent bloodborne diseases such as hepatitis C.

AndroGel and Androderm are topical forms that are more expensive than other testosterone preparations but may provide more consistent (though slower) results. A new topical form of the drug, Axiron, can be applied to the armpits to increase serum testosterone levels. For all topical testosterone preparations, be sure that the patient washes his hands between applications and covers the area with clothing.

Expected effects of testosterone therapy include deepening of the voice, increased libido (sex drive), increased body hair growth, breast and ovarian atrophy, clitoral enlargement, and cessation of menses (Aramburu Alegria, 2011; Jenner, 2010) (Table 73-4). Teach the patient taking testosterone that some of these changes take up to a year to appear. If menses does not stop in the first few months of drug therapy, the patient is placed on Depo-Provera (progesterone) every 3 months until the testosterone becomes effective.

Common side effects of testosterone therapy include edema, acne, seborrhea (oily skin), headaches, weight gain, and possible psychotic symptoms. Before taking this medication, the patient is screened for a history of liver and heart disease. Testosterone therapy can cause increased liver enzymes, increased low-density lipoproteins (LDLs, or "bad" cholesterol), and decreased high-density lipoproteins (HDLs, or "good" cholesterol). Increased blood glucose and decreased clotting factors can also occur when taking the drug (Aramburu Alegria, 2011). Teach patients that these changes can lead to diabetes, heart disease, and stroke. Therefore remind patients that they need to follow up with their health care providers for careful monitoring for these complications, including having extensive diagnostic and laboratory testing (see Table 73-4).

Reproductive Health Options. Using feminizing or masculinizing hormone therapy affects reproductive health, especially fertility. Therefore be sure that patients know their options for REPRODUCTION, if desired, *before* transition begins (Coleman et al., 2011). MtF patients may want to consider sperm banking prior to drug therapy or gender reassignment surgery if they desire to have a biologic child. FtM patients may want to consider oocyte (egg) or embryo freezing. These frozen gametes or embryo could be implanted in a surrogate woman to become pregnant and carry to birth. Inform patients that these options are expensive, but be sure all patients are informed. Be sure to include the patient's sexual partner, if any, in discussions related to reproductive options.

Voice and Communication Therapy. Communication is an essential aspect of human behavior and gender expression. Voice deepening for transgender people who are transitioning from female to male is accomplished by taking masculinizing hormones, such as testosterone. However, feminizing hormones have no effect on the adult MtF voice.

MtF patients may seek assistance from a voice and communication specialist to help them develop certain vocal characteristics, such as pitch and intonation. Vocal therapy can assist in management of gender dysphoria and be a positive step in the transition process. Specialists include speech-language pathologists and speech-voice clinicians. Remind patients to seek a specialist who is licensed, knowledgeable in transgender health, and has specialized training in assessment and development of communication skills for transgender patients (Coleman et al., 2011).

The purpose of vocal therapy is to help patients adapt their voice and communication such that it is authentic and reflects their gender identity. The voice therapist should take the patient's communication preferences and style into consideration as part of the assessment process to develop an individualized treatment plan. Some patients choose follow-up sessions for vocal therapy following voice feminization surgery, also called *feminization laryngoplasty*. This surgery is described in the next section.

Surgical Management. Many transgender people are satisfied with their gender identity, role, and self-expression without surgery. Surgery, particularly procedures that affect the external or internal genitalia, is usually the last and most carefully considered option for transitioning from one's natal sex to one's inner gender identity. These procedures are often referred to as gender or sex reassignment surgery (SRS). The patient has a number of surgical options to achieve either feminizing or masculinizing effects. Regardless of the procedure performed, the nurse collaborates with the patient, family, and health care team to promote positive outcomes for the transition process.

Gender reassignment surgeries are procedures that alter anatomically normal structures. Not all surgeons feel comfortable in performing procedures that could "harm" transgender patients. However, these procedures help treat gender dysphoria (discomfort with one's natal sex) (Coleman et al., 2011). Some patients elect to undergo the full range of surgeries, whereas others choose to have only some or none of them. Most health insurance plans do not cover their cost (Aramburu Alegria, 2011).

Genital surgeries "below the waist" are the most invasive procedures. The criteria for genital surgery depend on the type of surgery being requested. For example, most surgeons (usually urologists or plastic surgeons) require 12 months of hormone therapy plus one or two referrals from qualified psychotherapists for MtF patients who desire an orchiectomy (removal of testes). The same requirements are needed for FtM patients who desire a hysterectomy (uterus removal) and bilateral salpingo-oophorectomy (BSO, or removal of both fallopian tubes and ovaries) (Reed, 2011).

The psychotherapist assesses the patient's readiness for genital surgery and hormone therapy, including a discussion of risks and out-of-pocket costs. The patient's support system is assessed to ensure that the patient makes the best possible decision and achieves the desired outcomes.

For MtF patients requesting a vaginoplasty (creation of a vagina) or FtM patients desiring a phalloplasty (creation of a penis), the required criteria include 12 continuous months of living in a gender role that is congruent with the patient's gender identity. It is also recommended that these patients have regular visits with a mental health care professional (Coleman et al., 2011).

Feminizing Surgeries for MtF Patients. Feminizing surgeries are performed for MtF patients to create a functional and/or aesthetic (cosmetic) female anatomy, including (Brennan et al., 2012; Coleman et al., 2011):

- Breast/chest surgeries, such as breast augmentation (mammoplasty to increase breast tissue).
- Genital surgeries, such as partial penectomy (removal of the penis), orchiectomy (removal of the testes), vaginoplasty and labiaplasty vulvoplasty (creation of a vagina and labia/vulva), clitoroplasty (creation of a clitoris).
- Other surgeries, such as facial feminizing surgery (to achieve feminine facial contour), liposuction (fatty tissue removal), often from the waist or abdominal area, vocal feminizing surgery, gluteal augmentation (to enlarge buttocks), and other body-contouring procedures.

Breast augmentation creates breast tissue for the MtF patient through the use of silicone or saline implants. Although not a prerequisite, it is recommended that MtF patients take feminizing hormones for 12 months prior to surgery for the best results (Coleman et al., 2011). Perioperative care of any patient having this procedure is discussed in Chapter 70 on p. 1463.

Voice surgery, such as reduction thyroid chondroplasty, is performed to decrease the size of the "Adam's apple." The procedure is done through a bronchoscope for cosmetic purposes. Nursing care of the patient having a bronchoscopy is discussed in Chapter 27.

The most common "below the waist" genital surgeries for MtF patients are bilateral *orchiectomy* to remove the testes and vaginoplasty with partial penectomy. Orchiectomy procedures and associated nursing care are the same for the transgender patient as they are for other natal males (see Chapter 72 for a detailed discussion).

A vaginoplasty is the construction of a neovagina (new vagina) usually with inverted penile tissue (obtained during a partial penectomy) or a colon graft. The procedure also includes creating a clitoris and labia using scrotal or penile tissue and skin grafts. Using penile tissue creates a less appealing appearance and low patient satisfaction (Reed, 2011).

Preoperative Care. In addition to the required criteria to qualify for a vaginoplasty (also called *transvaginal surgery*), the transgender patient is medically evaluated like any other presurgical patient. Patients who have poorly controlled diabetes with vascular complications, coronary artery disease, or other systemic disease that limits functional ability are not candidates for gender reassignment surgery. Chapter 14 describes general preoperative care for any patient.

The surgeon explains the options for selected procedures, postoperative care expectations, and potential for complications after surgery. Postoperative recovery for transvaginal surgery takes a long time and has a high complication rate (Reed, 2011). Overweight patients have a higher incidence of wound infection and may have problems with adequate ventilation (breathing) and ambulation after surgery. Refer these patients for nutritional counseling as needed.

Written and verbal preoperative instructions are provided by the surgeon, including optional methods of body hair removal. A bowel preparation may be started 24 hours before surgery and includes a clear liquid diet, laxatives, and Fleet's enemas. Increased fluids are recommended until the patient goes to bed the night before surgery because the bowel "prep" can be very dehydrating. Antimicrobials such as neomycin sulfate and metronidazole (Flagyl) are typically given on the day of surgery to minimize the risk for infection.

Some surgeons require that the patient take supplements to prevent bruising and promote tissue healing, such as vitamin C. Patients who are very thin are encouraged to eat a high-protein diet. A powdered protein supplement with arginine (an amino acid) may also be prescribed to promote wound healing.

Patients have a number of laboratory tests to ensure they are healthy before surgery. Adequate hemoglobin and hematocrit (H&H) levels are especially important because some blood is lost during surgery. For patients who have low H&H levels, an erythropoietin such as epoetin alfa (Procrit) or IM testosterone with iron is given. Most patients choose testosterone because it is a lower-cost drug.

Operative Procedures. Because surgery requires multiple procedures to create a female anatomy, the patient is on the operating table for about 5 hours. The surgery may be performed in a hospital or specialized center for transgender surgeries. After general or epidural anesthesia is administered, the patient is placed in a lithotomy position (feet in stirrups) for the procedure. Epidural anesthesia is preferred for patients who are asthmatic or obese. The patient is transferred to the postanesthesia care unit (PACU) with a perineal dressing and packing, Jackson-Pratt drain, and indwelling urinary catheter.

Postoperative Care. Provide general postoperative care as described in Chapter 16. In addition, immediately after surgery, apply an ice pack to the perineum to decrease pain and bruising. Monitor the patient's pain level carefully, and offer analgesia as needed. Genital surgery is painful because there is a high concentration of nerve endings in the perineum.

Although not a common postoperative complication, monitor the patient for bleeding. Observe the surgical dressing and surrounding area for oozing or bright red blood. Report and document any indication of bleeding immediately to the surgeon, and keep the patient in bed.

Encourage the patient to drink liquids after surgery; discontinue the patient's IV line once oral fluids are tolerated. Evaluate the patient's intake and output every 8 to 12 hours.

! NURSING SAFETY PRIORITY (QSEN)

Action Alert

Patients are in a lithotomy position for an extended period during surgery. Therefore, after surgery, monitor lower extremity neurovascular status and encourage the patient to move the legs often during the first 24 hours after surgery. Report and document any unexpected findings, such as continued numbness or inability to move the lower legs or feet. Patients who had epidural anesthesia are not able to move their legs for several hours after surgery until the effect of the drug diminishes.

All patients stay in the hospital for at least one night after surgery, but some patients may stay longer depending on the number and complexity of the surgical procedures. Some agencies transfer the patient the day after surgery to a local hotel for continued follow-up and monitoring by a health care professional (usually a nurse) (Reed, 2011). Collaborate with the case manager for discharge planning and follow-up care.

The Jackson Pratt drain is removed typically in 3 to 5 days after surgery when drainage is less than 15 to 20 mL in a 24-hour period. In about a week after surgery, the surgical pressure dressing, packing, and external sutures are removed.

At this time, patients are taught how to douche and insert vaginal stents to dilate the vagina. Sexual intercourse also helps keep the vagina dilated. Remind patients that routine douching and douching after intercourse are needed to prevent infection in the new vagina. A solution of vinegar and water or a commercial product such as Massengill can be used. Vaginal stents (also called *dilators*) must be inserted several times a day for months after surgery. The stent should remain in the vagina for 30 to 45 minutes or as instructed by the surgeon. Teach patients the importance of using the stents with water-based lubrication. Collaborate with the surgeon to determine patient-specific instructions.

The urinary catheter is removed between postoperative day 7 and 12. Early removal can cause urinary retention (Reed, 2011).

TABLE 73-5 Postoperative Complications of Vaginoplasty Surgery
Most Serious Complications
• Vaginal-rectal fistula
• Rectal perforation
• Bleeding
Other Complications
• Surgical wound infection
• Urinary leakage/incontinence
• Chronic urinary tract infections
• Urinary meatus stenosis
• Vaginal stenosis
• Vaginal collapse
• Labial hematoma
• Inadequate vaginal length or width
• Lack of sensation
• Lack of sexual pleasure

Patients should continue follow-up visits with their health care provider for manifestations of complications. One of the worst complications is a vaginal-rectal fistula, which is caused by rectal perforation during surgery (Reed, 2011). Teach patients to report any leakage of stool into the vagina immediately to their surgeon. The treatment for this complication is a temporary colostomy and fistula wound management for many months. Other surgical complications of vaginoplasty are listed in Table 73-5.

In addition to physical complications after surgery, some MtF patients are not satisfied with the quality of the results. For example, the neovagina may not be functional for sexual intercourse. Some patients request another surgery to achieve more satisfying results.

? NCLEX EXAMINATION CHALLENGE

Physiological Integrity

A client is admitted to the postanesthesia care unit (PACU) following a vaginoplasty. Which nursing interventions are appropriate for this client? **Select all that apply.**
A. Irrigate the nasogastric tube every 4 hours.
B. Keep the client in a sitting position to facilitate breathing.
C. Apply an ice pack to the perineal area.
D. Monitor drainage from the Jackson-Pratt tube.
E. Perform frequent neurovascular assessments of the legs.

Masculinizing Surgeries for FtM Patients. Masculinizing surgeries are performed for FtM patients to create a functional and/or aesthetic male anatomy, including (Brennan et al., 2012; Coleman et al., 2011):
- Breast/chest surgeries, usually a bilateral mastectomy (removal of both breasts) and chest reconstruction.
- Genital surgeries, such as a hysterectomy and bilateral BSO, vaginectomy (removal of the vagina), phalloplasty (creation of an average-size male penis) with ureteroplasty (creation of a urethra) or metoidioplasty (creation of a small penis using hormone-enhanced clitoral tissue), and scrotoplasty (creation of a scrotum) with insertion of testicular prostheses.
- Other surgeries, such as liposuction, pectoral muscle implants, and other body-contouring procedures.

Care of transgender patients having a mastectomy, hysterectomy, and bilateral salpingo-oophorectomy (BSO) is similar to care for any patient having these procedures as described elsewhere in this text. If the transgender patient has not had previous abdominal surgery, a laparoscopic procedure is preferred for the hysterectomy and BSO surgery.

Surgery to create a penis has not been as successful as other gender reassignment procedures. Procedures to create a male anatomy are not performed as often as MtF surgeries. Phalloplasties are the most difficult reconstructive genital surgeries to perform and usually require several stages. Skin flaps from the radial forearm, anterior lateral thigh, or back are used to create the penis. Fat grafts may be needed to increase penile girth, and buccal mucosal tissue may be used to create the urethra. A penile prosthesis or implant is not inserted until months after surgery until the initial surgical healing has occurred.

Complications from phalloplasty include urinary tract stenosis, donor graft site scarring, and occasionally necrosis of the neopenis (new penis). In addition to these physical problems, the patient may not be satisfied with the results of the surgery, such as an inadequate length of the penis. For this reason, most FtM patients do not have this procedure and prefer to have only a laparoscopic hysterectomy and BSO (Coleman et al., 2011).

Community-Based Care

Transgender patients often take hormone therapy for many years. Teach them that ongoing follow-up with a qualified health care professional is needed to maintain health and detect any complications, such as diabetes or cardiovascular problems, as early as possible.

Long-term follow-up with the surgeon after gender reassignment is essential to detect and treat the frequent complications that occur. Assess the patient's support systems and coping strategies, including financial status and health insurance benefits. Collaborate with the case manager to ensure a smooth transition into the community, including the need for any ongoing mental health counseling or therapy.

Urogenital care is also needed for patients who have gender reassignment surgery. FtM patients usually do not have a vaginectomy and therefore may experience vaginal atrophy causing itching and burning. Recommend that they seek gynecologic care to treat this problem, although the examination can be physically and emotionally painful.

MtF patients need counseling about sexuality, genital hygiene, and prevention of sexually transmitted diseases. They are also at a high risk for frequent urinary tract infections as a result of a shortened urethra and urinary incontinence as a result of genital surgery (Coleman et al., 2011). Teach patients the importance of having follow-up care for these problems.

Preventive health care screenings for transgender patients are also important. For example, the MtF patient requires prostate health care screenings like natal males. Mammograms are also recommended to monitor for early signs of breast cancer.

A number of community resources and organizations are available for transgender support and information, such as:

- National Coalition for LGBT Health (http://lgbthealth.webolutionary.com/content/resources)
- National Resource Center for LGBT Aging (www.lgbtagingcenter.org)
- Services and Advocacy for Gay, Lesbian, Bisexual, and Transgender Elders (www.sageusa.org)
- University of San Francisco Center for Transgender Health (www.transhealth.ucsf.edu)
- World Professional Association for Transgender Health (www.wpath.org)

💡 CLINICAL JUDGMENT CHALLENGE

Patient-Centered Care; Teamwork and Collaboration QSEN

A 58-year-old male-appearing patient visits the gender identity clinic to discuss the desire to have sex reassignment surgery (SRS). As the clinical nurse, you take the patient's history and find that the patient was married to a woman for 30 years and had three children. The couple divorced 3 months ago when the patient's wife discovered that her husband identified as a woman. The couple's children have no contact with the patient since they found out that their father has been dressing as a woman for the past few weeks. The patient is employed as the vice-president of a large commercial construction company and has health insurance. The patient is interested in learning about his options for male-to-female transitioning.

1. How would you address this patient?
2. What other data do you need to collect for the patient's history and why?
3. What options for transitioning to a female does this patient have?
4. Is SRS the best first step for MtF patients? Why or why not?
5. After a physical examination, the clinic physician prescribed estrogen and spironolactone for the patient. What instructions will you provide for the patient before beginning drug therapy?
6. What health teaching does the patient need regarding ongoing follow-up and monitoring while taking these feminizing drugs?
7. With whom might you need to collaborate to manage the patient's care now and in the future?

GET READY FOR THE NCLEX® EXAMINATION!

KEY POINTS

Review these Key Points for each NCLEX Examination Client Needs Category.

Safe and Effective Care Environment

- Depending on identified health care needs, collaborate with the primary health care provider, mental health professional, surgeon, pharmacist, and/or vocal/speech specialist when caring for the transgender patient. **Teamwork and Collaboration** QSEN

- Advocate for the transgender patient who is often distrustful of health care professionals and fearful when seeking health care. **Patient-Centered Care** QSEN

Health Promotion and Maintenance

- Teach patients taking hormone therapy about the need for ongoing health care monitoring for adverse drug events and health complications. **Safety** QSEN

- Refer the transgender patient and significant others, as appropriate, to community resources for information and support, such as the University of San Francisco Center for Transgender Health and the Services and Advocacy for Gay, Lesbian, Bisexual, and Transgender Elders (SAGE) organization.

Psychosocial Integrity

- Use culturally sensitive and accurate language when communicating with transgender patients; use pronouns that match the patient's physical appearance and dress unless the patient requests a specific term (see Table 73-1). **Patient-Centered Care** QSEN
- Provide transgender care with dignity and respect for all patients.
- Be aware that transgender people often have gender dysphoria, which presents an inner conflict between the person's natal (birth) sex and perceived gender identity.
- Assess transgender patients for sources of stress in the community that can lead to health issues, such as depression, anxiety, and substance abuse.

- Be aware that transgender patients may avoid health care settings because they are often unemployed, have no health insurance, and/or fear lack of respect and understanding based on previous experiences. **Patient-Centered Care** QSEN

Physiological Integrity

- Monitor for expected, side, and adverse effects of hormone therapy as described in Tables 73-3 and 73-4.
- Recognize that patients receiving hormone therapy need to have periodic laboratory testing to monitor for complications as listed in Tables 73-3 and Table 73-4. **Evidence-Based Practice** QSEN
- Provide preoperative care for a patient having a vaginoplasty, including teaching about bowel preparation, food and fluid intake, hair removal methods, and the need for informed consent.
- Monitor for potentially life-threatening complications of sex reassignment surgery, such as fistula development, bleeding, and wound infection.

74 | CHAPTER

Care of Patients with Sexually Transmitted Disease

Shirley E. Van Zandt

 http://evolve.elsevier.com/Iggy/

PRIORITY CONCEPTS

- INFECTION
- PAIN
- SEXUALITY

LEARNING OUTCOMES

Safe and Effective Care Environment
1. Maintain patient confidentiality and privacy related to sexually transmitted diseases (STDs).

Health Promotion and Maintenance
2. Educate patients with STDs and their partners on self-care measures.
3. Describe the role of expedited partner therapy in reducing STD recurrence.
4. Develop a teaching plan for young adults and other at-risk people about risk factors, prevention, and treatment for STDs.
5. Explain the importance of respect for patients' personal values and beliefs regarding practices associated with SEXUALITY.

Psychosocial Integrity
6. Assess patients' and their partners' responses to a diagnosis of STD.

7. Reduce the psychological impact for the patient who has been diagnosed with STD.

Physiological Integrity
8. Compare the stages of syphilis.
9. Identify the role of drug therapy in managing patients with STDs.
10. Develop a health teaching plan for patients on how to self-manage their STD, including antibiotic therapy.
11. Describe the assessment findings, including PAIN, that are typical in patients with STDs.
12. Develop a collaborative plan of care for a patient with pelvic inflammatory disease (PID).
13. Identify three sexually transmitted vaginal INFECTIONS.

OVERVIEW

Sexually transmitted diseases (STDs) are caused by infectious organisms that have been passed from one person to another through intimate contact—usually oral, vaginal, or anal intercourse. Some organisms that cause these diseases are transmitted only through sexual contact. Other organisms are transmitted also by parenteral exposure to infected blood, fecal-oral transmission, intrauterine transmission to the fetus, and perinatal transmission from mother to neonate (Table 74-1). The term **sexually transmitted infections (STIs)** is used to describe the same group of health problems. This terminology is intended to focus on the management of acute INFECTIONS and to decrease the social stigma of labeling them as diseases. If the STI continues to recur and become chronic, the term *STD* is used. *STD continues to be the most acceptable term used by the Centers for Disease Control and Prevention (CDC) and is therefore used in this chapter.*

Improved diagnostic techniques, increased knowledge about organisms that can be sexually transmitted, and changes in sexual attitudes and practices have led to an increasing number of reported cases of STDs. *Sexual issues are often sensitive, personal, and controversial, and nurses must respect the patients' lifestyle. Providing confidentiality is essential for patients to receive correct information, make informed decisions, and obtain appropriate care.*

The prevalence of STDs is a major public health concern worldwide. Populations at greatest risk for acquiring STDs and suffering from their complications are pregnant women, adolescents, and men who have sex with men (MSM). External factors such as an increasing population, cultural factors (e.g., earlier first intercourse), political and economic policies, incidences of sexual abuse and sexual trafficking, and international travel and migration affect the prevalence of STDs.

TABLE 74-1   Sexually Transmitted Diseases

- Human immune deficiency virus infection
- Chancroid
- Syphilis
- Lymphogranuloma venereum
- Genital herpes simplex virus infection
- Genital warts
- Gonococcal infection
- Chlamydia infection
- Nongonococcal urethritis
- Mucopurulent cervicitis
- Epididymitis
- Pelvic inflammatory disease
- Sexually transmitted enteritis
- Sexually transmitted proctitis
- Trichomoniasis
- Candidal infection
- Bacterial vaginosis
- Viral hepatitis
- Cytomegalovirus infection
- Ectoparasitic infection:
  - Pediculosis pubis
  - Scabies

From Centers for Disease Control and Prevention (CDC). (2010). *Sexually transmitted diseases treatment guidelines, 2010. Morbidity and Mortality Weekly Report, 59*(RR-12), 1-110.

CONSIDERATIONS FOR OLDER ADULTS

Patient-Centered Care   QSEN

Another factor contributing to STD prevalence is the increasing number of older adults that will continue as the baby boomers age. People older than 50 years may not realize their risk for STDs or feel comfortable discussing their sexuality with health care providers. Providers may also lack awareness of the sexual activity of older adults. Be sure to teach older adults who are sexually active about their risk for developing STDs (Jeffers & DiBartolo, 2011).

In the United States, one of the greatest factors associated with STD prevalence is the secrecy that surrounds SEXUALITY, sexual behavior, and intimacy in the American culture. The stigma of STDs in the United States has been associated with higher rates of STDs as compared with rates in other developed countries. The prevalence of STDs is also affected by changing human physiology patterns such as earlier onset of menarche, comorbidities associated with human immune deficiency virus (HIV) and diabetes, treatments given for cancer or organ transplantation, and disparities in access to health care. Substance abuse has also been identified as a significant risk factor because of the effects illicit drugs have on sexual risk-taking behavior.

STDs cause complications that can contribute to severe physical and emotional suffering, including infertility, ectopic pregnancy, cancer, and death. Some of the most common complications caused by sexually transmitted organisms are listed in Table 74-2.

Chlamydia infection, gonorrhea, syphilis, chancroid, human immune deficiency virus (HIV) INFECTION, and acquired immune deficiency syndrome (AIDS) are reportable to local health authorities in every state (Centers for Disease Control and Prevention [CDC], 2013f). Other STDs such as genital herpes (GH) may or may not be reported, depending on local legal requirements. Positive results can be reported by clinicians and laboratories. Reports are kept strictly confidential.

Nurses in a variety of settings are responsible for identifying people at risk for STDs, caring for patients with diagnosed STDs, and preventing further cases through education and case finding. Nurses in primary care community settings and acute care settings have a responsibility to recognize patients who are at risk for or who have STDs, possibly while being treated for another unrelated health problem.

The CDC provides regularly updated guidelines for treatment of STDs. These best practice guidelines provide information, treatment standards, and counseling advice to help decrease the spread of these diseases and their complications (CDC, 2010b).

Evidence from the U.S. Preventive Services Task Force (USPSTF) has shown that education and counseling about STDs needs to be of high intensity and on multiple occasions for it to change behavior (USPSTF, 2014b). Health education messages that are short, nonspecific, and not related to the person's sexual behaviors have little effect in lowering the risk for acquiring STDs.

GENDER HEALTH CONSIDERATIONS

Patient-Centered Care   QSEN

Because of the very vascular and large surface area of the mucous membranes of the vagina, women are more easily infected with STDs and are at greater risk for STD-related health problems than are men. Young women who are sexually active with men have the greatest risk for contracting an STD. Younger adults have greater rates of sexual activity, including more partners and more unprotected sex than older adults. Women are more vulnerable to infections because of the exposure of cervical basal epithelium cells. Lesbian women have a decreased risk for STDs because of fewer partners, although many have or have had sex with men.

Some young women may also be at high risk because they:
- Lack knowledge about the risk for disease
- Believe that they are not vulnerable to disease
- Mistakenly believe that contraceptives also protect them from STDs
- Drink alcohol in binges, which promotes risky sexual behavior

Postmenopausal women also may be at risk for STDs because many perceive that pregnancy is no longer likely and thus do not use barrier protection. Changing social relationships (e.g., divorce and widowhood in the middle years) has changed risk for exposure to STDs. Physiologic changes during menopause such as mucosal tears from vaginal atrophy may also place them at risk.

Women have more asymptomatic infections that may delay diagnosis and treatment. Many STDs reside in the cervical os and cause little change in vaginal discharge or vulvar tissue so women are not aware that they are infected. This delay increases the likelihood of complications from STDs, including ascending infections that may cause reproductive organ damage and illness. Embarrassment, denial, or fear about STDs may further delay treatment, increasing the potential for serious complications.

INFECTIONS ASSOCIATED WITH ULCERS

SYPHILIS

❖ PATHOPHYSIOLOGY

Syphilis is a complex sexually transmitted disease (STD) that can become systemic and cause serious complications, including death. The causative organism is a spirochete called *Treponema pallidum*. Although the organism can be seen only with a darkfield microscope, several serologic tests are used to screen for the presence of syphilis antibody. *T. pallidum* is damaged by dry air or any known disinfectant. The organisms die within

TABLE 74-2   Complications Caused by Sexually Transmitted Organisms

COMPLICATION	CAUSATIVE ORGANISMS
Salpingitis, infertility, and ectopic pregnancy	*Neisseria gonorrhoeae* *Chlamydia trachomatis* *Mycoplasma hominis* *Ureaplasma urealyticum*
Reproductive loss (abortion/miscarriage)	*N. gonorrhoeae* *C. trachomatis* Herpes simplex virus *M. hominis* *U. urealyticum* *Treponema pallidum*
Puerperal infection	*N. gonorrhoeae* *C. trachomatis*
Perinatal infection	Hepatitis B virus Human immune deficiency virus Human papilloma virus *N. gonorrhoeae* *C. trachomatis* Herpes simplex virus *T. pallidum* Cytomegalovirus Group B streptococcus
Cancer of genital area	Human papilloma virus
Male urethritis	*M. hominis* Herpes simplex virus *N. gonorrhoeae* *C. trachomatis* *U. urealyticum*
Vulvovaginitis	Herpes simplex virus *Trichomonas vaginalis* Bacterial vaginosis *Candida albicans*
Cervicitis	*N. gonorrhoeae* *C. trachomatis* Herpes simplex virus
Proctitis	*N. gonorrhoeae* *C. trachomatis* Herpes simplex virus *Campylobacter jejuni* *Shigella* species *Entamoeba histolytica*
Hepatitis	*T. pallidum* Hepatitis A, hepatitis B, and hepatitis C viruses
Dermatitis	*Sarcoptes scabiei* *Phthirus pubis*
Genital ulceration or warts	*C. trachomatis* Herpes simplex virus Human papilloma virus *T. pallidum* *Haemophilus ducreyi* *Calymmatobacterium granulomatis*

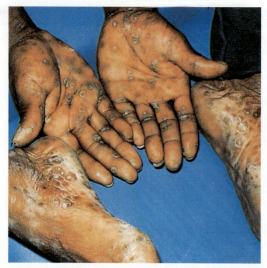

FIG. 74-1 Palmar and plantar secondary syphilis.

skin or mucous membranes but occur most often on the genitalia, lips, nipples, and hands and in the mouth, anus, and rectum.

During this highly infectious stage, the chancre begins as a small papule. Within 3 to 7 days, it breaks down into its typical appearance: a painless, indurated, smooth, weeping lesion. Regional lymph nodes enlarge, feel firm, and are not painful. Without treatment, the chancre usually disappears within 6 weeks. However, the organism spreads throughout the body and the patient is still infectious.

Secondary syphilis develops 6 weeks to 6 months after the onset of primary syphilis. During this stage, syphilis is a systemic disease because the spirochetes circulate throughout the bloodstream. Commonly mistaken for influenza, manifestations include flu-like symptoms (malaise, low-grade fever, headache, muscular aches, sore throat) and a generalized rash. There is no typical appearance of this rash except for its presence on the palms and soles of the feet and on mucous membranes. It can appear as diffuse macules (reddish brown), papules (usually less than 5 mm) or pustules, scaly psoriasis-like lesions (Fig. 74-1), or gray-white wart-like lesions (condylomata lata). *All of these lesions are highly contagious and should not be touched without gloves.* Patchy alopecia on the scalp or facial hair (missing part of the eyebrow, "moth-eaten" appearance) is another symptom. The rash subsides without treatment in 4 to 12 weeks.

After the second stage of syphilis, there is a period of latency. *Early latent* syphilis occurs during the first year after INFECTION, and infectious lesions can recur. *Late latent* syphilis is a disease of more than 1 year's duration after INFECTION. This stage is not infectious except to the fetus of a pregnant woman. Patients with latent syphilis may or may not have reactive serologic test (e.g., Venereal Disease Research Laboratory [VDRL]) findings.

Tertiary, or late, syphilis occurs after a highly variable period, from 4 to 20 years. This stage develops in untreated cases and can mimic other conditions because any organ system can be affected. Manifestations of late syphilis include:

- Benign lesions (gummas) of the skin, mucous membranes, and bones
- Cardiovascular syphilis, usually in the form of aortic valvular disease and aortic aneurysms
- Neurosyphilis, causing central nervous system symptoms (e.g., meningitis, hearing loss, generalized paresis [weakness])

hours at temperatures of 105.8° to 107.6°F (41° to 42°C) and are not airborne. *The INFECTION is usually transmitted by sexual contact and blood exposure, but transmission can occur through close body contact such as kissing.*

Syphilis progresses through four stages: primary, secondary, latent, and tertiary. The appearance of an ulcer called a **chancre** is the first sign of *primary* syphilis. It develops at the site of entry (inoculation) of the organism from 10 to 90 days after exposure (3 weeks is average). Chancres may be found on any area of the

🌐 CULTURAL CONSIDERATIONS
Patient-Centered Care QSEN

Disparity exists between racial and ethnic groups in the incidence of primary and secondary syphilis. In the most recent reports from 2011, the rates increased among Hispanics, American Indians/Alaska Natives (from 2.5 to 2.7 cases per 100,000 population), Euro-Americans (from 2.1 to 2.3 cases per 100,000 population), and most dramatically (33%) among Asian/Pacific Islanders but impressively have decreased among African Americans. Nevertheless, African Americans have a 7 times greater rate of acquiring syphilis than whites. Compared with Euro-Americans, the 2011 rate for Hispanics was 2 times higher (CDC, 2013a). The reason for these differences is unclear, but status of health literacy and lack of access to health care may be factors.

GENDER HEALTH CONSIDERATIONS
Patient-Centered Care QSEN

Unique needs regarding sexual health and prevention and treatment of sexually related infections of lesbian, gay, bisexual, transgender, and questioning (LGBTQ) patients should be identified and addressed by the nurse. Because of discrimination, health care inequities, and health care provider lack of understanding, the overall health status of people in these populations may be poor. LGBTQ people may have difficulty finding health care that identifies and addresses their particular risks and concerns. Taking a health history that provides opportunity for the patient to identify his or her sexual orientation, sexual identity, and sexual activity is crucial. Especially among transgender people, opportunities for physical examination are avoided or missed by both the patient and care provider because of fears of being misunderstood or inadequately prepared to give or receive appropriate care (Williamson, 2010).

The CDC does not currently collect or report the incidence or prevalence of STDs among transgender people. There have been estimates from self-report that 11% to 28% of the transgender community are infected with HIV (Cobos & Jones, 2009).

Men who have sex with men (MSM) are at greatest risk for contracting primary and secondary syphilis and made up 75% of cases of these diseases in 2012 (CDC, 2014a). These men are 17 times more likely to have anal cancer than heterosexual men, and those infected with HIV are at even greater risk. Infection with high-risk human papilloma virus (HPV) has been associated with greater risk for anal cancers among this population (CDC, 2012a).

A common perception that women who have sex with women (WSW) are at very low or no risk for getting STDs has not been supported in research because of the lack of data. Bacterial, viral, and protozoal infections have all been reported among WSW (CDC, 2014c). Identifying risk in this population may depend more on asking about sexual practices such as use of sex objects or oral-anal, digital-anal, or digital-vaginal sex. Being aware of these practices can increase the nurse's ability to identify risk factors for patients.

Assuming that lesbian women or gay men have sex only with same-gender partners or similarly assuming that heterosexual patients never have sexual encounters with partners of their same sex may limit the accuracy of the nurse's risk assessment. Nurses must be aware that patients may not reveal that they are bisexual. Establish a trusting relationship and be culturally sensitive and nonjudgmental when working with LGBTQ patients. Chapter 1 describes recommendations for communicating with this population. Chapter 73 discusses the special health care needs of transgender patients.

Health Promotion and Maintenance

One of the *Healthy People 2020* objectives is to completely eliminate syphilis in the United States (U.S. Department of Health and Human Services [USDHHS], 2014) (Table 74-3). One of the primary tools for prevention of sexually transmitted

TABLE 74-3 Meeting *Healthy People 2020* Objectives and Targets for Improvement: Sexually Transmitted Diseases

- Reduce the proportion of adolescents and young adults with *Chlamydia trachomatis* infections (by 10%).
- Reduce the proportion of females ages 15 to 44 years who have ever required treatment for pelvic inflammatory disease (by 10%).
- Reduce gonorrhea rates (by 10%).
- Reduce sustained domestic transmission of primary and secondary syphilis (by 10%).
- Reduce the proportion of females with human papilloma virus (HPV) infection (no specific target).
- Reduce the proportion of young adults with genital herpes due to herpes simplex type 2 (by 10%).

diseases (STDs), including syphilis, is education. All people, regardless of age, gender, ethnicity, socioeconomic status, education level, or sexual orientation, are susceptible to these diseases. Health literacy, motivation, and perceived risk can affect the health status of any patient. STDs are largely preventable through safer sex practices. *Do not assume that a person is not sexually active because of his or her age, education, marital status, profession, or religion.* Discuss prevention methods, including safer sex, with all patients who are or may become sexually active.

Safer sex practices are those that reduce the risk for nonintact skin or mucous membranes coming in contact with infected body fluids and blood. These practices include:

- Using a latex or polyurethane condom for genital and anal intercourse
- Using a condom or latex barrier (dental dam) over the genitals or anus during oral-genital or oral-anal sexual contact
- Wearing gloves for finger or hand contact with the vagina or rectum
- Abstinence
- Mutual monogamy
- Decreasing the number of sexual partners

❖ PATIENT-CENTERED COLLABORATIVE CARE
◆ Assessment

Assessment of the patient who has manifestations of syphilis begins with a history to gather information about any ulcers or rash. Take a sexual history and conduct a risk assessment to include whether previous testing or treatment for syphilis or other STDs has ever been done (Chart 74-1). Ask about allergic reactions to drugs, especially penicillin. A woman may report inguinal lymph node enlargement resulting from a chancre in the vagina or cervix that is not easily visible to her. She may state a history of sexual contact with a male partner who had an ulcer that she noticed during the encounter. Men usually discover the chancre on the penis or scrotum.

Conduct a physical examination, including inspection and palpation, to identify manifestations of syphilis. *Wear gloves while palpating any lesions because of the highly contagious treponemes that are present.* Observe for and document rashes of any type because of the variable presentation of secondary syphilis.

After the physical examination, the health care provider obtains a *specimen of the chancre* for examination under a

| CHART 74-1 | Focused Assessment |

The Patient with a Sexually Transmitted Disease

Assess history of present illness:
- Chief concern
- Onset
- Symptoms by quality and quantity, precipitating and palliative factors
- Any treatments taken (self-prescribed or over-the-counter products)

Assess past medical history:
- Major health problems—including any history of STDs/PID or immunosuppression
- Surgeries—obstetric and gynecologic, circumcision

Assess current health status:
- Menstrual history for irregularities
- Sexual history:
  - Type and frequency of sexual activity
  - Number of lifetime and past 6 months sexual contacts/partners; monogamous
  - Sexual orientation
- Contraception history
- Medications
- Allergies
- Lifestyle risks—drugs, alcohol, tobacco

Assess preventive health care practices:
- Papanicolaou (Pap) tests
- Regular STD screening
- Use of barrier contraceptives to prevent STDs and pregnancy

Assess physical examination findings:
- Vital signs
- Oropharyngeal findings
- Abdominal findings
- Genital or pelvic findings
- Anorectal findings

Assess laboratory data:
- Urinalysis
- Hematology
- ESR or CRP if PID is being considered
- Cervical, urethral, oral, rectal specimens
- Lesion samples for microbiology and virology
- Pregnancy testing

CRP, C-reactive protein; *ESR,* erythrocyte sedimentation rate; *PID,* pelvic inflammatory disease; *STDs,* sexually transmitted diseases.

darkfield microscope. Diagnosis of primary or secondary syphilis is confirmed if *T. pallidum* is present.

Blood tests are also used to diagnose syphilis. The usual screening and/or diagnostic nontreponemal tests are the *Venereal Disease Research Laboratory (VDRL)* serum test and the more sensitive *rapid plasma reagin (RPR)*. These tests are based on an antibody-antigen reaction that determines the presence and amount of antibodies produced by the body in response to an INFECTION by *T. pallidum.* They become reactive 2 to 6 weeks after infection. VDRL titers are also used to monitor treatment effectiveness. The antibodies are not specific to *T. pallidum,* and false-positive reactions often occur from such conditions as viral INFECTIONS, hepatitis, and systemic lupus erythematosus (SLE) (Pagana & Pagana, 2014).

If a VDRL result is positive, the health care provider requests or the laboratory may automatically perform a more specific treponemal test, such as the *fluorescent treponemal antibody absorption (FTA-ABS)* test or the *microhemagglutination assay for T. palladum (MHA-TP),* to confirm the infection. These tests are more sensitive for all stages of syphilis, although false-positive results may still occur. Patients who have a reactive test

will have this positive result for their entire life, even after sufficient treatment. This poses a challenge when receiving a positive result for a patient who denies a history of or does not know he or she had syphilis.

◆ Interventions

Patient-centered collaborative care includes drug therapy and health teaching to resolve the INFECTION and prevent infection transmission to others.

Drug Therapy. Benzathine penicillin G given IM as a single 2.4 million-unit dose is the evidence-based treatment for primary, secondary, and early latent syphilis (CDC, 2010b). Patients in the late latent stage receive the same dose every week for 3 weeks (CDC, 2010b). A different regimen, found in the CDC's *STD Treatment Guidelines,* is recommended for patients who are HIV-infected or pregnant.

! NURSING SAFETY PRIORITY (QSEN)

Drug Alert

Allergic reactions to benzathine penicillin G can occur. Monitor for allergic manifestations (e.g., rash, edema, shortness of breath, chest tightness, anxiety). Penicillin desensitization is recommended for penicillin-allergic patients. *Keep all patients at the health care agency for at least 30 minutes after they have received the antibiotic so that manifestations of an allergic reaction can be detected and treated. The most severe reaction is anaphylaxis. Treatment should be available and implemented immediately if symptoms occur.* Chapter 17 describes the management of drug allergies in detail.

After treatment, the CDC recommends follow-up evaluation including blood tests at 6, 12, and 24 months. Repeat treatment may be needed if the patient does not respond to the initial antibiotic.

The *Jarisch-Herxheimer reaction* may also follow antibiotic therapy for syphilis. This reaction is caused by the rapid release of products from the disruption of the cells of the organism. Symptoms include generalized aches, pain at the injection site, vasodilation, hypotension, and fever. They are usually benign and begin within 2 hours after therapy with a peak at 4 to 8 hours. This reaction may be treated symptomatically with analgesics and antipyretics.

Self-Management Education. Teach about the cause of INFECTION (sexual transmission); treatment, including side effects; possible complications of untreated or incompletely treated disease; and the need for follow-up care.

! NURSING SAFETY PRIORITY (QSEN)

Drug Alert

Discuss with the patient with syphilis the importance of partner notification and treatment, including the risk for re-infection if the partner goes untreated. All sexual partners must be prophylactically treated as soon as possible, preferably within 90 days of the syphilis diagnosis.

Inform the patient that the disease will be reported to the local health authority and that all information will be held in strict confidence. Encourage the patient to provide accurate information for this follow-up to ensure that all at-risk partners are treated appropriately. Provide a setting that offers privacy and encourages open discussion. Urge the patient to keep follow-up appointments. For primary and secondary syphilis, medication treatment will be completed at the first visit, which may suggest to the patient that no further visits are indicated or important. Remind the patient that follow-up for partners and assessment that symptoms have resolved are imperative and part of continuing care. Recommend sexual abstinence until the treatment of both the patient and partner(s) is completed.

The emotional responses to syphilis vary and may include feelings of fear, depression, guilt, and anxiety. Patients may experience guilt if they have infected others or anger if a partner has infected them. If further psychosocial interventions are needed, encourage the patient to discuss these feelings or refer him or her to other resources such as psychotherapy, self-help support groups, or STD clinics.

? NCLEX EXAMINATION CHALLENGE

Physiological Integrity

The nurse gives a client an IM dose of penicillin G for primary syphilis. Which client statement indicates a need for further teaching?
A. "I will wait in the clinic for 30 minutes to be sure I do not have a reaction."
B. "When I get home, I will call my partner to tell them about my diagnosis."
C. "If I have sex with someone, I do not have to worry about spreading the disease."
D. "I plan to return to see my primary care provider for follow-up in 6, 12, and 24 months."

GENITAL HERPES

❖ PATHOPHYSIOLOGY

Genital herpes (GH) is an acute, recurring, incurable viral disease. It is the most common STD in the United States, with 17.0% of Americans currently infected with herpes simplex virus type 2 (HSV-2) and 57.7% with type 1 (HSV-1) (Warren et al., 2011).

The prevalence among African Americans is 39.2%, disproportionately affecting African-American women (48.0%) (CDC, 2010a). These rates are based on the presence of HSV-2 antibodies in the blood of those tested, the majority of whom have had no symptoms and most have never received a diagnosis of GH INFECTION (CDC, 2010a).

Two serotypes of herpes simplex virus (HSV) affect the genitalia: type 1 (HSV-1) and type 2 (HSV-2). Most *nongenital* lesions such as cold sores are caused by HSV-1, transmitted via oral-oral contact. Historically, HSV-2 caused most of the genital lesions. However, this distinction is academic because the transmission, symptoms, diagnosis, and treatment are nearly identical for the two types. Either type can produce oral or genital lesions through oral-genital or genital-genital contact with an infected person. HSV-2 recurs and sheds asymptomatically more often than HSV-1. Most people with GH have not been diagnosed because they have mild symptoms and shed virus intermittently, with possibly only 10% to 25% of those with HSV-2 realizing they have GH (Patel & Rompalo, 2012).

The incubation period of genital herpes is 2 to 20 days, with the average period being 1 week. Many people do not have symptoms during the primary outbreak. When subsequent outbreaks of genital herpes occur, they are usually more severe and occasionally require hospitalization.

Recurrences are not caused by re-infection. Additional episodes are usually less severe and of shorter duration than the primary INFECTION episode. Some patients have no symptoms at all during recurrence or viral reactivation. *However, there is viral shedding and the patient is infectious.* Long-term complications of GH include the risk for neonatal transmission and an increased risk for acquiring HIV infection.

❖ PATIENT-CENTERED COLLABORATIVE CARE

◆ Assessment

The diagnosis of GH is based on the patient's history and physical examination (see Chart 74-1). Ask the patient if he or she felt itching or a tingling sensation in the skin 1 to 2 days before the outbreak, known as the *prodrome*. These sensations are usually followed by the appearance of **vesicles** (blisters) in a typical cluster on the penis, scrotum, vulva, vagina, cervix, or perianal region at the site of inoculation. The blisters rupture spontaneously in a day or two and leave painful ulcerations that can become extensive. Assess for other symptoms such as headaches, fever, general malaise, and swelling of inguinal lymph nodes. Ask if urination is painful. External dysuria is a painful symptom when urine passes over the eroded areas. Patients with urinary retention may need to be catheterized. Lesions resolve within 2 to 6 weeks.

After the lesions heal, the virus remains in a dormant state in the sacral nerve ganglia. Periodically, the virus may activate and symptoms recur. These recurrences may be triggered by many factors, including stress, fever, sunburn, poor nutrition, menses, and sexual activity. Assess the patient for these risk factors to provide anticipatory guidance for prevention of outbreaks.

GH is confirmed through a viral cell culture or polymerase chain reaction (PCR) assays of the lesions. PCR is the more sensitive test and is currently the gold standard; however, it is very expensive and usually not available. Fluid from inside the blister obtained within 48 hours of the first outbreak will yield the most reliable results because accuracy decreases as the blisters begin to heal (Patel & Rompalo, 2012). Serology testing, which is glycoprotein G antibody-based, can identify the HSV type, either 1 or 2. Serologic tests are used to identify INFECTION in high-risk groups such as HIV-positive patients, patients who have partners with HSV, or men who have sex with men (MSM) (CDC, 2010b). Antibodies may take up to 12 weeks to develop, so false-negative results can occur if tested too soon after the initial infection. Because 80% to 90% of the population will become positive over their lifetime, using the antibody serology test to screen for infection in the general population is not effective or appropriate (Patel & Rompalo, 2012).

◆ Interventions

The desired outcomes of treatment for HSV-infected patients are to decrease the discomfort from painful ulcerations, promote healing without secondary infection, decrease viral shedding, and prevent INFECTION transmission (Chart 74-2).

Drug Therapy. Antiviral drugs are used to treat GH. *The drugs decrease the severity, promote healing, and decrease the frequency of recurrent outbreaks but do not cure the infection.*

Drug therapy should be offered to anyone with an initial outbreak of GH regardless of the severity of the symptoms. Topical therapy is not recommended. Acyclovir (Zovirax, Avirax ✦), famciclovir (Famvir), or valacyclovir (Valtrex) may be prescribed. The main differences in these drugs are cost and

CHART 74-2 Best Practice for Patient Safety & Quality Care QSEN

Care of or Self-Management for the Patient with Genital Herpes

- Administer oral analgesics as prescribed.
- Apply local anesthetic sprays or ointments as prescribed.
- Apply ice packs or warm compresses to the patient's lesions.
- Administer sitz baths 3 or 4 times a day.
- Urge an increase in fluid intake to replace fluid lost through open lesions.
- Encourage frequent urination.
- Pour water over the patient's genitalia while voiding, or encourage voiding while the patient is sitting in a tub of water or standing in a shower.
- Catheterize the patient as necessary.
- Encourage genital hygiene, and encourage keeping the skin clean and dry.
- Wash hands thoroughly after contact with lesions, and launder towels that have had direct contact with lesions.
- Wear gloves when applying ointments or making any direct contact with lesions.
- Advise the patient to avoid sexual activity when lesions are present.
- Advise the patient to use latex or polyurethane condoms during all sexual exposures.
- Instruct the patient in the use, side effects, and risks versus benefits of antiviral agents.
- Advise the patient to discuss the diagnosis of genital herpes (GH) with current and new partners.

CHART 74-3 Patient and Family Education: Preparing for Self-Management

Use of Condoms

- Use latex or polyurethane condoms rather than natural membrane condoms.
- Use a condom with every sexual encounter (including oral, vaginal, and anal).
- Female condoms (Reality)—polyurethane or nitrile sheaths in the vagina—are effective in preventing transmission of viruses, including HIV.
- Condoms infrequently (2 per 100) break during sexual intercourse.
- Keep condoms (especially latex) in a cool, dry place, out of direct sunlight.
- Do not use condoms that are in damaged packages or that are brittle or discolored.
- Always handle a condom with care to avoid damaging it with fingernails, teeth, or other sharp objects.
- Put condoms on before any genital contact. Hold the condom by the tip and unroll it on the penis. Leave a space at the tip to collect semen.
- If you use a lubricant with condoms, make sure that the lubricant is water based and washes away with water. Oil-based products damage latex condoms.
- Use of spermicide (nonoxynol-9) with condoms, either lubricated condoms or vaginal application, has *not* been proven to be more or less effective against STDs than use without spermicide. Spermicide-coated condoms have been associated with *Escherichia coli* urinary tract infections in women. *Nonoxynol-9 may increase risk for transmission of HIV during vaginal intercourse and anal intercourse. Its use is discouraged.*
- If a condom breaks, replace it immediately.
- After ejaculation, withdraw the erect penis carefully, holding the condom at the base of the penis to prevent the condom from slipping off.
- Never use a condom more than once.

Modified from Centers for Disease Control and Prevention (CDC). (2010). Sexually transmitted diseases treatment guidelines, 2010. *Morbidity and Mortality Weekly Report, 59*(RR-12), 4-5.
HIV, Human immune deficiency virus; *STDs*, sexually transmitted diseases.

frequency of use. Dosage and length of treatment differ for primary outbreaks (7 to 10 days) and recurrent outbreaks (1 to 5 days). Therapy for recurrent outbreaks is most beneficial if it is started within 1 day of the appearance of lesions or during the period of itching or tingling before lesions appear. Intermittent or continuous (daily) suppressive antiviral therapy is offered to patients to lessen the severity and frequency of or prevent outbreaks, even for those with infrequent recurrent episodes.

Suppression reduces recurrences in most patients, but it does not prevent viral shedding, even when symptoms are absent (CDC, 2010b). Patients receiving continuous therapy should periodically (possibly once a year) be reassessed for recurrences, usually by stopping the antiviral drug temporarily.

IV acyclovir and hospitalization may be indicated for patients with severe HSV infections, such as disseminated disease or encephalitis. These are severe complications of genital herpes and may be fatal.

Self-Management Education. Nursing interventions focus on patient education about the INFECTION, sexual transmission, the potential for recurrent episodes, and the correct use and possible side effects of antiviral therapy. Frank discussion about sexual activity, including whether the patient has new or multiple partners, is an essential component of the nurse's intervention.

> **! NURSING SAFETY PRIORITY** QSEN
>
> **Action Alert**
>
> Remind patients to abstain from sexual activity while GH lesions are present. Sexual activity can be painful, and likelihood of viral transmission is higher. Urge condom use during all sexual exposures because of the increased risk for HSV transmission from viral shedding, which can occur even when lesions are not present. Teach the patient about how to use condoms (Chart 74-3).

Assess the patient's and partner's emotional responses to the diagnosis of genital herpes. Many people are initially shocked and need reassurance that they can manage the disease. Infected patients may have feelings of disbelief, uncleanness, isolation, and loneliness. They may also be angry at their partner(s) for transmitting the INFECTION or fear rejection because they have the infection. Help patients cope with the diagnosis by being sensitive and supportive during assessments and interventions. Encourage social support, and refer patients to support groups (e.g., local support groups of the National Herpes Resource Center [www.ashasexualhealth.org/std-sti/Herpes.html]) and therapists. Symptomatic care may include oral analgesics, topical anesthetics, sitz baths, and increased oral fluid intake (Bavis et al., 2009).

Emphasize the risk for neonatal INFECTION to all patients, both male and female. Men and women who have genital herpes need to inform their pregnancy care provider of their history. Uninfected women will be advised to avoid unprotected intercourse with infected partners during pregnancy to avoid the risk for a new primary infection and outbreak during pregnancy. People who have tested serology positive to HSV-1 or HSV-2 but have never had GH symptoms should be counseled with the same information as for those who have symptoms (CDC, 2010b).

INFECTIONS OF THE EPITHELIAL STRUCTURES

CONDYLOMATA ACUMINATA (GENITAL WARTS)

❖ PATHOPHYSIOLOGY

Condylomata acuminata (also known as *genital warts*) are caused by certain types of *human papilloma virus (HPV)*, 90% of which are types 6 and 11 or low-risk HPV (Datta et al., 2012; Mark et al., 2012). These types *rarely* result in invasive cancer of the genital tract such as cervical cancer. *However, HPV types 16, 18, 31, 33, and 35, considered high-risk HPV, can be found on the skin of the genitalia and increase the risk for genital cancers, especially cervical cancer.* INFECTION with several HPV types can occur at the same time. The presence of one strain increases the risk for acquiring a higher-risk strain. Genital warts are the most common viral disease that is sexually transmitted and are often seen with other infections. Among American women ages 14 to 59 years, 26.8% are infected with either high- or low-risk HPV (Datta et al., 2012).

HPV INFECTION has been established as the primary risk factor *for development of cervical cancer* (Datta et al., 2012). Sites commonly affected by INFECTION include the urinary meatus, labia, vagina, cervix, penis, scrotum, anus, and perineal area. The incubation period is usually 2 to 3 months. There is growing evidence that HPV infection through oral and anal sex, especially in men who have sex with men (MSM), may be a risk factor for developing oral and anal cancers (Kim, 2010).

❖ PATIENT-CENTERED COLLABORATIVE CARE

◆ Assessment

The diagnosis of condylomata acuminata is made by examination of the lesions. They are initially small, white or flesh-colored papillary growths that may grow into large cauliflower-like masses (Fig. 74-2). Multiple warts usually occur in the same area. Bleeding may occur if the wart is disturbed. Warts may disappear or resolve on their own without treatment. They may occur once or recur at the original site. Warts can

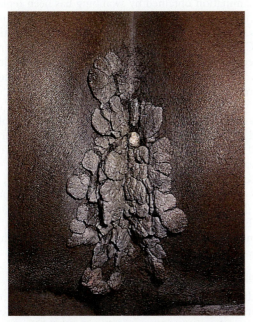

FIG. 74-2 Perianal condylomata acuminata.

occur on the external or internal surfaces of the genitalia, including the mucosal surfaces of the vagina and urethra.

Screening for HPV and dysplasia of the cervix is done by obtaining cervical specimens for Papanicolaou (Pap) and HPV DNA testing. The frequency of screening has changed significantly as new understanding about the course of HPV infection has evolved. Identifying high-risk strains of HPV and correlating with abnormal Pap smear findings is now the standard of care (Schiffman et al., 2011). High-risk HPV may coexist with low-risk HPV, the likely cause of the warts. The diagnosis should include consideration of condyloma lata or secondary syphilis since STDs frequently coexist. A VDRL test, HIV test, and cultures for chlamydia and gonorrhea infections are done. Condylomata lata (secondary syphilis) can resemble condylomata acuminata (genital warts). If a wartlike lesion bleeds easily, appears infected, is atypical, or persists, a biopsy of the lesion is performed to rule out other pathologic problems such as cancer. A biopsy of warts that are seen on the cervix should be performed prior to any treatment to eradicate them.

◆ Interventions

The outcome of treatment is to remove the warts. No current therapy eliminates the HPV infection, and recurrences after treatment are likely. It is not known whether removal of visible warts decreases the risk for disease transmission.

Drug Therapy. Patients may apply podofilox (Condylox) 0.5% cream or gel twice daily for 3 days with no treatment for the next 4 days. This regimen should be repeated for four cycles. Other options are imiquimod (Aldara) 5% cream applied topically at bedtime 3 times a week and sinecatechins 15% ointment (made from green tea extract) applied 3 times a day, both until the warts disappear or for up to 16 weeks. Imiquimod boosts the immune system rather than simply destroying the warts. These self-treatments are less expensive than those performed in the health care provider's office, but they take longer for healing. *Teach patients that over-the-counter (OTC) wart treatments should not be used on genital tissue (CDC, 2010b).*

Cryotherapy, trichloroacetic acid (TCA) or bichloroacetic acid (BCA), and podophyllin (Pododerm) are provider-applied treatments. **Cryotherapy** (freezing), usually with liquid nitrogen, can be used every 1 to 2 weeks until lesions are resolved. TCA/BCA (80% to 90%) can be applied weekly. Podophyllin resin can be applied weekly but needs to be washed off 1 to 4 hours after application. Extensive warts have been treated with the carbon dioxide laser, intra-lesion interferon injections, and surgical removal (CDC, 2010b).

Self-Management Education. *The priority nursing intervention is patient and sexual partner education about the mode of transmission, incubation period, treatment, and complications, especially the association with cervical cancer.* Reinforce instructions about local care of the lesions or patient-applied treatment for self-management.

> ❗ **NURSING SAFETY PRIORITY** (QSEN)
>
> ***Drug Alert***
>
> Teach patients that after treatment with cryotherapy, podophyllin, or TCA, they may experience discomfort, bleeding, or discharge from the site or sloughing of parts of warts. Instruct patients to keep the area clean (shower or bath) and dry. Teach them to be alert for any signs or symptoms of infection or side effects of the treatment.

Inform patients that recurrence is likely, especially in the first 3 months, and that repeated treatments may be needed. Urge all patients to have complete STD testing, since exposure to one STD may increase risk for contracting another. Sexual partners should also be evaluated and offered treatment if warts are present. Teach patients to avoid intimate sexual contact until external lesions are healed. Recommend condoms to help reduce transmission even after warts have been treated (see Chart 74-3). Encourage women to have a Pap test annually, starting at age 21 years; after they have had three normal smears, they should have a Pap test every 3 years if no new risk factors are present (e.g., new partner, other STDs) (Murphy & Mark, 2012). The presence of warts should increase suspicion that the patient may have had exposure to other STDs, which warrants additional testing.

Gardasil (Merck Sharpe & Dohme Corporation, 2014) is used to provide immunity for HPV types 6 and 11 (predominantly types causing warts, low risk for cervical cancer) and 16 and 18 (high risk for cervical cancer). Initially approved for females, the vaccine is now also recommended for males ages 9 to 26 years. Cervarix (GlaxoSmithKline, 2012) may be given to 9- to 25-year-old females and protects only against HPV types 16 and 18. Both vaccines are recommended before onset of sexual activity (and before age 26 years) and possible exposure to HPV. Because exposure to HPV is likely for most sexually active young adults, vaccination protects them against the strains to which they have not yet been exposed. Vaccination is also especially encouraged for MSM and immunocompromised young adults up to the age of 26 years (CDC, 2012a).

CHLAMYDIA INFECTION

❖ PATHOPHYSIOLOGY

Chlamydia trachomatis is an intracellular bacterium and the causative agent of genital chlamydia infections. It invades the epithelial tissues in the reproductive tract. The incubation period ranges from 1 to 3 weeks, but the pathogen may be present in the genital tract for months without producing symptoms.

C. trachomatis is reportable to local health departments in all states. Diagnosed cases continue to increase yearly, which reflects more sensitive screening tests and increased public health efforts to screen high-risk people. Each year there are an estimated 2.9 million new cases in the United States (CDC, 2013a), with 1.4 million reported to the CDC in 2011 (CDC, 2012c). Because it is frequently asymptomatic, the estimated incidence is about double of what is reported. African-American women between 15 and 24 years of age are at the highest risk for the disease (CDC, 2012c).

In women, 20% to 40% of those infected will develop pelvic inflammatory disease (PID) if not treated, discussed later in this chapter on p. 1541.

❖ PATIENT-CENTERED COLLABORATIVE CARE

◆ Assessment

Obtain a complete history including a genitourinary review of systems and psychosocial history. This will include a sexual history (see Chart 74-1). In particular, ask about:

- Presence of symptoms, including vaginal or urethral discharge, dysuria (painful urination), pelvic pain, irregular bleeding

- Any history of sexually transmitted diseases (STDs)
- Whether sexual partners have had symptoms or a history of STDs
- Whether patient has had a new or multiple sexual partner(s)
- Whether patient or partner has had unprotected intercourse

About 70% of chlamydia infections are asymptomatic in women. For men and women, their history may reveal only risk factors associated with *C. trachomatis,* such as new or multiple sexual partners, age younger than 26 years and female, or a male having sex with a male (MSM). As with all interviews concerning sexual behavior, use a nonjudgmental approach and provide privacy and confidentiality.

GENDER HEALTH CONSIDERATIONS
Patient-Centered Care QSEN

For men, ask about dysuria, frequent urination, and a mucoid discharge that is more watery and less copious than a gonorrheal discharge. *These manifestations indicate urethritis, the main symptom of chlamydia infection in men.* Some men have the discharge only in the morning on arising. Complications include epididymitis, prostatitis, infertility, and Reiter's syndrome, a type of connective tissue disease discussed in Chapter 18.

In contrast, many women have no symptoms. Those with symptoms have mucopurulent vaginal discharge (typically yellow and more opaque), urinary frequency, and abdominal discomfort or pain. Cervical bleeding, from infected and therefore fragile tissue, may present as spotting or bleeding between menses and frequently after intercourse. Complications of infection with *C. trachomatis* include salpingitis (inflammation of the fallopian tubes), PID, ectopic pregnancy, and infertility. These health problems are discussed in detail in maternal-child textbooks.

Diagnosis is made by sampling cells from the endocervix, urethra, or both, easily obtained with a swab. Because chlamydiae can reproduce only inside cells, cervical (or host) cells that harbor the organism (or parts of it) are required in the sample. Tissue culture (the gold standard) obtained from the cervical os during the female pelvic examination or male urethral examination obtained by swabbing has been replaced by genetic tests. As with gonorrhea, the nucleic acid amplification tests (NAATs) and gene amplification tests (ligand chain reaction [LCR] and polymerase chain reaction [PCR] transcription-mediated amplification) are the newest methods of detecting *Chlamydia* in endocervical samples, urethral swabs, and urine. They are more sensitive tests than the tissue culture. Samples can be obtained by swab by the examining clinician or by a patient-collected urine specimen. This urine self-collection method has been found to be more acceptable and highly sensitive and specific. The acceptability of urine testing has resulted in increased identification of asymptomatic people.

All sexually active women 24 years old or younger, and all women older than 25 years with new or multiple partners, should be screened annually for *Chlamydia* (CDC, 2010b; USPSTF, 2014a). There is no recommendation for or against screening asymptomatic men, regardless of age or other risk, and low-risk asymptomatic women.

◆ Interventions

The treatment of choice for chlamydia infections is azithromycin (Zithromax) 1 g orally in a single dose or doxycycline (Monodox, Doxy-Caps, Doxycin) 100 mg orally twice daily for 7 days. The one-dose course, although more expensive, is preferred because of the ease in completing the treatment. Directly observing the patient taking the medication in the health care setting assures the nurse of compliance. Drugs that are prescribed for patients with allergies to these drugs include erythromycin, ofloxacin, and levofloxacin, all for 7 days (CDC, 2010b).

Sexual partners should be treated and tested for other STDs. Expedited partner therapy, or patient-delivered partner therapy, shows signs of reducing chlamydia INFECTION rates (CDC, 2010b). **Expedited partner therapy (EPT)** is the practice of treating sexual partners of patients diagnosed with chlamydia infection or gonorrhea by providing prescriptions or medication to the patient, which they can take to their partner(s), without the health care provider examining the partner(s) (CDC, 2013c). Legal questions have arisen about whether a drug can be prescribed without a relationship between the health care provider and the patient, but many states have now ruled that this is appropriate and legal (CDC, 2013d). When patients have been given the drug to give to their partner, rates of infection have decreased and more partners have reported receiving treatment (CDC, 2013c; Trelle et al., 2007).

Patient and partner education is a crucial nursing intervention. Explain:

- The sexual mode of transmission
- The incubation period
- The high possibility of asymptomatic infections and the usual symptoms if present
- Treatment of infection with antibiotics and need for completion of course of treatment
- The need for abstinence from sexual intercourse until the patient and partner(s) have all completed treatment (7 days from the start of treatment, including a single-dose regimen)
- That women should be re-screened for re-infection 3 to 12 months after treatment because of the high risk for PID; also, that there is less evidence of the need for re-screening of treated men, but it should be considered
- The need to return for evaluation if symptoms recur or new symptoms develop (most recurrences are re-infections from a new or untreated partner)
- Complications of untreated or inadequately treated infection, which may include PID, ectopic pregnancy, or infertility

GONORRHEA

❖ PATHOPHYSIOLOGY

Gonorrhea is a sexually transmitted bacterial INFECTION that occurs in both men and women. The causative organism is *Neisseria gonorrhoeae,* a gram-negative intracellular diplococcus. It is transmitted by direct sexual contact with mucosal surfaces (vaginal intercourse, orogenital contact, or anogenital contact).

The first symptoms of gonorrhea may appear 3 to 10 days after sexual contact with an infected person. The disease can be present without symptoms and can be transmitted or progress without warning. In women, ascending spread of the organism can cause pelvic INFECTION **(pelvic inflammatory disease [PID]), endometritis** (endometrial infection), **salpingitis** (fallopian tube infection), and pelvic peritonitis. Rare complications of gonorrhea in adults include arthritis, meningitis, hepatitis, and disseminated infection (Bleich et al., 2012).

In 2011, 321,849 new gonococcal infections were diagnosed and reported, but the CDC estimates that this represents only about half of the cases that occurred (CDC, 2012c). Over the years, gonorrhea has become resistant to penicillin, tetracycline, and ciprofloxacin and recently to cefixime. Cefixime is no longer the drug of choice because of the development of oral cephalosporin-resistant *N. gonorrhoeae.* Intramuscular injection of Rocephin (ceftriaxone) 250 mg in a single dose is now the drug of choice (CDC, 2012d).

❖ PATIENT-CENTERED COLLABORATIVE CARE

◆ Assessment

A complete history includes reviewing the genitourinary systems, including taking a sexual history that includes sexual orientation and sites of sexual exposure or intercourse. Assess for allergies to antibiotics (see Chart 74-1). Establish a trusting relationship and use a nonjudgmental approach to gather more complete information. This approach may decrease the patient's anxiety and fear about having an STD.

The infection can be asymptomatic in both men and women, but women have asymptomatic, or "silent," infections more often than do men. If symptoms are present, men usually notice dysuria and a penile discharge that can be either profuse, yellowish green fluid or scant, clear fluid. The urethra is most commonly affected, but infection can extend to the prostate, the seminal vesicles, and the epididymis. Men seek curative treatment sooner, usually because they have symptoms, and thereby avoid some of the serious complications.

Women may report a change in vaginal discharge (yellow, green, profuse, odorous), urinary frequency, or dysuria. The cervix and urethra are the most common sites of infection.

Anal manifestations may include itching and irritation, rectal bleeding or diarrhea, and painful defecation. Assess the mouth for a reddened throat, ulcerated lips, tender gingivae, and lesions in the throat. Fig. 74-3 shows common sites of gonococcal infections.

If fever occurs, this may be a sign of an ascending (PID or epididymitis) or systemic infection (disseminated gonococcal infection). Symptoms could include joint or tendon pain, either in a single joint or as migratory arthralgias, especially of the knees, elbows, fingers or toes, and a rash usually on the palms and soles. The rash can be pustular or maculopapular (Bleich et al., 2012).

Clinical symptoms of gonorrhea can resemble those of chlamydia INFECTION and need to be differentiated. *Molecular testing for* N. gonorrhoeae *is currently the most widely used standard and preferred over cultures or microscopic examinations.* These nucleic acid amplification tests (NAATs) are highly sensitive and specific. During examination, providers can swab the male urethra or female cervix to obtain specimens. These specimens can be placed in medium for molecular testing, cultured

THROAT

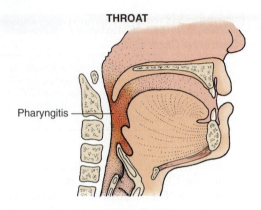

Pharyngitis

PELVIC/GENITAL

MEN

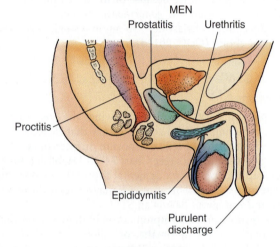

Prostatitis Urethritis

Proctitis

Epididymitis

Purulent discharge

WOMEN

Endometritis Salpingitis

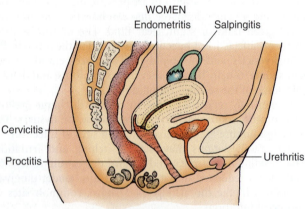

Cervicitis

Proctitis Urethritis

FIG. 74-3 Areas of involvement of gonorrhea in men and women.

on chocolate agar (gold standard), or viewed microscopically after Gram staining (male urethral specimens only). Patient-collected urine or vaginal swabs can also be used to diagnose both gonorrhea and chlamydia infections, allowing for testing without a full examination.

In men, gonorrhea can be diagnosed by Gram staining smears of urethral discharge that has been swabbed onto a glass slide, dried, and stained. The presence of gram-negative diplococci is diagnostic for gonococcal urethritis in men. If the man has symptoms, Gram stains are very sensitive and specific for gonorrhea and allow for immediate diagnosis and treatment in

the clinical setting. Without symptoms, Gram stains are less reliable. Smears do not confirm the diagnosis in women because the female genital tract normally harbors other *Neisseria* organisms that resemble *N. gonorrhoeae.*

All patients with gonorrhea should be tested for syphilis, chlamydia, hepatitis B and hepatitis C, and HIV infection and, if possible, examined for HSV and HPV, because they may have been exposed to these STDs as well. Sexual partners who have been exposed in the past 30 days should be examined, and specimens should be obtained.

◆ Interventions

Uncomplicated gonorrhea is treated with antibiotics. Chlamydia infection, which is 4 times more common, is frequently found in patients with gonorrhea. Because of this, patients treated for gonorrhea should also be managed with drugs that treat chlamydia infection.

Drug Therapy. Drug therapy recommended by the CDC is ceftriaxone (Rocephin) 250 mg IM *plus* azithromycin (Zithromax) 1 g orally in a single dose *or* doxycycline (Monodox, Doxy-Caps, Doxycin ✦) 100 mg orally twice daily for 1 week to treat a presumed co-infection with *Chlamydia* (up to 40%), unless a negative *Chlamydia* result has been obtained. These combinations seem to be effective for all mucosal gonorrheal infections; treatment failure is rare (CDC, 2012d). A test of cure is not required for treatment with ceftriaxone. Advise the patient to return for a follow-up examination if symptoms persist after treatment. Re-infection is usually the cause of these symptoms.

Sexual partners must be treated, not only evaluated, to prevent re-infection. Sexual partners also need to receive education about the INFECTION.

Because the best treatment for gonorrhea is injected Rocephin (ceftriaxone), expedited partner therapy (EPT) is not ideal for treating gonorrhea. If there is concern that the partner may not come to a health care facility for treatment, providing oral cefixime as an alternative has been recommended by the CDC. Because of the potential for resistance of gonorrhea to cefixime, a test of cure is recommended after treatment is completed.

Gonorrhea infection can become disseminated (disseminated gonococcal infection [DGI]), requiring hospitalization and IV or IM ceftriaxone 1 g every 24 hours. If symptoms resolve within 24 to 48 hours, the patient may be discharged to home to continue oral antibiotic therapy (cefixime 400 mg twice a day) for at least a week (CDC, 2010b).

Meningitis and endocarditis occur rarely. Hospitalization of patients with these problems is recommended for the initial treatment. Treatment includes IV antibiotic therapy, usually ceftriaxone 1 to 2 g every 12 hours. If meningitis or endocarditis is present, therapy is continued for 10 to 14 days for meningitis and at least 4 weeks for endocarditis. Collaborate with the infectious disease specialist for management of these INFECTIONS.

Self-Management Education. Teach the patient about transmission and treatment of gonorrhea. The use of medication to treat chlamydia infection at the same time as treating gonorrhea should be explained to the patient since the likelihood of co-infection is high. Discuss the possibility of re-infection, including the risk for pelvic inflammatory disease (PID), and resultant problems such as ectopic pregnancy, infertility, and chronic pelvic pain. Instruct patients to cease sexual activity until the antibiotic therapy is completed and they no longer have symptoms; but if abstinence is not possible, urge men and women to use condoms. Explain that gonorrhea is a *reportable disease.*

When a diagnosis of gonorrhea is made, patients may have feelings of fear or guilt. They may be concerned that they have contracted other STDs or see the disease as a punishment for promiscuity or "unnatural" sex acts. They may believe that acquiring gonorrhea (or any STD) is a risk that they must take to pursue their desired lifestyle. Such feelings can impair relationships with sexual partners. Encourage patients to express their feelings, and offer other information and professional resources to assist them in having a correct understanding of their diagnosis and treatment. Ensuring privacy during your discussion with them and maintaining confidentiality of personal health information are essential in meeting psychosocial needs.

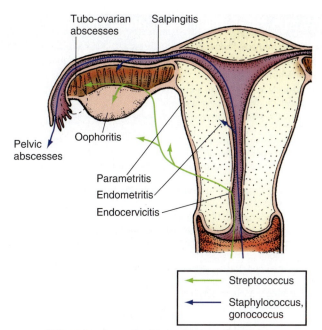

FIG. 74-4 The spread of pelvic inflammatory disease.

❓ CLINICAL JUDGMENT CHALLENGE

Patient-Centered Care; Teamwork and Collaboration ▮QSEN▮

A 39-year-old gay man has been diagnosed with a chlamydial infection and provided with treatment for the infection. After learning how the infection is transmitted, he states that he and his partner "broke up" briefly 3 months ago and he wonders if his partner became involved with someone who transmitted the infection to him. One week later, the patient and his partner return to the health care center. The partner states that he "slept with another man" during the break-up. As the nurse, you explain that medication treatment is available with expedited partner therapy (EPT) for the person the partner became involved with during the break-up. The patient becomes angry and tells his partner, "I don't want you ever speaking to him again!"

1. What is the best therapeutic approach for working with this patient and his partner?
2. How will you further explain to this couple the need for EPT for the other person?
3. In your presence, the patient tells his partner that he cannot imagine ever talking with "that jerk you slept with." What emotional feelings is this patient experiencing? How will you respond to the patient's statement?
4. Develop a collaborative plan of care for this patient to ensure that the needs of all involved parties will be met.

OTHER GYNECOLOGIC CONDITIONS

PELVIC INFLAMMATORY DISEASE

❖ PATHOPHYSIOLOGY

Pelvic inflammatory disease (PID) is a complex infectious process in which organisms from the lower genital tract migrate from the endocervix upward through the uterine cavity into the fallopian tubes. The spread of INFECTION to other organs and tissues of the upper genital tract occurs from direct contact with mucosal surfaces or through the fimbriated ends of the tubes to the ovaries, parametrium, and peritoneal cavity (Fig. 74-4). This may involve one or more pelvic structures, including the uterus, fallopian tubes, and adjacent pelvic structures. The most common site is the fallopian tube. Resulting infections include:

- Endometritis (infection of the endometrial cavity)
- Salpingitis (inflammation of the fallopian tubes)
- Oophoritis (ovarian infection)
- Parametritis (infection of the parametrium)

- Peritonitis (infection of the peritoneal cavity)
- Tubal or tubo-ovarian abscess

Usually multiple pathogens are involved in the development of PID. Sexually transmitted organisms are most often responsible, especially *C. trachomatis* and *N. gonorrhoeae*. Organisms that are part of the vaginal flora can also cause PID including *Gardnerella vaginalis, Haemophilus influenzae, Staphylococcus, Streptococcus, Mycoplasma, Escherichia coli,* and other aerobic and anaerobic organisms. There is increasing evidence that the anaerobes involved in bacterial vaginosis may have a role in the development of PID and increase the risk for INFECTION with HIV, *N. gonorrhoeae, C. trachomatis,* and HSV (CDC, 2010b; Sweet, 2012).

The organisms invade the pelvis from an infection ascending from the vagina or cervix. Infections are spread during sexual intercourse, during childbirth (including the postpartum period), and after abortion. *Sepsis and death can occur, especially if treatment is delayed or inadequate.*

PID is one of the leading causes of infertility and is related to the increase in the number of ectopic pregnancies reported in the United States. It is an acute syndrome resulting in tenderness in the tubes and ovaries (adnexa) and, typically, dull pelvic pain. However, many women experience only mild discomfort or menstrual irregularity, whereas others have acute pain, which can affect their gait. Others experience no symptoms at all—so-called "silent" or "subclinical" PID. The diagnosis and treatment of this disease are challenging. Irreversible scarring or stricture, causing sterility, may occur before it is diagnosed (Sweet, 2012).

Because of variations in patient manifestations, the diagnosis is difficult because women may have subtle symptoms not typical of the disease. Delay in diagnosis and treatment may add to complications of PID in the upper genital tract. The disease is usually diagnosed on the basis of clinical signs and symptoms. The Centers for Disease Control and Prevention (CDC) (2013e) has set minimum criteria for diagnosis, but no laboratory or physical examination techniques alone are both sensitive and specific (Table 74-4).

TABLE 74-4   Diagnostic Criteria For Pelvic Inflammatory Disease

Minimum Criteria for Initiating Empiric Treatment for Pelvic Inflammatory Disease

- Sexually active woman and at risk for STDs
- Pelvic or lower abdominal pain
- No other cause for illness can be found (e.g., appendicitis)

and

- Uterine tenderness *or*
- Adnexal tenderness *or*
- Cervical motion tenderness (chandelier sign)

Additional Criteria to Increase the Specificity of the Diagnosis of PID

- Oral temperature >101° F (>38.3° C)
- Abnormal cervical or vaginal mucopurulent discharge
- Presence of white blood cells on saline microscopy of vaginal secretions
- Elevated erythrocyte sedimentation rate
- Elevated C-reactive protein
- Laboratory documentation of cervical infection with *Neisseria gonorrhoeae* or *Chlamydia trachomatis*

Definitive Criteria for Diagnosing PID, Warranted in Selected Cases

- Histopathologic evidence of endometritis on endometrial biopsy
- Transvaginal sonography or MRI techniques showing thickened, fluid-filled tubes with or without free pelvic fluid or tubo-ovarian complex, or Doppler studies suggesting pelvic infection
- Laparoscopic abnormalities consistent with PID

Modified from Centers for Disease Control and Prevention (CDC). (2014). *Sexually transmitted diseases treatment guidelines, 2010: Pelvic inflammatory diseases.* Retrieved November 2014, from www.cdc.gov/std/treatment/2010/pid.htm
PID, Pelvic inflammatory disease; *STDs,* sexually transmitted diseases.

❖ PATIENT-CENTERED COLLABORATIVE CARE

◆ Assessment

History. Obtain a complete history of the symptoms with menstrual, obstetric, sexual, and family history and a history of previous episodes of pelvic inflammatory disease (PID) or other sexually transmitted diseases (see Chart 74-1). Assess for contraceptive use, a history of reproductive surgery, and other risk factors previously discussed. Ask the patient if sexual abuse has occurred. If so, encourage her to discuss what happened and whether she was seen by a health care provider.

Many of the same factors that place women at risk for STDs also place them at risk for PID. Risk factors for sexually active women include:

- Age younger than 26 years
- Multiple sexual partners
- Intrauterine device (IUD) placed within the previous 3 weeks
- Smoking
- A history of PID
- Chlamydial or gonococcal infection; bacterial vaginosis
- A history of sexually transmitted diseases (STDs)

Physical Assessment/Clinical Manifestations. *One of the most frequent symptoms of PID is lower abdominal or pelvic pain.* Conduct a complete pain assessment. Other symptoms include irregular vaginal bleeding (spotting or bleeding between periods), dysuria (painful urination), an increase or change in vaginal discharge, dyspareunia (painful sexual intercourse), malaise, fever, and chills.

Observe whether the patient has discomfort with movement. Often the patient has a hunched-over gait to protect her abdomen. She may find it difficult to independently get on the examination table or stretcher. Assess for lower abdominal tenderness, possibly with rigidity or rebound tenderness. A pelvic examination by the health care provider may reveal yellow or green cervical discharge and a reddened or **friable** cervix (a cervix that bleeds easily). Criteria for accurate diagnosis of PID are listed in Table 74-4. The diagnosis of PID is usually based on health history, physical examination, and laboratory tests. Imaging studies and laparoscopy are not generally used to make the diagnosis.

Psychosocial Assessment. The woman who has symptoms of PID is usually anxious and fearful of the examination and unknown diagnosis. She may need much reassurance and support during the physical examination because her abdomen may be very tender or painful. Explain what is taking place to help promote comfort during the examination.

Because PID is often associated with an STD, the woman may feel embarrassed or uncomfortable discussing her symptoms or history. Use a nonjudgmental approach, and encourage the patient to express her feelings and concerns. Determining the patient's ability to follow through with the treatment plan is essential in deciding whether hospitalization should be considered.

Laboratory Assessment. The health care provider obtains specimens from the cervix, urethra, and rectum to determine the presence of *N. gonorrhoeae* or *C. trachomatis.* The white blood cell (WBC) count, erythrocyte sedimentation rate (ESR), and C-reactive protein may be elevated but are not specific for PID. A sensitive test that detects human chorionic gonadotropin (hCG) in urine or blood should be performed to determine whether the patient is pregnant. Microscopic examination of vaginal discharge should be done to evaluate for the presence of more than 10 WBCs per high-power field, which correlates with infection. Bacterial vaginosis can be found by observing the diagnostic "clue" cells with microscopic examination of vaginal discharge.

Other Diagnostic Assessment. Abdominal *ultrasonography* may be used to determine the presence of appendicitis and tubo-ovarian abscesses that need to be ruled out when the diagnosis of PID is made. Transvaginal ultrasound and *MRI* are used in some cases to detect tubal wall thickening, fluid-filled tubes, and free pelvic fluid or a tubo-ovarian abscess, all associated with PID. *Endometrial biopsy* also has been used to increase the accuracy of the diagnosis.

◆ Analysis

The priority collaborative problem for patients with pelvic inflammatory disease (PID) is infection related to invasion of pelvic organs by pathogens.

◆ Planning and Implementation

Managing Infection

Planning: Expected Outcomes. The patient with PID is expected to have her infection resolved, be free of abdominal pain, and prevent re-infection.

Interventions. *Patient-centered collaborative care includes* antibiotic therapy and self-management measures.

Uncomplicated PID is usually treated on an ambulatory care basis. The CDC (2010b) recommends hospitalization for PID if the patient:

- Has appendicitis, ectopic pregnancy, or other surgical emergency that has not been excluded
- Is pregnant
- Does not respond to oral antibiotic therapy
- Is unable to follow or tolerate treatment on an ambulatory care basis
- Has severe illness, nausea and vomiting, or high fever
- Has a tubo-ovarian abscess

There are no recommendations about whether HIV-infected women should be hospitalized. Assess the ability of high-risk women for self-management at home. The patient's health status and availability of support systems are important considerations for home care. If the infection has not responded to treatment, the patient may need to be hospitalized for IV antibiotic therapy and further evaluation.

The CDC recommends oral and/or parenteral antibiotics for PID (CDC, 2010b). Drug therapy is required for 14 days. If the woman has not responded to oral antibiotics, she is hospitalized for IV antibiotic therapy and further evaluation. Inpatient therapy involves a combination of several IV antibiotics until the woman shows signs of improvement (e.g., decreased pelvic tenderness for at least 24 hours). Then oral antibiotics are continued at home until the course of treatment has lasted 14 days.

Antibiotic therapy relieves pain by destroying the pathogens and decreasing the inflammation caused by infection. Other pain-relief measures include taking mild analgesics and applying heat to the lower abdomen or back. As with any INFECTION, encourage the patient to increase her intake of fluids and to eat nutritious foods that can promote healing. *Teach the patient to rest in a semi-Fowler's position and encourage limited ambulation to promote gravity drainage of the infection that may help relieve pain.*

! NURSING SAFETY PRIORITY (QSEN)

Action Alert

Instruct women who are being treated for PID on an ambulatory care basis to avoid sexual intercourse for the full course of treatment and until their symptoms have resolved. Ask them to check their temperature twice a day. Teach them to report an increase in temperature to their health care provider. Remind them to be seen by the health care provider within 72 hours from starting antibiotic treatment and then 1 and 2 weeks from the time of the initial diagnosis.

In a small number of patients, the pain and tenderness may not be relieved by antibiotic therapy. The surgeon may perform a laparoscopy to remove an abscess through one or more subumbilical incisions to provide better access to the fallopian tubes. Before surgery, provide information about hospital routines and procedures. After surgery, the care of the woman with PID is similar to that of any patient after laparoscopic abdominal surgery. One difference is that she may have a wound drain for drainage of abscess fluid that may not have been completely removed during surgery. Observe, measure, and record wound drainage every 4 to 8 hours as requested.

Community-Based Care. If the woman is hospitalized, collaborate with the case manager or discharge planner before the woman is discharged to home. Teach the patient with PID to see her health care provider for follow-up to assess for complications and assess that the infection has resolved. The ongoing role of the nurse is to assess for any continued risk for

---

CHART 74-4 Patient and Family Education: Preparing for Self-Management

Oral Antibiotic Therapy for Sexually Transmitted Diseases

- Take your medicine for the number of times a day it is prescribed and until it is completed.
- Your sexual partner must be treated if you have a sexually transmitted disease (STD). Expedited partner therapy is one way to ensure partners are treated.
- Be sure to return for your follow-up appointment after completing your antibiotic treatment.
- Call if you have any questions or concerns.
- Do not have sex until after you and your partner complete your antibiotic therapy. This should be at least 7 days, even if treatment is one dose.
- Drink at least 8 to 10 glasses of fluid a day to help heal your infection, while taking your antibiotics.
- Do not take antacids containing calcium, magnesium, or aluminum, such as Tums, Maalox, or Mylanta, with your antibiotics. They may decrease the effectiveness of the antibiotic.
- Take your antibiotics on an empty stomach unless your health care provider instructs you to take them with food.

---

contracting PID again, signs of persistent or recurrent infection, and education to prevent exposure to and infection with all STDs (e.g., decrease the number of partners, consistently use condoms). Establish an atmosphere of trust that encourages the woman to return frequently, if needed, for education or reassurance.

Home Care Management. Parenteral antibiotic therapy may be given at home, but usually the health care provider changes the treatment regimen to oral antibiotics before hospital discharge.

Self-Management Education. Patient teaching focuses on providing information about PID, identifying symptoms that suggest persistent or recurrent infection (persistent pelvic pain, dysmenorrhea, low backache, fever), and urging completion of antibiotic treatment, rest, and healthy nutrition to resolve the infection and prevent complications. Review information for oral antibiotic therapy (Chart 74-4).

Counsel the patient to contact her sexual partner(s) for examination and treatment. All sexual partners should be treated for gonorrhea and chlamydia infection regardless of whether they have symptoms. Remind the patient about follow-up care, and counsel her about the complications that can occur after an episode of PID. These problems include increased risk for recurrence, ectopic pregnancy, and infertility. Chronic pelvic pain may also develop.

Discuss contraception and the patient's need or desire for it. This discussion includes the use of condoms that can decrease the risk for future episodes of PID. Consider the likelihood that the patient had unprotected (from pregnancy and STDs) intercourse, which resulted in PID. Contraception that includes the use of condoms is an important health message to be communicated. Help the patient understand that having sexual intercourse with multiple partners increases the risk for recurrent episodes. Douching has also been suggested as a risky behavior for development of PID and/or infection with *Chlamydia* or *N. gonorrhoeae.*

Psychosocial concerns may require counseling. A patient who has PID may exhibit a variety of feelings (guilt, disgust, anger) about having a condition that may have been transmitted to her sexually. These feelings may affect her relationship with significant others and future sexual partners. She may also have concerns about future fertility if PID has damaged or scarred the fallopian tubes and other reproductive organs. Provide nonjudgmental emotional support, and allow time for her to discuss her feelings. The primary provider of care may refer the patient to a mental health care provider as another appropriate option.

Health Care Resources. The cost of antibiotics for patients with PID and other STDs may be a concern for those who are uninsured, underinsured, or impoverished. In collaboration with the case manager or social worker, help locate community resources for free or discounted drugs for women who cannot afford them. Ask the patient directly if she has the ability to pay for the drug and her follow-up visits, regardless of her apparent financial status.

If infertility is a result of PID, the patient may need referral to a clinic specializing in infertility treatment and counseling. She can also contact support groups for infertile couples, which exist in many local communities.

◆ Evaluation: Outcomes

Evaluate the care of the patient with PID based on the identified priority patient problem. The expected outcomes include that the patient should:
- Show evidence that the infection has resolved
- Report or demonstrate that pain is relieved or reduced and that she feels more comfortable

- Demonstrate a plan for ensuring treatment of her partner, obtaining antibiotics, and returning for follow-up care

VAGINAL INFECTIONS

Vaginal INFECTION associated with sexual activity may produce vaginal discharge or vulvar irritation. The common causes of vaginal infection that can be but are not always sexually transmitted include:
- *Trichomonas vaginalis*
- *Candida,* primarily *Candida albicans*
- Bacteria that produce bacterial vaginosis, including *Gardnerella vaginalis, Mycoplasma hominis,* and anaerobes including *Prevotella* and *Mobiluncus* species

Men can also get these infections but are not always symptomatic.

Trichomoniasis and candida infections are limited to the vagina. They can be very irritating and bothersome but do not cause any long-term problems. The partner must also be treated for *trichomoniasis* for the infection to be resolved. *Candidiasis* does not usually require partner treatment. However, if the male partner is symptomatic (irritation of the genital skin), treatment is indicated. It is important to remember that *Candida* is a normal flora on the skin and vagina. Although it can be transmitted sexually, candidiasis occurs in women regardless of their sexual activity. Also, antibiotics that change the normal flora of the vagina contribute to infection.

Bacterial vaginosis (BV) has been implicated in upper genital tract infections. Women undergoing surgery of the upper genital tract should be evaluated and treated if BV is found. Chapter 71 describes the management of each of these infections.

OTHER SEXUALLY TRANSMITTED DISEASES

Less common diseases in the United States that are transmitted by sexual contact are lymphogranuloma venereum, chancroid, and granuloma inguinale. Like syphilis, all of these diseases are associated with ulcers but they are seen most often in less developed countries. As newcomers migrate into the United States and international travel increases, these STDs may become more common. Ask patients suspected of these infections whether they have traveled out of the United States and whether they had sexual contact with people who live in other countries.

NURSING CONCEPTS AND CLINICAL JUDGMENT REVIEW

What might you OBSERVE if the patient has altered SEXUALITY as a result of a sexually transmitted disease (STD)?
- Report of heavy and abnormal vaginal discharge
- Report of urinary frequency or dysuria
- Ulcers, blisters, or warts in the genital area
- Low-grade fever
- Report of malaise
- Report of vaginal, penile, or anal itching or irritation
- Report of abdominal pain (pelvic inflammatory disease [PID])
- Anxious behavior
- Depressive symptoms

- Report of disinterest in sexual activity
- Changes in relationships (e.g., ending a long-term relationship)

What should you INTERPRET and how should you RESPOND to a patient with altered SEXUALITY as a result of STD?

Perform and interpret focused physical assessment, including:
- Vital signs
- Pain intensity and quality
- Posture and mobility
- Skin inspection (genital area)

Respond by:
- Reporting and documenting all findings
- Helping patient with abdominal pain into a semi-Fowler's position
- Providing pain-control measures
- Teaching patient about prescribed antibiotic or antiviral therapy
- Teaching patient to avoid sexual intercourse while being treated
- Teaching patient the importance of treating all sexual partners
- Teaching patient and partner(s) about safer sex practices

- Providing support and listening to the patient and partner(s) without judgment

On what should you REFLECT?
- Examine your feelings about patients who make sexual choices different from your own.
- Think about what else you could do to help patients meet their physical and emotional needs during this time.
- Determine what other health teaching may be needed for this patient.
- Monitor the patient's response to pain-control interventions.

GET READY FOR THE NCLEX® EXAMINATION!

KEY POINTS

Review these Key Points for each NCLEX Examination Client Needs Category.

Safe and Effective Care Environment
- Maintain patient and partner confidentiality and privacy at all times. **Patient-Centered Care** QSEN
- Use gloves when examining the patient's genitalia or skin lesions. **Safety** QSEN

Health Promotion and Maintenance
- Teach patients to not have sexual intercourse during their treatment for sexually transmitted disease (STD). **Safety** QSEN
- Assume that all adult patients may be sexually active, regardless of age or stage of life. Sexually transmitted diseases are still spread within the older adult population because perception of risk is lower.
- Educate young women about increased vulnerability to STDs; women's vaginal mucous membranes place them at higher risk for contracting an STD, and young women statistically have more partners and more unprotected sex, which further increases their risk. **Safety** QSEN
- Teach the patient about the availability of expedited partner therapy; be sure that both the patient and the partner take all doses of the drug.
- Encourage all patients who are sexually active to use condoms during sexual intimacy (see Chart 74-3).
- Urge sexually active people, especially those younger than 26 years (or those older than 26 years if at high risk), to have STD screenings at least annually.
- Treat all patients, regardless of diagnosis, gender identity, or sexual orientation, with respect.

- Respect the sexual choices of all patients. **Patient-Centered Care** QSEN

Psychosocial Integrity
- Provide privacy for patients undergoing examination or testing for STDs.
- Allow the patient to express fears and/or anxiety regarding a diagnosis of STD. **Patient-Centered Care** QSEN
- Refer patients newly diagnosed with an STD to local resources and support groups as needed based on their response. **Teamwork and Collaboration** QSEN
- Encourage all patients who have an STD to inform their sexual partner(s) of their health status.

Physiological Integrity
- Assess patients with STD using the guidelines in Chart 74-1. **Evidence-Based Practice** QSEN
- Recognize that each stage of syphilis has unique symptoms and it is important to not overlook symptoms that resolve.
- Understand that patients without symptoms may still be infected with an STD.
- Encourage patients to adhere to their entire anti-infective drug regimen (see Chart 74-4), even after they begin to feel better.
- Teach patients the expected side effects and possible adverse reactions to prescribed drugs.
- Teach patients about the short-term and long-term complications of STD using the information in Table 74-2.
- Be aware that PID is diagnosed based on the criteria in Table 74-4. **Evidence-Based Practice** QSEN

BIBLIOGRAPHY

Asterisk indicates a classic or definitive work on this subject.

General References

This list represents references that are cited in the majority of chapters in this text.

Giddens, J. F. (2013). *Concepts for nursing practice.* St. Louis: Elsevier.

Jarvis, C. (2016). *Physical examination & health assessment* (7th ed.). St. Louis: Elsevier Saunders.

Lilley, L. L., Collins, S. R., & Snyder, J. S. (2014). *Pharmacology and the nursing process* (7th ed.). St. Louis: Mosby.

McCance, K., Huether, S., Brashers, V., & Rote, N. (2014). *Pathophysiology: The biologic basis for disease in adults and children* (7th ed.). St. Louis: Mosby.

Pagana, K. D., & Pagana, T. J. (2014). *Mosby's manual of diagnostic and laboratory tests* (5th ed.). St. Louis: Mosby.

Quality and Safety Education for Nurses (QSEN) (2014). *Pre-licensure KSAs (knowledge, skill, and attitudes).* Retrieved July 2014, from <http://qsen.org/competencies/pre-licensure-ksas/>.

Touhy, T., & Jett, K. (2014). *Ebersole and Hess' gerontological nursing healthy aging* (4th ed.). St. Louis: Mosby.

Chapter 1

Academy of Medical-Surgical Nurses (AMSN) (2012). *Scope and standards of medical-surgical nursing practice* (5th ed.). Pitman, NJ: Author.

Alfaro-LeFevre, R. (2012). *Critical thinking, clinical reasoning, and clinical judgment: A practical approach to outcome-focused thinking* (5th ed.). Philadelphia: Saunders.

American Nurses Association (ANA) (2010). *Code of ethics for nurses with interpretive statements.* Retrieved March 30, 2014, from <www.nursingworld.org/MainMenuCategories/EthicsStandards/CodeofEthicsforNurses>.

Benner, P. E., Malloch, K., & Sheets, V. (2010). *Nursing pathways for patient safety.* St. Louis: Mosby.

Bogert, S., Ferrell, C., & Rutledge, D. N. (2010). Experience with family activation of rapid response teams. *Medsurg Nursing, 19,* 215–222.

Burns, K. (2011). Nurse-physician rounds: A collaborative approach to improving communication, efficiencies, and perception of care. *Medsurg Nursing, 20,* 194–199.

*Donaldson, N., Shapiro, S., Scott, M., Foley, M., & Spetz, J. (2009). Leading successful rapid response teams: A multi-site implementation evaluation. *Journal of Nursing Administration, 39,* 176–181.

Evans, D., Grunawalt, J., McClish, D., Wood, W., & Friese, C. R. (2012). Bedside shift-to-shift nursing report: Implementation and outcomes. *Medsurg Nursing, 21*(5), 281–284, 292.

Flicek, C. L. (2012). Communication: A dynamic between nurses and physicians. *Medsurg Nursing, 21,* 385–386.

Furst, C. M., Finto, D., Malouf-Todaro, N., Moore, C., Orr, D., Santos, J., et al. (2013). Changing times: Enhancing clinical practice through evolving technology. *Medsurg Nursing, 22*(2), 131–134.

Gasarian, P. K., Henneman, E. A., & Chandler, G. E. (2010). Nurse decision making in the pre-arrest period. *Clinical Nursing Research, 19,* 21–37.

Hicks, D. (2012). Cultural competence and the Hispanic population. *Medsurg Nursing, 21,* 314–315.

*Institute for Healthcare Improvement (IHI) (2005). *Protecting 5 million lives from harm.* Accessed March 30, 2014, from <www.ihi.org>.

*Institute of Medicine (IOM) (2000). *To err is human: Building a safer health care system.* Washington, DC: National Academies Press.

*Institute of Medicine (IOM) (2003). *Health professions education: A bridge to quality.* Washington, DC: National Academies Press.

Institute of Medicine (IOM) (2011). *The health of lesbian, gay, bisexual, and transgender people: Building a foundation for better understanding.* Washington, DC: National Academies Press.

Joint Commission Center for Transforming Healthcare (2010). *Joint Commission Center for Transforming Healthcare tackles miscommunication among caregivers.* Accessed March 30, 2014, from <www.centerfortransforminghealthcare.org>.

Maklebust, J. (2011). Engaging the patient and family as partners in practice. *Nursing, 41*(6), 23–24.

Maxson, P. M., Derby, K. M., Wrobleski, D. M., & Foss, D. M. (2012). Bedside nurse-to-nurse handoff promotes patient safety. *Medsurg Nursing, 21,* 140–144.

Melnyk, B. M., & Fineout-Overholt, E. (2011). *Evidence-based practice in nursing and healthcare* (2nd ed.). Philadelphia: Lippincott Williams & Wilkins.

Morrison, D., & Sanders, C. (2011). Huddling for optimal care outcomes. *Nursing, 41*(12), 22–24.

Pettinato, M. (2012). Providing care for LGBTQ patients. *Nursing, 42*(12), 22–27.

Quality and Safety Education for Nurses (QSEN) (2011). *Competency KSAs (pre-licensure).* Accessed November 1, 2012, from <www.qsen.org>.

Robert, R. R., & Petersen, S. (2013). Critical thinking at the bedside. *Medsurg Nursing, 22*(2), 85–93.

Schneider, M. A. (2012). Nurse-physician collaboration: Its time has come. *Nursing, 42*(7), 50–53.

Shafer, L., & Aziz, M. G. (2013). Shaping a unit's culture through effective nurse-led quality improvement. *Medsurg Nursing, 22*(4), 229–236.

Sherwood, G., & Barnsteiner, J. (2012). *Quality and safety in nursing: A competency approach to improving outcomes.* Hoboken, NJ: Wiley-Blackwell.

The Joint Commission (TJC) (2011). *Speak Up initiatives: The Joint Commission's award-winning patient safety program.* Accessed March 30, 2014, from <www.jointcommission.org/speakup.aspx>.

Yoder-Wise, P. S. (2011). *Leading and managing in nursing* (5th ed.). St. Louis: Mosby.

Chapter 2

Berryman, S. N., Jennings, J., Ragsdale, S., Lofton, T., Huff, D. C., & Rooker, J. S. (2012). Beers criteria for potentially inappropriate medication use in older adults. *Medsurg Nursing, 21*(3), 129–133.

Brown-O'Hara, R. (2013). Geriatric syndromes and their implications for nursing. *Nursing, 43*(1), 1–3.

Dossa, A., Bokhour, B., & Hoenig, H. (2012). Care transitions from the hospital to home for patients with mobility impairments: Patient and family caregiver experiences. *Rehabilitation Nursing, 37,* 277–285.

Eldelman, M., & Ficorelli, C. T. (2012). Keeping older adults safe at home. *Nursing, 42,* 65–66.

Fink, A., Morton, S. C., Beck, J. C., Hays, R. D., Spritzer, K., Oishi, S., et al. (2002). The alcohol-related problems survey: Identifying hazardous and harmful drinking in older primary care patients. *Journal of the American Geriatrics Society, 50*(10), 1717–1722.

Fredriksen-Goldsen, K. I. (2011). Resilience and disparities among lesbian, gay, bisexual, and transgender older adults. *Public Policy and Aging Report, 21*(3), 3–7.

*Fulmer, T. (2007). How to try this: Fulmer SPICES. *American Journal of Nursing, 107*(10), 40–48.

Gerber, L. (2013). Bringing home effective nursing care for the homeless. *Nursing, 43*(3), 32–38.

Graham, B. C. (2012). Examining evidence-based interventions to prevent inpatient falls. *Medsurg Nursing, 21,* 267–270.

*Greenberg, S. A. (2007). How to try this: The Geriatric Depression Scale—Short Form. *The American Journal of Nursing, 107*(10), 60–69.

Lee, L. Y., Lee, D. T., & Woo, J. (2010). The psychosocial effect of Tai Chi on nursing home residents. *Journal of Clinical Nursing, 19*(7–8), 927–938.

McCaffrey, R., Hanson, C., & McCaffrey, W. (2010). Garden walking for depression: A research report. *Holistic Nursing Practice, 24*(5), 252–259.

Messina, B. A., & Escallier, L. A. (2011). Taking the "hyper" out of pharmacotherapy. *Nursing, 41*(7), 51–53.

National Institute on Alcohol Abuse and Alcoholism (NIAAA) (2011). *Older adults and alcohol problems*. Retrieved October 17, 2013, from <www.pubs.niaaa.nih.gov/publications/socialworkeducationmodule>.

National Institute of Mental Health (NIMH) (2011). *Older adults and depression*. Retrieved March 30, 2014, from <www.nimh.nih.gov/health/topics/depression>.

Phillips, L. A. (2013). Delirium in geriatric patients: Identification and prevention. *Medsurg Nursing, 22*, 9–12.

Planton, J., & Edlund, B. J. (2010). Strategies for reducing polypharmacy in older adults. *Journal of Gerontological Nursing, 36*(1), 8–12.

*Rocchiccioli, J. T., & Sanford, J. T. (2009). Revisiting geriatric failure to thrive. *Journal of Gerontological Nursing, 35*(1), 18–24.

Rogers, C., Keller, C., & Larkey, L. K. (2010). Perceived benefits of meditative movement in older adults. *Geriatric Nursing, 31*(1), 37–51.

*Sendelbach, S., & Guthrie, P. F. (2009). Evidence-based guideline—Acute confusion/delirium: Identification, assessment, treatment, and prevention. *Journal of Gerontological Nursing, 35*(11), 11–17.

Stark, S. (2012). Elder abuse: Screening, intervention, and prevention. *Nursing, 42*(10), 24–29.

Strunk, J., Townsend-Rocchiccioli, J., & Sanford, J. T. (2013). The aging Hispanic in America: Challenges for nurses in a stressed health care environment. *Medsurg Nursing, 22*, 45–50.

Swan, B. A., Becker, J., Brawer, R., & Sciamanna, C. N. (2011). Factors influencing the implementation of a point-of-care screening tool for delirium. *Medsurg Nursing, 20*, 318–322.

Swartzell, K. L., Fulton, J. S., & Friesth, B. M. (2013). Relationship between occurrence of falls and fall-risk scores in an acute care setting using the Hendrich II Fall Risk Model. *Medsurg Nursing, 22*(3), 180–187.

Toner, F., & Claros, E. (2012). Preventing, assessing, and managing constipation in older adults. *Nursing, 42*(12), 32–38.

Tzeng, H.-M., & Yin, C.-Y. (2010). Nurses response time to call lights and fall occurrences. *Medsurg Nursing, 19*(5), 266–272.

Tzeng, H.-M., & Yin, C.-Y. (2012). Toileting-related inpatient falls in adult acute care settings. *Medsurg Nursing, 21*, 372–377.

U.S. Census Bureau (2013). *Projections of the population by selected age groups and sex for the United States 2010 to 2050*. Retrieved March 30, 2014, from <http://www.census.gov/population/projections/data/national/2008/summarytables.html>.

Vitale, S. A. (2012). What your patient needs to know about CAM. *Nursing, 42*(8), 59–61.

Volkert, D., Saegitz, C., Gueldenzoph, H., Sieber, C. C., & Stehle, P. (2010). Underdiagnosed malnutrition and nutrition-related problems in geriatric patients. *Journal of Nutrition, Health & Aging, 14*(5), 387–392.

Williams, K. N., & Kemper, S. (2010). Interventions to reduce cognitive decline in aging. *Journal of Psychosocial Nursing and Mental Health Services, 48*(5), 42–51.

Wooten, A. C. (2010). An integrative review of Tai Chi research: An alternative form of physical activity to improve balance and prevent falls in older adults. *Orthopedic Nursing, 29*(2), 108–118.

Chapter 3

Allred, K. D., Byers, J., & Sole, M. L. (2010). The effect of music on postoperative pain and anxiety. *Pain Management Nursing, 11*, 15–25.

*American Geriatrics Society (AGS). (2009). The pharmacological management of persistent pain in older persons. *Journal of the American Geriatrics Society, 57*(8), 1331–1346.

American Society of Anesthesiologists (ASA) Task Force on Acute Pain Management. (2012). Practice guidelines for acute pain management in the perioperative setting: An updated report by the American Society of Anesthesiologists Task Force on Acute Pain Management. *Anesthesiology, 116*(2), 248–273.

Arnstein, P., Broglio, K., Wuhrman, E., & Kean, M. B. (2010). *American Society for Pain Management Nursing (ASPMN) position statement: Use of placebos in pain management* (revised). Retrieved November 15, 2013, from <http://aspmn.org/Organization/documents/Placebo_Position_FINAL.pdf>.

Bruckenthal, P. (2010). Integrating nonpharmacologic and alternative strategies into a comprehensive management approach for older adults with pain. *Pain Management Nursing, 11*(2), S23–S31.

Catterall, W. A., & Mackie, K. (2011). Local anesthetics. In L. L. Brunton, B. A. Chabner, & B. C. Knoolmann (Eds.), *Goodman & Gilman's pharmacologic basis of therapeutics* (12th ed., pp. 565–582). New York: McGraw-Hill.

Curtis, K., Osadchuk, A., & Katz, J. (2011). An eight-week yoga intervention is associated with improvements in pain, psychological functioning and mindfulness, and changes in cortisol levels in women with fibromyalgia. *Journal of Pain Research, 2011*(4), 189–201.

Dworkin, R. H., O'Connor, A. B., Audette, J., Baron, R., Gourlay, G. K., Haanpää, M. L., et al. (2010). Recommendations for pharmacological management of neuropathic pain. *Mayo Clinical Proceedings, 85*, S3–S14.

Fillingim, R. B., King, C. D., Ribeiro-Dasilva, M. C., Rahim-Williams, B., & Riley, J. L. (2009). Sex, gender, and pain: A review of recent clinical and experimental findings. *Journal of Pain, 10*(5), 447–485.

Fouladbakhsh, J. M., Szczesny, S., Jenuwine, E. S., & Vallerand, A. H. (2011). Nondrug therapies for pain management among rural older adults. *Pain Management Nursing, 12*(2), 70–81.

*Gordon, D. B., Dahl, J., Phillips, P., Frandsen, J., Cowley, C., Foster, R. L., et al. (2004). The use of "as needed" range orders for opioid analgesics in the management of acute pain: A consensus statement of the ASPMN and the APS. *Pain Management Nursing, 5*(2), 53–58.

Herr, K. (2010). Pain in the older adult: An imperative across all health care settings. *Pain Management Nursing, 11*(2), S1–S10.

Herr, K., Coyne, P. J., McCaffery, M., Manworren, R., & Merkel, S. (2011). *American Society for Pain Management Nursing position statement with clinical practice recommendations: Pain assessment in the patient unable to self report* (revised). Retrieved January 1, 2014, from <http://aspmn.org/Organization/documents/UPDATED_NonverbalRevisionFinalWEB.pdf>.

Ho, K. T., & Gan, T. J. (2009). Opioid-related adverse effects and treatment options. In R. S. Sinatra, O. A. de Leon-Casasola, B. Ginsberg, & E. R. Viscusi (Eds.), *Acute pain management* (pp. 406–415). New York: Cambridge University Press.

Institute of Medicine (IOM) (June 2011). *Relieving pain in America: A blueprint for transforming prevention, care, education, and research*. Retrieved November 15, 2013, from <www.iom.edu/~/media/Files/Report%20Files/2011/Relieving-Pain-in-America-A-Blueprint-for-Transforming-Prevention-Care-Education-Research/Pain%20Research%202011%20Report%20Brief.pdf>.

Jarzyna, D., Junquist, C., Pasero, C., Willens, J., Nisbet, A., Oakes, L., et al. (2011). American Society for Pain Management evidence-based guideline on monitoring for opioid-induced sedation and respiratory depression. *Pain Management Nursing, 12*(3), 118–145.

Kwekkeboom, K. L., Cherwin, C. H., Lee, J. W., & Wanta, B. (2010). Mind-body treatments for the pain-fatigue-sleep disturbance symptom cluster in persons with cancer. *Journal of Pain and Symptom Management, 39*, 126–138.

Liberto, L. A., & Fornili, K. S. (2013). Managing pain in opioid-dependent patients in general hospital settings. *Medsurg Nursing, 22*(1), 33–37.

*McCaffery, M. (1968). *Nursing practice and theories related to cognition, bodily pain, and man-environment interactions*. Los Angeles: University of California at Los Angeles Students' Store.

National Center for Complementary and Alternative Medicine (NCCAM) (2010). *What is CAM?* Retrieved November 15, 2013, from <http://nccam.nih.gov/health/whatiscam/>.

Nicolas, M. K., Asghari, A., Corbett, M., Smeets, R. J., Wood, B. M., Overton, S., et al. (2012). Is adherence to pain self-management strategies associated with improved pain, depression and disability in those with disabling chronic pain? *European Journal of Pain, 16*(1), 93–104.

Oliver, J., Coggins, C., Compton, P., Haggan, S., Matteliano, D., Stanton, M., et al. (2012). American Society for Pain Management Nursing position statement: Pain management in patients with substance use disorders. *Pain Management Nursing, 13*(3), 169–183. Retrieved November 15, 2013, from <http://aspmn.org/Organization/documents/PainManagementinPatientswithSubstanceAbuseDisorders.pdf>.

Pasero, C. (2011). Persistent post-surgical and post-trauma pain. *Journal of Perianesthesia Nursing, 26*(1), 38–41.

Pasero, C., & McCaffery, M. (2011). *Pain assessment and pharmacologic management.* St. Louis: Mosby.

Pasero, C., & Stannard, D. (2012). Role of IV acetaminophen in acute pain management: A case-illustrated review. *Pain Management Nursing, 13*(2), 107–124. Retrieved November 15, 2013, from <www.medscape.com/viewarticle/764841_5>.

Portenoy, R. K. (2011). Treatment of cancer pain. *The Lancet, 377*(9784), 2236–2247.

Quality and Safety Education for Nurses (QSEN) (2011). *Competency KSAs (pre-licensure).* Retrieved November 15, 2013, from <www.qsen.org>.

*Snidvongs, S. (2008). Gender differences in responses to medications and side effects of medications. *Pain Clinical Updates, 16*(5), 1–6.

Tate, J. A., Seaman, J. B., & Happ, M. B. (2012). Overcoming barriers to pain assessment: Communicating pain information with intubated older adults. *Geriatric Nursing, 33*(4), 310–313.

Turk, D. C., Wilson, H. D., & Cahana, A. (2011). Treatment of chronic non-cancer pain. *The Lancet, 377*(9784), 2226–2235.

Wu, C. L., & Raja, S. N. (2011). Treatment of acute postoperative pain. *The Lancet, 377*(9784), 2215–2225.

*Wuhrman, E., Cooney, M. F., Dunwoody, C. J., Eksterowicz, N., Merkel, S., Oakes, L. L., et al. (2007). Authorized and unauthorized ("PCA by Proxy") dosing of analgesic infusion pumps: Position statement with clinical practice recommendations. *Pain Management Nursing, 8*(1), 4–11.

Yaksh, T. L., & Wallace, M. S. (2011). Opioids, analgesia, and pain management. In L. L. Brunton, B. A. Chabner, & B. C. Knoolmann (Eds.), *Goodman & Gilman's pharmacologic basis of therapeutics* (12th ed., pp. 481–526). New York: McGraw-Hill.

Chapter 4

Badzek, L., Henaghan, M., Turner, M., & Monsen, R. (2013). Ethical, legal, and social issues in the translation of genomics into health care. *Journal of Nursing Scholarship, 45*(1), 15–24.

Beery, T., & Workman, M. L. (2012). *Genetics and genomics in nursing and health care.* Philadelphia: F.A. Davis.

Berkman, B., & Hull, S. (2014). The right not to know in the genomic era: Time to break from tradition? *American Journal of Bioethics, 14*(3), 28–31.

Bielinski, S., Olson, J., Pathak, J., Weinshilboum, R.M., Wang, L., Lyke, K.J., et al. (2014). Preemptive genotyping for personalized medicine: Design of the right drug, right dose, right time—using genomic data to individualize treatment protocol. *Mayo Clinic Proceedings, 89*(1), 25–33.

Calzone, K. A., Jenkins, J., Nicol, N., Skirton, H., Feero, W. G., & Green, E. D. (2013). Relevance of genomics to healthcare and nursing practice. *Journal of Nursing Scholarship, 45*(1), 1–2.

Cheek, D. (2013). What you need to know about pharmacogenomics. *Nursing, 43*(3), 44–48.

Conley, Y. P., Biesecker, L. G., Gonsalves, S., Merkle, C. J., Kirk, M., & Aouizerat, B. E. (2013). Current and emerging technology approaches in genomics. *Journal of Nursing Scholarship, 45*(1), 5–14.

Crockett-Maillet, G. (2010). Know the red flags of hereditary cancers. *The Nurse Practitioner Journal, 35*(7), 39–43.

Giarelli, E., & Reiff, M. (2012). Genomic literacy and competent practice: Call for research on genomics in nursing education. *Nursing Clinics of North America, 47*(4), 529–545.

Greco, K., & Mahon, S. (2012). Genomic health care has arrived, but are nurses competent to deliver it? *American Nurse Today, 7*(11), 37–38.

Kirk, M., Calzone, K., Arimori, N., & Tonkin, E. (2011). Genetic-genomics competencies and nursing regulation. *Journal of Nursing Scholarship, 43*(2), 107–116.

Manuck, S., & McCaffery, J. (2014). Gene environment interaction. *Annual Review of Psychology, 65*(1), 41–70.

Chapter 5

American Nurses Association (2010). *Nursing: Scope and standards of practice* (2nd ed.). Silver Spring, MD: Author.

Burnett, M., Lewis, M., Joy, T., & Jarrett, K. (2012). Participating in clinical nursing research: Challenges and solutions of the bedside nurse champion. *Medsurg Nursing, 21*(5), 309–311.

*Carlson, C. (2009). Use of three evidence-based postoperative pain assessment practices by registered nurses. *Pain Management Nursing, 10*(4), 174–187.

*Cronenwett, L., Sherwood, G., Barnsteiner, J., Disch, J., Johnson, J., Mitchell, P., et al. (2007). Quality and safety education for nurses. *Nursing Outlook, 55*(3), 122–131.

Fleming, K. (2008). Asking answerable questions. In N. Cullum, D. Ciliska, R. B. Haynes, & S. Marks (Eds.), *Evidence-based nursing.* Oxford, UK: Blackwell.

*DiCenso, A., Guyatt, G., & Ciliska, D. (2005). *Evidence-based nursing: A guide to clinical practice.* St. Louis: Mosby.

*Ervin, N. E. (2002). Evidence-based nursing practice: Are we there yet? *Journal of the New York State Nurses' Association, 33*(2), 11–16.

Fineout-Overholt, E., Melnyk, B. M., Stillwell, S. B., & Williamson, K. M. (2010). Critical appraisal of the evidence: Part 1—An introduction to gathering, evaluating, and recording the evidence. *The American Journal of Nursing, 110*(10), 47–52.

Fineout-Overholt, E., & Stillwell, S. B. (2011). Asking compelling clinical questions. In B. M. Melnyk & E. Fineout-Overholt (Eds.), *Evidence-based practice in nursing and healthcare: A guide to best practice* (2nd ed.). Philadelphia: Lippincott Williams & Wilkins.

Gélinas, C. (2010). Nurses' evaluation of the feasibility and the clinical utility of the critical-care pain observation tool. *Pain Management Nursing, 11*(2), 115–125.

*Hall, D. (2007). Evaluation of 3 pain assessment tools for use with critically ill adult patients. *American Journal of Critical Care, 16*(3), 309–310.

Institute of Medicine (IOM); Board on Health Care Services (2011). *Standards for developing trustworthy clinical practice guidelines: Clinical practice guidelines we can trust* (Report Brief). Washington, DC: National Academies Press. Available online at <www.nap.edu>.

*Institute of Medicine (IOM); Committee on the Health Professions Education Summit (2003). *Health professions education: A bridge to quality.* Washington, DC: National Academies Press.

*Institute of Medicine (IOM); Committee on Quality of Health Care in America (2001). *Crossing the quality chasm: A new health care system for the 21st century.* Washington, DC: National Academies Press.

Institute of Medicine (IOM); Committee on the Robert Wood Johnson Foundation Initiative on the Future of Nursing (2010). *The future of nursing: Leading change, advancing health* (Report Brief). Washington, DC: National Academies Press. Available online at <www.nap.edu>.

Keane, K. M. (2012). Validity and reliability of the critical care pain observation tool: A replication study. *Pain Management Nursing, 14*(4), e216–e225.

*Langley, G. J., Moen, R. G., Nolan, K. M., Nolan, T. W., Norman, C. L., & Provost, L. P. (2009). *The improvement guide: A practical approach to enhancing organizational performance* (2nd ed.). San Francisco: Jossey-Bass.

*Levin, R. F. (2008). Translating research evidence for WOCN practice—Evidence levels and quality ratings: What do they mean? *World Council of Enterostomal Therapists Journal, 28*(1), 30–31.

*Levin, R. F. (2009). Evidence-based practice—Implementing practice changes: Walk before you run. *Research and Theory in Nursing Practice, 23*(2), 85–87.

Levin, R. F. (2013). Formulating clinical questions: Follow my lips. In R. F. Levin & H. R. Feldman (Eds.), *Teaching evidence-based practice in nursing: A guide for academic and clinical settings* (pp. 75–83). New York: Springer.

Levin, R. F., Burke, R. E., & Kealey, S. B. (2013). Searching the sea of evidence: It takes a library. In R. F. Levin & H. R. Feldman (Eds.), *Teaching evidence-based practice in nursing: A guide for academic and clinical settings* (pp. 103–118). New York: Springer.

Levin, R. F., & Jacobs, S. K. (2012). Developing and evaluating clinical practice guidelines: A systematic approach. In M. Boltz, E. Capezuti, T. Fulmer, & D. Zwicker (Eds.), *Evidence-based geriatric nursing protocols* (4th ed.). New York: Springer.

Levin, R. F., Keefer, J. M., Marren, J., Vetter, M., Lauder, B., & Sobolewski, S. (2010). Evidence-based practice improvement: Merging 2 paradigms. *Journal of Nursing Care Quality, 25*(2), 117–126.

Levin, R. F., Melnyk, B. M., Fineout-Overholt, E., Barnes, M., & Vetter, M. (2011). Fostering evidence-based practice to improve nurse and cost outcomes in a community health setting: A pilot test of the ARCC model. *Nursing Administration Quarterly*, 35(1), 1–13.

Melnyk, B. M., & Fineout-Overholt, E. (2010). ARCC (Advancing Research and Clinical Practice through Close Collaboration): A model for system-wide implementation and sustainability of evidence-based practice. In J. Rycroft-Malone & T. Bucknall (Eds.), *Models and frameworks for implementing evidence-based practice: Linking evidence to action*. Oxford: Wiley-Blackwell.

Melnyk, B. M., & Fineout-Overholt, E. (2011). *Evidence-based practice in nursing and healthcare: A guide to best practice* (2nd ed.). Philadelphia: Lippincott Williams & Wilkins.

*Pravikoff, D. S., Tanner, A. B., & Pierce, S. T. (2005). Readiness of U.S. nurses for evidence-based practice: Many don't understand or value research and have had little or no training to help them find evidence on which to base their practice. *American Journal of Nursing*, 105(9), 40–52.

*Reavy, K., & Tavernier, S. (2008). Nurses reclaiming ownership of their practice: Implementation of an evidence-based practice model and process. *Journal of Continuing Education in Nursing*, 39(4), 166–172.

Rycroft-Malone, J., & Bucknall, T. (2010). Using theory and frameworks to facilitate the implementation of evidence into practice. *Worldviews on Evidence-Based Nursing*, 7(2), 57.

*Sackett, D. L., Straus, S. E., Richardson, W. S., Rosenberg, W., & Haynes, R. B. (2000). *Evidence-based medicine: How to practice and teach EBM* (2nd ed.). Edinburgh: Churchill Livingston.

Stetler, C. B. (2010). Stetler model. In J. Rycroft-Malone & T. Bucknall (Eds.), *Models and frameworks for implementing evidence-based practice: Linking evidence to action*. Oxford: Wiley-Blackwell.

Stillwell, S. B., Fineout-Overholt, E., Melnyk, B. M., & Williamson, K. M. (2010). Evidence-based practice, step by step: Asking the clinical question—A key step in evidence-based practice. *American Journal of Nursing*, 110(3), 58–61.

The Joint Commission (TJC) (2010). *Approaches to pain management* (2nd ed.). Oakbrook Terrace, IL: Author.

Titler, M. (2010). Iowa model of evidence-based practice. In J. Rycroft-Malone & T. Bucknall (Eds.), *Models and frameworks for implementing evidence-based practice: Linking evidence to action*. Oxford: Wiley-Blackwell.

*Wilding, J., Manias, E., & McCoy, D. (2009). Pain assessment and management in patients after abdominal surgery from PACU to the postoperative unit. *Journal of Perianesthesia Nursing*, 24(4), 233–240.

*Wolosin, R. (2008). Safety and satisfaction: Where are the connections? *Patient Safety & Quality Healthcare*, May/June, Available online at <www.psqh.com>.

*Worral, P. S., Levin, R. F., & Arsenault, D. C. (2009-2010). Documenting an EBP project: Guidelines for what to include and why. *Journal of the New York State Nurses Association*, 40(2), 12–19.

Chapter 6

American Nurses' Association (2012). *Safe patient handling practices*. Retrieved April 2014, from <www.anasafepatienthandling.org>.

*Association of Rehabilitation Nurses (ARN) (2002). *Practice guidelines for the management of constipation in adults*. Glenview, IL: Author.

*Association of Rehabilitation Nurses (ARN) (2008a). *Standards and scope of rehabilitation nursing practice*. Glenview, IL: Author.

*Association of Rehabilitation Nurses (ARN) (2008b). *The specialty practice of rehabilitation nursing: A core curriculum* (5th ed.). Skokie, IL: Author.

Coggrave, M. J., & Norton, C. (2010). The need for manual evacuation and oral laxatives in the management of neurogenic bowel dysfunction after spinal cord injury: A randomized controlled trial of a stepwise protocol. *Spinal Cord*, 48(6), 504–510.

Cournan, M. (2012). Bladder management in female stroke survivors: Translating research into practice. *Rehabilitation Nursing*, 37, 220–230.

Frisina, P. G., Guellnitz, R., & Alverzo, J. (2010). A time series of falls and injury in the inpatient rehabilitation setting. *Rehabilitation Nursing*, 35(4), 141–146, 166.

*Granger, C. V., & Gresham, G. E. (1984). *Functional assessment in rehabilitation medicine*. Baltimore: Williams & Wilkins.

Krebs, H. I. (2012). Robotic therapy: The tipping point. *American Journal of Physical Medicine and Rehabilitation*, 91(11 Suppl. 3), 290–297.

Pardee, C., Bricker, D., Rundquist, J., MacRae, C., & Tebben, C. (2012). Characteristics of neurogenic bowel in spinal cord injury and perceived quality of life. *Rehabilitation Nursing*, 37, 128–135.

Poslawsky, I. E., Schuurmans, M. J., Lindeman, E., & Hafsteinsdottir, T. B. (2010). A systematic review of nursing rehabilitation of stroke patients with aphasia. *Journal of Clinical Nursing*, 19(1–2), 17–32.

Pryor, J. (2010). Nurses create a rehabilitation milieu. *Rehabilitation Nursing*, 35(3), 123–128.

*Pullen, R. L. (2008). Transferring a patient from bed to wheelchair. *Nursing*, 38(2), 46–48.

*Rieg, L. S., Mason, C. H., & Preston, K. (2006). Spiritual care: Practical guidelines for rehabilitation nurses. *Rehabilitation Nursing*, 31(6), 249–256.

Sievert, K. D., Amend, B., Gakis, G., Toomey, P., Badke, A., Kaps, H. P., et al. (2010). Early sacral neuromodulation prevents urinary incontinence after complete spinal cord injury. *Annals of Neurology*, 67(1), 74–84.

Stein, J. (2012). Robotics in rehabilitation: Technology as destiny. *American Journal of Physical Medicine and Rehabilitation*, 91(11 Suppl. 3), S199–S203.

U.S. National Library of Medicine (NIH) (2011). *Cranberry*. Retrieved February 2013, from <www.nlm.nih.gov/medlineplus/druginfo/natural/958.html>.

Waters, T. R., & Rockefeller, K. (2010). Safe patient handling for rehabilitation professionals. *Rehabilitation Nursing*, 35(5), 216–222.

*Whipple, K. (2007). Therapeutic use of assistive technology: A clinical perspective. *Rehabilitation Nursing*, 32(2), 48–50.

Chapter 7

Abrahm, J. L. (2011). Advances in palliative medicine and end-of-life care. *Annual Review of Medicine*, 62, 187–199.

*American Association of Colleges of Nursing (2002). *Peaceful death competencies: Recommended competencies and curricular guidelines for end-of-life nursing care*. Washington, DC: Author.

Arnstein, P. R., & Robinson, E. M. (2011). Is palliative sedation right for your patient? *Nursing*, 41(8), 50–54.

Buck, H. G. (2012). Refusing artificial nutrition and hydration in advanced illness. *Nursing*, 42(9), 12–13.

Byock, I. (2012). *The best care possible*. New York: Avery.

Clabots, S. (2012). Strategies to help initiate and maintain the end-of-life discussion with patients and family members. *Medsurg Nursing*, 21(4), 197–204.

Clarke, V., & Holtslander, L. (2010). Incorporating the medicine wheel teaching in the care of Aboriginal people. *Journal of Palliative Care*, 26(1), 34–36.

Doka, K. J., & Tucci, A. S. (Eds.), (2011). *Spirituality and end-of-life care*. Washington, DC: Hospice Foundation of America.

Ferrell, B. (2010). Palliative care research: Nursing response to emergent society needs. *Nursing Science Quarterly*, 23(3), 221–225.

Ferrell, B., & Coyle, N. (Eds.), (2010). *Oxford textbook of palliative nursing* (3rd ed.). New York: Oxford University Press.

Giger, J. N. (2013). *Transcultural nursing: Assessment and intervention* (6th ed.). St. Louis: Mosby.

Gillick, M. R. (2010). Reversing the code status of advance directives? *New England Journal of Medicine*, 362, 1239–1240.

Goldstein, N. E., & Morrison, R. S. (2013). *Evidence-based practice of palliative medicine*. Philadelphia: Saunders.

Hoyert, D. L., & Xu, J. (2011). Deaths: Preliminary data for 2011. *National Vital Statistics Reports*, 61(6), 1–52. National Center for Health Statistics. Retrieved December 2013, from <www.cdc.gov/nchs/data/nvsr/nvsr61/nvsr61_06.pdf>.

Kazanowski, M. (2012). Suffering and palliative care at the end of life. In K. Perrin, C. Sheehan, M. Potter, & M. Kazanowski (Eds.), *Palliative care nursing: Caring for suffering patients* (pp. 119–159). New York: Springer.

Kelley, A. S., Deb, P., Du, Q., Aldridge Carlson, M. D., & Morrison, R. S. (2013). Hospice enrollment saves money for Medicare and improves care quality across a number of different lengths-of-stay. *Health Affairs, 32*(3), 552–561.

Kirk, T., Coyle, N., Poppito, S., & Bigoney, R. (2010). *Palliative sedation and existential suffering: A dialogue between medicine, nursing, philosophy, and psychology.* Boston: American Academy of Hospice and Palliative Medicine.

Lachman, V. (2010). Do-not-resuscitate orders: Nurse's role requires moral courage. *Medsurg Nursing, 19*(4), 249–251.

Lachman, V. D. (2011). Nurse's role in increasing patient access to hospice care. *Medsurg Nursing, 20*(4), 200–203.

Matzo, M. L., & Sherman, D. W. (Eds.), (2010). *Palliative care nursing: Quality care to the end of life* (3rd ed.). New York: Springer.

*National Consensus Project for Quality Palliative Care Task Force (2009). *Clinical practice guidelines for quality palliative care* (2nd ed.). Pittsburgh: Author.

*National Hospice and Palliative Care Organization. (2007). *Caring connections.* Retrieved February 2013, from <www. caringinfo.org>.

National Hospice and Palliative Care Organization (2012). *NHPCO facts and figures: Hospice care in America.* Author.

Peberdy, M. A., Ornato, J. P., Larkin, G. L., Braithwaite, R. S., Kashner, T. M., Carey, S. M., National Registry of Cardiopulmonary Resuscitation Investigators, et al. (2008). Survival from in-hospital cardiac arrest during nights and weekends. *Journal of the American Medical Association, 299*(7), 785–792.

Perrin, K. (2010). Communicating with seriously ill and dying patients, their families, and their healthcare providers. In M. Matzo & D. W. Sherman (Eds.), *Palliative care nursing* (3rd ed.). New York: Springer.

Perrin, K. (2012). Ethical responsibilities and issues in palliative care. In K. Perrin, C. Sheehan, M. Potter, & M. Kazanowski (Eds.), *Palliative care nursing: Caring for suffering patients* (pp. 77–117). New York: Springer.

Perrin, K. (2013). Caring for the ICU patient at the end of life. In K. Perrin & C. E. MacLeod (Eds.), *Understanding the essentials of critical care nursing* (pp. 510–530). Boston: Pearson.

Quill, T., Holloway, R., Shah, M. S., Caprio, T. V., Olden, A. M., & Storey, C. P. (2010). *Primer of palliative care* (5th ed.). Glenview, IL: American Academy of Hospice and Palliative Medicine.

Sessanna, L. (2010). End-of-life care needs and preferences among independent community dwelling older adults 65 years or older. *Journal of Hospice and Palliative Nursing, 12*(6), 360–369.

Silveira, M. J., Kim, S. Y. H., & Langa, K. M. (2010). Advance directives and outcomes of surrogate decision-making before death. *New England Journal of Medicine, 362,* 1211–1218.

Steed, M. (2012). Palliative care: Are you asking the right questions? *Nursing, 42*(10), 59–61.

*Support Study Principal Investigators. (1995). A controlled trial to improve care for seriously ill hospitalized patients: The Study to Understand Prognoses and Preferences for Outcomes and Risks of Treatments (SUPPORT). *Journal of the American Medical Association, 274,* 1591–1598.

Teno, J. M., Gozalo, P. L., Bynum, J. P., Leland, N. E., Miller, S., Morden, N. E., et al. (2013). Change in end-of-life care for Medicare beneficiaries' site of death, place of care, and health care transitions in 2000, 2005, and 2009. *Journal of the American Medical Association, 309*(5), 470–477.

Tian, J., Kaufman, D., Zarich, S., Ong, P., Amoateng-Adjepong, Y., & Manthous, C. (2010). Outcomes of critically ill patients who received cardiopulmonary resuscitation. *American Journal of Respiratory and Critical Care Medicine, 182*(4), 501–506.

Chapter 8

Aachargya, R. P., Gastmans, C., & Denier, Y. (2011). Emergency department triage: An ethical analysis. *BMC Emergency Medicine, 11*(16).

Alberts, M. J., Latchaw, R. E., Jagoda, A., Wechsler, L. R., Crocco, T., George, M. G., et al. (2011). Revised and updated recommendations for the establishment of primary stroke centers: A summary statement from the brain attack coalition. *Stroke, 42*(9), 2651–2665.

Alexander, D., Kinsley, T. L., & Waszinski, C. (2013). Journey to a safe environment: Fall prevention in an emergency department at a level I trauma center. *JEN: Journal of Emergency Nursing, 39*(4), 346–352.

American College of Surgeons Committee on Trauma (2006). *Resources for optimal care of the injured patient 2006.* Chicago: Author.

*American College of Surgeons Committee on Trauma (2008). *Advanced trauma life support course for doctors student manual* (8th ed.). Chicago: Author.

Blouin, A. S. (2011). Improving hand-off communication: New solutions for nurses. *Journal of Nursing Care Quality, 26*(2), 97–100.

Centers for Disease Control and Prevention (CDC) (2010). *FastStats: Emergency department visits.* Retrieved April 2014, from <www.cdc.gov/nchs/fastats/ervisits.htm>.

Centers for Medicare and Medicaid Services (2013). *Critical access hospitals.* Retrieved April 2014, from <www.cms.gov/Medicare/ Provider-Enrollment-and-Certification/ CertificationandComplianc/CAHs.html>.

*Cooper, G., & Laskowski-Jones, L. (2006). Development of trauma care systems. *Prehospital Emergency Care, 10*(3), 328–331.

Dateo, J. (2013). What factors increase the accuracy and inter-rater reliability of the emergency severity index among emergency nurses in triaging adult patients? *Journal of Emergency Nursing, 39*(2), 203–207.

Davis, D. T., Johannigman, J. A., & Pritts, T. A. (2012). New strategies for massive transfusion in the bleeding trauma patient. *Journal of Trauma Nursing, 19*(2), 69–75.

Desy, P., Howard, P. K., Perhats, C., & Li, S. (2010). Alcohol screening, brief intervention, and referral to treatment conducted by emergency nurses: An impact evaluation. *Journal of Emergency Nursing, 36*(6), 538–545.

Feagan, L. M., & Fisher, N. J. (2011). Impact of education on provider attitudes toward family witnessed resuscitation. *Journal of Emergency Nursing, 37*(3), 231–239.

Gerber, L. (2013). Bringing home effective nursing care for the homeless. *Nursing, 43*(3), 32–38.

Gurney, D., & Westergard, A. M. (2014). Chapter 5: Initial assessment. In D. Gurney (Ed.), *TNCC: Trauma nursing core course provider manual* (7th ed.). Des Plaines, IL: Emergency Nurses Association.

Harding, A. D. (2011). Education and culture: Mitigation for workplace violence. *Journal of Emergency Nursing, 37*(3), 256–257.

Hewitt, L. N., Bhavsar, P., & Phelan, H. (2011). The secrets women keep: Intimate partner violence screening in the female trauma patient. *The Journal of Trauma: Injury, Infection and Critical Care, 70*(2), 320–323.

*Howard, P. K. (2009). Crowding: A report of the ENA ED crowding work team. *Journal of Emergency Nursing, 35*(1), 55–56.

Institute of Medicine (IOM) Board on Health Care Services (2010). *Regionalizing emergency care workshop summary.* Washington, DC: National Academies Press. Retrieved April 2014, from <www.nap.edu/catalog. php?record_id=12872>.

*Johnson, D., & Parker, D. (2009). Managers Forum—Cutting-edge discussion of management, policy, and program issues in emergency care: Canine security (Solheim, J., & Papa, A. [Eds.]). *Journal of Emergency Nursing, 35*(5), 469–470.

Kisner, T., & Johnson-Anderson, H. (2010). Simulation on a shoestring budget. *Nursing, 40*(8), 32–35.

*Laskowski-Jones, L. (2008). Change management at the hospital front door: Integrating automatic patient tracking in a high volume emergency department and Level I trauma center. *Nurse Leader, 6*(2), 52–57.

Laskowski-Jones, L. (2009). Responding to trauma: Your priorities in the first hour. *Nursing, 39,* 7–12.

Moore, K. M. (2011). The four horsemen of the apocalypse of trauma. *Journal of Emergency Nursing, 37*(3), 294–295.

Mower-Wade, D., & Pirrung, J. M. (2010). Advanced practice nurses making a difference: Implementation of a formal rounding process. *Journal of Trauma Nursing, 17*(2), 69–71.

National Alliance to End Homelessness (2012). *The state of homelessness in America 2012.* Retrieved April 2014, from <www.endhomelessness .org/content/article/detail/4361>.

National Center for Injury Prevention and Control (NCIPC) (2012). *Injury prevention and control: Data & statistics* (WISQARS). Retrieved April 2014, from <www.cdc.gov/injury/wisqars/ index.html>.

Nikki, L., Lepisto, S., & Paavilainen, E. (2013). Experiences of family members of elderly patients in the emergency department: A qualitative study. *International Emergency Nursing, 20*(4), 193–200.

Nolan, M. R. (2009). Older patients in the emergency department: What are the risks? *Journal of Gerontological Nursing, 35*(12), 14–18.

Popovich, M. A., Boyd, C., Dachenhaus, T., & Kusler, D. (2012). Improving stable patient flow through the emergency department by utilizing evidence-based practice: One hospital's journey. *Journal of Emergency Nursing, 38*(5), 474–478.

Richardson, K. (2014). Front-gate triage. *JEN: Journal of Emergency Nursing, 40*(2), 198–200.

Robertson, D. J. (2013). An integrative review: Triage protocols and the effect on ED length of stay. *JEN: Journal of Emergency Nursing, 39*(4), 398–408.

Sadowski, L. S., Kee, R. A., VanderWeele, T. J., & Buchanan, D. (2009). Effect of a housing and case management program on emergency department visits and hospitalizations among chronically ill homeless adults. *The Journal of the American Medical Association, 301*(17), 1771–1778.

Shelton, R. (2010). ESI: A better triage system? *Nursing Critical Care, 5*(6), 34–37.

Strickler, J. (2010). Traumatic hypovolemic shock: Halt the downward spiral. *Nursing, 40*(10), 34–39.

The Joint Commission (TJC) (2013). *National Patient Safety Goals*. Retrieved April 2014, from <http://www.jointcommission.org/standards_information/npsgs.aspx>.

Touhy, T. A., & Jett, K. (2012). *Ebersole & Hess' toward healthy aging: human needs and nursing response* (8th ed.). St. Louis: Mosby.

U.S. Department of Health and Human Services (2013). *Read the law*. Retrieved April 2014, from <www.hhs.gov/healthcare/rights/law/index.html>.

Watkins, L. M., & Patrician, P. A. (2014). Handoff communication for the emergency department to primary care. *Advanced Emergency Nursing Journal, 36*(1), 44–51.

Chapter 9

*American Heart Association (2011). *Advanced cardiovascular life support provider manual*. Dallas: Author.

Arnold, T. C. (Last updated July 30, 2012). *Brown recluse spider envenomation treatment and management*. Retrieved April 2014, from *Medscape reference: drugs, diseases & procedures* <http://emedicine.medscape.com/article/772295-overview>.

*Auerbach, P. S. (2009). *Medicine for the outdoors: The essential guide to first aid and medical emergencies* (5th ed.). St. Louis: Mosby.

*Auerbach, P. S. (2012). *Wilderness medicine* (6th ed.). Philadelphia: Mosby.

Auerbach, P. S., Della-Giustina, D., & Ingebretsen, R. (2010). *Advanced wilderness life support* (4th ed.). Utah: AdventureMed.

*Auerbach, P. S., Donner, H. J., & Weiss, E. A. (2013). *Field guide to wilderness medicine* (4th ed.). St. Louis: Mosby.

*Bledsoe, G. H., Manyak, M. J., & Townes, D. A. (2009). *Expedition & wilderness medicine*. New York: Cambridge University Press.

Boyer, L. V., Binford, G. J., & Degan, J. A. (2012). Spider bites. In P. S. Auerbach (Ed.), *Wilderness medicine* (6th ed., pp. 975–996). Philadelphia: Mosby.

Bush, S. P. (2012). *Rattlesnake envenomation (updated November 14, 2012)*. Available on *Medscape website*. Retrieved April 2014, from <http://emedicine.medscape.com/article/771455-overview>.

Cardwell, M. D. (2011). Recognizing dangerous snakes in the United States and Canada: A novel 3-step identification method. *Wilderness & Environmental Medicine, 22*(4), 304–308.

Choo, K. J., Simons, F. E., & Sheikh, A. (2013). Glucocorticoids for the treatment of anaphylaxis. *Evidence-Based Child Health, 8*(4), 1279–1294.

Cusack, L., de Crespigny, C., & Athanasos, P. (2011). Heatwaves and their impact on people with alcohol, drug and mental health conditions: A discussion paper on clinical practice considerations. *Journal of Advanced Nursing, 67*(4), 915–922.

Davis, C., Engeln, A., Johnson, E., McIntosh, S. E., Zafren, K., Islas, A. A., et al. (2012). Wilderness Medical Society practice guidelines for the prevention and treatment of lightning injuries. *Wilderness & Environmental Medicine, 23*, 260–269.

Fougera Pharmaceuticals, Inc. (2008). *CroFab— Crotalidae Polyvalent Immune Fab (Ovine)*. Retrieved April 2014, from <www.savagelabs.com/Products/CroFab/Home/crofab_frame.htm>.

*Guoen, J., Shenghua, L., Rili, G., Mitchell, A., & Yanping, S. (2009). High altitude disease: Consequences of genetic and environmental interactions. *North American Journal of Medicine and Science, 2*(3), 74–80.

Hackett, P. H., & Roach, R. C. (2012). High altitude medicine and physiology. In P. S. Auerbach (Ed.), *Wilderness medicine* (6th ed., pp. 2–33). Philadelphia: Mosby.

Hausfater, P., Doumenc, B., Chopin, S., Le Manach, Y., Dautheville, S., Hericord, P., et al. (2010a). Elevation of cardiac troponin I during non-exertional heat-related illnesses in the context of a heat wave. *Critical Care, 14*(3), R99.

Hausfater, P., Megarbane, B., Dautheville, S., Patzak, A., Andronikof, M., Andre, S., et al. (2010b). Prognostic factors in non-exertional heatstroke. *Intensive Care Medicine, 36*, 272–280.

*Johnson, C., Anderson, S. R., Dallimore, J., Winser, S., & Warrell, D. A. (2008). *Oxford handbook of expedition and wilderness medicine*. New York: Oxford University Press.

Jones, P., Moran, K., & Webber, J. (2013). Drowning terminology: Not what it used to be. *New Zealand Medical Journal, 126*(1386), 114–116.

Krau, S. D. (2013). Bites and stings: Epidemiology and treatment. *Critical Care Nursing Clinics of North America, 25*(2), 143–150.

Krau, S. D. (2013). Heat-related illness: A hot topic in critical care. *Critical Care Nursing Clinics of North America, 25*(2), 251–262.

Krau, S. D. (2013). The impact of heat on morbidity and mortality. *Critical Care Nursing Clinics of North America, 25*(2), 243–250.

Laskowski-Jones, L. (2009). Winter emergencies: Managing ski and snowboard injuries. *Nursing, 39*(11), 24–30.

Laskowski-Jones, L. (2010). Summer emergencies: Can you take the heat? *Nursing, 40*(6), 24–32.

Leikin, S. M., Korley, F. K., Wang, E. E., & Leikin, J. B. (2012). The spectrum of hypothermia: From environmental exposure to therapeutic uses and medical simulation. *Disease-A-Month, 58*(1), 6–32.

Lin, C. J., Wu, C. J., Chen, H. H., & Lin, H. C. (2011). Multiorgan failure following mass wasp stings. *Southern Medical Journal, 104*(5), 378–379.

Mattis, J. G., & Yates, A. M. (2011). Heatstroke: Helping patients keep their cool. *Nurse Practitioner, 36*(5), 48–52.

*Mitchell, A. (2006). Africanized killer bees: A case study. *Critical Care Nurse, 26*(3), 23–32.

Norris, R. (2011). *Coral snake envenomation*. Retrieved April 2014 from *Medscape Reference: Drugs, Diseases & Procedures* <http://emedicine.medscape.com/article/771701-overview>.

Norris, R. L., Bush, S. P., & Smith, J. C. (2012). Bites by venomous reptiles in Canada, the United States, and Mexico. In P. S. Auerbach (Ed.), *Wilderness medicine* (6th ed., pp. 1011–1039). Philadelphia: Mosby.

O'Brien, K. K., Leon, L. R., & Kenefick, R. W. (2012). Clinical management of heat-related illnesses. In P. S. Auerbach (Ed.), *Wilderness medicine* (6th ed., pp. 232–238). Philadelphia: Mosby.

Paden, M., Franjic, L., & Halcomb, S. (2013). Hyperthermia caused by drug interactions and adverse reactions. *Emergency Medicine Clinics of North America, 31*(4), 1035–1044.

Simon, R. B., & Simon, D. A. (2014). Illness at high altitudes. *Nursing, 44*(7), 36–41.

Smallheer, B. A. (2013). Bee and wasp stings: Reactions and anaphylaxis. *Critical Care Nursing Clinics of North America, 25*(2), 151–164.

Suchard, J. R. (2011). "Spider bite" lesions are usually diagnosed as skin and soft tissue infections. *Journal of Emergency Medicine, 41*(5), 473–481.

*Suchard, J. R. (2012). Scorpion envenomation. In P. S. Auerbach (Ed.), *Wilderness medicine* (6th ed., pp. 996–1011). Philadelphia: Mosby.

Szpilman, D., Bierens, J. J., Handley, A. J., & Orlowski, J. P. (2012). Drowning. *New England Journal of Medicine, 366*, 2102–2110.

Vetter, R. S. (2013). Spider envenomation in North America. *Critical Care Nursing Clinics of North America, 25*(2), 205–223.

Weimer, S., Staubil, L., & Makic, M. B. F. (2013). Fending off disaster for a frostbite victim. *American Nurse Today, 8*(1), 20.

Wilbeck, J., & Gresham, C. (2013). North American snake and scorpion envenomations. *Critical Care Nursing Clinics of North America, 25*(2), 173–190.

Chapter 10

Adler, E., & Bauer, L. (2011). Condition gray: Inside the hospital as the Joplin tornado hit. *The Kansas City Star.* Retrieved April 2014, from <www.kansascity.com/2011/06/18/2959600/condition-gray-inside-the-hospital.html>.

*American Nurses Association (ANA) (2001). *Code of ethics for nurses with interpretive statements.* Washington, DC: Author.

Bulson, J. A., & Bulson, T. (2011). Nursing process and critical thinking linked to disaster preparedness. *Journal of Emergency Nursing, 37*(5), 477–483.

Busby, S., & Witucki-Brown, J. (2011). Theory development for situational awareness in multi-casualty incidents. *Journal of Emergency Nursing, 37*(5), 444–452.

Caramenico, A. (2013). In emergencies, hospital preparedness goes beyond planning. *FierceHealthcare.com.* Retrieved April 2014, from <www.fiercehealthcare.com/story/emergencies-hospital-preparedness-goes-beyond-planning/2013-04-18>.

Centers for Medicare and Medicaid Services (CMS) (2012). *Life safety code requirements.* Retrieved April 2014, from <www.cms.gov/Medicare/Provider-Enrollment-and-Certification/CertificationandComplianc/LSC.html>.

Chaffee, M. (2006). Making the decision to report to work in a disaster. *American Journal of Nursing, 106*(9), 54–57.

*Claudius, I., Behar, S., Ballow, S., Wood, R., Stevenson, K., Blake, N., et al. (2008). Disaster drill exercise documentation and management: Are we drilling to standard? *Journal of Emergency Nursing, 34*(6), 504–508.

Evans, M. (2012). Recovery mode. *Modern Healthcare, 42*(50), 6–7.

Federal Emergency Management Agency (FEMA) (2013). *Resources.* Retrieved April 2014, from <www.fema.gov/resources>.

Hyer, K., & Brown, L. M. (2008). The Impact of Event Scale—Revised. *American Journal of Nursing, 108*(11), 60–68.

International Critical Incident Stress Foundation, Inc. (2013). *Mission statement.* Retrieved April 2014, from <www.icisf.org/who-we-are>.

Kallman, M., & Feury, K. J. (2011). Preparing for patient surge in an emergency department during a disaster. *Journal of Emergency Nursing, 37*(2), 184–185.

*Laskowski-Jones, L. (2008). Change management at the hospital front door: Integrating automatic patient tracking in a high volume emergency department and Level I trauma center. *Nurse Leader, 6*(2), 52–57.

Laskowski-Jones, L. (2010). When disaster strikes: Ready, or not? (Editorial). *Nursing, 40*(4), 6.

Letner, J. (2011). A fist coming out of the sky: Six miles of terror. *The Joplin Globe.* Retrieved April 2014, from <www.joplinglobe.com/local/x564433625/A-fist-coming-out-of-the-sky-Six-miles-of-terror>.

Merchant, R. M., Leigh, J. E., & Lurie, N. (2010). Health care volunteers and disaster response: first, be prepared. *New England Journal of Medicine, 362*(10), 872–873.

National Fire Protection Association (2013). *Codes and standards.* Retrieved April 2014, from <www.nfpa.org/codes and standards.aspx>.

Olchin, L., & Krutz, A. (2012). Nurses as first responders to a mass casualty: Are you prepared? *Journal of Trauma Nursing, 19*(2), 122–129.

Smith, J. S. (2010). Mass casualty events: Are you prepared? *Nursing, 40*(4), 40–45.

Somes, J., & Donatelli, N. S. (2012). Disaster planning considerations involving the geriatric patient, Part I. *Journal of Emergency Nursing, 38*(5), 479–481.

The Joint Commission (2008). *Standards FAQs: Emergency management.* Retrieved April 2014, from <www.jointcommission.org/standards_information/jcfaqdetails.aspx?StandardsFaqId=392&ProgramId=47>.

U.S. Department of Health & Human Services (2013). *National Disaster Medical System.* Retrieved April 2014, from <www.phe.gov/Preparedness/responders/ndms/Pages/default.aspx>.

Wielawski, I. M. (2006). The health legacy of September 11: Five years later illness and memories haunt many. *American Journal of Nursing, 106*(9), 27–28.

Yin, H., He, H., Arbon, P., Zhu, J., Tan, J., & Zhang, L. (2012). Optimal qualifications, staffing and scope of practice for first responder nurses in disaster. *Journal of Clinical Nursing, 21*(1–2), 264–271.

Chapter 11

Collins, M., & Claros, E. (2011). Recognizing the face of dehydration. *Nursing, 41*(8), 26–31.

Cottrell, D. (2012). Managing acute hyperkalemia. *Nursing, 42*(10), 68.

Crawford, A., & Harris, H. (2011a). Balancing act: Hypomagnesemia and hypermagnesemia. *Nursing, 41*(10), 52–55.

Crawford, A., & Harris, H. (2011b). Balancing act: Na+ and K+. *Nursing, 41*(7), 44–50.

Crawford, A., & Harris, H. (2011c). IV fluids: What nurses need to know. *Nursing, 41*(5), 30–38.

Crawford, A., & Harris, H. (2012). Balancing act: Calcium and phosphorus. *Nursing, 42*(1), 36–42.

McGraw, M. (2012). Beer potomania: Drink in this atypical cause of hyponatremia. *Nursing, 42*(7), 24–30.

Nguyen, T., & Wang, A. (2012). Hyperphosphatemia: Consequences and management strategies. *The Journal for Nurse Practitioners, 8*(1), 56–60.

Schreiber, M. (2013a). Understanding hypernatremia. *Nursing Critical Care, 8*(3), 8–10.

Schreiber, M. (2013b). Understanding hyponatremia. *Nursing Critical Care, 8*(2), 8–10.

Scotto, C., Fridline, M., Menhart, C., & Klions, H. (2014). Preventing hypokalemia in critically ill patients. *American Journal of Critical Care, 23*(2), 145–149.

Stannard, D. (2012). Hypertonic saline for perioperative fluid management. *Journal of Perianesthesia Nursing, 27*(2), 115–117.

Thomsen, G., Berdjian, L., Rodriguez, L., & Hopkins, R. (2012). Clinical outcomes of a furosemide infusion protocol in edematous patients in the intensive care unit. *Critical Care Nurse, 32*(6), 25–33.

Trissel, L. (2013). *Handbook on injectable drugs* (17th ed.). Bethesda, MD: American Society of Hospital-System Pharmacists.

Chapter 12

Barnette, L., & Kautz, D. (2013). Creative ways to teach arterial blood gas interpretation. *Dimensions of Critical Care Nursing, 32*(2), 84–87.

Blevins, S. (2014). Making ABGs simple. *Medsurg Nursing, 23*(3), 185–186.

*Jones, M. (2010). Basic interpretation of metabolic acidosis. *Critical Care Nurse, 30*(5), 63–69.

Chapter 13

Aguiar, T. (2010). *Intraosseous access: Not just for emergencies anymore.* Presentation at the Infusion Nurses Society annual meeting: Las Vegas, NV.

Alekseyev, S., Byrne, M., Carpenter, A., Franker, C., Kidd, C., & Hulton, L. (2012). Prolonging the life of a patient's IV: An integrative review of intravenous securement devices. *Medsurg Nursing, 21*(5), 285–292.

Alexandrou, E., Ramjan, L. M., Spencer, T., Frost, S. A., Salamonson, Y., Davidson, P., et al. (2011). The use of midline catheters in the adult acute care setting: Clinical implications and recommendations for practice. *Journal for the Association of Vascular Access, 16*(1), 35–41.

*Almadrones, L. (2007). Evidence-based research for intraperitoneal chemotherapy in epithelial ovarian cancer. *Clinical Journal of Oncology Nursing, 11*(2), 211–216.

Bard Access Systems (2011). *PowerPICC Solo2 Catheter: Overview.* Retrieved December 2013, from <www.bardaccess.com/nurse-powerpiccsolo.php>.

Bard, C. R. (2013). *PowerGlide midline catheter.* Bard Access Systems. Retrieved December 2013, from <www.bardaccess.com/midline-powerglide.php>.

Breland, B. D. (2010). Continuous quality improvement using intelligent infusion pump data analysis. *American Journal of Health-System Pharmacy, 67,* 1446–1455.

Candon, H. L., Amirov, C., & Toen, J. V. (2010). A multifaceted intervention to address a case cluster of cellulitis associated with hypodermoclysis in a geriatric complex continuing care unit. *Canadian Journal of Infection Control, 25*(2), 101–106.

Centers for Disease Control and Prevention (CDC) (2011). *2011 guidelines for prevention of intravascular catheter-related infections.* Retrieved September 2013, from <www.cdc.gov/hicpac/bsi/07-bsi-background-info-2011.htmles-2011.html>.

Clemence, B. J., & Maneval, R. E. (2014). Risk factors associated with catheter-related upper extremity deep vein thrombosis in peripherally inserted central venous catheter: Literature review—Part 1. *Journal of Infusion Therapy, 37*(3), 187–196.

Connolly, S., Korzemba, H., Harb, G., Lebel, F., & Syltevik, C. (2011). Techniques for hyaluronidase-facilitated subcutaneous fluid administration with recombinant human hyaluronidase: The increased flow utilizing subcutaneously enabled administration technique (INFUSE AT) study. *Journal of Infusion Nursing, 43*(5), 300–307.

Crawford, A., & Harris, H. (2011). IV fluids: What nurses need to know. *Nursing, 41*(5), 30–39.

Davenport, D. E., & Utterback, V. A. (2011). Physics and flushes: The science supporting why we do what we do. *Nursing, 41*(8), 65–66.

Dumont, C., Getz, O., & Miller, S. (2014). Evaluation of midline vascular access: A descriptive study. *Nursing, 44*(10), 60–66.

*Earhart, A., & Kaminski, D. (2007). Evidence-based practice in infusion nursing: 2007 NACNS national conference abstracts. *Clinical Nurse Specialist, 21*(2), 107.

*Fowler, R., Gallagher, J. V., Isaacs, S. M., Ossman, E., Pepe, P., & Wayne, M. (2007). The role of intraosseous vascular access in the out-of-hospital environment. *Prehospital Emergency Care, 11*(1), 63–66.

Garcia, L. S., & Isenberg, H. D. (2010). *Clinical microbiology procedures handbook* (3rd ed.). Washington, DC: ASM Press.

Genentech USA, Inc. (2011). *Cathflo(r) Activase (r) (Alteplase).* Retrieved December 2013, from <www.cathflo.com>.

*Griswold-Theodorson, S., Hanna, H., Handly, N., Pugh, B., Fojtik, J., Saks, M., et al. (2009). Improving patient safety with ultrasonography guidance during internal jugular central venous catheter placement by novice practitioners. *Simulation in Healthcare, 4*(4), 212–216.

*Hadaway, L. C. (2009). Managing vascular access device occlusions, Part 1. *Nursing, 39*(1), 10.

Hadaway, L. C. (2010a). Infusion therapy equipment. In M. Alexander, A. Corrigan, L. Gorski, J. Hankins, & R. Perucca (Eds.), *Infusion nursing; An evidence-based approach* (3rd ed.). St. Louis: Saunders.

Hadaway, L. C. (2010b). Preventing and managing peripheral extravasation. *Nursing, 39*(10), 26–27.

Hayek, S. M., Deer, T. R., Pope, J. E., Panchal, S. J., & Patel, V. B. (2011). Intrathecal therapy for cancer and non-cancer pain. *Pain Physician, 14*(3), 219–248.

Infusion Nurses Society (INS). (2011). Infusion nursing standards of practice. *Journal of Infusion Nursing, 34*(1S), S8.

*Jarvis, W. R., Murphy, C., Hall, K. K., Fogle, P. J., Karchmer, T. B., Harrington, G., et al. (2009). Health care-associated bloodstream infections associated with negative- or positive-pressure or displacement mechanical valve needleless connectors. *Clinical Infectious Diseases, 49*(12), 1821–1827.

*Khalidi, N., Kovacevich, D. S., Papke-O'Donnell, L. F., & Btaiche, I. (2009). Impact of the positive pressure valve on vascular access device occlusions and bloodstream infections. *Journal of the Association for Vascular Access, 14*(2), 84–91.

*Macha, D. B., Nelson, R. C., Howle, L. E., Hollingsworth, J. W., & Schindera, S. T. (2009). Central venous catheter integrity during mechanical power injection of iodinated contrast medium. *Radiology, 253*(3), 870–878.

*Madigan, K. (2008). Now, intraosseous infusions for adults. *American Nurse Today, 3*(1), 11–12.

McGoldrick, M. (2010). Infection prevention and control. In M. Alexander, L. Gorski, J. Hankins, & R. Perucca (Eds.), *Infusion nursing: An evidence-based approach* (3rd ed.). St. Louis: Saunders.

McHugh, M. E., Miller-Saultz, D., Wuhrman, E., & Kosharskyy, B. (2012). Interventional pain management in the palliative care patient. *International Journal of Palliative Nursing, 18*(9), 426–433.

Mitchell, M. D., Anderson, B. J., Williams, K., & Umscheid, C. A. (2009). Heparin flushing and other interventions to maintain patency of central venous catheters: A systematic review. *Journal of Advanced Nursing, 65*(10), 2007–2021.

*Moran, J. E., Ash, S. R., & ASDIN Clinical Practice Committee. (2008). Locking solutions for hemodialysis catheters: Heparin and citrate—a position paper by ASDIN. *Seminars in Dialysis, 21*(5), 490–492.

Ness, K. K., Hudson, M. M., Pui, C. H., Green, D. M., Krull, K. R., Huang, T. T., et al. (2012). Neuromuscular impairments in adult survivors of childhood acute lymphoblastic leukemia: Associations with physical performance and chemotherapy doses. *Cancer, 118*(3), 828–838.

O'Grady, N. P., Alexander, M., Burns, L. A., Dellinger, E. P., Garland, J., Heard, S. O., et al. (2011). *Guidelines for the prevention of intravascular catheter-related infections.* Atlanta: Centers for Disease Control and Prevention.

Perucca, R. (2010). Peripheral venous access devices. In M. Alexander, A. Corrigan, L. Gorski, J. Hankins, & R. Perucca (Eds.), *Infusion nursing: An evidence-based approach* (3rd ed.). St. Louis: Saunders.

Phillips, L., Brown, L., Campbell, T., Miller, J., Proehl, J., & Youngberg, B. (2010). Recommendations for the use of intraosseous vascular access for emergent and nonemergent situations in various health care settings: A consensus paper. *Critical Care Nurse, 30*(6), e1–e7.

Santolim, T. Q., Santos, L. A., Giovani, A. M., & Dias, V. C. (2012). The strategic role of the nurse in the selection of IV devices. *British Journal of Nursing, 21*(21), S28–S32.

Scales, K. (2011). Use of hypodermoclysis to manage dehydration. *Nursing Older People, 23*(5), 16–22.

The Joint Commission (2014). *National Patient Safety Goals: NPSG.01.03.01 eliminate transfusion errors related to patient misidentification.* Retrieved April 2014, from <www.jointcommission.org/hap_2014_npsg/>.

Thompson, C. D., Vital-Carona, J., & Faustino, E. V. (2012). The effect of tubing dwell time on insulin absorption during intravenous insulin infusions. *Diabetes Technology & Therapeutics, 14*(10), 912–916.

Watts, D., & Kremer, M. J. (2011). Complex regional pain syndrome: A review of diagnostics, pathophysiologic mechanisms, and treatment implications for certified registered nurse anesthetists. *AANA Journal, 79*(6), 505–510.

Weeks, K. A. (2012). Intermittent IV infusions in acute care: Special considerations. *Nursing, 42*(11), 66–68.

White, A., Lopez, F., & Stone, P. (2010). Developing and sustaining an ultrasound-guided peripheral intravenous access program for emergency nurses. *Advanced Emergency Nursing Journal, 32*(2), 173–188.

Chapter 14

AmbulatorySurgeryCenter Association (2013). *Advancing surgical care.* Retrieved April 2014, <www.ascassociation.org/AdvancingSurgicalCare/AboutASCs/History>.

American Society of PeriAnesthesia Nurses (ASPAN) (2012). *2012-2014 Perianesthesia nursing standards, practice recommendations and interpretive statements.* Cherry Hill, NJ: Author.

Association of periOperative Registered Nurses (AORN) (2014a). Perioperative explications for the ANA code of ethics for nurses. In *Perioperative standards and recommended practices* (pp. 21–42). Denver: Author.

Association of periOperative Registered Nurses (AORN) (2014b). *Position statement on perioperative care of patients with do-not-resuscitate (DNR) orders.* Retrieved August 2014, from <http://www.aorn.org/Clinical_Practice/Position_Statements/Position_Statements.aspx>.

Association of periOperative Registered Nurses (AORN) (2014c). Position statement on verification of correct site, correct procedure, and correct patient. In *Perioperative standards and recommended practices* (pp. 640–643). Denver: Author.

Association of periOperative Registered Nurses (AORN) (2014d). Recommended practices for perioperative patient skin antisepsis. In *Perioperative standards and recommended practices* (pp. 73–85). Denver: Author.

Bradley, S. (2014). Infection prevention practices in ambulatory surgery centers. *The American Journal of Nursing, 114*(7), 64–67.

Crenshaw, J. (2011). Preoperative fasting: Will the evidence ever be put into practice? *American Journal of Nursing, 111*(10), 38–43.

*Doerflinger, D. (2009). Older adult surgical patients: Presentation and challenges. *AORN Journal, 90*(2), 223–240.

Elpern, E., Killeen, K., Patel, G., & Senecal, G. (2013). The application of intermittent pneumatic compression devices for thromboprophylaxis. *The American Journal of Nursing, 113*(4), 30–36.

Graham, D., Faggionato, E., & Timberlake, A. (2011). Preventing perioperative complications in the patient with a high body mass index. *AORN Journal, 94*(4), 334–344.

Johnson, J. (2011). Preoperative assessment of high-risk orthopedic surgery patients. *Nurse Practitioner, 36*(7), 40–47.

Larkin, B., Mitchell, K., & Petrie, K. (2012). Translating evidence to practice for mechanical venous thromboembolism prophylaxis. *AORN Journal, 96*(5), 513–527.

McEwen, D. (2011). Ambulatory surgery. In J. C. Rothrock (Ed.), *Alexander's care of the patient in surgery* (14th ed.). St. Louis: Mosby.

MDConsult (2012). *Propofol monograph*. Retrieved April 2014, from <www.mdconsult.com/das/pharm/body/407435066-4/0/full/519?infotype=2>.

Rock, M., & Hoebeke, R. (2014). Informed consent: Whose duty to inform? *Medsurg Nursing, 23*(3), 189–191, 194.

Rothrock, J. C. (2011). *Alexander's care of the patient in surgery* (14th ed.). St. Louis: Mosby.

*Sendelbach, S. (2010). Preoperative fasting doesn't mean nothing after midnight. *The American Journal of Nursing, 110*(9), 64–65.

Spruce, L., & Braswell, M. L. (2012). Implementing AORN recommended practices for electrosurgery. *AORN Journal, 95*(3), 373–387.

Tanner, J., Norrie, P., & Melen, K. (2011). Preoperative hair removal to reduce surgical site infection. *The Cochrane Library, 11*, 1–50.

The Joint Commission (2014). *National Patient Safety Goals*. Retrieved April 2014, from <www.jointcommission.org/patientsafety/nationalpatientsafetygoals/>.

Chapter 15

Adams, D., & Dervay, K. (2012). Pharmacology of procedural sedation. *AACN Advanced Critical Care, 23*(4), 349–354.

AmbulatorySurgeryCenter Association (2013). *Advancing surgical care*. Retrieved April 2014, <www.ascassociation.org/AdvancingSurgicalCare/AboutASCs/History>.

Association of periOperative Registered Nurses (AORN) (2014a). *Perioperative standards and recommended practices: For inpatient and ambulatory settings*. (2014 Ed.), Denver: Author.

Association of periOperative Registered Nurses (AORN) (2014b). *Position statement: AORN position statement on RN first assistants*. Retrieved August 2014, from <http://www.aorn.org/Clinical_Practice/Position_Statements/Position_Statements.aspx>.

Association of periOperative Registered Nurses (AORN) (2010c). *Position statement: Perioperative care of patients with do not resuscitate (DNR) orders*. Retrieved Augustl 2014, from <http://www.aorn.org/Clinical_Practice/Position_Statements/Position_Statements.aspx>.

Association of periOperative Registered Nurses (AORN) (2014d). Recommended practices for cleaning and care of surgical instruments and powered equipment. In *Perioperative standards and recommended practices* (pp. 541–560). Denver: Author.

Association of periOperative Registered Nurses (AORN) (2014e). Recommended practices for Disinfection, high-level. In *Perioperative standards and recommended practices* (pp. 515–528). Denver: Author.

Association of periOperative Registered Nurses (AORN) (2014f). Recommended practices for information management. In *Perioperative standards and recommended practices* (pp. 443–464). Denver: Author.

Association of periOperative Registered Nurses (AORN) (2014g). Recommended practices for environmental cleaning in the perioperative setting. In *Perioperative standards and recommended practices* (pp. 255–276). Denver: Author.

Association of periOperative Registered Nurses (AORN) (2014h). Recommended practices for laser safety in the practice settings. In *Perioperative standards and recommended practices* (pp. 141–154). Denver: Author.

Association of periOperative Registered Nurses (AORN) (2014i). Recommended practices for managing the patient receiving moderate sedation/analgesia. In *Perioperative standards and recommended practices* (pp. 471–480). Denver: Author.

Association of periOperative Registered Nurses (AORN) (2014j). Recommended practices for positioning the patient in the perioperative practice setting. In *Perioperative standards and recommended practices* (pp. 481–500). Denver: Author.

Association of periOperative Registered Nurses (AORN) (2014k). Recommended practices for preoperative patient skin antisepsis. In *Perioperative standards and recommended practices* (pp. 73–88). Denver: Author.

Association of periOperative Registered Nurses (AORN) (2014l). Recommended practices for sharps safety. In *Perioperative standards and recommended practices* (pp. 351–374). Denver: Author.

Association of periOperative Registered Nurses (AORN) (2014m). Recommended practices for sterile technique. In *Perioperative standards and recommended practices* (pp. 89–118). Denver: Author.

Association of periOperative Registered Nurses (AORN) (2014n). Recommended practices for sterilization. In *Perioperative standards and recommended practices* (pp. 575–602). Denver: Author.

Association of periOperative Registered Nurses (AORN) (2014o). Recommended practices for surgical attire. In *Perioperative standards and recommended practices* (pp. 49–60). Denver: Author.

Association of periOperative Registered Nurses (AORN) (2014p). Recommended practices for hand hygiene in the perioperative setting. In *Perioperative standards and recommended practices* (pp. 61–72). Denver: Author.

Association of periOperative Registered Nurses (AORN) (2014q). Recommended practices for traffic patterns in the perioperative practice setting. In *Perioperative standards and recommended practices* (pp. 110–122). Denver: Author.

Association of periOperative Registered Nurses (AORN) (2014r). Position statement on verification of correct site, correct procedure, and correct patient. In *Perioperative standards and recommended practices* (pp. 640–643). Denver: Author.

Centers for Disease Control and Prevention (2014). *National health statistics report: Surgical site infection (SSI) event*. Retrieved August 2014, from <www.cdc.gov/nhsn/pdfs/pscmanual/9pscssicurrent.pdf>.

*Dawson, R., von Fintel, N., & Naim, S. (2010). Sedation assessment using the Ramsay scale. *Emergency Nurse, 18*(3), 18–20.

DeLamar, L. (2011). Anesthesia. In J. C. Rothrock (Ed.), *Alexander's care of the patient in surgery* (14th ed.). St. Louis: Mosby.

Johnson, J. (2011). Preoperative assessment of high-risk orthopedic surgery patients. *Nurse Practitioner, 36*(7), 40–47.

Malignant Hyperthermia Association of the United States (2014). *Emergency therapy for MH acute phase treatment*. Retrieved August 2014, from <www.mhaus.org/healthcare-professionals/#.UPGIEGeN58F>.

Mitchell-Brown, F. (2012). Malignant hyperthermia: Turn down the heat. *Nursing, 42*(5), 38–44.

Norred, C. (2012). Anesthesia-induced anaphylaxis. *American Association of Nurse Anesthetists Journal, 80*(2), 129–140.

Online Mendelian Inheritance in Man (OMIM) (2013). *Malignant Hyperthermia, Susceptibility to, 1;MHS1*. Retrieved August 2014, from <www.omim.org/entry/145600>.

Rothrock, J. C. (2011). *Alexander's care of the patient in surgery* (14th ed.). St. Louis: Mosby.

The Joint Commission (TJC) (2014). *National Patient Safety Goals*. Retrieved August 2014, from <www.jointcommission.org/patientsafety/nationalpatientsafetygoals/>.

Tschannen, D., Bates, O., Talsma, A., & Guo, Y. (2012). Patient-specific and surgical characteristics in the documentation of pressure ulcers. *American Journal of Critical Care, 21*(2), 116–125.

*Ulmer, B. (2010). Best practices for minimally invasive procedures. *AORN Journal, 91*(5), 558–575.

World Health Organization (2014). *WHO: Good hand hygiene by health workers protects patients from drug resistant infections.* Retrieved August 2014, from <www.who.int/mediacentre/news/releases/2014/hand-hygiene/en/>.

Chapter 16

American Society of PeriAnesthesia Nurses (ASPAN) (2012). *2012-2014 Perianesthesia nursing standards, practice recommendations and interpretive statements.* Cherry Hill, NJ: Author.

Association of periOperative Registered Nurses (AORN) (2014f). Recommended practices for information management. In *Perioperative standards and recommended practices* (pp. 443–464). Denver: Author.

Brooks, P. (2012). Postoperative delirium in elderly patients. *American Journal of Nursing, 112*(9), 38–49.

Collins, A. (2011). Postoperative nausea and vomiting in adults: Implications for critical care. *Critical Care Nurse, 31*(6), 36–45.

Eby, A. (2012). Best practices in postoperative feeding. *Nursing, 42*(6), 20–22.

Kibler, V. A., Hayes, R. M., Johnson, D. E., Anderson, L. W., Just, S. L., & Wells, N. L. (2012). Early postoperative ambulation: Back to basics. *American Journal of Nursing, 112*(4), 63–69.

Massey, R. (2012). Return of bowel sounds indicating an end of postoperative ileus: Is it time to cease this long-standing nursing tradition? *Medsurg Nursing, 21*(3), 146–150.

Myles, M. (2012). Preventing postoperative complications: Surgical Care Improvement Project guidelines. *Medsurg Nursing, 21*(6), 383–384.

Rothrock, J. C. (2011). *Alexander's care of the patient in surgery* (14th ed.). St. Louis: Mosby.

Sullivan, J. M. (2011). Caring for older adults after surgery. *Nursing, 41*(4), 48–51.

The Joint Commission (2014). *National Patient Safety Goals.* Retrieved January 2013, from <www.jointcommission.org/patientsafety/nationalpatientsafetygoals/>.

Ward, C. (2012). Fast track program to prevent postoperative ileus. *Medsurg Nursing, 21*(4), 214–220.

Ward, C. (2014). Procedure-specific postoperative pain management. *Medsurg Nursing, 23*(2), 107–110.

Wronski, S. (2014). Chew on this: Reducing postoperative ileus with chewing gum. *Nursing, 44*(8), 19–23.

Chapter 17

Abbas, A., Lichtman, A., & Pillai, S. (2012). *Cellular and molecular immunology* (7th ed.). Philadelphia: Saunders.

Alexander, E., & Susla, G. (2013). Postoperative transplant immunosuppression in the critical care unit. *AACN Advanced Critical Care, 24*(4), 345–350.

Kaufman, C. (2011). The secret life of lymphocytes. *Nursing, 41*(6), 50–54.

Chapter 18

*Almada, P., & Archer, R. (2009). Planning ahead for better outcomes: Preparation for joint replacement surgery begins at home! *Orthopaedic Nursing, 28*(1), 3–8.

Antonelli, M. C., & Starz, T. W. (2012). Assessing for risk and progression of osteoarthritis: The nurse's role. *Orthopaedic Nursing, 31*(2), 98–102.

Arthritis Foundation (2013a). *Gout.* Retrieved December 2013, from <www.arthritis.org/conditions-treatments/disease-center/gout/>.

Arthritis Foundation (2013b). *Osteoarthritis.* Retrieved December 2013, from <www.arthritis.org/conditions-treatments/disease-center/osteoarthritis/>.

Arthritis Foundation (2013c). *Who gets rheumatoid arthritis?* Retrieved December 2013, from <www.arthritis.org/who-gets-rheumatoid-arthritis.php>.

*Barbay, K. (2009). Research evidence for the use of preoperative exercise in patients preparing for total hip or total knee arthroplasty. *Orthopaedic Nursing, 28*(3), 127–133.

Cranwell-Bruce, L. A. (2011). Biological disease modifying anti-rheumatic drugs. *Medsurg Nursing, 20*(3), 147–151.

Davies, P. S. (2011). New developments in the treatment of osteoarthritis. *Pain Management Nursing, 12*(1), 817–822.

Firestein, G. S., Budd, R. C., Gabriel, S. E., McInnes, I. B., & O'Dell, J. R. (2013). *Kelley's textbook of rheumatology* (9th ed.). Philadelphia: Saunders.

Fouladbakhsh, J. (2012). Complementary and alternative modalities to relieve osteoarthritis symptoms. *Orthopaedic Nursing, 31*(2), 115–121.

*Galimba, J. (2009). Promoting the use of periarticular modal drug injection for total knee arthroplasty. *Orthopaedic Nursing, 28*(5), 250–254.

Gillaspie, M. (2010). Better pain management after total joint arthroplasty: A quality improvement approach. *Orthopaedic Nursing, 29*(1), 20–24.

Horse, J. S. (2010). Improving clinical outcomes with continuous passive motion: An interactive educational approach. *Orthopaedic Nursing, 29*(1), 27–33.

Kim, I.-S., Chung, S.-H., Park, Y.-J., & Kang, H. Y. (2012). The effectiveness of an aquarobic exercise program for patients with osteoarthritis. *Applied Nursing Research, 25*(3), 181–189.

Lupus Foundation of America (2014). *What is lupus?* Retrieved June 2014, from <http://www.lupus.org/answers/entry/what-is-lupus>.

Marchese, N. M., & Primer, S. R. (2013). Targeting Lyme disease. *Nursing, 43*(5), 28–33.

Mazaleski, A. (2011). Postoperative total joint replacement class for support persons: Enhancing patient and family centered care using a quality improvement model. *Orthopaedic Nursing, 30*(6), 361–364.

McFadden, B. (2013). Is there a safe coital position after a total hip arthroplasty? *Orthopaedic Nursing, 32*(4), 223–228.

Nelson, D. E. (2011). Perioperative care of the patient with rheumatoid arthritis. *AORN Journal, 94*(3), 290–300.

*Nussbaum, R. L., McInnes, R., & Willard, H. (2007). *Thompson & Thompson genetics in medicine* (7th ed.). Philadelphia: Saunders.

Parker, R. J. (2011). Evidence-based practice: Caring for a patient undergoing total knee arthroplasty. *Orthopaedic Nursing, 30*(1), 4–8.

Pellatino, M. (2012). Providing care for GLBTQ patients. *Nursing, 42*(12), 22–28.

*Pullen, R. L., Jr., Brewer, S., & Ballard, A. (2009). Putting a face on systemic lupus erythematosus. *Nursing, 39*(8), 22–28.

Regan, E. R., Phillips, F., & Magri, T. (2013). Get a leg (or two) up on total knee arthroplasty. *Nursing, 43*(7), 32–37.

*Remadevi, R., & Szallisi, A. (2008). Adlea (ALGRX-4975), an injectable capsaicin (TRPV1 receptor agonist) formulation for long-lasting pain relief. *Drugs, 11*(2), 120–132.

*Rutledge, D. N., Mouttapa, M., & Wood, P. B. (2009). Symptom clusters in fibromyalgia: Potential utility in patient assessment and treatment evaluation. *Nursing Research, 58*, 359–366.

Scleroderma Foundation (2013). *What is scleroderma?* Retrieved December 2013, from <www.scleroderma.org/site/PageServer?pagename=patients_whatis#.Ur0aYbSJI5M>.

Simmons, S. (2011). Recognizing and managing rheumatoid arthritis. *Nursing, 41*(7), 34–40.

Thomas, K. M., & Sethares, K. A. (2010). Is guided imagery effective in reducing pain and anxiety in the postoperative total joint arthroplasty patient? *Orthopaedic Nursing, 29*(6), 393–399.

Valdes, A. M., & Spector, T. D. (2011). The genetic epidemiology of osteoarthritis. *Current Opinions in Rheumatology, 22*(2), 139–143.

Shin, S. Y., & Kolanowski, A. M. (2010). Best evidence of psychosocially focused nonpharmacologic therapies for symptom management in older adults with osteoarthritis. *Pain Management Nursing, 11*(4), 234–244.

Zhang, W. W., Nuki, G., Moskowitz, R., Abramson, S., Altman, R. D., Arden, N. K., et al. (2010). OARSI recommendations for the management of hip and knee osteoarthritis, Part III: Changes in evidence following systematic cumulative update of research published through January 2009. *Osteoarthritis and Cartilage, 18*(4), 476–499.

Chapter 19

American Academy of HIV Medicine (2012). *AAHIVM fundamentals of HIV medicine for the HIV specialist* (12th ed.). Washington, DC: Author.

Anastasi, J., Capili, B., & Chang, M. (2013). HIV peripheral neuropathy and foot care management: A review of assessment and relevant guidelines. *The American Journal of Nursing, 113*(12), 34–40.

Aschenbrenner, D. (2012). Truvada: The first drug approved to prevent HIV infection. *The American Journal of Nursing, 112*(11), 20–21.

Blanc, F., Sok, T., Laureillard, D., Borand, L., Rekacewicz, C., Nerrienet, E., et al. (2011). Earlier versus later start of antiretroviral therapy in HIV-infected adults with tuberculosis. *New England Journal of Medicine, 365*(16), 1471–1481.

Carr, R., & Traufler, R. (2011). Immune reconstitution inflammatory syndrome in HIV-infected patients: What a critical-care nurse needs to know. *Dimensions of Critical Care Nursing, 30*(3), 139–143.

*Centers for Disease Control and Prevention (CDC). (1987). Public Health Service guidelines for counseling and antibody testing to prevent HIV infection and AIDS. *Morbidity and Mortality Weekly Report, 36*(31), 509–515.

*Centers for Disease Control and Prevention (CDC). (1991). Recommendations for preventing transmission of human immunodeficiency virus and hepatitis B virus to patients during exposure-prone invasive procedures. *Morbidity and Mortality Weekly Report, 40*(RR–8), 1–9.

*Centers for Disease Control and Prevention (CDC). (2005). Updated Public Health Service guidelines for the management of health-care worker exposure to HIV and recommendations for postexposure prophylaxis. *Morbidity and Mortality Weekly Report, 54*(RR–9), 1–22.

*Centers for Disease Control and Prevention (CDC). (2008). Recommendations and reports: Appendix A—AIDS-defining conditions. *Morbidity and Mortality Weekly Report, 57*(RR–10), 9.

*Centers for Disease Control and Prevention (CDC). (2009). Guidelines for prevention and treatment of opportunistic infections in HIV infected adults and adolescents. *Morbidity and Mortality Weekly Report, 58*(RR–4), 1–207.

Centers for Disease Control and Prevention (CDC) (2013a). *HIV in the United States: At a glance.* Retrieved December 2013, from <www.cdc.gov/hiv/resources/factsheets/PDF/stats_basics_factsheet.pdf>.

Centers for Disease Control and Prevention (CDC) (2013b). *HIV surveillance report, 2011* (Vol. 23). Retrieved April 2014, from <www.cdc.gov/hiv/topics/surveillance/resources/reports/>.

Cohen, M., Chen, Y., McCauley, M., Gamble, T., Hosseinipour, M., Kumarasamy, N., et al. (2011). Prevention of HIV-1 infection with early antiretroviral therapy. *New England Journal of Medicine, 365*(6), 493–505.

Foster, V., Clark, P., Holstad, M., & Burgess, E. (2012). Factors associated with risky sexual behaviors in older adults. *Journal of the Association of Nurses in AIDS Care, 23*(6), 487–499.

Hoogbruin, A. (2011). Complementary and alternative therapy (CAT) use and highly active antiretroviral therapy (HAART): Current evidence in the literature, 2000-2009. *Journal of Clinical Nursing, 20*(7–8), 925–939.

Kaufman, C. (2011). The secret life of lymphocytes. *Nursing, 41*(6), 50–54.

Keithley, J., & Swanson, B. (2013). HIV-associated wasting. *Journal of the Association of Nurses in AIDS Care, 24*(1S), S103–S111.

Kirton, C. (2011). The changing HIV epidemic. *Nursing, 41*(1), 36–43.

Kuznar, W., & Kayyali, A. (2011). Tuberculosis prevention in HIV-positive adults with latent disease. *The American Journal of Nursing, 111*(11), 59.

Lanier, Y., & Sutton, M. (2013). Reframing the context of preventive health care services and prevention of HIV and other sexually transmitted infections for young men: New opportunities to reduce racial/ethnic sexual health disparities. *American Journal of Public Health, 103*(2), 262–269.

New York State Department of Health AIDS Institute (2014). *Free compilation of current guidelines for clinical practice.* Retrieved April 2014, from <www.hivguidelines.org>.

Nokes, K., Johnson, M. O., Webel, A., Rose, C. D., Phillips, J. C., Sullivan, K., et al. (2012). Focus on increasing treatment self-efficacy to improve human immunodeficiency virus treatment adherence. *Journal of Nursing Scholarship, 44*(4), 403–410.

Pettinato, M. (2012). Providing care for GLBTQ patients. *Nursing, 42*(12), 22–27.

Starr, M., & Bradley-Springer, L. (2014). Nursing in the fourth decade of the HIV epidemic. *The American Journal of Nursing, 114*(3), 38–47.

World Health Organization (WHO) (2013). *Global epidemic: HIV/AIDS online questions and answers.* Retrieved April 2014, from <www.who.int/features/qa/71/en/index.html>.

Chapter 20

Abbas, A., Lichtman, A., & Pillai, S. (2012). *Cellular and molecular immunology* (7th ed.). Philadelphia: Saunders.

Arnold, J., & Williams, P. (2011). Anaphylaxis: Recognition and management. *American Family Physician, 84*(10), 1111–1118.

Bostock-Cox, B. (2013). Dealing with emergencies in general practice: Anaphylaxis. *Practice Nurse, 43*(4), 24–26.

Catanzaro, J., & Dinkel, S. (2014). Sjogren's syndrome: The hidden disease. *Medsurg Nursing, 23*(4), 219–221.

Caton, E., & Flynn, M. (2013). Management of anaphylaxis in the ED: A clinical audit. *International Emergency Nursing, 21*(1), 64–70.

Holmes, S., & Scullion, J. (2012). Allergic rhinitis: Assessment and treatment. *Nurse Prescribing, 10*(5), 222–228.

Norred, C. (2012). Anesthesia-induced anaphylaxis. *AANA Journal, 80*(2), 129–150.

Poetzsch, B. (2012). Sjögren syndrome. *Journal of the American Academy of Physician Assistants, 25*(1), 67–68.

Ruiz, C. (2012). Act immediately against anaphylaxis. *American Nurse Today, 7*(7), 18.

Simons, E., Ardusso, L., Bilo, M. B., El-Gamal, Y., Ledford, D., Ring, J., et al. (2011). World Allergy Organization guidelines for the assessment and management of anaphylaxis. *The World Allergy Organization Journal, 4*(2), 13–37.

Vacca, V., & McMahon-Bowen, E. (2013). Anaphylaxis. *Nursing, 43*(11), 16–17.

Wade, J. (2012). Care of the type 1 latex allergy patient. *Australian Nursing Journal, 19*(9), 30–33.

Chapter 21

American Cancer Society (ACS) (2010). *Cancer prevention and early detection: Facts & figures—2010.* Report No. 8600.10. Atlanta: Author.

American Cancer Society (ACS) (2012). *Cancer facts and figures for Hispanics/Latinos—2012-2014.* Report No. 862313. Atlanta: Author.

American Cancer Society (ACS) (2013). *Cancer facts and figures for African Americans—2013-2014.* Report No. 861413. Atlanta: Author.

American Cancer Society (ACS) (2014). *Cancer facts and figures—2014.* Report No. 00-300M–No. 500814. Atlanta: Author.

Beery, T. A., & Workman, M. L. (2012). *Genetics and genomics in nursing and health care.* Philadelphia: F.A. Davis.

Calzone, K., Masny, A., &Jenkins, J. (Eds.). (2010). *Genetics and genomics in oncology nursing practice.* Pittsburgh: Oncology Nursing Society.

Canadian Cancer Society, Statistics Canada (2014). *Canadian Cancer Statistics, 2014.* Toronto: Canadian Cancer Society.

Feero, G., Guttmacher, E., & Collins, F. (2010). Genomic medicine: An updated primer. *New England Journal of Medicine, 362*, 2001–2011.

Santos, E. M., Edwards, Q. T., Floria-Santos, M., Rogatto, S. R., Achatz, M. I., & MacDonald, D. J. (2013). Integration of genomics in cancer care. *Journal of Nursing Scholarship, 45*(1), 43–51.

U.S. Department of Health and Human Services (USDHHS), Public Health Service, National Toxicology Program (2011). *Report on carcinogens* (12th ed.). Retrieved August 2014, from <http://ntp.niehs.nih.gov/go/roc12>.

Chapter 22

Abbas, A., Lichtman, A., & Pillai, S. (2012). *Cellular and molecular immunology* (7th ed.). Philadelphia: Saunders.

Agostinis, P., Berg, K., Cengel, K. A., Foster, T. H., Girotti, A. W., Gollnick, S. O., et al. (2011). Photodynamic therapy of cancer: An update. *CA: A Cancer Journal for Clinicians, 61*(4), 250–281.

American Cancer Society (2014). *Cancer facts and figures—2014.* Report No. 00-300M–No. 500814. Atlanta: Author.

Barak, F., Amoyal, M., & Kalichman, L. (2013). Using a simple diary for management of nausea and vomiting during chemotherapy. *Clinical Journal of Oncology Nursing, 17*(5), 479–481.

Beatty, K., Winkelman, C., Bokar, J., & Mazanec, P. (2011). Targeted therapies. *AACN Advanced Critical Care, 22*(4), 323–334.

Bergstrom, K. (2011). Development of a radiation skin care protocol and algorithm using the Iowa Model of Evidence-Based Practice.

Clinical Journal of Oncology Nursing, 15(5), 593–595.

Binner, M., Ross, D., & Browner, I. (2011). Chemotherapy-induced peripheral neuropathy: Assessment of oncology nurses' knowledge and practice. *Oncology Nursing Forum, 38*(4), 448–454.

Borsellino, M., & Young, M. (2011). Anticipatory coping: Taking control of hair loss. *Clinical Journal of Oncology Nursing, 15*(3), 311–315.

Boucher, J., Habin, K., & Underhill, M. (2014). Cancer genetics and genomics: Essentials for oncology nurses. *Clinical Journal of Oncology Nursing, 18*(3), 355–359.

Buck, H. (2012). Real-world symptom management. *Nursing, 42*(3), 18–19.

Byar, K., & Workman, M. (2012). Targeted therapies to treat cancer. In J. Kee, E. Hayes, & L. McCuistion (Eds.), *Pharmacology: A nursing process approach* (7th ed., pp. 543–567). St. Louis: Saunders.

Canadian Cancer Society, Statistics Canada (2014). *Canadian cancer statistics, 2014.* Toronto: Canadian Cancer Society.

Cherwin, C. (2012). Gastrointestinal symptom representation in cancer symptom clusters: A synthesis of the literature. *Oncology Nursing Forum, 39*(2), 157–165.

Dalby, C., Nesbitt, M., Frechette, C., Kennerley, K., Lacoursiere, L., & Buswell, L. (2013). Standardization of initial chemotherapy teaching to improve care. *Clinical Journal of Oncology Nursing, 17*(5), 472–475.

Davey, M. (2013). Improving adherence to oral anticancer therapy. *Nursing, 43*(9), 31–36.

Davidson, W., Teleni, L., Muller, J., Ferguson, M., McCarthy, A. L., Vick, J., et al. (2012). Malnutrition and chemotherapy-induced nausea and vomiting: Implications for practice. *Oncology Nursing Forum, 39*(4), E340–E345.

Denshar, R., Vanek, R., & Mazanec, P. (2011). Oncologic emergencies: New decade, new perspectives. *AACN Advanced Critical Care, 22*(4), 337–348.

Given, B. A., Given, C. W., & Sherwood, P. R. (2012). Family and caregiver needs over the course of the cancer trajectory. *Journal of Supportive Oncology, 10*(2), 57–64.

Gonzales, T. (2013). Chemotherapy extravasations: Prevention, identification, management, and documentation. *Clinical Journal of Oncology Nursing, 17*(1), 61–66.

Held-Warmkessel, J. (2011). Taming three high-risk chemotherapy complications. *Nursing, 41*(11), 30–37.

Kanaskie, M. (2012). Chemotherapy-related cognitive changes: A principle-based concept analysis. *Oncology Nursing Forum, 39*(3), E241–E248.

Limburg, C., Maxwell, C., & Mautner, B. (2014). Prevention and treatment of bone loss in patients with nonmetastatic breast or prostate cancer who receive hormone ablation therapy. *Clinical Journal of Oncology Nursing, 18*(2), 223–230.

Mackiewicz, T. (2012). Prevention of tumor lysis syndrome in an outpatient setting. *Clinical Journal of Oncology Nursing, 16*(2), 189–193.

Maloney, K., & Denno, M. (2011). Tumor lysis syndrome: Prevention and detection to enhance patient safety. *Clinical Journal of Oncology Nursing, 15*(6), 601–603.

Myers, J. (2012). Chemotherapy-related cognitive impairment: The breast cancer experience. *Oncology Nursing Forum, 39*(1), E31–E40.

Neuss, M., Polovich, M., McNiff, K., Esper, P., Gilmore, T., LeFebvre, K., et al. (2013). 2013 updated American Society of Clinical Oncology/Oncology Nursing Society chemotherapy safety standards including standards for the safe administration and management of oral chemotherapy. *Oncology Nursing Forum, 40*(3), 225–233.

Northouse, L. L. (2012). Helping patients and their family caregivers cope with cancer. *Oncology Nursing Forum, 39*(5), 500–506.

Poirier, P. (2011). The impact of fatigue on role functioning during radiation therapy. *Oncology Nursing Forum, 38*(4), 457–465.

Polovich, M., & Martin, S. (2011). Nurses' use of hazardous drug-handling precautions and awareness of national safety guidelines. *Oncology Nursing Forum, 38*(6), 718–726.

Proud, C. (2014). Radiogenomics: The promise of personalized treatment in radiation oncology? *Clinical Journal of Oncology Nursing, 18*(2), 185–189.

Running, A., & Turnbeaugh, E. (2011). Oncology pain and complementary therapy: A review of the literature. *Clinical Journal of Oncology Nursing, 15*(4), 374–379.

Ruppert, R. (2011). Radiation therapy 101: What you need to know to help cancer patients understand their treatment and cope with side effects. *American Nurse Today, 6*(1), 24–29.

Santos, E. M. M., Edwards, Q. T., Floria-Santos, M., Rogatto, S. R., Achatz, M. I. W., & MacDonald, D. J. (2013). Integration of genomics in cancer care. *Journal of Nursing Scholarship, 45*(1), 43–51.

Schulmeister, L. (2014). Safe management of chemotherapy: Infusion-related complications. *Clinical Journal of Oncology Nursing, 18*(3), 283–287.

Serra, D., Parris, C. R., Carper, E., Homel, P., Fleishman, S. B., Harrison, L. B., et al. (2012). Outcomes of guided imagery in patients receiving radiation therapy for breast cancer. *Clinical Journal of Oncology Nursing, 16*(6), 617–622.

Shaw, C., & Taylor, L. (2012). Treatment-related diarrhea in patients with cancer. *Clinical Journal of Oncology Nursing, 16*(4), 413–417.

Sheldon, L. K., Harris, D., & Arcieri, D. (2012). Psychosocial concerns in cancer care: The role of the oncology nurse. *Clinical Journal of Oncology Nursing, 16*(3), 316–319.

Tofthagen, C., McAllister, D., & McMillan, S. (2011). Peripheral neuropathy in patients with colorectal cancer receiving oxaliplatin. *Clinical Journal of Oncology Nursing, 15*(2), 182–188.

Vachani, C., Di Lullo, G., Hampshire, M. K., Hill-Kayser, C. E., & Metz, J. M. (2011). Nursing resources: Preparing patients for life after cancer treatment. *American Journal of Nursing, 111*(4), 51–55.

Walton, A. M., Mason, S., Busshart, M., Spruill, A. D., Cheek, S., Lane, A., et al. (2012). Safe handling: Implementing hazardous drug precautions. *Clinical Journal of Oncology Nursing, 16*(3), 251–254.

Wanchai, A., Armer, J., & Stewart, B. (2011). Nonpharmacologic supportive strategies to promote quality of life in patients experiencing cancer-related fatigue: A systematic review. *Clinical Journal of Oncology Nursing, 15*(2), 203–214.

Wiencek, C., Ferrell, B., & Jackson, M. (2011). The meaning of our work: Caring for the critically ill patient with cancer. *AACN Advanced Critical Care, 22*(4), 397–407.

Yagasaki, K., & Kumatsu, H. (2013). The need for a nursing presence in oral chemotherapy. *Clinical Journal of Oncology Nursing, 17*(5), 512–516.

Yu, H., Friedlander, D. R., Patel, S., & Hu, J. C. (2013). The current status of robotic oncologic surgery. *CA: A Cancer Journal for Clinicians, 63*(1), 45–56.

Chapter 23

Alspach, J. G. (2014). About that health care icon dangling around your neck: Do we have some cleaning up to do? *Critical Care Nurse, 34*(4), 11–14.

*Backman, C., Zoutman, D. E., & Marck, P. B. (2008). An integrative review of the current evidence on the relationship between hand hygiene interventions and the incidence of health care–associated infections. *American Journal of Infection Control, 36*(5), 333–348.

Barnes, B. E., & Sampson, D. A. (2011). A literature review on community-acquired methicillin-resistant *Staphylococcus aureus* in the United States: Clinical information for primary care nurse practitioners. *Journal of the Academy of Nurse Practitioners, 23*(1), 23–32.

*Centers for Disease Control and Prevention (CDC). (2002). Guideline for hand hygiene in health-care settings: Recommendations of the Healthcare Infection Control Practices Advisory Committee and the HICPAC/SHEA/APIC/IDSA Hand Hygiene Task Force. *Morbidity and Mortality Weekly Report, 51*(RR–16), 1–44.

Centers for Disease Control and Prevention (CDC) (2013). *2012 CRE toolkit: Guidance for control of carbapenem-resistant Enterobacteriaceae, Part 1: Facility-level CRE prevention.* Retrieved January 2014, from <www.cdc.gov/hai/organisms/cre/cre-toolkit/f-level-prevention-supmeasures.html>.

Centers for Disease Control and Prevention (CDC) (2014). *Ebola (Ebola virus disease).* Retrieved October 2014, from <www.cdc.gov/vhf/ebola/>.

*Childs, S. G. (2008). Biofilm: The pathogenesis of slime glycocalyx. *Orthopedic Nursing, 27*(6), 361–368.

Foulk, K. C., Tocydlowski, P., Snow, T. M., McCloud, K., Cuevas, M., Bishop, D., et al. (2012). Infusing fun into quality and safety initiatives. *Nursing, 41*(11), 14–16.

Grossman, S., & Mager, D. (2010). *Clostridium difficile:* Implications for nursing. *Medsurg Nursing, 19*(3), 155–158.

Kassakian, S. Z., Mermel, L. A., Jefferson, J. A., Parenteau, S. L., & Machan, J. T. (2011). Impact of chlorhexidine bathing on hospital-acquired infections among general medical patients. *Infection Control and Hospital Epidemiology, 32*(3), 238–243.

*Lo, S. F., Hayter, M., Change, C. J., Wu, W. Y., & Lee, L. L. (2008). A systematic review of silver-releasing dressings in the management of infected chronic wounds. *Journal of Clinical Nursing, 17*(15), 1973–1985.

Lopez-Bushnell, K., Demaroy, W. S., & Jaco, C. (2014). Reducing sepsis mortality. *Medsurg Nursing, 23*(1), 9–14.

Ly, E. (2013). A closer look at hantavirus. *Nursing, 43*(9), 65–66.

Mori, C. (2014). A-voiding catastrophe: Implementing a nurse-driven protocol. *Medsurg Nursing, 23*(1), 15–21, 28.

Myers, F. (2011). Beyond mainstream: Making the case for fecal bacteriotherapy. *Nursing, 41*(12), 50–53.

Palese, A., Buchini, S., Deroma, L., & Bartone, F. (2010). The effectiveness of the ultrasound bladder scanner in reducing urinary tract infections: A meta-analysis. *Journal of Clinical Nursing, 19*(21–22), 2970–2979.

*Parker, D., Callan, L., Harwood, J., Thompson, D. L., Wilde, M., & Gray, M. (2009). Nursing interventions to reduce the risk of catheter-associated urinary tract infection, Part 1: Catheter selection. *Journal of Wound, Ostomy, Continence Nursing, 36*(1), 23–34.

Powers, J., Peed, J., Burns, L., & Ziemba-Davis, M. (2012). Chlorhexidine bathing and microbial contamination in patients' bath basins. *American Journal of Critical Care, 21*(5), 338–342.

Powers, J., & Fortney, S. (2014). Bed baths: Much more than a basic nursing task. *Nursing, 44*(10), 67–68.

Ramage, G., Culshaw, S., Jones, B., & Williams, C. (2010). Are we any closer to beating the biofilm: Novel methods of biofilm control. *Current Opinion in Infectious Disease, 23*(6), 560–566.

Rosini, J. M., & Srivastava, N. (2013). Understanding vancomycin levels. *Nursing, 43*(11), 66–67.

*Siegel, J. D., Rhinehart, E., Jackson, M., Chiarello, L., & Healthcare Infection Control Practices Advisory Committee (2007). *Guidelines for isolation precautions: Preventing transmission of infectious agents in healthcare settings 2007.* Atlanta: CDC.

Simko, L. (2012). Breaking sterility: Dealing with procedural violations in health care. *Nursing, 42*(8), 22–26.

Snow, M. (2011). *Clostridium difficile:* Trouble for adults and children. *Nursing, 41*(8), 67–68.

Stickler, D. J., & Feneley, R. C. (2010). The encrustation and blockage of long-term indwelling catheters: A way forward in prevention and control. *Spinal Cord, 48*(11), 784–790.

Upshaw-Owens, M., & Bailey, C. A. (2012). Preventing hospital-associated infection: MRSA. *Medsurg Nursing, 21*(2), 77–80.

Chapter 24

American Cancer Society (2014). *Cancer facts and figures—2014.* Report No. 00-300M–No. 500814. Atlanta: Author.

Cross, H. H. (2014). Obtaining a wound swab culture specimen. *Nursing, 44*(7), 68–69.

*Gaskin, F. C. (1986). Detection of cyanosis in the person with dark skin. *Journal of National Black Nurses' Association, 1*(1), 52–60.

LeBlanc, K., & Baranowski, S. (2011). Skin tears: State of the science: Consensus statements for the prevention, prediction, assessment, and treatment of skin tears. *Advances in Skin & Wound Care, 24*(9), 2–15.

Marks, J., & Miller, J. (2013). *Lookingbill and Marks' principles of dermatology* (5th ed.). Philadelphia: Saunders.

McEnroe-Petitte, D. (2011). Melanoma. *Nursing, 41*(5), 45.

Siegel, V. (2012). Adding patient education of skin cancer and sun-protective behaviors to the skin assessment screening on admission to hospitals. *Medsurg Nursing, 21*(3), 183–184.

The Skin Cancer Foundation (2014). *Understanding melanoma—Warning signs: The ABCDEs of melanoma.* Retrieved September 2014, from <www.skincancer.org/skin-cancer-information/melanoma>.

Chapter 25

Ackerman, C. (2011). "Not on my watch": Treating and preventing pressure ulcers. *Medsurg Nursing, 20*(2), 86–93.

Adams, S., Sabesan, V., & Easley, M. (2012). Wound healing agents. *Critical Care Nursing Clinics of North America, 24*(2), 255–260.

Alderden, J., Whitney, J., Taylor, S., & Zaratkiewicz, S. (2011). Risk profile characteristics associated with outcomes of hospital-acquired pressure ulcers: A retrospective review. *Critical Care Nurse, 31*(4), 30–42.

Ambutas, S., Staffileno, B., & Fogg, L. (2014). Reducing nasal pressure ulcers with an alternative taping device. *Medsurg Nursing, 23*(2), 96–100.

American Cancer Society (ACS) (2014). *Cancer facts and figures 2014.* Report No. 00-300M– No. 500814. Atlanta: Author.

Armour-Burton, T., Fields, W., Outlaw, L., & Deleon, E. (2013). The healthy skin project: Changing nursing practice to prevent and treat hospital-acquired pressure ulcers. *Critical Care Nurse, 33*(3), 32–39.

Ayello, E., & Baranoski, S. (2014). Wound care and prevention. *Nursing, 44*(4), 32–40.

Barnes, E., & Murray, B. (2013). Bedbugs: What nurses need to know. *The American Journal of Nursing, 113*(10), 58–62.

Beitz, J. (2012). Wound debridement: Therapeutic options and care considerations. *Critical Care Nursing Clinics of North America, 24*(2), 239–253.

Bolton, L., Girolami, S., & Hurlow, J. (2013). The AAWC pressure ulcer guidelines. *The American Journal of Nursing, 113*(9), 58–63.

Bryce, J., & Passoni, C. (2013). Nursing management of patients with metastatic melanoma receiving ipilimumab. *Oncology Nursing Forum, 40*(3), 215–218.

Cooper, K. (2012). Drug reaction, skin care, skin loss. *Critical Care Nurse, 32*(4), 52–58.

Cowdell, F. (2011). Older people, personal hygiene, and skin care. *Medsurg Nursing, 20*(5), 235–240.

Cross, H. H. (2014). Obtaining a wound swab culture specimen. *Nursing, 44*(7), 68–69.

Demidova-Rice, T., Hamblin, M., & Herman, I. (2012a). Acute and impaired wound healing: Pathophysiology and current methods for drug delivery, Part 1: Normal and chronic wounds: Biology, causes, and approaches to care. *Advances in Skin & Wound Care, 25*(7), 304–314.

Demidova-Rice, T., Hamblin, M., & Herman, I. (2012b). Acute and impaired wound healing: Pathophysiology and current methods for drug delivery, Part 2: Role of growth factors in normal and pathological wound healing: Therapeutic potential and methods of delivery. *Advances in Skin & Wound Care, 25*(8), 349–370.

Estilo, M., Angeles, A., Perez, T., Hernandez, M., & Valdez, M. (2012). Pressure ulcers in the intensive care unit: New perspectives on an old problem. *Critical Care Nurse, 32*(3), 65–70.

Goldberg, S., & Diegelmann, R. (2012). Wound healing primer. *Critical Care Nursing Clinics of North America, 24*(2), 165–178.

LeBlanc, K., & Christensen, D. (2011). Demystifying skin tears, Part 2. *Nursing, 41*(7), 16–17.

LeBlanc, K., & Baranoski, S. (2014). Skin tears: Best practices for care and prevention. *Nursing, 44*(5), 36–46.

Li, D., & Korniewicz, D. (2013). Determination of the effectiveness of electronic health records to document pressure ulcers. *Medsurg Nursing, 22*(1), 17–25.

Lyder, C. H., Wang, Y., Metersky, M., Curry, M., Kliman, R., Verzier, N. R., et al. (2012). Hospital-acquired pressure ulcers: Results from the national Medicare Patient Safety Monitoring System study. *Journal of the American Geriatrics Society, 60*(9), 1603–1608.

Marks, J. G., Jr., & Miller, J. (2013). *Lookingbill & Mark's principles of dermatology* (5th ed.). Philadelphia: Saunders.

Mayo, T., & Cantrell, W. (2014). Putting onchomycosis under the microscope. *The Nurse Practitioner, 39*(5), 8–11.

Moreira, M., & Markovchick, M. (2012). Wound management. *Critical Care Nursing Clinics of North America, 24*(2), 215–237.

Napierkowski, D. (2013). Uncovering common bacterial skin infections. *The Nurse Practitioner, 38*(3), 30–37.

National Pressure Ulcer Advisory Panel, European Pressure Ulcer Advisory Panel, & Pan Pacific Pressure Injury Alliance (2014). *Prevention and treatment of pressure ulcers: Quick reference guide.* Perth, Australia: Cambridge Media. Retrieved Septermber 2014, from <www.npuap.org/wp-content/uploads/2014/08/Quick-Reference-Guide-DIGITAL-NPUAP-EPUAP-PPPIA.pdf>.

Nelson, M., & Harris, R. (2013). Pressure ulcer alert! *Nursing, 43*(11), 64–67.

Online Mendelian Inheritance in Man (OMIM) (2014a). *Melanoma, cutaneous malignant, Susceptibility to, 1; CMM1.* Retrieved September 2014, from <www.omim.org/entry/155600>.

Online Mendelian Inheritance in Man (OMIM) (2014b). Psoriasis, Susceptibility1; *PSORS1.* Retrieved September 2014, from <www.omim.org/entry/177900>.

Passalacqua, S., DiRocco, Z., DiPietro, C., Mozzetta, A., Tabolli, S., Scoppola, A., et al. (2012). Information needs of patients with melanoma: A nursing challenge. *Clinical Journal of Oncology Nursing, 16*(6), 625–632.

Posthauer, M. E. (2012). The role of nutrition in wound care. *Advances in Skin & Wound Care, 25*(2), 62–63.

Rock, R. (2011). Get positive results with negative-pressure wound therapy. *American Nurse Today, 6*(1), 49–51.

Rubin, K. (2012). Managing immune-related adverse events to ipilimumab: A nurse's guide. *Clinical Journal of Oncology Nursing, 16*(2), E69–E75.

Sardina, D. (2013). Is your wound-cleansing practice up to date? *American Nurse Today, 8*(7), 37–38.

Schaefer, P. (2011). Urticaria: Evaluation and treatment. *American Family Physician, 83*(9), 1078–1084.

The Skin Cancer Foundation (2014). *Understanding melanoma—Warning signs: The ABCDEs of melanoma.* Retrieved September 2014, from <www.skincancer.org/skin-cancer-information/melanoma>.

van Rijswijk, L. (2013). Measuring wounds to improve outcomes. *The American Journal of Nursing, 113*(8), 60–61.

Williams, J., & Barbul, A. (2012). Nutrition and wound healing. *Critical Care Nursing Clinics of North America, 24*(2), 179–200.

Wong, J., & Woo, J. Y. (2012). The safety of systemic treatments that can be used for geriatric psoriasis patients: A review. *Dermatology Research and Practice, 2012,* 1–4.

Woo, K., Coutts, P., & Sibbald, R. G. (2012). Continuous topical oxygen for the treatment of chronic wounds: A pilot study. *Advances in Skin & Wound Care, 25*(12), 543–547.

Yu, N., Long, X., Lujan-Hernandez, J., Hassan, K., Bai, M., Wang, Y., et al. (2013). Marjolin's ulcer: A preventable malignancy arising from scars. *World Journal of Surgical Oncology,* doi:10.1186/1477-7819-11-313; Retrieved September 2014, from <http://www.wjso.com/content/11/1/313>.

Chapter 26

Alharbi, Z., Piatkowski, A., Dembinski, R., Reckort, S., Grieb, G., Kauczok, J., et al. (2012). Treatment of burns in the first 24 hours: Simple and practical guide by answering 10 questions in a step-by-step form. *World Journal of Emergency Surgery, 7*(1), 13–22.

American Burn Association (ABA) (2012). *National Burn Repository: Summary of the findings 2002-2011.* Website <www.ameriburn.org>.

Aziz, Z., Abu, S. F., & Chong, N. J. (2012). A systematic review of silver-containing dressings and topical silver agents (used with dressings) for burn wounds. *Burns, 38*(3), 307–318.

Badger, K., & Royse, D. (2012). Describing compassionate care: The burn survivor's perspective. *Journal of Burn Care & Research, 33*(6), 772–780.

Bidwell, K., Miller, S., Coffey, R., Calvitti, K., Porter, K., & Murphy, C. (2013). Evaluation of the safety and efficacy of a nursing-driven midazolam protocol for management of procedural pain associated with burn injuries. *Journal of Burn Care & Research, 34*(1), 176–182.

Bishop, S., Walker, M., & Spivak, I. (2013). Family presence in the adult burn intensive care unit during dressing changes. *Critical Care Nurse, 33*(1), 14–23.

Brown-Guttovz, H. (2011). Burn injury. *Nursing, 41*(5), 72.

Butcher, M., & Swales, B. (2012). Assessment and management of patients with burns. *Nursing Standard, 27*(2), 50–56.

Carrougher, G., Martinez, E., McMullen, K., Fauerbach, J., Holavanahalli, R., Herndon, D., et al. (2012). Pruritus in adult burn survivors: Prevalence and risk factors associated with increased intensity. *Journal of Burn Care & Research, 34*(1), 94–101.

Coffey, R., & Murphy, C. (2012). Effects of alcohol use and abuse on critically ill burn patients. *Critical Care Nursing Clinics of North America, 24*(1), 1–7.

Culleiton, A., & Simko, L. (2013a). Caring for patients with burn injuries. *Nursing, 43*(8), 26–34.

Culleiton, A., & Simko, L. (2013b). Caring for patients with burn injuries. *Nursing Critical Care, 8*(1), 14–22.

Culleiton, A., & Simko, L. (2013c). Managing burn injuries in the ICU. *Nursing Critical Care, 8*(2), 22–30.

Dahl, O., Wickman, M., & Wengstrom, Y. (2012). Adapting to life after burn injury: Reflections on care. *Journal of Burn Care & Research, 33*(5), 595–605.

Fahlstrom, K., Boyle, C., & Makic, M. B. (2013). Implementation of a nurse-driven burn resuscitation protocol: A quality improvement project. *Critical Care Nurse, 33*(1), 25–35.

Hardwicke, J., Thomsom, R., Bamford, A., & Moiemen, N. (2013). A pilot evaluation study of high resolution digital thermal imaging in the assessment of burn depth. *Burns, 39*(1), 76–81.

Herndon, D. (2013). *Total burn care* (4th ed.). Philadelphia: Saunders.

Laing, C. (2013). Acute carbon monoxide toxicity: Be alert for this easy-to-miss illness. *Nursing Critical Care, 8*(1), 30–34.

Lewis, C. (2013). Stem cell application in acute burn care and reconstruction. *Journal of Wound Care, 11*(1), 7–16.

Murabit, A., & Tredget, E. (2012). Review of burn injuries secondary to home oxygen. *Journal of Burn Care & Research, 33*(2), 212–217.

Park, Y., Choi, Y., Lee, H., Moon, D., Kim, S., Lee, J., et al. (2013). The impact of laser Doppler imaging on the early decision-making process for surgical intervention in adults with indeterminate burns. *Burns, 39*(4), 655–661.

Silverstein, P., Heimbach, D., Meites, H., Latenser, B., Mozingo, D., Mullins, F., et al. (2011). An open, parallel, randomized, comparative, multicenter study to evaluate the cost-effectiveness, performance, tolerance, and safety of a silver-containing soft silicone foam dressing (intervention) vs sulfadiazine cream. *Journal of Burn Care & Research, 32*(6), 617–626.

Weimer, S., Staubli, L., & Makic, M. B. (2013). Fending off disaster for a frostbite victim. *American Nurse Today, 8*(1), 20.

Williams, F., Ludwik, K., Jeschke, M., & Herndon, D. (2011). What, how, and how much should burn patients be fed? *Surgical Clinics of North America, 91*(3), 609–629.

Chapter 27

American Lung Association (2012). *The LBGT community: A priority population for tobacco control.* Retrieved May 2014, from <www.lung.org/stop-smoking/tobacco-control-advocacy/reports-resources/tobacco-policy-trend>.

Baker, K., Barsamian, J., Leone, D., Donovan, B., Williams, D., Carnevale, K., et al. (2013). Routine dyspnea assessment on unit admission. *The American Journal of Nursing, 113*(11), 42–49.

Barnette, L., & Kautz, D. (2013). Creative ways to teach arterial blood gas interpretation. *Dimensions of Critical Care Nursing, 32*(2), 84–87.

Bauman, M., & Cosgrove, C. (2012). Understanding end-tidal CO2 monitoring. *American Nurse Today, 7*(11), 12–17.

Butler, K., Fallin, A., & Ridner, L. (2012). Evidence-based smoking cessation for college students. *Nursing Clinics of North America, 47*(1), 21–30.

Carlisle, H. (2014). The case for capnography in patients receiving opioids. *American Nurse Today, 9*(9), 22–26.

Fiala, S., Morris, D., & Pawlak, R. (2012). Measuring indoor air quality of hookah lounges. *American Journal of Public Health, 102*(11), 2043–2045.

Grief, S. (2011). Nicotine dependence: Health consequences, smoking cessation therapies, and pharmacotherapy. *Primary Care Clinics in Office Practice, 38*(1), 23–39.

Johnson, C., Anderson, M. A., & Hill, P. (2012). Comparison of pulse oximetry measures in a healthy population. *Medsurg Nursing, 21*(2), 70–75.

King, B. A., Dube, S. R., & Tynan, M. A. (2012). Current tobacco use among adults in the United States: Findings from the National Adult Tobacco Survey. *American Journal of Public Health, 102*, 93–100.

Lee, J., Blosnich, J., & Melvin, C. (2012). Up in smoke: Vanishing evidence of tobacco disparities in the Institute of Medicine's report on sexual and gender minority health. *American Journal of Public Health, 102*(11), 2041–2043.

MacIntyre, N. (2012). The future of pulmonary function testing. *Respiratory Care, 57*(1), 154–161.

Meridith, T., & Massey, D. (2011). Respiratory assessment 1: More key skills to improve care. *Journal of Cardiovascular Nursing, 6*(2), 63–68.

Murgu, S., Pecson, J., & Colt, H. (2011). Flexible bronchoscopy assisted by noninvasive positive pressure ventilation. *Critical Care Nurse, 31*(3), 70–76.

Passion, C., Matsumoto, K., & Day, D. (2011). Benzocaine puts a patient in a bind. *American Nurse Today, 6*(11), 25.

Riker, C., Lee, K., Darville, E., & Hahn, E. (2012). E-cigarettes: Promise or peril? *Nursing Clinics of North America, 47*(1), 159–171.

Ruppel, G., & Enright, P. (2012). Pulmonary function testing. *Respiratory Care, 57*(1), 165–175.

Wesley, C. (2014). Understanding acquired methemoglobinemia. *Nursing, 44*(2), 67.

Chapter 28

Abdo, W., & Heunks, L. (2012). Oxygen-induced hypercapnia in COPD: Myths and facts. *Critical Care, 16*(5), 323–326.

Ambutas, S., Staffileno, B., & Fogg, L. (2014). Reducing nasal pressure ulcers with an alternative taping device. *Medsurg Nursing, 23*(2), 96–100.

Bullard, D., Brothers, K., Davis, C., Kingsley, E., & Waters, J., III. (2012). Contraindications to nasopharyngeal airway insertion. *Nursing, 42*(10), 66–67.

Carlisle, H. (2014). The case for capnography in patients receiving opioids. *American Nurse Today, 9*(9), 22–26.

Dailey, C., Tola, D., & Kesten, K. (2012). Providing safe passage: Rapid sequence intubation for advanced practice nursing. *AACN Advanced Critical Care, 23*(3), 270–283.

Lamar, J. (2012). Relationship of respiratory care bundle with incentive spirometry to reduced pulmonary complications in a medical general practice unit. *Medsurg Nursing, 21*(1), 33–36.

Mac Sweeney, R., McAuley, D. F., & Matthay, M. A. (2011). Acute lung failure. *Seminars in Respiratory and Critical Care Medicine, 32*(5), 607–625.

Makic, M. B., Martin, S., Burns, S., Philbrick, D., & Rauen, C. (2013). Putting evidence into nursing practice: Four traditional practices not supported by the evidence. *Critical Care Nurse, 33*(2), 28–42.

Morris, L., McIntosh, E., & Whitmer, A. (2014). The importance of tracheostomy progression in the intensive care unit. *Critical Care Nurse, 34*(1), 40–48.

Morris, L., Whitmer, A., & McIntosh, E. (2013). Tracheostomy care and complications in the intensive care unit. *Critical Care Nurse, 33*(5), 18–30.

Murabit, A., & Tredget, E. (2012). Review of burn injuries secondary to home oxygen. *Journal of Burn Care & Research, 33*(2), 212–217.

Overdyk, F., & Guerra, J. (2011). Improving outcomes in med-surg patients with opioid-induced respiratory depression. *American Nurse Today, 6*(11), 26–30.

Rahu, M., Grap, M., Cohn, J., Munro, C., Lyon, D., & Sessler, C. (2013). Facial expression as an indicator of pain in critically ill intubated adults during endotracheal suctioning. *American Journal of Critical Care, 22*(5), 412–422.

Reed, C., Reineck, C., & Fonseca, I. (2011). Communicating with intubated patients: A new approach. *American Nurse Today, 6*(7), 34–35.

Simons, S., & Abdallah, L. (2012). Bedside assessment of enteral tube placement: Aligning practice with evidence. *American Journal of Nursing, 112*(2), 40–47.

Sole, M. L., Su, X., Talbert, S., Penover, D., Kalita, S., Jimenez, E., et al. (2011). Evaluation of an intervention to maintain endotracheal tube cuff pressure within therapeutic range. *American Journal of Critical Care, 20*(2), 109–118.

Stepter, C. (2012). Maintaining placement of temporary enteral feeding tubes in adults: A critical appraisal of the evidence. *Medsurg Nursing, 21*(2), 61–68.

Chapter 29

American Cancer Society (ACS) (2014). *Cancer facts and figures, 2014.* 01-300M–No. 500814. Atlanta: Author.

Ardilio, S. (2011). Calculating nutrition needs for a patient with head and neck cancer. *Clinical Journal of Oncology Nursing, 15*(5), 457–459.

Boucher, J., Olson, L., & Piperdi, B. (2011). Preemptive management of dermatologic toxicities associated with epidermal growth factor receptor inhibitors. *Clinical Journal of Oncology Nursing, 15*(5), 501–508.

Callaway, C. (2011). Rethinking the head and neck cancer population: The human papillomavirus association. *Clinical Journal of Oncology Nursing, 15*(2), 165–170.

Canadian Cancer Society, Statistics Canada (2014). *Canadian cancer statistics, 2014.* Toronto: Canadian Cancer Society.

Carlucci, M., Smith, M., & Corbridge, S. (2013). Poor sleep, hazardous breathing. *The Nurse Practitioner, 38*(3), 20–28.

Fletcher, B., Cohen, M., Schumacher, K., & Lydiatt, W. (2012). A blessing and a curse: Head and neck cancer survivors' experiences. *Cancer Nursing, 35*(2), 126–132.

Haisfield-Wolfe, M. E., McGuire, D., & Krumm, S. (2012). Perspectives on coping among patients with head and neck cancer receiving radiation. *Oncology Nursing Forum, 39*(3), E249–E257.

Happ, M. B., Garrett, K., Thomas, D., Tate, J., George, E., Houze, M., et al. (2011). Nurse-patient communication interactions in the intensive care unit. *American Journal of Critical Care, 20*(2), e28–e40.

Mannix, C., Bartholomay, M., Doherty, C., Lewis, M., & Bilodeau, M. L. (2012). A feasibility study of low-cost, self-administered skin care interventions in patients with head and neck cancer receiving chemoradiation. *Clinical Journal of Oncology Nursing, 16*(3), 278–285.

Mason, H., DeRubeis, M., Foster, J., Tayloe, J., & Worden, F. (2013). Outcomes evaluation of a weekly nurse practitioner-managed symptom management clinic for patients with head and neck cancer treated with chemotherapy. *Oncology Nursing Forum, 40*(6), 581–586.

McLaughlin, L. (2013). Taste dysfunction in head and neck cancer survivors. *Oncology Nursing Forum, 40*(1), E4–E13.

Nance-Floyd, B. (2011). Tracheostomy care: An evidence-based guide to suctioning and dressing changes. *American Nurse Today, 6*(7), 14–17.

National Comprehensive Cancer Network (2013). *Practice guidelines in oncology: Head and neck cancers.* (version 2.2013). Fort Washington, PA: Author.

Poetker, D. (2013). Adults with epistaxis. *Patient Management Perspectives in Otolaryngology, 42*(6), 1–26.

Reed, C., Reineck, C., & Fonseca, I. (2011). Communicating with intubated patients: A new approach. *American Nurse Today, 6*(7), 34–35.

Simmons, S., & Pruitt, B. (2012). Sounding the alarm for patients with obstructive sleep apnea. *Nursing, 42*(4), 35–41.

Suzuki, M. (2012). Quality of life, uncertainty, and perceived involvement in decision making in patients with head and neck cancer. *Oncology Nursing Forum, 39*(6), 541–548.

Vacca, V., & Poirier, W. (2013). Action STAT: Posterior epistaxis. *Nursing, 43*(1), 72.

Woidtke, R. (2013). Adult obstructive sleep apnea: Taking a patient-centered approach. *American Nurse Today, 8*(7), 12–15.

Zeien, J. (2011). Create your own tracheostomy and laryngectomy teaching aids. *Nursing, 41*(2), 17–18.

Chapter 30

Abdo, W., & Heunks, L. (2012). Oxygen-induced hypercapnia in COPD: Myths and facts. *Critical Care, 16*(5), 323–326.

American Cancer Society (ACS) (2014). *Cancer facts and figures—2014.* No. 01-300M–No. 500814. Atlanta: Author.

Bauman, M., & Handley, C. (2011). Chest-tube care: The more you know, the easier it gets. *American Nurse Today, 6*(9), 27–31.

Beery, T. A., & Workman, M. L. (2012). *Genetics and genomics in nursing and health care.* Philadelphia: F.A. Davis.

Burt, L., & Corbridge, S. (2013). COPD exacerbations: Evidence-based guidelines for identification, assessment, and management. *American Journal of Nursing, 113*(2), 34–43.

Cagle, P., & Chirieac, L. (2012). Advances in treatment of lung cancer with targeted therapy. *Archives of Pathology & Laboratory Medicine, 136*(5), 504–509.

Centers for Disease Control and Prevention (CDC). (2012). Summary of health statistics for U.S. adults: National Health Interview Survey, 2011. *Vital and Health Statistics, Series 10,* (256). Retrieved June 2014, from <www.cdc.gov/nchs/data/series/sr_10/sr10_256.pdf>.

Centers for Disease Control and Prevention (CDC) (2014a). *FastStats—Asthma.* Retrieved June 2014, from <www.cdc.gov/nchs/fastats/asthma.htm>.

Centers for Disease Control and Prevention (CDC) (2014b). *FastStats—Chronic obstructive pulmonary disease (COPD).* Retrieved June 2014, from <www.cdc.gov/nchs/fastats/copd.htm>.

Cystic Fibrosis Foundation (2014). *About cystic fibrosis.* Retrieved June 2014, from <www.cff.org/AboutCF/>.

Demerouti, E., Manginas, A., Athanassopoulis, G., Karatasakis, G., Leontiadis, E., & Pavlides, G. (2013). Successful epoprostenol withdrawal in pulmonary arterial hypertension: Case report and literature review. *Respiratory Care, 58*(2), e1–e5.

Esguerra-Gonzalez, A., Ilagan-Honorio, M., Fraschilla, S., Kehoe, P., Lee, A., Marcarian, T., et al. (2013). Pain after lung transplant: High frequency chest wall oscillation vs chest physiotherapy. *American Journal of Critical Care, 22*(2), 115–125.

Fuentes, A., Coralic, A., & Dawson, K. (2012). A new epoprostenol formulation for the treatment of pulmonary artery hypertension. *American Journal of Health-System Pharmacists, 69,* 1389–1393.

Global Initiative for Asthma (GINA) (2014). *Pocket guide for asthma management and prevention.* Retrieved June 2014, from <www.ginasthma.org/Guidelines/guidelines-resources.html>.

Global Initiative for Chronic Obstructive Lung Disease (GOLD) (2014). *Global strategy for the diagnosis, management, and prevention of chronic obstructive pulmonary disease.* Retrieved June 2014, from <www.goldcopd.org/>.

Grant, M., Sun, M., Fujinami, R., Sidhu, R., Otis-Green, S., Juarez, G., et al. (2013). Family caregiver burden, skills, preparedness, and quality of life in non–small cell lung cancer. *Oncology Nursing Forum, 40*(4), 337–346.

Held-Warmkessel, J., & Schiech, L. (2014). Non-small cell lung cancer: Recent advances. *Nursing, 44*(2), 32–42.

Kessenich, C., & Bacher, K. (2014). Alpha-1 antitrypsin deficiency. *The Nurse Practitioner, 39*(7), 12–14.

Kingman, M., & Chin, K. (2013). Safety recommendations for administering intravenous prostacyclins in the hospital. *Critical Care Nurse, 33*(5), 32–34, 36–41.

Lareau, S., & Hodder, R. (2012). Teaching inhaler use in chronic obstructive pulmonary disease patients. *Journal of the American Academy of Nurse Practitioners, 24*(2), 113–120.

Lehto, R. H. (2014). Lung cancer screening guidelines: The nurse's role in patient education and advocacy. *Clinical Journal of Oncology Nursing, 18*(3), 338–342.

Lewis, D., & Scullion, J. (2012). Palliative and end-of-life care for patients with idiopathic pulmonary fibrosis: Challenges and dilemmas. *International Journal of Palliative Nursing, 18*(7), 331–337.

Makic, M. B., Martin, S., Burns, S., Philbrick, D., & Rauen, C. (2013). Putting evidence into practice: Four traditional practices not supported by the evidence. *Critical Care Nurse, 33*(2), 28–42.

Nakano, S., & Tluczek, A. (2014). Genomic breakthroughs in the diagnosis and treatment of cystic fibrosis. *The American Journal of Nursing, 114*(6), 36–43.

Neufeld, K., & Keith, L. (2012). Care of patients with cystic fibrosis. *AORN Journal, 96*(5), 529–536.

O'Laughlen, M., & Rance, K. (2012). Update on asthma management in primary care. *The Nurse Practitioner, 37*(11), 32–40.

Online Mendelian Inheritance in Man (OMIM) (2013a). *Adenocarcinoma of the lung.* Retrieved June 2014, from <www.omim.org/entry/211980>.

Online Mendelian Inheritance in Man (OMIM) (2013b). *Asthma, susceptibility to.* Retrieved June 2014, from <www.omim.org/entry/600807>.

Online Mendelian Inheritance in Man (OMIM) (2013c). *Cystic fibrosis; CF.* Retrieved June 2014, from <www.omim.org/entry/219700>.

Online Mendelian Inheritance in Man (OMIM) (2013d). *Pulmonary hypertension, primary.* Retrieved June 2014, from <www.omim.org/entry/178600>.

Pruitt, B. (2011). Assessing and managing asthma: A global initiative for asthma update. *Nursing, 41*(5), 46–52.

Roberts-Collins, C., Tagney, J., Tulloh, R., & Garratt, V. (2013). Being mindful of pulmonary arterial hypertension. *British Journal of Cardiac Nursing, 8*(3), 127–133.

Smith, B., & Tasota, F. (2011). Smoking out the dangers of COPD. *Nursing, 41*(4), 32–39.

Weber, C., Silver, M., Cromer, D., Kaminski, S., Wirick, T., & Vallejo, J. (2011). Under pressure: Pulmonary arterial hypertension. *Critical Care Nurse, 31*(4), 87–94.

World Health Organization (WHO). (2011). Dasatinib: Pulmonary artery hypertension. *WHO Drug Information, 25*(4), 360.

World Health Organization (WHO). (2012). Ambrisentan: Idiopathic pulmonary fibrosis. *WHO Drug Information, 28*(3), 270.

Chapter 31

Acerra, J. (2014). Pharyngitis. *Medscape Reference.* Retrieved June 2014, from <http://emedicine.medscape.com/article/764304-overview>.

American Lung Association (ALA) (2010a). *Trends in pneumonia and influenza morbidity and mortality.* Retrieved June 2014, from <www.lungusa.org/finding-cures/our-research/trend-reports/pi-trend-report.pdf>.

American Lung Association (ALA) (2010b). *Trends in tuberculosis morbidity and mortality.* Retrieved June 2014, from <www.lungusa.org/finding-cures/our-research/trend-reports/TB-Trend-Report.pdf>.

Aung, K. (2013). Viral pharyngitis. *Medscape Reference.* Retrieved June 2014, from <http://emedicine.medscape.com/article/225362-overview#a0199>.

2012 Beers Criteria Update Expert Panel. (2012). American Geriatrics Society updated Beers criteria for potentially inappropriate medication use in older adults. *Journal of the American Geriatrics Society.* Retrieved June 2014, from <www.americangeriatrics.org/files/documents/beers/2012BeersCriteria_JAGS.pdf>.

Barclay, L. (2013). MERS-CoV: Different from SARS, comorbidities may be key. *Medscape Reference.* Retrieved June, 2014, from <http://www.medscape.com/viewarticle/808465>.

Bocka, J. J. (2014). Pertussis. *Medscape Reference.* Retrieved June 2014, from <http://emedicine.medscape.com/article/967268-overview>.

Brook, I. (2013). Acute sinusitis. *Medscape Reference.* Retrieved June 2014, from <http://emedicine.medscape.com/article/232670-overview>.

Buhrow, S. (2013). Coccidioidomycosis: A differential diagnosis for visitors to the southwest. *The American Journal of Nursing, 113*(11), 52–55.

CDC urges better flu, pertussis vaccination (2012). *Hospital Employee Health,* 3–4.

Centers for Disease Control and Prevention (CDC) (2010a). *Cover your cough.* Retrieved June 2014, from <www.cdc.gov/flu/protect/covercough.htm>.

Centers for Disease Control and Prevention (CDC) (2010b). *2009 H1N1: Overview of a pandemic.* Retrieved June 2014, from <www.cdc.gov/h1n1flu/yearinreveiw.htm>.

Centers for Disease Control and Prevention (CDC). (2010c). Prevention & control of influenza with vaccines: Recommendations of the Advisory Committee on Immunization Practices (ACIP). *Morbidity and Mortality Weekly Report, 59,* 1–62.

Centers for Disease Control and Prevention (CDC) (2012). *CDC fast facts: Pertussis.* Retrieved June 2014, from <www.cdc.gov/pertussis/fast-facts.html>.

Centers for Disease Control and Prevention (CDC) (2013). *HIV and tuberculosis.* Retrieved June 2014, from <www.cdc.gov/hiv/resources/factsheets/PDF/hivtb.htm>.

Centers for Disease Control and Prevention (CDC) (2014a). *Information on avian influenza.* Retrieved June 2014, from <www.cdc.gov/flu/avianflu/>.

Centers for Disease Control and Prevention (CDC) (2014b). *Key facts about seasonal flu vaccine.* Retrieved June 2014, from <www.cdc.gov/flu/protect/keyfacts.htm>.

Centers for Disease Control and Prevention (CDC) (2014c). *Global Tuberculosis.* Retrieved June, 2014, from <http://www.cdc.gov/tb/topic/globaltb/>.

Centers for Disease Control and Prevention (CDC) (2014d). Middle East Respiratory Syndrome (MERS). *Medscape Reference.* Retrieved June, 2014, from <http://www.cdc.gov/CORONAVIRUS/MERS/INDEX.HTML>.

Cunha, B. (2014). Anthrax. *Medscape Reference.* Retrieved June 2014, from <http://emedicine.medscape.com/article/212127-overview>.

Dambaugh, L. A. (2012). A review of influenza: Implications for the geriatric population. *Critical Care Nursing Clinics of North America, 24,* 573–580.

Echevarria, I., & Schwoebel, A. (2012). Development of an intervention model for the prevention of aspiration pneumonia in high-risk patients on a medical-surgical unit. *Medsurg Nursing, 21*(5), 303–308.

Gler, M., Skripconoka, V., Sanchez-Garavito, E., Xiao, H., Cabrera-Rivero, J., Vargas-Vasquez, D., et al. (2012). Delamanid for multidrug-resistant pulmonary tuberculosis. *The New England Journal of Medicine, 366*(23), 2151–2160.

Gould, D. (2011). The challenges of caring for patients with influenza. *Nursing Older People, 23*(10), 28–34.

Heavey, E. (2013). Does the BCG vaccine protect against TB? *Nursing, 43*(10), 62.

Kamangar, N. (2013). Lung abscess. *Medscape Reference.* Retrieved June 2014, from <http://emedicine.medscape.com/article/299425-overview>.

Krouse, H. J., & Krouse, J. (2014). Allergic rhinitis: Diagnosis through management. *The Nurse Practitioner, 39*(4), 20–29.

Medication Update. (2014). FDA approves first adjuvanted vaccine to prevent H5N1 avian flu. *The Nurse Practitioner, 39*(2), 56.

Ploskser, G. L. (2012). A/H5N1 prepandemic influenza vaccine (whole virion, vero cell-derived, inactivated) [Vepacel®]. *Drugs, 72*(11), 1543–1557.

Roark, D. C. (2012). Working toward perfection on the pneumonia core measure. *Journal of Emergency Nursing, 38,* 127–129.

Schweon, S. J. (2011). Pertussis: Not just for kids anymore. *Nursing, 41*(10), 61–62.

Scott, S., & Kardos, C. (2012). Community-acquired, health care-associated, and ventilator-associated pneumonia: Three variations of a serious disease. *Critical Care Nursing Clinics of North America, 24*(3), 431–441.

Shah, U. K. (2014a). Tonsillitis and peritonsillar abscess. *Medscape Reference.* Retrieved June 2014, from <http://emedicine.medscape.com/article/871977-overview>.

Shah, U. K. (2014b). Tonsillitis and peritonsillar abscess treatment and management. *Medscape Reference.* Retrieved June 2014, from <http://emedicine.medscape.com/article/871977-treatment>.

Sheikh, J. (2014). Allergic rhinitis. *Medscape Reference.* Retrieved June 2014, from <http://emedicine.medscape.com/article/134825-overview>.

Thornton, K., Alston, M., Dye, H., & Williamson, S. (2011). Are saline irrigations effective in relieving chronic rhinosinusitis symptoms? A review of the evidence. *The Journal for Nurse Practitioners, 7*(8), 680–686.

Todd, B. (2014). Middle east respiratory syndrome (MERS-CoV). *The American Journal of Nursing, 114*(1), 56–59.

World Health Organization (WHO) (2014a). *Global tuberculosis report 2013: Executive summary.* Retrieved June 2014, from <www.who.int/tb/data>.

World Health Organization (WHO) (2014b). *Global tuberculosis report 2013: Factsheet.* Retrieved June 2014, from <www.who.int/tb/publications/factsheets/en/index.html>.

World Health Organization (WHO) (2013). *What is multi-drug resistant tuberculosis and how do we treat it.* Retrieved June 2014, from <www.who.int/features/qu/79/en/>.

Zwanger, M. (2013). Empyema and abscess pneumonia. *Medscape Reference.* Retrieved June 2014, from <http://emedicine.medscape.com/article/807499-overview>.

Chapter 32

Amidei, C., & Sole, M. (2013). Physiological responses to passive exercise in adults receiving mechanical ventilation. *American Journal of Critical Care, 22*(4), 337–348.

ARDS Foundation (2013). *Facts about ARDS.* Retrieved June 2014, from <http://ardsfoundation.com>.

Aust, M. (2014). Compact clinical guide to mechanical ventilation: Foundations of practice for critical care nurses. *Critical Care Nurse, 34*(2), 80.

Bekken, N. (2011). Strategies for nursing care of adult patients with acute respiratory failure. *Mosby's Nursing Consult Clinical Updates.* Retrieved June 2014, from <www.nursingconsult.com/nursing/clinical-updates/full-text?clinical_update_id=203829&specId=0&sortBy=title-a&parentpage=search&sort_order=Relevance&contact_hours>.

Benson, A. B. (2012). Pulmonary complications of transfused blood components. *Critical Care Nursing Clinics of North America, 24,* 403–418.

Bjerke, H. S. (2012). Flail chest. *Medscape Reference.* Retrieved June 2014, from <http://emedicine.medscape.com/article/433779-overview>.

Booker, S., Murff, S., Kitko, L., & Jablonski, R. (2013). Mouth care to reduce ventilator-associated pneumonia. *The American Journal of Nursing, 113*(10), 24–30.

Bortolotto, S. J., & Makic, M. B. (2012). Understanding advanced modes of mechanical ventilation. *Critical Care Nursing Clinics of North America, 24*(4), 443–456.

Bull, A. (2014). Primary care of chronic dyspnea in adults. *The Nurse Practitioner, 39*(8), 34–40.

Carlisle, H. (2014). The case for capnography in patients receiving opioids. *American Nurse Today, 9*(9), 22–26.

Carroll, P., Shirato, S., & Beach, P. R. (2013). Acute respiratory distress syndrome/acute lung injury. *Mosby's Nursing Consult Evidence-Based Nursing Monographs.* Retrieved June 2014, from <www.nursingconsult.com/nursing/evidence-based-nursing/monograph?monograph_id=216675>.

Daley, B. (2014). Pneumothorax. *Medscape Reference.* Retrieved April 2013, from <http://emedicine.medscape.com/article/424547-overview>.

Day, M. (2011). On alert for iatrogenic pneumothorax. *Nursing, 41*(6), 66–67.

Dechert, R. E., Haas, C. F., & Ostwani, W. (2012). Current knowledge of acute lung injury and acute respiratory distress syndrome. *Critical Care Nursing Clinics of North America, 24,* 377–401.

Dennison, R. D., Johnson, J. M., & Blair, M. (2011). *Pass CEN!* Philadelphia: Elsevier.

Drumright, K., Jukenbeck, S., & Judd, C. (2013). The ABCs of acute PE. *Nursing Made Incredibly Easy, 11*(2), 45–49.

Duff, J., Walker, K., Omari, A., & Stratton, C. (2013). Prevention of venous thromboembolism in hospitalized patients: Analysis of reduced cost and improved clinical outcomes. *Journal of Vascular Nursing, 31,* 9–14.

Ferri, F. (2013). Acute respiratory distress syndrome. *Ferri's clinical advisor 2013.* St. Louis: Mosby.

Garg, K. (2013). Acute pulmonary embolism (Helical CT). *Medscape Reference.* Retrieved June 2014, from <http://emedicine.medscape.com/article/361131-overview>.

Golembiewski, J. A. (2011). Dabigatran: A new oral anticoagulant. *Journal of Perianesthesia Nursing, 26*(6), 420–423.

Grossbach, I., Chlan, L., & Tracy, M. (2011). Overview of mechanical ventilatory support and management of patient- and ventilator-related responses. *Critical Care Nurse, 31*(3), 30–44.

Grossbach, I., Stranberg, S., & Chlan, L. (2011). Promoting effective communication for patients receiving mechanical ventilation. *Critical Care Nurse, 31*(3), 46–60.

Hiller, B., Wilson, C., Chamberlain, D., & King, L. (2013). Preventing ventilator-associated pneumonia through oral care, product selection, and application method. *AACN Advanced Critical Care, 24*(1), 38–58.

Hussey, L. (2013). Reducing mortality in pulmonary embolism through prevention and careful management. *Mosby's Nursing Consult.* Retrieved June 2014, from <www.nursingconsult.com/nursing/clinical-updates/full-text?clinical_update_id=197598&specId=0&sortBy=title-a&parentpage=search&sort_order=Relevance&contact_hours>.

Kessenich, C., & Erigo-Backman, R. (2012). Computed tomography angiography and pulmonary embolism. *The Nurse Practitioner*, 37(10), 10–11.

Kiypshi-Teo, H., Cabana, M. O., Froelicher, E. S., & Blegen, M. A. (2014). Adherence to institution-specific ventilator-associated pneumonia prevention guidelines. *American Journal of Critical Care*, 23(3), 201–215.

Kydonaki, K., Huby, G., & Tocher, J. (2014). Difficult to wean patients: Cultural factors and their impact on weaning decision-making. *Journal of Clinical Nursing*, 23(5/6), 683–693.

Landeen, C., & Smith, H. L. (2014). Examination of pneumonia risks and risk levels in trauma patients with pulmonary contusion. *Journal of Trauma Nursing*, 21(2), 41–49.

Lee, A. (2014). Factor V Leiden. *Nursing*, 44(6), 10–12.

Lian, J. (2013). Using ABGs to optimize mechanical ventilation. *Nursing*, 43(6), 46–52.

Mancini, M. C. (2012a). Blunt chest trauma. *Medscape Reference*. Retrieved June 2014, from <http://emedicine.medscape.com/article/428723-overview>.

Mancini, M. C. (2012b). Hemothorax. *Medscape Reference*. Retrieved June 2014, from <http://emedicine.medscape.com/article/2047916-overview>.

Mathay, M. A., & Zemans, R. L. (2011). The acute respiratory distress syndrome: Pathogenesis and treatment. *Annual Review of Pathology*, 6, 147–163.

McLean, B. A. (2012). Acute respiratory failure and intensive measures. *Critical Care Nursing Clinics of North America*, 24, 361–375.

McLenon, M. (2012). Acute pulmonary embolism. *Critical Care Nursing Quarterly*, 35(2), 173–182.

Mellott, K. G., Grap, M., Munro, C. L., Sessler, C. N., Wetzel, P. A., Nilsestuen, J. O., et al. (2014). Patient ventilator asynchrony in critically ill adults: Frequency and types. *Heart and Lung*, 43(3), 231–243.

Mendez, M., Lazar, M., DiGiovine, B., Schuldt, S., Behrendt, R., Peters, M., et al. (2013). Dedicated multidisciplinary ventilator bundle team and compliance with sedation vacation. *American Journal of Critical Care*, 22(1), 54–60.

Messing, J. A., Gail, V., & Sarani, B. (2014). Successful management of severe flail chest via early operative intervention. *Journal of Trauma Nursing*, 21(2), 83–85.

Morris, P. E., Griffin, L., Berry, M., Thompson, C., Hite, R. D., Winkelman, C., et al. (2011). Receiving early mobility during an ICU admission is a predictor of improved outcomes in acute respiratory failure. *American Journal of Medical Sciences*, 341, 373–377.

Morton, P. G., & Fontaine, D. K. (2013). *Essentials of critical care nursing: A holistic approach*. Philadelphia: Lippincott Williams & Wilkins.

Munro, N., & Ruggiero, M. (2014). Ventilator-associated pneumonia bundle. *AACN Advanced Critical Care*, 25(2), 163–178.

Online Mendelian Inheritance in Man (OMIM) (2013). *Coagulation factor V; F5*. Retrieved July 2014, from <www.omim.org/entry/612309>.

Ouellette, D. R. (2014). Pulmonary embolism treatment and management. *Medscape Reference*. Retrieved June 2014, from <http://emedicine.medscape.com/article/300901-treatment>.

Poirier, W., & Vacca, V. (2013). Flail chest. *Nursing*, 43(12), 10–11.

Powers, K., & Talbot, L. (2011). Fat embolism syndrome after femur fracture with intramedullary nailing: Case report. *American Journal of Critical Care*, 20(3), 264–265, 267.

Riley, P. (2013). Measuring, monitoring heparin: A discussion of anti factorXa versus aPTT. *Advance for Medical Laboratory Professionals*, 25(2), 10–11.

Ruiz, C. (2011). Thwarting a pneumothorax. *American Nurse Today*, 6(5), 32.

Smithburger, P. L., Campbell, S., & Kane-Gill, S. L. (2013). Alteplase treatment of acute pulmonary embolism in the intensive care unit. *Critical Care Nurse*, 33(2), 17–26.

Urden, L. D., Stacy, K. M., & Lough, M. E. (2012). *Priorities in critical care nursing* (6th ed.). St. Louis: Mosby.

Warren, E. (2013). A practice guide to anticoagulation. *Prescribing Nurse*, 43(2), 29–33.

Williams, K. (2013). Extracorporeal membrane oxygenation for acute respiratory distress syndrome in adults. *AACN Advanced Critical Care*, 24(2), 149–158.

Wright, A. D., & Flynn, M. (2011). Using the prone position for ventilated patients with respiratory failure: A review. *Nursing in Critical Care*, 16(1), 19–27.

Chapter 33

American Heart Association (AHA) (2013). *Diet and lifestyle recommendations* (updated: March 19, 2013). Retrieved July 2014, from <www.heart.org/HEARTORG/GettingHealthy/Diet-and-Lifestyle-Recommendations_UCM_305855_Article.jsp>.

*Cheek, D., & Tester, J. (2008). Women and heart disease: What's new? *Nursing*, 38(1), 37–42.

Go, A. S., Mozaffarian, D., Roger, V. L., Benjamin, E. J., Berry, J. D., Borden, W. B., et al. (2013). Heart disease and stroke statistics—2014 update: A report from the American Heart Association. *Circulation*. Retrieved July 2014, from <http://circ.ahajournals.org/content/early/2013/12/18/01.Circ0000441139.102102.80.citation>.

*Howie-Esquivel, J., & White, M. (2008). Biomarkers in acute cardiovascular disease. *Journal of Cardiovascular Nursing*, 23(2), 124–131.

James, P. A., Oparil, S., Carter, B. L., Cushman, W. C., Dennison-Himmelfarb, C., Handler, J., et al. (2014). 2014 evidence-based guidelines for the management of high blood pressure in adults: report from the panel members appointed to the Eighth Joint National Committee (JNC 8). *The Journal of the American Medical Association*, 311(5), 507–520.

Johnson, C. J., Anderson, M. A., & Hill, P. D. (2012). Comparison of pulse oximetry in a health population. *Medsurg Nursing*, 21(2), 70–73.

Landgraf, J., Wishner, S. H., & Kloner, R. A. (2010). Comparison of automatic oscillometric versus auscultatory blood pressure measurement. *American Journal of Cardiology*, 106(3), 386–388.

Pearson, T. L. (2010). Ankle brachial index as a prognostic tool for women with coronary artery disease. *Journal of Cardiovascular Nursing*, 25(1), 20–24.

Sanborn, T. A., Ebrahimi, R., Manoukian, S. V., McLaurin, B. T., Cox, D. A., Feit, F., et al. (2010). Impact of femoral vascular closure devices and antithrombotic therapy on access site bleeding in acute coronary syndromes. *Circulation: Cardiovascular Interventions*, 3(1), 57–62.

Sulzbach-Hoke, L. M., Ratcliffe, S. J., Kimmel, S. E., Kolansky, D. M., & Polomano, R. (2010). Predictors of complications following sheath removal with percutaneous coronary intervention. *Journal of Cardiovascular Nursing*, 25(3), e1–e8.

*The New York Heart Association (1964). *Diseases of the heart and blood vessels: Nomenclature and criteria for diagnosis* (6th ed.). Boston: Little, Brown.

*Wright, J. D., Hirsch, R., & Wang, C. Y. (2009). One-third of U.S. adults embraced most heart healthy behaviors in 1999-2002. *National Center for Health Statistics Data Brief*, (17). Hyattsville, MD: National Center for Health Statistics. Retrieved July 2014, from <www.cdc.gov/nchs/data/databriefs/db17.htm>.

Chapter 34

American Heart Association (AHA) (2010). *Highlights of the 2010 American Heart Association Guidelines for CPR and ECC*. Retrieved June 2013, from <www.heart.org/idc/groups/heart-public/@wcm/@ecc/documents/downloadable/ucm_317350.pdf>.

Anderson, J., Halperin, J., Albert, N., Bozkurt, B., Brindis, R., Curtis, L., et al. (2013). Management of patients with atrial fibrillation (compilation of 2006 ACCF/AHA/ESC and 2011 ACCF/AHA/HRS recommendations). *Journal of the American College of Cardiology*, 61(18), 1935–1944.

Barekatain, A., & Razavi, M. (2012). Antiarrhythmic therapy in atrial fibrillation: Indications, guidelines and safety. *Texas Heart Institute*, 39(4), 532–534.

Batista, L., Lima, F., Januzzi, J., Donahue, V., Snydeman, C., & Greer, D. (2010). Feasibility and safety of combined percutaneous coronary intervention and therapeutic hypothermia following cardiac arrest. *Resuscitation*, 81(4), 398–403.

Berdowski, J., Blom, M., Bardai, A., Tan, H., Tijessen, J., & Koster, R. (2011). Impact of onsite or dispatched automated external defibrillator use on survival after out of hospital cardiac arrest. *Circulation, 124,* 2225–2232.

Berry, E., & Padgett, H. (2012). Management of patients with atrial fibrillation: Diagnosis and treatment. *Nursing Standard, 26*(22), 47–56.

Bosen, D. (2011). Pacing therapies for atrial fibrillation. *Nursing,* 11–12. doi:10.1097/01. NURSE.0000394518.21592.1a.

Buck, H. G. (2012). CPR in older adults: What's the evidence? *Nursing, 42*(5), 14–15.

Calkins, H., Kuck, K., Cappato, R., Brugada, J., Camm, A., Chen, S., et al. (2012). 2012 HRS/ EHRA/ECAS expert consensus statement on catheter and surgical ablation of atrial fibrillation: Recommendations for patient selection, procedural techniques, patient management and follow-up, definitions, endpoints and research trial design. *Heart Rhythm, 9*(4), 632–696.

Chalupka, A. N. (2010). Radiofrequency catheter ablation for atrial fibrillation. *American Association of Occupational Health Nurses, 58*(5), 220.

Cheng, J. M. (2010). New and emerging antiarrhythmic and anticoagulant agents for atrial fibrillation. *American Journal of Health-System Pharmacy, 67*(9), S26–S34.

Chilukuri, K., Dalal, D., Gadrey, S., Marine, J. E., MacPherson, E., Henrikson, C. A., et al. (2010). A prospective study evaluating the role of obesity and obstructive sleep apnea for outcomes after catheter ablation of atrial fibrillation. *Journal of Cardiovascular Electrophysiology, 21*(5), 521–525.

Chinitz, J., Halperin, J., Reddy, V., & Fuster, V. (2012). Rate or rhythm control for atrial fibrillation: Update and controversies. *The American Journal of Medicine, 125,* 1049–1056.

Craig, K. J., & Day, M. P. (2011). Are you up to date on the latest BLS and ACLS guidelines? *Nursing, 41*(5), 40–44.

Cronin, E., & Varma, N. (2012). Remote monitoring of cardiovascular implanted electronic devices: A paradigm shift for the 21st century. *Expert Reviews, 9*(4), 367–376.

Dagres, N., & Anastasiou-Nana, M. (2010). Atrial fibrillation and obesity: An association of increasing importance. *Journal of the American College of Cardiology, 55*(21), 2328–2329.

DeVon, H. A., Hogan, N., Ochs, A. L., & Shapiro, M. (2010). Time to treatment for acute coronary syndromes: The cost of indecision. *Journal of Cardiovascular Nursing, 25*(2), 106–114.

Dobromir, D., & Nattel, S. (2010). New antiarrhythmic drugs for treatment of atrial fibrillation. *The Lancet, 375*(9721), 1212–1223.

Franks, M., & Lawson, L. (2012). Body surface mapping improves diagnosis of acute myocardial infarction in the emergency department. *Advanced Emergency Nursing Journal, 34*(1), 32–40.

Garlitski, A. C., & Estes, N. A. I. I. I. (2010). Emerging therapies for atrial fibrillation: Is the paradigm shifting? *Journal of Interventional Cardiac Electrophysiology, 28*(1), 1–4.

Go, A., Mozaffarian, D., Roger, V., Benjamin, E., Berry, J., Borden, W., et al. (2013). Heart disease and stroke statistics—2013 update: A report from the American Heart Association. *Circulation, 127,* e6–e245.

Green, J. M., & Chiaramida, A. J. (2010). *12-lead EKG confidence: A step-by-step guide.* New York: Springer.

Hallas, C., Burke, J., White, D., & Connelly, D. (2010). A prospective 1-year study of changes in neuropsychological functioning after implantable cardioverter-defibrillator surgery. *Circulation: Arrhythmia and Electrophysiology, 3,* 170–177.

Harden, J. (2011). Taking a cool look at therapeutic hypothermia. *Nursing, 41*(9), 46–52.

*Hardin, S. R., & Steele, J. R. (2008). Atrial fibrillation among older adults: Pathophysiology, symptoms, and treatment. *Journal of Gerontological Nursing, 34*(7), 26–32.

Johnson, T., Jadick, E., & Knippers, L. (2011). Atrial fibrillation ablation. *American Journal of Nursing, 111*(2), 58–61.

Jost, D., Degrange, H., Verret, C., Hersan, O., Banville, I. L., Chapman, F. W., et al. (2010). A randomized controlled trial of the effect of automated external defibrillator cardiopulmonary resuscitation protocol on outcome from out-of-hospital cardiac arrest. *Circulation, 121,* 1614–1622.

Keseg, D. P. (2010). Reducing interruptions: Continuous compression CPR & minimally interrupted CPR result in improved survival. *A Journal of Emergency Medical Services, 35*(1), 14–17.

Kireyev, D., Fernandez, S., Gupta, V., Arkhipow, M., & Paris, J. (2012). Targeting tachycardia: Diagnostic tips and tools. *Journal of Family Practice, 61*(5), 258–263.

Lee, G., Sanders, P., & Kalman, J. (2012). Catheter ablation of atrial arrhythmias: State of the art. *Lancet, 380,* 1509–1519.

Link, M. (2012). Evaluation and initial treatment of supraventricular tachycardia. *New England Journal of Medicine, 367,* 1438–1448. doi:10.1056/NEJMcp1111259.

Marcus, G. M., Olgin, J. E., Whooley, M., Vittinghoff, E., Stone, K. L., Mehra, R., et al. (2010). Racial differences in atrial fibrillation prevalence and left atrial size. *American Journal of Medicine, 123*(4), 375.e1–375.e7.

Michaels, A. D., Spinler, S. A., Leeper, B., Ohman, E. M., Alexander, K. P., Newby, L. K., et al. (2010). Medication errors in acute cardiovascular and stroke patients: A scientific statement from the American Heart Association. *Circulation, 121,* 1664–1682.

Mooney, T. (2013). Use of dabigatran to prevent stroke in patients with atrial fibrillation. *Nursing Standard, 27*(27), 35–41.

Palmer, B. (2011). Systematic cardiac rhythm strip analysis. *Medsurg Nursing, 20*(2), 96–97.

Patel, M. R., Mahaffey, K. W., Garg, J., Pan, G., Singer, D. E., Hacke, W., ROCKET AF Steering Committee for the ROCKET AF Investigators, et al. (2011). Rivaroxaban versus warfarin in nonvalvular atrial fibrillation. *New England Journal of Medicine, 365*(10), 883–891.

Pelter, M. (2010). Time to treatment for acute coronary syndromes: The cost of indecision. *Journal of Cardiovascular Nursing, 25*(2), 115–116.

Richards, G. (2012). An overview of atrial fibrillation. *Nursing Standard, 26*(52), 47–56.

Rose, E., Chinitz, L. A., Holmes, D. S., & Aizer, A. (2010). A novel mechanism of failure to detect atrial arrhythmias by pacemakers and implantable cardioverter defibrillators. *Journal of Cardiovascular Electrophysiology, 21*(3), 325–328.

Ruiter, J. H., Mulder, E., Schuchert, A., Burri, H., Stuhlinger, M. C., Hartikainen, J., et al. (2010). The feasibility of fully automated pacemaker advice in treating atrial tachyarrhythmias. *Pacing & Clinical Electrophysiology, 33*(5), 605–614.

Sellers, M. B., & Newby, L. K. (2011). Atrial fibrillation, anticoagulants, fall risk, and outcomes in elderly patients. *American Heart Journal, 161*(2), 241–246.

Tedrow, U. B., Conen, D., Ridker, P. M., Cook, N. R., Koplan, B. A., Manson, J. E., et al. (2010). The long- and short-term impact of elevated body mass index on the risk of new atrial fibrillation: The WHS (Women's Health Study). *Journal of the American College of Cardiology, 55*(21), 2319–2327.

Tracy, C., Epstein, A., Darbar, D., DiMarco, J., Dunbar, S., Estes, M., et al. (2012). 2012 ACCF/AHA/HRS focused update of the 2008 guidelines for device based therapy of cardiac rhythm abnormalities. *Journal of the American College of Cardiology, 60*(14), 1247–1313. doi:10.1016/j.jacc2012.08.009.

Wann, L. S., Curtis, A. B., Ellenbogen, K. A., Estes, N. A., III, Ezekowitz, M. D., Jackman, W. M., et al. (2011). 2011 ACCF/AHA/HRS focused update on the management of patients with atrial fibrillation (update on dabigatran): A report of the American College of Cardiology Foundation/American Heart Association Task Force on Practice Guidelines. *Journal of the American College of Cardiology, 57*(11), 1330–1337.

Whinnett, Z., Sohaib, S., & Davies, D. (2012). Diagnosis and management of supraventricular tachycardia. *British Medical Journal, 345*(e7769), 1–9. doi:10.1136/bmj.e7769.

Wilber, D. J., Pappone, C., Neuzil, P., De Paola, A., Marchlinski, F., Natale, A., et al. (2010). Comparison of antiarrhythmic drug therapy and radiofrequency catheter ablation in patients with paroxysmal atrial fibrillation. *Journal of the American Medical Association, 303*(4), 333–340.

Wokhlu, A., Monahan, K. H., Hodge, D. O., Asirvatham, S. J., Friedman, P. A., Munger, T. M., et al. (2010). Long-term quality of life after ablation of atrial fibrillation: The impact of recurrence, symptom relief, and placebo effect. *Journal of the American College of Cardiology, 55*(21), 2308–2316.

Yeung, J., & Perkins, G. D. (2010). Timing of drug administration during CPR and the role of simulation. *Resuscitation, 81*(3), 265–266.

Zak, J. (2010). Ablation to treat atrial fibrillation: Beyond rhythm control. *Critical Care Nurse, 30*, 68–78. doi:10.4037/ccn2010335.

Zarraga, I., & Kron, I. (2013). Oral anticoagulation in elderly adults with atrial fibrillation: Integrating new options with old concepts. *Journal of the American Geriatrics Society, 61*, 143–150. doi:10.1111/jgs.12042.

Zishiri, E., Cronin, E., Williams, S., Blackstone, S., Ellis, S., Smedira, N., et al. (2011). Abstract 9816: Use of the wearable cardioverter defibrillator and survival after coronary artery revascularization in patients with left ventricular dysfunction. *Circulation, 124*, A9816.

Chapter 35

Albert, N. M. (2012). Fluid management strategies in heart failure. *Critical Care Nurse, 32*(2), 20–32.

Boyde, M., Turner, C., Thompson, D., & Stewart, S. (2011). Educational interventions for patients with heart failure: A systematic review of randomized controlled trials. *Journal of Cardiovascular Nursing, 26*(4), E27–E35.

Cary, T., & Pearce, J. (2013). Aortic stenosis: Pathophysiology, diagnosis, and medical management of nonsurgical patients. *Critical Care Nurse, 33*(2), 58–72.

Chen, W., Tran, K., & Maisel, A. (2010). Biomarkers in heart failure. *Heart, 96*, 314–320.

Christensen, D. (2012). Physiology of continuous-flow pumps. *Advanced Critical Care, 23*(1), 46–54.

Clerico, A., Giannoni, A., Vittorini, S., & Emdin, M. (2012). The paradox of low BNP levels in obesity. *Heart Failure Reviews, 17*(1), 81–96.

Cooper, K. L. (2011). Care of the lower extremities in patients with acute decompensated heart failure. *Critical Care Nurse, 31*(4), 21–29.

DeBeradinis, B., & Januzzi, J. L., Jr. (2012). Use of biomarkers to guide outpatient therapy of heart failure. *Current Opinion in Cardiology, 27*(6), 661–668.

DiSalvo, T., Acker, M., Dec, W., & Byrne, J. (2010). Mitral valve surgery in advanced heart failure. *Journal of the American College of Cardiology, 55*(4), 271–282.

Dudzinski, D., Mak, G., & Hung, J. (2012). Pericardial diseases. *Current Problems in Cardiology, 37*(3), 75–118.

Dworakowski, R., Prendergast, B., Wendler, O., & MacCarthy, P. (2010). Treatment of acquired valvular heart disease: Percutaneous alternatives. *Clinical Medicine, 10*(2), 181–187.

Eisen, H. J. (2014). *Prevention and treatment of cardiac allograft vasculopathy*. Retrieved December 8, 2014, from: <http://www.uptodate.com/content/prevention-and-1.com>.

Fard, A., Taub, P., Iqbal, N., & Maisel, A. (2012). Natriuretic peptides in the hospital: Risk stratification and treatment titration. In A.

Maisel (Ed.), *Cardiac biomarkers: Expert advice for clinicians* (pp. 128–139). London: JP Medical Publishers.

Go, A. S., Mozaffarian, D., Roger, V. L., Benjamin, E. J., Berry, J. D., Borden, W. B., et al. (2013). Heart disease and stroke statistics—2013 update: A report from the American Heart Association. *Circulation, 127*(1), 2–245.

Hannibal, G. (2012). ECG characteristics of acute pericarditis. *Advanced Critical Care, 23*(3), 341–344.

Hoen, B., & Duval, X. (2013). Clinical practice. Infective endocarditis. *The New England Journal of Medicine, 368*(15), 1425–1433.

*Hoercher, K. J., Vacha, C. J., & McCarthy, P. M. (2002). Left ventricular splints and wraps for end-stage heart failure: A new approach in the new millennium. *Journal of Cardiovascular Nursing, 16*(3), 82–86.

Hull, C. (2012). Treating calcific aortic stenosis: An evolving science. *Medsurg Nursing, 21*(2), 82–87.

Imazio, M., Brucato, A., Cemin, R., Ferrua, S., Belli, R., Maestroni, S., et al. (2011). Colchicine for recurrent pericarditis (CORP): A randomized trial. *Annals of Internal Medicine, 155*(7), 409–414.

Jacoby, D. L., DePasquale, E. C., & McKenna, W. J. (2013). Hypertrophic cardiomyopathy: Diagnosis, risk stratification and treatment. *Canadian Medical Association Journal, 185*(2), 127–134.

*Jessup, M., Abraham, W. T., Casey, D. E., Feldman, A. M., Francis, G. S., Ganiats, T. G., et al. writing on behalf of the 2005 guideline update for the diagnosis and management of chronic heart failure in the adult writing committee. (2009). 2009 Focused update: ACCF/AHA guidelines for the diagnosis and management of heart failure in adults: A report of the American College of Cardiology Foundation/American Heart Association Task Force on Practice Guidelines. *Circulation, 119*(14), 1977–2016.

Litton, K. (2011). Demystifying ventricular assist devices. *Critical Care Nursing Quarterly, 34*(3), 200–207.

Manning, S. (2011). Bridging the gap between hospital and home: A new model of care for reducing readmission rates in chronic heart failure. *Journal of Cardiovascular Nursing, 26*(5), 368–376.

McConaghy, J., & Oza, R. (2013). Outpatient diagnosis of acute chest pain in adults. *American Family Physician, 87*(3), 177–182.

*Nishimura, R., Carabello, B., Faxon, D., Freed, M., Lytle, B., O'Gara, P., et al. (2008). ACC/AHA 2008 guideline update on valvular heart disease: Focused update on infective endocarditis: A report of the American College of Cardiology/American Heart Association Task Force on Practice Guidelines: Endorsed by the Society of Cardiovascular Anesthesiologists, Society for Cardiovascular Angiography and Interventions, and Society of Thoracic Surgeons. *Circulation, 118*(8), 887–896.

Ramani, G., Uber, P., & Mehra, M. (2010). Chronic heart failure: Contemporary diagnosis

and management. *Mayo Clinic Proceedings, 85*(2), 180–195.

Ray, S. (2010). Changing epidemiology and natural history of valvular heart disease. *Clinical Medicine, 10*(2), 168–171.

Rogers, J., Aaronson, K., Boyle, A., Russell, S., Milano, C., Pagani, F., et al. (2010). Continuous flow left ventricular assist device improves functional capacity and quality of life of advanced heart failure patients. *Journal of the American College of Cardiology, 55*(17), 1826–1834.

Rowland, C. (2012). Pump it up with an LVAD left ventricular assist device. *Nursing, 42*(4), 47–50.

Saunders, M. (2010). A comparison of employed and unemployed caregivers of older heart failure patients. *Holistic Nursing Practice, 24*(1), 16–22.

Seward, J., & Casaclang-Verzosa, G. (2010). Infiltrative cardiovascular diseases. *Journal of the American College of Cardiology, 55*(17), 1769–1779.

Sherrid, M., & Arabadjian, M. (2012). A primer of disopyramide treatment of obstructive hypertrophic cardiomyopathy. *Progress in Cardiovascular Diseases, 54*(6), 483–492.

Streets, K., & Vickers, S. (2012). Is this patient with heart failure a candidate for ultrafiltration? *Nursing, 42*(6), 30–36.

Suter, P., Gorski, L., Hennessey, B., & Suter, W. (2012). Best practices for heart failure: A focused review. *Home Healthcare Nurse, 30*(7), 394–405.

Yancy, C., Jessup, M., Bozkurt, B., Butler, J., Casey, D., Drazner, M., et al. (2013). 2013 ACCF/AHA Guideline for the management of heart failure: Executive Summary: A report of the American College of Cardiology Foundation/American Heart Association Task Force on Practice Guidelines. *Journal of the American College of Cardiology, 62*(16), 1495–1539.

Chapter 36

*ALLHAT Officers and Coordinators for the ALLHAT Collaborative Research Group. (2002a). Major outcomes in high-risk hypertensive patients randomized to angiotensin-converting enzyme inhibitor or calcium channel blocker vs diuretic. The Antihypertensive and Lipid-Lowering Treatment to Prevent Heart Attack Trial (ALLHAT). *Journal of the American Medical Association, 288*(23), 2981–2997.

*ALLHAT Officers and Coordinators for the ALLHAT Collaborative Research Group. (2002b). Major outcomes in moderately hypercholesterolemic, hypertensive patients randomized to pravastatin vs usual care. The Antihypertensive and Lipid-Lowering Treatment to Prevent Heart Attack Trial (ALLHAT-LLT). *Journal of the American Medical Association, 288*(23), 2998–3007.

Anderson, D. J., Anderson, M. A., & Hill, P. D. (2010). Location of blood pressure measurement. *Medsurg Nursing, 19*(5), 287–294.

Anthony, M. (2013). Nursing assessment of deep vein thrombosis. *Medsurg Nursing, 22*(2), 95–98.

Armstrong, K. E. (2013). Stop the reflux: An update on treatment for symptomatic varicose veins. *Nursing, 43*(2), 27–34.

Bailey, D. G., Dresser, D., & Arnold, J. M. O. (2013). Grapefruit-medication interactions: Forbidden fruit or avoidable consequences. *CMAJ: Canadian Medical Association Journal, 185*, 309–316.

Baldwin, S. (2011). Helping patients manage hypertension. *Nursing, 41*(8), 60–63.

Braverman, A. C. (2010). Acute aortic dissection. *Circulation, 122*(2), 184.

Carlson, D. S. (2012). Action Stat: Acute aortic dissection. *Nursing, 42*(7), 72.

Coke, L. A. (2011). Vascular risk assessment of the older CV patient: The Ankle-Brachial Index (ABI). *Medsurg Nursing, 20*(1), 47–48.

Day, M. W. (2011). Action Stat: Hypertensive emergency. *Nursing, 41*(8), 11.

Eckel, R. H., Jakicic, J. M., Ard, J. D., Hubbard, V. S., de Jesus, J. M., Lee, I. M., et al. (2014). 2013 AHA/ACC guideline on lifestyle management to reduce cardiovascular risk: A report of the American College of Cardiology/American Heart Association Task Force on Practice Guidelines. *Circulation, 129*(25 Suppl. 2), S76–S99.

*Gay, V., Hamilton, R., Heiskell, S., & Sparks, A. M. (2009). Influence of bedrest or ambulation in the clinical treatment of acute deep vein thrombosis on patient outcomes: A review and synthesis of the literature. *Medsurg Nursing, 18*(5), 293–299.

Go, A. S., Mozaffarian, D., Roger, V. L., Benjamin, E. J., Berry, J. D., Borden, W. B., et al. (2013). Heart disease and stroke statistics—2013 update: A report from the American Heart Association. *Circulation, 127*(1), e6–e245.

Hiratzka, L. F., Bakris, G. L., Beckman, J. A., Bersin, R. M., Carr, V. F., Casey, D. E., et al. (2010). *Guidelines for the diagnosis and management of patients with thoracic aortic disease.* Philadelphia: Lippincott Williams & Wilkins.

James, P. A., Oparil, S., Carter, B. L., Cushman, W. C., Dennison-Himmelfarb, C., Handler, J., et al. (2014). 2014 evidence-based guidelines for the management of high blood pressure in adults: Report from the panel members appointed to the Eighth National Committee (JNC 8). *Journal of the American Medical Association, 311*(5), 507–520. Retrieved December 2013, from <http://jama.jamanetwork.com/article.aspx?articleid=1791497>.

Michaels, K., & Regan, N. (2013). Teaching patients INR self-management. *Nursing, 43*(5), 67–69.

National Center for Complementary and Alternative Medicine (2013). *Herbs at a glance: Garlic.* Retrieved June 2013, from <http://nccam.nih.gov/health/garlic/ataglance.htm>.

*National Cholesterol Education Program (2002). *Third Report of the Expert Panel on Detection, Evaluation, and Treatment of High Blood Cholesterol in Adults (Adult Treatment Panel III). NIH Publication No. 02-5215.* Bethesda, MD: National Heart, Lung, and Blood Institute.

National Heart, Lung, and Blood Institute (2012). *What is the DASH eating plan?* Retrieved December 2013, from <www.nhlbi.nih.gov/health/health-topics/topics/dash/>.

Pezzotti, W., & Freuler, M. (2012). Using anticoagulants to steer clear of clots. *Nursing, 42*(2), 26–34.

Stone, N. J., Robinson, J., Lichtenstein, A. H., Merz, N. B., Blum, C. B., Eckel, R. H., et al. (2014). 2013 ACC/AHA guidelines on the treatment of blood cholesterol to reduce atherosclerotic cardiovascular risk in adults: A report of the American College of Cardiology/American Heart Association Task Force on Practice Guidelines. *Circulation, 129*(25 Suppl. 2), S1–S45.

Van Tongeren, R., Bastiaansen, A., Van Wissen, R., Le Cessie, S., Hamming, J., & Van Bockel, J. (2010). A comparison of the Doppler-derived maximal systolic acceleration versus the ankle-brachial pressure index or detecting and quantifying peripheral arterial occlusive disease in diabetic patients. *Journal of Cardiovascular Surgery, 51*(3), 391–398.

*Verdecchia, P., Angeli, F., Mazzotta, G., Gentile, G., & Reboldi, G. (2009). Home blood pressure measurements will not replace 24-hour ambulatory blood pressure monitoring. *Hypertension, 54*, 188–195.

Woo, K. Y., & Gowie, B. G. (2013). Understanding compression for venous leg ulcers. *Nursing, 43*(1), 66–68.

Chapter 37

Abbas, A., Lichtman, A., & Pillai, S. (2012). *Cellular and molecular immunology* (7th ed.). Philadelphia: Saunders.

Bernstein, M., & Lynn, S. (2013). Helping patients survive sepsis. *American Nurse Today, 8*(1), 24–28.

Day, D., Matsumoto, K., & Passion, C. (2013). Acute traumatic coagulopathy: The latest intervention strategies. *American Nurse Today, 8*(11), 8–11.

Dellinger, R. P., Levy, M., Rhodes, A., Annane, D., Gerlach, H., Opal, S. M., et al. (2013). Surviving sepsis campaign: International guidelines for management of severe sepsis and septic shock: 2012. *Critical Care Medicine, 41*(2), 580–637.

Dumont, C., & Nesselrodt, D. (2012). Preventing CLABSI: Central line-associated bloodstream infections. *Nursing, 42*(6), 41–46.

Earhart, A. (2013). Recognizing, preventing, and troubleshooting central line complications. *American Nurse Today, 8*(11), 18–22.

Kilburn, F., Baily, P., & Price, D. (2013). Sepsis: Recognizing the next event. *Nursing, 43*(10), 14–16.

Kleinpell, R., Aitken, L., & Schorr, C. (2013). Implications of the new international sepsis guidelines for nursing care. *American Journal of Critical Care, 22*(3), 212–222.

Kleinpell, R., & Schorr, C. (2014). Targeting sepsis as a performance improvement metric: Role of the nurse. *AACN Advanced Critical Care, 25*(2), 179–180.

Lopez-Bushnell, K., Demaray, W., & Jaco, C. (2014). Reducing sepsis mortality. *Medsurg Nursing, 23*(1), 9–14.

Mann-Salinas, E., Engebretson, J., & Batchinsky, A. (2012). A complex systems review of sepsis: Implications for nursing. *Dimensions of Critical Care Nursing, 32*(1), 12–17.

Schell-Chaple, H., & Lee, M. (2014). Reducing sepsis deaths: A systems approach to early detection and management. *American Nurse Today, 9*(7), 26–30.

Walkey, A., Wiener, R., & Lindenauer, P. (2013). Utilization patterns and outcomes associated with central venous catheter in septic shock: A population-based study. *Critical Care Medicine, 41*(6), 1450–1457.

Chapter 38

Allen, J., & Dennison, C. (2010). Randomized trials of nursing interventions for secondary prevention in patients with coronary artery disease and heart failure. *Journal of Cardiovascular Nursing, 25*(3), 207–220.

American Heart Association (AHA) (2013). *Diet and lifestyle recommendations* (updated: March 19, 2013). Retrieved May 2013, from <www.heart.org/HEARTORG/GettingHealthy/Diet-and-Lifestyle-Recommendations_UCM_305855_Article.jsp>.

Berra, K., Fletcher, B., & Handberg, E. (2011). Antiplatelet therapy in acute coronary syndromes. *Journal of Cardiovascular Nursing, 26*(3), 239–249.

Cayla, G., Silvain, J., O'Connor, S., Collet, J., & Montalescot, G. (2012). Current antiplatelet options for NSTE-ACS patients. *QJM: Monthly Journal of the Association of Physicians, 105*, 935–948.

Cossette, S., Frasure-Smith, N., Dupuis, J., Juneau, M., & Guertin, M. (2012). Randomized control trial of tailored nursing interventions to improve cardiac rehabilitation enrollment. *Nursing Research, 61*(2), 111–120.

Crea, F., & Liuzzo, G. (2013). Pathogenesis of acute coronary syndromes. *Journal of the American College of Cardiology, 61*(1), 1–11.

Dechant, L. (2012). UA/NSTEMI: Are you following the latest guidelines? *Nursing, 42*(9), 26–33.

Dolansky, M. A., Xu, F., Zullio, M., Shishehbor, B., Moore, S. M., & Rimm, A. A. (2010). Post–acute care services received by older adults following a cardiac event: A population-based analysis. *Journal of Cardiovascular Nursing, 25*(4), 342–349.

Flicker, L. (2010). Cardiovascular risk factors, cerebrovascular disease burden and healthy brain aging. *Clinics in Geriatric Medicine, 26*(1), 17–27.

Gara, P., Kushner, F., Ascheim, D., Casey, D., Chung, M., de Lemos, J., et al. (2013). 2013 ACCF/AHA guideline for the management of ST-elevation myocardial infarction. *Circulation, 127*, e362–e425.

Go, A., Mozaffarian, D., Roger, V., Benjamin, E., Berry, J., Borden, W., et al. (2013). Heart disease and stroke statistics—2013 update: A report from the American Heart Association. *Circulation, 127,* e6–e245.

*Grundy, S. M., Cleeman, J. I., Daniels, S. R., Donato, K. A., Eckel, R. H., Franklin, B. A., et al. (2005). Diagnosis and management of the metabolic syndrome: An American Heart Association/National Heart, Lung, and Blood Institute scientific statement. *Circulation, 112*(17), 2735–2752.

*Harris, W. S., Mozaffarian, D., Rimm, E., Kris-Etherton, P., Rudel, L. L., Appel, L. J., et al. (2009). Omega-6 fatty acids and risk for cardiovascular disease: A science advisory from the American Heart Association Nutrition Subcommittee of the Council on Nutrition, Physical Activity and Metabolism; Council on Cardiovascular Nursing; and Council on Epidemiology and Prevention. *Circulation, 119*(6), 902–907.

Hillis, D., Smith, P., Anderson, J., Bittl, J., Bridges, C., Byrne, J., et al. (2011). 2011 ACCF/AHA guideline for coronary artery bypass graft surgery: Executive summary: A report of the American College of Cardiology Foundation/American Heart Association Task Force on Practice Guidelines. *Circulation, 124,* 2610–2642.

Housholder-Hughes, S. (2011). Non-ST-segment elevation acute coronary syndrome. *AACN Advanced Critical Care, 22*(2), 113–124.

Jneid, H., Anderson, J., Wright, R., Adams, C., Bridges, C., Casey, D., et al. (2012). 2012 ACCF/AHA focused update of the guideline for the management of patients with unstable angina/non-ST-elevation myocardial infarction (Updating the 2007 guideline and replacing the 2011 focused update). *Circulation, 126,* 875–910.

Leeper, B., Cyr, A., & Martin, K. (2011). Acute coronary syndrome. *Critical Care Nursing Clinics of North America, 23,* 547–557.

Lindholm, D., Varenhorst, C., Cannon, C., Harrington, R., Himmelmann, A., Maya, J., et al. (2013). Ticagrelor vs. clopidogrel in patients with non-ST-elevation acute coronary syndrome: Results from the PLATO trial. *Journal of the American College of Cardiology, 61*(10_Suppl).

McConaghy, J., & Oza, R. (2013). Outpatient diagnosis of acute chest pain in adults. *American Family Physician, 87*(3), 177–182.

McSweeney, J. C., O'Sullivan, P., Cleves, M. A., Lefler, L. L., Cody, M., Moser, D. K., et al. (2010). Racial differences in women's prodromal and acute symptoms of myocardial infarction. *American Journal of Critical Care, 19*(1), 63–73.

*NHLBI. (2004). *Third report of the national cholesterol education program expert panel on detection, evaluation and treatment of high blood cholesterol in adults (adult treatment panel III).* <www.nhlbi.nih.gov>.

Pettinato, M. (2012). Providing care for GLBTQ patients. *Nursing, 42*(12), 22–27.

Rowland, C. A. (2012). Pump it up with an LVAD. *Nursing, 42*(4), 47–50.

Sanz, J., Moreno, P. R., & Fuster, V. (2010). The year in atherothrombosis. *Journal of the American College of Cardiology, 55*(14), 1487–1498.

Scirica, B. (2010). Acute coronary syndrome: Emerging tools for diagnosis and risk assessment. *Journal of the American College of Cardiology, 55*(14), 1403–1415.

Sherrod, M. M., Sherrod, N. M., Spitzer, M. T., & Cheek, D. J. (2013). AHA recommendations for preventing heart disease in women. *Nursing, 43*(5), 61–66.

Shin, J., Martin, R., & Suls, J. (2010). Meta-analytic evaluation of gender differences and symptom measurement strategies in acute coronary syndromes. *Heart and Lung: The Journal of Critical Care, 39,* 283–295.

Summers, K., Martin, K., & Watson, K. (2010). Impact and clinical management of depression in patients with coronary artery disease. *Pharmacotherapy, 30*(3), 304–322.

Thygesen, K., Alpert, J., Jaffe, A., Simoons, M., Chaitman, B., White, H., et al. (2012). Third universal definition of myocardial infarction. *Circulation, 126,* 2020–2035.

Weustink, A. C., Mollet, N. R., Neefjes, L. A., Meijboom, W. B., Galema, T. W., van Mieghem, C. A., et al. (2010). Diagnostic accuracy and clinical utility of noninvasive testing for coronary artery disease. *Annals of Internal Medicine, 152*(10), 630–639.

Chapter 39

Karch, A. (2012). Pharmacology review: Drugs that alter blood coagulation. *American Nurse Today, 7*(11), 26–30.

Pezzotti, W., & Freuler, M. (2012). Using anticoagulants to steer clear of clots. *Nursing, 42*(2), 26–34.

Rauen, C. (2012). Beyond the bloody mess: Hematologic assessment. *Critical Care Nurse, 32*(5), 42–46.

Straznitskas, A., & Giarratano, M. (2014). Emergent reversal of oral anticoagulation: Review of current treatment strategies. *AACN Advanced Clinical Care, 25*(1), 5–12.

Chapter 40

AABB (2013). *Circular information for the use of human blood and blood components.* Retrieved July 2014, from <www.aabb.org/tm/coi/Documents/coi1113.pdf>.

Albrecht, T. (2014). Physiologic and psychological symptoms experienced by adults with acute leukemia: An integrative literature review. *Oncology Nursing Forum, 41*(3), 286–295.

American Cancer Society (ACS) (2014). *Cancer facts and figures 2014.* Report No. 01-300M–No. 500814. Atlanta: Author.

Baker, M., & McKiernan, P. (2011). Management of chronic graft-versus-host disease. *Clinical Journal of Oncology Nursing, 15*(4), 429–432.

Beery, T., & Workman, M. L. (2012). *Genetics and genomics in nursing and health care.* Philadelphia: F.A. Davis.

Byar, K., & Workman, M. (2012). Targeted therapies to treat cancer. In J. Kee, E. Hayes, & L. McCuistion (Eds.), *Pharmacology: A nursing process approach* (7th ed.). St. Louis: Saunders.

Card, E., Nelson, D., Jeskey, M., Miller, A., Michaels, D., Hardeman, W., et al. (2012). Early detection of a blood transfusion reaction utilizing a wireless remote monitoring device. *Medsurg Nursing, 21*(5), 299–302.

Chiffelle, R., & Kenny, K. (2013). Exercise for fatigue management in hematopoietic stem cell transplantation recipients. *Clinical Journal of Oncology Nursing, 17*(3), 241–242.

Elgin, K., Cozzi, K., Fowler, M., Perry, S., Davis, M., Conaway, M., et al. (2011). Maintaining patency with packed red blood cell infusions: Comparison of IV normal saline infusions vs. normal saline syringe method. *Medsurg Nursing, 20*(3), 134–138.

Hardwick, J., Osswald, M., & Walker, D. (2013). Acute pain transfusion reaction. *Oncology Nursing Forum, 40*(6), 543–545.

Hitch, D. (2013). What every nurse should know about hemophilia. *American Nurse Today, 8*(3), 22–26.

Jenerette, C., & Leak, A. (2012). The role of oncology nurses in the care of adults with sickle cell disease. *Clinical Journal of Oncology Nursing, 16*(6), 633–635.

Johnson, N. (2013). Ocular graft-versus-host disease after allogeneic transplantation. *Clinical Journal of Oncology Nursing, 17*(6), 621–626.

Kasberg, H., Brister, L., & Barnard, B. (2011). Aggressive disease, aggressive treatment: The adult hematopoietic stem cell transplant patient in the intensive care unit. *AACN Advanced Critical Care, 22*(4), 349–364.

Kessler, C. (2013). Priming blood transfusion tubing: A critical review of the blood transfusion process. *Critical Care Nurse, 33*(3), 80–83.

Kessler, D., Shaz, B., & Grima, K. (2012). Advances in blood transfusion. *American Nurse Today, 7*(3), 8–11.

Kurtin, S. (2012). Myelodysplastic syndromes: The challenge of developing clinical guidelines and supportive care strategies for a rare disease. *Clinical Journal of Oncology Nursing, S16*(3), S5–S7.

Kurtin, S., & Faiman, B. (2013). The changing landscape of multiple myeloma: Implications for oncology nurses. *Clinical Journal of Oncology Nursing, S17*(6), S2, S7–S11.

Ladizinski, B., Bazakas, A., Mistry, N., Alavi, A., Sibbald, R., & Salcido, R. (2012). Sickle cell disease and leg ulcers. *Advances in Skin & Wound Care, 25*(9), 420–428.

Leak, A., Smith, S., Crandell, J., Jenerette, C., Bailey, D., Zimmerman, S., et al. (2013). Demographic and disease characteristics associated with non-Hodgkin lymphoma survivors' quality of life: Does age matter? *Oncology Nursing Forum, 40*(2), 157–162.

Mangan, P., Gleason, C., & Miceli, T. (2013). Autologous hematopoietic stem cell transplantation for multiple myeloma. *Clinical Journal of Oncology Nursing, 17*(6), 43–47.

MD Consult. <www.mdconsult.com>.

Myers, F., & Reyes, C. (2011). Blood cultures: 5 steps to doing it right. *Nursing*, *41*(3), 62–63.

Myers, M., & Eckes, E. (2012). A novel approach to pain management in persons with sickle cell disease. *Medsurg Nursing*, *21*(5), 293–298.

National Hemophilia Foundation (2014). *MASAC recommendation regarding the use of recombinant clotting factor products with respect to pathogen transmission*. Retrieved July 2014, <www.hemophilia.org/Researchers-Healthcare-Providers/Medical-and-Scientific-Advisory-Council-MASC/All-MASAC-Recommendations/Rexommendation-Regarding-the-Use-of-recombinant-Clotting-Factor-Products-with-Respect-toPathogen-Transmission>.

Orton, C. (2012). Vitamin B12 (cobalamin) deficiency in the older adult. *The Journal for Nurse Practitioners*, *8*(7), 547–553.

Parsh, B., & Kumar, D. (2012). Understanding sickle cell disease. *Nursing*, *42*(8), 64.

Radovich, P. (2011). The multiple causes and myriad presentations of thrombocytopenia. *American Nurse Today*, *6*(1), 9–12.

Simmons, S. (2012). To B or not to B? The inside scoop on vitamin B12. *Nursing*, *42*(12), 55–59.

Simoneau, A. (2013). Treating chronic myeloid leukemia: Improving management through understanding of the patient experience. *Clinical Journal of Oncology Nursing*, *14*(3), 67–72.

Slater, S. (2012). Plerixafor. *Journal of the Advanced Practitioner in Oncology*, *3*(1), 49–54.

The Joint Commission (TJC) (2014). *Implementation guide for The Joint Commission patient blood management performance measures*. Retrieved July 2014, from <www.jointcommission.org/patient_blood_management_performance_measures_project/>.

Thoele, K. (2014). Engraftment syndrome in hematopoietic stem cell transplantations. *Clinical Journal of Oncology Nursing*, *18*(3), 349–354.

Tolich, D., Blackmur, S., Stahorsky, K., & Wabeke, D. (2013). Blood management: Best practice transfusion strategies. *Nursing*, *43*(1), 40–47.

United States National Library of Medicine (2014). *Genetics home reference: Sickle cell disease*. Retrieved October 2014, from <http://ghr.nlm.nih.gov/condition/sickle-cell-disease>.

Chapter 41

Adamis, D., Sharma, N., Whelan, P. J., & Macdonald, A. J. (2010). Delirium scales: A review of current evidence. *Aging & Mental Health*, *14*(5), 543–555.

Barr, J., Fraser, G. L., Puntillo, K., Ely, E. W., Gélinas, C., Dasta, J. F., et al. (2013). Clinical practice guidelines for the management of pain, agitation, and delirium in adult patients in the intensive care unit. *Critical Care Medicine*, *41*(1), 263–306.

Centers for Medicare & Medicaid (2014). *Recommend Core Measures*. Retrieved July 2014, from <http://www.cms.gov/Regulations-and-Guidance/Legislation/EHRIncentivePrograms/Recommended_Core_Set.html>.

Emmett, M., Fenves, A. Z., & Schwartz, J. C. (2012). Approach to the patient with kidney disease. In M. W. Taal, G. M. Chertow, P. A. Marsden, K. Skorecki, A. S. L. Yu, & B. M. Benner (Eds.), *Brenner and Rector's the kidney* (9th ed.). Philadelphia: Saunders.

Faraklas, I., Holt, B., Tran, S., Lin, H., Saffle, J., & Cochran, A. (2013). Impact of a nursing-driven sleep hygiene protocol on sleep quality. *Journal of Burn Care and Research*, *34*(2), 249–254.

Hickey, J. V. (2013). *The clinical practice of neurological and neuosurgical nursing* (7th ed.). Philadelphia: Lippincott Williams & Wilkins.

Holsinger, T., Plassman, B. L., Stechuchak, K. M., Burke, J. R., Coffman, C. J., & Williams, J. W. (2012). Screening for cognitive impairment: Comparing the performance of four instruments in primary care. *Journal of the American Geriatrics Society*, *60*(6), 1027–1036.

Iacono, L. A., Wells, C., & Mann-Finnerty, K. (2014). Standardizing neurological assessments. *The Journal of Neuroscience Nursing*, *46*(2), 125–132.

Iverson, D. J., Gronseth, G. S., Reger, M. A., Classen, S., Dubinsky, R. M., & Rizzo, M. (2010). Practice parameter update: Evaluation and management of driving risk in dementia: Report of the Quality Standards Subcommittee of the American Academy of Neurology. *Neurology*, *74*(16), 1316–1324.

Institute for magnetic resonance safety, education, and research (2014). *MRI Safety*. Retrieved July 2014. from, <http://www.mrisafety.com/>.

Rank, W. (2013). Performing a focused neurologic assessment. *Nursing*, *43*(12), 37–40.

Rattray, J. E., Lauder, W., Ludwick, R., Johnstone, C., Zeller, R., Winchell, J., et al. (2011). Indicators of acute deterioration in adult patients nursed in acute wards: A factorial survey. *Journal of Clinical Nursing*, *20*(5–6), 723–732.

Saliba, D., Buchanan, J., Edelen, M. O., Streim, J., Ouslander, J., Berlowitz, D., et al. (2012). Brief interview for mental status. *Journal of the American Medical Directors Association*, *13*(7), 611–617.

Schmidt, C. W. (2012). CT scans: Balancing health risks and medical benefits. *Environmental Health Perspectives*, *120*(3), A118–A121.

Wijdicks, E. F. M., Varelas, P. N., Gronseth, G. S., & Greer, D. M. (2010). Evidence-based guideline update: Determining brain death in adults. *Neurology*, *74*(23), 1911–1918.

Chapter 42

A.D.A.M. Medical Encyclopedia (2014). *Huntington's disease*. Retrieved July 2014, from <www.ncbi.nlm.nih.gov/pubmedhealth/PMH0001775/>.

Babtain, F. A. (2012). Management of women with epilepsy: Practical issues faced when dealing with women with epilepsy. *Neurosciences (Riyadh)*, *17*(2), 115–120.

Bettens, K., Sleegers, K., & Van Broeckhoven, C. (2013). Genetic insights in Alzheimer's disease. *Lancet Neurology*, *12*(1), 92–104.

Carod-Artel, F. J. (2014). Tackling chronic migraine: Current perspectives. *Journal of Pain Research*, *7*(online), 185–194.

Corbett, A., Stevens, J., Aarsland, D., Day, S., Moniz-Cook, E., Woods, R., et al. (2012). Systematic review of services providing information and/or advice to people with dementia and/or their caregivers. *International Journal of Geriatriatric Psychiatry*, *27*(6), 628–636.

Coskun, P., Wyrembak, J., Schriner, S. E., Chen, H. W., Marciniack, C., Laferla, F., et al. (2012). A mitochondrial etiology of Alzheimer and Parkinson disease. *Biochimica et Biophysica Acta*, *1820*(5), 553–564.

Cranwell-Bruce, L. A. (2010). Drugs for Parkinson's disease. *Medsurg Nursing*, *19*(6), 347–350.

D'Arcy, Y. (2014). Preventing migraine headaches in adults. *Nursing*, *44*(1), 58–61.

Diener, H. C., Dodick, D. W., Turkel, C. C., Demos, G., Degryse, R. E., Earl, N. L., et al. (2014). *European Jounal of Neurology*, *21*(6), 651–659.

Eggenberger, E., Heimerl, K., & Bennett, M. I. (2013). Communication skills training in dementia care: A systematic review of effectiveness, training content, and didactic methods in different care settings. *International Psychogeriatrics*, *25*(3), 345–358.

Ellison, D., Williams, M. L., Moodt, G., & Farrar, F. C. (2010). Electrodiagnostic studies. *Critical Care Nursing Clinics of North America*, *22*(1), 7–18.

Epilepsy Foundation. (2014). Retrieved July 2014 from <www.epilepsyfoundation.org/>.

Haahr, A., Kirkevold, M., Hall, E. O., & Ostergaard, K. (2011). Living with advanced Parkinson's disease: A constant struggle with unpredictability. *Journal of Advanced Nursing*, *67*(2), 408–417.

Hauser, L. (2012). Migraines and perimenopause: Helping women in midlife manage and treat migraine. *Nursing for Women's Health*, *16*(3), 247–250.

Heavey, E. (2010). An update on meningococcal meningitis. *Nursing*, *40*(10), 61–62.

Huntington's Disease Society of America (HDSA) (2014). *About Huntington disease*. Retrieved July 2014, from <www.hdsa.org/>.

Kropelin, T. F., Neyens, J. C., Halfens, R. J., Kempen, G. I., & Hamers, J. P. (2013). Fall determinants in older long-term care residents with dementia: A systematic review. *International Psychogeriatrics*, *25*(4), 549–563.

Johnson, D. K., Niedens, M., Wilson, J. R., Swartzendruber, L., Yeager, A., & Jones, K. (2013). Treatment outcomes of a crisis intervention program for dementia with severe psychiatric complications: The Kansas bridge project. *Gerontologist*, *53*(1), 102–112.

Kumar, K. R., Lohmann, K., & Klein, C. (2012). Genetics of Parkinson disease and other movement disorders. *Current Opinion in Neurology, 25*(4), 466–474.

Kwok, T., Bai, X., Chui, M. Y., Lai, C. K., Ho, D. W., Ho, F. K., et al. (2012). Effect of physical restraint reduction on older patients' hospital length of stay. *Journal of the American Medical Directors Association, 13*(7), 645–650.

Leuzy, A., & Gauthier, S. (2012). Ethical issues in Alzheimer's disease: An overview. *Expert Review of Neurotherapeutics, 12*(5), 557–567.

Lin, J. J., Mula, M., & Hermann, B. P. (2012). Uncovering the neurobehavioural comorbidities of epilepsy over the lifespan. *Lancet, 380*(9848), 1180–1192.

Marcus, D. A. (2014). *Tools for sufferers.* Retrieved July 2014, from <www.headaches.org/education/Tools_for_Sufferers>.

Mauskop, A. (2012). Nonmedication, alternative, and complementary treatments for migraine. *Continuum (Minneap Minn), 18*(4), 796–806.

Mayeux, R., & Stern, Y. (2012). Epidemiology of Alzheimer disease. *Cold Spring Harbor Perspectives in Medicine, 2*(8), 1–26.

Modgill, G., Jette, N., Wang, J. L., Becker, W. J., & Patten, S. B. (2012). A population-based longitudinal community study of major depression and migraine. *Headache, 52*(3), 422–432.

Mohler, R., Richter, T., Kopke, S., & Meyer, G. (2012). Interventions for preventing and reducing the use of physical restraints in long-term geriatric care: A Cochrane review. *Journal of Clinical Nursing, 21*(21–22), 3070–3081.

Moloney, M. F., & Cranwell-Bruce, L. A. (2010). Pharmacologic management of migraine headaches. *Nurse Practitioner, 35*(9), 16–22.

Moyle, W., Borbasi, S., Wallis, M., Olorenshaw, R., & Gracia, N. (2011). Acute care management of older people with dementia: A qualitative perspective. *Journal of Clinical Nursing, 20*(3–4), 420–428.

National Institute of Neurological Disorders and Stroke (NINDS) (2014). *Parkinson's disease.* Retrieved July 2014, from <www.ninds.nih.gov/disorders/parkinsons_disease/parkinsons_disease.htm>.

Niemeijer, A., Frederiks, B., Depla, M., Eefsting, J., & Hertogh, C. (2013). The place of surveillance technology in residential care for people with intellectual disabilities: Is there an ideal model of application. *Journal of Intellectual Disability Research, 57*(3), 201–215.

Overstreet, M. (2011). West Nile virus. *Nursing, 42*(6), 43.

Park, N. H. (2012). Parkinson disease. *JAAPA: Official Journal of the American Academy of Physician Assistants, 25*(5), 73–74.

Parkinson's Disease Foundation (2014). *About Parkinson's disease.* Retrieved July 2014, from <www.pdf.org/>.

Plesh, O., Adams, S. H., & Gansky, S. A. (2012). Self-reported comorbid pains in severe headaches or migraines in a U.S. national sample. *Headache, 52*(6), 946–956.

Rausa, M., Cevoli, S., Sancisi, E., Grimaldi, D., Pollutri, G., Casoria, M., et al. (2013). Personality traits in chronic daily headache patients with and without psychiatric comorbidity: An observational study in a tertiary care headache center. *Journal of Headache and Pain, 14*, 22.

Richter, T., Meyer, G., Mohler, R., & Kopke, S. (2012). Psychosocial interventions for reducing antipsychotic medication in care home residents. *Cochrane Database of Systematic Reviews,* (12), CD008634.

Roberts, B. R. (2010). Caring for patients with Parkinson's disease. *Nursing, 40*(7), 58–64.

Saliba, D., Buchanan, J., Edelen, M. O., Streim, J., Ouslander, J., Berlowitz, D., et al. (2012). MDS 3.0: Brief interview for mental status. *Journal of the American Medical Directors Association, 13*(7), 611–617.

Seitz, D. P., Brisbin, S., Herrmann, N., Rapoport, M. J., Wilson, K., Gill, S. S., et al. (2012). Efficacy and feasibility of nonpharmacological interventions for neuropsychiatric symptoms of dementia in long term care: A systematic review. *Journal of the American Medical Directors Association, 13*(6), 503–506.

Subramaniam, P., & Woods, B. (2012). The impact of individual reminiscence therapy for people with dementia: Systematic review. *Expert Review of Neurotherapeutics, 12*(5), 545–555.

Te Boekhorst, S., Depla, M. F., Francke, A. L., Twisk, J. W., Zwijsen, S. A., & Hertogh, C. M. (2012). Quality of life of nursing-home residents with dementia subject to surveillance technology versus physical restraints: An explorative study. *International Journal of Geriatric Psychiatry, 28*(4), 356–363.

The Joint Commission (2013). *2014 National Patient Safety Goals.* Retrieved July 2014, from <www.jointcommission.org/assets/1/18/NPSG_Chapter_Jan2014_OME.pdf>.

Tolson, D., & Morley, J. E. (2012). Physical restraints: Abusive and harmful. *Journal of the American Medical Directors Association, 13*(4), 311–313.

Van Mierlo, L. D., Meiland, F. J., Van der Roest, H. G., & Droes, R. M. (2012). Personalised caregiver support: Effectiveness of psychosocial interventions in subgroups of caregivers of people with dementia. *International Journal of Geriatric Psychiatry, 27*(1), 1–14.

Vasilevskis, E. E., Pandharipande, P. P., Girard, T. D., & Ely, E. W. (2010). A screening, prevention, and restoration model for saving the injured brain in intensive care unit survivors. *Critical Care Medicine, 38*(Suppl. 10), S683–S691.

Vervloet, M., Linn, A. J., van Weert, J. C. M., de Bakker, D. H., Bouvy, M. L., & van Dijk, L. (2012). The effectiveness of interventions using electronic reminders to improve adherence to chronic medication: a systematic review of the literature. *Journal of the American Medical Informatics Association, 19*(online), 696–704.

Weitzel, T., Robinson, S., Barnes, M. R., Berry, T. A., Holmes, J. M., Mercer, S., et al. (2011). The special needs of the hospitalized patient with dementia. *Medsurg Nursing, 20*(1), 13–18.

Yang, M. H., Wang, P. H., Wang, S. J., Sun, W. Z., Oyang, Y. J., & Fuh, J. L. (2012). Women with endometriosis are more likely to suffer from migraines: A population-based study. *PLoS ONE, 7*(3), e33941.

Zwijsen, S. A., Depla, M. F., Niemeijer, A. R., Francke, A. L., & Hertogh, C. M. (2012). Surveillance technology: An alternative to physical restraints? A qualitative study among professionals working in nursing homes for people with dementia. *International Journal of Nursing Studies, 49*(2), 212–219.

Chapter 43

Ahmad, F., Wang, M. Y., & Levi, A. D. (2013). Hypothermia for acute spinal cord injury: A review. *World Neurosurgery, S1878–8750*(13).

American Nurses Association (ANA) (2013). *Safe patient handling and mobility: interprofessional national standards across the care continuum.* Silver Spring, MD: ANA.

Andersen, P. M., Abrahams, S., Borasio, G. D., de Carvalho, M., Chio, A., Van Damme, P., et al. (2012). EFNS guidelines on the clinical management of amyotrophic lateral sclerosis (MALS): Revised report of an EFNS task force. *European Journal of Neurology, 19*(3), 360–375.

Bailey, J., Dijkers, M. P., Gassaway, J., Thomas, J., Lingefelt, P., Kreider, S. E., et al. (2012). Relationship of nursing education and care management inpatient rehabilitation interventions and patient characteristics to outcomes following spinal cord injury: The SCIRehab project. *Journal of Spinal Cord Medicine, 35*(6), 593–610.

Bergman, D., & Peterson, D. (2011). *Chiropractic technique* (3rd ed.). St. Louis: Mosby.

Costa-Black, K. M., Loisel, P., Anema, J. R., & Pransky, G. (2010). Back pain and work. *Best Practice & Research: Clinical Rheumatology, 24*(2), 227–240.

Courtois, F., Rodrigue, X., Cote, I., Boulet, M., Vezina, J. G., Charvier, K., et al. (2012). Sexual function and autonomic dysreflexia in men with spinal cord injuries: How should we treat? *Spinal Cord, 50*(12), 869–877.

de Carvalho, M., & Swash, M. (2011). Amyotrophic lateral sclerosis: An update. *Current Opinion in Neurology, 24*(5), 497–503.

Duddy, M., Haghikia, A., Cocco, E., Eggers, C., Drulovic, J., Carmona, O., et al. (2011). Managing MS in a changing treatment landscape. *Journal of Neurology, 258*(5), 728–739.

Forrest, G., Huss, S., Patel, V., Jeffries, J., Myers, D., Barber, C., et al. (2012). Falls on an inpatient rehabilitation unit: Risk assessment and prevention. *Rehabilitation Nursing, 37*(2), 56–61.

Frankel, D., & James, H. (2011). *Living with multiple sclerosis.* New York: National Multiple Sclerosis Society.

Furlan, J. C., Noonan, V., Singh, A., & Fehlings, M. G. (2011a). Assessment of disability in patients with acute traumatic spinal cord injury: A systematic review of the literature. *Journal of Neurotrauma, 28*(8), 1413–1430.

Furlan, J. C., Noonan, V., Singh, A., & Fehlings, M. G. (2011b). Assessment of impairment in patients with acute traumatic spinal cord injury: A systematic review of the literature. *Journal of Neurotrauma, 28*(8), 1445–1477.

Gunduz, H., & Binak, D. F. (2012). Autonomic dysreflexia: An important cardiovascular complication in spinal cord injury patients. *Cardiology Journal, 19*(2), 215–219.

Hart, E. S., & Puttaswamy, M. K. (2013). Epidural abscess with spinal cord compression. *Orthopaedic Nursing, 32*(4), 229–230.

Juknis, N., Cooper, J. M., & Volshteyn, O. (2012). The changing landscape of spinal cord injury. *Handbook of Clinical Neurology, 109,* 149–166.

Krassioukov, A. (2012). Autonomic dysreflexia: Current evidence related to unstable arterial blood pressure control among athletes with spinal cord injury. *Clinical Journal of Sport Medicine, 22*(1), 39–45.

Kuijpers, T., van Middelkoop, M., Rubinstein, S. M., Ostelo, R., Verhagen, A., Koes, B. W., et al. (2011). A systematic review on the effectiveness of pharmacological interventions for chronic non-specific low-back pain. *European Spine Journal, 20*(1), 40–50.

Lucas, S. M. (2012). Malignant spinal cord compression. *Nursing, 42*(2), 72.

Ludolph, A. C., Brettschneider, J., & Weishaupt, J. H. (2012). Amyotrophic lateral sclerosis. *Current Opinion in Neurology, 25*(5), 530–535.

*Miller, R. G., Jackson, C. E., Kasarskis, E. J., England, J. D., Forshew, D., Johnston, W., Quality Standards Subcommittee of the American Academy of Neurology, et al. (2009). Practice parameter update: The care of the patient with amyotrophic lateral sclerosis—Multidisciplinary care, symptom management, and cognitive/behavioral impairment (an evidence-based review): Report of the Quality Standards Subcommittee of the American Academy of Neurology. *Neurology, 73*(15), 1227–1233.

Miller, R. G., Mitchell, J. D., & Moore, D. H. (2012). Riluzole for amyotrophic lateral sclerosis (ALS)/motor neuron disease (MND). *Cochrane Database of Systematic Reviews,* (3), CD001447.

Mior, S., Gamble, B., Barnsley, J., Cote, P., & Cote, E. (2013). Changes in primary care physician's management of low back pain in a model of interprofessional collaborative care: An uncontrolled before-after study. *Chiropractic and Manual Therapies, 21*(1), 6.

National Multiple Sclerosis Society (2014a). *What we know about MS.* Retrieved July 20142013, from <www.nationalmssociety.org/about-multiple-sclerosis/what-we-know-about-ms/treatments/medications/tecfidera/index.aspx>.

National Multiple Sclerosis Society (2014b). *Who gets MS.* Retrieved July 2014, from <www.nationalmssociety.org/about-multiple-sclerosis/what-we-know-about-ms/who-gets-ms/index.aspx>.

National Spinal Cord Injury Statistical Center (2014). *Spinal cord injury facts and figures at a glance.* Retrieved July 2014, from <www.nscisc.uab.edu/PublicDocuments/fact_figures_docs/Facts2014.pdf>.

Nayduch, D. A. (2010). Back to basics: Identifying and managing acute spinal cord injury. *Nursing, 40*(9), 24–30.

*Nelson, A., Harwood, K. J., Tracey, C. A., & Dunn, K. L. (2008). Myths and facts about safe patient handling in rehabilitation. *Rehabilitation Nursing, 33*(1), 10–17.

Newland, P. K., Riley, M. A., Fearing, A. D., Neath, A. A., & Gibson, D. (2010). Pain in women with relapsing-remitting multiple sclerosis and healthy women: Relationship to demographic variables. *Medsurg Nursing, 19*(3), 177–182.

Newman, S. D. (2010). Evidence-based advocacy: using Photovoice to identify barriers and facilitators to community participation after spinal cord injury. *Rebailatation Nursing, 35*(2), 47–49.

Norton, C., & Chelvanayagam, S. (2010). Bowel problems and coping strategies in people with multiple sclerosis. *British Journal of Nursing, 19*(4), 220, 221–226.

Parkinson, L., Sibbritt, D., Bolton, P., van Rotterdam, J., & Villadsen, I. (2013). Well-being outcomes of chiropractic intervention for lower back pain: A systematic review. *Clinical Rheumatology, 32*(2), 167–180.

Patton, K. T., & Thibodeau, G. A. (2014). *The human body in health and disease* (6th ed.). St. Louis: Mosby.

Rubinstein, S. M., van Middelkoop, M., Kuijpers, T., Ostelo, R., Verhagen, A. P., de Boer, M. R., et al. (2010). A systematic review on the effectiveness of complementary and alternative medicine for chronic non-specific low-back pain. *European Spine Journal, 19*(8), 1213–1228.

Scherer, K., & Bedlack, R. S. (2012). Diaphragm pacing in amyotrophic lateral sclerosis: A literature review. *Muscle and Nerve, 46*(1), 1–8.

Stahel, P. F., VanderHeiden, T., & Finn, M. A. (2012). Management strategies for acute spinal cord injury: Current options and future perspectives. *Current Opinion in Critical Care, 18*(6), 651–660.

van Middelkoop, M., Rubinstein, S. M., Kuijpers, T., Verhagen, A. P., Ostelo, R., Koes, B. W., et al. (2011). A systematic review on the effectiveness of physical and rehabilitation interventions for chronic non-specific low back pain. *European Spine Journal, 20*(1), 19–39.

van Middelkoop, M., Rubinstein, S. M., Verhagen, A. P., Ostelo, R. W., Koes, B. W., & van Tulder, M. W. (2010). Exercise therapy for chronic nonspecific low-back pain. *Best Practice & Research: Clinical Rheumatology, 24*(2), 193–204.

Wegner, I., Widyahening, I. S., van Tulder, M. W., Blomberg, S. E., de Vet, H. C., Brønfort, G., et al. (2013). Traction of low-back pain with or without sciatica. *Cochrane Database of Systematic Reviews,* online doi:10.1002/14651858.CD003010.pub5.

Zychowicz, M. E. (2013). Pathophysiology of heterotopic ossification. *Orthopaedic Nursing, 32*(3), 173–177.

Chapter 44

Abbott, S. A. (2010). Diagnostic challenge: Myasthenia gravis in the emergency department. *Journal of the American Academy of Nurse Practitioners, 22*(9), 468–473.

Arcila-Londono, X., & Lewis, R. A. (2012). Guillain-Barré syndrome. *Seminars in Neurology, 32*(3), 179–186.

Centers for Disease Control and Prevention (CDC) (2014). *Guillain-Barré syndrome.* Retrieved July 2014, from <www.cdc.gov/flu/protect/vaccine/guillainbarre.htm>.

Cranwell-Bruce, L. A. (2011). Drug treatment for peripheral neuropathy. *Medsurg Nursing, 20*(5), 269–272.

Diaz-Manera, J., Rojas Garcia, R., & Illa, I. (2012). Treatment strategies for myasthenia gravis: An update. *Expert Opinion on Pharmacotherapy, 13*(13), 1873–1883.

Forrest, G., Huss, S., Patel, V., Jeffries, J., Myers, D., Barber, C., et al. (2012). Falls on an inpatient rehabilitation unit: Risk assessment and prevention. *Rehabilitation Nursing, 37*(2), 56–61.

Ibrahim, S. (2012). Trigeminal neuralgia: Diagnostic criteria, clinical aspects and treatment outcomes: A retrospective study. *Gerodontology, 31*(2), 89–94.

Kaplan, A. (2012). Complications of apheresis. *Seminars in Dialysis, 25*(2), 152–158.

Khan, F., & Amatya, B. (2012). Rehabilitation interventions in patients with acute demyelinating inflammatory polyneuropathy: A systematic review. *European Journal of Physical and Rehabilitation Medicine, 48*(3), 507–522.

Liang, C. L., & Han, S. (2013). Neuromuscular junction disorders. *Physical Medicine and Rehabilitation, 5*(Suppl. 5), S81–S88.

Lui, H., Li, H., Xu, M., Chung, K. F., & Zhang, B. P. (2010). A systematic review on acupuncture for trigeminal neuralgia. *Alternative Therapies in Health and Medicine, 16*(3), 30–35.

National Institute of Neurological Disease and Stroke (2014a). *Restless leg syndrome.* Retrieved July 2014, from <www.ninds.nih.gov/disorders/restless_legs/restless_legs.htm>.

National Institute of Neurological Disease and Stroke (2014b). *Trigeminal neuralgia information page.* Retrieved July 2014, from <www.ninds.nih.gov/disorders/trigeminal_neuralgia/trigeminal_neuralgia.htm>.

Novak, C. (2012). Peripheral nerve injuries. *MedScape Reference.* Retrieved April 2013, from <http://emedicine.medscape.com/article/1270360>.

Patwa, H. S., Chaudhry, V., Katzerg, H., Rae-Grant, A. D., & So, Y. T. (2012). Evidence-based guideline: Intravenous immunoglobulin in the treatment of nueromuscular disorders. *Neurology, 78*(13), 1009–1015.

Rajabally, Y. A. (2012). Treatment of Guillain-Barré syndrome: A review. *Inflammation and Allergy Drug Targets, 11*(4), 330–334.

Sejvar, J. J., Baughman, A. L., Wise, M., & Morgan, O. W. (2011). Population incidence of Guillain-Barré syndrome: A systematic review and meta-analysis. *Neuroepidemiology, 36*(2), 123–133.

Silber, M. H. (2013). Sleep-related movement disorders. *Continuum (Minneap Minn), 19*(1 Sleep Disorders), 170–184.

Simmons, S. (2010). Guillain-Barré syndrome. *Nursing, 40*(1), 24–29.

Walsh, M. T. (2012). Interventions in the disturbances in the motor and sensory environment. *Journal of Hand Therapy, 25*(2), 202–218.

Chapter 45

American Heart Association (2014). *Get with the guidelines® educational materials.* Retrieved August 2014, from <http://www.heart.org/HEARTORG/HealthcareResearch/GetWithTheGuidelines/Get-With-The-Guidelines-Educational-Materials_UCM_310980_Article.jsp>.

Aw, D., & Sharma, J. C. (2012). Antiplatelets in secondary stroke prevention: Should clopidogrel be the first choice? *Postgraduate Medical Journal, 88*(1035), 34–37.

Beal, C. C. (2010). Gender and stroke symptoms: A review of the current literature. *Journal of Neuroscience Nursing, 42*(2), 80–87.

Bousser, M. G. (2012). Stroke prevention: An update. *Frontiers of Medicine, 6*(1), 22–34.

Cahill, J. E., & Armstrong, T. S. (2011). Caring for an adult with a malignant primary brain tumor. *Nursing, 41*(6), 28–33.

Cameron, V. (2013). Best practices for stroke patient and family education in the acute care setting: A literature review. *Medsurg Nursing, 22*(3), 51–55.

Centers for Disease Control and Prevention (CDC) (2013a). *Injury prevention & control: Traumatic brain injury.* Retrieved Ocotber, 2014, from <www.cdc.gov/TraumaticBrainInjury>.

Centers for Disease Control and Prevention (CDC) (2013b). *Stroke.* Retrieved October, 2014, from <www.cdc.gov/stroke/>.

Courman, M. (2012). Bladder management in female stroke survivors: Translating research into practice. *Rehabilitation Nursing, 37*(5), 220–230.

Defazio, M. V., Rammo, R. A., Robles, J. R., Bramlett, H. M., Dietrich, W. D., & Bullock, M. R. (2013). The potential utility of blood-derived biochemical markers as indicators of early clinical trends following severe traumatic brain injury. *World Neurosurgery, 81*(1), 151–158.

Howard, G., Cushman, M., Kissela, B. M., Kleindorfer, D. O., McClure, L. A., Safford, M. M., Racial Differences in Stroke Investigators, et al. (2011). Traditional risk factors as the underlying cause of racial disparities in stroke: Lessons from the half-full (empty?) glass. *Stroke, 42*(12), 3369–3375.

Hughes, P. (2011). Comprehensive care of adults with acute ischemic stroke. *Critical Care Nursing Clinics of North America, 23*(4), 661–675.

Knauft, W., Chhabra, J., & McCullough, L. D. (2010). Emergency department arrival times, treatment, and functional recovery in women with acute ischemic stroke. *Journal of Woman's Health, 19*(4), 681–688.

Lakoski, S. G., Le, A. H., Muntner, P., Judd, S. E., Safford, M. M., Levine, D. A., et al. (2011). Adiposity, inflammation, and risk for death in black and white men and women in the United States: The Reasons for Geographic and Racial Differences in Stroke (REGARDS) study. *Journal of Clinical Endocrinology and Metabolism, 96*(6), 1805–1814.

Lee, L. K., Bateman, B. T., Wang, S., Schumacher, H. C., Pile-Spellman, J., & Saposnik, G. (2012). Trends in the hospitalization of ischemic stroke in the United States, 1998-2007. *International Journal of Stroke, 7*(3), 195–201.

Mink, J., & Miller, J. (2011a). Opening the window of opportunity for treating acute ischemic stroke. *Nursing, 41*(1), 24–32.

Mink, J., & Miller, J. (2011b). Stroke, Part 2: Respond aggressively to hemorrhagic stroke. *Nursing, 41*(3), 36–42.

Müller, B., Evangelopoulos, D. S., Bias, K., Wildisen, A., Zimmermann, H., & Exadaktylos, A. K. (2011). Can S-100B serum protein help to save cranial CT resources in a peripheral trauma centre? A study and consensus paper. *Emergency Medicine Journal, 28*(11), 938–940.

Muttikkal, T. J., & Wintermark, M. (2013). MRI patterns of global hypoxic-ischemic injury in adults. *Journal of Neuroradiology, 40*(3), 164–171.

Norton, C., Feltz, S. J., Brocker, A., & Granitto, M. (2013). Tackling long-term consequences of concussion. *Nursing, 43*(1), 50–55.

Oran, N. T., & Oran, I. (2010). Carotid angioplasty and stenting in carotid artery stenosis: Neuroscience nursing implications. *The Journal of Neuroscience Nursing, 42*(1), 3–11.

Perry, L., Hamilton, S., Williams, J., & Jones, S. (2013). Nursing interventions for improving nutritional status and outcomes of stroke patients: Descriptive reviews of processes and outcomes. *Worldviews on Evidence-based Nursing, 10*(1), 17–40.

Rank, W. (2012). Making repairs with endovascular surgical neuroradiology. *Nursing, 42*(12), 41–45.

Rank, W. (2013). Aneurysmal subarachnoic hemorrhage. *Nursing, 43*(5), 43–50.

Schnieder, M., & Schneider, M. D. E. (2012). Recognizing post stroke depression. *Nursing, 42*, 60–63.

Simmons, S. (2012). Recognizing stroke in women. *Nursing, 42*(3), 30–36.

Simpson, J. R., Zahuranec, D. B., Lisabeth, L. D., Sanchez, B. N., Skolarus, L. E., Mendizabal, J. E., et al. (2010). Mexican Americans with atrial fibrillation have more recurrent strokes than do non-Hispanic whites. *Stroke, 41*(10), 2132–2136.

Smania, N., Avesani, R., Roncari, L., Ianes, P., Girardi, P., Varalta, V., et al. (2013). Factors predicting functional and cognitive recovery following severe traumatic, anoxic, and cerebrovascular brain damage. *Journal of Head Trauma Rehabilitation, 28*(2), 131–140.

The Joint Commission (2014). *Stroke.* Retrieved October 2014, from <http://www.jointcommission.org/stroke/>.

Thompson, H. J., & Mauk, K. (2011). *Care of the patient with mild traumatic brain injury.* Retrieved October 2014, from <www.rehabnurse.org/uploads/files/cpgmtbi.pdf>.

Wijdicks, E. F., Varelas, P. N., Gronseth, G. S., Greer, D. M., & American Academy of Neurology. (2010). Evidence-based guideline update: Determining brain death in adults: Report of the Quality Standards Subcommittee of the American Academy of Neurology. *Neurology, 74*(23), 1911–1918.

Chapter 46

See General References.

Chapter 47

American Cancer Society (2014). *Cancer facts and figures 2014.* Report No. 00-300M–No. 500814. Atlanta: Author.

Corneal abrasion. (2013). Corneal abrasion. *Nursing, 43*(2), 49.

Foundation Fighting Blindness. (2012). Retrieved October 2014, from <www.blindness.org>.

Huber, M., Hofmann, W., & Drager, D. (2013). Ophthalmic drugs as part of polypharmacy in nursing home residents with glaucoma. *Drugs and Aging, 30*(1), 31–38.

Kerr, E. (2013). Back to basics: Age-related macular degeneration. *Nursing and Residential Care, 15*(7), 484–487.

National Eye Institute of the National Institutes of Health (2012). *Prevalence of adult vision impairment and age-related eye diseases in America.* Retrieved July 2014, from <www.nei.nih.gov/eyedata/adultvision_usa.asp>.

Newton, M., & Sanderson, A. (2013). The effect of visual impairment on patients' falls risk. *Nursing Older People, 25*(8), 16–21.

Online Mendelian Inheritance in Man (OMIM) (2014). *Retinitis pigmentosa.* Retrieved October 2014, from <www.omim.org/entry/268000>.

Russo, A., & Bowden, D. (2013). Visual impairment: Setting sights on an independent life. *Nursing & Residential Care, 15*(1), 38–40.

Warren, M. (2013). Promoting health literacy in older adults with low vision. *Topics in Geriatric Rehabilitation, 29*(2), 107–115.

Watkinson, S. (2013). Assessment and management of patients with acute red eye. *Nursing Older People, 25*(5), 27–34.

Chapter 48

Alm, M. (2012). Hope to cope. *Hearing Health, 28*(4), 14–15.

Barbara, M., Biagini, M., & Monini, S. (2011). The totally implantable middle ear device "Esteem" for rehabilitation of severe sensorineural hearing loss. *Acta Oto-Laryngologica, 131*(4), 399–404.

Bridges, J., Lataille, A., Buttorff, C., White, S., & Niparko, J. K. (2012). Consumer preferences for hearing aid attributes: A comparison of rating and conjoint analysis methods. *Trends in Amplification, 16*(1), 40–48.

Haynes, D. (2014). Defining Ménière's disease. *Hearing Health, Winter*, 34–37.

Holmes, A., Shrivastav, R., Krause, L., Siburt, H., & Schwartz, E. (2012). Speech based optimization of cochlear implants. *International Journal of Audiology, 51*(6), 806–816.

*National Institute on Deafness and other Communication Disorders (NIDCD) (2010). *Ménière's disease*. Retrieved October 2014, from <www.nidcd.nih.gov/health/balance/pages/meniere.aspx>.

National Institute on Deafness and other Communication Disorders (NIDCD) (2014). *Statistics about hearing, balance, ear infections and deafness*. Retrieved October 2014, from <www.nidcd.nih.gov/health/statistics/pages/hearing.aspx>.

National Institute on Deafness and other Communication Disorders (NIDCD) (2012). *Noise-induced hearing loss*. Retrieved October 2014, from <www.nidcd.nih.gov/health/statistics/pages/noise.aspx>.

Online Mendelian Inheritance in Man (OMIM) (2014). *Gap junction proteins, beta-2; GJB2*. Retrieved October 2014, from <www.omim.org/entry/121011>.

Oyler, A. (2012). The American hearing loss epidemic. *The American Speech-Language Hearing Association LEADER, 17*(2), 5–7.

Richardson, K. J. (2014). Deaf culture: Competencies and best practices. *The Nurse Practitioner, 39*(5), 20–28.

Ruppert, S., & Fay, V. (2012). Tinnitus evaluation in primary care. *The Nurse Practitioner, 37*(10), 20–26.

Shuler, G., Mistler, L., Torrey, K., & Depukat, R. (2013). Bridging communication gaps with the deaf. *Nursing, 43*(11), 24–30.

Spyridakou, C. (2012). Hearing loss: A health problem for all ages. *Primary Health Care, 22*(4), 16–20.

Chapter 49

Chou, R., Deyo, R. A., & Jarvik, J. G. (2012). Appropriate use of lumbar imaging for evaluation of low back pain. *Radiology Clinics of North America, 50*(4), entire issue.

*Collyott, C. L., & Brooke, M. V. (2008). Evaluation and management of joint pain. *Orthopaedic Nursing, 27*(4), 246–250.

Doheny, M. O., Sedlak, C. A., Estok, P. J., & Zeller, R. A. (2011). Bone density, health beliefs, and osteoporosis preventing behaviors in men. *Orthopaedic Nursing, 30*(4), 266–272.

Esoga, P. I., & Seidl, K. L. (2012). Best practices in orthopedic inpatient care. *Orthopaedic Nursing, 31*(4), 236–240.

Kamienski, M., Tate, D., & Vega, M. (2011). The silent thief: Diagnosis and management of osteoporosis. *Orthopaedic Nursing, 30*(3), 162–171.

*Kress, T., Krueger, D., & Ziccardi, S. (2008). Creatine kinase: An assay with muscle. *Nursing, 38*(10), 62.

Mosher, C. M. (2010). *An introduction to orthopaedic nursing* (4th ed.). Chicago: National Association of Orthopaedic Nurses.

*Nussbaum, R. L., McInnes, R. R., & Willard, H. F. (2007). *Thompson & Thompson genetics in medicine* (7th ed.). Philadelphia: Saunders.

Schoen, D. C. H. (2010). *Adult orthopaedic nursing*. Philadelphia: Lippincott-Williams-Wilkins.

Smith, M. A., & Smith, W. T. (2010). Rotator cuff tears: An overview. *Orthopaedic Nursing, 29*(5), 319–322.

Chapter 50

Chang, S. F., Yang, R. S., Chung, U. L., Chen, C. M., & Cheng, M. H. (2010). Perception of risk factors and DXA T-score among at-risk females of osteoporosis. *Journal of Clinical Nursing, 19*(13–14), 1795–1802.

Cohen, H. V. (2010). Bisphosphonate-associated osteonecrosis of the jaw—Patient care considerations: Overview for the orthopaedic nursing healthcare professional. *Orthopaedic Nursing, 29*(3), 176–180.

Crawford, A., & Harris, H. (2012). Balancing act: Calcium and phosphorus. *Nursing, 42*(1), 36–42.

Doheny, M. O., Sedlak, C. A., Estok, P. J., & Zeller, R. A. (2011). Bone density, health beliefs, and osteoporosis preventing behaviors in men. *Orthopaedic Nursing, 30*(4), 266–272.

Doheny, M. O., Sedlak, C. A., Zeller, R., & Estok, P. J. (2010). Validation of the Osteoporosis Smoking Health Belief instrument. *Orthopaedic Nursing, 29*(1), 11–16.

*Gloth, F. M., III, & Simonson, W. (2008). Osteoporosis is underdiagnosed in skilled nursing facilities: A large-scale heel BMD screening study. *Journal of the American Medical Directors Association, 9*(3), 190–193.

Greene, D., & Dell, R. M. (2010). Outcomes of an osteoporosis disease-management program managed by nurse practitioners. *Journal of the American Academy of Nurse Practitioners, 22*(6), 326–329.

Institute for Safe Medication Practices (2013). *ISMPs list of high-alert medications*. Retrieved June 2013, from <www.ismp.org/Tools/highalertmedications.pdf>.

*Johnson, M. A., Davery, A., Park, S., Hausman, D. B., & Poon, L. W. (2008). Age, race and season predict vitamin D status in African American and white octogenarians and centenarians. *Journal of Nutrition and Health Aging, 12*(10), 690–695.

Kamienski, M., Tate, D., & Vega, M. (2011). The silent thief: Diagnosis and management of osteoporosis. *Orthopaedic Nursing, 30*(3), 162–171.

*Lee, J. (2009). Complication related to bisphosphonate therapy: Osteonecrosis of the jaw. *Journal of Infusion Nursing, 32*(6), 330–335.

*Najat, D., Garner, T., Hagen, T., Shaw, B., Sheppard, P. W., Falchetti, A., et al. (2009). Characterization of a non-UBA domain missense mutation of sequestosome (SQSTM1) in Paget's disease of bone. *Journal of Bone and Mineral Research, 24*(4), 632–642.

National Institute of Arthritis and Musculoskeletal and Skin Diseases (2013). *Information for patients about Paget's disease of bone*. Retrieved June 2013, from <www.niams.nih.gov/Health_Info/Bone/pagets/patient_info.asp>.

National Osteoporosis Foundation (NOF) (2010). *Clinician's guide to prevention and treatment of osteoporosis*. Washington, DC: Author.

*Nussbaum, R., McInnes, R., & Willard, H. (2007). *Thompson & Thompson: Genetics in medicine* (7th ed.). Philadelphia: Saunders.

*Parikh, S., Avorn, J., & Solomon, D. H. (2009). Pharmacological management of osteoporosis in nursing home populations: A systematic review. *Journal of the American Geriatrics Society, 57*(2), 327–334.

*Sadler, C., & Huff, M. (2007). African-American women: Health beliefs, lifestyle, and osteoporosis. *Orthopaedic Nursing, 26*(2), 96–101.

Sambrook, P. N., Cameron, I. D., Chen, J. S., March, L. M., Simpson, J. M., Cumming, R. G., et al. (2010). Oral bisphosphonates are associated with reduced mortality in frail older people: A prospective five-year study. *Osteoporosis International, 21*(10), [Epub ahead of print].

Seton, M., Moses, A. M., Bode, R. K., & Schwartz, C. (2011). Paget's disease of bone: The skeletal distribution, complications, and quality of life as perceived by patients. *Bone, 48*(2), 281–285.

Sutcliffe, A. (2010). Paget's: The neglected bone disease. *International Journal of Orthopaedic and Trauma Nursing, 14*, 142–149.

Swislocki, A., Green, J. A., Heinrich, G., Barnett, C. A., Meadows, I. D., Harmon, E. B., et al. (2010). Prevalence of osteoporosis in men in a VA rehabilitation center. *American Journal of Managed Care, 16*(6), 427–433.

*Voda, S. C. (2009a). Dangerous curves: Treating adult idiopathic scoliosis. *Nursing, 39*(12), 42–46.

*Voda, S. C. (2009b). Help older men bone up on osteoporosis. *Nursing, 39*(12), 66–67.

Chapter 51

Al-Shaer, D., Hill, P. D., & Anderson, M. A. (2011). Nurses' knowledge and attitudes regarding pain assessment and intervention. *Medsurg Nursing, 20*(1), 7–12.

*Altizer, L. L. (2008). Colles' fracture. *Orthopaedic Nursing, 27*(2), 140–145.

Barry, M. (2010). Bringing Achilles tendinopathy to heel. *Nursing, 40*(10), 30–33.

Chang, H. J., Burke, A. E., & Glass, R. M. (2010). Achilles tendinopathy. *Journal of the American Medical Association, 303*(2), 188.

Friedrich, J. B., & Shin, A. Y. (2012). Management of forearm compartment syndrome. *Critical Care Nursing Clinics of North America, 24*(2), 261–274.

Guarin, P. L. B. (2013). How effective are nerve blocks after orthopedic surgery: A quality improvement study. *Nursing, 43*(6), 63–66.

*Herr, K., & Titler, M. (2009). Acute pain assessment and pharmacological management practices for the older adult with a hip fracture: Review of ED trends. *Journal of Emergency Nursing*, 35(4), 312–320.

Hershey, K. (2013). Fracture complications. *Critical Care Nursing Clinics of North America*, 25(2), 321–331.

*Hsu, E. (2009). Practical management of complex regional pain syndrome. *American Journal of Therapeutics*, 16(2), 147–154.

Huisstede, B. M., Randsdorp, M. S., Coert, J. H., Glerum, S., van Middlekoop, M., & Koes, B. W. (2010). Carpal tunnel syndrome, Part II— Effectiveness of surgical treatments: A systematic review. *Archives of Physical Medicine and Rehabilitation*, 91(7), 1005–1024.

*Ketz, A. K. (2008). Pain management in the traumatic amputee. *Critical Care Nursing Clinics of North America*, 20(1), 51–57.

*Lowe, J., & Tariman, J. D. (2008). Lower extremity amputations: Black men with diabetes overburdened. *Advance for Nurse Practitioners*, 16(11), 28.

Montana, C., & Kautz, D. D. (2011). Turning the nightmare of complex regional pain syndrome into a time of healing, renewal, and hope. *Medsurg Nursing*, 20(3), 139–142.

Nahm, E.-S., Resnick, B., Orwig, D., Magaziner, J., & Degrezia, M. (2010). Exploration of informal caregiving following hip fractures. *Geriatric Nursing*, 31(4), 254–262.

Nahm, E.-S., Resnick, B., Plummer, L., & Park, B. K. (2013). Use of discussion boards in an online hip fracture resource center for caregivers. *Orthopaedic Nursing*, 32(2), 89–96.

National Institute of Neurological Disorders and Stroke (2011). *Complex regional pain syndrome fact sheet*. Retrieved March 2011, from <www.ninds.nih.gov/disorders/reflex_sympathetic_dystrophy/detail.htm>.

Pirrung, J., & Mower-Wade, D. (2014). Early recognition and treatment of pelvic fractures. *Nursing*, 44(9), 38–46.

Pullen, R. L. (2010). Caring for a patient after amputation. *Nursing*, 40(1), 15.

Satryb, S. A., Wilson, T. J., & Patterson, M. M. (2011). Casting: All wrapped up. *Orthopedic Nursing*, 30(1), 37–41.

Smith, M. A., & Smith, W. T. (2010). Rotator cuff tears: An overview. *Orthopaedic Nursing*, 29(5), 319–322.

Sweitzer, V., Rondeau, D., Guido, V., & Rasmor, M. (2013). Interventions to improve outcomes in the elderly after hip fracture. *Journal for Nurse Practitioners*, 9(4), 238–242.

Uchiyama, S., Itsubo, T., Nakamura, K., Kato, H., Yasutomi, T., & Momose, T. (2010). Current concepts of carpal tunnel syndrome: Pathophysiology, treatment, and evaluation. *Journal of Orthopaedic Science*, 15(1), 1–13.

Voda, S. C. (2011). Bad breaks: A nurse's guide to distal radius fractures. *Nursing*, 41(8), 34–40.

Walsh, C. R. (2013). Wrist fractures in adults: Getting a grip. *Nursing*, 43(4), 38–44.

Chapter 52

American Cancer Society (2014). *American Cancer Society guidelines for the early detection of cancer*. Retrieved January 2014, from <www.cancer.org/healthy/findcancerearly/cancerscreeningguidelines/american-cancer-society-guidelines-for-the-early-detection-of-cancer>.

Bittler, R. D. (2011). Splenic injury due to colonoscopy: Nursing considerations. *Gastroenterology Nursing*, 34(5), 357–364.

Bjorkman, I., Karlsson, F., Lundberg, A., & Frisman, G. H. (2013). Gender differences when using sedative music during colonoscopy. *Gastroenterology Nursing*, 36(1), 14–20.

Bourque, A. L., Sullivan, M. E., & Winter, M. R. (2012). Reiki as a pain management adjunct in screening colonoscopy. *Gastroenterology Nursing*, 35(5), 308–312.

Bruesehoff, M. P. (2010). ERCP—Much ado about blockages: Update your knowledge about the diagnostic and therapeutic uses for endoscopic retrograde cholangiopancreatography. *Nursing*, 40(9), 46–50.

Devitt, J., Shellman, L., Gardner, K., & Nichols, L. W. (2011). Using positioning after a colonoscopy for patient comfort management. *Gastroenterology Nursing*, 34(2), 93–100.

Dudley-Brown, S. (2012). The importance of the physical examination. *Gastroenterology Nursing*, 35(5), 350–352.

Ellett, M. L. (2010). A literature review of the safety and efficacy of using propofol for sedation in endoscopy. *Gastroenterology Nursing*, 33(2), 113–117.

Hulse, R. S., Stuart-Shor, E. M., & Russo, J. (2010). Endoscopic procedure with a modified Reiki intervention: A pilot study. *Gastroenterology Nursing*, 33(1), 20–26.

Keske, L. A., & Letizia, M. (2010). *Clostridium difficile* infection: Essential information for nurses. *Medsurg Nursing*, 19(6), 329–333.

Mikocka-Walus, A. A., Moulds, L. G., Rollbusch, N., & Andrews, J. M. (2012). "It's a tube up your bottom: It makes people nervous": The experience of anxiety in initial colonoscopy patients. *Gastroenterology Nursing*, 35(6), 392–401.

Munson, G. W., Van Norstrand, M. D., O'Donnell, J. J., Hammes, N. L., & Francis, D. L. (2011). Intraprocedural evaluation of comfort for sedated outpatient upper endoscopy and colonoscopy: The La Crosse (WI) Intra-Endoscopy Sedation Comfort Score. *Gastroenterology Nursing*, 34(4), 296–301.

Muscarella, L. F. (2010). Evaluation of the risk of transmission of bacterial biofilms and *Clostridium difficile* during gastrointestinal endoscopy. *Gastroenterology Nursing*, 33(1), 28–35.

Tas, A. (2013). Periorbital ecchymosis following an upper gastrointestinal endoscopy. *Gastroenterology Nursing*, 36(1), 72.

Van Dongen, M. (2012). Enhancing bowel preparation for colonoscopy: An integrative review. *Gastroenterology Nursing*, 35(1), 36–44.

Welliver, M. (2012). Why capnography for procedural sedation? *Gastroenterology Nursing*, 35(6), 423–425.

Chapter 53

Agency for Toxic Substances and Disease Registry (2014). *ToxFAQs for polycyclic aromatic hydrocarbons (PAHs*. Retrieved July 2014, from <www.atsdr.cdc.gov/>.

AHFS® Consumer Medication Information (2013). *Thalidomide*. Retrieved July 2014, from <www.nlm.nih.gov/medlineplus/druginfo/meds/a699032.html>.

Alterburg, A., & Zouboulis, C. (2014). *Current concepts in the treatment of recurrent aphthous stomatitis*. Retrieved July 2014, from <www.skintherapyletter.com/2008/13.7/1.html>.

American Dietetic Association (2014). *Position of the American Dietetic Association: Oral health and nutrition*. Retrieved July 2014, from <www.eatright.org>.

Baldwin, C., Spiro, A., Ahern, R., & Emery, P. W. (2012). Oral nutritional interventions in malnourished patients with cancer: A systematic review and meta-analysis. *Journal of the National Cancer Institute*, 104(5), 371–385.

Broutian, T., Pickard, R., Tong, Z., Xiao, W., Kahle, L., Graubard, B., et al. (2012). Prevalence of oral HPV infection in the United States, 2009-2010. *Journal of the American Medical Association*, 307(7), 693–703.

Cancer Research UK (2014). *Types of mouth and oropharyngeal cancer*. Retrieved July 2014, from <www.cancerhelp.org.uk>.

Livestrong.com (2014). *Cautions for family members of persons receiving radiation treatment for cancer*. Retrieved July 2014, from <www.livestrong.com>.

Moriya, S., Tei, K., Murata, A., Muramatsu, M., Inoue, N., & Miura, H. (2012). Relationships between Geriatric Oral Health Assessment Index scores and general physical status in community-dwelling older adults. *Gerodontology*, 29(2), e998–e1004.

National Institutes of Health (2014). *Genetics home reference: TP53*. Retrieved July 2014, from <www.ghr.nlm.nih.gov/gene/TP53>.

North Carolina State Health Plan (2012). *Thalidomide*. Retrieved July 2014, from <www.shpnc.org/library/pdf/pharmacy/thalomid.pdf>.

Oral Cancer Foundation (OCF) (2014). *Oral cancer facts*. Retrieved July 2014, from <www.oralcancerfoundation.org>.

OralCDx (2013). *The OralCDx brush test*. Retrieved July 2014, from <www.sopreventable.com>.

Prendergast, V., Jakobsson, U., Renvert, S., & Hallberg, I. (2012). Effects of a standard versus comprehensive oral care protocol among intubated neuroscience ICU patients: Results of a randomized controlled trial. *Journal of Neuroscience Nursing*, 44(3), 134–146.

van der Meulen, I. C., de Leeuw, J. R. J., Gamel, C. J., & Hafsteinsdóttir, T. B. (2012). Educational intervention for patients with head and neck cancer in the discharge phase. *European Journal of Oncology Nursing*, 17(2), 220–227.

World Health Organization (2014). *Oral health.* Retrieved July 2014, from <www.who.int/mediacentre/factsheets/fs318/en/>.

Chapter 54

American Cancer Society (ACS) (2012). *Cancer facts and figures 2012.* Retrieved August 2014, from <www.cancer.org/acs/groups/content/@epidemiologysurveilance/documents/document/acspc-031941.pdf>.

American Cancer Society (ACS) (2014a). *Chemotherapy for cancer of the esophagus.* Retrieved August 2014, from <www.cancer.org/cancer/esophaguscancer/detailedguide/esophagus-cancer-treating-chemotherapy>.

American Cancer Society (ACS) (2014b). *Targeted therapy for cancer of the esophagus.* Retrieved June 2013, from <www.cancer.org/cancer/esophaguscancer/detailedguide/esophagus-cancer-treating-targeted-therapy>.

Buckley, F., & Roberts, K. (2014). *Laparoscopic Nissen fundoplication.* Retrieved August 2014, from <http://emedicine.medscape.com/article/1892517-overview>.

*Chait, M. M. (2010). Gastroesophageal reflux disease: Important considerations for older patients. *World Journal of Gastrointestinal Endoscopy, 2*(12), 388–396.

Harvard Health Publications (2011). *Proton-pump inhibitors.* Retrieved August 2014, from <www.health.harvard.edu/newsletters/Harvard_Health_Letter/2011/April/proton-pump-inhibitors>.

National Cancer Institute at the National Institutes of Health (2013). *A snapshot of esophageal cancer.* Retrieved August 2014, from <www.cancer.gov/researchandfunding/snapshots/esophageal>.

National Guideline Clearinghouse (NGC) (2013). *Guideline synthesis: Diagnosis and management of gastroesophageal reflux disease (GERD).* Retrieved August 2014, from <http://www.guideline.gov/content.aspx?id=43847&search=gerd>.

National Institutes of Health (2013). *Esophageal monometry.* Retrieved August 2014, from <www.nlm.nih.gov/medlineplus/ency/article/003884.htm>.

*Nussbaum, R. L., McInnes, R. R., & Willard, H. F. (2007). *Thompson and Thompson's genetics in medicine.* Philadelphia: Saunders.

Patel, D., & Siddiqui, R. (2013). Fully covered esophageal stents: Role in benign disease. *Practical Gastroenterology,* 39–46. Retrieved August 2014, from <www.practicalgastro.com/pdf/May13/D-Patel.pdf>.

Solomon, M., & Reynolds, J. C. (2012). Esophageal reflux disease and its complications. In *Geriatric gastroenterology.* New York: Springer.

The Ohio State University Wexner Medical Center (OSUWMC) (2014). *Diagnosing GERD.* Retrieved August 2014, from <http://medicalcenter.osu.edu/patientcare/healthcare_services/digestive_disorders/gerd_heartburn/diagnosing_treating_gerd/diagnosing_gerd/Pages/index.aspx>.

University of Michigan Health System (2012). *Gastroesophageal reflux disease (GERD).*

Retrieved August 2014, from <www.guideline.gov/content.aspx?id=37564>.

Chapter 55

Abe, N., Takeuchi, H., Yanagida, O., Sugiyama, M., & Atomi, Y. (2010). Surgical indications and procedures for bleeding peptic ulcer. *Digestive Endoscopy, 22*(Suppl. 1), S35–S37.

American Cancer Society (2014). *Stomach cancer.* Retrieved January 2014, from <www.cancer.org/acs/groups/cid/documents/webcontent/003141-pdf.pdf>.

Bailey, K. (2011). An overview of gastric cancer and its management. *Cancer Nursing Practice, 10*(6), 31–37.

Bosaeus, I., & Bergbom, I. (2010). Patients' experiences of the recovery period 12 months after upper gastrointestinal surgery. *Gastroenterology Nursing, 33*(6), 422–431.

DeRanieri, J. T. (2013). *Peptic ulcer disease.* Retrieved July 2013, from <www.nursingconsult.com/nursing/evidence-based-nursing/monograph?monograph_id=219951>.

Howlader, N., Noone, A. M., Krapcho, M., Neyman, N., Aminou, R., Altekruse, S. F., et al. (Eds.), (2012). *SEER cancer statistics review, 1975-2009 (Vintage 2009 Populations).* Bethesda, MD: National Cancer Institute. Retrieved July 2013, from <http://seer.cancer.gov/csr/1975_2009_pops09/>.

Jemal, A., Bray, F., Center, M. M., Ferlay, J., Ward, E., & Forman, D. (2011). Global cancer statistics. *CA: A Cancer Journal for Clinicians, 61,* 69–90.

Kwok, C. S., Yeong, J. K., & Loke, Y. K. (2010). Meta-analysis: Risk of fractures with acid-suppressing medication. *Bone, 48*(4), 768–776.

Mayhew, M. S. (2011). Long-term safety of proton pump inhibitors. *Journal for Nurse Practitioners, 7*(4), 323–324.

National Cancer Institute (2012). *Surveillance, epidemiology and end results (SEER) stat fact sheet: Cancer of the stomach.* Retrieved April 2013, from <http://seer.cancer.gov/statfacts/html/stomach.html#content>.

National Cancer Institute (2013). *Fact sheet: Helicobacter pylori and cancer.* Retrieved April 2013, from <www.cancer.gov/cancertopics/factsheet/Risk/h-pylori-cancer>.

National Digestive Diseases Information Clearinghouse (2012). *H. pylori and peptic ulcers. National Institute of Diabetes and Digestive and Kidney Diseases home page.* Retrieved April 2013, from <www.digestive.niddk.nih.gov/ddiseases/pubs/hpylori/index.aspx>.

Saif, W. W., Makrilia, N., Zalonis, A., Merikas, M., & Syrigos, K. (2010). Gastric cancer in the elderly: An overview. *European Journal of Surgical Oncology, 36*(8), 709–717.

Yang, D., Hendifar, A., Lenz, C., Togawa, K., Lurje, G., Pohl, A., et al. (2011). Survival of metastatic gastric cancer: Significance of age, sex and race/ethnicity. *Journal of Gastrointestinal Oncology, 2*(2), 77–84.

Zarowitz, B. J. (2011). The challenge of discontinuing proton pump inhibitors. *Geriatric Nursing, 32*(4), 276–278.

Chapter 56

American Cancer Society (ACS) (2014). *Cancer facts and figures 2014.* Atlanta: Author.

Barkhordari, E., Rezaei, N., Ansaripour, B., Larki, P., Alighardashi, M., Ahmad-Ashtiani, H. R., et al. (2010). Proinflammatory cytokine gene polymorphisms in irritable bowel syndrome. *Journal of Clinical Immunology, 30*(1), 74–79.

Bengtsson, M., Ulander, K., Borgdal, E. B., & Ohlsson, B. (2010). A holistic approach for planning care of patients with irritable bowel syndrome. *Gastroenterology Nursing, 33*(2), 98–108.

Berger, A. M., Grem, J. L., Visovsky, C., Marunda, H. A., & Yurkovich, J. M. (2010). Fatigue and other variables during adjuvant chemotherapy for colon and rectal cancer. *Oncology Nursing Forum, 37*(1), 59–69.

Carlsson, E., Berndtsson, I., Hallen, A. M., Lindholm, E., & Persson, E. (2010). Concerns and quality of life before surgery and during the recovery period in patients with rectal cancer and an ostomy. *Journal of Wound, Ostomy, and Continence Nursing, 37*(6), 654–661.

Good, K., Niziolek, J., Yoshida, C., & Rowlands, A. (2010). Insights into barriers that prevent African Americans from seeking colorectal screenings: A qualitative study. *Gastroenterology Nursing, 33*(3), 204–208.

Gwee, K. A., Bak, Y. T., Ghoshal, U. C., Gonlachanvit, S., Lee, O. Y., Fock, K. M., et al. (2010). Asian consensus on irritable bowel syndrome. *Journal of Gastroenterology and Hepatology, 25*(7), 1189–1205.

*Hamlyn, S. (2008). Reducing the incidence of colorectal cancer in African Americans. *Gastroenterology Nursing, 31*(1), 39–42.

Herman, J., Pokkunuri, V., Braham, L., & Pimentel, M. (2010). Gender distribution in irritable bowel syndrome is proportional to the severity of constipation relative to diarrhea. *Gender Medicine: The Journal for the Study of Sex & Gender Differences, 7*(3), 240–246.

Kapritsou, M., Korkolis, D. P., & Knostantinou, E. A. (2013). Open or laparoscopic surgery for colorectal cancer: A retrospective comparative study. *Gastroenterology Nursing, 36*(1), 37–41.

Kerckhoffs, A. P., Ben-Amor, K., Samsom, M., van der Rest, M. E., de Vogel, J., Knol, J., et al. (2011). Molecular analysis of faecal and duodenal samples reveals significantly higher prevalence and numbers of *Pseudomonas aeruginosa* in irritable bowel syndrome. *Journal of Medical Microbiology, 60,* 236–245.

Lee, R. K. (2012). Intra-abdominal hypertension and acute compartment syndrome: A comprehensive overview. *Critical Care Nurse, 22*(1), 19–32.

*Lindberg, D. A. (2009). Hydrogen breath testing in adults: What is it and why is it performed? *Gastroenterology Nursing, 32*(1), 19–24.

Lyra, A., Krogius-Kurikka, L., Nikkila, J., Malinen, E., Kajander, K., Kurikka, K., et al. (2010).

Effect of a multispecies probiotic supplement on quantity of irritable bowel syndrome-related intestinal microbial phylotypes. *BMC Gastroenterology, 10*, 110.

Malinen, E., Krogius-Kurikka, L., Lyra, A., Nikkila, J., Jaaskelainen, A., Rinttila, T., et al. (2010). Association of symptoms with gastrointestinal microbiota in irritable bowel syndrome. *World Journal of Gastroenterology, 16*(36), 4532–4540.

*Nicholl, B. I., Halder, S. L., Macfarlane, G. L., Thompson, D. G., O'Brien, S., Musleh, M., et al. (2008). Psychosocial risk markers for new onset irritable bowel syndrome: Results of a large prospective population-based study. *Pain, 137*(1), 147–155.

*Nussbaum, R. L., McInnes, R. R., & Willard, H. F. (2007). *Thompson and Thompson's genetics in medicine.* Philadelphia: Saunders.

Oliver, J. S., Worley, C. B., DeCoster, J., Palardy, L., Kim, G., Reddy, A., et al. (2012). Disparities in colorectal cancer screening behaviors: Implications for African American men. *Gastroenterology Nursing, 35*(2), 93–98.

Pimental, M., Lembo, A., Chey, W. D., Zakko, S., Ringel, Y., Yu, J., et al. (2011). Rifaximin therapy for patients with irritable bowel syndrome without constipation. *New England Journal of Medicine, 364*(1), 22–32.

*Pirotta, M. (2009). Irritable bowel syndrome: The role of complementary medicines in treatment. *Australian Family Physician, 389*(12), 966–968.

Rawl, S. N., Memon, U., Burness, A., & Breslau, E. S. (2012). Interventions to promote colorectal cancer screening: An integrative review. *Nursing Outlook, 60*(4), 172–181.

Russell, S., Champange, B., & Techner, L. (2012). Alvimopan for acceleration of GI recovery after bowel resection. *Medsurg Nursing, 21*(3), 151–157.

Stubenrauch, J. M. (2010). Rectal cancer rates rising in patients under 40. *The American Journal of Nursing, 110*(11), 15.

Walker, C. A., & Lochman, V. D. (2013). Gaps in the discharge process for patients with an ostomy: An ethical perspective. *Medsurg Nursing, 22*(1), 61–64.

Wilkes, G. (2013). *What's new in colon cancer: Update for the practicing nurse.* Retrieved July 2013, from <www.nursingconsult.com/nursing/clinical-updates/full-text?clinical_update_id=198216>.

Wilkes, G., & Hartshorn, K. (2012). Clinical update: Colon, rectal, and anal cancers. *Seminars in Oncology Nursing, 28*(4), 1–22.

Chapter 57

Centers for Disease Control and Prevention. (2014). *Parasites-American trypanosomiasis.* Retrieved from: <http://www.cdc.gov/parasites/chagas>; December 2014.

Cooper, J. M., Collier, J., James, V., & Hawkey, C. J. (2010). Beliefs about personal control and self-management in 30-40 year olds living with inflammatory bowel disease: A qualitative study. *International Journal of Nursing Studies, 47*(12), 1500–1509.

Cronin, E. (2010). Prednisolone in the management of patients with Crohn's disease. *British Journal of Nursing, 19*(21), 1333–1336.

*Crumbock, S. C., Loeb, S. J., & Fick, D. M. (2009). Physical activity, stress, disease activity, and quality of life in adults with Crohn disease. *Gastroenterology Nursing, 32*(3), 188–195.

Dolejs, S., Kennedy, G., & Heise, C. P. (2011). Small bowel obstruction following restorative proctocolectomy: Affected by a laparoscopic approach? *Journal of Surgical Research*, [Epub ahead of print].

*Dudley-Brown, S., Nag, A., Cullinan, C., Ayers, M., Hass, S., & Panjabi, S. (2009). Health-related quality-of-life evaluation of Crohn disease patients after receiving natalizumab therapy. *Gastroenterology Nursing, 32*(5), 327–339.

Fajardo, A. D., Dharmarajan, S., George, V., Hunt, S. R., Birnbaum, E. H., Fleshman, J. W., et al. (2010). Laparoscopic versus open 2-stage ileal pouch: Laparoscopic approach allows for faster restoration of intestinal continuity. *Journal of the American College of Surgeons, 211*(3), 377–383.

Grossman, V. A. (2011). Inflammatory bowel disease and MR enterography. *Journal of Radiology Nursing, 30*(1), 4–5.

Hall, M. A. (2011). Diagnosing diverticular disease. *Journal for Nurse Practitioners, 7*(7), 606–607.

Harris, H., & Jelemensky, L. (2014). Managing the ups and downs of ulcerative colitis. *Nursing, 44*(8), 36–43.

Kessler, H., Mudter, J., & Hohenberger, W. (2011). Recent results of laparoscopic surgery in inflammatory bowel disease. *World Journal of Gastroenterology, 17*(9), 1116–1125.

Krenzer, M. E. (2012). Viral gastroenteritis in the adult population. *Critical Care Nursing Clinics of North America, 24*(4), 541–553.

McMaster, K., Aguinaldo, L., & Parekh, N. K. (2012). Evaluation of an ongoing psychoeducational inflammatory bowel disease support group in an adult outpatient setting. *Gastroenterology Nursing, 35*(6), 383–390.

*Nussbaum, R. L., McInnes, R. R., & Willard, H. F. (2007). *Thompson & Thompson genetics in medicine* (7th ed.). Philadelphia: Saunders.

Pihl-Lesnovska, K., Hjortswang, H., Ek, A. C., & Frisman, G. H. (2010). Patients' perspective of factors influencing quality of life while living with Crohn disease. *Gastroenterology Nursing, 33*(1), 37–44.

Ryan, M., & Grossman, S. (2011). Celiac disease: Implications for patient management. *Gastroenterology Nursing, 34*(3), 225–228.

Smith, M. M., & Goodfellow, L. (2011). The relationship between quality of life and coping strategies of adults with celiac disease adhering to a gluten-free diet. *Gastroenterology Nursing, 34*(6), 460–468.

Spencer, C. (2010). Ulcerative colitis. *Nursing Standard, 24*(52), 59.

Strauch, K. A., & Cotter, V. T. (2011). Celiac disease: An overview and management for primary care nurse practitioners. *Journal for Nurse Practitioners, 7*(7), 588–594.

Chapter 58

Ahmed, N., & Vernick, J. (2011). Management of liver trauma in adults. *Journal of Emergencies, Trauma/Shock, 4*, 114–119.

American Liver Foundation (2010). *Hepatitis B.* New York: Author.

American Liver Foundation (2011). *Position statement on hepatitis A and vaccination.* New York: Author.

American Liver Foundation (2012). *Liver transplant.* Retrieved August 2014, from <www.liverfoundation.org/abouttheliver/info/transplant/>.

Augustin, S., Gonzalez, A., & Genesca, J. (2010). Acute esophageal variceal bleeding: Current strategies and new perspectives. *World Journal of Hepatology, 2*(7), 261–274.

Clayton, M. (2011). Assessing patients before and after a liver transplant. *Practice Nursing, 22*(5), 236–241.

Donnelly, G., Kent-Wilkinson, A., & Rush, A. (2012). The alcohol-dependent patient in the hospital: Challenges for nursing. *Medsurg Nursing, 21*(1), 9–14.

Elliott, D. T., Geyer, C., & Doty, L. (2012). Managing alcohol withdrawal in hospitalized patients. *Nursing, 42*(4), 22–30.

Felicilda-Reynaldo, R. F. D. (2012a). Ammonia abolishers: Antibiotics for hepatic encephalopathy. *Medsurg Nursing, 21*(3), 173–176.

Felicilda-Reynaldo, R. F. D. (2012b). Block the bleed: Pharmacologic therapies for gastroesophageal variceal bleeding. *Medsurg Nursing, 21*(2), 107–110.

Houghton-Rahrig, L., Schutte, D., Fenton, J. I., & Awad, J. (2014). Nonalcoholic fatty liver disease and the *PNPLA3* gene. *Medsurg Nursing, 23*(2), 101–106.

Lee, H., Park, W., Yang, J. H., & You, K. S. (2010). Management of hepatitis B virus infection. *Gastroenterology Nursing, 33*(2), 120–126.

*Lok, A. S. F., & McMahon, B. J. (2009). AASLD: Chronic hepatitis B: Update 2009. *Hepatology, 50*(3), 661–662.

Lucey, M. R., Terrault, N., Ojo, L., Hay, J. E., Neuberger, J., Blumberg, E., et al. (2013). Long-term management of the successful adult liver transplant: 2012 Practice Guideline by the American Association for the Study of Liver Diseases and the American Society of Liver Transplantation. *Liver Transplantation, 19*, 3–26.

Minano, C., & Garcia-Tsao, G. (2010). Clinical pharmacology of portal hypertension. *Gastroenterology Clinics of North America, 39*(3), 681–695.

Morrison, D., Sgrillo, J., & Daniels, L. H. (2014). Managing alcoholic liver disease. *Nursing, 44*(11), 30–40.

Richmond, J. A., Bailey, D. E., Jr., McHutchinson, J. G., & Muir, A. J. (2010). The use of mind-body medicine and prayer among adult patients with hepatitis C. *Gastroenterology Nursing, 33*(3), 201–216.

Rossi, L., Zoratto, F., Papa, A., Iodice, F., Minozzi, M., Frati, L., et al. (2010). Current approach in the treatment of hepatocellular carcinoma.

World Journal of Gastroenterology Oncology, 2(9), 348–359.

Rugari, S. M. (2010). Longitudinal quality of life in liver transplant recipients. *Gastroenterology Nursing, 33*(2), 219–230.

Sulkowski, M. S. (2013). Current management of hepatitis C virus infection in patients with HIV co-infection. *The Journal of Infectious Diseases, 207*(Suppl. 1), S26–S32.

Yee, H. S., Change, M. F., Pocha, C., Lim, J., Ross, D., Morgan, T. R., et al. (2012). Update on the management and treatment of hepatitis C virus infection: Recommendations from the Department of Veterans Affairs Hepatitis C Resource Center Program and the National Hepatitis C Program Office. *American Journal of Gastroenterology, 104,* 1–21.

World Gastroenterology Organisation (WGO) (2012). *World Gastroenterology Organisation global guidelines: Nonalcoholic fatty liver disease and nonalcoholic steatohepatitis.* Milwaukee, WI: Author.

Chapter 59

Agostino, D. I., Wang, D. Q., Bonfrate, L., & Portincasa, P. (2013). Current views on genetics and epigenetics of cholesterol gallstone disease. *Cholesterol,* [Epub ahead of print].

American Cancer Society (ACS) (2013). *Cancer facts and figures—2013.* Atlanta: Author.

Bharwani, N., Patel, S., Prabhusesal, S., Fortheringham, T., & Power, N. (2011). Acute pancreatitis: The role of imaging in diagnosis and management. *Clinical Radiology, 66*(2), 164–175.

Conwell, D. L., & Wu, B. U. (2012). Chronic pancreatitis: Making the diagnosis. *Clinical Gastroenterology and Hepatology, 10,* 1088–1095.

Culp, B. L., Cedillo, V. E., & Arnold, D. (2012). Single-incision laparoscopic cholecystectomy versus traditional four-port cholecystectomy. *Baylor University Medical Center Proceedings, 25*(4), 319–323.

Felicilda-Reynaldo, R. F. D. (2012). Oral gallstone dissolution therapies. *Medsurg Nursing, 21*(1), 41–44.

Fusaroli, P., Spada, A., Mancino, M. G., & Caletti, G. (2010). Contrast harmonic echo-endoscopic ultrasound improves accuracy in diagnosis of solid pancreatic masses. *Journal of Gastroenterology and Hepatology, 8*(7), 629–634.

Gee, C. (2011). Pancreatic cancer: A whistle-stop tour. *Gastrointestinal Nursing, 9*(7), 41–45.

Girometti, R., Brondani, G., Cereser, L., Como, G., Del Pin, M., Bazzocchi, M., et al. (2010). Post-cholecystectomy syndrome: Spectrum of biliary findings at magnetic resonance cholangiopancreatography. *The British Journal of Radiology, 83,* 351–361.

Griffin, N., Charles-Edwards, G., & Grant, L. (2011). Magnetic resonance cholangiopancreatography: The ABC of MRCP. *Insights Imaging, 3,* 11–21.

Grützmann, R., Post, S., Saeger, H. D., & Niedergethmann, M. (2011). Intraductal papillary mucinous neoplasia (IPMN) of the pancreas: Its diagnosis, treatment, and

prognosis. *Deutsches Ärzteblatt International, 108*(46), 788–794.

Huang, L., Ma, B., He, F., & Yang, S. (2012). Electrocardiographic, cardiac enzymes, and magnesium in patients with severe acute pancreatitis. *Gastroenterology Nursing, 35*(4), 256–260.

Hubb, H. A., & Saunders, M. (2011). The yellow bird of jaundice: Recognizing biliary obstruction. *Nursing, 41*(10), 28–36.

Huffman, J. L., & Schenker, S. (2010). Acute acalculous cholecystitis: A review. *Clinical Gastroenterology and Hepatology, 8,* 15–22.

Midha, S., Khajuria, R., Shastri, S., Kabra, M., & Garg, P. K. (2010). Idiopathic chronic pancreatitis in India: Phenotypic characterization and strong genetic susceptibility due to SPINK1 and CFTR gene mutations. *Gut, 59*(6), 800–807.

Navarra, G., La Malfa, G., Lazzara, S., Ullo, G., & Curro, G. (2010). SILS and NOTES cholecystectomy: A tailored approach. *Journal of Laparoendoscopic and Advanced Surgical Techniques, 20*(6), 511–514.

Novotny, I., Dite, P., Lata, J., Nechutova, H., & Klanicka, B. (2010). Autoimmune pancreatitis: Recent advances. *Digestive diseases, 28*(2), 334–338.

Pfadt, E., & Carlson, D. S. (2011). Sphincter of Oddi dysfunction. *Nursing, 41*(8), 42–45.

Salam, M. A. (2010). Single incision laparoscopic surgery. *Journal of Urology, 13,* 2.

Simmons, S. (2010). Gallstones. *Nursing, 37*(11), 37.

Society of American Gastrointestinal and Endoscopic Surgeons (SAGES) (2010). *Guidelines for the clinical application of laparoscopic biliary tract surgery.* Retrieved December 2013, from <www.sages.org/publications/guidelines/guidelines-for-the-clinical-application-of-laparoscopic-biliary-tract-surgery/>.

Targarona, E. M., Maldonado, M., Marzol, J. A., & Marinello, F. (2010). Natural orifice transluminal endoscopic surgery: The transvaginal route moving forward from cholecystectomy. *World Journal of Gastroenterology Surgery, 2*(6), 179–186.

Tonolini, M., Ravelli, A., Villa, C., & Bianco, R. (2012). Urgent MRI with MR cholangiopancreatography (MRCP) of acute cholecystitis and related complications: Diagnostic role and spectrum of imaging findings. *Emergency Radiology, 19,* 341–348.

Chapter 60

Academy of Nutrition and Dietetics (2013). *It's about eating right.* Retrieved September 2014, from <www.eatright.org/Public/content.aspx?id=6372>.

American Heart Association (2014). *Know your fats.* Retrieved September 2014, from <www.heart.org/HEARTORG/Conditions/Cholesterol/PreventionTreatmentofHighCholesterol/Know-Your-Fats_UCM_305628_Article.jsp>.

American Society for Bariatric Surgery (2011). *Longitudinal assessment of bariatric surgery.*

Retrieved September 2014, from <http://win.niddk.nih.gov/publications/labs.htm#howmany>.

American Society of Parenteral and Enteral Nutrition (ASPEN). (2011). Retrieved September 2014, from:< https://www.nutritioncare.org/Guidelines_and_Clinical_Practice/Clinical_Guidelines/>.

*Bankhead, R., Boullata, J., Brantley, S., Corkins, M., Guenter, P., Krenitsky, J., et al. (2009). Enteral nutrition administration. In A.S.P.E.N. enteral nutrition practice recommendations. *Journal of Parenteral Enteral Nutrition, 33*(2), 149–158.

*Bender, S., Pusateri, M., Cook, A., Ferguson, M., & Hall, J. C. (2000). Malnutrition: Role of the TwoCal® HN Med Pass Program. *Medsurg Nursing, 9*(6), 284–296.

Centers for Disease Control and Prevention (CDC) (2012). *About BMI for adults.* Retrieved January 2014, from <www.cdc.gov/healthyweight/assessing/bmi/adult_bmi/>.

Champion, A. (2011). Anorexia of aging. *Annals of Long Term Care, 19*(10), 18–24.

Grmec, Š., Lah, K., & Mally, Š. (2011). Capnometry/capnography in prehospital cardiopulmonary resuscitation. In A. Gullo (Ed.), *Anaesthesia, pharmacology, intensive care and emergency medicine APICE* (pp. 47–56). Milan: Springer.

Health Canada (2011). *Eating well with Canada's Food Guide: First Nations, Inuit, and Métis.* Retrieved September 2014, from <www.hc-sc.gc.ca/fn-an/food-guide-aliment/index_e.html>.

Kulie, T., Slattengren, A., Redmer, J., Counts, H., Eglash, A., & Schranger, S. (2011). Obesity and women's health: An evidence-based review. *Journal of the American Board of Family Medicine, 24*(1), 75–78.

*Lee, J., Visser, M., Tylavsky, F., Kritchevsky, S., Schwartz, A., Sahyoun, N., et al. (2010). Weight loss and regain and effects on body composition: The health, aging, and body composition study. *The Journals of Gerontology, Series A, 65*(1), 78–83.

Marchiondo, K. (2014). Stemming the obesity epidemic: Are nurses credible coaches? *Medsurg Nursing, 23*(3), 155–158.

Mayo Clinic (2014). *Obesity: Treatment and drugs.* Retrieved September 2014, from <www.mayoclinic.com/health/obesity/DS00314/DSECTION=treatments-and-drugs>.

*Mehanna, H. M., Moledina, J., & Travis, J. (2008). Refeeding syndrome: What it is, and how to prevent and treat it. *BMJ, 336,* 1495–1498.

Minister of Health Canada (2011). *Eating well with Canada's food guide.* Retrieved January 2014, from <www.hc-sc.gc.ca/fn-an/alt_formats/hpfb-dgpsa/pdf/food-guide-aliment/view_eatwell_vue_bienmang-eng.pdf>.

National Institute of Diabetes and Digestive and Kidney Diseases (2012). *Weight and waist measurement: Tools for adults.* Retrieved September 2014, from <https://fhs.umr.com/print/UM0868.pdf>.

National Institutes of Health (NIH) (2013a). *General information about parathyroid cancer.*

National Cancer Institute. Retrieved September 2014, from <http://www.cancer.gov/cancertopics/pdq/treatment/parathyroid/Patient/page1>.

National Institutes of Health (NIH) (2013b). *What are overweight and obesity*. National Heart, Lung, and Blood Institute. Retrieved September 2014, from <www.nhlbi.nih.gov/health/health-topics/topics/obe/>.

Tappenden, K. A., Quatrara, B., Parkhurst, M. L., Malone, A. M., Fanjiang, G., & Ziegler, T. R. (2013). Critical role of nutrition in improving quality of care: An interdisciplinary call to action to address adult hospital malnutrition. *Medsurg Nursing, 22*(3), 147–165.

The Institute of Medicine of the National Academies (2014). *Dietary references intakes and application tables*. Retrieved September 2014, from <www.iom.edu/Activities/Nutrition/SummaryDRIs/DRI-Tables.aspx>.

U.S. Department of Agriculture (USDA) (2010). *Dietary guidelines for Americans, 2010*. Retrieved September 2014, from <http://www.fns.usda.gov/dietary-guidelines-americans-2010>.

Virji, A. (2011). *Obesity and weight loss (bariatric surgery)*. Retrieved September 2014, from <www.essentialevidenceplus.com.ezproxy.midwives.org/content/eee/155>.

Yearwood, E., McCulloch, M., Tucker, M., & Riley, J. (2011). Care of the patient with Prader-Willi syndrome. *Medsurg Nursing, 20*(3), 113–122.

Chapter 61

Klee, G. (2011). Laboratory techniques for recognition of endocrine disorders. In S. Melmed, K. Polonsky, P. R. Larsen, & H. Kronenberg (Eds.), *Williams' textbook of endocrinology* (12th ed.). Philadelphia: Saunders.

Lamberts, S. (2011). Endocrinology and aging. In S. Melmed, K. Polonsky, P. R. Larsen, & H. Kronenberg (Eds.), *Williams' textbook of endocrinology* (12th ed.). Philadelphia: Saunders.

Melmed, S., Polonsky, K., Larsen, P. R., & Kronenberg, H. (Eds.), (2011). *Williams' textbook of endocrinology* (12th ed.). Philadelphia: Saunders.

Spiegel, A., Carter-Su, C., Taylor, S., & Kulkarni, R. (2011). Mechanism of action of hormones that act at the cell surface. In S. Melmed, K. Polonsky, P. R. Larsen, & H. Kronenberg (Eds.), *Williams' textbook of endocrinology* (12th ed.). Philadelphia: Saunders.

Chapter 62

Aschenbrenner, D. (2012). Drug watch: FDA approves first drug for endogenous Cushing's syndrome. *The American Journal of Nursing, 112*(6), 26–27.

Collins, M., & Claros, E. (2011). Recognizing the face of dehydration. *Nursing, 41*(8), 26–31.

Crawford, A., & Harris, H. (2011). Balancing act: Na+ and K+. *Nursing, 41*(7), 44–50.

Crawford, A., & Harris, H. (2012). SIADH: Fluid out of balance. *Nursing, 42*(9), 50–58.

Hunt, D. (2012). Is it Addison's disease or Cushing syndrome? *American Nurse Today, 7*(1), 8–11.

John, C., & Day, M. (2012). Central neurogenic diabetes insipidus, syndrome of inappropriate secretion of antidiuretic hormone, and cerebral salt-wasting syndrome in traumatic brain injury. *Critical Care Nurse, 32*(2), e1–e7.

Manchester, C. (2013). Multiple endocrine neoplasia: The enigma of MEN. *AACN Advanced Critical Care, 24*(3), 304–313.

McKeage, K. (2013). Pasireotide: A review of its use in Cushing's disease. *Drugs, 73*(6), 563–574.

Melmed, S., Kleinberg, D., & Ho, K. (2011). Pituitary physiology and diagnostic evaluation. In S. Melmed, K. Polonsky, P. R. Larsen, & H. Kronenberg (Eds.), *Williams' textbook of endocrinology* (12th ed.). Philadelphia: Saunders.

Melmed, S., Polonsky, K., Larsen, P. R., & Kronenberg, H. (Eds.), (2011). *Williams' textbook of endocrinology* (12th ed.). Philadelphia: Saunders.

Online Mendelian Inheritance in Man (OMIM) (2012). *Diabetes insipidus, nephrogenic, Autosomal*. Retrieved August 2014, from <www.omim.org/entry/125800>.

Online Mendelian Inheritance in Man (OMIM) (2011). *Diabetes insipidus, nephrogenic, X-linked*. Retrieved January 2014, from <www.omim.org/entry/304800>.

Online Mendelian Inheritance in Man (OMIM) (2014). *Pheochromocytoma, Susceptibility to*. Retrieved August 2014, from <www.omim.org/entry/171300>.

*Radovich, P. (2010). Primary adrenal insufficiency: Elusive and potentially life-threatening. *American Nurse Today, 5*(3), 37–39.

Robinson, A., & Verbalis, J. (2011). Posterior pituitary. In S. Melmed, K. Polonsky, P. R. Larsen, & H. Kronenberg (Eds.), *Williams' textbook of endocrinology* (12th ed.). Philadelphia: Saunders.

Stewart, P., & Krone, N. (2011). The adrenal cortex. In S. Melmed, K. Polonsky, P. R. Larsen, & H. Kronenberg (Eds.), *Williams' textbook of endocrinology* (12th ed.). Philadelphia: Saunders.

United States Food and Drug Administrations (USFDA) (2013). *Samsca (Tolvaptan): Drug Safety Communication-FDA limits duration and usage due to possible liver injury leading to organ transplant or death*. Retrieved August 2014, from <www.fda.gov/Safety/MedWatch/SafetyInformation/SafetyAlertsforHumanMedicalProducts/ucm350185>.

Yam, F., & Eraly, S. (2012). Syndrome of inappropriate antidiuretic hormone associated with moxifloxacin. *American Journal of Health-System Pharmacists, 69*(3), 217–220.

Young, W. (2011). Endocrine hypertension. In S. Melmed, K. Polonsky, P. R. Larsen, & H. Kronenberg (Eds.), *Williams' textbook of endocrinology* (12th ed.). Philadelphia: Saunders.

Chapter 63

American Cancer Society (2014). *Cancer facts and figures 2014*. Report No. 00-300M–No. 500814. Atlanta: Author.

Brent, G., & Davies, T. (2011). Hypothyroidism and thyroiditis. In S. Melmed, K. Polonsky, P. R. Larsen, & H. Kronenberg (Eds.), *Williams' textbook of endocrinology* (12th ed.). Philadelphia: Saunders.

Bringhurst, F. R., Demay, M., & Kronenberg, H. (2011). Hormones and disorders of mineral metabolism. In S. Melmed, K. Polonsky, P. R. Larsen, & H. Kronenberg (Eds.), *Williams' textbook of endocrinology* (12th ed.). Philadelphia: Saunders.

Burton, J. (2011). Hyperthyroidism. *Medsurg Nursing, 20*(3), 152–153.

Burton, J. (2012). Primary hypothyroidism. *Medsurg Nursing, 21*(3), 169–170.

Crawford, A., & Harris, H. (2011). Balancing act: Hypomagnesemia and hypermagnesemia. *Nursing, 41*(10), 52–55.

Crawford, A., & Harris, H. (2012). Thyroid imbalances: Dealing with disorderly conduct. *Nursing, 42*(11), 45–50.

Hampton, J. (2013). Thyroid gland emergencies: Thyroid storm and myxedema coma. *AACN Advanced Critical Care, 24*(3), 325–332.

Kapustin, J., & Schofield, D. (2012). Hyperparathyroidism: An incidental finding. *The Nurse Practitioner, 37*(11), 9–14.

Mandel, S., Larsen, P. R., & Davies, T. (2011). Thyrotoxicosis. In S. Melmed, K. Polonsky, P. R. Larsen, & H. Kronenberg (Eds.), *Williams' textbook of endocrinology* (12th ed.). Philadelphia: Saunders.

Melmed, S., Polonsky, K., Larsen, P. R., & Kronenberg, H. (Eds.), (2011). *Williams' textbook of endocrinology* (12th ed.). Philadelphia: Saunders.

Mosher, M. (2011). Amiodarone-induced hypothyroidism and other adverse effects. *Dimensions of Critical Care Nursing, 30*(2), 87–93.

Online Mendelian Inheritance in Man (OMIM) (2014). *Graves disease, susceptibility to, 1*. Retrieved November 2014, from <www.omim.org/entry/275000>.

Salvatore, D., Davies, T., Schlumberger, M., Hay, I., & Larsen, P. R. (2011). Thyroid physiology and diagnostic evaluation of patients with thyroid disorders. In S. Melmed, K. Polonsky, P. R. Larsen, & H. Kronenberg (Eds.), *Williams' textbook of endocrinology* (12th ed.). Philadelphia: Saunders.

Woodhouse, K. (2012). Thyrotoxicosis: Evaluation and treatment of a multinodular goiter. *The Nurse Practitioner, 37*(7), 6–10.

Chapter 64

Acee, A. (2012). Type 2 diabetes and vascular dementia: Assessment and clinical strategies of care. *Medsurg Nursing, 21*(6), 349–353.

American Association of Diabetes Educators (AADE) (2011). *AADE position statement:*

Diabetes and physical activity. <Diabeteseducator.org/>.

American Diabetes Association (ADA). (2013). Position statement: Standard of medical care in diabetes—2013. *Diabetes Care, 36*(Suppl. 1), S11–S66.

American Diabetes Association (ADA). (2014a). Diabetic retinopathy and other ocular findings in the Diabetes Control and Complications Trial/Epidemiology of Diabetes Interventions and Complications Study. *Diabetes Care, 37*(1), 17–23.

American Diabetes Association (ADA). (2014b). Kidney disease and related findings in the Diabetes Control and Complications Trial/Epidemiology of Diabetes Interventions and Complications Study. *Diabetes Care, 37*(1), 24–30.

American Diabetes Association (ADA). (2014c). National standards: National standards for diabetes self-management education and support. *Diabetes Care, 37*(Suppl. 1), S144–S153.

American Diabetes Association (ADA). (2014d). Position statement: Diagnosis and classification of diabetes mellitus. *Diabetes Care, 37*(Suppl. 1), S81–S90.

American Diabetes Association (ADA). (2014e). Position statement: Nutritional recommendations and interventions for diabetes. *Diabetes Care, 37*(Suppl. 1), S120–S143.

American Diabetes Association (ADA). (2014f). Update on cardiovascular outcomes at 30 years of the Diabetes Control and Complications Trial/Epidemiology of Diabetes Interventions and Complications Study. *Diabetes Care, 37*(Suppl. 1), S39–S43.

Aschenbrenner, D. (2012). First drug approved for treating diabetic macular edema. *The American Journal of Nursing, 112*(12), 20.

Bosak, K. (2012a). Managing metabolic syndrome in women. *The Nurse Practitioner, 37*(8), 14–20.

Bosak, K. (2012b). Managing metabolic syndrome: Focus on physical activity. *The Journal for Nurse Practitioners, 8*(3), 206–211.

Brady, V. (2013). Management of hyperglycemia in the intensive care unit: When glucose reaches critical levels. *Critical Care Nursing Clinics of North America, 25*(1), 7–13.

Carter, B., Barba, B., & Kautz, D. (2013). Culturally tailored education for African Americans with type 2 diabetes. *Medsurg Nursing, 22*, 105–109, 123.

Centers for Disease Control and Prevention (2011). *National diabetes fact sheet: National estimates and general information on diabetes and prediabetes in the United States.* Atlanta: U.S. Department of Health and Human Services.

Chou, C., Sherrod, C., Zhang, Z., Barker, L., Bullard, K., Crews, J., et al. (2014). Barriers to eye care among people aged 40 years and older with diagnosed diabetes, 2006-2010. *Diabetes Care, 37*(1), 180–188.

Chow, E., Foster, H., Gonzales, V., & McIver, L. (2012). The disparate impact of diabetes on racial/ethnic minority populations. *Clinical Diabetes, 30*(3), 130–133.

Crawford, K. (2013). Guidelines for care of the hospitalized patient with hyperglycemia and diabetes. *Critical Care Nursing Clinics of North America, 25*(1), 1–6.

Dokken, B. (2013). How insulin analogues can benefit patients. *The Nurse Practitioner, 38*(2), 44–48.

Freeland, B., & Funnell, M. (2012). Corticosteroid-induced hyperglycemia. *Nursing, 42*(11), 68–69.

Funnell, M. (2014). Managing the pain of diabetic peripheral neuropathy. *Nursing, 44*(7), 64–65.

Glover, T., & Galvan, E. (2013). Diabetes and heart failure. *Critical Care Nursing Clinics of North America, 25*(1), 93–99.

Hughes, L. (2012a). Assessing a patient with an insulin pump. *Nursing, 42*(9), 62–64.

Hughes, L. (2012b). Think "SAFE": Four crucial elements for diabetes education. *Nursing, 42*(1), 58–61.

Hunt, C., Sanderson, B., & Ellison, K. J. (2014). Support for diabetes using technology: A pilot study to improve self-management. *Medsurg Nursing, 23*(8), 231–237.

Kopecky, C. (2013). Use of noninsulin antidiabetic medications in hospitalized patients. *Critical Care Nursing Clinics of North America, 25*(1), 39–53.

Krolewski, A., Niewczas, M., Skupien, J., Gohda, T., Smiles, A., Eckfeldt, J., et al. (2014). Early progressive renal decline precedes the onset of microalbuminuria and its progression to macroalbuminuria. *Diabetes Care, 37*(Suppl. 1), S226–S234.

Kubacka, B. (2014). A balancing act: Achieving glycemic control in hospitalized patients. *Nursing, 44*(1), 30–37.

Levesque, C. (2013a). Management of hypertension in patients with diabetes. *Critical Care Nursing Clinics of North America, 25*(1), 71–91.

Levesque, C. (2013b). Perioperative care of patients with diabetes. *Critical Care Nursing Clinics of North America, 25*(1), 21–29.

Link, D. (2013). New paradigms in managing chronic kidney disease. *The Clinical Advisor, 16*(1), 18–23.

Martin, A. (2013). Intravenous insulin infusions: What nurses need to know. *Critical Care Nursing Clinics of North America, 25*(1), 15–20.

McCrea, D. (2013). Management of the hospitalized diabetes patient with an insulin pump. *Critical Care Nursing Clinics of North America, 25*(1), 111–121.

Mompoint-Williams, D., Watts, P., & Appel, S. (2012). Detecting and treating hypoglycemia in patients with diabetes. *Nursing, 42*(8), 50–52.

National Institute of Diabetes and Digestive and Kidney Diseases (NIDDK) of the National Institutes of Health (2011). *National Diabetes Information Clearing House: National diabetes statistics, 2011.* Retrieved September 2014, from <www.diabetes.niddk.nih.gov/statistics/>.

National Kidney Foundation. (2012). KDOQI clinical practice guidelines for diabetes and CKD: 2012 update. *American Journal of Kidney Diseases, 60*(5), 850–886.

Palmer, C., & Jessup, A. (2012). Ketoacidosis in patients with type 2 diabetes. *The Nurse Practitioner, 37*(5), 13–17.

Sacks, D., Arnold, M., Bakris, G., Bruns, D., Horvath, A., Kirkman, M., et al. (2011). Guidelines and recommendations for laboratory analysis in the diagnosis and management of diabetes mellitus. *Diabetes Care, 34*(6), 61–99.

Seaquist, E., Anderson, J., Childs, B., Cryer, P., Dagogo-Jack, S., Fish, L., et al. (2013). Hypoglycemia and diabetes: A report of a workgroup of the American Diabetes Association and the Endocrine Society. *Journal of Clinical Endocrinology and Metabolism, 98*(5), 1845–1859.

Sibbald, R., Ayello, E., Alavi, A., Ostrow, B., Lowe, J., Botros, M., et al. (2012). Screening for the high-risk diabetic foot: A 60-second tool. *Advances in Skin & Wound Management, 25*(10), 465–476.

Sisson, E., Mills, J., & Chin, L. (2012). Recent safety updates on type 2 diabetes medications. *The American Journal of Nursing, 112*(12), 49–53.

Smith, J., & Clinard, V. (2013). Diabetes and sudden cardiac death. *US Pharmacist, 38*(2), 38–42.

The Joint Commission (TJC) (2014). *Advanced certification in inpatient diabetes.* Retrieved September 2014, from <www.jointcommision.org/certification/inpatient_diabetes.aspx>.

Thomas, D. (2013). Clinical management of diabetic ulcers. *Clinics in Geriatric Medicine, 29*(2), 433–441.

Trotter, B., Conaway, M., & Burns, S. (2013). Relationship of glucose values to sliding scale insulin (correctional insulin) dose delivery and meal time in acute care patients with diabetes mellitus. *Medsurg Nursing, 22*(2), 99–104, 135.

Young, J. (2011). Educating staff nurses on diabetes: Knowledge enhancement. *Medsurg Nursing, 20*(3), 143–146, 150.

Zitkus, B. (2012). Type 2 diabetes mellitus: An evidence-based update. *The Nurse Practitioner, 37*(7), 28–37.

Chapter 65

Brenner, B. M. (Ed.), (2012). *Brenner & Rector's the kidney* (9th ed.). Philadelphia: Saunders.

Davenport, M., Khalatbari, S., & Ellis, J. (2014). The challenges in assessing contrast-induced nephropathy: Where are we now? *American Journal of Roentgenology, 202*(4), 784–789.

*Dong, K., & Quan, D. (2010). Appropriately assessing renal function for drug dosing. *Nephrology Nursing Journal, 37*(3), 304–308.

Gray, M. (2011). Traces: Making sense of urodynamics testing—part 3: Electromyography of the pelvic floor muscles. *Urologic Nursing, 31*(1), 31–38.

Gray, M. (2012a). Traces: Making sense of urodynamics testing—part 9: Evaluation of detrusor response to bladder filling. *Urologic Nursing, 32*(1), 21–28.

Gray, M. (2012b). Traces: Making sense of urodynamics testing—part 12: Videourodynamics testing. *Urologic Nursing, 32*(4), 193–202.

Lameire, N., & Kellum, J. (2013). Contrast-induced acute kidney injury and renal support for acute kidney injury: A KDIGO summary (Part 2). *Critical Care, 17*(1), 205.

National Kidney Disease Education Program (NKDEP) (2012). *GFR MDRD Calculator for adults (conventional units)*. Retrieved October 2014, from <nkdep.nih.gov/lab-evaluation/gfr-calculators/adults-conventional-unit.asp>.

Puzantian, H. V., & Townsend, R. R. (2013). Understanding kidney function assessment: The basics and advances. *Journal of the American Association of Nurse Practitioners, 25*(7), 334–341.

Society of Urologic Nurses and Associates (2014). *Patient Education*. Retrieved October 2014, from <https://www.suna.org/resource/patient-education>.

U.S. Renal Data Systems (2013). *USRDS 2013 annual data report: Atlas of chronic kidney disease and end-stage renal disease in the United States*. Bethesda, MD: The National Kidney and Urologic Diseases Information Clearinghouse (NKUDIC). National Institutes of Health.

Wood, S. (2012). Contrast-induced nephropathy in critical care. *Critical Care Nurse, 32*(6), 15–24.

Chapter 66

Agency for Healthcare Research and Quality (AHRQ) (2012). *Non-surgical treatments for urinary incontinence in adult women: Diagnosis and comparative effectiveness. AHRQ Comparative Effectiveness Reviews*. Rockville, MD: Author. Retrieved October 2014, from <http://effectivehealthcare.ahrq.gov/index.cfm/search-for-guides-reviews-and-reports/?productid=1021&pageaction=displayproduct>.

American Cancer Society (ACS) (2014). *Cancer facts and figures 2014*. Report No. 01-300M–No. 500814. Atlanta: Author.

Bagga, H. S., Tasian, G. E., Fisher, P. B., McCulloch, C. E., McAninch, J. W., & Breyer, B. N. (2013). Product related adult genitourinary injuries treated at emergency departments in the United States from 2002 to 2010. *Journal of Urology, 189*(4), 1362–1368.

Bernard, M. S., Hunter, K. F., & Moore, K. N. (2012). A review of strategies to decrease the duration of indwelling urethral catheters and potentially reduce the incidence of catheter-associated urinary tract infections. *Urologic Nursing, 32*(1), 29–37.

Brenner, B. (2012). *Brenner & Rector's the kidney* (9th ed.). Philadelphia: Saunders.

Brusch, J. L. (2013). *Cystitis in females*. emedicine, 5. Accessed October 2014, from <http://emedicine.medscape.com/article/233101-overview#showall>.

*Buckley, B. S., Lapitan, M. C., & Epidemiology Committee of the Fourth International Consultation on Incontinence, Paris. (2010). Prevalence of urinary incontinence in men, women, and children—current evidence: Findings of the Fourth International Consultation on Incontinence. *Urology, 76*(2), 265–270.

Canadian Cancer Society, Statistics Canada (2014). *Canadian Cancer Statistics, 2014*. Toronto: Canadian Cancer Society.

Centers for Disease Control and Prevention (CDC) (2013). *Guideline for prevention of catheter-associated urinary tract infections, 2013*. Retrieved February 2014, from <www.cdc.gov/>.

Christian, R. (2014). Do prophylactic antibiotics reduce UTI risk after urodynamic studies? *The American Journal of Nursing, 114*(2), 20.

Dowling-Castronovo, A., & Bradway, C. (2012). *Urinary incontinence. Nursing Standard of Practice Protocol: Urinary incontinence in older adults admitted to acute care. Evidence Based Geriatric Topics*. Retrieved October 2014, from <http://consultgerirn.org/topics/urinary_incontinence/want_to_know_more>.

DuBeau, C. B. (2013). *Approach to women with urinary incontinence. UpToDate*. Retrieved October 2014, from <www.uptodate.com/contents/clinical-presentation-and-diagnosis-of-urinary-incontinence>.

Dudeck, M. A., Horan, T. C., Peterson, K. D., Allen-Bridson, K., Morrell, G., Anttila, A., et al. (2013). National Healthcare Safety Network report, data summary for 2011, device-associated module. *American Journal of Infection Control, 41*(4), 286–300.

Fan, H. L., Chan, S. S., Law, T. S., Cheung, R. Y., & Chung, T. K. (2013). Pelvic floor muscle training improves quality of life of women with urinary incontinence: A prospective study. *The Australian and New Zealand Journal of Obstetrics & Gynaecology, 53*(3), 298–304.

Fink, H. A., Wilt, T. J., Eidman, K. E., Garimella, P. S., MacDonald, R., Rutks, I. R., et al. (2013). Medical management to prevent recurrent nephrolithiasis in adults: A systematic review for an American College of Physicians Clinical Guideline. *Annals of Internal Medicine, 158*(7), 535–543.

Fletcher, R. H. (2013). The risk of taking ascorbic acid. *JAMA Internal Medicine, 173*(5), 375–394.

*Foxman, B. (2010). The epidemiology of urinary tract infection. *Nature Reviews: Urology, 7*(12), 653–660.

Hooton, T. M. (2012). Clinical practice: Uncomplicated urinary tract infection. *New England Journal of Medicine, 366*(11), 1028–1037.

Hopkins, L., McCroskey, D., Reeves, G., & Tanabe, P. (2014). Implementing a urinary tract infection clinical practice guideline in an ambulatory urgent care practice. *The Nurse Practitioner, 39*(4), 50–54.

Jura, Y. H., Townsend, M. K., Curhan, G. C., Resnick, N. M., & Grodstein, F. (2011). Caffeine intake, and the risk of stress, urgency and mixed urinary incontinence. *Journal of Urology, 185*(5), 1775–1780.

Kannankeril, A., Lam, H., Reyes, E., & McCartney, J. (2011). Urinary tract infection rates associated with re-use of catheters in clean intermittent catheterization of male veterans. *Urologic Nursing, 31*(1), 41–48.

Li, K., Lin, T., Zhang, C., Fan, X., Xu, K., Bi, L., et al. (2013). Optimal frequency of shock wave lithotripsy in urolithiasis treatment: A systematic review and meta-analysis of randomized controlled trials. *Journal of Urology, 190*(4), 1260–1267.

Lowe, N. K., & Ryan-Wenger, N. A. (2012). Uncomplicated UTIs in women. *Nurse Practitioner, 37*(5), 41–48.

Mori, C. (2014). A-voiding catastrophe: Implementing a nurse-driven protocol. *Medsurg Nursing, 23*(1), 15–21, 28.

Myles, M. L. (2011). Urinary diversions. *Medsurg Nursing, 20*(2), 94–95.

Newman, D. K., & Willson, M. M. (2011). Review of intermittent catheterization and current best practices. *Urologic Nursing, 31*(1), 12–28, 48.

Pelvic Pain and Urgency Frequency symptom scale: PUF questionnaire. (2005). Retrieved October 2014, from <www.orthoelmiron.com/orthoelmiron/hcptools_puf.html?host>.

Quillin, R. B., & Erickson, D. R. (2012). Practical use of the new American Urological Association interstitial cystitis guidelines. *Current Urology Reports, 13*(5), 394–401.

Ragnarsdóttir, B., Lutay, N., Grönberg-Hernandez, J., Köves, B., & Svanborg, C. (2011). Genetics of innate immunity and UTI susceptibility. *Nature Reviews: Urology, 8*(8), 449–468.

*Richmond, C. F. (2010). Interstitial cystitis—chronic, common, and sometimes complicated to treat. *American Nurse Today, 5*(11), 19–24.

Rodgers, A. L. (2013). Race, ethnicity and urolithiasis: A critical review. *Urolithiasis, 41*(2), 99–103.

Rosa, M., Usai, P., Miano, R., Kim, F. J., Finazzi Agro, E., Bove, P., et al. (2013). Recent finding and new technologies in nephrolithiasis: A review of the recent literature. *BMC Urology, 13*, 10.

Scemons, D. (2013). Urinary incontinence in adults. *Nursing, 43*(11), 52–60.

Shultz, J. M. (2012). Rethink urinary incontinence in older women. *Nursing, 42*(11), 32–40.

Stapleton, A. E., Dziura, J., Hooton, T. M., Cox, M. E., Yarova-Yarovaya, Y., Chen, S., et al. (2012). Recurrent urinary tract infection and urinary *Escherichia coli* in women ingesting cranberry juice daily: A randomized controlled trial. *Mayo Clinic Proceedings, 87*(2), 143–150.

Sur, R. L., Masterson, J. H., Palazzi, K. L., L'Esperance, J. O., Auge, B. K., Chang, D. C., et al. (2013). Impact of statins on nephrolithiasis in hyperlipidemic patients: A 10-year review of an equal access health care system. *Clinical Nephrology, 79*(5), 351–355.

Townsend, M. K., Curhan, G. C., Resnick, N. M., & Grodstein, F. (2011). Original research: Rates of remission, improvement, and progression of urinary incontinence in Asian, Black, and White women. *American Journal of Nursing, 111*(4), 26–33.

Türk, C., Knoll, T., Petrik, A., Sarica, K., Straub, M., Seitz, C., et al. (2011). *Guidelines for urolithiasis.* Retrieved October 2014, from <www.uroweb.org/gls/pdf/18_Urolithiasis.pdf>.

U.S. Renal Data Systems (2012). *USRDS 2011 annual data report.* Bethesda, MD: The National Kidney and Urologic Diseases Information Clearinghouse (NKUDIC). National Institutes of Health.

Wagenlehner, F. M., Lichtenstern, C., Rolfes, C., Mayer, K., Uhle, F., Weidner, W., et al. (2013). Diagnosis and management for urosepsis. *International Journal of Urology, 20*(10), 963–970.

Wilde, M. L., Bliss, D., Booth, J., Cheater, F., & Tannenbaum, C. (2014). Self-management of urinary and fecal incontinence. *The American Journal of Nursing, 114*(1), 38–45.

Chapter 67

Aguiari, G., Catizone, L., & Del Senno, L. (2013). Multidrug therapy for polycystic kidney disease: A review and perspective. *American Journal of Nephrology, 37*(2), 175–182.

American Cancer Society (2014). *Cancer facts and figures 2014.* Report No. 00-300M–No. 500814. Atlanta: Author.

Aragona, F., Pepe, P., Patane, D., Malfa, P., D'Arrigo, L., & Pennisi, M. (2012). Management of severe blunt renal trauma in adult patients: A 10-year retrospective review from an emergency hospital. *BJU International, 110*(5), 744–748.

Aschenbrenner, D. (2012). New drug approved for advanced renal cell cancer. *American Journal of Nursing, 112*(5), 22–23.

Brenner, B. (Ed.), (2012). *Brenner & Rector's the kidney* (9th ed.). Philadelphia: Saunders.

Byar, K., & Workman, M. (2012). Targeted therapies to treat cancer. In J. Kee, E. Hayes, & L. McCuistion (Eds.), *Pharmacology: A nursing process approach* (7th ed.). St. Louis: Saunders.

Canadian Cancer Society, Statistics Canada (2014). *Canadian Cancer Statistics, 2014.* Toronto: Canadian Cancer Society.

Davies, H., & Leslie, G. (2012). Acute kidney injury and the critically ill patient. *Dimensions of Critical Care Nursing, 31*(3), 135–152.

Escobar, G. A., & Campbell, D. N. (2012). Randomized trials in angioplasty and stenting of the renal artery: Tabular review of the literature and critical analysis of their results. *Annals of Vascular Surgery, 26*(3), 434–442.

Fournier, M. (2013). Stemming the rising tide of acute kidney injury. *American Nurse Today, 8*(1), 12–16.

Hahn, B. H., McMahon, M. A., Wilkinson, A., Wallace, W. D., Daikh, D. I., Fitzgerald, J. D., et al. (2012). American College of

Rheumatology guidelines for screening, treatment, and management of lupus nephritis. *Arthritis Care & Research (Hoboken), 64*(6), 797–808.

Isaac, S. (2012). Contrast-induced nephropathy: Nursing implications. *Critical Care Nurse, 32*(3), 41–47.

Kidney stones. (2012). Kidney stones. *Nursing, 42*(12), 29.

National Kidney Foundation (2013). *Polycystic kidney disease.* Retrieved October 2014, from <www.kidney.org/atoz/content/polycystic.cfm>.

Online Mendelian Inheritance in Man (OMIM) (2014). *Polycystic kidney disease 1; PKD1.* Retrieved October 2014, from <www.omim.org/entry/173900>.

Patel, C., Ahmed, A., & Ellsworth, P. (2012). Renal cell carcinoma: A reappraisal. *Urologic Nursing, 32*(4), 182–190.

Pengo, M. F., Soloni, P., Cecchin, D., Maiolino, G., Rossi, G. P., & Caló, L. A. (2013). Pelvic-ureteric junction obstruction and hypertension with target organ damage: A case report and review of the literature. *Blood Pressure, 22*(5), 336–339.

U.S. Renal Data Systems (2012). *USRDS 2011 annual data report.* Bethesda, MD: The National Kidney and Urologic Diseases Information Clearinghouse (NKUDIC). National Institutes of Health.

Wood, S. (2012). Contrast-induced nephropathy in critical care. *Critical Care Nurse, 32*(6), 15–23.

Chapter 68

Akker, J. P., Egal, M., & Groeneveld, A. B. (2013). Invasive mechanical ventilation as a risk factor for acute kidney injury in the critically ill: A systematic review and meta-analysis. *Critical Care, 17*(3), R98.

Allegretti, A. S., Steele, D. J., David-Kasdan, J. A., Bajwa, E., Niles, J. L., & Bhan, I. (2013). Continuous renal replacement therapy outcomes in acute kidney injury and end stage renal disease: A cohort study. *Critical Care, 17*(3), R109.

American Nephrology Nurses Association (ANNA) (2011). *Nephrology Nursing Process of Care: Apheresis and Therapeutic Plasma Exchange and Continuous Renal Replacement Therapy.* Pitman, NJ: Author.

Beach, P. R., Hallett, A. M., & Zaruca, K. (2011). Organ donation after circulatory death: Vital partnerships. *The American Journal of Nursing, 111*(5), 32–38.

Beal-Lloyd, D., & Groh, C. J. (2012). Dialysis and sexuality. *Nephrology Nursing Journal, 39*(4), 281–283.

Berger, J. C., Muzaale, A. D., James, N., Hoque, M., Wang, J. M., Montgomery, R. A., et al. (2011). Living kidney donors ages 70 and older: Recipient and donor outcomes. *Clinical Journal of the American Society of Nephrology, 6*(12), 2887–2893.

Davies, H., & Leslie, G. (2012). Acute kidney injury and the critically ill patient. *Dimensions of Critical Care Nursing, 31*(3), 135–152.

Dutka, P. (2012). Erythropoiesis-stimulating agents for the management of anemia of chronic kidney disease: Past advancements and current innovations. *Nephrology Nursing Journal, 39*(6), 447–457.

Elliott, R. W. (2012). Demographics of the older adult and chronic kidney disease: A literature review. *Nephrology Nursing Journal, 39*(6), 491–496.

Elseviers, M. M., Lins, R. L., Van der Niepen, P., Hoste, E., Malbrain, M. L., Damas, P., et al. (2010). Renal replacement therapy is an independent risk factor for mortality in critically ill patients with acute kidney injury. *Critical Care, 14*(6), R221.

Ficorelli, C. T., Edelman, M., & Weeks, B. H. (2013). Living donor renal transplant: A gift of life. *Nursing, 43*(1), 58–62.

Fournir, M. (2013). Stemming the rising tide of acute kidney injury. *American Nurse Today, 8*(1), 12–16.

Fukagawa, M., Komaba, H., & Kakuta, T. (2013). Hyperparathyroidism in chronic kidney disease patients: An update on current pharmacotherapy. *Expert Opinion on Pharmacotherapy, 14*(7), 863–871.

Gentry, S. E., Montgomery, R. A., & Segev, D. L. (2011). Kidney paired donation: Fundamentals, limitations, and expansions. *American Journal of Kidney Diseases, 57*(1), 144–151.

Golestaneh, L., Richter, B., & Amato-Hayes, M. (2012). Logistics of renal replacement therapy: Relevant issues for critical care nurses. *American Journal of Critical Care, 21*(2), 126–130.

Horigan, A., Rocchiccioli, J., & Trimm, D. (2012). Dialysis and fatigue: Implications for nurses—A case study analysis. *Medsurg Nursing, 21*(3), 158–163, 175.

Lewis, R. (2012). Mineral and bone disorders in chronic kidney disease: New insights into mechanism and management. *Annals of Clinical Biochemistry, 49*(Pt. 5), 432–440.

Moore, E. M., Bellomo, R., & Nichol, A. D. (2012). The meaning of acute kidney injury and its relevance to intensive care and anaesthesia. *Anaesthesia and Intensive Care, 40*(6), 929–948.

Obermüller, N., Geiger, H., Weipert, C., & Urbschat, A. (2014). Current developments in early diagnosis of acute kidney injury. *International Urology and Nephrology, 46*(1), 1–7.

Prescott, A. M., Lewington, A., & O'Donoghue, D. (2012). Acute kidney injury: Top ten tips. *Clinical Medicine, 12*(4), 328–332.

Puzantian, H. V., & Townsend, R. R. (2013). Understanding kidney function assessment: The basics and advances. *Journal of the American Association of Nurse Practitioners, 25*(7), 334–341.

Ralib, A. M., Pickering, J. W., Shaw, G. M., & Endre, Z. H. (2013). The urine output definition of acute kidney injury is too liberal. *Critical Care, 17*(3), R112.

Ricci, Z., Cruz, D. N., & Ronco, C. (2011). Classification and staging of acute kidney injury: Beyond the RIFLE and AKIN criteria. *Nature Reviews. Nephrology, 7*(4), 201–208.

Ryan, E. J. (2012). When do (or don't) you administer drugs to patients on hemodialysis? *Nursing, 42*(8), 47–49.

Saccomano, S. J., & DeLuca, D. A. (2012). Living with chronic kidney disease: Related issues and treatment. *Nurse Practitioner, 37*(8), 32–38.

Streets, K. W., & Vickers, S. M. (2012). Is this patient with heart failure a candidate for ultrafiltration? *Nursing, 42*(6), 30–36.

Taal, M. W. (2012). Risk factors and chronic kidney disease. In M. W. Taal, G. M. Chertow, K. Skorecki, A. S. L. Yu, & B. M. Brenner (Eds.), *Brenner and Rector's the kidney* (9th ed.). Philadelphia: Saunders.

Taal, M. W., Chertow, G. M., Skorecki, K., Yu, A. S. L., & Brenner, B. M. (2012). *Brenner and Rector's the kidney* (9th ed.). Philadelphia: Saunders.

Uchino, S., Bellomo, R., Bagshaw, S. M., & Goldsmith, D. (2010). Transient azotaemia is associated with a high risk of death in hospitalized patients. *Nephrology, Dialysis, Transplantation, 25*(6), 1833–1839.

United Network for Organ Sharing online (UNOS). (2014). Retrieved October 2014, from <www.unos.org>.

U.S. Renal Data Systems (USRDS) (2014). *USRDS 2013 annual data report.* Bethesda, MD: The National Kidney and Urologic Diseases Information Clearinghouse (NKUDIC). National Institutes of Health. Retrieved October 2014, from <http://kidney.niddk.nih.gov/statistics/index.aspx>.

Vanmassenhove, J., Vanholder, R., Nagler, E., & Van Biesen, W. (2013). Urinary and serum biomarkers for the diagnosis of acute kidney injury: An in-depth review of the literature. *Nephrology, Dialysis, Transplantation, 28*(2), 254–273.

Wilson, B., & Lawrence, J. (2013). Implementation of a foot assessment program in a regional satellite hemodialysis setting. *Canadian Association of Nephrology Nurses and Technologists Journal, 23*(2), 41–47.

Wong, L. P., Yamamoto, K. T., Reddy, V., Cobb, D., Chamberlin, A., Pham, H., et al. (2014). Patient education and care for peritoneal dialysis catheter placement: A quality improvement study. *Peritoneal Dialysis International, 34*(1), 12–23.

Wynne, J., Narveson, S. Y., & Littmann, L. (2012). Cardiorenal syndrome. *Heart and Lung: The Journal of Critical Care, 41*(2), 157–160.

Yeun, J. Y., Ornt, D., & Depner, T. A. (2012). Hemodialysis. In M. W. Taal, G. M. Chertow, K. Skorecki, A. S. L. Yu, & B. M. Brenner (Eds.), *Brenner and Rector's the kidney* (9th ed.). Philadelphia: Saunders.

Chapter 69

American Cancer Society (ACS) (2014a). *Cancer facts and figures 2013-2014.* Retrieved October 2014, from <www.cancer.org/acs/groups/content/@epidemiologysurveillance/documents/document/acspc-036845.pdf>.

American Cancer Society (ACS) (2014b). *Mammograms.* Retrieved October 2014, from <www.cancer.org/cancer/breastcancer/moreinformation/breastcancerearlydetection/breast-cancer-early-detection-acs-recs-mammograms>.

American Cancer Society (ACS) (2014c). *American Cancer Society recommendations for early breast cancer detection in women without breast symptoms.* Retrieved October 2014, from <www.cancer.org/cancer/breastcancer/moreinformation/breastcancerearlydetection/breast-cancer-early-detection-acs-recs>.

American Congress of Obstetricians and Gynecologists (ACOG) (2011). *Hysterosalpingography.* Retrieved October 2014, from <www.acog.org/~/media/For%20Patients/faq143.pdf?dmc=1&ts=20130827T1635426695>.

Cleveland Clinic (2013). *What is hysteroscopy?* Retrieved October 2014, from <http://my.clevelandclinic.org/services/hysteroscopy/hic_what_is_hysteroscopy.aspx>.

Johns Hopkins Medicine (2014). *Cervical biopsy.* Retrieved October 2014, from <www.hopkinsmedicine.org/healthlibrary/test_procedures/gynecology/cervical_biopsy_92,P07767/>.

Levin, K. (2012). *Transvaginal ultrasound.* Retrieved October 2014, from <www.nlm.nih.gov/medlineplus/ency/article/003779.htm>.

Lowdermilk, D. L., & Perry, S. E. (2014). *Maternity and women's health care* (11th ed.). St. Louis: Mosby.

Mayo Clinic (2013). *Prostate biopsy.* Retrieved October 2014, from <www.mayoclinic.com/health/prostate-biopsy/MY00182/DSECTION=what-you-can-expect>.

National Cancer Institute at the National Institutes of Health (2014). *General information about male breast cancer.* Retrieved October 2014, from <www.cancer.gov/cancertopics/pdq/treatment/malebreast/Patient/page1#Keypoint3>.

*Ruhl, C. (2010). Sleep is a vital sign: Why assessing sleep is an important part of women's health. *Nursing for Women's Health, 14*(3), 243–247.

Susan G. Komen (2013). *Accuracy of mammograms.* Retrieved October 2014, from <http://ww5.komen.org/BreastCancer/AccuracyofMammograms.html>.

Taş, B., Donatsky, A. M., & Gögenur, I. (2013). Techniques to reduce shoulder pain after laparoscopic surgery for benign gynaecological disease: A systematic review. *Gynecological Surgery, 10*(3), 169–175.

U.S. Preventive Services Task Force (2013). *Screening for HIV.* Retrieved October 2014, from <www.uspreventiveservicestaskforce.org/uspstf/uspshivi.htm>.

Chapter 70

Alakhras, M. M., Bourne, R. R., Rickard, M. M., Ng, K. H., Pietrzyk, M. M., & Brennan, P. C. (2013). Digital tomosynthesis: A new future for breast imaging? *Clinical Radiology, 68*(5), e225–e236.

American Cancer Society (ACS) (2013a). *Breast cancer detailed guide.* Atlanta: Author.

American Cancer Society (ACS) (2013b). *Breast cancer facts & figures 2011-2012.* Atlanta: Author.

American College of Obstetricians and Gynecologists (ACOG). (2011). Annual mammogram should start at age 40 years. *Contemporary OB/GYN, 56*(9), 20.

Amin, A. L., Purdy, A. C., Mattingly, J. D., Kong, A. L., & Termuhlen, P. M. (2013). Multidisciplinary breast management benign breast disease. *Surgical Clinics of North America, 93*(2), 299–308.

Association of Women's Health, Obstetric, and Neonatal Nursing (AWHONN). (2010). Breast cancer screening: A AWHONN position statement. *Journal of Obstetric, Gynecologic, & Neonatal Nursing, 39*(5), 608–610.

Beredjick, C. (2012). The lesbian breast cancer link. *Advocate, 1062,* 16.

Bryan, T., & Snyder, E. (2013). The clinical breast exam: A skill that should not be abandoned. *JGIM: Journal of General Internal Medicine, 28*(5), 719–722.

Davies, C., Hongchao, P., Godwin, J., Gray, R., Arriagada, R., Raina, V., et al. (2013). Long-term effects of continuing adjuvant tamoxifen to 10 years versus stopping at 5 years after diagnosis of oestrogen receptor-positive breast cancer: ATLAS, a randomised trial. *Lancet, 381*(9869), 805–816.

Edwards, J., Herzberg, S., Shook, J., Beirne, T., & Schomas, D. (2013). Breast conservation therapy utilizing partial breast brachytherapy for early-stage cancer of the breast: A retrospective review from the Saint Luke's Cancer Institute. *American Journal of Clinical Oncology,* [epub ahead of print].

Greif, J. M., Pezzi, C. M., Klimberg, S., Bailey, L., & Zuraek, M. (2012). Gender differences in breast cancer: Analysis of 13,000 breast cancers in men from the National Cancer Data Base. *Annals of Surgical Oncology, 19,* 3199–3204.

Jankowitz, R. C., & Lee, A. V. (2013). The evolving role of multi-gene tests in breast cancer management. *Oncology, 27*(3), 210–214.

Johnson, R. H., Chien, F. L., & Bleyer, A. (2013). Incidence of breast cancer with distant involvement among women in the United States, 1976-2009. *Journal of the American Medical Association, 309*(8), 800–805.

Justice, M., Greenburg, G., Hernick, A. D., & Monroe, P. (2012). Disseminating research findings to the community: Breast cancer advocates conduct education forums. *Environmental Justice, 5*(3), 128–132.

Kamdar, B., Tergas, A., Mateen, F., Bhayani, N., & Oh, J. (2013). Night-shift work and risk of breast cancer: A systematic review and meta-analysis. *Breast Cancer Research and Treatment, 138*(1), 291–301.

Kedde, H., Wiel, H. B., Weijmar Schultz, W. C., & Wijsen, C. (2013). Sexual dysfunction in young women with breast cancer. *Supportive Care in Cancer, 21*(1), 271–280.

Khatcheressian, J., Hurley, P., Bantug, E., Esserman, L., Grunfeld, E., Halberg, F., et al.

(2013). Breast cancer follow-up and management after primary treatment: American Society of Clinical Oncology clinical practice guideline update. *Journal of Clinical Oncology, 31*(7), 961–965.

Klaeson, K. K., Sandell, K. K., & Bertero, C. M. (2011). To feel like an outsider: Focus group discussions regarding the influence on sexuality caused by breast cancer treatment. *European Journal of Cancer Care, 20*(6), 728–737.

Lavigne, E., Holowaty, E. J., Pan, S. Y., Villeneuve, P. J., Johnson, K. C., Furgusson, D. A., et al. (2013). Breast cancer detection and survival among women with cosmetic breast implants: Systematic review and meta-analysis of observational studies. *British Medical Journal, 346*(f2399), 1–12.

Mattarella, A. (2010). Breast cancer in men. *Radiologic Technology, 81*(4), 361M–378M.

McLaughlin, S. (2013). Surgical management of the breast: Breast conservation therapy and mastectomy. *The Surgical Clinics of North America, 93*(2), 411–428.

Mohler, E., & Mondry, T. (2013). *Patient education: Lymphedema after breast cancer surgery (Beyond the basics).* Retrieved January 2014, from <www.uptodate.com>.

Morgan, S. D., Redman, S., D'Este, C., & Rogers, K. (2011). Knowledge, satisfaction with information, decisional conflict and psychological morbidity amongst women diagnosed with ductal carcinoma in situ (DCIS). *Patient Education and Counseling, 84*, 62–68.

National Breast Cancer Coalition (NBCC) (2012). *Breast cancer deadline 2020: 2nd annual progress report.* Washington, DC: Author.

National LGBT Cancer Network (2013). *About us.* New York: Author.

Ooi, S., Martinez, M., & Li, C. (2011). Disparities in breast cancer characteristics and outcomes by race/ethnicity. *Breast Cancer Research and Treatment, 127*(3), 729–738.

Pollán, M. (2010). Epidemiology of breast cancer in young women. *Breast Cancer Research and Treatment, 123*(Suppl.), 3–6. doi:10.1007/s10549-010-1098-2.

Quinn, E., Corrigan, M., McHugh, S., Murphy, D., O'Mullane, J., Hill, A., et al. (2013). Who's talking about breast cancer? Analysis of daily breast cancer posts on the internet. *Breast, 22*(1), 24–27.

Ridner, S. H., Sinclair, V., Deng, J., Bonner, C. M., Kidd, N., & Dietrich, M. S. (2012). Breast cancer survivors with lymphedema. *Clinical Journal of Oncology Nursing, 16*(6), 609–614.

Saquib, J., Parker, B., Natarajan, L., Madlensky, L., Saquib, N., Patterson, R., et al. (2012). Prognosis following the use of complementary and alternative medicine in women diagnosed with breast cancer. *Complementary Therapies in Medicine, 20*(5), 283–290.

Schmidt, C. (2012). IOM issues report on breast cancer and the environment. *Environmental Health Perspectives, 120*(2), a60–a61.

Soran, A., Ibrahim, A., Kanbour, M., McGuire, K., Balci, F., Polat, A., et al. (2013). Decision

making and factors influencing long-term satisfaction with prophylactic mastectomy in women with breast cancer. *American Journal of Clinical Oncology*, [epub ahead of print].

*U.S. Preventive Services Task Force (USPSTF). (2009). Screening for breast cancer: U.S. Preventive Services Task Force recommendations statement. *Annals of Internal Medicine, 151*, 716–726.

Wanchai, A., Armer, J. M., & Stewart, B. R. (2010). Complementary and alternative medicine use among women with breast cancer: A systematic review. *Clinical Journal of Oncology Nursing, 14*(4), 45–55.

Weigelt, B., Geyer, F., & Reis-Filho, J. (2010). Histological types of breast cancer: How special are they? *Molecular Oncology, 4*(3), 192–208.

Williams, A. F. (2012). Living with and beyond breast cancer. *Journal of Community Nursing, 26*(1), 6.

Wyatt, G., Sikorskii, A., Wills, C., & Su, H. (2010). Complementary and alternative medicine use, spending, and quality of life in early stage breast cancer. *Nursing Research, 59*(1), 58–66.

Zakhireh, J., Fowble, B., & Esserman, L. (2010). Application of screening principles to the reconstructed breast. *Journal of Clinical Oncology, 28*(1), 173–180.

Chapter 71

American Cancer Society (ACS) (2014a). *Cancer facts and figures 2013-2014.* Retrieved November 2014, from <www.cancer.org/acs/groups/content/@epidemiologysurveilance/documents/document/acspc-036845.pdf>.

American Cancer Society (ACS) (2014b). *Cervical cancer prevention and early detection.* Retrieved November 2014, from <http://www.cancer.org/acs/groups/cid/documents/webcontent/003167-pdf.pdf>.

American Cancer Society (ACS) (2012). *New screening guidelines for cervical cancer.* Retrieved January 2014, from <www.cancer.org/cancer/news/new-screening-guidelines-for-cervical-cancer>.

American Cancer Society (ACS) (2013a). *Cancer facts and figures 2013.* Retrieved November 2014, from <www.cancer.org/acs/groups/content/@epidemiologysurveilance/documents/document/acspc-036845.pdf>.

American Cancer Society (ACS) (2013b). *Sex and pelvic radiation therapy.* Retrieved November 2014, from <www.cancer.org/treatment/treatmentsandsideeffects/physicalsideeffects/sexualsideeffectsinwomen/sexualityforthewoman/sexuality-for-women-with-cancer-pelvic-rad>.

American Cancer Society (ACS) (2014). *Ovarian cancer prevention.* Retrieved November 2014, from <www.cancer.gov/cancertopics/pdq/prevention/ovarian/Patient/page3>.

American Congress of Obstetricians and Gynecologists (ACOG) (2011). *Sonohysterography FAQ.* Retrieved November 2014, from <www.acog.org/~/media/For%20

Patients/faq175.pdf?dmc=1&ts=20130830T2133066904>.

American Congress of Obstetricians and Gynecologists (ACOG) (2013). *Statement on robotic surgery by ACOG.* Retrieved November 2014, from <www.acog.org/About_ACOG/News_Room/News_Releases/2013/Statement_on_Robotic_Surgery>.

Bradley, L. (2013). *Hysteroscopic myomectomy.* Retrieved November 2014, from <www.uptodate.com/contents/hysteroscopic-myomectomy>.

Braun, R. (2014). *Bartholin cyst.* Retrieved November 2014, from <www.emedicinehealth.com/bartholin_cyst/page3_em.htm#bartholins_cyst_symptoms>.

Centers for Disease Control and Prevention (CDC) (2014a). *Cervical cancer statistics.* Retrieved November 2014, from <www.cdc.gov/cancer/cervical/statistics/>.

Centers for Disease Control and Prevention (CDC) (2014b). *Genital HPV infection: Fact sheet.* Retrieved November 2014, from <www.cdc.gov/std/hpv/stdfact-hpv.htm>.

Falcone, T. (2014). *Overview of hysterectomy.* Retrieved November 2014, from <www.uptodate.com/contents/overview-of-hysterectomy?detectedLanguage=en&source=search_result&search=hysterectomy+robotic&selectedTitle=3~7&provider=noProvider>.

Gallo, T., Kashani, S., Patel, D. A., Elsahwi, K., Silasi, D. A., & Azodi, M. (2012). Robotic-assisted laparoscopic hysterectomy: Outcomes in obese and morbidly obese patients. *Journal of the Society of Laparoendoscopic Surgeons, 16*(3), 421.

GlaxoSmithKline (2012). *Cervarix.* Retrieved November 2014, from <http://www.cervarix.ca/>.

Lazarou, G. (2012). *Pelvic organ prolapse treatment and management.* Retrieved November 2014, from <http://emedicine.medscape.com/article/276259-treatment#a1134>.

Low, D. (2013). Toxic shock syndrome: Major advances in pathogenesis, but not treatment. *Critical Care Clinics, 29*, 651–675.

Mayo Clinic (2011). *Endometriosis: Definition.* Retrieved January 2014, from <www.mayoclinic.com/health/ca-125-test/MY00590>.

Mayo Clinic (2013). *Endometriosis: Causes.* Retrieved January 2014, from <www.mayoclinic.com/health/endometriosis/DS00289/DSECTION=causes>.

Merck Sharpe & Dohme Corporation (2014). *Gardasil.* Retrieved November 2014, from <http://www.gardasil.com/>.

National Cancer Institute (NCI) (2013a). *Endometrial cancer treatment: Endometrial cancer prevention.* Retrieved November 2014, from <www.cancer.gov/cancertopics/pdq/prevention/endometrial/Patient/page3>.

National Cancer Institute (NCI) (2013b). *A snapshot of endometrial cancer: Incidence and mortality.* Retrieved November 2014, from <http://www.cancer.gov/researchandfunding/snapshots/endometrial>.

Nguyen, M., LaFargue, C., Pua, T., & Tedjarati, S. (2013). Grade 1 endometrioid endometrial carcinoma presenting with pelvic bone metastasis: A case report and review of the literature. *Case Reports in Obstetrics and Gynecology*, *2013*, doi:10.1155/2013/807205.

Northwest Radiology Associates (2014). *Uterine fibroid embolization: FAQ*. Retrieved November 2014, from <www.fibroiddoc.com/faq/>.

Saul, T. (2013). *Emergent treatment of endometriosis*. Retrieved November 2014, from <http://emedicine.medscape.com/article/795771-overview>.

Storck, S. (2012). *Uterine artery embolization*. Retrieved November 2014, from <www.nlm.nih.gov/medlineplus/ency/article/007384.htm>.

Storck, S. (2014). *Cervical polyps*. Retrieved November 2014, from <www.nlm.nih.gov/medlineplus/ency/article/001494.htm>.

Turandot, S. (2013). *Emergent treatment of endometriosis*. Retrieved November 2014, from <http://emedicine.medscape.com/article/795771-overview>.

U.S. Food and Drug Administration (USFDA) (2011). *Urogynecologic surgical mesh: Update on the safety and effectiveness of transvaginal placement for pelvic organ prolapse*. Retrieved November 2014, from <www.fda.gov/downloads/MedicalDevices/Safety/AlertsandNotices/UCM262760.pdf>.

Chapter 72

American Cancer Society (ACS) (2014a). *Prostate cancer*. Retrieved November 2014, from <www.cancer.org/cancer/prostatecancer/detailedguide/prostate-cancer-key-statistics>.

American Cancer Society (ACS) (2014b). *Testicular cancer*. Retrieved November 2014, from <www.cancer.org/cancer/testicularcancer/detailedguide/testicular-cancer-key-statistics>.

Barry, M. J., Meleth, S., Lee, J. Y., Kreder, K. J., Avins, A. A., Nickel, J. C., et al. (2011). Effect of increasing doses of saw palmetto extract on lower urinary tract symptoms: A randomized trial. *Journal of the American Medical Association*, *306*, 1344–1351.

*Bohenkamp, S., & Yoder, L. H. (2009). The medical-surgical nurse's guide to testicular cancer. *Medsurg Nursing*, *18*(2), 116–124.

Carmody, J. F., Olendzki, B. C., Merriam, P. A., Liu, Q., Qiao, Y., & Ma, Y. (2012). A novel measure of dietary change in a prostate cancer dietary program incorporating mindfulness training. *Journal of the Academy of Nutrition and Dietetics*, *112*(11), 1822–1827.

Chitlik, A. (2011). Safe positioning for robotic-assisted laparoscopic prostatectomy. *AORN Journal: Association of periOperative Registered Nurses*, *94*(1), 37–48.

Cranwell-Bruce, L. A. (2010). Drugs for erectile dysfunction. *Medsurg Nursing*, *19*(3), 185–187.

Dunn, M. W., & Kazer, M. W. (2011). Prostate cancer overview. *Seminars in Oncology Nursing*, *27*(4), 244–250.

Eltabey, M. A., Sherif, H., & Hussein, A. A. (2010). Holmium laser enucleation versus transurethral resection of the prostate. *Canadian Journal of Urology*, *17*(6), 5447–5452.

Galbraith, M. E., Fink, R., & Wilkins, G. G. (2011). Couples surviving prostate cancer: Challenges in their lives and relationships. *Seminars in Oncology Nursing*, *27*(4), 300–308.

Hegarty, J., & Bailey, D. E. (2011). Active surveillance as a treatment option for prostate cancer. *Seminars in Oncology Nursing*, *27*(4), 260–266.

Johnson, T. V., Abbasi, A., Ehrlich, S. S., Kleris, R. S., Chirumamilla, S. L., Schoenberg, E. D., et al. (2010). Major depression drives severity of American Urological Association Symptom Index. *Urology*, *76*(6), 1317–1320.

King, D. (2012). Benign prostatic hyperplasia. *Nursing*, *42*(5), 37.

*Leman, E. S., Cannon, G. W., Trock, B. J., Sokoll, L. J., Chan, D. W., Mangold, R., et al. (2007). EPCA-2: A highly specific serum marker for prostate cancer. *Urology*, *69*(4), 714–720.

Maliski, S. L., Connor, S. E., Oduro, C., & Litwin, M. S. (2011). Access to health care and quality of life for underserved men with prostate cancer. *Seminars in Oncology Nursing*, *27*(4), 267–277.

O'Rourke, M. E. (2011). The prostate-specific antigen screening conundrum: Examining the evidence. *Seminars in Oncology Nursing*, *27*(4), 251–259.

Perlman, G., & Drescher, J. (2011). *A gay man's guide to prostate cancer*. Binghamton, NY: Haworth Medical Press.

Roehrborn, C. G. (2011). Male lower urinary tract symptoms (LUTS) and benign prostatic hyperplasia (BPH). *Medical Clinics of North America*, *95*(1), 87–100.

*Tackland, J., MacDonald, R., Rutks, I., & Wilt, T. J. (2009). *Serenoa repens* for benign prostatic hyperplasia. *Cochrane Database of Systematic Reviews*, (2), CD001423. Retrieved August 24, 2013, from <www.ncbi.nlm.nih.gov/pubmed/19370565>.

Viatori, M. (2012). Testicular cancer. *Seminars in Oncology Nursing*, *28*(3), 180–189.

Wang, C. J., Lin, Y. N., Huang, S. W., & Chang, C. H. (2011). Low dose oral desmopressin for nocturnal polyuria in patients with benign prostatic hyperplasia: A double-blind, placebo controlled, randomized study. *Journal of Urology*, *185*(1), 219–223.

Zarowitz, B. J. (2010). Opportunity to optimize management of benign prostatic hyperplasia. *Geriatric Nursing*, *31*(6), 441–445.

Chapter 73

*American Nurses Association (ANA) (2001). *Code of ethics for nurses*. Washington, DC: Author.

American Psychiatric Association (APA) (2013). *Diagnostic and statistical manual of mental disorders* (5th ed.). Washington, DC: Author.

Aramburu Alegria, C. (2011). Transgender identity and health care: Implications for psychosocial and physical evaluation. *Journal of the American Academy of Nurse Practitioners*, *23*, 175–182.

Brennan, A. M., Barnsteiner, J., Siantz, M. L., Cotter, V. T., & Everett, J. (2012). Lesbian, gay, bisexual, transgendered, or intersexed content for nursing curricula. *Journal of Professional Nursing*, *28*(2), 96–104.

Chestnut, S., Dixon, E., & Jindasurat, C. (2013). *Lesbian, gay, bisexual, transgender, queer, and HIV-affected hate violence in 2012*. National Coalition of Anti-Violence Programs. Retrieved September 2014, from <www.avp.org/storage/documents/ncavp_2012_hvreport_final.pdf>.

Coleman, E., Bockting, W., Botzer, M., Cohen-Kettenis, P., DeCuypere, G., Fladman, J., et al. (2011). Standards of care for the health of transsexual, transgender, and gender-nonconforming people (Version 7). *International Journal of Transgenderism*, *13*, 165–232.

Conron, K. J., Mimiago, M. J., & Landers, S. J. (2010). A population-based study of sexual orientation identity and gender differences in African Americans. *American Journal of Public Health*, *100*, 1953–1960.

Edwards-Leeper, L., & Spack, N. P. (2013). Psychological evaluation and medical treatment of transgender youth in an interdisciplinary "Gender Management Services" (GeMS) in a major pediatric center. In J. Drescher & W. Byne (Eds.), *Treating transgender children and adolescents: An interdisciplinary discussion*. New York: Routledge.

Eliason, M. J., Chinn, P., Dibble, S. L., & DeJoseph, J. (2013). Open the door for LGBTQ patients. *Nursing*, *43*(8), 44–50.

Gates, G. (2011). *How many people are gay, lesbian, bisexual, or transgender?* Williams Institute on Sexual Orientation and Gender Identify Law and Public Policy at UCLA School of Law. Retrieved September 2014, from <http://wiwp.law.ucla.edu/wp-content/uploads/Gates-How-Many-People-LGBT-Apr-2011.pdf>.

Grant, J. M., Mottet, L. A., & Tanis, J. (2010). *National transgender discrimination survey report on health and health care*. National Center for Transgender Equality and National Gay and Lesbian Task Force. Retrieved September 2014, from <http://transequality.org/PDFs/NTDSReportonHealth_final.pdf>.

Grant, J. M., Mottet, L. A., & Tanis, J. (2011). *Injustice at every turn: A report of the national transgender discrimination survey*. National Center for Transgender Equality and National Gay and Lesbian Task Force. Retrieved September 2014, from <http://transequality.org/PDFs/Executive_Summary.pdf>.

Institute of Medicine (IOM) (2011). *The health of LGBT people: Building a foundation for better understanding*. Washington, DC: National Academies Press.

Jenner, C. O. (2010). Transsexual primary care. *Journal of the American Academy of Nurse Practitioners, 22,* 403–408.

Lombardi, E. (2010). Transhealth: A review and guidance for future research—Proceedings from The Summer Institute at the Center for Research on Health and Sexual Orientation, University of Pittsburgh. *Journal of Transgenderism, 12,* 211–229.

Pettinato, M. (2012). Providing care for GLBTQ patients. *Nursing, 42*(12), 22–27.

Reed, H. M. (2011). Aesthetic and functional male to female genital and perineal surgery: Feminizing vaginoplasty. *Seminars in Plastic Surgery, 25*(2), 163–174.

Rounds, K. E., McGrath, B. B., & Walsh, E. (2013). Perspectives on provider behaviors: A qualitative study of sexual and gender minorities regarding quality of care. *Contemporary Nurse, 44*(1), 99–110.

Shipherd, J. C., Maguen, S., Skidmore, W. C., & Abramovitz, S. M. (2011). Potentially traumatic events in a transgender sample: Frequency and associated symptoms. *Traumatology, 17,* 56–67.

Spack, N. P. (2013). Management of transgenderism. *Journal of the American Medical Association, 309,* 478–484.

The Joint Commission (TJC) (2011). *Advancing effective communication, cultural competence, and patient- and family-centered care for the lesbian, gay, bisexual, and transgender community.* Retrieved September 2014, from <www.jointcommission.org/lgbt>.

Chapter 74

Augenbraum, M. (2012). Genital ulcer disease. In M. J. Zenilman & M. Shahmanesh (Eds.), *Sexually transmitted infections: Diagnosis, management and treatment* (pp. 155–163). Sudbury, MA: Jones & Bartlett Learning.

*Bavis, M. P., Smith, D. Y., & Siomos, M. Z. (2009). Genital herpes: Diagnosis, treatment, and counseling in the adolescent patient. *Journal for Nurse Practitioners, 5*(6), 415–420.

Bleich, A. T., Sheffield, J. S., Wendel, G. D., Sigman, A., & Cunningham, G. (2012). Disseminated gonococcal infection in women. *Obstetrics and Gynecology, 119*(3), 597–602.

Centers for Disease Control and Prevention (CDC). (2010a). Seroprevalence of herpes simplex virus type 2 among persons aged 14-49 years—United States, 2005-2008. *Morbidity and Mortality Weekly Report, 59*(15), 456–459.

Centers for Disease Control and Prevention (CDC). (2010b). Sexually transmitted diseases treatment guidelines, 2010. *Morbidity and Mortality Weekly Report, 59*(RR–12), 1–110.

Centers for Disease Control and Prevention (CDC) (2012a). *HPV vaccine information for clinicians—Fact sheet.* Retrieved November 2014, from <www.cdc.gov/std/hpv/stdfact-hpv-vaccine-hcp.htm>.

Centers for Disease Control and Prevention (CDC). (2012b). National and state vaccination coverage among adolescents aged 13-17 years—United States, 2011. *Morbidity and Mortality Weekly Report, 61*(34), 671–677. Retrieved November 2014, from <www.cdc.gov/mmwr/preview/mmwrhtml/mm6134a3.htm>.

Centers for Disease Control and Prevention (CDC) (2012c). *Sexually transmitted disease surveillance 2011.* Atlanta: U.S. Department of Health and Human Services. Retrieved November 2014, from <www.cdc.gov/std/stats11/Surv2011.pdf>.

Centers for Disease Control and Prevention (CDC). (2012d). Update to CDC's sexually transmitted diseases treatment guidelines, 2010: Oral cephalosporins no longer a recommended treatment for gonococcal infections. *Morbidity and Mortality Weekly Report, 61*(31), 590–594.

Centers for Disease Control and Prevention (CDC) (2013a). *CDC fact sheet: Incidence, prevalence, and cost of sexually transmitted infections in the United States.* Retrieved November 2014, from <www.cdc.gov/std/stats/STI-Estimates-Fact-Sheet-Feb-2013.pdf>.

Centers for Disease Control and Prevention (CDC) (2013c). *Guidance on the use of expedited partner therapy in the treatment of gonorrhea.* Retrieved November 2014, from <www.cdc.gov/std/ept/GC-Guidance.htm>.

Centers for Disease Control and Prevention (CDC) (2013d). *Legal status of expedited partner therapy (EPT).* Retrieved November 2014, from <www.cdc.gov/std/ept/legal/default.htm>.

Centers for Disease Control and Prevention (CDC) (2013e). *Pelvic inflammatory disease treatment: Guidelines, research, & updates.* Retrieved November 2014, from <www.cdc.gov/std/PID/treatment.htm>.

Centers for Disease Control and Prevention (CDC). (2013f). Summary of notifiable diseases, United States, 2011. *Morbidity and Mortality Weekly Report, 60*(53), 1–118. Retrieved November 2014, from <www.cdc.gov/mmwr/PDF/wk/mm6053.pdf>.

Centers for Disease Control and Prevention (CDC) (2014a). *Expedited partner therapy.* Atlanta: U.S. Department of Health and Human Services. Retrieved November 2014, from <www.cdc.gov/std/ept/>.

Centers for Disease Control and Prevention (CDC) (2014b). *Gay and bisexual men's health: Sexually transmitted diseases.* Retrieved November 2014, from <www.cdc.gov/msmhealth/STD.htm>.

Centers for Disease Control and Prevention (CDC). (2014c). *Sexually transmitted diseases: Treatment Guidelines 2010, Special populations.* Retrieved November 2014, from <www.cdc.gov/std/treatment/2010/specialpops.htm#wsw>.

Centers for Disease Control and Prevention (CDC). (2014d). *Syphilis: CDC Fact Sheet.* Retrieved November 2014, from <www.cdc.gov/std/syphilis/stdfact-syphilis-detailed.htm>.

*Cobos, D. G., & Jones, J. (2009). Moving forward: Transgender persons as change agents in health care access and human rights. *Journal of the Association of Nurses in AIDS Care, 20*(5), 341–347.

Datta, D., Dunne, E. F., Saraiya, M., & Markowitz, L. (2012). Human papillomaviruses. In M. J. Zenilman & M. Shahmanesh (Eds.), *Sexually transmitted infections: Diagnosis, management and treatment.* Sudbury, MA: Jones & Bartlett Learning.

Fenton, K. A., & French, P. (2012). Infectious syphilis. In M. J. Zenilman & M. Shahmanesh (Eds.), *Sexually transmitted infections: Diagnosis, management and treatment* (pp. 80–82). Sudbury, MA: Jones & Bartlett Learning.

GlaxoSmithKline. (2012). *Cervarix.* Retrieved November 2014, from <http://www.cervarix.ca/>.

Holmes, K. K., Sparling, P. F., Stamm, W. E., Wasserheit, J. N., Corey, L., et al. (Eds.), (2008). *Sexually transmitted diseases* (4th ed.). New York: McGraw-Hill.

Jeffers, L. A., & DiBartolo, M. C. (2011). Raising health care provider awareness of sexually transmitted disease in patients over 50. *Medsurg Nursing, 20*(6), 285–290.

Johns Hopkins Point of Care-IT Center (2014). *Antibiotic guide.* Retrieved November 2014, from <www.hopkinsguides.com/hopkins/ub>.

Kim, J. J. (2010). Targeted human papillomavirus vaccination of men who have sex with men in the USA: A cost-effectiveness modeling analysis. *The Lancet Infectious Diseases, 10*(12), 845–852.

Koester, K. A., Collins, S. P., Fuller, S. M., Galindo, G. R., Gibson, S., & Steward, W. T. (2013). Sexual healthcare preferences among gay and bisexual men: A qualitative study in San Francisco, California. *PLoS ONE, 8*(8), e71546.

Mark, H., Jordan, E. T., Cruz, J., & Warren, N. (2012). What's new in sexually transmitted infection management: Changes in the 2010 guidelines from the Centers for Disease Control and Prevention. *Journal of Midwifery & Women's Health, 57*(3), 276–284.

Markowitz, L. E., Hariri, S., Lin, C., Dunne, E. F., Steinau, M., McQuillan, G., et al. (2013). Reduction in human papillomavirus (HPV) prevalence among young women following HPV vaccine introduction in the United States, National Health and Nutrition Examination Surveys, 2003-2010. *Journal of Infectious Diseases, 208*(3), 385–393.

Merck Sharpe & Dohme Corporation (2014). *Gardasil.* Retrieved November 2014, from <http://www.gardasil.com/>.

Murphy, J., & Mark, H. (2012). Cervical cancer screening in the era of human papillomavirus testing and vaccination. *Journal of Midwifery & Women's Health, 57*(6), 569–576.

Owusu-Edusei, K., Chesson, H. W., Gift, T. L., Tao, G., Mahajan, R., Ocfemia, M. C., et al. (2013). The estimated direct medical cost of selected sexually transmitted infections in the United States, 2008. *Sexually Transmitted Diseases, 40*(3), 197–201.

Patel, R., & Rompalo, A. (2012). Genital herpes infections. In M. J. Zenilman & M.

Shahmanesh (Eds.), *Sexually transmitted infections: Diagnosis, management and treatment* (pp. 165–176). Sudbury, MA: Jones & Bartlett Learning.

Satterwhite, C. L., Torrone, E., Meites, E., Dunne, E. F., Mahajan, R., Banez Ocfemia, M. C., et al. (2013). Sexually transmitted infections among U.S. women and men: Prevalence and incidence estimates, 2008. *Sexually Transmitted Diseases, 40*(3), 187–193.

Schiffman, M., Wentzensen, N., Wacholder, S., Kinney, W., Gage, J. C., & Castle, P. E. (2011). Human papillomavirus testing in the prevention of cervical cancer. *Journal of the National Cancer Institute, 103*, 368–383.

*Spinola, S. M. (2008). Chancroid and *Haemophilus ducreyi*. In K. K. Holmes, P. F. Sparling, W. E. Stamm, P. Piot, J. N. Wasserheit, L. Corey, et al. (Eds.), *Sexually transmitted diseases* (4th ed., pp. 689–699). New York: McGraw-Hill.

Sweet, R. L. (2012). Pelvic inflammatory disease: Current concepts of diagnosis and management. *Current Infectious Diseases Reports*, [epub ahead of print].

*Trelle, S., Shang, A., Nartey, L., Cassell, J. A., & Low, N. (2007). Improved effectiveness of partner notification for patients with sexually transmitted infections: Systematic review. *BMJ, 334*(7589), 354.

U.S. Department of Health and Human Services (USDHHS), Office of Disease Prevention and Health Promotion (2014). *Healthy People 2020*. Retrieved November 2014, from <www.healthypeople.gov/hp2020/>.

U.S. Preventive Services Task Force (USPSTF) (2014a). *Guide to clinical preventive services, 2014: Recommendations of the U.S. Preventive Services Task Force*. Rockville, MD: Agency for Healthcare Research and Quality. Retrieved November 2014, from <http://www.ahrq .gov/professionals/clinicians-providers/ guidelines-recommendations/guide/index .html>.

U.S. Preventive Services Task Force (USPSTF) (2014b). *Sexually transmitted infections: Behavioral Counseling. U.S. Preventive Services Task Force recommendation statement*. AHRQ Publication. 08-05123-EF-2. Retrieved November 2014, from <www .uspreventiveservicestaskforce.org/uspstf08/ sti/stirs.htm>.

Warren, T., Gilbert, L., & Mark, H. (2011). Availability of serologic and virologic testing for herpes simplex virus in the largest sexually transmitted disease clinics in the United States. *Sexually Transmitted Diseases, 38*(4), 267–269.

Williamson, C. (2010). Providing care to transgender persons: A clinical approach to primary care, hormones, and HIV management. *Journal of the Association of Nurses in AIDS Care, 21*(3), 221–229.

Zenilman, M. J., & Shahmanesh, M. (2012). *Sexually transmitted infections: Diagnosis, management and treatment*. Sudbury, MA: Jones & Bartlett Learning.

GLOSSARY

A

abdominal acute compartment syndrome (AACS) A complication after abdominal trauma that occurs when the intraabdominal pressure is sustained at greater than 200 mm Hg.

abdominoperineal (AP) resection The surgical removal of the sigmoid colon, rectum, and anus through combined abdominal and perineal incisions. This resection is performed when rectal tumors are present.

ablative The process or act of removing.

abscess A localized collection of pus caused by an inflammatory response to bacteria in tissues or organs.

absolute neutrophil count (ANC) The percentage and actual number of mature circulating neutrophils; used to measure a patient's risk for infection. The higher the numbers, the greater the resistance to infection.

absorption The uptake from the intestinal lumen of nutrients produced by digestion.

acalculia Difficulty with math calculations; caused by brain injury or disease.

acalculous cholecystitis Inflammation of the gallbladder occurring in the absence of gallstones; typically associated with biliary stasis caused by any condition that affects the regular filling or emptying of the gallbladder.

acclimatization The process of adapting to a high altitude; involves physiologic changes that help the body compensate for less available oxygen in the atmosphere.

accommodation The process of maintaining a clear visual image when the gaze is shifted from a distant object to a near object. The eye adjusts its focus by changing the curvature of the lens.

achlorhydria The absence of hydrochloric acid from gastric secretions.

acid A substance that releases hydrogen ions when dissolved in water. The strength of an acid is measured by how easily it releases hydrogen ions in solution.

acidosis An acid-base imbalance in which blood pH is below normal.

acinus The structural unit of the lower respiratory tract consisting of a respiratory bronchiole, an alveolar duct, and an alveolar sac.

Acorn cardiac support device A polyester mesh jacket that is placed over the ventricles to provide support and avoid overstretching the myocardial muscle in the patient with heart failure; reduces heart muscle hypertrophy and assists with improvement of ejection fraction.

acoustic neuroma A benign tumor of cranial nerve VIII; symptoms include damage to hearing, facial movements, and sensation. The tumor can enlarge into the brain, damaging structures in the cerebellum.

active euthanasia Purposeful action that directly causes death; not supported by most professional organizations, including the American Nurses Association.

active immunity Resistance to infection that occurs when the body responds to an invading antigen by making specific antibodies against the antigen. Immunity lasts for years and is natural by infection or artificial by stimulation (e.g., vaccine) of the body's immune defenses.

active surveillance (AS) Observation for cancer, without immediate active treatment.

activities of daily living (ADLs) The activities performed in the course of a normal day, such as bathing, dressing, feeding, and ambulating.

activity therapist See *recreational therapist*.

acute Having relatively greater intensity; marked by a sudden onset and short duration.

acute adrenal insufficiency A life-threatening event in which the need for cortisol and aldosterone is greater than the available supply. Also called "addisonian crisis."

acute arterial occlusion The sudden blockage of an artery, typically in the lower extremity, in the patient with chronic peripheral arterial disease.

acute compartment syndrome (ACS) A complication of a fracture characterized by increased pressure within one or more compartments and causing massive compromise of circulation to the area. Compartments are sheaths of inelastic fascia that support and partition muscles, blood vessels, and nerves in the body.

acute coronary syndrome (ACS) A disorder, including unstable angina and myocardial infarction, that results from obstruction of the coronary artery by ruptured atherosclerotic plaque and leads to platelet aggregation, thrombus formation, and vasoconstriction.

acute gastritis Inflammation of the gastric mucosa or submucosa after exposure to local irritants. Various degrees of mucosal necrosis and inflammatory reaction occur in acute disease. Complete regeneration and healing usually occur within a few days.

acute hematogenous infection An infection resulting from bacteremia, disease, or nonpenetrating trauma that is disseminated by the blood through the circulation.

acute kidney injury (AKI) A rapid decrease in kidney function, leading to the collection of metabolic wastes in the body; formerly called "acute renal failure (ARF)."

acute-on-chronic kidney disease A condition in which acute kidney injury occurs in addition to chronic kidney disease.

acute pain The unpleasant sensory and emotional experience associated with tissue damage that results from acute injury, disease, or surgery.

acute pancreatitis A serious inflammation of the pancreas characterized by a sudden onset of abdominal pain, nausea, and vomiting. It is caused by premature activation of pancreatic enzymes that destroy ductal tissue and pancreatic cells and results in autodigestion and fibrosis of the pancreas.

acute paronychia Inflammation of the skin around the nail, which usually occurs with a torn cuticle or an ingrown toenail.

acute pericarditis An inflammation or alteration of the pericardium, the membranous sac that encloses the heart; may be fibrous, serous, hemorrhagic, purulent, or neoplastic.

acute pyelonephritis Active bacterial infection in the kidney.

acute respiratory distress syndrome (ARDS) Respiratory failure marked by hypoxemia that persists even when 100% oxygen is given, as well as decreased pulmonary compliance, dyspnea, noncardiac-associated bilateral pulmonary edema, and dense pulmonary infiltrates on x-ray.

acute sialadenitis Inflammation of a salivary gland; can be caused by infectious agents, irradiation, or immunologic disorders.

adaptive immunity The immunity that a person's body makes (or can receive) as an adaptive response to invasion by organisms or foreign proteins; occurs either naturally or artificially through lymphocyte responses and can be either active or passive.

addisonian crisis Acute adrenal insufficiency; a life-threatening event in which the need for cortisol and aldosterone is greater than the available supply.

adenocarcinoma Tumor that arises from the glandular epithelial tissue.

adenohypophysis The anterior lobe of the pituitary gland, which makes up about 70% of the gland.

adiponectin An anti-inflammatory and insulin sensitizing hormone.

adipose Fatty.

adjuvant A substance that aids another substance, such as a cancer treatment that uses chemotherapy in addition to surgery.

adjuvant therapy Chemotherapy that is used along with surgery or radiation.

adrenal crisis Acute adrenocortical insufficiency, which can be life threatening.

adrenal Cushing's disease An excess of glucocorticoids caused by a problem in the adrenal cortex, usually a benign tumor (adrenal adenoma). This usually occurs in only one adrenal gland.

advance directive (AD) A written document prepared by a competent person to specify what, if any, extraordinary actions he or she would want when no longer able to make decisions about personal health care.

adverse drug event (ADE) An unintended harmful reaction to an administered drug.

aerosolization Transmission via fine airborne droplets.

aesthetic plastic surgery Plastic surgery that is cosmetic and aims to alter a person's physical appearance.

afferent arteriole The smallest, most distal portion of the renal arterial system that supplies blood to the nephron. From the afferent arteriole, blood flows into the glomerulus, a series of specialized capillary loops.

after-drop A continued decrease in core body temperature after a victim is removed from a cold environment; results from equilibration of core and peripheral blood temperature and counter-current cooling of the blood perfusing cold tissue.

afterload The pressure or resistance that the ventricles must overcome to eject blood through the semilunar valves and into the peripheral blood vessels; the amount of resistance is directly related to arterial blood pressure and blood vessel diameter.

agglutination A clumping action that results during the antibody-binding process when antibodies link antigens together to form large and small immune complexes.

agnosia A general term for a loss of sensory comprehension; may include an inability to write, comprehend reading material, or use an object correctly.

agraphia Loss of the ability to write; caused by brain injury or disease.

Airborne Precautions Infection control guidelines from the Centers for Disease Control and Prevention; used for patients with infections spread by the airborne transmission route, such as tuberculosis. Negative airflow rooms are required to prevent the airborne spread of microbes.

akinesia Slow or no movement, as seen in a patient with Parkinson disease. Also called "bradykinesia."

albuminuria The presence of albumin in the urine.

alcoholic hepatitis Liver inflammation caused by the toxic effect of alcohol on hepatocytes. The liver becomes enlarged, with cellular degeneration and infiltration by fat, leukocytes, and lymphocytes.

aldosterone The chief mineralocorticoid produced by the adrenal cortex. Aldosterone increases kidney reabsorption of sodium and water, thus restoring blood pressure, blood volume, and blood sodium levels. Aldosterone secretion is regulated by the renin-angiotensin system, serum potassium ion concentration, and adrenocorticotropic hormone.

alexia Complete inability to understand written language; caused by brain injury or disease.

alkaline reflux gastropathy A complication of gastric surgery in which the pylorus is bypassed or removed. Endoscopic examination reveals regurgitated bile in the stomach and mucosal hyperemia. Symptoms include early satiety, abdominal discomfort, and vomiting. Also called "bile reflux gastropathy."

alkalosis An acid-base imbalance in which blood pH is above normal.

allele An alternate form (or variation) of a gene.

allergen A foreign protein that is capable of causing a hypersensitivity response, or allergy, that ranges from uncomfortable (itchy, watery eyes or sneezing) to life threatening (allergic asthma, anaphylaxis, bronchoconstriction, or circulatory collapse); causes a release of natural chemicals, such as histamine, in the body.

allergy An increased or excessive response to the presence of a foreign protein or allergen (antigen) to which the patient has been previously exposed.

allogeneic bone marrow transplantation The transplantation of bone marrow from a sibling.

allograft A graft of tissue or bone between individuals of the same species but a different genotype; the donor may be a cadaver or a living person, either related or unrelated. Also called "homograft."

alopecia Hair loss.

alveolitis Inflammation of the alveoli.

amaurosis fugax A transient, brief episode of blindness in one eye.

ambulatory A term that refers to a patient who goes to the hospital or physician's office for treatment and returns home on the same day.

ambulatory aid Assistive device such as a cane or a walker.

ambulatory pump Infusion therapy pump generally used with a home care patient to allow a return to his or her usual activities while receiving infusion therapy.

amenorrhea The absence of menstrual periods in women.

amnesia Loss of memory.

amputation The removal of a limb or other appendage of the body.

amyotrophic lateral sclerosis (ALS) A progressive and degenerative disease of the motor system that is characterized by atrophy of the hands, forearms, and legs and results in paralysis and death. There is no known cause, no cure, no specific treatment, no standard pattern of progression, and no method of prevention. Also called "Lou Gehrig's disease."

anaerobic Lacking adequate oxygen.

anaerobic cellular metabolism Metabolism without oxygen.

anal fissure A painful ulcer at the margin of the anus.

analgesia Pain relief or pain suppression.

anaphylaxis The widespread reaction that occurs in response to contact with a substance to which the person has a severe allergy (antigen); characterized by blood vessel and bronchiolar smooth muscle involvement causing widespread blood vessel dilation, decreased cardiac output, and bronchoconstriction; results in cell damage and the release of large amounts of histamine, severe hypovolemia, vascular collapse, decreased cardiac contraction, and dysrhythmias and causes extreme whole-body hypoxia.

anasarca Generalized edema.

anastomosis Surgical reattachment. Also a general term meaning "a connection."

anatomic dead space Places in which air flows but the structures are too thick for gas exchange.

anemia A clinical sign of some abnormal condition related to a reduction in one of the following: number of red blood cells, amount of hemoglobin, or hematocrit (percentage of packed red blood cells per deciliter of blood).

anergy The inability to mount an immune response to an antigen.

anesthesia An induced state of partial or total loss of sensation with or without loss of consciousness.

aneuploid (aneuploidy) An abnormal karyotype with more or fewer than 23 pairs of chromosomes.

aneurysm A permanent localized dilation of an artery (to at least 2 times its normal diameter) that forms when the middle layer (media) of the artery is weakened, stretching the inner (intima) and outer (adventitia) layers. As the artery widens, tension in the wall increases and further widening occurs, thus enlarging the aneurysm.

aneurysmectomy A surgical procedure performed to excise an aneurysm.

angina pectoris Literally, "strangling of the chest"; a temporary imbalance between the ability of the coronary arteries to supply oxygen and the demand for oxygen by the cardiac muscle. As a result, the patient experiences chest discomfort.

angioedema Diffuse swelling resulting from a vascular reaction in the deep tissues; can occur in a patient having an anaphylactic reaction.

anion Ion that has a negative charge.

anisocoria A difference in the size of the pupils.

ankle-brachial index (ABI) A ratio derived by dividing the ankle blood pressure by the brachial blood pressure; this calculation is used to assess the vascular status of the lower extremities. To obtain the ABI, a blood pressure cuff is applied to the lower extremities just above the malleoli. The systolic pressure is measured by Doppler ultrasound at both the dorsalis pedis and posterior tibial pulses. The higher of these two pressures is then divided by the higher of the two brachial pulses.

anomia Inability to find words.

anorectal abscess A localized induration and fluctuance that is caused by inflammation of the soft tissue near the rectum or anus and is most often the result of obstruction of the ducts of glands in the anorectal region by feces, foreign bodies, or trauma.

anorectic drugs Drugs that suppress appetite, which reduces food intake and, over time, may result in weight loss; may be prescribed for obese patients in a comprehensive weight reduction program.

anorexia The loss of appetite for food.

anorexia nervosa An eating disorder of self-induced starvation resulting from a fear of fatness, even though the patient is underweight.

anorexin Neuropeptide that decreases appetite.

anoxic Completely lacking oxygen.

antalgic (gait) A term that refers to an abnormality in the stance phase of gait. When part of one leg is painful, the person shortens the stance phase on the affected side.

anterior colporrhaphy Surgery for severe symptoms of cystocele in which the pelvic muscles are tightened for better bladder support.

anterior nares The nostrils or external openings into the nasal cavities.

antibody-mediated immunity (AMI) or antibody-mediated immune system The defense response that produces antibodies directed against certain pathogens. The antibodies inactivate the pathogens and protect against future infection from that microorganism.

antidepressants A group of drugs that help manage clinical depression.

antiepileptic drugs (AEDs)   A class of drugs used to control seizures. Also called "anticonvulsants."

antigen   A foreign protein or allergen that is capable of causing an immune response; protein on the surface of a cell.

anuria   Complete lack of urine output; usually defined as less than 100 mL/24 hr.

aortic regurgitation   The flow of blood from the aorta back into the left ventricle during diastole; occurs when the aortic valve leaflets do not close properly during diastole and the annulus (the valve ring that attaches to the leaflets) is dilated or deformed.

aortic stenosis   Narrowing of the aortic valve orifice and obstruction of left ventricular outflow during systole.

aphasia   Inability to use or comprehend spoken or written language due to brain injury or disease.

apheresis   A procedure in which whole blood is withdrawn from the patient, a blood component (e.g., stem cells) is filtered out, and the plasma is returned to the patient.

aphonia   Inability to produce sound; complete but temporary loss of the voice.

aphthous stomatitis   Noninfectious stomatitis.

apical impulse   The pulse located at the left fifth intercostal space in the midclavicular line in the mitral area (the apex of the heart). Also called the "point of maximal impulse."

apolipoprotein E   One of several regulators of lipoprotein metabolism.

appendectomy   Surgical removal of the inflamed appendix.

appendicitis   Acute inflammation of the vermiform appendix, which is the blind pouch attached to the cecum of the colon, usually located in the right iliac region just below the ileocecal valve.

approximated   In a clean laceration or a surgical incision to be closed with sutures or staples, the act of bringing together the wound edges with the skin layers lined up in correct anatomic position so they can be held in place until healing is complete.

apraxia   The loss of the ability to carry out a purposeful motor activity.

aqueous humor   The clear, watery fluid that is continually produced by the ciliary processes and fills the anterior and posterior chambers of the eye. This fluid drains through the canal of Schlemm into the blood to maintain balanced intraocular pressure (pressure within the eye).

arcus senilis   An opaque ring within the outer edge of the cornea caused by fat deposits. Its presence does not affect vision.

areflexic bladder   Urinary retention and overflow (dribbling) caused by injuries to the lower motor neuron at the spinal cord level of S2 to S4 (e.g., multiple sclerosis and spinal cord injury below T12). Bladder emptying may be achieved by performing a Valsalva maneuver or tightening the abdominal muscles. The effectiveness of these maneuvers should be ascertained by catheterizing the patient for residual urine after voiding. Also called "flaccid bladder."

arrhythmogenic right ventricular cardiomyopathy (dysplasia)   A form of cardiomyopathy that results from the replacement of myocardial tissue with fibrous and fatty tissue.

arterial revascularization   The surgical procedure most commonly used to increase arterial blood flow in the affected limb of a patient with peripheral arterial disease.

arterial ulcers   A painful complication in the patient with peripheral arterial disease. Typically, the ulcer is small and round, with a "punched out" appearance and well-defined borders. Ulcers develop on the toes (often the great toe), between the toes, or on the upper aspect of the foot. With prolonged occlusion, the toes can become gangrenous.

arteriography   Angiography of the arterial vessels; this invasive diagnostic procedure involves fluoroscopy and the use of a contrast medium and is performed when an arterial obstruction, narrowing, or aneurysm is suspected.

arteriosclerosis   A thickening, or hardening, of the arterial wall.

arteriotomy   A surgical opening into an artery.

arteriovenous malformation (AVM)   An abnormality that occurs during embryonic development, resulting in a tangled mass of malformed, thin-walled, dilated vessels. The congenital absence of a capillary network in these vessels forms an abnormal communication between the arterial and venous systems and increases the risk that the vessels may rupture, causing bleeding, such as into the subarachnoid space or into the intracerebral tissue with brain AVMs. In the absence of the capillary network, the thin-walled veins are subjected to arterial pressure.

arthralgia   Pain in a joint.

arthritis   Inflammation of one or more joints.

arthrodesis   The surgical fusion of a joint.

arthrogram   An x-ray study of a joint after contrast medium (air or solution) has been injected to enhance its visualization.

arthroscopy   Procedure in which a fiberoptic tube is inserted into a joint for direct visualization of the ligaments, menisci, and articular surfaces of the joint.

articulations   Joint surfaces.

artifact   In the electrocardiogram, interference that is seen on the monitor or rhythm strip and may look like a wandering or fuzzy baseline; can be caused by patient movement, loose or defective electrodes, improper grounding, or faulty equipment.

ascending tracts   Groups of nerves that originate in the spinal cord and end in the brain.

ascites   The accumulation of free fluid within the peritoneal cavity. Increased hydrostatic pressure from portal hypertension causes this fluid to leak into the peritoneal cavity.

assistive/adaptive device   Any item that enables the patient to perform all or part of an activity independently.

assistive technology   Electronic equipment that increases the ability of disabled patients to care for themselves.

asterixis   A coarse tremor characterized by rapid, nonrhythmic extensions and flexions in the wrists and fingers; a motor disturbance seen in portal-systemic encephalopathy. Also called a "liver flap" or "flapping tremor."

asthma   A chronic respiratory condition in which reversible airflow obstruction in the airways occurs intermittently.

astigmatism   A refractive error caused by unevenly curved surfaces on or in the eye (especially of the cornea) that distort vision.

ataxia   Gait disturbance or loss of balance.

atelectasis   Collapse of alveoli.

atelectrauma   Shear injury to alveoli from opening and closing.

atherectomy   An invasive nonsurgical technique in which a high-speed, rotating metal burr uses fine abrasive bits to scrape plaque from inside an artery while minimizing damage to the vessel surface.

atherosclerosis   A type of arteriosclerosis that involves the formation of plaque within the arterial wall; the leading contributor to coronary artery and cerebrovascular disease.

atrial fibrillation (AF)   A cardiac dysrhythmia in which multiple rapid impulses from many atrial foci, at a rate of 350 to 600 times per minute, depolarize the atria in a totally disorganized manner, with no P waves, no atrial contractions, a loss of the atrial kick, and an irregular ventricular response.

atrial gallop   An abnormal fourth heart sound that occurs as blood enters the ventricles during the active filling phase at the end of ventricular diastole; may be heard in patients with hypertension, anemia, ventricular hypertrophy, myocardial infarction, aortic or pulmonic stenosis, and pulmonary emboli.

atrioventricular (AV) junction   In the cardiac conduction system, the area consisting of a transitional cell zone, the atrioventricular (AV) node itself, and the bundle of His. The AV node lies just beneath the right atrial endocardium, between the tricuspid valve and the ostium of the coronary sinus.

attenuated   The quality of making a substance weaker; for example, antigens that are used to make vaccines are specially processed to make them less likely to grow in the body.

atypical angina   Angina that manifests itself as indigestion, pain between the shoulders, an aching jaw, or a choking sensation that occurs with exertion. Many women experience atypical angina.

atypical migraine   The least common of the three types of migraine headaches, after migraines with aura and migraines without aura; the atypical category includes menstrual and cluster migraines.

aura   A sensation that signals the onset of a headache or seizure; the patient may experience visual changes, flashing lights, or double vision.

autoamputation of the distal digits   A condition in which the tips of the digits fall off spontaneously; can occur in severe cases of Raynaud's phenomenon.

autoantibodies   Antibodies directed against self tissues of cells.

autocontamination   The occurrence of infection in which the patient's own normal flora overgrows and penetrates the internal environment.

autodigestion Self-digestion. Specifically, the process of the stomach digesting itself if there is a break in its protective mucosal barrier.

autogenous Belonging to the person, such as a person's vein being moved from one part of the body to another.

autoimmune pancreatitis A chronic inflammatory form of pancreatitis that can also affect the bile ducts, kidneys, and other major connective tissues.

autologous blood transfusion Reinfusing the patient's own blood during surgery.

autologous bone marrow transplantation A type of bone marrow transplant in which patients receive their own stem cells, which were collected before high-dose chemotherapy.

autologous donation The donation of a patient's own blood before scheduled surgery for use, if needed, during the surgery to eliminate transfusion reactions and reduce the risk of bloodborne disease.

autolysis The spontaneous disintegration of tissue by the action of the patient's own cellular enzymes.

automaticity The ability of a cell to initiate an impulse spontaneously and repetitively; in cardiac electrophysiology, the ability of primary pacemaker cells (SA node, AV junction) to generate an electrical impulse.

autonomic dysreflexia (AD) A syndrome that affects the patient with an upper spinal cord injury; characterized by severe hypertension and headache, bradycardia, nasal stuffiness, and flushing; caused by a noxious stimulus, usually a distended bladder or constipation. This is a neurologic emergency and must be promptly treated to prevent a hypertensive brain attack.

autonomic nervous system (ANS) The part of the nervous system that is not under conscious control; consists of the sympathetic nervous system and the parasympathetic nervous system.

autonomy Ethical principle that implies a person's self-determination and self-management.

autosome Any of the 22 pairs of human chromosomes containing genes that code for all the structures and regulatory proteins needed for normal function but do not code for the sexual differentiation of a person.

axial loading A mechanism of injury that involves vertical compression. An example is a diving accident, in which the blow to the top of the head causes the vertebrae to shatter and pieces of bone enter the spinal canal and damage the cord.

azoospermia The absence of living sperm in the semen.

azotemia An excess of nitrogenous wastes (urea) in the blood.

B

B-type natriuretic peptide (BNP) A peptide produced and released by the ventricles when the patient has fluid overload as a result of heart failure (HF).

Babinski's sign Dorsiflexion of the great toe and fanning of the other toes, which is an abnormal reflex in response to testing the plantar reflex with a pointed (but not sharp) object; indicates the presence of central nervous system disease. The normal response is plantar flexion of all toes.

bacteremia The presence of bacteria in the bloodstream.

bacteriuria Bacteria in the urine.

bad death A death embodied by pain, not having one's wishes followed at the end of one's life, isolation, abandonment, and constant agonizing about losses associated with death.

Baker's cyst Enlarged popliteal bursa.

banding See *endoscopic variceal ligation.*

barbiturate coma The use of drugs such as pentobarbital sodium or sodium thiopental at dosages to maintain complete unresponsiveness; used for patients whose increased intracranial pressure cannot be controlled by other means. These drugs decrease the metabolic demands of the brain and cerebral blood flow, stabilize cell membranes, decrease the formation of vasogenic edema, and produce a more uniform blood supply. The patient in a barbiturate coma requires mechanical ventilation, sophisticated hemodynamic monitoring, and intracranial pressure monitoring.

bariatrics Branch of medicine that manages obesity and its related diseases.

baroreceptors Sensory receptors in the arch of the aorta and at the origin of the internal carotid arteries that are stimulated when the arterial walls are stretched by an increased blood pressure.

Barrett's epithelium Columnar epithelium (instead of the normal squamous cell epithelium) that develops in the lower esophagus during the process of healing from gastroesophageal reflux disease. It is considered premalignant and is associated with an increased risk of cancer in patients with prolonged disease.

Barrett's esophagus Ulceration of the lower esophagus caused by exposure to acid and pepsin, leading to the replacement of normal distal squamous mucosa with columnar epithelium as a response to tissue injury.

base A substance that binds (reduces) free hydrogen ions in solution. Strong bases bind hydrogen ions easily; weak bases bind less readily.

Basic Cardiac Life Support (BCLS) Procedure that involves ventilating the patient who has stopped breathing, as well as giving chest compressions in the absence of a carotid pulse. Also known as "cardiopulmonary resuscitation (CPR)."

Bell's palsy Acute paralysis of cranial nerve VII; characterized by a drawing sensation and paralysis of all facial muscles on the affected side. The patient cannot close the eye, wrinkle the forehead, smile, whistle, or grimace. The face appears masklike and sags. Also called "facial paralysis."

beneficence The ethical principle of preventing harm and ensuring the patient's well-being.

benign Altered cell growth that is harmless and does not require intervention.

benign tumor cells Normal cells growing in the wrong place or at the wrong time.

bereavement Grief and mourning experienced by the survivor before and after a death.

bicaval technique Surgical technique in heart transplantation in which the intact right atrium of the donor heart is preserved by anastomoses at the recipient's superior and inferior vena cavae.

bifurcation The point of division of a single structure into two branches.

bigeminy A type of premature complex that exists when normal complexes and premature complexes occur alternately in a repetitive two-beat pattern, with a pause occurring after each premature complex so that complexes occur in pairs.

bilateral orchiectomy The surgical removal of both testes, typically performed as palliative surgery in patients with prostate cancer. It is not intended to cure the prostate cancer but to arrest its spread by removing testosterone.

bilateral salpingo-oophorectomy (BSO) Surgical removal of both fallopian tubes and both ovaries.

biliary colic Intense pain due to obstruction of the cystic duct of the gallbladder from a stone moving through or lodged within the duct. Tissue spasm occurs in an effort to mobilize the stone through the small duct.

biliary stent A plastic or metal device that is placed percutaneously to keep a duct of the biliary system open in patients experiencing biliary obstruction.

biofilm A complex group of microorganisms that functions within a "slimy" gel coating on medical devices.

biological response modifiers (BRMs) A class of immunomodulating drugs that attempt to modify the course of disease. Also called "biologics."

biologics See *biological response modifiers.*

biomedical technician Member of the health care team who maintains the safety of adaptive and electronic devices by monitoring their function and making repairs as needed.

biotrauma Inflammatory response–mediated damage to alveoli.

bivalve To cut a cast lengthwise into two equal pieces.

black box warning A governmental designation indicating that a drug has at least one serious side effect and must be used with caution.

bladder ultrasound Less invasive test to determine postvoiding residual urine volumes for the patient with a reflex (upper motor neuron) or uninhibited bladder; often used to measure residual urine in the bladder of patients with spinal cord injury.

blanch To whiten or lighten.

blast phase cell Immature cell that divides.

bloodborne metastasis The release of tumor cells into the blood; the most common cause of cancer spread.

blood pressure (BP) The force of blood exerted against the vessel walls.

blood stem cells Immature, unspecialized (undifferentiated) cells that are capable of becoming any type of blood cell, depending on the body's needs.

Blumberg's sign Pain felt on abrupt release of steady pressure (rebound tenderness) over the site of abdominal pain.

body mass index (BMI) A measure of nutritional status that does not depend on frame size;

indirectly estimates total fat stores within the body by the relationship of weight to height.

bolus feeding A method of tube feeding that involves intermittent feeding of a specified amount of enteral product at specified times during a 24-hour period, typically every 4 hours.

bone biopsy Procedure in which the physician extracts a specimen of bone tissue for microscopic examination to confirm the presence of infection or neoplasm; not commonly done today.

bone mineral density (BMD) The quality of bone that determines bone strength. It peaks between 30 and 35 years of age, when both bone resorption activity and bone-building activity occur at a constant rate. When bone resorption activity exceeds bone-building activity, bone density decreases.

bone reduction Realignment of fractured bone ends for proper healing.

bone resorption Loss of bone density due to demineralization resulting from the release of calcium from storage areas in bones.

bone scan A radionuclide test in which radioactive material is injected for visualization of the entire skeleton; used to detect tumors, arthritis, osteomyelitis, osteoporosis, vertebral compression fractures, and unexplained bone pain.

borborygmus (borborygmi) Bowel sounds, especially loud gurgling sounds, resulting from hypermotility of the bowel.

boring In pain, the type of intense pain that feels like it is going through the body.

Bouchard's nodes Swelling at the proximal interphalangeal joints in osteoarthritis involving the hands.

bowel retraining A program for patients with neurologic problems that is designed to include a combination of suppository use and a consistent toileting schedule.

bradycardia Slowness of the heart rate; characterized as a pulse rate less than 50 to 60 beats/min.

bradydysrhythmia An abnormal heart rhythm characterized by a heart rate less than 60 beats/min.

bradykinesia Slow or no movement, as seen in a patient with Parkinson disease. Also called "akinesia."

brain abscess A collection of pus that forms in the extradural, subdural, or intracerebral area of the brain as a result of a purulent infection, usually due to bacteria invading the brain directly or indirectly.

brain attack Stroke; disruption in the normal blood supply to the brain, either as an interruption in blood flow (ischemic stroke) or as bleeding within or around the brain (hemorrhagic stroke). A medical emergency that occurs suddenly, a stroke should be treated immediately to prevent neurologic deficit and permanent disability. Formerly called "cerebrovascular accident," the National Stroke Association now uses the term "brain attack" to describe stroke.

brain herniation syndrome In the patient with untreated increased intracranial pressure, protrusion (herniation) of the brain downward toward the brainstem or laterally from a unilateral lesion within one cerebral hemisphere, causing irreversible brain damage and possibly death.

breakthrough pain Additional pain that "breaks through" the pain that is being managed by mainstay analgesic drugs.

breast augmentation Cosmetic surgical procedure to enhance the size, shape, or symmetry of the breasts.

breast-conserving surgery Surgical method for breast cancer that removes the bulk of the tumor rather than the entire breast.

Broca's aphasia See *expressive aphasia.*

Broca's area An important speech area of the cerebrum. It is located in the frontal lobe and is composed of neurons responsible for the formation of words, or speech.

bronchoscopy Insertion of a tube in the airway, usually as far as the secondary bronchi, for the purpose of visualizing airway structures and obtaining tissue samples for biopsy or culture.

bruit Swishing sound in the larger arteries (carotid, aortic, femoral, and popliteal) that can be heard with a stethoscope or Doppler probe; may indicate narrowing of the artery and is usually associated with atherosclerotic disease.

bulbar Pertaining to the muscles involved in facial expression, chewing, and speech.

bulimia nervosa An eating disorder that is characterized by episodes of binge eating in which the patient ingests a large amount of food in a short time, followed by purging behavior such as self-induced vomiting or excessive use of laxatives and diuretics.

bunion Hallux valgus deformity of the foot in which lateral deviation of the great toe causes the first metatarsal head to become enlarged.

bunionectomy Surgical removal of the hallux valgus deformity (bunion) of the foot.

butterfly rash A dry, scaly, raised rash on the face; the major skin manifestation of systemic lupus erythematosus.

C

cachexia Extreme body wasting and malnutrition that develop from an imbalance between food intake and energy use.

calciphylaxis A condition of thrombosis and skin necrosis that can occur in stage 5 chronic kidney disease.

calculi Abnormal formations of a mass of mineral salts that can occur in the body; forms in the kidney when excess calcium precipitates out of solution. Also called "stones."

calculous cholecystitis Inflammation of the gallbladder usually following and created by obstruction of the cystic duct by a stone (calculus).

callus The loose, fibrous, vascular tissue that forms at the site of a fracture as the first phase of healing and is normally replaced by hard bone as healing continues.

calyx The anatomic term for a cuplike structure.

Canadian Triage Acuity Scale (CTAS) A standardized model for triage in which lists of descriptors are used to establish the triage level.

cancellous The softer tissue inside bones that contains large spaces, or trabeculae, that are filled with red and yellow marrow.

candidiasis An infection caused by the fungus *Candida albicans.*

canthus The place where the upper and lower eyelids meet at the corner of either side of the eye.

capillary closing pressure The amount of pressure needed to occlude skin capillary blood flow.

capillary leak syndrome The response of capillaries to the presence of biologic chemicals (mediators) that change blood vessel integrity and allow fluid to shift from the blood in the vascular space into the interstitial tissues.

Caplan's syndrome The presence of pneumoconiosis and rheumatoid nodules in the lungs; noted primarily in coal miners and asbestos workers.

capsule The layer of fibrous tissue on the outer surface of the kidney, which provides protection and support. The renal capsule itself is surrounded by layers of fat and connective tissue.

carboxyhemoglobin Carbon monoxide on oxygen-binding sites of the hemoglobin molecule.

carcinoembryonic antigen (CEA) An oncofetal antigen that may be elevated in 70% of people with colorectal cancer. CEA is not specifically associated with the colorectal cancer and may be elevated in the presence of other benign or malignant diseases and in smokers. CEA is often used to monitor the effectiveness of treatment and to identify disease recurrence.

carcinogen Any substance that changes the activity of the genes in a cell so that the cell becomes a cancer cell.

carcinogenesis Cancer development.

cardiac axis In electrocardiography (ECG), the direction of electrical current flow in the heart. The relationship between the cardiac axis and the lead axis is responsible for the deflections seen on the ECG pattern.

cardiac catheterization The most definitive but most invasive test in the diagnosis of heart disease; involves passing a small catheter into the heart and injecting contrast medium.

cardiac index A calculation of cardiac output requirements to account for differences in body size; determined by dividing the cardiac output by the body surface area.

cardiac markers Serum studies that include troponin, creatine kinase–MB, and myoglobin.

cardiac output (CO) The volume of blood ejected by the heart each minute; normal range in adults is 4 to 7 L/min.

cardiac rehabilitation The process of actively assisting the patient with cardiac disease to achieve and maintain a productive life while remaining within the limits of the heart's ability to respond to increases in activity and stress. *Phase 1* begins with the acute illness and ends with discharge from the hospital. *Phase 2* begins after discharge and continues through convalescence at home. *Phase 3* refers to long-term conditioning.

cardiac resynchronization therapy (CRT) In patients with some types of heart failure, the use of a permanent pacemaker alone or in combination with an implantable cardioverter-defibrillator to provide biventricular pacing.

cardiac tamponade Compression of the myocardium by fluid that has accumulated around the heart; this compresses the atria and ventricles, prevents them from filling adequately, and reduces cardiac output.

cardiogenic shock Post–myocardial infarction heart failure in which necrosis of more than 40% of the left ventricle has occurred. Also called "class IV heart failure."

cardiomegaly Enlarged heart.

cardiomyopathy A subacute or chronic disease of cardiac muscle; classified into four categories based on abnormalities in structure and function: dilated, hypertrophic, restrictive, and arrhythmogenic.

cardiopulmonary bypass (CPB) Diversion of the blood from the heart to a bypass machine, where it is heparinized, oxygenated, and returned to the circulation through a cannula placed in the ascending aortic arch or femoral artery to provide oxygenation, circulation, and hypothermia during induced cardiac arrest for coronary artery bypass surgery. This process ensures a motionless operative field and prevents myocardial ischemia.

cardioversion A synchronized countershock that may be performed in emergencies for hemodynamically unstable ventricular or supraventricular tachydysrhythmias or electively for stable tachydysrhythmias that are resistant to medical therapies. The shock depolarizes a critical mass of myocardium simultaneously during intrinsic depolarization and is intended to stop the re-entry circuit and allow the sinus node to regain control of the heart.

carina The point at which the trachea branches into the right and left mainstem bronchi.

carpal tunnel syndrome (CTS) A common condition in which the median nerve in the wrist becomes compressed, causing pain and numbness.

carrier (1) A person who harbors an infectious agent without symptoms of active disease; (2) in genetics, a person who has one mutated allele for a recessive genetic disorder. A carrier does not usually have any manifestations of the disorder but can pass the mutated allele to his or her children.

case management The process of assessment, planning, implementation, evaluation, and interaction for patients who have complex health problems and incur a high cost to the health care system. Goals include promoting quality of life, decreasing fragmentation and duplication of care across health care settings, and maintaining cost-effectiveness.

caseation necrosis A type of necrosis in which tissue is turned into a granular mass.

cast A rigid device that immobilizes the affected body part while allowing other body parts to move. It is most commonly used for fractures but may also be applied to correct deformities (e.g., clubfoot) or to prevent deformities (e.g., those seen in some patients with rheumatoid arthritis).

cataract A lens opacity that distorts the image projected onto the retina.

catechol O-methyltransferases (COMTs) Enzymes that inactivate dopamine.

catecholamines Hormones (dopamine, epinephrine, and norepinephrine) released by the adrenal medulla in response to stimulation of the sympathetic nervous system.

cation Ion that has a positive charge.

cell-mediated immunity Microbial resistance that is mediated by the action of specifically sensitized T-lymphocytes.

cellulitis An acute, spreading, edematous inflammation of the deep subcutaneous tissues; usually caused by infection of a wound or burn.

central IV therapy IV therapy in which a vascular access device (VAD) is placed in a central blood vessel, such as the superior vena cava.

cerebral angiography (arteriography) Visualization of the cerebral circulation (carotid and vertebral arteries) after injecting a contrast medium into an artery (usually the femoral).

cerebral blood flow (CBF) Useful in evaluating cerebral vasospasm; can be measured in many areas of the brain with the use of radioactive substances.

cerebral perfusion pressure (CPP) The pressure gradient over which the brain is perfused. It is influenced by oxygenation, cerebral blood volume, blood pressure, cerebral edema, and intracranial pressure (ICP) and is determined by subtracting the mean ICP from the mean arterial pressure. A cerebral perfusion pressure above 70 mm Hg is generally accepted as an appropriate goal of therapy.

cerebral salt wasting (CSW) The primary cause of hyponatremia in the neurosurgical population; characterized by hyponatremia, decreased serum osmolality, and decreased blood volume. It is thought to result from the extrarenal influence of atrial natriuretic factor.

cerumen The wax produced by glands within the external ear canal; helps protect and lubricate the ear canal.

cervical polyp Tumor that arises from the mucosa and extends to the opening of the cervical os. Polyps result from hyperplasia of the endocervical epithelium, inflammation, or an abnormal local response to hormonal stimulation or localized vascular congestion of the cervical blood vessels. Polyps are the most common benign growth of the cervix.

CHADS₂ scoring system Acronymn for Congestive heart failure, Hypertension, Age ≥ 75 years, Diabetes mellitus, Stroke. Determines if a patient with atrial fibrillation needs preventive anticoagulant therapy.

chalazion An inflammation of a sebaceous gland in the eyelid.

chancre The ulcer that is the first sign of syphilis. It develops at the site of entry (inoculation) of the organism, usually 3 weeks after exposure. The lesion may be found on any area of the skin or mucous membranes but occurs most often on the genitalia, lips, nipples, and hands and in the oral cavity, anus, and rectum.

chemotherapy The treatment of cancer with chemical agents that have systemic effects; used to cure and to increase survival time.

chemotherapy-induced peripheral neuropathy (CIPN) The loss of sensory or motor function of peripheral nerves associated with exposure to certain anticancer drugs.

chest tube A drain placed in the pleural space to allow closed–chest drainage, which restores intrapleural pressure and allows re-expansion of the lung after surgery in patients who have undergone thoracotomy (incision of the chest wall).

Cheyne-Stokes respirations Common sign of nearing death in which apnea alternates with periods of rapid breathing.

choked disc See *papilledema*.

cholecystectomy The surgical removal of the gallbladder.

cholecystitis Inflammation of the gallbladder.

cholecystokinin A hormone that stimulates digestive juices and may work with leptin to increase or decrease appetite.

choledochojejunostomy Surgical anastomosis of the common bile duct with the jejunum.

cholelithiasis The presence of gallstones.

cholesteatoma A benign overgrowth of squamous cell epithelium.

cholesterol Serum lipid that includes high-density lipoproteins and low-density lipoproteins.

cholinergic crisis Overmedication with cholinesterase inhibitors.

cholinesterase inhibitors Drugs that improve cholinergic neurotransmission in the central nervous system by delaying the destruction of acetylcholine by acetylcholinesterase, thus delaying the onset of cognitive decline. These are approved for symptomatic treatment of Alzheimer's disease but do not affect the course of the disease.

chondroitin A supplement that may play a role in strengthening cartilage.

choreiform movement Rapid, jerky movement.

chronic Having a slow onset and symptoms that persist for an extended period.

chronic calcifying pancreatitis (CCP) Alcohol-induced chronic pancreatitis that is characterized by protein precipitates that plug the ducts and lead to ductal obstruction, atrophy, and dilation. The epithelium of the ducts undergoes histologic changes, resulting in metaplasia (cell replacement) and ulceration. This inflammatory process causes fibrosis of the pancreatic tissue.

chronic constrictive pericarditis A fibrous thickening of the pericardium that prevents adequate filling of the ventricles and eventually results in cardiac failure; caused by chronic pericardial inflammation due to tuberculosis, radiation therapy, trauma, kidney failure, or metastatic cancer.

chronic fatigue syndrome (CFS) A chronic illness characterized by severe fatigue for 6 months or longer, usually following flu-like symptoms. At least four of the following criteria are required for diagnosis: sore throat; substantial impairment in short-term memory or concentration; tender lymph nodes; muscle pain;

multiple joint pain with redness or swelling; headaches of a new type, pattern, or severity; unrefreshing sleep; and postexertional malaise lasting more than 24 hours.

chronic gastritis A patchy, diffuse inflammation of the mucosal lining of the stomach. Chronic gastritis usually heals without scarring but can progress to hemorrhage and ulcer formation.

chronic health problem A condition that has existed for at least 3 months.

chronic hepatitis Chronic liver inflammation that usually occurs as a result of hepatitis B or C. Superimposed infection with hepatitis D virus (HDV) in patients with chronic hepatitis B may also result in chronic hepatitis. Can lead to cirrhosis and liver cancer.

chronic kidney disease (CKD) A condition characterized by loss of kidney function over time.

chronic obstructive pancreatitis Pancreatitis that develops from inflammation, spasm, and obstruction of the sphincter of Oddi. Inflammatory and sclerotic lesions occur in the head of the pancreas and around the ducts, causing obstruction and backflow of pancreatic secretions.

chronic osteomyelitis Bone infection that persists over a long time due to misdiagnosis or inadequate treatment. Also called "subchronic osteomyelitis."

chronic pain Pain that persists or recurs for indefinite periods (usually more than 3 months), often involves deep body structures, is poorly localized, and is difficult to describe. Also called "persistent pain."

chronic pancreatitis A progressive, destructive disease of the pancreas characterized by remissions and exacerbations. Inflammation and fibrosis of the tissue contribute to pancreatic insufficiency and diminished function of the organ.

chronic paronychia Inflammation of the skin around the nail that persists for months. People at risk for chronic paronychia are those with frequent exposure to water, such as homemakers, bartenders, and laundry workers.

chronic pyelonephritis A kidney disorder that results from repeated or continued upper urinary tract infections or the effects of such infections.

chronic stable angina (CSA) Type of angina characterized by chest discomfort that occurs with moderate to prolonged exertion and in a pattern that is familiar to the patient.

chyme The liquid formed when food is transformed during the digestion process in the gastrointestinal tract.

circle of Willis At the base of the brain, the ring formed by the anterior, middle, and posterior cerebral arteries where they are joined together by small communicating arteries.

circumcision The surgical removal of the prepuce or foreskin of the penis.

circumferential Referring to something that completely surrounds an extremity or the thorax.

cirrhosis Liver disease that is characterized by extensive scarring of the liver and is usually caused by a chronic irreversible reaction to hepatic inflammation and necrosis; disease typically develops insidiously and has a prolonged, destructive course.

classic heat stroke A form of heat stroke in which the body's ability to dissipate heat is significantly impaired; occurs over time as a result of long-term exposure to a hot, humid environment such as a home without air-conditioning in the high heat of the summer.

clinical practice guideline An "official recommendation" based on evidence to diagnose and/or manage a health problem (e.g., pain management).

clinical psychologist Member of the health care team who counsels patients and families on their psychological problems and on strategies to cope with disability.

clinically competent The condition of being legally competent and having decisional capacity.

clonic (rhythmic) Pertaining to a state of alternating muscle stiffness followed by rhythmic jerking motions, as in a tonic-clonic seizure.

clonus The sudden, brief, jerking contraction of a muscle or muscle group often seen in seizures. Also called "myoclonus."

closed fracture A fracture that does not extend through the skin and therefore has no visible wound. Also called "simple fracture."

closed reduction A nonsurgical method for managing a simple fracture. While applying a manual pull, or traction, on the bone, the health care provider manipulates the bone ends so they realign.

closed traumatic brain injury A type of traumatic primary brain injury that occurs as the result of blunt trauma; the integrity of the skull is not violated, and damage to brain tissue depends on the degree and mechanisms of injury.

***C. difficile*–associated disease (CDAD)** Clinical manifestations that are caused by *Clostridium difficile* as a potential result of antibiotic therapy use, especially in older adults.

clubbing Changes in the tissue beds of the fingers and toes, with the base of the nail becoming spongy; results from chronic oxygen deprivation in the tissue beds.

cluster headache A type of oculotemporal or oculofrontal headache marked by unilateral, excruciating, nonthrobbing pain that is felt deep in and around the eye and may radiate to the forehead, temple, cheek, ear, occiput, or neck. Average duration is 10 to 45 minutes. Headaches occur every 8 to 12 hours and up to 24 hours daily at the same time for about 6 to 8 weeks (hence the term "cluster"), followed by remission for 9 months to a year. Cause and mechanism are unknown but have been attributed to vasoreactivity and oxyhemoglobin desaturation.

clysis See *hypodermoclysis.*

coagulopathy Clotting abnormalities.

cognition The ability of the brain to process, store, retrieve, and manipulate information.

cognitive therapist A member of the rehabilitative health care team, usually a neuropsychologist, who works primarily with patients who have experienced head injuries and have cognitive impairments.

cohorting The practice of grouping patients who are colonized or infected with the same pathogen.

cold antibody anemia A form of immunohemolytic anemia (in which the immune system attacks a person's own red blood cells for unknown reasons) that occurs with complement protein fixation on immunoglobulin M (IgM). In this condition, the arteries in the hands and feet constrict profoundly in response to cold temperatures or stress.

cold phase A phase after peripheral nerve trauma resulting in complete denervation in which the skin appears cyanotic, mottled, or reddish blue and feels cool compared with the contralateral unaffected extremity. The cold phase follows the warm phase, which lasts 2 to 3 weeks after injury.

colectomy Surgical removal of part or all of the colon.

collaboration The planning, implementing, and evaluation of patient care using an interdisciplinary (ID) plan of care.

collateral circulation Circulation that provides blood to an area with altered tissue perfusion through smaller vessels that develop and compensate for the occluded vessels.

colon interposition A surgical procedure that may be performed in patients with an esophageal tumor when the tumor involves the stomach or the stomach is otherwise unsuitable for anastomosis. In colon interposition, a section of right or left colon is removed and brought up into the thorax to substitute for the esophagus.

colon resection Surgery performed for colorectal cancer in which the tumor and regional lymph nodes are removed.

colonoscopy The endoscopic examination of the entire large bowel.

colostomy The surgical creation of an opening between the colon and the surface of the abdomen.

colposcopy Examination of the cervix and vagina using a colposcope, which allows three-dimensional magnification and intense illumination of epithelium with suspected disease. This procedure can locate the exact site of precancerous and malignant lesions for biopsy.

command center See *emergency operations center.*

commando procedure Mnemonic for combined neck dissection, mandibulectomy, and oropharyngeal resection—a procedure in which the surgeon removes a segment of the mandible with the oral lesion and performs a radical neck dissection.

communicable The ability of an infection, such as influenza, to be transmitted from person to person.

communicating hydrocephalus Form of hydrocephalus that occurs when the flow of cerebrospinal fluid (CSF) is blocked after it exits the ventricles; this form is "communicating" because CSF can still flow between the ventricles, which remain open.

compartment syndrome A condition in which increased tissue pressure in a confined anatomic space causes decreased blood flow to the area, leading to hypoxia and pain.

compensated cirrhosis A form of cirrhosis in which the liver has significant scarring but is still able to perform essential functions without causing significant symptoms.

compensatory mechanism The means of producing compensation. Also called "adaptive mechanism."

complement activation and fixation Actions triggered by some classes of antibodies that can remove or destroy antigen.

complete spinal cord injury An injury in which the spinal cord has been severed or damaged in a way that eliminates all innervation below the level of the injury.

complex regional pain syndrome (CRPS) A complex disorder that includes debilitating pain, atrophy, autonomic dysfunction (excessive sweating, vascular changes), and motor impairment (most notably muscle paresis), probably caused by an abnormally hyperactive sympathetic nervous system. This syndrome most often results from traumatic injury and commonly occurs in the feet and hands; formerly called "reflex sympathetic dystrophy (RSD)."

compliance In respiratory physiology, a measure of elasticity within the lung. Also, a patient's fulfillment of a caregiver's prescribed course of treatment.

compound fracture See *open fracture.*

compression fracture A fracture that is produced by a loading force applied to the long axis of cancellous bone. These fractures commonly occur in the vertebrae of patients with osteoporosis.

computed tomography coronary angiography (CTCA) 64-slice diagnostic scan used to diagnose coronary artery disease in symptomatic patients.

conductive hearing loss Hearing loss that results from any physical obstruction of sound wave transmission (e.g., a foreign body in the external canal, a retracted or bulging tympanic membrane, or fused bony ossicles).

conductivity The ability of a cell to transmit an electrical stimulus from cell membrane to cell membrane.

congestive heart failure (CHF) Former term for "left-sided heart failure." Categorized as either systolic heart failure or diastolic heart failure, which may be acute or chronic and mild to severe.

conization The removal of a cone-shaped sample of tissue from the cervix for cytologic study.

conjunctivae The mucous membranes of the eye that line the undersurface of the eyelids (palpebral conjunctiva) and cover the sclera (bulbar conjunctiva).

connective tissue disease (CTD) A group of diseases that are the major focus of rheumatology (the study of rheumatic diseases); most are musculoskeletal disorders.

consensual response In assessing pupillary reaction to light, a slight constriction of the pupil of the eye not being tested when a penlight is brought in from the side of the patient's head and shined into the eye being tested as soon as the patient opens his or her eyes.

consolidation Solidification; lack of air spaces in the lung, such as occurs in pneumonia.

constipation The passage of hard, dry stool fewer than 3 times a week (as defined by the Association of Rehabilitation Nurses).

contact laser prostatectomy (CLP) Procedure for treating benign prostatic hyperplasia that uses laser energy to coagulate excess tissue. Also called "interstitial laser coagulation (ILC)."

Contact Precautions Infection control guidelines from the Centers for Disease Control and Prevention; used for patients with infections spread by direct contact or contact with items in the patient's environment, such as pediculosis.

contiguous Something in direct contact with, or adjacent to, another area or structure.

continence The ability to voluntarily control emptying the bladder and colon. Continence is a learned behavior whereby a person can suppress the urge to urinate until a socially appropriate location is available.

continuous feeding A method of tube feeding in which small amounts of enteral product are continuously infused (by gravity drip or by a pump or controller device) over a specified time.

continuous positive airway pressure (CPAP) A respiratory treatment that improves obstructive sleep apnea in patients with heart failure.

contractility The ability of a cell to contract in response to an impulse. In cardiac electrophysiology, the ability of atrial and ventricular muscle cells to shorten their fiber length in response to electrical stimulation, generating sufficient pressure to propel blood forward. Contractility is the mechanical activity of the heart.

contraction The closure of a wound as new collagen replaces damaged tissue, pulling the wound edges inward along the path of least resistance.

contralateral Pertaining to the opposite side.

contrecoup injury Bruising of the brain tissue, with damage occurring on the side opposite the site of impact.

control therapy drugs Drugs used every day, regardless of symptoms, to reduce airway responsiveness to prevent asthma attacks from occurring.

contusion A bruise; when referring to closed head injury, a bruising of brain tissue usually found at the site of impact (coup injury). Compare with *contrecoup injury.*

cor pulmonale Right-sided heart failure caused by pulmonary disease.

cordectomy Excision of a vocal cord in surgery for laryngeal cancer.

cornea The clear layer that forms the external coat on the front of the eye.

corneal abrasion Scrape or scratch of the cornea that disrupts its integrity.

corneal ulceration Deep disruption of the corneal epithelium that extends into the stromal layer and is caused by bacteria, protozoa, or fungi.

coronary artery bypass graft (CABG) A surgical procedure in which occluded coronary arteries are bypassed with the patient's own venous or arterial blood vessels or synthetic grafts.

coronary artery disease (CAD) Disease affecting the arteries that provide blood, oxygen, and nutrients to the myocardium; partial or complete blockage of the blood flow through the coronary arteries, causing ischemia and infarction of the myocardium, angina pectoris, and acute coronary syndromes. Also known as "coronary heart disease" or simply "heart disease."

coronary artery vasculopathy (CAV) A form of coronary artery disease that presents as diffuse plaque in the arteries of the donor heart in patients who have received a heart transplant.

cortisol The main glucocorticoid produced by the adrenal cortex.

coryza The common cold, or acute viral rhinitis.

cough assist A technique for assisting the tetraplegic patient to cough. Place his or her hands on either side of the rib cage or upper abdomen below the diaphragm; then, as the patient inhales, push upward to help expand the lungs and cough.

craniotomy Surgical incision into the cranium.

creatine kinase (CK) An enzyme specific to cells of the brain, myocardium, and skeletal muscle. Its appearance in the blood indicates tissue necrosis or injury, with levels following a predictable rise and fall during a specified period.

Credé maneuver A technique used to assist in urination in which a patient places his or her hand in a cupped position directly over the bladder area and pushes inward and downward gently as if massaging the bladder to empty.

crepitus A continuous grating sensation caused when irregular cartilage or bone fragments rub together and which may be felt or heard as a joint is put through passive range of motion; also, a crackling sensation that can be felt on a patient's chest, indicating that air is trapped within the tissues.

CREST syndrome In patients with systemic sclerosis, the combination of calcinosis (calcium deposits), Raynaud's phenomenon, esophageal dysmotility, sclerodactyly (scleroderma of the digits), and telangiectasia (spiderlike hemangiomas).

cricothyroidotomy Surgical procedure in which an opening is made between the thyroid cartilage and cricoid cartilage ring and results in a tracheostomy. Also called "cricothyrotomy." The procedure is used in an emergency for access to the lower airways.

crises In the patient with sickle cell disease, periodic episodes of extensive cellular sickling that have a sudden onset and can occur as often as weekly or as seldom as once a year.

critical access hospital A small rural facility of 15 or fewer inpatient beds that provides around-the-clock emergency care services 7 days per week. Considered a necessary provider of health care to community residents who are not close to other hospitals in a given region.

cross-contamination A type of contamination in which organisms from another person or from the environment are transmitted to the patient.

cryotherapy (1) A way of decreasing muscle pain by "cooling down" the area with a local, short-acting gel or cream, such as after physical therapy; (2) in ophthalmologic surgery, use of a freezing probe to repair retinal detachment.

cryptorchidism Failure of the testes to descend into the scrotum.

culture A procedure for identifying a microorganism by cultivating and isolating it in tissue cultures or artificial media.

Curling's ulcer Acute ulcerative gastroduodenal disease, which may develop within 24 hours of a severe burn injury because of reduced gastrointestinal blood flow and mucosal damage.

Cushing's disease (Cushing's syndrome) Hypercortisolism caused by oversecretion of hormones by the adrenal cortex.

Cushing's triad A classic yet late sign of increased intracranial pressure (ICP) manifested by severe hypertension with a widened pulse pressure and bradycardia. As ICP increases, the pulse becomes thready, irregular, and rapid. Cerebral blood flow increases in response to hypertension.

Cushing's ulcer Acute ulcerative gastroduodenal disease that may develop as a result of increased intracranial pressure.

cutaneous (superficial) reflexes Superficial reflexes. Usually the plantar and abdominal reflexes are tested.

cyanosis Bluish or darkened discoloration of the skin and mucous membranes; results from an increased amount of deoxygenated hemoglobin.

cyclic feeding A method of tube feeding similar to continuous feeding (see definition of *continuous feeding*) except the infusion is stopped for a specified time in each 24-hour period ("down time"); the down time typically occurs in the morning to allow bathing, treatments, and other activities.

cystitis Inflammation of the bladder.

cystocele Herniation of the bladder into the vagina.

cytokines Small protein hormones produced by white blood cells.

cytotoxic Having cell-damaging effects.

D

dandruff An accumulation of patchy or diffuse white or gray scales on the surface of the scalp.

death When illness or trauma overwhelms the compensatory mechanisms of the body and the lungs and heart cease to function.

death rattle Loud, wet respirations caused by secretions in the respiratory tract and oral cavity of a patient who is near death.

débridement The removal of infected tissue from a healing wound.

debriefing After a mass casualty incident or disaster, (1) the provision of sessions for small groups of staff in which teams are brought in to discuss effective coping strategies (critical incident stress debriefing), and (2) the administrative review of staff and system performance during the event to determine opportunities for improvement in the emergency management plan.

debris Dead cells and tissues in a wound.

decerebrate posturing Abnormal posturing and rigidity characterized by extension of the arms and legs, pronation of the arms, plantar flexion, and opisthotonos; usually associated with dysfunction in the brainstem area. Also called "decerebration."

decerebration See *decerebrate posturing.*

decompensated cirrhosis A form of cirrhosis in which liver function is significantly impaired with obvious manifestations of liver failure.

decompressive craniectomy Removal of a section of the skull in the patient with uncontrolled intracranial pressure (ICP); allows for additional space for edema without increasing ICP.

decorticate posturing Abnormal posturing seen in the patient with lesions that interrupt the corticospinal pathways. The arms, wrists, and fingers are flexed with internal rotation and plantar flexion of the legs. Also called "decortication."

decortication See *decorticate posturing.*

deep tendon reflexes Tested as part of the neurologic assessment. An intact reflex arc is indicated when the muscle contracts in response to the tendon being struck with a reflex hammer.

deep vein thrombophlebitis Presence of a thrombus associated with inflammation in the deep veins, usually in the legs. Compared with superficial thrombophlebitis, it presents a greater risk for pulmonary embolism. Also called "deep vein thrombosis."

deep vein thrombosis (DVT) Common term for "deep vein thrombophlebitis."

defibrillation An asynchronous countershock that depolarizes a critical mass of myocardium simultaneously to stop the re-entry circuit, allowing the sinus node to regain control of the heart.

dehiscence A partial or complete separation of the outer layers of a wound, sometimes described as a "splitting open" of the wound.

dehydration Fluid intake less than what is needed to meet the body's fluid needs.

delayed union Term describing a fracture that has not healed within 6 months of injury.

delegation The process of transferring to a competent person the authority to perform a selected nursing task or activity in a selected patient care situation.

delirium An acute state of confusion, usually short-term and reversible within 3 weeks. Often seen among older adults in a hospital or other unfamiliar setting.

dementia A syndrome of slowly progressive cognitive decline with global impairment of intellectual function. The most common type is Alzheimer's disease.

demyelination Destruction of myelin between the nodes of Ranvier; a major pathologic finding in multiple sclerosis or Guillain-Barré syndrome.

depolarization The ability of a cell to respond to a stimulus by initiating an impulse. Also called "excitability."

depression A response to multiple life stresses, a single situation, a primary disorder, or a problem associated with dementia; this response can range from mild, transient feelings of sadness to a severe sense of helplessness and hopelessness.

dermal papillae Fingerlike projections of dermal tissue that anchor the epidermis to the dermis.

dermatomes Specific areas of the skin that receive sensory input from spinal nerves.

descending tracts Groups of nerves that begin in the brain and end in the spinal cord.

desquamation The shedding or peeling of skin.

diabetic peripheral neuropathy (DPN) A progressive deterioration of nerves that results in loss of nerve function (sensory perception). A common complication of diabetes, it often involves all parts of the body.

diagnostic peritoneal lavage (DPL) Test that determines the presence of internal bleeding following abdominal trauma.

dialysate The solution used in dialysis. It is composed of water, glucose, sodium chloride, potassium, magnesium, calcium, and bicarbonate; dialysate composition may be altered according to the patient's needs for treatment of electrolyte imbalances.

dialyzer The apparatus used to perform hemodialysis. Also known as the "artificial kidney," it has four parts: a blood compartment, a dialysate compartment, a semipermeable membrane, and an enclosed structure to support the membrane.

diaphragmatic pacing A pacemaker for the phrenic nerve to cause the diaphragm to contract (leading to inhalation). Also known as "phrenic nerve pacing."

diastole The phase of the cardiac cycle that consists of relaxation and filling of the atria and ventricles; normally about two thirds of the cardiac cycle.

diastolic blood pressure The amount of pressure/force against the arterial walls during the relaxation phase of the heart.

diastolic heart failure Heart failure that occurs when the left ventricle is unable to relax adequately during diastole, which prevents the ventricle from filling with sufficient blood to ensure adequate cardiac output.

Dietary Guidelines for Americans Recommendations made by the USDA and U.S. Department of Health and Human Services to help people maintain nutritional health; updated every 5 years.

Dietary Reference Intakes (DRIs) Nutrition guide developed by the Institute of Medicine of the National Academies that provides a scientific basis for food guidelines in the United States and Canada.

diffuse axonal injury (DAI) A type of closed head injury that is usually related to high-speed acceleration/deceleration, as with motor vehicle crashes. There is significant damage to axons in the white matter, and there are lesions in the corpus callosum, midbrain, cerebellum, and upper brainstem. Patients with severe injury may present with immediate coma, and most survivors require long-term care.

diffuse cutaneous systemic sclerosis Skin thickening on the trunk, face, and proximal and distal extremities in patients with systemic sclerosis.

diffuse light reflex A description of a light reflex that is spotty or multiple because of a changed eardrum shape from either retraction or bulging.

diffusion The spontaneous, free movement of particles (solute) across a permeable membrane down a concentration gradient; that is, from an area of higher concentration to an area of lower concentration.

digestion The mechanical and chemical process in which complex foodstuffs are broken down into simpler forms that can be used by the body.

digoxin toxicity A reaction to therapy with digitalis derivatives (digoxin) that is identified by monitoring serum digoxin and potassium levels (hypokalemia potentiates digitalis toxicity). Signs of toxicity are nonspecific (anorexia, fatigue, changes in mental status). Toxicity may cause dysrhythmia, most commonly premature ventricular contractions.

dilated cardiomyopathy (DCM) A type of cardiomyopathy that involves extensive damage to the myofibrils and interference with myocardial metabolism. There is normal ventricular wall thickness but dilation of both ventricles and impairment of systolic function.

dilation Increase in the diameter of blood vessels.

diplopia Double vision.

direct current stimulation (DCS) The placement of an implantable device to promote bone fusion; used as an adjunct for patients for whom spinal fusion may be difficult.

direct inguinal hernia A sac formed from the peritoneum that contains a portion of the intestine and passes through a weak point in the abdominal wall.

direct response Pupil constriction in response to bringing a penlight in from the side of the patient's head and shining the light in the eye being tested as soon as the patient opens his or her eyes.

directly observed therapy (DOT) A technique in which a health care professional watches the patient swallow prescribed drugs.

disabling health problem Any physical or mental health problem that can cause disability.

disaster A mass casualty incident in which the number of casualties exceeds the resource capabilities of a particular community or hospital facility.

disaster triage tag system A system that categorizes triage priority by colored and numbered tags.

discoid lesion Round lesion in patients who have discoid lupus erythematosus; evident when exposed to sunlight or ultraviolet light.

disease-modifying antirheumatic drugs (DMARDs) Drugs prescribed to slow the progression of mild rheumatoid disease before it worsens, such as hydroxychloroquine, sulfasalazine, or minocycline.

disequilibrium A condition in which the hydrostatic pressure is not the same in the two fluid spaces on either side of a permeable membrane.

disinfection A method of infection control in which the level of disease-causing organisms is reduced but the organisms are not killed; adequate when an item is entering a body area that has resident bacteria or normal flora, such as the respiratory tract.

diskitis Disk inflammation.

dislocation of a joint Occurrence of the articulating surfaces of two or more bones moving away from each other.

dissociate The act of separating and releasing ions.

diverticula Sacs resulting from the herniation of the mucosa and submucosa of a tubular organ into surrounding tissue.

diverticulitis The inflammation of one or more diverticula.

diverticulosis The presence of many abnormal pouchlike herniations (diverticula) in the wall of the intestine.

dizziness A disturbed sense of a person's relationship to space.

DNR Do not resuscitate; order from a physician or other authorized health care provider who instructs that CPR not be attempted in the event of cardiac or respiratory arrest.

dopamine agonist A class of drugs that mimic dopamine. Dopamine agonists stimulate dopamine receptors and are typically the most effective during the first 3 to 5 years of use. Prescribed for the patient with Parkinson disease to reduce dyskinesias (problems with movement).

dose-dense chemotherapy Chemotherapy that uses higher doses more often for aggressive cancer treatment, especially breast cancer.

double-barrel stoma The least common type of colostomy, which is created by dividing the bowel and bringing both the proximal and distal portions to the abdominal surface to create two stomas.

doubling time The amount of time it takes for a tumor to double in size.

Droplet Precautions Infection control guidelines from the Centers for Disease Control and Prevention; used for patients with infections spread by the droplet transmission route, such as influenza.

drug holiday Period of time lasting up to 10 days in which the patient with Parkinson disease receives no drug therapy.

dual x-ray absorptiometry (DXA or DEXA) A type of radiographic scan that measures bone mineral density in the hip, wrist, or vertebral column; used as a screening and diagnostic tool for diagnosis and for follow-up evaluation of treatment of osteoporosis.

ductal carcinoma in situ (DCIS) An early, non-invasive form of breast cancer in which cancer cells are located within the duct and have not invaded the surrounding fatty breast tissue.

ductal ectasia A benign breast disease caused by dilation and thickening of the collecting ducts in the subareolar area. The ducts become distended and filled with cellular debris, which activates an inflammatory response. It is usually seen in women approaching menopause.

dumping syndrome A constellation of vasomotor symptoms that typically occur within 30 minutes after eating; believed to occur as a result of the rapid emptying of gastric contents into the small intestine, which shifts fluid into the gut and causes abdominal distention. Early manifestations include vertigo, tachycardia, syncope, sweating, pallor, and palpitations.

Dupuytren's contracture A slowly progressive contracture of the palmar fascia that results in flexion of the fourth or fifth digit of the hand and occasionally affects the third digit. Although a fairly common problem, the cause is unknown. It usually occurs in older men, tends to occur in families, and can be bilateral.

durable power of attorney for health care (DPOAHC) A legal document in which a person appoints someone else to make health care decisions in the event he or she becomes incapable of making decisions.

dysarthria Slurred speech.

dysfunctional uterine bleeding (DUB) A nonspecific term to describe bleeding that is excessive or abnormal in amount or frequency without predisposing anatomic or systemic conditions. Such bleeding occurs most often at either end of the span of a woman's reproductive years, when ovulation is becoming established or when it is becoming irregular at menopause.

dyskinesia Difficulty with movement.

dyslexia Problems understanding written language; caused by brain injury or disease.

dysmetria The inability to direct or limit movement.

dyspareunia Painful sexual intercourse.

dyspepsia Indigestion or heartburn following meals.

dysphagia Difficulty in swallowing.

dysphasia Slurred speech.

dyspnea Difficulty in breathing or breathlessness.

dyspnea on exertion (DOE) Dyspnea that is associated with activity, such as climbing stairs.

dysrhythmia A disorder of the heartbeat involving a disturbance in cardiac rhythm; irregular heartbeat.

dystrophic Pertaining to or characterized by dystrophy; abnormal.

dystrophin A muscle protein that maintains muscle integrity by sending signals to coordinate smooth, synchronous muscle fiber contraction. Faulty action of this protein causes muscular dystrophy.

dysuria Painful urination.

E

Eaton-Lambert syndrome A form of myasthenia gravis that affects the muscles of the trunk and the pelvic and shoulder girdles; often observed in combination with small cell carcinoma of the lung. Although weakness increases after exertion, there may be a temporary increase in muscle strength during the first few contractions, followed by a rapid decline.

ecchymoses Large purple, blue, or yellow bruises of the skin resulting from small hemorrhages; these bruises are larger than petechiae.

ecchymotic Pertaining to a bruise.

ECG caliper A measurement tool used in analysis of an electrocardiographic (ECG) rhythm strip.

echocardiography In cardiovascular assessment, the use of ultrasound waves to assess cardiac structure and mobility, particularly of the valves; a noninvasive, risk-free test that is easily performed at the bedside or on an ambulatory care basis.

echolalia Automatic repetition of what another person says.

ectopic Out of place.

ectropion A turning outward and sagging of the eyelid, which is caused by relaxation of the orbicular muscle.

edema Tissue swelling as a result of the accumulation of excessive fluid in the interstitial spaces.

edentulous Without teeth.

efferent arterioles The extremely small blood vessels that carry the remaining blood out of the glomerulus (once the glomerulus has filtered the blood to make urine) and into one of two additional capillary systems (the peritubular capillaries or the vasa recta).

effluent Drainage.

effusion An accumulation of fluid, such as in a joint (where it may limit movement).

ejection fraction The percentage of blood ejected from the heart during systole.

electrical bone stimulation The use of an electronic device (e.g., magnetic coils applied on the skin or over a cast to deliver a pulsed magnetic field) to promote bone union after a fracture. The exact mechanism of action is unknown, but this procedure is based on research showing that bone has inherent electrical properties that are used in healing.

electrocardiogram (ECG) A graphic recording of the electrical current generated by the heart. The ECG provides information about cardiac dysrhythmias, myocardial ischemia, site and extent of myocardial infarction, cardiac hypertrophy, electrolyte imbalances, and effectiveness of cardiac drugs. It is a routine part of cardiovascular evaluation and is a valuable diagnostic test.

electroencephalography (EEG) A recording of the electrical activity of the cerebral hemispheres; it represents the voltage changes in various areas of the brain as determined by recording the difference between two electrodes.

electrolyte A substance in body fluids that carries an electrical charge. Also called an "ion."

electromyography (EMG) A recording of the electrical activity of peripheral nerves by testing muscle activity.

electrophysiologic study (EPS) In cardiovascular assessment, an invasive procedure performed in a catheterization laboratory during which programmed electrical stimulation of the heart is used to induce and evaluate lethal dysrhythmias and conduction abnormalities to permit accurate diagnosis and effective treatment. The study is used in patients who have survived cardiac arrest, have recurrent tachydysrhythmias, or experience unexplained syncopal episodes.

electrovaporization of the prostate (EVAP) Procedure for treating benign prostatic hyperplasia with high-frequency electrical current to cut and vaporize excess tissue.

embolectomy Removal of a blood clot.

embolic stroke Damage to the brain when a blood clot forms somewhere in the body (usually the heart) and travels through the bloodstream to block one or more of the arteries supplying the brain.

embolus The occurrence of inflammation and thickening of the vein wall around a clot (thrombus).

emergence Recovery from anesthesia.

emergency medical technician (EMT) Prehospital care provider who supplies basic life-support interventions such as oxygen, basic wound care, splinting, spinal immobilization, and monitoring of vital signs.

emergency medicine physician A member of the emergency health care team with education and training in the specialty of emergency patient management.

emergency operations center (EOC) A designated location in the Hospital Incident Command System (HICS) with accessible communication technology. Also called the "command center."

emergency preparedness A goal or plan to meet the extraordinary need for hospital beds, staff, drugs, personal protective equipment, supplies, and medical devices such as mechanical ventilators.

Emergency Severity Index (ESI) A standardized model for triage that categorizes both patient acuity and resource utilization into five levels, from most urgent to least urgent.

emergent triage In a three-tiered triage scheme, the category that includes any condition or injury that poses an immediate threat to life or limb, such as crushing chest pain or active hemorrhage.

emetogenic A substance that induces nausea and vomiting.

emmetropia The state of perfect refraction of the eye; with the lens at rest, light rays from a distant source are focused into a sharp image on the retina.

emotional abuse The intentional use of threats, humiliation, intimidation, and isolation to another person.

emotional lability Having uncontrollable emotions; for example, the patient laughs and then cries unexpectedly for no apparent reason.

empyema A collection of pus in the pleural space.

encephalitis An inflammation of the brain parenchyma (brain tissue) and meninges that affects the cerebrum, brainstem, and cerebellum; usually caused by a virus.

endometrial ablation Procedure for dysfunctional uterine bleeding that removes a built-up uterine lining using a laser, roller ball, or balloon.

endometrial cancer Cancer of the inner uterine lining.

endometriosis The abnormal occurrence of endometrial tissue outside the uterine cavity.

endometritis An infection of the endometrium.

endoscope A tube that allows viewing and manipulation of internal body areas.

endoscopic retrograde cholangiopancreatography (ERCP) The visual and radiographic examination of the liver, gallbladder, bile ducts, and pancreas by means of an endoscope and the injection of radiopaque dye to identify the cause and location of obstruction.

endoscopic variceal ligation (EVL) The application of small "O" bands around the base of the esophageal varices to cut off their blood supply. Also called "banding."

endoscopy The direct visualization of the gastrointestinal tract by means of a flexible fiberoptic endoscope.

endothelin A secretion produced by the endothelial cells when they are stretched.

endovascular stent graft The repair of an abdominal aortic aneurysm using a stent made of flexible material; the stent is inserted through a skin incision into the femoral artery by way of a catheter-based system.

end-stage kidney disease (ESKD) Acute renal failure combined with chronic renal insufficiency, resulting in the inability of the kidney to excrete waste products normally. The patient may need hemodialysis or a kidney transplant.

energy conservation Strategies to reduce the fatigue associated with chronic and disabling conditions, such as allowing rest periods and setting priorities.

engraftment The successful transplantation of cells in the patient's bone marrow.

enophthalmos Backward displacement of the eyeball into the orbit so that the eye appears sunken.

enteroscopy Visualization of the small intestine.

enterostomal feeding tube A tube used for patients who need long-term enteral feeding; the physician directly accesses the gastrointestinal tract using surgical, endoscopic, or laparoscopic techniques.

entropion The turning inward of the eyelid, causing the eyelashes to rub against the eye.

enucleation The surgical removal of the entire eyeball.

envenomation Venom injection from a snakebite.

epididymitis Inflammation of the epididymis.

epidural Term for the space between the dura mater and vertebrae; it consists of fat, connective tissue, and blood vessels.

epidural hematoma An accumulation of clotted blood resulting from arterial bleeding into the space between the dura and the skull; a neurosurgical emergency.

epiglottis A leaf-shaped, elastic structure that is attached along one edge to the top of the larynx; it closes over the glottis during swallowing to prevent food from entering the trachea and opens during breathing and coughing.

epiglottitis Infection or inflammation of the epiglottis and supraglottic structures that results in swelling. If swelling is great enough, the airway can be obstructed.

epilepsy A chronic disorder characterized by recurrent, unprovoked seizure activity; may be caused by an abnormality in electrical neuronal activity, an imbalance of neurotransmitters, or a combination of both.

epistaxis Nosebleed.

erectile dysfunction (ED) The inability to achieve or maintain a penile erection sufficient for sexual intercourse.

ergonomics An applied science in which the workplace is designed to increase worker comfort (thus reducing injury) while increasing efficiency and productivity.

erosion Ulceration.

eructation The act of belching.

erythema Redness of the skin.

erythema migrans A round or oval flat or slightly raised rash.

erythrocyte A red blood cell (RBC). Red blood cells are the major cells in the blood and are responsible for tissue oxygenation.

erythroplakia A velvety red mucosal lesion, most often occurring in the oral cavity.

erythropoiesis The selective maturation of stem cells into mature erythrocytes.

eschar The crust of dead tissue that forms from coagulated particles of destroyed dermis in a patient with a full-thickness burn injury.

escharotomy Incision made through tight eschar to relieve pressure and allow normal blood flow and breathing.

esophageal stricture Narrowing of the esophageal opening.

esophageal varices The distention of fragile, thin-walled esophageal veins due to increased pressure; the increased pressure is a result of portal hypertension, in which the blood backs up from the liver and enters the esophageal and gastric vessels that carry it into the systemic circulation.

esophagectomy The surgical removal of all or part of the esophagus.

esophagitis Inflammation of the esophagus.

esophagogastroduodenoscopy (EGD) The visual examination of the esophagus, stomach, and duodenum by means of a fiberoptic endoscope.

esophagogastrostomy The surgical creation of a communication between the stomach and the esophagus; it involves the removal of part of the esophagus and proximal stomach.

essential hypertension Elevated blood pressure that is not caused by a specific disease. The major risk factor is a family history of hypertension. Also called "primary hypertension."

euploid Having the correct number of chromosome pairs for the species.

euploidy The normal diploid number for a cell.

eustachian tube Tube that connects the nasopharynx with the middle ear and opens during swallowing to equalize pressure within the middle ear.

euthyroid Having normal thyroid function.

euvolemia A state of balanced fluid intake and output.

evidence-based practice (EBP) A QSEN competency in which the nurse integrates best current evidence with clinical expertise and patient/family preferences and values for delivery of optimal health care.

evisceration The total separation of all layers of a wound and the protrusion of internal organs through the open wound.

evoked potentials Tests to measure the electrical signals to the brain generated by hearing, touch, or sight. Also called "evoked response."

exacerbation An increase in severity of a disease. Also called "flare-up."

excitability The ability of a cell to respond to a stimulus by initiating an impulse. Also called "depolarization." In cardiac electrophysiology, it is the ability of non-pacemaker myocardial cells to respond to an electrical impulse generated from pacemaker cells and to depolarize.

exercise electrocardiography In cardiovascular assessment, a test that assesses cardiovascular response to an increased workload. Also called "exercise tolerance" or a "stress test." Exercise electrocardiography helps determine the functional capacity of the heart, screens for coronary artery disease, and identifies dysrhythmias that develop during exercise. It also aids in evaluating the effectiveness of antidysrhythmic drugs.

exercise tolerance See *exercise electrocardiography*.

exertional dyspnea Breathlessness or difficulty breathing that develops during activity or exertion.

exertional heat stroke A form of heat stroke with a sudden onset, typically due to strenuous physical activity in hot, humid conditions. Lack of acclimatization to hot weather and wearing clothing too heavy for the environment are common contributing factors.

exogenous Originating outside the body.

exogenous hyperthyroidism Hyperthyroidism caused by excessive use of thyroid replacement hormones.

exophthalmos Abnormal protrusion of the eyeball (proptosis).

expedited partner therapy (EPT) Therapy used to treat chlamydia in which patients are given a drug or prescription with specific instructions for administration to their partners without direct evaluation by a health care provider. Also called "patient-delivered partner therapy."

exploratory laparotomy A surgical opening of the abdominal cavity to investigate the cause of an obstruction or peritonitis.

exposure (1) The final component of the primary survey that allows for thorough assessment of the trauma patient; (2) in radiation therapy, the amount of radiation that is delivered to a tissue.

expressed gene When a particular gene has been "turned on."

expressive aphasia A type of aphasia resulting from damage in Broca's area of the frontal lobe of the brain. A motor speech problem in which the patient understands what is said but is unable to communicate verbally and has difficulty writing; rote speech and automatic speech, such as responses to a greeting, are often intact. The patient is aware of the deficit and may become frustrated and angry. Also called "Broca's aphasia" or "motor aphasia."

expressivity In genetics, the degree of expression a person has when a specific autosomal dominant gene is present. The gene is always expressed, but some people have more severe results.

external fixation A system in which pins or wires are passed through skin and bone and connected to a rigid external frame to immobilize a fracture during healing.

external fixator See *external fixation*.

external hemorrhoid A hemorrhoid that lies below the anal sphincter and can be seen on inspection of the anal region.

external otitis A painful irritation or infection of the skin of the external ear, with resulting allergic response or inflammation. When it occurs in patients who participate in water sports, external otitis is called "swimmer's ear."

external urethral sphincter The sphincter composed of the skeletal muscle that surrounds the urethra.

extracapsular Located outside the joint capsule.

extracellular fluid (ECF) The portion of total body water (about one third) that is in the space outside the cells. This space also includes interstitial fluid, blood, lymph, bone, and connective tissue water, and the transcellular fluids.

extracranial-intracranial bypass A surgical procedure in which the surgeon performs a craniotomy and bypasses the blocked artery by making a graft (bypass) from the first artery to the second artery to establish blood flow around the blocked artery and re-establish blood flow to the involved areas.

extramedullary tumor A tumor found within the spinal dura but outside the cord.

extrapulmonary Involving nonpulmonary tissues.

extravasation Escape of fluids or drugs into the subcutaneous tissue; a complication of intravenous infusion.

extrinsic factor In hematology, an event (e.g., trauma) that occurs outside the blood to cause platelet plugs to form.

extubation The removal of an endotracheal tube.

F

facial paralysis See *Bell's palsy*.

facilitated diffusion Diffusion across a cell membrane that requires the assistance of a transport system or membrane-altering system. Also called "facilitated transport."

facilitated transport See *facilitated diffusion*.

failed back surgery syndrome (FBSS) A combination of organic, psychological, and socioeconomic factors in patients for whom back surgery is not successful. Discouraged by repeated surgical procedures, these patients must continue long-term nonsurgical management of pain, including nerve blocks.

fall An unintentional change in body position that results in the patient's body coming to rest on the floor or ground.

fallophobia In some older adults, the fear of falling and sustaining a serious injury.

far point (of vision) The farthest point at which the eye can see an object.

fascia An inelastic tissue that surrounds groups of muscles, blood vessels, and nerves in the body.

fasciculation Abnormal, involuntary twitching of a muscle.

fasciotomy A surgical procedure in which an incision is made through the skin and subcutaneous tissues into the fascia of the affected compartment to relieve the pressure in and restore circulation to the affected area in the patient with acute compartment syndrome.

fat embolism syndrome (FES) A serious complication, usually resulting from a fracture, in which fat globules are released from the yellow bone marrow into the bloodstream. This syndrome usually occurs within 48 hours of the fracture and can result in respiratory failure or death, often from pulmonary edema.

fatigue (stress) fracture A fracture that results from excessive or repeated strain and stress on a bone.

fatty liver Caused by the accumulation of fats in and around the hepatic cells. It may be caused by alcohol abuse or other factors. Also known as "steatosis."

fecal occult blood test (FOBT) A diagnostic test that measures the presence of blood in the stool from gastrointestinal bleeding; this is a common finding associated with colorectal cancer.

Felty's syndrome The combination of rheumatoid arthritis, hepatosplenomegaly (enlarged liver and spleen), and leukopenia.

femoral hernia A hernia that protrudes through the femoral ring.

fetor hepaticus The distinctive fruity or musty breath odor of chronic liver disease and portal-systemic encephalopathy.

fibrinolysis The breakdown of a clot.

fibrinolytic Drug that targets the fibrin component of the coronary thrombosis; used to dissolve thrombi in the coronary arteries and restore myocardial blood flow; examples include tissue plasminogen activator, anisoylated plasminogen-streptokinase activator complex, and reteplase.

fibroadenoma A solid, slowly enlarging, benign mass of connective tissue that is unattached to the surrounding breast tissue and is typically discovered by the patient herself. The mass is usually round, firm, easily movable, nontender, and clearly delineated from the surrounding tissue.

fibrocystic breast condition (FBC) Physiologic nodularity of the breast that is thought to be caused by an imbalance in the normal estrogen-to-progesterone ratio. It is the most common breast problem of women between 20 and 30 years of age.

fibroids See *leiomyomas*.

fibromyalgia syndrome (FMS) A chronic pain syndrome characterized by pain and tenderness at specific sites in the back of the neck, upper chest, trunk, low back, and extremities along with fatigue, sleep disturbances, and headache.

fibrosis Replacement of normal cells with connective tissue and collagen (scar tissue).

fidelity Ethical principle that refers to the agreement that nurses will keep their obligations or promises to patients to follow through with care.

filter The movement of fluid from the space with higher hydrostatic pressure through the membrane into the space with lower hydrostatic pressure.

filtration The movement of fluid through a cell or blood vessel membrane because of hydrostatic pressure differences on both sides of the membrane.

financial abuse Mismanagement or misuse of the patient's property or resources.

first heart sound (S₁) Sound created by the closure of the mitral and tricuspid valves (atrioventricular valves).

first intention Healing in which the wound can be easily closed and dead space eliminated without granulation, which thus shortens the phases of tissue repair. Inflammation resolves quickly, and connective tissue repair is minimal, resulting in a thin scar.

fistula An abnormal opening between two adjacent organs or structures.

five cardinal manifestations of inflammation Warmth, redness, swelling, pain, and decreased function.

fixed occlusion Wiring the jaws together in the mouth closed position.

flaccid bladder See *areflexic bladder*.

flaccid paralysis Paralysis of a part of the body that is characterized by loss of muscle tone due to hypotonia; may be seen in the patient who has experienced a brain attack.

flail chest Inward movement of the thorax during inspiration, with outward movement during expiration; results from multiple rib fractures caused by blunt chest trauma that leaves a segment of the chest wall loose.

flatulence The presence of an excessive amount of gas in the stomach or intestines.

fluid overload An excess of body fluid. Also called "overhydration."

folliculitis A superficial bacterial infection involving only the upper portion of the hair follicle.

forensic nurse examiner (RN-FNE) Emergency department specialist who is trained to recognize evidence of abuse and to intervene on the patient's behalf and who obtains patient histories, collects forensic evidence, and offers counseling and follow-up care for victims of rape, child abuse, and domestic violence.

fracture A break or disruption in the continuity of a bone.

fremitus Vibration.

frequency (1) The highness or lowness of tones (expressed in hertz). The greater the number of vibrations per second, the higher the frequency (pitch) of the sound; the fewer the number of vibrations per second, the lower the pitch; (2) an urge to urinate frequently in small amounts.

fresh frozen plasma (FFP) Plasma that is frozen immediately after donation so that the clotting factors are preserved.

friable Easily crumbled or damaged.

frostbite A cold injury characterized by the degree of tissue freezing and the resultant damage it produces. Frostbite injuries can be superficial, partial, or full thickness.

frostnip A form of superficial frostbite (typically on the face, fingers, or toes) that produces pain, numbness, and pallor but is easily remedied with the application of warmth and does not induce tissue injury.

Fulmer SPICES A framework that identifies six serious "marker conditions" that can lead to longer hospital stays for patients, higher medical costs, and deaths.

fulminant hepatitis A severe acute and often fatal form of hepatitis caused by failure of the liver cells to regenerate, with progression to necrosis.

furuncle A localized inflammation of the skin caused by bacterial infection, usually *Staphylococcus*, of a hair follicle. Also called "a boil."

G

gallium scan A test that is similar to the bone scan but uses the radioisotope *gallium citrate* and

is more specific and sensitive in detecting bone problems. This substance also migrates to brain, liver, and breast tissue and therefore is used to examine these structures when disease is suspected.

gamma globulin See *immunoglobulin*.

ganglion A round, cystlike lesion, often overlying a wrist joint or tendon.

gastrectomy The surgical removal of part or all of the stomach.

gastric bypass A type of gastric restriction surgery in which gastric resection is combined with malabsorption surgery. The patient's stomach, duodenum, and part of the jejunum are bypassed so that fewer calories can be absorbed. Also known as a "Roux-en-Y gastric bypass," or "RNYGB."

gastric lavage Procedure of irrigating the stomach in which a large-bore nasogastric tube is inserted into the stomach and room-temperature solution is instilled in volumes of 200 to 300 mL. The solution and blood are repeatedly withdrawn manually until returns are clear or light pink and without clots.

gastritis An inflammation of the gastric mucosa (stomach lining).

gastroenteritis An increase in the frequency and water content of stools or vomiting as a result of inflammation of the mucous membranes of the stomach and intestinal tract. It affects primarily the small bowel and can be of either viral or bacterial origin.

gastroesophageal reflux (GER) Condition that occurs as a result of backward flow of stomach contents into the esophagus.

gastroesophageal reflux disease (GERD) An upper gastrointestinal disease caused by the backward flow (reflux) of gastrointestinal contents into the esophagus.

gastrojejunostomy Surgical anastomosis of the stomach to the jejunum.

gastroparesis Delay in gastric emptying.

gastrostomy A stoma created from the abdominal wall into the stomach.

gel phenomenon In patients with rheumatoid arthritis, morning stiffness that lasts between 45 minutes and several hours after awakening.

gender dysphoria Discomfort with one's natal sex.

gender identity A person's inner sense of maleness or femaleness not related to reproductive anatomy.

gender reassignment surgery See *sex reassignment surgery*.

gene The deoxyribonucleic acid (DNA) in the form of chromosomes within the nucleus of each cell that contains the instructions for making all the different proteins any organism makes. Every human cell with a nucleus contains the entire set of human genes.

general anesthesia A reversible loss of consciousness induced by inhibiting neuronal impulses in the central nervous system.

generalized seizure One of the three broad categories of seizure disorders along with partial seizures and unclassified seizures. There are six types: tonic-clonic, tonic, clonic, absence, myoclonic, and atonic (akinetic).

genetics The science concerned with the general mechanisms of heredity and the variation of inherited traits.

genital herpes (GH) An acute, recurring, incurable viral disease of the genitalia caused by the herpes simplex virus and transmitted through contact with an infected person. An outbreak typically is preceded by a tingling sensation of the skin followed by the appearance of vesicles (blisters) on the penis, scrotum, vulva, perineum, vagina, cervix, or perianal region. The blisters rupture spontaneously, leaving painful erosions. After the lesions heal, the virus remains dormant, periodically reactivating with a recurrence of symptoms.

genome The complete set of human genes. Each human cell with a nucleus contains the entire set of human genes. The human genome contains about 35,000 individual genes.

genomic health care The application of known genetic variation to enhance health care to individuals and their families.

genomics The science focusing on the function of all of the human DNA, including genes and noncoding DNA regions.

genotype The actual alleles for a genetic trait, not just what can be observed.

genu valgum A deformity in which the knees are abnormally close together and the space between the ankles is increased. Also called "knock-knee."

genu varum A deformity in which the knees are abnormally separated and the lower extremities are bowed inward. Also called "bowleg."

Geriatric Depression Scale—Short Form (GDS-SF) A valid and reliable screening tool to help determine if an older patient has clinical depression.

geriatric failure to thrive (GFTT) A complex syndrome including under-nutrition, impaired physical functioning, depression, and cognitive impairment.

geriatric syndromes Major health issues that are associated with late adulthood in community and inpatient settings.

ghrelin The "hunger hormone" that is secreted in the stomach; increases in a fasting state and decreases after a meal.

Glasgow Coma Scale (GCS) An objective and widely accepted tool for neurologic assessment and documentation of level of consciousness. It establishes baseline data for eye opening, motor response, and verbal response. The patient is assessed and assigned a numeric score for each of these areas. A score of 15 represents normal neurologic functioning, and a score of 3 represents a deep coma state.

glaucoma A group of ocular diseases resulting in increased intraocular pressure, causing reduced blood flow to the optic nerve and retina and followed by tissue damage.

glomerulus A series of specialized capillary loops that receive blood from the afferent arteriole and then filter water and small particles from the blood to make urine. The remaining blood leaves the glomerulus via the efferent arteriole.

glossectomy The partial or total surgical removal of the tongue.

glossitis A smooth, beefy red tongue.

glottis The opening between the true vocal cords inside the larynx.

glucagon A hormone secreted by the pancreas that increases blood glucose levels. It is a "counterregulatory" hormone that has actions opposite those of insulin. It causes the release of glucose from cell storage sites whenever blood glucose levels are low.

gluconeogenesis The conversion of proteins and amino acids to glucose in the body.

glucosamine A supplement that may decrease inflammation.

glycemic A term referring to blood glucose.

glycogenesis The production of glycogen in the body.

glycogenolysis The breakdown of glycogen into glucose.

glycoprotein (GP) IIb/IIIa inhibitors Drugs that target the platelet component of the thrombus. They are administered intravenously to prevent fibrinogen from attaching to activated platelets at the site of a thrombus and are given to patients with acute coronary syndromes (especially unstable angina and non–Q-wave myocardial infarction). Examples include abciximab, eptifibatide, and tirofiban.

glycosylated hemoglobin (A1C) A standardized test that measures how much glucose permanently attaches to the hemoglobin molecule. A1C levels greater than 6.5% are diagnostic of diabetes mellitus.

"go bag" See *personal readiness supplies.*

goiter Enlargement of the thyroid gland.

gonadotropins Hormones that stimulate the ovaries and testes to produce sex hormones.

gonads The male and female reproductive endocrine glands. Male gonads are the testes, and female gonads are the ovaries.

goniometer An instrument for measuring angles; also refers to a tool used to measure joint range of motion.

good death A death that is free from avoidable distress and suffering for patients, families, and caregivers; in agreement with patients' and families' wishes; and consistent with clinical practice standards.

gout A systemic disease in which urate crystals deposit in the joints and other body tissues, causing inflammation.

grading System of classifying cellular aspects of a cancer tumor.

granulation The formation of scar tissue for wound healing to occur.

granuloma Growth that develops in the lungs of patients with sarcoidosis and contains lymphocytes, macrophages, epithelioid cells, and giant cells; scar tissue.

Graves' disease Toxic diffuse goiter characterized by hyperthyroidism, enlargement of the thyroid gland, abnormal protrusion of the eyes, and dry, waxy swelling of the front surfaces of the lower legs.

gray (gy) Unit of measurement for an absorbed radiation dose.

gray matter In the spinal cord, neuron cell bodies.

grief The emotional feeling related to the perception of loss.

grommet A polyethylene tube that is surgically placed through the tympanic membrane to allow continuous drainage of middle-ear fluids in the patient with otitis media.

ground substance A lubricant composed of protein and sugar groups that surrounds the dermal cells and fibers and contributes to the skin's normal suppleness and turgor.

guardian A person appointed to make health care decisions for a patient who is determined to not be legally competent.

Guillain-Barré syndrome (GBS) An acute autoimmune disorder characterized by varying degrees of motor weakness and paralysis. It may be referred to by a variety of other names, such as "acute idiopathic polyneuritis" and "polyradiculoneuropathy."

gynecomastia Abnormal enlargement of the breasts in men.

H

H₂-receptor antagonists A group of drugs that inhibit gastric acid secretion by blocking the effects of histamine on parietal cell receptors in the stomach.

half-life Time it takes for the amount of drug in the body to be reduced by 50%.

halitosis A foul odor of the mouth.

hallux valgus A common deformity of the foot that occurs when the great toe deviates laterally at the metatarsophalangeal joint; sometimes referred to as a "bunion."

halo fixator A static traction device used for immobilization of the cervical spine. Four pins or screws are inserted into the skull, and a metal halo ring is attached to a plastic vest or cast when the spine is stable, allowing increased patient mobility.

hammertoe The dorsiflexion of any metatarsophalangeal joint with plantar flexion of the adjacent proximal interphalangeal joint. The second toe is most often affected.

hand hygiene Infection control protocol that refers to both handwashing and alcohol-based hand rubs.

health care–associated infection (HAI) Infections associated with the provision of health care; for example, microorganisms can enter the body through the genitourinary tract in patients with indwelling urinary catheters.

heart failure A general term for the inadequacy of the heart to pump blood throughout the body, causing insufficient perfusion of body tissues with vital nutrients and oxygen. Also called "pump failure."

heart rate (HR) Term referring to the number of times the ventricles contract each minute.

heart transplantation A surgical procedure in which a heart from a donor with a comparable body weight and ABO compatibility is transplanted into a recipient less than 6 hours after procurement. It is the treatment of choice for patients with severe dilated cardiomyopathy and may be considered for patients with restrictive cardiomyopathy.

heat exhaustion A syndrome primarily caused by dehydration from heavy perspiration and inadequate fluid and electrolyte consumption during heat exposure over hours to days; if left untreated, can be a precursor to heat stroke.

heat stroke A true medical emergency in which the victim's heat regulatory mechanisms fail and are unable to compensate for a critical elevation in body temperature; if uncorrected, organ dysfunction and death will ensue.

Heberden's nodes Swelling at the distal interphalangeal joints in osteoarthritis that involves the hands.

hematemesis The vomiting of blood.

hematochezia The passage of red blood via the rectum.

hematocrit The percentage of packed red blood cells per deciliter of blood.

hematogenous tuberculosis A form of tuberculosis that spreads throughout the body when a large number of organisms enter the blood. Also called "miliary tuberculosis."

hematopoiesis The production of blood cells, which occurs in the red marrow of bones.

hematuria Blood in the urine.

hemianopsia Blindness in half of the visual field of one or both eyes. Also called "hemianopia."

hemiarthroplasty Surgical replacement of part of the shoulder joint, typically the humeral component, as an alternative to total shoulder arthroplasty.

hemiparesis Weakness on one side of the body.

hemiplegia Paralysis on one side of the body.

hemoconcentration Elevated plasma levels of hemoglobin, hematocrit, serum osmolarity, glucose, protein, blood urea nitrogen, and electrolytes that occur when only the water is lost and other substances remain.

hemodilution Excessive water in the vascular space.

hemoglobin A (HbA) Normal adult hemoglobin. The molecule has two alpha chains and two beta chains of amino acids.

hemoglobin S (HbS) An abnormal beta chain of hemoglobin associated with sickle cell disease that is sensitive to low oxygen content of red blood cells.

hemolytic The characteristic of destroying red blood cells.

hemolytic anemia Anemia caused by the destruction of red blood cells.

hemoptysis Coughing up blood or blood-stained sputum.

hemorrhoid Unnaturally swollen or distended vein in the anorectal region.

hemorrhoidectomy The excision of a hemorrhoid.

hemostasis The multi-step process of controlled blood clotting.

heparin-induced thrombocytopenia (HIT) The aggregation of platelets into "white clots" that can cause thrombosis, usually in the form of an acute arterial occlusion; occurs with heparin administration. Also called "white clot syndrome."

hepatic encephalopathy See *portal-systemic encephalopathy.*

hepatitis The widespread inflammation of liver cells.

hepatitis A Hepatitis that is caused by the hepatitis A virus (HAV) and is characterized by a mild course similar to that of a typical viral syndrome

and often goes unrecognized. It is spread via the fecal-oral route by oral ingestion of fecal contaminants. Sources of infection include contaminated water, shellfish caught in contaminated water, and food contaminated by infected food handlers. The virus may also be spread by oral-anal sexual activity. The incubation period is usually 15 to 50 days. The disease is usually not life threatening but may be more severe in people older than 40 years. It can also complicate pre-existing liver disease.

hepatitis B A form of hepatitis that is caused by the hepatitis B virus (HBV), which is shed in the body fluids of infected people and asymptomatic carriers. It is spread through unprotected sexual intercourse with an infected partner, needle sharing, blood transfusions, and other modes. Symptoms usually occur within 25 to 180 days of exposure and include nausea, fever, fatigue, joint pain, and jaundice. Most adults who get hepatitis B recover, clear the virus from their body, and develop immunity; however, up to 10% of patients with the disease do not develop immunity and become carriers.

hepatitis C Hepatitis that is caused by the hepatitis C virus (HCV). Transmission is blood to blood, most commonly by needle sharing or needle stick injury with contaminated blood. The rate of sexual transmission is very low; it is not spread by casual contact and is rarely transmitted from mother to fetus. The average incubation period is 7 weeks. Most people are asymptomatic and are not diagnosed until long after the initial exposure when an abnormality is detected during a routine laboratory evaluation or when symptoms of liver impairment appear. Hepatitis C causes chronic inflammation in the liver that eventually causes the hepatocytes to scar and may progress to cirrhosis.

hepatitis carrier Person who has had hepatitis B but has not developed immunity. Hepatitis carriers can infect others even though they are not sick and demonstrate no obvious signs of disease. Chronic carriers are at high risk for cirrhosis and liver cancer.

hepatitis D The hepatitis D virus (HDV) co-infects with hepatitis B virus (HBV) and needs the presence of HBV for viral replication. HDV can co-infect a patient with HBV or can occur as a superinfection in a patient with chronic HBV. Superinfection usually develops into chronic HDV infection. The incubation period is 14 to 56 days. As with HBV, the disease is transmitted primarily by parenteral routes.

hepatitis E Hepatitis E virus (HEV) was originally identified by its association with waterborne epidemics of hepatitis in the Indian subcontinent. Since then, it has occurred in epidemics in Asia, Africa, the Middle East, Mexico, and Central and South America, typically after heavy rains and flooding. In the United States, hepatitis E has been found only in travelers returning from endemic areas. The virus is transmitted via the fecal-oral route, and the clinical course resembles that of hepatitis A. HEV has an incubation period of 15 to 64 days. There is no evidence at this time of a chronic form of hepatitis E.

hepatocyte Liver cell.

hepatomegaly Enlargement of the liver.

hepatorenal syndrome (HRS) A state of progressive oliguric renal failure associated with hepatic failure, resulting in functional impairment of kidneys with normal anatomic and morphologic features. It indicates a poor prognosis for the patient with hepatic failure and is often the cause of death in patients with cirrhosis.

hereditary chronic pancreatitis Pancreatitis that may be associated with *SPINK1* and *CFTR* gene mutations.

heritability The risk that a disorder can be transmitted to one's children in a recognizable pattern.

hernia A weakness in the abdominal muscle wall through which a segment of the bowel or other abdominal structure protrudes.

herniated nucleus pulposus (HNP) The protrusion (herniation) of the pulpy material from the center of a vertebral disk; herniated disks occur most often between the fourth and fifth lumbar vertebrae (L4-5) but may occur at other levels. A herniation in the lumbosacral area can press on the adjacent spinal nerve (usually the sciatic nerve), causing severe burning or stabbing pain into the leg or foot, or it may press on the spinal cord itself, causing leg weakness and bowel and bladder dysfunction. The specific area of pain depends on the level of herniation.

hernioplasty Surgical repair of a hernia in which the surgeon reinforces the weakened outside muscle wall with a mesh patch.

herniorrhaphy The surgical repair of a hernia.

heterotopic ossification Abnormal bony overgrowth, often into muscle; seen as a complication of prolonged immobility in patients with spinal cord injury.

hiatal hernia Protrusion of the stomach through the esophageal hiatus of the diaphragm and into the thorax. Also called "diaphragmatic hernia."

high-alert drug A drug that has an increased risk for causing patient harm if given in error.

high altitude disease (HAD) See *high altitude illnesses.*

high altitude illnesses Pathophysiologic responses in the body caused by exposure to low partial pressure of oxygen at high elevations.

high altitude pulmonary edema (HAPE) A form of acute mountain sickness often seen with high altitude cerebral edema. Clinical indicators include persistent dry cough, cyanosis of the lips and nail beds, tachycardia and tachypnea at rest, and rales auscultated in one or both lungs. Pink, frothy sputum is a late sign.

high-density lipoproteins (HDLs) Part of the total cholesterol value that should be more than 45 mg/dL for men and more than 55 mg/dL for women; "good" cholesterol.

highly sensitive C-reactive protein (hsCRP) A serum marker of inflammation and a common and critical component to the development of atherothrombosis.

high-output heart failure Heart failure that occurs when cardiac output remains normal or above normal. It is usually caused by increased metabolic needs or hyperkinetic conditions such as septicemia (fever), anemia, and hyperthyroidism. This type of heart failure is different from left- and right-sided heart failure, which are typically low-output states, and is not as common as other types.

hilum The area of the kidney in which the renal artery and nerve plexus enter and the renal vein and ureter exit. This area is not covered by the renal capsule.

hirsutism Abnormal growth of body hair, especially on the face, chest, and the linea alba of the abdomen of women.

homeostasis The narrow range of normal conditions (e.g., body temperature, blood electrolyte values, blood pH, blood volume) in the human body; the tendency to maintain a constant balance in normal body states.

homeostatic mechanism A safeguard or control mechanism within the human body that prevents dangerous changes.

homocysteine An essential sulfur-containing amino acid that is produced when dietary protein breaks down; elevated values (greater than 15 mmol/L) may be a risk factor for the development of cardiovascular disease.

homonymous hemianopsia Condition in which there is blindness in the same side of both eyes.

hordeolum An infection of the sweat glands in the eyelid.

hormone Chemical produced in the body that exerts its effects on specific tissues known as "target tissues."

hospice An interdisciplinary approach to facilitate quality of life and a "good" death for patients near the end of their lives, with care provided in a variety of settings.

Hospital Incident Command System (HICS) An organizational model for disaster management in which roles are formally structured under the hospital or long-term care facility incident commander, with clear lines of authority and accountability for specific resources.

hospital incident commander As defined in a hospital's emergency response plan, the person (either an emergency physician or administrator) who assumes overall leadership for implementing the institutional plan at the onset of a mass casualty incident. The hospital incident commander has a global view of the entire situation, facilitates patient movement through the system, and brings in resources to meet patient needs.

hospitalist Family practitioner or internist employed by a hospital.

human leukocyte antigen (HLA) Antigen that is present on the surfaces of nearly all body cells as a normal part of the person and acts as an antigen only if it enters another person's body.

human papilloma virus (HPV) test A test that can identify many high-risk types of HPV associated with the development of cervical cancer.

humoral immunity A type of immunity provided by antibodies circulating in body fluids.

Huntington disease (HD) A hereditary disorder transmitted as an autosomal dominant trait at the time of conception (formerly called "Huntington chorea"). Men and women between 35 and 50 years of age are affected; clinical onset is gradual. The two main symptoms are progressive mental status changes (leading to dementia) and choreiform movements (rapid, jerky movements) in the limbs, trunk, and facial muscles.

hydrocephalus The abnormal accumulation of cerebrospinal fluid within the skull.

hydronephrosis Abnormal enlargement of the kidney caused by a blockage of urine lower in the tract and filling of the kidney with urine.

hydrophilic Tending to absorb water readily.

hydrophobic Not readily absorbing water; waterproof.

hydrostatic pressure The force of the weight of water molecules pressing against the confining walls of a space.

hydrotherapy The application of water for treatment of injury or disease.

hydroureter Abnormal distention of the ureter.

hyperacusis An intolerance for sound levels that do not bother other people.

hyperaldosteronism Excessive mineralocorticoid production.

hypercalcemia A total serum calcium level above 10.5 mg/dL or 2.75 mmol/L, which can cause fatigue, anorexia, nausea and vomiting, constipation, polyuria, and serious damage to the urinary system.

hypercapnia Increased arterial carbon dioxide levels.

hypercarbia Increased partial pressure of arterial carbon dioxide ($PaCO_2$) levels.

hypercellularity An abnormal number of cells.

hyperemia Increased blood flow to an area.

hyperesthesia Abnormally increased sensation.

hyperextension A mechanism of injury that occurs when a part of the body is suddenly accelerated and then decelerated, causing extreme extension.

hyperflexion A mechanism of injury that occurs when a part of the body is suddenly and forcefully accelerated forward, causing extreme flexion.

hyperglycemia Abnormally high levels of blood glucose.

hyperinsulinemia Chronic high blood insulin levels.

hyperkalemia An elevated level of potassium in the blood.

hyperlipidemia An elevation of serum lipid (fat) levels in the blood.

hypermagnesemia A serum magnesium level above 2.1 mEq/L.

hypernatremia An excessive amount of sodium in the blood.

hyperopia An error of refraction that occurs when the eye does not refract light enough, causing images to fall (converge) behind the retina and resulting in poor near vision. Also called "farsightedness."

hyperosmotic Describes fluids with osmolarities (solute concentrations) greater than 300 mOsm/L; hyperosmotic fluids have a greater osmotic pressure than do isosmotic fluids and tend to pull water from the isosmotic fluid space into the hyperosmotic fluid space until an osmotic balance occurs. Also called "hypertonic."

hyperpharmacy See *polypharmacy*.

hyperphosphatemia A serum phosphorus level above 4.5 mg/dL.

hyperpituitarism Hormone oversecretion that occurs with pituitary tumors or hyperplasia.

hyperplasia Growth that causes tissue to increase in size by increasing the number of cells; abnormal overgrowth of tissue.

hyperpnea An abnormal increase in the depth of respiratory movements.

hypersensitivity An overreaction to a foreign substance.

hypertension A cardiovascular condition pertaining to people who have a systolic blood pressure of 140 mm Hg or higher or a diastolic blood pressure of 90 mm Hg or higher or who take medication to control blood pressure; approximately 1 of every 5 Americans has hypertension.

hypertensive crisis A severe elevation in blood pressure (greater than 180/120 mm Hg) that can cause damage to organs such as the kidneys or heart.

hyperthermia Elevated body temperature; fever.

hyperthyroidism A condition caused by excessive production of thyroid hormone.

hypertonia A condition of excessive muscle tone, which tends to cause fixed positions or contractures of the involved extremities and restricted range of motion of the joints.

hypertonic See *hyperosmotic*.

hypertriglyceridemia Elevated levels (150 mg/dL or above) of triglyceride in the blood.

hypertrophic cardiomyopathy (HCM) A type of cardiomyopathy that involves disarray of the myocardial fibers and asymmetric ventricular hypertrophy; leads to a stiff left ventricle that results in diastolic filling abnormalities.

hypertrophy The enlargement or overgrowth of an organ; tissue increases in size by the enlargement of each cell.

hyperuricemia An excess of uric acid in the blood.

hyperventilation A state of increased rate and depth of breathing.

hyperviscous The quality of being thicker than normal.

hypervolemia Increased plasma volume; or fluid excess.

hypocalcemia A total serum calcium level below 9.0 mg/dL or 2.25 mmol/L.

hypocapnia Decreased arterial carbon dioxide levels.

hypodermoclysis The slow infusion of isotonic fluids into subcutaneous tissue.

hypoesthesia Abnormally decreased sensation.

hypoglycemia Abnormally low levels of glucose in the blood.

hypokalemia A decreased serum potassium level; a common electrolyte imbalance.

hyponatremia A serum sodium level below 136 mEq/L (mmol/L).

hypo-osmotic Describes fluids with osmolarities of less than 270 mOsm/L. Hypo-osmolar fluids have a lower osmotic pressure than isosmotic fluids, and water tends to be pulled from the hypo-osmotic fluid space into the isosmotic fluid space until an osmotic balance occurs. Also called "hypotonic."

hypophonia Soft voice.

hypophosphatemia Inadequate levels of phosphate in the blood (below 3.0 mg/dL).

hypophysectomy Surgical removal of the pituitary gland.

hypoproteinemia A decrease in serum proteins.

hypothalamic-hypophysial portal system The small, closed circulatory system that the hypothalamus shares with the anterior pituitary gland, which allows hormones produced in the hypothalamus to travel directly to the anterior pituitary gland.

hypothalamus A structure within the brain; an integral part of autonomic nervous system control (controlling temperature and other functions) that is essential in intellectual function.

hypothermia A core body temperature less than 95° F (35° C).

hypotonia An abnormal condition of inadequate muscle tone, with an inability to maintain balance.

hypotonic See *hypo-osmotic.*

hypoventilation A state in which gas exchange at the alveolar-capillary membrane is inadequate so that too little oxygen reaches the blood and carbon dioxide is retained.

hypovolemia Abnormally decreased volume of circulating fluid in the body; fluid deficit.

hypoxemia (hypoxemic) Decreased blood oxygen levels; hypoxia.

hypoxia A reduction of oxygen supply to the tissues.

hysterosalpingogram An x-ray of the cervix, uterus, and fallopian tubes that is performed after injection of a contrast medium. This test is used in infertility workups to evaluate tubal anatomy and patency and uterine problems such as fibroids, tumors, and fistulas.

hysteroscopy Examination of the interior of the uterus and cervical canal using an endoscope.

I

icterus Yellow discoloration of the sclerae.

idiopathic chronic pancreatitis Pancreatitis that may be associated with *SPINK1* and *CFTR* gene mutations.

idiopathic seizure See *unclassified seizure.*

ileostomy The surgical creation of an opening into the ileum, usually by bringing the end of the terminal ileum through the abdominal wall and forming a stoma, or ostomy.

immediate memory Short-term or new memory. Test by asking the patient to repeat two or three unrelated words to make sure they were heard; after about 5 minutes, while continuing the examination, ask the patient to repeat the words.

immunity Resistance to infection; usually associated with the presence of antibodies or cells that act on specific microorganisms.

immunocompetent Having proper functioning of the body's ability to maintain itself and defend against disease.

immunoglobulin Antibody. Also called "gamma globulin."

impermeable Not porous.

implanted port A device used for long-term or frequent infusion therapy; consists of a portal body, a dense septum over a reservoir, and a catheter that is surgically implanted on the upper chest or upper extremity.

inactivation The process of binding an antibody to an antigen to cover the antigen's active site and to make the antigen harmless without destroying it. Also called "neutralization."

incisional hernia Protrusion of the intestine at the site of a previous surgical incision resulting from inadequate healing. Most often caused by postoperative wound infections, inadequate nutrition, and obesity. Also called "ventral hernia."

incomplete spinal cord injury An injury in which the spinal cord has been damaged in a way that allows some function or movement below the level of the injury.

incontinence Involuntary loss of urine or stool severe enough to cause social or hygienic problems.

independent living skills See *instrumental activities of daily living (IADLs).*

indirect inguinal hernia A sac formed from the peritoneum that contains a portion of the intestine or omentum. The hernia pushes downward at an angle into the inguinal canal. In males, indirect inguinal hernias can become large and often descend into the scrotum.

indolent Slow-growing.

induration Hardening.

infarction Necrosis, or cell death.

infective endocarditis A microbial infection (e.g., viruses, bacteria, fungi) involving the endocardium; previously called "bacterial endocarditis."

inferior vena cava filtration Surgical procedure in which the surgeon inserts a filter device percutaneously into the inferior vena cava of a patient with recurrent deep vein thrombosis (to prevent pulmonary emboli) or pulmonary emboli that do not respond to medical treatment. The device is meant to trap emboli in the inferior vena cava before they progress to the lungs. Holes in the device allow blood to pass through, thus not significantly interfering with the return of blood to the heart.

inferior wall myocardial infarction A type of myocardial infarction that occurs in patients with obstruction of the right coronary artery, causing significant damage to the right ventricle.

infiltrating ductal carcinoma The most common type of breast cancer; it originates in the mammary ducts and grows in the epithelial cells lining these ducts.

infiltration The leakage of IV solution into the tissues around the vein.

inflammatory breast cancer A rare but highly aggressive form of invasive breast cancer. Symptoms include swelling, skin redness, and pain in the breasts.

inflammatory cytokines Proteins produced primarily by white blood cells that assist in the inflammatory and immune responses of the body (e.g., tumor necrosis factor, interleukins).

inflow disease Chronic peripheral arterial disease with obstruction at or above the common iliac artery, abdominal aorta, or profunda femoris artery. The patient experiences discomfort in the lower back, buttocks, or thighs after walking a certain distance. The pain usually subsides with rest.

informatics A QSEN competency in which the nurse uses information and technology to communicate, manage knowledge, mitigate error, and support decision making.

infratentorial Located below the tentorium of the cerebellum.

infusate A solution that is infused into the body.

infusion therapy The delivery of parenteral medications and fluids through a variety of catheter types and locations using multiple techniques and procedures, such as intravenous and intra-arterial therapy to deliver solutions into the vascular system.

inpatient A patient who is admitted to a hospital.

inpatient rehabilitation facilities (IRFs) Free-standing rehabilitation hospitals, rehabilitation or skilled units within hospitals (e.g., transitional care units), and skilled nursing facilities to which the patient is typically admitted for 1 to 3 weeks or longer.

insensible water loss Water loss from the skin, lungs, and stool that cannot be controlled.

instrumental activities of daily living (IADLs) Special activities performed in the course of a day such as using the telephone, shopping, preparing food, and housekeeping. Also called "independent living skills."

insufflation The practice of injecting gas or air into a cavity before surgery to separate organs and improve visualization.

intensity A quality of sound that is expressed in decibels; generally, having a high degree of energy or activity.

intensivist A physician who specializes in critical care.

intention tremor A tremor that occurs when performing an activity.

interbody cage fusion Cagelike spinal device that is implanted into the space where a disk was removed. Bone graft tissue grows into and around the cage and creates a stable spine at that level.

intercostally Located between the ribs.

intermittent claudication A characteristic leg pain experienced by patients with chronic peripheral arterial disease. Typically, patients can walk only a certain distance before a cramping muscle pain forces them to stop. As the disease progresses, the patient can walk only shorter and shorter distances before pain recurs. Ultimately, pain may occur even at rest.

internal derangement A broad term for disturbances of an injured knee joint.

internal fixation The use of metal pins, screws, rods, plates, or prostheses to immobilize a fracture during healing. The surgeon makes an incision (open reduction) to gain access to the broken bone and implants one or more devices.

internal hemorrhoid A hemorrhoid that is located above the anal sphincter and cannot be seen on inspection of the perineal area.

internal urethral sphincter The smooth detrusor muscle that lines the interior of the bladder neck.

interstitial cystitis A bladder inflammation of unknown etiology that occurs predominantly in women and is characterized by urinary frequency and pain on bladder filling.

interstitial fluid A portion of the extracellular fluid that is between cells, sometimes called the "third space."

interstitial laser coagulation (ILC) Procedure for treating benign prostatic hyperplasia that uses laser energy to coagulate excess tissue. Also called "contact laser prostatectomy (CLP)."

intra-abdominal hypertension (IAH) Condition of sustained or repeated intra-abdominal pressure of 12 mm Hg or higher.

intra-abdominal pressure Pressure contained within the abdominal cavity.

intra-aortic balloon pump (IABP) An intra-aortic counterpulsation device. It may be used as an invasive intervention to improve myocardial perfusion during an acute myocardial infarction, reduce preload and afterload, and facilitate left ventricular ejection. It is also used when patients do not respond to drug therapy with improved tissue perfusion, decreased workload of the heart, and increased cardiac contractility.

intra-arterial infusion therapy The use of catheters placed into arteries to obtain repeated arterial blood samples, to monitor various hemodynamic pressures continuously, and to infuse chemotherapy agents or fibrinolytics.

intracapsular Located within the joint capsule.

intracellular fluid (ICF) The portion of total body water (about two thirds) that is found inside the cells.

intracerebral hemorrhage Bleeding within the brain tissue caused by the tearing of small arteries and veins in the subcortical white matter.

intracorporeal Situated or occurring inside the body.

intramedullary tumor Tumor originating within the spinal cord in the central gray matter and anterior commissure. It is often malignant.

intraocular pressure (IOP) Pressure of the fluid within the eye; may be measured by methods that involve direct contact with the eye or by noncontact techniques.

intraoperative During surgery.

intraosseous (IO) therapy Infusion therapy that is delivered to the vascular network in the long bones.

intraperitoneal (IP) infusion therapy The administration of antineoplastic agents into the peritoneal cavity.

intrapulmonary Within the respiratory tract.

intrarenal/intrinsic renal failure Decreased renal function resulting from damage to the glomeruli, interstitial tissue, or tubules. It can contribute to acute renal failure.

intrathecal Referring to the spine.

intravascular ultrasonography (IVUS) In cardiac catheterization, the use of a flexible catheter with a miniature transducer that emits sound waves. Sound waves are reflected off the plaque and the arterial wall, creating an image of the blood vessel; used as an alternative to injecting a contrast medium into the coronary arteries.

intravenous (systemic) fibrinolytic therapy The intravenous administration of thrombolytic agents to dissolve a thrombus.

intravesical Situated inside the bladder.

intrinsic factor A substance normally secreted by the gastric mucosa and needed for intestinal absorption of vitamin B_{12}. A deficiency of intrinsic factor and the resulting failure to absorb vitamin B_{12} lead to pernicious anemia.

intussusception The telescoping of a segment of the intestine within itself.

invasive hemodynamic monitoring System used in critical care areas to provide quantitative information about vascular capacity, blood volume, pump effectiveness, and tissue perfusion. It directly measures pressures in the heart and great vessels.

ion A substance found in body fluids that carries an electrical charge. Also called "electrolyte."

iontophoresis A treatment for lower back pain in which a small electrical current and dexamethasone are typically used.

ipsilateral Occurring on the same side.

iris The colored portion of the external eye; its center opening is the pupil. Muscles of the iris contract and relax to control pupil size and the amount of light entering the eye.

irreducible hernia A hernia that cannot be reduced or placed back into the abdominal cavity; requires immediate surgical evaluation.

irritability An overresponse to stimuli.

irritable bowel syndrome (IBS) A chronic gastrointestinal disorder characterized by chronic or recurrent diarrhea, constipation, and/or abdominal pain and bloating. Also called "spastic colon," "mucous colon," or "nervous colon."

ischemia Blockage of blood flow through a blood vessel resulting in a lack of oxygen. Prolonged severe ischemia can cause irreversible damage to tissue.

ischemic Cell dysfunction or death from a lack of oxygen resulting from decreased blood flow in a body part.

ischemic stroke A type of brain attack caused by occlusion of a cerebral artery by either a thrombus or an embolus. About 80% of all brain attacks are ischemic.

isoelectric Having equal electric potentials, such as in the heart.

isosmotic Having the same osmotic pressures. Also called "isotonic" or "normotonic."

isotonic See *isosmotic*.

J

jaundice A syndrome characterized by excessive circulating bilirubin levels. Liver cells cannot effectively excrete bilirubin, and skin and mucous membranes become characterized by a yellow coloration.

jejunostomy The surgical creation of an opening between the jejunum and the surface of the abdominal wall.

joint The place at which two or more bones come together. Also referred to as "articulation" of the joint. The primary function is to provide movement and flexibility in the body.

jugular venous distention (JVD) Enlargement of the jugular vein of the neck; caused by an increase in jugular venous pressure.

juxtaglomerular complex Specialized cells that produce and store renin in the afferent arteriole, efferent arteriole, and distal collecting tubule; taken together, the juxtaglomerular cells and the macula densa.

K

karyotype Technique used to make an organized arrangement of all the chromosomes within one cell during the metaphase section of mitosis.

keratin The protein produced by keratinocytes; makes the outermost skin layer waterproof.

keratinocytes Basal skin cells attached to the basement membrane of the epidermis that undergo cell division and differentiation to continuously renew skin tissue integrity and maintain optimal barrier function. As basal cells divide, keratinocytes are pushed upward and flattened to form the stratified layers of the epithelium (malpighian layers).

keratoconjunctivitis sicca A condition of the eyes that results from changes in tear composition, lacrimal gland malfunction, or altered tear distribution. Also called "dry eye syndrome."

keratoconus The degeneration of the corneal tissue resulting in abnormal corneal shape.

keratoplasty Corneal transplant. The surgical removal of diseased corneal tissue and replacement with tissue from a human donor cornea.

ketogenesis The conversion of fats to acids in the body.

ketone bodies Substances, including acetone, that are produced as by-products of the incomplete metabolism of fatty acids. When insulin is not available (as in uncontrolled diabetes mellitus), they accumulate in the blood and cause metabolic acidosis. Also called "ketones."

knee height caliper Device that uses the distance between the patella and heel to estimate height.

Kupffer cells Phagocytic cells that are part of the body's reticuloendothelial system and are involved in the protective function of the liver. Kupffer cells engulf harmful bacteria and anemic red blood cells.

Kussmaul respiration A type of breathing that occurs when excess acids caused by the absence of insulin increase hydrogen ion and carbon dioxide levels in the blood. This state triggers an increase in the rate and depth of respiration in an attempt to excrete more carbon dioxide and acid.

kwashiorkor Lack of protein quantity and quality in the presence of adequate calories. Body weight is somewhat normal, and serum proteins are low.

kyphoplasty A minimally invasive surgery for managing vertebral fractures in patients with osteoporosis. Bone cement is injected into the fracture site to provide pain relief, and an inflated balloon is used to restore height to the vertebra.

L

labyrinthectomy Surgical removal of the labyrinth; used as a radical treatment of Ménière's disease when medical therapy is ineffective and the patient already has significant hearing loss.

labyrinthitis An infection of the labyrinth of the ear; may occur as a complication of acute or chronic otitis media.

laceration A type of wound characterized by tearing or mangling and usually caused by sharp objects and projectiles.

lacrimal gland A small gland that produces tears; located in the upper outer part of each ocular orbit.

lacto-ovo-vegetarian A vegetarian diet pattern in which milk, cheese, eggs, and dairy foods are eaten but meat, fish, and poultry are avoided.

lactose intolerance The inability to convert lactose (found in milk and dairy products) to glucose and galactose in the body.

lacto-vegetarian A vegetarian diet pattern in which milk, cheese, and dairy foods are eaten but meat, fish, poultry, and eggs are avoided.

laparoscopy A minimally invasive procedure in which the surgeon makes several small incisions near the umbilicus through which a small endoscope is placed to examine the abdomen; direct examination of the pelvic cavity through an endoscope.

laparotomy An open surgical approach in which a large abdominal incision is made.

laryngectomee A person who has had a laryngectomy.

laryngopharynx The area behind the larynx that extends from the base of the tongue to the esophagus. It is the critical dividing point at which solid foods and fluids are separated from air.

larynx The "voice box"; it is composed of several cartilages and is located above the trachea and just below the throat at the base of the tongue; part of the upper respiratory tract.

laser An acronym for light amplification by stimulated emission of radiation. As a surgical tool, a laser emits a high-powered beam of light that cuts tissue more cleanly than do scalpel blades. A laser creates intense heat, rapidly clots blood vessels or tissue, and turns target tissue (e.g., a tumor) into vapor.

latency period The time between the initiation of a cell and the development of an overt tumor.

latex allergy Reactions to exposure to latex in gloves and other medical products; reactions include rashes, nasal or eye symptoms, and asthma.

latrodectism A syndrome caused by the venom of a black widow spider bite in which neurotransmitter releases from nerve terminals to cause severe abdominal pain, muscle rigidity and spasm, hypertension, and nausea and vomiting.

lead In an ECG, the provider of one view of the heart's electrical activity.

lead axis In electrocardiography, the imaginary line that joins the positive and negative poles of the lead systems.

left shift An increase in the band cells (immature neutrophils) in the white blood cell differential count; an early indication of infection.

left-sided heart (ventricular) failure Inadequacy of the left ventricle of the heart to pump adequately; results in decreased tissue perfusion from poor cardiac output and pulmonary congestion from increased pressure in the pulmonary vessels; typical causes include hypertensive, coronary artery, or valvular disease involving the mitral or aortic valve. Most heart failure begins with failure of the left ventricle and progresses to failure of both ventricles.

legally competent A person 18 years of age or older, a pregnant or a married minor, a legally emancipated (free) minor who is self-supporting, or a person not declared incompetent by a court of law.

leiomyomas Benign, slow-growing solid tumors of the uterine myometrium (muscle layer). These are the most commonly occurring pelvic tumors. Also called "myomas" and "fibroids."

lens The circular, convex structure of the eye that lies behind the iris and in front of the vitreous body. Normally transparent, the lens bends the rays of light entering through the pupil so they focus on the retina. The curve of the lens changes to focus on near or distant objects.

leptin A hormone that is released by fat cells and possibly by gastric cells; it also acts on the hypothalamus to control appetite.

leukemia A type of cancer with uncontrolled production of immature white blood cells in the bone marrow; the bone marrow becomes overcrowded with immature, nonfunctional cells, and the production of normal blood cells is greatly decreased.

leukocyte White blood cell (WBC); this immune system cell protects the body from the effects of invasion by organisms.

leukopenia A reduction in the number of white blood cells.

leukoplakia White, patchy lesions on a mucous membrane.

levels of evidence Term used to refer to the status, rank, or strength of evidence.

LGBTQ Acronym for "lesbian, gay, bisexual, transgender, and queer/questioning" culture.

libido Sexual desire.

lichenified An abnormal thickening of the skin to a leathery appearance; can occur in patients with chronic dermatitis because of their continual rubbing of the area to relieve itching.

Lichtenberg figures Branching or ferning marks that appear on the skin as a result of a lightning strike. Also called "keraunographic markings" or "erythematous arborization."

life review A structured process of reflecting on one's life that is often facilitated by an interviewer.

light reflex The reflection of the otoscope's light off the eardrum in the form of a clearly demarcated triangle of light in the normal ear.

limited cutaneous systemic sclerosis Thick skin that is usually limited to sites distal to the elbow and knee but also involves the face and neck.

lipid Fat, including cholesterol and triglycerides, that can be measured in the blood.

lipolysis The decomposition or splitting up of fat to provide fuel for energy when liver glucose is unavailable.

liposuction A cosmetic procedure to reduce the amount of adipose tissue in selected areas of the body.

lithotripsy The use of sound, laser, or dry shock wave energy to break a kidney stone into small fragments. Also called "extracorporeal shock wave lithotripsy."

living will A legal document that instructs physicians and family members about what life-sustaining treatment is wanted (or not wanted) if the patient becomes unable to make decisions.

lobectomy Surgical removal of an entire lung lobe.

lobular carcinoma in situ (LCIS) A noninvasive form of breast cancer that does not show up as a calcified cluster on a mammogram and is therefore most often diagnosed incidentally during a biopsy for another problem.

local anesthesia Anesthesia that is delivered by applying it to the skin or mucous membranes of the area to be anesthetized or by injecting it directly into the tissue around an incision, wound, or lesion.

locus The specific chromosome location for a gene.

log rolling Turning technique in which the patient turns all at once while his or her back is kept as straight as possible.

loop electrosurgical excision procedure (LEEP) Diagnostic procedure/treatment in which a thin loop-wire electrode that transmits a painless electrical current is used to cut away affected cervical cancer tissue.

lordosis The anterior concavity in the curvature of the lumbar and cervical spine when viewed from the side; a common finding in pregnancy and abdominal obesity.

Lou Gehrig's disease See *amyotrophic lateral sclerosis (ALS)*.

low back pain (LBP) Pain in the lumbosacral region of the back caused by muscle strain or spasm, ligament sprain, disk degeneration, or herniation of the nucleus pulposus from the center of the disk. Herniated disks occur most often between the fourth and fifth lumbar vertebrae (L4-5) but may occur at other levels.

low-density lipoproteins (LDLs) Part of the total cholesterol value that should be less than 130 mg/dL; "bad" cholesterol.

lower esophageal sphincter (LES) The portion of the esophagus proximal to the gastroesophageal junction; when at rest, the sphincter is closed to prevent reflux of gastric contents into the esophagus.

low-intensity pulsed ultrasound A method using ultrasonic waves to promote bone union in slow-healing fractures or for new fractures as an alternative to surgery.

low-profile gastrostomy device (LPGD) A gastrostomy device that uses a firm or balloon-style internal bumper or retention disk; an anti-reflux valve keeps gastric contents from leaking onto the skin.

loxoscelism Systemic effects from the injected toxin of a spider bite.

lumbar puncture (spinal tap) The insertion of a spinal needle into the subarachnoid space between the third and fourth (sometimes the fourth and fifth) lumbar vertebrae to withdraw spinal fluid for analysis.

lumen   The inside cavity of a tube or tubular organ, such as a blood vessel or airway.

lung compliance   The quality of elasticity of the lungs.

lunula   The white crescent-shaped portion of the nail at the lower end of the nail plate.

lurch   An abnormality in the swing phase of gait; occurs when the muscles in the buttocks or legs are too weak to allow the person to change weight from one foot to the other.

Lyme disease   A systemic infectious disease that is caused by the spirochete *Borrelia burgdorferi* and results from the bite of an infected deer tick. Signs and symptoms include a large "bull's-eye" circular rash, malaise, fever, headache, and muscle or joint aches.

lymphadenopathy   Persistently enlarged lymph nodes.

lymphedema   Abnormal accumulation of protein fluid in the subcutaneous tissue of the affected limb after a mastectomy.

lymphoblastic   Pertaining to abnormal leukemic cells that come from the lymphoid pathways and develop into lymphocytes.

lymphocytic   Pertaining to abnormal leukemic cells that come from the lymphoid pathways.

lymphokine   Cytokine produced by T-cells.

lysis   Breakage, for example, of a cell membrane.

M

macrocytic anemia   A form of vitamin B_{12} deficiency anemia characterized by abnormally large precursor cells.

macrovascular   Referring to large blood vessels.

macular   Referring to a macula, a discolored spot on the skin that is not raised above the surface.

macular degeneration   The deterioration of the macula, the area of central vision.

magnesium (Mg^{2+})   A mineral that forms a cation when dissolved in water.

magnetoencephalography (MEG)   A noninvasive imaging technique that measures the magnetic fields produced by electrical activity in the brain via extremely sensitive devices such as superconducting quantum interference devices (SQUIDs).

malabsorption   A syndrome associated with a variety of disorders and intestinal surgical procedures and characterized by impaired intestinal absorption of nutrients.

malignant   Referring to cancer.

malignant cell growth   Altered cell growth that is serious and, without intervention, leads to death; cancer.

malignant hypertension   A severe type of elevated blood pressure that rapidly progresses, with systolic blood pressure greater than 200 mm Hg and diastolic blood pressure greater than 150 mm Hg (greater than 130 mm Hg when there are pre-existing complications).

malignant transformation   The process of changing a normal cell into a cancer cell.

mammography   An x-ray of the soft tissue of the breast.

mandibulectomy   Surgical removal of the jaw.

marasmic-kwashiorkor   A combined protein and energy malnutrition that often presents clinically when metabolic stress is imposed on a chronically starved patient.

marasmus   A calorie malnutrition in which body fat and protein are wasted but serum proteins are often preserved.

marsupialization   Surgical formation of a pouch that is a new duct opening.

mass casualty event   A situation affecting the public health that is defined based on the resource availability of a particular community or hospital facility. When the number of casualties exceeds the resource capabilities, a disaster situation is recognized to exist.

mastication   The process of chewing.

mastoiditis   An acute or chronic infection of the mastoid air cells caused by untreated or inadequately treated otitis media.

maze procedure   An open chest surgical technique often performed with coronary artery bypass grafting for patients in atrial fibrillation with decompensation.

mean arterial pressure (MAP)   The arterial blood pressure (between 60 and 70 mm Hg) necessary to maintain perfusion of major body organs, such as the kidneys and brain.

mechanical débridement   Method of débriding a wound by mechanical entrapment and detachment of dead tissue.

mechanical obstruction   The physical obstruction of the bowel by disorders outside the intestine (e.g., adhesions or hernias) or by blockages in the lumen of the intestine (e.g., tumors, inflammation, strictures, or fecal impactions).

mediastinal shift   A shift of central thoracic structures toward one side; seen on chest x-ray.

mediastinitis   Infection of the mediastinum.

medical command physician   As defined in a hospital's emergency response plan, the person responsible for determining the number, acuity, and medical resource needs of victims arriving from the incident scene and for organizing the emergency health care team response to injured or ill patients.

medical harm   Physician incidents and all errors caused by members of the health care team or system that lead to patient injury or death.

medical nutrition supplements (MNSs)   Enteral products taken by patients who cannot consume enough nutrients in their usual diet (e.g., Ensure, Boost).

medication overuse headache   See *rebound headache.*

medulla   A general term for the most interior portion of an organ or structure.

melena   Blood in the stool, with the appearance of black tarry stools.

memory cell   A type of B-lymphocyte that remains sensitized but does not start to produce antibodies until the next exposure to the same antigen.

Ménière's disease   Tinnitus, one-sided sensorineural hearing loss, and vertigo that is related to overproduction or decreased reabsorption of endolymphatic fluid and causes a distortion of the entire inner canal system.

meninges   The immediate protective covering of the brain and the spinal cord.

meningioma   A type of benign brain tumor that arises from the coverings of the brain (the meninges) and causes compression and displacement of adjacent brain tissue.

meningitis   Inflammation, usually bacterial or viral, of the arachnoid and pia mater of the brain and spinal cord and the cerebrospinal fluid. May be caused by bacteria or viruses; symptoms are the same regardless of the causative organism.

meniscectomy   Surgical excision of a meniscus, as in a knee joint.

menses   The monthly flow of blood from the genital tract of women.

metabolic syndrome   A collection of related health problems with insulin resistance as a main feature. Other features include obesity, low levels of physical activity, hypertension, high blood levels of cholesterol, and elevated triglyceride levels. Metabolic syndrome increases the risk for coronary heart disease. Also called "syndrome X."

metastasis   The growth and spread of cancer.

metastasize   To spread cancer from the main tumor site to many other body sites.

metastatic   Referring to disease, such as cancer, that transfers from one organ to another organ or part not directly connected; pertains to additional tumors that form after cancer cells move from the primary location by breaking off from the original group and establishing remote colonies.

methemoglobinemia   The conversion of normal hemoglobin to methemoglobin.

microalbuminuria   The presence of very small amounts of albumin in the urine that are not measurable by a urine dipstick or usual urinalysis procedures. Specialized assays are used to analyze a freshly voided urine specimen for microscopic levels of albumin.

microcytic   Abnormally small in size, such as an abnormally small red blood cell.

microvascular   Referring to small blood vessels.

microvascular decompression   A surgical procedure to relieve the pain of trigeminal neuralgia by relocating a small artery that compresses the trigeminal nerve as it enters the pons. The surgeon carefully lifts the loop of the artery off the nerve and places a small silicone sponge between the vessel and the nerve.

midline catheter   A type of catheter that is 6 to 8 inches long and inserted through the veins of the antecubital fossa; used in therapies lasting from 1 to 4 weeks.

migraine headache   An episodic familial disorder manifested by a unilateral, frontotemporal, throbbing pain that is often worse behind one eye or ear. It is often accompanied by a sensitive scalp, anorexia, photophobia, and nausea with or without vomiting. Three categories of migraine headache are migraines with aura, migraines without aura, and atypical migraines.

migratory arthritis   In the early stage of rheumatoid arthritis, symptoms that are migrating or involve more joints.

miliary tuberculosis   See *hematogenous tuberculosis.*

minimally invasive direct coronary artery bypass (MIDCAB)   Surgical procedure that does not require cardiopulmonary bypass and may be used for patients with a lesion of the left anterior descending artery. Also known as "keyhole" surgery.

minimally invasive esophagectomy (MIE)   A laparoscopic surgical procedure to remove part of the esophagus; may be performed in patients with early-stage cancer.

minimally invasive inguinal hernia repair (MIIHR)   Surgical repair of an inguinal hernia through a laparoscope, which is the treatment of choice.

minimally invasive surgery (MIS)   A general term for any surgery performed using laparoscopic technique.

Minimum Data Set (MDS) 3.0   Interdisciplinary tool required by the U.S. Centers for Medicare and Medicaid Services (CMS) to assess patients (residents) in nursing homes.

miosis   Constriction of the pupil of the eye.

mitosis   Cell division.

mitotic index   The percentage of actively dividing cells within a tumor.

mitral regurgitation   Inability of the mitral valve to close completely during systole, which allows the backflow of blood into the left atrium when the left ventricle contracts; usually due to fibrosis and calcification caused by rheumatic disease. Also called "mitral insufficiency."

mitral stenosis   Thickening of the mitral valve due to fibrosis and calcification and usually caused by rheumatic fever. The valve leaflets fuse and become stiff, the chordae tendineae contract, and the valve opening narrows, preventing normal blood flow from the left atrium to the left ventricle. As a result, left atrial pressure rises, the left atrium dilates, pulmonary artery pressures increase, and the right ventricle hypertrophies.

mitral valve prolapse (MVP)   Dysfunction of the mitral valve that occurs because the valvular leaflets enlarge and prolapse into the left atrium during systole; usually benign but may progress to pronounced mitral regurgitation.

mixed conductive-sensorineural hearing loss   A profound hearing loss that results from a combination of both conductive and sensorineural types of hearing loss.

modifiable risk factor   A factor in disease development that can be altered or controlled by the patient. Examples include elevated serum cholesterol levels, cigarette smoking, hypertension, impaired glucose tolerance, obesity, physical inactivity, and stress.

monokine   Cytokine made by macrophages, neutrophils, eosinophils, and monocytes.

morbid obesity   A weight that has a severely negative effect on health; usually more than 100% above ideal body weight or a body mass index greater than 40.

morbidity   An illness or an abnormal condition or quality.

mortality   Death.

Morton's neuroma   Plantar digital neuritis, a condition in which a small tumor grows in a digital nerve of the foot. The patient usually describes the pain as an acute, burning sensation in the web space that involves the entire surface of the third and fourth toes.

motor   Facilitating movement.

motor aphasia   See *expressive aphasia.*

motor cortex   Area in the frontal lobe of the brain that controls voluntary movement.

mourning   The outward social expression of loss.

mucositis   Open sores on mucous membranes.

multi-casualty event   A disaster event in which a limited number of victims or casualties are involved and can be managed by a hospital using local resources.

multigated blood pool scanning   In nuclear cardiology, cardiac blood pool imaging is a non-invasive test to evaluate cardiac motion and calculate ejection fraction by using a computer to synchronize the patient's electrocardiogram with pictures obtained by a gamma-scintillation camera. In multigated blood pool scanning, the computer breaks the time between R waves into fractions of a second, called "gates." The camera records blood flow through the heart during each gate. By analyzing information from multiple gates, the computer can evaluate ventricular wall motion and calculate ejection fraction (percentage of the left ventricular volume that is ejected with each contraction) and ejection velocity.

multiple organ dysfunction syndrome (MODS)   The sequence of inadequate blood flow to body tissues, which deprives cells of oxygen and leads to anaerobic metabolism with acidosis, hyperkalemia, and tissue ischemia; this is followed by dramatic changes in vital organs and leads to the release of toxic metabolites and destructive enzymes.

multiple sclerosis (MS)   A chronic autoimmune disease that affects the myelin sheath and conduction pathway of the central nervous system. It is one of the leading causes of neurologic disability in persons 20 to 40 years of age.

murmur   Abnormal heart sound that reflects turbulent blood flow through normal or abnormal valves; murmurs are classified according to their timing in the cardiac cycle (systolic or diastolic) and their intensity depending on their level of loudness.

muscle biopsy   The extraction of a muscle specimen for the diagnosis of atrophy (as in muscular dystrophy) and inflammation (as in polymyositis).

muscular dystrophy (MD)   A group of degenerative myopathies characterized by weakness and atrophy of muscle without nervous system involvement. At least nine types have been clinically identified and can be broadly categorized as slowly progressive or rapidly progressive.

mutation   A change in deoxyribonucleic acid (DNA) that is passed from one generation to another.

myalgia   Muscle aches/muscle pain.

myasthenia gravis (MG)   A chronic autoimmune disease of the neuromuscular junction. It is characterized by remissions and exacerbations, with fatigue and weakness primarily in the muscles innervated by the cranial nerves and in the skeletal and respiratory muscles. It ranges from mild disturbances of the ocular muscles to a rapidly developing, generalized weakness that may lead to death from respiratory failure.

myasthenic crisis   Undermedication with cholinesterase inhibitors.

mydriasis   Dilation of the pupil of the eye.

myelin sheath   A white, lipid covering of the axon.

myelocytic   Pertaining to leukemias in which the abnormal cells come from the myeloid pathways.

myelogenous   Pertaining to leukemias in which the abnormal cells come from the myeloid pathways.

myelography   Radiography of the spine after injection of contrast medium into the subarachnoid space of the spine; used to visualize the vertebral column, intervertebral disks, spinal nerve roots, and blood vessels.

myocardial hypertrophy   Enlargement of the myocardium.

myocardial infarction (MI)   Injury and necrosis of myocardial tissue that occurs when the tissue is abruptly and severely deprived of oxygen; usually caused by atherosclerosis of a coronary artery, rupture of the plaque, subsequent thrombosis, and occlusion of blood flow.

myocardial nuclear perfusion imaging (MNPI)   The use of radionuclide techniques in which radioactive tracer substances are used to view, record, and evaluate cardiovascular abnormalities; useful for detecting myocardial infarction and decreased myocardial blood flow and for evaluating left ventricular ejection.

myocardium   The heart muscle.

myoglobin   A low–molecular-weight heme protein found in cardiac and skeletal muscle; an early marker of myocardial infarction.

myoglobinuria   The release of muscle myoglobulin into the urine.

myomas   See *leiomyomas.*

myomectomy   The surgical removal of leiomyomas with preservation of the uterus.

myopathy   A problem in muscle tissue.

myopia   An error of refraction that occurs when the eye over-refracts or over-bends the light and focuses images in front of the retina; this results in normal near vision but poor distance vision. Also called "nearsightedness."

myositis   Inflammation of a muscle.

myosplint   Electrical stimulation of tension splints in the heart to help the ventricle change to a more normal shape in the patient with heart failure; under investigation in Europe and the United States.

myringoplasty   Surgical reconstruction of the eardrum.

myringotomy   The surgical creation of a hole in the eardrum; performed to drain middle-ear fluids and relieve pain in the patient with otitis media (middle-ear infection).

myxedema   Dry, waxy swelling of the skin that is accompanied by nonpitting edema (especially around the eyes, in the hands and feet, and between the shoulder blades) and is associated with primary hypothyroidism.

myxedema coma   A rare, serious complication of untreated or poorly treated hypothyroidism in which decreased metabolism causes the heart muscle to become flabby and the chamber size to increase, resulting in decreased cardiac output and decreased perfusion to the brain and other vital organs.

N

nadir In cancer treatment therapy, the period of greatest bone marrow suppression, when the patient's platelet count may be very low.

nasoduodenal tube (NDT) A tube that is inserted through a nostril and into the small intestine.

nasoenteric tube (NET) Any feeding tube that is inserted nasally and then advanced into the gastrointestinal tract.

nasogastric (NG) tube A tube that is inserted through a nostril and into the stomach for liquid feeding or for withdrawing gastric contents.

nasotracheal The route for inserting a tube into the trachea via the nose.

natal sex A person's genital anatomy present at birth. Also known as "biological sex."

National Patient Safety Goals (NPSGs) Goals published by The Joint Commission that require health care organizations to focus on specific priority safety practices.

natural chemical débridement Method of débriding a wound by creating an environment that promotes self-digestion of dead tissues by bacterial enzymes.

near point of vision The closest distance at which the eye can see an object clearly.

near-drowning Recovery after submersion in a liquid medium (usually water); this term is no longer used because language that describes drowning incidents has been standardized.

near-syncope Dizziness with an inability to remain in an upright position.

necrotizing hemorrhagic pancreatitis (NHP) Inflammation of the pancreas that is characterized by diffusely bleeding pancreatic tissue with fibrosis and tissue death. This form affects about 20% of patients with pancreatitis.

needle thoracostomy A quick, temporary method of chest decompression in which a large-bore needle is used to vent trapped air pending chest tube insertion.

negative deflection In electrocardiography, the flow of electrical current in the heart (cardiac axis) away from the positive pole and toward the negative pole.

negative feedback control mechanism The condition of maintaining a constant output of a system by exerting an inhibitory control on a key step by a product of that system. Used in a series of reactions that control hormone secretion and cellular activity based on responses to correct any movement away from normal function. An example of a simple negative feedback hormone response is the control of insulin secretion in which the action of insulin (decreasing blood glucose levels) is the opposite of the condition that stimulated insulin secretion (elevated blood glucose levels).

negative nitrogen balance A net loss of protein that occurs when the breakdown (degradation) of protein exceeds buildup (synthesis).

neglect In nursing, failure to provide for a patient's basic needs.

neoadjuvant therapy Treatment of a cancerous tumor with chemotherapy to shrink the tumor before it is surgically removed.

neoplasia Any new or continued cell growth not needed for normal development or replacement of dead and damaged tissues.

nephrectomy The surgical removal of the kidney.

nephrolithiasis The formation of stones in the kidney.

nephron The "working" unit of the kidney where urine is formed from blood. Each kidney consists of about 1 million nephrons, and each nephron separately makes urine. There are two types of nephrons: cortical and juxtamedullary.

nephropathy Pathologic change in the kidney that reduces kidney function and leads to renal failure.

nephrosclerosis Thickening in the nephron blood vessels that results in narrowing of the vessel lumen, with decreased renal blood flow and chronically hypoxic kidney tissue.

nephrostomy The surgical creation of an opening directly into the kidney; performed to divert urine externally and prevent further damage to the kidney when a stricture is causing hydronephrosis and cannot be corrected with urologic procedures.

nephrotic syndrome (NS) A condition of increased glomerular permeability that allows larger molecules to pass through the membrane into the urine and be removed from the blood. This process causes massive loss of protein into the urine, edema formation, and decreased plasma albumin levels.

neuraxial Referring to the epidural or spinal area.

neuritic plaques Degenerating nerve terminals found particularly in the hippocampus, an important part of the limbic system, and marked by increased amounts of an abnormal protein called "beta amyloid"; a characteristic change of the brain found in patients with Alzheimer's disease.

neurofibrillary tangles Tangled masses of fibrous elements throughout the neurons; a classic finding at autopsy in the brains of patients with Alzheimer's disease.

neurogenic shock Hypotension and bradycardia associated with cervical spinal injuries and caused by a loss of autonomic function. The patient is at greatest risk in the first 24 hours after injury.

neuroglia cells Cells of varying size and shape that provide protection, structure, and nutrition for the neurons.

neurohypophysis The posterior lobe of the pituitary gland that stores hormones produced in the hypothalamus.

neuroma A sensitive tumor consisting of nerve cells and nerve fibers.

neuron Excitable nerve cell that processes and transmits information through electrical and chemical signals.

neuropathic pain A type of chronic non-cancer pain that results from a nerve injury. Examples of causes include diabetic neuropathy, postherpetic neuralgia, radiculopathy (spinal nerve damage), and trigeminal neuralgia. Neuropathic pain is described as burning, shooting, stabbing, and the sensation of "pins and needles."

neurotransmitter Regulatory chemical that exerts inhibitory (slowing down) or excitatory (speeding up) activity at postsynaptic nerve cell membranes. Acetylcholine, norepinephrine, epinephrine, dopamine, and serotonin are neurotransmitters.

neurovascular assessment Assessment of the neuromuscular system that includes inspection of skin color, temperature, and capillary refill distal to an injury, surgical procedure, or cast. Palpation of pulses in the extremities below level of injury and assessment of sensation, movement, and pain in the injured part give a complete assessment.

neutralization See *inactivation*.

neutropenia Decreased numbers of leukocytes, especially neutrophils, which causes immunosuppression.

neutrophilia Increased number of circulating neutrophils.

nevus A mole; a benign skin growth of the pigment-forming cells.

new-onset angina Cardiac chest pain that occurs for the first time.

nitroglycerin (NTG) A drug prescribed for patients with angina. It increases collateral blood flow, redistributes blood flow toward the subendocardium, and causes dilation of the coronary arteries.

nits Lice eggs.

N-methyl-D-aspartate (NMDA) receptor antagonist A group of drugs that block excess amounts of glutamate, which damages nerve cells in the brain; used to treat Alzheimer's disease.

nociception Term used to describe how pain becomes a conscious experience.

nociceptive pain Pain related to the skin, musculoskeletal structures, or body organs.

nociceptors Sensory neurons that respond to pain or other noxious stimuli.

nocturia The need to urinate excessively at night. Also called "nocturnal polyuria."

nocturnal polyuria See *nocturia*.

nonadherence In health care, accidental failure by a patient to take medication.

noncompliance In health care, deliberate failure by a patient to take medication.

nonmaleficence Ethical principle that emphasizes the importance of preventing harm and ensuring the patient's well-being.

nonmechanical obstruction Intestinal obstruction that does not involve a physical obstruction in or outside the intestine. Instead, decreased or absent peristalsis results in a slowing of the movement or a backup of intestinal contents. This is also known as "paralytic ileus" or "adynamic ileus" because it is a result of neuromuscular disturbance.

nonmodifiable risk factor Factor in disease development that cannot be altered or controlled by the patient. Examples include age, gender, family history, and ethnic background.

non–ST-segment elevation myocardial infarction (NSTEMI) Myocardial infarction in which the patient typically has ST and T-wave changes on a 12-lead ECG; this indicates myocardial ischemia.

nonsustained ventricular tachycardia (NSVT) Occurrence of three or more successive premature ventricular complexes.

nontunneled percutaneous central venous catheter (CVC) A type of catheter, usually 15 to 20 cm long and with dual or triple lumens, that is inserted through the subclavian vein in the upper chest or through the jugular veins in the neck using sterile technique.

nonurgent In a three-tiered triage scheme, the category that includes patients who can generally tolerate waiting several hours for health care services without a significant risk of clinical deterioration, such as those with sprains, strains, or simple fractures.

normal flora The microorganisms living in or on the human host without causing disease; the bacteria that are characteristic of each body location. Normal flora often compete with and prevent infection from unfamiliar microorganisms attempting to invade a body site.

normal sinus rhythm (NSR) The rhythm originating from the sinoatrial node (dominant pacemaker), with atrial and ventricular rates of 60 to 100 beats/min and regular atrial and ventricular rhythms.

normotonic See *isosmotic.*

North American pit vipers The Crotalidae, one of two families of indigenous poisonous snakes in North America; named for the characteristic depression between each eye and nostril. They include rattlesnakes, copperheads, and water moccasins and account for most poisonous snakebites in the United States.

nosocomial (infection) Acquired in an inpatient health care setting; for example, infections that were not present at hospital admission. Also called "hospital-acquired infections" and "health care–associated infections."

nothing by mouth (NPO) No eating, drinking (including water), or smoking.

nuchal rigidity Stiff neck, which can be a sign of cerebrospinal fluid leak; nuchal rigidity is not checked until a spinal cord injury has been ruled out.

nucleotide The final form of a base that actually gets put into the strand of deoxyribonucleic acid. A nucleoside becomes a complete nucleotide by the attachment of phosphate groups.

nursing assistant A member of the rehabilitative health care team who assists the registered nurse in the care of patients.

nursing technician See *nursing assistant.*

nutritional screening A screening by the health care provider that includes visual inspection, measured height and weight, weight history, usual eating habits, ability to chew and swallow, and any recent changes in appetite or food intake. The screening is a way to determine which patients need more extensive nutritional assessment.

nutritional status Reflects the balance between nutrient requirements and intake.

nystagmus Involuntary, rapid eye movements.

O

obesity An increase in body weight at least 20% above the upper limit of the normal range for ideal body weight, with an excess amount of body fat; in an adult, a body mass index greater than 30.

obligatory urine output The minimum amount of urine per day needed to dissolve and excrete toxic waste products.

obstipation The inability to pass stool; intractable constipation.

obstruction Blockage.

obstructive jaundice Jaundice caused by an impediment to the flow of bile from the liver to the duodenum; may be caused by edema of the ducts or gallstones.

obstructive sleep apnea A breathing disruption during sleep that lasts at least 10 seconds and occurs a minimum of 5 times in an hour.

Occupational Safety and Health Administration (OSHA) A federal agency that protects workers from injury or illness at their place of employment.

occupational therapist (OT, OTR) A member of the rehabilitation health care team who works to develop the patient's fine motor skills used for activities of daily living and the skills related to coordination and cognitive retraining.

odynophagia Pain on swallowing.

oligomenorrhea Scant or infrequent menses.

oligospermia Low sperm count.

oliguria Decreased excretion of urine in relation to amount of fluid intake; usually defined as urine output less than 400 mL/day.

oncogene Proto-oncogene that has been "turned on" and can cause cells to change from normal cells to cancer cells.

oncogenesis Cancer development.

oncovirus Virus that causes cancer.

oophorectomy Surgical removal of the ovary.

open fracture A fracture in which the skin surface over the broken bone is disrupted, causing an external wound. Also called "compound fracture."

open reduction The reduction of a fracture after surgical incision into the site to allow direct visualization of the fracture. See *internal fixation.*

open traumatic brain injury A type of traumatic primary brain injury that occurs with a skull fracture or when the skull is pierced by a penetrating object. The integrity of the brain and the dura is violated and there is exposure to outside contaminants, with damage to the underlying vessels, dural sinus, brain, and cranial nerves.

opportunistic infection Infection caused by organisms that are present as part of the normal environment and would be kept in check by normal immune function.

optic disc The point at the inside back of the eye where the optic nerve enters the eyeball. It appears as a creamy pink to white depressed area in the retina and contains only nerve fibers and no photoreceptor cells.

optic fundus The area at the inside back of the eye that can be seen with an ophthalmoscope.

optic nerve The nerve of sight; connects the optic disc to the brain.

orbit The bony socket of the skull that surrounds and protects the eye along with the attached muscles, nerves, vessels, and tear-producing glands.

orchiectomy The surgical removal of one or both testes.

orchitis An acute testicular inflammation resulting from trauma or infection.

orexin Neuropeptide that is an appetite stimulant.

orotracheal The route for inserting a tube into the trachea via the mouth.

orthopnea Shortness of breath that occurs when lying down but is relieved by sitting up.

orthostatic Pertaining to or caused by standing erect.

orthostatic hypotension A decrease in blood pressure (20 mm Hg systolic and/or 10 mm Hg diastolic) that occurs during the first few seconds to minutes after changing from a sitting or lying position to a standing position. Also called "postural hypotension."

orthotopic The most common type of transplantation procedure in which a diseased organ is removed and a donor organ is grafted in its place. For example, during heart transplantation, the surgeon removes the diseased heart and leaves the posterior walls of the patient's atria, which serve as the anchor for the donor heart; anastomoses are made between the recipient and donor atria, aorta, and pulmonary arteries.

osmolality The number of milliosmoles in a kilogram of solution.

osmolarity The number of milliosmoles in a liter of solution.

osmosis The movement of a solvent across a semipermeable membrane (a membrane that allows the solvent but not the solute to pass through) from a lesser to a greater concentration.

ossiculoplasty Replacement of the ossicles within the middle ear.

osteitis deformans See *Paget's disease.*

osteoarthritis Noninflammatory form of arthritis characterized by the progressive deterioration and loss of cartilage in one or more joints; most common form of arthritis.

osteoblast Cell associated with formation of bone.

osteoclast Cell associated with destruction or resorption of bone.

osteocyte Bone cell.

osteomalacia Abnormal softening of the bone tissue characterized by inadequate mineralization of osteoid. It is the adult equivalent of rickets (vitamin D deficiency) in children.

osteomyelitis An inflammation of bone tissue caused by pathogenic microorganisms; produces an increased vascularity and edema often involving the surrounding soft tissues.

osteonecrosis The death of bone tissue, usually because the blood supply to the bone is disrupted. Usually a complication of a hip fracture or any fracture in which there is displacement of bone.

osteopenia A condition of low bone mass that occurs when there is a disruption in the bone remodeling process.

osteophyte Bone spur.

osteoporosis A metabolic disease in which bone demineralization results in decreased density and subsequent fractures.

osteotomy Surgical resection of bone.

ostomate   A patient with an ostomy.

ostomy   The surgical creation of an opening, usually referring to an opening in the abdominal wall; stoma.

otorrhea   Ear discharge.

otosclerosis   Irregular bone growth around the ossicles.

otoscope   An instrument used to examine the ear; consists of a light, a handle, a magnifying lens, and a pneumatic bulb for injecting air into the external canal to test mobility of the eardrum.

ototoxic   Having a toxic effect on the inner ear structures.

outflow disease   Chronic peripheral arterial disease with obstruction at or below the superficial femoral or popliteal artery. The patient experiences burning or cramping in the calves, ankles, feet, and toes after walking a certain distance; the pain usually subsides with rest.

outpatient   A patient who goes to the hospital for treatment and returns home on the same day.

overflow urinary incontinence   The involuntary loss of urine when the bladder is overdistended.

overweight   An increase in body weight for height compared with a reference standard (e.g., the Metropolitan Life height and weight tables) or 10% greater than ideal body weight. However, this weight may not reflect excess body fat, which in an adult is a body mass index of 25 to 30.

ovoid pupil   In evaluating pupils for size and reaction to light, the midstage between a normal-size pupil and a dilated pupil; indicates the development of increased intracranial pressure.

oxygen concentrator   A machine that removes nitrogen, water vapor, and hydrocarbons from room air. Also known as "oxygen extractor."

oxygen dissociation   The transfer of oxygen from hemoglobin to tissues.

P

P wave   In the electrocardiogram, the deflection representing atrial depolarization.

pack-years   The number of packs of cigarettes per day multiplied by the number of years the patient has smoked; used in recording the patient's smoking history.

Paget's disease   A metabolic disorder of bone remodeling, or turnover, in which increased resorption or loss results in bone deposits that are weak, enlarged, and disorganized. Also known as "osteitis deformans."

pain   An unpleasant sensory and emotional experience associated with actual or potential tissue damage; the most reliable indication of pain is the patient's self-report.

palliation   Relieving symptoms.

palliative care   A compassionate and supportive approach to patients and families who are living with life-threatening illnesses; involves a holistic approach that provides relief of symptoms experienced by the dying patient.

palpitations   A feeling of fluttering in the chest, an unpleasant awareness of the heartbeat, and an irregular heartbeat; may result from a change in heart rate or rhythm or from an increase in the force of heart contractions.

pancreatic abscess   A collection of purulent material that results from extensive inflammatory necrosis of the pancreas after infection by organisms such as *Escherichia coli*; the most serious complication of pancreatitis. It is fatal if left untreated.

pancreatic pseudocyst   A false cyst, so named because, unlike a true cyst, it does not have an epithelial lining. It is an encapsulated saclike structure that forms on or surrounds the pancreas and develops as a complication of acute or chronic pancreatitis. It may contain up to several liters of straw-colored or dark-brown viscous fluid, the enzymatic exudate of the pancreas.

pancreaticojejunostomy   Surgical anastomosis of the pancreatic duct with the jejunum.

pancytopenia   A deficiency of all three cell types (red blood cells, white blood cells, and platelets) of the blood.

pandemic   A general epidemic spread over a wide geographic area and affecting a large proportion of the population.

panniculectomy   The surgical removal of any panniculus, most often the abdominal apron; usually done as a follow-up to bariatric surgery in an obese patient.

panniculitis   Infection of the panniculus.

panniculus   A layer of membrane; also used to refer to skinfold areas in the obese patient.

pannus   Vascular granulation tissue composed of inflammatory cells that forms in a joint space; erodes articular cartilage and eventually destroys bone.

Papanicolaou test (Pap smear)   A cytologic study that is effective in detecting precancerous and cancerous cells obtained from the cervix.

papilla   The anatomic term for a small, nipple-shaped projection or structure.

papilledema   Edema and hyperemia of the optic disc; a sign of increased intracranial pressure found on ophthalmoscopic examination. Also called a "choked disc."

papilloma   A pedunculated outgrowth of tissue.

papillotomy   An incision of a papilla, a small nipple-shaped projection or structure.

papular   Referring to a papule, a small, solid elevation of the skin.

paracentesis   A procedure in which the physician inserts a trocar catheter into the abdomen to remove and drain ascitic fluid from the peritoneal cavity.

paradoxical blood pressure   An exaggerated decrease in systolic pressure by more than 10 mm Hg during the inspiratory phase of the respiratory cycle (normal is 3 to 10 mm Hg); clinical conditions that may produce a paradoxical blood pressure include pericardial tamponade, constrictive pericarditis, and pulmonary hypertension. Also known as "paradoxical pulse" and "pulsus paradoxus."

paradoxical chest wall movement   The "sucking inward" of the loose chest area during inspiration and a "puffing out" of the same area during expiration in a patient with a flail chest.

paradoxical pulse   See *paradoxical blood pressure*.

paradoxical splitting   Abnormal splitting of the S_2 heart sound heard in patients with severe myocardial depression; causes early closure of the pulmonic valve or a delay in aortic valve closure.

paralysis   Absence of movement.

paralytic ileus   Absence of peristalsis.

paramedic   Prehospital care provider for patients who require care that exceeds basic life support resources. Advanced life support (ALS) may include cardiac monitoring, advanced airway management and intubation, establishing IV access, and administering drugs en route to the emergency department.

paranasal sinuses   The air-filled cavities within the bones that surround the nasal passages. Lined with ciliated membrane, the sinuses provide resonance during speech and decrease the weight of the skull.

paraparesis   Weakness that involves only the lower extremities, as seen in lower thoracic and lumbosacral injuries or lesions.

paraplegia   Paralysis that involves only the lower extremities, as seen in lower thoracic and lumbosacral injuries or lesions.

paresis   Weakness.

paresthesia   Abnormal or unusual nerve sensations of touch, such as tingling and burning.

parietal cells   Cells lining the wall of the stomach that secrete hydrochloric acid and produce intrinsic factor.

Parkinson disease (PD)   A debilitating neurologic disease that affects motor ability and is characterized by four cardinal symptoms: tremor, rigidity, akinesia (slow movement), and postural instability. It is the third most common neurologic disorder of older adults. Also called "paralysis agitans."

parotidectomy   The surgical removal of the parotid glands.

paroxysmal nocturnal dyspnea (PND)   In the patient with heart disease, difficulty breathing that develops after lying down for several hours and causes the patient to awaken abruptly with a feeling of suffocation and panic. Occurs because the heart is unable to compensate for the increased volume when blood from the lower extremities is redistributed to the venous system, which increases venous return to the heart. A diseased heart is ineffective in pumping the additional fluid into the circulatory system, and pulmonary congestion results.

paroxysmal supraventricular tachycardia (PSVT)   A form of supraventricular tachycardia that occurs when the rhythm is intermittent, initiated suddenly by a premature complex such as a premature atrial complex, and terminated suddenly with or without intervention.

partial left ventriculectomy (PLV)   A ventricular reconstructive procedure that involves removing a triangle-shaped section of the weakened heart in the left lateral ventricle to reduce the ventricle's diameter and decrease wall tension. Also known as "heart reduction surgery" and "Batista procedure."

partial seizure   One of the three broad categories of seizure disorders along with generalized seizure and unclassified seizure. Partial seizures are of two types: complex and simple. Partial seizures begin in a part of one cerebral hemisphere; some can evolve into generalized tonic-clonic, tonic, or clonic seizures. They are most often seen in adults and in general are less responsive to medical treatment. Also called "focal seizures" or "local seizures."

passive euthanasia See *withdrawing or withholding life-sustaining therapy.*

passive immunity Resistance to infection that is of short duration (days or months) and either natural by transplacental transfer from the mother or artificial by injection of antibodies (e.g., immunoglobulin).

patellofemoral pain syndrome (PFPS) A health problem that occurs most often in people who are runners or who overuse their knee joints. For that reason, it is sometimes referred to as "runner's knee." These patients describe pain as being behind or around their patella (knee cap) in one or both knees.

pathogen Any microorganism capable of producing disease.

pathogenicity The ability to cause disease.

pathologic (spontaneous) fracture A fracture that occurs after minimal trauma to a bone that has been weakened by a disease such as bone cancer or osteoporosis.

patient-centered care A QSEN competency in which the nurse recognizes the patient or designee as the source of control and full partner in providing compassionate and coordinated care based on respect for the patient's preferences, values, and needs.

patient-controlled analgesia A method that allows the patient to control the dosage of opioid analgesic received by using an infusion pump to deliver the desired amount of medication through a conventional IV route.

PDSA Acronym for plan, do, study, act, which is one of the steps of the evidence-based practice improvement (EBPI) model.

pedal Pertaining to the feet.

pediculosis An infestation by human lice.

pedigree A graph of a family history for a specific trait or health problem over several generations.

pelvic inflammatory disease (PID) Any infection of the pelvis involving the upper genital tract beyond the cervix in women. It occurs when organisms from the lower genital tract migrate from the endocervix upward through the uterine cavity into the fallopian tubes.

pelvic organ prolapse (POP) Condition in which the sling of muscles and tendons that support the pelvic organs becomes weak and is no longer able to hold them in place.

penetrance In genetics, how often or how well a gene is expressed when it is present within a population.

penetrating trauma Injuries caused by piercing; classified by the velocity of the vehicle (e.g., knife or bullet) causing the injury. Low-velocity injuries from knife wounds cause damage directly at the site; high-velocity injuries from gunshot wounds cause both direct and indirect damage. Also called "penetrating injury."

peptic ulcer A mucosal lesion of the stomach or duodenum.

peptic ulcer disease (PUD) The impairment of gastric mucosal defenses so they no longer

protect the epithelium from the effects of acid and pepsin.

percutaneous Performed through the skin and other tissues.

percutaneous alcohol septal ablation Surgical procedure for hypertrophic cardiomyopathy (HCM) in which alcohol is injected into a target septal branch of the left anterior descending coronary artery to produce a small septal infarction. This procedure also widens the left ventricular outflow tract.

percutaneous coronary intervention (PCI) See *percutaneous transluminal coronary angioplasty (PTCA).*

percutaneous endoscopic gastrostomy (PEG) A stoma created from the abdominal wall into the stomach for insertion of a short feeding tube.

percutaneous stereotactic rhizotomy (PSR) Procedure performed under general anesthesia to treat trigeminal neuralgia; a hollow needle is passed through the inside of the patient's cheek into the trigeminal nerve fibers, and a heating current (radiofrequency thermocoagulation) goes through the needle to destroy some of the fibers.

percutaneous transhepatic cholangiography (PTC) The radiographic study of the biliary duct system using an iodinated dye instilled via a percutaneous needle inserted through the liver into the intrahepatic ducts. It may be performed when a patient has jaundice or persistent upper abdominal pain, even after cholecystectomy, but it is rarely performed as a diagnostic procedure.

percutaneous transluminal coronary angioplasty (PTCA) A nonsurgical method of improving arterial flow by opening the vessel lumen and creating a smooth inner vessel surface. One or more arteries are dilated with a balloon catheter advanced through a cannula, which is inserted into or above an occluded or stenosed artery. Also called "percutaneous vascular intervention" and "percutaneous coronary intervention (PCI)."

percutaneous vascular intervention See *percutaneous transluminal coronary angioplasty.*

pericardial effusion Complication of pericarditis that occurs when the space between the parietal and visceral layers of the pericardium fills with fluid.

pericardial friction rub An abnormal sound that originates from the pericardial sac and occurs with the movements of the heart during the cardiac cycle; usually transient and a sign of inflammation, infection, or infiltration; may be heard in patients with pericarditis resulting from myocardial infarction, cardiac tamponade, or post-thoracotomy.

pericardiectomy Surgical excision of the pericardium (the sac around the heart).

pericardiocentesis Withdrawal of pericardial fluid through a catheter inserted into the pericardial space to relieve the pressure on the heart.

pericarditis An inflammation of the tissue (pericardium) surrounding the heart.

perichondrium A tough, fibrous tissue layer that surrounds the ear cartilage and gives shape to the pinna.

periodontal disease Gum disease in which mandibular bone loss has occurred.

perioperative The operative experience consisting of the preoperative, intraoperative, and post-operative time periods.

peripheral blood stem cells (PBSCs) Stem cells that are collected from peripheral blood for transplantation into the patient.

peripheral chemoreceptors Several 1- to 2-mm collections of tissue identified in the carotid arteries and along the aortic arch.

peripheral IV therapy IV therapy in which a vascular access device (VAD) is placed in a peripheral vein, usually in the arm.

peripheral vascular disease (PVD) Any disorder that alters the natural flow of blood through the arteries and veins of the peripheral circulation.

peripherally inserted central catheter (PICC) A long catheter inserted through a vein of the antecubital fossa (inner aspect of the bend of the arm) or the middle of the upper arm.

peritonitis Acute inflammation of the visceral/parietal peritoneum and endothelial lining of the abdominal cavity, or peritoneum.

peritonsillar abscess (PTA) A complication of acute tonsillitis. The infection spreads from the tonsil to the surrounding tissue, which forms an abscess.

periungual lesion Skin lesion around the nail bed.

permeable The quality of being porous.

pernicious anemia A form of megaloblastic anemia caused by failure to absorb vitamin B_{12} because of a deficiency of intrinsic factor (normally secreted by the gastric mucosa) needed for intestinal absorption of vitamin B_{12}.

PERRLA An acronym that stands for the phrase "Pupils should be equal in size, round and regular in shape, and react to light and accommodation."

personal emergency preparedness plan An individual plan that outlines specific arrangements in the event of disaster, such as childcare, pet care, and older adult care.

personal protective equipment (PPE) Infection control protocol that refers to the use of gloves, isolation gowns, face protection, and respirators with N95 or higher filtration.

personal readiness supplies A preassembled disaster supply kit for the home and/or automobile that contains clothing and basic survival supplies. Also called a "go bag."

petechiae Pinpoint red spots on the mucous membranes, palate, conjunctivae, or skin.

pH A measure of the free hydrogen ion level in body fluid.

pH monitoring examination The most accurate testing method of diagnosing GERD, accomplished by placing a small catheter into the distal esophagus or esophageal wall (depending on the specific technique). The patient then records a diary of activities and symptoms over a 24- to 48-hour period while pH is continuously monitored.

phagocytosis The process of engulfing, ingesting, killing, and disposing of an invading organism by neutrophils and macrophages; a key process of inflammation.

Phalen's maneuver Test to determine the presence of carpal tunnel syndrome (CTS); a positive test for CTS causes paresthesia in the medial nerve distribution of the palm of the hand in 60 seconds.

phantom limb pain (PLP) A frequent complication of amputation in which the patient perceives sensation in the absent (amputated) foot or hand. This sensation usually diminishes over time.

pharmacist Member of the health care team who oversees the prescription and preparation of medications and provides the team with essential information regarding drug safety.

pharmacologic stress echocardiogram A form of echocardiography in which either dobutamine (increases heart's contractility) or adenosine (dilates coronary arteries) is given to the patient; usually used when patients cannot tolerate exercise.

phenotype Any genetic characteristic that can actually be observed or, in some cases, determined by laboratory test.

pheochromocytoma A tumor of the adrenal medulla, which can cause excessive secretion of catecholamines.

phlebitis Inflammation of a vein, which can predispose patients to thrombosis.

phlebothrombosis Presence of a thrombus in a vein without inflammation.

phonophobia Abnormal sensitivity to sound.

phonophoresis Treatment for back pain in which a topical drug (e.g., lidocaine, hydrocortisone) is applied followed by continuous ultrasound for 10 minutes.

photophobia Abnormal sensitivity to light.

photopsia The appearance of bright flashes of light due to the onset of retinal detachment.

physiatrist A physician who specializes in rehabilitative medicine.

physical abuse The use of a physical force, such as hitting, burning, pushing, and molesting the patient, that results in bodily injury.

physical therapist (PT, RPT) A member of the rehabilitation health care team who helps the patient achieve mobility and who teaches techniques for performing certain activities of daily living.

piggyback set See *secondary administration set.*

pitting Indentation of the skin; often occurs with edema.

pituitary Cushing's disease Oversecretion of ACTH by the anterior pituitary gland, which causes hyperplasia of the adrenal cortex in both adrenal glands and an excess of most hormones secreted by the adrenal cortex.

plantar fasciitis An inflammation of the plantar fascia, which is located in the area of the arch of the foot. It is often seen in athletes, especially runners.

plasma cell A short-lived B-lymphocyte that begins functioning immediately to produce antibodies against sensitizing antigens.

plasmapheresis The separation of plasma from whole blood, after which the blood cells are returned to the patient without the plasma to eliminate antibodies.

plethoric A flushed appearance of the skin.

pleura The continuous smooth membrane composed of two surfaces that totally enclose the lungs.

pleural effusion Fluid in the pleural space.

pleuritic chest pain A stabbing pain on taking a deep breath.

plexus Cluster of nerves.

ploidy The number and appearance of chromosomes; used to describe cancer cells.

pluripotent stem cell The precursor cell involved in the production of red blood cells.

pneumonectomy Removal of an entire lung, including all blood vessels.

pneumonia Excess fluid in the lungs resulting from an inflammatory process that can include infection.

pneumothorax Air in the pleural (chest) cavity.

podagra Inflammation of the metatarsophalangeal joint of the great toe.

point of maximal impulse (PMI) See *apical impulse.*

polycystic kidney disease (PKD) An inherited disorder in which fluid-filled cysts develop in the kidneys.

polycythemia vera (PV) A disease that involves massive production of red blood cells, leukocytes, and platelets.

polydipsia Excessive intake of water.

polymorphism A variation in form.

polyp An abnormal outgrowth from a mucous membrane.

polyphagia Excessive eating.

polypharmacy The use of many drugs to treat multiple health problems for older adults. Also known as "hyperpharmacy."

polyuria Frequent and excessive urination.

pores Openings or spaces.

portal hypertension An abnormal persistent increase in pressure within the portal vein; a major complication of cirrhosis.

portal hypertensive gastropathy A complication that can occur in patients with portal hypertension, with or without esophageal varices. Slow gastric mucosal bleeding may result in chronic slow blood loss, occult positive stools, and anemia.

portal-systemic encephalopathy (PSE) A clinical disorder seen in hepatic failure and cirrhosis; it is manifested by neurologic symptoms and is characterized by an altered level of consciousness, impaired thinking processes, and neuromuscular disturbances. Also called "hepatic encephalopathy" and "hepatic coma."

positive deflection In electrocardiography, the flow of electrical current in the heart (cardiac axis) toward the positive pole.

positive inotropic agents Drugs that increase myocardial contractility and are prescribed to improve cardiac output.

postanesthesia care unit (PACU) Recovery room.

postcholecystectomy syndrome (PCS) The occurrence of the clinical manifestations of biliary tract disease following cholecystectomy; caused by residual or recurring calculi, inflammation, or stricture of the common bile duct.

post-concussion syndrome A group of clinical manifestations following a concussion that

consist of personality changes, irritability, headaches, dizziness, restlessness, nervousness, insomnia, memory loss, and depression. The prolonged pattern is classified as post-trauma syndrome.

posterior colporrhaphy The surgical procedure to repair a rectocele by strengthening pelvic supports and reducing the bulging.

posteroanterior Back to front; position for standard chest x-rays.

postherpetic neuralgia Pain that persists after herpes zoster lesions have resolved.

postictal stage Referring to the time immediately after a seizure.

postoperative period After surgery.

postpericardiotomy syndrome Symptoms, including pericardial and pleural pain, pericarditis, friction rub, elevated temperature and white blood cell count, and dysrhythmias, that occur in patients after cardiac surgery; may occur days to weeks after surgery and seems to be associated with blood that remains in the pericardial sac.

postrenal failure Decrease in renal function related to an obstruction in the flow of urine. It can progress to acute renal failure.

postural hypotension See *orthostatic hypotension.*

posture A person's body build and alignment when standing and walking.

post-void residual (PVR) The amount of urine remaining in the bladder within 20 minutes after voiding.

power air purifying respirator (PAPR) Device with a high efficiency particulate air (HEPA) filter and battery to promote positive pressure air flow; more effective than an N95 respirator.

PQRST A mnemonic (memory device) that may help in the current problem assessment of patients with gastrointestinal tract disorders. The letters represent these areas: P, precipitating or palliative (What brings it on? What makes it better or worse?); Q, quality or quantity (How does it look, feel, or sound?); R, region or radiation (Where is it? Does it spread anywhere?); S, severity scale (How bad is it [on a scale of 0 to 10]? Is it getting better, worse, or staying the same?); T, timing (Onset, duration, and frequency?).

PR interval In the electrocardiogram, the interval measured from the beginning of the P wave to the end of the PR segment; represents the time required for atrial depolarization as well as impulse delay in the atrioventricular node and travel time to the Purkinje fibers.

PR segment In the electrocardiogram, the isoelectric line from the end of the P wave to the beginning of the QRS complex, when the electrical impulse is traveling through the atrioventricular node, where it is delayed.

Prader-Willi syndrome (PWS) A complex neurodevelopmental genetic disorder that results from a hypothalamic-pituitary dysfunction that prevents appetite control. Patients with this syndrome are typically morbidly obese.

prandial (insulin secretion) The increased levels of insulin that are secreted after eating. Within 10 minutes of eating, an early burst of insulin secretion occurs, which is followed by an increasing insulin release that lasts as long as hyperglycemia is present.

prealbumin (PAB) A protein secreted by the liver that binds thyroxine.

precipitation The formation of large, insoluble antigen-antibody complexes during the antibody-binding process.

prediabetes An impaired fasting glucose (IFG) or impaired glucose tolerance (IGT).

prehospital care provider Typically, any of the first caregivers encountered by the patient if he or she is transported to the emergency department by an ambulance or helicopter.

preictal phase Referring to events that a patient experiences before a seizure, such as the presence of an aura.

pre-infarction angina Chest pain that occurs in the days or weeks before a myocardial infarction.

preload The degree of myocardial fiber stretch at the end of diastole and just before contraction; determined by the amount of blood returning to the heart from both the venous system (right heart) and the pulmonary system (left heart).

premature atrial complex (contraction) (PAC) In the electrocardiogram, an early complex that occurs when atrial tissue becomes irritable. This ectopic focus fires an impulse before the next sinus impulse is due, thus usurping the sinus pacemaker. The premature P wave from the atrial focus is early and has a shape different from that of the P wave generated from the sinus node.

premature complex In the electrocardiogram, an early complex that occurs when a cardiac cell or cell group other than the sinoatrial node becomes irritable and fires an impulse before the next sinus impulse is generated. After the premature complex, there is a pause before the next normal complex, which creates an irregularity in the rhythm.

premature ventricular complex (PVC) In the electrocardiogram, an early ventricular complex is followed by a pause that results from increased irritability of ventricular cells. The QRS complexes may be unifocal or uniform (of the same shape), or multifocal or multiform (of different shapes).

preoperative Before surgery.

prerenal failure Condition that causes inadequate kidney perfusion; can progress to acute renal failure.

presbycusis The loss of hearing, especially for high-pitched sounds; occurs as a result of aging.

presbyopia An age-related impairment of vision characterized by a loss of lens elasticity and the ability of the eye to accommodate. The near point of vision increases, and near objects must be placed farther from the eye to be seen clearly.

presence A type of communication that consists of listening and acknowledging the legitimacy of the patient's and/or family's pain.

pressure ulcer Tissue damage caused when the skin and underlying soft tissue are compressed between a bony prominence and an external surface for an extended period; commonly occurs over the sacrum, hips, and ankles.

pretibial Pertaining to the front of the leg below the knee.

pretibial myxedema Dry, waxy swelling of the front surfaces of the lower legs.

primary angle-closure glaucoma A form of glaucoma characterized by a narrowed angle and forward displacement of the iris so that movement of the iris against the cornea narrows or closes the chamber angle, obstructing the outflow of aqueous humor. It can have a sudden onset and is an emergency. Also called "closed-angle glaucoma," "narrow-angle glaucoma," or "acute glaucoma."

primary arthroplasty A total joint arthroplasty procedure that has been performed for the first time.

primary gout The most common type of gout; results from one of several inborn errors of purine metabolism.

primary lesions In describing skin disease, the initial reaction to a problem that alters one of the structural components of the skin.

primary open-angle glaucoma (POAG) The most common form of primary glaucoma; characterized by reduced outflow of aqueous humor through the chamber angle. Because the fluid cannot leave the eye at the same rate it is produced, intraocular pressure gradually increases.

primary prevention Strategies used to avoid or delay the actual occurrence of a specific disease.

primary progressive multiple sclerosis (PPMS) A type of multiple sclerosis (MS) that involves a steady and gradual neurologic deterioration without remission of symptoms. Patients with this type of MS are usually between 40 and 60 years of age at onset of the disease and experience progressive disability with no acute attacks.

primary survey Priorities of care addressed in order of immediate threats to life as part of the initial assessment in the emergency department. Survey is based on an "ABC" mnemonic with "D" and "E" added for trauma patients: airway/cervical spine (A), breathing (B), circulation (C), disability (D), and exposure (E).

primary tumor The original tumor, usually identified by the tissue from which it arose (parent tissue), such as in breast cancer or lung cancer.

progressive multifocal leukoencephalopathy (PML) Rare disease affecting the white matter of the brain caused by a virus that attacks the cells that make myelin; occurs most often in patients who are immunosuppressed.

progressive-relapsing multiple sclerosis (PRMS) A type of multiple sclerosis (MS) that occurs in only 5% of patients with MS. It is characterized by the absence of periods of remission, and the patient's condition does not return to baseline. Progressive cumulative symptoms and deterioration occur over several years.

proliferative diabetic retinopathy A form of retinopathy associated with diabetes mellitus in which a network of fragile new blood vessels develops, leaking blood and protein into surrounding tissue. The new blood vessels are stimulated by retinal hypoxia that results from poor capillary perfusion of the retinal tissues. New blood vessels grow in the retina, onto the iris, and into the back of the vitreous. The vitreous contracts and pulls away from the retina, causing blood vessels to break and bleed into the vitreous.

promoter In oncology, a substance that promotes or enhances growth of the initiated cancer cell; may be a hormone, drug, or chemical.

pronator drift Occurs in a patient with muscle weakness due to cerebral or brainstem reasons. The arm on the weak side tends to fall, or "drift," with the palm pronating (turning inward) after the patient has closed his or her eyes and held the arms perpendicular to the body with the palms up for 15 to 30 seconds; part of the neurologic assessment.

prophylactic mastectomy Highly controversial practice of surgically removing the breast in order to reduce the risk of breast cancer.

proportionate palliative sedation A care management approach involving the administration of drugs such as benzodiazepines for the purpose of lowering patient consciousness.

proprioception (proprioceptive) Awareness of body position and movement.

prosopagnosia The inability to recognize oneself and other familiar faces; occurs in patients in the later stages of Alzheimer's disease.

prostaglandins Chemicals that are produced in the cells and cause inflammation and swelling.

prostate-specific antigen (PSA) A glycoprotein produced solely by the prostate. The normal blood level of PSA is less than 4 ng/mL; levels are higher in patients with increased prostatic tissue as a result of benign prostatic hyperplasia, prostatic infarction, prostatitis, and prostate cancer. Levels associated with prostate cancer are usually much higher than those occurring with other prostate tissue enlargement.

prostatitis Inflammation of the prostate.

protein-calorie malnutrition (PCM) A disorder of nutrition that may present in three forms: marasmus, kwashiorkor, and marasmic-kwashiorkor. Also called "protein-energy malnutrition."

protein-energy malnutrition (PEM) See *protein-calorie malnutrition.*

protein synthesis The process by which genes are used to make the proteins needed for physiologic function.

proteinuria The presence of protein in the urine.

proteolysis The breakdown of proteins to provide fuel for energy when liver glucose is unavailable.

proton pump inhibitor (PPI) A group of drugs that inhibit the proton pump in the stomach to decrease gastric acid production.

pruritus An unpleasant itching sensation.

psoriasis A chronic, autoimmune disorder of the skin with exacerbations and remissions. It results from overstimulation of the immune system (Langerhans' cells) in the skin that activates T-lymphocytes. The features include increased skin cell division in patchy areas forming scaly plaques.

psoriatic arthritis (PsA) A syndrome of inflammatory arthritis associated with psoriasis, the skin condition characterized by a scaly, itchy rash.

psychiatric crisis nurse team An emergency department specialty team whose nurses interact with patients and families in crisis.

psychotropic drugs Antipsychotic and neuroleptic drugs. These are appropriately given to patients with emotional and behavioral health problems (e.g., hallucinations and delusions) that accompany dementia but are sometimes inappropriately used for agitation, combativeness, or restlessness. They are considered chemical restraints because they decrease mobility and patients' ability to care for themselves.

ptosis Drooping of the eyelid.

pulmonary artery occlusive pressure (PAOP) See *pulmonary artery wedge pressure.*

pulmonary artery wedge pressure (PAWP) Measurement of pressure in the left atrium using a balloon-tipped catheter introduced into the pulmonary artery. When the balloon at the catheter tip is inflated, the catheter advances and wedges in a branch of the pulmonary artery. The tip of the catheter is able to sense pressures transmitted from the left atrium, which reflect left ventricular end-diastolic pressure. Also called "pulmonary artery occlusive pressure."

pulmonary autograph The relocation of the patient's own pulmonary valve to the aortic position for aortic valve replacement (Ross procedure).

pulmonary embolism (PE) A collection of particulate matter, most commonly a blood clot, that enters venous circulation and lodges in the pulmonary vessels, obstructing pulmonary blood flow and leading to decreased systemic oxygenation, pulmonary tissue hypoxia, and potential death.

pulmonary empyema A collection of pus in the pleural space most commonly caused by a pulmonary infection.

pulse deficit The difference between the apical and peripheral pulses.

pulse pressure The difference between the systolic and diastolic pressures.

pulse therapy Any therapy given at a high dose for a short duration.

pulsus alternans A type of pulse in which a weak pulse alternates with a strong pulse despite a regular heart rhythm; seen in patients with severely depressed cardiac function.

punctum The opening through which tears drain; located at the nasal side of the eyelid edges.

pupil The opening through which light enters the eye; located in the center of the iris of the eye.

Purkinje cells In the cardiac conduction system, the cells that make up the bundle of His, bundle branches, and terminal Purkinje fibers. These cells are responsible for the rapid conduction of electrical impulses throughout the ventricles, leading to ventricular depolarization and subsequent ventricular muscle contraction.

purpura Purple patches on the skin that may be caused by blood disorders, vascular abnormalities, or trauma.

pyelolithotomy The surgical removal of a stone from the kidney.

pyelonephritis A bacterial infection in the kidney and renal pelvis (the upper urinary tract).

pyloromyotomy An incision through the serosa and muscularis of the pylorus, down to the mucosa; created to prevent gastric motility

disturbances in patients who have undergone esophagectomy.

pyuria The presence of white blood cells (pus) in the urine.

Q

QRS complex In the electrocardiogram, the portion consisting of the Q, R, and S waves, representing ventricular depolarization.

QRS duration In the electrocardiogram, the time required for depolarization of both ventricles; measured from the beginning of the QRS complex to the J point (the junction where the QRS complex ends and the ST segment begins).

QT interval In the electrocardiogram, the time from the beginning of the QRS complex to the end of the T wave. It represents the total time required for ventricular depolarization and repolarization.

quadriceps-setting exercise Postoperative leg exercise performed by straightening the legs and pushing the back of the knees into the bed.

quadrigeminy A type of premature complex consisting of a repetitive four-beat pattern; usually occurs as three sequential normal complexes followed by a premature complex and a pause, with the same pattern repeating itself in a four-beat pattern.

quadriparesis Weakness that involves all four extremities; seen with cervical spinal cord injury.

qualitative question A clinical question that focuses on the meanings and interpretations of human phenomena or experience of people and usually analyzes the content of what a person says during an interview or what a researcher observes.

quality improvement A QSEN competency in which the nurse uses data to monitor the outcomes of care processes and uses improvement methods to design and test changes to continuously improve the quality and safety of health care systems.

quantitative question A clinical question that asks about the relationship between or among defined, measurable phenomena and includes statistical analysis of information that is collected to answer a question.

R

radiation dose The amount of radiation absorbed by the tissue.

radiation proctitis Rectal mucosa inflammation that results from external beam radiation therapy.

radical cystectomy Removal of the bladder and surrounding tissue with urinary diversion.

radicular Referring to a nerve root.

radiculopathy Referring to radicular pain; spinal nerve root involvement.

radiofrequency catheter ablation An invasive procedure that uses radiofrequency waves to abolish an irritable focus that is causing a supraventricular or ventricular tachydysrhythmia.

Rapid Response Team Team of critical care experts who save lives and decrease the risk for harm by providing care to patients before a respiratory or cardiac arrest occurs. Also called "Medical Emergency Team."

RBC Red blood cell.

rebound headache Headache that occurs as a side effect of a drug that has relieved an initial migraine headache. Also called "medication overuse headache."

recall memory Recent memory, which can be tested during the history taking by asking about items such as the dates of clinic or physician appointments.

receptive aphasia A type of aphasia caused by injury to Wernicke's area in the temporoparietal area of the brain and characterized by an inability to understand the spoken and written word; both reading and writing ability are equally affected. Although the patient can talk, the language is often meaningless and neologisms (made-up words) are common parts of speech. Also called "Wernicke's aphasia" or "sensory aphasia."

reconstructive plastic surgery Type of plastic surgery that corrects or improves functional defects that have occurred as a result of congenital problems, trauma and scarring, or other types of therapy.

recreational therapist A member of the health care team who works to help patients continue or develop hobbies or interests. Also called "activity therapist."

rectocele A protrusion of the rectum through a weakened vaginal wall.

red reflex A reflection of light on the retina seen as a red glare during ophthalmoscopic examination. An absent red reflex may indicate a lens opacity or cloudiness of the vitreous.

redirection An intervention to help with communication problems in patients with dementia; consists of attracting the patient's attention before conversing, keeping the environment as free of distractions as possible, and speaking directly to the patient in a distinct manner using clear and short sentences.

reducible hernia A hernia that can be placed back into the abdominal cavity by gentle pressure.

reduction mammoplasty Breast reduction surgery in which the surgeon removes excess breast tissue and then repositions the nipple and remaining skin flaps to produce an optimal cosmetic effect.

Reed-Sternberg cell A specific cancer cell type, found in lymph nodes, that is a marker for Hodgkin's lymphoma.

re-epithelialization In partial-thickness (superficial) wounds involving damage to the epidermis and upper layers of the dermis, a form of healing by means of the production of new skin cells by undamaged epidermal cells in the basal layer of the dermis.

refeeding syndrome Life-threatening metabolic complication that can occur when nutrition is restarted for a patient who is in a starvation state.

reflex arc A closed circuit of spinal and peripheral nerves that requires no control by the brain.

reflex sympathetic dystrophy (RSD) See *complex regional pain syndrome.*

reflux Reverse or backward flow.

reflux esophagitis Damage to the esophageal mucosa, often with erosion and ulceration, in patients with gastroesophageal reflux disease.

refraction The bending of light rays.

refractory hypoxemia Low blood oxygen levels that persist even when 100% oxygen is given.

regional anesthesia A type of local anesthesia that blocks multiple peripheral nerves in a specific body region.

registered dietitian (RD) Member of the health care team who ensures patients meet their nutritional needs. Also called "nutritionist."

regurgitation Flowing in the opposite direction from normal, as the occurrence of warm fluid traveling up the throat, unaccompanied by nausea, in the patient with gastroesophageal reflux disease.

rehabilitation The process of learning to live with chronic and disabling conditions by returning the patient to the fullest possible physical, mental, social, vocational, and economic capacity.

rehabilitation case manager Nurse or other health care professional who coordinates health care for patients undergoing rehabilitation in home or acute care settings.

rehabilitation nurse Nurse who coordinates the efforts of health care team members for patients undergoing rehabilitation in the inpatient setting; may be designated as the patient's case manager.

relapsing-remitting multiple sclerosis (RRMS) A type of multiple sclerosis that occurs in 85% of cases and is characterized by a mild or moderate course, depending on the degree of disability. Relapses develop over 1 to 2 weeks and resolve over 4 to 8 months, after which the patient returns to baseline.

reliever drugs Drugs used in asthma therapy to stop an asthma attack once it has started.

religions Formal belief systems that provide a framework for making sense of life, death, and suffering and responding to universal spiritual questions; a formal expression of spirituality.

relocation stress syndrome Physiologic or psychosocial distress following transfer from one environment to another, such as after admission to a hospital or nursing home. Also called "relocation trauma."

reminiscence The process of randomly reflecting on memories of events in one's life.

remote memory Long-term memory of events; can be tested by asking patients about their birth date, schools attended, city of birth, or anything from the past that can be verified.

renal colic Severe pain associated with distention or spasm of the ureter, such as with an obstruction or the passing of a stone; the pain radiates into the perineal area, groin, scrotum, or labia. Pain may be intermittent or continuous and may be accompanied by pallor, diaphoresis, and hypotension.

renal columns Cortical tissue that dips into the interior of the kidney and separates the pyramids in the medulla. Also called "columns of Bertin."

renal cortex The outermost layer of functional kidney tissue lying beneath the renal capsule.

renal osteodystrophy The problems in bone metabolism and structure caused by renal failure–induced hypocalcemia and hyperphosphatemia.

renal pelvis The expansion from the upper end of the ureter into which the calices of the kidney open.

renal threshold The limit to the amount of glucose that the kidney can reabsorb as glucose is filtered from the blood. Also called the "transport maximum."

renin A hormone that is produced in the juxtaglomerular complex of the kidney and helps regulate blood flow, glomerular filtration rate, and blood pressure. Renin is secreted when sensing cells (macula densa) in the distal convoluted tubule sense changes in blood volume and pressure.

repetitive stress injury (RSI) Injury caused by repeated movements of the same part of the body (e.g., carpal tunnel syndrome).

replicate The reproduction of DNA that occurs each time a cell divides.

resident An individual who lives in an inpatient facility and has all the rights of anyone living in his or her home.

residuals Amount of feeding that remains in the stomach after enteral nutrition.

resistin A hormone produced by fat cells that creates resistance to insulin activity.

resorption In referring to bone, the loss of bone minerals and density; the release of free calcium from bone storage sites directly into the extracellular fluid.

restorative aide A member of the health care team, often with the nursing department, who assists the therapists, especially in the long-term care setting.

restraint Any device (physical restraint) or drug (chemical restraint) that prevents the patient from moving freely.

restrictive cardiomyopathy A form of cardiomyopathy that restricts the filling of the ventricles; a type of lung disease that prevents good expansion and recoil of the gas exchange unit.

restrictive (lung disorder) Any lung disorder that prevents good expansion and recoil of the gas exchange unit.

resurfacing Regrowth of new skin cells across the open area of a wound as it heals.

resuscitation phase The first phase of a burn injury, beginning at the onset of injury and continuing to about 48 hours.

rete pegs The fingers of epidermal tissue that project into the dermis.

reticular activating system (RAS) Special cells throughout the brainstem that constitute the system that controls awareness and alertness.

retina The innermost layer of the eye, made up of sensory receptors that transmit impulses to the optic nerve. It contains blood vessels and two types of photoreceptors called "rods" and "cones." Rods work at low light levels and provide peripheral vision; cones are active at bright light levels and provide color and central vision.

retinal detachment Separation of the retina from the epithelium.

retinal hole A break in the retina; can be caused by trauma or can occur with aging.

retinal tear Jagged and irregularly shaped break in the retina resulting from traction on the retina.

retinopathy Inflammation of the retina. Also used as a general term for vision problems.

retrograde Going against the normal direction of flow.

retroviruses The family of viruses that includes the human immune deficiency virus.

revision arthroplasty Surgical replacement of a prosthesis that has loosened and is causing pain.

rhabdomyolysis The breakdown or disintegration of muscle tissue; associated with excretion of myoglobin in the urine.

rheumatic carditis Inflammatory lesions in the heart due to a sensitivity response that develops after an upper respiratory tract infection with group A beta-hemolytic streptococci, which occurs in about 40% of patients with rheumatic fever. Inflammation results in impaired contractile function of the myocardium, thickening of the pericardium, and valvular damage. Also called "rheumatic endocarditis."

rheumatic disease Any disease or condition involving the musculoskeletal system.

rheumatoid arthritis (RA) A chronic, progressive, systemic, inflammatory autoimmune disease process that primarily affects the synovial joints; one of the most common connective tissue diseases and the most destructive to the joints.

rhinitis An inflammation of the nasal mucosa.

rhinoplasty A surgical reconstruction of the nose done for cosmetic purposes and improvement of airflow.

rhinorrhea Watery drainage from the nose; a "runny" nose.

rickets Vitamin D deficiency in children.

right-sided heart (ventricular) failure The inability of the right ventricle to empty completely, resulting in increased volume and pressure in the systemic veins and systemic venous congestion with peripheral edema.

robotic technology Technology that provides mechanical parts for extremities when they are not functional or have been amputated.

Romberg sign Swaying or falling when the patient is standing with arms at the sides, feet and knees close together, and eyes closed; a test of equilibrium in neurologic assessment.

rotation A mechanism of injury in which the head is turned excessively beyond the normal range.

rubor Dusky red discoloration of the skin.

rugae Folds, as of a mucous membrane.

S

S₃ gallop The third heart sound; an early diastolic filling sound that indicates an increase in left ventricular pressure and may be heard on auscultation in patients with heart failure.

safety A QSEN competency in which the nurse minimizes risk of harm to patients and providers through both system effectiveness and individual performance.

Salem sump tube Tube inserted through the nose and placed into the stomach that is attached to low continuous suction. It has a vent ("pigtail") that prevents the stomach mucosa from being pulled away during suctioning.

salpingitis Infection of the fallopian tube.

sanguineous Having a bloody appearance.

sarcoidosis A granulomatous disorder of unknown cause that can affect any organ but most often involves the lung.

SBAR Acronym for a formal method of communication between two or more members of the health care team. It is used most often when there is an unmet patient need or problem but can also be used to communicate continuing care issues when a patient is discharged from one agency to another. It consists of four steps: Situation, Background, Assessment, Recommendation.

scabies A contagious skin disease caused by mite infestations.

sclera The external white layer of the eye.

scleroderma See *systemic sclerosis*.

sclerotherapy The injection of a sclerosing agent via a catheter, usually in an endoscopic procedure, to stop variceal bleeding.

sclerotic Hard, or hardening.

scoliosis An abnormal lateral curve in the spine, which normally should be a straight vertical line.

scotomas Changes in peripheral vision.

sebum A mildly bacteriostatic, fat-containing substance produced by the sebaceous glands. Sebum lubricates the skin and reduces water loss from the skin surface.

second intention Healing of deep tissue injuries or wounds with tissue loss in which a cavity-like defect requires gradual filling of the dead space with connective tissue, which prolongs the repair process.

secondary administration set A short conduit that is attached to the primary administration set at a Y-injection site and is used to deliver intermittent medications. Also called a "piggyback set."

secondary gout Gout involving hyperuricemia.

secondary hypertension Elevated blood pressure that is related to a specific disease (e.g., kidney disease) or medication (e.g., estrogen).

secondary lesion Describing skin disease in terms of changes in the appearance of the primary lesion. These changes occur with progression of an underlying disease or in response to a topical or systemic therapeutic intervention.

secondary prevention Early detection of a disease or condition, sometimes before signs and symptoms are evident, to prevent or limit permanent disability or death.

secondary progressive multiple sclerosis (SPMS) A type of multiple sclerosis that begins with a relapsing-remitting course and later becomes steadily progressive. Attacks and partial recoveries may continue to occur.

secondary survey In the emergency department, a more comprehensive head-to-toe assessment performed to identify other injuries or medical issues that need to be managed or that might impact the course of treatment.

secondary tumor Additional tumor that is established when cancer cells move from the primary location to another area in the body. Also called "metastatic tumor."

seizure An abnormal, sudden, excessive, uncontrolled electrical discharge of neurons within the brain that may result in an alteration in consciousness, motor or sensory ability, and/or behavior. A single seizure may occur for no known reason; however, seizures may be due to a pathologic condition of the brain, such as a tumor.

self-tolerance In immunology, the ability to recognize self cells versus non-self cells, which is necessary to prevent healthy body cells from being destroyed along with invading cells.

Sengstaken-Blakemore tube Tube similar to a nasogastric tube that is placed through the nose and into the stomach in which an attached balloon is inflated to apply pressure to bleeding variceal areas of the esophagus.

sensitivity The likelihood that infecting bacterial organisms will be killed or stopped by a particular antibiotic drug. Sensitivity is determined by testing different antibiotics against the organisms. Organisms are "sensitive" if the antibiotic is effective in stopping their growth; organisms are "resistant" if the antibiotic is not effective.

sensorineural hearing loss Hearing loss that results from a defect in the cochlea, the eighth cranial nerve, or the brain itself. Exposure to loud noises and music may cause this type of hearing loss as a result of damage to the cochlear hair cells.

sensory Facilitating sensation.

sensory aphasia See *receptive aphasia*.

sentinel event As defined by The Joint Commission, an unexpected occurrence involving serious physical or psychological injury or the risk thereof and requiring an intense analysis of the contributing factors and corrective action.

sepsis Systemic infection.

septic shock The type of shock that occurs when large amounts of toxins and endotoxins produced by bacteria are released into the blood, causing a whole-body inflammatory reaction.

septicemia Systemic disease associated with sepsis; the presence of pathogens in the blood.

sequestrum A piece of necrotic bone that has separated from surrounding bone tissue; a common complication of osteomyelitis.

serologic testing Laboratory testing that is performed to identify pathogens by detecting antibodies to the organism.

serositis Inflammation of a serous membrane, such as the pleura or peritoneum.

serous Having a serum-like appearance, or yellow color.

serum sickness A type III hypersensitivity reaction that develops first as a skin rash and occurs within 3 to 21 days of the administration of antivenin (Crotalidae) polyvalent. This allergic response is often accompanied by other manifestations such as fever, arthralgias (joint pains), and pruritus (itching).

severe acute respiratory syndrome (SARS) An easily spread respiratory infection first identified in China in November 2002. At first appearing as an atypical pneumonia, it is caused by a new, more virulent form of coronavirus, and there is no known effective treatment.

severe sepsis The progression of sepsis with an amplified inflammatory response.

sex chromosomes The pair of chromosomes containing the genes for sexual differentiation in humans. In males, the sex chromosomes are an X and a Y; in females, the sex chromosomes are two Xs.

sex reassignment surgery (SRS) Surgery, particularly procedures that affect the external or internal genitalia, that transitions an individual from one's natal sex to one's inner gender identity. Also known as "gender reassignment surgery."

sexually transmitted infections (STIs) Any of a group of diseases caused by infectious organisms that have been passed from one person to another through intimate contact. Some organisms that cause these diseases are transmitted only through sexual contact. Other organisms are transmitted by parenteral exposure to infected blood, fecal-oral transmission, intrauterine transmission to the fetus, and perinatal transmission from mother to neonate. Also known as "sexually transmitted diseases (STDs)."

SHARE Acronym standing for Standardize critical content, Hardwire within your system, Allow opportunity to ask questions, Reinforce quality and measurement, Educate and coach.

shift to the left An increased number of immature neutrophils found on a differential count in patients with infections; can be characterized by changes in percentages of different types of leukocytes. Also known as "left shift."

shock The whole-body response to poor tissue oxygenation. Any problem that impairs oxygen delivery to tissues and organs can start the syndrome of shock and lead to a life-threatening emergency.

short peripheral catheter A catheter that consists of a plastic cannula built around a sharp stylet for venipuncture, which extends slightly beyond the cannula and is advanced into the vein.

sialagogue An agent that stimulates the flow of saliva.

simple fracture See *closed fracture*.

single-photon emission computed tomography (SPECT) A diagnostic tool using a radiopharmaceutical (agent that enables radioisotopes to cross the blood-brain barrier) that is administered by IV injection, after which the patient is scanned.

sinoatrial (SA) node In the cardiac conduction system, the primary pacemaker of the heart; located close to the epicardial surface of the right atrium near its junction with the superior vena cava. It can spontaneously and rhythmically generate electrical impulses at a rate of 60 to 100 beats/min. Also called the "sinus node."

sinus arrhythmia A variant of normal sinus rhythm that results from changes in intrathoracic pressure during breathing; heart rate increases slightly during inspiration and decreases slightly during exhalation. Atrial and ventricular rates are between 60 and 100 beats/min, and atrial and ventricular rhythms are irregular.

sinus bradycardia A cardiac dysrhythmia caused by a decreased rate of sinus node discharge, with a heart rate that is less than 60 beats/min.

sinus tachycardia A cardiac dysrhythmia caused by an increased rate of sinus node discharge, with a heart rate that is more than 100 beats/min.

sinusitis An inflammation of the mucous membranes of the sinuses.

SIRS Acronym for systemic inflammatory response syndrome, an inflammatory state affecting the whole body.

Sjögren's syndrome In patients with advanced rheumatoid arthritis, the triad of dry eyes, dry mouth, and dry vagina caused by the obstruction of secretory ducts and glands by inflammatory cells and immune complexes.

skilled nursing facility (SNF) Part of either a hospital or long-term care (nursing home) setting in which care is reimbursed through Medicare Part A for the first 21 days after admission.

skinfold measurement Measurement that estimates body fat.

smart pump An infusion pump with dosage calculation software.

social justice Ethical principle that refers to equality and fairness—that all patients should be treated equally and fairly, regardless of age, gender, religion, race, ethnicity, or education.

social worker Member of the health care team who helps patients identify support services and resources and who coordinates transfers to or discharges from the rehabilitation setting.

sodium (Na⁺) A mineral that is the major cation in the extracellular fluid and maintains extracellular fluid (ECF) osmolarity.

solute A particle dissolved or suspended in the water portion (solvent) of body fluids; a solution consists of a solute and a solvent.

solvent The water portion of fluids.

spastic bladder Incontinence characterized by sudden, gushing voids, usually without completely emptying the bladder; caused by neurologic problems affecting the upper motor neuron, such as with spinal cord injuries above the twelfth thoracic vertebra.

spastic paralysis Paralysis of a part of the body that is characterized by spasticity of muscles due to hypertonia; may be seen in the patient who has experienced a brain attack.

specialized nutrition support (SNS) Total nutritional intake orally or intravenously with commercially prepared products (either total enteral nutrition or total parenteral nutrition).

speech-language pathologist (SLP) A member of the rehabilitation health care team who evaluates and retrains patients with speech, language, or swallowing problems.

sphincter of Oddi The sheath of muscle fibers surrounding the papillary opening of the duodenum.

sphincterotomy A procedure for opening a sphincter.

spider angiomas See *telangiectasias.*

spinal fusion (arthrodesis) A surgical procedure to stabilize the spine after repeated laminectomies have been unsuccessful. Chips of bone are removed (typically from the iliac crest) or are obtained from donor bone; the chips are grafted between the vertebrae for support and to strengthen the back.

spinal shock See *spinal shock syndrome.*

spinal shock syndrome Loss of reflex activity below the level of a spinal lesion; occurs immediately after injury as a result of disruption in the communication pathways between the upper motor neurons and the lower motor neurons. Also called "spinal shock."

spinal stenosis Narrowing of the spinal canal; typically seen in people older than 60 years.

spirituality The connection to self, others, the environment, and a "higher power."

spiritual counselor Counselor who specializes in spiritual assessments and care, usually a member of the clergy.

splenectomy Surgical removal of the spleen.

splenomegaly Enlargement of the spleen.

splint Any object or device that extends to the joints above and below a fracture to immobilize it.

splinter hemorrhage Black longitudinal line or small red streak on the distal third of the nail bed; seen in patients with infective endocarditis.

spondee Two-syllable words in which there is generally equal stress on each syllable, such as *airplane, railroad,* and *cowboy;* used in testing speech reception threshold.

spondylolisthesis Condition in which one vertebra slips forward on the one below it, often as a result of spondylolysis. This problem causes pressure on the nerve roots, leading to pain in the lower back and into the buttocks.

spondylolysis A defect in one of the vertebrae; usually found in the lumbar spine.

spontaneous bacterial peritonitis (SBP) Bacterial infection of the abdominal peritoneum caused by ascites; often seen in patients with cirrhosis of the liver.

spore An encapsulated, inactive organism.

sprain Excessive stretching of a ligament.

ST segment In the electrocardiogram, the line (normally isoelectric) representing early ventricular repolarization. It occurs from the J point to the beginning of the T wave.

ST-elevation myocardial infarction (STEMI) Myocardial infarction in which the patient typically has ST elevation in two contiguous leads on a 12-lead ECG; this indicates myocardial infarction/necrosis.

staging System of classifying clinical aspects of a cancer tumor.

Standard Precautions Infection control guidelines from the Centers for Disease Control and Prevention stating that all body excretions, secretions, and moist membranes and tissues are potentially infectious; combines protective measures from Universal Precautions and Body Substance Isolation.

stasis dermatitis In patients with venous insufficiency, discoloration of the skin along the ankles, which extends up to the calf.

stasis ulcer In patients with long-term venous insufficiency, ulcer formed as a result of edema or minor injury to the limb; typically occurs over the malleolus.

status epilepticus Prolonged seizures lasting more than 5 minutes or repeated seizures over the course of 30 minutes; a potential complication of all types of seizures.

steatorrhea An excessive amount of fat in the stool.

stem cell An immature, undifferentiated cell produced by the bone marrow.

stent A small tube that is placed in a tubular structure to dilate it; a wirelike device that may be used along with percutaneous transluminal angioplasty to help keep the vessel open.

stereotactic pallidotomy A surgical treatment for the patient with Parkinson disease when drugs are ineffective in symptom management. An electrode is used to create a lesion in a targeted area within the pallidum, with the goal of reducing tremor and rigidity.

sterilization A method of infection control in which all living organisms and bacterial spores are destroyed; used on items that invade human tissue where bacteria are not commonly found.

stoma The surgical creation of an opening; usually refers to an opening in the abdominal wall.

stomatitis Inflammation of the oral mucosa; characterized by painful single or multiple ulcerations that impair the protective lining of the mouth. The ulcerations are commonly referred to as "canker sores."

strain Excessive stretching of a muscle or tendon when it is weak or unstable; sometimes referred to as "muscle pulls."

strangulated hernia A tightly constricted hernia that compromises the blood supply to the herniated segment of the bowel as a result of pressure from the hernial ring (the band of muscle around the hernia); leads to ischemia and obstruction of the bowel loop, with necrosis of the bowel and possibly bowel perforation.

strangulated obstruction Intestinal obstruction with compromised blood flow.

stratum corneum The outermost layer of the skin.

stress test See *exercise electrocardiography.*

stress ulcers Multiple shallow erosions of the proximal stomach and occasionally the duodenum.

stress urinary incontinence (SUI) Loss of urine during activities that increase intraabdominal pressure, such as laughing, coughing, sneezing, or lifting heavy objects.

striae Reddish purple streaks on the skin. Also called "stretch marks."

stricture Narrowing.

stridor A high-pitched crowing sound caused by laryngospasm or edema above or below the glottis; heard during respiration.

stroke See *brain attack.*

stroke volume (SV) The amount of blood ejected by the left ventricle during each heartbeat.

subarachnoid space Term for the space between the arachnoid mater and pia mater of the spinal cord. Also called "subarachnoid."

subcutaneous emphysema The presence of bubbles under the skin because of air trapping; an uncommon late complication of fracture.

subcutaneous infusion therapy Infusion therapy that is delivered under the skin when patients cannot tolerate oral medications, when intramuscular injections are too painful, or when vascular access is not available.

subcutaneous nodule Characteristic round, movable, nontender swelling under the skin of the arm or fingers in patients with severe rheumatoid arthritis.

subdural hematoma (SDH) The collection of clotted blood that typically results from venous bleeding into the space beneath the dura and above the arachnoid.

subdural space Term for the space between the dura mater and the middle layer (arachnoid).

subluxation Partial joint dislocation.

submucous resection (SMR) Surgical procedure to straighten a deviated septum when chronic symptoms or discomfort occur. Also called "nasoseptoplasty."

substernally Located below the ribs.

subtotal thyroidectomy The surgical removal of part of the thyroid tissue.

sundowning In patients with Alzheimer's disease, increased confusion at night or when excessively fatigued.

superinfection Reinfection or a second infection of the same type.

supervision Guidance or direction, evaluation, and follow-up by the nurse to ensure that the task or activity is performed appropriately.

supratentorial Located within the cerebral hemispheres, in the area above the tentorium of the cerebellum; the tentlike fold of dura that surrounds the cerebellar hemisphere and supports the occipital lobe.

supraventricular tachycardia (SVT) A form of tachycardia that involves the rapid stimulation of atrial tissue at a rate of 100 to 280 beats/min. It is most often due to a re-entry mechanism in which one impulse circulates repeatedly throughout the atrial pathway, re-stimulating the atrial tissue at a rapid rate.

surfactant A fatty protein secreted by type II pneumocytes to reduce surface tension in the alveoli.

surveillance Term used to describe the tracking of infections by health care agencies.

susceptibility The risk of the host to infection; may be increased by the breakdown of host defenses against pathogens.

swimmer's ear See *external otitis*.

sympathectomy Surgical cutting of the sympathetic nerve branches via endoscopy through a small axillary incision.

sympathetic tone A state of partial blood vessel constriction caused when nerves from the sympathetic division of the autonomic nervous system continuously stimulate vascular smooth muscle.

synapse The area through which impulses are transmitted to their eventual destination.

syncope Transient loss of consciousness (blackouts), most commonly caused by decreased perfusion to the brain.

syndrome of inappropriate antidiuretic hormone (SIADH) Persistent hyponatremia, hypovolemia, and inappropriately elevated urine osmolality that occurs when vasopressin (antidiuretic hormone) is secreted even when plasma osmolarity is low or normal.

synovectomy The surgical removal of synovium.

synovial joint Type of joint lined with synovium, a membrane that secretes synovial fluid for lubrication and shock absorption.

synovitis Inflammation of synovial membrane.

syphilis A complex sexually transmitted disease that can become systemic and cause serious complications and even death. It is caused by the spirochete *Treponema pallidum,* which is found in the mouth, intestinal tract, and genital areas of people and animals. The infection is usually transmitted by sexual contact, but transmission can occur through close body contact and kissing.

syringe pump Pump for infusion therapy that uses a battery-powered piston to push the plunger continuously at a selected mL/hr rate; limited to small-volume continuous or intermittent infusions.

systemic Affecting the body system as a whole.

systemic lupus erythematosus (SLE) A chronic, progressive, inflammatory connective tissue disorder that can cause major body organs and systems to fail; characterized by spontaneous remissions and exacerbations.

systemic sclerosis (SSc) A chronic connective tissue disease characterized by inflammation, fibrosis, and sclerosis of the skin and vital organs. Also called "scleroderma" and formerly called "progressive systemic sclerosis."

systole The phase of the cardiac cycle that consists of the contraction and emptying of the atria and ventricles.

systolic blood pressure The amount of pressure/force generated by the left ventricle to distribute blood into the aorta with each contraction of the heart.

systolic heart failure (systolic ventricular dysfunction) Heart failure that results when the heart is unable to contract forcefully enough during systole to eject adequate amounts of blood into the circulation.

T

T wave In the electrocardiogram, the deflection that follows the ST segment and represents ventricular repolarization.

tachycardia An excessively fast heart rate; characterized as a pulse rate greater than 100 beats/min.

tachydysrhythmia An abnormal heart rhythm with a rate greater than 100 beats/min.

tactile (vocal) fremitus A vibration of the chest wall produced when the patient speaks; can be palpated on the chest wall.

target tissues The tissues that respond specifically to a given hormone.

taut Tightly stretched.

teamwork and collaboration A QSEN competency in which the nurse functions effectively within nursing and interprofessional teams, fostering open communication, mutual respect, and shared decision making to achieve quality patient care.

telangiectasias Vascular lesions with a red center and radiating branches. Also called "spider angiomas," "spider nevi," or "vascular spiders."

telemetry In electrocardiography (ECG), the use of a battery-powered transmitter system for monitoring an ambulatory patient; allows freedom of movement within a certain radius without losing transmission of the ECG.

temporal field blindness A decrease in lateral peripheral vision.

temporary pacing A nonsurgical intervention for cardiac dysrhythmia that provides a timed electrical stimulus to the heart when either the impulse initiation or the intrinsic conduction system of the heart is defective.

tendon Any one of many bands of tough, fibrous tissue that attach muscles to bones.

tendon transplant Removal of a tendon from one part of the body and transplantation into the affected area to replace a ruptured tendon that cannot be repaired surgically.

tenesmus Straining, especially painful straining to defecate.

teratogenic Tending to produce birth defects.

tetany Continuous contractions of muscle groups; hyperexcitability of nerves and muscles.

tetraplegia Another term for *quadriplegia* (paralysis that involves all four extremities).

thalamotomy An alternative to stereotactic pallidotomy as a surgical treatment for the patient with Parkinson disease; uses thermocoagulation of brain cells to reduce tremor. Usually only unilateral surgery is performed to benefit the side of the body most affected by the disease.

thalamus A structure within the brain; functions as the "central switchboard" for the central nervous system.

thallium scan A test that is similar to the bone scan but uses the radioisotope *thallium* and is more sensitive in diagnosing the extent of disease in patients with osteosarcoma.

The Joint Commission An organization that offers peer evaluation for accreditation every 3 years for all types of health care agencies that meet their standards. Formerly known as the *Joint Commission for Accreditation of Healthcare Organizations (JCAHO).*

therapeutic hypothermia Treatment that lowers the body core temperature to reduce the risk of cell, tissue, and organ damage from a low or absent blood flow. Usually follows cardiac arrest.

thermotherapy Technique for treating benign prostatic hyperplasia that uses a variety of heat methods to destroy excess prostate tissue.

third intention Delayed primary closure of a wound with a high risk for infection. The wound is intentionally left open for several days until inflammation has subsided and is then closed by first intention.

thoracentesis The aspiration of pleural fluid or air from the pleural space.

threshold In evaluating hearing, the lowest level of intensity at which pure tones and speech are heard by a patient; in general, the lowest level at which a stimulus is perceived.

thrombectomy Removal of a clot (thrombus) from a blood vessel.

thrombocytopenia A reduction in the number of blood platelets below the level needed for normal coagulation, resulting in an increased tendency to bleed.

thrombophlebitis   The presence of a thrombus associated with inflammation; usually occurs in the deep veins of the lower extremities.

thrombosis   The formation of a blood clot (thrombus) within a blood vessel.

thrombotic stroke   Damage to the brain when blood flow is impaired from a clot, resulting in blockage to one or more of the arteries supplying blood to the brain.

thrombus   A blood clot believed to result from an endothelial injury, venous stasis, or hypercoagulability.

thymectomy   Removal of the thymus gland.

thymoma   An encapsulated tumor of the thymus gland.

thyrocalcitonin (TCT)   A hormone produced and secreted by the parafollicular cells of the thyroid gland to help regulate serum calcium levels; secreted in response to excess plasma calcium.

thyroiditis   Inflammation of the thyroid gland.

thyroid storm (thyroid crisis)   A life-threatening event that occurs in patients with uncontrolled hyperthyroidism and is usually caused by Graves' disease. Key manifestations include fever, tachycardia, and systolic hypertension.

thyrotoxicosis   The condition caused by excessive amounts of thyroid hormones.

thyroxine (T_4)   A hormone that is produced by the follicular cells of the thyroid gland and increases metabolism.

Tinel's sign   Test that confirms a diagnosis of carpal tunnel syndrome; a positive test causes palmar paresthesias when the area of the median nerve is tapped lightly.

tinnitus   A continuous ringing or noise perception in the ears.

titration   Adjustment of IV fluid rate on the basis of the patient's urine output plus serum electrolyte values.

TNM (tumor, node, metastasis)   System developed by the American Joint Committee on Cancer to describe the anatomic extent of cancers.

toe brachial pressure index (TBPI)   Toe systolic pressure divided by brachial (arm) systolic pressure; may be performed instead of or in addition to ankle-brachial index to determine arterial perfusion in the feet and toes.

tonic phase   Pertaining to a state of stiffening or rigidity of the muscles, particularly of the arms and legs, and immediate loss of consciousness of a tonic-clonic seizure.

tonsillitis   An inflammation and infection of the tonsils and lymphatic tissues located on each side of the throat.

tophi   A collection of uric acid crystals that form hard, irregular, painless nodules on the ears, arms, and fingers of patients with gout.

topical chemical débridement   Method of débriding a wound by applying topical enzyme preparations to loosen necrotic tissue.

torn meniscus   Tear of the knee meniscus (medial or lateral) in which the patient typically has pain, swelling, and tenderness in the knee.

torsades de pointes   A type of ventricular tachycardia that is related to a prolonged QT interval.

total hysterectomy   Removal of the uterus and cervix; the procedure may be vaginal or abdominal.

total joint arthroplasty (TJA)   Surgical creation of a joint, or total joint replacement; commonly performed in patients with osteoarthritis. Also called "total joint replacement (TJR)."

total joint replacement (TJR)   See *total joint arthroplasty.*

total parenteral nutrition (TPN)   Provision of intensive nutritional support for an extended time; delivered to the patient through access to central veins, usually the subclavian or internal jugular veins.

total thyroidectomy   The surgical removal of all of the thyroid tissue.

touch discrimination   Part of the neurologic examination. The patient closes his or her eyes while the practitioner touches the patient with a finger and asks that the patient point to the area touched.

toxic and drug-induced hepatitis   Liver inflammation resulting from exposure to hepatotoxins (e.g., industrial toxins, alcohol, and medications).

toxic epidermal necrolysis (TEN)   A rare acute drug reaction of the skin that results in diffuse erythema and blister formation, with mucous membrane involvement and systemic toxicity.

toxic megacolon   Acute enlargement of the colon along with fever, leukocytosis, and tachycardia; usually associated with ulcerative colitis.

toxic multinodular goiter   Hyperthyroidism caused by multiple thyroid nodules, which may be enlarged thyroid tissues or adenomas, and a goiter that has been present for several years.

toxic shock syndrome (TSS)   A severe illness caused by a toxin produced by certain strains of *Staphylococcus aureus*. It was first recognized in 1980 as related to menstruation and tampon use. It is characterized by abrupt onset of a high fever and headache, sore throat, vomiting, diarrhea, generalized rash, and hypotension. The most common manifestations are skin changes (initially a rash that resembles a severe sunburn and changes to a macular erythema similar to a drug-related rash).

toxidrome   A syndrome related to drug toxicity.

toxin   Protein molecule released by bacteria that affects host cell at a distant site. Continued multiplication of a pathogen is sometimes accompanied by toxin production.

trabeculation   An abnormal thickening of the bladder wall caused by urinary retention and obstruction.

tracheostomy   The (tracheal) stoma, or opening, that results from a tracheotomy.

tracheotomy   The surgical incision into the trachea for the purpose of establishing an airway.

trachoma   A chronic conjunctivitis caused by *Chlamydia trachomatis*.

traction   The application of a pulling force to a part of the body to provide reduction, alignment, and rest.

transcellular fluid   Any of the fluids in special body spaces, including cerebrospinal fluid, synovial fluid, peritoneal fluid, and pleural fluid.

transcutaneous pacing   Temporary pacing that is accomplished through the application of two large external electrodes.

transesophageal echocardiography (TEE)   A form of echocardiography performed transesophageally (through the esophagus); an ultrasound transducer is placed immediately behind the heart in the esophagus or stomach to examine cardiac structure and function.

transferrin   An iron-transport protein that can be measured directly or calculated as an indirect measurement of total iron-binding capacity.

transgender   Patients who self-identify as the opposite gender or a gender that does not match their natal sex.

transient ischemic attack (TIA)   A brief attack (lasting a few minutes to less than 24 hours) of focal neurologic dysfunction caused by a brief interruption in cerebral blood flow, possibly resulting from cerebral vasospasm or transient systemic arterial hypertension. Repeated attacks may damage brain tissue; multiple attacks indicate significant increased risk for brain attack.

transmyocardial laser revascularization   A new surgical procedure for patients with unstable angina and inoperable coronary artery disease with areas of reversible myocardial ischemia. After a single-lung intubation, a left anterior thoracotomy is performed and the heart is visualized. A laser is used to create 20 to 24 long, narrow channels through the left ventricular muscle to the left ventricle. The channels eventually allow oxygenated blood to flow from the left ventricle during diastole to nourish the muscle.

transport maximum   See *renal threshold.*

transsexual   A person who has modified his or her natal body to match the appropriate gender identity, either through cosmetic, hormonal, or surgical means.

transurethral microwave therapy (TUMT)   Procedure for treating benign prostatic hyperplasia using high temperatures to heat and destroy excess tissue.

transurethral needle ablation (TUNA)   Procedure for treating benign prostatic hyperplasia using low radiofrequency energy to shrink the prostate.

transurethral resection of the prostate (TURP)   The traditional "closed" surgical procedure for removal of the prostate. In this procedure, the surgeon inserts a resectoscope (an instrument similar to a cystoscope, but with a cutting and cauterizing loop) through the urethra. The enlarged portion of the prostate gland is then resected in small pieces.

trauma   Bodily injury.

trauma center   Specialty care facility that provides competent and timely trauma services to patients depending on its designated level of capability.

trauma system   An organized and integrated approach to trauma care designed to ensure that all critical elements of trauma care delivery are aligned to meet the injured patient's needs.

triage   In the emergency department, sorting or classifying patients into priority levels depending on illness or injury severity, with the highest acuity needs receiving the quickest evaluation and treatment.

triage officer In a hospital's emergency response plan, the person who rapidly evaluates each patient who arrives at the hospital. In a large hospital, this person is generally a physician who is assisted by triage nurses; however, a nurse may assume this role when physician resources are limited.

trigeminy A type of premature complex consisting of a repetitive three-beat pattern; usually occurs as two sequential normal complexes followed by a premature complex and a pause, with the same pattern repeating itself in triplets.

trigger points In patients with fibromyalgia syndrome, tender areas that can typically be palpated to elicit pain in a predictable, reproducible pattern.

triglycerides Serum lipid profile that includes the measurement of cholesterol and lipoproteins.

triiodothyronine (T₃) A hormone produced by the follicular cells of the thyroid gland.

troponin A myocardial muscle protein released into the bloodstream after injury to myocardial muscle. Because it is not found in healthy patients, any rise in values indicates cardiac necrosis or acute myocardial infarction.

truss A device, usually a pad made with firm material, that is held in place over the hernia with a belt to keep the abdominal contents from protruding into the hernial sac.

tuberculosis (TB) A highly communicable disease caused by *Mycobacterium tuberculosis*. It is the most common bacterial infection worldwide.

tumescence The condition of being swollen.

tunneled central venous catheter A type of catheter used for long-term infusion therapy in which a portion of the catheter lies in a subcutaneous tunnel, separating the points where the catheter enters the vein from where it exits the skin.

turbidity Cloudiness of a solution.

turbinates Three bony projections that protrude into the nasal cavities from the walls of the internal portion of the nose.

turgor The condition of being swollen and congested; indicates the amount of skin elasticity; the normal resiliency of a pinched fold of skin.

tyrosine kinase inhibitors (TKIs) Drugs with the main action of inhibiting activation of tyrosine kinases. There are many different TKIs. Some are unique to the cell type; others may be present only in cancer cells that express a specific gene mutation. As a result, the different TKI drugs are effective in disrupting the growth of some cancer cell types and not others.

U

U wave In the electrocardiogram, the deflection that follows the T wave and may result from slow repolarization of ventricular Purkinje fibers. When present, it is of the same polarity as the T wave, although generally smaller. Abnormal prominence of the U wave suggests an electrolyte abnormality or other disturbance.

ulcerative colitis (UC) A chronic inflammatory process that affects the mucosal lining of the colon or rectum; one of a group of bowel diseases of unknown etiology characterized by remissions and exacerbations. It can result in loose stools containing blood and mucus, poor absorption of vital nutrients, and thickening of the colon wall.

umbilical hernia Protrusion of the intestine at the umbilicus; can be congenital or acquired. Congenital umbilical hernias appear in infancy. Acquired umbilical hernias directly result from increased intra-abdominal pressure and are most commonly seen in obese people.

unclassified seizure One of the three broad categories of seizure disorders along with partial seizure and generalized seizure. They occur for no known reason, do not fit into the generalized or partial classifications, and account for about half of all seizure activity. Also called "idiopathic seizures."

uncus The inner part of the temporal lobe of the brain that can move downward and cause pressure on the brainstem; the vital sign center.

undermining Separation of the skin layers at the wound margins from the underlying granulation tissue.

unilateral body neglect syndrome In the patient who has had a brain attack, an unawareness of the existence of the paralyzed side. For example, the patient may believe he or she is sitting up straight when actually he or she is leaning to one side. Another typical example is the patient who washes or dresses only one side of the body.

Unna boot A wound dressing constructed of gauze moistened with zinc oxide; used to promote venous return in the ambulatory patient with a stasis ulcer and to form a sterile environment for the ulcer. The boot is applied to the affected limb, from the toes to the knee, after the ulcer has been cleaned with normal saline solution and covered with an elastic wrap. The dressing hardens like a cast.

upper endoscopy See *esophagogastroduodenoscopy*.

upper esophageal sphincter (UES) The ring-like band of muscle fibers at the upper end of the esophagus. When at rest, the sphincter is closed to prevent air from entering into the esophagus during respiration.

upper GI (gastrointestinal) radiographic series The radiographic visualization of the gastrointestinal tract from the oral part of the pharynx to the duodenojejunal junction; used to detect disorders of structure or function of the esophagus (barium swallow), stomach, or duodenum.

uremia The accumulation of nitrogenous wastes in the blood (azotemia); a result of renal failure, with clinical symptoms including nausea and vomiting.

uremic frost A layer of urea crystals from evaporated sweat; may appear on the face, eyebrows, axilla, and groin in patients with advanced uremic syndrome.

uremic syndrome The systemic clinical and laboratory manifestations of end-stage kidney disease.

ureterolithiasis Formation of stones in the ureter.

ureteropelvic junction (UPJ) The narrow area in the upper third of the ureter at the point at which the renal pelvis becomes the ureter.

ureteroplasty Surgical repair of the ureter.

ureterovesical junction (UVJ) The point at which each ureter becomes narrow as it enters the bladder.

urethral meatus The opening at the endpoint of the urethra.

urethral stricture An obstruction that occurs low in the urinary tract due to decreased diameter of the urethra, causing bladder distention before hydroureter and hydronephrosis.

urethritis An inflammation of the urethra that causes symptoms similar to urinary tract infection.

urethroplasty Surgical treatment of the urethral stricture to remove the affected area with or without grafting to create a larger opening.

urgency The feeling that urination will occur immediately.

urgent triage In a three-tiered triage scheme, the category that includes patients who should be treated quickly but in whom an immediate threat to life does not currently exist, such as those with abdominal pain or displaced fractures or dislocations.

urinary tract infection (UTI) An infection in the normally sterile urinary system. The unobstructed and complete passage of urine from the renal and urinary systems is critical in maintaining a sterile urinary tract. When any structural abnormality is present, the risk for damage as a result of infection is greatly increased.

urolithiasis The presence of calculi (stones) in the urinary tract.

urosepsis The spread of an infection from the urinary tract to the bloodstream, resulting in systemic infection accompanied by fever, chills, hypotension, and altered mental status.

urticaria A transient vascular reaction of the skin marked by the development of wheals (hives).

uterine artery embolization Treatment for leiomyomas in which a radiologist uses a percutaneous catheter inserted through the femoral artery to inject polyvinyl alcohol pellets into the uterine artery. The resulting blockage starves the tumor of circulation, allowing it (or them) to shrink.

uterine prolapse Downward displacement of the uterus into the vagina.

uvea The middle layer of the eye, which consists of the choroid, ciliary body, and iris. The choroid has many blood vessels that supply nutrients to the retina.

V

vagal maneuver Nonsurgical management of cardiac dysrhythmias that is intended to induce vagal stimulation of the cardiac conduction system, specifically the sinoatrial and atrioventricular nodes. Vagal maneuvers may be attempted to terminate supraventricular tachydysrhythmia.

vaginoplasty The construction of a new vagina in a male-to-female patient, usually with inverted penile tissue or a colon graft, and the creation of a clitoris and labia using scrotal or penile tissue and skin grafts.

validation therapy For the patient with moderate or severe Alzheimer's disease, the process of recognizing and acknowledging the patient's feelings and concerns without reinforcing an erroneous belief (e.g., if the patient is looking for his or her deceased mother).

Valsalva maneuver A form of vagal stimulation of the cardiac conduction system in which the health care provider instructs the patient to bear down as if straining to have a bowel movement.

valvular regurgitation Regurgitation of any heart valve. See also *mitral regurgitation*.

variant (Prinzmetal's) angina A type of angina caused by coronary vasospasm (vessel spasm); usually associated with elevation of the ST segment on an electrocardiogram obtained during anginal attacks.

varicose veins Distended, protruding veins that appear darkened and tortuous; common in patients older than 30 years whose occupations require prolonged standing. As the vein wall weakens and dilates, venous pressure increases and the valves become incompetent (defective). The incompetent valves enhance the vessel dilation, and the veins become tortuous and distended.

vascular access device (VAD) A catheter; a plastic tube placed in a blood vessel to deliver fluids and medications.

vasculitis Blood vessel inflammation.

vasoconstriction Decrease in diameter of blood vessels.

vasopressin Secretion of the posterior pituitary gland. Also known as "antidiuretic hormone" or "ADH."

vasospasm A sudden and transient constriction of a blood vessel.

Vaughn-Williams classification System used to categorize antidysrhythmic agents according to their effects on the action potential of cardiac cells.

vegan A vegetarian diet pattern in which only foods of plant origin are eaten.

venous beading A complication of diabetes; the abnormal appearance of retinal veins in which areas of swelling and constriction along a segment of vein resemble links of sausage. Such bleeding occurs in areas of retinal ischemia and is a predictor of proliferative diabetic retinopathy.

venous insufficiency Alteration of venous efficiency by thrombosis or defective valves; caused by prolonged venous hypertension, which stretches the veins and damages the valves, resulting in further venous hypertension, edema, and, eventually, venous stasis ulcers, swelling, and cellulitis.

venous thromboembolism (VTE) A term that refers to both deep vein thrombosis and pulmonary embolism; obstruction by a thrombus.

ventilator-associated lung injury (VALI) Damage from prolonged ventilation causing loss of surfactant, increased inflammation, fluid leakage, and noncardiac pulmonary edema. Also known as "ventilator-induced lung injury."

ventilator-induced lung injury (VILI) See *ventilator-associated lung injury*.

ventral hernia See *incisional hernia*.

ventricular asystole The complete absence of any ventricular rhythm. There are no electrical impulses in the ventricles and therefore no ventricular depolarization, no QRS complex, no contraction, no cardiac output, and no pulse, respirations, or blood pressure. The patient is in full cardiac arrest.

ventricular fibrillation (VF) A cardiac dysrhythmia that results from electrical chaos in the ventricles; impulses from many irritable foci fire in a totally disorganized manner so that ventricular contraction cannot occur; there is no cardiac output or pulse and therefore no cerebral, myocardial, or systemic perfusion. This rhythm is rapidly fatal if not successfully terminated within 3 to 5 minutes.

ventricular gallop An abnormal third heart sound that arises from vibrations of the valves and supporting structures and is produced during the rapid passive filling phase of ventricular diastole when blood flows from the atrium to a noncompliant ventricle. In patients older than 35 years, it is an early sign of heart failure or ventricular septal defect.

ventricular remodeling (1) Progressive myocyte (myocardial cell) contractile dysfunction over time; results from activation of the renin-angiotensin system caused by reduced blood flow to the kidneys, a common occurrence in low-output states; (2) after a myocardial infarction, permanent changes in the size and shape of the left ventricle due to scar tissue; such remodeling may decrease left ventricular function, cause heart failure, and increase morbidity and mortality.

ventricular tachycardia (VT) An abnormal heart rhythm that occurs with repetitive firing of an irritable ventricular ectopic focus, usually at a rate of 140 to 180 beats/min or more.

ventriculomyomectomy The surgical excision of a portion of the hypertrophied ventricular septum to create a widened outflow tract in patients with obstructive hypertrophic cardiomyopathy. Also called "ventricular septal myectomy."

veracity Ethical principle that requires that the nurse is obligated to tell the truth to the best of his or her knowledge.

vertebroplasty A minimally invasive surgery for managing vertebral fractures in patients with osteoporosis. Bone cement is injected directly into the fracture site to provide immediate pain relief.

vertigo A sense of spinning movement that may result from diseases of the inner ear.

vesicants Chemicals or drugs that cause tissue damage on direct contact or extravasation.

vesicle In health care, a small bladder or blister.

vestibule A longitudinal area between the labia minora, the clitoris, and the vagina that contains Bartholin glands and the openings of the urethra, Skene's glands (paraurethral glands), and vagina.

viral hepatitis Inflammation of the liver that results from an infection caused by one of five major categories of viruses (hepatitis A, B, C, D, or E). Viral hepatitis is the most common type and can be either acute or chronic.

viral load testing Test that measures the presence of human immune deficiency virus genetic material (ribonucleic acid) or other viral proteins in the patient's blood.

Virchow's triad The occurrence of stasis of blood flow, endothelial injury, or hypercoagulability; often associated with thrombus formation.

viremia The presence of viruses in the blood.

virilization The presence of male secondary sex characteristics.

virtual colonoscopy A noninvasive alternative to the colonoscopy procedure. A scanner is used to view the colon.

virulence A term used to describe the frequency with which a pathogen causes disease (degree of communicability) and its ability to invade and damage a host. Virulence can also indicate the severity of the disease; often used as a synonym for *pathogenicity*.

visceral proteins Proteins such as albumin that circulate in the bloodstream and may be produced by the liver.

vitiligo An abnormality of the skin characterized by patchy areas of pigment loss with increased pigmentation at the edges. It is seen with primary hypofunction of the adrenal glands and is due to autoimmune destruction of melanocytes in the skin.

vitreous body The clear, thick gel that fills the vitreous chamber of the eye (the space between the lens and the retina). This gel transmits light and shapes the eye.

vocational counselor A member of the rehabilitative health care team who assists the patient with job placement, training, or further education.

volutrauma Damage to the lung by excess volume delivered to one lung over the other.

volvulus Obstruction of the bowel caused by twisting of the bowel.

vulvovaginitis Inflammation of the lower genital tract resulting from a disturbance of the balance of hormones and flora in the vagina and vulva.

W

warm antibody anemia A form of immunohemolytic anemia (in which the immune system attacks a person's own red blood cells for unknown reasons) that occurs with immunoglobulin G antibody excess and may be triggered by drugs, chemicals, or other autoimmune problems.

warm phase A phase lasting 2 to 3 weeks after peripheral nerve trauma resulting in complete denervation; the extremity is warm, and the skin appears flushed or rosy. The warm phase is gradually superseded by a cold phase.

water brash Reflex salivary hypersecretion that occurs in response to reflux in the patient with gastroesophageal reflux disease.

WBC White blood cell.

weaning The process of going from ventilatory dependence to spontaneous breathing.

wedge resection Removal of small, localized areas of disease.

Wernicke's aphasia See *receptive aphasia*.

Wernicke's area An important speech area of the cerebrum. It is located in the temporal lobe and plays a significant role in higher-level brain function. It enables the processing of words into coherent thought and recognition of the idea behind written or printed words (language).

Whipple procedure (radical pancreaticoduodenectomy) A surgical treatment for cancer of the head of the pancreas. The procedure entails removal of the proximal head of the pancreas, the duodenum, a portion of the jejunum, the stomach (partial or total gastrectomy), and the gallbladder, with anastomosis of the pancreatic duct (pancreaticojejunostomy), the common bile duct (choledochojejunostomy), and the stomach (gastrojejunostomy) to the jejunum.

white matter In the spinal cord, myelinated axons that surround the gray matter (neuron cell bodies).

Williams position A position in which the patient lies in the semi-Fowler's position and flexes the knees to relax the muscles of the lower back and relieve pressure on the spinal nerve root. This is typically more comfortable and therapeutic for the patient with low back pain.

withdrawing or withholding life-sustaining therapy The withdrawal or withholding of one or more therapies that might prolong the life of a person who cannot be cured by the therapy; the withdrawal of therapy does not directly cause death. Formerly called "passive euthanasia."

work-related musculoskeletal disorders (MSDs) Disorders caused by heavy lifting and dependent transfers by staff members.

X

xenograft Tissue transplanted (grafted) from another species; for example, a heart valve transplanted from a pig to a human.

xerostomia Abnormal dryness of the mouth caused by a severe reduction in the flow of saliva.

x-ray Radiation that is generated by machine.

NCLEX® EXAMINATION CHALLENGES—ANSWER KEY

Chapter 2
p. 12   C
p. 15   C
p. 21   D

Chapter 3
p. 33   A, B, E
p. 34   B
p. 37   C
p. 41   0.4 mL
p. 44   B

Chapter 4
p. 62   D

Chapter 6
p. 79   D
p. 88   A

Chapter 7
p. 97   A, B, D, E
p. 99   A, B, C, E

Chapter 8
p. 112   A
p. 118   C

Chapter 9
p. 122   B
p. 132   A, B, C, D, E
p. 135   C

Chapter 10
p. 141   D
p. 144   A, B, E

Chapter 11
p. 158   D
p. 163   D
p. 165   B
p. 170   D

Chapter 12
p. 183   C

Chapter 13
p. 190   D, A, C, B
p. 193   100

Chapter 14
p. 216   C
p. 222   A
p. 225   C

Chapter 15
p. 244   D
p. 248   C

Chapter 16
p. 261   C
p. 263   D
p. 271   A

Chapter 17
p. 281   B

Chapter 18
p. 294   B, C, E
p. 300   B, D, E
p. 302   A
p. 308   B, C, E, F
p. 317   A, B, C, E
p. 320   C

Chapter 19
p. 332   B
p. 332   C
p. 340   D
p. 342   A

Chapter 20
p. 354   B
p. 355   D

Chapter 21
p. 365   C
p. 369   D

Chapter 22
p. 377   A
p. 383   C
p. 387   B
p. 394   C

Chapter 23
p. 405   C
p. 406   B, E

Chapter 24
p. 424   C
p. 430   B

Chapter 25
p. 453   B
p. 458   D
p. 461   C

Chapter 26
p. 475   D
p. 479   B
p. 485   A

Chapter 27
p. 500   C
p. 503   A
p. 506   C

Chapter 28
p. 516   D
p. 522   C
p. 527   A

Chapter 29
p. 533   C
p. 537   C
p. 539   D

Chapter 30
p. 557   B
p. 564   D
p. 569   D
p. 579   C

Chapter 31
p. 587   B
p. 593   A
p. 598   A, B, D

Chapter 32
p. 608   A, E
p. 616   A
p. 619   D

Chapter 33
p. 634   D
p. 645   C

Chapter 34
p. 663   C
p. 668   A, D
p. 669   C
p. 673   D

Chapter 35
p. 683   B, C, E
p. 686   D
p. 687   B
p. 697   B

Chapter 36
p. 709   A
p. 717   C
p. 722   B
p. 733   D
p. 735   A

Chapter 37
p. 746   C
p. 749   B
p. 753   D

Chapter 38
p. 761   B, D, F
p. 768   79
p. 778   C

Chapter 39
p. 792   B
p. 795   C

Chapter 40
p. 801   D
p. 806   A
p. 809   B
p. 814   C
p. 826   B

Chapter 41
p. 839   B
p. 848   A

Chapter 42
p. 857   C
p. 862   A, B, D
p. 876   C
p. 879   D

Chapter 43
p. 891   D
p. 897   A

Chapter 44
p. 916   A, C, D
p. 928   C

Chapter 45
p. 933   A, B, E
p. 938   B, A, D, C
p. 942   D
p. 953   D
p. 961   C

Chapter 46
p. 971   C

Chapter 47
p. 985   D
p. 989   C
p. 989   A
p. 994   C

Chapter 48
p. 1002   D
p. 1008   A
p. 1009   A

Chapter 49
p. 1023   B, E
p. 1027   D

Chapter 50
p. 1034   B
p. 1039   C

Chapter 51
p. 1061   A, C, D
p. 1066   A
p. 1073   C
p. 1075   A, B, E

Chapter 52
p. 1091   C
p. 1093   A, D, E

Chapter 53
p. 1102   A
p. 1105   C
p. 1107   A, E, F

Chapter 54
p. 1114   A
p. 1118   A, B, C, E

Chapter 55
p. 1130   C, B, A, D
p. 1131   A, C, E
p. 1141   D

Chapter 56
p. 1148   A
p. 1155   B, C, D
p. 1163   C

Chapter 57
p. 1172   C
p. 1176   A
p. 1179   D
p. 1188   C

Chapter 58
p. 1196   A, D, E
p. 1200   D
p. 1203   A

Chapter 59
p. 1218   B
p. 1220   C
p. 1226   C, E
p. 1230   A, C, D, E

Chapter 60
p. 1236   45.9
p. 1241   C, D, E, F

Chapter 61
p. 1259   D
p. 1264   C

Chapter 62
p. 1268   C
p. 1273   B
p. 1280   A

Chapter 63
p. 1288   A, D, E, F, G
p. 1291   C
p. 1298   D

Chapter 64
p. 1302   D
p. 1306   C
p. 1317   A
p. 1328   B

Chapter 65
p. 1354   B
p. 1359   D
p. 1363   C

Chapter 66
p. 1372   D
p. 1383   C
p. 1388   C
p. 1389   A

Chapter 67
p. 1397   B
p. 1399   A
p. 1406   C

Chapter 68
p. 1416   A
p. 1418   C
p. 1423   B

Chapter 69
p. 1456   B
p. 1459   A

Chapter 70
p. 1467   D
p. 1474   C

Chapter 71
p. 1485   C, D, E
p. 1490   B

Chapter 72
p. 1505   725
p. 1506   B
p. 1513   D
p. 1515   B

Chapter 73
p. 1524   C
p. 1527   C, D, E

Chapter 74
p. 1535   C
p. 1544   B

Chapter 1

1-1, From Potter, P., Perry, A., Stocker, P., & Hall, A. (2011). *Basic nursing* (7th ed.). St. Louis: Mosby; 1-2, from Sorrentino, S. (2011). *Mosby's textbook for long-term care nursing assistants* (6th ed.). St. Louis: Mosby.

Chapter 2

2-3, From the Aging Clinical Research Center (ACRC), a joint project of Stanford University and the VA Palo Alto Health Care System, Palo Alto, CA, funded by the National Institute of Aging and the Department of Veterans Affairs.

Chapter 3

3-1, Modified from Pasero, C., & McCaffery, M. (2011). *Pain assessment and pharmacologic management.* St. Louis: Mosby; 3-2, from Melzack, R. (1975). The McGill Pain Questionnaire: Major properties and scoring methods. *Pain, 1,* 272-281; 3-3, Copyright 1983 Wong-Baker FACES Foundation.

Chapter 4

4-2, Modified from Nussbaum, R., McInnes, R., & Willard, H. (2007). *Thompson & Thompson: Genetics in medicine* (7th ed.). Philadelphia: Saunders; 4-5, modified from Jorde, L., Carey, J., Bamshad, M., & White, R. (2000). *Medical genetics* (2nd ed.). St. Louis: Mosby; 4-8, modified from Jorde, L., Carey, J., & Bamshad, M. (2010). *Medical genetics* (4th ed.). St. Louis: Mosby.

Chapter 5

5-1, © 2010. Rona F. Levin & Jeffrey M. Keefer; 5-2, © 2010. R.E. Burke & R.F. Levin; 5-3, © 2007. Visiting Nurse Service of New York and Rona F. Levin.

Chapter 6

6-1, From Scott, K., Webb, M., & Sorrentino, S. (2011). *Long-term caring* (2nd ed.). Sydney: Mosby Australia; 6-5, from Potter, P., Perry, A., Stockert, P., & Hall, A. (2013). *Fundamentals of nursing* (8th ed.). St. Louis: Mosby.

Chapter 7

7-1, © 2005. National Hospice and Palliative Care Organization, 2007 Revised. All rights reserved. Reproduction and distribution by an organization or organized group without the written permission of the National Hospice and Palliative Care Organization is expressly forbidden. Visit caringinfo.org for more information.

Chapter 9

9-1, From Auerbach, P. S. (2012). *Wilderness medicine* (6th ed.). Philadelphia: Mosby; courtesy Michael Cardwell & Carl Barden Venom Laboratory; 9-2, from Auerbach, P. S. (2012). *Wilderness medicine* (6th ed.).

Philadelphia: Mosby; courtesy Sherman Minton, MD; 9-3, from Auerbach, P. S. (2012). *Wilderness medicine* (6th ed.). Philadelphia: Mosby; courtesy Michael Cardwell & Jude McNally; 9-4, from Auerbach, P. S. (2012). *Wilderness medicine* (6th ed.). Philadelphia: Mosby; courtesy Indiana University Medical Center; 9-5, from Auerbach, P. S. (2012). *Wilderness medicine* (6th ed.). Philadelphia: Mosby; courtesy Paul S. Auerbach, MD; 9-6, from Auerbach, P. S. (2012). *Wilderness medicine* (6th ed.) Philadelphia: Mosby; 9-7, from Auerbach, P. S. (2008). *Wilderness medicine* (5th ed.). Philadelphia: Mosby; courtesy Cameron Bangs, MD.

Chapter 10

10-2, Courtesy Meg Blair, PhD, RN; 10-3, courtesy Jeanne McConnell, MSN, RN.

Chapter 11

11-2, 11-7, 11-9, ©1992 by M. Linda Workman. All rights reserved.

Chapter 12

12-3, 12-12, ©1992 by M. Linda Workman. All rights reserved.

Chapter 13

13-1, From Perry, A., Potter, P., & Ostendorf, W. (2014). *Clinical nursing skills & techniques* (8th ed.). St. Louis: Mosby; 13-2, 13-16, courtesy and © Becton, Dickinson and Company; 13-3, courtesy AccuVein, LLC; 13-7, courtesy Edwards Lifesciences, Irvine, CA; 13-11, courtesy NowMedical, Chadds Ford, PA; 13-12, from Lilley, L., Collins, S., & Snyder, J. (2014). *Pharmacology and the nursing process* (7th ed.). St. Louis: Mosby; 13-14, courtesy Kimberly-Clark Corporation; 13-15, courtesy Venetec International, San Diego, CA; 13-17, courtesy I.V. House, Hazelwood, MO; 13-18, from Lopez, J. H., & Reyes-Ortiz, A. (2010). Subcutaneous hydration by hypodermoclysis. *Reviews in Clinical Gerontology, 20,* 105-113.

Chapter 14

14-1, From World Health Organization: Surgical safety checklist, ed 1. Available at www.who.int/patientsafety/safesurgery/en/. © World Health Organization, 2009. 14-2, courtesy Christiana Care Health Services, Newark, DE; 14-4, from Perry, A. G., & Potter, P. A. (2010). *Clinical nursing skills and techniques* (7th ed.). St. Louis: Mosby; 14-5, from Angelo, R., Ryu, R., & Esch, J. (2010). *AANA advanced arthroscopy: the shoulder.* Philadelphia: Saunders.

Chapter 15

15-1, Courtesy Christiana Care Health Services, Newark, DE; 15-3, A, from Patell, A., Whang, P., & Vaccaro, A. (2008). Overview of computer-assisted image-guided surgery of the spine.

Seminars in Spine Surgery, 20(3), 186-194; 15-3, B, from Miller, R., & Pardo, M. (2011). *Basics of anesthesia* (6th ed.). Philadelphia: Saunders; 15-5, redrawn with permission by Intuitive Surgical, Inc., 2007.

Chapter 16

16-1, Courtesy Forrest General Hospital, Hattiesburg, MS; 16-2, 16-4, from Harkreader, H., Hogan, M. A., & Thobaben, M. (2007). *Fundamentals of nursing: Caring and clinical judgment* (3rd ed.). Philadelphia: Saunders; 16-3, A, from Sirois, M. (2011). *Principles and practice of veterinary technology* (3rd ed.). St. Louis: Mosby; 16-3, B, courtesy 2014 C. R. Bard, Inc. Covington, GA. Used with permission; 16-3 C, D, courtesy C.R. Bard, Inc., Covington, GA.

Chapter 17

17-3, Modified from Goldman, L., & Schafer, A. (Eds.). (2012). *Goldman's Cecil medicine* (24th ed.). Philadelphia: Saunders.

Chapter 18

18-2, From Sainani, G. S. (2010). *Manual of clinical and practical medicine.* New Delhi: Elsevier India; 18-3, A, from Jebson, L.R., & Coons, D.D. (1998). Total hip arthroplasty. *Surgical Technologist, 30*(10), 12-21; B, from Mercier, L.R. (2000). *Practical orthopaedics* (5th ed.). St. Louis: Mosby; 18-6, from Damjanov, I. (2006). *Pathophysiology for the health professions* (3rd ed.). Philadelphia: Saunders; 18-9, from Goldman, L., & Ausiello, D. (2007). *Cecil medicine* (23rd ed.). Philadelphia: Saunders; 18-10, from Currie, G., & Douglas, G. (2011). *Flesh and bones of medicine.* Edinburgh: Mosby Ltd.

Chapter 19

19-1, From Kumar, V., Abbas, A., & Fausto, N. (2010). *Robbins & Cotran pathologic basis of disease* (8th ed.). Philadelphia: Saunders; 19-3, from McCance, K.L., & Huether, S.E. (2002). *Pathophysiology: The biologic basis for disease in adults and children* (4th ed.). St. Louis: Mosby; 19-4A, adapted from New York State Department of Health AIDS Institute. Clinical Guidelines Development Program. (2013). Recommendations for non-occupational post-exposure prophylaxis for HIV infection. New York: Author. www.hivguidelines.org.; 19-4B, adapted from New York State Department of Health AIDS Institute. Clinical Guidelines Development Program. (2012). Recommendations for occupational post-exposure prophylaxis for HIV infection. New York: Author. www.hivguidelines.org.; 19-5, from Marks, J., & Miller, J. (2006). *Lookingbill & Marks' principles of dermatology* (4th ed.). Philadelphia: Saunders; 19-6, from Leonard, P. C. (2012). *Building a medical vocabulary* (8th ed.). St. Louis: Saunders.

Chapter 20

20-2, Courtesy Dey, Napa, CA; **20-3,** from Auerbach, P. (2008). *Wilderness medicine* (5th ed.). Philadelphia: Mosby; courtesy Sheryl Olson.

Chapter 22

22-2, From Weinzweig, J., & Weinzweig, N. (2005). *The mutilated hand,* St. Louis: Mosby; **22-3,** from Workman, M.L., & LaCharity, L. (2011). *Understanding pharmacology: Essentials for medication safety.* St. Louis: Saunders; **22-4,** from Kee, J., Hayes, E., & McCuistion, L. (2012). *Pharmacology: A nursing process approach,* St. Louis: Saunders; **22-6,** from Forbes, C.D., & Jackson, W.F. (2003). *Colour atlas and text of clinical medicine* (3rd ed.). London: Mosby.

Chapter 23

23-1, A, From deWit, S.C. (2014). *Fundamental concepts and skills for nursing* (4th ed.). Philadelphia: Saunders; **B,** from Currance, P. (2006). *Medical response to weapons of mass destruction.* Philadelphia: Mosby/JEMS.

Chapter 24

24-10, Modified from Marks, J., & Miller, J. (2013). *Lookingbill and Marks' principles of dermatology* (5th ed.). Philadelphia: Saunders.

Chapter 25

25-3, Modified from Swaim, S.F. (1980). *Surgery of traumatized skin.* Philadelphia: Saunders; **25-5,** from Barbara Braden & Nancy Bergstrom. © 1988. Reprinted with permission; **25-6,** illustrations from the National Pressure Ulcer Advisory Panel and European Pressure Ulcer Advisory Panel. (2009). *Pressure ulcer prevention and treatment: Clinical practice guideline.* Washington, DC: NPUAP. Used with permission; **25-9,** from The Centers for Disease Control and Prevention, Atlanta, GA (www.bt.cdc.gov/agent/anthrax/anthrax-images/); **25-15,** courtesy Stevens Johnson Syndrome Foundation, Littleton, CO.

Chapter 26

26-15, from Herndon, D. N. (2012). *Total burn care* (4th ed.). Philadelphia: Saunders.

Chapter 27

27-12, From Young, A.P., & Proctor, D. (2008). *Kinn's the medical assistant: An applied learning approach* (10th ed.). St. Louis: Saunders; **27-13,** from Harkreader, H., Hogan, M.A., & Thobaben, M. (2007). *Fundamentals of nursing: Caring and clinical judgment* (3rd ed.). Philadelphia: Saunders.

Chapter 28

28-3, 28-9, 28-10, From Perry, A. G., Potter, P. A., & Ostendorf, W. R. (2014). *Clinical nursing skills and techniques* (8th ed.). St. Louis: Mosby; **28-11,** courtesy Chad Therapeutics, Chatsworth, CA; **28-13,** courtesy Mallinckrodt, Inc., Shiley Tracheostomy Products, St. Louis, MO; **28-14,** courtesy J.T. Posey Company,

Arcadia, CA; **28-15,** courtesy Dale Medical Products, Inc., Plainville, MA.

Chapter 29

29-1, From Tardy, M.E. (1997). *Rhinoplasty: The art and science.* Philadelphia: Saunders. Used with permission; **29-2, A,** courtesy Invotec International, Jacksonville, FL.

Chapter 30

30-3, From Jarvis, C. (2012). *Physical examination and health assessment* (6th ed.). Philadelphia: Saunders; **30-4,** from Aehlert, B. (2011). *Paramedic practice today: Above and beyond.* St. Louis: Mosby; **30-9,** modified from Gift, A. (1989). A dyspnea assessment guide. *Critical Care Nurse,* 9(8), 79. Used with permission; **30-10,** from Swartz, M.H. (2009). *Textbook of physical diagnosis: History and examination* (6th ed.). Philadelphia: Saunders; **30-11,** courtesy Axcan Pharma, Mont-Saint-Hilaire, Quebec, Canada; **30-12,** modified © 2015 Hill-Rom Services, Inc. Reprinted With Permission—All Rights Reserved; **30-16,** courtesy Atrium Medical Corporation, Hudson, NH.

Chapter 31

31-1, Courtesy Covidien, AG, Switzerland; **31-2,** illustration from Workman, M.L., & LaCharity, L. (2011). *Understanding pharmacology.* St. Louis: Saunders; photo from Kumar, V., Abbas, A., Fausto, N., & Aster, J. (2009). *Robbins and Cotran pathologic basis for disease* (8th ed.). Philadelphia: Saunders; **31-3,** from Zitelli, B.J., McIntire, S. C., & Nowalk, A. J. (2012). *Zitelli and Davis' atlas of pediatric physical diagnosis* (6th ed.). Philadelphia: Saunders; courtesy Kenneth Schuitt, MD.

Chapter 32

32-2, A, courtesy Sims Porter, Inc.; **32-3,** © Dräger Medical AG & Co. KG, Lübeck, Germany. All rights reserved. No portion hereof may be reproduced, saved or stored in a data processing system, electronically or mechanically copied or otherwise recorded by any other means without express prior written permission; **32-4,** from McCance, K.L. Huether S.E., Brashers, V.L., & Rote, N.S. (2010). *Pathophysiology: The biologic basis for disease in adults and children* (6th ed.). St. Louis: Mosby.

Chapter 33

33-5, From Sahrmann, S. (2011). *Movement system impairment syndromes of the extremities, cervical and thoracic spines.* St. Louis: Mosby; **33-9,** From Baker, T., Nikolic, G., & O'Connor, S. (2008). *Practical cardiology,* ed 2, Sydney: Churchill Livingstone Australia.

Chapter 34

34-10, Reproduced with permission of Medtronic, Inc., Minneapolis, MN; **34-15,** courtesy Philips Medical Systems, Andover, MA.

Chapter 35

35-1, From McCance, K.L., & Huether, S.E. (2002). *Pathophysiology: The biologic basis for*

disease in adults and children (4th ed.). St. Louis: Mosby; **35-2,** courtesy Abiomed, Inc., Danvers, MA; **35-4, A, B,** courtesy Medtronic, Inc., Minneapolis, MN; **C** courtesy Baxter Healthcare Corporation, Edwards CVS Division, Santa Ana, CA.

Chapter 36

36-4, From Brooks, M., & Jenkins, M.P. (2008). Acute and chronic ischaemia of the limb. *Surgery* 26(1), 17-20; **36-8,** from Forbes, C.D., & Jackson, W.F. (2003). *Colour atlas and text of clinical medicine* (3rd ed.). London: Mosby.

Chapter 38

38-1, From Huether S.E., McCance, K.L., Brashers, V.L., & Rote, N.S. (2012). *Understanding pathophysiology* (5th ed.). St. Louis: Mosby.

Chapter 40

40-3, From Feldman, M., Friedman, L., & Brandt, L. (2010). *Sleisenger and Fordtran's gastrointestinal and liver disease* (9th ed.). Philadelphia: Saunders; **40-4,** from Leonard, P.C. (2012). *Building a medical vocabulary: With Spanish translations* (8th ed.). St. Louis: Saunders; **40-7,** from deWit, S.C., & O'Neill, P. (2014). *Fundamental concepts and skills for nursing* (4th ed.). St. Louis: Saunders.

Chapter 41

41-3, Modified from Thibodeau, G.A., & Patton, K.T. (2007). *Anatomy and physiology* (6th ed.). St. Louis: Mosby.

Chapter 42

42-1, From Salvo, S.G. (2014). *Mosby's pathology for massage therapists* (3rd ed.). St. Louis: Mosby; **42-2, A,** from Mini-Mental State Examination © 1975, 1998, 2001 by MiniMental, LLC. All rights reserved. Published 2001 by Psychological Assessment Resources, Inc. May not be reproduced in whole or in part in any form or by any means without written permission of Psychological Assessment Resources, Inc., 16204 N. Florida Ave., Lutz, FL 33549; (800) 331-8378, www4.parinc.com/. **B,** from Seidel, H.M., Ball, J.W., Dains, J.E., Benedict, G.W. (2003). *Mosby's guide to physical examination* (5th ed.). St. Louis: Mosby.

Chapter 43

43-1, From Patton, K.T., & Thibodeau, G.A. (2014). *The human body in health & disease* (6th ed.). St. Louis: Mosby; **43-5,** from Harkreader, H. (2007). *Fundamentals of nursing: Caring and clinical judgment* (3rd ed.). Philadelphia: Saunders.

Chapter 45

45-3, From Seidel, H.M., Ball, J.W., Dains, J.E., Flynn, J.A., Solomon, B.S., & Stewart, R.W. (2011). *Mosby's guide to physical examination* (7th ed.). St. Louis: Mosby; **B,** modified from Stein, H.A., Slatt, B.J., & Stein, R.M. (1994). *The ophthalmic assistant* (6th ed.). St. Louis: Mosby. **45-10,** from Flint, P.W., Haughey, B.H., Lund, V.J., Niparko, J.K., Richardson, M.A.,

Robbins, K.T., et al. (2010). *Cummings otolaryngology: Head & neck surgery* (5th ed.). Philadelphia: Mosby; courtesy Elekta, Inc.

Chapter 46

46-11, Courtesy Medtronic Ophthalmics, Minneapolis, MN.

Chapter 47

47-5, from Patton, K.T., & Thibodeau, G.A. (2010). *Anatomy and physiology* (7th ed.). St. Louis: Mosby; **47-8,** from Workman, M.L., LaCharity, L., & Kruchko, S.C. (2011). *Understanding pharmacology.* St. Louis: Saunders.

Chapter 50

50-3, From Johal, S., Sawalha, S., & Pasapula, C. (2010). Post-traumatic acute hallux valgus: A case report. *The Foot, 29*(2), 87-89; **50-4,** from Hochberg, M., Silman, A., Smolen, J., Weinblatt, M., & Weisman, M. (2011). *Rheumatology* (5th ed). Philadelphia: Mosby.

Chapter 51

51-3, 51-5, 51-10, Courtesy Smith & Nephew, Inc., Orthopaedics Divisions, Memphis, TN; **51-4,** from Perry, A.G., Potter, P.A., & Elkin, M.K. (2012). *Nursing interventions & clinical skills* (5th ed.). St. Louis: Mosby; **51-6,** from McCance, K.L., Huether, S.E., Brashers, V.L., & Rote, N.S. (2010). *Pathophysiology: The biologic basis for disease in adults and children* (6th ed.). St. Louis: Mosby; **51-8,** from Douglas, G., Robertson, C., & Nicol, F. (2011). *Macleod exploración clínica* (12th ed.). Barcelona: Elsevier; **51-14,** courtesy Zimmer, Inc., Warsaw, IN; **51-15,** from Darby, M., & Walsh, M. (2010). *Dental hygiene: theory and practice* (3rd ed.). St. Louis: Saunders.

Chapter 53

53-1, From Friedman-Kien, A.E., & Cockerell, C.J. (1996). *Color atlas of AIDS* (2nd ed.). Philadelphia: Saunders.

Chapter 56

56-6, From Evans, S. (2009). *Surgical pitfalls.* Philadelphia: Saunders.

Chapter 57

57-3, B, From Perry, A.G., & Potter, P.A. (2006). *Clinical nursing skills & techniques* (6th ed.). St. Louis: Mosby; courtesy ConvaTec, Princeton, NJ; **57-5,** courtesy ConvaTec, a Bristol-Myers Squibb Company, Princeton, NJ.

Chapter 58

58-1, From Leonard, P. (2011). *Quick & easy medical terminology* (6th ed.). St. Louis: Saunders; **58-2,** from Talley, N., & O'Connor, S. (2010). *Clinical examination: a systematic guide to physical diagnosis* (6th ed.). Sydney: Churchill Livingstone Australia.

Chapter 60

60-1, From U.S. Department of Agriculture, 2011, www.ChooseMyPlate.gov; **60-2,** ® Société des Produits Nestlé S.A., Vevey, Switzerland, Trademark Owners; **60-3, A,** from Lilley, L., Rainforth Collins, S., Harrington, S., & Snyder, J. (2011). *Pharmacology and the nursing process* (6th ed.). St. Louis: Mosby; **B,** from Harkreader, H. (2007). *Fundamentals of nursing* (3rd ed.). St. Louis: Saunders; courtesy C.R. Bard, Inc., Billerica, MA; **C,** from Harkreader, H. (2007). *Fundamentals of nursing* (3rd ed.). St. Louis: Saunders; courtesy Ballard Medical Products, Draper, UT.

Chapter 61

61-4, From Guyton, A., & Hall, J. (2006). *Textbook of medical physiology* (11th ed.). Philadelphia: Saunders.

Chapter 62

62-1, Courtesy of the Group for Research in Pathology Educations (GRIPE), Oklahoma City, OK; **62-2,** from Wilson J.D., Foster, D., Kronenberg, H., & Larsen, P.R. (1998). *Williams textbook of endocrinology* (9th ed.). Philadelphia: Saunders; courtesy Dr. H. Patrick Higgins; **62-3,** from Wenig B.M., Heffess, C.S., & Adair, C.F. (1997). *Atlas of endocrine pathology.* Philadelphia: Saunders.

Chapter 64

64-4, Courtesy Medtronic Diabetes, Northridge, CA; **64-5,** courtesy Becton, Dickinson and Company, Franklin Lakes, NJ; **64-6,** from Frykberg, R.G., Zgonis, T., Armstrong, D.G., Driver, V.R., Giurini, J.M., Kravitz, S.R., et al. (2006). Diabetic foot disorders: A clinical practice guideline—2006 revision. *The Journal of Foot and Ankle Surgery, 45*(5), S1-S66.

Chapter 65

65-3, From Patton, K.T., & Thibodeau, G.A. (2014). *The human body in health & disease* (6th ed.). St. Louis: Mosby; **65-8,** modified from Patton, K.T., & Thibodeau, G.A. (2013).

Anatomy & physiology (8th ed.). St. Louis: Mosby; **65-10,** Courtesy Verathon Corporation, Bothell, WA.

Chapter 66

66-1, A, Courtesy ConvaTec, A Bristol-Meyers Squibb Company, a Division of E.R. Squibb & Sons, Inc., Princeton, NJ; **66-2,** from Pollack, H.M. (2000). *Clinical urography* (2nd ed.). Philadelphia: Saunders; **66-3,** modified from Singal, R.K., & Denstedt, J.D. (1997). Contemporary management of ureteral stones. *The Urologic Clinics of North America, 24*(1), 59-70.

Chapter 67

67-2, From Kumar, V., Abbas, A., Fausto, N., & Aster, J. (2010). *Robbins and Cotran pathologic basis of disease* (8th ed.). Philadelphia: Saunders.

Chapter 68

68-1, Courtesy Kendall Company, Bothell, WA; **68-3, 68-4,** from Feehally, J., Floege, J., & Johnson, R. (2007). *Comprehensive clinical nephrology* (3rd ed.). Philadelphia: Mosby; **68-5,** courtesy Gambro Lundia AB, Lund, Sweden; **68-8, A,** from Geary, D.F., & Schaefer, F. (2008). *Comprehensive pediatric nephrology.* Philadelphia: Mosby; **68-12,** courtesy Baxter International, Inc., Deerfield, IL.

Chapter 70

70-1, From Swartz, M.H. (2009). *Textbook of physical diagnosis: History and examination* (6th ed.). Philadelphia: Saunders; **70-2,** from Mansel, R., & Bundred, N. (1995). *Color atlas of breast disease.* St. Louis: Mosby; **70-3,** from Gallager, H.S., Leis, H.P. Jr., Snyderman, R.K., & Urban, J.A. (1978). *The breast.* St. Louis: Mosby; **70-4, 70-5,** © 2010 Terese Winslow. U.S. Govt. has certain rights.

Chapter 72

72-2, Adapted from the American Urological Association Practice Guidelines Committee. (2003). Guideline on the management of benign prostatic hyperplasia (BPH). *Journal of Urology, 170*(2 Pt 1), 530-547.

Chapter 74

74-1, 74-2, From Morse, S., Ballard, R., Holmes, K., & Moreland, A. (2003). *Atlas of sexually transmitted diseases and AIDS* (3rd ed.). Edinburgh: Mosby.

A

AAAs. *See* Abdominal aortic aneurysms (AAAs).
AAT deficiency. *See* Alpha₁-antitrypsin (AAT) deficiency.
Abatacept, 309b, 311
ABCDE skin assessment, 421
Abdominal aortic aneurysms (AAAs), 726
Abdominal assessment, 793, 793b
Abdominal herniation, 1146-1148, 1146f, 1148b
Abdominal pain, 315
Abdominal surgery, skin preparation for, 229f
Abdominal trauma, 1161-1163, 1162b
Abducens nerve, 835t
ABGs. *See* Arterial blood gases (ABGs).
ABHRs. *See* Alcohol-based hand rubs (ABHRs).
ABI. *See* Ankle-brachial index (ABI).
AbioCor Implantable Replacement Heart, 688f
Ablative surgery, 702
Abnormal heart sounds, 640
Abortive therapy in migraines, 855-856
ABPM. *See* Ambulatory blood pressure monitoring (ABPM).
Abscesses
  anorectal, 1188, 1188b
  brain, 962-964, 963b
  lung, 599
  pancreatic, 1226
  peritonsillar, 586
Absolute neutrophil count (ANC), 279
Absorbable sutures, 253
Absorption atelectasis, 516, 516b
Acalculia, 934
Acalculous cholecystitis, 1214
ACC/AHA staging system, 679
Accelerated graft atherosclerosis (AGA), 287
Acceleration-deceleration injuries, 116
Accessory muscles of respiration, 499
Accessory nerve, 835t
Acclimatization, 134
Accommodation, 969
AccuVein AV 300, 190, 191f
ACDF. *See* Anterior cervical diskectomy and fusion (ACDF).
ACE inhibitors. *See* Angiotensin-converting enzyme (ACE) inhibitors.

Acebutolol hydrochloride, 658b-662b
Acetaminophen, 35
  live damage and, 293b
Acetazolamide, 134, 134b
Achlorhydria, 1138
Acid deficit, 184, 184f
Acid suppression in peptic ulcer disease, 1137
Acid-base assessment, 177b
Acid-base balance, 174-179
  acids and, 175, 175f
  bases and, 175
  bicarbonate ions and, 176, 176f
  buffers and, 175-176, 175f
  carbon dioxide and hydrogen ions and, 176, 176f-177f
  postoperative assessment of, 262
  regulatory actions and mechanisms in, 177-179, 177b, 178t
  chemical, 177, 178t
  compensation process and, 179
  kidney and, 178-179, 178t
  respiratory, 177-178, 178f
  sources of acids and bicarbonate, 176-177
Acid-base imbalances, 179-185
  acidosis, 179-183, 179b, 180t
    combined metabolic and respiratory, 181
    history in, 181
    laboratory assessment in, 182-183, 182b, 182f
    metabolic, 180, 180t, 183
    physical assessment in, 181-182, 181b
    psychosocial assessment in, 182
    respiratory, 180-181, 180t, 183
  alkalosis, 179, 183-185, 183t, 184b-185b, 184f
  in chronic kidney disease, 1420
Acidosis, 179-183, 179b, 180t, 185-186
  in chronic obstructive pulmonary disease, 558, 560f
  combined metabolic and respiratory, 181, 182b
  in diabetic ketoacidosis, 1334, 1334b
  history in, 181
  in hypovolemic shock, 743
  laboratory assessment in, 182-183, 182b, 182f
  metabolic, 180, 180t, 183
  physical assessment in, 181-182, 181b
  psychosocial assessment in, 182
  respiratory, 180-181, 180t, 183

Acids, 175, 175f, 186
  kidney formation of, 179
  sources of, 176-177
Acinus, 499, 499f
Acitretin, 321, 458b
ACLS. *See* Advanced Cardiac Life Support (ACLS).
Acorn cardiac support device, 688
Acoustic neuromas, 958, 1009
Acquired hypoxic-anoxic brain injury, 964
Acquired immune deficiency syndrome (AIDS), 326-345
  antibody tests in, 336-337
  classification of, 328, 329t
  community-based care in, 343-344, 343b-344b
  complementary and alternative therapies for, 340-341
  confusion in, 342-343, 342b
  cultural considerations in, 329b
  diarrhea in, 341-342, 342b
  drug therapy for, 332b, 338-341, 339b-340b
  endocrine complications in, 335-336
  evaluation of care of patient with, 344
  gender health considerations in, 329b
  genetic considerations in, 329b, 337b
  health care resources for, 344
  history in, 333
  HIV genotype test in, 337b
  home care management in, 343, 343b
  immune enhancement for, 340
  incidence and prevalence of, 328-329, 329b
  infection prevention in, 337-340, 338b-340b
  infectious process of, 327-328, 327f-328f
  key features of, 334b
  lymphocyte counts in, 336
  malignancies in, 334b, 335, 335f
  mortality rate of, 329-333
  nutrition and, 341
  older adults and, 329b-330b
  opportunistic infections in, 328, 333-335, 334b-335b, 334f
  outcomes for care of patients with, 329b
  oxygenation enhancement in, 340
  pain management in, 340-341
  parenteral transmission of, 331-332
  perinatal transmission of, 332
  progression of, 328
  psychosocial assessment in, 336
  psychosocial preparation in, 343

Acquired immune deficiency syndrome (AIDS) *(Continued)*
  self-esteem and, 343
  self-management education in, 343, 344b
  sexual transmission of, 330-331, 331f, 332b
  skin integrity and, 342
  testing for, 333-337, 333b, 337b
  transmission and health care workers, 332, 332b
  viral load testing in, 337
Acromegaly, 1268, 1268f, 1269b
Actemra. *See* Tocilizumab.
Acticoat, 486b
Actinic keratoses, 458, 459t
Activated partial thromboplastin time (aPTT), 223b-224b
Active euthanasia, 103, 103t
Active immunity, 284-285, 398
Activities of daily living (ADLs)
  dyspnea and, 503t
  rehabilitation and, 79
  spinal cord injury and, 901
Activity
  after total hip arthroplasty, 297-300, 297b, 299b-300b
  in asthma, 535
  in atherosclerosis, 708
  coronary artery disease and, 768-769, 769b, 781b
  heart failure and, 690-691
  leukemia and, 814, 815b
  older adults and, 11-12, 12b, 12f
Activity therapists, 77
Activity tolerance, 565
Acupressure, 856-857
Acupuncture, 856-857
Acute adrenal insufficiency, 1274
Acute cardiac tamponade, 699-700
Acute cholecystitis, 1213-1214, 1214f
Acute compartment syndrome, 1053-1054, 1054b
Acute coronary syndrome, 640-641, 758-760, 758f-759f
Acute gastritis, 1126-1127
Acute glomerulonephritis, 1397-1399, 1402t, 1403b
Acute hematogenous infection, 1040
Acute inflammatory bowel disorders, 1168-1173
  appendicitis, 1168-1170, 1169b, 1169f
  gastroenteritis, 1172-1173, 1172t, 1173b
  peritonitis, 1170-1172, 1170b-1171b
Acute kidney injury (AKI), 1412-1419
  assessment in, 1414-1416, 1415b
  characteristics of, 1412t

Page numbers followed by "f" indicate figures, "t" indicate tables, and "b" indicate boxes.

Acute kidney injury (AKI)
(Continued)
drug therapy for, 1416-1417
health promotion and
maintenance in, 1414, 1414b
nutrition therapy for, 1417
pathophysiology of, 1412-1414,
1412t, 1413t
posthospital care in, 1418-1419
renal replacement therapy for,
1417-1418, 1417f
in tumor lysis syndrome, 394
Acute leukemia, 810
Acute low back pain, 887
Acute lymphocytic leukemia (ALL),
807t
Acute mountain sickness (AMS), 134
Acute myelogenous leukemia (AML),
807t
Acute pain, 25-26
characteristics of, 25t, 28t
in coronary artery disease,
764-766, 764b-766b
in peptic ulcer disease, 1132-1136,
1132b, 1135b-1136b
Acute pancreatitis, 1218-1223
assessment in, 1220-1221, 1221b,
1221t
community-based care in, 1223
evaluation of care of patient with,
1223
nutrition in, 1222-1223
pain management in, 1221-1222,
1222b
pathophysiology of, 1218-1220,
1219f, 1219t
Acute paronychia, 427
Acute pericarditis, 699
Acute peripheral arterial occlusion,
725, 725b-726b
Acute pharyngitis, 584
Acute phase of burns, 481-488
burn wound infections and, 485,
485b-486b
cardiopulmonary assessment in,
481
immune assessment in, 481, 482t
maintenance of mobility in,
487-488, 487b, 488f
musculoskeletal assessment in,
482
neuroendocrine assessment in,
481
supporting self-image in, 488
weight loss control in, 486-487
wound care in, 482-488, 483f-484f
Acute promyelocytic leukemia
(APL), 807t
Acute pyelonephritis, 1399
Acute rehabilitation, 90
Acute rejection, 287
Acute respiratory distress syndrome
(ARDS), 612-614, 613b-614b,
613t
burn-related, 481b, 487-488

Acute respiratory failure (ARF),
610-612, 611t-612t
Acute sialadenitis, 1107-1108
Acute thyroiditis, 1295
Acute transfusion reactions, 824-825
Acute viral rhinitis, 583
Acute-on-chronic kidney disease, 1411
Acyclovir, 453
Adalimumab, 309b, 310, 458b
Adam's apple, 497
Adaptive devices for functional
ability, 84, 84t
Adaptive immunity, 284
Addiction, opioid, 40, 50
Addisonian crisis, 1274
Add-on devices in infusion therapy,
197-198
A-delta fibers, 26-28, 29f
Adenocard. See Adenosine.
Adenohypophysis, 1257
Adenosine, 658b-662b, 662, 666b
ADEs. See Adverse drug events
(ADEs).
ADH. See Antidiuretic hormone
(ADH).
Adipose tissue, 222, 416, 416f
Adjuvant analgesics, 35, 36t, 45,
45b-46b, 50
Adjuvant therapy
for breast cancer, 1476
for cancer, 377
ADLs. See Activities of daily living
(ADLs).
Administration sets, 197-198,
197f-198f, 202
Administrative review after critical
events, 145-146
Adrenal cortex, 1258-1259, 1258t
hormones secreted by, 1256t
Adrenal glands, 1256f, 1257-1259,
1259t
hyperfunction of, 1276-1283
hyperaldosteronism, 1282
hypercortisolism, 1276-1281,
1277f, 1277t, 1278b-1279b,
1281b
pheochromocytoma, 1282-1283,
1283b
hypofunction of, 1273-1276
assessment in, 1274-1275,
1274b-1275b, 1275f
interventions in, 1275-1276,
1276b
pathophysiology of, 1273-1274,
1274b, 1274t
Adrenal medulla, 1259, 1259t
Adrenalin. See Epinephrine.
Adrenocorticotropic hormone
deficiency of, 1267b
overproduction of, 1269b
Adult health nursing. See Medical-
surgical nursing.
Advance directives, 92-94, 93f, 95b,
103, 250, 250b
heart failure and, 691

Advanced Cardiac Life Support
(ACLS), 111, 111t, 672, 672b
Advancing Research and Clinical
Practice through Close
Collaboration (ARCC) model,
69-70
Adventitious breath sounds, 506,
507t
Adverse drug effects in older adults,
14, 14t
Adverse drug events (ADEs), 189
Adverse events during emergency
care, 109b
AEDs. See Automated external
defibrillators (AEDs).
Aerosol masks, 519t
Aerosolization of Mycobacterium
tuberculosis, 595, 595f
Aesthetic plastic surgery, 462-463
Afferent arterioles, 1345
Afferent neurons, 830
Afinitor. See Everolimus.
Africanized bees, 128
Afterdrop in hypothermia, 132
Afterload, 631, 680
AGA. See Accelerated graft
atherosclerosis (AGA).
Age
cancer development and, 367,
367b, 367t
increased surgical risk with, 219t
Agglutination, 283-284
Aging
cardiovascular changes with, 632,
633b
endocrine changes with,
1260-1261, 1261b
eye changes with, 969-970,
970b
gastrointestinal changes with,
1087, 1088b
hearing changes with, 998, 999b
hematologic changes with, 788,
790b
immune function changes with,
276, 277b, 289
increasing complications in burns
and, 474b
integumentary changes with,
398b, 418b-419b
musculoskeletal changes with,
1020, 1020b
neurologic changes with, 836-837,
836b-837b
renal changes with, 1351, 1351b
reproductive system changes in,
1452, 1452b
respiratory changes with, 500,
500b-501b
skin changes associated with,
417-420, 417f, 418b-419b,
419f-420f
with spinal cord injury, 901b
Agitation management in end-of-life
care, 99-100, 99b

Agnosia
in Alzheimer's disease, 873
in stroke, 934-936
Agraphia, 934
AIDS. See Acquired immune
deficiency syndrome (AIDS).
AIDS dementia complex, 336
AIDS wasting syndrome, 336
Air embolism, 202
Air warming and humidification in
tracheostomy, 525, 525b
Airborne Precautions, 404t, 405
in tuberculosis, 335b
Airborne transmission, 400
Airway, 498-499, 498f-499f
gender and, 500b
primary survey and, 116, 117b,
118t
Airway assessment in traumatic
brain injury, 951
Airway management
in burn injury, 477-478, 478b
postoperative, 266
in spinal cord injury, 896, 896b
Airway obstruction, 536-537,
536b-537b, 537f
burn-related, 474t, 477
in head and neck cancer, 539-542,
540b-541b, 541t, 542f
in pneumonia, 593
respiratory acidosis and, 181
Airway pressure-release ventilation
(APRV), 614
AIs. See Aromatase inhibitors (AIs).
AKI. See Acute kidney injury (AKI).
Akinesia, 867
Alarm system of ventilators, 619, 620t
Albumin, 477b, 786
Albuminuria, 1303
Albuterol, 539b
Alcohol, 18-19, 19b, 23
Alcohol-based hand rubs (ABHRs),
402, 402b
Alcohol-Related Problems Survey
(ARPS), 19
Aldosterone, 153-155, 1258
Aldosterone receptor antagonists,
715b-716b, 717
Alefacept, 458b
Alexia, 934
Aliskiren, 715b-716b
Alkali burns, 471
Alkaline reflux gastropathy, 1141
Alkalosis, 179, 183-186, 183t,
184b-185b, 184f
metabolic, 183t, 184
respiratory, 183t, 184
Alkylating agents, 377, 378t, 380t
ALL. See Acute lymphocytic
leukemia (ALL).
Alleles, 54-55, 55f
Allerdryl. See Diphenhydramine.
Allergens in allergic rhinitis, 349
Allergic rhinitis, 349-351, 349f, 351b,
583

Allergic transfusion reactions, 825
Allergies, 348-356, 349t
    to antibiotics, 409b, 409t
    cytotoxic reactions, 355
    delayed reactions, 355-356
    immune complex reactions, 355, 355f
    integumentary assessment and, 420
    intraoperative care and, 251
    to latex in gloves and other medical products, 402-403
    to monoclonal antibodies, 388
    rapid hypersensitivity reactions, 348-355
        allergic rhinitis in, 349-351, 349f, 351b
        anaphylaxis in. See Anaphylaxis.
        latex allergy in, 354-355, 355b
        respiratory assessment and, 502, 502b
Allergy testing, 350
Allogeneic bone marrow transplantation, 811, 812f
Allogeneic transplant, 811t
Allografts
    in bone cancer, 1044
    for burn wounds, 483
Allowing natural death, 103
Alopecia, chemotherapy-related, 381, 384-385, 576, 810
Aloxil. See Palonosetron.
Alpha particles, 374, 374f
Alpha$_1$-antitrypsin (AAT) deficiency, 558
Alpha-glucosidase inhibitors, 1312b, 1313
ALS. See Amyotrophic lateral sclerosis (ALS).
Alteplase, 607b, 939b
Altitude-related illnesses, 133-135, 133b-135b
Alveolar ducts, 498f-499f, 499
Alveolar-capillary diffusion, 181
Alveoli, 498f, 499, 501b
Alveolitis, 571
Alzheimer's disease, 871-881
    caregiver role strain in, 879, 880b
    chronic confusion in, 875-878, 875t, 876b-877b
    evaluation of care of patient with, 880-881
    genetic considerations in, 872b
    health care resources for, 880
    history in, 872-873, 873t
    home care management in, 879-880
    imaging assessment in, 875
    injury prevention in, 878-879, 878b, 879t
    laboratory assessment in, 875
    pathophysiology of, 871-872
    physical assessment in, 873-875, 873b, 874f
    psychosocial assessment in, 34b, 875
    self-management education in, 880

Amantadine, 869
Amaurosis fugax, 936
Ambulation after burns, 487
Ambulatory aids, 81, 83b
Ambulatory blood pressure monitoring (ABPM), 718
Ambulatory pumps, 199
Ambulatory surgery, 218
Amenorrhea, 1452
American Cancer Society, 368
American College of Cardiology staging system, 679
American College of Rheumatology, 320
American Heart Association staging system, 679
American Nurses Association's Code of Ethics, 1519
American Society of Anesthesiologists (ASA), 244
American Society of Clinical Oncologists (ASCO), 378-379
Americans with Disabilities Act, 80
Amevive. See Alefacept.
AMI. See Antibody-mediated immunity (AMI).
Amiodarone, 188b, 658b-662b
AML. See Acute myelogenous leukemia (AML).
Amlodipine, 715b-716b
Ammonia, kidney formation of, 179
Amnesia, 245
    in traumatic brain injury, 950
Amputations, 1069-1075
    community-based care in, 1074-1075, 1074f, 1075b
    complications of, 1071
    cultural considerations in, 1071b
    interventions in, 1072-1074, 1072b, 1074f
    levels of, 1070-1071, 1070f
AMS. See Acute mountain sickness (AMS).
Amylin analogs, 1312b-1313b, 1313
Amyotrophic lateral sclerosis (ALS), 910-911, 910b-911b
ANA. See Antinuclear antibody (ANA).
Anaerobic metabolism, 176, 180
Anakinra, 309b, 310-311
Anal disorders, 1188-1189, 1188b
Anal fissure, 1188-1189
Anal fistula, 1189
Analgesia, 245
Analgesics
    adjuvant, 35, 36t, 45, 45b-46b, 50
    epidural, 42-43, 42b, 269
    intrathecal, 42, 50
        in spinal fusion, 888
    non-opioid, 35-37, 36t, 37b
    opioid. See Opioid analgesics.
    patient-controlled, 35, 35b, 269
    preemptive, 34

Anaphylaxis, 348-349, 741
    assessment of, 352-353, 352f, 353b
    in bee stings, 129
    interventions, 353-354, 353b-354b
    pathophysiology of, 351-352, 351t, 352b, 352f
Anasarca, 637
Anastomosis, 263b
Anatomic dead space, 517
ANC. See Absolute neutrophil count (ANC).
Androgens, 391t
Anemias, 798
    after total hip arthroplasty, 299
    aplastic, 799t, 805
    chemotherapy-related, 381-383
    common causes of, 798-799, 799t
    folic acid deficiency, 799t, 804
    glucose-6-phosphate dehydrogenase deficiency anemia, 799t, 803
    immunohemolytic, 803-804
    key features of, 799b
    macrocytic, 804
    microcytic, 804
    in older adults, 804b
    pernicious, 804
    resulting from decreased production of red blood cells, 804-805, 804b, 804f
    sickle cell disease, 799-804, 799t
        community-based care in, 803
        etiology and genetic risk in, 800, 800f, 804b
        history in, 800-801
        imaging assessment in, 801
        incidence and prevalence of, 800
        infection prevention in, 802-803
        laboratory assessment in, 801
        pain in, 801-802, 802b
        pathophysiology of, 799-800, 799f
        physical assessment in, 800-801
        pregnancy in, 803b
        psychosocial assessment in, 801
Anergy, 334-335, 596
Aneroid pressure manometers, 525, 525f
Anesthesia, 244-249, 246t
    allergies to, 251
    general, 245-248, 246t, 247b-248b
    local or regional, 45, 248-249, 248f-249f, 248t
    moderate sedation, 249, 250t
    neuraxial, 296
Anesthesiologists, 239
Aneuploid, 54
Aneuploidy, 362, 365
Aneurysmectomy, 727
Aneurysms
    of central arteries, 726-728, 726f, 727b
    of peripheral arteries, 726f, 728
    stroke and, 932, 940t

Angina, 636t, 762b
Angina pectoris, 757
Angioedema, 352, 352f
Angiogenesis inhibitors, 380t, 390, 390t
Angiography
    in cardiovascular assessment, 643
    cerebral, 845, 845b, 846t-847t
Angiomas, senile, 420f
Angiotensin II, 154-155, 154f
Angiotensin-converting enzyme, 154
Angiotensin-converting enzyme (ACE) inhibitors
    for heart failure, 684-685, 685b
    for hypertension, 717b
Angiotensinogen, 154
Angiotensin-receptor blockers (ARBs)
    for heart failure, 684-685, 685b
    for hypertension, 715b-716b
Anions, 160
Anisocoria, 972
Ankle-brachial index (ABI), 638, 720
Ankles
    arthroplasty of, 303
    positioning to prevent contractures, 487b
    skin preparation for surgery of, 229f
Ankylosing spondylitis, 323t
Ann Arbor Staging Criteria for Hodgkin's Lymphoma, 817t
Annular lesions, 422t
Anomia, 873, 877
Anorectal abscesses, 1188, 1188b
Anorectic drugs, 1249, 1250b
Anorexia nervosa, 1238
ANS. See Autonomic nervous system (ANS).
Anterior cerebral artery strokes, 934b
Anterior cervical diskectomy and fusion (ACDF), 428b, 891-892, 892b
Anterior colporrhaphy, 1487
Anterior nares, 496
Anterior pituitary gland
    disorders of
        hyperpituitarism, 1268-1271, 1268b-1270b, 1268f
        hypopituitarism, 1266-1268, 1267b-1268b
    hormones of, 1256t, 1258t
Anthrax, 411t
    cutaneous, 453, 453b, 454f
    inhalation, 599-600, 599b-600b
Anthropometric measurements, 1234-1236, 1236b
Antiandrogens, 391t
Antibiotics
    allergic reactions to, 409b, 409t
    for anthrax, 453
    antitumor, 378, 378t
    for eye inflammation and infection, 979b
    inadequate therapy with, 407-411

Antibiotics (Continued)
  for sexually transmitted disease, 1543b
Antibodies, 282
Antibody tests, 336-337
Antibody-antigen binding, 282-283, 283f
Antibody-mediated immunity (AMI), 281-285, 282f, 400
  acquiring of, 284-285, 289
  age-related changes in, 277b
  antibody classification and, 284, 284t
  antigen-antibody interactions in, 281-284, 283f
  immune functions of leukocytes in, 278t
  role of leukocytes in, 787t
Anticholinergic drugs, 99
Anti-clotting forces, 788, 790f
Anticoagulants
  for atrial fibrillation, 668b
  blood tests for monitoring of, 608b
  continuous negative pressure wound therapy and, 447b
  in hemodialysis, 1432-1433
  patient safety and, 609b
Antidepressants
  for Alzheimer's disease, 877
  older adults and, 16, 16b, 45b
  for pain management, 45
Antidiabetic drugs, 1310-1319, 1310b, 1312b-1313b
Antidiuretic hormone (ADH), 153
Antiembolism stockings, 232
Antiemetics, 383-384, 384b-385b
Antiepileptic drugs, 859, 859b
  for pain management, 45
Antiestrogens, 391t
Anti-factor Xa test, 795
Antifungals, 409, 453
  for eye inflammation and infection, 979b
Antigen-antibody interactions, 281-284, 283f
Antigens, 276
  human leukocyte, 276, 276f, 289
  hypersensitivity and, 348
  in leukemia, 808-809
Antihemophilic drugs, 821t
Antihistamines
  for allergic rhinitis, 351
  for anaphylaxis, 354, 354b
  for bee stings, 129
  for itching in skin inflammation, 456
  older adults and, 584b
  for pruritus, 433
Antihypertensives, 712-717, 714b-717b
Anti-infective agents. See Antimicrobial therapy.
Anti-inflammatory drugs, 534-535, 539b
Antimetabolites, 378, 378t, 380t

Antimicrobial therapy
  inadequate, 407-411
  for infection, 409, 409b, 409t
Antimitotic agents, 378, 378t
Antinuclear antibody (ANA), 307, 307b, 314
Antiplatelet agents
  for coronary artery disease, 765b-766b
  patient safety and, 609b
Antiproliferatives, 287b-288b
Antipsychotics as chemical restraints, 22, 22b
Antipyretics, 409, 414
Antitumor antibiotics, 378, 378t
Antivenom
  for coral snake envenomation, 126
  for pit viper envenomation, 125
Antivirals, 409
  for eye inflammation and infection, 979b
Anuria, 1385
Anxiety
  chest pain in, 636t
  in chronic kidney disease, 1430
  in chronic obstructive pulmonary disease, 565
  in head and neck cancer, 543-544
  preoperative, 233
  in pulmonary embolism, 609-610
Anzemet. See Dolasetron.
Aortic dissection, 728
Aortic regurgitation, 692b, 693
Aortic stenosis, 692b, 693
Aortoiliac bypass surgery, 723, 723f
Aphasia, 78
  in Alzheimer's disease, 873, 877
  in stroke, 934, 943, 943t
Apheresis, 812
Aphonia, 536
Apical impulse, 639
APL. See Acute promyelocytic leukemia (APL).
Aplastic anemia, 799t, 805
Apnea, obstructive sleep, 534-535
Apocrine sweat glands, 417, 418b-419b
Apoptosis, 360-361
Appendectomy, 1175
Appendicitis, 1168-1170, 1169b, 1169f
Approximated wounds, 435
Apraxia
  in Alzheimer's disease, 873, 877
  in stroke, 934-936
Aprepitant, 385b
APRV. See Airway pressure-release ventilation (APRV).
APTT. See Activated partial thromboplastin time (aPTT).
Aquacel Ag, 486b
Aqueous humor, 967, 968f
Aranesp. See Darbepoetin alfa.
Arava. See Leflunomide.
Arboviruses, 865

ARBs. See Angiotensin-receptor blockers (ARBs).
ARCC model. See Advancing Research and Clinical Practice through Close Collaboration (ARCC) model.
Arcus senilis, 417f, 969
ARDS. See Acute respiratory distress syndrome (ARDS).
Areflexic bladder, 86-87, 86t
ARF. See Acute respiratory failure (ARF).
Arms as sites for peripheral catheter placement, 192f
Aromatase inhibitors (AIs), 1478
Aromatherapy, 97, 99
ARPS. See Alcohol-Related Problems Survey (ARPS).
Arrhythmias, 656. See also Dysrhythmias.
Arrhythmogenic right ventricular cardiomyopathy, 702
Arterial blood gases (ABGs)
  in burn assessment, 477b
  in heart failure, 683-684
  in pneumonia, 592
  in pulmonary embolism, 605
  in respiratory assessment, 507, 508b
Arterial pulses, 638-639, 638f
Arterial revascularization, 723
Arterial system, 631-632
Arterial therapy, 214
Arterial ulcers, 720, 721b
Arteriography
  in cardiovascular assessment, 644
  renal, 1361
Arteriosclerosis, 706-709
  complementary and alternative therapies for, 709
  drug therapy for, 708-709, 709b, 709t
  laboratory assessment in, 708
  nutrition therapy for, 708
  pathophysiology of, 706-707, 707f, 707t
  physical assessment in, 707-708, 708b
Arteriotomy, 725
Arteriovenous fistula, 1435t
Arteriovenous graft, 1435t
Arteriovenous malformations (AVMs), 932, 932f, 940t, 941f
Arthralgias, 1021
Arthritis, 291
  common disorders associated with, 322, 323t
  infectious, 320
  osteoarthritis, 291-304
    chronic pain in, 293-303
      complementary and alternative medicine for, 294-295, 295b
      drug therapy for, 293-294, 293b-294b

Arthritis (Continued)
      nonpharmacologic interventions for, 294, 294b
    etiology and genetic risk for, 300-301, 304b
    health care resources for, 304
    health promotion and maintenance in, 301
    history in, 292
    home care management in, 304
    imaging assessment in, 293
    improving mobility in, 303, 303b
    incidence and prevalence of, 291
    laboratory assessment in, 293
    pathophysiology of, 291, 291f
    physical assessment in, 292-293, 292f, 292t
    psychosocial assessment in, 293
    self-management education in, 304, 304b
    surgical management of, 295-303
      hand and ankle arthroplasties in, 303
      total elbow arthroplasty in, 303
      total hip arthroplasty in, 295-300, 297b-300b, 297f-298f, 297t
      total knee arthroplasty in, 300-302, 301f, 302b
      total shoulder arthroplasty in, 303
  psoriatic, 321, 456
  rheumatoid, 304-313
    arthrocentesis in, 308, 308b
    body image and, 312
    complementary and alternative therapies for, 312
    fatigue in, 312, 312b
    health care resources for, 313
    home care management in, 313, 313f
    inflammation and pain management in, 308-312, 308b-310b
    laboratory assessment in, 307, 307b
    nonpharmacologic interventions in, 311
    pathophysiology of, 304-305, 305b
    patient and family education in, 313
    physical assessment in, 295b, 305-306, 305b-306b
    psychosocial assessment in, 306-307
    self-management in, 312, 312b
Arthritis Foundation, 292, 316-317
Arthrocentesis, 308, 308b
Arthrodesis
  spinal, 888

Arthrogram, 1025
Arthroplasty
　hand and ankle, 303
　total elbow, 303
　total hip, 295-300, 300b
　　infection prevention after, 297t, 299, 299b
　　mobility and activity after, 297-300, 297b, 299b-300b
　　older adults and, 297b
　　operative procedures in, 296-297, 297f
　　pain management after, 299
　　postoperative care in, 297-300, 297b, 297t
　　preoperative care in, 296
　　prevention of hip dislocation after, 297t, 298, 298b
　　self-management after, 298b
　　venous thromboembolism after, 296, 297t, 298-299
　total knee, 300-302, 301f, 302b
　total shoulder, 303
Arthropod bites and stings, 126-129
　bees and wasps, 128-129, 129b
　black widow spider, 127-128, 127b
　brown recluse spider, 126-127, 126f-127f, 137
　prevention of, 126b
　scorpion, 128, 128f
Arthroscopy, 1026-1027, 1027b, 1027f
Articulations, 303
Artifacts in electrocardiogram, 653-654
Artificial active immunity, 285, 289
Artificial airway. See Tracheostomy.
Artificial fingernails, 402, 414
Artificial skin, 483
Arytenoid cartilage, 497, 498f
ASA. See American Society of Anesthesiologists (ASA).
Asbestosis, 573b
Ascending tracts, 833, 833f
Ascites, 1193
ASCO. See American Society of Clinical Oncologists (ASCO).
Asepsis in burns, 485
Aspiration
　bone marrow, 795-796, 796b
　in head and neck cancer, 543, 543b
　in stroke, 942, 942b
Aspirin, 765b-767b, 766-767
Assay, 1263
Assist-control ventilation, 616-617
Assistive devices, 84, 84t
Assistive technology, 84
Asthma, 531-534
　drug therapy for, 534, 535b, 539b-541b, 543b
　exercise and activity in, 535
　history in, 532
　laboratory assessment in, 532
　levels of control in, 534b
　occupational, 573b

Asthma (Continued)
　oxygen therapy for, 535, 543b
　pathophysiology of, 531-532, 532f-533f
　　etiology and genetic risk in, 531-532, 532b
　　incidence and prevalence of, 531-532, 533b
　physical assessment in, 532-533
　pulmonary function tests in, 532-533
　self-management education in, 534, 536b-537b, 542f
　status asthmaticus and, 535
　step system for medication use in, 535b
　using peak flowmeter in, 536b, 542f, 552-553
Astigmatism, 969, 991
Asystole, ventricular, 671-673, 671f-672f, 672b
Ataxia, 934, 952
Atelectasis
　oxygen therapy-related, 516, 516b
　surfactant and, 499
　surgery in older adults and, 219-220
Atelectrauma, 620
Atenolol, 715b-716b
Atherectomy, 722, 722b, 775
Atherosclerosis, 706-709
　complementary and alternative therapies for, 709
　coronary artery disease and, 758f
　drug therapy for, 708-709, 709b, 709t
　laboratory assessment in, 708
　nutrition therapy for, 708
　pathophysiology of, 706-707, 707f, 707t
　physical assessment in, 707-708, 708b
Ativan. See Lorazepam.
Atopic allergy, 348-349
Atopic dermatitis, 455, 455b
Atrial dysrhythmias, 665-669
　atrial fibrillation in, 666-669, 666b-668b, 667f, 667t
　premature atrial complexes in, 665
　supraventricular tachycardia in, 665-666, 666b
Atrial fibrillation, 666-669, 666b-668b, 667f, 667t
Atrial gallop, 640
Atrial natriuretic peptide, 153-154
Atrioventricular junctional area, 650
Atrioventricular valve, 628
Atrophic gastritis, 1127
Atrophy, 423f
Atropine sulfate, 658b-662b, 662
Atrovent. See Ipratropium.
Atypical migraines, 854, 855b
Audiometry, 1002-1003, 1002t
Audioscopy, 1001

Auditory brainstem-evoked response, 1003
Augmentation mammoplasty, 462t
Auras in migraine, 854, 855b
Auscultation
　in endocrine assessment, 1263
　in gastrointestinal assessment, 1090
　for normal breath sounds, 505-506, 505f, 506b, 506t-507t
　in precordial assessment, 639
Autoamputation of distal digits, 317
Autoantibodies, 356
Autocontamination
　in burns, 484
　in leukemia, 809
Autodigestion, 1126
Autografts
　for burn wounds, 484-485, 484f
　pulmonary, 696
Autoimmune disorders, 356t
　chronic fatigue syndrome, 322
　fibromyalgia syndrome, 321-322
　Goodpasture's syndrome, 357
　lupus erythematosus, 313-317, 314b, 314f, 316b-317b
　multiple sclerosis. See Multiple sclerosis (MS).
　myasthenia gravis. See Myasthenia gravis (MG).
　psoriasis, 456-458, 456b-458b, 457f
　rheumatoid arthritis. See Rheumatoid arthritis (RA).
　Sjögren's syndrome, 306, 356-357
Autoimmune hemolytic anemia, 799t
Autoimmune pancreatitis, 1224
Autoimmune responses, 348
Autoimmune thrombocytopenic purpura, 820
Autoimmunity, 356-357, 356b-357b, 356t
Autologous blood donations, 220-221
Autologous blood transfusions, 250, 251b, 825-826
Autologous bone marrow transplantation, 1478
Autologous transplant, 811t
Automated external defibrillators (AEDs), 672-673, 672f
Automatic epinephrine injectors, 352b
Automatic external defibrillation, 107
Automaticity of heart, 649
Autonomic dysreflexia, 899, 899b
Autonomic nervous system (ANS), 835-836
Autonomy, patient, 4
Autosomal dominant pattern of inheritance, 57-58, 57t
Autosomal recessive pattern of inheritance, 57t, 58, 58f
Autosomes, 54

Avandamet, 384b
Avian influenza, 140
AVMs. See Arteriovenous malformations (AVMs).
Avoidance therapy, 350
Axial loading injury of spine, 893, 893f
Axilla, positioning to prevent contractures, 487b
Axillofemoral bypass surgery, 723, 723f
Azathioprine
　for lupus, 316
　to prevent transplant rejection, 287b-288b
Azoospermia, 1514

B
Babinski's sign, 841
Bacillus anthracis, 411t, 453
Back pain, 885-892
　cervical neck pain and, 891-892, 891b-892b
　low, 885-891
　　health care resources for, 891
　　health promotion and maintenance in, 886, 886b
　　home care management in, 890
　　imaging assessment in, 886-887
　　nonsurgical management of, 887-888, 887b
　　pathophysiology of, 885-886, 885f, 886b
　　physical assessment in, 886
　　self-management education in, 890, 890b-891b
　　surgical management of, 888-890, 889b
Bacteremia, 399
Bacteria, normal flora, 397, 398t
Bacterial infections
　after burn injury, 516-517, 530, 530t-531t
　AIDS and, 334
　cultures for, 429
　cutaneous, 450-451, 450b, 451f, 453
　in cystitis. See Cystitis.
　in inhalation anthrax, 599-600, 599b-600b
　in lung abscesses, 599
　oxygen therapy-related, 516, 516b
　in pertussis, 600
　in pharyngitis, 584-586, 585b
　in pneumonia. See Pneumonia.
　in pulmonary empyema, 599
Bacterial transfusion reactions, 825
Bacterial vaginosis, 1544
Bacteriuria, 1366
Bad death, 91
Baker's cysts, 306
Balance testing, 1003
Bandemia, 279
Barbiturate coma, 955
BARD PowerPort, 195

Bariatrics, 1250-1252, 1251b-1252b, 1251f
Bark scorpion, 128, 128f
Baroreceptors, 631, 633b
Barotrauma, 612, 620
Barrett's epithelium, 1111
Barrett's esophagus, 1117-1118
Bartholin cysts, 1491
Basal cell carcinomas, 459, 459f, 459t
Base pairs, 53, 53f
Bases, 175
  of DNA, 53, 53f
Basic Cardiac Life Support (BCLS), 671-672
Basic Life Support (BLS), 107, 111, 111t
Basiliximab, 287b-288b
Basophils, 279-280, 787t
  immune function of, 278t
  in white blood cell differential count, 508b
BBB. See Blood-brain barrier (BBB).
B-cell lymphomas, 335
B-cells in antibody-mediated immunity, 281, 282f
BCLS. See Basic Cardiac Life Support (BCLS).
Beau's grooves, 427t
Bedbugs, 454-455
Bedside sonography, 1359-1360, 1359f
Bee stings, 128-129, 129b
Beers criteria, 15t
Behavior
  Alzheimer's disease and, 874
  hypokalemia and, 164
  traumatic brain injury and, 955-956
Behavioral health problems
  older adults and, 16-19
  sexual health and, 1448
Behavioral management
  of obesity, 1250
  of urge incontinence, 1380-1381, 1381b
Belimumab, 316
Bell's palsy, 927-928
Benadryl. See Diphenhydramine.
Beneficence, 4
Benemid. See Probenecid.
Benign breast disorders, 1461-1464, 1462t
  ductal ectasia, 1462-1463, 1462t
  fibroadenomas, 1461, 1462t
  fibrocystic breast condition, 1462, 1462b, 1462t
  gynecomastia, 1463-1464, 1464f
  intraductal papilloma, 1462t, 1463
  issues of large-breasted women, 1463
  issues of small-breasted women, 1463, 1463b
Benign cell growth, 359

Benign neoplasms, 1487-1491
  Bartholin cysts, 1491
  cervical polyps, 1491
  ovarian cysts, 1487
  uterine leiomyomas, 1487-1491, 1488f, 1489b-1490b, 1489t
Benign prostatic hyperplasia, 1499-1506
  assessment in, 1500-1502, 1501f-1502f
  community-based care in, 1506
  complementary and alternative therapies for, 1503
  concept map for, 1504f
  drug therapy for, 1503, 1503b
  pathophysiology of, 1499-1500, 1500f
  surgical management of, 1505-1506, 1505b-1506b
Benign tumor cells, 361, 361t
Benlysta. See Belimumab.
Benuryl. See Probenecid.
Benzocaine spray, 510
Benzodiazepines
  for chemotherapy-induced nausea and vomiting, 385b
  end-of-life care and, 99b
  for heat stroke, 122
  overdose of, 266, 266b
Bereavement, 96, 96b
Berylliosis, 573b
Beta particles, 374, 374f
Beta-adrenergic blockers
  for coronary artery disease, 767, 767b
  for heart failure, 687
  for hypertension, 715b-716b, 717
  for migraines, 856b
Betamethasone, 979b
Betapace. See Sotalol.
Bexarotene, 458b
Bicarbonate, 176, 176f
  acid-base assessment and, 177b
  kidney movement of, 178-179
  sources of, 176-177
Bicaval technique in heart transplantation, 682, 703f
Bifurcation, 931
Bigeminy, 657
Biguanides, 1310, 1310b
Bilateral orchiectomy, 1509
Bilateral salpingo-oophorectomy, 1489t
  in endometrial cancer, 1492
  in ovarian cancer, 1496
Bi-level positive airway pressure (BiPAP), 520, 617
  in obstructive sleep apnea, 535
Biliary colic, 1215, 1215b
Biliary obstructions, 1193
Biliary problems
  cholecystitis, 1213-1218
    assessment in, 1215-1216, 1215b-1216b

Biliary problems (Continued)
    nonsurgical management of, 1216-1217
    pathophysiology of, 1213-1214, 1214f, 1215b, 1215t
  cholecystitis
    surgical management of, 1217-1218, 1217b, 1218t
Biofilms, 405, 414
Biologic dressings, 483, 483f
Biological response modifiers (BRMs)
  for cancer, 387-388, 387t
  for infection risk in neutropenia, 381
  for psoriasis, 458, 458b
  for rheumatoid arthritis, 309b, 310-311
Biomedical technicians, 77
Biopsies
  of bacterial infections, 429
  bone marrow, 795-796, 796b
  breast, 1458-1459
  cervical, 1458, 1458b
  endometrial, 1458
  kidney, 1363
  lung, 511-512
  muscle, 850, 1026
  in musculoskeletal assessment, 1026, 1026b
  in neurologic assessment, 850
  in reproductive assessment, 1458-1459, 1458b
  skin, 429, 461
Biorhythms, 837
Biosynthetic wound dressings, 483
Bioterrorism, 411-413, 411t, 453b
Biotherapy
  for head and neck cancer, 540
  for skin cancer, 461
Biotrauma, 620
BiPAP. See Bi-level positive airway pressure (BiPAP).
Bird fancier's lung, 573b
Bisacodyl, 88
Bisphosphonates, 1034, 1034b
Bites and stings, 126-129
  bees and wasps, 128-129, 129b
  black widow spider, 127-128, 127b
  brown recluse spider, 126-127, 126f-127f, 137
  prevention of, 126b
  scorpion, 128, 128f
Black box warning, 1310
Black Lung disease, 573b
Black widow spiders, 127-128, 127b
Black-tagged patients, 141b
Bladder
  assessment of, 1346f, 1353-1354
  dysfunction of
    in spinal cord injury, 899-900
    in stroke, 943-944
    trauma, 1391-1392
Bladder cancer, 367b

Bladder outlet obstruction, 1500, 1500f
Bladder scanners, 1359-1360, 1359f
Bladder ultrasonography, 900
BladderScan, 86
Blanching, 441-443
Blast effect, 116
Blast phase cells, 808-809
Bleeding
  after coronary artery bypass graft, 778b
  in peptic ulcer disease, 1136-1137, 1136b-1137b
  postoperative, 297t, 299
  in pulmonary embolism, 609, 609b
  risk in leukemia, 816b
  in ulcerative colitis and Crohn's disease, 1179-1180, 1180b
Blepharoplasty, 462t
Blisters in frostbite, 133f
Blood, 786-787, 787f, 787t
  accessory organs in formation of, 787
Blood clotting, 787-788, 789f, 790t
Blood disorders. See Hematologic problems.
Blood donation, 220-221
Blood glucose, 1308b
Blood glucose management in diabetes mellitus, 1317-1319, 1318b, 1328-1329
  diabetic ketoacidosis and, 1333
  hospitalized patient and, 1322-1323
  hypoglycemia and, 1330-1331
Blood pressure (BP), 631
  in cardiovascular assessment, 637-638
  hypertension and. See Hypertension.
  measurement during infusion therapy, 200b
  mechanisms influencing, 710
Blood replacement therapy, 188-189, 189f, 821-826
  acute transfusion reactions in, 824-825
  autologous, 825-826
  indications for, 822t
  older adults and, 823b
  pretransfusion responsibilities, 821-823, 822b-823b, 823f
  red blood cell, 824, 824b, 824t
  in sepsis and septic shock, 754
Blood samples from central venous catheters, 202-203, 203f
Blood stem cells, 785, 786f
Blood tests
  to monitor anticoagulation therapy, 608b
  in renal assessment, 1354-1355, 1354b-1355b
  in respiratory assessment, 508b

Blood urea nitrogen (BUN), 1354, 1355b
  perioperative assessment of, 223b-224b
Bloodborne metastasis, 363
Blood-brain barrier (BBB), 832
Blood-producing functions, cancer and, 372
Bloodstream infection (BSI)
  in cancer, 392
  inadequate antimicrobial therapy and, 407
  indwelling urinary catheters and, 399
BLS. See Basic Life Support (BLS).
Blunt trauma, 116
B-lymphocytes, 278t, 282f, 787t
BMI. See Body mass index (BMI).
BMPR2 gene, 569b
Body defenses, immunity and, 275
Body fluids, 152-153, 152b
  abnormal electrolyte values in, 152t
  age-related changes in, 153b
  pH of, 174
Body image
  amputation and, 1073-1074
  breast cancer and, 1479-1480
  rheumatoid arthritis and, 312
Body lice, 453-454
Body mass index (BMI), 1236
  obesity and, 1249
  older adults and, 1236b
  preoperative assessment of, 222b
Boils, 450, 450b, 451f
Bolus feeding, 1241-1242
Bone cancer, 372, 1042-1045, 1044b
Bone marrow, 276
Bone marrow aspiration and biopsy, 795-796, 796b
Bone marrow harvesting, 811b
Bone marrow suppression in chemotherapy, 381-383, 381b-384b
Bone marrow transplantation, 808f, 811-814, 811b-812b, 811t, 812f
Bone mineral density in osteoporosis, 1030
Bone reduction, 1058
Bone remodeling, 1030
Bone scans
  in musculoskeletal assessment, 1025
  in rheumatoid arthritis, 308
Bone spurs. See Osteophytes.
Bone tumors, benign, 1042
Bones, 1017-1019
  fracture of. See Fractures.
  healing of, 1052-1053, 1053b, 1053f
  Paget's disease of, 1037-1039, 1037b-1038b
  types and structure of, 1017-1018, 1018f
Bony ossicle, 996-997, 997f
BOOP. See Bronchiolitis obliterans organizing pneumonia (BOOP).

Bordetella pertussis, 600
Borrelia burgdorferi, 320
Bortezomib, 390
Botulism, 411t
Bouchard's node, 292, 292f
Bowel dysfunction
  rehabilitation and, 87-88, 87b-88b, 87t
  in spinal cord injury, 899-900
  in stroke, 943-944
Bowel elimination, 1082
  rehabilitation setting and, 78, 88
Bowel retraining, 88, 88b
Bowel sounds, postoperative, 262
Bowlegged deformity, 1023
BP. See Blood pressure (BP).
Brachial plexus complications, 253b
Brachytherapy, 375
  for breast cancer, 1476b
  for uterine cancer, 1492-1493, 1493b
Braden Scale, 437-438, 439f
Bradycardia, 655
  sinus, 663-665, 664f-665f
Bradydysrhythmias, 657, 657b
Bradykinesia in Parkinson disease, 867
Brain
  stroke and pathophysiologic changes in, 931
  structure and function of, 830-832, 831f-832f, 831t-832t
  traumatic injury of. See Traumatic brain injury (TBI).
Brain abscesses, 962-964, 963b
Brain attack. See Stroke.
Brain death, 954
Brain herniation syndromes, 948, 950
Brain natriuretic peptide, 153-154
Brain tumors, 957-962
  assessment of, 958-959, 959b
  classification of, 958, 958t
  community-based care in, 962
  interventions for, 959-962, 959f, 960b-961b, 961t
  pathophysiology of, 957-958
Brainstem
  functions of, 832t
  tumors of, 959b
BRCA1 and BRCA2 gene mutations, 369
Breakthrough pain, 34-35
Breast augmentation surgery, 462t, 1463, 1463b
Breast biopsy, 1458-1459
Breast cancer, 1464-1480
  adjuvant therapy for, 1476
  assessment in, 1469, 1469b-1470b
  chemotherapy for, 1476-1477, 1477b, 1477t
  complementary and alternative therapies for, 1471-1472, 1471t, 1472b
  coping strategies in, 1470-1471, 1471b

Breast cancer (Continued)
  cultural considerations in, 1466b, 1469b
  health care resources for, 1480
  health promotion and maintenance and, 369, 369b, 1465-1468, 1467b-1468b, 1481
  home care management in, 1478, 1478b-1479b
  hormonal therapy for, 1477-1478, 1477t
  metastasis in, 1471-1478
  pathophysiology of, 1464-1465
    etiology and genetic risk in, 1465, 1465b-1466b, 1466t, 1470b
    incidence and prevalence of, 1465
    invasive, 1464-1465, 1464f-1465f
    in men, 1465
    noninvasive, 1464
    in young women, 1465
  psychosocial support in, 1479-1480
  radiation therapy for, 1476, 1476b
  self-management education in, 1478-1479, 1479b
  stem cell transplantation for, 1478
  surgical management of, 1472-1478, 1472f-1473f, 1474b, 1475t, 1476b, 1478b
  targeted therapy for, 1477, 1477t
Breast disorders, 1461-1481
  benign breast disorders, 1461-1464, 1462t
    ductal ectasia, 1462-1463, 1462t
    fibroadenomas, 1461, 1462t
    fibrocystic breast condition, 1462, 1462b, 1462t
    gynecomastia, 1463-1464, 1464f
    intraductal papilloma, 1462t, 1463
    issues of large-breasted women, 1463
    issues of small-breasted women, 1463, 1463b
  breast cancer. See Breast cancer.
Breast reconstruction, 1474-1476, 1475t, 1476b
Breast reduction surgery, 462t
Breast self-examination (BSE), 1467, 1468b
Breast-conserving surgery, 1473
Breasts, 1450-1451, 1451f
  clinical examination of, 1467-1468
  disorders of. See Breast disorders.
  mammography and, 1456, 1467, 1470
  self-examination of, 1467, 1468b
Breath sounds
  adventitious, 506, 507t
  normal, 505-506, 506t

Breathing
  difficulties in lung cancer, 575
  primary survey and, 116-117, 118t
  purpose of, 496
Breathing exercises
  for chronic obstructive pulmonary disease, 562, 563b
  patient and family education in, 230b
  postoperative, 266-267
Breathing management in spinal cord injury, 896, 896b
Brevibloc. See Esmolol.
BRMs. See Biological response modifiers (BRMs).
Broca's aphasia, 943, 943t
Broca's area, 831
Bromocriptine, 869
Bronchi, 498-499, 498f
Bronchial breath sounds, 505-506, 506t
Bronchial hygiene in tracheostomy, 527-528
Bronchioles, 498f-499f, 499
Bronchiolitis obliterans organizing pneumonia (BOOP), 572-573
Bronchodilators
  for asthma, 534, 539b-541b, 543b
  for bronchospasm near death, 98
Bronchoscopy, 510-511
  in burn injury, 477
Bronchospasm
  in asthma, 550
  in bee stings, 129
  during suctioning of tracheostomy, 527
Bronchovesicular breath sounds, 505-506, 506t
Brown recluse spider, 126-127, 126f-127f, 137
Bruising. See Ecchymosis.
Bruits, 639
  in leukemia, 808
Bruton's agammaglobulinemia, 346
BSE. See Breast self-examination (BSE).
BSI. See Bloodstream infection (BSI).
B-type natriuretic peptide, 681, 683
Bubble humidifier in oxygen therapy, 516f
Buffers, 175-177, 175f
Bulbar involvement in myasthenia gravis, 918
Bulimia nervosa, 1238
Bullae, 557
BUN. See Blood urea nitrogen (BUN).
Bundle of His, 650
Bunions, 1046, 1046f
Bupropion, 495, 496b
Burn wound sepsis, 481, 482b, 482t
Burns, 465-491
  acute phase of, 481-488
    burn wound infection and, 485, 485b-486b

Burns (*Continued*)
cardiopulmonary assessment in, 481
immune assessment in, 481, 482t
maintenance of mobility in, 487-488, 487b, 488f
musculoskeletal assessment in, 482
neuroendocrine assessment in, 481
supporting self-image in, 488
weight loss control in, 486-487
wound care in, 482-488, 483f-484f
evaluation of care of patient with, 489
health promotion and maintenance in, 472-473
pathophysiology of, 465-472
cardiac changes resulting from, 470
compensatory responses to, 470, 471f
depth of, 466-469, 466t-467t, 467f
deep full-thickness wounds, 466, 469, 469f
full-thickness wounds, 466, 468-469, 468f
partial-thickness wounds, 466-468, 468f
superficial-thickness wounds, 466-467
etiology of burns injuries, 470-472, 471f-472f
gastrointestinal changes resulting from, 470
immunologic changes resulting from, 470
incidence and prevalence of burn injuries, 472
metabolic changes resulting from, 470
pulmonary changes resulting from, 470
skin changes resulting from, 465-466
vascular changes resulting from, 469, 469f
rehabilitative phase of, 488-489, 489t
health care resources for, 489
home care management in, 489
psychosocial support during, 489
self-management education in, 489
resuscitation phase of, 473-481, 473b
acute respiratory distress syndrome and, 481b, 487-488
age-related changes increasing complications in, 474b, 479b

Burns (*Continued*)
airway management in, 477-478, 478b
carbon monoxide poisoning and, 474, 475t
cardiovascular assessment in, 475
fluid resuscitation in, 478-479, 479b
gastrointestinal assessment in, 476
history in, 473
hypovolemic shock and, 478-479, 479b, 480f
imaging assessment in, 476-477
kidney/urinary assessment in, 475-476
laboratory assessment in, 476, 476b-477b
pain management during, 479-480, 480b
pulmonary fluid overload in, 475, 475b
respiratory assessment in, 473-474, 474b, 474t
skin assessment in, 476, 476f
surgical management in, 478-480, 480f
Butorphanol, 270b
Butterfly needles, 191, 210
Butterfly rash, 314, 314f
Buttonhooks, 84t

C
C. difficile–associated disease (CDAD), 413
C fibers, 26-28, 29f
CABG surgery. *See* Coronary artery bypass graft (CABG) surgery.
Cachexia, 372, 1237
CAD. *See* Coronary artery disease (CAD).
CAGE questionnaire, 19
CAL. *See* Chronic airflow limitation (CAL).
Calan. *See* Verapamil.
Calcineurin inhibitors
for transplant rejection, 287b-288b
Calcium, 167-170
abnormal values of, 152t
hypercalcemia and, 169-170, 169t, 170b
hypocalcemia and, 167-169, 168b, 168f, 168t
osteoporosis and, 1034
plasma values in older adults, 152b
Calcium channel blockers (CCBs), 714-717, 715b-716b
Calculus cholecystitis, 1213-1214
Calyx, 1345, 1345f
CA-MRSA. *See* Community-associated methicillin-resistant *Staphylococcus aureus* (CA-MRSA).

Canada Food Guide, 1233
Canadian Triage Acuity Scale (CTAS), 112
Cancellous tissue, 1018
Cancer, 359-370, 372t
AIDS-related, 335, 335f
bladder, 367b
bone, 1042-1045, 1044b
breast. *See* Breast cancer.
cervical, 1494-1495, 1495b
chemotherapy for. *See* Chemotherapy.
classification by tissue type, 363, 364f, 364t
colorectal. *See* Colorectal cancer.
development of, 362-368
cancer classification and, 363, 364f, 364t
cancer grading, ploidy, and staging in, 365, 365b, 365t
carcinogenesis/oncogenesis and, 362-363
cultural considerations in, 368b
external factors in, 366-367, 366t, 367b
genetic considerations in, 367b, 368t
metastasis and, 362-363, 363t
older adults and, 367b
personal factors in, 367-368, 367b, 367t
disease-related consequences of, 371-372
altered gastrointestinal structure and function in, 372
motor and sensory deficits in, 372
reduced gas exchange in, 372
reduced immunity and blood-producing functions in, 372
endometrial, 1491-1494, 1492t, 1493b
esophageal, 1117-1123
assessment in, 1118, 1118b
community-based care, 1122
evaluation of care of patient with, 1123
nutrition considerations in, 1119, 1119b
pathophysiology of, 1117-1118, 1117b
surgical management of, 1120-1122, 1121b-1122b, 1121f
gastric, 1138-1139, 1139b, 1140f, 1141t
grading of, 365, 365t
head and neck. *See* Head and neck cancer.
HIV-related, 335
hormonal manipulation for, 391-392, 391t
immunotherapy for, 387-388, 387t
leukemia. *See* Leukemia.
liver, 1208-1209

Cancer (*Continued*)
lung. *See* Lung cancer.
molecularly targeted therapy for, 388-391, 389f, 390t
angiogenesis inhibitors in, 390, 390t
epidermal growth factor/receptor inhibitors in, 390, 390t
multikinase inhibitors in, 390, 390t
proteasome inhibitors in, 390, 390t
tyrosine kinase inhibitors in, 390, 390t
vascular endothelial growth factor/receptor inhibitors in, 390, 390t
nose and sinus, 533-534
oncologic emergencies in, 392-394
hypercalcemia, 393
sepsis and disseminated intravascular coagulation, 392
spinal cord compression, 393
superior vena cava syndrome, 393-394, 393f-394f, 394b
syndrome of inappropriate antidiuretic hormone, 392-393, 392b
tumor lysis syndrome, 394, 394f
oral, 1102-1103
assessment of, 1103-1104, 1103b, 1103f
health care resources for, 1107
home care management in, 1106
interventions for, 1104, 1104b-1105b
pathophysiology of, 1102-1103, 1103b
self-management education in, 1106-1107, 1107b
ovarian, 1495-1497, 1496t
pancreatic, 1226-1230, 1227b, 1229f, 1229t, 1230b
pathophysiology of, 359-362, 360f
abnormal cell biology and, 361-362, 361t
normal cell biology and, 360-361, 360f-361f
photodynamic therapy for, 391
prevention of, 368-369
prostate. *See* Prostate cancer.
radiation therapy for, 374-377, 374f
delivery methods and devices in, 375, 376b
sealed implants of radioactive sources in, 376b
side effects of, 375-376, 376t
skin protection during, 376, 376b-377b

Cancer (Continued)
  skin, 458-461
    drug therapy for, 461
    etiology and genetic risk in, 458-460, 459f, 460b
    incidence and prevalence of, 460
    older adults and, 367b
    pathophysiology of, 458-460, 459t
    prevention of, 460, 460b
    surgical management of, 460-461
  surgery for, 373-374, 374b
  testicular, 1513-1516
    assessment in, 1514, 1514b
    chemotherapy for, 1515-1516
    community-based care in, 1516, 1516b
    external beam radiation therapy for, 1516
    pathophysiology of, 1513, 1513b, 1513t
    sperm banking and, 1514-1515, 1514b
    surgical management of, 1515, 1515b
  thyroid, 1295-1296
  urothelial, 1369b, 1388-1390, 1390b
  uterine, 1491-1494, 1492t, 1493b
Cancer control surgery, 373
Cancer therapy symptom distress, 381
Candida albicans, 334, 334f, 451-452
Candida infections, 450b
  in human immune deficiency virus infection, 334, 334f
  sexually-transmitted, 1544
  in stomatitis, 1100, 1100f
Canes, 81, 83b, 83f
Canthus, 967
Capillaries, 150f, 416
Capillary closing pressure, pressure ulcers and, 440
Caplan's syndrome, 306
Capnography, 509
Capnometry, 509
Capsaicin, 294
Capsule, 1345, 1345f
Carbapenem-resistant Enterobacteriaceae (CRE), 406
Carbohydrate counting, 1320
Carbon dioxide, 494
  hydrogen ions and, 176, 176f-177f
  perioperative assessment of, 223b-224b
  respiratory acid-base control and, 177-178, 178f
Carbon monoxide poisoning, 474, 475t
Carbonic anhydrase equation, 176, 176f
Carboxyhemoglobin, 219-220
  in burn assessment, 477b
Carcinoembryonic antigen, 1151

Carcinogenesis, 362-363, 365
Carcinogens, 362
Carcinomas
  basal cell, 459, 459f, 459t
  renal cell, 1406-1408, 1407t
  squamous cell, 458-459, 459f, 459t
Cardiac arrest, 249
Cardiac axis, 650-651
Cardiac catheterization, 643-644, 643t, 644b, 644f
Cardiac conduction system, 649-650, 650f
Cardiac cycle, 629-630, 630f
Cardiac dysrhythmias. See Dysrhythmias.
Cardiac index, 630
Cardiac markers, 640-641
Cardiac monitoring
  in hypercalcemia, 170
  in hyperkalemia, 167, 167b
Cardiac output (CO), 630
  after burn injuries, 470
  chronic kidney disease and, 1427
  heart failure and, 679-680, 684-688, 684t, 685b, 687b, 688f
Cardiac rehabilitation, 768, 769b
Cardiac resynchronization therapy (CRT), 687
Cardiac tamponade
  after coronary artery bypass graft, 778
  in pericarditis, 699-700
Cardiac valves, 628, 629f, 633b
Cardiogenic shock, 740, 741t, 772
Cardiomyopathies, 701-704, 701t, 703b, 703f
Cardiopulmonary bypass (CPB), 776
  in hypothermia rewarming, 132
Cardiopulmonary resuscitation (CPR), 671-672, 672b
  DNR orders and, 92-94
Cardiovascular assessment, 627-648
  arteriography in, 644
  in burns, 475
  cardiac catheterization in, 643-644, 643t, 644b, 644f
  current health problems in, 634-636, 634b, 636t
  echocardiography in, 645-646
  electrocardiogram in, 644-645
  electrophysiologic studies in, 645
  exercise electrocardiography in, 645, 645f
  family history and genetic risk in, 634, 634b
  functional history in, 636, 636t
  gender health considerations in, 632b, 634b-635b
  in hematologic assessment, 792
  laboratory assessment in, 640-642, 641b
  magnetic resonance imaging in, 647
  myocardial nuclear perfusion imaging in, 646-647

Cardiovascular assessment (Continued)
  nutrition history in, 634
  older adults and, 635b
  patient history in, 632-634
  physical assessment in, 636-640
    blood pressure in, 637-638
    extremities and, 637, 637f
    general appearance and, 637
    precordium and, 639-640, 639f, 640t
    skin and, 637
    venous and arterial pulses in, 638-639, 638f
  postoperative, 260
  psychosocial assessment in, 640
  in rehabilitation setting, 77-78, 78t
  in spinal cord injury, 895
  in stroke, 936-937
  transesophageal echocardiography in, 646
Cardiovascular disease (CVD), 627
Cardiovascular disease risk in diabetes mellitus, 1303
Cardiovascular problems. See Dysrhythmias; Heart failure (HF); Vascular problems.
Cardiovascular status, preoperative assessment of, 221
Cardiovascular system
  acidosis and, 181, 181b
  alkalosis and, 184, 184b
  anatomy and physiology of, 627-632
    changes associated with aging, 632, 633b
    heart, 627-631
      conduction system of, 649-650, 650f
      function of, 629-631, 630f
      structure of, 627-629, 629f
    vascular system, 631-632
      arterial system, 631-632
      venous system, 632
  assessment of. See Cardiovascular assessment.
  chronic kidney disease and, 1421
  complications of immobility and, 83t
  dehydration and, 156
  fluid overload and, 159b
  hypercalcemia and, 169
  hyperkalemia and, 166
  hypernatremia and, 163
  hypocalcemia and, 168
  hypokalemia and, 164
  hyponatremia, 162
  potential complications of surgery and, 258t
Cardioversion, 668, 668b
Cardizem. See Diltiazem.
Caregiver role strain in Alzheimer's disease, 879, 880b
Carina, endotracheal intubation and, 615, 615f

Carotid artery angioplasty with stenting, 939
Carotid artery rupture after head and neck surgery, 541, 541b
Carotid sinus massage, 666
Carpal tunnel syndrome (CTS), 1077-1078, 1077b
Carrier testing, 59t
Carriers, 58, 398
Carvedilol, 765b-766b
Case management, 5
  in acute respiratory distress syndrome, 614
  in emergency care, 113
Caseation necrosis in tuberculosis, 595
Casts, 1058-1060, 1059b-1060b, 1059f, 1060t, 1065b
Catabolism after burn injury, 470
Cataracts, 982-985
  home care management in, 984, 984b, 984f
  pathophysiology of, 982, 982f, 982t
  physical assessment in, 983, 983f
  self-management education in, 984, 984b
  surgery for, 983, 983f
Catechol O-methyltransferases (COMTs), 869
Catecholamine receptors, 1259t
Catecholamines, 470, 1259
Catheter embolism, 207t
Catheter maze procedure, 669
Catheter-associated urinary tract infections (CAUTIs), 399, 405
Catheterized urine specimens, 1357t
Catheter-related infections, 204, 204t
  central venous catheters and, 208t
  reducing, 399b
Catheters
  central venous
    blood samples from, 202-203, 203f
    home care of, 815b
    nontunneled percutaneous, 194-195, 194f
    peripherally inserted, 193-194, 193f, 194b
    tunneled, 195, 195f
  epistaxis, 533, 533f
  hemodialysis, 196
  intraventricular, 956t
  migration of, 208t
  for monitoring intracranial pressure, 956t
  older adults and, 209, 209b
  in peripheral infusion therapy
    flushing of, 202, 202b
    midline, 192-193, 192f, 201
    short, 190-192, 190f-192f, 190t, 191b, 201b
  peritoneal dialysis, 1440b
  securement of, 200-201, 201b
  subdural, 956t
  urinary
    infection and, 399, 405
    intermittent, 86

Cations, 160

CAUTIs. See Catheter-associated urinary tract infections (CAUTIs).

CAV. See Coronary artery vasculopathy (CAV).

Caval-atrial junction (CAJ). See Superior vena cava (SVC).

CBC. See Complete blood count (CBC).

CBE. See Clinical breast examination (CBE).

CCBs. See Calcium channel blockers (CCBs).

CD4 + T-cell count, 336

CD8 + T-cell count, 336

CD4+ T-cells, 327-328, 327f

CDAD. See C. difficile–associated disease (CDAD).

CDC. See Centers for Disease Control and Prevention (CDC).

Celiac disease, 1188, 1188b

Cell biology
  abnormal, 361-362, 361t
  normal, 360-361, 360f-361f

Cell cycle, 360, 361f

Cell division, 360, 361f

CellCept. See Mycophenolate.

Cell-mediated immunity (CMI), 285-286, 400
  age-related changes in, 277b
  cell types involved in, 285-286
  cytokines and, 286, 286t
  immune functions of leukocytes in, 278t
  protection provided by, 286
  role of leukocytes in, 787t

Cellulitis, 443, 450, 450b

Centers for Disease Control and Prevention (CDC)
  on bioterrorism agents, 411t
  classification of AIDS-defining conditions, 328, 329t
  on hand hygiene, 401
  recommendations for HIV testing, 333b
  on Standard Precautions, 402
  in tracking of infections, 397-398
  transmission-based guidelines of, 402, 405

Centers for Medicare & Medicaid (CMS), 6

Central artery aneurysms, 726-728
  community-based care in, 727-728, 727b
  imaging assessment in, 727
  nonsurgical management of, 727
  pathophysiology of, 726, 726f
  physical assessment in, 726-727
  surgical management of, 727

Central intravenous (IV) therapy, 193-196
  hemodialysis catheters in, 196
  implanted ports in, 195-196, 195f-196f, 196b

Central intravenous (IV) therapy (Continued)
  nontunneled percutaneous central venous catheters in, 194-195, 194f
  peripherally inserted central catheters in, 193-194, 193f, 194b
  tunneled central venous catheters in, 195, 195f

Central nervous system
  acidosis and, 181, 181b
  alkalosis and, 184, 184b
  in hematologic assessment, 793
  structure and function of, 829-833
    brain, 830-832, 831f-832f, 831t-832t
    spinal cord, 832-833, 833f

Central nervous system problems
  Alzheimer's disease. See Alzheimer's disease.
  amyotrophic lateral sclerosis, 910-911, 910b-911b
  back pain. See Back pain.
  cervical neck pain, 891-892, 891b-892b
  dementia. See Dementia.
  encephalitis, 865-867, 866b
  headaches, 853-858, 854b
    cluster, 857-858
    migraine, 854-857, 855b-857b, 855t
  Huntington disease (HD), 881-882, 881b
  meningitis, 863-867, 863b-865b, 864t
  multiple sclerosis, 904-910, 905b, 907f, 908b-909b
  Parkinson disease, 867-871, 867t, 868b-869b, 868f
    drug therapy for, 868-870, 869b
    genetic considerations in, 867b
    psychosocial support in, 870-871
    surgical management of, 871
  seizures and epilepsy
    drug therapy for, 859, 859b-860b
    emergency care in, 861-862, 862b
    etiology and genetic risk in, 858-859
    older adults and, 858b
    seizure precautions and management in, 860-861, 860b-861b
    self-management education in, 859, 861b
    surgical management of, 862-863
    types of, 858
  spinal cord injury. See Spinal cord injury (SCI).
  spinal cord tumors, 902-904, 903b

Central venous catheters (CVCs)
  blood samples from, 202-203, 203f
  complications of, 208t
  home care of, 815b
  nontunneled percutaneous, 194-195, 194f
  peripherally inserted, 193-194, 193f, 194b
  tunneled, 195, 195f

Centriacinar emphysema, 532f

Centrilobular emphysema, 532f

Cerebellar function assessment, 842-843

Cerebellum, 830-831

Cerebral angiography, 845, 845b, 846t-847t

Cerebral blood flow evaluation, 849

Cerebral cortex, 831

Cerebral perfusion, 938-942, 938b-939b, 940t, 941b, 941f

Cerebral perfusion pressure, 948-949

Cerebral salt wasting (CSW), 962

Cerebral tumors, 959b. See also Brain tumors.

Cerebrospinal fluid (CSF), 829-830, 832, 849-850, 850t
  in meningitis, 864, 864t

Cerebrospinal fluid leak
  after lumbar spinal surgery, 889b

Cerebrovascular disease risk in diabetes mellitus, 1303

Cerebrum, 831, 831t

Certification in emergency care, 111, 111t

Certified registered nurse anesthetists (CRNAs), 239

Certified registered nurse infusion (CRNI), 188

Certified surgical technologists (CSTs), 239

Cerumen
  cultural considerations in, 1001b
  impaction of, 1004-1005, 1005b, 1005f
  removal of, 999b

Cervarix vaccine, 368-369

Cervical biopsy, 1458, 1458b

Cervical cancer, 1494-1495, 1495b

Cervical disease, 306b

Cervical polyps, 1491

Cervical spine
  neck pain and, 891-892, 891b-892b
  primary survey and, 118t

Cervix, 1450, 1450f

CF. See Cystic fibrosis (CF).

CFS. See Chronic fatigue syndrome (CFS).

CGM. See Continuous blood glucose monitoring (CGM).

CHADS2 scoring system, 667, 667t

Chalazion, 978

Chancre, 1532

Chancroid, 1544

Chantix. See Varenicline.

Charcot foot, 1325, 1325f

Chart review, preoperative, 233-234

Checklist of Nonverbal Pain Indicators, 34

Chemical acid-base control, 177, 178t

Chemical burns, 471

Chemical carcinogenesis, 366

Chemical debridement of pressure ulcers, 444-446

"Chemo brain", 372, 386

Chemotherapy, 377-387
  alopecia in, 381, 384-385
  for bone cancer, 1044
  bone marrow suppression in, 381-383, 381b-384b
  for brain tumors, 959
  for breast cancer, 1476-1477, 1477b, 1477t
  categories of drugs in, 377-378, 378t
  cognitive changes in, 372, 385-386
  for colorectal cancer, 1151-1152
  combination, 378
  for esophageal cancer, 1119
  for head and neck cancer, 539
  infection prevention in, 382b
  for liver cancer, 1209
  for lung cancer, 576
  mucositis in, 384, 386b, 576
  nausea and vomiting in, 383-384, 384b-385b
  oral agents in, 380, 380t
  peripheral neuropathy in, 386-387, 386b-387b
  preventing injury or bleeding in, 384b
  for prostate cancer, 1510-1511
  side effects of, 381
  for skin cancer, 461
  for spinal cord tumors, 903
  for testicular cancer, 1515-1516
  thrombocytopenia in, 381-383
  treatment issues in, 378-381, 379b, 379f, 380t

Chemotherapy-induced peripheral neuropathy (CIPN), 386-387, 386b-387b

Chemotherapy-nausea and vomiting (CINV), 383-384, 384b-385b

Cherry angiomas, 420f

Chest
  expansion in respiratory acidosis, 180-181
  inspection of, 503-504, 504f
  palpation of, 504
  percussion of, 504, 504f, 505t
  positioning to prevent contractures, 487b

Chest fractures, 1069

Chest pain, 634-635
  in coronary artery disease, 782b
  respiratory assessment and, 502
  types of, 636t

Chest physiotherapy, 568, 568f

Chest radiography, 507
Chest surgery, skin preparation for, 229f
Chest trauma, 622-624
 flail chest, 623, 623f
 hemothorax, 624
 pneumothorax, 623-624
 pulmonary contusions, 622-623
 rib fractures, 623
 tension pneumothorax, 624
 tracheobronchial trauma, 624
Chest tubes, 577-579, 577f, 579b
Chest wall changes with aging, 501b
Cheyne-Stokes respirations, 95
CHF. See Congestive heart failure (CHF).
Chlamydia infections, 1538-1539, 1538b
Chlamydia trachomatis, 1538
Chloride, 172
 abnormal values of, 152t
 levels in burn assessment, 477b
 perioperative assessment of, 223b-224b
 plasma values in older adults, 152b
Chlorpheniramine, 129
Chlor-Trimeton. See Chlorpheniramine.
Choked disc, 952
Cholecystectomy, 1217-1218, 1218t
Cholecystitis, 1213-1218
 assessment in, 1215-1216, 1215b-1216b
 nonsurgical management of, 1216-1217
 pathophysiology of, 1213-1214, 1214f, 1215b, 1215t
 surgical management of, 1217-1218, 1217b, 1218t
Choledochojejunostomy, 1229, 1229f
Cholelithiasis, 1213-1214
Cholesterol, 641-642, 641b
Cholinergic antagonists, 539b, 556
Cholinergic crisis, 919-920, 920t
Cholinesterase inhibitors
 for Alzheimer's disease, 877
 for myasthenia gravis, 920, 920b
Chondroitin, 294-295
Choreiform movements, 881
Christianity, end of life and death rituals in, 100t
Chromosomes, 52-54, 52f, 54f
Chronic airflow limitation (CAL), 532f, 548. See also Asthma; Chronic obstructive pulmonary disease (COPD).
Chronic bronchitis, 532f, 536-545
Chronic calcifying pancreatitis, 1223
Chronic cholecystitis, 1214
Chronic confusion in Alzheimer's disease, 875-878, 875t, 876b-877b
Chronic constrictive pericarditis, 699
Chronic fatigue syndrome (CFS), 322
Chronic gastritis, 1127

Chronic glomerulonephritis, 1403-1404
Chronic health problems, rehabilitation for, 74-90
 community-based care and, 88-89
 complications of immobility and, 83, 83t
 establishing bowel continence and, 87-88, 87b-88b, 87t
 establishing urinary continence and, 85-87, 86b-87b, 86t
 evaluation of, 89
 functional assessment in, 79-80, 80t
 gait training and, 81-84, 83b, 83f, 83t
 health care resources for, 89
 history in, 77
 home care management and, 88-89
 improving physical mobility and, 80-84, 81b, 82f-83f, 83b, 83t
 increasing functional ability and, 84, 84t, 85b
 maintaining skin integrity and, 85
 NANDA-I and, 80
 older adults and, 77b, 87b
 physical assessment in, 77-79, 78t, 79b, 90
 psychosocial assessment in, 80, 90
 rehabilitation team and, 75-77, 76f, 76t
 self-management education and, 89
 settings for, 75, 75f
 vocational assessment in, 80
Chronic hepatitis, 1204
Chronic inflammatory bowel disease, 1173-1188
 Crohn's disease. See Crohn's disease.
 ulcerative colitis, 1173-1188, 1173t
 assessment in, 1175
 community-based care in, 1180-1181, 1181b
 drug therapy for, 1176-1177, 1176b, 1176t
 evaluation of care of patient with, 1181
 lower gastrointestinal bleeding in, 1179-1180, 1180b
 pain in, 1179, 1179b
 pathophysiology of, 1174-1181, 1174t, 1175b
 surgical management of, 1177-1179, 1177b, 1178f
Chronic kidney disease (CKD), 1419-1446
 anxiety in, 1430-1431
 assessment in, 1422-1424, 1423b
 cardiac output in, 1427-1428
 characteristics of, 1412t
 community-based care in, 1444-1446
 concept map for, 1425f
 evaluation of care of patient with, 1446
 fatigue in, 1430
 focused assessment in, 1445

Chronic kidney disease (CKD) (Continued)
 health promotion and maintenance in, 1421-1422
 hemodialysis in, 1431-1437
 anticoagulation in, 1432-1433
 complications of, 1433-1437, 1435t
 dialysis settings in, 1432
 older adults and, 1437b
 patient selection for, 1431
 post-dialysis care and, 1436
 procedure in, 1433f, 1436t
 vascular access in, 1432-1435, 1432f, 1434f, 1435b, 1435f, 1436b
 infection prevention in, 1428
 injury prevention in, 1428-1430, 1428b
 kidney transplantation
 candidate selection criteria in, 1441-1442
 complications of, 1443-1444, 1444t
 donors in, 1441-1442, 1442f
 immunosuppressive drug therapy in, 1408
 operative procedures in, 1442, 1443f
 postoperative care in, 1442-1443
 preoperative care in, 1442
 management of fluid volume in, 1424-1427, 1426b
 nutrition and, 1427-1428, 1427t
 pathophysiology of, 1419-1422, 1419b
 cardiac changes in, 1421
 etiology and genetic risk in, 1421, 1422t
 gastrointestinal changes in, 1421
 hematologic changes in, 1421
 incidence and prevalence of, 1421, 1422b
 kidney changes in, 1420
 metabolic changes in, 1420-1421, 1420f
 stages of, 1419, 1419b, 1419t
 peritoneal dialysis in, 1437-1441, 1431t
 complications in, 1440-1441, 1440b
 dialysate additives for, 1438
 nursing care in, 1441
 patient selection for, 1437
 procedure in, 1437-1438, 1438f
 types of, 1438-1440, 1438f, 1439f, 1440f
 pulmonary edema in, 1426-1427
Chronic leukemia, 806
 drug therapy for, 810
Chronic low back pain, 887-888, 887b
Chronic lymphocytic leukemia (CLL), 807t
Chronic myelogenous leukemia (CML), 807t

Chronic obstructive pulmonary disease (COPD), 535-536
 activity tolerance and, 565
 anxiety in, 565
 breathing techniques for, 562, 563b
 chronic bronchitis in, 536
 complications of, 536-537, 545b
 concept map for respiratory acidosis in, 560f
 drug therapy for, 563-564, 564b
 effective coughing for, 563
 emphysema in, 536-545
 etiology and genetic risk in, 536-537, 545b
 evaluation of care of patient with, 566-567
 exercise conditioning in, 564
 health care resources for, 566, 566b
 health promotion and maintenance in, 537
 history in, 538
 home care management in, 566
 hydration in, 564
 imaging assessment in, 561
 incidence and prevalence of, 536
 laboratory assessment in, 561
 lung transplantation for, 564-565
 monitoring for respiratory status changes in, 562
 oxygen therapy for, 563
 physical assessment in, 559-561, 559f, 561f
 positioning for, 562-563
 positive expiratory pressure device for, 564, 564f
 psychosocial assessment in, 561
 respiratory infections and, 565-566
 self-management education in, 566
 severity classification in, 562t
 suctioning in, 564
 weight loss in, 565
Chronic osteomyelitis, 1040
Chronic pain, 26
 in cancer, 26
 characteristics of, 25-26
 in osteoarthritis, 293-303
 complementary and alternative therapies for, 294-295, 295b
 drug therapy for, 293-294, 293b-294b
 nonpharmacologic interventions for, 294, 294b
 psychosocial assessment in, 32-33
Chronic pancreatitis, 1223-1226, 1224b-1225b
Chronic paronychia, 427
Chronic peripheral arterial disease, 719b
Chronic pyelonephritis, 1399, 1400b

Chronic rejection of transplant, 287
Chronic renal failure. *See* Chronic kidney disease (CKD).
Chronic stable angina pectoris, 757-758
Chronic thyroiditis, 1295
Chvostek's sign, 168, 168f
Cimex lectularius, 454-455
CINV. *See* Chemotherapy-nausea and vomiting (CINV).
CIPN. *See* Chemotherapy-induced peripheral neuropathy (CIPN).
Ciprofloxacin, 188b
Circadian rhythm disorders, 837
Circinate lesions, 422t
Circle of Willis, 832, 832f
Circulating nurses, 239
Circulation
    of the brain, 832, 832f
    primary survey and, 117, 118t
    pulmonary, 499, 499f
Circulatory overload, 207t
Circumcision, 1451
Circumferential burn injuries, 468
Circumscribed lesions, 422t
Cirrhosis, 1192-1202
    assessment in, 1195-1197, 1196f, 1197t
    bleeding episodes in, 1200
    community-based care, 1201-1202, 1202b
    concept map for, 1198f
    evaluation of care of patient with, 1202
    management of fluid volume in, 1197-1200, 1199b
    pathophysiology of, 1192-1195, 1193t
    complications of, 1193-1194, 1194f, 1194t
    etiology and genetic risk in, 1194-1195, 1195b
    incidence and prevalence of, 1195
CK. *See* Creatine kinase (CK).
CKD. *See* Chronic kidney disease (CKD).
Class I antidysrhythmic drugs, 658, 658b-662b
Class I antigens, 276
Class II antidysrhythmic drugs, 658-662, 658b-662b
Class III antidysrhythmic drugs, 658b-662b, 662
Class IV antidysrhythmic drugs, 658b-662b, 662
Classic heat stroke, 121
Clean-catch urine specimen, 1357t
Clinical breast examination (CBE), 1467-1468, 1467b
Clinical practice guidelines, 67, 68f
Clinical psychologists, 77
Clinical questions, 65-66, 73
Clinical staging, 365
Clinically competent, definition of, 16

CLL. *See* Chronic lymphocytic leukemia (CLL).
Clonus, 841
Clopidogrel, 765b-766b
Closed fractures, 1051-1052, 1052f
Closed reduction, 1058-1060, 1058f-1059f, 1059b-1060b, 1060t
    of nasal fractures, 532
Closed traumatic brain injury, 946-947, 947f, 948b
Clostridium botulinum, 411t
Clostridium difficile, 413
Clostridium tetani, 485
Clotting, 787-788, 789f, 790t
Clotting factor disorders, 820-821, 821b, 821t
Clubbing, 426, 427t, 637
    in chronic obstructive pulmonary disease, 561, 561f
Cluster headaches, 857-858
Clustered lesions, 422t
CMI. *See* Cell-mediated immunity (CMI).
CML. *See* Chronic myelogenous leukemia (CML).
CMS. *See* Centers for Medicare & Medicaid (CMS).
CMV. *See* Cytomegalovirus (CMV).
CO. *See* Cardiac output (CO).
Coagulation disorders
    autoimmune thrombocytopenic purpura, 820
    hemophilia, 820-821, 821b, 821t
Coal Miner's Disease, 573b
Coalesced lesions, 422t
Co-analgesics. *See* Adjuvant analgesics.
Coarse crackles, 507t
Coccidioidomycosis, 600-601
Cochlea, 998
Code Blue, 257b
Codeine, 42, 270b
Cognition, 828
    in neurologic assessment, 839, 839b
Cognitive function
    after stroke, 934, 936b
    Alzheimer's disease and, 873t
    chemotherapy-related changes in, 372, 385-386
    diabetes mellitus and, 1306
    hypothyroidism and, 1293-1294
    multiple sclerosis and, 909, 909b
    older adults and, 398b
    traumatic brain injury and, 955-956
Cognitive rehabilitation in traumatic brain injury, 955-956
Cognitive therapists, 77
Cognitive-behavioral pain management, 47-48
Cohorting, 403-405
Cold antibody anemia, 804
Cold application
    for osteoarthritis pain, 294, 294b
    for pain management, 46-47

Cold-related injuries, 131-133, 136-137
    frostbite, 122b, 132-133, 132b-133b
    hypothermia, 131-132, 131b-132b
Collaboration, 4-6, 5t, 6b, 8
Collagen, 416
Collagenase, 483
Collateral circulation, peripheral arterial disease and, 721
Colon interposition, 1121, 1121f
Colonization of bacteria, 397
Colonoscopy, 1095-1096, 1096b
Color
    of nails, 426, 426f, 426t
    of skin, 421
        common alterations in, 422t
        cultural considerations in, 427b
Color vision, 970b, 973, 973f
Colorectal cancer, 1148-1157
    assessment in, 1150-1151, 1150f
    community-based care in, 1155-1157, 1155b-1156b
    evaluation of care of patient with, 1157
    grieving in, 1155, 1155b
    health promotion and maintenance in, 1149, 1150b
    metastasis in, 1151-1154
    nonsurgical management of, 1151-1152
    older adults and, 367b
    pathophysiology of, 1148-1149, 1148f, 1149b
    surgical management of, 1152-1154, 1152t, 1153f-1154f, 1154b
Colostomy, 1152-1154, 1152t, 1153f-1154f, 1154b, 1156, 1156b
Colposcopy, 1457, 1495
Combination drug therapy
    for diabetes mellitus, 1312b, 1313
    for HIV infection, 339b
    for tuberculosis, 596-597, 597b
Combined metabolic and respiratory acidosis, 181, 182b
Combined metabolic and respiratory alkalosis, 182b
Combined ventilatory and oxygenation failure, 611-612
Command center in emergency, 142-143
Commando procedure, 1105
Common variable immune deficiency, 346
Communicable infections, 397
Communicating hydrocephalus, 949-950
Communication
    after laryngectomy, 545
    collaboration and, 5-6, 5t, 6b, 8
    emergency care and, 110-111, 114
    in genetic counseling, 61-62
    in Guillain-Barré syndrome, 917
    hand-off communication in emergency care, 107-108

Communication (*Continued*)
    hearing loss and, 1014, 1014b
    in minimizing preoperative anxiety, 233
    with patient unable to speak, 540b
    stroke and, 943, 943t
    tracheostomy and, 528
Community Emergency Response Team, 142
Community relations officers, 143, 143t
Community-acquired pneumonia, 590t
Community-associated methicillin-resistant *Staphylococcus aureus* (CA-MRSA), 406
Community-based care
    in acute pancreatitis, 1223
    in AIDS and HIV infection, 343-344, 343b-344b
    in Alzheimer's disease, 879-880, 880b
    in amputations, 1074-1075, 1074f, 1075b
    in aneurysms, 727-728, 727b
    in back surgery, 890-891, 890b-891b
    in benign prostatic hyperplasia, 1506
    in bone cancer, 1045
    in breast cancer, 1478-1480, 1478b-1479b
    in burns, 489, 489t
    in cataracts, 984-985, 984b, 984f
    in chronic kidney disease, 1444-1446, 1445b
    in chronic obstructive pulmonary disease, 566, 566b
    in chronic pancreatitis, 1225-1226
    in cirrhosis, 1201-1202, 1202b
    in colorectal cancer, 1155-1157, 1155b-1156b
    in coronary artery disease, 779-782, 780b-782b
    in Crohn's disease, 1185-1186
    in cystitis, 1373
    in diabetes mellitus, 1337-1339, 1337t, 1339b, 1339t
    in diverticular disease, 1187-1188
    in dysrhythmias, 673-676, 673b-675b
    in endometrial cancer, 1493-1494
    in esophageal cancer, 1122
    in fractures, 1065
    in gastric cancer, 1141-1142
    in Guillain-Barré syndrome, 917
    in head and neck cancer, 544-545, 544b-545b
    in hearing loss, 1014
    in heart failure, 689-692, 689b-691b, 690t
    in hepatitis, 1207-1208, 1208b
    in hypercortisolism, 1281, 1281b
    in hypertension, 718
    in hypothyroidism, 1294-1295, 1294b-1295b

Community-based care *(Continued)*
  in hypovolemic shock, 748
  in infection, 410
  in infective endocarditis, 698-699,
    699b
  in intestinal obstruction, 1161
  in kidney trauma, 1409
  in leukemia, 815-816, 815b-816b
  in lupus, 316-317, 316b
  in malnutrition, 1245-1246
  in multiple sclerosis, 909-910
  in myasthenia gravis, 922-923,
    922b, 922t
  in obesity, 1252, 1252b
  in oral cancer, 1106-1107, 1107b
  in osteoarthritis, 304, 304b
  in osteoporosis, 1036
  in ovarian cancer, 1497
  in oxygen therapy, 521, 521f, 522b
  in pain, 48-49
  in pancreatic cancer, 1230
  in pelvic inflammatory disease,
    1543-1544, 1543b
  in peptic ulcer disease, 1137-1138,
    1138b
  in peripheral arterial disease,
    724-725, 724b-725b
  in peritonitis, 1171-1172
  in pneumonia, 593-594, 594b
  postoperative, 271-272, 272b
  in pressure ulcers, 447-449, 449b
  in prostate cancer, 1511, 1511b
  in pulmonary embolism, 609-610,
    610b
  in pyelonephritis, 1401
  rehabilitation and, 88-89
  in rheumatoid arthritis, 313, 313b,
    313f
  in sepsis, 754, 754b
  in sickle cell disease, 803
  in spinal cord injury, 900-902,
    901b, 902f
  in spinal cord tumors, 904
  in stroke, 944-945, 945b, 945f
  in systemic sclerosis, 319
  in testicular cancer, 1516, 1516b
  in tracheostomy, 529
  for transgender patients, 1528
  in traumatic brain injury, 956-957,
    957b
  in tuberculosis, 598-599
  in ulcerative colitis, 1180-1181,
    1181b
  in urinary incontinence, 1383,
    1383b
  in urothelial cancer, 1390, 1390b
  in uterine leiomyomas, 1490-1491,
    1490b
  in valvular heart disease, 696-697,
    697b
  in venous insufficiency, 735
  in venous thromboembolism,
    733-734, 733b
Compartment syndrome
  intraosseous therapy-related,
    211-212

Compensated cirrhosis, 1193
Compensation, 179
Compensatory mechanisms
  in burn injuries, 470, 471f
  in heart failure, 679-681, 680f
  in hypovolemic shock, 744
Complement activation fixation,
  284
Complementary and alternative
    therapies
  for AIDS and HIV infection,
    340-341
  for allergic rhinitis, 351
  for atherosclerosis, 709
  for back pain, 888
  for benign prostatic hyperplasia,
    1503
  for breast cancer, 1471-1472,
    1471t, 1472b
  for coronary artery disease, 781
  end-of-life care and, 104
    nausea and vomiting
      management and, 99
    pain management and, 97
    restlessness and agitation
      management and, 100
  for gastritis and peptic ulcer
      disease, 1129t
  for hepatitis, 1206b
  for hypertension, 712
  for migraines, 856-857
  for multiple sclerosis, 909
  for obesity, 1250
  older adults and, 15
  for osteoarthritis, 294-295, 295b
  for pain management
    after total knee arthroplasty,
      301
    in burns, 480
    postoperative, 271, 271b
  for peptic ulcer disease, 1129t,
    1136, 1136b
  for preventing coronary artery
      disease, 761
  for rheumatoid arthritis, 312
  for sickle cell disease, 802
  for ulcerative colitis, 1177
Complementary base pairs, 53, 53f
Complete blood count (CBC)
  in respiratory assessment, 508b
Complete fractures, 1051
Complete partial seizures, 861b
Complete spinal cord injury, 892
Complex inheritance and familial
    clustering, 57t, 59
Complex partial seizures, 858, 858b
Complex regional pain syndrome
    (CRPS), 1075
Composite resection in head and
    neck cancer, 542
Composite urine collection, 1357t,
    1358, 1359b
Compound fractures, 1051-1052,
    1052f
Compression dressings, 487-488,
    488f

Compression fractures, 1052
  of spine, 1069
Computed tomography (CT)
  in gastrointestinal assessment,
    1093
  in infection diagnosis, 408
  in neurologic assessment, 845-847,
    846t-847t
  in renal assessment, 1360-1361,
    1360t, 1361b
  in reproductive assessment, 1456
  in respiratory assessment,
    507-508
  in spinal cord injury, 895
  in vision assessment, 973
Computed tomography coronary
    angiography (CTCA), 763
COMTs. *See* Catechol
    O-methyltransferases
    (COMTs).
Concept maps
  for benign prostatic hyperplasia,
    1504f
  for chronic kidney disease, 1426f
  for cirrhosis, 1198f
  for diabetes mellitus, 1311f
  for glaucoma, 986f
  for hypertension, 713f
  for hypovolemic shock, 745f
  for multiple sclerosis, 907f
  for pneumonia, 591f
  for pressure ulcers, 445f
  for respiratory acidosis in COPD,
    560f
Condom, 1536b
Conduction system, 633b, 649-650,
    650f
Conductive hearing loss, 1001
  sensorineural versus, 1009t
Conductivity of heart cells, 649
Condylomata acuminata, 1537-1538,
    1537b, 1537f
Confidentiality in genetic testing,
    61-62
Confusion
  in AIDS and HIV infection,
    342-343, 342b
  in Alzheimer's disease, 875-878,
    875t, 876b-877b
  hospitalized older adults and,
    20-22
Confusion Assessment Method, 18,
    18t, 90
Congenital immune deficiencies,
    345-346
Congestive heart failure (CHF), 679.
    See also Heart failure (HF).
Conization, 1458
Conjunctiva, 967
Conjunctival disorders, 978-980,
    980b
Conjunctivitis, 979-980
Connective tissue diseases (CTDs),
    290-325
  ankylosing spondylitis, 323t
  chronic fatigue syndrome, 322

Connective tissue diseases (CTDs)
    (Continued)
  common disorders associated with
    arthritis, 322, 323t
  fibromyalgia syndrome, 321-322
  gout, 319-320, 319f
  infectious arthritis, 320
  lupus erythematosus, 313-317,
    314b, 314f, 316b-317b
  Lyme disease in, 320-321, 321b
  Marfan syndrome, 323t
  mixed connective tissue disease,
    322-323
  osteoarthritis, 291-304
    chronic pain in, 293-303
      complementary and
        alternative medicine for,
        294-295, 295b
      drug therapy for, 293-294,
        293b-294b
      nonpharmacologic
        interventions for, 294,
        294b
    etiology and genetic risk for,
      300-301, 304b
    health care resources for, 304
    health promotion and
      maintenance in, 301
    history in, 292
    home care management in, 304
    imaging assessment in, 293
    improving mobility in, 303,
      303b
    incidence and prevalence of,
      291
    laboratory assessment in, 293
    pathophysiology of, 291, 291f
    physical assessment in, 292-293,
      292f, 292t
    psychosocial assessment in, 293
    self-management education in,
      304, 304b
    surgical management of,
      295-303
      hand and ankle arthroplasties
        in, 303
      total elbow arthroplasty in,
        303
      total hip arthroplasty in,
        295-300, 297b-300b,
        297f-298f, 297t
      total knee arthroplasty in,
        300-302, 301f, 302b
      total shoulder arthroplasty
        in, 303
  polymyalgia rheumatica and
    temporal arteritis, 323t
  polymyositis/dermatomyositis,
    323t
  psoriatic arthritis, 321
  Reiter's syndrome, 323t
  rheumatoid arthritis, 304-313
    arthrocentesis in, 308, 308b
    body image and, 312
    complementary and alternative
      therapies for, 312

Connective tissue diseases (CTDs) (Continued)
fatigue in, 312, 312b
health care resources for, 313
home care management in, 313, 313f
inflammation and pain management in, 308-312, 308b-310b
laboratory assessment in, 307, 307b
nonpharmacologic interventions in, 311
pathophysiology of, 304-305, 305b
patient and family education in, 313
physical assessment in, 295b, 305-306, 305b-306b
psychosocial assessment in, 306-307
self-management in, 312, 312b
systemic necrotizing vasculitis, 323t
systemic sclerosis, 314b, 317-319, 318b, 318f
Consciousness, loss of. See Syncope.
Consensual response of pupil, 840, 972
Consolidation in lobar pneumonia, 589
Consolidation therapy in leukemia, 810
Constipation
end-of-life care and, 99
opioid-induced, 43, 43t
in polycystic kidney disease, 1397
postoperative, 263
rehabilitation setting and, 78, 88
Contact burns, 470-471
Contact dermatitis, 455, 455b
Contact inhibition in cell division, 360
Contact laser prostatectomy, 1503
Contact Precautions, 404t, 405
Contact transmission, 399
Containers in infusion systems, 196-197, 197b
Contamination
of food, 413
of pressure ulcers, 444
Continence, 1350, 1373
rehabilitation and, 85-87, 86b-87b, 86t
stroke and, 943-944
Continuous blood glucose monitoring (CGM), 1319
Continuous electrocardiographic monitoring, 652, 653f
Continuous feeding, 1241-1242
Continuous negative pressure wound therapy
anticoagulant therapy and, 447b
Continuous passive motion (CPM) machines, 301, 301f, 302b

Continuous positive airway pressure (CPAP), 520, 520f, 618
for heart failure, 687
for obstructive sleep apnea, 535
Continuous renal replacement therapy, 1418
Continuous subcutaneous infusion of insulin, 1315, 1316f
Continuous sutures, 254f
Continuous wet gauze dressing, 446t
Contractility of heart muscle, 650
Contraction in wound healing, 434f-435f, 436
Contracture, positioning to prevent, 487b
Contrecoup injuries, 947, 947f
Control therapy drugs for asthma, 553
Contusions, 947
Convergence, 969
Coomb's test, 794
COPD. See Chronic obstructive pulmonary disease (COPD).
Coping
in breast cancer, 1470-1471, 1471b
in coronary artery disease, 769
in endometrial cancer, 1493
Cor pulmonale
in chronic obstructive pulmonary disease, 545b, 558
in sarcoidosis, 571
Coral snakes, 125-126, 125f, 126b
Cord blood harvesting, 812
Cordarone. See Amiodarone.
Cordectomy, 540, 541t
Core competencies, 3-6, 8
in emergency nursing, 110-111
evidence-based practice in, 6, 8
informatics in, 7-8, 7f
patient-centered care in, 3-4, 3t, 5t, 8
quality improvement in, 6-8
safety in, 7
teamwork and collaboration in, 4-6, 5t, 6b, 8
Core Measures, 6
Corium. See Dermis.
Cornea, 967, 967f
changes with aging, 970b
Corneal disorders, 980-982
corneal abrasion, ulceration, and infection, 980-981, 980b
keratoconus and corneal opacities, 981-982, 981f, 982t
Corneal light reflex, 973, 973f
Corneal staining, 974
Coronary arteriography, 644
Coronary artery bypass graft (CABG) surgery, 774-779, 777f
neurologic status after, 779b
postoperative care in, 776-779, 778b-779b
preoperative care in, 775-776

Coronary artery disease (CAD), 757-784
activity tolerance and, 768-769, 769b
cardiopulmonary tissue perfusion in, 766-768, 767b-768b, 768t
complementary and alternative therapies and, 761, 781
coping with, 769
cultural considerations in, 760b, 762b
drug therapy for chest pain, 764-766, 764b-766b
dysrhythmias in, 769
emergency care in chest pain and, 764, 764b
evaluation of care of patient with, 782
gender health considerations in, 632b, 759b-760b, 762b
health care resources for, 782
health promotion and maintenance and, 760-761, 761b, 761t, 783
history in, 762
home care management in, 779-781, 780b
imaging assessment in, 763
laboratory assessment in, 763
metabolic syndrome and, 761, 761t
monitoring/managing heart failure in, 769-772, 770b, 771f, 771t, 772b-773b
monitoring/managing recurrent symptoms and extension of myocardial injury in, 772-779, 774f, 775b, 776f-777f, 778b-779b
older adults and, 760b, 762b, 769b, 780b
pathophysiology of, 757-760
acute coronary syndrome and, 758-760, 758f-759f, 759b
chronic stable angina pectoris and, 757-758
etiology and genetic risk in, 760, 760b
incidence and prevalence in, 760, 760b
physical assessment in, 762-763, 762b
psychosocial assessment in, 763
self-management education in, 781-782, 781b-782b
Coronary artery vasculopathy (CAV), 703-704
Coronary heart disease. See Coronary artery disease (CAD).
Corticosteroids
for allergic rhinitis, 351
for anaphylaxis, 354b
for asthma, 539b, 556
for bee stings, 129
for chemotherapy-induced nausea and vomiting, 385b

Corticosteroids (Continued)
immune deficiency and, 345
for psoriasis, 457
for skin inflammation, 455-456, 456b
for transplant rejection, 287b-288b
Cortisol replacement therapy, 1281b
Corvert. See Ibutilide.
Coryza, 583
Cosmetic surgery, 218t, 462-463
after burns, 488
common procedures in, 462t
Cottonmouth water moccasins, 123, 123f
Cough
in pneumonia, 592t
respiratory assessment and, 502
Cough assist technique, 896
Coughing exercises
for chronic obstructive pulmonary disease, 563
to prevent postoperative respiratory complications, 230-231
Coumadin. See Warfarin.
Counseling, genetic, 60-63, 60b, 62b
Counterimmunoelectrophoresis in meningitis, 864
COX-2 inhibiting drugs, 294b
CPAP. See Continuous positive airway pressure (CPAP).
CPB. See Cardiopulmonary bypass (CPB).
CPM machines. See Continuous passive motion (CPM) machines.
CPR. See Cardiopulmonary resuscitation (CPR).
Crackles in pneumonia, 592
Cranial nerve diseases, 926-928
facial paralysis, 927-928
trigeminal neuralgia, 926-927, 926f, 927b
Cranial nerves, 834, 835t
assessment of, 840
stroke and, 936
Craniotomy for brain tumors, 960-962, 960b-961b, 961t
CRE. See Carbapenem-resistant Enterobacteriaceae (CRE).
Creatine kinase (CK), 641
Creatinine, 223b-224b
Creatinine clearance, 1358
older adults and, 14
Credé maneuver, 86
Crepitus
in neck trauma, 537
in osteoarthritis, 291-292
palpation of chest and, 504
CREST syndrome, 317
Cricoid cartilage, 497, 498f
Cricothyroid membrane, 497, 498f

Cricothyroidotomy, 497
    in facial trauma, 534
    in upper airway obstruction, 536
Critical access hospitals, 105
Critical incident stress debriefing, 145, 145b
Critically ill patients
    acquired hypoxic-anoxic brain injury in, 964
    acute respiratory distress syndrome in, 612-614, 613b-614b, 613t
    acute respiratory failure in, 610-612, 611t-612t
    brain abscesses in, 962-964, 963b
    brain tumors in, 957-962
        assessment of, 958-959, 959b
        classification of, 958, 958t
        community-based care in, 962
        interventions for, 959-962, 959f, 960b-961b, 961t
        pathophysiology of, 957-958
    burns in. See Burns.
    chest trauma in, 622-624, 623f
        flail chest, 623, 623f
        hemothorax, 624
        pneumothorax, 623-624
        pulmonary contusions, 622-623
        rib fractures, 623
        tension pneumothorax, 624
        tracheobronchial trauma, 624
    mechanical ventilation for. See Mechanical ventilation.
    pulmonary embolism in. See Pulmonary embolism.
    stroke in. See Stroke.
    transient ischemic attack in, 930-931, 931b
    traumatic brain injury in. See Traumatic brain injury (TBI).
CRNAs. See Certified registered nurse anesthetists (CRNAs).
CRNI. See Certified registered nurse infusion (CRNI).
Crohn's disease, 1173t, 1181-1186
    assessment in, 1182-1183, 1183b
    community-based care in, 1185-1186
    drug therapy for, 1183, 1183b
    fistula management in, 1184b, 1185f
    pathophysiology of, 1174t, 1181-1182, 1182f
    surgical management of, 1185
Cromones, 539b, 556
Cross-contamination
    in burns, 484
    in leukemia, 809
CRPS. See Complex regional pain syndrome (CRPS).
CRT. See Cardiac resynchronization therapy (CRT).
Crusts and oozing, 423f
Cryosurgery for skin cancer, 460

Cryotherapy
    for genital warts, 1537
    for pain management, 46-47
Cryptococcosis, 334
Cryptorchidism, 1513
Cryptosporidiosis, 334
Cryptosporidium, 1189
CSF. See Cerebrospinal fluid (CSF).
CSTs. See Certified surgical technologists (CSTs).
CSW. See Cerebral salt wasting (CSW).
CT. See Computed tomography (CT).
CTAS. See Canadian Triage Acuity Scale (CTAS).
CTCA. See Computed tomography coronary angiography (CTCA).
CTDs. See Connective tissue diseases (CTDs).
CTS. See Carpal tunnel syndrome (CTS).
Cultural competence, 4
Cultural considerations
    in bone marrow donation, 811b
    in breast cancer, 1466b, 1469b
    in burns, 476b
    in cancer, 368b
    in cerumen, 1001b
    in coronary artery disease, 760b, 762b
    in emergency care, 110b, 113b
    in end-of-life care, 95b
    in end-stage kidney disease, 1405b
    in food preferences, 1233b
    in gastrointestinal assessment, 1088b
    in genetic biology, 56b
    in glomerular filtration rate, 1351b
    in gonorrhea, 1539b
    in hematologic assessment, 792b
    in HIV infection, 329b
    in hypertension, 711b
    in lupus, 314b
    in malnutrition, 1237b
    in older adults, 20b
    in osteoporosis, 1031b
    in peripheral arterial disease, 720b
    in prostate cancer, 1507b
    in reproductive assessment, 1453b
    in respiratory assessment, 500b
    in sickle cell disease, 476b
    in skin color, 427b
    in smoking, 496b
    in stroke, 933b
    in syphilis, 1533b
    in ulcerative colitis, 1175b
    in urinary incontinence, 1382b
    in urolithiasis, 1385b
Culture and sensitivity, 408
    urine for, 1358
Cultured skin for burn wounds, 483
Curative surgery, 218t, 373

Curettage and electrodesiccation for skin cancer, 460
Curling's ulcers, 1130
Cushing's disease. See Hypercortisolism.
Cushing's triad, 951-952
Cushing's ulcers, 1130
Cutaneous anthrax, 453, 453b, 454f
Cutaneous infections, 449-453, 450b
    in anthrax, 453, 453b, 454f
    bacterial, 450-451, 450b, 451f, 453
    fungal, 450b, 451-452
    laboratory assessment in, 452
    physical assessment in, 450b, 452
    prevention of, 452, 452b
    viral, 450b, 451, 451f
Cutaneous reflexes, 841
Cutaneous stimulation for pain management, 46-47
Cuticles, 417, 417f
CVCs. See Central venous catheters (CVCs).
CVD. See Cardiovascular disease (CVD).
Cyanide poisoning, 478
Cyanosis, 428, 428b
    assessment of, 792b
    cardiovascular assessment and, 637
Cyclic feeding, 1241-1242
Cyclosporine
    immune deficiency and, 345
    to prevent transplant rejection, 287b-288b
CYP2C19 gene, 608b
Cystectomy, 1388
Cystic fibrosis (CF), 567-569
    genetic considerations in, 567b
    nonsurgical management of, 568, 568f
    pathophysiology of, 567-569, 1368b
    surgical management of, 569
Cystitis, 1367-1373
    assessment in, 1369-1370, 1370b
    community-based care in, 1373
    health promotion and maintenance in, 1369, 1369b
    interventions for, 1370-1373, 1370b-1372b
    pathophysiology of, 1367-1369, 1369b
    prostatitis and, 1512
Cystocele, 1376, 1486, 1486f
Cystography, 1360t, 1362
Cystoscopy, 1360t, 1361-1362
Cystourethrography, 1360t, 1362
Cystourethroscopy, 1361-1362
Cysts, 423f
    Baker's, 306
    Bartholin cysts, 1491
    ovarian, 1487
Cytokines, 286, 286t
Cytomegalovirus (CMV), 335
Cytoreductive surgery, 373

Cytotoxic hypersensitivity reactions, 355
Cytotoxic systemic agent therapy, 377-392
    chemotherapy. See Chemotherapy.
    hormonal manipulation, 391-392, 391t
    immunotherapy: biological response modifiers, 387-388, 387t
    molecularly targeted therapy, 388-391, 389f, 390t
    photodynamic therapy, 391
Cytotoxic/cytolytic T-cells, 278t, 285, 787t

D
Daclizumab, 287b-288b
DAIs. See Diffuse axonal injuries (DAIs).
Dandruff, 425
Darbepoetin alfa, 383, 387t
Darker skinned patients, integumentary assessment in, 427b-428b, 428
Dawn phenomenon, 1315, 1315f
DBS. See Deep brain stimulation (DBS).
DCIS. See Ductal carcinoma in situ (DCIS).
DCM. See Dilated cardiomyopathy (DCM).
DCT. See Distal convoluted tubule (DCT).
Death and dying, 91-104
    advance directives and, 92-94, 93f, 95b, 103
    agitation and delirium management in, 99-100, 99b
    cultural considerations in end-of-life care, 95b
    desired outcomes for end-of-life care in, 96
    DNR directives and, 92-94
    durable power of attorney and, 92, 93f
    dyspnea management in, 98-99, 98b-99b
    in emergency department, 114
    euthanasia and, 103, 103t
    hospice and palliative care and, 94-95, 94b, 95t, 97b, 103
    leading causes of, 91, 92t
    nausea and vomiting management in, 99
    older adults and, 92b, 94b, 97b
    pain management in, 97, 97b
    pathophysiology of, 92
    physical assessment in, 95, 96b
    postmortem care and, 102, 102b
    psychosocial assessment in, 95-96, 96b, 103
    psychosocial management in, 100-102, 100t, 101b-102b, 101f

Death and dying *(Continued)*
refractory symptoms of distress
management in, 100
religious death rituals and, 100t
seizure management in, 100
signs and symptoms at end of life,
95-96, 96b
weakness management in, 98, 98b
Death rattle, 99
Debridement
in burns, 482-483, 483f-484f
of pressure ulcers, 444-446, 446t
of surgical wounds, 268
Debriefing after disasters, 144-146,
145b
Debris from wounds, 435
Decadron. *See* Dexamethasone.
Decannulation of tubes, accidental,
522, 527b
Decerebrate posturing, 841, 841f,
952
Decibel intensity of sounds,
1002-1003, 1002t
Decompensated cirrhosis, 1193
Decompressive craniectomy, 956
Decongestants, 351
Decorticate posturing, 841, 841f, 952
Deep brain stimulation (DBS), 871
Deep breathing exercises, 230b
Deep full-thickness wounds, 466,
469, 469f
Deep partial-thickness wounds,
467-468, 468f
Deep tendon reflexes, 841, 842f
Deep vein thrombophlebitis. *See*
Deep vein thrombosis (DVT).
Deep vein thrombosis (DVT),
618-619, 737
postoperative assessment for, 260
Defibrillation, 672, 672b
Degenerative joint disease. *See*
Osteoarthritis.
Degenerative kidney disorders,
1405-1406
diabetic nephropathy, 1306, 1406
nephrosclerosis, 1405
renovascular disease, 1405-1406,
1405b
Dehiscence, 264, 264f, 268
Dehydration, 155-158, 155b, 155t
changes in fluid compartment
volumes with, 155f
health promotion and
maintenance in, 156
history in, 156
interventions for, 157-158,
157b-158b, 158t
laboratory assessment in, 157
older adults and, 230b, 409b,
424b
physical assessment in, 156-157,
156b, 156f
Delayed healing, 267-269, 267b-
269b, 267f
Delayed hypersensitivity reactions,
355-356

Delayed union, 1055
Delegation, 6, 8
Delirium, 840
dementia versus, 18t
end-of-life care and, 99-100
in older adults, 18, 18b, 18t, 23
Deltasone. *See* Prednisone.
Dementia, 16, 23, 840
in Alzheimer's disease, 871-881
caregiver role strain in, 879,
880b
chronic confusion in, 875-878,
875t, 876b-877b
evaluation of care of patient
with, 880-881
genetic considerations in, 872b
health care resources for, 880
history in, 872-873, 873t
home care management in,
879-880
imaging assessment in, 875
injury prevention in, 878-879,
878b, 879t
laboratory assessment in, 875
pathophysiology of, 871-872
physical assessment in, 873-875,
873b, 874f
psychosocial assessment in, 34b,
875
self-management education in,
880
delirium versus, 18t
pain in, 34
Demerol. *See* Meperidine.
Demyelination
in Guillain-Barré syndrome,
913-914
in multiple sclerosis, 904
Deoxyribose sugar, 53
Depolarization, 649
Depression, older adults and, 16,
16b-17b, 17f, 23
Dermabrasion, 462t
Dermal papillae, 416
Dermatitis
atopic, 455, 455b
contact, 455, 455b
nonspecific eczematous, 455, 455b
Dermatomes, 834, 834f
Dermatomyositis, 323t
Dermatophytes, 450b, 451, 453
Dermis, 415-416, 416f
changes resulting from burns, 466,
467f
changes with aging, 418b-419b
function of, 418t
Deronil. *See* Dexamethasone.
Descending tracts, 833, 833f
Desensitization therapy, 351
Detrusor hyperreflexia, 1374t
Detrusor muscle, 1351
Dexamethasone
for acute mountain sickness, 134
for anaphylaxis, 354b
for chemotherapy-induced nausea
and vomiting, 385b

Dexamethasone *(Continued)*
for eye inflammation and
infection, 979b
Diabetes insipidus, 1271-1272,
1271b-1272b
Diabetes mellitus (DM), 1300-1341
absence of insulin in, 1302-1303,
1302t
acute complications of, 1303
adjustments for complications in,
1321
blood glucose control in
hospitalized patient,
1322-1323
blood glucose monitoring in,
1317-1319, 1318b, 1328-1329
chronic complications of,
1303-1306
cardiovascular disease, 1303
cerebrovascular disease, 1303
cognitive dysfunction, 1306
diabetic nephropathy, 1306
diabetic peripheral neuropathy,
1305-1306, 1305t
eye and vision, 1303-1304,
1305b
male erectile dysfunction, 1306
classification of, 1300-1301,
1301t
concept map for, 1311f
cultural considerations in, 1307b,
1307t
diabetic ketoacidosis in,
1332-1335, 1333f, 1334b-
1335b, 1334t
drug therapy for, 1310-1319,
1310b, 1312b-1313b
endocrine pancreas and, 1301,
1301f
etiology and genetic risk in,
1306-1307, 1306t, 1307b
evaluation of care of patient with,
1339, 1339t
exercise therapy in, 1321-1322,
1322b
focused assessment in, 1339b
glucose homeostasis and,
1301-1302
health promotion and
maintenance in, 1307-1308,
1340
history in, 1308
home care management in, 1339
hyperglycemic-hyperosmolar state
in, 1334t, 1335-1337,
1335b-1336b, 1336f
hypoglycemia in, 1330-1332, 1330t
blood glucose management
and, 1330-1331
drug therapy for, 1331, 1331b
establishing treatment plans,
1332
hyperglycemia vs., 1330t
nutrition therapy for, 1331,
1331b
older adults and, 1332b

Diabetes mellitus (DM) *(Continued)*
patient and family education in,
1332
prevention strategies, 1332
incidence and prevalence of, 1307
insulin therapy for, 1313-1319
alternative methods of insulin
administration in,
1315-1316, 1316f
complications of, 1315, 1315f
factors influencing absorption
in, 1314-1315, 1314f,
1315b
mixing of insulins in, 1315,
1315b
patient education in, 1316-
1317, 1316b, 1317f
regimens in, 1313-1314
subcutaneous administration
of, 1316b
types of insulin in, 1313, 1314t
laboratory assessment in,
1308-1309, 1308b,
1308t-1309t
nutrition therapy in, 1319-1321,
1319t, 1320b-1321b,
1329-1330
older adults and
activity program for, 1322b
diabetic retinopathy and, 1305b
hypoglycemia in, 1332b
nutrition and, 1321b
pain in, 1328
peripheral neuropathy injury
prevention in, 1325-1327,
1325f-1327f, 1326b-1327b,
1326t
preventing injury from reduced
vision in, 1328-1329
psychosocial preparation in,
1338-1339
reducing kidney disease risk in,
1329-1330
safety assessment in, 1321-1322,
1322b
screening for, 1309
self-management education in,
1337-1338, 1337t
sick-day rules in, 1335b
surgical management of, 1323-1324
intraoperative care in, 1324
postoperative care in,
1324-1325
preoperative care in, 1324
urine tests in, 1309
wound care in, 1327
Diabetic ketoacidosis, 1332-1335,
1333f, 1334b-1335b, 1334t
Diabetic nephropathy, 1306, 1406
Diabetic peripheral neuropathy
(DNP), 1305-1306, 1305t
Diabetic ulcers, 721b
*Diagnostic and Statistical Manual of
Mental Disorders*, 1520
Diagnostic peritoneal lavage (DPL),
1162

Diagnostic surgery, 373
Dialysate, 1432
Dialysate additives, 1438
Dialyzer, 1432, 1432f
Diamox. *See* Acetazolamide.
Diaphragmatic breathing
    in chronic obstructive pulmonary
        disease, 563b
    patient and family education in,
        230b
Diaphragmatic pacing, 911
Diarrhea
    in AIDS and HIV infection,
        341-342, 342b
    in malabsorption syndrome,
        1166b
    in ulcerative colitis, 1175-1179,
        1176b, 1176t
Diascopy, 429
Diastole, 629, 630f
Diastolic blood pressure, 631
Diastolic heart failure, 679
Diazepam, 122
DIC. *See* Disseminated intravascular
    coagulation (DIC).
Diencephalon, 830-831, 831f
Diet
    after burns, 486
    in chronic kidney disease,
        1427-1428, 1427t
    obesity and, 1248-1249
    preoperative restrictions in, 228,
        228b
Dietary Guidelines for Americans,
    1232-1233, 1233t
Dietary Reference Intakes (DRIs),
    1232-1233
Dietary supplements, 294-295
Differentiated function, 360
Diffuse axonal injuries (DAIs), 947
Diffuse cutaneous systemic sclerosis,
    317
Diffuse interstitial fibrosis, 573b
Diffuse lesions, 422t
Diffuse nail pigmentation, 426f
Diffusion, 150, 150f
    in dialysis, 1432
Diffusion capacity of the lung for
    carbon monoxide (DLCO),
    510t
Digestion, 1099
Digital mammography, 1470
Digoxin, 658b-662b, 662
    for heart failure, 686, 687b, 691b
Dilated cardiomyopathy (DCM),
    701, 701t
Dilaudid. *See* Hydromorphone.
Diltiazem, 658b-662b
Diphenhydramine
    for anaphylaxis, 354, 354b
    for bee stings, 129
Diplopia
    in migraines, 854
    in myasthenia gravis, 918
    in traumatic brain injury, 952
Direct contract transmission, 399

Direct current stimulation device,
    889
Direct inguinal hernias, 1147
Direct response of pupil, 840
Directly observed therapy (DOT),
    407, 598-599
Disability, primary survey and, 117,
    118t
Disabling health problems,
    rehabilitation for, 74-90
    community-based care and, 88-89
    complications of immobility and,
        83, 83t
    establishing bowel continence and,
        87-88, 87b-88b, 87t
    establishing urinary continence
        and, 85-87, 86b-87b, 86t
    evaluation of, 89
    functional assessment in, 79-80,
        80t
    gait training and, 81-84, 83b, 83f,
        83t
    health care resources for, 89
    history in, 77
    home care management and,
        88-89
    improving physical mobility and,
        80-84, 81b, 82f-83f, 83b, 83t
    increasing functional ability and,
        84, 84t, 85b
    maintaining skin integrity and, 85
    NANDA-I and, 80
    older adults and, 77b, 87b
    physical assessment in, 77-79, 78t,
        79b, 90
    psychosocial assessment in, 80, 90
    rehabilitation team and, 75-77,
        76f, 76t
    self-management education and,
        89
    settings for, 75, 75f
    vocational assessment in, 80
Disaster Medical Assistance Team,
    142
Disaster Mortuary Operational
    Response Team, 142
Disaster preparedness. *See*
    Emergency and disaster
    preparedness.
Disaster triage tag system, 140
Discharge instructions, 272b
    in bariatric surgery, 1252b
    in burns, 489, 489t
    from emergency department,
        113-114, 113b
Discharge planning, 221
Discoid lupus erythematosus (DLE),
    313-314
Disease-modifying antirheumatic
    drugs (DMARDs)
    immune deficiency and, 345
    for rheumatoid arthritis, 308-311,
        308b-309b
Disequilibrium, 149
Disinfection, 402
Diskitis, 888

Dislocations, 1079
    after total hip arthroplasty, 297t,
        298b
    after total knee arthroplasty, 302
Dislodgement and accidental
    decannulation of tubes, 522,
        523b
Dislodgement of central venous
    catheters, 208t
Disopyramide phosphate, 658b-662b
Disseminated intravascular
    coagulation (DIC), 392
Dissociation of hemoglobin, 499
Distal convoluted tubule (DCT),
    1348, 1349f
Distraction
    for pain management, 47
    for preoperative anxiety, 233
Distributive shock, 740-741, 741t
Diuretics
    for heart failure, 685-686,
        685b-686b, 715b-716b
    for hypertension, 714, 714b-716b
Diverticula, esophageal, 1123
Diverticular disease, 1186-1188,
    1186b-1187b, 1186f
Diverticulitis, 1186, 1187b
Diverticulosis, 1186
Dizziness, 1008
DLCO. *See* Diffusion capacity of the
    lung for carbon monoxide
    (DLCO).
DLE. *See* Discoid lupus
    erythematosus (DLE).
DM. *See* Diabetes mellitus (DM).
DMARDs. *See* Disease-modifying
    antirheumatic drugs
    (DMARDs).
DNA, 52-54
    chromosomes and, 52f, 53-54,
        54f
    replication of, 53, 53f
    structure of, 52-53, 52f-53f
DNP. *See* Diabetic peripheral
    neuropathy (DNP).
DNR directives. *See* Do-not-
    resuscitate (DNR) directives.
Documentation
    of infusion therapy, 203
    of seizures, 861b
DOE. *See* Dyspnea on exertion
    (DOE).
Dofetilide, 658b-662b
Dolasetron, 384b-385b
Dolophine. *See* Methadone.
Donors in kidney transplantation,
    1441-1442, 1442f
Do-not-resuscitate (DNR) directives,
    92-94, 250, 251b
Dopamine
    for anaphylaxis, 354b
    for hypovolemic shock, 748b
    Parkinson disease and, 867
Dopamine agonists, 869, 869b
Doppler-derived maximal systolic
    acceleration, 720

Dorsal recumbent position during
    surgery, 252-253, 252f
Dose-dense chemotherapy, 378
Dose-track technology, 199
DOT. *See* Directly observed therapy
    (DOT).
Double effect, principle of, 103t
Double gloves, 379-380
Double-barrel stoma, 1153
Doubling time of tumors, 365
DPL. *See* Diagnostic peritoneal
    lavage (DPL).
DPP-4 inhibitors, 1312b-1313b, 1313
Drainage
    from nasogastric tubes, calculation
        of, 263t
    from wounds, 264
Drains
    postoperative care of, 268
    preoperative preparation for, 230
    for surgical wounds, 264, 265f
Dressings
    after burn injury skin grafts,
        487-488, 488f
    for burn wounds, 483, 483f-484f
    in infusion therapy, 200-201, 201b
    postoperative changing of,
        267-268, 267f
    for pressure ulcers, 444-446, 446b,
        446t
    for tracheostomy, 527, 528f
DRIs. *See* Dietary Reference Intakes
    (DRIs).
Driving safety, 13, 14b
Dronedarone, 658b-662b
Droplet Precautions, 404t, 405
    in meningitis, 865b
Drowning, 135-137, 136b
Droxia. *See* Hydroxyurea.
Drug abuse, increased risk for
    surgical complications and, 219
Drug history in vision assessment,
    971, 971t
Drug therapy
    for acute kidney injury, 1416-1417
    for acute respiratory distress
        syndrome, 614
    for adrenal insufficiency,
        1275-1276, 1276b
    for AIDS and HIV infection, 332b,
        338-341, 339b-340b
    for allergic rhinitis, 350-351,
        351b
    for Alzheimer's disease, 877-878
    for anaphylaxis, 354b
    for asthma, 534, 535b, 539b-541b,
        543b
    for atherosclerosis, 708-709, 709b,
        709t
    for atrial fibrillation, 667, 667t,
        668b
    for back pain, 887, 887b, 891b
    for benign prostatic hyperplasia,
        1503, 1503b
    for bone cancer, 1043-1044
    for brain tumors, 959

Drug therapy (Continued)
  for burns
    for infection prevention in, 485,
      486b
    for mechanical ventilation in,
      478, 478b
    for pain management in, 480,
      480b
    for shock prevention in, 479
  for chemotherapy-induced nausea
    and vomiting, 383-384,
    384b-385b
  for chest pain, 764-766, 764b-766b
  for cholecystitis, 1216
  for chronic kidney disease,
    1428-1430, 1429b, 1430b
  for chronic obstructive pulmonary
    disease, 563-564, 564b
  for cirrhosis, 1199-1201
  for coronary artery disease,
    766-767, 767b-768b, 768t,
    772, 773b
  for Crohn's disease, 1183, 1183b
  for cystitis, 1370-1372,
    1370b-1372b
  for dehydration, 157-158
  for diabetes mellitus, 1310-1319,
    1310b, 1312b-1313b
    and prevention of
      hypoglycemia, 1331, 1331b
    to reduce kidney disease risk,
      1329
  for diabetic ketoacidosis, 1334
  for dysrhythmias, 657-662,
    658b-662b
  for endometrial cancer, 1493
  for epilepsy, 859, 859b-860b
  for eye inflammation and
    infections, 979b
  for eye problems, 978b, 978f, 988b
  for fever, 409, 409b, 409t
  for fluid overload, 159b
  for fracture pain, 1061-1062
  for gastritis, 1128, 1128b,
    1133b-1134b
  for gastroesophageal reflux
    disease, 1113, 1113b
  for genital herpes, 1535-1536
  for genital warts, 1537, 1537b
  for gonorrhea, 1540
  for Goodpasture's syndrome, 357
  for gout, 320
  for Guillain-Barré syndrome, 915,
    915b
  for hearing loss, 1011
  for heart failure
    ACE inhibitors and angiotensin
      receptor blockers in,
      684-685, 685b
    beta-adrenergic blockers in, 687
    digoxin in, 686, 687b, 691b
    diuretics in, 685-686, 685b-686b
    human B-type natriuretic
      peptides in, 685, 689b
    inotropic drugs in, 686-687

Drug therapy (Continued)
  for hemophilia, 821t
  for human immune deficiency
    virus infection, 332b
  for hypercalcemia, 169-170
  for hyperkalemia, 166
  for hypernatremia, 163
  for hypertension, 712-717,
    714b-717b
  for hyperthyroidism, 1288,
    1288b-1289b
  for hypocalcemia, 169
  for hypokalemia, 164-165, 165b
  for hyponatremia, 162
  for hypophosphatemia, 170
  for hypovolemic shock, 748, 748b
  for inhalation anthrax, 600b
  intravenous, 189, 189b
  for kidney transplantation, 1444
  for leukemia, 810-811
  for lung cancer, 580
  for lupus, 315-316, 316b
  for malnutrition, 1240
  for migraines, 855-857, 855t, 856b
  for multiple sclerosis, 906-908, 908b
  for myasthenia gravis, 920, 920b,
    920t, 922b
  for obesity, 1249, 1250b
  for older adults, 13-16
  for osteoporosis, 1034-1035,
    1034b-1035b
  for Paget's disease of the bone,
    1039
  for pain management, 34-45
    adjuvant analgesics in, 35, 36t,
      45, 45b-46b
    around-the-clock dosing in,
      34-35
    multimodal analgesia in, 34, 49
    non-opioid analgesics in, 35-37,
      36t, 37b
    older adults and, 37b-38b
    opioid analgesics in. See Opioid
      analgesics.
    patient-controlled analgesia in,
      35, 35b
    postoperative, 269-270,
      269b-271b
    routes of administration in, 34
  for Parkinson disease, 868-870,
    869b
  for peptic ulcer disease, 1132-
    1135, 1132b-1135b
  for peripheral arterial disease, 722
  preoperative, 228, 234
  for pressure ulcers, 446
  for psoriasis, 457-458, 457b-458b
  for pulmonary arterial
    hypertension, 570-571,
    570b-571b
  for pulmonary embolism, 606,
    606b-608b, 608-610
  for respiratory acidosis, 183
  for rheumatoid arthritis, 308-312,
    308b-310b

Drug therapy (Continued)
  for rhinitis, 584
  for sepsis and septic shock, 754
  for sickle cell crisis, 802, 802b
  for skin cancer, 461
  for skin infections, 453
  for skin inflammation, 455-456,
    456b
  for smoking cessation, 495, 496b
  for spinal cord injury, 898, 901b
  for stomatitis, 1101
  for stroke, 941-942
  for syphilis, 1534, 1534b
  for systemic sclerosis, 318-319
  for transgender patients,
    1524-1525
    patients transition from female
      to male, 1525, 1525t
    patients transition from male to
      female, 1524-1525, 1524t,
      1525b
  for transplant rejection, 287,
    287b-288b, 289
  for traumatic brain injury,
    954-955
  for trigeminal neuralgia, 926-927
  for tuberculosis, 596-598,
    597b-598b
  for urinary incontinence, 1377,
    1378b, 1379-1380, 1380b
  for valvular heart disease, 694,
    694b
  for venous thromboembolism,
    731-733, 731b-732b
  for wound infections, 268
Drug-induced disorders, immune
  deficiencies in, 344-345
Dry heat injuries, 470
Dry mouth
  radiation therapy-related, 376-377
  in Sjögren's syndrome, 306
Dry powder inhalers, 541b, 555
Dry skin, 421-422, 433b
DUB. See Dysfunctional uterine
  bleeding (DUB).
Ductal carcinoma in situ (DCIS),
  1464
Ductal ectasia, 1462-1463, 1462t
Dulcolax. See Bisacodyl.
Dull percussion note, 505t
Dumping syndrome, 1140, 1141t,
  1252
Duodenal ulcers, 1132t
Dupuytren's contracture, 1045-1046
Durable power of attorney for health
  care, 92, 93f
DVT. See Deep vein thrombosis
  (DVT).
Dying patients. See Death and
  dying.
Dysarthria in stroke, 943
Dysfunctional uterine bleeding
  (DUB), 1483-1484, 1484t
Dyskinesias, 869, 871
Dyslexia, 934

Dysmetria, 905
Dyspareunia in endometriosis, 1483
Dyspepsia
  in gastroesophageal reflux disease,
    1111
  in peptic ulcer disease, 1131
Dysphagia, 78
  end-of-life care and, 98, 98b
  in myasthenia gravis, 918
  in stroke, 936
  in systemic sclerosis, 317
Dyspnea
  activities of daily living and, 503t
  in acute respiratory failure, 612
  in asthma, 550-551
  cardiovascular assessment and, 635
  in chronic obstructive pulmonary
    disease, 565
  end-of-life care and, 98-99,
    98b-99b
  in heart failure, 682
  in laryngeal trauma, 536
  in lung cancer, 580
  in pneumonia, 592t
  respiratory assessment and, 502,
    503t
Dyspnea on exertion (DOE), 612,
  635
Dysrhythmias, 649-677
  atrial, 665-669
    atrial fibrillation in, 666-669,
      666b-668b, 667f, 667t
    premature atrial complexes in,
      665
    supraventricular tachycardia in,
      665-666, 666b
  cardiac conduction system and,
    649-650, 650f
  community-based care in,
    673-676
    health care resources for, 676
    home care management in, 673
    self-management education in,
      673-675, 673b-675b
  in coronary artery disease, 769
  drug therapy for, 657-662,
    658b-662b
  electrocardiography and, 650-656,
    651f
    complexes, segments, and
      intervals in, 652-654, 654f
    continuous electrocardiographic
      monitoring and, 652, 653f
    heart rate determination using,
      654-655
    heart rhythm analysis using,
      655-656
    lead systems in, 650-652, 651t
    normal sinus rhythm and, 656,
      656f
    older adults and, 674b
    patient safety in, 658b
  sinus, 662-665
    bradycardia in, 663-665,
      664f-665f

Dysrhythmias (Continued)
  tachycardia in, 662-663, 663b,
      663f
  sustained tachydysrhythmias and
      bradydysrhythmias in, 657,
      657b
  ventricular, 669-673
    premature ventricular
        complexes in, 669-670,
        669f, 670b
    ventricular asystole in, 671-673,
        671f-672f, 672b
    ventricular fibrillation in,
        670-671, 671f
    ventricular tachycardia in, 670,
        670b, 670f
Dystrophic nails, 425-426
Dysuria, preoperative assessment of,
    221-222

E
Ear problems, 996-1016
  external ear conditions, 1003-
      1005, 1004b-1005b, 1005f
  hearing loss. See Hearing loss.
  inner ear, 1007-1009
  middle ear, 1005-1007, 1006f,
      1007b
Eardrops, 1004b, 1005f
Eardrum, 996-997, 997f
Ears
  anatomy and physiology of,
      996-998
    function of, 998
    structure, 996-998
      external, 996, 997f
      inner, 997-998, 997f
      middle, 996-997, 997f-998f
  hearing assessment and
      audiometry in. See Hearing
      assessment.
  hearing changes associated with
      aging, 998, 999b
Eating disorders, 1238
Eaton-Lambert syndrome, 918
EBP. See Evidence-based practice
    (EBP).
EBPI model. See Evidence-based
    practice improvement (EBPI)
    model.
EBRT. See External beam radiation
    therapy (EBRT).
Ecchymosis, 424
  in autoimmune thrombocytopenic
      purpura, 820
  intravenous therapy-related,
      204t-206t
  in pit viper envenomation, 124
Eccrine sweat glands, 417,
    418b-419b
ECF. See Extracellular fluid (ECF).
ECG. See Electrocardiography
    (ECG).
Echocardiography, 645-646
E-cigarettes, 495

ECMO. See Extracorporeal membrane
    oxygenation (ECMO).
Ectopic heart rhythms, 673b
Ectropion, 977-978, 978b-979b, 978f
Eczema, 455, 455b
Edema, 150
  cardiovascular assessment and, 635
  in frostbite, 133f
  in inflammation, 280
  palpation of, 425t
  pitting, 158, 159f, 637, 637f
  pulmonary
    in burns, 475, 475b
    in chronic kidney disease,
        1426-1427
    in heart failure, 688-689,
        688b-689b
  taut skin in, 421
EDs. See Emergency departments
    (EDs).
Edwards Lifescience PreSep central
    venous catheters, 194f
EEG. See Electroencephalography
    (EEG).
Efferent arteriole, 1346
Effusions, 305
EGD. See
    Esophagogastroduodenoscopy
    (EGD).
EGFRIs. See Epidermal growth factor
    receptor inhibitors (EGFRIs).
Ejection fraction, 679
Elbow surgery
  skin preparation for, 229f
  total elbow arthroplasty in, 303
Elbows, 487b
Elder neglect and abuse, 19, 19t, 23
Elderly. See Older adults.
Elective surgery, 218t
Electrical bone stimulation, 1063
Electrical burns, 471-472, 471f-472f,
    481b
Electrical stimulation for pressure
    ulcers, 446
Electrocardiograph calipers, 655-656
Electrocardiography (ECG), 650-656,
    651f
  in cardiovascular assessment,
      644-645
  complexes, segments, and intervals
      in, 652-654, 654f
  continuous electrocardiographic
      monitoring and, 652, 653f
  heart rate determination using,
      654-655
  heart rhythm analysis using,
      655-656
  lead systems in, 650-652, 651t
  preoperative, 225
  in sickle cell disease, 801
Electrodesiccation for skin cancer, 460
Electroencephalography (EEG)
  in Alzheimer Æ s disease, 950
  in neurologic assessment,
      846t-847t, 849

Electrolarynges, 542, 542f
Electro-Larynx, 542f
Electrolyte balance, 148, 160-161
  body fluids and, 160, 160f
  homeostasis and, 148, 149f
  levels in burn assessment, 477b
  physiologic influences on, 148-152
    diffusion, 150, 150f
    filtration, 149-150, 149f-150f
    osmosis, 151-152, 151f
  postoperative assessment of, 262
  preoperative assessment of, 223b
  in traumatic brain injury, 955
Electrolyte imbalances, 160
  abnormal electrolyte values, 152t
  after craniotomy, 962
  calcium, 167-170
    hypercalcemia and, 169-170,
        169t, 170b
    hypocalcemia and, 167-169,
        168b, 168f, 168t
  chloride, 172
  in coronary artery bypass graft,
      777
  in diabetic ketoacidosis,
      1333-1334
  in enteral nutrition, 1244
  in intestinal obstructions, 1160
  magnesium, 171-172
    hypermagnesemia and, 171-172,
        171t
    hypomagnesemia and, 171, 171t
  older adults and, 161b
  phosphorus, 170-171
    hyperphosphatemia and, 171
    hypophosphatemia and, 170,
        170t
  potassium, 163-167
    hyperkalemia and, 166-167,
        166t, 167b
    hypokalemia and, 163-165,
        164b-165b, 164t
  sodium, 161-163
    hypernatremia and, 162-163,
        162t, 163b
    hyponatremia and, 161-162,
        161t, 162b
  in total parenteral nutrition, 1245
Electromyography (EMG)
  in musculoskeletal assessment,
      1026
  in neurologic assessment, 848
Electronic health record, 7, 7f
Electronic infusion devices, 199
Electrophysiologic studies (EPS)
  in cardiovascular assessment, 645
  in Guillain-Barré syndrome,
      914-915
Electroretinography, 975
Electrovaporization of prostate,
    1503
ELISA. See Enzyme-linked
    immunosorbent assay (ELISA).
Elite old, 9
E-mail, 5

Embolectomy
  in pulmonary embolism, 608
  in stroke, 938-939
Embolic stroke, 931, 931f, 932t
Embolism
  air
    central venous catheter-related,
        207t
  pulmonary. See Pulmonary
      embolism.
Embolization of arteriovenous
    malformation, 941f
Embolus, 618, 931
Emend. See Aprepitant.
Emergence from general anesthesia,
    245
Emergency and disaster
    preparedness, 138-147
  event resolution and debriefing
      and, 144-146, 145b
  hospital incident command
      system and, 142-143, 143t
  impact of disasters and, 139-140,
      140f
  mass casualty triage and, 140-141,
      141b, 141t
  notification and activation of
      emergency plans in, 141-142
  personal preparedness and, 143,
      143t
  psychosocial response of survivors
      and, 146-147, 146b-147b
  role of nurse in, 143-144, 144b,
      144t, 146
    responding to health care
        facility fires, 139b
  types of disasters, 138-139, 139f
Emergency care, 105
  in abdominal trauma, 1162, 1162b
  in acute cardiac tamponade,
      699-700
  in amputations, 1072
  in burns. See Burns.
  in cholinergic crisis, 920, 920t
  endotracheal intubation in, 615b
  in environmental emergencies. See
      Environmental emergencies.
  in fractures, 1058, 1058b
  in malignant hyperthermia, 247b
  in myasthenic crisis, 920, 920t
  nursing concepts in
    case management and, 113
    core competencies, 110-111
    cultural considerations and,
        110b, 113b
    death in emergency department
        and, 114
    patient and family education
        and, 113-114
    patient disposition and, 112-114
    scope of emergency nursing
        practice, 109-111
    training and certification in,
        111, 111t
    triage and, 111-112, 111t, 112b

Emergency care *(Continued)*
  in oncologic emergencies, 392-394
    hypercalcemia, 393
    sepsis and disseminated
        intravascular coagulation,
        392
    spinal cord compression, 393
    superior vena cava syndrome,
        393-394, 393f-394f, 394b
    syndrome of inappropriate
        antidiuretic hormone,
        392-393, 392b
    tumor lysis syndrome, 394, 394f
  in status epilepticus, 861-862,
      862b
  trauma nursing principles in,
      106-108
    mechanism of injury and, 116
    patient disposition and, 118
    primary survey and resuscitation
        interventions in, 116-117,
        117b-118b, 118t
    secondary survey and
        resuscitation interventions
        in, 118
    trauma centers and, 115-116,
        115f, 115t
    trauma systems and, 116
  in upper gastrointestinal bleeding,
      1136, 1136b
  in ventricular fibrillation, 671
Emergency departments (EDs),
    105-106
  death in, 114
  environment of, 106-108, 118-119
    demographic data and
        vulnerable populations
        and, 106
    interdisciplinary team
        collaboration and,
        106-108, 107f
    patient safety and, 108-109,
        108b-109b
    special nursing teams and, 106
    staff safety and, 108, 108b
  homeless patients and, 114
  improving flow of patients
      through, 113b
  older adults and, 106b, 109b-110b,
      112b
Emergency management plans, 138
Emergency medical technicians
    (EMTs), 107
Emergency medicine physicians, 107
Emergency nurses, 107-111
Emergency operations center,
    142-143
Emergency preparedness, 140
Emergency Severity Index (ESI), 112
Emergent surgery, 218t
Emergent triage, 111-112, 111t
Emerging infections, 411-413, 412t
Emetogenic drugs, 383
EMG. *See* Electromyography (EMG).
Emmetropia, 968-969
Emotional abuse of older adult, 19

Emotional lability after stroke, 937
Emphysema, 532f, 536-545
Empyema, pulmonary, 599
Emtricitabine/tenofovir, 332b
EMTs. *See* Emergency medical
    technicians (EMTs).
Enalapril, 715b-716b
Enbrel. *See* Etanercept.
Encephalitis, 865-867, 866b
Encephalopathy, hepatic, 1193-1194,
    1194t
Endocrine assessment, 1255-1265
  current health problems in, 1262
  family history and genetic risk in,
      1262
  imaging assessment in, 1264
  laboratory assessment in,
      1263-1264, 1263b
  nutrition history in, 1261-1262
  patient history in, 1261-1262
  physical assessment in, 1262-1263,
      1263b
  psychosocial assessment in, 1263
Endocrine disorders in HIV disease,
    335-336
Endocrine pancreas, 1301, 1301f
Endocrine system, 1255
  anatomy and physiology of,
      1256-1261
    adrenal glands, 1256f,
        1257-1259, 1259t
    glands, 1255, 1256f
    gonads, 1256f, 1257
    hormones, 1255-1256, 1256f,
        1256t
    hypothalamus and pituitary
        glands, 1256f-1257f, 1256t,
        1257, 1258t
    pancreas, 1260, 1260f
    parathyroid glands, 1260, 1260f
    thyroid gland, 1259-1260, 1259f
  changes associated with aging,
      1260-1261, 1261b
End-of-life care, 91-104
  advance directives and, 92-94, 93f,
      95b, 103
  agitation and delirium
      management in, 99-100, 99b
  cultural considerations in, 95b
  desired outcomes for, 96
  DNR directives and, 92-94
  durable power of attorney and, 92,
      93f
  dyspnea management in, 98-99,
      98b-99b
  in emergency department, 114
  euthanasia and, 103, 103t
  hospice and palliative care in,
      94-95, 94b, 95t, 97b, 103
  nausea and vomiting management
      in, 99
  older adults and, 92b, 94b, 97b
  pain management in, 97, 97b
  pathophysiology of dying and, 92
  physical assessment in, 95, 96b
  postmortem care and, 102, 102b

End-of-life care *(Continued)*
  psychosocial assessment in, 95-96,
      96b, 103
  psychosocial management in,
      100-102, 100t, 101b-102b,
      101f
  refractory symptoms of distress
      management in, 100
  religious death rituals and, 100t
  seizure management in, 100
  signs and symptoms at end of life,
      95-96, 96b
  weakness management in, 98, 98b
Endometrial biopsy, 1458
Endometrial cancer, 1491-1494,
    1492t, 1493b
Endometriosis, 1482-1483, 1483f
Endoscopes, 242, 242f
Endoscopic retrograde
    cholangiopancreatography
    (ERCP), 1094-1095, 1095b
  in cirrhosis, 1197
Endoscopic sclerotherapy for
    bleeding esophageal varices,
    1200
Endoscopic ultrasonography, 1097
Endoscopic variceal ligation, 1200
Endoscopy
  in bleeding esophageal varices,
      1200
  in gastroesophageal reflux disease,
      1114, 1114b
  in gastrointestinal assessment,
      1093
  in peptic ulcer disease, 1136-1137,
      1137b
  in respiratory assessment,
      509-511, 510b
Endothelin, 681
Endothelin receptor antagonists, 318
Endotracheal intubation, 615-616,
    615b-616b, 615f
  complications during
      intraoperative period,
      247-248
  in upper airway obstruction, 536
Endotracheal tubes, 615, 615f
Endovascular interventions in stroke,
    938-939, 939b
Endovascular stent grafts, 727
Endovascular vessel harvesting, 779
End-stage kidney disease (ESKD),
    1411
  chronic kidney disease and, 1423b
  cultural considerations in, 1405b
  nephrosclerosis and, 1405
  polycystic kidney disease and,
      1397, 1397b
  pyelonephritis and, 1401
Energy balance, 1232
Energy conservation
  in leukemia, 814, 815b
  in rheumatoid arthritis, 312, 312b
Engraftment in stem cell
    transplantation, 812-813
Enophthalmos, 972

Enoxaparin, 607, 607b
Enterococcus, 398
  vancomycin-resistant, 403, 406
Enterostomal feeding tubes, 1241
Entropion, 977-978, 978b-979b, 978f
Entry inhibitors, 339b
Envenomation
  bees and wasps, 128
  black widow spider, 127-128
  brown recluse spider, 126-127, 127f
  coral snake, 125
  pit vipers, North American,
      123-125, 124b, 124t
  prevention of, 123b, 126b
  scorpion, 128, 128f
Environmental control
  for pain in burns, 480
  standard precautions and, 403t
Environmental emergencies, 120-137
  altitude-related illnesses, 133-135,
      133b-135b
  arthropod bites and stings, 126-129
    bees and wasps, 128-129, 129b
    black widow spider, 127-128,
        127b
    brown recluse spider, 126-127,
        126f-127f, 137
    prevention of, 126b
    scorpion, 128, 128f
  cold-related, 131-133, 136-137
    frostbite, 122b, 132-133,
        132b-133b
    hypothermia, 131-132,
        131b-132b
  drowning, 135-137, 136b
  heat-related, 120-122
    heat exhaustion, 121
    heat stroke, 121-122, 122b-123b
    older adults and, 121,
        121b-122b
  lightning injuries, 129-131, 130b
  snakebites, 123-126, 123f
    coral snakes and, 125-126, 125f,
        126b
    North American pit vipers and,
        123-125, 124b, 124t, 137
    prevention of, 123, 123b
Enzymatic debridement
  in burns, 483
Enzyme-linked immunosorbent
    assay (ELISA)
  for hepatitis C, 1206
  for HIV infection, 336-337
Enzymes, 641b
Eosinophils, 280, 787t
  in differential white blood cell
      count, 508b
  immune function of, 278t
Ephedrine sulfate, 354t
Epidermal growth factor receptor
    inhibitors (EGFRIs), 390, 390t
Epidermis, 415-416, 416f
  changes resulting from burn, 465,
      467f
  changes with aging, 418b-419b
  functions of, 418t

Epididymis, 1451-1452, 1451f
Epididymitis, 1512
Epidural analgesics, 42-43, 42b, 269
    patient-controlled, 35
Epidural anesthesia, 248t
    administration of, 249f
    complications of, recognizing,
        261b
Epidural hematomas, 261b, 949, 949f
Epiglottis, 497-498, 498f
Epilepsy, 858-863
    drug therapy for, 859, 859b-860b
    emergency care in, 861-862, 862b
    etiology and genetic risk in,
        858-859
    gender health considerations in,
        859b
    older adults and, 858b
    seizure precautions and
        management in, 860-861,
        860b-861b
    self-management education in,
        859, 861b
    surgical management of, 862-863
    types of seizures and, 858
Epinephrine, 352-353, 352b-354b,
    352f
EpiPen, 352f
Epistaxis, 532-533, 532b-533b, 533f
    in Sjögren's syndrome, 356
Epithelial cells, 417
Epitympanum, 996-997, 997f
Eplerenone, 717b
Epoetin alfa, 383, 387t
Epogen. See Epoetin alfa.
EPS. See Electrophysiologic studies
    (EPS).
Epworth Sleepiness Scale (ESS), 535
Equianalgesia, 40, 50
Equilibrium, 149
ERCP. See Endoscopic retrograde
    cholangiopancreatography
    (ERCP).
Erectile dysfunction, 1512-1513, 1512b
    in diabetes mellitus, 1306
Ergonomics, 886
Ergotamine preparations, 856
Erosions, 423f
Eructation in gastroesophageal
    reflux disease, 1112
Erythema, 422t
Erythema migrans, 320-321
Erythrocyte count. See Red blood
    cell count.
Erythrocyte sedimentation rate
    (ESR), 408
    in rheumatoid arthritis, 307, 307b
Erythrocytes. See Red blood cells
    (RBCs).
Erythroplakia, 538
Erythropoiesis, 786-787
Erythropoiesis-stimulating agents
    (ESAs), 383
Erythropoietin, 276, 1349, 1349t
ESAs. See Erythropoiesis-stimulating
    agents (ESAs).

Eschar
    in brown recluse spider bite, 126,
        127f
    in cutaneous anthrax, 453, 454f
    in pressure ulcers, 443
Escharotomies, 468, 479, 480f
ESI. See Emergency Severity Index
    (ESI).
ESKD. See End-stage kidney disease
    (ESKD).
Esmolol, 658b-662b
Esophageal dilation in esophageal
    cancer, 1120
Esophageal diverticula, 1123
Esophageal problems, 1110-1125
    esophageal diverticula, 1123
    esophageal trauma, 1123-1124,
        1123t
    gastroesophageal reflux disease,
        1110-1114, 1111b-1113b,
        1111t
    health promotion and
        maintenance in, 1124
    hiatal hernias. See Hiatal hernias.
    tumors in. See Esophageal tumors.
Esophageal speech, 542
Esophageal stricture, 1111
Esophageal trauma, 1123-1124, 1123t
Esophageal tumors, 1117-1123
    assessment in, 1118, 1118b
    community-based care, 1122
    evaluation of care of patient with,
        1123
    nutrition considerations in, 1119,
        1119b
    pathophysiology of, 1117-1118,
        1117b
    surgical management of,
        1120-1122, 1121b-1122b,
        1121f
Esophageal varices, 1193
Esophageal-gastric pain, 636t
Esophagectomy, 1120
Esophagitis, 318b
Esophagogastroduodenoscopy
    (EGD), 1093-1094, 1094b, 1094f
    in cirrhosis, 1197
Esophagogastrostomy, 1120
Esophagus, 1085
ESR. See Erythrocyte sedimentation
    rate (ESR).
ESS. See Epworth Sleepiness Scale
    (ESS).
Essential hypertension, 710
Estrogen agonist/antagonists, 1034
Estrogens, 391t
Etanercept
    for psoriasis, 458b
    for rheumatoid arthritis, 309b, 310
Ethambutol, 597b
Ethical issues
    in euthanasia, 103t
    in genetic testing, 61, 61b
Euploid, 54
Euploidy, 361, 365
Eustachian tubes, 497

Euthanasia, 103, 103t
Evacuation plans, 139
Everolimus, 287b-288b
Eversion, eyelid, 419f
Evidence-based practice (EBP), 6, 8,
    64-73
    annual eye care in diabetes
        mellitus, 1304b
    best position after colonoscopy,
        1096b
    chronic hepatitis C and
        complementary and
        alternative therapies, 1206b
    colorectal cancer screening, 1150b
    complementary and alternative
        methods to relieve
        osteoarthritis symptoms, 295b
    critical role of nutrition in
        improving quality of care,
        1237b
    definitions of, 64-65
    electrical burn injury, 481b
    exercise for less fatigue, 816b
    how to know when suctioning is
        painful to patients, 526b
    manual bowel disimpaction in
        spinal cord injury, 87t
    Medicare patients use of hospice
        services, 94b
    men's knowledge about
        osteoporosis risk, 1031b
    models and frameworks for
        implementation of, 68-70
        ARCC model, 69-70
        improvement (EBPI) model,
            70-73, 70f, 72t
        Iowa model, 68
        Reavy and Tavernier model, 69,
            69t
    most effective education method
        to provide heart failure
        patients, 690b
    night-shift work and breast cancer
        risk, 1466b
    nursing interventions and
        enrollment in cardiac
        rehabilitation, 780b
    obesity and atrial fibrillation,
        666b
    older adults at risk for HIV
        infection, 330b
    online resources for caregivers of
        patients after hip fracture,
        1068b
    oral hygiene during critical illness,
        1101b
    oral hygiene to prevent ventilator-
        associated pneumonia, 621b
    pain and multiple sclerosis, 906b
    pain management in older adults
        in rural communities, 46b
    prediction of non-exertional heat
        stroke, 122b
    process of, 65-68
        asking "burning" clinical
            questions, 65-66, 66t, 73

Evidence-based practice (EBP)
    (Continued)
    critically appraising and
        synthesizing evidence,
        67
    evaluating outcomes, 68
    finding best evidence, 66-67,
        66f, 67t-68t, 68f
    implementing
        recommendations,
        67-68
    making recommendations and
        improving practice, 67
    prostate-specific antigen screening
        recommendations for
        prostate cancer, 1507b
    reflective activities and depression
        in older adults, 17b
    return of bowel function after
        postoperative ileus, 263b
    securing a patient's peripheral IV
        line, 201b
    skin protection in lupus, 316b
    support group for patients with
        inflammatory bowel disease,
        1181b
    teaching patients and families
        about strokes, 945b
    use of sitters in care of older
        adults with dementia in acute
        care settings, 877b
    VTE prevention beyond the SCIP,
        232b
    what people with reduced hearing
        want most from hearing aids,
        1012b
Evidence-based practice
    improvement (EBPI) model,
    70-73, 70f, 72t
Evisceration, 264, 264f, 268,
    268b-269b
Evoked potentials, 849
Exacerbation therapy in cystic
    fibrosis, 568
Exacerbations
    in multiple sclerosis, 904
    in rheumatoid arthritis, 306
    in systemic lupus erythematosus,
        313-314
Excisional biopsy, 429
    in skin cancer, 461
Excitability of heart cells, 649
Exercise
    in asthma, 535
    in chronic obstructive pulmonary
        disease, 564
    in diabetes mellitus, 1321-1322,
        1322b
    in fibromyalgia, 322
    in leukemia, 816b
    obesity and, 1249
    older adults and, 11-12, 12b, 12f
    in osteoarthritis, 299
    in peripheral arterial disease,
        721-722
    post-mastectomy, 1474b

Exercise (Continued)
preoperative instructions for postoperative procedures and, 230b
in urinary incontinence, 1377, 1377b
Exercise electrocardiography, 645, 645f
in respiratory assessment, 509
Exercise tolerance test. See Exercise electrocardiography.
Exertional dyspnea, 682
Exertional heat stroke, 121
Exfoliative psoriasis, 456
Exogenous hyperthyroidism, 1286
Exophthalmos, 972
Exotoxins, 398
Expansion breathing, 230b
Expedited partner therapy, 1539
Exploratory laparotomy, 1160-1161
Exposure
primary survey and, 117, 117b, 118t
to radiation, 374
Expressive aphasia, 943, 943t
Expressivity of genes, 58
Extended-care environment, 256-257
Extension exercises, 887b
Extension sets, 197-198
External beam radiation therapy (EBRT)
in endometrial cancer, 1493
in testicular cancer, 1516
External disasters, 138-140, 140f
External ear problems, 1003-1005
cerumen or foreign bodies, 1004-1005, 1005b, 1005f
external otitis, 1003-1004, 1004b
perichondritis, 1004
External ears, 1000
External fixation of fractures, 1062, 1062f
External genitalia, female, 1449-1450
External hemorrhoids, 1164, 1164f
External otitis, 1003-1004, 1004b
External urethral sphincter, 1350
Extracellular fluid (ECF), 148
electrolytes in, 160, 160f
normal pH of, 185
sodium in, 161
Extracorporeal membrane oxygenation (ECMO), 614
Extracranial-intracranial bypass, 942
Extramedullary spinal cord tumors, 902
Extraocular muscles, 967-968, 968f, 969t
function testing of, 973, 973f
Extrapulmonary ventilatory failure, 611, 611t
Extravasation
during chemotherapy, 379, 379f
in intravenous therapy, 188b, 204t-206t
vesicant medications and, 192

Extremities, cardiovascular assessment and, 637, 637f
Extrinsic allergic alveolitis, 573b
Extrinsic factors, 788
Extubation in mechanical ventilation, 622, 622b
Exudate in pressure ulcers, 443t
Eye problems, 977-995
cataracts, 982-985
home care management in, 984, 984b, 984f
pathophysiology of, 982, 982f, 982t
physical assessment in, 983, 983f
self-management education in, 984, 984b
surgery for, 983, 983f
conjunctival disorders, 978-980, 980b
corneal disorders, 980-982, 980b, 981f, 982t
in diabetes mellitus, 1303-1304, 1305b, 1328-1329
drug therapy for, 988b
eyelid disorders, 977-978, 978b-980b, 978f
glaucoma, 985-989
concept map for, 986f
drug therapy for, 988b
nonsurgical management of, 987-988, 987b-988b, 989f
pathophysiology of, 985, 985t
surgical management of, 988-989
health promotion and maintenance in, 994-995
keratoconjunctivitis sicca, 978
ocular melanomas, 992
reduced visual sensory perception, 992-994, 993b
refractive errors, 991
retinal disorders, 989-991, 990b
trauma in, 991-992, 991b-992b
Eyedrops, 970b, 975b
Eyelid disorders, 977-978
chalazion, 978
entropion and ectropion, 977-978, 978b-979b
hordeolum, 978
instillation of ophthalmic ointment for, 978b, 978f
Eyelids, eversion of, 419f
Eyes. See also Vision assessment.
anatomy and physiology of, 966-971
function of, 968-969, 969f
structure, 966-968
external structures, 967, 968f
layers of the eyeball, 966-967, 967f
muscles, nerves, and blood vessels, 967-968, 968f, 969t
refractive structures and media, 967, 967f-968f

Eyes (Continued)
changes with aging, 417f, 969-970, 970b
health promotion and maintenance of, 970-971, 970b-971b, 976
using eyedrops and, 970b, 975b
Ezetimibe, 709

F
Facelift, 462t
Facemasks, 517t, 518-519, 518f-519f, 519b
Faces Pain Scale-Revised, 30
Facial nerve, 835t
Facial paralysis, 927-928
Facial trauma, 534, 534b
Facilitated diffusion, 150
Facilitated transport, 150
Factor V Leiden, 605b
Failed back surgery syndrome (FBSS), 890
Fainting. See Syncope.
Fallophobia, 13, 1032
Fallopian tubes, 1450, 1450f
Falls
hospitalized older adults and, 20-22, 21b-22b
prevention of, 13, 21b, 69b, 885b
in emergency room, 109
Famciclovir, 453
Familial clustering, 57t, 59
Family history
in cardiovascular assessment, 634, 634b
in endocrine assessment, 1262
in gastrointestinal assessment, 1089
in hearing assessment, 1000, 1000b
in hematologic assessment, 791
increased surgical risk and, 219t
in integumentary assessment, 421
in musculoskeletal assessment, 1021
in renal assessment, 1353
in reproductive assessment, 1453
in respiratory assessment, 502
of skin problems, 420b
in vision assessment, 971
Famvir. See Famciclovir.
Far point of vision, 970
Farmer's lung, 573b
Fasciculations
in pit viper envenomation, 124
tensilon testing-related, 919, 919b
Fasciotomies, 468, 479
Fasting blood glucose, 1308-1309
Fat embolism syndrome
after lumbar spinal surgery, 889b
in fractures, 1054, 1055b
Fatigue
cardiovascular assessment and, 635
in chronic kidney disease, 1430
in heart failure, 688
in leukemia, 816b
in rheumatoid arthritis, 312, 312b

Fatigue fractures, 1052
Fatty liver, 1208
FBC. See Fibrocystic breast condition (FBC).
FBSS. See Failed back surgery syndrome (FBSS).
Febrile transfusion reaction, 825
Febuxostat, 320
Fecal impaction, 1161b
Fecal occult blood test, 1151
Federal Emergency Management Agency, 142
Feet
in diabetes mellitus, care of, 1325-1327, 1325f-1327f, 1326b-1327b, 1326t
disorders, 1046-1047
foot deformities, 1046, 1046f
Morton's neuromas, 1047
plantar fasciitis, 1047
skin preparation for surgery of, 229f
treatment of, 1047t
FEF$_{25\%-75\%}$, 510t
Felty's syndrome, 306
Female reproductive system
anatomy and physiology of, 1449-1451
breasts, 1450-1451, 1451f
external genitalia, 1449-1450
internal genitalia, 1450, 1450f
changes with aging, 1452b
physical assessment of, 1454
Feminizing surgeries for male to female patients, 1526-1527, 1527b, 1527t
Femoral hernias, 1147
Fentanyl, 41, 41t
transdermal, 41b
Fetal tissue transplantation, 871
FEV$_1$. See Forced expiratory volume in 1 second (FEV$_1$).
Fever
in infection, 407b
in pneumonia, 592t
FEV$_1$/FVC, 510t
Fiberoptic transducer-tipped catheters, 956t
Fibrillation
atrial, 666-669, 666b-668b, 667f, 667t
ventricular, 670-671, 671f
Fibrin clot formation, 788
Fibrinogen, 790t
Fibrinolysis, 788, 790f
Fibrinolytics, 726b
for coronary artery disease, 767-768
for pulmonary embolism, 606, 608, 609b
for stroke, 938, 938b
Fibroadenomas, 1461, 1462t
Fibroblasts, 416, 436
Fibrocystic breast condition (FBC), 1462, 1462b, 1462t

Fibroids, uterine. *See* Uterine leiomyomas.
Fibromyalgia syndrome (FMS), 321-322
Fibrosis in sarcoidosis, 571
Fidelity, 4
Field block, 248t
Filgrastim, 381b, 387t
Filters in infusion therapy, 198
Filtration, 149-150, 149f-150f
FIM. *See* Functional Independence Measure (FIM).
Financial abuse of older adults, 19
Fine crackles, 507t
Fine rales, 507t
Finger positioning to prevent contractures, 487b
Fingolimod, 908
Fio₂. *See* Fraction of inspired oxygen (Fio₂).
Fire risk assessment, 240f
Fires in health care facilities, 139b
First aid
    in bee stings, 129
    in black widow spider bites, 127, 127b
    in brown recluse spider bites, 127
    in coral snake envenomation, 125
    in frostbite, 133
    in heat stroke, 122
    in high altitude-related illness, 134
    in hypothermia, 131-132
    in lightning strike injuries, 130
    in near-drowning, 136
    in pit viper envenomation, 124
First heart sound, 639
First intention healing, 434f, 435
First-degree frostbite, 132-133
Fissures, 423f
    anal, 1188-1189
Fistula
    anal, 1189
    arteriovenous, 1435b
    in Crohn's disease, 1184b, 1185f
    tracheoesophageal, 523t
    tracheo-innominate artery, 523t
Fixed occlusion in facial trauma, 534
Flaccid bladder, 86-87, 86t, 900
Flaccid bowel, 87t
Flaccid paralysis in stroke, 934-936
Flail chest, 623, 623f
Flash burns, 472
Flat bones, 1017-1018
Flecainide acetate, 658b-662b
Flexion exercises, 887b
Flora, normal, 397, 398t, 415
Flovent. *See* Fluticasone.
Flow rate, 618
Fluid balance
    body fluids and, 152-153, 152b
        abnormal electrolyte values in, 152t
        age-related changes in, 153b
        homeostasis and, 148, 149f
        hormonal regulation of, 153-154

Fluid balance (*Continued*)
    in hypercortisolism, 1278-1280, 1279b
    physiologic influences on, 148-152
        diffusion, 150, 150f
        filtration, 149-150, 149f-150f
        osmosis, 151-152, 151f
    postoperative assessment of, 262
    renin-angiotensin II pathway and, 154-155, 154f
        clinical application of, 155
    in traumatic brain injury, 955
Fluid imbalances, 155-160
    after craniotomy, 962
    in burns, 469, 475
    in chronic kidney disease, 1424, 1426, 1426b
    in cirrhosis, 1197-1200, 1199b
    in coronary artery bypass graft, 777
    dehydration and, 155-158, 155b, 155t
        changes in fluid compartment volumes with, 155f
        health promotion and maintenance in, 156
        history in, 156
        interventions for, 157-158, 157b-158b, 158t
        laboratory assessment in, 157
        physical assessment in, 156-157, 156b, 156f
    in diabetic ketoacidosis, 1333-1334
    fluid overload in, 155t, 158, 158f-159f, 159b-160b
    in total parenteral nutrition, 1245
Fluid intake, 153, 153t
    in cystitis, 1372
Fluid loss, 153, 153t
Fluid overload, 155t, 158, 158f-159f, 159b-160b
    in enteral nutrition, 1244
    in syndrome of inappropriate antidiuretic hormone, 392b
Fluid replacement
    in acute respiratory distress syndrome, 614
    in burns, 478-479, 479b
    in dehydration, 157, 157b
    in hyperglycemic-hyperosmolar state, 1336-1337, 1336b
    in intestinal obstructions, 1160
Fluid retention
    fluid overload and, 160
    in mechanical ventilation, 620
Fluid shift
    in burn injuries, 469, 469f
Fluid volume deficit after lumbar spinal surgery, 889b
Fluorescein angiography, 975
Fluorometholone, 979b

Flushing
    of catheters in infusion therapy, 202, 202b
    of peripherally inserted central catheter, 194b
Fluticasone, 539b
Flutter valve mucus clearance device, 564, 564f
FMS. *See* Fibromyalgia syndrome (FMS).
Foam buildups, 84t
Focused assessment
    in acquired immune deficiency syndrome, 343b
    in chronic kidney disease, 1445b
    in diabetes mellitus, 1339b
    in hearing loss, 1010b
    in patients with leukemia at risk for infections, 809b
    in pneumonia, 594, 594b
    postoperative, 258b
    preoperative, 225, 225b
    in sexually transmitted disease, 1534b
    in testicular lump, 1514b
    in total abdominal hysterectomy, 1490b
    in tracheostomy, 527, 527b
    in urinary incontinence, 1376b
Folic acid deficiency anemia, 799t, 804
Folliculitis, 450, 450b
Food
    contaminated, 413
    cultural considerations in, 1233b
    warfarin and, 733b
Food intake, preoperative, 228, 228b
Footwear for diabetic patients, 1327
Forced expiratory volume in 1 second (FEV₁), 510t
Forced vital capacity (FVC), 510t
Forearms, skin preparation for surgery of, 229f
Forebrain, 830
Foreign bodies
    in ear, 1004-1005, 1005b, 1005f
    in eye, 991-992, 991b
Forensic nurse examiners, 106
Fraction of inspired oxygen (Fio₂), 514-515, 618
Fractures, 1051-1066
    chest, 1069
    classification of, 1051-1052, 1052f
    community-based care in, 1065
    complications of, 1053-1055
        acute compartment syndrome, 1053-1054, 1054b
        fat embolism syndrome, 1054, 1055b
        hypovolemic shock, 1054
        infection, 1054-1055
        venous thromboembolism, 1054
    emergency care of, 1058, 1058b
    etiology and genetic risk in, 1055

Fractures (*Continued*)
    evaluation of care of patient with, 1065-1066
    health care resources for, 1065
    health promotion and maintenance in, 1055
    history in, 1055-1057
    home care management in, 1065
    imaging assessment in, 1057
    improving physical mobility in, 1064-1065, 1065f
    incidence and prevalence of, 1055
    infection prevention in, 1064, 1064b
    laboratory assessment in, 1057
    lower extremity, 1066-1068
        hip, 1066-1068, 1067b-1068b, 1067f
        other fractures of, 1068-1069
    mandibular, 534
    monitoring for neurovascular compromise, 1063-1064, 1064b
    nasal, 531-532, 532b, 532f
    nonsurgical management of, 1058-1062, 1058f-1059f, 1059b-1060b, 1060t-1061t, 1061f
    pain in, 1057-1063
    pelvic, 1069
    physical assessment in, 1055-1057, 1056b-1057b
    physical therapy for, 1063
    procedures for nonunion of, 1063
    psychosocial assessment in, 1057
    rib, 623
    self-management education in, 1065, 1065b
    stages of bone healing and, 1052-1053, 1053b, 1053f
    surgical management of, 1062-1063, 1062f
    traction for, 1060b, 1061f, 1061t
    upper extremity, 1066-1069, 1066f
    vertebral, 1069, 1070b
Frail elderly, 9-10
FRC. *See* Functional residual capacity (FRC).
Fremitus, 504
    in lung cancer, 575
Friction, pressure ulcers and, 437, 437f
Frontal lobe, 831t
Frostbite, 122b, 132-133, 132b-133b
Frostnip, 132
Fructosamine, 1309
Full-thickness wounds, 435-436, 435f, 466, 468-469, 468f
Fulmer SPICES framework, 20
Fulminant hepatitis, 1204
Functional assessment
    of mobility, 1022, 1022f
    in rehabilitation, 79-80, 80t
Functional history in cardiovascular assessment, 636, 636t

Functional incontinence, 1374t, 1375
Functional Independence Measure
    (FIM), 79, 90
Functional residual capacity (FRC),
    510t
Functional urinary incontinence,
    1382
Fungal infections
    after burn injury, 481, 482t
    in Coccidioidomycosis, 600-601
    cultures for, 429
    cutaneous, 450b, 451-452
    in human immune deficiency
        virus infection, 334, 334f
Furacin. See Nitrofurazone.
Furosemide, 715b-716b
Furuncles, 450-451, 450b, 451f
Fusion inhibitors, 339b
FVC. See Forced vital capacity
    (FVC).

G
Gabapentin, 45
Gait assessment, 1021-1022, 1022f
Gait training, 81-84, 83b, 83f, 83t
Gallbladder, 1086-1087
Gallium scans, 1025
Gamma globulins, 284
Gamma knife, 959-960, 959f
Gamma rays, 374, 374f
Ganglion, 1046
Garamycin. See Gentamicin sulfate.
Gardasil vaccine, 368-369
Gas exchange, 514
    after burn injury, 478
    cancer and, 372
    combined ventilatory and
        oxygenation failure, 611-612
    failure and, 611, 612t
    in heart failure, 684, 684b
    hematologic system's role in, 785,
        786f
    pneumonia and, 593
    respiratory problems and, 603,
        604f
    respiratory system's role in, 494,
        495f
    shock and, 739-740, 740f, 742f
Gastrectomy, 1229
Gastric analysis, 1097
Gastric bypass, 1250, 1251f
Gastric cancer, 1138-1139, 1139b,
    1140f, 1141t
Gastric lavage, 1136
Gastric surgery, 263b
Gastric ulcers, 1132t
Gastritis, 1126-1128, 1127b-1128b,
    1133b-1134b
Gastroenteritis, 1172-1173, 1172t,
    1173b
Gastroesophageal reflux, 1110
Gastroesophageal reflux disease
    (GERD), 1203-1208
    diagnosis of, 1112
    drug therapy for, 1113, 1113b

Gastroesophageal reflux disease
    (GERD) (Continued)
    nonsurgical management of,
        1112-1114, 1113b
    older adults and, 1112b
    physical assessment in, 1111-1112,
        1111b
    surgical management of, 1114
Gastrointestinal assessment,
    1084-1098
    in burns, 476
    colonoscopy in, 1095-1096, 1096b
    current health problems in, 1089
    endoscopic retrograde
        cholangiopancreatography in,
        1094-1095, 1095b
    endoscopic ultrasonography in,
        1097
    esophagogastroduodenoscopy in,
        1093-1094, 1094b, 1094f
    family history and genetic risk in,
        1089
    gastric analysis in, 1097
    health promotion and
        maintenance in, 1098
    imaging assessment in, 1093
    laboratory assessment in,
        1091-1093, 1092b
    liver-spleen scan in, 1097
    nutrition history in, 1087-1089,
        1088b
    patient history in, 1087, 1088b
    physical assessment in, 1089-1091,
        1089f, 1090b, 1090t
    postoperative, 262-263, 263b, 263t
    psychosocial assessment in, 1091
    in rehabilitation setting, 78, 78t
    sigmoidoscopy in, 1096
    small bowel capsule endoscopy in,
        1095
    in spinal cord injury, 895
    ultrasonography in, 1097
    virtual colonoscopy in, 1096
Gastrointestinal bleeding
    lower, 1179-1180, 1180b
    upper, 1136-1137, 1136b-1137b
Gastrointestinal system
    anatomy and physiology of,
        1084-1087, 1085f
    function of, 1084-1087
        esophagus, 1085
        large intestine, 1087
        liver and gallbladder,
            1086-1087
        oral cavity, 1085
        pancreas, 1086, 1086f
        small intestine, 1087
        stomach, 1085-1086
    structure of, 1084
    cancer and, 372
    changes associated with aging,
        1087, 1088b
    changes resulting from burns,
        470
    chronic kidney disease and, 1424

Gastrointestinal system (Continued)
    complications of immobility and,
        83t
    fluid overload and, 159b
    older adults and, 398b
    potential complications of surgery
        and, 258t
Gastrojejunostomy, 1229, 1229f
Gastroparesis, 1305
Gastrostomy, 1241
Gate control theory, 26, 29f
GBS. See Guillain-Barré syndrome
    (GBS).
GCS. See Glasgow Coma Scale (GCS).
GDS-SF. See Geriatric Depression
    Scale-Short Form (GDS-SF).
Gel pads, 84t
Gel phenomenon, 305
Gender
    cancer incidence and death by, 364f
    human immune deficiency virus
        transmission and, 330
Gender dysphoria, 1520, 1520t
Gender health considerations
    in autoimmune disorders, 356b
    in body fluids, 152b
    in breast cancer, 1470b
    in cardiovascular assessment,
        632b, 634b-635b
    in chlamydia infections, 1538b
    in cholecystitis, 1215b
    in chronic calcium loss, 152b
    in cirrhosis, 1195b
    in coronary artery disease, 632b,
        759b-760b, 762b
    in epilepsy, 859b
    in hematologic assessment, 789b
    in HIV infection, 329b
    in hypertension, 711b
    in LGBTQ older adults, 269b
    in nonopioid analgesics, 38b
    in osteoarthritis, 291b
    in osteoporosis, 1031b
    in renal assessment, 1354b
    in reproductive assessment, 1453b
    in respiratory assessment, 500b
    in sexually transmitted diseases,
        1531b
    in sickle cell disease, 803b
    smoking and, 495b
    in stroke, 938b
    in syphilis, 1533b
Gender identity, 1519-1520, 1520t
Genderqueer, 1520t
Gene expression, 51-52, 55
Gene mutations, 56
    cultural considerations in, 56b
General anesthesia, 245-248
    administration of, 245-246
    complications from, 246-248,
        247b-248b
    stages of, 245, 246t
General appearance, cardiovascular
    assessment and, 637
Generalized seizures, 858

Genes, 51
    expressivity of, 58
    structure and function of, 54-55,
        55f
Genetic biology, 51-63
    DNA in, 52-54
        chromosomes and, 52f, 53-54,
            54f
        replication of, 53, 53f
        structure of, 52-53, 52f-53f
    essential genetic competencies
        and, 52t
    gene expression in, 51-52, 55
    gene mutations in, 56, 56b
    gene structure and function in,
        54-55, 55f
    genetic counseling and, 60-63,
        60b, 62b
    genetic testing and, 59-61, 59t,
        60b
    patterns of inheritance in, 56-59
        autosomal dominant, 57-58, 57t
        autosomal recessive, 57t, 58, 58f
        complex inheritance and
            familial clustering and, 57t,
            59
        pedigree and, 57, 57f, 57t
        sex-linked recessive, 57t, 58-59,
            59f
    protein synthesis in, 55-56, 56f
Genetic considerations
    in acute respiratory distress
        syndrome, 613b
    in altitude-related illnesses, 133b
    in Alzheimer's disease, 872b
    in asthma, 531-532, 532b
    in cancer, 367b, 368t
        breast, 1465, 1465b
        colorectal, 1149b
        esophageal, 1117b
        in lung, 574, 574b
        oral, 1103b
        pancreatic, 1227b
        skin, 460b
    in cardiovascular assessment, 634,
        634b
    in chronic obstructive pulmonary
        disease, 545b
    in cystic fibrosis, 567b
    in diabetes insipidus, 1271b
    in diabetes mellitus, 1306-1307,
        1307b
    in endocrine assessment, 1262
    in gastrointestinal assessment,
        1089
    in hearing assessment, 1000, 1000b
    in hematologic assessment, 791
    in hemophilia, 821b
    in HIV infection, 329b, 337b
    in Huntington disease, 881b
    in hyperpituitarism, 1268b
    in hyperthyroidism, 1286b
    in integumentary assessment, 421
    in malignant hyperthermia, 247b
    in multiple sclerosis, 905b

Genetic considerations (Continued)
in muscular dystrophy, 1049b
in musculoskeletal assessment, 1021
in obesity, 1247b
in opioid administration, 37b
in osteoporosis, 1030b
in Paget's disease of the bone, 1037b
in Parkinson disease, 867b
in polycystic kidney disease, 1396b
in prostate cancer, 1507b
in psoriasis, 456b
in pulmonary arterial hypertension, 569b
in pulmonary embolism, 605b, 608b
in renal assessment, 1353
in reproductive assessment, 1453
in retinitis pigmentosa, 990b
in rheumatoid arthritis, 305, 305b
in testicular cancer, 1513b
in urolithiasis, 1384b
in vision assessment, 971
Genetic counseling, 60-63, 60b, 62b
Genetic testing, 59-61, 59t, 60b
for cancer predisposition, 368
Genetics, 51
Genital herpes, 1535-1536, 1536b
Genital warts, 1537-1538, 1537b, 1537f
Genitalia
female
external, 1449-1450
internal, 1450, 1450f
male, 1451, 1451f
Genitourinary assessment, 895
Genitourinary surgery, skin preparation for, 229f
Genome, 51-52
Genome-wide association studies (GWAS), 532b
Genomic health care, 51
Genomics, 51
Genotype, 55
Gentamar. See Gentamicin sulfate.
Gentamicin sulfate, 486b
Genu valgum, 1023
Genu varum, 1023
GERD. See Gastroesophageal reflux disease (GERD).
Geriatric Depression Scale-Short Form (GDS-SF), 15f, 16, 17f
Geriatric failure to thrive (GFTT), 11
Geriatric syndromes, 9-10
Germinative layer, 416
Germline mutations, 56
GFR. See Glomerular filtration rate (GFR).
GFTT. See Geriatric failure to thrive (GFTT).
Glasgow Coma Scale (GCS)
rapid neurologic assessment and, 843, 843f, 844b
in spinal cord injury, 894

Glass bottles, 196
Glaucoma, 985-989
concept map for, 986f
drug therapy for, 988b
nonsurgical management of, 987-988, 987b-988b, 989f
pathophysiology of, 985, 985t
surgical management of, 988-989
Gleevec. See Imatinib mesylate.
Global bioterrorism, 411-413, 411t
Globulins, 786
Glomerular filtration, 1347
Glomerular filtration rate (GFR), 1347
cultural considerations in, 1351b
Glomerulonephritis
acute, 1397-1399, 1402t, 1403b
chronic, 1403-1404
rapidly progressive, 1403
Glomerulus, 1346
Glossectomy, 1105
Glossitis, 804, 804f
Glossopharyngeal nerve, 835t
Glottis, 497-498
Gloves and gloving, 244, 245f
for infection control, 402b
latex allergies and, 402-403
Glucagon, 1301
Glucocorticoids, 1258, 1258t
for rheumatoid arthritis, 311
Gluconeogenesis, 1301-1302
Glucophage. See Metformin.
Glucosamine, 294-295, 295b
Glucose
burn assessment and, 477b
homeostasis of, 1301-1302
perioperative assessment of, 223b-224b
renal threshold for reabsorption of, 1348
testing in endocrine assessment, 1264
Glucose-6-phosphate dehydrogenase deficiency anemia, 799t, 803
Glycocalyx, 405, 414
Glycogenesis, 1301-1302
Glycoprotein IIb/IIIa inhibitors, 767, 767b
Glycosylated hemoglobin assay, 1308
Goiters
classification of, 1287t
in hyperthyroidism, 1285-1286
Golimumab
for psoriatic arthritis, 321
for rheumatoid arthritis, 309b
Gonadotropins
deficiency of, 1267, 1267b
overproduction of, 1269b
Gonads, 1257. See also Ovaries; Testes.
Goniometer, 1022
Gonioscopy, 975
Gonorrhea, 1539-1541, 1539b, 1540f
Good death, 91
Goodpasture's syndrome, 357
Gout, 319-320, 319f

Gowning, 244, 245f
Gradient, 150
Grading of cancer, 365, 365t
Graft occlusion, 724b
Grafts
arteriovenous, 1435b
endovascular stent, 727
Graft-versus-host disease (GVHD)
in stem cell transplantation, 812-813, 813f
Granisetron, 385b
Granulation in wound healing, 434f, 435-436
Granulocyte transfusions, 824
Granuloma inguinale, 1544
Granulomas, 571
Granulomatous thyroiditis, 1295
Graves' disease, 1286
Gravity drains, 265f
Gray (gy), 374
Gray matter, 830, 832-833
Grief, 100
Grieving process, 100-101, 1155, 1155b
Ground substance, 416
Growth factor therapy, 383, 387
Growth factors, 286t
Growth hormone
deficiency of, 1267b
oversecretion of, 1269b
Guardians, 16
Guillain-Barré syndrome (GBS), 913-917, 914b-916b
GVHD. See Graft-versus-host disease (GVHD).
GWAS. See Genome-wide association studies (GWAS).
Gy. See Gray (gy).
Gynecologic problems, 1482-1498
benign neoplasms, 1487-1491
Bartholin cysts, 1491
cervical polyps, 1491
ovarian cysts, 1487
uterine leiomyomas, 1487-1491, 1488f, 1489b-1490b, 1489t
dysfunctional uterine bleeding, 1483-1484, 1484t
endometriosis, 1482-1483, 1483f
gynecologic cancers, 1491-1497
cervical cancer, 1494-1495, 1495b
endometrial cancer, 1491-1494, 1492t, 1493b
ovarian cancer, 1495-1497, 1496t
pelvic inflammatory disease, 1539, 1541, 1541f, 1542t, 1543b
pelvic organ prolapse, 1485-1487, 1486f, 1487b
toxic shock syndrome, 1485, 1485b
vulvovaginitis, 1484-1485, 1485b
Gynecologic surgery, skin preparation for, 229f
Gynecomastia, 1463-1464, 1464f
cancer therapy-related, 392
in testicular cancer, 1513

H
HAART. See Highly active antiretroviral therapy (HAART).
HACE. See High altitude cerebral edema (HACE).
HAI. See Health care-associated infection (HAI).
Hair, 415
assessment of, 424-425
changes with aging, 418b-419b
structure of, 417
Hair follicles, 417
Hair loss, 425
chemotherapy-related, 381, 384-385
Half-life, definition of, 40-41
Hallux valgus deformity, 1046, 1046f
Halo fixators, 897, 897b-898b, 897f
Hammertoes, 1046, 1046f
HA-MRSA. See Health care-associated methicillin-resistant Staphylococcus aureus (HA-MRSA).
Hand hygiene
catheter-related bloodstream infection and, 204t
in infection control, 401-402, 401b-402b
standard precautions and, 402b, 403t
Hand surgery, skin preparation for, 229f
Hand-off communication in emergency care, 107-108
Hand-off reports, postoperative, 257, 257b
Hands
arthroplasty of, 303
disorders of, 1045-1046
Dupuytren's contracture, 1045-1046
ganglion, 1046
Handwashing, 401-402, 402b
Hantavirus pulmonary syndrome, 407
HAPE. See High altitude pulmonary edema (HAPE).
Hashimoto's disease, 1295
Haversian system, 1018f
Hay fever, 349-351, 349f, 351b
Hazardous materials (HAZMAT) training, 139, 140f
HAZMAT training. See Hazardous materials (HAZMAT) training.
HbA. See Hemoglobin A (HbA).
HBOT. See Hyperbaric oxygen therapy (HBOT).
HbS. See Hemoglobin S (HbS).
HCM. See Hypertrophic cardiomyopathy (HCM).
HD. See Huntington disease (HD).
HDLs. See High-density lipoproteins (HDLs).

Head
  hematologic assessment and, 792
  positioning to prevent
    contractures, 487b
Head and neck cancer, 537-545
  anxiety in, 543-544
  aspiration prevention in, 543, 543b
  etiology of, 538
  evaluation of care of patient with,
    545
  health care resources for, 545
  history in, 538
  home care management in, 544,
    544b
  imaging assessment in, 538
  incidence and prevalence of, 538
  laboratory assessment in, 538
  physical assessment in, 538, 538t
  preventing respiratory obstruction
    in, 539-542, 540b-541b, 541t,
    542f
  psychosocial assessment in, 538
  psychosocial support in, 545
  self-concept in, 544
  self-management education in,
    544-545, 545b
  surgery for, 540-542, 541b, 541t,
    542f
Head lice, 453-454
Head surgery, skin preparation for,
  229f
Headaches, 853-858, 854b
  cluster, 857-858
  migraine, 854-857, 855b-857b, 855t
  postdural puncture, 261b
Healing
  delayed, 267-269, 267b-269b, 267f
  phases of, 433-435, 433t,
    434f-435f, 436t
Health care facility, fires in, 139b
Health care personnel, transmission
  of HIV and, 332, 332b
Health care resources
  after hospital discharge, 272
  for AIDS and HIV infection, 344
  for Alzheimer's disease, 880
  for back pain, 891
  for bone cancer, 1045
  for breast cancer, 1480
  for burns, 489
  for cataracts, 985
  for chronic kidney disease,
    1445-1446
  for chronic obstructive pulmonary
    disease, 566, 566b
  for cirrhosis, 1202
  for colorectal cancer, 1157
  for coronary artery disease, 782
  for dysrhythmias, 676
  for endometrial cancer, 1494
  for esophageal cancer, 1122
  for fractures, 1065
  for gastric cancer, 1142
  for head and neck cancer, 545
  for hearing loss, 1014

Health care resources (Continued)
  for heart failure, 691-692
  for hypertension, 718
  for hypothyroidism, 1294-1295,
    1295b
  for infection, 410
  for intestinal obstruction, 1161
  for leukemia, 816
  for malnutrition, 1246
  for multiple sclerosis, 909-910
  for myasthenia gravis, 922-923
  for oral cancer, 1107
  for osteoarthritis, 304
  for pain management, 48-49
  in pelvic inflammatory disease,
    1544
  for peptic ulcer disease, 1138
  for pneumonia, 594
  for polycystic kidney disease, 1397
  for pressure ulcers, 449, 449b
  for prostate cancer, 1511
  for pulmonary embolism, 610,
    611b
  for pyelonephritis, 1401
  for rehabilitation, 89
  for rheumatoid arthritis, 313
  for spinal cord injury, 901-902,
    902f
  for stroke, 945
  for traumatic brain injury, 957
  for tuberculosis, 599
  for ulcerative colitis, 1180-1181
  for urinary incontinence, 1383
  for urothelial cancer, 1389-1390
  for valvular heart disease, 697
Health care-associated infection
  (HAI), 400-401
Health care-associated methicillin-
  resistant *Staphylococcus aureus*
  (HA-MRSA), 405-406, 406b
Health Professions Education (IOM),
  3
Health promotion and maintenance
  in acute kidney injury, 1414, 1414t
  in acute respiratory distress
    syndrome, 613
  in Alzheimer's disease, 872
  in amputation, 1071
  in back pain, 886, 886b
  in breast cancer, 369, 369b,
    1465-1468, 1467b-1468b,
    1481
  in burns, 472-473
  in carpal tunnel syndrome, 1077
  in cervical cancer, 1494
  in chronic kidney disease,
    1421-1422
  in chronic obstructive pulmonary
    disease, 537
  in cold-related injuries, 131, 132b
  in colorectal cancer, 1149, 1150b
  in coronary artery disease,
    760-761, 761b, 761t, 783
  in cystitis, 1369, 1369b
  in dehydration, 156

Health promotion and maintenance
  (Continued)
  in diabetes mellitus, 1307-1308,
    1340
  in dysrhythmias, 676
  in esophageal problems, 1124
  in eye problems, 994-995
  in fractures, 1055
  in gastritis, 1127, 1127b
  in gastrointestinal assessment,
    1098
  in hearing loss, 1010, 1010b
  in heart failure, 704
  in heat-related illnesses, 121, 121b
  in hematologic assessment, 797
  in hemorrhoids, 1164
  in hepatitis, 1204, 1205b
  in human immune deficiency
    virus infection, 329-333,
    330b, 331f, 332b-333b, 347
  in hypersensitivity, 358
  in hypertension, 711, 711t
  in hypovolemic shock, 744
  in inflammatory intestinal
    disorders, 1191
  in influenza
    pandemic, 587-588
    seasonal, 587
  in kidney disorders, 1410
  in lightning strike prevention, 130,
    130b
  in liver problems, 1211
  in lung cancer, 574
  in musculoskeletal problems, 1050
  in musculoskeletal trauma, 1080
  in neurologic assessment, 851
  in noninflammatory intestinal
    disorders, 1167
  nutrition standards for, 1232-
    1233, 1233b, 1233f, 1233t
  in obesity, 1247-1248, 1247t
  in older adults, 10, 10b, 12b, 23
  in oral cavity problems, 1109
  in osteoarthritis, 301
  in osteomalacia, 1036-1037
  in osteoporosis, 1031-1032
  in ovarian cancer, 1496
  in peripheral nervous system
    problems, 928
  in pneumonia, 589-590,
    589b-590b
  in pressure ulcers, 437-441, 438b,
    439f
  in prevention of anaphylaxis, 352,
    352b, 352f
  in prevention of drowning, 135
  in prostate cancer, 1507, 1507b
  in pulmonary embolism, 604,
    604b
  in renal assessment, 1364
  in respiratory problems, 494-496
  in sepsis and septic shock,
    751-752, 751b
  in sexually transmitted diseases,
    1545

Health promotion and maintenance
  (Continued)
  in shock, 755
  in skin cancer, 460, 460b
  in skin infections, 452, 452b
  in smoking cessation, 495,
    495b-496b, 512b
  in snakebite prevention, 123, 123b
  in stomach disorders, 1142-1143
  in stroke, 933, 933b
  in syphilis, 1533, 1533t
  in traumatic brain injury, 950
  in urinary problems, 1392
  in vascular problems, 709
  in venous thromboembolism, 730
  in vision, 970-971, 970b-971b, 976
Health teaching. *See* Patient and
  family education.
Healthy People 2020 initiative
  on heart disease and stroke, 711t
  on LGBTQ population, 4
  on older adults, 15
  heart failure and, 681t
Healthy People 2020 objectives
  for sexually transmitted disease,
    1533t
*Healthy People 2020 objectives for
  Nutrition and Weight Status,*
  1247-1248, 1247t
Hearing aid, 1011-1012,
  1011b-1012b
Hearing assessment, 998-1003
  audiometry in, 1002-1003, 1002t
  auditory brainstem-evoked
    response in, 1003
  balance testing in, 1003
  current health problems in, 1000
  external ear and mastoid
    assessment in, 1000
  family history and genetic risk in,
    1000, 1000b
  general auditory assessment in,
    1001-1002
  history in, 998-1000, 999b
  imaging assessment in, 1002
  laboratory assessment in, 1002
  otoscopic assessment in,
    1000-1001, 1000b-1001b,
    1001f
  psychosocial assessment in, 1002
  tympanometry in, 1003
Hearing loss, 1009-1015
  communication and, 1014, 1014b
  community-based care in, 1014
  conductive versus sensorineural,
    1001, 1009t
  drug therapy for, 1011
  evaluation of care of patient with,
    1015
  health promotion and
    maintenance in, 1010, 1010b
  hearing aid for, 1011-1012,
    1011b-1012b
  history in, 1010
  imaging assessment in, 1011

Hearing loss (Continued)
  laboratory assessment in, 1011
  pathophysiology of, 1009-1010, 1009t
  physical assessment in, 1010
  psychosocial assessment in, 1010
  stapedectomy for, 1013, 1013b, 1013f
  totally implanted device for, 1013-1014
  tympanoplasty for, 1012-1013, 1012f
Hearing problems. See Ear problems.
Heart, 627-631
  conduction system of, 649-650, 650f
  function of, 629-631, 630f
  mechanical properties of, 630-631
  structure of, 627-629, 629f
Heart disease. See Coronary artery disease (CAD).
Heart failure (HF), 678-705
  cardiac resynchronization therapy for, 687
  in cardiomyopathies, 701-704, 701t, 703b, 703f
  in chronic kidney disease, 1421
  in chronic obstructive pulmonary disease, 558
  classification and staging of, 679
  compensatory mechanisms in, 679-681, 680f
  continuous positive airway pressure for, 687
  in coronary artery disease, 769-772, 770b, 771f, 771t, 772b-773b
  drug therapy for
    ACE inhibitors and angiotensin receptor blockers in, 684-685, 685b
    beta-adrenergic blockers in, 687
    digoxin in, 686, 687b, 691b
    diuretics in, 685-686, 685b-686b
    human B-type natriuretic peptides in, 685, 689b
    inotropic drugs in, 686-687
  etiology of, 681, 681t
  evaluation of care of patient with, 692
  fatigue and weakness in, 688
  health care resources for, 691-692
  Healthy People 2020 objectives for, 681t
  history in, 681-684
  home care management in, 689, 690b
  imaging assessment in, 684
  improving gas exchange in, 684, 684b
  incidence and prevalence of, 681
  in infective endocarditis, 697-699, 697b, 699b
  laboratory assessment in, 683-684, 683b

Heart failure (HF) (Continued)
  nutrition therapy for, 685
  older adults and, 681b, 681t, 683b, 685b
  in pericarditis, 699-700, 700b
  physical assessment in, 682-683, 682b-683b
  psychosocial assessment in, 683
  pulmonary edema in, 688-689, 688b-689b
  in rheumatic carditis, 700-701
  self-management education in, 689-691, 690b-691b, 690t
  surgical management of, 687-688, 688f
  types of, 679
Heart murmurs, 640, 640t
  in leukemia, 808
Heart rate, 630
  after burn injury, 470
  determination using electrocardiography, 654-655
Heart rhythm analysis, 655-656
Heart sounds
  abnormal, 640
Heart transplantation, 702-704, 703b, 703f
Heart valve reparative procedures, 695
Heart valve replacement procedures, 695-696, 696b, 696f
Heat application
  for osteoarthritis pain, 294
  for pain management, 46-47
  for rheumatoid arthritis, 311
Heat energy, 1082
Heat exhaustion, 121, 121b
Heat stroke, 121-122, 122b-123b
Heat-related illnesses, 120-122, 121b-123b
Heberden's node, 292, 292f
Helper/inducer T-cells, 278t, 285, 327-328, 327f, 787t
Hematocrit, 798
  in burn assessment, 477b
  in cardiovascular assessment, 642
  in hypovolemic shock, 747b
  perioperative assessment of, 223b-224b
  in respiratory assessment, 508b
Hematogenous tuberculosis, 595
Hematologic assessment, 785-797
  bone marrow aspiration and biopsy in, 795-796, 796b
  cultural considerations in, 792b
  current health problems in, 792
  family history and genetic risks in, 791
  gender health considerations in, 789b
  health promotion and maintenance in, 797
  history in, 788-791, 791t
  imaging assessment in, 795
  laboratory assessment in, 793-796, 794b

Hematologic assessment (Continued)
  nutrition status in, 791
  older adults and, 790b
  physical assessment in, 792-793, 792b-793b, 796
  psychosocial assessment in, 793
Hematologic problems, 798-827
  coagulation disorders, 819-821
    autoimmune thrombocytopenic purpura, 820
    hemophilia, 820-821, 821b, 821t
  red blood cell disorders. See Red blood cell disorders.
  transfusion therapy for, 821-826
    acute transfusion reactions in, 824-825
    autologous, 825-826
    indication for, 822t
    older adults and, 823b
    pretransfusion responsibilities, 821-823, 822b-823b, 823f
    red blood cell, 824, 824b, 824t
  white blood cell disorders
    leukemia. See Leukemia.
    malignant lymphomas, 817-819
      Hodgkin's lymphoma, 817, 817t
      multiple myeloma, 818-819
      non-Hodgkin lymphoma, 818
Hematologic system
  anatomy and physiology of, 785-788
    accessory organs of blood formation, 787
    anti-clotting forces, 788, 790f
    blood components, 786-787, 787f, 787t
    hemostasis and, 787-788, 789f, 790t
  assessment of. See Hematologic assessment.
  changes associated with aging, 788, 790b
  chronic kidney disease and, 1421
  disorders of. See Hematologic problems.
  drugs impairing function of, 791t
  oxygenation and, 785, 786f
Hematomas
  epidural, 261b, 949, 949f
  intravenous therapy-related, 204t-206t
  subdural, 949, 949f
Hematopoietic stem cell transplantation
  in leukemia, 808f, 811-814, 811b-812b, 811t, 812f
Hematuria
  after pancreas transplantation, 1323
  in benign prostatic hyperplasia, 1500
  in polycystic kidney disease, 1396

Hemianopsia, 936
Hemiarthroplasty, 303
Hemilaryngectomy, 541t
Hemiparesis, 934
Hemiplegia, 934
Hemoconcentration, 157
  in burns, 469
Hemodialysis
  in acute kidney injury, 1417-1418, 1417f
  in chronic kidney disease, 1431-1437
    anticoagulation in, 1432-1433
    complications of, 1433-1437, 1435t, 1436b
    dialysis settings in, 1432
    nursing care in, 1436
    older adults and, 1437b
    patient selection for, 1431
    peritoneal dialysis vs., 1431t
    post-dialysis care and, 1436, 1436b
    procedure in, 1432, 1432f, 1433f
    vascular access in, 1433, 1434f, 1434t, 1435f
Hemodialysis catheters, 196
Hemodilution, 158
Hemodynamic monitoring, 770-771, 770b, 771f
Hemoglobin
  in burn assessment, 477b
  in hypovolemic shock, 747b
  oxygen-hemoglobin dissociation curve and, 499-500, 500f
  perioperative assessment of, 223b-224b
Hemoglobin A (HbA), 799
Hemoglobin electrophoresis, 793
Hemoglobin S (HbS), 799
Hemolytic anemia
  in brown recluse spider bite, 127
  in sickle cell disease, 800
Hemolytic transfusion reaction, 825
Hemophilia, 820-821, 821b, 821t
Hemoptysis
  in laryngeal trauma, 536
  in pulmonary embolism, 604
  respiratory assessment and, 502
Hemorrhage
  brain hematoma and, 949, 949b, 949f
  of esophageal varices, 1200
Hemorrhagic stroke, 931f-932f, 932, 932t
Hemorrhoidectomy, 1164, 1165b
Hemorrhoids, 1164-1165, 1164f, 1165b
Hemostasis, 787-788, 789f, 790t
Hemothorax, 624
Hemovac drains, 264, 265f, 268
Heparin, 606-607, 606b-607b
Heparin-induced thrombocytopenia (HIT), 821

Hepatic encephalopathy, 1193-1194, 1194t
Hepatitis, 1203-1208
    assessment in, 1204-1206
    community-based care in, 1207-1208, 1208b
    health promotion and maintenance in, 1204, 1205b
    interventions for, 1206-1208, 1206b-1207b, 1207t
    pathophysiology of, 1203-1204
Hepatitis A, 1203
Hepatitis B, 1203
    cirrhosis in, 1194
Hepatitis C, 1203-1204
    cirrhosis and liver failure in, 1194
    combination drug therapy for, 1207t
    laboratory assessment in, 1206
Hepatitis D, 1194, 1204
Hepatitis E, 1204
Hepatomegaly, 1090
    in pancreatic cancer, 1227
Hepatorenal syndrome, 1194
Hereditary hemochromatosis, 806
Heritability, 51
Hernia
    abdominal, 1146-1148, 1146f, 1148b
    hiatal, 1111, 1114-1115
        assessment in, 1115, 1115b
        community-based care in, 1117
        interventions for, 1115-1117, 1115b-1116b, 1116f
        pathophysiology of, 1114-1115, 1114b, 1114f
Hernioplasty, 1147
Herniorrhaphy, 1147
Herpes simplex virus (HSV), 1535
    in HIV or AIDS, 335, 342
    in skin infections, 450b, 451, 451f
Herpes simplex virus type 2 (HSV-2), 1535
Herpes zoster, 450b, 452
Herpetic whitlow, 451
Heterografts, 483, 483f
Heterotropic ossification, 895, 898
HF. See Heart failure (HF).
HFCWO. See High-frequency chest wall oscillation (HFCWO).
H5N1, 587-588
Hiatal hernias, 1111, 1114-1115
    assessment in, 1115, 1115b
    community-based care in, 1117
    interventions for, 1115-1117, 1115b-1116b, 1116f
    pathophysiology of, 1114-1115, 1114b, 1114f
HICS. See Hospital Incident Command System (HICS).
Hierarchy of Pain Measures, 33-34, 33t
High altitude cerebral edema (HACE), 134-135
High altitude illnesses, 133-135, 133b-135b

High altitude pulmonary edema (HAPE), 134-135
High blood pressure. See Hypertension.
High-alert drugs, 1316-1317
High-density lipoproteins (HDLs), 641-642, 641b
High-efficiency particulate air respirator, 657, 657f
High-flow oxygen delivery systems, 519-520, 519f-520f, 519t
High-frequency chest wall oscillation (HFCWO), 568, 568f
Highly active antiretroviral therapy (HAART), 338-340, 339b, 342
Highly sensitive C-reactive protein (hsCRP), 642
High-output heart failure, 679
High-pitched rales, 507t
High-pressure alarm of ventilators, 620t
High-sensitivity C-reactive protein, 307, 307b
Hilum, renal, 1345, 1345f
Hips
    positioning to prevent contractures, 487b
    skin preparation for surgery of, 229f
    total hip arthroplasty and, 295-300, 300b
        infection prevention after, 297t, 299, 299b
        mobility and activity after, 297-300, 297b, 299b-300b
        older adults and, 297b
        operative procedures in, 296-297, 297f
        pain management after, 299
        postoperative care in, 297-300, 297b, 297t
        preoperative care in, 296
        prevention of hip dislocation after, 297t, 298, 298b
        self-management after, 298b
        venous thromboembolism after, 296, 297t, 298-299
Hirsutism, 425
    endocrine dysfunction and, 1262
Histamine, 349, 349f
Histone inhibitor, 380t
Histoplasmosis, 334
History
    in acidosis, 181
    in acute glomerulonephritis, 1402
    in acute kidney injury, 1412
    in acute pancreatitis, 1220
    in adrenal insufficiency, 1274-1275
    in allergic rhinitis, 349
    in Alzheimer's disease, 872-873, 873t
    in asthma, 532
    in benign prostatic hyperplasia, 1500, 1501f-1502f
    in breast cancer, 1469, 1469b

History (Continued)
    in burns, 473
    in cardiovascular assessment, 632-634
    in chronic glomerulonephritis, 1404
    in chronic kidney disease, 1422-1423
    in chronic obstructive pulmonary disease, 538
    in cirrhosis, 1195
    in colorectal cancer, 1150
    in coronary artery disease, 762
    in dehydration, 156
    in diabetes mellitus, 1308
    in endocrine assessment, 1261-1262
    in esophageal tumors, 1118
    in fractures, 1055-1057
    in gastrointestinal assessment, 1087, 1088b
    in head and neck cancer, 538
    in hearing assessment, 998-1000, 999b
    in hearing loss, 1010
    in heart failure, 681-684
    in hematologic assessment, 788-791, 791t
    in hepatitis, 1204-1205
    in HIV infection, 333
    in hypercortisolism, 1277
    in hyperthyroidism, 1286, 1287f
    in hypothyroidism, 1292
    in hypovolemic shock, 744
    in infection, 407
    in integumentary assessment, 420, 420b
    intraoperative care and, 250, 250b
    in leukemia, 807-808
    in lung cancer, 574-575, 575t
    in malnutrition, 1238, 1238b
    in multiple sclerosis, 905
    in musculoskeletal assessment, 1020-1021
    in neurologic assessment, 837-850, 838b
    in obesity, 1248
    in osteoarthritis, 292
    in pelvic inflammatory disease, 1542
    in peptic ulcer disease, 1131
    in pneumonia, 589t, 590-592
    in polycystic kidney disease, 1396
    postoperative plan of care and, 257, 258t
    preoperative, 219-221, 219t, 220b
    in pressure ulcers, 441
    in prostate cancer, 1508
    in psoriasis, 456
    in pyelonephritis, 1400
    in rehabilitation, 77
    in renal assessment, 1352-1353
    in renal cell carcinoma, 1407
    in reproductive assessment, 1452-1454
    in respiratory assessment, 500-503, 502b, 502t

History (Continued)
    in sepsis, 752, 752b
    in sickle cell disease, 800-801
    in skin infection, 452-453
    in spinal cord injury, 894
    in stroke, 933
    in traumatic brain injury, 950-953, 951b
    in tuberculosis, 596
    in ulcerative colitis, 1175
    in urinary incontinence, 1376, 1376b
    in vision assessment, 971-975, 971b, 971t
HIT. See Heparin-induced thrombocytopenia (HIT).
HIV infection. See Human immune deficiency virus (HIV) infection.
Hives, 433
    in bee stings, 129
    in serum sickness, 125
HLAs. See Human leukocyte antigens (HLAs).
HMG-CoA reductase inhibitors, 709t
Hodgkin's lymphoma, 335, 817, 817t
Holding area nurses, 239, 240f
Home care management
    in acquired immune deficiency syndrome, 343, 343b
    after rehabilitation, 88-89
    in Alzheimer's disease, 879-880
    in amputations, 1075b
    in back pain, 890
    in bone cancer, 1045
    in breast cancer, 1478, 1478b-1479b
    in burns, 489
    in cataracts, 984, 984b, 984f
    in chronic kidney disease, 1444-1445, 1445b
    in chronic obstructive pulmonary disease, 566
    in cirrhosis, 1201-1202
    in colorectal cancer, 1155, 1156b
    in coronary artery disease, 779-781, 780b
    in diabetes mellitus, 1339, 1339b
    in dysrhythmias, 673
    in endometrial cancer, 1493
    in esophageal cancer, 1122
    in fractures, 1065
    in gastric cancer, 1141-1142
    in head and neck cancer, 544, 544b
    for hearing loss, 1014
    in heart failure, 689, 690b
    in hypertension, 718
    in hypothyroidism, 1294
    in infection, 410
    in intestinal obstruction, 1161, 1161b
    in leukemia, 815
    in malnutrition, 1246
    in multiple sclerosis, 909

Home care management (Continued)
  in myasthenia gravis, 922
  in oral cancer, 1106
  in osteoarthritis, 304
  in oxygen therapy, 521
  in pain, 48, 50
  in pelvic inflammatory disease, 1543
  in peptic ulcer disease, 1137-1138, 1138b
  in peripheral arterial disease, 724b
  in pneumonia, 593-594, 594b
  postoperative, 271-272
  in pressure ulcers, 447-449
  in prostate cancer, 1511
  in pulmonary embolism, 610, 611b
  in pyelonephritis, 1401
  in rheumatoid arthritis, 313, 313f
  in sepsis, 754, 754b
  in spinal cord injury, 900
  in stroke, 944
  in traumatic brain injury, 956
  in tuberculosis, 598
  in ulcerative colitis, 1180-1181
  in urinary incontinence, 1383
  in valvular heart disease, 696
Home hospice symptom relief kit, 97b
Home infusion therapy for pain management, 48
Homeless patients
  emergency care for, 114
  older adults, 10
Homeostasis, 148, 149f, 1255
  glucose, 1301-1302
  skin's role in, 418t
Homeostatic mechanisms, 148
Homocysteine, 642
Homografts, 483
Homonymous hemianopsia, 936
Hook and loop fasteners, 84t
Hookah smoking, 495
Hordeolum, 978
Hormone antagonists, 391, 391t
Hormone inhibitors, 391t
Hormone therapy
  for breast cancer, 1477-1478, 1477t
  for cancer, 391-392, 391t
  for prostate cancer, 1510, 1510b
  for transgender patients, 1524-1525
    patients transition from female to male, 1525, 1525t
    patients transition from male to female, 1524-1525, 1524t, 1525b
Hormones, 1255, 1256f, 1256t
  adrenal medullary, 1259t
  glucocorticoids, 1258t
  in regulation of fluid balance, 153-154
  renal, 1349-1350, 1349t
Hospice care, 94-95, 94b, 95t, 97b, 103
  for lung cancer, 580

Hospital Incident Command System (HICS), 142-143, 143t
Hospital incident commanders, 143, 143t
Hospital-acquired infection
  emergency care and, 109
  infection control and, 400-401
Hospital-acquired pneumonia, 590t
Hospitalists, 3
Host factors in infection, 398, 398t
HPV. See Human papilloma virus (HPV).
HsCRP. See Highly sensitive C-reactive protein (hsCRP).
HSV. See Herpes simplex virus (HSV).
HSV-2. See Herpes simplex virus type 2 (HSV-2).
Huber implanted ports, 195-196
Human B-type natriuretic peptides, 685, 689b
Human immune deficiency virus (HIV) infection, 326-345
  antibody tests in, 336-337
  classification of, 328, 329t
  community-based care in, 343-344, 343b-344b
  complementary and alternative therapies for, 340-341
  confusion in, 342-343, 342b
  cultural considerations in, 329b
  diarrhea in, 341-342, 342b
  drug therapy for, 332b, 338-341, 339b-340b
  endocrine complications in, 335-336
  evaluation of care of patient with, 344
  gender health considerations in, 329b
  genetic considerations in, 329b, 337b
  health care resources for, 344
  history in, 333
  HIV genotype test in, 337b
  home care management in, 343, 343b
  immune enhancement for, 340
  incidence and prevalence of, 328-329, 329b
  infection prevention in, 337-340, 338b-340b
  infectious process of, 327-328, 327f-328f
  key features of, 334b
  lymphocyte counts in, 336
  malignancies in, 334b, 335, 335f
  nutrition and, 341
  older adults and, 329b-330b
  opportunistic infections in, 328, 333-335, 334b-335b, 334f
  oxygenation enhancement in, 340
  pain management in, 340-341
  parenteral transmission of, 331-332
  perinatal transmission of, 332

Human immune deficiency virus (HIV) infection (Continued)
  progression of, 328
  psychosocial assessment in, 336
  psychosocial preparation in, 343
  self-esteem and, 343
  self-management education in, 343, 344b
  sexual transmission of, 330-331, 331f, 332b
  skin integrity and, 342
  testing for, 333-337, 333b, 337b
  transmission and health care workers, 332, 332b
  viral load testing in, 337
Human leukocyte antigens (HLAs), 276, 276f, 289
  rheumatoid arthritis and, 305b
Human papilloma virus (HPV)
  in HIV infection, 335
  testing for, 1454-1455
  vaccination for, 368-369
Human waste management after emergency event, 146
Humidification in tracheostomy care, 525
Humira. See Adalimumab.
Humoral immunity. See Antibody-mediated immunity (AMI).
Huntington disease (HD), 881-882, 881b
Hyaluronidase, 210
Hydration
  in chronic obstructive pulmonary disease, 564
  older adults and, 11, 11b
  postoperative assessment of, 262
  skin health and, 421
  in tumor lysis syndrome, 394
Hydrocele, 1516, 1516f
Hydrocephalus
  in meningitis, 864
  in stroke, 941
  traumatic brain injury and, 949-950
Hydrochlorothiazide
  for hypertension, 715b-716b
Hydrocodone, 41
Hydrocortisone, 354b
Hydrogen ions, 174-176, 175f
  carbon dioxide and, 176, 176f-177f
Hydromorphone, 41, 41t
  for postoperative pain, 269, 269b-270b
Hydronephrosis, 1397-1399, 1398f, 1399b
  in benign prostatic hyperplasia, 1500
Hydrophilic dressings, 446
Hydrophobic dressings, 446
Hydrostatic pressure, 149, 149f, 632
Hydrotherapy, 482-483
Hydroureter, 1397-1399, 1398f, 1399b, 1500

Hydroxychloroquine
  for lupus, 316
  for rheumatoid arthritis, 310b
Hydroxyurea, 802, 802b
Hygiene
  hand, 401-402, 401b-402b
  of surgical team, 242-243
Hyperactive delirium, 18
Hyperacute rejection, 286-287
Hyperaldosteronism, 1282
Hyperbaric oxygen therapy (HBOT), 447
Hypercalcemia, 169-170, 169t, 170b
  in cancer, 393
Hypercapnia, 631
  in hypokalemia, 165
Hypercarbia
  in chronic obstructive pulmonary disease, 561
  in facial trauma, 534
  oxygen therapy for, 514-515
Hypercellularity, 805
Hypercortisolism, 1276-1281
  assessment in, 1277-1278, 1277f, 1278b
  community-based care in, 1281, 1281b
  evaluation of care of patient with, 1281
  interventions in, 1278-1281, 1279b, 1281b
  pathophysiology of, 1276-1281, 1277f, 1277t
Hyperemia, 132-133, 280
Hyperesthesia, 894
Hyperextension injury of cervical spine, 892-893, 893f
Hyperflexion injury of cervical spine, 892, 893f
Hyperfunction of adrenal glands, 1276-1283
  hyperaldosteronism, 1282
  hypercortisolism, 1276-1281, 1277f, 1277t, 1278b-1279b, 1281b
  pheochromocytoma, 1282-1283, 1283b
Hyperglycemia
  absence of insulin and, 1302
  in diabetes mellitus, 1310-1324
    drug therapy for, 1310-1319, 1310b, 1312b-1313b
  in hyperthyroidism, 1285
  hypoglycemia vs., 1330t
Hyperglycemic-hyperosmolar state, 1334t, 1335-1337, 1335b-1336b, 1336f
Hyperinsulinemia, 1320
Hyperkalemia, 166-167, 166t, 167b
  in burns, 469
  in chronic kidney disease, 1420
  in diabetes mellitus, 1302-1303
  in hypovolemic shock, 743
  preoperative assessment of, 223
  surgery for diabetes mellitus and, 1325
  in tumor lysis syndrome, 394

Hyperkinetic pulse, 639
Hyperlipidemia
  atherosclerosis and, 707
  in chronic kidney disease, 1421
  diabetes mellitus and, 1300
Hypermagnesemia, 171-172, 171t
Hypernatremia, 162-163, 162t, 163b
  changes associated with aging, 1351
Hyperopia, 969, 969f, 991
Hyperosmotic fluid, 151
Hyperparathyroidism, 1296-1298, 1296t, 1297b
Hyperpharmacy, 13
Hyperphosphatemia, 171
Hyperpituitarism, 1268-1271, 1268b-1270b, 1268f
Hyperplasia, 359, 360f
Hyperresonance percussion note, 505t
Hypersensitivities, 348-356, 349t
  suppressor T-cells and, 285
  types of
    cytotoxic reactions, 355
    delayed reactions, 355-356
    immune complex reactions, 355, 355f
    rapid reactions, 348-355
      allergic rhinitis in, 349-351, 349f, 351b
      anaphylaxis in. See Anaphylaxis.
      latex allergy in, 354-355, 355b
Hypertension, 637-638, 709-718
  adherence to plan of care in, 717-718, 718b
  classifications of, 710
  complementary and alternative therapies for, 712
  concept map for, 713f
  cultural considerations in, 711b
  diagnostic assessment in, 712
  drug therapy for, 712-717, 714b-717b
  etiology and genetic risk in, 710-711, 710t, 711b
  evaluation of care of patient with, 718
  health care resources for, 718
  health promotion and maintenance in, 711, 711t
  health teaching in, 712-717
  Healthy People 2020 objectives for, 711t
  home care management in, 718
  incidence and prevalence of, 711, 711b
  lifestyle changes for, 712
  mechanisms influencing blood pressure and, 710
  physical assessment in, 711-712, 712f

Hypertension (Continued)
  in polycystic kidney disease, 1397
  psychosocial assessment in, 712
  pulmonary arterial, 569-571, 569b-571b, 570t
  renin-angiotensin II pathway and, 155
  self-management education in, 718
Hypertensive crisis, 717-718, 718b
Hyperthermia, 407b
  malignant, 246-247, 247b-248b
  managing, 409, 409b, 409t
Hyperthyroidism, 1285-1291
  assessment in, 1286-1287, 1287f, 1287t, 1288b
  nonsurgical management for, 1288-1289, 1288b-1289b
  pathophysiology of, 1285-1286, 1286b
  surgical management of, 1289-1291, 1290b-1291b
Hypertonia, 934-936
Hypertonic solutions, 151, 188
Hypertriglyceridemia, 708
Hypertrophic cardiomyopathy (HCM), 701, 701t
Hypertrophy, 359, 360f
Hyperuricemia, 319
  in Paget's disease of the bone, 1038
Hyperventilation, 178
Hyperviscosity of blood, 805
Hypervolemia, 158, 162
Hypoactive delirium, 18
Hypocalcemia, 167-169, 168b, 168f, 168t
  alkalosis and, 184
Hypocapnia, 134
Hypodermoclysis, 210
Hypoesthesia, 894
Hypofunction of adrenal glands, 1273-1276
  assessment in, 1274-1275, 1274b-1275b, 1275f
  interventions in, 1275-1276, 1276b
  pathophysiology of, 1273-1274, 1274b, 1274t
Hypogammaglobulinemia, 346
Hypoglossal nerve, 835t
Hypoglycemia
  in diabetes mellitus, 1330-1332, 1330t
    blood glucose management and, 1330-1331
    drug therapy for, 1331, 1331b
    establishing treatment plans, 1332
    hyperglycemia vs., 1330t
    nutrition therapy for, 1331, 1331b
    older adults and, 1332b
    patient and family education in, 1332
    prevention strategies, 1332

Hypokalemia, 163-165, 164b-165b, 164t
  alkalosis and, 184
  in burns, 469
  in diabetes mellitus, 1302-1303
  preoperative assessment of, 223
  surgery for diabetes mellitus and, 1325
Hypokinetic pulse, 639
Hypomagnesemia, 171, 171t
  in hypoparathyroidism, 1298
Hyponatremia, 161-162, 161t, 162b
  in burns, 469
Hypo-osmotic fluid, 151
Hypoparathyroidism, 1296t, 1298
Hypophosphatemia, 170, 170t
Hypophysis, 831
Hypopituitarism, 1266-1268, 1267b-1268b
Hypoproteinemia, 1237
Hypotension
  in hypothyroidism, 1293
  orthostatic, 638
    in dehydration, 156
  in pulmonary embolism, 609
  in total hip arthroplasty, 297t
  in traumatic brain injury, 948
Hypothalamic-hypophysial portal system, 1257
Hypothalamus, 830, 831f, 1256f-1257f, 1256t, 1257
  hormones secreted by, 1256t
Hypothermia
  after coronary artery bypass graft, 777
  environmental, 131-132, 131b-132b
Hypothyroidism, 1291-1295
  assessment in, 1292-1293
  community-based care, 1294-1295, 1294b-1295b
  evaluation of care of patient with, 1295
  interventions in, 1293-1294, 1294b
  pathophysiology of, 1291-1295, 1292b, 1292f, 1292t
Hypotonia, 934-936
Hypotonic solutions, 151, 188
Hypoventilation
  acid-base balance and, 178
  anesthesia-induced, 247
  in combined ventilatory and oxygenation failure, 721
  oxygen-induced, 515
  prevention of, during surgery, 253-254
Hypovolemia
  in dehydration, 155-156
  hyponatremia and, 162
Hypovolemic shock, 740, 741t, 742-748
  in burns, 475, 478-479, 479b, 480f
  community-based care in, 748
  concept map for, 745f
  fracture-related, 1054

Hypovolemic shock (Continued)
  health promotion and maintenance in, 744
  history in, 744
  laboratory assessment in, 746-747, 747b
  management of, 747-748, 747b-748b
  pathophysiology of, 742-744, 742f
  physical assessment in, 744-746, 744b
  psychosocial assessment in, 746
  stages of, 742-744, 743b, 743t
Hypoxemia
  in acute respiratory failure, 611
  in asthma, 552
  in chronic obstructive pulmonary disease, 558, 561
  in hypokalemia, 165
  oxygen therapy for, 514
  in pneumonia, 592-593
  postoperative, 266-267, 266b
  in pulmonary embolism, 603, 605-610, 606b-608b, 606t
  in sickle cell crisis, 800
Hypoxia, 948
  erythropoietin and, 786-787
  in near-drowning, 135
  oxygen therapy for, 514
  tracheostomy and, 526
  in vaso-occlusive event, 799
Hysterectomy
  in cervical cancer, 1495
  in uterine leiomyomas, 1489-1490, 1489t, 1490b
Hysterosalpingography, 1456
Hysteroscopy, 1458

I
IABP. See Intra-aortic balloon pump (IABP).
Iatrogenic hypoparathyroidism, 1298
IBS. See Irritable bowel syndrome (IBS).
Ibuprofen for postoperative pain, 270b
Ibutilide, 658b-662b
ICDs. See Implantable cardioverter/defibrillators (ICDs).
ICF. See Intracellular fluid (ICF).
ICH. See Intracerebral hemorrhage (ICH).
ICPs. See Infection control practitioners (ICPs).
Idiopathic hypoparathyroidism, 1298
Idiopathic pulmonary fibrosis, 571-572
Idiopathic seizures, 858
IFNs. See Interferons (IFNs).
IHI. See Institute for Healthcare Improvement (IHI).
Ileostomy, 1177
ILs. See Interleukins (ILs).
Imagery, 47

Imaging assessment
  in acute kidney injury, 1416
  in acute pancreatitis, 1221
  in adrenal insufficiency, 1275
  in Alzheimer's disease, 875
  in aneurysms, 727
  in back pain, 886-887
  in breast cancer, 1470
  in burns, 476-477
  in chronic obstructive pulmonary
    disease, 561
  in cirrhosis, 1197
  in coronary artery disease, 763
  in endocrine assessment, 1264
  in fractures, 1057
  in gastrointestinal assessment, 1093
  in head and neck cancer, 538
  in hearing assessment, 1002
  in hearing loss, 1011
  in heart failure, 684
  in hematologic assessment, 795
  in hypercortisolism, 1278
  in infection, 408
  in leukemia, 809
  in musculoskeletal assessment,
    1025-1026
  in neurologic assessment, 844-848
    cerebral angiography in, 845,
      845b
    computed tomography in,
      845-847, 846t-847t
    electroencephalography in,
      846t-847t, 849
    electromyography in, 848
    evoked potentials in, 849
    magnetic resonance imaging in,
      846t-847t, 847-848
    magnetoencephalography in,
      848
    plain x-rays in, 844-845
    positron emission tomography
      in, 846t-847t, 848
    single-photon emission
      computed tomography in,
      846t-847t, 848
    transcranial Doppler
      ultrasonography in, 850
  in osteoarthritis, 293
  in osteoporosis, 1033
  in peripheral arterial disease, 720
  preoperative, 224-225
  in pulmonary embolism, 605
  in pyelonephritis, 1400
  in renal assessment, 1360-1362,
    1360t, 1361b
  in reproductive assessment, 1456
  in respiratory assessment, 507-508
  in sickle cell disease, 801
  in spinal cord injury, 895
  in stroke, 937
  in traumatic brain injury, 953
  in urinary incontinence, 1376
  in vision assessment, 973
Imatinib mesylate, 390
Immediate memory, 839

Immobility
  complications of, 83, 83t
  in Guillain-Barré syndrome, 916
Immobilization
  of fractures, 1058-1060,
    1058f-1059f, 1059b-1060b,
    1060t
  in spinal cord injury, 897,
    897b-898b, 897f
Immune complex hypersensitivity
  reactions, 355, 355f
Immune deficiencies, 326-347
  Bruton's agammaglobulinemia, 346
  common variable immune
    deficiency, 346
  congenital, 345-346
  drug-induced, 344-345
  HIV infection and AIDS, 326-345
    antibody tests in, 336-337
    classification of, 328, 329t
    community-based care in,
      343-344, 343b-344b
    complementary and alternative
      therapies for, 340-341
    confusion in, 342-343, 342b
    cultural considerations in, 329b
    diarrhea in, 341-342, 342b
    drug therapy for, 332b, 338-341,
      339b-340b
    endocrine complications in,
      335-336
    evaluation of care of patient
      with, 344
    gender health considerations in,
      329b
    genetic considerations in, 329b,
      337b
    health care resources for, 344
    history in, 333
    HIV genotype test in, 337b
    home care management in, 343,
      343b
    immune enhancement for, 340
    incidence and prevalence of,
      328-329, 329b
    infection prevention in,
      337-340, 338b-340b
    infectious process of, 327-328,
      327f-328f
    key features of, 334b
    lymphocyte counts in, 336
    malignancies in, 334b, 335, 335f
    nutrition and, 341
    older adults and, 329b-330b
    opportunistic infections in, 328,
      333-335, 334b-335b, 334f
    oxygenation enhancement in,
      340
    pain management in, 340-341
    parenteral transmission of,
      331-332
    perinatal transmission of, 332
    progression of, 328
    psychosocial assessment in, 336
    psychosocial preparation in, 343

Immune deficiencies (Continued)
    self-esteem and, 343
    self-management education in,
      343, 344b
    sexual transmission of, 330-331,
      331f, 332b
    skin integrity and, 342
    testing for, 333-337, 333b, 337b
    transmission and health care
      workers, 332, 332b
    viral load testing in, 337
  radiation-induced, 345
  selective immunoglobulin A
    deficiency, 345-346, 346b
  therapy-induced, 344-345
Immune enhancement in acquired
  immune deficiency syndrome,
  340
Immune function
  aging and, 276, 277b, 289,
    418b-419b
  assessment after burn injury, 481,
    482t
  cancer development and, 367
Immune response
  aging-related changes in, 277b
  self versus non-self and, 276, 276f
Immune system, 275, 326
  aging-related changes in, 276,
    277b
  changes resulting from burns, 470
  older adults and, 398b
  organization of, 276-277,
    277f-278f, 278t
  recognition of self versus non-self
    proteins and cells, 276, 276f
Immunity, 275, 281-287, 282f, 326
  antibody-mediated, 281-285, 282f,
    400
    acquiring of, 284-285, 289
    age-related changes in, 276,
      277b
    antigen-antibody interactions
      in, 281-284, 283f
    immune functions of leukocytes
      in, 278t
    role of leukocytes in, 787t
  cancer and, 372
  cell-mediated, 285-286, 400
    age-related changes in, 277b
    cell types involved in, 285-286
    cytokines and, 286, 286t
    immune functions of leukocytes
      in, 278t
    protection provided by, 286
    role of leukocytes in, 787t
  infection risk and, 398, 398t
  purpose of, 274-276
  transplant rejection and, 286-287,
    289
    acute, 287
    chronic, 287
    hyperacute, 286-287
    management of, 287, 287b-288b
Immunocompetence, 275, 278f, 289

Immunoglobulin A (IgA), 284, 284t
  selective immunoglobulin A
    deficiency and, 345-346, 346b
Immunoglobulin D (IgD), 284, 284t
Immunoglobulin E (IgE), 284, 284t
Immunoglobulin G (IgG), 284, 284t
Immunoglobulin M (IgM), 284, 284t
Immunoglobulins, 284, 284t
Immunohemolytic anemia, 803-804
Immunologic kidney disorders,
  1401-1405, 1402t
  acute glomerulonephritis,
    1397-1399, 1402t, 1403b
  chronic glomerulonephritis,
    1403-1404
  interstitial and tubulointerstitial,
    1405
  nephrotic syndrome, 1404-1405,
    1404b
  rapidly progressive
    glomerulonephritis, 1403
Immunosuppressants
  for kidney transplantation, 1444
  for lupus, 316, 316b
  for myasthenia gravis, 920
  to prevent transplant rejection,
    287, 287b-288b, 289
  for rheumatoid arthritis, 311
Immunotherapy in cancer, 387-388,
  387t
Implantable cardioverter/
  defibrillators (ICDs), 673-675,
  675b
Implanted ports, 195-196, 195f-196f,
  196b
IMRT. See Intensity modulated
  radiation therapy (IMRT).
Imuran. See Azathioprine.
Inactivation process in immunity,
  284
INCC. See Infusion Nurses
  Certification Corporation
  (INCC).
Incentive spirometry
  in pneumonia, 593
  to prevent postoperative
    respiratory complications,
    230, 231f
Incisional hernias, 1147
Incomplete fractures, 1051
Incomplete spinal cord injury, 892
Incontinence. See Urinary
  incontinence.
Increased intracranial pressure
  in stroke, 939-941, 939b, 941b
  in traumatic brain injury, 948-949
Incretin mimetics, 1312b-1313b,
  1313
Incus, 996-997, 997f
Indacaterol, 539b
Independent living skills,
  rehabilitation and, 79
Inderal. See Propranolol.
Indirect contact transmission,
  399-400

Indirect inguinal hernias, 1146-1147
Inducer T-cells, 285
Induration, 596, 596f
Indwelling urinary catheters, 399, 405
Infection, 397-414
    acute hematogenous, 1040
    after burns, 481, 482t, 485, 485b-486b
    allergic reactions to antibiotics and, 409b, 409t
    bioterrorism and, 411-413, 411t
    burn-related, 481, 482t
    in chronic obstructive pulmonary disease, 558, 565-566
    in Coccidioidomycosis, 600-601
    community-based care in, 410
    control and prevention. See Infection control and prevention.
    in cornea, 980-981
    emerging, 411-413, 412t
    in encephalitis, 865-867, 866b
    evaluation of care of patient with, 411
    fever in, 409, 409b, 409t
    fracture and, 1054-1055
    health care resources for, 410
    health teaching in, 410
    history in, 407
    home care management in, 410
    human immune deficiency virus (HIV) infection. See Human immune deficiency virus (HIV) infection.
    imaging assessment in, 408
    inadequate antimicrobial therapy and, 407-411
    in infective endocarditis, 697-699, 697b, 699b
    inflammation in, 278
    in influenza
        pandemic, 587-588
        seasonal, 586-587
    in inhalation anthrax, 599-600, 599b-600b
    laboratory assessment in, 408
    in lung abscesses, 599
    mechanical ventilation-related, 621
    in meningitis, 863-867, 863b-865b, 864t
    multidrug-resistant organisms and, 403, 405-406
        carbapenem-resistant Enterobacteriaceae, 406
        methicillin-resistant Staphylococcus aureus, 403, 405-406, 406b, 451
        vancomycin-resistant Enterococcus, 403, 406
    occupational exposure to, 406-407, 407b
    older adults and, 398, 398b, 407b
    opportunistic, 328, 333-335, 334b-335b, 334f

Infection (Continued)
    oxygen therapy-related, 516, 516b
    pandemics, 413
    in peritonsillar abscesses, 586
    in pertussis, 600
    in pharyngitis, 584-586, 585b-586b, 585t
    physical assessment in, 407-408
    physiologic defenses against, 400
    in pneumonia. See Pneumonia.
    psychosocial assessment in, 408
    in pulmonary empyema, 599
    in pyelonephritis, 1372b, 1399-1401, 1399f, 1400b
    respiratory, 583-602
        COPD and, 558, 565-566
    in rheumatic carditis, 700-701
    in rhinitis, 583-584, 584b
    in rhinosinusitis, 584
    in septic shock, 749, 749f
    in severe acute respiratory syndrome, 594-595, 595b
    sexually transmitted. See Sexually transmitted diseases (STDs).
    skin, 449-453, 450b
        in anthrax, 453, 453b, 454f
        bacterial, 450-451, 450b, 451f
        fungal, 450b, 451-452
        history in, 452-453
        interventions in, 452-453, 452b
        laboratory assessment in, 452
        physical assessment in, 450b, 452
        prevention of, 452, 452b
        viral, 450b, 451, 451f
    social isolation and, 410
    in tonsillitis, 586, 586b
    tracheostomy-related, 523b, 526, 527b
    transmission of infectious agents in, 398b-399b, 398t, 406-407
    in tuberculosis, 595-599
        in AIDS, 334-335
        diagnosis of, 596, 596f
        directly observed therapy for, 407
        drug therapy for, 596-598, 597b-598b
        health care resources for, 599
        history in, 596
        home care management in, 598
        pathophysiology of, 595-596, 595f
            etiology of, 595
            incidence and prevalence of, 596
        physical assessment in, 596
        self-management education in, 598-599
    urinary tract. See Urinary tract infections (UTIs).
    wound
        drug therapy for, 268
        prevention of, 267-269, 267b-269b, 267f

Infection control and prevention, 400-405, 401b
    in acquired immune deficiency syndrome, 337-340, 338b-340b
    after burns, 485, 485b-486b
    during chemotherapy, 382b
    in chronic kidney disease, 1428-1430
    in chronic obstructive pulmonary disease, 565-566
    in fractures, 1064, 1064b
    in health care settings, 400-401
    in hypercortisolism, 1280-1281
    during intraoperative care, 253, 254f
    in leukemia, 809-814, 809b-813b, 811t, 812f-813f, 816b
    methods of, 401-402
        hand hygiene, 401-402, 401b-402b
        staff and patient placement and cohorting, 403-405
        Standard Precautions, 402-403, 402b, 403t, 404f
        sterilization and disinfection, 402
        transmission-based precautions, 403, 404t
    in pressure ulcers, 447, 448b
    in sickle cell disease, 802-803
    social isolation and, 410
    in total hip arthroplasty, 297t, 299, 299b
    in urolithiasis, 1387
Infection control practitioners (ICPs), 397-398
Infectious arthritis, 320
Infective endocarditis, 697-699, 697b, 699b
Inferior oblique muscle, 968f, 969t
Inferior rectus muscle, 968f, 969t
Inferior vena cava filtration
    in pulmonary embolism, 608-609
    in venous thromboembolism, 733
Inferior wall myocardial infarction (IWMI), 760
Infiltrating ductal carcinoma, 1464-1465
Infiltration, intravenous therapy-related, 188, 204t-206t
Infiltration scale, 209t
Inflammation, 275, 277-281, 279f
    after burns, 470
    age-related changes in, 277b
    in asthma, 550
    basophils in, 279-280
    in dark skinned patient, 428, 428b
    as defense against infection, 400
    eosinophils in, 280
    in gout, 319
    macrophages in, 279, 279t, 281
    neutrophils in, 278-279, 279f, 279t, 281

Inflammation (Continued)
    in pericarditis, 699-700, 700b
    phagocytosis and, 280, 280f
    in pharyngitis, 584
    purpose of, 275-276
    in rheumatoid arthritis, 308-312, 308b-310b
    sequence of, 280-281
    skin, 455-456, 455b-456b
    tissue mast cells in, 280
    in tonsillitis, 586
    in urethra, 1373
Inflammatory breast cancer, 1465
Inflammatory intestinal disorders, 1168-1191
    acute inflammatory bowel disorders, 1168-1173
        appendicitis, 1168-1170, 1169b, 1169f
        gastroenteritis, 1172-1173, 1172t, 1173b
        peritonitis, 1170-1172, 1170b-1171b
    anal fissure, 1188-1189
    anal fistula, 1189
    anorectal abscesses, 1188, 1188b
    celiac disease, 1188, 1188b
    chronic inflammatory bowel disease
        Crohn's disease. See Crohn's disease.
        ulcerative colitis. See Ulcerative colitis.
    diverticular disease, 1186-1188, 1186b-1187b, 1186f
    health promotion and maintenance in, 1191
Inflammatory phase of healing, 433, 433t
Infliximab
    for psoriasis, 458b
    for rheumatoid arthritis, 309b-310b, 310
Inflow disease, 720
Influenza
    pandemic, 413, 587-588
    seasonal, 586-587
Informatics, 7-8, 7f
Informed consent
    surgical, 226, 226b, 227f, 228b, 250b
Infratentorial brain tumors, 958
Infusate, 188
Infusion nurses, 188
Infusion Nurses Certification Corporation (INCC), 188
Infusion Nurses Society (INS), 188
Infusion pressure, 202
Infusion systems, 196-200
    administration sets in, 197-198, 197f-198f
    containers in, 196-197, 197b
    rate-controlling infusion devices in, 198-200, 199f

Infusion therapy, 187-214
  blood and blood components in, 188-189, 189f
  blood pressure measurement and, 200b
  central, 193-196
    hemodialysis catheters in, 196
    implanted ports in, 195-196, 195f-196f, 196b
    nontunneled percutaneous central venous catheters in, 194-195, 194f
    peripherally inserted central catheters in, 193-194, 193f, 194b
    tunneled central venous catheters in, 195, 195f
  changing administration sets and needleless connectors in, 202
  complications of, 204-207
    catheter-related bloodstream infections, 204, 204t
    infiltration scale and, 209t
    insertion-related, 208t
    local, 204-207, 204t-206t
    phlebitis scale and, 209t
    systemic, 204-207, 207t
  controlling infusion pressure in, 202
  documentation of, 203
  extravasation in, 188b
  flushing catheters in, 202, 202b
  infusion systems in, 196-200
    administration sets in, 197-198, 197f-198f
    containers in, 196-197, 197b
    rate-controlling infusion devices in, 198-200, 199f
  intra-arterial, 212, 212b
  intraosseous, 211-212, 211f, 214
  intraperitoneal, 212, 214
  intraspinal, 212-213
  intravenous drugs and, 189, 189b
  intravenous solutions for, 188
  nursing assessment in, 200
  obtaining blood samples from central venous catheters in, 202-203, 203f
  older adults and, 207-210
    cardiac and renal status changes and, 209-210
    catheter securement and, 209b, 210f
    skin care in, 207-209
    vein and catheter selection in, 209
  patient education in, 200
  peripheral, 190-193
    midline catheters in, 192-193, 192f
    short peripheral catheters in, 190-192, 190f-192f, 190t, 191b
  prescribing of, 189, 189b

Infusion therapy (Continued)
  removal of vascular access device and, 203
  securing and dressing the catheter in, 200-201, 201b
  subcutaneous, 210-211
  vascular access devices in, 189-190
INH. See Isoniazid.
Inhalation anthrax, 599-600, 599b-600b
Inhalation burn injuries, 470
Inhalers
  for asthma, 540b-541b, 543b
  for chronic obstructive pulmonary disease, 564
Inheritance patterns, 56-59
  autosomal dominant, 57-58, 57t
  autosomal recessive, 57t, 58, 58f
  complex inheritance and familial clustering and, 57t, 59
  pedigree and, 57, 57f, 57t
  sex-linked recessive, 57t, 58-59, 59f
Injury prevention
  after spinal cord injury, 896-898, 897b-898b, 897f
  in Alzheimer's disease, 878-879, 878b, 879t
  during chemotherapy, 383b
  in chronic kidney disease, 1428-1430, 1429b
  in hypercortisolism, 1280
  in hypocalcemia, 169
  during intraoperative care, 252-253, 252f, 253b
  in leukemia, 814, 814b
Innate-native immunity, 277
Inner ear problems, 1007-1009
  acoustic neuromas, 1009
  labyrinthitis, 1008
  Ménière's disease, 1008
  tinnitus, 1007-1008
  vertigo and dizziness, 1008
Inotropic drugs
  for heart failure, 686-687
  for hypovolemic shock, 748b
Inpatient rehabilitation facilities (IRFs), 75
Inpatient surgery, 218
INR. See International normalized ratio (INR).
INS. See Infusion Nurses Society (INS).
Insensible water loss, 153
Inspection
  in cardiovascular assessment, 639, 639f
  in endocrine assessment, 1262
  of eyes, 972
  in gastrointestinal assessment, 1090, 1090b
  of skin, 421-424, 422t, 423f-424f, 424b

Institute for Healthcare Improvement (IHI)
  on health care errors in hospitals, 2
Institute of Medicine (IOM)
  on competencies to ensure patient safety and quality care, 3
  development of Dietary Reference Intakes, 1232-1233
  on patient deaths from preventable errors, 2
  on use of and evidence-based practice approach to practice, 64
Instrumental activities of daily living rehabilitation and, 79
Insufflation, 242
Insulin, 55-56
  absence in diabetes mellitus, 1302-1303, 1302t
Insulin sensitizers, 1310, 1312b
Insulin therapy, 1313-1319
  alternative methods of insulin administration in, 1315-1316, 1316f
  complications of, 1315, 1315f
  factors influencing absorption in, 1314-1315, 1314f, 1315b
  mixing of insulins in, 1315, 1315b
  patient education in, 1316-1317, 1316b, 1317f
  regimens in, 1313-1314
  subcutaneous administration of, 1316b
  types of insulin in, 1313, 1314t
Integrase inhibitors, 339b
Integumentary assessment, 415-431
  common alterations in skin color and, 422t
  family history and genetic risk in, 421
  hair assessment in, 424-425
  history in, 420, 420b
  inspection of skin in, 421-424, 422t, 423f-424f, 424b
  laboratory assessment in, 429
  nail assessment in, 425-427, 426f, 426t-427t
  nutrition status in, 420-421
  palpation of skin in, 424, 424b, 425t
  patients with darker skin and, 427b-428b, 428
  psychosocial assessment in, 428
  skin lesions and, 421, 422t, 423f
Integumentary system. See also Skin.
  acidosis and, 181b
  complications of immobility and, 83t
  older adults and, 398b, 418b-419b
  structure of skin appendages, 417, 417f
Intensity modulated radiation therapy (IMRT), 375

Intensivists, 3
Intention tremor, 905
Interbody cage fusion, 888-889
Intercostal retraction, 613
Intercostal space, 504
Interdisciplinary teams in emergency care, 106-108, 107f
Interferons (IFNs), 387
Interleukins (ILs), 387
Intermittent administration sets, 197
Intermittent catheterization, 86
Intermittent claudication
  cardiovascular assessment and, 636
  in peripheral arterial disease, 719
Intermittent renal replacement therapy, 1418
Internal carotid artery strokes, 934b
Internal derangement of knee, 1076
Internal disasters, 138-139
Internal fixation of fractures, 1062
Internal genitalia
  female, 1450, 1450f
  male, 1451, 1451f
Internal hemorrhoids, 1164, 1164f
Internal urethral sphincter, 1350
International Medical Surgical Response Teams, 142
International normalized ratio (INR), 608b, 795
  perioperative assessment of, 223b-224b
International Prostate Symptom Score (I-PSS), 1500, 1501f-1502f
International Society of Blood Transfusion (ISBT) universal bar-coding system, 188, 189f
Interrupted sutures, 254f
Interstitial cystitis, 1367-1368
Interstitial fluid, 148
Interstitial immunologic renal disease, 1405
Interstitial laser coagulation, 1503
Interstitial pulmonary diseases, 571-572
Interventional radiologic procedures, 1137
Interventional radiology, 1044
Intestinal disorders
  abdominal trauma, 1161-1163, 1162b
  acute inflammatory bowel disorders, 1168-1173
    appendicitis, 1168-1170, 1169b, 1169f
    gastroenteritis, 1172-1173, 1172t, 1173b
    peritonitis, 1170-1172, 1170b-1171b
  anal fissure, 1188-1189
  anal fistula, 1189
  anorectal abscesses, 1188, 1188b
  celiac disease, 1188, 1188b
  chronic inflammatory bowel disease

Intestinal disorders (Continued)
Crohn's disease. See Crohn's disease.
ulcerative colitis. See Ulcerative colitis.
colorectal cancer. See Colorectal cancer.
diverticular disease, 1186-1188, 1186b-1187b, 1186f
hemorrhoids, 1164-1165, 1164f, 1165b
herniation, 1146-1148, 1146f, 1148b
intestinal obstructions, 1157-1161, 1158f, 1159b, 1161b
intestinal polyps, 1163-1164
irritable bowel syndrome, 1144-1146, 1145f, 1146b
malabsorption syndrome, 1165-1166, 1166b
parasitic infections, 1189-1190, 1190b
Intestinal obstructions, 1157-1161, 1158f, 1159b, 1161b
Intestinal peristalsis, postoperative, 262, 263b
Intestinal polyps, 1163-1164
Intestinal preparation, preoperative, 228
Intra-abdominal pressure monitoring, 1163
Intra-aortic balloon pump (IABP), 772
Intra-arterial chemotherapy, 378
Intra-arterial infusion therapy, 212, 212b
Intracellular fluid (ICF), 148
dehydration and, 155-156, 155f
electrolytes in, 160, 160f
sodium in, 161
Intracerebral hemorrhage (ICH), 932, 949, 949f
Intracranial pressure, increased
stroke and, 939-941, 939b, 941b
traumatic brain injury and, 948-949
Intradermal testing, 350
Intraductal papilloma, 1462t, 1463
Intramedullary tumors, 902
Intramural leiomyomas, 1487
Intraocular pressure, 967
Intraoperative care, 238-255
anesthesia and, 244-249, 246t
general, 245-248, 246t, 247b-248b
local or regional, 248-249, 248f-249f, 248t
moderate sedation, 249, 250t
evaluation of, 254
history and, 250, 250b
hypoventilation prevention and, 253-254
identification of patient, procedure, and surgical side/sites, and fire risk assessment, 240f

Intraoperative care (Continued)
infection prevention and, 253, 254f
injury prevention and, 252-253, 252f, 253b
medical record review and, 250-251, 250b-251b
older adults and, 251b
in surgery for diabetes mellitus, 1324
surgical suite preparation and team safety in, 241-244
health and hygiene of surgical team and, 242-243
layout of suite and, 241-242, 241f
minimally invasive and robotic surgery and, 242, 242f-243f
surgical attire and, 243, 244f
surgical scrub and, 243-244, 244b, 245f
surgical team members and, 238-241, 241f
Intraosseous infusion therapy, 211-212, 211f, 214
Intraperitoneal chemotherapy, 378
Intraperitoneal infusion therapy, 212, 214
Intrapulmonary ventilatory failure, 611, 611t
Intraspinal analgesia, 42-43, 42b, 50
Intraspinal infusion therapy, 212-213
Intrathecal analgesia, 42, 50
in spinal fusion, 888
Intrathecal chemotherapy, 378
Intrathecal infusion, 214
Intravascular ultrasonography (IVUS), 644
Intravenous drugs, 189, 189b
Intravenous fibrinolytic therapy, 938
Intravenous solutions, 188
Intravenous therapy, 187-214
blood and blood components in, 188-189, 189f
blood pressure measurement and, 200b
central, 193-196
hemodialysis catheters in, 196
implanted ports in, 195-196, 195f-196f, 196b
nontunneled percutaneous central venous catheters in, 194-195, 194f
peripherally inserted central catheters in, 193-194, 193f, 194b
tunneled central venous catheters in, 195, 195f
changing administration sets and needleless connectors in, 202
complications of, 204-207
catheter-related bloodstream infections, 204, 204t
infiltration scale and, 209t
insertion-related, 208t

Intravenous therapy (Continued)
local, 204-207, 204t-206t
phlebitis scale and, 209t
systemic, 204-207, 207t
controlling infusion pressure in, 202
for dehydration, 157-158, 158t
documentation of, 203
extravasation in, 188b
flushing catheters in, 202, 202b
infusion systems in, 196-200
administration sets in, 197-198, 197f-198f
containers in, 196-197, 197b
rate-controlling infusion devices in, 198-200, 199f
intravenous drugs and, 189, 189b
intravenous solutions for, 188
nursing assessment in, 200
obtaining blood samples from central venous catheters in, 202-203, 203f
older adults and, 207-210
cardiac and renal status changes and, 209-210
catheter securement and, 209b, 210f
skin care in, 207-209
vein and catheter selection in, 209
patient education in, 200
peripheral, 190-193
midline catheters in, 192-193, 192f
short peripheral catheters in, 190-192, 190f-192f, 190t, 191b
postoperative assessment of, 262
prescribing of, 189, 189b
for pulmonary embolism, 609
removal of vascular access device and, 203
securing and dressing the catheter in, 200-201, 201b
vascular access devices in, 189-190
Intraventricular catheters, 956t
Intraventricular chemotherapy, 378
Intravesicular chemotherapy, 378
Intrinsic factors, 788, 789f, 804
Intropin. See Dopamine.
Intubation
complications during intraoperative period, 247-248
endotracheal, 615-616, 615b-616b, 615f
in upper airway obstruction, 536
Intussusception, 1158, 1158f
Invasive breast cancers, 1464-1465, 1464f-1465f
Invasive hemodynamic monitoring, 684
Inverse square law of radiation exposure, 374-375
Involuntary active euthanasia, 103t

IOM. See Institute of Medicine (IOM).
Ions, 160
Iontophoresis, 887, 1063
Iowa model of evidence-based practice, 68
Ipratropium, 539b
I-PSS. See International Prostate Symptom Score (I-PSS).
IRFs. See Inpatient rehabilitation facilities (IRFs).
Iris, 966, 967f
arcus senilis of, 417f
changes with aging, 970b
Iron deficiency anemia, 799t
Irregular bones, 1017-1018
Irrigation, ocular, 991b
Irritability, 162
Irritable bowel syndrome (IBS), 1144-1146, 1145f, 1146b
Irritant-induced asthma, 573b
ISBT universal bar-coding system. See International Society of Blood Transfusion (ISBT) universal bar-coding system.
Ischemia
myocardial, 757
in pressure ulcers, 443
Ischemic heart disease, 673b
Ischemic stroke, 931-932, 931f, 932t
Islam, end of life and death rituals in, 100t
Islet cell transplantation, 1324
Isoelectric line, 650-651
Isolation precautions, 403, 404t
Isolation therapy, 485
Isoniazid, 596-597, 597b
Isoproterenol, 354b
Isoptin. See Verapamil.
Isosmotic fluid, 151
Isosorbide dinitrate, 765b-766b
Isosorbide mononitrate, 765b-766b
Isotonic infusate, 188
Isotonic solutions, 151, 188
Isuprel. See Isoproterenol.
Itching. See Pruritus.
Itch-scratch-itch cycle, 433
IVUS. See Intravascular ultrasonography (IVUS).
IWMI. See Inferior wall myocardial infarction (IWMI).

J
Jackson-Pratt drains, 264, 265f, 268
Jaundice
in cholecystitis, 1214
in cirrhosis, 1193, 1194f
in dark skinned patient, 428, 428b
in hepatitis, 1203
Jejunostomy, 1241
in Whipple procedure, 1228
Joint Commission, The (TJC)
on assessing for pressure ulcers risk, 437-438
Core Measures and, 6

Joint Commission, The (TJC) (Continued)
  on creating a safe, welcoming environment for LGBT patients, 1522, 1522b
  on informed consent, 225-226
  on marking of surgical site, 226
  on mechanical ventilation and neuromuscular blockers, 478b
  on pain assessment, 264
  on patient identification, 250, 250b, 510b
  patient safety and, 2, 8, 108, 189
  Speak-Up campaign and, 4
  Surgical Care Improvement Project of, 216, 217t, 260
  on use of physical restraints in hospitals and nursing homes, 21
Joint disorders. See Connective tissue diseases (CTDs).
Joint effusions, 292-293
Joints, 1019, 1019f
  dislocation of, 1079
Judaism, end of life and death rituals in, 100t
Jugular venous distention (JVD), 392b, 638
Juxtaglomerular complex, 1346, 1346f
JVD. See Jugular venous distention (JVD).

K

Kaposi's sarcoma, 335, 335f, 342
Karyotype, 54, 54f
Kegel exercises, 1377, 1377b
Keratin, 416-417
Keratinocytes, 416
Keratoconjunctivitis sicca, 978
Keratoconus, 981-982, 981f, 982t
Keratoses, actinic, 458, 459t
Ketoconazole, 717b
Ketogenesis, 1301-1302
Ketone bodies, 1302
Ketorolac, 270b
Kidney, ureter, and bladder (KUB) x-rays, 1360, 1360t
Kidney biopsy, 1363
Kidney compensation, 179
Kidney disorders, 1394, 1395f
  acute kidney injury. See Acute kidney injury (AKI).
  chronic kidney disease. See Chronic kidney disease (CKD).
  degenerative, 1405-1406
    diabetic nephropathy, 1306, 1406
    nephrosclerosis, 1405, 1405b
    renovascular disease, 1405-1406, 1405b
  in diabetes mellitus, 1329-1330
  health promotion and maintenance in, 1410

Kidney disorders (Continued)
  hydronephrosis, hydroureter, and urethral stricture, 1397-1399, 1398f, 1399b
  immunologic, 1401-1405, 1402t
    acute glomerulonephritis, 1397-1399, 1402t, 1403b
    chronic glomerulonephritis, 1403-1404
    interstitial and tubulointerstitial, 1405
    nephrotic syndrome, 1404-1405, 1404b
    rapidly progressive glomerulonephritis, 1403
  kidney trauma, 1408-1409, 1408b-1409b
  polycystic kidney disease, 1394-1397, 1395f-1396f, 1396b-1397b
  pyelonephritis, 1372b, 1399-1401, 1399f, 1400b
  renal cell carcinoma, 1406-1408, 1407t
Kidney stones. See Urolithiasis.
Kidney transplantation, 1441-1444
  candidate selection criteria in, 1441
  complications of, 1443-1444, 1444t
  donors in, 1441-1442, 1442f
  immunosuppressive drug therapy in, 1444
  operative procedures in, 1442, 1443t
  postoperative care in, 1442-1443
  preoperative care in, 1442
Kidneys
  in acid-base balance, 178-179, 178t
  assessment of, 1346f, 1353-1354
  burn injury and, 475-476
  changes associated with aging, 1351, 1351b
  changes in chronic kidney disease, 1420
  dehydration and, 157
  function of, 1342, 1344, 1346-1350, 1348t-1349t, 1349b, 1349f, 1394
  hematologic assessment and, 792-793
  hormonal functions of, 1349-1350, 1349t
  hypovolemic shock and, 746
  postoperative assessment of, 262
  potential complications of surgery and, 258t
  preoperative assessment of, 221-222
  structure of, 1345-1346, 1345f-1347f
  trauma to, 1408-1409, 1408b-1409b
Killer bees, 128
Killip classification of heart failure, 771, 771t
Kineret. See Anakinra.

Knee height calipers, 1234-1236
Knee immobilizer, 1076f
Knee injuries, 1075-1077, 1076b, 1076f
Knees, 300-302, 301f, 302b
Knock-knee deformity, 1023
Knowledge, skills, and attitudes (KSAs), 3, 3t
KSAs. See Knowledge, skills, and attitudes (KSAs).
KUB x-rays. See Kidney, ureter, and bladder (KUB) x-rays.
Kupffer cells, 1086
Kussmaul respiration
  in acidosis, 181
  in chronic kidney disease, 1420
  in diabetes mellitus, 1302
  in diabetic ketoacidosis, 1333
Kwashiorkor, 1236
Kyphoplasty, 1069, 1070b
Kytril. See Granisetron.

L

LABA. See Long-acting beta$_2$ agonists (LABA).
Labia majora, 1449-1450
Labia minora, 1450
Laboratory assessment
  in acid-base assessment, 177b
  in acidosis, 182-183, 182b, 182f
  in acute glomerulonephritis, 1403
  in acute kidney injury, 1415-1416, 1415b
  in allergic rhinitis, 350
  in Alzheimer's disease, 875
  in asthma, 532
  in atherosclerosis, 708
  in benign prostatic hyperplasia, 1500
  in breast cancer, 1470
  in burns, 476, 476b-477b
  in cardiovascular assessment, 640-642, 641b
  in chronic kidney disease, 1424
  in chronic obstructive pulmonary disease, 561
  in cirrhosis, 1196-1197, 1197t
  in colorectal cancer, 1151
  in coronary artery disease, 763
  in cystitis, 1369-1370
  in dehydration, 157
  in diabetes mellitus, 1308-1309, 1308b, 1308t-1309t
  in endocrine assessment, 1263-1264, 1263b
  in endometrial cancer, 1492
  in fractures, 1057
  in gastrointestinal assessment, 1091-1093, 1092b
  in head and neck cancer, 538
  in hearing assessment, 1002
  in hearing loss, 1011
  in heart failure, 683-684, 683b
  in hematologic assessment, 793-796, 794b

Laboratory assessment (Continued)
  in hepatitis, 1205-1206
  in HIV infection and AIDS, 336-337, 337b
  in hypercortisolism, 1278
  in hyperthyroidism, 1287, 1288b
  in hypothyroidism, 1293
  in hypovolemic shock, 746-747, 747b
  in infection, 408
  in integumentary assessment, 429
  intraoperative care and, 251
  in leukemia, 808-809, 808f
  in lupus, 315
  in malnutrition, 1238-1239
  in multiple sclerosis, 906
  in musculoskeletal assessment, 1024-1025, 1024b
  in neurologic assessment, 844
  in osteoarthritis, 293
  in osteoporosis, 1032-1033
  in pelvic inflammatory disease, 1542
  in peptic ulcer disease, 1132
  in pneumonia, 592, 592f
  postoperative, 265-266
  preoperative, 223, 223b-224b, 236
  in pressure ulcers, 444
  in prostate cancer, 1508
  in pulmonary embolism, 605
  in pyelonephritis, 1400
  in renal assessment, 1354-1360
    bedside sonography and bladder scan in, 1359-1360, 1359f
    blood tests in, 1354-1355, 1354b-1355b
    urine tests in, 1355-1359, 1356b, 1357t, 1359b
  in reproductive assessment, 1454-1459, 1455b
  in respiratory assessment, 507, 508b
  in rheumatoid arthritis, 307, 307b
  in sepsis and septic shock, 753
  in sickle cell disease, 801
  in skin infections, 452
  in spinal cord injury, 895
  in stroke, 937
  in systemic sclerosis, 318
  in testicular cancer, 1514
  in traumatic brain injury, 953
  in ulcerative colitis, 1175
  in urinary incontinence, 1376
  in vision assessment, 973
Labyrinthitis, 1008
Lacerations
  of cerebral cortex, 947
  ocular, 992, 992b
Lacrimal gland, 967, 968f
Lactate, 177b
Lactic acidosis, 180
Lacto-ovo-vegetarians, 1233
Lactose intolerance, 1233b
Lacto-vegetarians, 1233
Lanoxin. See Digoxin.

Laparoscopic cholecystectomy, 1217, 1217b
Laparoscopic Nissen fundoplication (LNF), 1116b
Laparoscopic radical prostatectomy, 1509
Laparoscopy
  in appendicitis, 1175
  in reproductive assessment, 1457-1458, 1457f
Laparotomy, 1160-1161
Large intestine, 1087
Laryngectomy, 541t
  home care management in, 544, 544b-545b
Laryngofissure, 541t
Laryngopharynx, 497, 497f
Larynx, 497-498, 498f
  cancer of. See Head and neck cancer.
  changes with aging, 501b
  physical assessment of, 503
  trauma to, 536, 536b
  vocal cord paralysis and, 535, 535b
Laser imaging of retina and optic nerve, 975
Laser-assisted laparoscopic lumbar diskectomy, 888
Late adulthood, 9-10
Latency period in carcinogenesis, 362
Lateral position during surgery, 252-253, 252f
Lateral rectus muscle, 968f, 969t
Latex allergies, 251, 354-355, 355b, 402-403
Latrodectism, 127
Laundry, standard precautions and, 403t
Laxatives, 88
Layout of surgical suites, 241-242, 241f
LCIS. See Lobular carcinoma in situ (LCIS).
LDLs. See Low-density lipoproteins (LDLs).
Le Fort fractures, 534
LEAD. See Lower extremity arterial disease (LEAD).
Lead axis, 650-651
Lead systems in electrocardiography, 650-652, 651t
Leave-of-absence visit, 89
LEEP procedure, 1495
Leflunomide, 308-310
Left atrium, 628, 629f
Left shift, 279
Left-sided heart failure, 679
  history in, 682
  physical assessment in, 682-683, 682b
Left ventricle, 633b
Left ventricular failure, 770-772, 770b, 771f, 771t, 772b-773b
Legally competent, definition of, 16

Legs
  positioning to prevent contractures, 487b
  postoperative exercises for, 231b, 232
Leiomyomas, uterine, 1487-1491, 1488f, 1489b-1490b, 1489t
Lens, 967, 967f
  changes with aging, 970b
Lesbian, gay, bisexual, transgender, and queer and/or questioning (LGBTQ) population, 1519. See also Transgender patients.
  breast cancer and, 1470b
  osteoarthritis and, 291b
  patient-centered care for, 20b
  smoking and, 495b
  special needs of, 4, 5t, 8
  terminology associated with transgender health of, 1520t
Lesions, 421, 422t
  around nails, 427
  classification of, 423f
Leukemia, 806-817
  conserving energy in, 814, 815b
  drug therapy for, 810-811
  evaluation of care of patient with, 817
  health care resources for, 816
  history in, 807-808
  home care management in, 815
  imaging assessment in, 809
  infection prevention in, 809-814, 809b-813b, 811t, 812f-813f
  injury prevention in, 814, 814b
  laboratory assessment in, 808-809, 808f
  older adults and, 367b
  pathophysiology of, 806-807
    etiology and genetic risk in, 807
    incidence and prevalence of, 807, 807t
  physical assessment, 808, 808b
  psychosocial assessment in, 808
  psychosocial preparation for, 815-816
  risk for bleeding in, 816b
  self-management education in, 815, 815b-816b
Leukine. See Sargramostim.
Leukocyte count. See White blood cell (WBC) count.
Leukocytes. See White blood cells (WBCs).
Leukoesterase in urine, 1357-1358
Leukopenia, 805
Leukoplakia, 538
Leukotriene antagonists, 351
Leukotriene modifiers, 539b, 556
Level I trauma centers, 115, 115t
Level II trauma centers, 115, 115t
Level III trauma centers, 115-116, 115t
Level IV trauma centers, 115-116, 115t

Level of consciousness in neurologic assessment, 838, 838b
Levels of evidence (LOE), 66-67, 66f, 67t
Levodopa-carbidopa, 869
Levophed. See Norepinephrine.
LGBTQ population. See Lesbian, gay, bisexual, transgender, and queer and/or questioning (LGBTQ) population.
Libido, 1452
Lice, 403, 425, 453-454
Lichenifications, 421, 423f
Lichtenberg figures, 130
Lidocaine, 658b-662b
  for pain management, 45
Life review at end of life, 101
Lifestyle changes
  after amputation, 1073-1074
  after spinal cord injury, 900
  for gout, 320
  for hypertension, 712
  for osteoporosis, 1033
  to promote wellness, 10b
Ligaments, 1020
Light reflex, 1001
Light therapy for psoriasis, 457
Lightning injuries, 129-131, 130b
Limb leads, 651
Limbic lobe, 831t
Limited cutaneous systemic sclerosis, 317
Linear lesions, 422t
Linear nail pigmentation, 426f
Lipids, 707
Lipoatrophy, 335-336
  insulin injection-related, 1315
Lipodystrophy, 335-336
Lipolysis, 1302
Liposuction, 462t, 1250
Liquid oxygen, 521, 521f
Lithotomy position during surgery, 252-253, 252f
Lithotripsy, 1386
Liver, 1086-1087
  as accessory organ of blood formation, 787
  acetaminophen and, 293b
Liver biopsy, 1206
Liver cancer, 1208-1209
Liver problems
  cirrhosis. See Cirrhosis.
  fatty liver, 1208
  health promotion and maintenance in, 1211
  hepatitis, 1203-1208
    assessment in, 1204-1206
    community-based care in, 1207-1208, 1208b
    health promotion and maintenance in, 1204, 1205b
    interventions for, 1206-1208, 1206b-1207b, 1207t
    pathophysiology of, 1203-1204

Liver problems (Continued)
  liver cancer, 1208-1209
  liver trauma, 1208, 1208b
Liver transplantation, 1208-1211, 1208b, 1210b, 1210t
Liver-spleen scan, 1097
Living will, 92-94
LNF. See Laparoscopic Nissen fundoplication (LNF).
Lobar pneumonia with consolidation, 589
Lobectomy, 576
Lobular carcinoma in situ (LCIS), 1464
Local anesthesia, 248-249
Local anesthetics, 45
Local complications of infusion therapy, 204-207, 204t-206t
Locus, 52
LOE. See Levels of evidence (LOE).
Log rolling after back surgery, 889
Long bones, 1017-1018
Long-acting beta$_2$ agonists (LABA), 539b, 555-556
Long-handled reachers, 84t
Longitudinal ridges and thickening of nails, 417f
Long-term memory, 839
Long-term nonprogressors (LTNPs), 329b
Loop diuretics
  heart failure, 685b
  for hypertension, 714, 714b
Loop electrosurgical excision procedure (LEEP), 1495
Lorazepam, 385b
Lordosis, 1023
  in scoliosis, 1047
Losartan, 715b-716b
Loss, older adults and, 12
Lou Gehrig's disease. See Amyotrophic lateral sclerosis (ALS).
Lovenox. See Enoxaparin.
Low back pain, 885-891
  health care resources for, 891
  health promotion and maintenance in, 886, 886b
  home care management in, 890
  imaging assessment in, 886-887
  nonsurgical management of, 887-888, 887b
  pathophysiology of, 885-886, 885f, 886b
  physical assessment in, 886
  self-management education in, 890, 890b-891b
  surgical management of, 888-890, 889b
Low-density lipoproteins (LDLs), 641-642, 641b, 709b
Low-dose brachytherapy, 1510
Lower esophageal sphincter, 1085
  gastroesophageal reflux disease and, 1110, 1111t

Lower extremity arterial disease (LEAD), 718-719
Lower extremity fractures, 1066-1068, 1067b-1068b, 1067f
Lower extremity ulcers, 721b
Lower gastrointestinal bleeding, 1179-1180, 1180b
Lower motor neuron diseases, 87
Lower respiratory problems, 532f, 548-582
　asthma. See Asthma.
　bronchiolitis obliterans organizing pneumonia, 572-573
　chronic obstructive pulmonary disease. See Chronic obstructive pulmonary disease (COPD).
　cystic fibrosis, 567-569
　　genetic considerations in, 567b
　　nonsurgical management of, 568, 568f
　　pathophysiology of, 567-569
　　surgical management of, 569
　interstitial pulmonary diseases, 571-572
　lung cancer. See Lung cancer.
　occupational pulmonary disease, 572, 573b
　pneumonia. See Pneumonia.
　pulmonary arterial hypertension, 569-571, 569b-571b, 570t
Lower respiratory tract, 498-499
　accessory muscles of respiration in, 499
　airways in, 498-499, 498f-499f
　lungs in, 499, 499f
Low-flow oxygen delivery systems, 517-519, 517t, 518f, 519b
　facemasks in, 517t, 518-519, 518f, 519b
　nasal cannula in, 517-518, 518f
Low-intensity pulsed ultrasound, 1063
Low-molecular-weight heparin, 732
Low-pitched crackles, 507t
Low-profile gastrostomy device (LPGD), 1241, 1242f
Loxoscelism, 126
LPGD. See Low-profile gastrostomy device (LPGD).
LTNPs. See Long-term nonprogressors (LTNPs).
Luer-Lok devices, 197-198, 212b
Lukens tube for sputum specimen, 592f
Lumbar puncture, 846t-847t, 849-850, 849b, 850t
Lumbar spinal surgery, 889-890, 889b
Lumen occlusion in central venous catheters, 208t
Lung biopsy, 511-512
Lung cancer, 573-580
　chemotherapy for, 576
　chest tube for, 577-579, 577f, 579b
　diagnosis of, 575

Lung cancer (Continued)
　health promotion and maintenance in, 574
　history in, 574-575, 575t
　hospice care and, 580
　older adults and, 367b
　pain management in, 579-580
　pathophysiology of, 573-580, 574t
　　etiology and genetic risk in, 574, 574b
　　incidence and prevalence of, 574
　photodynamic therapy for, 576
　physical assessment in, 575
　pneumonectomy care in, 580
　psychosocial assessment in, 575
　radiation therapy for, 576, 580
　respiratory management in, 579-580
　surgical management of, 576-580, 577b, 577f-578f, 579b-580b
Lung compliance
　in acute respiratory distress syndrome, 612-613
　in sarcoidosis, 571
Lung transplantation
　in chronic obstructive pulmonary disease, 564-565
　in cystic fibrosis, 569
Lung volume, 561-562
Lungs, 499, 499f
　abscesses of, 599
　changes with aging, 501b
　injury of
　　from inhalation burns, 470
　　systemic sclerosis and, 317-318
Lunula, 417, 417f
Lupus erythematosus, 313-317, 314b, 314f, 316b-317b
Lurch, 1021-1022
Luteinizing hormone-releasing hormone, 425t
Lyme disease, 320-321, 321b, 407
Lymphadenopathy, 408
Lymphedema after breast cancer surgery, 1479, 1479b
Lymphoblastic leukemia, 806-807
Lymphocytes
　count in AIDS, 336
　in differential white blood cell count, 508b
Lymphocytic leukemia, 806-807
Lymphogranuloma venereum, 1544
Lymphokines, 286
Lymphomas, malignant, 817-819
　in AIDS, 335
　Hodgkin's lymphoma, 817, 817t
　multiple myeloma, 818-819
　non-Hodgkin lymphoma, 818
Lysis, 284

M

Machine Operator's Lung, 573b
Macitentan, 570
Macrocytic anemia, 804

Macrophages, 278t-279t, 279, 281, 787t
Macrovascular complications in diabetes mellitus, 1303
Macular degeneration, 989
Macular rash, 424
Macules, 423f
Mafenide acetate, 486b
Magnesium, 171-172
　abnormal values of, 152t
　hypermagnesemia and, 171-172, 171t
　hypomagnesemia and, 171, 171t
　plasma values in older adults, 152b
Magnesium sulfate, 658b-662b
Magnetic resonance angiography in neurologic assessment, 846t-847t
Magnetic resonance imaging (MRI)
　in cardiovascular assessment, 647
　in musculoskeletal assessment, 1025-1026, 1026b
　in neurologic assessment, 846t-847t, 847-848
　in renal assessment, 1360-1361, 1360t
　in spinal cord injury, 895
　in vision assessment, 973
Magnetic resonance spectroscopy, 846t-847t
Magnetoencephalography, 848
Mainstem bronchi, 498-499, 498f
Maintenance therapy
　in leukemia, 810
　in transplantation, 287
Major burns, 467t
Major histocompatibility complex (MHC), 276
Major surgery, 218t
Malabsorption syndrome, 1165-1166, 1166b
Male reproductive problems, 1499-1518
　benign prostatic hyperplasia, 1499-1506
　　assessment in, 1500-1502, 1501f-1502f
　　community-based care in, 1506
　　complementary and alternative therapies for, 1503
　　concept map for, 1504f
　　drug therapy for, 1503, 1503b
　　pathophysiology of, 1499-1500, 1500f
　　surgical management of, 1505-1506, 1505b-1506b
　erectile dysfunction, 1512-1513, 1512b
　hydrocele, 1516, 1516f
　prostate cancer, 1506-1511
　　assessment in, 1508, 1508b
　　chemotherapy for, 1510-1511
　　community-based care in, 1511, 1511b

Male reproductive problems (Continued)
　　health promotion and maintenance in, 1507, 1507b
　　hormone therapy for, 1510, 1510b
　　older adults and, 367b
　　pathophysiology of, 1506-1511, 1507b, 1507f
　　radiation therapy in, 1510
　　surgical management of, 1509-1510, 1509b
　prostatitis, 1500, 1512
　spermatocele, 1516, 1516f
　testicular cancer, 1513-1516
　　assessment in, 1514, 1514b
　　chemotherapy for, 1515-1516
　　community-based care in, 1516, 1516b
　　external beam radiation therapy for, 1516
　　pathophysiology of, 1513, 1513b, 1513t
　　sperm banking and, 1514-1515, 1514b
　　surgical management of, 1515, 1515b
　varicocele, 1516, 1516f
Male reproductive system, 1451-1452, 1451f
　changes with aging, 1452b
　physical assessment of, 1454
Malignancies. See Cancer.
Malignant cell growth, 359
Malignant hypertension, 710
Malignant hyperthermia (MH), 246-247, 247b-248b
Malignant lymphomas, 817-819
　Hodgkin's lymphoma, 817, 817t
　multiple myeloma, 818-819
　non-Hodgkin lymphoma, 818
Malignant transformation, 362
Malleus, 996-997, 997f
Malnutrition, 1236-1246.
　See also Obesity.
　assessment in, 1238-1239, 1238b, 1239t
　community-based care in, 1245-1246
　cultural considerations, 1237b
　drug therapy for, 1240
　evaluation of care of patient with, 1246
　nutrition management in, 1239-1240, 1240b, 1244b
　older adults and, 1237b-1238b, 1240b
　parenteral nutrition in, 1244-1245, 1245b
　　total parenteral nutrition in, 1245, 1245b
　pathophysiology of, 1236-1238, 1237b

Malnutrition (*Continued*)
  total enteral nutrition in, 1240-1244, 1242b-1244b, 1242f
Mammalian target of rapamycin (mTOR), 391
Mammography, 1456, 1467, 1470
Mandibular fractures, 534
Mandibulectomy, 1105
MAOIs. *See* Monoamine oxidase inhibitors (MAOIs).
MAP. *See* Mean arterial pressure (MAP).
Marasmic-kwashiorkor, 1236
Marasmus, 1236
Marfan syndrome, 323t
Marsupialization, 1491
Masculinizing surgeries for female to male patients, 1527-1528
Mass casualty events, 138-139, 145b
  psychosocial response of survivors to, 146-147, 146b-147b
Mass casualty triage, 140-141, 141b, 141t
Massage, 97
Mast cell stabilizers, 351
Mastectomy, 1472-1480, 1472f-1473f, 1474b, 1475t, 1476b
Mastication, 1085
Mastoid assessment, 1000
Mastoid process, 996, 997f
Mastoiditis, 1007
Maturation phase of healing, 433, 433t
Maximal barrier precautions, 204t
Maximum mandatory ventilation, 617
Maze procedure, 669
MD. *See* Muscular dystrophy (MD).
MDRO infections. *See* Multidrug-resistant organism (MDRO) infections.
MDS. *See* Minimum Data Set (MDS).
Meal planning strategies, 1320-1321
Mean arterial pressure (MAP), 628
  shock and, 742-744, 742f
  calculation of, 1416t
Mechanical debridement
  in burns, 482-483
  in pressure ulcer, 444-446
Mechanical energy, 1082
Mechanical forces in pressure ulcers, 437, 437f
Mechanical obstruction, 1157
Mechanical ventilation, 614-622
  after burn injury, 478, 478b
  after coronary artery bypass graft, 778-779
  complications in, 620-622, 621b
  endotracheal intubation in, 615-616, 615b-616b, 615f
  extubation in, 622, 622b
  managing the ventilator system in, 619, 619b
  modes of ventilation in, 616-617
  monitoring in, 618-619, 619b

Mechanical ventilation (*Continued*)
  nursing management in, 618-622, 618b
  oral care during, 621b
  pain assessment and, 34
  patient safety in, 617b
  types of ventilators in, 616, 617f
  ventilator alarms and, 619, 620t
  ventilator controls and settings in, 618
  weaning from, 622, 622b, 622t
Mechanically regulated devices, 199
Medial nerve complications, 253b
Medial rectus muscle, 968f, 969t
Mediastinal shift, 511
Mediastinitis, 779
Medical command physicians, 143, 143t
Medical harm, 2-3
Medical history. *See* History.
Medical nutritional supplements (MNSs), 1240
Medical record review during intraoperative period, 250-251, 250b-251b
Medical Reserve Corps, 142
Medical-surgical nursing, 1-8
  essential genetic competencies for, 52t
  National Patient Safety Goals and, 2
  patient safety and, 2-7, 2t
  Quality and Safety Education for Nurses (QSEN) core competencies and, 3-6, 8
  evidence-based practice in, 6, 8
  informatics in, 7-8, 7f
  observe for slow and sudden changes in patient condition, 3b, 8
  patient-centered care in, 3-4, 3t, 5t, 8
  quality improvement in, 6-8
  safety in, 7
  teamwork and collaboration in, 4-6, 5t, 6b, 8
  scope of, 1-2, 2f
Medicare, 94, 94b
Medication history
  in renal assessment, 1352
  in skin problems, 420b
Medication overuse headaches, 856
Medications, increased surgical risk and, 219t
Medicine wheel, 101b, 101f
Medulla
  functions of, 832t
  renal, 1345, 1345f
Meglitinide analogs, 1312b
Melanocytes, 417
Melanomas, 459, 459f, 459t
  ocular, 992
Memory cells, 278t, 282, 787t
Memory in neurologic assessment, 839

Ménière's disease, 1008
Meninges, 830
Meningiomas, 958
Meningitis, 863-867, 863b-865b, 864t
  after craniotomy, 962
Meniscectomy, 1076
Menses, 1483
Mental health disorders, older adults and, 16-19
Mental status assessment, 838-840, 838b-839b
Mental status changes in pressure ulcers, 438
Meperidine, 42, 49
Mepilex Ag, 486b
Metabolic acidosis, 180, 180t, 183
  in burns, 469
  combined metabolic and respiratory acidosis and, 181, 182b
  laboratory assessment in, 182, 182b
Metabolic alkalosis, 183t, 184
Metabolic bone diseases, 1029-1039
  osteomalacia, 1036-1037, 1036t
  osteoporosis, 1029-1036
    community-based care in, 1036
    drug therapy for, 1034-1035, 1034b-1035b
    health promotion and maintenance in, 1031-1032
    imaging assessment in, 1033
    laboratory assessment in, 1032-1033
    osteomalacia vs., 1036t
    pathophysiology of, 1029-1031, 1030b-1031b, 1030t
    physical assessment in, 1032, 1032f
    psychosocial assessment in, 1032
  Paget's disease of the bone, 1037-1039, 1037b-1038b
Metabolic syndrome, 761, 761t
Metabolism, 1082
  changes resulting from burns, 470
  chronic kidney disease and, 1420, 1420f
  as source of acids and bicarbonate, 176
Metastasis, 362-363, 363t, 371-372, 377
  in breast cancer, 1471-1478
  in colorectal cancer, 1151-1154
  in endometrial cancer, 1492-1493
  in head and neck cancer, 538
  in lung cancer, 574
  in thyroid cancer, 1295
Metformin, 1310, 1310b, 1361b
Methadone, 41-42
Methemoglobinemia, 510, 510b
Methicillin-resistant *Staphylococcus aureus* (MRSA), 403, 405-406, 406b
  preventing spread of, 452, 452b
  in skin infections, 451

Methimazole, 1288b-1289b
Methotrexate
  for lupus, 316
  for rheumatoid arthritis, 293, 308, 308b
Methylprednisolone, 354b
Metoclopramide, 385b
Metoprolol
  for coronary artery disease, 765b-766b
  for hypertension, 715b-716b
Mexiletine hydrochloride, 658b-662b
MG. *See* Myasthenia gravis (MG).
MH. *See* Malignant hyperthermia (MH).
MHC. *See* Major histocompatibility complex (MHC).
Microalbuminuria, 642, 1356
  in diabetes mellitus, 1306
Microcytic anemia, 804-805
Microdiskectomy, 888
Microprocessor ventilators, 616
Microvascular complications in diabetes mellitus, 1303-1306, 1304b-1305b, 1305t
Microvascular decompression in trigeminal neuralgia, 927
Micturition, 1350
Midarm circumference, 1236
Midbrain, 832t
MIDCAB. *See* Minimally invasive direct coronary artery bypass (MIDCAB).
Middle cerebral artery, 832
  strokes, 934b
Middle ear problems, 1005-1007
  mastoiditis, 1007
  neoplasms, 1007
  otitis media, 1005-1006, 1006f, 1007b
  trauma, 1007
Middle old, 9
Midline catheters, 192-193, 192f, 201
  older adults and, 209
  removal of, 203
Midrin, 856
Migraine headaches, 854-857, 855b-857b, 855t
  drug therapy for, 855-857, 855t, 856b
Migratory arthritis, 305
Mild traumatic brain injuries (MTBI), 947, 948b
Miliary tuberculosis, 595
Milrinone, 748b
Mineralocorticoids, 1258
Mini Nutritional Assessment (MNA), 1234, 1235f
Mini-Cog, 18
Minimally invasive direct coronary artery bypass (MIDCAB), 779
Minimally invasive esophagectomy, 1120
Minimally invasive inguinal repair, 1147

Minimally invasive surgery (MIS), 218t, 221
  in back pain, 889
  in pancreatic cancer, 1228
  in peptic ulcer disease, 1137
  in prostate cancer, 1509
  surgical suites for, 242, 242f-243f
  in total hip arthroplasty, 296
  in total knee arthroplasty, 301
  in urolithiasis, 1386-1387
MiniMed Paradigm insulin pump, 1316f
Mini-Mental State Examination (MMSE), 873-874, 874f
Minimum Data Set (MDS), 79-80, 80t, 90
Minor burns, 467t
Minor surgery, 218t
Miosis, 969, 969f
MIS. See Minimally invasive surgery (MIS).
Mitosis, 360, 361f
Mitotic index, 365
Mitoxantrone, 908
Mitral regurgitation, 692b, 693
Mitral stenosis, 692, 692b, 696b
Mitral valve, 628, 629f
Mitral valve prolapse (MVP), 692b, 693
Mixed agonists antagonists, 38
Mixed conductive-sensorineural hearing loss, 1001
Mixed connective tissue disease, 322-323
Mixed delirium, 18
Mixed incontinence, 1374t, 1375
Mixed urinary incontinence, 1382
Mixing of insulins, 1315, 1315b
MMSE. See Mini-Mental State Examination (MMSE).
MNA. See Mini Nutritional Assessment (MNA).
MNPI. See Myocardial nuclear perfusion imaging (MNPI).
MNSs. See Medical nutritional supplements (MNSs).
Mobility, 828
  after burns, 487-488, 487b, 488f
  assessment of, 1022, 1022f
  fractures and, 1064-1065, 1065f
  multiple sclerosis and, 908-909
  myasthenia gravis and, 919-920
  older adults and, 11-12, 12b, 12f
  osteoarthritis and, 303, 303b
  postoperative, 232-233
    in amputation, 1073
    in total hip arthroplasty, 297-300, 297b, 299b-300b
  pressure ulcers and, 438-440
  rehabilitation and
    physical, 80-84, 81b, 82f-83f, 83b, 83t
  spinal cord injury and, 898-899
  stroke and, 942-943, 943b
Moderate burns, 467t
Moderate sedation, 249, 250t

Moderate traumatic brain injury, 948
Modifiable risk factors, 760
MODS. See Multiple organ dysfunction syndrome (MODS).
Modulation of pain, 28, 29f
Mohs' surgery, 461
Moist heat injuries, 470
Moisture content of skin, 421, 425t
Moisture-retentive dressing for pressure ulcers, 446t
Molecularly targeted therapy for cancer, 388-391, 389f, 390t
  angiogenesis inhibitors in, 390, 390t
  epidermal growth factor/receptor inhibitors in, 390, 390t
  multikinase inhibitors in, 390, 390t
  proteasome inhibitors in, 390, 390t
  tyrosine kinase inhibitors in, 390, 390t
  vascular endothelial growth factor/receptor inhibitors in, 390, 390t
Moles, 459
Monitoring
  blood glucose, 1317-1319, 1318b
  continuous electrocardiographic, 652, 653f
  in fluid overload, 160
  hemodynamic, 770-771, 770b, 771f
  in hyperkalemia, 165
  of intracranial pressure, 939-941, 939b, 941b
  of mechanical ventilation, 618-619, 619b
  postoperative, 260, 266, 266b
  of pressure ulcers, 447, 448b
  in pulmonary embolism, 606, 609
  for respiratory status changes in COPD, 562
  in surgery for diabetes mellitus, 1324-1325, 1325b
Monoamine oxidase inhibitors (MAOIs), 869, 869b
Monoclonal antibodies
  for cancer, 388, 390t
  for osteoporosis, 1034-1035
  to prevent transplant rejection, 287b-288b
  for skin cancer, 461
Monocytes, 787t
  in differential white blood cell count, 508b
Monokines, 286
Montelukast, 539b
Montgomery straps, 267, 267f
Morbidity, 221
Morphine, 41, 41b, 41t
  for postoperative pain, 270b
Mortality, 221
Morton's neuromas, 1047

Motor aphasia, 943, 943t
Motor cortex, 831
Motor end plate, 1020
Motor function
  after stroke, 934-936
  in cancer, 372
  in spinal cord injury, 894-895
Motor function assessment, 840-841, 841f
Motor neurons, 830, 830f
Mourning, 100
Movement, postoperative, 267
MRI. See Magnetic resonance imaging (MRI).
MRSA. See Methicillin-resistant Staphylococcus aureus (MRSA).
MS. See Multiple sclerosis (MS).
MTBI. See Mild traumatic brain injuries (MTBI).
MTOR. See Mammalian target of rapamycin (mTOR).
Mu opioid agonists, 38, 40, 40t, 49
Mucositis, chemotherapy-related, 381, 384, 386b, 576
Mucous membranes
  as defense against infection, 400
  fluid overload and, 159b
  oxygen therapy drying of, 516, 516f
  respiratory assessment and, 506
Multaq. See Dronedarone.
Multi-casualty events, 138-139
Multidrug-resistant organism (MDRO) infections, 403, 405-406
  carbapenem-resistant Enterobacteriaceae, 406
  methicillin-resistant Staphylococcus aureus, 403, 405-406, 406b, 451
  vancomycin-resistant Enterococcus, 403, 406
Multigated blood pool scanning, 646
Multikinase inhibitors, 390, 390t
Multimodal analgesia, 34, 49
Multiple myeloma, 818-819
Multiple organ dysfunction syndrome (MODS), 92
  refractory stage of shock and, 743-744
  in sickle cell disease, 802-803
Multiple sclerosis (MS), 904-910
  cognitive impairment and, 909, 909b
  complementary and alternative therapies for, 909
  concept map for, 907f
  drug therapy for, 906-908, 908b
  genetic considerations in, 905b
  health care resources for, 909-910
  history in, 905
  home care management in, 909
  laboratory assessment in, 906
  mobility problems in, 908-909, 909b
  pathophysiology of, 904-905
  physical assessment in, 905-906, 905b-906b

Multiple sclerosis (MS) (Continued)
  psychosocial assessment in, 906
  self-management education in, 909-910
Murmurs, 640, 640t
  in leukemia, 808
Muromonab-CD3, 287b-288b
Muscle biopsies, 850, 1026
Muscle strain, 1079
Muscle strength, grading, 1024, 1024t
Muscle weakness
  in hyponatremia, 162b
  mechanical ventilation-related, 621-622
Muscular dystrophy (MD), 1048-1049, 1048t, 1049b
Muscular system, 1019-1020
  assessment of, 1023-1024, 1024t
Musculoskeletal assessment, 1017-1028
  arthroscopy in, 1026-1027, 1027b, 1027f
  biopsies in, 1026, 1026b
  in burns, 482
  current health problems in, 1021
  electromyography in, 1026
  family history and genetic risk in, 1021
  in hematologic assessment, 793
  imaging assessment in, 1025-1026
  laboratory assessment in, 1024-1025, 1024b
  magnetic resonance imaging in, 1025-1026, 1026b
  mobility and functional assessment in, 1022, 1022f
  muscular system and, 1023-1024, 1024t
  neurovascular assessment in, 1023, 1023b
  nutrition history in, 1021
  patient history in, 1020-1021
  posture and gait in, 1021-1022, 1022f
  preoperative, 222
  psychosocial assessment in, 1024
  in rehabilitation setting, 78-79, 78t
  specific areas in, 1023, 1023f
Musculoskeletal problems, 1029-1050
  benign bone tumors, 1042
  bone cancer, 1042-1045, 1044b
  disorders of the foot, 1046-1047, 1046f
  disorders of the hand, 1045-1046
  health promotion and maintenance in, 1050
  metabolic bone diseases, 1029-1039
    osteomalacia, 1036-1037, 1036t
    osteoporosis. See Osteoporosis.
  Paget's disease of the bone, 1037-1039, 1037b-1038b
  osteomyelitis, 1039-1041, 1040b-1041b, 1040f

Musculoskeletal problems (Continued)
  progressive muscular dystrophies, 1048-1049, 1048t, 1049b
  scoliosis, 1047-1048, 1048b
Musculoskeletal system
  anatomy and physiology of, 1017-1020
    muscular system, 1019-1020
    skeletal system, 1017-1019, 1018t
      bones, 1017-1019, 1018f
      joints, 1019, 1019f
  changes related to aging, 1020, 1020b
  complications of immobility and, 83t
  hypokalemia and, 164
  hypophosphatemia and, 170
Musculoskeletal trauma, 1051-1081
  amputations, 1069-1075
    community-based care in, 1074-1075, 1074f, 1075b
    complications of, 1071
    cultural considerations in, 1071b
    interventions in, 1072-1074, 1072b, 1074f
    levels of, 1070-1071, 1070f
  carpal tunnel syndrome, 1077-1078, 1077b
  complex regional pain syndrome, 1075
  fractures in. See Fractures.
  health promotion and maintenance in, 1080
  knee injuries, 1075-1077, 1076b, 1076f
  rotator cuff injuries, 1079
  strains and sprains, 1079
  tendinopathy and joint dislocation, 1079
Music therapy in end-of-life care, 97, 100
Mutation, 56
MVP. See Mitral valve prolapse (MVP).
Myalgia in meningitis, 863
Myasthenia gravis (MG), 917-923
  diagnostic assessment in, 918-919, 919b
  drug therapy for, 920, 920b, 920t, 922b
  health care resources for, 922-923
  home care management in, 922
  myasthenic and cholinergic crises in, 920, 920t
  pathophysiology of, 917-918
  physical assessment in, 918-919, 918b
  respiratory support in, 919, 919b
  self-management education in, 922, 922b, 922t
  surgical management of, 921, 922b

Myasthenic crisis, 919-920, 919b, 920t
Mycobacterium avium complex, 339-340
Mycobacterium tuberculosis, 399, 595, 595f
Mycophenolate, 287b-288b
Mydriasis, 969, 969f
Myelin sheath, 830
Myelocytic leukemia, 806-807
Myelodysplastic syndromes, 806
Myelogenous leukemia, 806-807
Myelography, 1025
Myelosuppression, 381, 382b
Myfortic. See Mycophenolate.
Myocardial hypertrophy, 681
Myocardial infarction, 759-760, 759f
  chest pain in, 636t, 764
  emergency care in, 764
  home care management after, 780b
  inferior wall, 760
  key features of, 762b
Myocardial nuclear perfusion imaging (MNPI), 646-647
Myoglobin, 641
Myoglobinuria
  in coral snake envenomation, 125
  in malignant hyperthermia, 246-247
Myomas. See Uterine leiomyomas.
Myomectomy, 702-704, 1489
Myopathy, 1021
Myopia, 969, 991
Myositis, 315
Myosplint, 688
MyPlate, 1233, 1233f
Myxedema, 1291, 1292f
Myxedema coma, 1291, 1292f, 1294, 1294b

N
NAAT. See Nucleic acid amplification test (NAAT).
Nadir, 377, 814
Nails, 415
  artificial, 402, 414
  assessment of, 425-427, 426f, 426t-427t
  changes with aging, 417f, 418b-419b
  common variations in, 427t
  cultural considerations in, 500b
  structure of, 417, 417f
Naloxone, 44b
Narcan. See Naloxone.
Nasal cannula, 517-518, 517t, 518f
Nasal fractures, 531-532, 532b, 532f
Nasoduodenal tubes, 1241, 1242f
Nasoenteric tubes, 1241
Nasogastric tubes
  after head and neck surgery, 543
  calculation of drainage from, 263t
  for enteral nutrition, 1241

Nasogastric tubes (Continued)
  in esophageal surgery, 1122, 1122b
  in intestinal obstructions, 1159, 1159b
  irrigation of, after gastric surgery, 263b
  in peptic ulcer disease, 1136
Nasoseptoplasty, 532
Nasotracheal intubation, 536
Natal sex, 1520, 1520t
National Council of State Boards of Nursing (NCSBN), 7
National Institutes of Health Stroke Scale (NIHSS), 933-934, 935t-936t
National Patient Safety Goals (NPSGs), 2, 21, 108
  medication safety and, 189
  verifying patient identity, 510b
National Psoriasis Foundation, 321
National Veterinary Response Team, 142
Natrecor. See Nesiritide.
Natriuretic peptides, 153-154
Natural active immunity, 285, 289
Natural chemical debridement of pressure ulcers, 444-446
Natural immunity, 277, 398t
Natural killer cells, 278t, 285-286, 787t
  transplant rejection and, 286
Natural passive immunity, 285
Nausea
  chemotherapy-related, 383-384, 384b-385b
  in enteral nutrition, 1244
  management at end of life, 99
NCSBN. See National Council of State Boards of Nursing (NCSBN).
Near point of vision, 970
Near vision, 972
Near-drowning, 135
Nearsightedness, 969
Near-syncope, 635
Neck
  cancer of, 537-545
    anxiety in, 543-544
    aspiration prevention in, 543, 543b
    etiology of, 538
    evaluation of care of patient with, 545
    health care resources for, 545
    history in, 538
    home care management in, 544, 544b
    imaging assessment in, 538
    incidence and prevalence of, 538
    laboratory assessment in, 538
    physical assessment in, 538, 538t
    preventing respiratory obstruction in, 539-542, 540b-541b, 541t, 542f

Neck (Continued)
    psychosocial assessment in, 538
    psychosocial support in, 545
    self-concept in, 544
    self-management education in, 544-545, 545b
    surgery for, 540-542, 541b, 541t, 542f
  hematologic assessment and, 792
  positioning to prevent contractures, 487b
  trauma to, 537
Neck pain, 891-892, 891b-892b
Neck vein distention, 156
Necrotizing hemorrhagic pancreatitis, 1218
Necrotizing vasculitis, 323t
Nedocromil, 539b
NEECHAM Confusion Scale, 18
Needle stick injuries, HIV transmission and, 331f, 332
Needle thoracostomy, 624
Needleless connection devices, 198, 198f, 202
Needles, Standard Precautions and, 403t
Needlestick Safety and Prevention Act, 198
Negative deflection, 651, 651f
Negative feedback control mechanism of endocrine system, 1256, 1257f
Negative nitrogen balance, 1285
Negative pressure wound therapy (NPWT), 447
Neisseria meningitidis, 398
Neoplasia, 360
Neoplasms, 1007
Nephrectomy, 1401
Nephrolithiasis, 1384
Nephrons, 1346, 1346f
  vascular and tubular components of, 1348t
Nephropathy, diabetic, 1303, 1306
Nephrosclerosis, 1405, 1405b
Nephrostomy tubes, 1398-1399, 1399b
Nephrotic syndrome, 1404-1405, 1404b
Nerve biopsies, 850
Nerve block, 45, 248t
  for pain after total knee arthroplasty, 302
Nerve damage, intravenous therapy-related, 204t-206t
Nervous system
  anatomy and physiology of, 829-837
    autonomic nervous system, 835-836
    central nervous system, 829-833
      brain, 830-832, 831f-832f, 831t-832t
      spinal cord, 832-833, 833f
    nervous system cells, 830, 830f

Nervous system *(Continued)*
  peripheral nervous system, 830, 833-834, 834f-835f, 835t
  assessment of. *See* Neurologic assessment.
  changes associated with aging, 836-837, 836b-837b
  complications of immobility and, 83t
  dehydration and, 157
  disorders of. *See* Neurologic problems.
  fluid overload and, 159b
  hypokalemia and, 164
  systemic lupus erythematosus and, 315
Nesiritide, 685
Neulasta. *See* Pegfilgrastim.
Neumega. *See* Oprelvekin.
Neupogen. *See* Filgrastim.
Neuroaxial anesthesia, 296
Neuroendocrine assessment, 481
Neurogenic bladder, 86-87, 86t
Neurogenic bowel, 87t
Neurogenic shock in spinal cord injury, 896, 896b
Neuroglia cells, 830
Neurohypophysis, 1257
Neurokinin receptor antagonists, 385b
Neurologic assessment, 829-852
  cerebellar function assessment in, 842-843
  cerebral blood flow evaluation in, 849
  cranial nerves assessment in, 840
  health promotion and maintenance in, 851
  imaging assessment in, 844-848
    cerebral angiography in, 845, 845b
    computed tomography in, 845-847, 846t-847t
    electroencephalography in, 846t-847t, 849
    electromyography in, 848
    evoked potentials in, 849
    magnetic resonance imaging in, 846t-847t, 847-848
    magnetoencephalography in, 848
    plain x-rays in, 844-845
    positron emission tomography in, 846t-847t, 848
    single-photon emission computed tomography in, 846t-847t, 848
    transcranial Doppler ultrasonography in, 850
  laboratory assessment in, 844
  lumbar puncture in, 846t-847t, 849-850, 849b, 850t
  mental status assessment in, 838-840, 838b-839b
  motor function assessment in, 840-841, 841f

Neurologic assessment *(Continued)*
  muscle and nerve biopsies in, 850
  patient history in, 837-850, 838b
  postoperative, 260-261, 260t, 261b
  preoperative, 222
  psychosocial assessment in, 844
  rapid, 843-844, 843f, 844b
  reflex activity assessment in, 841, 842f
  in rehabilitation setting, 78-79, 78t
  sensory assessment in, 841-842
  in traumatic brain injury, 952, 952b
Neurologic problems
  acquired hypoxic-anoxic brain injury, 964
  Alzheimer's disease. *See* Alzheimer's disease.
  amyotrophic lateral sclerosis, 910-911, 910b-911b
  back pain. *See* Back pain.
  brain abscesses, 962-964, 963b
  brain tumors, 957-962
    assessment of, 958-959, 959b
    classification of, 958, 958t
    community-based care in, 962
    interventions for, 959-962, 959f, 960b-961b, 961t
    pathophysiology of, 957-958
  cranial nerve diseases, 926-928
    facial paralysis, 927-928
    trigeminal neuralgia, 926-927, 926f, 927b
  dementia. *See* Dementia.
  encephalitis, 865-867, 866b
  Guillain-Barré syndrome, 913-917, 914b-916b
  headaches, 853-858, 854b
    cluster, 857-858
    migraine, 854-857, 855b-857b, 855t
  Huntington disease (HD), 881-882, 881b
  meningitis, 863-867, 863b-865b, 864t
  multiple sclerosis, 904-910, 905b, 907f, 908b-909b
  myasthenia gravis. *See* Myasthenia gravis (MG).
  Parkinson disease, 867-871, 867t, 868b-869b, 868f
    drug therapy for, 868-870, 869b
    genetic considerations in, 867b
    psychosocial support in, 870-871
    surgical management of, 871
  peripheral nerve trauma, 923-925, 923f-924f, 925b
  restless legs syndrome, 925-926
  seizures and epilepsy, 858-863
    drug therapy for, 859, 859b-860b
    emergency care in, 861-862, 862b

Neurologic problems *(Continued)*
    etiology and genetic risk in, 858-859
    gender health considerations in, 859b
    older adults and, 858b
    seizure precautions and management in, 860-861, 860b-861b
    self-management education in, 859, 861b
    surgical management of, 862-863
    types of seizures and, 858
  spinal cord injury. *See* Spinal cord injury (SCI).
  spinal cord tumors, 902-904, 903b
  stroke. *See* Stroke.
  transient ischemic attack, 930-931, 931b
  traumatic brain injury. *See* Traumatic brain injury (TBI).
Neuromas
  acoustic, 958, 1009
  Morton's, 1047
Neuromuscular blockers, 481
Neuromuscular changes
  in acidosis, 181, 181b
  in alkalosis, 184, 184b
  in hypercalcemia, 169
  in hyperkalemia, 166
  in hypermagnesemia, 171
  in hypocalcemia, 168
  in hypomagnesemia, 171
  in hyponatremia, 161-162
Neurons, 830, 830f
Neurontin. *See* Gabapentin.
Neuropathic pain, 28, 28t
Neurotoxin, 411t
Neurotransmitters, 830
Neurovascular assessment
  after total hip arthroplasty, 299, 299b
  after total knee arthroplasty, 302, 302b
  in musculoskeletal assessment, 1023, 1023b
Neutralization, 284
Neutropenia
  chemotherapy-related, 381-382, 381b-382b
  in myelodysplastic syndromes, 806
Neutrophils, 278-279, 279f, 279t, 281, 787t
  in differential white blood cell count, 508b
  immune function of, 278t
Nevus, 459
New York Heart Association Functional Classification, 636, 636t
New-onset angina, 759
NICHE project. *See* Nurses Improving Care for Healthsystem Elders (NICHE) project.

Nicotine replacement therapies (NRTs), 495, 495b, 594b
NIHSS. *See* National Institutes of Health Stroke Scale (NIHSS).
Nitrates, 765b-766b
Nitrofurazone, 486b
Nitroglycerin, 764, 764b-766b
Nitroglycerin patch, 765b-766b
Nitrolingual translingual spray, 765b-766b
NMDA receptor antagonist. *See* N-methyl-D-aspartate (NMDA) receptor antagonist.
N-methyl-D-aspartate (NMDA) receptor antagonist, 877
NNRTIs. *See* Non-nucleoside reverse transcriptase inhibitors (NNRTIs).
Nociceptive pain, 26-28, 28t, 29f
Nocturia
  hospitalized older adults and, 21
  preoperative assessment of, 221-222
Nocturnal polyuria, 1351
Nodules, 423f
Nonabsorbable sutures, 253
Nonadherence, 407
Noncompliance, 407
Noncoring needles, 195, 196f
Non-exertional heat stroke, 122b
Non-Hodgkin's lymphoma, 335, 818
Noninflammatory intestinal disorders, 1144-1167
  abdominal trauma, 1161-1163, 1162b
  colorectal cancer. *See* Colorectal cancer.
  health promotion and maintenance in, 1167
  hemorrhoids, 1164-1165, 1164f, 1165b
  intestinal obstructions, 1157-1161, 1158f, 1159b, 1161b
  intestinal polyps, 1163-1164
  irritable bowel syndrome, 1144-1146, 1145f, 1146b
  malabsorption syndrome, 1165-1166, 1166b
Noninvasive breast cancers, 1464
Noninvasive heart valve reparative procedures, 694-695, 695b, 695f
Noninvasive positive-pressure ventilation (NPPV), 520, 520f
Nonmaleficence, 4
Nonmechanical obstruction, 1157
Nonmodifiable risk factors, 760
Non-nucleoside reverse transcriptase inhibitors (NNRTIs), 327, 339, 339b
Non-opioid analgesics, 35-37, 36t, 37b
Nonpharmacologic interventions for pain, 46-48, 46b, 48b, 50
Non-rebreather masks, 517t, 518, 518f, 519b

Non-self versus self, 276, 276f, 277b
Nonspecific eczematous dermatitis, 455, 455b
Nonsteroidal anti-inflammatory drugs (NSAIDs), 35, 37
    adverse effects of, 37, 37b, 49
    for eye inflammation and infection, 979b
    for rheumatoid arthritis, 310
Nonsustained ventricular tachycardia (NSVT), 669-670
Nontunneled percutaneous central venous catheters, 194-195, 194f
    removal of, 203
Nonunion, 1063
Nonurgent triage, 111t, 112
Norepinephrine
    for anaphylaxis, 354b
    for hypovolemic shock, 748b
Normal breath sounds, 505-506, 506t
Normal flora, 397, 398t, 415
Normal sinus rhythm (NSR), 656, 656f
Normeperidine, 42
Normotonic fluid, 151
Norpace. See Disopyramide phosphate.
North American pit vipers, 123-125, 124b, 124t, 137
Nose, 496-497, 497f
    cancer of, 533-534
    fracture of, 531-532, 532b, 532f
    physical assessment of, 503, 503b
    rhinitis and, 583-584, 584b
        allergic, 349-351, 349f, 351b
Nosebleed, 532-533, 532b-533b, 533f
    in Sjögren's syndrome, 356
Nosocomial infections, 243
Novantrone. See Mitoxantrone.
NPO status, 228, 228b
NPPV. See Noninvasive positive-pressure ventilation (NPPV).
NPSGs. See National Patient Safety Goals (NPSGs).
NPWT. See Negative pressure wound therapy (NPWT).
NRTIs. See Nucleoside reverse transcriptase inhibitors (NRTIs).
NRTs. See Nicotine replacement therapies (NRTs).
NSAIDs. See Nonsteroidal anti-inflammatory drugs (NSAIDs).
NSR. See Normal sinus rhythm (NSR).
NSVT. See Nonsustained ventricular tachycardia (NSVT).
Nuchal rigidity, 863
Nuclear, biologic, and chemical threats, 139
Nuclear scans, 1018
Nucleic acid amplification test (NAAT), 334-335
Nucleoside reverse transcriptase inhibitors (NRTIs), 327, 339, 339b

Nucleotides, 53, 53f
Nucynta. See Tapentadol.
Nurses Improving Care for Healthsystem Elders (NICHE) project, 20
Nurse's role in emergency and disaster preparedness, 143-144, 144b, 144t, 146
Nursing assistants, 76
Nursing technicians, 76
Nutrient deficiencies, 1239t
Nutrition, 1082, 1082f
    acquired immune deficiency syndrome and, 341
    acute pancreatitis and, 1222-1223
    after burns, 486-487
    after head and neck cancer surgery, 542
    chronic kidney disease and, 1427-1428, 1427t
    myasthenia gravis and, 921b
    older adults and, 10-11, 11b, 1233b
    pressure ulcer prevention and, 440
    standards for health promotion and maintenance, 1232-1233, 1233b, 1233f, 1233t
    tracheostomy and, 528, 528b
Nutrition assessment, 1233-1236
    anthropometric measurements in, 1234-1236, 1236b
    initial screening in, 1234, 1234b, 1235f
    in rehabilitation setting, 78, 78t
Nutrition history
    in cardiovascular assessment, 634
    in endocrine assessment, 1261-1262
    in gastrointestinal assessment, 1087-1089, 1088b
    in musculoskeletal assessment, 1021
    in renal assessment, 1352
    in reproductive assessment, 1453, 1453b
    in vision assessment, 971
Nutrition screening, initial, 1234, 1234b, 1235f
Nutrition therapy
    in acute kidney injury, 1417
    in acute respiratory distress syndrome, 614
    in AIDS and HIV infection, 341
    in atherosclerosis, 708
    in cancer, 372
    in chronic obstructive pulmonary disease, 565
    in cirrhosis, 1199, 1201
    in Crohn's disease, 1183-1184
    in diabetes mellitus, 1319-1321, 1319t, 1320b-1321b, 1329-1331, 1331b
    in esophageal tumors, 1119, 1119b, 1122
    in fluid overload, 159-160
    in gout, 320
    in heart failure, 685, 691

Nutrition therapy (Continued)
    in hyperkalemia, 167b
    in hypernatremia, 163
    in hypocalcemia, 169
    in hypokalemia, 165
    in hyponatremia, 162
    in hypophosphatemia, 170
    in leukemia, 814
    in malnutrition, 1239-1240, 1240b
    in obesity, 1249
    in osteoporosis, 1033
    in peptic ulcer disease, 1135
    postoperative
        in diabetes mellitus, 1325
        in pressure ulcers, 438b, 446
    in ulcerative colitis, 1177
    in urge incontinence, 1380
    in urinary incontinence, 1377
    in urolithiasis, 1387, 1388t
Nutritional status, 1233
    in hematologic assessment, 791
    in integumentary assessment, 420-421
    preoperative assessment of, 222
    in pressure ulcers, 440
    in respiratory assessment, 502
    in traumatic brain injury, 955
Nutritional supplements, 1240
Nystagmus, 905, 936, 973, 973f

O
Obesity, 1246-1252. See also Malnutrition.
    assessment in, 1248
    atrial fibrillation and, 666b
    behavioral management of, 1250
    community-based care in, 1252, 1252b
    complementary and alternative therapies for, 1250
    diet programs for, 1248-1249
    drug therapy for, 1249, 1250b
    exercise program for, 1249
    health promotion and maintenance in, 1247-1248, 1247t
    nutrition therapy for, 1248-1249
    pathophysiology of, 1246-1247, 1247b, 1247t
    preoperative assessment of, 222
    surgical management of, 1250-1252, 1251b-1252b, 1251f
Obligatory urine output, 153
Obstructions
    airway, 536-537, 536b-537b, 537f
        in head and neck cancer, preventing, 539-542, 540b-541b, 541t, 542f
        in pneumonia, 593
    biliary, 1193
    bladder outlet, 1500, 1500f
    intestinal, 1157-1161, 1158f, 1159b, 1161b
    urinary
        in urolithiasis, 1387-1388, 1388b, 1388t

Obstructive jaundice, 1214
Obstructive shock, 741
Obstructive sleep apnea (OSA), 534-535
Occipital lobe, 831t
Occupational exposure to infection, 406-407, 407b
Occupational pulmonary disease, 572, 573b
Occupational Safety and Health Administration (OSHA), 379-380, 406
Occupational therapists, 76, 76f
Ocular irrigation, 991b
Ocular melanomas, 992
Ocular muscles, 967-968, 969t, 970b
Oculomotor nerve, 835t
Odynophagia
    in esophageal tumors, 1118
    in gastroesophageal reflux disease, 1112
Off-pump coronary artery bypass (OPCAB), 779
Old old, 9-10
Older adults, 9-23
    acid-base imbalances in, 179b
    acute glomerulonephritis in, 1403b
    Alzheimer's disease in. See Alzheimer's disease.
    anemia in, 804b
    antihistamines and, 584b
    appendicitis in, 1169b
    asthma in, 533b
    benign prostatic hyperplasia and, 1505b
    body weight and body mass index of, 1236b
    bone healing in, 1053b
    burns in, 474b, 479b
    cancer in
        bladder, 367b
        chemotherapy-induced nausea and vomiting and, 384b
        chemotherapy-induced neutropenia and, 381b
        colorectal, 367b
        leukemia in, 367b
        lung, 367b
        prostate, 367b
    cardiovascular assessment in, 635b
    cholecystitis in, 1215b-1216b
    chronic respiratory problems in, 532b
    clinical breast examination in, 1467b
    coronary artery disease in, 760b, 762b, 769b, 780b
    cultural considerations in, 20b
    decreased mobility in, 11-12, 12b, 12f
    decreased nutrition and hydration in, 10-11, 11b
    dehydration in, 155b-156b, 156f, 230b, 424b

Older adults *(Continued)*
  diabetes mellitus in
    activity program for, 1322b
    diabetic retinopathy and, 1305b
    hypoglycemia in, 1332b
    nutrition and, 1321b
  diverticular disease in, 1186b
  diverticulitis in, 1187b
  driving safety and, 13, 14b
  drug use and misuse and, 13-16, 23
    adverse drug events and, 14
    medication assessment and
      health teaching in, 15-16,
      15b, 15t
    self-administration of drugs
      and, 14-15, 15f
  dysrhythmias in, 674b
  elder neglect and abuse and, 19,
    19t, 23
  electrolyte imbalances and, 161b
  emergency care of, 106b
    discharge from emergency
      department and, 112b
    patient assessment and,
      109b-110b
  endocrine system of, 1260-1261,
    1261b
  end-of-life care for, 92b
    hospice and, 94b
    pain management in, 97b
  eye problems in, 970b
  fall prevention and, 13
  fecal impaction in, 1161b
  fluid balance and, 153b
  fractures in, 1064b, 1067b
  gastroesophageal reflux disease in,
    1112b-1113b
  gastrointestinal changes in, 1087,
    1088b
  geriatric syndromes and, 9-10
  health promotion and, 10, 10b, 23
  hearing changes in, 999b
  heart failure in, 681b, 681t, 683b,
    685b
  heat-related illness in, 121b-122b
  hematologic assessment in, 790b
  hemodialysis and, 1437b
  HIV infection in, 329b-330b
  homeless, 10
  hospitalized or institutionalized
    confusion, falls, and skin
      breakdown in, 20-22,
      21b-22b
    sleep, nutrition, and
      incontinence issues in, 20
  immune function and, 276, 277b
  impaired vision in, 987b
  infection risk in, 398, 398b, 407b
  infusion therapy in, 207-210
    cardiac and renal status changes
      and, 209-210
    catheter securement and, 209b,
      210f
    skin care in, 207-209
    vein and catheter selection in,
      209

Older adults *(Continued)*
  integumentary system and, 398b,
    418b-419b
  loop diuretics and, 714b
  low back pain in, 886b
  malnutrition in, 1237b-1238b,
    1240b, 1244b
  mental health and behavioral
    health problems in, 16-19
    alcohol use and abuse, 18-19,
      19b
    delirium, 18, 18b, 18t, 23
    dementia, 16, 18t, 23
    depression, 16, 16b-17b, 17f, 23
  musculoskeletal changes in, 1020,
    1020b
  neurologic changes in, 836b
  normal plasma electrolyte values
    for, 152b
  nutritional recommendations for,
    1233b
  pain and, 32b, 37b, 46b
    adjuvant analgesics and, 45b
    opioid analgesics and, 38b-39b,
      44b
  peptic ulcer disease and, 1132b
  pneumonia in, 592b
  pressure ulcers in, 437b
  rehabilitation and, 77b, 87b
  renal changes associated with
    aging in, 1351, 1351b
  reproductive system of, 1452b
  seizures in, 858b
  sexually transmitted diseases and,
    1531b
  shingles and, 452
  shock in, 752b
  skin of, 418b-419b, 419f, 424b, 432
  stomatitis and, 1100b
  stress and loss and, 12-13, 13b, 23
  surgery and
    increased risk for surgical
      complications and, 219,
      220b
    intraoperative care and, 251b
    postoperative care and, 261b,
      267b
    preoperative care and, 219,
      220b-221b, 230b
    total hip arthroplasty in, 297b
  thyroid problems and, 1294b
  tracheostomy in, 529b
  transfusion therapy in, 823b
  as transgender patients, 1523b
  transition from hospital or
    long-term care setting to
    home, 22
  urinary incontinence in, 1375b
  urinary tract infections in, 1369b
  ventilator dependence and, 622b
  wound healing in, 436b
Olfactory nerve, 496, 835t
Oligospermia, 1514
Oliguria
  preoperative assessment of, 221-222
  in renal colic, 1385

Oncogene activation, 365-366
Oncogenes, 362, 366
Oncogenesis, 362-363
Oncologic emergencies, 392-394
  hypercalcemia, 393
  sepsis and disseminated
    intravascular coagulation, 392
  spinal cord compression, 393
  superior vena cava syndrome,
    393-394, 393f-394f, 394b
  syndrome of inappropriate
    antidiuretic hormone,
    392-393, 392b
  tumor lysis syndrome, 394, 394f
Oncology Nursing Society (ONS),
  378-379
Oncoviruses, 366, 366t
Ondansetron, 385b
On-Q PainBuster pump, 199-200,
  199f
ONS. *See* Oncology Nursing Society
  (ONS).
Onychomycosis, 427
Opacities, corneal, 981-982, 981f,
  982t
OPCAB. *See* Off-pump coronary
  artery bypass (OPCAB).
Open fractures, 1051-1052, 1052f
Open orchiectomy, 1515, 1515b
Open radical prostatectomy, 1509,
  1509b
Open reduction with internal
  fixation, 1062
Open traumatic brain injury,
  946-947, 947f, 948b
Operating room technicians (ORTs),
  239
Operating rooms, 241-244
  health and hygiene of surgical
    team and, 242-243
  layout of, 241-242, 241f
  minimally invasive and robotic
    surgery and, 242, 242f-243f
  patient transfer to, 234-236, 235f,
    251b
  surgical attire and, 243, 244f
  surgical scrub and, 243-244, 244b,
    245f
Ophthalmic ointment, 978b, 978f
Ophthalmoscopy, 974-975, 974f,
  975b, 975t
Opioid analgesics, 35, 36t, 37-44.
  *See also specific opioid
  analgesics.*
  adverse effects of, 43-44, 43t-44t,
    44b
  for burns, 480, 480b
  for dyspnea near death, 98
  equianalgesia and, 40, 50
  gender considerations in, 38b
  genetic considerations in
    administration of, 37b
  for lung cancer, 580
  modified-release, 40-41, 41b
  older adults and, 38b-39b, 44b
  overdose of, 271b

Opioid analgesics *(Continued)*
  physical dependence, tolerance,
    addition, and, 38-40, 49-50
  for postoperative pain, 269,
    269b-270b
Opioid antagonists, 38, 44b
Opportunistic infections in HIV
  infections, 328, 333-335,
    334b-335b, 334f
Oprelvekin, 383, 387t
Optic disc, 967, 967f
Optic fundus, 967, 967f
Optic nerve, 835t, 968
Oral cancer, 1102-1103
  assessment of, 1103-1104, 1103b,
    1103f
  health care resources for, 1107
  home care management in, 1106
  interventions for, 1104,
    1104b-1105b
  pathophysiology of, 1102-1103,
    1103b
  self-management education in,
    1106-1107, 1107b
Oral candidiasis, 452
Oral cavity, 1085, 1100b
Oral cavity problems, 1099-1109
  health promotion and
    maintenance in, 1109
  oral care in, 1100b
  oral tumors. *See* Oral tumors.
  salivary gland disorders,
    1107-1108
  stomatitis, 1100-1102, 1100b-
    1102b, 1100f
Oral food challenges, 350
Oral hygiene
  during chemotherapy, 384,
    386b
  during mechanical ventilation,
    621b
  tracheostomy and, 527-528
Oral rehydration solutions (ORS),
  157
Oral tumors, 1102-1107
  oral cancer, 1102-1103
    assessment of, 1103-1104,
      1103b, 1103f
    health care resources for, 1107
    home care management in,
      1106
    interventions for, 1104,
      1104b-1105b
    pathophysiology of, 1102-1103,
      1103b
    self-management education in,
      1106-1107, 1107b
  premalignant lesions, 1102
Orbit, 966
Orchiectomy, 1515, 1515b
Orchitis, 1452
Orencia. *See* Abatacept.
Organ of Corti, 998
Orotracheal intubation, 536
ORS. *See* Oral rehydration solutions
  (ORS).

Orthopnea, 503
in acute respiratory failure, 612
cardiovascular assessment and, 635
in chronic obstructive pulmonary disease, 538
in heart failure, 682
Orthostatic hypotension, 638
in dehydration, 156
in hypertension, 711
in rehabilitation setting, 81b
Orthotopic heart transplantation, 702, 703f
ORTs. See Operating room technicians (ORTs).
OSA. See Obstructive sleep apnea (OSA).
Oseltamivir, 588
OSHA. See Occupational Safety and Health Administration (OSHA).
Osmolality, 151
Osmolarity, 151
of urine, 1358-1359
Osmoreceptors, 151
Osmosis, 151-152, 151f
Osteoarthritis, 291-304
chronic pain in, 293-303
complementary and alternative medicine for, 294-295, 295b
drug therapy for, 293-294, 293b-294b
nonpharmacologic interventions for, 294, 294b
etiology and genetic risk for, 300-301, 304b
health care resources for, 304
health promotion and maintenance in, 301
history in, 292
home care management in, 304
imaging assessment in, 293
improving mobility in, 303, 303b
incidence and prevalence of, 291
laboratory assessment in, 293
pathophysiology of, 291, 291f
physical assessment in, 292-293, 292f, 292t
psychosocial assessment in, 293
self-management education in, 304, 304b
surgical management of, 295-303
hand and ankle arthroplasties in, 303
total elbow arthroplasty in, 303
total hip arthroplasty in, 295-300, 297b-300b, 297f-298f, 297t
total knee arthroplasty in, 300-302, 301f, 302b
total shoulder arthroplasty in, 303
Osteoblasts, 1018
Osteoclasts, 1018
Osteocytes, 1018

Osteomalacia, 1036-1037, 1036t
Osteomyelitis, 1039-1041, 1040b-1041b, 1040f
Osteonecrosis, 1034
in systemic lupus erythematosus, 315
total joint arthroplasty for, 295
Osteopenia, 1030
Osteophytes, 291, 291f
Osteoporosis, 1029-1036
community-based care in, 1036
drug therapy for, 1034-1035, 1034b-1035b
health promotion and maintenance in, 1031-1032
imaging assessment in, 1033
laboratory assessment in, 1032-1033
lifestyle changes for, 1033
nutrition therapy in, 1033
osteomalacia vs., 1036t
pathophysiology of, 1029-1031, 1030b-1031b, 1030t
physical assessment in, 1032, 1032f
psychosocial assessment in, 1032
Osteotomies, 1046
Ostomate, 1177
Ostomy, 1152t
Otitis media, 1005-1006, 1006f, 1007b
Otorrhea, 863
Otoscopic examination, 1000-1001, 1000b-1001b, 1001f
Outflow disease, 720
Outpatient surgery, 218-219
Ovarian cancer, 1495-1497, 1496t
Ovarian cysts, 1487
Ovarian hormones, 1256t
Ovaries, 1450, 1450f
Overactive bladder, 87
Overdose of anesthesia, 247
Overflow incontinence, 1373, 1374t, 1375
in benign prostatic hyperplasia, 1500
Overhydration, 158
Overweight, 633
Ovoid pupil in traumatic brain injury, 952
Oxycodone, 41, 270b
Oxygen concentrator, 521
Oxygen delivery systems, 516-520
high-flow, 519-520, 519t
face tent, aerosol mask, tracheostomy collar, and T piece in, 519-520, 520f
Venturi masks in, 519, 519f
low-flow, 517-519, 517t, 518f, 519b
nasal cannula in, 517-518, 518f
non-rebreather masks in, 518, 518f, 519b
partial rebreather masks in, 518, 518f
simple facemasks in, 518, 518f
respiratory problems and, 603, 604f
Oxygen dissociation, 786

Oxygen saturation
cultural considerations in, 500b
in sepsis and septic shock, 754
Oxygen therapy, 514-521, 515f
in acute respiratory failure, 612
in asthma, 535, 543b
in burns, 478
in chronic obstructive pulmonary disease, 563
in dyspnea near death, 98, 98b
hazards and complications of, 515-516
absorption atelectasis in, 516, 516b
bacterial contamination of oxygen delivery system in, 516, 516b
drying of mucous membranes in, 516, 516f
oxygen toxicity in, 516
oxygen-induced hypoventilation in, 515
high-flow delivery systems for, 519-520, 519f-520f, 519t
home care management in, 521
home care preparation for, 521, 521f, 522b
low-flow delivery systems for, 517t
facemasks in, 518-519, 518f, 519b
nasal cannula in, 517-518, 518f
in lung cancer, 579-580
noninvasive positive-pressure ventilation in, 520, 520f
patient safety in, 515b
in pneumonia, 593
pneumonia and, 593
postoperative, 266
in respiratory acidosis, 183
self-management education in, 521
transtracheal, 520, 522b
Oxygen toxicity, 516
Oxygenation, 492-493, 514
AIDS/HIV infection and, 340
cancer and, 372
hematologic system's role in, 785, 786f
oxygen therapy and, 514, 515f
pneumonia and, 593
respiratory problems and, 603, 604f
respiratory system's role in, 494, 495f
shock and, 739-740, 740f, 742f
Oxygenation failure, 610-611, 612t
combined ventilatory and, 611-612
Oxygen-hemoglobin dissociation curve, 499-500, 500f
Oxygen-induced hypoventilation, 515

P
P waves, 652, 654f, 655
PAC. See Premature atrial complexes (PAC).

Pacemakers, 664, 664f-665f, 674, 674b-675b
Pack-years, 494-495, 632
Paco$_2$. See Partial pressure of arterial carbon dioxide (Paco$_2$).
PACU. See Postanesthesia care unit (PACU).
PACU nurses. See Postanesthesia care unit (PACU) nurses.
PAD. See Peripheral arterial disease (PAD).
Paget's disease of the bone, 1037-1039, 1037b-1038b
PAH. See Pulmonary arterial hypertension (PAH).
Pain, 24-50
abdominal, 315
acute, 25-26
characteristics of, 25t, 28t
in coronary artery disease, 764-766, 764b-766b
in acute pancreatitis, 1221-1222, 1222b
in AIDS and HIV infection, 340-341
assessment of, 28-34, 49-50
challenges in, 33-34, 33t, 34b
comprehensive, 29-32, 30t, 31f-32f
postoperative, 264-265
psychosocial, 32-33, 33b
back. See Back pain.
in bone cancer, 1045
in burns, 479-480, 480b
categorization of
by duration, 25-26, 25t
by underlying mechanisms, 26-28, 28t, 29f
chest, 634-635
in coronary artery disease, 782b
in lung cancer, 579-580
respiratory assessment and, 502
types of, 636t
chronic, 26
in cancer, 26
in osteoarthritis, 293-303
complementary and alternative therapies for, 294-295, 295b
nonpharmacologic interventions for, 294, 294b
psychosocial assessment in, 32-33
definitions of, 25
in diabetes mellitus, 1328
drug therapy for, 34-45, 49-50
adjuvant analgesics in, 35, 36t, 45, 45b-46b
around-the-clock dosing in, 34-35
multimodal analgesia in, 34, 49
non-opioid analgesics in, 35-37, 36t, 37b
older adults and, 37b-38b

Pain (Continued)
  opioid analgesics in. See Opioid
    analgesics.
  in osteoarthritis, 293-294,
    293b-294b
  patient-controlled analgesia in,
    35, 35b
  routes of administration in, 34
  in fractures, 1057-1063
  in Guillain-Barré syndrome, 916,
    916b
  home care management in, 48,
    50
  management at end of life, 97,
    97b
  neck, 891-892, 891b-892b
  nonpharmacologic interventions
    for, 46-48, 46b, 48b, 50
  older adults and, 32b, 37b
  in peptic ulcer disease, 1132-1136,
    1132b, 1135b-1136b
  in pericarditis, 699
  in polycystic kidney disease, 1397,
    1397b
  postoperative
    in amputation, 1072-1073,
      1072b
    in coronary artery bypass graft,
      778
    drug therapy for, 269-270,
      269b-271b
    in head and neck cancer
      surgery, 542
    management of, 269-271,
      269b-271b
  in total hip arthroplasty, 299
  in pyelonephritis, 1401
  in rheumatoid arthritis, 308-312,
    308b-310b
  scope of problem, 25, 25t
  in sickle cell disease, 801-802,
    802b
  in ulcerative colitis, 1179, 1179b
  in urolithiasis, 1385-1387
Pain rating scales, 30-32, 30t
Palliation, 94, 574, 580
Palliative care, 94-95, 95t, 97b
  for amyotrophic lateral sclerosis,
    911b
Palliative sedation, 100
Palliative surgery, 218t, 373
Pallor, 422t
  assessment of, 792b
  in darker skinned patient, 428
Palmoplantar pustulosis (PPP), 456
Palonosetron, 385b
Palpation
  in abdominal assessment,
    1090-1091
  of chest, 504
  in endocrine assessment,
    1262-1263, 1263b
  of kidney, 1353, 1354f
  of skin, 424, 424b, 425t
  of spleen, 793b

Palpitations, 635, 656-657
PALS. See Pediatric Advanced Life
  Support (PALS).
Panacinar emphysema, 532f
Pancreas, 1086, 1086f, 1260, 1260f
  diabetes mellitus and, 1301, 1301f
  hormones secreted by, 1256t
Pancreas transplantation, 1323-1324
Pancreatic abscesses, 1226
Pancreatic cancer, 1226-1230, 1227b,
  1229f, 1229t, 1230b
Pancreatic problems
  acute pancreatitis, 1218-1223
    assessment in, 1220-1221,
      1221b, 1221t
    community-based care in, 1223
    evaluation of care of patient
      with, 1223
    nutrition in, 1222-1223
    pain management in,
      1221-1222, 1222b
    pathophysiology of, 1218-1220,
      1219f, 1219t
  chronic pancreatitis, 1223-1226,
    1224b-1225b
  pancreatic abscesses, 1226
  pancreatic cancer, 1226-1230,
    1227b, 1229f, 1229t, 1230b
  pancreatic pseudocysts, 1226
Pancreatic pseudocysts, 1226
Pancreaticoduodenectomy, 1229,
  1229f
Pancreatitis
  acute, 1218-1223
    assessment in, 1220-1221,
      1221b, 1221t
    community-based care in, 1223
    evaluation of care of patient
      with, 1223
    nutrition in, 1222-1223
    pain management in,
      1221-1222, 1222b
    pathophysiology of, 1218-1220,
      1219f, 1219t
  chronic, 1223-1226, 1224b-1225b
Pancytopenia
  after transplantation, 813
  in aplastic anemia, 805
  in lupus, 315
  in myelodysplastic syndromes, 806
Pandemic influenza, 587-588
Pandemics, 140, 413
Panhysterectomy, 1489t
Panlobular emphysema, 532f
Panniculectomy, 1252
Panniculus, 1252
Pannus, 305
PAOP. See Pulmonary artery
  occlusive pressure (PAOP).
Papanicolaou test, 1454, 1459
Papilla, renal, 1345, 1345f
Papilledema
  in brain tumors, 958
  in traumatic brain injury, 952
Papilloma, intraductal, 1462t, 1463

Papillotomy, 1094
PAPR. See Powered air purifying
  respirator (PAPR).
Papular rash, 424
Papules, 423f
Paracentesis for ascites, 1199,
  1199b
Paradoxical blood pressure, 638
Paradoxical chest movement, 623,
  623f
Paradoxical pulse, 699
Paradoxical splitting, 640
Paraffin dip in rheumatoid arthritis,
  311
Paralysis
  assessment in rehabilitation
    setting, 78-79
  facial, 927-928
  in lightning strike injury, 130
  vocal cord, 535, 535b
Paralytic ileus, 1157
  after lumbar spinal surgery, 889b
  in hypokalemia, 164
Paramedics, 107
Paranasal sinuses, 497, 497f
Paraneoplastic syndromes, 574, 574t
Paraparesis, 894
Paraplegia, 894
Parasitic disorders, 453-455
  bedbugs, 454-455
  intestinal infections, 1189-1190,
    1190b
  pediculosis, 453-454
  scabies, 454, 454f
Parathyroid glands, 1260, 1260f
  hormones secreted by, 1256t
Parathyroid problems, 1296-1298
  hyperparathyroidism, 1296-1298,
    1296t, 1297b
  hypoparathyroidism, 1296t, 1298
Parenteral nutrition, 1244-1245,
  1245b
  after burns, 487
  total parenteral nutrition in, 1245,
    1245b
Parenteral transmission of human
  immune deficiency virus,
  331-332
Paresis, 78-79
Paresthesia
  in back pain, 886
  in black widow spider bites, 127
  in Guillain-Barré syndrome, 914
  in hyperkalemia, 166
  in rheumatoid arthritis, 306
Parietal cells, 1086
Parietal lobe, 831t
Parkinson disease (PD), 867-871,
  867t, 868b-869b, 868f
  drug therapy for, 868-870, 869b
  genetic considerations in, 867b
  psychosocial support in, 870-871
  surgical management of, 871
Paronychia, 427
Parotidectomy, 1108

Paroxysmal nocturnal dyspnea
  (PND), 503
  cardiovascular assessment and,
    635
  in heart failure, 682
Paroxysmal supraventricular
  tachycardias (PSVT), 665
Partial agonist opioids, 38
Partial pressure of arterial carbon
  dioxide (Paco₂), 514-515
Partial rebreather masks, 517t, 518,
  518f
Partial seizures, 858
Partial thromboplastin time (PTT),
  606, 608b, 795
Partial-breast irradiation, 1476
Partial-pressure of end-tidal carbon
  dioxide (PETCO₂), 509
Partial-thickness wounds, 435, 435f,
  466-468, 468f
Pasero Opioid-Induced Sedation
  Scale (POSS), 44t
Passive euthanasia, 103
Passive immunity, 285, 398
Passive smoking, 495
Patch testing, 356
Patches, 423f, 456
Patellofemoral pain syndrome
  (PFPS), 1076
Pathogenicity, 397
Pathogens, 397-400
  bioterrorism agents, 411t
  routes of transmission and, 399
Pathologic fractures, 372, 1052
Patient and family education
  in advance directives, 103
  in AIDS and HIV infection
    HIV testing and, 333b
    preventing transmission by
      health care workers, 332b
    prevention of infection, 338,
      338b, 343, 344b
  in Alzheimer's disease, 880
  in arthropod bite/sting
    prevention, 126b
  in asthma, 534
    self-management and, 537b
    using inhalers, 540b-541b, 543b
    using peak flow meters, 536b,
      542f, 552-553
  in automatic epinephrine
    injectors, 352b
  in back pain, 886b
    exercises for chronic or
      postoperative low back
      pain, 887b
  in bariatric surgery, 1252b
  in burns, 489
  in cancer
    in breast, 1478-1479, 1479b
    chemotherapy-induced
      peripheral neuropathy,
      386b
    in colorectal, 1155-1157,
      1155b-1156b

Patient and family education
(Continued)
  dietary habits to reduce risk of,
    367b
  infection prevention during
    chemotherapy and, 382b
  mouth care for mucositis and,
    386b
  prevention of injury or bleeding
    and, 384b
  prevention of skin cancer and,
    460b
  in cataracts, 984, 984b
  in cerumen removal, 999b
  in cervical ablation therapies,
    1495b
  in cervical biopsy, 1458b
  in chronic kidney disease, 1445
  in chronic obstructive pulmonary
    disease, 563b
  in chronic pancreatitis, 1225b
  in cirrhosis, 1202, 1202b
  in coronary artery disease,
    781-782, 781b-782b
  in cortisol replacement therapy,
    1281b
  in diabetes mellitus
    blood glucose monitoring,
      1317-1319
    diabetic ketoacidosis and,
      1335b
    exercise and, 1322b
    foot care and, 1327b
    hypoglycemia and, 1331,
      1331b
    insulin administration,
      1316-1317, 1316b
    nutrition plan and, 1320
  in dysrhythmias, 673-676,
    673b-675b
  in emergency care, 113-114
  in emotional signs of approaching
    death, 96b
  in energy conservation in arthritis,
    312b
  in epilepsy, 859, 861b
  in fractures, 1065, 1065b
  in gastric cancer, 1142
  in gastritis prevention, 1127b
  in gastroesophageal reflux disease,
    1113b-1114b
  in genital herpes, 1536, 1536b
  in glucosamine supplements, 295b
  in gonorrhea, 1540-1541
  in head and neck cancer, 544-545,
    545b
  in heart failure, 691, 691b
  in hiatal hernias, 1114b, 1116b
  in home care of central venous
    catheter, 815b
  in hyperkalemia, 167, 167b
  in hypersensitivity, 358
  in hypertension, 712-717
  in implantable cardioverter/
    defibrillator, 675b
  in infection, 410

Patient and family education
(Continued)
  in infection control and
    prevention, 410, 816b
    MRSA and, 452b
  in infusion therapy, 200
  in insulin therapy, 1316-1317,
    1316b, 1317f
  in kidney and genitourinary
    trauma, 1408b
  in kidney and urinary problems,
    1422b
  in lightning strike prevention, 130b
  in Lyme disease, 321b
  in magnetic resonance imaging,
    1026b
  in maintaining healthy oral cavity,
    1100b
  in malnutrition, 1246
  in multiple sclerosis, 909-910
  in myasthenia gravis, 922, 922b,
    922t
  in oral cancer, 1106-1107, 1107b
  in osteoarthritis, 303-304,
    303b-304b
  in oxygen therapy, 521
  in pain management, 37, 46b, 48
  in pelvic inflammatory disease,
    1543-1544, 1543b
  in pelvic muscle exercises, 1377b
  in peptic ulcer disease, 1138,
    1138b
  in peripheral arterial disease, 725b
  in permanent pacemakers,
    674b-675b
  in pneumonia, 589-590, 589b, 594
  in polycystic kidney disease, 1397b
  in polycythemia vera, 805b
  in post-mastectomy exercises,
    1474b
  postoperative, 272-273, 272b
  preoperative, 225-233, 226t,
    230b-231b, 231f, 236
  in preparing for self-management,
    10, 10b
  in pressure ulcers, 443
  in prevention of ear infection or
    trauma, 1013b
  in prostate cancer, 1511, 1511b
  in psoriasis, 457
  in pulmonary embolism, 610,
    610b
  in recovery from ear surgery, 1007b
  in rehabilitation, 89
  in rheumatoid arthritis, 313
  in risk for bleeding in leukemia,
    816b
  in sickle cell crisis, 803b
  in signs and symptoms of
    approaching death, 96b
  in signs that death has occurred,
    102b
  in skin problems
    in lupus, 316b
    prevention of dry skin and,
      433b

Patient and family education
(Continued)
  in smoking cessation, 496b
  in spinal cord injury, 898b,
    900-901, 901b
  in stroke, 933b, 944-945, 945b,
    945f
  in total hip arthroplasty, 298b,
    300b
  in toxic shock syndrome, 1485b
  in traumatic brain injury, 956-957,
    957b
  in ulcerative colitis, 1180, 1181b
  in urinary calculi, 1388b
  in urinary incontinence, 1383,
    1383b
  in urinary tract infection
    prevention, 1369b
  in using eyedrops, 970b, 975b
  in vaginal infections, 1485b
  in valvular heart disease, 696-697,
    697b
  in venous insufficiency, 734b
  in viral hepatitis, 1205b, 1208b
  in vulvovaginitis, 1485b
  in warfarin, 733b
  in West Nile virus, 866b
Patient autonomy, 4
Patient disposition
  after emergency care, 112-114
  in trauma care, 118
Patient history. See History.
Patient identification
  in emergency care, 108b, 109
  Joint Commission on, 250,
    250b
Patient placement, infection control
  and, 405
Patient preparation
  for arthroscopy, 1026
  for bone marrow aspiration and
    biopsy, 795-796
  for bronchoscopy, 510, 510b
  for cardiac catheterization, 643,
    643t
  for colonoscopy, 1095-1096
  for cystography and
    cystourethrography, 1362
  for cystoscopy or
    cystourethroscopy, 1361-1362
  for endoscopic surgery, 242
  for exercise electrocardiography,
    645
  for kidney biopsy, 1363
  for lung biopsy, 511-512
  for nephrostomy, 1398
  preoperative, 234
  for renal scan, 1361
  for thoracentesis, 511, 511f
Patient safety, 2-7
  after anterior cervical diskectomy
    and fusion, 428b
  allergic reactions to bee or wasp
    stings and, 129b
  in Alteplase, 939b
  in anticoagulant therapy, 609b

Patient safety (Continued)
  in arteriovenous fistula or graft,
    1435b
  aspiration prevention, 543b
  in assessing breast mass, 1469b
  in assessing changes in dark skin,
    428b
  in bladder training and habit
    training, 1381b
  in brachytherapy, 1493b
  care of hospitalized
    immunosuppressed patients,
    338b
  in carpal tunnel syndrome, 1077b
  in chemotherapy-related
    neutropenia, 382b
  in chemotherapy-related
    thrombocytopenia, 383b
  in chest tube drainage systems,
    579b
  in cognition assessment, 540b
  in colonoscopy, 1096b
  in colorectal cancer, 1150b, 1154b
  in communication with patient
    with advanced dementia or
    Alzheimer's disease, 877b
    unable to speak, 540b
  in conserving energy, 815b
  in continuous passive motion
    machines, 302b
  dehydration and, 157, 157b
  in dysrhythmias, 658b
  emergency care and, 108-109,
    108b-109b, 112
    of burns, 473b
    of patient experiencing
      benzodiazepine overdose,
      266b
    of patient experiencing chest
      pain, 764b
    of patient experiencing opioid
      overdose, 271b
    of patient experiencing surgical
      wound evisceration, 269b
    of patient with acute adrenal
      insufficiency, 1274b
    of patient with anaphylaxis,
      353b
    of patient with anterior
      nosebleed, 532b
    of patient with extremity
      fracture, 1058b
    of patient with hypertensive
      urgency or crisis, 718b
    of patient with sports-related
      injuries, 1076b
  in endocrine testing, 1263b
  in esophagitis and systemic
    sclerosis, 318b
  establishing a nursing database:
    history, 838b
  fluid overload and, 158-159, 160b
  fluid resuscitation of burn patient,
    479b
  frostbite and, 133b
  gait training and, 83b

Patient safety (Continued)
  in gastrointestinal assessment, 1088b
  health care facility fires and, 139b
  heat stroke and, 123b
  history of patient of with skin problem and, 420b
  in hospitalized patients with Alzheimer's disease, 878b
  in hypovolemic shock, 747b
  in infection control for home care of person with AIDS, 344b
  in instillation of eardrops, 1004b, 1005f
  in instillation of eyedrops, 975b
  in instillation of ophthalmic ointment, 978b
  in interventions for patients at risk for infection, 401b
  in intraoperative autologous blood salvage and transfusion, 251b
  intraoperative care and
    advance directives and, 250b
    malignant hyperthermia and, 247b
    intraoperative positioning and, 253b
  iodine-based contrast agent and, 845b
  in kidney tests or procedures using contrast medium, 1361b
  in lumbar spinal surgery, 889b
  in management of fluid volume in chronic kidney disease, 1426b
  in mechanical ventilation, 617b
  in meningitis, 865b
  in myasthenia gravis, 921b
  in myxedema coma, 1294b
  in ocular compresses, 980b
  in ocular irrigation, 991b
  in older adult receiving transfusion, 823b
  in open radical prostatectomy, 1509b
  in oral hygiene, 1101b
  in osteoporosis, 1030b
  in oxygen therapy, 515b
  in paracentesis, 1199b
  in Parkinson disease, 869b
  in pericarditis, 700b
  perineal wound care and, 1154b
  in peritoneal dialysis, 1440b
  in positioning to prevent contractures, 487b
  postmortem care and, 102b
  postoperative
    complications in hiatal hernia surgery, 1116b
    in complications of spinal and epidural anesthesia, 261b
    hand-off reports and, 257b
    in heart transplantation rejection, 703b
    in hernia repair, 1148b
    in hypophysectomy, 1270b

Patient safety (Continued)
    in nasogastric tube after esophageal surgery, 1122b
    in nonpharmacologic pain reduction, 271b
    in swallowing after laryngectomy, 543b
  in pressure ulcers
    monitoring of, 448b
    prevention of, 438b
    wound management of, 444b
  pronouncement of death and, 102b
  in psychosocial interventions for dying patients and families, 101b
  in pulmonary embolism, 604b, 606b, 609b
  in reduced vision, 993b
  reducing caregiver stress, 880b
  in reproductive health problems, 1453b
  in sealed implants of radioactive sources, 376b
  in seizures, 861b
  severe hypothermia and, 132b
  in sickle cell crisis, 802b
  in skin care in chronic diarrhea, 1166b
  in spinal cord injury, 897b
  in symptom relief kit for patients in home hospice, 97b
  in thrombocytopenia, 814b
  in thyroid storm, 1291b
  in total parenteral nutrition, 1245b
  in tracheostomy care, 525b, 527b-528b
  in transfusion therapy, 822b
  in transurethral resection of prostate, 1506b
  in tube feeding care and maintenance, 1243b
  in unsealed radioactive isotope for hyperthyroidism, 1290b
  in vertebroplasty and kyphoplasty, 1070b
  in viral hepatitis, 1205b
Patient selection
  for hemodialysis, 1431
  for peritoneal dialysis, 1437
Patient Self-Determination Act, 92, 228
Patient transfer
  infection control principles for, 405
  to surgical suites, 234-236, 235f, 251b
Patient-controlled analgesia (PCA), 35, 35b
  postoperative, 269
Patterns of inheritance. See Inheritance patterns.
PAWP. See Pulmonary artery wedge pressure (PAWP).
PBSC harvesting. See Peripheral blood stem cell (PBSC) harvesting.

PCA. See Patient-controlled analgesia (PCA).
PD. See Parkinson disease (PD).
PDSA cycles, 70, 70f, 72-73
PDT. See Photodynamic therapy (PDT).
Peak airway pressure, 618
Peak expiratory flow (PEF), 552
Peak flow meters, 536b, 542f, 552-553
Peak levels, 409
Pediatric Advanced Life Support (PALS), 111, 111t
Pediculosis, 403, 453-454
Pedigree, 57, 57f, 57t
PEEP. See Positive end-expiratory pressure (PEEP).
PEF. See Peak expiratory flow (PEF).
PEG. See Percutaneous endoscopic gastrostomy (PEG).
Pegfilgrastim, 387t
Pelvic floor exercise therapy, 1377, 1377b
Pelvic fractures, 1069
Pelvic inflammatory disease (PID), 1539, 1541, 1541f, 1542t, 1543b
Pelvic organ prolapse, 1485-1487, 1486f, 1487b
Penetrance, 58
Penetrating trauma, 116
  ocular, 992
  of spinal cord, 893
Penile implants, 1513
Penrose drains, 264, 265f, 268
Peptic ulcer disease (PUD), 1128-1138
  acid suppression for, 1137
  assessment in, 1131-1132, 1132t
  community-based care, 1137-1138, 1138b
  complementary and alternative therapies for, 1129t, 1136, 1136b
  complications of, 1130-1131, 1130b, 1130f
  drug therapy for, 1132-1135, 1132b-1135b
  endoscopic therapy for, 1136-1137, 1137b
  etiology and genetic risk in, 1131
  evaluation of care of patient with, 1138
  incidence and prevalence of, 1131
  interventional radiologic procedures for, 1137
  pain in, 1132-1136, 1132b, 1135b-1136b
  surgical management of, 1137
  types of ulcers in, 1129-1130, 1129f
  upper gastrointestinal bleeding in, 1136-1137, 1136b-1137b
Perception of pain, 28, 29f
Percussion
  of chest, 504, 504f, 505t
  in gastrointestinal assessment, 1090

PCA. See Patient-controlled analgesia (PCA).
Percutaneous alcohol septal ablation, 702
Percutaneous endoscopic gastrostomy (PEG), 1241
Percutaneous lung biopsy, 511-512
Percutaneous stereotactic rhizotomy (PSR), 926-927, 927b
Percutaneous transhepatic cholangiography (PTC), 1093
Percutaneous transluminal angioplasty (PTCA), 722
Perennial rhinitis, 583
Pericardial effusion, 699
Pericardial friction rub, 640
Pericardiectomy, 699
Pericardiocentesis, 700, 700b
Pericarditis, 699-700, 700b
  chest pain in, 636t
  in systemic lupus erythematosus, 315
Perichondritis, 1004
Perinatal transmission of human immune deficiency virus, 332
Perioperative nursing staff, 239-241, 240f-241f
Peripheral arterial disease (PAD), 718-725
  community-based care in, 724-725, 724b-725b
  cultural considerations in, 720b
  imaging assessment in, 720
  nonsurgical management of, 721-723, 722b
  pathophysiology of, 718-719, 719f
  physical assessment in, 719-720, 720f, 721b
  stages of, 719b
  surgical management of, 723-724, 723f, 724b
Peripheral artery aneurysms, 726f, 728
Peripheral blood stem cell (PBSC) harvesting, 811-812
Peripheral chemoreceptors, 631
Peripheral intravenous (IV) therapy, 190-193
  midline catheters in, 192-193, 192f
  short peripheral catheters in, 190-192, 190f-192f, 190t, 191b, 201b
Peripheral nerve blockades (PNBs), 302
Peripheral nerve trauma, 923-925, 923f-924f, 925b
Peripheral nervous system (PNS), 830, 833-834, 834f-835f, 835t
Peripheral nervous system problems, 913-929
  cranial nerve diseases, 926-928
    facial paralysis, 927-928
    trigeminal neuralgia, 926-927, 926f, 927b
  Guillain-Barré syndrome, 913-917, 914b-916b
  myasthenia gravis. See Myasthenia gravis (MG).

Peripheral nervous system problems (Continued)
  peripheral nerve trauma, 923-925, 923f-924f, 925b
  restless legs syndrome, 925-926
Peripheral neuropathy
  chemotherapy-related, 386-387, 386b-387b
  in diabetes mellitus, 1325-1327, 1325f-1327f, 1326b-1327b, 1326t
Peripheral vascular assessment, 260
Peripheral vascular disease (PVD), 718
Peripheral venous disease
  varicose veins in, 735-736
  vascular trauma and, 736
  venous insufficiency in, 734-735, 734b-735b
  venous thromboembolism in. See Venous thromboembolism (VTE).
Peripherally inserted central catheters (PICCs), 193-194, 193f, 194b
Peristalsis, 262
Peritoneal dialysis, 1437-1441
  complications in, 1440-1441, 1440b
  dialysate additives for, 1438
  hemodialysis vs., 1431t
  nursing care in, 1441
  patient selection for, 1437
  procedure in, 1437-1438, 1438f
  types of, 1438-1440, 1438f, 1439f, 1440f
Peritonitis, 1170-1172, 1170b-1171b
Peritonsillar abscesses, 586
Periungual lesions
  in rheumatoid arthritis, 306
  in systemic sclerosis, 317
Permanent pacemaker insertion, 664-665, 665f
Pernicious anemia, 804
PERRLA mnemonic, 840
Persistent pain. See Chronic pain.
Personal emergency preparedness plan, 144, 144t
Personal protective equipment (PPE), 402
  standard precautions and, 403t, 404f
Personal readiness supplies, 144b
Person-to-person transmission, 399
Pertussis, 600
PET. See Positron emission tomography (PET).
PETCO$_2$. See Partial-pressure of end-tidal carbon dioxide (PETCO$_2$).
Petechiae, 422-424, 424f, 792
  in infective endocarditis, 698
PFPS. See Patellofemoral pain syndrome (PFPS).
PFTs. See Pulmonary function tests (PFTs).
PH, 174
  of intravenous solutions, 188

Phagocytosis, 280, 280f, 398t, 400
Phagosome formation, 280
Phalen's maneuver, 1077
Pharmacists, 77
Pharmacologic stress echocardiogram, 646
Pharyngitis, 584-586, 585b-586b, 585t
Pharynx, 497, 1099
  changes with aging, 501b
  physical assessment of, 503
Phenotype, 55
Pheochromocytoma, 1282-1283, 1283b
Phlebitis, 618-619
  catheter-related, 209t
  intravenous therapy-related, 188, 188b, 204t-206t
Phlebothrombosis, 618
Phonophobia, 854, 855b
  in meningitis, 863
Phonophoresis, 887
Phosphorus, 170-171
  abnormal values of, 152t
  hyperphosphatemia and, 171
  hypophosphatemia and, 170, 170t
  plasma values in older adults, 152b
Photodynamic therapy (PDT), 391
  for esophageal cancer, 1120
  for lung cancer, 576
Photophobia
  drug-induced, 971
  in meningitis, 863
  in migraines, 854, 855b
  in stroke, 940
Photovoice, 901-902
Phrenic nerve pacing, 911
Physiatrists, 76
Physical abuse of older adults, 19, 19t
Physical activity in atherosclerosis, 708
Physical assessment
  in acidosis, 181-182, 181b
  in acute glomerulonephritis, 1402, 1403b
  in acute kidney injury, 1415
  in acute pancreatitis, 1220-1221, 1221b
  in acute respiratory distress syndrome, 613
  in adrenal insufficiency, 1274-1275, 1274b, 1275f
  in allergic rhinitis, 349
  in Alzheimer's disease, 873-875, 873b, 874f
  in aneurysms, 726-727
  in asthma, 532-533
  in atherosclerosis, 707-708, 708b
  in back pain, 886
  in benign prostatic hyperplasia, 1503
  in brain abscesses, 963
  in breast cancer, 1469-1470, 1469b
  in burns, 473-476
    airway obstruction and, 474t
    cardiopulmonary assessment and, 481

Physical assessment (Continued)
    cardiovascular assessment and, 475
    direct airway injury and, 473-474, 474b, 474t
    gastrointestinal system and, 476
    immune assessment and, 481, 482t
    kidney/urinary assessment and, 475-476
    musculoskeletal assessment and, 482
    neuroendocrine assessment and, 481
    skin assessment and, 476, 476f
  in cardiovascular assessment, 636-640
    blood pressure in, 637-638
    extremities and, 637, 637f
    general appearance and, 637
    precordium and, 639-640, 639f, 640t
    skin and, 637
    venous and arterial pulses in, 638-639, 638f
  in cataracts, 983, 983f
  in cervical cancer, 1494-1495
  in cholecystitis, 1215-1216, 1215b-1216b
  in chronic glomerulonephritis, 1404
  in chronic kidney disease, 1423, 1423b
  in chronic obstructive pulmonary disease, 559-561, 559f, 561f
  in cirrhosis, 1195-1196, 1197t
  in colorectal cancer, 1150-1151, 1150f
  in coronary artery disease, 762-763, 762b
  in cystitis, 1369, 1370b
  in dehydration, 156-157, 156b, 156f
  in endocrine assessment, 1262-1263, 1263b
  in end-of-life care, 95, 96b
  in endometrial cancer, 1492
  in esophageal tumors, 1118, 1118b
  in fractures, 1055-1057, 1056b-1057b
  in gastroesophageal reflux disease, 1111-1112, 1111b
  in gastrointestinal assessment, 1089-1091, 1089f, 1090b, 1090t
  in glaucoma, 985
  in head and neck cancer, 538, 538t
  in hearing loss, 1010
  in heart failure, 682-683, 682b-683b
  in hematologic assessment, 792-793, 792b-793b, 796
  in hepatitis, 1205
  in HIV infection, 333-336, 334b-335b, 334f-335f, 346

Physical assessment (Continued)
  in hypercortisolism, 1277-1278, 1277f, 1278b
  in hypertension, 711-712, 712f
  in hyperthyroidism, 1286-1287, 1287f, 1287t
  in hypothyroidism, 1293
  in hypovolemic shock, 744-746, 744b
  in infection, 407-408
  in infective endocarditis, 698
  intraoperative care and, 251
  in leukemia, 808, 808b
  in lung cancer, 575
  in lupus, 314-315, 314f
  in malnutrition, 1238
  in multiple sclerosis, 905-906, 905b-906b
  in myasthenia gravis, 918-919, 918b
  in obesity, 1248
  in osteoarthritis, 292-293, 292f, 292t
  in osteoporosis, 1032, 1032f
  in Paget's disease of the bone, 1038, 1038b
  in pelvic inflammatory disease, 1542, 1542t
  in peptic ulcer disease, 1131, 1132t
  in peripheral arterial disease, 719-720, 720f, 721b
  in pneumonia, 590-592, 592t
  in polycystic kidney disease, 1396, 1396b
  postoperative, 257-265, 258b, 259f
    cardiovascular system and, 260
    dressings and drains and, 264, 265f
    fluid, electrolyte, acid-base balance and, 262
    gastrointestinal system and, 262-263, 263b, 263t
    impaired wound healing and, 264, 264f
    kidneys/urinary system, 262
    neurologic system and, 260-261, 260t, 261b
    pain and, 264-265
    respiratory system and, 257b, 258-260, 259b
    skin and, 263-264, 264f-265f
  preoperative, 221-222, 221b-222b, 236
  in pressure ulcers, 441
  in prostate cancer, 1508
  in psoriasis, 456, 457f
  in pulmonary embolism, 604-605, 605b
  in pyelonephritis, 1400, 1400b
  in rehabilitation, 77-79, 78t, 90
  in renal assessment, 1346f, 1353-1354, 1354b
  in renal cell carcinoma, 1407
  in reproductive assessment, 1454
  in respiratory assessment, 503-506

Physical assessment (Continued)
auscultation in, 505-506, 505f, 506b, 506t-507t
for indicators of respiratory adequacy, 506
inspection of thorax in, 503-504, 504f
palpation of chest in, 504
percussion of chest in, 504, 504f, 505t
of pharynx, trachea, and larynx, 503
in rheumatoid arthritis, 295b, 305-306, 305b-306b
in sepsis and septic shock, 752
in sickle cell disease, 800-801
in skin infections, 450b, 452
in spinal cord injury, 894-895
in stroke, 933-937, 934b, 935t-936t, 936b, 937f
in systemic sclerosis, 317-318, 318f
in testicular cancer, 1514, 1514b
of transgender patients, 1522-1524, 1523b
in traumatic brain injury, 951-952, 951b-952b
in tuberculosis, 596
in ulcerative colitis, 1175
in urinary incontinence, 1376
in urothelial cancer, 1389
Physical carcinogenesis, 366
Physical dependence, 38-39, 49-50
Physical mobility. See Mobility.
Physical modalities for reducing pain, 46-47
Physical status, 244
Physical therapists, 76, 76f
Physical therapy
for fibromyalgia, 322
in fractures, 1063
in pressure ulcers, 446
Physician-assisted suicide, 103t
Physiologic defenses against infection, 400
Physiotherapists, 76, 76f
PICCs. See Peripherally inserted central catheters (PICCs).
PICO(T) format, 65-66, 66t, 68f
PID. See Pelvic inflammatory disease (PID).
Piercings, 424
Piggyback sets, 197, 197f
Pigmentation, nail, 426, 426f, 426t
Pinna, 996, 997f
Pit vipers, North American, 123-125, 124b, 124t
Pitting edema, 158, 159f, 637, 637f
Pitting nails, 427t
Pituitary gland, 1256f-1257f, 1257
hormones secreted by, 1256t, 1258t
Pituitary gland problems
diabetes insipidus, 1271-1272, 1271b-1272b

Pituitary gland problems (Continued)
hyperpituitarism, 1268-1271, 1268b-1270b, 1268f
hypopituitarism, 1266-1268, 1267b-1268b
syndrome of inappropriate antidiuretic hormone, 1272-1273, 1272t
after craniotomy, 962
in cancer, 392-393, 392b
Pituitary tumors, 958
PKD. See Polycystic kidney disease (PKD).
Placebos, 45, 46b
Plague, 411t, 413
Plantar fasciitis, 1047
Plaquenil. See Hydroxychloroquine.
Plaques, 423f
Plasma, electrolytes in, 152b
Plasma cells, 282, 787t
immune function of, 278t
Plasma exchange in rheumatoid arthritis, 311
Plasma high-density lipoproteins, 641b
Plasma low-density lipoproteins, 641b
Plasma transfusions, 736-737
Plasmapheresis
in acute glomerulonephritis, 1403
in Guillain-Barré syndrome, 915, 915b
in myasthenia gravis, 920
in rheumatoid arthritis, 311
Plastic containers, 196-197
Plastic surgery, 462-463
after burns, 488
common procedures in, 462t
Plate guards and sporks, 84t
Platelet aggregation, 788, 795
Platelet count, 793
Platelet disorders, 819-820
Platelet inhibitors, 726b
Platelet transfusions, 824, 824b
Platelets, 787
Plethoric appearance in polycythemia vera, 805
Pleura, 499
Pleural effusion, 504
in systemic lupus erythematosus, 315
Pleural friction rub, 507t
Pleur-evac drainage system, 578f
Pleuritic pain
in lung abscesses, 599
in pneumonia, 592t
Pleuropulmonary pain, 636t
Plexuses, 834
Ploidy, 365
Pluripotent stem cells, 276
PMI. See Point of maximal impulse (PMI).
PML. See Progressive multifocal leukoencephalopathy (PML).

PMR. See Polymyalgia rheumatica (PMR).
PNBs. See Peripheral nerve blockades (PNBs).
PND. See Paroxysmal nocturnal dyspnea (PND).
Pneumatic compression devices, 232
Pneumoconiosis, 573b
Pneumonectomy, 576, 577f, 580
Pneumonia, 588-594
with AIDS, 335
airway obstruction in, 593
bronchiolitis obliterans organizing =, 572-573
concept map for, 591f
evaluation of care of patient with, 594
health care resources for, 594
history in, 589t, 590-592
home care management in, 593-594, 594b
improving gas exchange in, 593
laboratory assessment in, 592, 592f
older adults and, 592b
pathophysiology of, 588-589
etiology of, 589, 589t-590t
incidence and prevalence of, 589
physical assessment in, 590-592, 592t
prevention of, 589-590, 589b-590b
psychosocial assessment in, 592
self-management education in, 594, 594b
sepsis in, 593
ventilator-associated, 590t, 621, 621b
Pneumothorax, 511, 623-624
tension, 624
tracheostomy-related, 523
PNS. See Peripheral nervous system (PNS).
POAG. See Primary open-angle glaucoma (POAG).
Podagra, 319
POI. See Postoperative ileus (POI).
Point of maximal impulse (PMI), 639
Poisoning
carbon monoxide, 474, 475t
cyanide, 478
smoke, 475
Polyclonal antibodies, 287b-288b
Polycystic kidney disease (PKD), 1394-1397, 1395f-1396f, 1396b-1397b
Polycythemia, 561
Polycythemia vera (PV), 805-806, 805b
Polydipsia, 1302
Polymedicine, 13
PolyMem, 486b
Polymorphism, 56
Polymorphonuclear neutrophils, 278
Polymyalgia rheumatica (PMR), 323t

Polymyositis, 323t
Polymyxin, 486b
Polyphagia, 1302
Polypharmacy, 13
Polyps
cervical polyps, 1491
intestinal, 1163-1164
Polyuria, 1302
Pons, 832t
PONV. See Postoperative nausea and vomiting (PONV).
Pores, 149, 150f
Portable chest drainage system, 578f
Portal hypertension, 1201
Portal of exit, 400
Portal-systemic encephalopathy, 1193-1194, 1194t
Positioning
in acute respiratory distress syndrome, 614
after burns, 478, 487, 487b
in chronic obstructive pulmonary disease, 562-563
in osteoarthritis, 294, 297b
in peripheral arterial disease, 722, 722b
postoperative, 266
in preventing pressure ulcers, 438b
during surgery, 252-253, 252f
Positive deflection, 651, 651f
Positive end-expiratory pressure (PEEP), 481, 613-614, 618
Positive inotropic drugs, 609
Positron emission tomography (PET)
in cardiovascular assessment, 646-647
in neurologic assessment, 846t-847t, 848
POSS. See Pasero Opioid-Induced Sedation Scale (POSS).
Postanesthesia care unit (PACU), 256
assessment of readiness for discharge from, 258, 258b, 259f
pain assessment in, 264-265
purpose of, 257
Postanesthesia care unit (PACU) nurses, 257
Postcholecystectomy syndrome, 1218, 1218t
Postdural puncture headaches, 261b
Posterior cerebral artery strokes, 934b
Posterior colporrhaphy, 1487
Posterior pituitary gland hormones of, 1258t
Posterior pituitary gland problems
diabetes insipidus, 1271-1272, 1271b-1272b
syndrome of inappropriate antidiuretic hormone, 1272-1273, 1272t
after craniotomy, 962
in cancer, 392-393, 392b

Posteroanterior chest x-rays, 507

Postexposure prophylaxis to human immune deficiency virus, 331f

Postherpetic neuralgia, 451

Posthospital care in acute kidney injury, 1418-1419

Postictal stage, 858

Post-irradiation sialadenitis, 1108

Post-mastectomy exercises, 1474b

Postmortem care, 102, 102b

Postoperative care, 256-273
  in back surgery, 889-890, 889b
  in bariatric surgery, 1250-1252, 1251b
  in benign prostatic hyperplasia, 1505-1506, 1505b-1506b
  in bone cancer, 1044-1045, 1044b
  in colorectal cancer, 1154, 1154b, 1154f
  in coronary artery bypass graft, 776-779, 778b-779b
  in craniotomy, 960-962, 960b
  evaluation of, 272
  focused assessment in, 258b
  in fracture surgery, 1062-1063
  in gastric cancer, 1140-1141
  health care resources and, 272
  in heart transplantation, 702-704, 703b
  in hiatal hernias, 1114b, 1116-1117, 1116b
  history review in, 257, 258t
  home care management and, 271-272
  in hypercortisolism, 1280
  in hyperpituitarism, 1270-1271, 1270b
  hypoxemia prevention and, 266-267, 266b
  in hysterectomy, 1489-1490, 1490b
  in intestinal obstruction, 1160-1161
  in kidney transplantation, 1442-1443
  laboratory assessment in, 265-266
  in lung transplantation, 565, 569
  in mastectomy, 1473-1478, 1473f, 1474b, 1475t, 1476b
  older adults and, 261b, 267b
  in open ureterolithotomy, 1387
  in oral cancer, 1105-1106, 1106b
  pain management in, 269-271, 269b-271b
  patient and family education and, 272-273, 272b
  in peripheral arterial disease, 723-724, 724b
  physical assessment in, 257-265, 258b, 259f
    cardiovascular system and, 260
    dressings and drains and, 264, 265f
    fluid, electrolyte, acid-base balance and, 262
    gastrointestinal system and, 262-263, 263b, 263t

Postoperative care (Continued)
    impaired wound healing and, 264, 264f
    kidneys/urinary system, 262
    neurologic system and, 260-261, 260t, 261b
    pain and, 264-265
    respiratory system and, 257b, 258-260, 259b
    skin and, 263-264, 264f-265f
  postoperative hand-off reports and, 257, 257b
  preventing wound infection and delayed healing in, 267-269, 267b-269b, 267f
  in prostatectomy, 1509-1510, 1509b
  psychosocial assessment in, 265
  in renal cell carcinoma, 1408
  in retinal detachment, 990
  in stapedectomy, 1013
  in stress incontinence surgery, 1379
  in surgery for diabetes mellitus, 1324-1325
  in testicular cancer, 1515, 1515b
  in thyroid surgery, 1290-1291, 1290b
  in total knee arthroplasty, 301-302, 301f, 302b
  in tracheostomy, 522
  in tympanoplasty, 1013
  in ulcerative colitis, 1178-1179
  in urothelial cancer, 1390
  in in vaginoplasty, 1527, 1527b, 1527t
  in Whipple procedure, 1229-1230, 1229t, 1230b

Postoperative hand-off reports, 257, 257b

Postoperative ileus (POI), 263b

Postoperative nausea and vomiting (PONV), 43, 43t, 262

Postoperative pain, acute, 28t

Postpericardiotomy syndrome, 779

Post-traumatic stress disorder (PTSD), 145, 145b

Postural hypotension, 638
  in dehydration, 156

Posture assessment, 1021-1022, 1022f

Posturing, 841, 841f, 952

Post-void residual, 86

Potassium, 163-167
  abnormal values of, 152t
    in chronic kidney disease, 1420
  hyperkalemia and, 166-167, 166t, 167b, 469
  hypokalemia and, 163-165, 164b-165b, 164t
  levels in burn assessment, 477b
  perioperative assessment of, 223b-224b
  plasma values in older adults, 152b

Potassium-sparing diuretics, 714

Powered air purifying respirator (PAPR), 400, 404f

PowerGlide, 193

PPE. See Personal protective equipment (PPE).

PPMS. See Primary progressive multiple sclerosis (PPMS).

PPP. See Palmoplantar pustulosis (PPP).

PQRST mnemonic, 1089

PR interval, 653, 654f, 655

PR segments, 652, 654f

Prasugrel, 765b-766b

Precipitation, 284

Precordium assessment, 639-640, 639f, 640t

Prediabetes, 1307

Prednisolone, 979b

Prednisone
  for asthma, 539b
  to prevent transplant rejection, 287b-288b

Preemptive analgesia, 34

Pregnancy
  methotrexate use during, 308
  sickle cell disease and, 803b
  urinary tract infection during, 1372b

Prehospital care providers, 107, 107f

Preictal phase, 859

Pre-infarction angina, 759

Preload, 630

Premalignant oral lesions, 1102

Premature atrial complexes (PAC), 665

Premature complexes, 656-657

Premature ventricular complexes (PVCs), 669-670, 669f, 670b

Preoperative anxiety, 233

Preoperative care, 215-237
  in back surgery, 888
  in bariatric surgery, 1250
  in benign prostatic hyperplasia, 1505
  in bone cancer, 1044
  in cataract surgery, 983
  categories and purposes of surgery and, 217, 218t
  in colorectal cancer, 1152-1153, 1152t
  in coronary artery bypass graft surgery, 775-776
  in craniotomy, 960
  dietary restrictions and, 228, 228b
  in esophageal cancer, 1120
  evaluation of, 236
  focused assessment in, 225, 225b
  in fracture surgery, 1062
  in gastric cancer surgery, 1140
  in head and neck cancer surgery, 540
  in heart transplantation, 702
  in hiatal hernias, 1115
  history in, 219-221, 219t, 220b
  in hypercortisolism, 1279
  in hyperpituitarism, 1270
  imaging assessment in, 224-225

Preoperative care (Continued)
  informed consent and, 226, 226b, 227f, 228b
  in intestinal obstruction, 1160
  intestinal preparation in, 228
  in kidney transplantation, 1442
  laboratory assessment in, 223, 223b-224b, 236
  in lung cancer, 576
  in lung transplantation, 564, 569
  in mastectomy, 1472-1473, 1474b
  minimizing anxiety in, 233
  older adults and, 219, 220b-221b, 230b
  in open ureterolithotomy, 1387
  in oral cancer, 1105
  in pancreatic cancer, 1228-1229
  patient education and, 225-233, 226t, 230b-231b, 231f, 236
  patient self-determination and, 228
  patient transfer to surgical suite, 234-236, 235f
  in peripheral arterial disease, 723
  physical assessment in, 221-222, 221b-222b, 236
  preoperative chart review and, 233-234
  preoperative checklist and, 235f
  preoperative drugs and, 234
  preoperative patient preparation and, 225-234, 226b
  preparation for tubes, drains, and vascular access in, 229-230
  in prostate cancer, 1509
  psychosocial assessment in, 222-223
  regularly scheduled drugs and, 228
  in renal cell carcinoma, 1408
  in retinal detachment surgery, 990
  risk for postoperative complications and, 219, 219t
  skin preparation in, 228-229, 229f
  in stapedectomy, 1013, 1013b
  in stress incontinence surgery, 1379
  in surgery for diabetes mellitus, 1324
  surgical settings and, 218-219
  teaching postoperative procedures and exercises, 230b
  in testicular cancer, 1515
  in thyroid surgery, 1289
  in total hip arthroplasty, 296
  in total knee arthroplasty, 300-301
  in tracheostomy, 522
  in tympanoplasty, 1012
  in ulcerative colitis, 1177
  in urothelial cancer, 1389-1390
  in vaginoplasty, 1526

Preoperative chart review, 233-234

Presbycusis, 1010

Presbyopia, 13, 970, 991

Prescribing of infusion therapy, 189, 189b

Presence at end of life, 100-101

Pressure support ventilation, 622t
Pressure ulcers, 436-449
  concept map for, 445f
  evaluation of care of patient with, 449
  health care resources for, 449, 449b
  history in, 441
  home care management in, 447-449
  identification of high-risk patients, 437-440, 439f
  incidence and prevalence of, 437
  infection prevention in, 447, 448b
  laboratory assessment in, 444
  massage and, 440b
  mechanical forces in, 437, 437f
  nutrition therapy and, 438b, 446
  older adults and, 437b
  pathophysiology of, 436-449
  physical assessment in, 441
  from positioning during surgery, 268-269
  pressure-relieving and pressure-reducing techniques for, 440-441
  prevention of, 437-441, 438b
  psychosocial assessment in, 443
  rehabilitation setting and, 79
  self-management education in, 449
  stages of, 433-436
  surgical management of, 447
  wound assessment in, 441-443, 441b, 442f, 443t
  wound care in, 444-447, 444b, 445f, 446b-447b, 446t
Pressure-cycled ventilators, 616
Pressure-reducing techniques, 440-441
Pressure-relieving techniques, 440-441
Preventive therapy for migraines, 856, 856b
Priapism, 800
Primary adrenal insufficiency, 1274t
Primary arthroplasty, 295-296
Primary brain injury, 946-948, 947f, 948b
Primary glomerular diseases and syndromes, 1402t
Primary gout, 319
Primary immune deficiencies, 345-346
Primary lesions, 421, 423f
Primary open-angle glaucoma (POAG), 985
Primary osteoarthritis, 291
Primary prevention, 368-370
Primary progressive multiple sclerosis (PPMS), 904
Primary survey, 116-117, 117b-118b, 118t
Primary tumors, 362, 365t
Prinzmetal's angina, 759
Priority setting in emergency care, 110

Privacy in genetic counseling, 62
PRMS. See Progressive-relapsing multiple sclerosis (PRMS).
Proaccelerin, 790t
Probenecid, 320
Pro-cell division signal transduction pathway, 389f
Proconvertin, 790t
Procrit. See Epoetin alfa.
Progestin, 391t
Prograf. See Tacrolimus.
Progressive multifocal leukoencephalopathy (PML), 908
Progressive muscular dystrophies, 1048-1049, 1048t, 1049b
Progressive-relapsing multiple sclerosis (PRMS), 904
Pro-inflammatory cytokines, 286t
Prokine. See Sargramostim.
Prokinetic agents, 385b
Prolactin, 1269b
Proliferative diabetic retinopathy, 1304
Proliferative phase of healing, 433, 433t
Promotors, carcinogenesis and, 362
Pronator drift, 841
Prone position during surgery, 252-253, 252f
Propafenone hydrochloride, 658b-662b
Proparacaine hydrochloride, 979b
Prophylactic surgery, 373
Propranolol, 658b-662b
Proprioception, 833, 842
  after stroke, 934
Prosopagnosia, 876
Prostacyclin, 571b
Prostaglandins, 1349, 1349t
  migraine and, 854
Prostate cancer, 1506-1511
  assessment in, 1508, 1508b
  chemotherapy for, 1510-1511
  community-based care in, 1511, 1511b
  health promotion and maintenance in, 1507, 1507b
  hormone therapy for, 1510, 1510b
  older adults and, 367b
  pathophysiology of, 1506-1511, 1507b, 1507f
  radiation therapy in, 1510
  surgical management of, 1509-1510, 1509b
Prostate gland, 1451f, 1452
Prostate-specific antigen (PSA), 1507b, 1508
Prostatic stents, 1503
Prostatitis, 1500, 1512
Prosthesis, 1073, 1074f
Protease inhibitors, 327, 339b
Proteases, 557
Proteasome inhibitors, 390, 390t
Protective environment, 405
Protective genes, 56

Protein synthesis, 55-56, 56f
Protein-calorie malnutrition, 1236
Protein-energy malnutrition, 1236
Proteinuria, 1356
  in polycystic kidney disease, 1396
Proteolysis, 1302
Prothrombin, 790t
Prothrombin time (PT)
  for monitoring of anticoagulation therapy, 608b
  perioperative assessment of, 223b-224b
Proton pump inhibitors, 1113, 1113b
Protozoal infections, 334
Provenge. See Sipuleucel-T-T.
Proventil. See Albuterol.
Pruritus, 421, 432-433
  dry skin and, 433b
  opioid-induced, 43
  in serum sickness, 125
PSA. See Prostate-specific antigen (PSA).
Pseudoaddiction, 40
Pseudocysts, pancreatic, 1226
Psoralen and ultraviolet radiation treatment, 457
Psoriasis, 456-458, 456b-458b, 457f
Psoriasis vulgaris, 456, 457f
Psoriatic arthritis, 321, 456
PSR. See Percutaneous stereotactic rhizotomy (PSR).
PSVT. See Paroxysmal supraventricular tachycardias (PSVT).
Psychiatric crisis nurse teams, 106
Psychosocial assessment
  in acidosis, 182
  in acquired immune deficiency syndrome, 336
  in adrenal insufficiency, 1275
  in Alzheimer's disease, 875
  in amputations, 1071-1072
  in benign prostatic hyperplasia, 1500
  in breast cancer, 1469-1470, 1470b
  in cardiovascular assessment, 640
  in cataracts, 983
  in chronic kidney disease, 1424
  in chronic obstructive pulmonary disease, 561
  in cirrhosis, 1196
  in colorectal cancer, 1151
  in coronary artery disease, 763
  in endocrine assessment, 1263
  in end-of-life care, 95-96, 96b, 103
  in endometrial cancer, 1492
  in esophageal tumors, 1118
  in fractures, 1057
  in gastrointestinal assessment, 1091
  in head and neck cancer, 538
  in hearing assessment, 1002
  in hearing loss, 1010
  in heart failure, 683
  in hematologic assessment, 793
  in hepatitis, 1205

Psychosocial assessment (Continued)
  in hypercortisolism, 1278
  in hypertension, 712
  in hyperthyroidism, 1287
  in hypothyroidism, 1293
  in hypovolemic shock, 746
  in infection, 408
  in integumentary assessment, 428
  in leukemia, 808
  in lung cancer, 575
  in lupus, 315
  in malnutrition, 1238
  in multiple sclerosis, 906
  in musculoskeletal assessment, 1024
  in neurologic assessment, 844
  in obesity, 1248
  in osteoarthritis, 293
  in osteoporosis, 1032
  in pain, 32-33, 33b
  in pelvic inflammatory disease, 1542
  in peptic ulcer disease, 1131
  in pneumonia, 592
  in polycystic kidney disease, 1396
  postoperative, 265
  preoperative, 222-223
  in pressure ulcers, 443
  in prostate cancer, 1508
  in pulmonary embolism, 605
  in rehabilitation, 80, 90
  in renal assessment, 1354
  in reproductive assessment, 1454
  in respiratory assessment, 506
  in rheumatoid arthritis, 306-307
  in sepsis, 753
  in sickle cell disease, 801
  in stroke, 937
  in testicular cancer, 1514
  of transgender patients, 1524
  in traumatic brain injury, 952-953
  in ulcerative colitis, 1175
  in urothelial cancer, 1389
  in vision assessment, 973
Psychosocial response of survivors to mass casualty events, 146-147, 146b-147b
Psychosocial support
  in acquired immune deficiency syndrome, 343
  in breast cancer, 1479-1480
  in burns, 489
  in chronic kidney disease, 1445
  in colorectal cancer, 1156-1157
  in diabetes mellitus, 1338-1339
  in end-of-life care, 100-102, 100t, 101b-102b, 101f
  in Guillain-Barré syndrome, 917
  in head and neck cancer, 545
  in leukemia, 815-816
  in Parkinson disease, 870-871
  in tracheostomy, 528-529
  in urinary incontinence, 1383
Psychotropic drugs, 877-878
PT. See Prothrombin time (PT).

PTC. *See* Percutaneous transhepatic cholangiography (PTC).

PTCA. *See* Percutaneous transluminal angioplasty (PTCA).

Ptosis, 972
in black widow spider bites, 127
in myasthenia gravis, 918
in stroke, 936

PTSD. *See* Post-traumatic stress disorder (PTSD).

PTT. *See* Partial thromboplastin time (PTT).

Public information officers, 143, 143t

PUD. *See* Peptic ulcer disease (PUD).

Pulmonary arterial hypertension (PAH), 569-571, 569b-571b, 570t

Pulmonary artery occlusive pressure (PAOP), 770

Pulmonary artery wedge pressure (PAWP), 770

Pulmonary autografts, 696

Pulmonary circulation, 499, 499f

Pulmonary edema
in burns, 475, 475b
in chronic kidney disease, 1426-1427
in heart failure, 688-689, 688b-689b
in syndrome of inappropriate antidiuretic hormone, 392b

Pulmonary embolism, 603-610
anxiety in, 609-610
bleeding in, 609, 609b
drug therapy for, 606, 606b-608b, 608-610
evaluation of care of patient with, 610
genetic considerations in, 605b, 608b
health care resources for, 610, 611b
health promotion and maintenance in, 604, 604b
home care management in, 610, 611b
hypotension in, 609
hypoxemia in, 603, 605-610, 606b-608b, 606t
imaging assessment in, 605
laboratory assessment in, 605
pathophysiology of, 603-604
physical assessment in, 604-605, 605b
psychosocial assessment in, 605
self-management education in, 610, 610b
surgical management of, 608-609

Pulmonary empyema, 599

Pulmonary function tests (PFTs), 509, 510t
in asthma, 532-533

Pulmonary tuberculosis, 595-599
diagnosis of, 596, 596f
drug therapy for, 596-598, 597b-598b
health care resources for, 599
history in, 596
home care management in, 598
pathophysiology of, 595-596, 595f
etiology of, 595
incidence and prevalence of, 596
physical assessment in, 596
self-management education in, 598-599

Pulmonic valve, 628

Pulse, hypernatremia and, 163

Pulse deficit, 260, 652

Pulse oximetry, 508-509, 509f
cultural considerations in, 500b
in pneumonia, 592

Pulse pressure, 638

Pulsus alternans, 682-683

Pump failure. *See* Heart failure (HF).

Punch biopsy, 429

Punctum, 967, 968f

Pupils, 966, 967f
assessment of, 972
changes in traumatic brain injury, 952b
changes with aging, 970b

Pure-tone audiometry, 1002-1003

Purkinje cells, 650

Pursed-lip breathing, 563b

Purulent exudate, 443t

Pustules, 423f

PV. *See* Polycythemia vera (PV).

PVCs. *See* Premature ventricular complexes (PVCs).

PVD. *See* Peripheral vascular disease (PVD).

Pyelolithotomy, 1401

Pyelonephritis, 1372b, 1399-1401, 1399f, 1400b
pregnancy and, 1372b

Pyloric obstruction, 1137

Pyloromyotomy, 1120

Pyrazinamide, 597b

PZA. *See* Pyrazinamide.

Q

QRS complex, 653, 654f

QRS duration, 653, 654f, 655-656

QSEN core competencies. *See* Quality and Safety Education for Nurses (QSEN) core competencies.

QT interval, 653, 654f

Quadriceps-setting exercises, 299

Quadrigeminy, 657

Qualitative questions, 65, 67, 73

Quality and Safety Education for Nurses (QSEN) core competencies, 3-6, 3t, 5t, 6b, 7f, 8

Quality improvement, 6-8

Quantitative questions, 65, 67, 73

Quantitative RNA assays, 337

R

RA. *See* Rheumatoid arthritis (RA).

Radial nerve complications, 253b

Radiation dose, 374

Radiation injuries, 472

Radiation proctitis, 1510

Radiation therapy, 374-377, 374f
for bone cancer, 1044
for breast cancer, 1476, 1476b
delivery methods and devices in, 375, 376b
for endometrial cancer, 1492-1493, 1493b
for esophageal cancer, 1119
for head and neck cancer, 539
for lung cancer, 576, 580
for prostate cancer, 1510
sealed implants of radioactive sources in, 376b
side effects of, 375-376, 376t
for skin cancer, 461
skin protection during, 376, 376b-377b
for spinal cord tumors, 903

Radiation-induced immune deficiencies, 345

Radical cystectomy, 1388

Radical hysterectomy, 1489t

Radical pancreaticoduodenectomy, 1229, 1229f

Radical surgery, 218t

Radicular pain, 902

Radiculopathy, 887

Radio frequency identification, 7

Radioactive iodine (RAI) therapy, 1289

Radiofrequency catheter ablation, 668-669

Radiography
chest
in cardiovascular assessment, 642-643
in pneumonia, 592
in gastrointestinal assessment, 1093
in musculoskeletal assessment, 1025
in neurologic assessment, 844-845

Radioisotope scan, 973

Radionuclide studies, 684

Radiosurgery
in brain tumors, 959-960, 959f
in trigeminal neuralgia, 926-927

RAI therapy. *See* Radioactive iodine (RAI) therapy.

Ramsay Sedation Scale (RSS), 249, 250t

Range of motion in rehabilitation setting, 83-84, 83t

Range-of-motion exercises after burns, 487

Rapamune. *See* Sirolimus.

Rapid hypersensitivity reactions, 348-355
allergic rhinitis in, 349-351, 349f, 351b
anaphylaxis in, 348-349, 351-354
assessment of, 352-353, 352f, 353b
in bee stings, 129
interventions, 353-354, 353b-354b
pathophysiology of, 351-352, 351t, 352b, 352f
latex allergy in, 354-355, 355b

Rapid neurologic assessment, 843-844, 843f, 844b

Rapid Response Teams, 3, 8

Rapidly progressive glomerulonephritis, 1403

Rash
macular vs. papular, 424
in systemic lupus erythematosus, 314, 314f

Rate-controlling infusion device, 198-200, 199f

Raynaud's phenomenon/disease, 729t
in systemic lupus erythematosus, 315
in systemic sclerosis, 317

RBCs. *See* Red blood cells (RBCs).

RCC. *See* Renal cell carcinoma (RCC).

Reavy and Tavernier model of evidence-based practice, 69, 69t

Rebound headaches, 856

Recall memory, 839

Receptive aphasia, 943, 943t

Reconstructive plastic surgery, 373, 462-463
after burns, 488
common procedures in, 462t

Recreational therapists, 77

Red blood cell count
in cardiovascular assessment, 642
in respiratory assessment, 508b

Red blood cell disorders, 798-806
anemias, 799b
glucose-6-phosphate dehydrogenase deficiency anemia, 799t, 803
immunohemolytic anemia, 803-804
in older adults, 804b
resulting from decreased production of red blood cells, 804-805, 804b, 804f
sickle cell disease, 799-804, 799t
community-based care in, 803
etiology and genetic risk in, 476b, 800, 800f
history in, 800-801
imaging assessment in, 801
incidence and prevalence of, 800

Red blood cell disorders (Continued)
  infection prevention in, 802-803
  laboratory assessment in, 801
  pain in, 801-802, 802b
  pathophysiology of, 799-800, 799f
  physical assessment in, 800-801
  pregnancy in, 803b
  psychosocial assessment in, 801
  myelodysplastic syndromes, 806
  polycythemia vera, 805-806, 805b
Red blood cell transfusions, 824, 824b, 824t
Red blood cells (RBCs), 786-787, 787f, 798
  growth factor for, 276
Redirection in Alzheimer's disease, 877
Reduced visual sensory perception, 992-994, 993b
Reduction mammoplasty, 462t, 1463
Reed Sternberg cell, 817
Re-epithelialization, 435-436, 435f
Refeeding syndrome, 1242, 1242b
Reflex arc, 834
Reflex bowel, 87t
Reflex sympathetic dystrophy. See Complex regional pain syndrome (CRPS).
Reflexes, 834, 841, 842f
Reflux esophagitis, 1110
Reflux urinary incontinence, 1381-1382
Refraction, 968-969, 969f
Refractive errors, 991
Refractory symptoms of distress management in end-of-life care, 100
Regional anesthesia, 45, 248-249, 248f-249f, 248t
Registered dietitians, 77
Reglan. See Metoclopramide.
Regurgitation in gastroesophageal reflux disease, 1111
Rehabilitation, 74-90
  after total knee arthroplasty, 302
  bowel continence and, 87-88, 87b-88b, 87t
  in burns, 488-489, 489t
    health care resources for, 489
    home care management in, 489
    psychosocial support during, 489
    self-management education in, 489
  cardiac, 302
  community-based care and, 88-89
  complications of immobility and, 83, 83t
  evaluation of, 89
  functional assessment in, 79-80, 80t

Rehabilitation (Continued)
  gait training and, 81-84, 83b, 83f, 83t
  health care resources for, 89
  history in, 77
  home care management after, 88-89
  improving physical mobility and, 80-84, 81b, 82f-83f, 83b, 83t
  increasing functional ability and, 84, 84t, 85b
  maintaining skin integrity during, 85
  NANDA-I and, 80
  older adults and, 77b, 87b
  physical assessment in, 77-79, 78t, 79b, 90
  psychosocial assessment in, 80, 90
  self-management education and, 89
  settings, 75, 75f
  team, 75-77, 76f, 76t
  urinary continence and, 85-87, 86b-87b, 86t
  vocational assessment in, 80
Rehabilitation case managers, 76
Rehabilitation nurses, 76, 76t
Rehabilitation team, 75-77, 76f, 76t
Rehabilitative surgery. See Reconstructive plastic surgery.
Reiter's syndrome, 323t
Rejection of pancreas transplant, 1323
Relapsing-remitting multiple sclerosis (RRMS), 904
Relaxation techniques for pain management, 48
Reliever drugs for asthma, 534
Religion
  death rituals and, 100t
  end-of-life care and, 101-102
Relocation stress syndrome, 12, 13b, 23
Remicade. See Infliximab.
Reminiscence at end of life, 101
Remote memory, 839
Renal arteriography, 1361
Renal assessment, 1344-1365
  current health problems in, 1353
  family history and genetic risk in, 1353
  gender health considerations, 1354b
  health promotion and maintenance in, 1364
  imaging assessment in, 1360-1362, 1360t, 1361b
  kidney biopsy in, 1363
  laboratory assessment in, 1354-1360
    bedside sonography and bladder scan in, 1359-1360, 1359f
    blood tests in, 1354-1355, 1354b-1355b
    urine tests in, 1355-1359, 1356b, 1357t, 1359b
  medication history in, 1352

Renal assessment (Continued)
  nutrition history in, 1352
  patient history in, 1352-1353
  physical assessment in, 1346f, 1353-1354, 1354b
  psychosocial assessment in, 1354
  in rehabilitation setting, 78, 78t
  urodynamic studies in, 1362-1363
Renal cell carcinoma (RCC), 1406-1408, 1407t
Renal colic, 1385
Renal columns, 1345, 1345f
Renal cortex, 1345, 1345f
Renal osteodystrophy, 1421
Renal pelvis, 1345
Renal replacement therapies (RRTs), 1431-1446
  for acute kidney injury, 1417-1418, 1417f
  hemodialysis in acute kidney injury, 1431
    anticoagulation in, 1432-1433
    complications of, 1433-1435
    dialysis settings in, 1432
    patient selection for, 1431
    peritoneal dialysis vs., 1431t
    post-dialysis care and, 1436, 1436t
    procedure in, 1432, 1432f, 1433f
    vascular access in, 1433-1436, 1434f, 1434t, 1435b, 1435f
  peritoneal dialysis in chronic kidney disease, 1437-1441
    complications in, 1440, 1441, 1441b
    dialysate additives for, 1432
    nursing care in, 1438
    patient selection for, 1437
    procedure in, 1438, 1438f
    types of, 1438-1439, 1438f, 1439f, 1440f
Renal scan, 1360t, 1361
Renal system
  anatomy and physiology of, 1344-1351
    kidneys. See also Kidneys.
      function of, 1342, 1344, 1346-1350, 1348t-1349t, 1349b, 1349f, 1394
      structure of, 1345-1346, 1345f-1347f
    ureters, 1350
    urinary bladder, 1350, 1350f
  changes associated with aging, 1351, 1351b
  complications of immobility and, 83t
Renal threshold for glucose reabsorption, 1348
Renin, 1258, 1346, 1346f, 1349, 1349t
Renin inhibitors, 715b-716b, 717
Renin-angiotensin II pathway, 154-155, 154f
Renovascular disease, 1405-1406, 1405b

Reperfusion therapy, 767-768
Repetitive nerve stimulation, 919
Repetitive stress injury, 1077
Replication of DNA, 53, 53f
Repositioning patients in wheelchairs, 85
Reproductive assessment, 1449-1460
  biopsy studies in, 1458-1459, 1458b
  cultural considerations in, 1453b
  current health problems in, 1453-1454, 1453b
  family history and genetic risk in, 1453
  gender health considerations in, 1453b
  imaging assessment in, 1456
  laboratory assessment in, 1454-1459, 1455b
  nutrition history in, 1453, 1453b
  patient history in, 1452-1454
  physical assessment in, 1454
  psychosocial assessment in, 1454
Reproductive system
  anatomy and physiology of, 1449-1452
    female, 1449-1451
      breasts, 1450-1451, 1451f
      external genitalia, 1449-1450
      internal genitalia, 1450, 1450f
      physical assessment of, 1454
    male, 1451-1452, 1451f
      physical assessment of, 1454
  changes associated with aging, 1452, 1452b
Rescue therapy
  in bleeding esophageal varices, 1200
  in transplant rejection, 287
Residents, 75
Residual volume (RV), 510t
Resistance genes, 56
Resonance, percussion note, 505t
Resorption of bone, 1018
Respiration
  accessory muscles of, 499
  purpose of, 496
Respiratory acid-base control, 177-178, 178f, 178t
Respiratory acidosis, 180-181, 180t, 183
  combined metabolic and respiratory acidosis and, 181, 182b
  concept map for, 560f
  laboratory assessment in, 182, 182b
Respiratory alkalosis, 183t, 184
Respiratory anthrax, 599-600, 599b-600b
Respiratory assessment, 494-513
  in burns, 473-474, 474b, 474t
  capnometry and capnography in, 509
  cultural considerations in, 500b
  current health problems in, 502-503, 503t

Respiratory assessment *(Continued)*
  endoscopic examinations in, 509-511, 510b
  exercise testing in, 509
  family history and genetic risk in, 502
  gender health considerations in, 500b
  in hematologic assessment, 792
  imaging assessment in, 507-508
  laboratory assessment in, 507, 508b
  lung biopsy in, 511-512
  nutrition status in, 502
  patient history in, 500-503, 502b, 502t
  physical assessment in, 503-506
    auscultation in, 505-506, 505f, 506b, 506t-507t
    for indicators of respiratory adequacy, 506
    inspection of thorax in, 503-504, 504f
    of nose and sinuses, 503, 503b
    palpation of chest in, 504
    percussion of chest in, 504, 504f, 505t
    of pharynx, trachea, and larynx, 503
  postoperative, 257b, 258-260, 259b
  psychosocial assessment in, 506
  pulmonary function tests in, 509, 510t
  pulse oximetry in, 508-509, 509f
  in rehabilitation setting, 77-78, 78t
  skin tests in, 509
  in spinal cord injury, 895
  thoracentesis in, 511, 511f
Respiratory care, patient and family education in, 230-231, 230b, 231f
Respiratory compensation, 179
Respiratory depression
  opioid-induced, 43t, 44, 44b
  in respiratory acidosis, 180
Respiratory distress during mechanical ventilation, 619b
Respiratory failure, acute, 610-612, 611t-612t
Respiratory hygiene/cough etiquette, 403
Respiratory problems
  acute respiratory distress syndrome, 612-614, 613b-614b, 613t
  burn-related, 481b, 487-488
  acute respiratory failure, 610-612, 611t-612t
  asthma. *See* Asthma.
  bronchiolitis obliterans organizing pneumonia, 572-573
  burn-related, 470
  chest trauma, 622-624
    flail chest, 623, 623f
    hemothorax, 624
    pneumothorax, 623-624

Respiratory problems *(Continued)*
    pulmonary contusions, 622-623
    rib fractures, 623
    tension pneumothorax, 624
    tracheobronchial trauma, 624
  chronic obstructive pulmonary disease. *See* Chronic obstructive pulmonary disease (COPD).
  Coccidioidomycosis, 600-601
  cystic fibrosis, 567-569
    genetic considerations in, 567b
    nonsurgical management of, 568, 568f
    pathophysiology of, 567-569
    surgical management of, 569
  head and neck cancer. *See* Head and neck cancer.
  inhalation anthrax, 599-600, 599b-600b
  interstitial pulmonary diseases, 571-572
  larynx disorders
    laryngeal trauma, 536, 536b
    vocal cord paralysis, 535, 535b
  lung abscesses, 599
  lung cancer. *See* Lung cancer.
  mechanical ventilation for. *See* Mechanical ventilation.
  neck trauma, 537
  nose and sinus disorders, 531-534
    epistaxis, 532-533, 532b-533b, 533f
    facial trauma, 534, 534b
    nasal fractures, 531-532, 532b, 532f
    nose and sinus cancer, 533-534
    rhinitis, 583-584, 584b
      allergic, 349-351, 349f, 351b
    rhinosinusitis, 584
  obstructive sleep apnea, 534-535
  occupational pulmonary disease, 572, 573b
  older adults and chronic respiratory problems in, 532b
  oxygen delivery systems and, 603, 604f
  oxygen therapy for. *See* Oxygen therapy.
  pandemic influenza, 587-588
  pertussis, 600
  pharynx and tonsils disorders
    peritonsillar abscesses, 586
    pharyngitis, 584-586, 585b-586b, 585t
    tonsillitis, 586, 586b
  pneumonia. *See* Pneumonia.
  pulmonary arterial hypertension, 569-571, 569b-571b, 570t
  pulmonary embolism. *See* Pulmonary embolism.
  pulmonary empyema, 599
  seasonal influenza, 586-587
  severe acute respiratory syndrome, 594-595, 595b

Respiratory problems *(Continued)*
  tracheostomy for. *See* Tracheostomy.
  tuberculosis, 595-599
    in AIDS, 334-335
    diagnosis of, 596, 596f
    directly observed therapy for, 407
    drug therapy for, 596-598, 597b-598b
    etiology of, 595
    health care resources for, 599
    history in, 596
    home care management in, 598
    incidence and prevalence of, 596
    pathophysiology of, 595-596, 595f
    physical assessment in, 596
    self-management education in, 598-599
  upper airway obstruction, 536-537, 536b-537b, 537f
Respiratory rate in pneumonia, 592t
Respiratory status
  in chronic obstructive pulmonary disease, 562
  preoperative assessment of, 221
Respiratory support
  in ascites, 1199-1200, 1199b
  in myasthenia gravis, 919, 919b
Respiratory system, 494
  acidosis and, 181, 181b
  alkalosis and, 184, 184b
  anatomy and physiology of, 496-500
    lower respiratory tract, 498-499
      accessory muscles of respiration, 499
      airways, 498-499, 498f-499f
      lungs, 499, 499f
    upper respiratory tract, 496-498, 497f
      larynx, 497-498, 498f
      nose and sinuses, 496-497, 497f
      pharynx, 497
  assessment of. *See* Respiratory assessment.
  changes associated with aging, 500, 500b-501b
  complications of immobility and, 83t
  dehydration and, 156
  disorders of. *See* Respiratory problems.
  fluid overload and, 159b
  hypokalemia and, 164, 164b
  older adults and, 398b
  oxygen delivery and oxygen-hemoglobin dissociation curve and, 499-500, 500f
  potential complications of surgery and, 258t
  role in oxygenation and tissue perfusion, 494, 495f, 514
Respiratory tract, 399

Rest, preoperative anxiety and, 233
Rest pain, 720
Restless legs syndrome (RLS), 925-926
Restorative aides, 77
Restorative proctocolectomy with ileo pouch-anal anastomosis, 1177, 1177b, 1178f
Restorative surgery, 218t
Restraints
  chemical, 22, 22b
  hospitalized older adults and, 21-22, 22b
Restrictive cardiomyopathy, 701-702
Resurfacing of skin in wounds, 435
Resuscitation phase of burns, 473-481, 473b
  acute respiratory distress syndrome and, 481b, 487-488
  age-related changes increasing complications in, 474b, 479b
  airway management in, 477-478, 478b
  carbon monoxide poisoning and, 474, 475t
  cardiovascular assessment in, 475
  fluid resuscitation in, 478-479, 479b
  gastrointestinal assessment in, 476
  history in, 473
  hypovolemic shock and, 478-479, 479b, 480f
  imaging assessment in, 476-477
  inflammatory compensation during, 470
  kidney/urinary assessment in, 475-476
  laboratory assessment in, 476, 476b-477b
  pain management during, 479-480, 480b
  pulmonary fluid overload in, 475, 475b
  respiratory assessment in, 473-474, 474b, 474t
  skin assessment in, 476, 476f
  surgical management in, 478-480, 480f
Rete pegs, 416
Retention bridge skin closure, 254f
Reticular activating system, 832
Reticulocyte count, 793
Retina, 966, 967f
Retinal disorders, 989-991, 990b
  macular degeneration, 989
  retinal holes, tears, and detachments, 989-990
  retinitis pigmentosa, 990-991, 990b
Retinitis pigmentosa, 990-991, 990b
Retinopathy, diabetic, 1303
Retrograde procedures, 1362
Retroviruses, 327
Reverse transcriptase, 327
Revision arthroplasty, 295-296

Rewarming methods
in frostbite, 133b
in hypothermia, 132
RF. See Rheumatoid factor (RF).
Rhabdomyolysis, 130-131, 170
Rheumatic carditis, 700-701
Rheumatic disease, 290
Rheumatic endocarditis, 700
Rheumatoid arthritis (RA), 304-313
arthrocentesis in, 308, 308b
body image and, 312
complementary and alternative
therapies for, 312
fatigue in, 312, 312b
health care resources for, 313
home care management in, 313,
313f
inflammation and pain
management in, 308-312,
308b-310b
laboratory assessment in, 307,
307b
nonpharmacologic interventions
in, 311
pathophysiology of, 304-305, 305b
patient and family education in,
313
physical assessment in, 295b,
305-306, 305b-306b
psychosocial assessment in,
306-307
self-management in, 312, 312b
Rheumatoid factor (RF), 307, 307b
Rheumatology, 290
Rheumatrex. See Methotrexate.
Rhinitis, 583-584, 584b
allergic, 349-351, 349f, 351b
Rhinoplasty, 462t, 532, 532b, 532f
Rhinorrhea
in allergic rhinitis, 349-350, 583
in meningitis, 863
Rhinosinusitis, 584
Rhonchus, 507t
Rhytidectomy, 462t
Rib fractures, 623
Rifampin, 596-597, 597b
Right atrium, 628, 628f
Right coronary artery, 629
Right ventricle, 628, 628f
Right-sided heart failure, 679
history in, 682
physical assessment in, 682b, 683
Rinne tuning fork test, 1002
Rituxan. See Rituximab.
Rituximab, 309b
RLS. See Restless legs syndrome
(RLS).
Robotic surgery
cardiac, 779
surgical suites for, 242, 243f
Robotic technology, 84
Romberg sign, 842
Rotation injury of neck, 893
Rotator cuff injuries, 1079
Roux-en Y gastric bypass, 1250,
1251f

RRMS. See Relapsing-remitting
multiple sclerosis (RRMS).
RRTs. See Renal replacement
therapies (RRTs).
RSS. See Ramsay Sedation Scale
(RSS).
Rubor, 637
Rubor, 720, 720f
Rugae, 1126-1127
Rupture of central venous catheters,
208t
RV. See Residual volume (RV).
Rythmol. See Propafenone
hydrochloride.

S
SA node. See Sinoatrial (SA) node.
SABA. See Short-acting beta$_2$
agonists (SABA).
Safe patient handling practices,
80-81, 81b, 82f-83f
Safe sex practices, 330
Safety. See Patient safety.
Saline lock, 191
Salivary gland disorders, 1107-1108
Salivary gland tumors, 1108
Salmeterol, 539b
Salpingitis, 1452
gonorrhea and, 1539
Same-day admission, 218
Same-day surgery, 218
Sanguineous drainage, 264
Sarcoidosis, 571
Sarcomas, Kaposi's, 335, 335f, 342
Sargramostim, 387t
SARS. See Severe acute respiratory
syndrome (SARS).
SBAR communication technique, 5,
8
SBRT. See Stereotactic body
radiotherapy (SBRT).
Scabies, 403, 454, 454f
Scald injuries, 470
Scales, 423f
Scars, 424
SCI. See Spinal cord injury (SCI).
SCIP. See Surgical Care Improvement
Project (SCIP).
Sclera, 966, 967f
Scleroderma, 317
Scoliosis, 1023, 1047-1048, 1048b
Scorpions, 128, 128f
Scotomas, 905
Screening for diabetes mellitus, 1309
Scrotum, 1451
Scrub attire, 244f
Scrub nurses, 239, 241f, 245f
Sealed implants of radioactive
sources, 376b
Seasonal influenza, 586-587
Sebaceous glands, 417
Sebum, 417
Second heart sound, 639
Second intention healing, 434f, 435
Secondary administration sets, 197,
197f

Secondary adrenal insufficiency,
1274t
Secondary brain injury, 948-950,
949b, 949f-950f
Secondary glomerular diseases and
syndromes, 1402t
Secondary gout, 319
Secondary hypertension, 710
Secondary lesions, 421, 423f
Secondary osteoarthritis, 291
Secondary osteoporosis, 1030t
Secondary prevention, 368-370
Secondary progressive multiple
sclerosis (SPMS), 904
Secondary survey, 118
Secondary syphilis, 1532, 1532f
Secondary tuberculosis, 595
Secondary tumors, 362-363
Second-degree frostbite, 132-133
Secondhand smoke, 495
Second-look surgery, 373
Sectral. See Acebutolol
hydrochloride.
Securing catheter in infusion
therapy, 200-201, 201b
Sedation
moderate, 249, 250t
opioid-induced, 43-44, 43t-44t
palliative, 100
Sedentary lifestyle, risk for heart
disease and, 632-633
Segmental systolic blood pressure
measurements, 720
Seizures, 858-863
drug therapy for, 859, 859b
emergency care in, 861-862,
862b
etiology and genetic risk in,
858-859
management in end-of-life care,
100
older adults and, 858b
seizure precautions and
management in, 860-861,
860b-861b
self-management education in,
859, 861b
surgical management of, 862-863
types of, 858
Selective estrogen receptor
modulators (SERMs), 1478
Selective immunoglobulin A
deficiency, 345-346, 346b
Selective serotonin reuptake
inhibitors (SSRIs), 16
Self versus non-self, 276, 276f, 277b
Self-care deficit in spinal cord injury,
898-899
Self-ear irrigation, 999b
Self-esteem
acquired immune deficiency
syndrome and, 343
burns and, 488
head and neck cancer and, 544
mastectomy and, 1479-1480
tracheostomy and, 528-529

Self-management
in acquired immune deficiency
syndrome, 343, 344b
in Alzheimer's disease, 874-875,
880
in asthma, 534, 536b-537b, 542f
in back pain, 890, 890b-891b
in breast cancer, 1478-1479, 1479b
in burns, 489
in cataracts, 984, 984b
in chronic kidney disease, 1445
in chronic obstructive pulmonary
disease, 563b, 566
in cirrhosis, 1202, 1202b
in colorectal cancer, 1155-1157,
1155b-1156b
in coronary artery disease,
781-782, 781b-782b
in diabetes mellitus, 1337-1338,
1337t
in endometrial cancer, 1494
in epilepsy, 859, 861b
in esophageal cancer, 1122
in fractures, 1065, 1065b
in gastric cancer, 1142
in genital herpes, 1536, 1536b
in genital warts, 1537-1538,
1537b
in gonorrhea, 1540-1541
in head and neck cancer, 544-545,
545b
in heart failure, 689-691,
690b-691b, 690t
in hypertension, 718
in hypothyroidism, 1294, 1294b
in infection, 410
in intestinal obstruction, 1161
in leukemia, 815, 815b-816b
lifestyles and practices to promote
wellness and, 10, 10b
in lupus, 316b-317b
in malnutrition, 1246
in multiple sclerosis, 909-910
in myasthenia gravis, 922, 922b,
922t
in oral cancer, 1106-1107, 1107b
in osteoarthritis, 304, 304b
in oxygen therapy, 521
in pain, 48
in pelvic inflammatory disease,
1543-1544, 1543b
in peptic ulcer disease, 1138,
1138b
in pneumonia, 594, 594b
postoperative, 272, 272b
in pressure ulcers, 449
in prostate cancer, 1511, 1511b
in pulmonary embolism, 610,
610b
in pyelonephritis, 1401
in rheumatoid arthritis, 312, 312b
in sepsis, 754
in spinal cord injury, 900-901,
901b
in stroke, 942-943, 943b, 945b,
945f

Self-management (Continued)
in syphilis, 1534-1535, 1534b
in total hip arthroplasty, 298b,
300, 300b
in tracheostomy, 529, 529b
in traumatic brain injury, 956-957,
957b
in tuberculosis, 598-599
in ulcerative colitis, 1180, 1181b
in urinary incontinence, 1383,
1383b
in urothelial cancer, 1390, 1390b
in valvular heart disease, 696-697,
697b
Self-monitoring of blood glucose
(SMBG), 1317-1319, 1318b
Self-tolerance, 276, 289
Semilunar valves, 628
Sengstaken-Blakemore tube, 1200
Senile angiomas, 420f
Sensitivity, culture and, 408
Sensorineural hearing loss, 1001
conductive versus, 1009t
Sensory aphasia, 943, 943t
Sensory assessment in spinal cord
injury, 894-895
Sensory function
cancer and, 372
neurologic assessment of, 841-842
stroke and, 936, 937f, 944
traumatic brain injury and,
955-956
Sensory neurons, 830, 830f
Sensory perception, 828
Sensory receptors, 834
Sepsis, 741
burn wound, 481, 482t
in cancer, 392
etiology of, 751, 751t
evaluation of care of patient with,
754
history in, 752, 752b
home care management in, 754,
754b
incidence and prevalence of, 751
infection and, 749, 749f
interventions for, 753-754, 753t
laboratory assessment in, 753
physical assessment in, 752
in pneumonia, 590b, 593
prevention of, 751-752, 751b
psychosocial assessment in, 753
self-management education in,
754
severe, 750-751
systemic inflammatory response
syndrome and, 749, 750b,
750f, 750t
Sepsis-induced distributive shock,
407
Septic shock, 741, 749
in bloodstream infection, 407
etiology of, 751, 751t
evaluation of care of patient with,
754

Septic shock (Continued)
incidence and prevalence of, 751
infection in, 749, 749f
interventions for, 753-754, 753t
laboratory assessment in, 753
physical assessment in, 752
prevention of, 751-752
psychosocial assessment in, 753
Septicemia
in cancer, 392
inadequate antimicrobial therapy
and, 407
Sequestrectomy, 1041, 1041b
Serevent. See Salmeterol.
SERMs. See Selective estrogen
receptor modulators (SERMs).
Serologic testing, 408
Serosanguineous exudate, 443t
Serositis, 315
Serotonin antagonists, 385b
Serous, 264
Serpiginous lesions, 422t
Serum cardiac enzymes, 641b
Serum creatinine, 1354,
1354b-1355b
Serum lipids, 641-642, 641b
Serum markers of myocardial
damage, 640-641, 641b
Serum sickness, 125, 355
Serum studies
in burn assessment, 477b
in gastrointestinal assessment, 1091
Severe acute respiratory syndrome
(SARS), 594-595, 595b
Severe sepsis, 750-751, 753t
Severe traumatic brain injury, 948
Sex chromosomes, 54, 54f
Sex reassignment surgery, 1526-1528
feminizing surgeries for male to
female patients, 1526-1527,
1527b, 1527t
masculinizing surgeries for female
to male patients, 1527-1528
Sex-linked recessive pattern of
inheritance, 57t, 58-59, 59f
Sexual activity, coronary artery
disease and, 781
Sexual assault forensic examiners,
106
Sexual assault nurse examiners, 106
Sexual transmission of human
immune deficiency virus,
330-331, 331f, 332b
Sexuality, 1448, 1519
Sexually transmitted diseases
(STDs), 1530-1545
chlamydia infections, 1538-1539,
1538b
complications of, 1532t
focused assessment in, 1534b
gender health considerations in,
1531b
genital herpes, 1535-1536, 1536b
genital warts, 1537-1538, 1537b,
1537f

Sexually transmitted diseases (STDs)
(Continued)
gonorrhea, 1539-1541, 1539b,
1540f
health promotion and
maintenance in, 1545
human immune deficiency virus
(HIV) infection. See Human
immune deficiency virus
(HIV) infection.
older adults and, 1531b
oral antibiotic therapy for, 1543b
pelvic inflammatory disease, 1539,
1541, 1541f, 1542t, 1543b
syphilis, 1531-1535, 1532f,
1533b-1534b, 1533t
vaginal infections, 1544
SHARE acronym, 5-6, 5t, 6b
SHARPS. See Short ARPS (sHARPS).
Sharps injuries, HIV transmission
and, 332
Shave biopsies, 429
Shear, pressure ulcers and, 437, 437f
Shift to left, 408
Shingles, 451-452, 451f
Shivering, 409
Shock, 739-756
cardiogenic, 740, 741t, 772
health promotion and
maintenance in, 755
hypovolemic. See Hypovolemic
shock.
key features of, 741b
oxygenation and tissue perfusion
in, 739-740, 740f, 742f
sepsis and septic shock, 749-754,
749f
etiology of, 751, 751t
evaluation of care of patient
with, 754
history in, 752, 752b
home care management in, 754,
754b
infection in, 749
interventions for, 753-754,
753t
laboratory assessment in, 753
physical assessment in, 752
prevention of, 751-752, 751b
psychosocial assessment in, 753
self-management education in,
754
severe sepsis, 750-751
systemic inflammatory response
syndrome and, 749, 750b,
750f, 750t
spinal, 894
types of, 740-741, 741t
Shoe closures, velcro, 84t
Shoehorns, 84t
Shoehorns, extended, 84t
Shoelaces, elastic, 84t
Shoes for diabetic patients, 1327
Short ARPS (sHARPS), 19
Short bones, 1017-1018

Short Michigan Alcoholism
Screening Test-Geriatric Version
(SMAST-G), 18-19
Short peripheral catheters, 190-192,
190f-192f, 190t, 191b, 201b
Short-acting beta$_2$ agonists (SABA),
539b, 555
Shortness of breath. See Dyspnea.
Shoulders
positioning to prevent
contractures, 487b
total shoulder arthroplasty and,
303
SIADH. See Syndrome of
inappropriate antidiuretic
hormone (SIADH).
Sick-day rules in diabetes mellitus,
1335b
Sickle cell crisis, 800
Sickle cell disease, 799-804, 799t
community-based care in, 803
etiology and genetic risk in, 476b,
800, 800f
history in, 800-801
imaging assessment in, 801
incidence and prevalence of, 800
infection prevention in, 802-803
laboratory assessment in, 801
pain in, 801-802, 802b
pathophysiology of, 799-800, 799f
physical assessment in, 800-801
pregnancy in, 803b
psychosocial assessment in, 801
Sigmoidoscopy, 1096
Silicosis, 573b
Silvadene. See Silver sulfadiazine.
Silver sulfadiazine, 486b
Simple facemasks, 517t, 518, 518f
Simple fractures, 1051-1052
Simple surgery, 218t
Simponi. See Golimumab.
Simulect. See Basiliximab.
Single nucleotide polymorphism, 56
Single-fiber electromyography, 919
Single-photon emission computed
tomography (SPECT)
in neurologic assessment,
846t-847t, 848
Singulair. See Montelukast.
Sinoatrial (SA) node, 650
Sinus arrhythmias, 656
Sinus bradycardia, 663-665,
664f-665f
Sinus dysrhythmias, 662-665
bradycardia in, 663-665, 664f-665f
tachycardia in, 662-663, 663b,
663f
Sinus tachycardia, 662-663, 663b,
663f
Sinuses, 497, 497f
cancer of, 533-534
physical assessment of, 503
rhinitis and, 583-584, 584b
allergic, 349-351, 349f, 351b
rhinosinusitis and, 584

Sinusitis. *See* Rhinosinusitis.
Sipuleucel-T-T, 387t
Sirolimus, 287b-288b
SIRS. *See* Systemic inflammatory response syndrome (SIRS).
Site infection, intravenous therapy-related, 204t-206t
Sjögren's syndrome (SS), 306, 356-357
Skeletal muscle
    alkalosis and, 184, 184b
    hypernatremia and, 162-163
    hypocalcemia and, 169
Skeletal system, 1017-1019, 1018t
    assessment of, 1021-1023, 1022f-1023f, 1023b
    bones, 1017-1019, 1018f
Skilled nursing facilities (SNFs), 75, 75f
Skin, 415
    age-related changes in, 417-420, 417f, 418b-419b, 419f-420f
    breakdown in hospitalized older adults, 22, 22b
    burn injury of. *See* Burns.
    cardiovascular assessment and, 637
    changes in HIV infection, 334b
    dehydration and, 156, 156b, 156f
    fluid overload and, 159b
    functions of, 417, 418t
    hypovolemic shock and, 746
    lupus and, 314-316, 314f, 316b
    potential complications of surgery and, 258t
    respiratory assessment and, 506
    role in body protection, 415, 416f
    structure of, 415-417, 416f
Skin appendages, 417, 417f
Skin assessment, 421-424
    in burns, 476, 476f
    in darker skinned patients, 427b-428b, 428
    in hematologic assessment, 792, 792b
    inspection in, 421-424, 422t, 423f-424f, 424b
    palpation in, 424, 424b, 425t
    postoperative, 263-264, 264f-265f
    preoperative, 222
    in rehabilitation setting, 78t, 79, 79b
Skin barrier, 415
Skin biopsy, 429
Skin cancer, 458-461
    drug therapy for, 461
    older adults and, 367b
    pathophysiology of, 458-460, 459t
        etiology and genetic risk in, 458-460, 459f, 460b
        incidence and prevalence of, 460
    prevention of, 460, 460b
    surgical management of, 460-461

Skin care
    in chronic diarrhea, 1166b
    in infusion therapy, 207-209
    postoperative, 267b
    in preventing pressure ulcers, 438b
    during radiation therapy, 376, 376b-377b
    in skin infections, 453
Skin closures, 253, 254f
Skin color, 421
    common alterations in, 422t
    cultural considerations in, 427b
Skin grafting, 483-485, 484f
Skin integrity, 415, 432
    in acquired immune deficiency syndrome, 342
    assessment of, 424
    during emergency care, 109
    during rehabilitation, 85
Skin lesions, 421, 422t
    classification of, 423f
Skin preparation
    for peripheral catheter placement, 191-192
    preoperative, 228-229, 229f
Skin problems, 432-464
    common infections, 449-453, 450b
        bacterial, 450-451, 450b, 451f
        fungal, 450b, 451-452
        history in, 452-453
        interventions in, 452-453, 452b
        laboratory assessment in, 452
        physical assessment in, 450b, 452
        prevention of, 452, 452b
        viral, 450b, 451, 451f
    common inflammations, 455-456, 455b-456b
    cutaneous anthrax, 453, 453b, 454f
    minor skin irritations, 437-441
        pruritus, 432-433
            dry skin and, 433b
            urticaria, 433
    parasitic disorders, 453-455
        bedbugs, 454-455
        pediculosis, 453-454
        scabies, 454, 454f
    plastic surgery for, 462-463
        common procedures in, 462t
    pressure ulcers, 436-449
        concept map for, 445f
        evaluation of care of patient with, 449
        health care resources for, 449, 449b
        history in, 441
        home care management in, 447-449
        identification of high-risk patients, 437-440, 439f
        incidence and prevalence of, 437
        infection prevention in, 447, 448b

Skin problems (Continued)
        laboratory assessment in, 444
        massage and, 440b
        mechanical forces in, 437, 437f
        nutrition therapy and, 438b, 446
        older adults and, 437b
        pathophysiology of, 436-449
        physical assessment in, 441
        pressure-relieving and pressure-reducing techniques for, 440-441
        prevention of, 437-441, 438b
        psychosocial assessment in, 443
        self-management education in, 449
        stages of, 433-436
        surgical management of, 447
        wound assessment in, 441-443, 441b, 442f, 443t
        wound care in, 444-447, 444b, 445f, 446b-447b, 446t
    psoriasis, 456-458, 456b-458b, 457f
    Stevens-Johnson syndrome, 461-462, 461f
    toxic epidermal necrolysis, 461
    trauma, 433-436
        burns in. *See* Burns.
        full-thickness wounds in, 435-436, 435f
        partial-thickness wounds in, 435, 435f
        phases of wound healing in, 433-435, 433t, 434f-435f, 436t
Skin self-examination, 421
Skin stimulation for pain management, 46-47
Skin substitutes, 447
Skin tests for allergies, 350
Skin tests in respiratory assessment, 509
Skinfold measurements, 1236
SLE. *See* Systemic lupus erythematosus (SLE).
Sleep apnea, obstructive, 534-535
Sleep deprivation, 837
Sleep disorders and hospitalized older adults, 20
Slip lock, 197-198
Slit-lamp examination, 974, 974f
SLP. *See* Speech and language pathologist (SLP).
Small bowel capsule endoscopy, 1095
Small intestine, 1087
Smallpox, 411t
Smart pumps, 199
SMAST-G. *See* Short Michigan Alcoholism Screening Test-Geriatric Version (SMAST-G).
SMBG. *See* Self-monitoring of blood glucose (SMBG).
Smoke poisoning, 475

Smoking
    after laryngectomy, 545
    cancer and, 574
    cultural considerations in, 496b
    gender considerations and, 495b, 500b
    hookah, 495
    oxygen therapy and, 522b
    passive, 495
    respiratory assessment and, 494-495
    social, 495
Smoking cessation, 495, 495b-496b, 512b
SMR. *See* Submucous resection (SMR).
Snakebites, 123-126, 123f
    coral snakes and, 125-126, 125f, 126b
    North American pit vipers and, 123-125, 124b, 124t, 137
    prevention of, 123, 123b
SNFs. *See* Skilled nursing facilities (SNFs).
Social history in skin problems, 420b
Social isolation, infection and, 410
Social justice, 4
Social smoking, 495
Social workers, 77
Socks for diabetic patients, 1327
Sodium, 161-163
    abnormal values of, 152t
    hypernatremia and, 162-163, 162t, 163b
    hyponatremia and, 161-162, 161t, 162b
    in burns, 469
    levels in burn assessment, 477b
    perioperative assessment of, 223b-224b
    plasma values in older adults, 152b
Sodium nitroprusside, 748b
Solu-Cortef. *See* Hydrocortisone.
Solu-Medrol. *See* Methylprednisolone.
Solutes, 148-149
Solvents, 148-149
Somatic mutations, 56
Somatic pain, 28
Somogyi phenomenon, 1315, 1315f
Sonoran coral snake, 125f
Sore throat, 584-586, 585b-586b, 585t
Soriatane. *See* Acitretin.
Sotalol, 658b-662b
Southern copperhead snakes, 123, 123f
Spastic bladder, 85-87, 86t
Spastic paralysis, 934-936
Speak-Up campaign, 4
Specialized nutrition support, 1240
Specialty beds, 85
Specialty nurses, 239

SPECT. *See* Single-photon emission computed tomography (SPECT).

Speech, head and neck cancer and, 542, 542f

Speech and language pathologist (SLP), 542

Speech audiometry, 1003

Speech-language pathologists, 77

Speed shock in intravenous therapy, 207t

Sperm banking
   before gender reassignment surgery, 1525
   in testicular cancer, 1514-1515, 1514b

Spermatocele, 1516, 1516f

Sphincter of Oddi, 1087

Spider veins, 735

Spinal anesthesia, 248t
   administration of, 249f
   complications of, recognizing, 261b

Spinal cord, 832-833, 833f
   compression in cancer, 393

Spinal cord injury (SCI), 892-902
   adjustment to major life changes in, 900
   airway management in, 896, 896b
   autonomic dysreflexia in, 899, 899b
   bowel disimpaction in, 87t
   drug therapy for, 898
   etiology of, 894
   evaluation of care of patient with, 902
   health care resources for, 901-902, 902f
   history in, 894
   home care management in, 900
   imaging assessment in, 895
   impaired mobility and self-care deficit in, 898-899
   incidence and prevalence of, 894
   injury prevention in, 896-898, 897b-898b, 897f
   laboratory assessment in, 895
   mechanism of injury in, 892-893, 893f
   neurogenic shock in, 896, 896b
   physical assessment in, 894-895
   self-management in, 900-901, 901b
   surgical management in, 898, 898b
   urinary and bowel elimination and, 899-900

Spinal cord stimulation for pain management, 47, 890, 891b

Spinal cord tumors, 902-904, 903b

Spinal fusion, 888, 898, 898b

Spinal nerves, 833-834, 834f

Spinal shock syndrome, 894

Spinal tap, 846t-847t, 849-850, 849b, 850t

Spine, compression fractures of, 1069

Spinous layer, 416

Spiritual counselors, 77

Spirituality, 101-102, 101b, 101f

Spironolactone, 715b-716b

Spleen
   in blood cell regulation, 787
   liver-spleen scan and, 1097
   palpation of, 793b

Splinting of surgical incisions, 230-231, 230b

Splints for fractures, 1058, 1058f

SPMS. *See* Secondary progressive multiple sclerosis (SPMS).

Spontaneous bacterial peritonitis, 1199

Spontaneous fractures, 1052

Spoon nails, 427t

Spore, anthrax, 599-600

Sports-related musculoskeletal trauma, 1076b

Sprains, 1079

Sputum analysis
   in chronic obstructive pulmonary disease, 561
   in pneumonia, 592, 592f
   in respiratory assessment, 502, 507
   in tuberculosis, 596

Squamous cell carcinomas, 458-459, 459f, 459t

Squamous metaplasia, 538

SS. *See* Sjögren's syndrome (SS).

SSc. *See* Systemic sclerosis (SSc).

SSRIs. *See* Selective serotonin reuptake inhibitors (SSRIs).

ST segment, 653, 654f, 656

Staff safety in emergency care, 108, 108b

Staging
   of cancer, 365, 365t
   of heart failure, 679

Standard Precautions, 402-403, 402b, 403t-404t, 404f

Stapedectomy, 1013, 1013b, 1013f

Stapes, 996-997, 997f

Staphylococcus, 450, 453

Staphylococcus aureus, 398
   methicillin-resistant, 405-406

Staples, 254f

Stasis dermatitis, 734

Stasis ulcers, 734

Stationary chest tube drainage system, 577

StatLock IV stabilization device, 200, 201f

Status asthmaticus, 535

Status epilepticus, 861-862, 862b

Stay sutures, 254f

STDs. *See* Sexually transmitted diseases (STDs).

Steatorrhea, 1091
   in Crohn's disease, 1182
   in cystic fibrosis, 567

Steatosis, 1208

Stelara. *See* Ustekinumab.

Stem cell transplantation
   in breast cancer, 1478
   in leukemia, 808f, 811-814, 811b-812b, 811t, 812f

Stem cells, 276, 277f, 785, 786f

Stenosis
   aortic, 692b, 693
   mitral, 692, 692b, 696b
   tracheal, 523t

Stents
   cardiac, 774, 774f
   prostatic, 1503
   for urolithiasis, 1386

Stereotactic body radiotherapy (SBRT), 375

Stereotactic pallidotomy/thalamotomy, 871

Stereotactic radiosurgery, 959-960, 959f

Sterile table, 241f

Sterilization, 402

Steroid therapy
   for eye inflammation and infection, 979b
   for lupus, 316b
   for rheumatoid arthritis, 311
   for skin inflammation, 455

Stevens-Johnson syndrome, 461-462, 461f

S_3 gallop, 683

Stimulation tests in endocrine assessment, 1263-1264

Stings. *See* Bites and stings.

Stoma care after total laryngectomy, 545

Stomach, 1085-1086

Stomach disorders, 1126-1143
   gastric cancer, 1138-1139, 1139b, 1140f, 1141t
   gastritis, 1126-1128, 1127b-1128b, 1133b-1134b
   health promotion and maintenance in, 1142-1143
   peptic ulcer disease. *See* Peptic ulcer disease (PUD).

Stomatitis, 1100-1102, 1100b-1102b, 1100f
   chemotherapy-related, 384, 810

Stool tests, 1091-1093

Strains, 1079

Strangulated obstruction, 1157-1158

Stratum corneum, 416, 416f

Stratum germinativum, 416

Stratum lucidum, 416

Stratum spinosum, 416

Streptococcal infections, 585t

Stress
   in health of transgender patients, 1521
   older adults and, 12-13, 13b

Stress fractures, 1052

Stress test. *See* Exercise electrocardiography.

Stress ulcers, 1130

Stress urinary incontinence (SUI), 1374t, 1375, 1486

Striae, 1262

Stridor
   after extubation in mechanical ventilation, 622, 622b

Stridor (*Continued*)
   in pharyngitis, 586b
   postoperative, 260

Stroke, 931-946
   bladder and bowel continence in, 943-944
   cardiovascular assessment in, 936-937
   cerebral perfusion and, 938-942, 938b-939b, 940t, 941b, 941f
   communication and, 943, 943t
   cultural considerations in, 933b
   dysphagia in, 936
   endovascular interventions in, 938-939, 939b
   etiology and genetic risk in, 932
   evaluation of care of patient with, 945-946
   gender health considerations in, 938b
   health care resources for, 945
   health promotion and maintenance in, 933, 933b
   history in, 933
   home care management in, 944
   imaging assessment in, 937
   impaired swallowing and, 942, 942b
   incidence and prevalence of, 932-933
   increased intracranial pressure in, 939-941, 939b, 941b
   laboratory assessment in, 937
   mobility and self-care in, 942-943, 943b
   monitoring complications in, 941
   National Institutes of Health Stroke Scale in, 933-934, 935t-936t
   ongoing drug therapy for, 941-942
   pathophysiologic changes in brain in, 931
   physical assessment in, 933-937, 934b, 935t-936t, 936b, 937f
   psychosocial assessment in, 937
   self-management education in, 944-945, 945b, 945f
   sensory perception and, 944
   surgical management of, 940t, 942
   types of, 931-932, 931f-932f, 932t
   unilateral body neglect and, 944

Stroke volume (SV)
   heart failure and, 680
   hypovolemic shock and, 744

Subacute thyroiditis, 1295

Subarachnoid bolt, 956t

Subarachnoid space, 830

Subclavian steal, 729t

Subcutaneous emphysema, 504
   in laryngeal trauma, 536
   in pneumothorax, 624
   tracheostomy-related, 523

Subcutaneous fat, 416, 416f

Subcutaneous infusion therapy, 210-211

Subcutaneous nodules, 306

Subcutaneous tissue, 415, 416f
  changes resulting from burns, 467f
  changes with aging, 418b-419b
  function of, 418t
Subdural catheters, 956t
Subdural hematoma, 949, 949f
Subdural space, 830
Sublimaze. See Fentanyl.
Subluxations
  after total hip arthroplasty, 297
  after total shoulder arthroplasty,
    303
Submucous resection (SMR), 532
Substance abuse, 219
Substernal retraction, 613
Subtotal thyroidectomy, 1289
Suction lipectomy, 462t
Suctioning
  in chronic obstructive pulmonary
    disease, 564
  in severe acute respiratory
    syndrome, 595b
  of tracheostomy, 525-527,
    525b-527b
SUI. See Stress urinary incontinence
  (SUI).
Suicide, physician-assisted, 103t
Sulfamylon. See Mafenide acetate.
Sundowning, 874
Superficial partial-thickness wounds,
  467, 468f
Superficial-thickness wounds,
  466-467
Superinfection, 410
Superior oblique muscle, 968f, 969t
Superior rectus muscle, 968f, 969t
Superior vena cava (SVC), 193
Superior vena cava syndrome,
  393-394, 393f-394f, 394b
Supervision, 6
Supine position during surgery, 252,
  252f
Suppression tests, 1263-1264
Suppressor T-cells, 285
Supraglottic partial laryngectomy,
  541t
Supratentorial brain tumors, 958
Supraventricular tachycardia (SVT),
  665-666, 666b
Surfactant, 499
Surgeons, 238-239
Surgery
  in abdominal herniation,
    1147-1148, 1148b
  in abdominal trauma, 1163
  in acute pancreatitis, 1222
  anesthesia and, 244-249, 246t
    general, 245-248, 246t,
      247b-248b
    local or regional, 248-249,
      248f-249f, 248t
    moderate sedation, 249, 250t
  in appendicitis, 1175
  in back pain, 888-890, 889b
  in benign prostatic hyperplasia,
    1505-1506, 1505b-1506b

Surgery (Continued)
  in brain tumors, 960-962,
    960b-961b, 961t
  in burns, 478-480, 480f, 483-485,
    484f
  in cancer, 373-374, 374b
    bone, 1044-1045, 1044b
    breast, 1472-1478, 1472f-1473f,
      1474b, 1475t, 1476b, 1478b
    cervical, 1495
    colorectal, 1152-1154, 1152t,
      1153f-1154f, 1154b
    endometrial, 1492
    esophageal, 1120-1122,
      1121b-1122b, 1121f
    gastric, 1139-1141
    head and neck, 540-542, 541b,
      541t, 542f
    lung, 576-580, 577b, 577f-578f,
      579b-580b
    oral, 1105-1106, 1106b
    ovarian, 1496-1497
    pancreatic, 1228-1230, 1229f,
      1229t, 1230f
    prostate, 1509-1510, 1509b
    skin, 460-461
    testicular, 1515, 1515b
  in cardiomyopathy, 702-704, 703b,
    703f
  categories and purposes of, 217,
    218t
  in cholecystectomy, 1217-1218,
    1217b, 1218t
  in chronic obstructive pulmonary
    disease, 564-565
  in chronic pancreatitis, 1225
  in Crohn's disease, 1185
  in cystic fibrosis, 569
  in cystitis, 1372-1373
  in diabetes mellitus, 1323-1324
    intraoperative care in, 1324
    postoperative care in,
      1324-1325
    preoperative care in, 1324
  in diverticular disease, 1187
  in dysfunctional uterine bleeding,
    1484
  ear
    myringotomy in, 1006, 1006f,
      1007b
    stapedectomy in, 1013, 1013b,
      1013f
    tympanoplasty in, 1012-1013,
      1012f
  in endometriosis, 1483
  eye
    for glaucoma, 988-989
    for refractive errors, 991
  in fracture, 1062-1063, 1062f
  in gastroesophageal reflux disease,
    1114
  in heart failure, 687-688, 688f
  in hiatal hernias, 1115-1117,
    1115b-1116b, 1116f
  history and, 250, 250b
  in hypercortisolism, 1279-1280

Surgery (Continued)
  in hyperparathyroidism,
    1297-1298
  in hyperpituitarism, 1270-1271,
    1270b
  in hyperthyroidism, 1289-1291,
    1290b-1291b
  hypoventilation prevention and,
    253-254
  identification of patient,
    procedure, and surgical site
    in, 226, 226b, 240f, 250
  infection prevention and, 253, 254f
  in infective endocarditis, 698
  injury prevention and, 252-253,
    252f, 253b
  in intestinal obstructions,
    1160-1161
  medical record review and,
    250-251, 250b-251b
  in myasthenia gravis, 921, 922b
  in obesity, 1250-1252, 1251b-
    1252b, 1251f
  in osteomyelitis, 1041, 1041b
  in Parkinson disease, 871
  patient self-determination and, 228
  patient transfer to surgical suites,
    234-236, 235f, 251b
  in pelvic organ prolapse, 1487,
    1487b
  in peptic ulcer disease, 1137
  in peripheral arterial disease,
    723-724, 723f, 724b
  in peritonitis, 1171, 1171b
  preoperative care in. See
    Preoperative care.
  in pulmonary embolism, 608-609
  in pyelonephritis, 1401
  reconstructive, 462-463
  in renal cell carcinoma, 1408
  risk for postoperative
    complications, 219, 219t
  safety checklist for, 216f
  in seizures and epilepsy, 862-863
  settings for, 218-219
  in spinal cord injury, 898, 898b
  in stress incontinence, 1379, 1380t
  in stroke, 940t, 942
  surgical suite preparation for,
    241-244
    health and hygiene of surgical
      team and, 242-243
    layout of suite and, 241-242,
      241f
    minimally invasive and robotic
      surgery and, 242,
      242f-243f
    surgical attire and, 243, 244f
    surgical scrub and, 243-244,
      244b, 245f
    surgical team members and,
      238-241, 241f
  in transgender patients, 1526-1528
    feminizing surgeries for male to
      female patients, 1526-1527,
      1527b, 1527t

Surgery (Continued)
  masculinizing surgeries for
    female to male patients,
    1527-1528
  in traumatic brain injury, 956, 956t
  in trigeminal neuralgia, 926-927,
    927b
  in ulcerative colitis, 1177-1179,
    1177b, 1178f
  in urolithiasis, 1386-1387
  in urothelial cancer, 1389-1390,
    1391f
  in uterine leiomyomas, 1489-1490,
    1489b-1490b, 1489t
  in valvular heart disease, 695-696,
    696b, 696f
  in venous thromboembolism, 733
Surgical assistants, 238-239
Surgical attire, 243, 244f
Surgical Care Improvement Project
  (SCIP), 216, 217t, 260
Surgical excision of burn wounds,
  484
Surgical safety checklist, 215-216,
  216f
Surgical scrub, 243-244, 244b, 245f
Surgical site
  identification of, 240f
  marking of, 226, 226b
  patient transfer to, 234-236, 235f
Surgical staging, 365
Surgical suites, 241-244
  health and hygiene of surgical
    team and, 242-243
  layout of, 241-242, 241f
  minimally invasive and robotic
    surgery and, 242, 242f-243f
  patient transfer to, 234-236, 235f,
    251b
  surgical attire and, 243, 244f
  surgical scrub and, 243-244, 244b,
    245f
Surgical teams, 238-241, 241f
  anesthesia providers in, 239
  health and hygiene of, 242-243
  perioperative nursing staff in,
    239-241, 240f-241f
  surgeons and surgical assistants in,
    238-239
Surgical technologists, 239
Surgical wound infections, 264
Surveillance in infection control,
  397-398
Survivor response to mass casualty
  events, 146-147, 146b-147b
Susceptibility genes, 56
Susceptibility to infection, 398
Sustained immunity, 284
Sutures, 253, 254f
SV. See Stroke volume (SV).
SVC. See Superior vena cava (SVC).
SVT. See Supraventricular
  tachycardia (SVT).
Swallowing
  after laryngectomy, 543, 543b
  difficulty in stroke, 942, 942b

Swallowing (Continued)
head and neck cancer and, 543, 543b
supraglottic method of, 543b
Sweat glands, 417
changes with aging, 418b-419b
Sympathetic nervous system, 470, 471f
Synapse, 830
Synchronized intermittent mandatory ventilation, 617, 622t
Syncope
cardiovascular assessment and, 635, 635b
in complex partial seizure, 858
in pulmonary embolism, 605
Syndrome of inappropriate antidiuretic hormone (SIADH), 1272-1273, 1272t
after craniotomy, 962
in cancer, 392-393, 392b
Syngeneic transplant, 811t
Synovectomy, 308
Synovial joints, 1019, 1019f
Synthetic dressings, 446b, 483, 484f
Syphilis, 1531-1535, 1532f, 1533b-1534b, 1533t
Syringe pumps, 199
Syringes, insulin, 1316
Systemic complications of infusion therapy, 204-207, 207t
Systemic inflammatory response syndrome (SIRS)
sepsis and, 749, 750b, 750f, 750t
Systemic lupus erythematosus (SLE), 313-317, 314b, 314f, 316b-317b
Systemic necrotizing vasculitis, 323t
Systemic sclerosis (SSc), 314b, 317-319, 318b, 318f
Systole, 629, 630f
Systolic blood pressure, 631
Systolic heart failure, 679
Systolic ventricular dysfunction, 679

T

T waves, 167b, 653, 654f
TAAs. See Thoracic aortic aneurysms (TAAs).
Tachycardia, 655
sinus, 662-663, 663b, 663f
supraventricular, 665-666, 666b
ventricular, 670, 670b, 670f
Tachydysrhythmias, 657, 657b
Tacrolimus, 287b-288b
Tactile fremitus, 504
Tactile stimulation for pain in burns, 480
Talcosis, 573b
Tambocor. See Flecainide acetate.
Tamiflu. See Oseltamivir.
Tape skin closure, 254f
Tapentadol, 42
Tar preparations for psoriasis, 457
Target tissues, 1255
Taste alteration, radiation therapy-related, 375-376

Tattoos, 424
TAVR. See Transcatheter aortic valve replacement (TAVR).
Tazarotene, 457, 457b
Tazorac. See Tazarotene.
TB. See Tuberculosis (TB).
TBB. See Transbronchial biopsy (TBB).
TBI. See Traumatic brain injury (TBI).
TBNA. See Transbronchial needle aspiration (TBNA).
TBPI. See Toe brachial pressure index (TBPI).
TBSA. See Total body surface area (TBSA).
TCD. See Transcranial Doppler ultrasonography (TCD).
T-cells, 278t, 285-286, 787t
TEA. See Total elbow arthroplasty (TEA).
Teamwork, 4-6, 5t, 6b, 8
Tears, 970b
TEE. See Transesophageal echocardiography (TEE).
TEF. See Tracheoesophageal fistula (TEF).
Telangiectasias, 735
Telemetry system of electrocardiogram, 652
Teletherapy, 375
Temporal arteritis, 323t
Temporal field blindness, 963
Temporal lobe, 831t
Temporary pacing, 664, 664f
Temsirolimus, 391
TEN. See Toxic epidermal necrolysis (TEN).
Tendinopathy, 1079
Tendon transplant, 1079
Tendons, 1020
TENS. See Transcutaneous electrical nerve stimulation (TENS).
Tensilon testing, 919, 919b
Tension pneumothorax, 624
Terminal delirium, 104
Terminology, patient-centered, 1519-1520, 1520t
Testes, 1451, 1451f
hormones secreted by, 1256t
hydrocele and, 1516, 1516f
self-examination of, 1513, 1513b
spermatocele and, 1516, 1516f
varicocele and, 1516, 1516f
Testicular cancer, 1513-1516
assessment in, 1514, 1514b
chemotherapy for, 1515-1516
community-based care in, 1516, 1516b
external beam radiation therapy for, 1516
pathophysiology of, 1513, 1513b, 1513t
sperm banking and, 1514-1515, 1514b

Testicular cancer (Continued)
surgical management of, 1515, 1515b
Testicular self-examination (TSE), 1513, 1513b
Tetany, thyroid surgery-related, 1290
Tetracaine hydrochloride, 979b
Tetraplegia, 894
Texture of skin, 425t
THA. See Total hip arthroplasty (THA).
Thalamotomy, 871
Thalamus, 830, 831f
Thallium imaging scans, 1025
Therapeutic hypothermia, 953-954
Therapeutic touch for dying patient, 97
Therapy-induced immune deficiencies, 344-345
Thermal injuries, 472, 474. See also Burns.
electrical, 518-519
Thermazene. See Silver sulfadiazine.
Thermotherapy for benign prostatic hyperplasia, 1503
Thiazide diuretics, 714, 714b
Thigh and leg surgery, skin preparation for, 229f
Third intention healing, 434f, 435
Third-degree frostbite, 132-133
Thirdhand smoke, 495
Thoracentesis, 511, 511f, 580
Thoracic aortic aneurysms (TAAs), 726
Thoracic outlet syndrome, 729t
Thoracoabdominal surgery, skin, preparation for, 229f
Thoracoscopy, 575
Thorax, 503-504, 504f
Thorough skin self-examination (TSSE), 421
Threshold of hearing, 1002, 1002t
Throat, sore, 584-586, 585b-586b, 585t
Thrombectomy
in acute peripheral arterial occlusion, 725b
in peripheral arterial disease, 724
in venous thromboembolism, 733
Thrombin, 788
Thrombocytopenia, 819
in aplastic anemia, 805
in brown recluse spider bites, 127
cancer and, 372
chemotherapy-related, 381-383
in myelodysplastic syndromes, 806
patient safety in, 814b
Thrombolytic drugs
for coronary artery disease, 767-768, 768b, 768t
for venous thromboembolism, 733
Thrombophlebitis, 618
intravenous therapy-related, 204t-206t
Thrombopoietin, 787

Thrombosis
intravenous therapy-related, 188, 204t-206t
in polycythemia vera, 805
Thrombotic stroke, 931, 931f, 932t
Thrombotic thrombocytopenia purpura, 820
Thrombus, 618, 931
Thrush, 452
Thymectomy, 921, 922b
Thyrocalcitonin, 1259
Thyroid cancer, 1295-1296
Thyroid cartilage, 497
Thyroid crisis, 1290, 1290b
Thyroid gland, 1259-1260, 1259f
hormones secreted by, 1256t, 1259t
Thyroid problems, 1285-1296
hyperthyroidism, 1285-1291
assessment in, 1286-1287, 1287f, 1287t, 1288b
nonsurgical management for, 1288-1289, 1288b-1289b
pathophysiology of, 1285-1286, 1286b
surgical management of, 1289-1291, 1290b-1291b
hypothyroidism, 1291-1295
assessment in, 1292-1293
community-based care in, 1294-1295, 1294b-1295b
evaluation of care of patient with, 1295
interventions in, 1293-1294, 1294b
pathophysiology of, 1291-1295, 1292b, 1292f, 1292t
thyroid cancer, 1295-1296
thyroiditis, 1295
Thyroid storm, 1290, 1291b
Thyroiditis, 1295
Thyroid-stimulating hormone, deficiency of, 1267b
Thyrotoxicosis, 1285
Thyrotropin, 1269b
Thyroxine, 1259
TIA. See Transient ischemic attack (TIA).
Tidal volume, 618
Tight adherence, 360-361
Tikosyn. See Dofetilide.
Tilade. See Nedocromil.
Time-cycled ventilators, 616
Tinea infections, 451-452
Tinel's sign, 1078
Tinnitus, 958, 1007-1008
Tissue mast cells, 280
Tissue perfusion
after amputations, 1072-1073
coronary artery disease and, 766-768, 767b-768b, 768t
hematologic system's role in, 785, 786f
oxygen therapy and, 514, 515f
respiratory problems and, 603, 604f

Tissue perfusion (Continued)
　respiratory system's role in, 494, 495f
　shock and, 739-740, 740f, 742f
Tissue thromboplastin, 790t
TJA. See Total joint arthroplasty (TJA).
TJC. See Joint Commission, The (TJC).
TKA. See Total knee arthroplasty (TKA).
TKIs. See Tyrosine kinase inhibitors (TKIs).
TKs. See Tyrosine kinases (TKs).
TLC. See Total lung capacity (TLC).
TLS. See Tumor lysis syndrome (TLS).
T-lymphocytes, 282f, 787t
TNM system. See Tumor, node, metastasis (TNM) system.
To Err Is Human (IOM), 2
Tobacco use, cancer and, 366, 366t, 370
Tocainide hydrochloride, 658b-662b
Tocilizumab, 309b, 311
Toe brachial pressure index (TBPI), 638
Toes, surgery, skin preparation for, 229f
Tofacitinib, 311
Tolerance, 39-40, 50
Tonic-clonic seizures, 861b
Tonocard. See Tocainide hydrochloride.
Tonometry, 974, 974f
Tonsillitis, 586, 586b
Tophi, 319-320, 319f
Topical chemical debridement of pressure ulcers, 444-446
Topical drugs for eye inflammation and infection, 979b
Topical enzyme preparations for pressure ulcers, 446t
Topical growth factors, 447
Topoisomerase inhibitors, 378, 378t, 380t
Torisel. See Temsirolimus.
Torsades de pointes, 662
Total abdominal hysterectomy, 1489
Total body surface area (TBSA), 476, 476f
Total body water, 148, 149f, 155b
Total elbow arthroplasty (TEA), 303
Total enteral nutrition, 1240-1244, 1242b-1244b, 1242f
Total hemoglobin in respiratory assessment, 508b
Total hip arthroplasty (THA), 295-300, 300b
　infection prevention after, 297t, 299, 299b
　mobility and activity after, 297-300, 297b, 299b-300b
　older adults and, 297b
　operative procedures in, 296-297, 297f

Total hip arthroplasty (THA) (Continued)
　pain management after, 299
　postoperative care in, 297-300, 297b, 297t
　preoperative care in, 296
　prevention of hip dislocation after, 297t, 298, 298b
　self-management after, 298b
　venous thromboembolism after, 296, 297t, 298-299
Total hysterectomy, 1489t
　in endometrial cancer, 1492
Total joint arthroplasty (TJA), 295
Total joint replacement (TJR). See Total hip arthroplasty (THA).
Total knee arthroplasty (TKA), 300-302, 301f, 302b
Total laryngectomy, 541t
Total lung capacity (TLC), 510t
Total parenteral nutrition (TPN), 1245, 1245b
　after surgery for diabetes mellitus, 1325
Total protein in burn assessment, 477b
Total shoulder arthroplasty (TSA), 303
Total thyroidectomy, 1289
Total urinary incontinence, 1382
Total vaginal hysterectomy, 1489
Totally implanted device for hearing loss, 1013-1014
Touch discrimination, 842
Toxic epidermal necrolysis (TEN), 461
Toxic megacolon, 1176-1177
Toxic multinodular goiters, 1286
Toxic shock syndrome (TSS), 1485, 1485b
Toxidrome, 844
Toxins, 398
Toxoplasma gondii, 334
Toxoplasmosis encephalitis, 334
T-piece, 519-520, 519t, 520f
T-piece technique in weaning from ventilators, 622t
TPN. See Total parenteral nutrition (TPN).
Trachea, 498, 498f
　physical assessment of, 503
Tracheal stenosis, 523t
Tracheobronchial trauma, 624
Tracheobronchial tree, 498
Tracheoesophageal fistula (TEF), 523t
Tracheoesophageal puncture (TEP), 542
Tracheo-innominate artery fistula, 523t
Tracheomalacia, 523t
Tracheostomy, 522-529
　care issues for patients with, 525-529, 527b
　bronchial and oral hygiene, 527-528

Tracheostomy (Continued)
　communication and, 528
　ensuring air warming and humidification, 525, 525b
　focused assessment of patient, 527, 527b
　nutrition and, 528, 528b
　preventing tissue damage, 525, 525f
　psychosocial needs and self-image and, 528-529
　suctioning, 525-527, 525b-527b
　weaning from, 529
　community-based care in, 529
　complications of, 522-524, 523b, 523t
　older adults and, 529b
　postoperative care in, 522
　preoperative care in, 522
Tracheostomy button, 529
Tracheostomy collar, 519-520, 520f
Tracheostomy tubes, 524, 524f, 525b
　correct placement of, 527, 528f
　dislodgement and accidental decannulation of, 522, 523b, 527b
　obstruction of, 522
　weaning from, 529
Tracheotomy
　in facial trauma, 534
　in head and neck cancer, 542
　in upper airway obstruction, 536-537
Trachoma, 980, 980b
Traction, 1060b, 1061f, 1061t
Training and certification in emergency care, 111, 111t
Tramadol, 42, 270b
Transbronchial biopsy (TBB), 511
Transbronchial needle aspiration (TBNA), 511
Transcatheter aortic valve replacement (TAVR), 695, 695f
Transcellular fluids, 148
Transcervical endometrial resection, 1489
Transcranial Doppler ultrasonography (TCD), 850
Transcription factors, 388
Transcutaneous electrical nerve stimulation (TENS), 47
Transcutaneous pacing, 664, 664f
Transduction of pain, 26, 29f
Transesophageal echocardiography (TEE)
　in cardiovascular assessment, 646
Transfer of patients, 81b
　to surgical suites, 234-236, 235f, 251b
Transfusion therapy, 188-189, 189f, 821-826
　acute transfusion reactions in, 824-825
　allergies to, 251
　autologous, 825-826

Transfusion therapy (Continued)
　indications for, 822t
　in leukemia, 814
　older adult and, 823b
　pretransfusion responsibilities, 821-823, 822b-823b, 823f
　red blood cell, 824, 824b, 824t
Transgender patients, 1519-1529
　community-based care for, 1528
　drug therapy for, 1524-1525
　　patients transition from female to male, 1525, 1525t
　　patients transition from male to female, 1524-1525, 1524t, 1525b
　health issues of, 1520-1521
　history of, 1522-1523
　need to improve health care for, 1521-1528, 1522b, 1522f, 1522t
　older adults as, 1523b
　patient-centered terminology and, 1519-1520, 1520t
　physical assessment of, 1522-1524, 1523b
　pronoun usage and, 1523
　psychosocial assessment of, 1524
　reproductive health options, 1525
　sex reassignment surgery for, 1526-1528
　　feminizing surgeries for male to female patients, 1526-1527, 1527b, 1527t
　　masculinizing surgeries for female to male patients, 1527-1528
　stress and health of, 1521
　vocal and communication therapy for, 1525-1526
Transient ischemic attack (TIA), 930-931, 931b
Transjugular intrahepatic portal-systemic shunts, 1200
Transmission of pain, 26-28, 29f
Transmission-based precautions, 403, 404t
　in skin infections, 453
　social isolation and, 410
Transmyocardial laser revascularization, 779
Transoral cordectomy, 541t
Transplant rejection, 286-287, 289
　acute, 287
　chronic, 287
　hyperacute, 286-287
　management of, 287, 287b-288b, 289
Transplantation
　fetal tissue, 871
　heart, 702-704, 703b, 703f
　islet cell, 1324
　kidney, 1441-1444
　　candidate selection criteria in, 1441
　　complications of, 1443, 1444t

Transplantation (Continued)
- donors in, 1441-1442, 1442f
- immunosuppressive drug therapy in, 1444
- operative procedures in, 1442, 1443f
- postoperative care in, 1442-1443
- preoperative care in, 1442
- liver, 1208-1211, 1208b, 1210b, 1210t
- lung, 564-565, 569
- pancreas, 1323-1324
- stem cell
  - in breast cancer, 1478
  - in leukemia, 808f, 811-814, 811b-812b, 811t, 812f
Transport maximum for glucose reabsorption, 1348
Transrectal ultrasonography (TRUS), 1508, 1508b
Transsexuals, 1520, 1520t. See also Lesbian, gay, bisexual, transgender, and queer and/ or questioning (LGBTQ) population; Transgender patients.
Transtracheal oxygen therapy (TTO), 520, 522b
Transurethral microwave therapy, 1503
Transurethral needle ablation, 1503
Transurethral resection of prostate (TURP), 1505-1506, 1505b-1506b
Trauma, 114-115
- abdominal, 1161-1163, 1162b
- bladder, 1391-1392
- burns. See Burns.
- chest, 622-624
  - flail chest, 623, 623f
  - hemothorax, 624
  - pneumothorax, 623-624
  - pulmonary contusions, 622-623
  - rib fractures, 623
  - tension pneumothorax, 624
  - tracheobronchial trauma, 624
- ear, 1007
- esophageal, 1123-1124, 1123t
- eye, 991-992, 991b-992b
- facial, 534, 534b
- to kidneys, 1408-1409, 1408b-1409b
- laryngeal, 536, 536b
- musculoskeletal. See Musculoskeletal trauma.
- neck, 537
- peripheral nerve, 923-925, 923f-924f, 925b
- skin, 433-436
  - full-thickness wounds in, 435-436, 435f
  - partial-thickness wounds in, 435, 435f

Trauma (Continued)
- phases of wound healing in, 433-435, 433t, 434f-435f, 436t
- vascular, 736
Trauma centers, 115-116, 115f, 115t
Trauma nursing, 106-108
- mechanism of injury and, 116
- patient disposition in, 118
- primary survey and resuscitation interventions in, 116-117, 117b-118b, 118t
- secondary survey and resuscitation interventions in, 118
- trauma centers and, 115-116, 115f, 115t
- trauma systems and, 116
Trauma systems, 116
Traumatic brain injury (TBI), 946-957
- determining brain death in, 954
- drug therapy for, 954-955
- fluid and electrolyte management in, 955
- health care resources for, 957
- health promotion and maintenance in, 950
- history in, 950-953, 951b
- home care management in, 956
- imaging assessment in, 953
- inducing barbiturate coma, 955
- laboratory assessment in, 953
- nutritional status in, 955
- pathophysiology of, 946-950, 946f
  - etiology of, 950
  - incidence and prevalence of, 950
  - primary, 946-948, 947f, 948b
  - secondary, 948-950, 949b, 949f-950f
- physical assessment in, 951-952, 951b-952b
- preventing and detecting secondary brain injury in, 953-954, 954b
- psychosocial assessment in, 952-953
- self-management education in, 956-957, 957b
- sensory, cognitive, and behavioral changes in, 955-956
- surgical management of, 956, 956t
Triage, 111-112, 111t, 112b
- mass casualty, 140-141, 141b, 141t
Triage officers, 143, 143t
Trichomoniasis, 1544
Tricyclic antidepressants
- for fibromyalgia, 322
- older adults and, 16b
Trigeminal nerve, 835t
Trigeminal neuralgia, 926-927, 926f, 927b
Trigeminy, 657
Trigger points in fibromyalgia, 321

Triglycerides, 641-642, 641b
Triptans, 856, 856b
Trochlear nerve, 835t
Troponins, 641
Trough levels, 409
TRUS. See Transrectal ultrasonography (TRUS).
Truss for abdominal herniation, 1147
Truvada. See Emtricitabine/tenofovir.
TSA. See Total shoulder arthroplasty (TSA).
TSE. See Testicular self-examination (TSE).
TSS. See Toxic shock syndrome (TSS).
TSSE. See Thorough skin self-examination (TSSE).
TTO. See Transtracheal oxygen therapy (TTO).
T-tube drains, 264, 265f
Tube feeding, 1240-1244, 1242b-1244b, 1242f
Tuberculin test, 596, 596f
Tuberculosis (TB), 595-599
- in AIDS, 334-335
- diagnosis of, 596, 596f
- directly observed therapy for, 407
- drug therapy for, 596-598, 597b-598b
- health care resources for, 599
- history in, 596
- home care management in, 598
- pathophysiology of, 595-596, 595f
  - etiology of, 595
  - incidence and prevalence of, 596
- physical assessment in, 596
- self-management education in, 598-599
Tubes. See also Nasogastric tubes.
- endotracheal, 615, 615f
- preoperative preparation for, 230
- tracheostomy, 524, 524f
Tubular filtrate, 1347
Tubular reabsorption, 1347
Tubular secretion, 1349
Tubulointerstitial immunologic renal disease, 1405
Tumor, node, metastasis (TNM) system, 365, 365t
Tumor lysis syndrome (TLS), 394, 394f
Tumors. See also Cancer.
- bone
  - benign, 1042
- brain. See Brain tumors.
- esophageal. See Esophageal tumors.
- oral. See Oral tumors.
- pituitary, 958
- in renal cell carcinoma, 1406-1408, 1407t
- salivary gland, 1108
- spinal cord, 902-904, 903b

Tuning fork test, 1001
Tunneled central venous catheters, 195, 195f
Turbidity, 197b
Turbinates, 496, 497f
Turgor, 424, 424b, 425t
TURP. See Transurethral resection of prostate (TURP).
Tympanic membrane, 996, 997f
Tympanometry, 1003
Tympanoplasty, 1012-1013, 1012f
Tympany percussion note, 505t
Type A chronic gastritis, 1127
Type B gastritis, 1127
Type I diabetes mellitus, 1306, 1306t
- genetic considerations in, 1307b
- type 2 versus, 1306t
Type I rapid hypersensitivity reactions, 348-355
- allergic rhinitis in, 349-351, 349f, 351b
- anaphylaxis in, 348-349, 351-354
  - assessment of, 352-353, 352f, 353b
  - in bee stings, 129
  - interventions, 353-354, 353b-354b
  - pathophysiology of, 351-352, 351t, 352b, 352f
- latex allergy in, 354-355, 355b
Type II cytotoxic hypersensitivity reactions, 355
Type II diabetes mellitus, 1306-1307, 1306t
- lifestyle changes in, 1320-1321
- testing for, 1307t
- type 1 versus, 1306t
Type III immune complex reactions, 355, 355f
Type IV delayed hypersensitivity reactions, 355-356
Tyrosine kinase inhibitors (TKIs), 318, 380t, 390, 390t
Tyrosine kinases (TKs), 388, 390

U
U waves, 653, 654f
UAP. See Unlicensed assistive personnel (UAP).
Ulcerative colitis, 1173-1188, 1173t
- assessment in, 1175
- community-based care in, 1180-1181, 1181b
- drug therapy for, 1176-1177, 1176b, 1176t
- evaluation of care of patient with, 1181
- lower gastrointestinal bleeding in, 1179-1180, 1180b
- pain in, 1179, 1179b
- pathophysiology of, 1174-1181, 1174t, 1175b
- surgical management of, 1177-1179, 1177b, 1178f

Ulcers, 423f
arterial, 720, 721b
corneal, 980-981
Curling's, 470
diabetic, 721b
lower extremity, 721b
pressure. See Pressure ulcers.
venous, 721b
Ulnar nerve complications, 253b
Uloric. See Febuxostat
Ultram. See Tramadol.
Ultrasonography
of bladder, 900
of breast, 1470
in gastrointestinal assessment, 1097
in musculoskeletal assessment, 1026
in neurologic assessment, 850
in renal assessment, 1359-1361, 1360t
in reproductive assessment, 1456-1457
in vision assessment, 973
Ultrasound-guided peripheral IV insertion, 191
Ultra-Stat epistaxis catheter, 533f
Ultraviolet light therapy for psoriasis, 457
Umbilical herniation, 1147
Unclassified seizures, 858
Uncus, 950
Undermining in pressure ulcers, 443
Unfractionated heparin, 731-732, 731b
Unilateral body neglect syndrome, 936, 944
Unintentional injury, 114-115
Universal lesions, 422t
Unlicensed assistive personnel (UAP), 6
neutropenic patients and, 382
Unstable angina pectoris, 758-759
Upper airway obstruction, 536-537, 536b-537b, 537f
Upper esophageal sphincter, 1085
Upper extremity fractures, 1066-1069, 1066f
Upper gastrointestinal bleeding, 1136-1137, 1136b-1137b
Upper gastrointestinal radiographic series, 1093
Upper motor neuron diseases, 87
Upper respiratory problems, 531-547
facial trauma in, 534, 534b
head and neck cancer. See Head and neck cancer.
larynx disorders
laryngeal trauma, 536, 536b
vocal cord paralysis, 535, 535b
neck trauma, 537
nose and sinus disorders, 531-534
epistaxis, 532-533, 532b-533b, 533f

Upper respiratory problems (Continued)
nasal fractures, 531-532, 532b, 532f
nose and sinus cancer, 533-534
rhinitis, 583-584, 584b
allergic, 349-351, 349f, 351b
rhinosinusitis, 584
upper airway obstruction, 536-537, 536b-537b, 537f
obstructive sleep apnea in, 534-535
Upper respiratory tract, 496-498, 497f
larynx in, 497-498, 498f
nose and sinuses in, 496-497, 497f
pharynx in, 497
Urea nitrogen in burn assessment, 477b
Uremia, 1353
in chronic kidney disease, 1419, 1419b
Uremic frost, 1424
Ureterolithiasis, 1384
Ureteropelvic junction, 1350
Ureteroplasty, 1401
Ureterovesical junction, 1350
Ureters, 1350
assessment of, 1353-1354
Urethra
assessment of, 1354
Urethral strictures, 1373, 1397-1399, 1399b
Urethritis, 1373
Urethroplasty, 1373
Urge incontinence, 1374t, 1375, 1380b-1381b
Urgency
changes associated with aging, 1351
in urinary tract infection, 1369
Urgent surgery, 218t
Urgent triage, 111t, 112
Urinalysis, 1355-1358, 1356b, 1357t
in heart failure, 683
Urinary assessment
in hematologic assessment, 792-793
in rehabilitation setting, 78, 78t
Urinary bladder, 1350, 1350f
benign prostatic hyperplasia and, 1503-1506, 1503b
dysfunction of
in spinal cord injury, 899-900
in stroke, 943-944
Urinary catheterization
home care management of, 1511b
intermittent, 86
Urinary continence, rehabilitation and, 85-87, 86b-87b, 86t
Urinary diversion procedures, 1389-1390, 1391f
Urinary elimination, 1342-1343, 1342f

Urinary incontinence, 1373-1384
assessment in, 1376, 1376b
community-based care in, 1383, 1383b
cultural considerations in, 1382b
drug therapy for, 1377, 1378b, 1379-1380, 1380b
evaluation of care of patient with, 1384
functional, 1382
hospitalized older adults and, 20
mixed, 1382
nonsurgical management of, 1377-1379, 1377b-1378b, 1379f
in older adults, 1375b
pathophysiology of, 1373-1376, 1374t
pressure ulcers and, 440
reflux, 1381-1382
surgical management of, 1379, 1380t
total, 1382
urge, 1380b-1381b
Urinary problems, 1366-1393
bladder trauma, 1391-1392
health promotion and maintenance in, 1392
infectious disorders, 1366-1373, 1367t
cystitis, 1367-1373
assessment in, 1369-1370, 1370b
community-based care in, 1373
health promotion and maintenance in, 1369, 1369b
interventions for, 1370-1373, 1370b-1372b
pathophysiology of, 1367-1369, 1369b
urethritis, 1373
urethral strictures, 1373
urinary incontinence. See Urinary incontinence.
urolithiasis, 1384-1388
assessment in, 1385, 1385f
pathophysiology of, 1384-1385, 1384b-1385b, 1384t
urothelial cancer, 1369b, 1388-1390, 1390b
Urinary retention after lumbar spinal surgery, 889b
Urinary system
changes associated with aging, 1351, 1351b
postoperative assessment of, 262
Urinary tract infections (UTIs), 1366-1373
cystitis, 1367-1373
assessment in, 1369-1370, 1370b
community-based care in, 1373
health promotion and

Urinary tract infections (UTIs) (Continued)
maintenance in, 1369, 1369b
interventions for, 1370-1373, 1370b-1372b
pathophysiology of, 1367-1369, 1369b
management of, 87
older adults and, 1369b
pregnancy and, 1372b
prevention of, 86b, 87, 399b
pyelonephritis, 1372b, 1399-1401, 1399f, 1400b
risk factors associated with, 1367t
urethritis, 1373
Urine electrolytes, 1358
Urine osmolarity, 1358-1359
Urine specimen collection, 1357t
Urine tests, 1355-1359, 1356b, 1357t, 1359b
in diabetes mellitus, 1309
in endocrine assessment, 1264
in gastrointestinal assessment, 1091
Urodynamic studies, 1362-1363
Urolithiasis, 1384-1388
assessment in, 1385, 1385f
interventions for, 1385-1388, 1386f, 1388b, 1388t
pathophysiology of, 1384-1385, 1384b-1385b, 1384t
Urosepsis, 1368-1369
Urothelial cancer, 1369b, 1388-1390, 1390b
Urticaria, 433
in bee stings, 129
in serum sickness, 125
Ustekinumab, 321, 458b
Uterine artery embolization, 1488, 1489b
Uterine cancer. See Endometrial cancer.
Uterine leiomyomas, 1487-1491, 1488f, 1489b-1490b, 1489t
Uterine prolapse, 1485-1486, 1486f
Uterus, 1450, 1450f
dysfunctional bleeding of, 1483-1484, 1484t
endometriosis and, 1482-1483, 1483f
UTIs. See Urinary tract infections (UTIs).
Uvea, 966

V
Vaccination
for cancer, 368-369
for human papilloma virus, 368-369
Vacuum constriction devices, 1513
VADs. See Vascular access devices (VADs).
Vagal maneuvers for dysrhythmias, 665-666
Vagal nerve stimulation (VNS), 862

Vagina, 1450, 1450f
Vaginal cone therapy, 1377-1379, 1379f
Vaginal infections, 1544
Vaginoplasty, 1526-1527, 1527b, 1527t
Vagus nerve, 835t
Valacyclovir, 453
Validation therapy, 876
Valium. See Diazepam.
VALI/VILI. See Ventilator-associated lung injury/Ventilator-induced lung injury (VALI/VILI).
Valtrex. See Valacyclovir.
Valvular heart disease, 692-697, 692b
    aortic regurgitation in, 692b, 693
    aortic stenosis in, 692b, 693
    drug therapy for, 694, 694b
    health care resources for, 697
    home care management in, 696
    mitral regurgitation in, 692b, 693
    mitral stenosis in, 692, 692b, 696b
    mitral valve prolapse in, 692b, 693
    noninvasive heart valve reparative procedures for, 694-695, 695b, 695f
    self-management education in, 696-697, 697b
    surgical management of, 695-696, 696b, 696f
Valvular regurgitation, 628
Vancocin. See Vancomycin.
Vancomycin, 188b
Vancomycin-resistant Enterococcus (VRE), 403, 406
VAP. See Ventilator-associated pneumonia (VAP).
Varenicline, 495, 496b
Variant angina, 759, 763
Varicella-zoster virus (VZV), 335, 450b
Varicocele, 1516, 1516f
Varicose veins, 735-736
Variola virus, 411t
Vas deferens, 1451-1452, 1451f
Vascular access devices (VADs), 189-190, 214
    preoperative preparation for, 230
    removal of, 203
Vascular access in hemodialysis, 1433-1435, 1434f, 1434t, 1435b, 1435f
    complications of, 1433, 1435f
    precautions in, 1433
Vascular endothelial growth factor receptor inhibitors (VEGFRIs), 390, 390t
Vascular leak syndrome, 279-280
Vascular problems, 706-738
    acute peripheral arterial occlusion, 725, 725b-726b
    aneurysms
        of central arteries, 726-728, 726f, 727b
        of peripheral arteries, 726f, 728

Vascular problems (Continued)
    aortic dissection, 728
    arteriosclerosis and atherosclerosis, 706-709
        complementary and alternative therapies for, 709
        drug therapy for, 708-709, 709b, 709t
        laboratory assessment in, 708
        nutrition therapy for, 708
        pathophysiology of, 706-707, 707f, 707t
        physical assessment in, 707-708, 708b
    Buerger's disease, 729t
    health promotion and maintenance in, 709
    hypertension. See Hypertension.
    peripheral arterial disease, 718-725
        community-based care in, 724-725, 724b-725b
        cultural considerations in, 720b
        imaging assessment in, 720
        nonsurgical management of, 721-723, 722b
        pathophysiology of, 718-719, 719f
        physical assessment in, 719-720, 720f, 721b
        stages of, 719b
        surgical management of, 723-724, 723f, 724b
    peripheral venous disease. See Peripheral venous disease.
    Raynaud's phenomenon/disease. See Raynaud's phenomenon/disease.
    subclavian steal, 729t
    thoracic outlet syndrome, 729t
Vascular system, 631-632
    arterial system, 631-632
    changes resulting from burns, 469, 469f
    peripheral, 706
    venous system, 632
Vascular trauma, 736
Vasculitis
    in lupus, 314
    in rheumatoid arthritis, 305
    systemic necrotizing, 323t
Vasoconstriction in shock, 739-740
Vasoconstrictors, 748b
Vasodilation promotion in peripheral arterial disease, 722
Vaso-occlusive event, 799
Vasopressin, 1266
    deficiency of, 1267b
Vasopressors, 354b
Vasospasms in stroke, 932
Vasovagal attacks, 673b
Vatronal. See Ephedrine sulfate.
Vaughn-Williams classification, 657-658
Vegans, 1233

Vegetarians, 1233
VEGFRIs. See Vascular endothelial growth factor receptor inhibitors (VEGFRIs).
Velcade. See Bortezomib.
Velcro straps, 84t
Venous beading, 1304
Venous insufficiency, 734-735, 734b-735b
Venous pulses, 638-639
Venous sampling, 1264
Venous spasm, intravenous therapy-related, 204t-206t
Venous stasis, 231-232
Venous system, 632
Venous thromboembolism (VTE), 626
    after hip surgery, 296, 297t, 298-299
    community-based care in, 733-734, 733b
    fracture-related, 1054
    nonsurgical management of, 731-733, 731b-732b
    postoperative assessment for, 260
    prevention of, 231-233, 232b, 730
    pulmonary embolism and, 603
    surgical management of, 733
Venous ulcers, 721b
Ventilation assistance
    after burn injury, 477
    in respiratory acidosis, 183
Ventilator dependence, 622, 622b
Ventilator-associated lung injury/ Ventilator-induced lung injury (VALI/VILI), 620
Ventilator-associated pneumonia (VAP), 590t, 621, 621b
Ventilators, 619, 619b
    alarm systems of, 619, 620t
    controls and settings of, 618
Ventilatory failure, 610-611, 611t
    combined oxygenation and, 611-612
Ventolin. See Albuterol.
Ventricular assist devices, 687-688, 688f
Ventricular asystole, 671-673, 671f-672f, 672b
Ventricular dysrhythmias, 669-673
    premature ventricular complexes in, 669-670, 669f, 670b
    ventricular asystole in, 671-673, 671f-672f, 672b
    ventricular fibrillation in, 670-671, 671f
    ventricular tachycardia in, 670, 670b, 670f
Ventricular fibrillation (VF), 670-671, 671f
Ventricular gallop, 640
Ventricular remodeling, 759
Ventricular tachycardia (VT), 670, 670b, 670f
Ventriculomyectomy, 702

Venturi masks, 519, 519f, 519t
Veracity, 4
Verapamil, 658b-662b, 715b-716b
Verbal Descriptor Scale, 30-32
Vertebrobasilar artery strokes, 934b
Vertebroplasty, 1069, 1070b
Vertical laryngectomy, 541t
Vertigo, 1008
Vesicants, 192
    extravasation of, 379, 379f
Vesicles, 423f
Vesicular breath sounds, 505-506, 506t
Vestibule of inner ear, 998
Vestibulocochlear nerve, 835t
VF. See Ventricular fibrillation (VF).
Vibratory positive expiratory pressure device, 564, 564f
Viral carcinogenesis, 366, 366t
Viral infections
    cultures for, 429
    cutaneous, 450b, 451, 451f
    in hepatitis. See Hepatitis.
    human immune deficiency virus infection. See Human immune deficiency virus (HIV) infection.
    in pharyngitis, 584-586, 585b
    in severe acute respiratory syndrome, 594-595, 595b
    in tonsillitis, 586, 586b
Viral load testing, 337
Virchow's triad, 729
Viremia, 330
Virtual colonoscopy, 1096
Virulence, 397
Visceral pain, 28
Vision, 966
Vision assessment, 966-976
    fluorescein angiography in, 975
    imaging assessment in, 973
    inspection of eyes in, 972
    laboratory assessment in, 973
    ophthalmoscopy in, 974-975, 974f, 975b, 975t
    patient history in, 971-975, 971b, 971t
    psychosocial assessment in, 973
    slit-lamp examination in, 974, 974f
    tonometry in, 974, 974f
    vision testing in, 972-973, 973f
Vision loss, older adults and, 970b
Vision problems. See also Eye problems.
    in diabetes mellitus, 1303-1304, 1305b, 1328-1329
    older adults and, 970b
    reduced visual sensory perception, 992-994, 993b
Vision testing, 972-973, 973f
Visual acuity tests, 972
Visual Analog Dyspnea Scale, 561, 561f
Visual field testing, 972-973

Vital signs in traumatic brain injury, 951-952
Vitamin B 12 deficiency, 799t
Vitamin D
    activation in kidney, 1349-1350, 1349t
    in epidermis, 416
Vitiligo, 1262
Vitreous body, 967
VKORC1 gene, 608b
VNS. *See* Vagal nerve stimulation (VNS).
Vocal cord paralysis, 535, 535b
Vocal fremitus, 504
Vocal resonance, 506
Vocal therapy for transgender patients, 1525-1526
Vocational assessment in rehabilitation, 80
Vocational counselors, 77
Voice box. *See* Larynx.
Voice sounds, 506
Voided urine specimen, 1357t
Volume-cycled ventilators, 616, 617f
Voluntary active euthanasia, 103t
Volutrauma, 620
Volvulus, 1158, 1158f
Vomiting
    chemotherapy-related, 383-384, 384b-385b
    in enteral nutrition, 1244
    management at end of life, 99
VRE. *See* Vancomycin-resistant *Enterococcus* (VRE).
VT. *See* Ventricular tachycardia (VT).
VTE. *See* Venous thromboembolism (VTE).
Vulva, 1449
Vulvovaginitis, 1484-1485, 1485b
VZV. *See* Varicella-zoster virus (VZV).

W
Walkers, 83b, 83f
Warfarin
    cultural considerations in use of, 56b
    foods and drugs interfering with, 733b

Warfarin *(Continued)*
    for pulmonary embolism, 607b
    for venous thromboembolism, 732, 732b
Warm antibody anemia, 804
Wasp stings, 128-129, 129b
Water, homeostasis and, 148, 149f, 418t
Water brash, 1111
Water pipe smoking, 495
WBC count. *See* White blood cell (WBC) count.
WBCs. *See* White blood cells (WBCs).
Weakness
    in heart failure, 688
    management in end-of-life care, 98, 98b
Weaning
    from mechanical ventilation, 622, 622b, 622t
    from tracheostomy tube, 529
Weapons of mass destruction, 139, 142
Wedge resection in lung cancer, 576
Weight gain in rehabilitation setting, 81
Weight loss
    after burns, 486-487
    in chronic obstructive pulmonary disease, 565
Wernicke's aphasia, 943, 943t
Wernicke's area, 831
West Nile virus, 865-866, 866b
Western blot analysis for HIV infection, 336-337
Wet-to-damp saline-moistened gauze dressing, 446t
Wheals, 423f
Wheelchairs, 81
    repositioning patients in, 85
Wheezing, 507t
Whipple procedure, 1228-1229, 1229f
White blood cell (WBC) count
    in cardiovascular assessment, 642
    with differentiation, 408, 414
    perioperative assessment of, 223b-224b
    in respiratory assessment, 508b

White blood cell disorders
    leukemia. *See* Leukemia.
    malignant lymphomas, 817-819
        Hodgkin's lymphoma, 817, 817t
        multiple myeloma, 818-819
        non-Hodgkin lymphoma, 818
White blood cell transfusions, 824
White blood cells (WBCs), 277, 787, 787t
    immune functions of, 278t
    inflammation and, 278-281
        basophils in, 279-280
        eosinophils in, 280
        macrophages in, 279, 279t
        neutrophils in, 278-279, 279f, 279t
    leukemia and. *See* Leukemia.
White matter, 830, 832-833
WHO. *See* World Health Organization (WHO).
Whole-pancreas transplantation, 1323-1324
Wide excision surgery in skin cancer, 461
Wigs, 385
Wild-type gene sequence, 56
Williams position for acute low back pain, 887
Winged needles, 191, 210
Withdrawing or withholding life-sustaining therapy, 103, 103t
Women's health considerations. *See* Gender health considerations.
Wong-Baker FACES Pain Rating Scale, 30, 32f
Wood's light examination, 429
Work-related musculoskeletal disorders, 81
World Health Organization (WHO), 215-216, 216f
Wound care
    in burn injury, 482-488, 483f-484f
    in colostomy, 1154, 1154b
    in diabetes mellitus, 1327
    in pressure ulcers, 444-447, 444b, 445f, 446b-447b, 446t

Wound dressings, 483
Wound healing, 264
    in full-thickness wounds, 435-436, 435f
    impaired, 264, 264f
    in older adults, 436b
    in partial-thickness wounds, 435, 435f
    phases of, 433-435, 433t, 434f-435f, 436t
Wound infections
    postoperative, 272
        assessment of, 272-273
        prevention of, 267-269, 267b-269b, 267f
Wrist drop, 253b
Wrists
    arthroplasty of, 303
    positioning to prevent contractures, 487b

X
Xanthines, 556
Xeljanz. *See* Tofacitinib.
Xenografts, 696, 696f
Xeroform dressing, 484f
Xerostomia
    in post-irradiation sialadenitis, 1108
    radiation therapy-related, 376-377, 539
    in Sjögren's syndrome, 306
X-rays. *See* Radiography.
Xylocaine. *See* Lidocaine.

Y
Yersinia pestis, 411t
Young old, 9

Z
Zenapax. *See* Daclizumab.
Zetia. *See* Ezetimibe.
Ziconotide, 890, 891b
Zofran. *See* Ondansetron.
Zostavax, 452, 452b
Zovirax. *See* Acyclovir.
Zyban. *See* Bupropion.